# CLINICAL GYNECOLOGY

**Eric J. Bieber, MD, MHCM**
Chair, Department of Obstetrics and Gynecology
Medical Director, Women's Service Line
Chief Medical Officer, Geisinger Wyoming Valley and
    Geisinger South Wilkes-Barre
Senior Vice President
Geisinger Health Systems
Wilkes-Barre and Danville, PA

**Joseph S. Sanfilippo, MD, MBA**
Vice Chair, Reproductive Sciences
Director, Division of Reproductive Endocrinology and Infertility
University of Pittsburgh School of Medicine
Pittsburgh, PA

**Ira R. Horowitz, MD, MHCM**
Willaford Ransom Leach Professor and Vice Chair
Department of Obstetrics and Gynecology
Director, Division of Gynecologic Oncology
Assistant Dean of Clinical Affairs
Emory University School of Medicine
Associate Director, Emory Clinic
Atlanta, GA

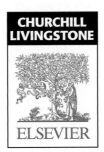

CHURCHILL
LIVINGSTONE

ELSEVIER

## CHURCHILL
## LIVINGSTONE
### ELSEVIER

1600 John F. Kennedy Blvd.
Ste 1800
Philadelphia, PA 19103–2899

CLINICAL GYNECOLOGY

ISBN-13: 978-0-443-06691-7
ISBN-10: 0-443-06691-4

**Library of Congress Cataloging-in-Publication Data**

Clinical gynecology/[edited by] Eric J. Bieber, Joseph S. Sanfilippo, Ira R. Horowitz.
    p.; cm.
    ISBN 0-443-06691-4
    1. Gynecology. 2. Clinical medicine. 3. Generative organs, Female—Diseases. I. Bieber, Eric J.
II. Horowitz, Ira R. III. Sanfilippo, J. S. (Joseph S.)
    [DNLM: 1. Genital Diseases, Female. 2. Gynecologic Surgical Procedures—methods.
3. Gynecology—methods. WP 140 C6408 2006]
RG101.C677 2006
618.1—dc22

2005041448

*Acquisitions Editor:* Rebecca Gaertner
*Developmental Editor:* Dee Simpson
*Project Manager:* Mary Stermel
*Design Director:* Gene Harris
*Marketing Manager:* Matt Latuchie

Printed in Canada.

Last digit is the print number: 9  8  7  6  5  4  3  2  1

To our patients whom we treat as family, and to our families for their patience.

I would like to thank my wife, Edie, and our sons, Brandon and Andrew, for continuing to support my academic endeavors and for providing a loving environment from which to grow professionally and personally. Also to my parents, George and Audrey, who taught me to "reach for the stars." To the many mentors who have had such a profound impact on my life—to them I am forever indebted. Finally, I would like to recognize my coeditors, IH and JS. Their friendship has made this project enjoyable from the onset; their exemplary professionalism is a credit to our field of medicine.

—EB

I dedicate this book to my family: Patricia, my wife, and our children, Angela, Andrea, and Luke for their unending enthusiasm and support for all my academic ventures. To my mother, who in her ninetieth year continues to remind me how "she is responsible for it all." Finally as noted in the preface, behind every successful professional is one other key person, *viz.* their Administrative Assistant. This book could not have been completed without the capable assistance of Doreen Smith, whose tireless hours addressed the entire "attention to detail" prerequisite to what you have in your hands today.

—JS

I dedicate this text to my wife, Julie, and daughters, Andrea and Rebecah. It is through their support and sacrifice that I have been able to pursue my academic career. In addition to my family, I would like to recognize the mentors who have assisted me in my academic pursuits. As mentioned in the preface, my participation in preparing this text would not have been possible without my Administrative Assistant, Julie Cook. It is my hope that this text will provide physicians with an evidence-based approach to gynecology.

—IH

# Contributors

**Rony A. Adam, MD**
Director, Division of Gynecologic
Specialties, Department of
Gynecology and Obstetrics,
Emory University School of Medicine,
Atlanta, GA
*Diagnosis and Treatment of Fistulas;*
*Nonsurgical Treatment of Urinary*
*Incontinence*

**Raedah Al-Fadhli, MD**
Fellow, Reproductive Endocrinology
and Infertility, McGill University,
Montreal, Quebec, Canada
*Laparoscopic Instrumentation*

**Zoyla Almeida-Parra, MD**
Gynecologic Oncologist, Department of
Obstetrics and Gynecology, Memorial
Miramar Hospital; Gynecologic
Oncologist, Department of Obstetrics
and Gynecology, Memorial West
Hospital, Miramar, FL
*Cervical Carcinoma*

**Rudi Ansbacher, MD, MS**
Professor Emeritus, Obstetrics and
Gynecology, University of Michigan
Medical Center, Ann Arbor, MI
*Geriatric Gynecology*

**Gloria Bachmann, MD**
Professor, Departments of
Obstetrics and Gynecology and
Medicine; Associate Dean for
Women's Health, Women's Health
Institute; UMDNJ–Robert Wood
Johnson Medical School; Attending,
Obstetrics and Gynecology, Robert
Wood Johnson University Hospital,
New Brunswick, NJ
*Sexual Function and Disorders*

**Patricia E. Bailey-Sarnelli, MD**
Department of Obstetrics and
Gynecology, Baystate Health Systems,
Longmeadow, MA
*Contraception*

**Randall B. Barnes, MD**
Associate Professor, Department of
Obstetrics and Gynecology,
Northwestern University, Chicago, IL
*Abnormal Uterine Bleeding*

**Jack Basil, MD**
Associate Director, Department of
Gynecologic Oncology, TriHealth,
Tristate Gynecologic Oncology,
Cincinnati, OH
*Vaginal Carcinoma*

**John Bennett, MD**
Department of Radiology,
St. Joseph's Health Care, London,
Ontario, Canada
*Uterine Leiomyomas*

**Inbar Ben-Shachar, MD**
Lecturer, Faculty of Medicine,
Hebrew University; Attending,
Division of Gynecologic Oncology,
Department of Obstetrics and
Gynecology, Hadassah University
Medical Center, Jerusalem, Israel
*Gestational Trophoblastic Disease*

**Jonathan S. Berek, MD, MMSc**
Professor and Chair, College of Applied
Anatomy; Executive Vice Chair,
Department of Obstetrics and
Gynecology; Chief, Division of
Gynecologic Oncology and Gynecology
Service; Director, UCLA Women's
Reproductive Cancer Program, David
Geffen School of Medicine at UCLA,
UCLA Center for the Health Sciences,
Los Angeles, CA
*Cancer Genetics*

**Sarah L. Berga, MD**
James Robert McCord Professor and
Chair, Department of Gynecology and
Obstetrics, Emory University School of
Medicine; Department of Gynecology
and Obstetrics, Emory Healthcare,
Atlanta, GA
*Physiology of the Menstrual Cycle*

**Eric J. Bieber, MD, MHCM**
Chair, Department of Obstetrics and
Gynecology; Medical Director,
Women's Service Line; Chief Medical
Officer, Geisinger Wyoming Valley
and Geisinger South Wilkes-Barre;
Senior Vice President; Geisinger
Health Systems; Wilkes-Barre and
Danville, PA
*Hysteroscopic Instrumentation;*
*Hysteroscopic Procedures; Laparoscopic*
*and Hysteroscopic Complications;*
*Laparoscopic Instrumentation*

**Anita Blanchard, MD**
Assistant Professor, Department of
Obstetrics and Gynecology, University
of Chicago Pritzker School of Medicine,
Chicago, IL
*Benign Vulvar Diagnosis*

**Thèrése E. Bocklage, MD**
Associate Professor, Department
of Pathology, University of
New Mexico School of Medicine;
Associate Professor, Department of
Pathology, University of New Mexico
Health Sciences Center,
Albuquerque, NM
*Fallopian Tube Carcinoma*

**Candace Brown, MSN, PharmD**
Professor, Departments of Pharmacy,
Obstetrics and Gynecology, and
Psychiatry, University of Tennessee
Health Science Center, Memphis, TN
*Premenstrual Syndrome/Premenstrual*
*Dysphoric Disorder*

**Colleen Buggs, MD, PhD**
Assistant Professor, Department of
Pediatrics, University of Chicago
Pritzker School of Medicine;
Assistant Professor, Pediatrics
Section of Pediatric Endocrinology,
University of Chicago Children's
Hospital, Chicago IL
*Delayed Puberty and Primary*
*Amenorrhea*

**Ronald T. Burkman, MD**
Deputy Chair and Professor, Department of Obstetrics and Gynecology, Tufts University School of Medicine, Boston; Chair, Department of Obstetrics and Gynecology, Baystate Medical Center, Springfield, MA
*Contraception*

**John E. Buster, MD**
Professor and Director, Division of Reproductive Endocrinology and Infertility, Department of Obstetrics and Gynecology, Baylor College of Medicine; Professor and Director, Division of Reproductive Endocrinology and Infertility, Department of Obstetrics and Gynecology, Methodist Hospital; Professor and Director, Division of Reproductive Endocrinology and Infertility, Department of Obstetrics and Gynecology, St. Luke's Episcopal Hospital, Houston, TX
*Polycystic Ovary Syndrome*

**Michael Byas-Smith, MD**
Associate Professor, Department of Anesthesiology, Emory University School of Medicine; Department of Anesthesiology, Emory University Hospital; Department of Anesthesiology, Crawford Long Hospital; Department of Anesthesiology/Pain, Winship Cancer Institute of Emory University, Atlanta, GA
*Cancer Pain*

**Alexandra S. Carey, MD**
Department of Adolescent Medicine, Children's Hospital of Pittsburgh, Pittsburgh, PA
*Puberty and Precocious Puberty*

**Sandra A. Carson, MD**
Professor, Department of Obstetrics and Gynecology, Baylor College of Medicine; Attending Physician, Obstetrics and Gynecology, St. Luke's Episcopal Hospital; Attending Physician, Obstetrics and Gynecology, Methodist Hospital; Attending Physician, Obstetrics and Gynecology, Ben Taub Hospital, Houston, TX
*Female Infertility and Evaluation of the Infertile Couple*

**Judy C. Chang, MD, MPH**
Assistant Professor, Department of Obstetrics, Gynecology, and Reproductive Sciences, University of Pittsburgh; Junior Investigator, BIRCWH Scholar, Magee-Women's Research Institute, Pittsburgh, PA
*Domestic Violence*

**Alice W. Chuang, MD**
Assistant Professor, Department of Obstetrics and Gynecology, University of North Carolina–Chapel Hill School of Medicine, Chapel Hill, NC
*Preventive Health*

**Daniel L. Clarke-Pearson, MD**
James M. Ingram Professor of Gynecologic Oncology, Department of Obstetrics and Gynecology, Duke University School of Medicine; Director of Gynecologic Oncology, Department of Obstetrics and Gynecology, Duke University Hospital, Durham, NC
*Preoperative Evaluation and Postoperative Management*

**Larry J. Copeland, MD**
Professor and William Greenville Pace III and Joann Norris Collins Pace Chair, Department of Obstetrics and Gynecology, The Ohio State University College of Medicine; Professor, Gynecologic Oncology, James Cancer Hospital and Solove Research Institute, Columbus, OH
*Gestational Trophoblastic Disease*

**Susannah D. Copland, MD**
Fellow, Reproductive Endocrinology and Infertility, Department of Obstetrics and Gynecology, Emory University School of Medicine, Atlanta, GA
*Physiology of the Menstrual Cycle*

**Bryan D. Cowan, MD**
Professor and Chair, Department of Obstetrics and Gynecology, University of Mississippi Medical Center, Jackson, MS
*Assisted Reproductive Technologies/ In Vitro Fertilization*

**Kristin L. Dardano, MD**
Assistant Professor, Department of Obstetrics and Gynecology, Tufts University School of Medicine, Boston; Assistant Professor, Department of Obstetrics and Gynecology, Baystate Medical Center, Springfield, MA
*Contraception*

**Michael P. Diamond, MD**
Kamran S. Moghissi Professor and Associate Chair, Department of Obstetrics and Gynecology, Wayne State University; Director, Division of Reproductive Endocrinology and Infertility, Department of Obstetrics and Gynecology, Detroit Medical Center, Detroit, MI
*Uterine Leiomyomas*

**Concepcion Diaz-Arrastia, MD**
Associate Professor, Department of Obstetrics and Gynecology, University of Texas Medical Branch, Galveston, TX
*Human Papillomaviruses*

**Oliver Dorigo, MD, PhD**
Assistant Professor, Department of Gynecologic Oncology, David Geffen School of Medicine at UCLA, Los Angeles, CA
*Cancer Genetics*

**Steven C. Eberhardt, MD**
Assistant Professor, Department of Radiology, University of New Mexico, Albuquerque, NM
*Fallopian Tube Carcinoma*

**Philip N. Eskew, Jr., MD**
Clinical Professor, Department of Obstetrics and Gynecology, Indiana University School of Medicine; Director, Physician and Patient Relations, Department of Medical Affairs, St. Vincent Hospital, Indianapolis, IN
*Coding Tips for the Busy Physician*

**Sebastian Faro, MD, PhD**
Clinical Professor, Department of Obstetrics, Gynecology, and Reproductive Sciences, The University of Texas–Houston Health Sciences Center; Attending Physician, Departments of Obstetrics and Gynecology and Surgery, The Woman's Hospital of Texas, Houston, TX
*Gynecologic and Surgical Sepsis; Pelvic Inflammatory Disease; Vulvovaginal Infections*

**Murray J. Favus, MD**
Professor, Department of Medicine, University of Chicago Pritzker School of Medicine; Attending Physician and Director, Bone Program, Department of Medicine, University of Chicago Hospitals, Chicago, IL
*Osteoporosis*

**Lisa Flowers, MD**
Assistant Professor, Department of Obstetrics and Gynecology, Emory University School of Medicine, Atlanta, GA
*Colposcopy*

**Thomas P. Foley, Jr., MD**
Professor Emeritus, Department of Pediatrics and Epidemiology, University of Pittsburgh; Professor Emeritus, Division of Endocrinology, Department of Pediatrics, Children's Hospital of Pittsburgh, Pittsburgh, PA
*Thyroid Function and Disorders*

**Jennifer S. Gell, MD**
Associate, Department of Obstetrics and Gynecology, Division of Reproductive Endocrinology, Geisinger Wyoming Valley Hospital, Wilkes-Barre, PA
*Alternative Medicine*

**Karen Godette, MD**
Assistant Professor, Department of Radiation Oncology, Emory University School of Medicine, Atlanta, GA
*Breast Carcinoma*

**Alan N. Gordon, MD**
Clinical Professor, Department of Obstetrics and Gynecology, University of Arizona, Phoenix; Department of Obstetrics and Gynecology, Banner Good Samaritan Medical Center; Department of Obstetrics and Gynecology, St. Joseph's Hospital and Medical Center, Phoenix, AZ
*Vulvar Carcinoma*

**Victoria L. Green, MD, MBA, JD**
Associate Professor, Department of Obstetrics and Gynecology; Winship Cancer Institute of Emory University, Cancer Control and Population Sciences, Emory University School of Medicine, Atlanta, GA
*Breast Cancer Screening*

**Nidhi Gupta, MD**
Departments of Obstetrics and Gynecology and Medicine, UMDNJ–Robert Wood Johnson Medical School, New Brunswick, NJ
*Sexual Function and Disorders*

**Enrique Hernandez, MD, FACOG, FACS**
The Abraham Roth Professor and Chair, Department of Obstetrics, Gynecology and Reproductive Sciences, Temple University School of Medicine; Chair, Department of Obstetrics and Gynecology, Temple University Hospital, Philadelphia, PA
*Endometrial Carcinoma*

**S. Paige Hertweck, MD**
Associate Professor, Pediatric and Adolescent Gynecology, Department of Obstetrics, Gynecology and Women's Health, University of Louisville School of Medicine; Chief of Gynecologic Surgery, Kosair Children's Hospital, Louisville, KY
*Medical Management of Gynecologic Problems in the Pediatric and Adolescent Patient*

**Randall S. Hines, MD**
Associate Professor and Director, Division of Reproductive Endocrinology and Infertility, Department of Obstetrics and Gynecology, University of Mississippi Medical Center, Jackson, MS
*Assisted Reproductive Technologies/ In Vitro Fertilization*

**Ira R. Horowitz, MD, MHCM**
Willaford Ransom Leach Professor and Vice Chair, Department of Obstetrics and Gynecology; Director, Division of Gynecologic Oncology; Assistant Dean of Clinical Affairs, Emory University School of Medicine; Associate Director, Emory Clinic, Atlanta, GA
*Federal Regulations*

**Karen L. Houck, MD**
Assistant Professor, Department of Obstetrics, Gynecology and Reproductive Services, Temple University Hospital, Philadelphia, PA
*Endometrial Carcinoma*

**Fred M. Howard, MS, MD**
Professor and Associate Chair, Department of Obstetrics and Gynecology, University of Rochester School of Medicine and Dentistry, Rochester, NY
*Chronic Pelvic Pain*

**Denise J. Jamieson, MD, MPH**
Clinical Associate Professor, Department of Gynecology and Obstetrics, Emory University School of Medicine, Atlanta, GA
*Human Immunodeficiency Virus*

**Mohit Khera, MD, MBA, MPH**
Urology Resident, Scott Department of Urology, Baylor College of Medicine, Houston, TX
*Male Infertility*

**Jeremy A. King, MD**
Instructor, Division of Reproductive Endocrinology, Department of Gynecology and Obstetrics, The Johns Hopkins Hospital, Baltimore, MD
*Hyperprolactinemia*

**Ira J. Kodner, MD**
Solon and Bettie Gershman Professor of Colon and Rectal Surgery, Department of Surgery, Washington University School of Medicine, St. Louis, MO
*Treatment of Fecal Incontinence*

**Athena P. Kourtis, MD, PhD, MPH**
Associate Professor, Department of Obstetrics and Gynecology, Eastern Virginia Medical School, Norfolk, VA
*Human Immunodeficiency Virus*

**S. Robert Kovac, MD**
Distinguished Professor of Gynecologic Surgery, Department of Gynecology and Obstetrics, Emory University School of Medicine, Atlanta, GA
*Surgical Treatment of Urinary Incontinence; Diagnosis and Treatment of Fistulas*

**Ertug Kovanci, MD**
Fellow, Department of Obstetrics and Gynecology, Division of Reproductive Endocrinology and Infertility, Baylor College of Medicine, Houston, TX
*Female Infertility and Evaluation of the Infertile Couple; Polycystic Ovary Syndrome*

**William H. Kutteh, MD, PhD, HCLD**
Professor and Director of Reproductive Endocrinology, Obstetrics and Gynecology, University of Tennessee, Memphis; Director, Reproductive Endocrinology; Director, Reproductive Immunology, Fertility Associates of Memphis, Memphis, TN
*Recurrent Pregnancy Loss*

**Eduardo Lara-Torre, MD**
Chair, Obstetrics and Gynecology, Milford Memorial Hospital; Medical Director, Sexual Assault Nurse Examiner Program, Bayhealth Medical Center; Private Practice, Pediatric and Adolescent Gynecology, Milford Memorial Hospital, Milford, DE
*Medical Management of Gynecologic Problems in the Pediatric and Adolescent Patient*

**Herschel W. Lawson, MD**
Clinical Assistant Professor, Department of Gynecology and Obstetrics, Emory University School of Medicine; Senior Medical Advisor, Division of Cancer Prevention and Control, Centers for Disease Control and Prevention, Atlanta, GA
*Cervical Cancer Screening*

**Paula S. Lee, MD, MPH**
Clinical Associate, Department of Obstetrics and Gynecology, Duke University Medical Center, Durham, NC
*Preoperative Evaluation and Postoperative Management*

**Ronald L. Levine, MD**
Professor and Chief, Gynecologic Endoscopy Section, Department of Obstetrics, Gynecology, and Women's Health, University of Louisville School of Medicine; Director, Outpatient Gynecologic Surgery, Department of Obstetrics, Gynecology, and Women's Health, University of Louisville Hospital, Louisville, KY
*Surgical Setup for Minimally Invasive Surgery*

**Frank W. Ling, MD**
Clinical Professor, Department of Obstetrics and Gynecology, Vanderbilt University School of Medicine, Nashville; Partner, Women's Health Specialists, PLLC, Memphis, TN
*Premenstrual Syndrome/Premenstrual Dysphoric Disorder; Preventive Health*

**Larry I. Lipshultz, MD**
Professor of Urology; Lester and Sue Smith Chair in Reproductive Medicine; Chief, Division of Male Reproductive Medicine and Surgery; Scott Department of Urology, Baylor College of Medicine, Houston, TX
*Male Infertility*

**Christopher V. Lutman, MD, FACOG**
Clincal Instructor, Department of Obstetrics and Gynecology, Ohio State University College of Medicine; Attending Gynecologic Oncologist, Department of Obstetrics and Gynecology, Columbus, OH
*Preoperative Evaluation and Postoperative Management*

**Ali Mahdavi, MD, FACOG**
Minimally Invasive Surgery Fellow, Division of Gynecologic Oncology, Department of Obstetrics and Gynecology, Mount Sinai School of Medicine, New York, NY
*Laparoscopic Procedures*

**Suketu Mansuria, MD**
Assistant Professor; Coordinator of Gynecologic Minimally Invasive Surgery Fellowship, Department of Obstetrics, Gynecology and Reproductive Sciences, University of Pittsburgh and Magee-Womens Hospital, Pittsburgh, PA
*Surgical Problems in the Pediatric Patient*

**Robert McLellan, MD**
Chair, Department of Gynecology, Lahey Clinic Foundation, Inc., Burlington, MA; Clinical Professor of Obstetrics and Gynecology, Boston University School of Medicine, Boston, MA
*Uterine Sarcomas*

**Luis E. Mendez, MD**
South Florida Gynecologic Oncology, Miami, FL
*Cervical Carcinoma*

**Pamela J. Murray, MD, MPH**
Associate Professor and Division Chief, Adolescent Medicine, Department of Pediatrics, University of Pittsburgh School of Medicine; Director, Adolescent Medicine, Children's Hospital of Pittsburgh, Pittsburgh, PA
*Puberty and Precocious Puberty*

**Padma C. Nadella, MD**
Assistant Professor, Department of Hematology and Oncology, Emory University School of Medicine; Attending Physician, Department of Internal Medicine, Veterans Medical Center; Attending Physician, Department of Medical Oncology, Winship Cancer Institute of Emory University, Atlanta, GA
*Breast Carcinoma*

**Farr Nezhat, MD, FACOG, FACS**
Professor, Department of Obstetrics, Gynecology, and Reproductive Science, Mount Sinai Medical Center, New York, NY
*Laparoscopic Procedures*

**Peggy A. Norton, MD**
Chief, Urogynecology and Reconstructive Pelvic Surgery, Department of Obstetrics and Gynecology, University of Utah School of Medicine, Salt Lake City, UT
*Nonsurgical Treatment of Urinary Incontinence*

**Ruth M. O'Regan, MD**
Assistant Professor, Department of Hematology and Oncology, Emory University School of Medicine; Emory University Hospital; Director, Translational Breast Cancer Research Program, Department of Hematology/Oncology/Breast, Winship Cancer Institute of Emory University, Atlanta, GA
*Breast Carcinoma*

**Mitesh Parekh, MD**
Chief of Urogynecology; Director of Undergraduate Medical Education; Director of 3rd Year Obstetrics and Gynecology Clerkship, Departments of Obstetrics and Gynecology and Urogynecology, Geisinger Health System, Danville, PA
*Urogynecologic Workup and Testing*

**Kristiina Parviainen, MD**
Fellow, Maternal-Fetal Medicine, Department of Obstetrics, Gynecology and Reproductive Sciences, University of Pittsburgh; Fellow, Maternal-Fetal Medicine, Department of Obstetrics, Gynecology and Reproductive Sciences, Magee-Womens Hospital, Pittsburgh, PA
*Thyroid Function and Disorders*

**Resad Pasic, MD, PhD**
Associate Professor, Department of
Obstetrics, Gynecology, and
Women's Health, University of
Louisville School of Medicine,
Louisville, KY
*Surgical Setup for Minimally Invasive
Surgery*

**Tanja Pejovic, MD, PhD**
Assistant Professor, Department of
Obstetrics and Gynecology,
Division of Gynecologic Oncology,
Oregon Health and Science University,
Portland, OR
*Laparoscopic Procedures*

**Manuel Peñalver, MD**
Medical Director, South Florida
Gynecologic Oncology,
Coral Gables, FL
*Cervical Carcinoma*

**Elizabeth E. Puscheck, MD**
Associate Professor, Department of
Obstetrics and Gynecology, Division of
Reproductive Endocrinology and
Infertility, Wayne State University
School of Medicine; Hutzel Women's
Hospital, Detroit; IVF Director and
Gynecologic Ultrasound Director,
University Women's Care in Southfield,
Southfield, MI
*Secondary Amenorrhea*

**David B. Redwine, MD**
Private Practice, Endometriosis
Treatment Program, St. Charles Medical
Center–Bend, Bend, OR
*Endometriosis*

**Robert L. Reid, MD, FRCSC**
Professor, Department of Obstetrics
and Gynecology; Chair, Division of
Reproductive Endocrinology and
Infertility, Queen's University; Deputy
Head, Obstetrics and Gynecology,
Kingston General Hospital, Kingston,
Ontario, Canada
*Menopause*

**Monica Rizzo, MD**
Assistant Professor, Department of
Surgery, Emory University School of
Medicine, Atlanta, GA
*Breast Carcinoma*

**Carla P. Roberts, MD, PhD**
Assistant Professor, Division of
Reproductive Endocrinology and
Infertility, Department of Gynecology
and Obstetrics, Emory University
School of Medicine; Emory University
Hospital; Emory Crawford Long
Hospital, Atlanta, GA
*Disorders of the Adrenal Gland*

**Robert M. Rogers, Jr., MD**
Attending Gynecologist, Department
of Obstetrics and Gynecology,
Reading Hospital and Medical Center,
Reading, PA
*The Anatomic Basis of Normal and
Abnormal Pelvic Support*

**Walter Romano, MD, FRCPC**
Associate Professor, Department of
Radiology, University of Western
Ontario; Director of Ultrasound,
Department of Radiology, St. Joseph's
Health Centre, London, Ontario, Canada
*Uterine Leiomyomas*

**Peter G. Rose, MD**
Professor of Surgery, Reproductive
Biology, and Oncology, Case Western
Reserve University; Director,
Gynecologic Onclogy, Cleveland Clinic,
Cleveland, OH
*Ovarian Carcinoma*

**Robert L. Rosenfield, MD**
Professor of Pediatrics and Medicine,
Department of Pediatrics, The
University of Chicago Pritzker School
of Medicine; Attending Physician,
Section of Pediatric Endocrinology,
The University of Chicago Children's
Hospital, Chicago, IL
*Delayed Puberty and Primary
Amenorrhea*

**Mack T. Ruffin IV, MD, MPH**
Professor and Assistant Chair for
Research, Department of Family
Medicine, University of Michigan,
Ann Arbor, MI
*Human Papillomaviruses*

**Joseph S. Sanfilippo, MD, MBA**
Vice Chair, Reproductive Sciences;
Director, Division of Reproductive
Endocrinology and Infertility,
University of Pittsburgh School of
Medicine, Pittsburgh, PA
*Federal Regulations Surgical Problems in
the Pediatric Patient*

**Brook A. Saunders, MD**
Resident, Department of Obstetrics
and Gynecology, University of
Tennessee Health Science Center,
Memphis, TN
*Ectopic Pregnancy*

**Hyagriv N. Simhan, MD, MSCR**
Assistant Professor, Division of
Maternal-Fetal Medicine, Department of
Obstetrics, Gynecology, and
Reproductive Sciences, University of
Pittsburgh School of Medicine;
Magee-Womens Hospital, Pittsburgh, PA
*Thyroid Function and Disorders*

**Harriet O. Smith, MD**
Professor, Department of Obstetrics
and Gynecology, Cancer Research and
Treatment Center, University of New
Mexico Health Sciences Center,
Albuquerque, NM
*Fallopian Tube Carcinoma*

**Thomas E. Snyder, MD**
Associate Professor, Department of
Obstetrics and Gynecology, University
of Kansas School of Medicine; Associate
Professor, Department of Obstetrics
and Gynecology, University of Kansas
Hospital, Kansas City, KS
*Perimenopause*

**Valena Soto-Wright, MD**
Assistant Professor, Department of
Obstetrics and Gynecology, Boston
University School of Medicine, Boston;
Director, Gynecologic Oncology,
Department of Gynecology, Lahey
Clinic Foundation, Inc., Burlington, MA
*Uterine Sarcomas*

**Monique A. Spillman, MD, PhD**
Gynecologic Oncology Fellow, Division
of Gynecologic Oncology, Duke
University Medical Center, Durham, NC
*Preoperative Evaluation and
Postoperative Management*

**Mary D. Stephenson, MD, MSc**
Professor, Department of Obstetrics
and Gynecology, Section of
Reproductive Endocrinology and
Infertility, University of Chicago
Pritzker School of Medicine; Director,
Recurrent Pregnancy Loss Program,
University of Chicago Hospitals,
Chicago, IL
*Recurrent Pregnancy Loss*

**Thomas G. Stovall, MD**
Clinical Professor, Department of
Obstetrics and Gynecology, Vanderbilt
University School of Medicine,
Nashville; Clinical Professor,
Department of Obstetrics and
Gynecology, University of Tennessee;
Partner, Women's Health Specialists,
PLLC, Memphis, TN
*Ectopic Pregnancy*

**Toncred M. Styblo, MD, FACS**
Associate Professor, Department of
Surgery, Emory University School of
Medicine, Atlanta, GA
*Breast Carcinoma*

**Richard L. Sweet, MD**
Professor and Vice Chair,
Department of Obstetrics and
Gynecology, University of California,
Davis; Director, Women's Center for
Health, University of California,
Davis Health System,
Sacramento, CA
*Sexually Transmitted Diseases*

**Togas Tulandi, MD, MHCM, FRCSC,
FACOG**
Professor and Milton Leong Chair in
Reproductive Medicine, Department
of Obstetrics and Gynecology,
McGill University; Department Chief,
Obstetrics and Gynecology, The Sir
Mortimer B. Davis, Jewish General
Hospital; Associate Medical Director,
McGill Reproductive Center, McGill
University Health Center, Montreal,
Quebec, Canada
*Laparoscopic Instrumentation*

**Elizabeth R. Unger, MD, PhD**
Team Leader, Human Papillomavirus
Laboratory, Division of Viral and
Rickettsial Diseases, National Center for
Infectious Diseases, Centers for Disease
Control and Prevention, Atlanta, GA
*Human Papillomaviruses*

**Denise Uyar, MD**
Assistant Professor, Department of
Obstetrics and Gynecology, Division of
Gynecology and Oncology, Medical
College of Wisconsin; Department of
Obstetrics and Gynecology, Division of
Gynecology and Oncology, Froedtert
Memorial Lutheran Hospital,
Milwaukee, WI
*Ovarian Carcinoma*

**Marion S. Verp, MD**
Associate Professor, Obstetrics and
Gynecology, and Human Genetics,
University of Chicago Pritzker School of
Medicine; Chicago Lying-In Hospital,
Chicago, IL
*Preconception Counseling*

**Claire F. Verschraegen, MD, FACP**
Associate Professor, Division of
Hematology Oncology, Cancer Research
and Treatment Center, Albuquerque, NM
*Fallopian Tube Carcinoma*

**Rahi Victory, MD, FRCSC**
Fellow, Reproductive Endocrinology and
Infertility, Department of Obstetrics and
Gynecology, Wayne State University;
Fellow, Reproductive Endocrinology
and Infertility, Department of Obstetrics
and Gynecology, Detroit Medical
Center, Detroit, MI
*Uterine Leiomyomas*

**Tamara J. Vokes, MD**
Associate Professor of Medicine,
Department of Endocrinology,
University of Chicago Pritzker School of
Medicine; Associate Professor of
Medicine, Endocrinology, University of
Chicago Hospitals, Chicago, IL
*Osteoporosis*

**Paul E. Wise, MD**
Assistant Professor of Surgery,
Department of Colon and Rectal
Surgery, Division of General Surgery,
Vanderbilt University, Nashville, TN
*Treatment of Fecal Incontinence*

**Frank M. Wittmaack, MD**
Director, Fertility Center, Geisinger
Health System, Danville, PA
*Hysteroscopic Instrumentation*

**Howard A. Zacur, MD, PhD**
Theodore and Ingrid Baramki Professor
and Director of Reproductive
Endocrinology and Infertility,
Department of Gynecology and
Obstetrics, The Johns Hopkins
University School of Medicine,
Baltimore, MD
*Hyperprolactinemia*

# Preface

The stage is set as this segment of a textbook is always written, but may not always be read. The editors conceptualized this textbook almost a decade ago. While several popular gynecologic texts existed, we were unable to find a substantive reference text that had all of the qualities we envisioned. We spent many months debating format options that we believed would optimize the educational experience of you our audience. This final version is the distillation of those many discussions.

The three editors come from distinct and vastly different backgrounds: Eric Bieber's greatest interest lies in minimally invasive surgery (MIS), reproductive endocrinology and infertility (REI), and general gynecology; Ira Horowitz is interested in gynecologic oncology, pelvic surgery, and anatomy; and Joseph Sanfilippo is integrally involved with REI, MIS, and pediatric and adolescent gynecology. Each of us has directed fellowships, residencies, and departments over the years and each of us has also completed master's degrees in business administration or healthcare management. These disparate, yet singularly motivated interests, were an excellent nidus and most appropriate prerequisite for the text genesis.

The planning of this book has the basic tenets of combing the literature, pursuing the shelves of libraries, and arriving at a conclusion focused on what is needed for all sectors of female healthcare provision. The editors felt it was of paramount importance to provide for our readers a well-illustrated text in full color that was visually interesting but that also spanned the spectrum of gynecology. The text is thus divided into the following sections:

1 Ambulatory office practice
2 General gynecology
3 Gynecologic infectious disease
4 Urogynecology
5 Pediatric and adolescent gynecology
6 Minimal invasive surgery
7 Gynecologic oncology
8 Reproductive endocrinology and infertility
9 Coding and office management

We tapped into the expertise of leading authorities to provide the most current information in a succinct and easily understood format. This allows each chapter to be a "stand alone" entity, although there is continuity of style from chapter to chapter. However, given how we have intentionally structured the text, there are areas where we have allowed seeming incongruencies to stand as written. This allows the reader a panoramic understanding regarding some topics where there are inherent multiplicities of opinions and data.

The reader will note the increased breadth given to the topic of minimal invasive surgery. In addition, we address other areas such as compliance and the regulatory environment that are typically not covered in other texts.

In an effort to bring the most up-to-date and relevant information to the reader, we asked the chapter authors to provide references with coding of the level of strength of study design. Furthermore, they were requested to limit their citations to references that were particularly important. While several quality-of-evidence paradigms exist, we chose one that has been internationally accepted and widely used for evaluating strength of data. This format will help the reader who desires to pursue more in-depth information on a particular topic. We have also asked each chapter author to highlight key points that are presented at the beginning of each chapter.

Clinical decision making represents collating the clinical circumstance, research evidence, and patient preference after learning alternative management strategies. Back in 1992, evidence-based medicine proponents focused on a new paradigm in which provision was made how to best utilize research in clinical correlation. We have requested all contributors to grade the strength of the study design and its implementation. This classification is as follows:

**Quality of evidence**

Ia   Evidence obtained from meta-analysis of randomized controlled trials
Ib   Evidence obtained from at least one randomized controlled trial
IIa  Evidence obtained from at least one well-designed controlled study without randomization
IIb  Evidence obtained from at least one other type of well-designed quasi-experimental study
III  Evidence obtained from well-designed non-experimental descriptive studies, such as comparative studies, correlation studies, and case studies
IV   Evidence obtained from expert committee reports or opinions and/or clinical experience of respected authorities

**Strength of recommendation**

A   At least one randomized controlled trial as part of a body of literature of overall good quality and consistency addressing the specific recommendation (Evidence levels Ia, Ib)
B   Well-controlled clinical studies available but no randomized clinical trials on the topic of recommendations (Evidence levels IIa, IIb, III)
C   Evidence obtained from expert committee reports or opinions and/or clinical experiences of respected authorities. Indicates an absence of directly applicable clinical studies of good quality (Evidence level IV)

Haynes RB: What kind of evidence is it that evidence-based medicine advocates want health care providers and consumers to pay attention to? http://www.biomedcentral.com/1472–6963/2/3. Accessed Feb. 8, 2004

We want to express our appreciation to the administrative and secretarial staff for the tireless effort in seeing the textbook to completion. We are indebted to Doreen Smith and Julie Cook among many individuals who were helpful in this regard. We would also like to thank Elsevier for their incredible effort in seeing this very large project from genesis to completion. Without their belief in the project we would be unable to produce this heavily illustrated text. Specifically, we would like to thank Dee Simpson, Todd Hummel, and Mary Stermel.

We hope for you, as the reader, that we have accomplished our goal of providing a single authoritative reference text for the broad area of gynecology. Significant effort has been put into making this the most visually interesting and distinct text available. We hope this aids you in managing your patients and continuing to be enthusiastic about providing them with the latest gynecologic care.

Happy reading and care providing!

EB, JS, IH

# Contents

# Contents

## SECTION 9  CODING AND OFFICE MANAGEMENT

# CLINICAL GYNECOLOGY

# Chapter 1

# Osteoporosis

## Tamara J. Vokes, MD, and Murray J. Favus, MD

## KEY POINTS

- Osteoporosis is asymptomatic until a fracture occurs; making the diagnosis and initiating treatment in the presymptomatic stage may prevent fractures.
- Measurement of bone mineral density (BMD) is a good but not prefect predictor of fractures; additional risk factors, such as previous fractures (particularly vertebral), family history of osteoporosis and fractures, and presence of other diseases or use of medications that affect bone, should be considered in assessing fracture risk and making therapeutic decisions.
- Secondary causes of osteoporosis (such as osteomalacia or hyperparathyroidism) should be considered in the evaluation of a patient with low BMD and fractures.
- Several effective therapies that improve BMD and reduce fracture risks are available; the choice of the drug should be individualized.
- The T-score is the number of standard deviations (SD) above or below the young adult mean. It is a better measure than the Z-score for predicting fracture risk.
- Pregnancy and lactation are associated with demineralization of the mother's skeleton, which is fully restored after weaning; consequently, multiparity is not a risk factor for osteoporosis.

## INTRODUCTION

Osteoporosis is a systemic skeletal disorder characterized by low bone mass and microarchitectural deterioration of bone tissue (Fig. 1-1), with a consequent increase in bone fragility and susceptibility to fracture.[1] The definition encompasses several essential characteristics of this disease: one is the susceptibility to fractures that occur at considerably lower levels of trauma in osteoporotic subjects than in those with normal bone. Although the typical osteoporotic fractures are those of the wrist, vertebrae, and hip, almost any fracture is dependent on the quantity and quality of bone.[2,3] The problem with the fracture-based definition of osteoporosis is that fractures occur relatively late in the course of the disease and have long-term consequences that are largely irreversible. This leads to recognition of the other aspect of osteoporosis that is captured by the current definition: the finding of low bone mass, which usually is present during the long asymptomatic phase of the disease. Introducing this concept into the definition and understanding of osteoporosis

allows recognition of the disease before fracture occurs and the use of bone density–based diagnostic criteria for osteoporosis[4] (Table 1-1). The third aspect of the osteoporosis definition is the microarchitectural deterioration of bone tissue. Changes in bone microarchitecture cannot be assessed easily using currently available methods, yet represent an important aspect of this disease and an active area of research.[5]

The evolution of the human skeleton has resulted in bones that are light enough to allow adequate mobility and strong enough to avoid disabling fractures during the reproductive years. However, with advancing age in both sexes, and particularly after the menopause in women, bone becomes weaker and neuromuscular function declines. These changes produce a dramatic increase in the risk of fracture, which is the only symptom of osteoporosis. Osteoporotic fractures are a major public health problem as they are a significant cause of disability in the aging population and a major contributor to the cost of health care in many countries.[6]

## EPIDEMIOLOGY AND CLINICAL PRESENTATION

Osteoporosis is a common disease. Approximately 44 million persons in the United States have low bone mass, and the number is likely to increase substantially during the next several decades as the proportion of elderly people in the population increases.[6] It is estimated that a Caucasian woman aged 50 years has a 40% chance of having at least one of the typical osteoporotic fractures during her lifetime and a 70% chance if fractures other than spine, hip, and wrist are considered (such as pelvic, humeral, tibial, and other fractures). The probability of fracture in men is about one third that of women. Because women have a higher fracture risk and because they live longer, they account for 80% of all hip fractures. Osteoporosis occurs more frequently with increasing age as bone tissue is progressively lost. In women, there is accelerated bone loss after menopause such that most women meet the World Health Organization (WHO) bone density criteria for osteoporosis (see Table 1-1) by age 70 years.

Hip fractures are the most devastating and costly consequence of osteoporosis. Most hip fractures occur in individuals with reduced bone mass, after a fall from standing height or less. Most require hospitalization and surgical intervention, which are often associated with thromboembolic, cardiovascular, and infectious complications. The high rate of these complications is due at least in part to the advanced age of the subjects who sustain hip fractures. As a result, during the first year following

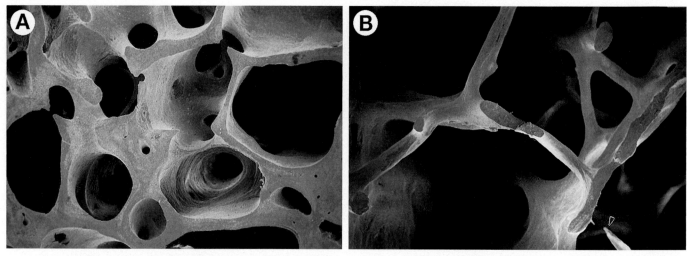

Figure 1-1    Scanning electron micrographs of normal *(A)* and osteoporotic *(B)* cancellous bone from human iliac crest. Note that the osteoporotic bone has both lower mass and altered bone microarchitecture. (From Dempster DW: The contribution of trabecular architecture to cancellous bone quality. J Bone Miner Res 2000;15:20–23. Reproduced with permission from the American Society for Bone and Mineral Research.)

hip fractures there is an increase in mortality of about 36% in men and 21% in women, greater in older men and in persons with higher level of comorbidities or declining cognitive function. In those who survive, there is often residual disability or decline in functional status, resulting in loss of independence that necessitates nursing home admission in almost 50% of patients. The degree of functional recovery is inversely proportionate to age and prefracture functional status.

The incidence of hip fractures increases exponentially with age[6] (Fig. 1-2). Worldwide, an estimated 1.66 million hip fractures occurred in 1990. In the United States, about 300,000 hip fractures occur annually, most of which require hospital admission and surgical intervention. The current cost resulting from hip fractures is more than $11.5 billion per year in the United States alone. There is significant geographic variation in the rates of hip fractures (Fig. 1-3). In addition, the rates are higher in urban than in rural areas, probably because urbanization results in decline in physical activity and because change from softer ground to hardwood, tile, concrete, and asphalt surfaces

increases the impact of falling. The rates of hip fracture are increasing worldwide, because of the aging population and because of an absolute increase in age-adjusted hip fracture rates.[7] The most likely explanation for this is a decline in physical activity and possibly increased frailty of the aging population.

Vertebral fractures usually occur in the course of routine daily activities, with only one quarter resulting from a fall. Although approximately 500,000 vertebral fractures occur each year in the United States, most are asymptomatic; only about one third of fractures that are found on radiographs come to medical attention and less than 10% require hospital admission. Interestingly, even when a vertebral fracture is present on the

| Table 1-1 WHO Definition of Osteoporosis Based on BMD Measurement | | |
|---|---|---|
| **Category** | **Defined as BMD That Is** | **T-Score** |
| Normal | No more than 1 SD below the young adult mean | >–1 |
| Osteopenia | Between 1 and 2.5 SD below the young adult mean | –1 to –2.5 |
| Osteoporosis | More than 2.5 SD below the young adult mean | <–2.5 |
| Severe (established) osteoporosis | More than 2.5 SD below the young adult mean and at least one fragility fracture | <–2.5 |

BMD, bone mineral density.
From Consensus Development Conference: Diagnosis, prophylaxis, and treatment of osteoporosis. Am J Med 1993;94:646–650.

**Age-related fractures**

Incidence/ 100,000 person-year

Men        Women

4000
3000
2000
1000

35–39        85        85
Age group (yr)

— Hip    — Vertebra    — Colles'

Figure 1-2    Age-specific incident rates for hip, vertebral, and distal forearm fractures in men and women. (From Melton LJ: Epidemiology of fractures. In Riggs BL, Melton LJ [eds]: Osteoporosis: Etiology, Diagnosis and Management. New York, Raven Press, 1988, pp 133–154.)

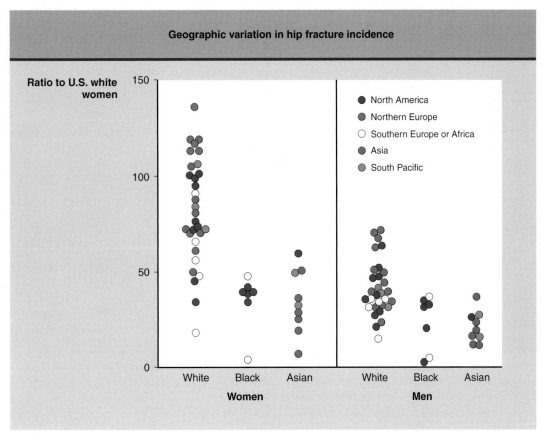

**Figure 1-3　Geographic variation in hip fracture incidence.** (From Melton LJ III: Differing patterns of osteoporosis across the world. In Chesnut CH III [ed]: New dimensions in osteoporosis in the 1990s—proceedings of the Second Asian Symposium on Osteoporosis, Nov 10, 1990. Hong Kong, Asia Pacific Congress Series No. 125, Excerpta Medica, 1991, pp 13–18.)

radiograph it often is not mentioned by the radiologist, is not noted in the chart, and does not lead to diagnosis or treatment of osteoporosis. Although vertebral fractures are often undiagnosed, they are commonly associated with significant morbidity and increased mortality.[8] Multiple fractures lead to height loss and kyphosis, chronic pain resulting from altered biomechanics of the kyphotic back, restrictive lung disease resulting from decreased thoracic cavity, and digestive complaints of early satiety, gastroesophageal reflux, and constipation resulting from decreased volume of the abdominal cavity[8] (Fig. 1-4). Vertebral fractures should be suspected in older people with kyphosis or height loss of at least 4 to 5 cm (1.5 to 2 in.), changes that many patients and physicians fail to recognize as a sign of disease and erroneously attribute to effects of aging. Although often asymptomatic, vertebral fractures are associated with a significant risk of additional vertebral and nonvertebral fractures.[8,9]

Because vertebral fractures are often asymptomatic, their epidemiology is less clear than that of hip fractures. In addition, studies of prevalence of radiographic vertebral fractures have been complicated by lack of consensus about what constitutes a vertebral fracture. It is clear, nevertheless, that the incidence of vertebral fractures increases with age, with the curve being steeper in women (see Fig. 1-2). Although the risk of vertebral fractures is about three times higher in women over age 65, the prevalence is similar in men and women aged 50 to 60 years,

possibly reflecting a higher risk of traumatic vertebral fractures in younger men as a result of greater occupational and recreational physical activity. There is less geographic variability in the risk of vertebral fractures compared with hip fractures.[6]

Distal forearm fractures almost always follow a fall on the outstretched arm. Because this pattern of falling is seen in younger people (in comparison with the elderly, who tend to fall to the side or backward and sustain a hip fracture), the peak incidence of these fractures in Caucasian women is between ages 40 and 65 (see Fig. 1-2). The main importance of wrist fracture is that it often is a first manifestation of osteoporosis, which should prompt appropriate evaluation and therapy.

### Risk Factors

Many conditions increase the risk of fracture by either causing decreased bone mass or increasing the risk of falling (Table 1-2). Among these, the most significant are the history of fracture as an adult, maternal history of hip fracture (or other fractures), cigarette smoking, and low body weight (below 58.5 kg [129 lb]).[10]

## PATHOGENESIS

Osteoporosis or low bone mass can result from inadequate accumulation of bone in young adulthood (low peak bone mass)

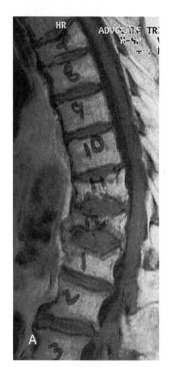

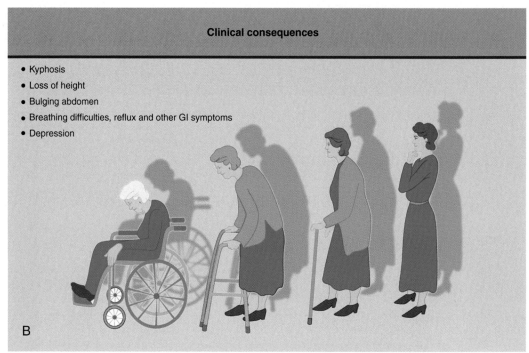

**Clinical consequences**

- Kyphosis
- Loss of height
- Bulging abdomen
- Breathing difficulties, reflux and other GI symptoms
- Depression

**Figure 1-4    Vertebal fractures.** *A,* MRI of the thoracic and lumbar spine showing multiple vertebral fractures (T7, T11, T12, L1, and L2). *B,* Clinical consequences of vertebral fractures. (*B,* From Gallagher JC, Hedlund LR, Stone S, et al: Vertebral morphometry: normative data. Bone Miner 1988;4:189–196.)

or excessive bone loss later in life[11,12] (Fig. 1-5). The increase in bone mass that occurs during childhood and puberty results from a combination of bone growth at the endplates (endochondral bone formation) and change in bone shape (modeling). The rapid increase in bone mass during puberty associated with an increase in sex hormone levels continues for 3 to 4 years and then slows down with the closure of growth plates. Further increase in BMD in the next several years is relatively modest and the consequence of periosteal apposition (modeling). The peak bone mass is achieved by age 20 to 30 and is greater in men than in women and greater in African American than in Caucasian, Asian, or Hispanic populations. Genetic factors are

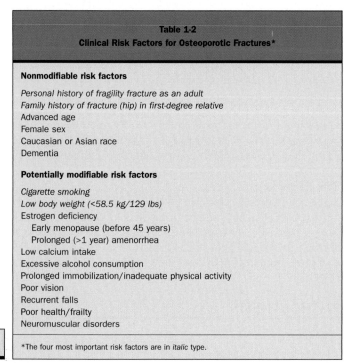

**Table 1-2**
**Clinical Risk Factors for Osteoporotic Fractures\***

**Nonmodifiable risk factors**

*Personal history of fragility fracture as an adult*
*Family history of fracture (hip) in first-degree relative*
Advanced age
Female sex
Caucasian or Asian race
Dementia

**Potentially modifiable risk factors**

*Cigarette smoking*
*Low body weight (<58.5 kg/129 lbs)*
Estrogen deficiency
    Early menopause (before 45 years)
    Prolonged (>1 year) amenorrhea
Low calcium intake
Excessive alcohol consumption
Prolonged immobilization/inadequate physical activity
Poor vision
Recurrent falls
Poor health/frailty
Neuromuscular disorders

*\*The four most important risk factors are in italic type.*

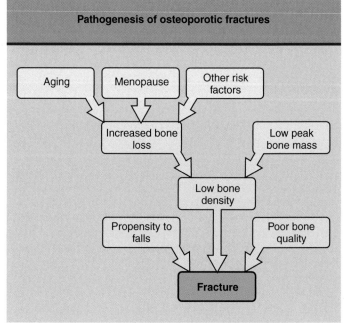

**Pathogenesis of osteoporotic fractures**

Aging — Menopause — Other risk factors → Increased bone loss

Low peak bone mass

Increased bone loss + Low peak bone mass → Low bone density

Propensity to falls

Poor bone quality

Low bone density + Propensity to falls + Poor bone quality → **Fracture**

**Figure 1-5    Pathogenesis of osteoporotic fractures.**

the main determinants of peak bone mass and account for 50% to 85% of the variance in bone density and size. It is likely that several genes regulate bone mass, each with modest effect. Nongenetic factors associated with low peak bone mass include low calcium intake during childhood, low body weight, sedentary lifestyle, chronic disease, and delayed puberty.

After the peak bone mass is attained, further changes in bone, including bone loss associated with aging and menopause, are determined by bone remodeling (Fig. 1-6). Bone remodeling is responsible for repair of microdamage of bone, maintenance of skeletal strength, and supply of calcium from the skeleton when needed to maintain normal serum calcium. Bone remodeling involves osteoclast-mediated bone resorption followed by

osteoblastic bone formation. The initial stimulus is often a micro-crack, which leads to *activation*—recruitment and fusion of osteoclast precursors into mature osteoclast. The mature osteoclast then attaches to the bone surface by binding with the ruffled border. *Resorption* of bone trapped by the osteoclast produces a cutting cone (cortical bone) or a trench (trabecular bone). Bone resorption is followed by *bone formation*, the process during which osteoblasts synthesize bone matrix that subsequently mineralizes. After the matrix fills a resorption cavity, osteoblasts remain trapped in the bone and become osteocytes. The latter are believed to be responsible for mechanotransduction and bone response to mechanical loading. While the process of osteoclastic bone resorption of a single

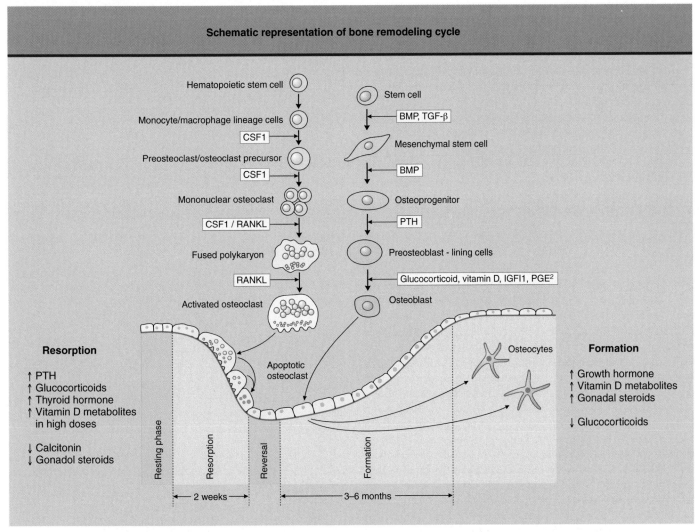

**Schematic representation of bone remodeling cycle**

**Figure 1-6  Bone remodeling.** Note that the resorption phase lasts approximately 2 weeks, whereas the formation phase requires 3 to 6 months for completion. As a result, conditions associated with increased bone turnover often result in a net loss of bone. Osteoclast is a tissue-specific macrophage polykaryon created by the differentiation of the monocyte/macrophage precursor cells at or near bone surface. One of the main physiologic regulators of osteoclast differentiation and function is RANKL, which binds to RANK on the surface of the osteoclast and its precursors. RANKL is transmembrane protein expressed on osteoblasts, which also produce a soluble factor osteoprotegerin (OPG), which acts as a decoy receptor for RANKL and decreases osteoclast-mediated bone resorption. OPG is under investigation as a possible pharmacologic agent for treatment of osteoporosis. BMP, bone morphogenic protein; CSF, colony stimulating factor; IGF-I, insulin-like growth factor–I; $PGE_2$, prostaglandin $E_2$, PTH, parathyroid hormone; RANKL, receptor activator of nuclear factor kappaB ligand; TGF-β, transforming growth factor–β.

cavity usually takes approximately 2 weeks, osteoblastic bone formation requires 3 to 6 months to fill in a resorption pit. Consequently, any physiologic or pathologic process (such as decrease in estrogen level during menopause) that increases activation frequency (rate of initiation of new bone remodeling cycle) results in a net loss of bone. Numerous circulating or locally produced factors influence bone remodeling (see Fig. 1-6). Imbalance in bone remodeling, i.e., greater resorption than formation, results in bone loss. This manifests as increased cortical porosity in cortical bone and perforation of trabecular plates in trabecular bone. These processes greatly diminish the biomechanical competence of the aging skeleton. Multiple diseases and medications are associated with these processes (Table 1-3). Therapeutic agents used to treat osteoporosis act primarily by either decreasing bone resorption ("antiresorptive agents") or increasing bone formation ("anabolic agents").

## DIAGNOSIS

Because osteoporosis is largely asymptomatic, it is necessary to diagnose bone fragility before fractures occur. This can be approached through assessment of bone mass (widely used in clinical practice and in research), assessment of bone structure (used only in research), and assessment of bone turnover (widely used in research, beginning to be used in clinical practice).

### Assessment of Bone Mass

Currently available methods used to assess bone mass can be grouped according to the site scanned or the scanning method used (Table 1-4). There are multiple indications to assess bone mass, which continue to be reevaluated on the basis of new information and studies (Table 1-5).

The standard method used for assessment of bone mass in both clinical practice and the research setting is dual energy x-ray absorptiometry (DXA) of the central sites, i.e., lumbar spine and proximal femur.[13,14] Measuring bone mass at peripheral sites such as distal radius, calcaneus, and phalanges are widely available and less costly.[13] Although peripheral measurements can be used for assessment of fracture risks in population studies, their use in making a diagnosis of osteoporosis in an individual is problematic because their fracture prediction ability is lower than that of central BMD and because the proportion of patients with T-score less than –2.5 varies considerably from one type of device to another (Fig. 1-7).[15] Peripheral measurements are best used as screening tools to identify patients who are unlikely to have osteoporosis at central sites or increased fragility. To properly select patients who do not need further testing by central densitometry device, specific cut-off points should be established for each device. It should be noted, however, that subjects with significant risk factors such as chronic corticosteroid therapy or history of fractures, should have central densitometry regardless of the results of peripheral testing. Because of lower precision and lack of adequate prospective data, peripheral measurements should not be used for monitoring therapy.[16]

Quantitative computed tomography (CT) scans of the spine can also be used for assessing bone mass.[13] The advantage of CT scans is that they are three-dimensional, permitting a separate assessment of trabecular and cortical bone. In addition, arthritic

---

**Table 1-3**
**Diseases and Medications Associated with Osteoporosis/Low Bone Mass**

**Hypogonadal states (primary or secondary)**

Amenorrhea
Hyperprolactinemia
Anorexia nervosa
Turner's syndrome
Kleinfelter's syndrome

**Endocrine disorders**

Cushing's syndrome
Hyperparathyroidism, primary
Thyrotoxicosis
Idiopathic hypercalciuria
Insulin-dependent diabetes mellitus
Adrenal insufficiency
Acromegaly
Hypopituitarism

**Nutritional and gastrointestinal disorders**

Malnutrition
Parenteral nutrition
Malabsorption syndromes
Crohn's disease
Gastrectomy
Liver diseases (biliary cirrhosis)

**Rheumatologic disorders**

Rheumatoid arthritis
Ankylosing spondylitis

**Malignant and hematologic disorders**

Multiple myeloma
Lymphoma and leukemia
Tumors with ectopic PTHrP production
Mastocytosis
Thalassemia
Hemophilia

**Inherited and other miscellaneous conditions**

Pregnancy and lactation (transient)
Osteogenesis imperfecta
Scoliosis
Marfan syndrome
Hemochromatosis
Hypophosphatasia
Glycogen storage diseases
Immobilization
Multiple sclerosis
Weight loss
Porphyria

**Medications**

Corticosteroids
Anticonvulsants
Alcohol
Chemotherapy/immunosuppression
Cyclosporine
Excess thyroid hormone
GnRH agonists
Heparin
Lithium
Aluminum
Excess vitamin A
Tobacco
Tamoxifen (premenopausal women)
?Bile acid–binding resins

**Table 1-4**
**Classification of Tests Used for Assessment of Bone Mass**

**According to site**

Central (hip and spine)
Peripheral (forearm, heel, phalanges)

**According to method**

DXA (spine, hip, heel, forearm)
Ultrasound (heel)
qCT—quantitative CT (spine, radius)
Radio-absorptiometry (phalanges)

**Table 1-5**
**Indications for Bone Mineral Density Testing\*†**

- Women aged 65 and older
- Postmenopausal women under age 65 with risk factors
- Men aged 70 and older
- Adults with a fragility fracture
- Adults with a disease or condition associated with low bone mass or bone loss
- Adults taking medications associated with low bone mass or bone loss
- Anyone being considered for pharmacologic therapy for bone loss
- Anyone being treated for bone loss, to monitor treatment effect
- Anyone not receiving therapy in whom evidence of bone loss would lead to treatment

\*Women discontinuing estrogen should be considered for bone density testing according to the indications listed in the table.
† As recommended by International Society for Clinical Densitometry (ISCD), 2003 consensus conference.[16]

changes of the spine, which falsely elevate DXA, do not affect CT measurement. The disadvantages of CT include high cost and high radiation exposure, and its ability to predict fracture is not well studied. Applying WHO BMD criteria for osteopenia and osteoporosis to CT measurements leads to a tendency to overdiagnose osteoporosis in younger women. All the difficulties associated with CT measurements largely limit its application to that of a research tool. When CT measurements are used in clinical practice, care should be taken that WHO criteria are not strictly applied.

Numerous studies have documented a strong inverse relationship between fracture risk and central, particularly hip, BMD, making DXA measurement the gold standard for assessing bone mass and predicting fracture risk (Table 1-6).[13,14] BMD is measured at the lumbar spine and proximal femur.

Spine DXA measures BMD of the L1–L4 vertebrae. Since vertebrae are composed primarily of metabolically active trabecular bone, this site is more likely to show the earliest

changes in menopause, during exposure to corticosteroids, and in response to therapy. A potentially limiting factor of spine DXA is that spine BMD is measured in the anteroposterior projection, which includes the mineral in the posterior elements and facet joints and calcifications in the abdominal aorta, none of which contribute to the mechanical strength of the vertebrae.[13,14] For this reason, the spine BMD is often artifactually elevated in elderly subjects, which is only partly remedied by exclusion of artifact laden vertebrae when interpreting it (see Table 1-6).[16]

**Table 1-6**
**Use of Central DXA for Diagnosis of Osteoporosis\***

**Skeletal sites to measure**

Measure BMD at both posteroanterior spine and hip in all patients
Forearm BMD should be measured under the following circumstances:
  Hip or spine cannot be measured or interpreted
  Patient has hyperparathyroidism
  Very obese patient (over weight limit for DXA table)

**Spine region of interest**

Use posteroanterior L1–L4 for spine BMD measurement
Use all evaluable vertebrae and exclude only vertebrae affected by local structural change or artifact; use three vertebrae if four cannot be used, and two if three cannot be used
Lateral spine should not be used for diagnosis, but may have a role in monitoring

**Hip region of interest**

Use total proximal femur, femoral neck, or trochanter, whichever is lowest
BMD may be measured at either hip
Do not use Ward's area for diagnosis
There are insufficient data to determine whether mean T-scores for bilateral hip BMD can be used for diagnosis
The mean hip BMD can be used for monitoring, with total hip being preferred

**Forearm region of interest**

Use 33% radius (sometimes called one-third radius) of the nondominant forearm for diagnosis
Other forearm regions of interest are not recommended

BMD, bone mineral density; DXA, dual energy x-ray absorptiometry.
\*As recommended by International Society for Clinical Densitometry (ISCD), 2003 consensus conference.[16]

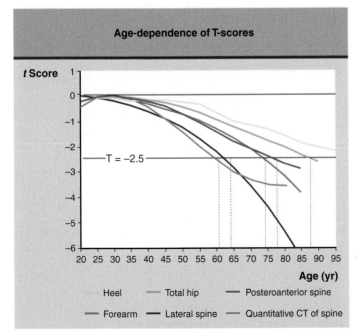

**Age-dependence of T-scores**

Figure 1-7   Prevalence of osteoporosis, defined as T-score of −2.5 and below, depends on the site and technique used to assess bone mass. (From Faulkner KG, von Stetten E, Miller P: Discordance in patient classification using T-scores. J Clin Densitom 1999;2:343–350.)

The proximal femur (hip) is composed of more cortical bone than the spine is, and it is less likely to show large changes with therapy. Since hip BMD is not affected by the artifacts that may affect spine BMD, it may be a more reliable site for measuring BMD in patients over 65 years of age. Bone density of the hip is the best predictor of the risk of hip fractures and indeed of overall fracture risk.[13,14] Several regions of interest of the proximal femur can be used for diagnosis (see Table 1-6).[16]

For each patient, BMD is compared with two sets of normative data. First, it is compared with BMD obtained in the healthy young adult Caucasian population, which yields a T-score (the number of standard deviations above or below the young adult mean). The T-score is used for diagnosing osteopenia and osteoporosis because it is the best predictor of fracture risk. The second comparison is to age, race, and sex-matched population and is the basis for calculating the Z-score (the number of standard deviations above or below the mean of age, race, and sex-matched population). While a low Z-score (below −1.5 or −2) is thought to suggest the presence of secondary causes of osteoporosis, no studies support that belief.

WHO criteria for diagnosing osteoporosis and osteopenia based on BMD measurements (see Table 1-1) is applicable only to postmenopausal women (see Table 1-7 for BMD interpretation in other populations[16]). In premenopausal women with low bone mass, particularly if associated with fracture, a thorough search for secondary causes should be undertaken.

### Assessing Non–Bone Mineral Density Aspects of Fragility

BMD accounts for 85% of fracture risk in population studies, and in vitro biomechanical testing confirms the importance of bone mass in determining bone strength. However, BMD is not the sole predictor of fragility, as evidenced by a large overlap in BMD values between subjects with and without fractures (Fig. 1-8). Among the non-BMD factors that predict fragility, the paramount variable is age (Fig. 1-9): at any level of BMD, fracture risk is considerably higher in older subjects.[17]

Vertebral fractures, and to a lesser degree other low trauma fractures, also strongly predict future fractures.[2,9] Although vertebral fractures herald future fractures, they often are asymptomatic and require radiographs for detection. However, radiographs usually are not a part of standard patient evaluation for osteoporosis. Recently, imaging of the thoracic and lumbar spine has become possible using the same DXA equipment used for measuring BMD (Fig. 1-10). With this methodology, termed vertebral fracture assessment (VFA), detection of vertebral fractures and measurement of BMD is possible at the same visit.[18] The presence of atraumatic vertebral fractures, even in a patient who does not have BMD criteria for osteoporosis, is considered diagnostic of osteoporosis and should prompt a more aggressive evaluation and treatment.

### Assessment of Bone Structure

Assessment of bone structure is not available clinically at present but has significant potential as a tool for determining non-BMD aspects of bone fragility. The methods under development include three-dimensional evaluations using magnetic resonance imaging (MRI) and micro-CT, and two-dimensional techniques such as fractal analysis of bone radiographs.[5]

**Table 1-7**

**Definition of T-Scores and Diagnosis of Osteoporosis in Various Populations***

**Reference database for T-scores**

Use a uniform Caucasian (non-race-adjusted) female normative database for women of all ethnic groups

Use a uniform Caucasian (non-race-adjusted) male normative database for men of all ethnic groups

**Diagnosis in postmenopausal women**

Use the WHO criteria (normal, T-score −1.0 or above; osteoporosis, T-score −2.5 or below; osteopenia, t score between −1.0 and −2.5)

Select the lowest T-score of posteroanterior spine, femoral neck, total hip, trochanter, or the 33% radius, if measured

**Diagnosis in men (aged 20 yr and older)**

The WHO criteria should not be applied in their entirety to men

In men aged 65 yr and older, T-scores should be used and osteoporosis diagnosed if the T-score is at or below −2.5

Between ages 50 and 65 yr, T-scores may be used and osteoporosis diagnosed if the T-score is at or below −2.5 and other risk factors for fracture are identified

Men at any age with secondary causes of low BMD (e.g., glucocorticoid therapy, hypogonadism, hyperparathyroidism) may be diagnosed clinically with osteoporosis supported by findings of low BMD

The diagnosis of osteoporosis in men under age 50 yr should not be made on the basis of densitometric criteria alone

**Diagnosis in premenopausal women (aged 20 yr to menopause)**

The WHO criteria should not be applied to healthy premenopausal women

Z-scores rather than T-scores should be used

Osteoporosis may be diagnosed if there is low BMD with secondary causes (e.g., glucocorticoid therapy, hypogonadism, hyperparathyroidism) or with risk factors for fracture

The diagnosis of osteoporosis in premenopausal women should not be made on the basis of densitometric criteria alone

**Diagnosis in children (male or female < aged 20 yr)**

T-scores should not be used in children; Z-scores should be used instead

T-scores should not appear in reports or on DXA printouts in children

The diagnosis of osteoporosis in children should not be made on the basis of densitometric criteria alone

Terminology such as low bone density for chronologic age may be used if the Z-score is below −2.0

Z-scores must be interpreted in light of the best available pediatric databases of age-matched controls; the reference database should be cited in the report

Spine and total body are the preferred skeletal sites for measurement

The value of BMD to predict fractures in children is not clearly determined

There is no agreement on standards for adjusting BMD or bone mineral content (BMC) for factors such as bone size, pubertal stage, skeletal maturity, and body composition; if adjustments are made, they should be clearly stated in the report

Serial BMD studies should be done on the same machine using the same scanning mode, software, and analysis method when appropriate; changes may be required with growth of the child

Any deviation from standard adult acquisition protocols, such as use of low-density software and manual adjustment of region of interest, should be stated in the report

*As recommended by International Society for Clinical Densitometry (ISCD), 2003 consensus conference.[16]

### Biochemical Markers of Bone Turnover

Biochemical markers of bone turnover also assess non-BMD aspects of bone fragility.[19] Currently available markers of bone formation and resorption are listed in Table 1-8. Because bone formation and resorption usually are coupled, measuring any

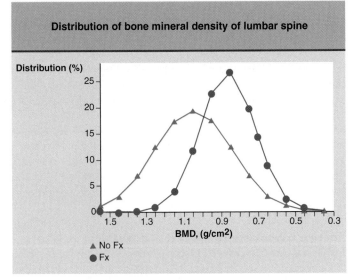

**Figure 1-8   Distribution of bone mineral density (BMD) of the lumbar spine in women with and without vertebral fractures.** (From Melton LJ III, Kan SH, Frye MA, et al: Epidemiology of vertebral fractures in women. Am J Epidemiol 1989;129:1000–1011.)

marker is likely to yield similar information. In epidemiologic studies, markers of bone resorption are more consistent predictors of future fractures. Biochemical markers of bone turnover may be useful in clinical evaluation of osteoporosis as a way of predicting fracture risk. Thus, subjects with high markers of bone resorption have higher fracture risk than those with similar BMD and low levels of bone markers (Fig. 1-11). Although widely used in research, biochemical markers are of limited use in clinical practice at present because of relatively

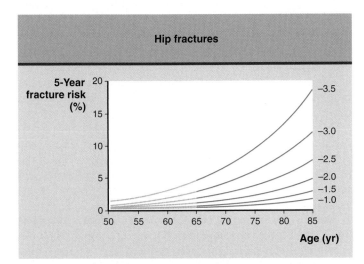

**Figure 1-9   Five-year risk of hip fractures as a function of age and bone mineral density (BMD).** Note that at any level of BMD, the fracture risk is considerably higher in older than in younger subjects. The hip fracture risk for women over age 65 is observed in Study of Osteoporotic Fractures (SOF), which included women over age 65 only. The fracture risk in younger women is extrapolated. (From Cummings SR, Bates D, Black DM: Clinical use of bone densitometry: scientific review. JAMA 2002;288:1889–1897.)

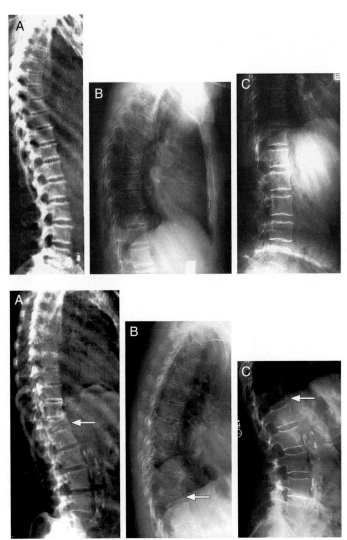

**Figure 1-10** Vertebral fracture assessment (VFA) image from the densitometer *(A)* and radiographs of the thoracic *(B)* and lumbar spine *(C)* in a patient without fractures *(top)* and a patient with T12 fracture indicated by arrows *(bottom)*. (From Vokes TJ, Dixon LB, Favus MJ: Clinical utility of dual-energy vertebral assessment [DVA]. Osteoporos Int 2003;14:871–878.)

high analytical and biological variability and the lack of guidelines regarding the selection of markers and their practical application. The potential application of bone markers is in patients who have borderline BMD values in whom finding a high marker will prompt a therapeutic intervention. Bone markers are also used to assess response to therapy. Changes in bone markers during therapy predict subsequent increase in bone density and reduction in fracture rate. In the future, it also may be possible to use biochemical markers of bone turnover to select therapeutic agents that either reduce bone resorption or stimulate bone formation.

## Monitoring Changes in Bone Status

BMD can be used to monitor bone loss in early menopause, during corticosteroid therapy, or in the course of diseases that may have detrimental effects on bone. Increased bone mass occurs in response to osteoporosis therapy, during the resolution

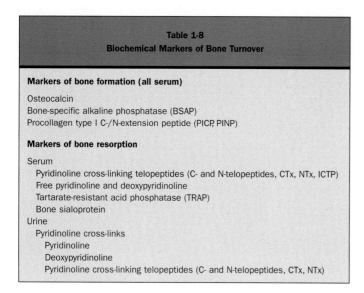

**Table 1-8**
**Biochemical Markers of Bone Turnover**

**Markers of bone formation (all serum)**

Osteocalcin
Bone-specific alkaline phosphatase (BSAP)
Procollagen type I C-/N-extension peptide (PICP, PINP)

**Markers of bone resorption**

Serum
  Pyridinoline cross-linking telopeptides (C- and N-telopeptides, CTx, NTx, ICTP)
  Free pyridinoline and deoxypyridinoline
  Tartarate-resistant acid phosphatase (TRAP)
  Bone sialoprotein
Urine
  Pyridinoline cross-links
    Pyridinoline
    Deoxypyridinoline
  Pyridinoline cross-linking telopeptides (C- and N-telopeptides, CTx, NTx)

of a disease, and upon discontinuing medications associated with bone loss. The frequency with which bone density testing should be repeated depends on the expected rate of change in bone mass and the precision of the DXA instrument.[16] The "least significant change," which is the smallest difference between two measurements that can be considered a true change with 95% confidence, is calculated as 2.7 (approximated to 3) times the precision error of the measurement. Since the precision of the lumbar spine BMD measurement is 1%, the least significant change is 3%. Hip precision of 1.5% requires the least significant change to be greater than 4.5% to 5%. On the basis of this information, bone density can be repeated every 1 to 2 years in early menopause, when the rate of bone loss is the greatest. In

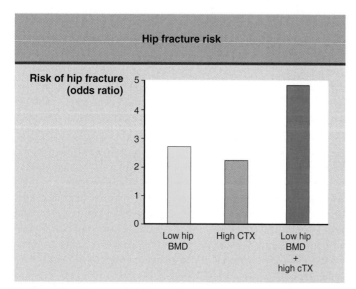

**Hip fracture risk**

**Figure 1-11** **Hip fracture risk is better assessed by a combination of bone mineral density (BMD) and bone resorption rate in a cohort of elderly (mean age, 82.5 years) French women.** Low BMD was defined by a value below 2.5 SD of the young adult mean and high bone resorption by urinary CTx values above 2.0 SD of the young adult mean. CTx, C-terminal telopeptide of type I collagen.

late menopause, the time between two BMD measurements should be at least 2 years. Corticosteroid therapy induces rapid bone loss during the first 6 months of therapy, which can be monitored by repeating BMD at 6 to 12 months after long-term treatment is begun, and yearly thereafter. Pharmacologic treatment of osteoporosis can be monitored by repeating BMD 1 year after the initiation of therapy and every 2 years thereafter. Stable or increased BMD, greater than the least significant change, indicates a satisfactory response to therapy. A decrease in BMD greater than the least significant change should prompt a search for secondary causes, particularly if this was not done prior to initiation of therapy, and a reassessment of the patient's compliance, including adequate intake of calcium and vitamin D.

### Routine Laboratory Evaluation and Workup for Secondary Causes of Osteoporosis

No laboratory abnormalities are diagnostic of postmenopausal osteoporosis. However, laboratory evaluation might be helpful in determining whether the patient has secondary causes of osteoporosis, i.e., conditions other than age and menopause that contribute to bone loss. There are no clear guidelines regarding screening for secondary causes of osteoporosis, primarily because there is relatively little information regarding the proportion of patients with osteoporosis who have evidence of secondary causes.[20] In a study from a tertiary referral center in Canada,[21] more than half of patients with a T-score less than −2.5 had a history of diseases or medications contributing to bone loss (Table 1-9). Among the 173 women with no history of any bone-related disorder or medication, more than 30% were found to have secondary causes on laboratory testing (see Table 1-9). Interestingly, there was no significant difference in T-scores or Z-scores between patients with and without secondary causes. The authors of that study concluded that the most cost-effective approach is to measure 24-hour urine calcium, serum calcium, and parathyroid hormone (PTH) in all patients and thyroid-stimulating hormone (TSH) in those receiving exogenous thyroid hormone. It is also reasonable to obtain a chemistry panel, looking for evidence of renal or hepatic disease or elevation of alkaline phosphatase. Low urinary calcium suggests deficient intake or absorption of calcium or vitamin D. Idiopathic hypercalciuria and primary hyperparathyroidism both are associated with high urinary calcium, and can be differentiated by serum calcium and PTH, which are normal in the former disease and elevated in the latter. In all patients with elevated PTH, renal function should be assessed to exclude renal insufficiency and accompanying secondary hyperparathyroidism and renal osteodystrophy.

While some secondary causes of low bone mass explain low BMD, other causes have important therapeutic implications. For example, osteomalacia often presents with low BMD and fractures. Osteomalacia results from vitamin D deficiency, which decreases calcium absorption and induces secondary hyperparathyroidism, which in turn increases excretion of phosphate and decreases excretion of calcium in the urine. Consequently, hypophosphatemia is more common than hypocalcemia, which is seen only in advanced cases. High PTH increases bone turnover, which raises serum alkaline phosphatase, particularly its bone fraction, which is normal in postmenopausal osteoporosis.

## TREATMENT

### Lifestyle Changes

The goal of treating osteoporosis is prevention of fractures. Since most fractures are associated with trauma, it is important to prevent falls by adapting the environment (removing loose carpeting, cables, and other objects that increase the risk of falling), avoiding medication that is associated with orthostatic hypotension or sedation, and correcting visual problems. Smoking and excessive alcohol intake should also be discouraged.[10]

### Nutritional Recommendations

Adequate calcium intake is a necessary part of the treatment plan for all patients with osteoporosis and for postmenopausal women and other patients at risk of developing osteoporosis. Recommended calcium intake is a 1000 mg/day for premenopausal women and 1200 to 1500 mg/day for postmenopausal women.[10] Calcium can be taken from food or from calcium supplements (Table 1-10). It is important to limit the amount of elemental calcium taken at one time to no more than 600 mg, since the calcium absorption fraction decreases with higher doses. Calcium supplements are best taken with food, particularly in the case of calcium carbonate, which requires an acid environment for the dissociation of calcium from carbonate and for its absorption. For this reason, patients who take proton pump inhibitors or have low gastric acid production should receive calcium citrate. Calcium citrate may be also preferable for patients who are prone to constipation, which tends to worsen with carbonate preparations.

Vitamin D, which is necessary for intestinal calcium absorption, is synthesized in the skin under the influence of ultraviolet light. Vitamin D insufficiency is common particularly among the elderly and in those living in northern latitudes. Because few food sources contain a significant amount of vitamin D, it often is necessary to use vitamin D supplementation at the recommended dose of 200 IU for adults less than 50 years of age, 400 IU for adults between 50 and 70 years of age, and 600 to 800 IU for adults over 70 years of age. A multivitamin tablet usually contains 200 to 400 units, as do many calcium supplements. Patients who have very low serum levels of 25-OH-vitamin D should be treated with high vitamin D doses (50,000 IU/wk) until the deficiency is corrected. In the frail elderly, it also is important to provide adequate caloric and protein intake. Caffeine and salt intake should be limited because they increase urinary calcium excretion.

### Exercise

By itself, exercise can not maintain or increase bone mass in postmenopausal women. However, regular physical activity should be a part of the therapeutic approach because it is beneficial to patients with osteoporosis.[11,12] Since gravity enhances bone formation, weight-bearing exercise (e.g., walking, dancing, cross country skiing) is thought to decrease bone loss in the elderly and promote maintenance of peak bone mass in younger subjects. In addition, exercise improves muscle strength and coordination, thereby decreasing the risk of falling and minimizing the severity of injury upon a fall. Even for those who cannot walk, swimming and water exercise are beneficial for improving muscle function. Exercising at least three times a week should be a consistent and long-term habit.

| Table 1-9 Secondary Causes of Osteoporosis and Their Frequency in a Tertiary Referral Center | |
| --- | --- |
| **Known history of disorders or medications among 355 (53%) of 664 women with bone mineral density (BMD) T-score <−2.5** | |
| **Disorder** | **No. (%)** |
| Oral glucocorticoid use | 129 (36) |
| Premature ovarian failure | 76 (21) |
| Weight loss | 37 (10) |
| Alcoholism | 34 (10) |
| Liver disease | 34 (10) |
| Immobility (>3 months) | 33 (9) |
| Chemotherapy | 27 (8) |
| Hyperthyroidism | 22 (6) |
| Current anticonvulsant use | 19 (5) |
| Rheumatoid arthritis or systemic lupus erythematosus | 18 (5) |
| Hyperparathyroidism | 18 (5) |
| Malabsorption | 14 (4) |
| Other known metabolic or bone disorders | 12 (3) |
| Other medications known to affect bone | 11 (3) |
| **Secondary causes of osteoporosis found among 173 women who had no history of disorders or medications known to affect bone** | |
| **Disorder** | **No. (%)** |
| Hypercalciuria | 17 (10) |
| Malabsorption | 14 (8) |
| Hyperparathyroidism | 12 (7) |
| Primary (1) | |
| Secondary due to low calcium intake (6) | |
| Unexplained secondary (5) | |
| Vitamin D deficiency (<30 nM/L or 12 ng/mL) | 7 (4) |
| Thyroid hormone overtreatment | 4 (2) |
| Cushing's disease | 1 (1) |
| Patients with at least one new diagnosis | 55 (32) |

From Tannenbaum C, et al: Yield of laboratory testing to identify contributors to osteoporosis in otherwise healthy women. J Clin Endocrinol Metab 2002;87:4431–4437.

Osteomalacia requires treatment with calcium and vitamin D to normalize bone mass and structure. Importantly, the ensuing increase in BMD is far greater than observed with antiresorptive therapy in osteoporosis. Use of potent antiresorptive agents such as bisphosphonates is contraindicated in osteomalacia and may result in severe hypocalcemia caused by inhibition of osteoclastic bone resorption, which previously had maintained eucalcemia in the face of deficient intestinal absorption.

Idiopathic hypercalciuria is also important to detect because it may explain in part the low BMD and because it requires a different therapeutic approach. Calcium intake should be limited to 600 to 800 mg/day (rather than the 1500 recommended for postmenopausal women) and be supplied by food. Higher intake of calcium, particularly if obtained from calcium supplements, aggravates hypercalciuria and increases risk of kidney stones. On the other hand, severe restriction in calcium intake (as was recommended in the past to patients with kidney stones) does not eliminate hypercalciuria but increases calcium recruitment from bone, resulting in further bone loss. Hypercalciuria may be controlled by administration of thiazide diuretics, particularly the longer acting chlorthalidone.

### Table 1-10
### Calcium Content of Food and Supplements

#### Calcium Content of Some Common Food Items

| Food | Portion | Amount of Calcium (mg) |
|---|---|---|
| **Milk and milk products** | | |
| Yogurt, plain, low fat | 1 cup/175 mL | 292 |
| Ice cream | 1/2 cup/125 mL | 93 |
| Milk—whole, 2%, 1%, skim | 1 glass/250 mL | 315 |
| Cheese—Swiss, Gruyère | 1.75 oz/50 g | 493 |
| Cheese—brick, cheddar, colby, edam, gouda | 1.75 oz/50 g | 353 |
| Cheese—mozzarella | 1.75 oz/50 g | 269 |
| Cheese—cottage, creamed, 2%, 1% | 1/2 cup/125 mL | 87 |
| | | |
| **Breads and cereals** | | |
| Total cereal 100% calcium | 3/4 cup | 1,000 |
| Muffin, bran | 1/35 g | 50 |
| Bread, white and whole wheat | 1 slice/30 g | 25 |
| | | |
| **Meat, fish, poultry, and alternatives** | | |
| Sardines, with bones | 8 small | 153 |
| Salmon, with bones, canned | 213 g | 242 |
| Almonds | 1/2 cup/125 mL | 200 |
| Sesame seeds | 1/2 cup/125 mL | 100 |
| Beans, cooked—kidney, navy, pinto, garbanzo | 1 cup/250 mL | 90 |
| Soybeans, cooked | 1 cup/250 mL | 175 |
| Chicken, roasted | 3 oz/90 g | 13 |
| Beef, roasted | 3 oz/90 g | 7 |
| Tofu with calcium sulfate | 1.5 cup/125 mL | 130 |
| | | |
| **Fruits and vegetables** | | |
| Broccoli, raw | 1 cup | 76 |
| Broccoli, cooked | 1 cup | 94 |
| Kale, cooked | 1 cup | 179 |
| Collards, cooked | 1 cup | 357 |
| Orange | 1 medium | 52 |
| Banana | 1 medium | 10 |
| Lettuce | 2 large leaves | 8 |
| Figs | 10 | 270 |

#### Some Commonly Used Calcium Supplements

| Type and Brand Name | Per Tablet (mg) | Elemental Calcium Tablet (mg) |
|---|---|---|
| **Calcium carbonate** | | |
| Alka Mints | 850 | 340 |
| Caltrate | 1600 | 600 |
| OsCal | 625 or 1250 | 250 or 500 |
| Rolaids | 550 | 220 |
| Titralac | 420 | 168 |
| Titralac Liquid | 1000 | 400 |
| Tums/Tums E-X | 500 or 750 | 200 or 300 |
| Tums Ultra/Tums 500 | 1000 or 1250 | 400 or 500 |
| Viactive chewable candy | | 500 |
| | | |
| **Calcium citrate** | | |
| Citracal | 950 | 200 |
| Citracal Caplets + D | 1500 | 315 + 200 IU vitamin D |

Hip protectors decrease the risk of hip fractures and should be recommended to all frail elderly subjects who are at high risk of hip fracture.[22]

## Pharmacologic Therapies

Selection of patients for pharmacologic therapy should be based on their risk of fracture and the efficacy of the proposed therapy. National Osteoporosis Foundation (NOF) guidelines recommend pharmacologic therapy in postmenopausal women based on BMD measurement, as follows: initiate therapy if the T-score is below –2.0 by hip DXA with no risk factors, if the T-score is below –1.5 by hip DXA with one or more risk factors, or if there is a prior vertebral or hip fracture.[10] The most important risk factors are chronic corticosteroid therapy, older age, history of osteoporotic fracture in a first-degree relative, personal history of fracture as an adult, smoking, and low body weight. The best time to start therapy is a subject of debate. Because age is an independent risk factor for fractures, the short-term risk of fractures is considerably higher in older than in younger subjects at any level of BMD. Consequently, treatment is likely to result in greater appreciable short-term fracture reduction in older subjects. Younger postmenopausal women with low bone density do not need to be treated urgently because their immediate fracture risk is low. However, because they have a higher lifetime risk of fractures and many more years during which further bone loss may occur, intervention that would prevent bone loss is warranted at some point. Patients with high markers of bone resorption also have an increased fracture risk and may be considered for antiresorptive therapy at higher BMD levels (T-score –1.5).

Pharmacologic agents used to treat osteoporosis (Table 1-11) can be classified based on their mechanism of action as antiresorptive or anabolic agents.[23] The former reduce fractures by inhibiting bone resorption, which usually is increased in postmenopausal osteoporosis. They produce modest increases in the measured BMD, primarily by promoting greater mineralization of existing bone. The only currently available anabolic agent is 1–34 fragment of human PTH (teriparatide), which stimulates bone formation and increases bone size. Despite the difference in their mechanism of action, the antifracture efficacy of anabolic and the more potent antiresorptive agents is similar. The choice of therapy should be individualized according to the patient's BMD, fracture history, and other health problems.[24,25] Very few studies have performed a head-to-head comparison of the effects of different agents on BMD, and none have done so in terms of fracture efficacy. Consequently, a meaningful comparison of relative potency of different agents is not possible. Indirectly, some conclusions about relative efficacy may be arrived at by meta-analyses of the published trials, such as shown in Figures 1-12 to 1-15.[25]

### Bisphosphonates

Bisphosphonates are bone-specific agents that bind to hydroxylapatite crystals on the bone surface, particularly at the site of bone remodeling, and inhibit bone resorption by reducing activity of osteoclasts in part by accelerating their apoptosis. Two bisphosphonates (alendronate and risedronate) have been approved for treatment of postmenopausal and steroid-induced osteoporosis and osteoporosis in men. In addition, ibandronate

**Table 1-11**
**Pharmacologic Agents for Osteoporosis Approved for Use in the United States**

| Pharmacologic | Dosing | Cost* | Advantages | Disadvantages |
|---|---|---|---|---|
| **Antiresorptive agents** | | | | |
| Bisphosphonates | | | Bone specific (no effects on other organs) Reduces vertebral and other fractures Easy weekly or monthly dosing Long duration of effect in bone | GI upset (infrequent) Cannot be used in renal insufficiency (creatinine clearance <35 mL/min) Dosing regimen (on an empty stomach with nothing by mouth and upright posture for at least 30 minutes) |
| Alendronate (Fosamax) | 70 mg/wk | $67 | | |
| Risedronate (Actonel) | 35 mg/wk | $68 | | |
| Ibandronate (Boniva) | 150 mg/mo | $76 | | |
| Estrogen, various | | | Improves hot flashes Reduces vertebral and nonvertebral fractures | Increases risk of breast cancer Increases risk of thromboembolic events Increases risk of cardiovascular events |
| CEE, oral | 0.625 mg/day | $28 | | |
| Estradiol, oral | 0.5 mg/day | $8 | | |
| Transdermal | 0.05 mg/day | $20 | | |
| Raloxifene (Evista) | 60 mg/day | $85 | Reduces vertebral fractures | No effect on nonvertebral fractures Increases hot flashes Increases risk of thromboembolic events Not as potent as estrogen and bisphosphonates |
| Calcitonin (Miacalcin) | 200 IU/day nasally | $93 | Reduces vertebral fractures Well tolerated Pain relief in some patients | No effect on nonvertebral fractures Low potency |
| **Anabolic agents** | | | | |
| 1,34 rh PTH teriparatide (Forteo) | 20 µg/day SC injection | $590 | Builds new bone rather than mineralizes existing bone Greater increase in BMD than with antiresorptive agents Reduces vertebral and nonvertebral fractures | Has to be taken by daily injection High cost Associated with osteosarcoma in rats |

*Approximate retail price in U.S. $/mo in 2005 from www.drugstore.com.

given once a month has recently been approved for postmenopausal osteoporosis. Bisphosphonates increase BMD of the spine and to a lesser degree of the hip (see Figs. 1-12 and 1-13) and decrease bone turnover, thereby reducing the risk of vertebral and nonvertebral fractures (see Figs. 1-14 and 1-15). The antifracture effect is demonstrable after only 6 to 12 months of therapy. Alendronate and risedronate are generally well tolerated, but gastrointestinal side effects such as heartburn, abdominal pain, and nausea may occur. Because of poor absorption rates and high affinity for foods, liquids, and medications, bisphosphonates are taken on an empty stomach with 150 to 250 mL (6 to 8 oz) of water followed by no other food or drink for 30 to 60 minutes. During this time, the patient should remain upright to prevent movement of the bisphosphonate tablet into the esophagus, where it can cause perforation or ulceration. The inconvenience associated with the use of oral bisphosphonates is minimized by the once weekly or monthly dosing regimen, which is associated with a lower incidence of gastrointestinal side effects. In an occasional patient who cannot take one of the approved oral bisphosphonates, oral etidronate (400 mg/day for 14 days every 3 months) or intravenous pamidronate (30 to 60 mg infused over 1 to 2 hours

every 3 months) or zoledronate (4 mg infused over 10 minutes once a year) are used, although they have not been approved for osteoporosis by the U.S. Food and Drug Administration (FDA).

Bisphosphonates are the first choice for treatment of osteoporosis in most patients because they are bone specific-agents that have no other hormonal or metabolic effects, are easy to take, and have documented antifracture efficacy and long-term safety. The duration of therapy is debatable. A recent analysis of 10-year treatment with alendronate showed a progressive increase in BMD for all 10 years. In those patients who stopped alendronate after 5 years, there was preservation of bone mass in the spine but not at the hip during the next 5 years. This observation raises the possibility of a "drug holiday" for patients who have taken bisphosphonates for several years. There is no information regarding the effect of either prolonged therapy or periodic discontinuation of bisphosphonates on fracture rates.

### Estrogen and Selective Estrogen Receptor Modulators
For many years estrogen was the sole therapeutic agent available for postmenopausal osteoporosis. Estrogen was a logical choice

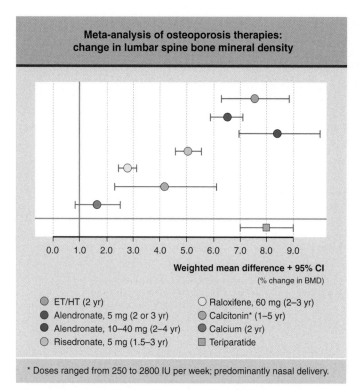

**Figure 1-12  Changes in lumbar spine bone mineral density (BMD) during treatment with currently available pharmacologic agents.** Changes are expressed relative to placebo controls. The effects of antiresorptive agents are taken from the meta-analysis,[25] which was performed before teriparatide was available. The effect of teriparatide is from a single randomized placebo controlled trial.[27] Please note that meta-analysis is not to be used for direct comparison of different agents, which is only possible from head-to-head trials. Such trials have not been performed. ET/HT, estrogen therapy/hormone therapy. (From Cranney A, Guyatt G, Griffith L, et al: Meta-analyses of therapies for postmenopausal osteoporosis IX: summary of meta-analyses of therapies for postmenopausal osteoporosis. Endocr Rev 2002;23:570–578; and Neer RM, Arnaud CD, Zanchetta JR, et al: Effect of parathyroid hormone [1–34] on fractures and bone mineral density in postmenopausal women with osteoporosis. N Engl J Med 2001;344:1434–1441.)

estrogen. On the basis of currently available information, the use of estrogen for osteoporosis should be limited to a short course (a few years) given to early postmenopausal women who have hot flashes (hot flushes) and are at low risk of breast cancer and other undesirable effects of estrogen. This recommendation may change as information regarding lower doses or alternative delivery becomes available. Estrogen may be a reasonable therapeutic alternative for women who cannot tolerate oral bisphosphonates. It should be noted, however, that the effect of estrogen on bone is lost rapidly upon its discontinuation, in contrast to the bisphosphonates, whose effect may persist for several years. In women who are discontinuing estrogen therapy, BMD should be measured, and in those found to be at risk for osteoporotic fractures, the use of other bone active agents, such as bisphosphonates, should be considered.

Two selective estrogen receptor modulators (SERMs) are available in the United States: tamoxifen and raloxifene. Tibolone is available in several European countries. Tamoxifen, which is approved for prevention and treatment of breast cancer, has a mild antiresorptive effect that prevents bone loss at the lumbar spine. No studies have been undertaken to assess its effect on fractures. Tamoxifen is not as potent as estrogen in preventing bone loss. However, it causes less bone loss than the

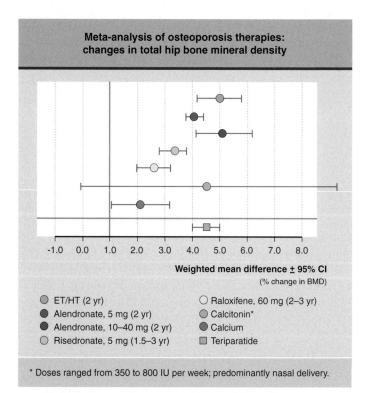

**Figure 1-13  Changes in hip bone mineral density (BMD) during treatment with currently available pharmacologic agents.** For explanation, see Figure 1-12. (From Cranney A, Guyatt G, Griffith L, et al: Meta-analyses of therapies for postmenopausal osteoporosis IX: summary of meta-analyses of therapies for postmenopausal osteoporosis. Endocr Rev 2002;23:570–578; and Neer RM, Arnaud CD, Zanchetta JR, et al: Effect of parathyroid hormone [1–34] on fractures and bone mineral density in postmenopausal women with osteoporosis. N Engl J Med 2001;344:1434–1441.)

based on the observation that bone loss accompanied menopause as well as conditions associated with estrogen loss in younger women. In postmenopausal women, estrogen produces dose-dependent increases in BMD. The high dose of estradiol is 2 mg orally or 100 µg transdermally, and for conjugated equine estrogen (CCE) 1.25 mg orally. The intermediate dose is 1 mg of oral or 50 µg of transdermal estradiol, and 0.625 mg of CEE. The low dose corresponds to 0.5 mg of oral or 25 µg of transdermal estradiol, and 0.3 mg of CEE. Addition of progesterone does not have an appreciable effect on bone.

In the Women's Health Initiative (WHI) trial, the intermediate dose reduced vertebral and hip fractures by 34% and all osteoporotic fractures by 23%[26] (Fig. 1-16). The fracture protection of estrogen in the WHI trial is particularly significant, since the study population was not selected for osteoporosis. However, the WHI trial revealed that estrogen/progestin therapy was associated with increases in breast cancer and cardiovascular morbidity,[26] which has led to a significant decrease in the use of aromatase inhibitors. The bone actions of these agents should be considered when deciding which drug to choose for prevention and treatment of breast cancer.

Raloxifene is the first SERM that received FDA approval for the treatment of postmenopausal osteoporosis. While raloxifene has estrogen-like effects on the bone, its effect on the breast is antiestrogenic, which accounts for the observed decrease in the risk of estrogen receptor–positive breast cancer in subjects receiving raloxifene for the treatment of osteoporosis. The skeletal effect of raloxifene is less potent than that of estrogen, as evidenced by the effects on BMD (see Figs. 1-12 and 1-13). Raloxifene reduces bone markers by about 34% compared with a decrease of 50% with an intermediate dose of estrogen and a 60% to 75% decrease with alendronate. Raloxifene reduces vertebral fractures but not nonvertebral fractures (see Figs. 1-14 and 1-15). The side effects of raloxifene include an increase in hot flashes, muscle cramps, and thromboembolic events. The effect of raloxifene on cardiovascular risk is under study. It appears that good candidates for raloxifene therapy are women with a family history or risk of breast cancer and moderate osteoporosis of the spine (since raloxifene reduces vertebral but not nonvertebral, particularly hip, fractures). Raloxifene may

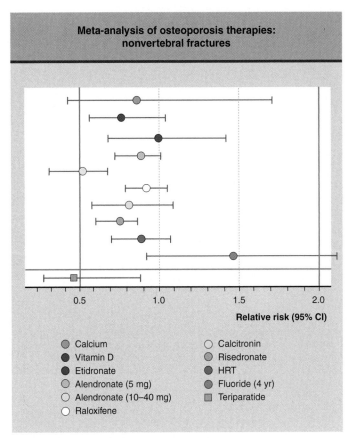

**Meta-analysis of osteoporosis therapies: nonvertebral fractures**

**Relative risk (95% CI)**

- Calcium
- Vitamin D
- Etidronate
- Alendronate (5 mg)
- Alendronate (10–40 mg)
- Raloxifene
- Calcitronin
- Risedronate
- HRT
- Fluoride (4 yr)
- Teriparatide

**Figure 1-15   Effects of different agents on nonvertebral fracture.** For explanation, see Figure 1-12. (From Cranney A, Guyatt G, Griffith L, et al: Meta-analyses of therapies for postmenopausal osteoporosis IX: summary of meta-analyses of therapies for postmenopausal osteoporosis. Endocr Rev 2002;23:570–578; and Neer RM, Arnaud CD, Zanchetta JR, et al: Effect of parathyroid hormone [1–34] on fractures and bone mineral density in postmenopausal women with osteoporosis. N Engl J Med 2001;344:1434–1441.)

not be a good choice for women with hot flashes or those who are discontinuing estrogen and likely to develop hot flashes.

### Calcitonin

Calcitonin, a hormone secreted by the C cells of the thyroid gland, is used for treatment of hypercalcemia and osteoporosis because it inhibits osteoclastic bone resorption. It has mild anti-resorptive activity and only minor effects on BMD (see Figs. 1-12 and 1-13) and only a 12% reduction in bone resorption markers. Calcitonin reduces vertebral fractures by about 30% to 40% (see Fig. 1-14), but the effect may be highly variable. Calcitonin does not reduce the rates of hip and other nonvertebral fractures (see Fig. 1-15). Calcitonin causes mild side effects usually limited to occasional irritation of the nasal mucosa and facial flushing. In some patients calcitonin has an analgesic effect, making it particularly suitable for patients with painful acute vertebral fractures who cannot or should not receive other pharmacologic agents for osteoporosis.

The beneficial effects of estrogen, SERMs, and calcitonin on bone are likely to dissipate quickly after their discontinuation, suggesting that these drugs need to be taken either indefinitely or, if stopped, replaced by another active agent.

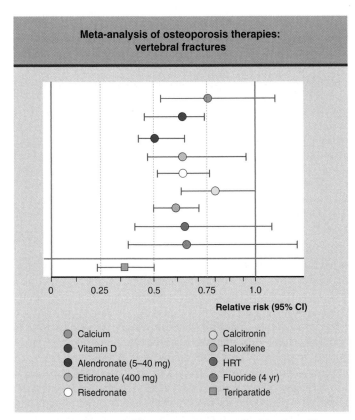

**Meta-analysis of osteoporosis therapies: vertebral fractures**

**Relative risk (95% CI)**

- Calcium
- Vitamin D
- Alendronate (5–40 mg)
- Etidronate (400 mg)
- Risedronate
- Calcitronin
- Raloxifene
- HRT
- Fluoride (4 yr)
- Teriparatide

**Figure 1-14   Effects of different agents on vertebral fracture.** Meta-analysis of effects of different agents on nonvertebral fracture. For explanation, see Figure 1-12. (From Cranney A, Guyatt G, Griffith L, et al: Meta-analyses of therapies for postmenopausal osteoporosis IX: summary of meta-analyses of therapies for postmenopausal osteoporosis. Endocr Rev 2002;23:570–578; and Neer RM, Arnaud CD, Zanchetta JR, et al: Effect of parathyroid hormone [1–34] on fractures and bone mineral density in postmenopausal women with osteoporosis. N Engl J Med 2001;344:1434–1441.)

Ambulatory Office Practice

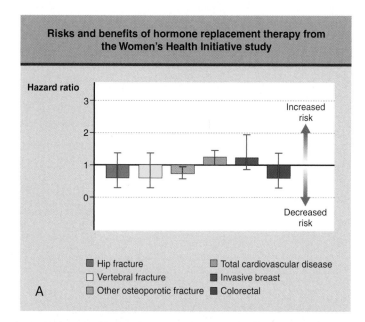

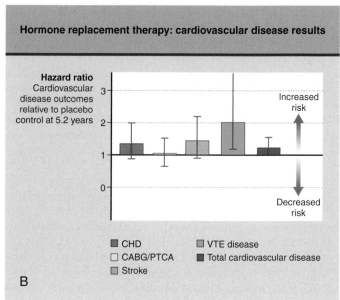

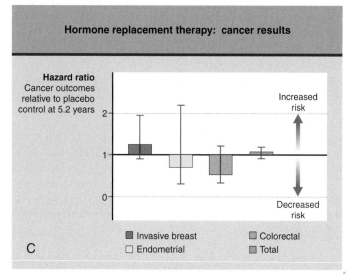

**Figure 1-16    Risks and benefits of hormone replacement therapy (HRT) from the Women's Health Initiative study.** CABG/PTCA, coronary artery bypass graft/percutaneous transluminal coronary angioplasty; CHD, coronary heart disease; HRT, hormone replacement therapy; VTE, venous thrombosis and embolism. (From Rossouw JE, Anderson GL, Prentice RL, et al: Risks and benefits of estrogen plus progestin in healthy postmenopausal women: principal results from the Women's Health Initiative randomized controlled trial. JAMA 2002;288:321–333.)

### Teriparatide (rhPTH [1–34])

Chronic elevation of PTH such as occurs in hyperparathyroidism typically is associated with decreased bone mass and increased risk of fracture. In contrast, intermittent daily injection of small doses of PTH activates bone formation without concurrent activation of bone resorption. Teriparatide, given by subcutaneous injection, produces a dramatic increase in BMD, particularly at the spine (see Fig. 1-12).[27] This anabolic therapy also increases bone size, which is not reported with antiresorptive agents. During an 18 month clinical trial, teriparatide reduced the rate of vertebral fractures by 60% to 65% and nonvertebral fractures to a lesser extent (see Figs. 1-14 and 1-15).[27] The effect of teriparatide on hip fractures specifically is not known. The increase in osteosarcoma in rats given teriparatide raises some concerns. However, the higher doses and longer duration of treatment may be responsible for this effect. While the appearance of osteosarcoma remains a theoretical concern in human use, it is reassuring that there have not been reports of osteosarcoma in humans treated to date and no increased incidence of these tumors in subjects with chronic elevation of endogenous PTH

of primary, secondary, or tertiary hyperparathyroidism. The subcutaneous injections are generally well tolerated with the most common side effects being nausea, dizziness, and mild transient hypercalcemia, and hypercalciuria. Teriparatide is contraindicated in patients with hypercalcemia or hypercalciuria, renal insufficiency, Paget's disease, or history of bone tumors. It currently is not clear who are the best candidates for treatment with teriparatide or how it should be added to or combined with other agents. A reasonable suggestion is to reserve teriparatide for patients who cannot tolerate bisphosphonates or show inadequate response to antiresorptive agents (i.e., fracturing during bisphosphonate therapy). Since the anabolic response to teriparatide is diminished in subjects pretreated with alendronate,[28,29] it may also be reasonable (although no data support this position) to use teriparatide in previously untreated subjects with very low bone density of the spine or prevalent vertebral fractures. The effect of teriparatide dissipates upon its discontinuation, suggesting that this treatment should be followed by an antiresorptive agent such as a bisphosphonate to preserve the increases in bone mass.

### Combination Therapy

The combination of antiresorptive agents such as estrogen or raloxifene and alendronate produces only a slightly greater increase in BMD than alendronate alone.[29] Although there are no clear guidelines, it seems prudent to use one antiresorptive agent and to add a second only if there is documented lack of response to the first. The theoretical concern about combining several antiresorptive agents is that profound suppression of bone resorption may lead to "dead bone," which theoretically may increase the risk of fracture because of failure to repair microcracks. Although no increase in fractures has been observed with prolonged use of a single agent (alendronate) for up to 10 years, it is not clear if a combination of antiresorptive drugs increases fracture risk. A combination of teriparatide and bisphosphonate is not recommended, since it has been shown that the increase in bone density seen with teriparatide is attenuated by concurrent or prior administration of alendronate.[28]

### Skeletal Changes during Pregnancy and Lactation

Pregnancy and lactation place a demand on the calcium homeostasis of the mother. During pregnancy, the increased demand for calcium necessary for formation of the fetal skeleton is met primarily by increased intestinal absorption.[30] This is due to the increased circulating levels of 1,25-dihydroxyvitamin D, probably mediated by increased renal or placental 25(OH)-vitamin $D_{1\alpha}$-hydroxylase under the influence of the PTH-related protein (PTHrP), estradiol, prolactin, or placental lactogen. Little information is available regarding the changes in bone mass during pregnancy because of the need to avoid ionizing radiation. However, one study found proximal femur BMD to decline during pregnancy and then rapidly increase in the months following delivery. Thus, it seems that pregnancy itself is not associated with dramatic bone loss. In contrast, a significant bone loss of 3% to 10% may occur after 2 to 6 months of lactation. The bone loss is primarily due to the increased maternal bone resorption necessary to provide 300 to 400 mg, and up to 1000 mg, of calcium that is secreted in the milk daily. The main mediator of lactation-related changes in calcium homeostasis appears to be PTHrP, which is produced by the lactating breast. PTHrP makes more calcium available for milk production by increasing bone resorption and decreasing urinary calcium excretion. In contrast to pregnancy, there is no elevation of serum 1,25-dihydroxyvitamin D during lactation and no increase in intestinal calcium absorption. Thus, loss of calcium from the mother's skeleton is not prevented by increasing dietary calcium and vitamin D intake beyond the usual requirements. The loss of bone mass resulting from lactation is rapidly reversed upon weaning with an increase in BMD of 0.5% to 2% per month. Consequently, multiparity or breastfeeding does not increase the risk of osteoporosis and fracture.

Fragility fractures and low BMD have been reported during pregnancy and during lactation. It is likely that many of these women had low BMD before pregnancy, with further bone loss due to increased bone turnover in pregnancy and particularly during lactation. An exaggeration of normal lactation-associated skeletal effects might cause excessive demineralization and increased bone fragility. No specific treatment for bone loss under these conditions exists; however, it is important to exclude secondary causes of osteoporosis, provide adequate calcium and vitamin D intake, and consider discouraging breastfeeding to allow restoration of the mother's skeletal health.

## CONTROVERSY AND FUTURE CHALLENGES

Recent years have seen dramatic increases in the understanding of the pathophysiology of osteoporosis, the development of diagnostic modalities, and more effective treatment options. However, several challenges remain in approaching this disease. One is the economic issue.[7] With the number of patients with osteoporosis increasing as a result of the aging population and the increased secular trend in fracture incidence, the financial challenge of diagnosing and treating osteoporosis needs to be addressed on a national scale. In developing countries, health care resources likely will best be used for large population measures to prevent osteoporosis and fractures. In more developed countries, a case finding approach such as that used in the United States is more likely to predominate. With increased health care expenditure and competition with other significant diseases, allocation of resources for diagnosing and treating osteoporosis will most certainly generate intense debate.

The second challenge in osteoporosis therapy is that even the most potent currently available therapeutic agents reduce fracture risk by only half. It is not clear whether earlier diagnosis and treatment of patients with low bone mass will prevent subsequent bone loss and osteoporotic fractures. If that is the case, it might be more economical to treat patients earlier and thereby prevent development of very low levels of bone mass. However, identifying patients who would most benefit from treatment requires identifying which factors other than BMD predict fracture, since nonselectively treating everyone with osteopenia is likely to be prohibitively expensive. Finally, it will be necessary to develop treatment strategies that are individualized according to a patient's specific clinical characteristics to ensure tolerability and efficacy of the chosen therapy. Further exploration of the effects of combination therapy is necessary to determine how to optimize currently available agents. Despite these challenges, it is possible that in the future osteoporosis will no longer be considered an inevitable feature of aging and prevention and treatment will reduce it to an infrequent disorder.

## REFERENCES

1. Consensus development conference: diagnosis, prophylaxis, and treatment of osteoporosis. Am J Med 1993;94:646–650. (IV, C, consensus statement)
2. Klotzbuecher CM, Ross PD, Landsman PB, et al: Patients with prior fractures have an increased risk of future fractures: a summary of the literature and statistical synthesis. J Bone Miner Res 2000;15:721–739. (IV, C)
3. Wu F, Mason B, Horne A, et al: Fractures between the ages of 20 and 50 years increase women's risk of subsequent fractures. Arch Intern Med 2002;162:33–36. (IIb, B, cross-sectional study)
4. Kanis JA, Melton LJ III, Christiansen C, et al: The diagnosis of osteoporosis. J Bone Miner Res 1994;9:1137–1141. (WHO consensus statement) (IV, C)
5. Link TM, Bauer JS: Imaging of trabecular bone structure. Semin Musculoskelet Radiol 2002;6:253–262. (IV, C)

6. Cummings SR, Melton LJ: Epidemiology and outcomes of osteoporotic fractures. Lancet 2002;359:1761–1767. **(IV, C)**

7. Melton LJ III, Johnell O, Lau E, et al: Osteoporosis and the global competition for health care resources. J Bone Miner Res 2004; 19:1055–1058. **(IV, C)**

8. Genant HK, Delmas P: Osteoporosis education programme to improve the recognition and reporting of vertebral fractures by radiologists. Created by International Osteoporosis Foundation. Available at http://www.osteofound.org/health_professionals/education_radiologists/index.html. Accessed 9/13/05. (Review: excellent overall resource on diagnosis of vertebral fractures) **(IV, C)**

9. Melton LJ III, Atkinson EJ, Cooper C, et al: Vertebral fractures predict subsequent fractures. Osteoporos Int 1999;10:214–221. **(IIb, B)**

10. National Osteoporosis Foundation: Physician's Guide to Prevention and Treatment of Osteoporosis. Belle Mead, NJ, Excerpta Medica, 1998. **(IV, C practice recommendations)**

11. Mundy GR: Osteoporosis: pathophysiology and non-pharmacological management. Best Pract Res Clin Rheumatol 2001;15:727–745. **(IV, C)**

12. Seeman E: Pathogenesis of bone fragility in women and men. Lancet 2002;359:1841–1850. **(IV, C)**

13. Cummings SR, Bates D, Black DM: Clinical use of bone densitometry: scientific review. JAMA 2002;288:1889–1897. **(IV, C)**

14. Kanis JA: Diagnosis of osteoporosis and assessment of fracture risk. Lancet 2002;359:1929–1936. **(IV, C)**

15. Faulkner KG, von Stetten E, Miller P: Discordance in patient classification using T-scores. J Clin Densitom 1999;2:343–350. **(IIb, B)**

16. ISCD 2003 position statements are published in J Clin Densitom 2004;7. Available at http://www.iscd.org/Visitors/official.cfm. Accessed 9/13/05. **(IV, C)**

17. Kanis JA, Johnell O, Oden A, et al: Ten year probabilities of osteoporotic fractures according to BMD and diagnostic thresholds. Osteoporos Int 2001;12:989–995. **(IIb, B)**

18. Genant HK, Li J, Wu CY, Shepherd A: Vertebral fractures in osteoporosis: a new method for clinical assessment. J Clin Densitom 2000;3:281–290. **(IV, C)**

19. Ebeling PR, Akesson K: Role of biochemical markers in the management of osteoporosis. Best Pract Res Clin Rheumatol 2001;15:385–400. (Very good review) **(IV, C)**

20. Fitzpatrick LA: Secondary causes of osteoporosis. Mayo Clin Proc 2002;77:453–468. **(IV, C)**

21. Tannenbaum C, Clark J, Schwartzman K, et al: Yield of laboratory testing to identify secondary contributors to osteoporosis in otherwise healthy women. J Clin Endocrinol Metab 2002;87:4431–4437. **(IIb, B)**

22. van Schoor NM, Smit JH, Twisk JW et al: Prevention of hip fractures by external hip protectors: a randomized controlled trial. JAMA 2003; 289:1957–1962. **(Ib, A)**

23. Delmas PD: Treatment of postmenopausal osteoporosis. Lancet 2002; 359:2018–2026. **(IV, C)**

24. Cranney A: Treatment of postmenopausal osteoporosis. BMJ 2003; 327:355–356. **(IV, C)**

25. Cranney A, Guyatt G, Griffith L, et al: Meta-analyses of therapies for postmenopausal osteoporosis. 9. Summary of meta-analyses of therapies for postmenopausal osteoporosis. Endocr Rev 2002; 23:570–578. **(Ia, A)**

26. Rossouw JE, Anderson GL, Prentice RL, et al: Risks and benefits of estrogen plus progestin in healthy postmenopausal women: principal results from the Women's Health Initiative randomized controlled trial. JAMA 2002;288:321–333. **(Ib, A)**

27. Neer RM, Amaud CD, Zanchetta JR, et al: Effect of parathyroid hormone (1–34) on fractures and bone mineral density in postmenopausal women with osteoporosis. N Engl J Med 2001;344:1434–1441. **(Ib, A)**

28. Khosla S: Parathyroid hormone plus alendronate—a combination that does not add up. N Engl J Med 2003;349:1277–1279. **(Ib, A)**

29. Johnell O, Scheele WH, Lu Y, et al: Additive effects of raloxifene and alendronate on bone density and biochemical markers of bone remodeling in postmenopausal women with osteoporosis. J Clin Endocrinol Metab 2002;87:985–992. **(Ib, A)**

30. Kovacs CS: Calcium and bone metabolism in pregnancy and lactation. J Clin Endocrinol Metab 2001;86:2344–2348. **(IV, C)**

# Premenstrual Syndrome/Premenstrual Dysphoric Disorder

## Candace Brown, MSN, PharmD, and Frank W. Ling, MD

## KEY POINTS

- Premenstrual syndrome (PMS) is characterized by psychological and physical symptoms occurring before menses; premenstrual dysphoric disorder (PMDD) is a more severe form of PMS with significant mood symptoms and disability.
- Standard criteria and prospective symptom calendars should be used in diagnosing women with PMS or PMDD.
- Lifestyle changes such as diet, exercise, sleep hygiene, stress reduction, and patient education should be a part of treatment regimens.
- SSRIs and venlafaxine are the treatments of choice for severe PMS and PMDD.
- Oral contraceptives and GnRH agonists are second-line agents used when first-line agents are ineffective or when symptoms are primarily physical.
- Scientific evidence does not support the use of natural progesterone and primrose oil, and the risks of surgical oophorectomy outweigh its benefits.
- The most crucial factor in establishing the diagnosis of PMS/PMDD is ascertaining that the patient does not have another underlying medical or psychiatric diagnosis that is showing premenstrual exacerbation in symptoms.

## EPIDEMIOLOGY

PMS is a condition of recurrent physical and psychological symptoms occurring in a cyclic fashion during the 1- to 2-week period preceding a woman's menstrual period. Most surveys find that as many as 85% of menstruating women report one or more mild premenstrual symptoms. Severe symptoms that meet the criteria for PMS, however, are much less common, with only 10% of women reporting significant impairment in lifestyle.[1] PMDD, a variant of PMS that entails more severe psychologic symptoms and impairment of functioning, occurs in 2% to 9% of women of reproductive age.[2]

## RISK FACTORS

The only proven risk factor for PMS and PMDD is ovulatory cycles. Women with a prior history of a depressive disorder, including postpartum depression, or with a family history of PMS may represent high-risk groups.[3] There appears to be an increased risk with age and increased parity.[4] Dalton proposed that tubal ligation, oral contraceptive use, pre-eclampsia, and

absence of dysmenorrhea were associated with increased risk for premenstrual symptoms.[5] However, none of these factors have been shown empirically to have an association. PMS has been reported among women in diverse geographic locations, cultural and ethnic groups, and historical periods. Racial, socioeconomic, or marital status differences have not been identified. Finally, risk factors such as increased imposed stress and specific personality profiles are not helpful in differentiating women with PMS/PMDD from those without the disorder.[1]

## PATHOGENESIS

Although the etiology of PMS is incompletely understood, considerable progress has been made in understanding its pathophysiology. The most common theories are serotonergic dysregulation, fluctuating sex steroid levels, and genetic predisposition.[1] Most likely, central nervous system neurotransmitters, such as serotonin, interact with sex steroids in genetically vulnerable women.[6]

### Serotonin

A number of experimental models have consistently demonstrated an important role for serotonin in the pathophysiology of PMS/PMDD. PMS/PMDD patients have lower whole blood serotonin levels[7] and lower platelet serotonin uptake[8] during the premenstrual phase. Challenges with serotonergic agents, such as L-tryptophan, fenfluramine, and buspirone, also have provided evidence of serotonin dysfunction in women with PMS/PMDD.[9–11] Finally, the finding that serotonergic drugs, particularly the selective serotonin reuptake inhibitors (SSRIs), rapidly treat PMS/PMDD and at low doses, strongly supports the hypothesis that serotonin is involved in the etiology of PMS/PMDD. However, it is notable that only 60% of PMS/PMDD patients respond to treatment with SSRIs,[12] suggesting that serotonin may not be the primary etiologic variable in all PMS/PMDD patients.

### Sex Steroids

Although there is a temporal relationship between symptoms of PMS/PMDD, female sex hormones, and phases of the menstrual cycle, the relationship is unclear. Women with PMS/PMDD show no consistent diagnosis-related differences in basal levels of ovarian hormones.[13] However, suppression of ovarian function by pharmacotherapy or through surgical menopause eliminates the symptoms of PMS/PMDD.[14] The most likely explanation is that women with PMS/PMDD are in some way vulnerable to the normal physiologic changes associated with the menstrual cycle.[13] This hypothesis is supported in one study in which women with PMS/PMDD developed depressed mood in response to challenge with physiologic levels of estrogen and progesterone compared with controls.[15]

Allopregnanolone, a centrally active progesterone metabolite, has been implicated in PMS/PMDD. Though the results have been contradictory, there is some evidence that low plasma allopregnanolone concentrations are correlated with depressive symptoms during the luteal phase.[16] Changes in allopregnanolone concentrations have also been associated with improvement in response to pharmacotherapy for PMDD.[17] Allopregnanolone's hypothesized site of action is the $GABA_A$ receptor, the receptor that also affects the pharmacologic activity of benzodiazepines. PMS/PMDD patients have been shown to be more sensitive than control subjects to the anxiogenic effects of the benzodiazepine antagonist flumazenil[18] and less sensitive than controls to a number of benzodiazepines.[19]

Androgens have been investigated in PMD/PMDD because of the prominence of irritability in the symptom profile. Elevated testosterone levels have been reported in women with severe premenstrual irritability,[20] and a positive correlation has been observed between free testosterone concentrations and irritability.[21] Moreover, some success has been reported in treating PMS/PMDD with androgen antagonists.[20]

### Genetic Risk

Genetics appears to play a role in PMS. The concordance rate of PMS is twice as high among monozygotic twins as among dizygotic twins.[22] A study including more than 1000 female twins estimated heritability of premenstrual symptoms at approximately 56%, with no substantial role for familial environmental factors.[23]

## CLINICAL FEATURES

More than 150 different symptoms have been attributed to PMS.[4] Psychological symptoms are the most common reason for seeking help, and the hallmark symptom is irritability. Others include easily precipitated crying spells, low self-esteem, anxiety, and depression. The full range of depressive symptoms, including low mood, sleep disturbance, and abnormal eating are more commonly encountered with PMDD. The cognitive problems, although less frequently reported, can have a significant impact, particularly on a woman's work efficiency. These symptoms include short-term memory problems, difficulty concentrating, and "fuzzy" thinking. Finally, the somatic, or physical, symptoms are more characteristic of PMS than PMDD, and include breast tenderness, bloating, fluid retention, hot flashes (hot flushes), headaches, and musculoskeletal discomfort (Table 2-1).

No feature of the definition of PMS/PMDD is more important to a clinically useful understanding than the level of severity. The majority of menstruating women experience symptoms that are qualitatively similar to those associated with "mild" PMS. The difference between these normal symptoms, also referred to as "molimina," and PMS or PMDD, is quantitative. Molimina symptoms are typically present for a few days prior to the onset of menses and do not interfere with daily functioning. Severe PMS and PMDD, in contrast, begin 2 weeks or so before menses and result in difficulties with daily function-

| Table 2-1 | | |
|-----------|---|---|
| **Symptoms of Premenstrual Syndrome/Premenstrual Dysphoric Disorder** | | |
| **Psychological Symptoms** | **Cognitive Symptoms** | **Physical Symptoms** |
| Irritability | Forgetfulness | Breast tenderness |
| Mood swings | Decreased concentration | Bloating |
| Depressed mood | | Fluid retention |
| Crying spells | | Weight gain |
| Low self-esteem | | Constipation |
| Anxiety | | Hot flashes |
| Sleep disturbance | | Headaches |
| Increased appetite | | Musculoskeletal |
| Lethargy or fatigue | | discomfort |
| | | Acne |
| | | Rhinitis |
| | | Palpitations |

ing. PMDD is most likely to present with mood symptoms and the most severe disability. The percentage of women reporting mood symptoms in one study of PMDD was as follows: anger/irritability (76%), anxiety/tension (71%), tired/lethargic (58%), mood swings (58%), sad/depressed (54%), interpersonal conflicts (54%), bloated/breast swelling (54%), less interested in activities (49%), sensitive to rejection (47%), and poor concentration (43%).[24] Although most women clearly fall into one of these three groups, there is a spectrum of experience in between.

In this chapter, the term *PMS/PMDD* refers to the more severe premenstrual symptoms that interfere with functioning and require medical management.

## DIAGNOSIS

The key clinical features of both PMS and PMDD include (1) restriction of symptoms to the luteal phase of the menstrual cycle, (2) affective and somatic symptoms, (3) impairment in function, and (4) exclusion of other diagnoses that may better explain the symptoms.[1] PMDD represents the more severe end of the diagnostic spectrum of premenstrual syndromes and is characterized by severe mood symptoms. This difference is observed by comparing the diagnostic criteria for PMDD created by the American Psychiatric Association to the diagnostic criteria for PMS developed by the American College of Obstetricians and Gynecologists (Table 2-2). To be diagnosed with PMDD, a woman must have at least five affective symptoms, of which one must be irritability, affective lability (mood swings), depressed mood, or anxiety.[25] In PMS, only one symptom (either an affective or a somatic symptom) is necessary to meet diagnostic criteria.[1]

The diagnosis of PMS/PMDD should be based on prospective symptom diaries, because as many as half of women reporting a luteal-phase pattern will be found to have some other pattern when the diaries are examined. Because some women experience cycle-to-cycle variability in symptoms, reviewing 2 to 3 months of prospective charting is preferable to reviewing a single cycle.[26] A number of valid and reliable diagnostic instruments are available to document symptoms in PMS/PMDD, including the Calendar of Premenstrual Experiences[27] and the Daily Record of Severity of Problems.[28] Patients record emotional,

**Table 2-2**
**Comparison of Diagnostic Criteria for Premenstrual Syndrome/Premenstrual Dysphoric Disorder**

| ACOG Diagnostic Criteria for Premenstrual Syndrome | DSM-IV Criteria for Premenstrual Dysphoric Disorder |
|---|---|
| Patient reports at least one affective and/or somatic symptom:<br>Affective<br>    Depression<br>    Angry outbursts<br>    Irritability<br>    Anxiety<br>    Confusion<br>    Social withdrawal<br>Somatic<br>    Breast tenderness<br>    Abdominal bloating<br>    Headache<br>    Swelling extremities | Patient reports at least five emotional symptoms, with at least one of four specific symptoms (indicated with asterisk):<br>Emotional<br>    Depressed mood*<br>    Irritability, anger*<br>    Anxiety, tension*<br>    Increased sensitivity*<br>    Decreased concentration<br>    Decreased interest<br>    Lethargy, lack of energy<br>    Change in appetite<br>    Insomnia or hypersomnia<br>    Overwhelmed or out of control<br>Physical<br>    Breast tenderness or swelling<br>    Headaches<br>    Joint or muscle pain<br>    Weight gain<br>    "Bloated" feeling |
| Symptoms occur 5 days before menses, remit within 4 days of menses onset, and do not reoccur until at least cycle day 13 | Symptoms occur a week before menses and remit within a few days after the onset of menses<br>Symptoms are experienced in most of the menstrual cycle for the past year |
| Symptoms present in the absence of any pharmacologic therapy, hormone ingestion, or drug or alcohol use | Symptoms are discretely related to menstrual cycle and are not merely worsening of pre-existing depression, anxiety, or personality disorder |
| Symptoms occur reproducibly during two cycles of prospective recording | Symptoms occur for at least two consecutive menstrual cycles of prospective daily ratings |
| Symptoms cause identifiable dysfunction in social or economic performance | Symptoms interfere with social, occupational, sexual, or school functioning |

From American College of Obstetricians and Gynecologists (ACOG): Premenstrual Syndrome. ACOG Practice Bulletin No. 15, Apr 2000, and American Psychiatric Association Diagnostic and Statistical Manual of Mental Disorders, 4th ed DSM-IV, text revision. Washington, DC, American Psychiatric Association, 2000.

physical, and functional symptoms daily using one of these tools to assess the presence, timing, and severity of symptoms. The diagnosis of PMS/PMDD is confirmed if there is evidence of a relative absence of symptoms during the follicular phase of the menstrual cycle; a substantial increase in emotional symptoms, physical symptoms, or both during the luteal phase of the menstrual cycle; and functional impairment during the luteal phase.[29]

### Differential Diagnosis

Establishing a diagnosis of PMS/PMDD can be difficult because of the wide and variable range of symptoms and because there are no confirmatory laboratory tests or signs on physical examination. Nevertheless, a comprehensive history and physical examination are required to rule out other possible causes of the emotional and physical symptoms.

The most crucial factor in establishing the diagnosis of PMS/PMDD is making sure that the patient does not have another underlying medical or psychiatric diagnosis that is showing premenstrual exacerbation in symptoms. More than 50% of patients suffering from major depression report a clear-cut premenstrual exacerbation in their depressive symptoms.[30] Other psychiatric conditions that may be magnified are bipolar disorder (manic-depressive illness), panic disorder, generalized anxiety disorder, eating disorders, and psychosocial conditions resulting from sexual and physical abuse. Prospective rating

of daily diaries can facilitate making a differential diagnosis. Women who report symptoms across all phases of the cycle, but with increasing severity during the premenstrual period, should be treated for the underlying disorder.

Table 2-3 summarizes the medical and psychiatric conditions that most frequently present with premenstrual exacerbation, or whose symptoms mimic some of the typical symptoms of PMS/PMDD. Medical disorders that may mimic premenstrual syndromes include hypothyroidism, diabetes, autoimmune conditions, anemia, chronic fatigue syndrome, and endometriosis. As a rule, these disorders should be treated first before treatment of PMS/PMDD is initiated, unless one drug has proven efficacy in both conditions.

Other medical disorders subject to premenstrual exacerbation are migraine and seizure disorders, irritable bowel syndrome, asthma, chronic fatigue syndrome, and allergies. The diagnosis of these conditions usually is straightforward because the symptoms are not part of the typical PMS/PMDD symptom set and emotional symptoms are not prominent, as they are in PMS/PMDD.

Finally, women in the period of transition to menopause may have symptoms typical of PMS/PMDD, especially mood disturbance, fatigue, and hot flashes. Because menstrual periods are often less predictable, these women may be less aware of the relationship of the symptoms to the menstrual cycle. Considering the patient's age, a history of recent menstrual cycle changes,

**Table 2-3**
**Differential Diagnosis of Premenstrual Syndrome/**
**Premenstrual Dysphoric Disorder**

**Psychiatric disorders**

Major depression
Bipolar disorder
Generalized anxiety disorder
Psychosocial (physical abuse/sexual abuse)
Bipolar depression
Eating disorder
Panic disorder

**Medical disorders**

Hypothyroidism
Diabetes
Autoimmune disorder
Collagen vascular disorder
Anemia
Chronic fatigue syndrome
Endometriosis
Migraine
Seizure disorder
Irritable bowel syndrome
Asthma
Allergies
Perimenopause

From American College of Obstetricians and Gynecologists: Premenstrual Syndrome. ACOG Practice Bulletin No. 15, Apr 2000, and Freeman EW, Sondheimer SJ: Premenstrual dysphoric disorder: recognition and treatment. J Clin Psychiatry 2003;5:30–39.

and a symptom diary showing sporadic or daily occurrence of symptoms usually can help make the correct diagnosis.

## Clinical Course and Progression

Little is known about the natural history of PMS/PMDD. Most women who seek help for premenstrual symptoms are in their mid-thirties, although often symptoms have been present for several years.[3] The longitudinal course of PMS/PMDD is not well defined, particularly the extent to which spontaneous remissions occur. Clinical experience suggests that many women have recurrent symptoms until menopause.

## NONPHARMACOLOGIC TREATMENT

A wide variety of supportive, lifestyle, and dietary supplementation approaches have been recommended to treat premenstrual symptoms, and some have demonstrated real benefit. Therefore, these strategies can be recommended to women with mild to moderate symptoms as primary therapy and to women with severe symptoms as adjunctive therapy. Table 2-4 lists these nonpharmacologic treatments and the evidence supporting their efficacy and safety.

### Lifestyle

For women with mild symptoms, education about the condition, supportive counseling, and general healthy lifestyle measures, such as a regular exercise and healthy diet, may be sufficient to

**Table 2-4**
**Nonpharmacologic Treatment of Premenstrual Syndrome/Premenstrual Dysphoric Disorder**

| Treatment | Strength of Recommendation* | Quality of Evidence† | Efficacy† | Adverse Events§ |
|---|---|---|---|---|
| **Lifestyle changes** | | | | |
| Exercise (daily, moderate aerobic) | B | Ib | A | A |
| Dietary modifications | C | IV | C | A |
| Sleep hygiene | C | IV | C | A |
| Stress reduction | C | IV | C | A |
| **Psychotherapy and group support** | | | | |
| Supportive therapy and patient education | B | Ib | C | A |
| Cognitive-behavioral therapy | B | Ib | C | A |
| **Dietary supplements** | | | | |
| Calcium 1000–1200 mg/day | A | Ib | A | A |
| Magnesium 200–360 mg/day 14 days before menses | B | IIb | C | A |
| Vitamin E 400–800 IU/day | B | Ib | C | A |
| Vitamin B$_6$ 100–200 mg/day | B | Ib | C | C |
| **Herbal products** | | | | |
| Chasteberry (Vitex Agnus-castus) | B | Ib | B | D |
| St. John's wort (Hypericum perforatum) | B | Ib | C | D |
| Black cohosh (Cimicifuga racemosa) | C | III | C | D |
| Evening primrose oil | B | Ib | D | D |

*Strength of recommendation: A, at least one randomized controlled trial as part of a body of literature of overall good quality and consistency addressing the specific recommendation; B, well-controlled clinical studies available but no randomized clinical trials on the topic of recommendations; C, evidence obtained from expert committee reports or opinions and/or clinical experiences of respected authorities; indicates an absence of directly applicable clinical studies of good quality.

†Quality of evidence: Ia, evidence obtained from meta-analysis of randomized controlled trials; Ib, evidence obtained from at least one randomized controlled trial; IIb, evidence obtained from at least one other type of well-designed quasi-experimental study; III, evidence obtained from well-designed nonexperimental descriptive studies, such as comparative studies, correlation studies, and case studies; IV, evidence obtained from expert committee reports or opinions and/or clinical experience of respected authorities.

†Efficacy: A, effective; B, conflicting data; C, insufficient data; D, ineffective.

§Adverse effects: A, minimal/mild; B, moderate; C, major; D, unknown.

result in symptom improvement. Lifestyle modifications should be the first approach taken in all women with premenstrual complaints and can be conveniently given during a 2-month trial while the patient completes the prospective daily ratings necessary to confirm the diagnosis of PMS/PMDD.[12,31,32]

## Exercise

Several studies support the efficacy of exercise in reducing PMS/PMDD symptoms. In a 3-month randomized trial of 23 women with prospectively diagnosed PMS/PMDD, the group taking regular moderate aerobic exercise reported more improvement than the control group, who did nonaerobic exercise.[33] In another small prospective but not randomized study, two groups of women who exercised aerobically reported fewer premenstrual symptoms at the end of a 6-month trial than did a nonexercising comparison group.[34] Therefore, aerobic exercise for 20 to 30 minutes, three to four times per week, is recommended.[32] Reduction of body weight to within 20% of ideal, where possible, is an appropriate goal.[14]

## Diet

Dietary modification can have a noticeable impact on symptom severity. Women should be encouraged to reduce or eliminate intake of salty foods, sugar, caffeine (especially coffee), and alcohol. Increased consumption of fruits, vegetables, legumes, whole grains, and water is recommended. Finally, eating smaller, more frequent meals that are high in carbohydrates may specifically improve symptoms of tension and depression.[32]

## Sleep Hygiene

For many women, PMS/PMDD is associated with sleep irregularities.[35] To alleviate the associated distress and discomfort, adoption of a regular sleep-wake pattern may be helpful. Women should be encouraged to adhere to consistent bedtime and waking times during the premenstrual period and ideally across the menstrual cycle.[32]

## Stress Reduction

Encouraging women to avoid planning stressful activities for the premenstrual period whenever possible can be helpful. Women should be encouraged to review their own daily diaries and identify triggers for symptom exacerbation.[14]

## Psychotherapy and Group Support

### Supportive Therapy and Patient Education

Group support can be effective in managing PMS and PMDD. A recent controlled trial of psychoeducational group intervention with a focus on positive reframing of women's perceptions of their menstrual cycles found that women with PMS/PMDD who received the intervention had reduced premenstrual symptoms and premenstrual impairment, though there were no differences in posttreatment depression or anxiety scores.[36] Several other studies also noted efficacy of group support in managing symptoms of PMS/PMDD.[37]

### Cognitive Behavioral Therapy

Several small studies have investigated the effectiveness of cognitive therapy in alleviating negative symptoms in women with PMS/PMDD. A 12-week study comparing women randomized to weekly cognitive behavioral therapy (CBT) with a group of controls allocated to a waiting group list found CBT was significantly more effective in reducing psychological and somatic symptoms as well as impairment of functioning.[38] In another study,[39] women using CBT with relaxation instructions had significantly reduced PMS symptoms compared with women randomized to a nonactive control group during two menstrual cycles. In a study[40] of 367 women with severe premenstrual symptoms randomly assigned to CBT, a nonspecific treatment, or a waiting-list group, CBT significantly reduced premenstrual symptoms compared with both control groups at posttreatment and at the 9-month follow-up evaluation. However, lack of a true placebo group makes these results difficult to interpret.

One randomized 6-month trial showed equal efficacy of CBT compared with fluoxetine (20 mg) in treating 60 women with PMS/PMDD.[41] However, women responded more quickly to fluoxetine but had better maintenance of treatment effects at 1-year follow-up with CBT. Fluoxetine was more effective in alleviating symptoms of anxiety, whereas CBT was associated with increased use of more effective coping strategies.[42] There was no apparent benefit of combining the treatments.[41] The results of this study support earlier findings that individual CBT is of benefit for women with PMS in improving partner relationships, daily functioning, and mood.[38]

## Dietary Supplements

### Calcium

A 3-month multicenter trial of 497 women reported that calcium carbonate 1200 mg/day was significantly more effective than placebo in reducing premenstrual symptoms.[43] Several similar clinical trials have suggested that calcium supplementation can improve mood and somatic symptoms in PMS/PMDD.[44] Moreover, increased calcium intake has benefits beyond those associated with reduction of premenstrual symptoms, particularly with respect to prevention of osteoporosis, and is not associated with adverse effects with doses of up to 1500 mg/day.[32]

### Magnesium

Two small trials have found that magnesium 200 to 400 mg may decrease premenstrual pain.[45,46] A possible biological rationale for the effectiveness of magnesium is the inhibition of $PGF_{2\alpha}$ and the promotion of muscle relaxation and vasodilatation.[47]

### Vitamin E

Vitamin E has been recommended as a treatment for mastalgia. Vitamin E 400 IU/day significantly improved affective and somatic symptoms in PMS/PMDD patients in one randomized, double-blind, controlled study.[48] Although its effectiveness probably is minimal, no serious side effects are reported with vitamin E 400 IU/day, and as an antioxidant it has other beneficial effects.

### Vitamin B$_6$ (Pyridoxine)

Vitamin B$_6$ is a water-soluble vitamin that may improve premenstrual symptoms by its effects on serotonin.[47] Results of a systematic review suggest that doses of up to 100 mg/day may improve premenstrual symptoms, including depression. Higher doses have been associated with peripheral neuropathy.[49]

### Herbal Products
#### Chasteberry (Vitex agnus-castus)
The fruit of the chasteberry tree is a botanical commonly used for PMS/PMDD. Active constituents in chasteberries are the essential oils, iridoid glycosides, and flavonoids.[44] The mechanism of action is unclear, but it may involve decreasing estrogen and increasing progesterone, prolactin, and dopamine levels.[47] In a study of 1542 women with PMS/PMDD, 33% reported total relief of their symptoms and 57% reported partial relief. A 3-month, randomized, double-blind, placebo-controlled study of 217 PMS/PMDD subjects found chasteberry (600 mg 3 times daily) alleviated only restlessness.[50] Another study showed that chasteberry and vitamin B$_6$ groups had similar reductions in PMS scores (77% and 66%, respectively).[51] In general, the data show conflicting results but appear promising.

#### St. John's Wort (Hypericum perforatum)
The use of serotonin reuptake inhibitors for the mood symptoms of PMS/PMDD is well established.[52] Consequently, St. John's wort is often used as a botanical alternative for treating premenstrual mood symptoms. A number of reviews have suggested that St. John's wort can be useful for mild depression but not severe depression.[53] In a pilot study, 19 women with PMS/PMDD were treated with 300 mg of hypericin standardized to 0.3% hypericin. The results showed a reduction of 51% in PMS/PMDD scores between baseline and the end of the trial, with more than two thirds showing at least a 50% decrease in symptom severity.[54] Patients taking protease inhibitors (for HIV), cyclosporine, or other medications that are metabolized by the cytochrome P-450 enzyme system should avoid using St. John's wort because it reduces serum levels of these medications.[44] The dose recommended for mild depression in most clinical trials is 300 mg of a standardized product to hypericin at 0.3% three times daily.[44]

#### Black Cohosh (Cimicifuga racemosa)
Most studies looking at black cohosh have been for treatment of menopausal symptoms. The mechanism of action is somewhat unclear but may involve suppressing luteinizing hormone secretion.[47] A number of studies using Remifemin, a proprietary extract of black cohosh, show efficacy in treating menopausal symptoms (hot flashes, profuse sweating, sleep disturbance, and depressive moods).[52] Because women with PMS/PMDD often have these symptoms, many clinicians have recommended the use of black cohosh in this population. Further clinical studies are needed to determine its efficacy. The recommended dose is 40 to 80 mg of a standardized extract twice daily providing 4 to 8 mg of triterpene glycosides.[52]

#### Evening Primrose Oil (Oenothera)
Seven clinical trials have been conducted to determine the efficacy of evening primrose in PMS/PMDD.[47] Five of the seven trials were randomized studies, but none found a beneficial effect. However, the sample sizes in all might have been too small to detect a modest benefit.[55] Nevertheless, at this time it does not appear that evening primrose improves premenstrual symptoms.

## PHARMACOLOGIC TREATMENT

Women with severe symptoms or symptoms resistant to non-medical approaches should be considered for drug therapy. Table 2-5 lists pharmacologic agents used to treat PMS/PMDD and the evidence supporting their efficacy and safety.

### Selective Serotonin Reuptake Inhibitors
#### Efficacy
Selective serotonin reuptake inhibitors (SSRIs) are the initial choice for severe PMS/PMDD. Both continuous and intermittent dosing are effective. A recent meta-analysis of 15 randomized, placebo-controlled trials of the use of SSRIs for PMS/PMDD found no significant difference in symptom reduction between the two dosing methods.[56] Intermittent administration has many advantages. It is less expensive, reduces the overall rate of side effects, limits exposure to medications, may reduce tolerance, and is more acceptable to many women. Moreover, no studies have reported discontinuation symptoms with the luteal-phase regimen in PMS/PMDD. The drug is started between 7 and 14 days before the next menstrual period, with the start day individualized to begin at or just before the expected onset of symptoms.

#### Fluoxetine
Fluoxetine has U.S. Food and Drug Administration (FDA) approval for continuous and luteal-phase administration for PMS/PMDD and is sold as Sarafem for this use. One large, multicenter trial[57] and six smaller randomized, double-blind, placebo-controlled studies[58–63] have reported efficacy for fluoxetine administered daily for the treatment of PMS/PMDD. Luteal-phase administration with fluoxetine was recently reported in a large, multicenter study[64] in which 260 women were randomly assigned to receive fluoxetine either 10 or 20 mg/day from ovulation (midcycle) to menses for three menstrual cycles. Fluoxetine 20 mg/day was superior to placebo in reducing the total symptoms, depressed mood, and physical symptom clusters and improving social functioning as assessed by daily ratings. The 10 mg/day dose improved mood and social functioning but not the physical symptom cluster. In the first month after stopping the medication, there was no longer a drug-placebo difference, which was interpreted as an indication of the rapid return of symptoms when mediation was discontinued.

Another large, multicenter, randomized, placebo-controlled study examined the efficacy of enteric-coated fluoxetine 90 mg administered once on day 14 and/or at day 21 of the menstrual cycle for PMS/PMDD.[65] Women who received both doses of fluoxetine showed significant improvement compared with placebo as assessed by total daily symptom scores, the mood symptom cluster, functioning, and several other outcome measures. The single dose of fluoxetine at day 21 was not significantly better than placebo. Fluoxetine was well tolerated; only 5 of 257 subjects (2%) discontinued, all as a result of nonserious adverse events.

A nonrandomized study compared fluoxetine 20 mg/day as continuous and luteal-phase administration in a group of 48 women with PMS/PMDD.[66] Seventy-five percent of the

**Table 2-5**
**Pharmacologic and Surgical Treatments for Premenstrual Syndrome/Premenstrual Dysphoric Disorder**

| Class | Specific Agent | Strength of Recommendation* | Quality of Evidence† | Efficacy‡ | Adverse Effects§ |
|---|---|---|---|---|---|
| Selective serotonergic reuptake inhibitors (SSRIs) | Fluoxetine | A | Ia | A | A |
| | Sertraline | A | Ib | A | A |
| | Paroxetine | A | Ib | A | A |
| | Citalopram | B | Ib | C | A |
| | Fluvoxamine | B | Ib | C | C |
| Other serotonergic antidepressants | Venlafaxine | A | Ib | A | A |
| | Buspirone | B | Ib | C | A |
| | Clomipramine | B | Ib | C | B |
| Ovulation suppression | Oral contraceptive | B | Ib | C | A |
| | Estrogen patch | B | III | C | B |
| | Progesterone | A | Ib | D | A |
| | Danazol | A | Ib | A | C |
| | GnRH agonist | A | Ib | A | C |
| | Ovariectomy | A | IIb | A | C |
| Miscellaneous drugs | Alprazolam | A | Ib | B | B |
| | NSAID | B | IIb | C | A |
| | Spironolactone | A | Ib | B | A |

*Strength of recommendation: A, at least one randomized controlled trial as part of a body of literature of overall good quality and consistency addressing the specific recommendation; B, well-controlled clinical studies available but no randomized clinical trials on the topic of recommendations; C, evidence obtained from expert committee reports or opinions and/or clinical experiences of respected authorities; indicates an absence of directly applicable clinical studies of good quality.

†Quality of evidence: Ia, evidence obtained from meta-analysis of randomized controlled trials; Ib, evidence obtained from at least one randomized controlled trial; IIb, evidence obtained from at least one other type of well-designed quasi-experimental study; III, evidence obtained from well-designed nonexperimental descriptive studies, such as comparative studies, correlation studies, and case studies; IV, evidence obtained from expert committee reports or opinions and/or clinical experience of respected authorities.

‡Efficacy: A, effective; B, conflicting data; C, insufficient data; D, ineffective.

§Adverse effects: A, minimal/mild; B, moderate; C, major.

continuous administration group and 67% of the luteal-phase administration group were rated as responders, a nonsignificant difference. Reported adverse events included headache, insomnia, muscle pain, and nausea. The results suggested that the regimens were similarly effective, although nonrandomization limited the conclusions that can be drawn from these data. A more extensive review of fluoxetine and its applications to PMS/PMDD concluded that fluoxetine is generally a well-tolerated treatment for PMS/PMDD.[67]

*Sertraline*

Sertraline has been used in a number of luteal-phase administration studies[68-73] and has FDA approval for continuous and luteal-phase administration for PMS/PMDD. In a 3-month, double-blind, placebo-controlled trial in 281 women with PMS/PMDD, sertraline (50–100 mg/day) administered for the last 2 weeks of the menstrual cycle was significantly more effective than placebo in reducing premenstrual symptoms.[73] The superiority of sertraline compared with placebo was shown in the endpoint daily symptom rating scores, Clinical Global Impression (CGI) improvement ratings, and measures of functioning and quality of life. However, premenstrual physical symptoms did not improve significantly more with sertraline compared with placebo in this study. The luteal-phase administration regimen was well tolerated, with only 8% (11/142) of subject discontinuing as a result of adverse events. There were no reports of discontinuation symptoms.

Multiple preliminary studies of luteal-phase administration of sertraline were consistent with the above results. In a double-blind crossover study, 79% (11/14) of women with PMS/PMDD who had responded to continuous treatment with sertraline 100 mg/day responded equally well to the same dosage administered only in the luteal phase.[68] In another double-blind crossover study of 11 women, sertraline at a dosage of 50 mg/day in the luteal phase was significantly better than placebo as assessed by daily symptom scores. Both the behavioral and physical symptom clusters improved with sertraline significantly more than with placebo.[70] In a third crossover study of 57 women with PMS/PMDD, which used a flexible dosage of sertraline 50 to 100 mg/day only in the luteal phase, improvement was significantly greater with sertraline compared with placebo for total symptoms and behavioral and physical symptom clusters as assessed by daily symptom reports.[69] This study showed that most of the women improved at the 50 mg/day dosage although 25% had greater improvement with 100 mg/day dosage. Insomnia was the only adverse event reported by 10% or more of the women in the sertraline group.

In a preliminary double-blind study to compare continuous and luteal-phase administration, 31 subjects with PMS/PMDD were randomized to receive either full-cycle or luteal-phase sertraline.[71] The results showed no statistically significant difference between the two administration regimens for the total daily symptom report scores, although the mood factor was significantly more improved in the luteal-phase administration group. Flexible dosages ranged from 50 to 150 mg per luteal day, but 42% remained at the 50 mg/day dosage after three cycles of treatment. Adverse events did not differ between the two administration regimens; no subjects reported discontinuation symptoms. These preliminary studies consistently indicated that luteal-phase administration of sertraline was more effective than placebo and that response was achieved with dosages of 50 to 100 mg/day. Some studies reported an improvement in physical as well as emotional symptoms.

### Paroxetine

A controlled-release formulation of paroxetine was recently approved by the FDA for continuous (daily) and intermittent (each day for 2 weeks before menses) administration for PMS/PMDD. As yet, there are no fully published studies of luteal-phase administration of paroxetine for the treatment of PMS/PMDD. However, data presented in abstracts indicate that both continuous and intermittent administration of the controlled-release formulation at dosages of 12.5 and 25 mg/day were more effective than placebo in the treatment of PMS/PMDD.[74,75] In addition, the efficacy of continuous administration of immediate-release paroxetine (10 to 30 mg/day) was reported in one controlled trial of 65 women with PMS/PMDD[76] and in an unblended study of 14 women with PMS/PMDD at average dosage of 22 ± 10 mg/day.[77]

### Citalopram

Luteal-phase administration of citalopram was reported in one randomized, placebo-controlled trial.[78] Sixty-seven women with PMS/PMDD were randomized to one of four parallel treatment arms: continuous, luteal-phase, or low follicular dose increased in the luteal-phase administration of citalopram or placebo. The luteal-phase administration group received citalopram 10 to 30 mg per luteal day for the 3 months of treatment. Both the continuous administration group and the luteal-phase administration group reported significantly more improvement compared with placebo. Ratings of irritability, which the researchers considered the cardinal symptom of PMS/PMDD, were superior in all drug-treated groups compared with placebo. These data indicated that luteal-phase administration of citalopram was more effective than either continuous or semi-intermittent administration for PMS/PMDD. The researchers suggested that the intermittent administration regimen, with its regular and repeated drug-free intervals, averted the possible development of tolerance to the medication, thus favoring luteal-phase administration of the drug.[78]

Citalopram was well tolerated. Adverse events were generally mild and transient. Only 8 of the 67 subjects (12%) discontinued, all as a result of nonserious adverse events. The three most frequently reported adverse events in the citalopram-treated group were reduced libido, dry mouth, and sweating. The reports of reduced libido decreased by the third treatment cycle (39% [in the first treatment cycle] and 6% [in the third treatment cycle]), in contrast to previous reports indicating that the sexual adverse effects of other SSRIs do not decrease with time.[76,79] Whether this was related to intermittent administration or other unidentified factors could not be determined. It is noteworthy that the subjects included in the trial had marked irritability as the cardinal symptom of the PMS/PMDD and no major depression or dysthymia (which can affect sexual function) within the previous 2 years.

A small preliminary study of citalopram compared luteal-phase with continuous administration in 17 women who had not

improved with an initial SSRI for the treatment of severe PMS/PMDD.[80] Flexible dosages ranged from 20 to 40 mg/day. Both administration regimens significantly improved symptoms as assessed by total premenstrual scores from daily symptom reports. The majority of subjects (59%) responded at the 20 mg/day dosage. Reported adverse events were mild and transient and did not differ between the full-cycle and luteal-phase administration groups. There were no reports of discontinuation symptoms with luteal-phase administration.

### Fluvoxamine

At present, no studies of luteal-phase administration of fluvoxamine have been reported. Information on continuous administration is limited to two very small studies with conflicting results. In open-label treatment with fluvoxamine at 100 mg/day, 10 women with PMS/PMDD showed significant improvement from baseline.[81] In a randomized study of 20 women with self-described PMS/PMDD, fluvoxamine at 150 mg/day did not differ significantly from placebo.[82] The latter is the only negative report in the literature of SSRIs for PMS/PMDD; however, the small sample size and likelihood of type II error, the lack of daily symptom ratings and other screening criteria to confirm the diagnosis, and the low dose of fluvoxamine may have contributed to the results.

### Adverse Effects

The adverse events associated with SSRIs when administered in the luteal phase are similar to those that occur with continuous administration. Overall in the treatment of PMS/PMDD, adverse events that occur with SSRIs are generally mild and transient and decrease or abate with adjustment of the medication. In controlled clinical trials, discontinuation rates of SSRIs due to nonserious adverse effects ranged from 2% to 12%.[64,65,73,78,83,84] A meta-analysis of SSRI treatments for PMS/PMDD indicated that the most common adverse effects are nausea, insomnia, dizziness/lightheadedness, fatigue, dry mouth, gastrointestinal problems, sweating, headache, and decreased libido/delayed orgasm.[56] Although no studies have directly compared the adverse effects among SSRIs and venlafaxine in the treatment of PMS/PMDD, the comparative effects in depressive disorders are known (Table 2-6).[85]

#### Sexual Side Effects

Decreased libido or sexual dysfunction was reported as an adverse event by about 9% to 16% of participants receiving SSRIs in PMS/PMDD studies. This is notably lower than the rates in the population of SSRI users in trials of the use of the drugs in depression, which were recently reported to be 36% to 43%.[86] This same study also examined the prevalence of decreased libido or sexual dysfunction in the subpopulation of SSRI users deemed unlikely to have predisposing factors for these conditions and found a much lower rate of 7% to 30%. This latter group may be a more appropriate comparator for PMS/PMDD patients who do not have a history of depressive disorders and are otherwise healthy.

A baseline assessment of sexual function rarely is available prior to the use of treatments for PMS/PMDD, which makes it difficult to determine the actual extent of disturbance in sexual functioning that results from the medication. The importance

| Table 2-6 Adverse Effects of Antidepressants* | | | | | | | |
| --- | --- | --- | --- | --- | --- | --- | --- |
| Medication | Sedation | Agitation | Orthostatus | Seizures | Weight Gain | ACH[†] | GI[†] |
| Fluoxetine | –/+ | ++ | – | –/+ | + | – | +++ |
| Sertraline | – | ++ | – | – | + | – | +++ |
| Paroxetine | ++ | ++ | – | – | + | + | +++ |
| Fluvoxamine | ++ | – | – | – | + | + | ++++ |
| Citalopram | –/+ | + | – | – | + | – | +++ |
| Venlafaxine | +/++ | ++ | + | + | – | + | ++ |

*Risk of adverse effect: –, unlikely; –/+, minimally likely; +, mildly likely; ++, moderately likely; +++, very likely; ++++, highly likely.

[†]ACH, anticholinergic side effects: dry mouth, constipation, urinary retention.

[†]GI, gastrointestinal side effects: nausea, vomiting.

From Wells BG, Mandos LA, Hayes PE: Depressive disorders. In Dipiro JT, Talbert RL, Yee GC, et al (eds): Pharmacotherapy: A Pathophysiologic Approach. Stamford, Conn, Appleton & Lange, 1999, pp 1141–1160.

of baseline information was shown in a study of luteal-phase administration of fluoxetine, where fluoxetine-treated subjects were significantly more likely than placebo-treated subjects to report decreased libido as an adverse effect (9% vs. 0% for placebo-treated patients), but an analysis of change from baseline sexual functioning to treatment endpoint showed no statistically significant differences in libido among the study groups.[64] For patients who experience sexual dysfunction when receiving an SSRI, a shift to another SSRI may be beneficial[80] although there are no scientific guidelines. Bupropion is associated with lower rates of sexual dysfunction than SSRIs or venlafaxine,[85] and buspirone may also be a useful alternative[87]; however, the efficacy of these medications for PMS/PMDD is less studied and appears to be modest. Some other management strategies for sexual dysfunction have been reviewed,[88] but none have consistent evidence of efficacy.

Intermittent administration may reduce troublesome adverse effects compared with continuous administration, possibly owing to lower exposure or reduced risk of development of tolerance[89] although there is no conclusive evidence for this at present. However, in support of this possibility, fewer subjects reported treatment-emergent adverse events with luteal administration[73] than with continuous administration[83] in multicenter studies of sertraline for PMS/PMDD, although the study designs and samples were not directly comparable and the studies were not designed to definitively answer questions about adverse effects. In contrast, in a randomized, double-blind, placebo-controlled study that compared luteal-phase and continuous administration for PMS/PMDD, adverse events that commonly diminish with adjustment to medication were more likely to decrease in the continuous administration group than in the luteal administration group.[72] In a study of luteal-phase administration with fluoxetine, only decreased libido was reported significantly more frequently with active medication compared with placebo.[64] With luteal-phase administration of weekly fluoxetine, nausea, diarrhea, and breast pain were reported significantly more often with the drug than with placebo, possibility a result of the higher dose used in the weekly regimen.[65]

### Discontinuation Effects

Discontinuation symptoms have been reported after SSRI therapy is interrupted in patients with depression. However, there have been no reports of discontinuation symptoms in the published studies of luteal-phase administration of SSRIs for PMS/PMDD. A recent study specifically monitored discontinuation symptoms with luteal-phase administration with sertraline, but none were identified during the 3-month course of intermittent treatment.[72] In a secondary analysis of symptoms reported during the first 3 days after stopping luteal-phase doses of sertraline, no discontinuation symptoms were identified.[90] Possible reasons for the absence of discontinuation symptoms in patients with PMS/PMDD who are treated with SSRIs are the lower doses that typify luteal-phase treatment of PMS/PMDD; the short interval of each drug treatment (2 weeks); insufficient monitoring of discontinuation effects, which could be confused with re-emergence of premenstrual symptoms; and the short course of therapy that has been studied in PMS/PMDD (about 3 months), which may be too brief to determine the long-term effects of medication and discontinuation.

There is no evidence in the PMS/PMDD literature that the likelihood of discontinuation symptoms varies among the SSRIs. This may, in part, be a result of the absence of sufficient data that address this question in PMS/PMDD studies, but it is also possible that the likelihood of discontinuation symptoms is lower in PMS/PMDD treatment for the reasons noted above. Although claims are made that discontinuation symptoms may be less frequent or severe with fluoxetine because of the long half-life of its metabolite norfluoxetine, this assertion is not supported in studies of its use in other depressive disorders, which identified discontinuation symptoms after a longer time interval than was consistent with its longer half-life.[91] Furthermore, other factors in addition to the half-life of the medication may effect discontinuation reactions, for example, the metabolism of the agent or other elements such as anticholinergicity (e.g., paroxetine has shown a greater propensity to produce discontinuation symptoms than fluvoxamine, an SSRI with a similarly short half-life).[91] Nonetheless, discontinuation reactions are an important clinical issue, particularly because they may be confused with the re-emergence of the treated symptoms and the reinstatement or expansion of drug therapy. It is clinically important to carefully evaluate complaints of follicular phase symptoms after stopping medication.

On the basis of limited evidence, improvement is maintained with the long-term use of SSRIs and PMS/PMDD symptoms

| | | Table 2–7 | |
| | | **Drug Interactions of SSRIs** | |

| SSRI | Half-life (hr) | Active Metabolite | Cytochrome P-450 System Significantly Inhibited (expect to see > 50% increase in plasma levels) |
|---|---|---|---|
| Fluoxetine | 96–144 (fluoxetine) 96–384 (metabolite) | Norfluoxetine | 2C19*, 2D6†, 3A† |
| Sertraline | 26 (sertraline) 66–80 (metabolite) | Desmethylsertraline | None |
| Paroxetine | 17–22 | None | 2D6† |
| Fluvoxamine | 16 | None | 1A2§, 2C19*, 3A† |
| Citalopram | 33–37 | None | None |

SSRI, selective serotonin reuptake inhibitor.

*CYP2C19 substrates: citalopram, diazepam, hexobarbital, mephobarbital, moclobemide, tertiary amine tricyclic antidepressants, omeprazole

†CYP2D6 substrates: codeine, fluoxetine, haloperidol, paroxetine, secondary (nortriptyline, desipramine, protriptyline) and tertiary amine tricyclic antidepressants, type 1C antiarrhythmics (encainide, flecainide), beta-blockers

†CYP3A3/4 substrates: alprazolam, carbamazepine, clonazepam, codeine, diazepam, diltiazem, midazolam, sertraline, tertiary amine tricyclic antidepressants, erythromycin, lidocaine, loratadine, lovastatin, quinidine

§CYP1A substrates: clozapine, caffeine, tertiary amine tricyclic antidepressants (amitriptyline, clomipramine, doxepin, imipramine, trimipramine), propranolol, theophylline

From Harvey AT, Preskorn SH: Cytochrome P-450 enzymes: interpretation of their interactions with selective serotonin reuptake inhibitors. Pts I and II. J Clin Psychopharmacol 1996;6:273–285, 345–355.

return swiftly when medication is discontinued.[92–94] The appropriate duration of treatment for patients with PMS/PMDD that has responded to medication and the cost/benefit ratio of long-term treatment are important clinical issues that warrant further study.

### Pregnancy and Breastfeeding

By definition, women being treated for PMS/PMDD are of reproductive age and the possibility of pregnancy is a consideration. Data obtained from pharmaceutical registries and SSRI studies have shown no increased incidence of fetal teratogenic risk during any trimester[95] and no effect on global development in infants and preschool-aged children.[96] Infant exposure to SSRIs through breastfeeding was low in most studied cases, with no evidence of long-term complications in exposed infants.[97] However, the small numbers studied limit definitive conclusions about infant exposure through breastfeeding.

### Drug-Drug Interactions

Drug-drug interactions (particularly with drugs metabolized by the same microsomal system in the liver) remain as potentially serious during intermittent therapy as when used daily. Table 2-7 provides a list of drugs that interact with specific SSRIs according to the pathway in which they are metabolized.[98,99]

### General Guidelines for Treating PMS/PMDD with SSRIs

The effective dosage range for treatment of PMS/PMDD with SSRIs appears to be somewhat lower than that used in other psychiatric disorders such as major depression or obsessive-compulsive disorder. Many clinicians initiate fluoxetine treatment at 10 mg and sertraline at 25 mg. For sertraline, there is evidence from a large crossover study[100] that the 25 mg dose is as effective in treating the PMS/PMDD spectrum as the 50 mg dose, using either dosing strategy. A distinctive feature of PMS/PMDD treatment with SSRIs is the rapid response, which occurs within 2 to 3 days in the majority of patients.[69,70,71,73] It is this rapid response that makes intermittent premenstrual dosing an effective treatment strategy.

The decision about which dosing strategy to choose for a patient with PMS/PMDD must be individualized. Table 2-8 lists commonly used dosage regimens. Certainly if PMS/PMDD is complicated by another comorbid depressive or anxiety disorder, then continuous dosing is indicated. Similarly, if the duration of symptoms is highly variable, then continuous dosing may also be indicated. In most patients presenting with only PMS/PMDD, intermittent premenstrual dosing is highly effective, very well tolerated, and likely to be the treatment of choice.

Data still are insufficient to guide physicians about the appropriate duration of treatment in women with PMS/PMDD who have successfully responded to a course of SSRIs. Preliminary studies of sertraline and fluoxetine[93,101] suggest that treatment prevention studies have not been reported for either continuous or premenstrual dosing. It seems reasonable to recommend occasional one- or two-cycle treatment "holidays" to permit reassessment of the ongoing need for treatment. Premenstrual dosing lends itself particularly well to this empirical approach.

### Other Serotonergic Antidepressants

#### Venlafaxine

Venlafaxine increases the central activity of both serotonin and noradrenaline (norepinephrine). Venlafaxine (50 to 200 mg/day) was significantly more effective than placebo for mood, function,

| | Table 2-8 | |
| | **Dosage Regimens for Commonly Used Agents in Premenstrual Syndrome/Premenstrual Dysphoric Disorder** | |

| Medication | Dosage | Dosing Strategy |
|---|---|---|
| Fluoxetine (Sarafem) | 20 mg once daily 90 mg enteric-coated on days 14 and 7 | Continuous, luteal Luteal (days 14 and 7 only) |
| Sertraline (Zoloft) | 50–150 mg once daily | Continuous, luteal |
| Paroxetine (Paxil) | 20–30 mg once daily | Continuous, luteal |
| Citalopram (Celexa) | 10–20 mg once daily | Continuous |
| Venlafaxine (Effexor) | 37.5–150 mg twice daily | Continuous |

pain, and physical symptoms in a 4-month randomized trial in 164 women with PMS/PMDD.[84] Improvement was relatively swift, with approximately 80% symptom reduction in the first treatment cycle. Adverse events—primarily nausea, insomnia, and dizziness—were mild and transient. There are no published studies of luteal-phase administration of venlafaxine. It would be important to know whether similar efficacy is maintained with intermittent administration of this medication, which is now available as an extended-release formulation.

### Buspirone

Buspirone is a partial 5-hydroxytryptamine receptor 1A (5-HT1A) agonist. While it can be administered in the symptomatic luteal phase, its effect appears to be modest. Improvement of the mood symptoms of PMS/PMDD is inconsistent, although evidence is limited to several preliminary studies. Buspirone administration (10 to 30 mg/day) in the luteal phase was compared with nefazodone and placebo in a 2-month randomized, double-blind, placebo-controlled trial with 63 PMS/PMDD subjects.[87] Response to buspirone was significantly greater than to placebo for patients' self-rated global improvement but did not reach significance in any of the mood symptom scores. There were no differences in frequency of adverse effects between the buspirone, nefazodone, and placebo-treated groups.

In another randomized, double-blind, 3-month study of 34 patients with PMS/PMDD, buspirone (25 mg/day) administered during the luteal phase[102] produced a significantly greater decrease in total PMS symptoms than did placebo. However, in item analysis only physical symptoms of aches, fatigue, cramps, and impaired social interaction significantly improved, whereas changes in mood symptoms did not reach statistical significance. Because of its modest effects and its requirement for multiple daily doses, buspirone should be limited to second-line treatment.

### Clomipramine

Clomipramine is a tricyclic antidepressant (TCA) that is a potent but a relatively nonselective inhibitor of serotonin reuptake. Clomipramine (50 to 75 mg/day) was significantly more effective than placebo when administered during the luteal phase in a 3-month randomized study of 29 women with PMS/PMDD.[103] Adverse events reported by more than 10% of the subjects and more frequently with clomipramine than placebo included dry mouth, fatigue, vertigo, nausea, headache, and constipation. This was the first study to demonstrate that the clinical effect of serotonergic antidepressants occurred more rapidly when used for premenstrual syndrome than for other depressive disorders.

### Ovulation Suppression

#### Oral Contraceptives

Although oral contraceptives (OCs) are widely prescribed for the treatment of PMS/PMDD, efficacy studies have shown mixed results. In one randomized trial, a triphasic formulation reduced physical symptoms but not mood alterations.[104] In another study comparing triphasic and monophasic regimens, the monophasic formulation was less likely to cause mood alterations.[105]

The major trend in the formulation of OCs over the last 40 years has been a reduction in the doses of both the estrogen and the progestin components, and more recently, chemical alterations of the progestins to provide fewer androgenic compounds. Ethinyl estradiol doses have decreased from 100 µg to 20 to 30 µg. The dose of the progestin component has also decreased. All but one currently prescribed OC still contains a progestin derived from 19-nortestosterone. Table 2-9 summarizes the pharmacologic profile of progesterone, 19-nortestosterone, and a new progestin derived from spironolactone called drospirenone. Drospirenone has antiandrogenic and antimineralocorticoid activity.[106] One 6-month open-label study of drospirenone and ethinyl estradiol (30 µg) in 326 women with PMS/PMDD showed significant decreases in negative affect, water retention, and appetite.[107]

Numerous health advantages are afforded by OC intake. The OCs provide effective, reversible contraception but also have other known benefits including prevention of bone loss and decreased risk for ovarian and endometrial cancer, anemia, abnormal uterine bleeding, pelvic inflammatory disease, as well as complications of unplanned pregnancy, such as ectopic

---

**Table 2-9**
**Pharmacologic Profile of Progestins (in Animal Models)**

| Progestins | Pharmacologic Activity* | | | |
|---|---|---|---|---|
| | Progestogenic | Antiandrogenic | Antimineralocorticoid | Androgenic |
| Progesterone | + | (+) | + | – |
| Drospirenone | + | + | + | – |
| Norgestimate[†] | + | – | – | (+) |
| Levonorgestrel | + | – | – | (+) |
| Desogestrel | + | – | – | (+) |
| Norethindrone | + | – | – | (+) |
| Cyproterone acetate[†] | + | + | – | – |

*+, distinct effect; (+), negligible effect at therapeutic doses; –, no effect.
[†]Metabolized to levonorgestrel-3-oxime and levonorgestrel.
[†]Not available in the United States.
From Fuhrmann U, Krattenmacher R, Slater EP, et al: The novel progestin drospirenone and its natural counterpart progesterone: biochemical profile and antiandrogenic potential. Contraception 1996;54:243–251.

pregnancy and molar gestation. The most bothersome physical side effects of OCs are bloating and breast tenderness, and these symptoms are at least in part attributable to water retention, probably related to their estrogenic component.

Current evidence suggests that OCs should be considered if symptoms are primarily physical but may not be effective if mood symptoms are more prevalent. More controlled studies are needed to evaluate the efficacy of antiandrogenic progestins, such as drospirenone. Studies are also needed to determine whether continuous OCs are more likely to ameliorate premenstrual symptoms.[108]

### Transdermal Estradiol

High-dose transdermal estradiol 200 µg provided via patch can prevent ovulation and reduce symptoms of PMS/PMDD.[109] However, this high-dose estrogen therapy with cyclic low-dose progestin supplementation for the last 7 days of the cycle has not been clearly demonstrated to eliminate the risk of endometrial hyperplasia associated with estrogen administration.

### Progesterone

Historically, natural progesterone has been one of the most commonly employed therapies in women with PMS/PMDD, but careful scientific scrutiny has not supported an overall benefit of this hormone when compared with placebo, whether administered as a vaginal suppository[110] or as oral micronized progesterone.[111] Evidence from a large, placebo-controlled study,[111] as well as a recent meta-analysis,[112] suggests that micronized progesterone has no efficacy in the treatment of PMDD.

### Danazol

The synthetic steroid danazol appears to reduce affective and physical symptoms of PMS/PMDD[113]; however, its practical use is limited by the need for concurrent administration of a reliable contraceptive method. At 200 mg/day dosage, ovulation and thus conception are still possible, and danazol can cause virilization of the fetus. Doses sufficient to inhibit ovulation (600 to 800 mg/day) have been associated with undesirable side effects, including weight gain, mood changes, and acne.[12]

### Gonadotropin-Releasing Hormone Agonists

Improvement in PMS/PMDD symptoms with gonadotropin-releasing hormone (GnRH) agonists has been reported in the majority of well-designed studies[114,115] but not in all of them.[116] Like oral contraceptives, GnRH agonists appear to be less effective in treating affective symptoms than physical symptoms in PMS/PMDD.[114] The hypoestrogenic side effects and cost of GnRH agonists limit their usefulness except in severe cases of PMS/PMDD unresponsive to other treatment. Oral contraceptives may provide a safer means of inhibiting ovulation and reducing physical symptoms in PMS/PMDD patients.

If GnRH agonists are to be used for more than a few months, bone loss becomes a concern. The most commonly used approach is add-back estrogen therapy (with progestin if indicated). Add-back therapy also may result in return of symptoms, although studies are limited and sometimes confusing. In a double-blind, placebo-controlled study, both estrogen add-back therapy alone and progesterone therapy alone were associated with significant

recurrence of symptoms.[117] Another small, rigorous study evaluated eight women with PMS. Administration of the GnRH agonist resulted in an improvement of approximately 75% in luteal-phase symptom scores. The addition of estrogen as well as progesterone was associated with worsening symptoms, but a similar worsening also was seen with placebo.[118] If hormone therapy results in a return of symptoms, alendronate should be considered for osteoporosis prevention.

### Bilateral Salpingo-Oophorectomy

The final treatment option for women with severe PMS/PMDD symptoms and no response to other therapies is permanent suppression of ovulation through bilateral salpingo-oophorectomy. Bilateral ovariectomy with hysterectomy was highly effective in permanently eliminating symptoms of PMS/PMDD in two studies.[60,119] However, surgery for PMS/PMDD is controversial because it is irreversible. It is associated with morbidity and mortality, and the resulting hypoestrogenemia must be addressed to prevent long-term complications. This approach should be reserved for those severely affected patients who meet strict diagnostic criteria and who do not respond to any potentially effective therapy other than GnRH agonists.[120] These limitations are critical, because a major cause of therapy failure with any of the described treatments is an incorrect diagnosis of PMS/PMDD. It is advisable to perform a diagnostic trial with an agonist for a minimum of 3 months to determine whether oophorectomy will be effective. An additional advantage to extended use of an agonist is the opportunity to assess the woman's tolerance for estrogen replacement therapy.

### *Other Medications*

#### Alprazolam

Alprazolam, a benzodiazepine, has been studied in PMS/PMDD with some[111,121-123] but not all reports[124] indicating greater improvement with alprazolam compared with placebo. Study dosages ranged from 0.25 mg twice daily to 0.5 mg three times daily, administered during the luteal phase. A benzodiazepine such as alprazolam, with its swift onset of action and short half-life, lends itself to the treatment of luteal-phase symptoms, but the problems of dependence and tolerance that occur with benzodiazepines require careful diagnosis and monitoring with ongoing use. One study found no withdrawal symptoms when alprazolam administration was strictly limited to the luteal phase in patients clearly diagnosed with PMS/PMDD.[125] Nevertheless, patients whose symptoms are not strictly limited to the premenstrual phase and patients who are at risk for addiction are not appropriate candidates for this class of medication. Benzodiazepines may also be sedating and worsen symptoms in patients who are depressed. Conversely, alprazolam may be useful if agitation and anxiety are the primary premenstrual symptoms. The modest efficacy of alprazolam shown in the studies of PMS/PMDD, coupled with the potential for physical dependence and withdrawal, makes this drug a second-line treatment for PMDD.

#### Nonsteroidal Anti-Inflammatory Drugs

Few studies of nonsteroidal anti-inflammatory drugs (NSAIDs) were identified. On the whole, studies of mefenamic acid[126-130] and naproxen sodium[131] provide insufficient data to determine effectiveness, but NSAIDs are considered to be potentially useful, practical, and of low risk.

### Spironolactone

Because complaints of fluid retention are common in the luteal phase, diuretic therapy has been advocated. No evidence exists that thiazide diuretics are of benefit. Spironolactone, an aldosterone antagonist with antiandrogenic properties, is the only diuretic that has been shown to be of benefit in PMS/PMDD. Several randomized, double-blind, placebo-controlled trials have shown a significant reduction in somatic and affective complaints.[132-136] Usual dosage in most studies is 100 mg/day in the morning during the 14-day luteal phase. However, not all reports evaluating spironolactone for PMS/PMDD have shown benefit.

## TREATMENT GUIDELINES

The treatment guidelines presented in Table 2-10 emphasize the availability of multiple treatment options and the need for reassessment following initiation of therapy. Any first-line treatment or combination of first-line treatments is considered appropriate for the management of PMS/PMDD. First-line options include nonpharmacologic treatments (exercise, diet modification, sleep hygiene, stress reduction, and patient education), psychotropics (SSRIs and venlafaxine), and other pharmacologic therapies (calcium, NSAIDs, and transdermal estradiol combined with oral progestin).

Once treatment is initiated, reevaluation should include measurement of luteal-phase symptoms using a standardized instrument. Failure to achieve a 50% or greater reduction in symptoms and either a resolution of interference with daily activities or the conclusion by the patient and clinician that overall the symptoms are at least moderately improved should lead to a modification in the management strategy.

Second-line treatments should be considered only for individuals who have failed to respond to various combinations of first-line options, as they tend to be less efficacious or impractical or to have significant potential side effects. Second-line treatment options include nonpharmacologic treatments (cognitive-behavioral therapy), psychotropics (fluvoxamine, buspirone, clomipramine, and alprazolam), other pharmacologic treatments (oral contraceptives, danazol, GnRH agonists, alprazolam, and spironolactone), and herbal products (chasteberry and black cohosh).

Evening primrose oil and progesterone are not recommended because there is no evidence to prove that they are effective. St. John's wort is not recommended primarily out of concern for potential drug interactions.

Bilateral ovariectomy with hysterectomy is highly effective in permanently eliminating symptoms of PMS/PMDD. However, because of the extreme nature of this treatment method, it is recommended only in the most recalcitrant of cases when future fertility is not an issue. It is possible that the sudden change in hormonal milieu associated with surgical menopause could also be a trigger for mood problems in vulnerable women.

## FURTHER RESEARCH

Because SSRIs are first-line therapy for severe premenstrual symptoms that require medical management, most research questions pertain to this class of agents. Whether SSRIs remain effective when used as long-term maintenance treatment is a major question that warrants further study. It is particularly important to determine whether the long-term use of intermittent administration differs from long-term continuous administration. The rate and extent of which symptoms return after stopping medication for one or more menstrual cycles is not clear.

Another unanswered question is whether SSRIs with longer half-lives (e.g., fluoxetine) provide ongoing, rather than

| Table 2-10 Treatment Guidelines for Premenstrual Syndrome/Premenstrual Dysphoric Disorder | | | |
|---|---|---|---|
| **Treatment** | **First Line** | **Second Line** | **Not Recommended** |
| Nonpharmacologic | Exercise Diet modification Sleep hygiene Stress reduction Patient education | Cognitive-behavioral therapy (CBT) | |
| Dietary supplements | Calcium | Magnesium Vitamin E Vitamin B$_6$ | |
| Psychotropics | Fluoxetine Sertraline Paroxetine Citalopram Venlafaxine | Fluvoxamine Buspirone Clomipramine Alprazolam | |
| Other pharmacologics | Estrogen patch NSAIDs | Oral contraceptives Danazol GnRH agonists Spironolactone | Progesterone Ovariectomy |
| Herbal products | | Chasteberry Black cohosh | St. John's wort Evening primrose |

intermittent, medication effects and whether such medications enable a swifter adjustment to adverse events than do short half-life medications when intermittently administered. Whether SSRIs with short half-lives (e.g., paroxetine) are more likely to manifest discontinuation symptoms, as has been observed in the treatment of major depressive disorder, remains in question although there is no evidence for this in currently available studies of paroxetine in the treatment of PMS/PMDD.

Another major gap in our knowledge of the treatment for PMS/PMDD is availability of data to guide the treatment of patients whose symptoms do not respond to SSRIs. Whether such patients will respond to anxiolytic or other classes of medication that have been studied for PMS/PMDD is not known. The treatment of PMS/PMDD with comorbid conditions also has not been studied and lacks guidelines. Predictors of response to SSRIs or other treatments for PMS/PMDD have not been identified.

Finally, the role of newer OCs with antiandrogenic properties, and continuous dosing of OCs, require further study. More research is necessary on nonpharmacologic treatments. The role of cognitive functioning in PMS/PMDD and the efficacy of cognitive therapy have been suggested, but data are sparse. Exercise provides promising preliminary data and warrants more investigation.

# REFERENCES

1. American College of Obstetricians and Gynecologists: Premenstrual Syndrome. ACOG Practice Bulletin No. 15, Apr 2000. **(IV, C)**

2. Freeman EW: Luteal phase administration of agents for the treatment of premenstrual dysphoric disorder. CNS Drugs 2004;18:453–468. **(IV, C)**

3. Johnson SR: Premenstrual syndrome: In Wallis LA (ed): Textbook of Women's Health. Philadelphia, Lippincott-Raven, 1998, pp 691–697. **(IV, C)**

4. Robinson GE, Stewart DF: Psychological aspects of premenstrual syndrome. In Wallis LA (ed): Textbook of Women's Health. Philadelphia, Lippincott-Raven, 1998, pp 699–701. **(IV, C)**

5. Dalton K: The premenstrual syndrome and progesterone therapy, 2nd ed. Chicago, Year Book, 1984. **(IV, C)**

6. Steiner M, Pearlstein T: Premenstrual dysphoria and the serotonin system: pathophysiology and treatment. J Clin Psychiatry 2000; 61(Suppl 12):17–21. **(IV, C)**

7. Rapkin AJ, Edelmuth E, Chang LC, et al: Whole-blood serotonin in premenstrual syndrome. Obstet Gynecol 1987;70:533–537. **(Ib, A)**

8. Taylor DL, Mathew RJ, Ho BT, et al: Serotonin levels and platelet uptake during premenstrual tension. Neuropsychobiology 1984; 12:16–18. **(Ib, A)**

9. Rasgon N, Serra M, Biggio G, et al: Neuroactive steroid-serotonergic interaction: responses to an intravenous L-tryptophan challenge in women with premenstrual syndrome. Eur J Endocrinol 2001; 145:25–33. **(IIa, B)**

10. FitzGerald M, Malone KM, Li S, et al: Blunted serotonin response to fenfluramine challenge in premenstrual dysphoric disorder. Am J Psychiatry 1997;154:556–558. **(Ib, A)**

11. Yatham LN: Is 5HT1α receptor subsensitivity a trait marker for late luteal phase dysphoric disorder? A pilot study. Can J Psychiatry 1993; 38:662–664. **(IIa, B)**

12. Mitwally MF, Kahn LS, Halbreich U: Pharmacotherapy of premenstrual syndromes and premenstrual dysphoric disorder: current practices. Expert Opin Pharmacother 2002;3:1577–1590. **(IV, C)**

13. Roca CA, Schmidt PJ, Bloch M, et al: Implications of endocrine studies of premenstrual syndrome. Psychiatr Ann 1996;26:576–580. **(IV, C)**

14. Ross LE, Steiner M: A biopsychosocial approach to premenstrual dysphoric disorder. Psychiatr Clin North Am 2003;26:529–546. **(IV, C)**

15. Rapkin AJ: A review of treatment of premenstrual syndrome and premenstrual dysphoric disorder. Psychoneuroendocrinology 2003; 28(Suppl 3):39–53. **(IV, C)**

16. Rapkin AJ, Morgan M, Goldman L, et al: Progesterone metabolite allopregnanolone in women with premenstrual syndrome. Obstet Gynecol 1997;90:709–714. **(IIa, B)**

17. Freeman EW, Frye CA, Rickels K, et al: Allopregnanolone levels and symptom improvement in severe premenstrual syndrome. J Clin Psychopharmacol 2002;22:516–520. **(IIa, B)**

18. Le Melledo JM, Van Driel M, Coupland NK, et al: Response to flumazenil in women with premenstrual dysphoric disorder. Am J Psychiatry 2000;157:821–823. **(Ib, A)**

19. Sundstrom I, Nyberg S, Backstrom T: Patients with premenstrual syndrome have reduced sensitivity to midazolam compared to control subjects. Neuropsychopharmacology 1997;17:370–381. **(Ib, A)**

20. Eriksson E, Sundblad C, Landen M, et al: Behavioral effects of androgens in women. In Steiner M, Yonkers KA, Ericksson E (eds): Mood Disorders in Women. London, Martin Dunitz, 2000, pp 233–246. **(IV, C)**

21. Steiner M, Dunn EJ, MacDougall M, et al: Serotonin transporter gene polymorphism, free testosterone, and symptoms associated with premenstrual dysphoric disorder. Biol Psychiatry 2002;51:91S. **(IIa, B)**

22. Condon JT: The premenstrual syndrome: a twin study. Br J Psychiatry 1993;162:481–486. **(IV, C)**

23. Kendler KS, Karkowski LM, Corey LA, et al: Longitudinal population-based twin study of retrospectively reported premenstrual symptoms and lifetime major depression. Am J Psychiatry 1998;155:1234–1240. **(IIa, B)**

24. Halbreich U, Bergeron R, Yonkers KA, et al: Efficacy of intermittent, luteal phase sertraline treatment of premenstrual dysphoric disorder. Poster presented at the 39th annual meeting of the American College of Neuropsychopharmacology. San Juan, Puerto Rico, Dec 10–14, 2000. **(Ib)**

25. American Psychiatric Association Diagnostic and Statistical Manual of Mental Disorders, 4th ed, text revision. Washington, DC, American Psychiatric Association, 2000. **(IV, C)**

26. Hart WG, Coleman GJ, Russell JW: Assessment of premenstrual symptomatology: a re-evaluation of the predictive validity of self-report. J Psychosom Res 1987;31:185–190. **(III)**

27. Thys-Jacobs, A, Fratarcangelo P: Comparative analysis of three PMS assessment instruments—the identification of premenstrual syndrome with core symptoms. Psychopharmacol Bull 1995;31:389–396. **(IIa, B)**

28. Endicott J: Severe premenstrual dysphoria: differential diagnosis and treatment. J Am Med Womens Assoc 1998;53:170–175. **(IV, C)**

29. Smith MJ, Schmidt PJ, Rubinow DR: Operationalizing DSM-IV criteria for PMDD: selecting symptomatic an asymptomatic cycles for research. J Psychiatr Res 2003;37:75–83. **(IV, C)**

30. Endicott J: The menstrual cycle and mood disorders. J Affect Disord 1993;29:193–200. **(IV, C)**

31. Freeman EW, Sondheimer SJ: Premenstrual dysphoric disorder: recognition and treatment. J Clin Psychiatry 2003;5:30–39. **(IV, C)**

32. Frackiewicz EJ, Shiovitz TM: Evaluation and management of premenstrual syndrome and premenstrual dysphoric disorder. J Am Pharm Assoc 2001;41:437–47. **(IV, C)**

33. Steege JF, Blumenthal JA: The effects of aerobic exercise on premenstrual symptoms in middle-aged women: a preliminary study. J Psychosom Res 1993;37:127–133. **(Ib, A)**

34. Prior JC, Vigna Y, Sciarretta DS, et al: Conditioning exercise decreases premenstrual symptoms: a prospective, controlled 6-month trial. Fertil Steril 1987;47:402–408. **(IIa, B)**

35. Sundstrom I, Backstrom T: Patients with premenstrual syndrome have decreased saccadic eye velocity compared to control subjects. Biol Psychiatry 1998;44:755–764. **(Ib, A)**

36. Morse G: Positively reframing perceptions of the menstrual cycle among women with premenstrual syndrome. J Obstet Gynecol Neonatal Nurs 1999;28:165–174. **(IIa, B)**

37. Taylor D: Effectiveness of professional-peer group treatment: symptom management for women with PMS. Res Nurs Health 1999; 22:496–511. **(IIa, B)**

38. Blake F, Salkovskis P, Gath D, et al: Cognitive therapy for premenstrual syndrome: a controlled trial. J Psychosom Res 1998; 45:307–318. **(Ib, A)**

39. Morse CA, Dennerstein L, Farrell E, et al: A comparison of hormone therapy, coping skills training, and relaxation for the relief of premenstrual syndrome. Behav Med 1991;14:469–489. **(Ib, A)**

40. Kirkby RJ: Changes in premenstrual symptoms and irrational thinking following cognitive-behavioral coping skills training. J Consult Clin Psychol 1994;62:1026–1032. **(Ib, A)**

41. Hunter MS, Ussher JM, Browne SJ, et al: A randomized comparison of psychological (cognitive behavior therapy), medical (fluoxetine) and combined treatment for women with premenstrual dysphoric disorder. J Psychosom Obstet Gynaecol 2002;23:193–199. **(Ib, A)**

42. Hunter MS, Ussher JM, Cariss M, et al: Medical (fluoxetine) and psychological (cognitive-behavioral therapy) treatment for premenstrual dysphoric disorder: a study of treatment processes. J Psychosom Res 2002;53:811–817. **(Ib, A)**

43. Thys-Jacobs, Starkey P, Bernstein D, et al: Calcium carbonate and the premenstrual syndrome: effects on premenstrual and menstrual symptoms. Premenstrual Syndrome Study Group. Am J Obstet Gynecol 1998;179:444–452. **(Ib, A)**

44. Blumenthal M, Busse WR, Goldberg A, et al: The complete German Commission E monographs: therapeutic guide to herbal medicines. Austin, Tex, American Botanical Council, 1998, p 1694. **(IV, C)**

45. Walker AF, De Souza MC, Vickers MF, et al: Magnesium supplementation alleviates premenstrual symptoms of fluid retention. J Womens Health 1998;7:1157–1165. **(IIb, B)**

46. Facchinetti F, Borella P, Sances G, et al: Oral magnesium successfully relieves premenstrual mood changes. Obstet Gynecol 1991; 78:177–181. **(IIb, B)**

47. Girman A, Lee R, Kligler B: An integrative medicine approach to premenstrual syndrome (editorial). Am J Obstet Gynecol 2003;188 (Suppl 5, pt 2): S56–S65. **(IV, C)**

48. London BS, Murphy L, Kitlowski KE, et al: Efficacy of alpha-tocopherol in the treatment of the premenstrual syndrome. J Reprod Med 1987;32:400–404. **(Ib, A)**

49. Wyatt RM, Dimmock PW, Jones PW, et al: Efficacy of vitamin B-6 in the treatment of premenstrual syndrome: systematic review. BMJ 1999;318:1375–1381. **(Ia, A)**

50. Dittmar G, Bohnert K: Premenstrual syndrome: treatment with phytopharmaceutical. TW Gynakol 1992;5:60–68. **(Ib, A)**

51. Schellenberg R: Treatment for the premenstrual syndrome with agnus castus fruit extract: prospective, randomized, placebo-controlled study. BMJ 2001;322:134–137. **(Ib, A)**

52. Williams JW, Mulrow CD, Chiquette E, et al: A systematic review of newer pharmacotherapies for depression in adults: evidence report summary. Ann Intern Med 2000;132:743–756. **(IV, C)**

53. Shelton RC, Keller MB, Gelenberg A, et al: Effectiveness of St. John's wort in major depression: a randomized placebo controlled trial. JAMA 2001;285:1978–1986. **(Ib, A)**

54. Stevinson C, Ernst E: A pilot study of hypericum perforatum for the treatment of premenstrual syndrome. BJOG 2000;107:870–876. **(IIb, B)**

55. Horribin DF, Manku MS, Brush M, et al: Abnormalities in plasma essential fatty acid levels in women with premenstrual syndrome and nonmalignant breast disease. J Nutr Med 1991;2:259–264. **(IIa, B)**

56. Dimmock PW, Wyatt KM, Jones PW, et al: Efficacy of selective serotonin-reuptake inhibitors in premenstrual syndrome: a systematic review. Lancet 2000;356:1131–1136. **(Ia, A)**

57. Steiner M, Steinberg S, Stewart D, et al: Fluoxetine in the treatment of premenstrual dysphoria. Canadian Fluoxetine/Premenstrual Dysphoria Collaborative Study Group. N Engl J Med 1995; 332:1529–1534. **(Ib, A)**

58. Wood SH, Mortola JF, Chan YF, et al: Treatment of premenstrual syndrome with fluoxetine: a double-blind, placebo-controlled, cross-over study. Obstet Gynecol 1992;80:339–344. **(Ib, A)**

59. Ozeren S, Corakci A, Yucesoy I, et al: Fluoxetine in the treatment of premenstrual syndrome. Eur J Obstet Gynecol Reprod Biol 1997; 73:167–170. **(Ib, A)**

60. Pearlstein TB, Stone AB, Lund S: Comparison of fluoxetine, bupropion, and placebo in the treatment of premenstrual dysphoric disorder. J Clin Psychopharmacol 1997;17:261–266. **(Ib, A)**

61. Su TP, Schmidt PJ, Danaceau MA, et al: Fluoxetine in the treatment of premenstrual dysphoria. Neuropsychopharmacology 1997; 16:346–356. **(Ib, A)**

62. Stone AB, Pearlstein TB, Brown WA: Fluoxetine in the treatment of late luteal phase dysphoric disorder. J Clin Psychiatry 1991; 52:290–293. **(Ib, A)**

63. Menkes DB, Taghavi E, Mason PA, et al: Fluoxetine's spectrum of action in premenstrual syndrome. Int Clin Psychopharmacol 1993; 8:95–102. **(Ib, A)**

64. Cohen LS, Miner C, Brown E, et al: Premenstrual daily fluoxetine for premenstrual dysphoric disorder: a placebo-controlled clinical trial using computerized diaries. Obstet Gynecol 2002;100;435–444. **(Ib, A)**

65. Miner C, Brown E, McCray S, et al: Weekly luteal-phase dosing with enteric-coated fluoxetine 90 mg in premenstrual dysphoric disorder: a randomized, double-blind, placebo-controlled clinical trial. Clin Ther 2002;24:417–433. **(Ib, A)**

66. Steiner M, Korzekwa M, Lamont J, et al: Intermittent fluoxetine dosing in the treatment of women with premenstrual dysphoria. Psychopharmacol Bull 1997;33:771–774. **(III, B)**

67. Pearlstein T, Yonkers K: Review of fluoxetine and its clinical applications in premenstrual dysphoric disorder. Expert Opin Pharmacother 2002;3:979–991. **(IV, C)**

68. Halbreich U, Smoller JW: Intermittent luteal phase sertraline treatment of dysphoric premenstrual syndrome. J Clin Psychiatry 1997; 58:399–402. **(III, B)**

69. Jermain DM, Preece CK, Sykes RL, et al: Luteal phase sertraline treatment for premenstrual dysphoric disorder: results of a double-blind, placebo-controlled, crossover study. Arch Fam Med 1999; 8:328–332. **(Ib, A)**

70. Young SA, Hurt PH, Benedek DM, et al: Treatment of premenstrual dysphoric disorder with sertraline during the luteal phase: a randomized, double-blind, placebo-controlled crossover trial. J Clin Psychiatry 1998;59:76–80. **(Ib, A)**

71. Freeman EW, Rickels K, Arredondo F, et al: Full-or half-cycle treatment of severe premenstrual syndrome with a serotonergic antidepressant. J Clin Psychopharmacol 1999;19:3–8. **(III, B)**

72. Freeman EW, Rickels K, Sondheimer SJ, et al: Continuous or intermittent dosing with sertraline for severe premenstrual syndrome/premenstrual dysphoric disorder. Am J Psychiatry 2004;161:343–351. **(III, B)**

73. Halbreich M, Bergeron R, Yonkers KA, et al: Efficacy of intermittent, luteal phase sertraline treatment of premenstrual dysphoric disorder. Obstet Gynecol 2002;100;1219–1229. **(Ib, A)**

74. Cohen LS, Soares CN, Yonkers KA, et al: Paroxetine controlled release is effective in treating premenstrual dysphoric disorder [abstract]. Obstet Gynecol 2003; 101(Suppl 4):111S. **(Ib, A)**

75. Gee M, Bellew KM, Holland FJ, et al: Luteal phase dosing of paroxetine controlled release is effective in treating PMDD [abstract No. NR760 plus poster]. American Psychiatric Association 2003 annual meeting. San Francisco, May 17–22, 2003. **(Ib, A)**

76. Eriksson E, Hedberg A, Andersch B, Sunblad C: The SSRI paroxetine is superior to the noradrenaline reuptake inhibitor maprotiline in the treatment of premenstrual syndrome. Neuropsychopharmacol 1995; 12:167–176. **(Ib, A)**

77. Yonkers KA, Gullion C, Williams A, et al: Paroxetine as a treatment for premenstrual dysphoric disorder. J Clin Psychopharmacol 1996;16:3–8. **(Ib, A)**

78. Wikander I, Sundblad C, Andersch B, et al: Citalopram in premenstrual dysphoria: is intermittent treatment during luteal phase more effective than continuous medication throughout the menstrual cycle? J Clin Psychopharmacol 1998;18:390–398. **(Ib, A)**

79. Sundblad C, Wikander I, Andersch B, et al: A naturalistic study of paroxetine in premenstrual syndrome: efficacy and side effects during ten cycles of treatment. Eur Neuropsychopharmacol 1997;7:201–206. **(III, B)**

80. Freeman EW, Jabara S, Sondheimer SF, et al: Citalopram in PMS patients with prior SSRI treatment failure: a preliminary study. J Womens Health Gend Based Med 2002;11:459–464. **(III, B)**

81. Freeman EW, Rickels K, Sondheimer SJ: Fluvoxamine for premenstrual dysphoric disorder: a pilot study. J Clin Psychiatry 1996;57(Suppl 8):56–60. **(IIb, B)**

82. Veeninga AT, Westenberg HG, Weusten JT: Fluvoxamine in the treatment of premenstrually related mood disorders. Psychopharmacology (Berl) 1990;102:414–416. **(Ib, A)**

83. Yonkers KA, Halbreich U, Freeman E, et al: Symptomatic improvement of premenstrual dysphoric disorder with sertraline treatment: a randomized controlled trial. Sertraline Premenstrual Dysphoric Collaborative Study Group. JAMA 1997;278:983–988. **(Ib, A)**

84. Freeman EW, Rickels K, Yonkers KA, et al: Venlafaxine in the treatment of premenstrual dysphoric disorder. Obstet Gynecol 2001; 98:737–744. **(Ib, A)**

85. Wells BG, Mandos LA, Hayes PE: Depressive disorders. In Dipiro JT, Talbert RL, Yee GC, et al (eds): Pharmacotherapy: A Pathophysiologic Approach. Stamford, Conn, Appleton & Lange, 1999, pp 1141–1160. **(IV, C)**

86. Clayton AH, Pradko JF, Croft HA, et al: Prevalence of sexual dysfunction among newer antidepressants. J Clin Psychiatry 2002; 63:357–366. **(IV, C)**

87. Landen M, Eriksson O, Sundblad C, et al: Compounds with affinity for serotonergic receptors in the treatment of premenstrual dysphoria: a comparison of buspirone, nefazodone and placebo. Psychopharmacology (Berl) 2001;155:292–298. **(Ib, A)**

88. Rothschild AJ: Sexual side effects of antidepressants. J Clin Psychiatry 2000;61:28–36. **(IV, C)**

89. Eriksson E: Serotonin reuptake inhibitors for the treatment of premenstrual dysphoria. Int Clin Psychopharmacol 1999;14(Suppl 2): S27–S33. **(IV, C)**

90. Pearlstein T, Gillespie JA: When should premenstrual dosing in PMDD end? Poster presentation, 155th Annual APA American Psychiatric Association meeting. Philadelphia, 2002. **(III, B)**

91. Goldstein BJ, Goodnick PJ: Selective serotonin reuptake inhibitors in the treatment of affective disorders. 3. Tolerability, safety and pharmacoeconomics. J Psychopharmacol 1998;12(3 Suppl B): S55–S87. **(IV, C)**

92. Freeman EW, Sondheimer SJ, Rickels K, et al: A pilot naturalistic follow-up of extended sertraline treatment for severe premenstrual syndrome. J Clin Psychopharmacol 2004;24:1–2. **(III, B)**

93. Pearlstein TB, Stone AB: Long-term fluoxetine treatment of late luteal phase dysphoric disorder. J Clin Psychiatry 1994;55:332–335. **(IIb, B)**

94. Yonkers KA, Barnett LK, Carmody T, et al: Serial discontinuation of SSRI treatment for PMDD. Biol Psychol 1998;43(Suppl 8):358. **(IIb, B)**

95. Kulin NA, Pastuszak A, Sager S, et al: Pregnancy outcome following maternal use of the new selective serotonin reuptake inhibitors. JAMA 1998;279:609–610. **(IIa, B)**

96. Nulman I, Rovet J, Stewart DE, et al: Neurodevelopment of children exposed in vitro to antidepressant drugs. N Engl J Med 1997; 336:258–262. **(IIa, B)**

97. Hendrick V, Fukuchi A, Altshuler L, et al: Use of sertraline, paroxetine and fluvoxamine by nursing women. Br J Psychiatry 2001;179:163–166. **(III, B)**

98. Harvey AT, Preskorn SH: Cytochrome P450 enzymes: interpretation of their interactions with selective serotonin reuptake inhibitors. Pt 1. J Clin Psychopharmacol 1996;6:273–285. **(IV, C)**

99. Harvey AT, Preskorn SH: Cytochrome P450 enzymes: interpretation of their interactions with selective serotonin reuptake inhibitors. Pt 11. J Clin Psychopharmacol 1996;16:345–355. **(IV, C)**

100. Kornstein S, Pearlstein T, Farfel G, et al: Efficacy of sertraline in the treatment of premenstrual syndrome. Poster presented at the 41st annual meeting of the New Clinical Drug Evaluation Unit. Phoenix, Ariz, May 28–31, 2001. **(Ib, A)**

101. Freeman EW, Sondheimer SJ, Rickels K, et al: A pilot study of extended sertraline treatment for severe PMS. Poster presented at the 155th annual meeting of the American Psychiatric Association. Philadelphia, May 18–23, 2002. **(IIb, B)**

102. Rickels K, Freeman E, Sondheimer S: Buspirone in treatment of premenstrual syndrome [letter]. Lancet 1989;1:777. **(Ib, A)**

103. Sundblad C, Hedberg M, Eriksson E: Clomipramine administered during the luteal phase reduces the symptoms of premenstrual syndrome: a placebo controlled trial. Neuropsychopharmacology 1993;9:133–145. **(Ib, A)**

104. Graham CA, Sherwin BB: A prospective treatment study of premenstrual symptoms using a triphasic oral contraceptive. Psychosom Res 1992;36:257–266. **(Ib, A)**

105. Backstrom T, Hansson-Malmstrom Y, Lindhe BA, et al: Oral contraceptives in premenstrual syndrome: a randomized comparison of triphasic and monophasic preparations. Contraception 1992; 36:257–266. **(III, B)**

106. Fuhrmann U, Krattenmacher R, Slater EP, et al: The novel progestin drospirenone and its natural counterpart progesterone: biochemical profile and antiandrogenic potential. Contraception 1996;54:243–251. **(IV, C)**

107. Parsey KS, Pong A: An open-label multicenter study to evaluate Yasmin, a low-dose combination oral contraceptive containing drospirenone, a new progestogen. Contraception 2000;61:105–111. **(III, B)**

108. Sulak PJ, Scow RD, Preece D, et al: Hormone withdrawal symptoms in oral contraceptive users, continuous use. Obstet Gynecol 2000; 95:261–266. **(IV, C)**

109. Watson NR, Studd JWW, Savvas M, et al: Treatment of severe premenstrual syndrome with oestradiol patches and cyclical oral norethisterone. Lancet 1989;2:730–732. **(III, B)**

110. Freeman E, Rickels K, Sondheimer SJ, et al: Ineffectiveness of progesterone suppository treatment for premenstrual syndrome. JAMA 1990;264:349–353. **(Ib, A)**

111. Freeman EW, Rickels K, Sondheimer SJ, et al: A double-blind trial of oral progesterone, alprazolam, and placebo in treatment of severe premenstrual syndrome. JAMA 1995;274:51–57. **(Ib, A)**

112. Wyatt K, Dimmock P, Jones P, et al: Efficacy of progesterone and progestogens in management of premenstrual syndrome: systematic review. BMJ 2001;323:776–780. **(Ia, A)**

113. O'Brien PMS, Abukhalil I: Randomized controlled trial of the management of premenstrual mastalgia using luteal phase only Danazol. Am J Obstet Gynecol 1999;180:18–23. **(Ib, A)**

114. Freeman EW, Sondheimer SJ, Rickels K: Gonadotropin-releasing hormone agonist in treatment of premenstrual symptoms with and without ongoing dysphoria: a controlled study. Psychopharmacol Bull 1997;33:303–309. **(Ib, A)**

115. Johnson SR: Premenstrual syndrome therapy. Clin Obstet Gynecol 1998;41:405–421. **(IV, C)**

116. West CP, Hillier H: Ovarian suppression with the gonadotropin-releasing hormone agonist goserelin (Zoladex) in management of the premenstrual tension syndrome. Hum Reprod 1994;9:1058–1063. **(Ib, A)**

117. Schmidt PJ, Nieman LK, Danaceau MA, et al: Differential behavioral effects of gonadal steroids in women with and in those without premenstrual syndrome. N Engl J Med 1998;338:209–216. **(Ib, A)**

118. Mortola AJF, Girton L, Fischer U: A successful treatment of severe premenstrual syndrome by combined use of gonadotropin-releasing hormone agonist and estrogen/progestin. J Clin Endocrinol Metab 1991;72:252A–252F. **(Ib, A)**

119. Casper RF, Heart MT: The effect of hysterectomy and bilateral oophorectomy in women with severe premenstrual syndrome. Am J Obstet Gynecol 1990;162:105–109. **(IIb, B)**

120. Casson P, Hahn PM, Van Vugt DA, et al: Lasting response to ovariectomy in severe intractable premenstrual syndrome. Am J Obstet Gynecol 1990;162:99–105. **(IIb, B)**

121. Berger CP, Presser B: Alprazolam in the treatment of two subsamples of patients with late luteal phase dysphoric disorder: a double-blind, placebo-controlled crossover study. Obstet Gynecol 1994;84:379–385. **(Ib, A)**

122. Harrison WM, Endicott J, Nee J: Treatment of premenstrual dysphoria with alprazolam: a controlled study. Arch Gen Psychiatry 1990;47:270–275. **(Ib, A)**

123. Smith S, Rinehart JS, Ruddock VE, et al: Treatment of premenstrual syndrome with alprazolam: results of a double-blind, placebo-controlled, randomized crossover clinical trial. Obstet Gynecol 1987;70:37–43. **(Ib, A)**

124. Schmidt PJ, Grover GN, Rubinow DR: Alprazolam in the treatment of premenstrual syndrome: a double-blind, placebo-controlled trial. Arch Gen Psychiatry 1993;50:467–473. **(Ib, A)**

125. Rickels K, Freeman EW: Prior benzodiazepine exposure and benzo-diazepine treatment outcome. J Clin Psychiatry 2000;61:409–413. **(IIb, B)**

126. Gunston KD: Premenstrual syndrome in Cape Town. 2. A double-blind placebo-controlled study of the efficacy of mefenamic acid. S Afr Med J 1986;70:159–160. **(Ib, A)**

127. Jakubowicz DL, Godard E, Dewhurst J: The treatment of pre-menstrual tension with mefenamic acid: analysis of prostaglandin concentrations. Br J Obstet Gynaecol 1984;91:78–84. **(IIa, B)**

128. Rees MCP, Randle J, Yudkin P: Mefenamic acid and the premenstrual syndrome. J Obstet Gynaecol 1991;11:359–360. **(IIa, B)**

129. Wood C, Jakubowicz D: The treatment of premenstrual symptoms with mefenamic acid. Br J Obstet Gynaecol 1980;87:627–630. **(IIa, B)**

130. Mira M, McNeil D, Fraser IS, et al: Mefenamic acid in the treatment of premenstrual syndrome. Obstet Gynecol 1986;68:395–398. **(IIa, B)**

131. Facchinetti F, Fioroni L, Sances G, et al: Naproxen sodium in the treatment of premenstrual symptoms: a placebo-controlled study. Gynecol Obstet Invest 1989;28:205–208. **(Ib, A)**

132. Burnet RB, Radden HS, Easterbrook EG, et al: Premenstrual syndrome and spironolactone. Aust N Z J Obstet Gynaecol 1991;31:366–368. **(Ib, A)**

133. Hellberg D, Claesson B, Nilsson S: Premenstrual tension: a placebo-controlled efficacy study with spironolactone and medroxyprogesterone acetate. Int J Gynaecol Obstet 1991;34:243–248. **(Ib, A)**

134. O'Brien PM, Craven D, Selby C, et al: Treatment of premenstrual syndrome by spironolactone. Br J Obstet Gynaecol 1979;86:142–147. **(Ib, A)**

135. Vellacott ID, Schroff NE, Pearce MH, et al: A double-blind, placebo-controlled evaluation of spironolactone in the premenstrual syndrome. Curr Med Res Opin 1987;10:450–456. **(Ib, A)**

136. Wang M, Hammarback S, Lindhe BA, et al: Treatment of premenstrual syndrome by spironolactone: a double-blind placebo controlled study. Acta Obstet Gynecol Scand 1995;74:803–808. **(Ib, A)**

# Chapter 3

## Geriatric Gynecology

### Rudi Ansbacher, MD, MS

**KEY POINTS**

- The physiologic condition of the woman is more important than her chronologic age.
- Listening to what is said by the patient helps derive the maximum benefit for her.
- The periodic assessment guidelines in Table 3-1 are essential in evaluating women 65 years of age and older.

The word *geriatric* is derived from Greek words *geras* meaning old age and *iatrike* meaning surgery or medicine. Thus, it pertains to the aged or their characteristic afflictions. Gerontology is the study of normal aging, whereas geriatrics is the medical study of the physiology and pathology of old age. Geriatric gynecology includes preventive care for and diagnosis and treatment of illnesses and disabilities in older women. Interest in this medical field intensified after World War II. The first issue of the journal *Geriatrics* appeared in 1945.

Stenchever[1] coined the word *gynogeriatrics* in a 1997 editorial focusing on health maintenance by paying attention to screening for acute and chronic illnesses in women over the age of 65. No one to date has identified a specific age when this period of life begins. Many use the age of 65, since this is the eligible age for Medicare, Social Security payments often begin, and retirement may occur. However, the age of 65 is arbitrary because the genetic background of an individual is more important in determining the impact of disease processes with aging than is a specific age limit.

The Committee on Gynecologic Practice of the American College of Obstetricians and Gynecologists (ACOG) outlined what should be emphasized as part of the periodic assessment of women over 65 years of age,[2] as modified in Table 3-1. This is an excellent guide to what should be covered and accomplished during a patient's initial and follow-up visits. There is a mixture of primary and specialty care, which typifies how a gynecologist should practice the specialty in an office setting.

## DEMOGRAPHICS

At present, the expected life span for a woman is around 80 years, almost double what it was at the beginning of the 20th century. Whether the increase occurred owing to genetic predisposition or better nutrition and environmental conditions, or to a combination of these and other factors, is undetermined. The population of developed countries such as the United States is graying. The physician must become familiar with the aging process in order to provide good health care for those rapidly gaining entrance to the geriatric population. By the year 2050 it is estimated that 25% of the U.S. population will be over age 65.

## PHYSIOLOGY OF AGING

A person's physiologic condition is more important than chronologic age because the former monitors how the body reacts to both internal and external stimuli. Most older persons maintain adequate though diminished reserves. As a person ages, there is a generalized functional decline with subsequent physiologic changes. These affect multiple organ systems and may result in a decreased response to inflammatory diseases, probably owing to lowered immune response, diminished neuroendocrine response to stimuli, and inability to maintain homeostasis.

Visual impairments are frequently encountered as a result of loss of visual acuity secondary to conditions such as cataract, diabetic retinopathy, glaucoma, macular degeneration, and retinal degeneration. Hearing impairment is due to diminished ability to discriminate frequency changes and to delays in the processing of auditory messages.

The cardiovascular system loses the elasticity of its blood vessels secondary to intimal thickening, and hypertrophy of smooth muscle cells occur, leading to decreased blood flow to the heart, gastrointestinal tract, kidneys, liver, and brain. There is an increase in the systolic component of the blood pressure, whereas the diastolic component remains the same or slightly decreases. Orthostatic hypotension is more common and can result in syncope and falls.

The respiratory system experiences a loss of lung elasticity resulting in a decrease in vital capacity and expiratory rates. The cough reflex is less vigorous, which may lead to a decrease in the evacuation of mucous secretions. As a result, older individuals are more susceptible to pulmonary infections such as pneumonia and influenza, thus the emphasis on annual influenza vaccination and the one-time administration of pneumococcal vaccine after age 65. According to the University of Michigan Immunization Clinic, the latter should be repeated after 5 years if the patient develops a chronic illness or debilitating disease.

The gastrointestinal tract loses motility. Dentition and mastication decrease, hepatic clearance is diminished, and the coordination required in swallowing is reduced. Therefore, there is less absorption of nutrients. Constipation may result, especially when activity is curtailed or in conjunction with poor nutritional habits. Fecal incontinence also can occur and causes much embarrassment.

The renal/urinary system is characterized by a decrease in kidney mass, loss of nephrons, and a decrease in creatinine clearance although creatinine levels remain in the normal range. The

## Ambulatory Office Practice

### Table 3-1
### Periodic Assessment for Women Aged 65 Years and Older

**History**

Reason for visit
Health status
   Medical
   Surgical
   Family
Dietary/nutritional assessment
Physical activity
Prescribed medications
Use of complementary and alternative medications
Use of tobacco, alcohol, street drugs
Abuse/neglect
Sexual practices
Urinary and fecal incontinence

**Physical examination**

Height
Weight
Blood pressure
Oral cavity
Neck: lymph nodes, thyroid
Breasts
Axillae
Abdomen
Pelvic and rectal examination
Extremities
Skin

**Annually assess**

Cardiovascular risk factors
Fitness and nutrition
Health risk behaviors
Psychosocial interactions
Sexuality

**Laboratory testing**

Pap smear
Mammography
Complete blood count
Urinalysis
Cardiac (lipid) profile every 5 years
Fasting blood glucose every 3 years
Thyroid screen after age 55
Fecal occult blood yearly
Flexible sigmoidoscopy every 5 years or colonoscopy every 10 years
Bone mineral density of spine and hip

**Immunizations**

Tetanus-diphtheria booster every 10 years
Influenza vaccine yearly
Pneumococcal vaccine

From Committee on Gynecologic Practice of the American College of Obstetricians and Gynecologists: Committee Opinion, No. 292, Nov 2003.

### Table 3-2
### Types of Urinary Incontinence

Stress
Urge
Overflow
Functional
Mixed
Transient (temporary, due to infection or medication)

by holding hands, caressing, and kissing or the intimacy of intercourse.

The musculoskeletal system is characterized by a loss in muscle mass, osteoarthritis, osteopenia, and osteoporosis. Lean body mass decreases and total body fat increases.

Counseling should include discussions about appropriate exercise, adequate nutrition, and supplements such as calcium and vitamin D when indicated, the latter being especially necessary in areas with inadequate sunshine or for women in nursing homes unable to partake in outdoor activities.

Central nervous system changes are highlighted by a decrease in memory, cognition, and attention deficits. Anxiety, confusion, and depression are not uncommon and may lead to aggression, fearfulness, overcompliance, or withdrawal. Changes in affect and cognition, decreased involvement in the basic activities of everyday living, gait disorders or a tendency to fall, and a lessened desire to partake in activities that require the use of instruments occur as one ages.

The endocrine system is characterized by diminished thyroid function and a slight increase in fasting glucose levels. The former should be evaluated yearly.

Healing takes longer because of physiologic changes that decrease the body's response to injury. Aging skin is result of both intrinsic (time elapsed) and extrinsic (sun, smoking, deficient nutrition) factors, which lead to declining epidermal cell repair. The accompanying loss of elastin and collagen in the dermis leads to laxity of the overlying epidermis, wrinkling, and eventually to dermatitis and skin breakdown even with minor trauma.

The main causes of morbidity in women over 65 years of age are listed in Table 3-3.[2]

The leading causes of mortality in women over 65 years of age are given in Table 3-4.[2]

### Table 3-3
### Leading Causes of Morbidity in Women Greater Than 65 Years of Age

| | |
|---|---|
| Arthritis | Hypertension |
| Back symptoms | Hypothyroidism |
| Breast cancer | Influenza |
| Chronic obstructive pulmonary disease | Respiratory infections |
| Cardiovascular diseases | Osteoporosis |
| Deformity or orthopedic impairments | Skin lesions |
| Macular degeneration | Urinary incontinence |
| Diabetes | Urinary tract infections |
| Hearing and visual impairments | Vertigo |

From Committee on Gynecologic Practice of the American College of Obstetricians and Gynecologists: Committee Opinion, No. 292, Nov 2003.

bladder capacity is diminished and urinary frequency is a common sequela. The intake of cranberry juice will reverse diminished urine acidity. Calcium absorption is decreased as is vitamin D hydroxylation. The various forms of incontinence are listed in Table 3-2 and discussed in urogynecology sections of this book.

The pelvic floor is prone to relaxation, which may result in uterine prolapse, cystocele, rectocele, and enterocele. The production of moisture by the mucosal lining of the vagina is enhanced by coital activity. Sexual function may decrease, but most women with a partner still enjoy the closeness provided

**Table 3-4**
**Leading Causes of Mortality in Women Greater Than 65 Years of Age***

Heart diseases
Cancer
Cerebrovascular diseases
Chronic obstructive pulmonary diseases
Pneumonia and influenza
Diabetes mellitus
Accidents
Alzheimer's disease

*Listed by most to least frequent.
From Committee on Gynecologic Practice of the American College of Obstetricians and Gynecologists: Committee Opinion, No. 292, Nov 2003.

## COMMUNICATION

To establish rapport, the physician has to develop both verbal and nonverbal communication skills. The physician must become a good listener to derive the most benefit from talking with patients. To do so requires a quiet, neutral setting. It is preferable to be face to face, without anything in between. Sitting behind a desk implies a superior attitude or authority. The discourse should remain focused and the time spent uninterrupted in order to maximize attention. An unemotional, undemonstrative, neutral attitude enhances the stature of the listener, exhibits support, and creates the trust needed to proceed with medical interventions when indicated. Remember that a person cannot learn anything while talking!

Seventy-six percent of a diagnosis comes from a properly taken history (listen to what the patient tells you and watch her body language), 12% from an appropriately performed physical examination (physical diagnosis is an extremely important component in the evaluation of a patient), and 12% from laboratory or ancillary studies.[3]

## HISTORY

The physician must be diligent in assessing the patient's current and past medical and surgical history. The review of systems should be specific, with directed questions such as "do you have diabetes?" The importance of the family history cannot be overemphasized. As the author has often stated, "you have to pick the right parents," meaning that much of what happens to a person is genetically determined. This aspect will be better clarified when personal genomes have been determined.

The nutritional status of the individual must be determined, as well as what may be needed to round out a person's diet. Nutritional requirements are not met by those who partake of only one meal a day. The best source of nutrients still is food, although supplements may be needed.

Daily activities and exercise should be explored and the latter encouraged when indicated. Medications the person is taking should be documented, side effects discussed, and interactions with proposed additional drugs evaluated. Micromedix Healthcare Services on the Internet and The United States Pharmacopeial *Drug Information for the Health Care Professional* are good resources for such information. The physician should also ask

about the use of tobacco, alcohol, and over-the-counter or street drugs in order to help stop their intake.

The possibility of domestic and elderly violence or abuse should be evaluated. Abandonment, financial exploitation, and neglect are frequently encountered, especially in women who are living alone. Emotional, physical, and sexual abuse must be addressed during history taking.

Malnutrition, dehydration, hypothermia, hyperthermia, decubitus ulcers, general health deterioration, lack of hygiene, and misuse of medications are all problems that may be encountered.

## PHYSICAL EXAMINATION

The height, weight, and blood pressure should be recorded yearly. The first indication of loss of bone mass, osteopenia, and eventually osteoporosis is decreased height. Have a height scale chart attached to a wall in your office or clinic so that actual height can be determined. The height measurements attached to weight scales are inaccurate. A thorough physical examination should be performed and recorded and is essential to the primary care evaluation of the patient.

## LABORATORY TESTING

The guidelines listed in Table 3-1 should be followed, with a Papanicolaou (Pap) smear and mammography performed on a yearly basis, although some suggest that this may not be necessary. In late 2003, a 65-year-old in a monogamous relationship for 25 years, with 15 consecutive years of negative Pap smears, had a report of a low-grade intraepithelial lesion (LGSIL) and subsequent human papillomavirus (HPV) testing positive for types 16, 18, and others (high risk). Because the sixth is the second most common decade in which to find abnormal Pap smears and cervical lesions, since 25% of cervical cancer occurs after age 65,[4] and because of the preceding case, the author still performs yearly Pap smears until age 75.

A cervical Pap smear may be reported as abnormal or with too few cells to evaluate if there is estrogen deficiency. Type-specific HPV testing enables the clinician to properly triage patients with abnormal Pap smears for further evaluation.

A woman should still perform breast self-examination if culturally acceptable. The advice to not do so is based on the lack of finding a benefit in a randomized controlled trial performed in China. Whether this finding is applicable to white and African American women in the United States, where there is a higher incidence of breast cancer than in Asia, is unclear. Mammography may be performed 6 months after the woman's office visit and breast examination, thereby giving her two breast evaluations per year, 6 months apart.

## IMMUNIZATIONS

In addition to one-time immunization with the pneumococcal vaccine, the yearly need for the influenza vaccine, and the tetanus-diphtheria booster every 10 years, patients who frequently travel are encouraged to receive hepatitis A (two doses) and hepatitis B (three doses). The hepatitis A infections that occurred in November 2003 in more than 500 people eating tainted green onions from Mexico emphasizes the need for protection secondary to consumption of imported foods.

## FREQUENTLY ENCOUNTERED CONDITIONS

### Estrogen Deficiency

Hot flashes (hot flushes) are one of the symptoms of estrogen deficiency. The etiology of hot flashes is undetermined. Many women who were placed on hormonal therapy to relieve this symptom and discontinued it as a result of reports from the Women's Health Initiative had recurrences and needed to be re-placed on estrogen therapy. The oldest woman reporting such problems in the author's practice was 73. The use of alternative and complementary medicines such as herbal products, phytoestrogens, and soy, to date in the majority of randomized controlled trials, have not been more effective than placebos in relieving hot flashes, and no long-term data support their use to prevent osteoporosis.[5]

After menopause, estrogen deficiency can be a frequent cause of discomfort with intercourse. The epidermis of the vulva thins, making the labial folds less prominent. Elastic fibers decrease, and hair thins. There is a loss of elasticity in the rugal folds of the vagina, which can appear shiny or slightly reddened. The vaginal pH rises from below 4.5 to above 6.5, and the rate of production and volume of vaginal fluid is reduced. Döderlein bacilli are diminished. The genital tissues become atrophic, and fissures or ulcerations can occur. Symptoms of genital atrophy include the feeling of burning, dryness, irritation, soreness, and tightness. Dyspareunia, especially on insertion of the penis or with deep thrusting, and postcoital spotting can occur.

Local therapy with estrogen creams (e.g., Premarin or Estrace vaginal creams) or estrogen vaginal rings (Estring), releasing estrogen in a measured amount daily, are effective in restoring tissues to a premenopausal state. Advise the patient to use estrogen cream after intercourse to decrease absorption of estrogen by the skin or genitalia of her partner. Vaginal lubricants such as Astroglide, Gyne-Moistrin, K-Y Jelly, Lubrin, Moist Again, Replens, Surgilube, Today Personal Lubricant, and Vagisil counteract vaginal dryness and thereby reduce the incidence of dyspareunia. Some women prefer to use virgin olive oil.

Androgen supplementation for women as they age is still controversial, mainly because of lack of data derived in a scientific fashion to prove its efficacy in enhancing sexual responsiveness. It has long been thought that androgen supplementation in a woman enhances her feelings of well being. The need for libido-enhancing medications for women is important because such items are supplied to their male partners.

The use of DHEA, DHEAS, and melatonin have not been proved to be beneficial.

Selective estrogen receptor modulators (SERMs) are being developed and most likely will replace many items in current use for hormone therapy in postmenopausal women.

The future preferred avenue for hormonal therapy will be through the vagina. The use of the tampon has desensitized women to the use of medications intravaginally.

### Vaginitis

Women with symptomatic vaginal discharge are frequently seen by their health care providers. Atrophic vaginitis is characterized by a watery discharge, as opposed to the characteristic malodorous white-to-yellow discharge of bacterial vaginosis, the white cottage cheese–like discharge of candidal infections, and the yellow-to-green frothy discharge of trichomoniasis. The last is rarely seen in postmenopausal women. Candidal infections should alert the health care provider to the patient's use of antibiotic or immunosuppressive agents, or the presence of diabetes or human immunodeficiency virus (HIV).

The vaginal pH should be checked in patients complaining of vaginal discharge. The proper area to obtain the pH is the upper lateral third of the vagina. Microscopic examination of the secretions should be performed with both saline and potassium hydroxide. This helps distinguish among the various forms of vaginitides encountered.

Atrophic vaginitis results from the lack of estrogen or is secondary to the intake of antiestrogenic medications. Symptoms may include vaginal discomfort and dyspareunia. The epithelium is thin and friable and may bleed after minimal trauma (e.g., intercourse or vaginal or speculum examination). Small epithelial tears, erosions, or ulcers may be noted. Concomitant capillary fragility results in punctuate hemorrhages or hemosiderin deposits. Cell maturation from parabasal to superficial cells does not occur. On microscopic examination, numerous white blood cells are noted in the thin watery discharge, making Pap smear evaluation difficult to interpret. Vaginal estrogen cream will thicken the epithelium, and the maturation of parabasal to intermediate and subsequently to superficial squamous cells will recur. Occasionally a woman on adequate exogenous estrogen therapy, given either orally or transdermally, will still have atrophic vaginal epithelium.

Proper perineal hygiene should be emphasized, including wiping from front to back to exclude rectal organisms from the vulva and vagina, wearing 100% cotton underwear, and discontinuing the use of abrasive soaps or laundry detergents, scented vaginal products, and occlusive sleepwear, which keeps the vulvar area moist at night.

### Vulvar Conditions

Lichen sclerosus is the next most frequently encountered vulvar condition after atrophy and is typified by whitening of the epidermis. Microscopically, a thin keratin layer, loss of the rete pegs, and thinning of the dermal layer are noted, although hyperkeratosis may be present secondary to scratching. Various treatment regimens are utilized for vulvar lichen sclerosus.

Generally, a class 1 topical corticosteroid ointment such as clobetasol propionate 0.05% twice a day for 1 month, then once a day for 2 months, is prescribed. This may be followed by the daily application of a less potent corticosteroid such as 0.1% triamcinolone acetonide ointment (a class 4 topical corticosteroid) with a gradual reduction in strength and frequency. Some health care providers prefer to prescribe a class 1 corticosteroid on an as-needed basis after the first 3 months of use.

There should be increased surveillance for vulvar carcinoma (Fig. 3-1). Any lesion that appears thickened, with ulcerations or increased punctation and vessel ingrowth, irregular borders, and increased pigmentation should be sampled by biopsy to rule out vulvar intraepithelial neoplasia, invasive squamous cell carcinoma, melanoma, and Paget's disease.

Sixty-five percent of vulvar cancers occur in the elderly.[6] Brown spots (lentigines) must not be confused with melanomas,

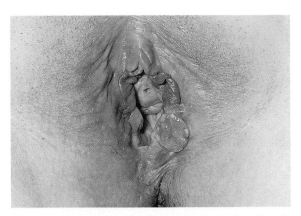

**Figure 3-1   Small carcinoma of the left vulva that is less than 2 cm in size.** (From DiSaia PJ, Creasman WT: Clinical Gynecologic Oncology, 6th ed. St. Louis, Mosby, 2002, color plate 8-1.)

and if the distinction is unclear, a biopsy specimen with adequate margins should be studied. Other suspicious skin lesions should be excised under local analgesia.

A woman may become more susceptible to recurrence of herpes virus and HPV infections or to HIV because of the decrease in responsiveness of her immune system.

### Urinary Tract Conditions
A urinary tract infection is due to bacterial invasion of the urothelium. It presents with the classic symptoms of frequency, urgency, and dysuria, associated with microscopic evidence of pyuria and bacteriuria. A clean-catch urine culture aids in determining the antimicrobial agent with the best sensitivity to eradicate the offending organism. Elderly women are more susceptible to urinary tract infections; if left untreated, they may be a source of bacteremia. For those with recurrent cystitis, emphasis should be placed on proper perineal hygiene, as previously discussed.

Fever and flank pain are suggestive of a kidney infection (i.e., pyelonephritis). Hematuria is associated with some urinary tract infections but is more likely present with kidney or ureteral stones.

Urethritis is rare. A history of dribbling may signal a urethral diverticulum. A caruncle is an eversion of the urethral mucosa at the orifice of the urethra. It is a frequent finding in elderly women and requires no therapy.

### Other Conditions
Urinary and rectal incontinence are frequently encountered, and to a lesser extent cystocele, rectocele, and enterocele. The reader is referred to the chapters on urogynecology for discussions of pelvic floor support, alterations in urinary bladder and rectal functions, and appropriate therapies. However, surgery can be obviated in some estrogen-deficient patients by the use of vaginal estrogen plus Kegel exercises. Women who are not candidates for surgery, usually because of the anesthetic risk in associated chronic medical conditions, can be fitted with an appropriate pessary. For further information on indications for use, types available, and complications of pessaries, please refer to the article by Bash.[7]

The woman's views concerning sexual matters should be explored. Reticence to do so usually implies that the medical caregiver is uncomfortable discussing sex despite the importance of this subject to many women as they age. Moreover, male libido-enhancing agents have stimulated greater demands on the older woman by her male partner. There is an urgent need to develop a corresponding female libido-enhancing agent.

## CONCOMITANT CONDITIONS

Osteoporosis is covered in Chapter 1.

Cancer is worrisome to many women in their waning years. Therefore, appropriate screening (see Table 3-1) should be undertaken for the more common cancers (breast, colon, and genital tract, which includes the cervix, endometrium, ovaries, vagina, and vulva).

Cardiovascular changes occur with aging, and the signs of impending myocardial infarction in a woman are more subtle than those in men. Therefore, evaluation of cardiac status by an internist is often indicated. Death due to heart disease leads all other causes of death in women by tenfold.

Sinusitis and upper respiratory conditions are not infrequent complaints, especially during the winter months, and should be treated accordingly.

Lung cancer in present or past smokers must be sought for those with a chronic cough.

Gastrointestinal complaints can be evaluated. Indigestion and abdominal discomfort are common, and these symptoms must be evaluated to rule out a cardiac condition or pneumonia.

Gait disturbances, incontinence of urine, malnutrition, osteoporosis, and sleep disturbances often generate an office visit. Since seniors are more sensitive to medications for pain and sleep, the minimal effective dose to obtain the desired result should be prescribed.

Persistent adenopathy, fever, night sweats, and weight loss should alert the physician to the possibility of lymphoma or leukemia.

Changes in mentation, including delirium, dementia, and depression, must be recognized. Often, these conditions are secondary to malnutrition or substance abuse and are associated with gait disturbances.

## OFFICE PROCEDURES

The physical examination can be augmented by in-office procedures including, when indicated, colposcopy; endocervical curettage; cervical, endometrial, vaginal, and vulvar biopsy; and transvaginal ultrasound. Office transvaginal ultrasound is complementary to the pelvic and rectal examinations. Transvaginal ultrasounds allow visualization of endometrial stripes and masses felt, such as leiomyomata and ovarian enlargement. Rarely does an endometrial stripe of 5 mm or less indicate intrauterine disease. Office sonohysterograms help determine uterine intracavitary polyps and leiomyomata. It is important to remember that tamoxifen therapy can induce hyperplasia of the endometrium and endometrial polyps.[8]

Any woman exhibiting postmenopausal bleeding must undergo appropriate evaluation including endometrial sampling. Forty-five percent of endometrial cancers occur in the elderly.[7]

Abdominal discomfort may occur secondary to hematometra or hydrometra, secondary to cervical stenosis, and although rare, tubal carcinoma must also be ruled out if there is fluid discharge. If needed, paracervical block and subsequent dilation of the cervical canal can be performed to enhance outpatient endometrial biopsy, and the use of a nonsteroidal analgesic 1 hour prior to the procedure helps diminish the cramping associated with the procedure.

Transvaginal ultrasound is helpful in the evaluation of adnexal masses. Forty-three percent of epithelial ovarian carcinomas occur in the elderly.[7] The majority of unilocular ovarian cysts having a diameter of less than 5 cm in postmenopausal women are benign. Expectant management can be advised if there is no increase in the ovarian cyst diameter and the serum CA 125 concentration remains normal.[9] Persistent adnexal masses greater than 5 cm should be evaluated surgically.

Nipple discharge should be sampled for cytologic screening. Breast aspiration can be performed in the office after proper training, or women requiring this procedure can be referred to a breast care specialist.

## ADDITIONAL PREVENTIVE CARE

Senior citizens are more sensitive to medications, especially those for pain and sleep. The minimal effective dose to obtain the desired result should be prescribed.

Adverse drug reactions are not infrequent in those taking multiple medications, and the central nervous system and gastrointestinal tract manifestations are listed in Table 3-5.[10] The physician should review all the medications that a woman is taking and ensure that she knows the proper dosage for each. Drug interactions can be identified, and she can be informed of possible side effects.

The functional status should be ascertained (i.e., activities of daily living). These include the ability to bathe, dress, prepare meals, eat, take medicine, ambulate, urinate, and defecate. A review of systems, physical assessment, support systems, and vaccination history should all be evaluated. Pertinent laboratory and radiologic imaging studies are ordered as needed.

Advanced directives, available systems of care, living wills, and end-of-life care needs should be discussed well in advance of the development of adverse conditions and are explained by Finnerty and colleagues for the primary care obstetrician/gynecologist.[11]

All women over the age of 65 should have access to comprehensive and, at times, multidisciplinary geriatric care. Therefore, the physician needs to be aware of the social and community resources available for caring for the aging woman.

Clinical experience will help the physician make decisions. Every patient is different, and each may respond differently to a particular therapy.

Know your limitations. Make referrals to those who have more experience with medical conditions that you are uncomfortable evaluating and treating. This is particularly important for gynecologists as the attempt is under way to define and integrate primary care and specialist activities.

---

**Table 3-5**
**Adverse Drug Events**

| Central Nervous System | | Gastrointestinal Tract | |
|---|---|---|---|
| *Symptom* | *Possible Cause* | *Symptom* | *Possible Cause* |
| Confusion | Narcotics | Anorexia | Antidepressants |
| Drowsiness | Antidepressants | Constipation | Narcotics |
| Restlessness | Theophylline | Diarrhea | Antibiotics |
| Nausea | Various medications | | |

From Nardo LG, Kroon ND, Reginald PW: Persistent unilocular ovarian cysts in a general population of post menopausal women: is there a place for expectant management? Obstet Gynecol 2003;102:589–593.

---

## REFERENCES

1. Stenchever MA: Gynogeriatrics: a challenge for the 21st century (editorial). Obstet Gynecol 1997;90:632–633. **(IV, C)**
2. Committee on Gynecologic Practice of the American College of Obstetricians and Gynecologists: Committee Opinion, No. 292, Nov 2003;113. **(IV, C)**
3. Peterson MC, Holbrook JM, Von Hales D, et al: Contributions of the history, physical examination and laboratory investigation in making medical diagnoses. West J Med 1992;156:163–167. **(III, B)**
4. Fletcher A: Screening for cancer of the cervix in elderly women. Lancet 1990;335:97–99. **(III, B)**
5. Kang HJ, Ansbacher R, Hammoud MM: Use of alternative and complementary medicine in menopause. Int J Gynecol Obstet 2002;79:195–207. **(III, B)**
6. Lawton FG, Hacker NF: Surgery for invasive gynecologic cancer in the elderly female population. Obstet Gynecol 1990;76:287–289. **(III, B)**
7. Bash K: Review of vaginal pessaries. Obstet Gynecol Surv 2000;55:455–460. **(III, B)**
8. Ansbacher R, Advincula AP: Images in reproductive medicine: endometrial polyp secondary to tamoxifen therapy. Fertil Steril 2003;80:216–217. **(III, B)**
9. Nardo LG, Kroon ND, Reginald PW: Persistent unilocular ovarian cysts in a general population of post menopausal women: is there a place for expectant management? Obstet Gynecol 2003;102:589–593. **(III, B)**
10. Walley T, Scott AK: Prescribing in the elderly. Postgrad Med J 1995;71:466–471. **(III, B)**
11. Finnerty JF, Fuerst CW, Karns LB, et al: End-of-life discussions for the primary care obstetrician/gynecologist. Am J Obstet Gynecol 2002;187:296–301. **(IV, C)**

# Chronic Pelvic Pain

## Fred M. Howard, MS, MD

## EPIDEMIOLOGY

Chronic pelvic pain is a far more common affliction of women than is generally recognized. One study from the United Kingdom found a prevalence of 3.8% in women age 15 to 73. This was higher than the prevalence of migraine (2.1%) and was similar to that of asthma (3.7%) and back pain (4.1%).[1] Similarly a study in Seveso, Italy, found that 4% of all women had moderate to severe, noncyclic pelvic pain.[2] A U.S. study using telephone polling suggested a higher prevalence. It found that 15% of women reported pelvic pain, with a mean average pain score of 5 (on a 0 to 10 scale), and 4% had pain severe enough to cause them to miss work.[3] This study estimated that 9.2 million U.S. women suffer from chronic pelvic pain.

Chronic pelvic pain is the indication for 12% of all hysterectomies and more than 40% of gynecologic diagnostic laparoscopies. It is estimated that direct and indirect costs of chronic pelvic pain in the United States are over $2 billion per year.[3] At an individual level, chronic pelvic pain frequently leads to years of disability and suffering, with loss of employment, marital discord, and divorce, as well as numerous untoward and unsuccessful medical interventions. Clearly, pelvic pain is an important issue in the health care of women.

*Chronic pelvic pain* may be defined as nonmenstrual pain of 6 or more months' duration that localizes to the anatomic pelvis, anterior abdominal wall below the umbilicus, or the lumbosacral back and causes functional disability or requires medical or surgical treatment. This definition excludes vulvar pain and the cyclical pain of dysmenorrhea. These exclusions are somewhat arbitrary. In fact, women with chronic pelvic pain often have vulvar pain or dysmenorrhea as part of their symptom complex.

## RISK FACTORS

### Age
Women of all ages may experience chronic pelvic pain, but it tends to be more common in women of reproductive age. Otherwise, patient age does not appear to be a specific risk factor for chronic pelvic pain.

### Physical and Sexual Abuse
There is a significant association of physical and sexual abuse with various chronic pain disorders, including chronic pelvic pain. Of women with chronic pelvic pain, 40% to 60% have a history of abuse. Whether physical or sexual abuse specifically causes chronic pelvic pain is not clear.

### Pelvic Inflammatory Disease
It is estimated that 18% to 35% of all women with acute pelvic inflammatory disease (PID) develop chronic pelvic pain. The actual mechanisms by which chronic pelvic pain results from PID are not known, nor is it clear why some, but not all, women with reproductive organ damage secondary to acute PID develop chronic pelvic pain. Whether acute PID is treated with outpatient or inpatient regimens does not appear to significantly alter the odds of developing subsequent chronic pelvic pain (34% with outpatient therapy vs. 30% with inpatient therapy).[4]

### Endometriosis
Although endometriosis may be a direct cause of dysmenorrhea and chronic pelvic pain, it may also indirectly place women at increased risk of chronic pelvic pain. For example, human and animal experimental data show that women with dysmenorrhea or endometriosis have increased episodes and severity of pain related to urinary calculi than women without dysmenorrhea or endometriosis. Similar results have been experimentally demonstrated for vaginal pain, as well. Such viscerovisceral interactions may have a significant role in chronic pelvic pain in women and may explain why some women with a past history of endometriosis have persistent pelvic pain after their endometriosis is gone.

### Obstetrical History
Pregnancy and childbirth may lead to chronic pelvic pain, possibly due to musculoskeletal trauma, particularly to the pelvis and back. Historical risk factors associated with pregnancy and pain include lumbar lordosis, delivery of a large infant, muscle weakness and poor physical conditioning, a difficult delivery,

vacuum or forceps delivery, and use of gynecologic stirrups for delivery. Conversely, women with a history of no pregnancies may have disorders that cause infertility and chronic pelvic pain, such as endometriosis, chronic PID, or pelvic adhesive disease.

### Past Surgery

A history of abdominopelvic surgery is associated with chronic pelvic pain. In some cases the relationship is relatively clear, such as unrecognized spillage of gallstones at the time of cholecystectomy, or osteitis pubis or osteomyelitis after a Marshall-Marchetti-Krantz procedure. Prior cervical surgery for dysplasia may cause cervical stenosis, and there is a reported high association of cervical stenosis and endometriosis. Additionally, in women without preoperative pelvic pain, 3% to 9% develop pelvic pain or back pain in the 2 years after hysterectomy.[5,6] A recent case-control study suggests that cesarean section may also be a risk factor for chronic pelvic pain (odds ratio [OR] = 3.7).[7]

## PATHOGENESIS

Pain is "an unpleasant sensory and emotional experience primarily associated with tissue damage or described in terms of such damage, or both."[8] Pain is defined in this way to make it clear that pain is a personal subjective experience, not an objective physiological event. No objective tests allow measurement, characterization, or confirmation of the patient's pain. Many patients report pain in the absence of tissue damage or any likely pathophysiological cause. If patients regard their experience as pain and report it in the same ways as pain caused by tissue damage, it should be accepted as pain. This definition of pain avoids tying pain to the stimulus.

Pain may be of central or peripheral origin (Table 4-1). Central pain may be due to psychogenic or neurogenic mechanisms. *Neurogenic* refers to pain caused by a primary lesion or lesions, or intrinsic dysfunction, in the central nervous system. Peripheral pain may be neurogenic or nociceptive. *Nociceptive pain* is caused by stimulation of nociceptors, neurons or neuroreceptors that

are sensitive to a noxious stimulus (Table 4-2). Both visceral and somatic structures have nerves that function as nociceptors. Neuropathic or neurogenic pain is caused by a primary lesion or dysfunction in the peripheral nervous system, meaning the nerve or nerves themselves are the pain generators. Such lesions or dysfunctions may be due to injury, disease, or localized insult or injury due to infection or surgery, for example.

In women with chronic pelvic pain, pain is thought usually to be of peripheral, not central, origin. Clinically, chronic pelvic pain is not commonly diagnosed as being primarily due to psychological or central neurologic disorders. Many visceral and somatic disorders are thought to cause or precipitate chronic pelvic pain (Table 4-3), but the mechanisms that cause these diseases to result in chronic pain are not well understood. Pain may become chronic because there is no known cure for the etiologic disease; for example, interstitial cystitis or irritable bowel syndrome (IBS). In other cases, it may be that the development of neurogenic pain is responsible or that pain becomes "centralized" and is maintained by central nervous system dysfunction.

Potential visceral sources of chronic pelvic pain include disorders of the reproductive, urinary, and gastrointestinal tracts. Potential somatic sources include the pelvic bones, ligaments, muscles, and fascia. Although it is helpful to the gynecologist to classify potential etiologies into gynecologic and nongynecologic causes, clearly knowledge and familiarity with all visceral and somatic diagnoses are crucial to the clinician evaluating and treating a woman with chronic pelvic pain.

Realistically, not many of the diseases thought to cause chronic pelvic pain fulfill traditional epidemiologic criteria of causality. Sufficient evidence strongly suggests that several of the most common disorders in women with chronic pelvic pain are causal, such as endometriosis, interstitial cystitis, and IBS (see Table 4-3). For many of the diseases often listed as causes of chronic pelvic pain, only limited evidence or expert opinion supports an etiologic relationship.

---

**Table 4-1**
**Classification of the Pathophysiologic Origins of Chronic Pain**

**Central**

Neurogenic
Psychogenic

**Peripheral**

Somatic
  Neuropathic
  Nociceptive
    Myofascial
    Skeletal
    Cutaneous
Visceral
  Neuropathic
  Nociceptive
    Gynecologic
    Urologic
    Gastrointestinal

---

**Table 4-2**
**General Classification of Noxious Stimuli That Can Cause Pain**

**Mechanical**

Crushing*
Cutting*
Distention of hollow viscus
Distention of capsule of solid viscus
Traction of mesentery of viscus

**Thermal**

Burning*
Cold*

**Chemical**

Hemorrhage
Infection
Inflammation
Neoplasm

*Do not appear to cause pain in viscera, only in somatic tissues.

---

**Table 4-3**
**Disorders Associated with Chronic Pelvic Pain in Women**

**Gynecologic disorders with causal relationship to chronic pelvic pain based on good and consistent scientific evidence**

Endometriosis
Gynecologic malignancies (especially late stage)
Ovarian retention syndrome (residual ovary syndrome)
Ovarian remnant syndrome
Pelvic congestion syndrome
Pelvic inflammatory disease
Tuberculous salpingitis

**Gynecologic disorders with causal relationship to chronic pelvic pain based on limited or inconsistent scientific evidence**

Adhesions
Benign cystic mesothelioma
Leiomyomata
Postoperative peritoneal cysts

**Gynecologic disorders with causal relationship to chronic pelvic pain based on expert opinions**

Adenomyosis
Atypical dysmenorrhea or ovulatory pain
Adnexal cysts (nonendometriotic)
Cervical stenosis
Chronic ectopic pregnancy
Chronic endometritis
Endometrial or cervical polyps
Endosalpingiosis
Intrauterine contraceptive system
Ovarian ovulatory pain
Residual accessory ovary
Symptomatic pelvic relaxation (genital prolapse)

**Nongynecologic disorders with causal relationship to chronic pelvic pain based on good and consistent scientific evidence**

Urologic
  Bladder malignancy
  Interstitial cystitis
  Radiation cystitis
  Urethral syndrome
Gastrointestinal
  Carcinoma of the colon
  Constipation
  Inflammatory bowel disease
  Irritable bowel syndrome
Musculoskeletal
  Abdominal wall myofascial pain (trigger points)
  Chronic coccygeal or back pain
  Faulty or poor posture
  Fibromyalgia
  Neuralgia of iliohypogastric, ilioinguinal, and/or genitofemoral nerves

  Pelvic floor myalgia (levator ani or piriformis syndrome)
  Peripartum pelvic pain syndrome
Other
  Abdominal cutaneous nerve entrapment in surgical scar
  Depression
  Somatization disorder

**Nongynecologic disorders with causal relationship to chronic pelvic pain based on limited or inconsistent scientific evidence**

Urologic
  Stone/urolithiasis
  Uninhibited bladder contractions (detrusor dyssynergia)
  Urethral diverticulum
Musculoskeletal
  Herniated nucleus pulposus
  Low back pain
  Neoplasia of spinal cord or sacral nerve
Other
  Celiac disease
  Neurologic dysfunction
  Porphyria
  Shingles
  Sleep disturbances

**Nongynecologic disorders with causal relationship to chronic pelvic pain based on expert opinions**

Urologic
  Chronic urinary tract infection
  Recurrent, acute cystitis
  Recurrent, acute urethritis
  Stone/urolithiasis
  Uninhibited bladder contractions (destrusor dyssynergia)
  Urethral caruncle
Gastrointestinal
  Colitis
  Chronic intermittent bowel obstruction
  Diverticular disease
Musculoskeletal
  Compression of lumbar vertebrae
  Degenerative joint disease
  Hernias: ventral, inguinal, femoral, Spigelian
  Muscular strains and sprains
  Rectus tendon strain
  Spondylosis
Other
  Abdominal epilepsy
  Abdominal migraine
  Bipolar personality disorders
  Familial Mediterranean fever

## CLINICAL FEATURES

More than 80% of women with chronic pelvic pain have had pain for longer than 1 year when they seek medical care, and about one third have had pain for longer than 5 years.[9] About one half of women with chronic pelvic pain have either urinary or gastrointestinal symptoms, or both, in addition to their pelvic pain. Reproductive tract symptoms are also common. For example, dysmenorrhea is present in more than 80% of women with chronic pelvic pain (in contrast to about 50% in the general population).

Dyspareunia is also more common in women with chronic pelvic pain, being present in at least 40% (in comparison to 10% to 15% in the general population). Most women with dyspareunia and chronic pelvic pain report the pain is deep and occurs both during and after intercourse. Dyspareunia is more severe and disabling in women with IBS and urinary symptoms, when compared to women with chronic pelvic pain and no gastrointestinal or urinary symptoms.

Women with nociceptive, somatic pain usually describe pain that is well localized to the area of disease. This is not always the case, however. For example, sometimes with levator ani pain the symptoms are described as deep, aching, heavy pain and the patient cannot accurately localize the pain to the pelvic floor muscles. With nociceptive, visceral pain there is almost always poor localization and usually a description of deep, dull, and cramping pain.

## DIAGNOSIS

Making an accurate diagnosis in the woman with chronic pelvic pain can be difficult. The number of potential diagnoses, the variety of anatomic sources of pain, the likelihood that the patient may have more than one diagnosis, and the potential that pain itself may need to be considered a diagnosis are only a few of the issues that make diagnostic evaluation challenging.

The history and physical examination are powerful diagnostic and therapeutic tools in chronic pelvic pain. As diagnostic tools, a thorough history and examination may lead to accurate diagnosis, minimizing the need for expensive laboratory or imaging testing or risky operative interventions. As therapeutic tools, a compassionately taken history, during which the patient talks and the physician listens, and a sensitively performed examination establish rapport and trust that the physician is caring and competent and allow the patient to leave the physician's office feeling better. Because the examination is often painful for the woman with chronic pelvic pain, it is important that the physician remember that even a "routine" pelvic examination is emotionally stressful for many patients with chronic pelvic pain.

The diversity of potential etiologic or associated diagnoses demands a multidisciplinary approach to diagnostic evaluation. Referrals to and consultations with other specialists may be needed. The history of the patient's pain must be thoroughly obtained, as must the review of systems, with particular attention to the gastrointestinal, reproductive, urologic, and musculoskeletal systems. Because of the complexity of the history in most patients, intake questionnaires are extremely helpful in obtaining details of the history (see, for example, www.pelvicpain.org). However, they should not replace allowing the patient to tell her story.

Establishing the location of the patient's pain can be crucial to accurate diagnosis. An ideal way to do this is to have the patient mark the location(s) of her pain on a pain map (Fig. 4-1). Pain maps frequently reveal that the patient has other areas of pain. For example, up to 60% of women with chronic pelvic pain also have headaches, and up to 90% have backaches. A pain map may show both ventral and dorsal pain, suggesting intrapelvic pathology, whereas one showing only dorsal lower back pain suggests an orthopedic or musculoskeletal origin. A pain map may show a dermatomal distribution of pain, suggesting a central neurologic source, or it may show a unilateral cutaneous distribution along the anterior lower abdominal wall into the labia or upper inner aspect of the thigh, suggesting neuropathic pain of the iliohypogastric or ilioinguinal nerves. A pain map may show a very diffuse distribution, consistent with visceral pain. Visceral pain is not as well localized as somatic or dermatomal pain, so patients with chronic pain and visceral pathology may have trouble localizing their pain. Furthermore, because the cervix, uterus, and adnexae have the same metameric innervation as the bladder, distal ureter, lower ileum, colon, and rectosigmoid, it is often difficult to determine if visceral abdominopelvic pain is of gynecologic, urologic, or intestinal origin.

The patient should also be questioned about radiation of pain. It is not uncommon for the lateral pain of adnexal origin to radiate down the anterior or anteromedial thigh. Pain of uterine or cervical origin, including dysmenorrhea, may also radiate down the anteromedial thigh. Radiation down the posterior thigh is often associated with musculoskeletal problems. Sciatica associated with lumbosacral disease is a classic example of this.

Asking about the severity of pain is less useful diagnostically in chronic pain than it is in acute pain. It is still important, because it is one of the major measures of response to any treatment. In clinical practice, a simple rating system of "no pain, mild pain, moderate pain, severe pain" is often used, but this is not very sensitive to changes in pain severity and may not be very useful in following patients' responses during treatment. For endometriosis-associated pain the American Fertility Society (now the Society for Reproductive Medicine, Birmingham, Ala.) has suggested rating pain as "mild," "discomforting," "distressing," "horrible," and "excruciating" (this is the same rating as that of the McGill Pain Questionnaire). Numerical scales may be more useful and reliable. The best-studied numerical scale is the visual analog scale, which uses a 10-cm line with descriptive labels of pain severity at the ends. The patient marks the line at the point that best represents the severity of her pain (Fig. 4-2). The distance in centimeters from the beginning of the line to the patient's mark is a measure of her pain severity. A numerical

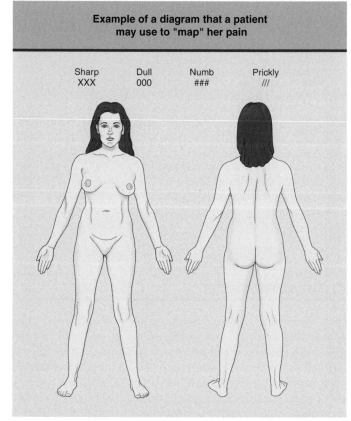

**Figure 4-1    Example of a diagram that a patient may use to "map" her pain.**

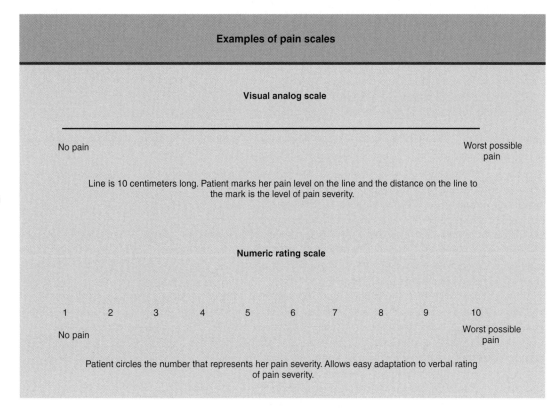

**Figure 4-2    Examples of pain scales.**

rating scale is a commonly used adaptation of the visual analog scale. This allows the patient to directly give a numerical rating to her pain and facilitates conversion to a verbal numerical rating system. Whatever pain severity scale is used, it is important to be consistent.

Exploring the nature of the onset of pain may aid in diagnosis. For example, an immediately antecedent trauma, such as a fall, surgery, or motor vehicle accident, suggests a musculoskeletal cause. Pain that started with a pregnancy or immediately post-partum may suggest peripartum pelvic pain syndrome. Pain that started at or soon after menarche as dysmenorrhea, progressed to premenstrual pain, and then became constant suggests endo-metriosis. If pain started soon after a physical or sexual assault, it may have significant musculoskeletal or psychological components.

Finding out if there is any temporal pattern to the pain may be helpful. Cyclicity related to menses suggests gynecologic pain, but is not pathognomonic of gynecologic disease. The same pattern may occur with pain of intestinal, urologic, or musculo-skeletal origin also. For example, symptoms of IBS or interstitial cystitis frequently increase premenstrually. A history of pain or increased pain with coitus is frequently present and may be due to a variety of disorders, including psychological disease, marital problems, endometriosis, vulvodynia, interstitial cystitis, and IBS. If intercourse is painful, it is important to find out if pain is with entry at the outermost part of the vagina or if it is with deeper penetration high in the vagina or pelvis, or both. Diseases associated with chronic pelvic pain do not generally cause entry dyspareunia, except as vaginismus secondary to deep dyspareunia.

The quality or nature of pain should be sought, because such descriptors may have diagnostic value. The McGill Pain Questionnaire short form (Table 4-4) is helpful in assessing the quality of pain. For example, neuropathic pain is often described as burning or sharp and piercing, with an electric shock-like quality. Muscular pain may be aching in quality, with sharp, lancinating pain with changes in position. Similar qualities of aching with occasional intermittent sharp and radiating pains may also be described with visceral pain.

**Table 4-4**
**McGill Pain Questionnaire Short Form**

| Type of Pain | What does your pain feel like? | | | |
|---|---|---|---|---|
| | None (0) | Mild (1) | Moderate (2) | Severe (3) |
| Throbbing | _____ | _____ | _____ | _____ |
| Shooting | _____ | _____ | _____ | _____ |
| Stabbing | _____ | _____ | _____ | _____ |
| Sharp | _____ | _____ | _____ | _____ |
| Cramping | _____ | _____ | _____ | _____ |
| Gnawing | _____ | _____ | _____ | _____ |
| Hot–Burning | _____ | _____ | _____ | _____ |
| Aching | _____ | _____ | _____ | _____ |
| Heavy | _____ | _____ | _____ | _____ |
| Tender | _____ | _____ | _____ | _____ |
| Splitting | _____ | _____ | _____ | _____ |
| Tiring–Exhausting | _____ | _____ | _____ | _____ |
| Sickening | _____ | _____ | _____ | _____ |
| Fearful | _____ | _____ | _____ | _____ |
| Punishing–Cruel | _____ | _____ | _____ | _____ |

# Ambulatory Office Practice

Finding out about any prior treatments for chronic pelvic pain and the response to those treatments is a crucial part of the history. It may be important to know about any prior surgery, not just surgical treatment for pain, because pain may be a risk factor for or cause of chronic pelvic pain.

Ideally a thorough psychosocial history should be obtained on every patient with chronic pelvic pain. An extensive evaluation by a psychologist or similarly educated professional cannot always be done—nor is it always necessary. However, a basic psychosocial history is always important, especially asking about depression. Depression is one of several predictors of pain severity in women with chronic pelvic pain, and it is also a significant indicator of responsiveness to treatment. Using a screening tool such as the Zung or Beck depression inventories or HANDS questionnaire is helpful. Asking about abuse is another important part of the psychosocial history. There is a significant association between physical and sexual abuse and the development of chronic pelvic pain.

The physical examination should seek to find the exact anatomic locations of any areas of tenderness and, as much as possible, correlate these with areas of pain. This type of "pain mapping" examination requires a systematic and methodical attempt to duplicate the patient's pain by palpation, positioning, or bodily movement. At any tender areas or painful positions, the patient should be asked whether the pain produced is the same as her chronic pain. The examination should evaluate the musculoskeletal, gastrointestinal, urinary, and neurological systems, not just the reproductive tract. It facilitates the examination to divide it into standing, sitting, supine, and lithotomy components. Tables 4-5 to 4-8 summarize some of the evaluations that may be helpful, as well as some of the potential diagnoses that may be suggested.

One of the aspects of the pain mapping examination that differs from the traditional examination is the use of single-digit palpation of the back, abdomen, and pelvis. The single-digit examination is particularly useful when looking for myofascial or trigger point pain. The abdominal wall tenderness test (Carnett's test) is also a useful technique in pain mapping and may be used to distinguish abdominal wall tenderness from visceral tenderness. In this test, while the area of abdominal tenderness is palpated, the patient voluntarily tenses the abdominal muscles, which is readily accomplished by having her raise her head or legs. If the pain is increased, it suggests that the pain is of abdominal wall origin. If the pain is decreased or unchanged, it suggests that the pain is most likely of visceral origin.

A single-digit examination, using only one hand, is also how the pelvic examination should be initiated. The introital bulbo-carvenosus and transverse perineal muscles, then the levator ani muscles, should be palpated for tone, spasm, and tenderness. In patients with pelvic floor pain this may cause pain consistent with at least part of the patient's clinical pain symptoms. Pelvic floor pain may also result from trigger points of one or more of the muscles of the pelvis. The piriformis, coccygeal, and internal obturator muscles should be thoroughly evaluated using single-digit examination. The piriformis muscles can be difficult to evaluate transvaginally, however. Rectal examination may allow an easier evaluation than vaginal examination. Transvaginally or transrectally the examining finger is pressed posterolaterally just superior to the ischial spine. In the lithotomy position, if the

patient is asked to abduct the thigh against resistance as the piriform muscle is palpated, the muscle may be more easily palpated, and there is exquisite tenderness of the muscle if there is spasm or tension myalgia involving the piriform muscle (piriformis syndrome).

The anterior vaginal, urethral, and trigonal areas should be palpated to elicit any areas of tenderness, induration, discharge, or thickening suggestive of chronic urethritis, chronic urethral syndrome, urethral diverticulum, vaginal wall cyst, trigonitis, or interstitial cystitis. With deeper palpation the cervix, paracervical areas, and vaginal fornices should be palpated with the single digit for tenderness or trigger points suggestive of problems such as repeated cervical trauma (usually from intercourse), pelvic infection, endometriosis, ureteral pain, or trigger points.

**Table 4-5**
**Components of the Standing Physical Examination of the Woman with Chronic Pelvic Pain**

| Standing Examination | Possible Problems |
|---|---|
| Gait | Short leg syndrome; herniated disk; general musculoskeletal problems |
| Posture with and without forward | Typical pelvic pain posture; scoliosis; one-leg standing |
| Standing on one leg with and without hip flexion | Laxity of the pubic symphysis; laxity of pelvic girdle; weakness of the hip and pelvis |
| Iliac crest symmetry | Short leg syndrome; one-leg standing |
| Groin evaluation with and without Valsalva maneuver | Inguinal hernia; femoral hernia |
| Pubic symphysis evaluation, including trigger points | Peripartum pelvic pain syndrome; trigger points; osteitis pubis; osteomyelitis pubis |
| Hip and sacroiliac evaluation, including trigger points | Arthritis of hip; trigger points |
| Buttocks (gluteus and piriformis) evaluation, including trigger points | Piriformis syndrome; pelvic floor pain syndrome; gluteal trigger points |
| Fibromyalgia tender point evaluation | Fibromyalgia |

**Table 4-6**
**Components of the Sitting Physical Examination of the Woman with Chronic Pelvic Pain**

| Sitting Examination | Possible Problems Diagnosed |
|---|---|
| Posture | Levator ani spasm; pelvic floor pain syndrome |
| Palpation of the upper and lower back | Trigger points; myalgia; arthritis |
| Palpation of sacrum | Trigger points; sacroiliitis |
| Palpation of gluteal and piriform muscles | Trigger points; myalgia |
| Palpation of the posterior superior iliac crests | Peripartum pelvic pain syndrome |
| Basic sensory testing to sharpness, dullness, and light touch | Herniated disk |
| Muscle strength testing and deep tendon | Herniated disk |

cotton-tipped swab also can elicit allodynia in a neural distribution in women with pudendal neuralgia. A cotton-tipped swab can be used to evaluate the cervical os and the paracervical and cervical tissues for tenderness. In posthysterectomy patients the full vaginal cuff should be similarly palpated for tenderness with a cotton-tipped swab.

The traditional visual, speculum, and bimanual examinations are still needed for a thorough evaluation, but they should usually follow the single-digit examination. The pain or tenderness

**Table 4-7**
**Components of the Supine Physical Examination of the Woman with Chronic Pelvic Pain**

| Supine Examination | Possible Problems Diagnosed |
| --- | --- |
| Active leg flexion, knee to chest | Low back dysfunction; low back pain; abdominal muscle weakness; deconditioning |
| Obturator and psoas sign testing | Shortening, dysfunction, or spasm of the obturator or iliopsoas muscles or fascia |
| Head raise and leg raise | Herniated disk; abdominal muscle weakness; deconditioning |
| Light abdominal palpation | Referred visceral pain; nerve entrapment; neuropathy |
| Gentle pinching | Referred visceral pain; nerve entrapment; neuropathy |
| Head's maneuver | Referred visceral pain; nerve entrapment; neuropathy |
| Dermographism evaluation | Referred visceral pain; nerve entrapment; neuropathy |
| Single-digit palpation | Trigger points; myofascial pain; hernias; nerve entrapments |
| Abdominal wall tenderness test | Abdominal wall pain; visceral pain |
| Groin and abdominal evaluation with and without Valsalva maneuver | Inguinal hernia; Spigelian hernia; epigastric hernia; diastasis recti |
| Incisional evaluation with and without Valsalva maneuver | Incisional hernia |
| Pubic symphysis evaluation | Trigger points; osteitis pubis; osteomyelitis pubis |
| Traditional abdominal examination for distention, masses, ascites, bowel sounds, shifting dullness, vascular bruits, deep tenderness, guarding, or rigidity | Acute disease |

The uterus usually can be adequately evaluated for tenderness by direct palpation with a single digit. Significant uterine tenderness may be consistent with diseases such as adenomyosis, pelvic congestion syndrome, pelvic infection sequelae, endometriosis, or premenstrual syndrome. A uterus that is immobile and fixed in position, especially a retroflexed one, may suggest endometriosis or adhesions. The coccyx should also be palpated with the single digit, and an attempt should be made to move it 30 degrees or less. This may be easier to evaluate during the rectovaginal examination. Normally the coccyx moves 30 degrees without eliciting pain, but in patients with coccydynia this movement elicits pain. The ureteral and the adnexal areas should be palpated next, still using a single digit without the use of the abdominal hand. All of the preceding evaluations are "monomanual-monodigital"—that is, only one finger of one hand is used. No abdominal palpation with the other hand is involved.

Examination with a moistened cotton-tipped swab may be more useful than the single-digit examination to evaluate the vulva and the vulvar vestibule for tenderness. This is particularly useful in patients with localized vulvodynia (vulvar vestibulitis), who have exquisite tenderness in localized areas at the minor vestibular glands just external to the hymen, with normal sensation in adjacent vulvar areas. Sometimes palpation with a

**Table 4-8**
**Components of the Lithotomy Physical Examination of the Woman with Chronic Pelvic Pain**

| Lithotomy Examination | Possible Problems Diagnosed |
| --- | --- |
| Visual inspection of the external genitalia | Inflammatory and infectious disease; vulvar abscess; trauma; fistula; ulcerative disease; pigmented lesions (neoplasias); condylomata; atrophic changes; fissure |
| Basic sensory testing to sharpness, dullness, and light touch | Nerve entrapment; neuropathy; spinal cord lesion |
| Cotton-tipped swab evaluation of the vestibule | Vulvar vestibulitis |
| Single-digit palpation of vulva and pubic arch | Trigger points |
| Colposcopic evaluation of the vulva and vestibule | Neoplasia |
| Sims retractor or single-blade speculum examination of vagina and pelvic muscles | Enterocele; cystocele; rectocele; uterine descensus |
| Cotton-tipped swab evaluation of cervical os, paracervical and cervical tissues | Trigger points |
| Cotton-tipped swab evaluation of vaginal cuff | Trigger points; neuroma |
| Single-digit pelvic examination of introitus | Vulvar vestibulitis; vaginismus; trigger points |
| Single-digit pelvic examination of levator ani | Pelvic floor pain syndrome, trigger points |
| Single-digit pelvic examination of coccygeus | Pelvic floor pain syndrome; trigger points |
| Single-digit pelvic examination of piriformis with and without abduction | Piriformis syndrome |
| Single-digit pelvic examination of anterior vaginal urethral and trigonal evaluation | Chronic urethral syndrome; urethritis; cystitis; interstitial cystitis; trigonitis; urethral diverticulum; vaginal wall cyst |
| Single-digit pelvic examination of cervix, paracervical areas, and vaginal fornices | Trigger points; endometriosis; cervicitis; repeated cervical trauma; pelvic infection; ureteral pain |
| Single-digit pelvic examination of uterus | Adenomyosis; pelvic congestion syndrome; pelvic infection; premenstrual syndrome; adhesions |
| Single-digit pelvic examination of coccyx | Coccydynia |
| Single-digit pelvic examination of adnexa | Pelvic congestion syndrome; endometriosis |
| Bimanual pelvic examination | See text |
| Rectovaginal examination | See text |

| Table 4-9 Diagnostic Tests Useful in the Evaluation of Women with Chronic Pelvic Pain | |
| --- | --- |
| Symptom, Finding, or Suspected Diagnosis | Potentially Useful Tests |
| Adenomyosis | Ultrasonography; hysterosalpingography, MRI |
| Chronic urethral syndrome | Urodynamic testing |
| Compression or entrapment neuropathy | Nerve conducting velocities; needle electromyographic studies |
| Constipation | Anorectal balloon manometry; colonic transit time |
| Diarrhea | Stool specimens for ova and parasites; stool polymorphonuclear leukocytes and red blood cells; stool cultures; stool for *C. difficile* toxin; stool guiaic testing; barium enema radiography; colonoscopy; upper gastrointestinal series with follow-through; CT |
| Diverticular disease | Barium enema radiograph |
| Dyspareunia | Urethral and cervical gonorrhea and chlamydia cultures; chlamydial PCR testing; vaginal cultures; urine cultures; vaginal wet preparations; vaginal pH |
| Endometriosis | Ca-125; ultrasonography; barium enema radiography; hysterosalpingography; CT; MRI |
| Hernias | Abdominal wall ultrasonography; CT; herniography |
| Interstitial cystitis | Cystourethroscopy; KCl bladder challenge test; urine culture; urine cytologies; urodynamic testing; bladder biopsy |
| Ovarian remnant syndrome | Follicle-stimulating hormone; estradiol; gonadotropin releasing hormone agonist stimulation test; ultrasonography ± clomiphene stimulation; barium enema radiography; CT |
| Ovarian retention syndrome | Ultrasonography; CT |
| Pelvic congestion syndrome | Pelvic venography; ultrasonography ± Doppler |
| Pelvic tuberculosis | Chest x-ray; PPD skin test |
| Porphyria | Urine porphobilinogen |
| Urethral diverticulum | Vaginal sonography; voiding cystourethrography; double balloon cystourethrography; MRI |

CT, computed tomography; KCl, potassium chloride; MRI, magnetic resonance imaging; PCR, polymerase chain reaction; PPD, purified protein derivative.

diagnostic laparoscopies are done for chronic pelvic pain. It is important to remember that a negative laparoscopy is not synonymous with no diagnosis or no disease and does not mean that a woman has no physical basis for her pain. Discriminative use of laparoscopy, carefully based on the patient's history, physical examination, laboratory, and imaging findings might decrease the rate of negative laparoscopies from 39% to 4%.

Diagnostic laparoscopy under local anesthesia, termed *conscious laparoscopic pain mapping* or *patient-assisted laparoscopy*, has been suggested as a way to improve the diagnostic capability of laparoscopy.[10,11] The stimulus used with conscious laparoscopic pain mapping is a gentle probing or tractioning of tissues, lesions, and organs with a blunt probe or forceps passed through a secondary trocar site. Diagnosis of an etiologic lesion or organ is based on the severity of pain elicited and on replication of the pain that is the patient's presenting symptom. Chronic pelvic pain, however, is a multifaceted and complicated problem, and it is not established that the findings with mechanically elicited pain at conscious pain mapping directly translate into cause and cure. Published data from an observational controlled study failed to show any improvement in outcome.[10]

## Irritable Bowel Syndrome

Irritable bowel syndrome appears to be the most common diagnosis in women with chronic pelvic pain,[12] with symptoms suggestive of IBS in 50% to 80%. The diagnosis is based on the history (Table 4-10); usually extensive laboratory and radiologic tests are not necessary. In the patient with suspected IBS a complete blood cell count with differential, chemistry profile, and sedimentation rate are suggested. The complete blood cell count helps rule out anemia and inflammation or infection. The sedimentation rate similarly helps rule out an inflammatory process. The white blood cell differential is useful in evaluating parasitic infection (which often causes eosinophilia), tuberculosis (which causes monocytosis), and inflammation (which may cause toxic granulation). With IBS the chemistry profile should be normal, whereas in inflammatory bowel disease electrolyte abnormalities are more likely. To rule out infection with *Giardia*, amoeba, and other parasites, three stool specimens should be sent for ova and parasite testing.

| Table 4-10 Rome II Criteria for the Diagnosis of Irritable Bowel Syndrome |
| --- |
| At least 12 weeks, which need not be consecutive, in the preceding 12 months of abdominal discomfort or pain that has two or three features: |
| 1. relieved with defecation, and/or |
| 2. onset associated with a change in frequency of stool, and/or |
| 3. onset associated with a change in form (appearance) of stool |
| Supportive symptoms of irritable bowel syndrome: |
| <3 bowel movements/week |
| >3 bowel movements/day |
| Hard or lumpy stools |
| Loose or watery stools |
| Straining during a bowel movement |
| Urgency |
| Feeling of incomplete bowel movements |
| Passing mucus |
| Abdominal fullness, bloating, or swelling |

elicited with the bimanual examination is less specific, because it involves stimulation of all layers of the abdominal wall, the parietal peritoneum, and the palpated organ or organs. Including the rectovaginal examination is important in most women with chronic pelvic pain, looking particularly for nodularity and tenderness, suggesting endometriosis.

A thorough history and examination often are diagnostic. Further diagnostic testing may or may not be deemed necessary. Table 4-9 lists some of the diagnostic tests that may be helpful in the evaluation of women with chronic pelvic pain.

Laparoscopy is a particularly important diagnostic test in the evaluation of pelvic pain—more than 40% of gynecologic

Stool also should be checked for occult blood; results should be negative in IBS patients. Similarly, methylene blue stain of stool to look for white blood cells should be negative with IBS, because the presence of large numbers of white blood cells is diagnostic of inflammation. A Sudan stain for fat can be performed to exclude severe steatorrhea, if suspected. Stools should be checked for *Clostridium difficile* toxin if there has been antibiotic exposure within the past 6 weeks.

The possibility of lactose intolerance can be formally tested with a hydrogen breath test if there is any question. The breath test is much more sensitive than the blood test.

Some of the findings that mandate more extensive diagnostic testing to rule out more serious pathology are blood in stool, weight loss, ascites, watery bowel movements more than three times per day, an abdominal mass, or fever.

### Interstitial Cystitis

Interstitial cystitis is a chronic inflammatory condition of the bladder of unknown etiology. The criteria to diagnose interstitial cystitis are controversial, but most often it is defined clinically by the following triad: urinary urgency and frequency, pelvic pain, and mucosal hemorrhages with cystoscopic hydrodistention. Hunner's ulcer at the time of cystoscopy is considered pathognomic but is not a common finding. Voiding frequency with interstitial cystitis is usually every 2 hours or less during the day and two or more times at night. Incontinence is not a common symptom. Evaluation should show the absence of objective evidence of another urinary tract disease that could cause the symptoms. Bladder tumors, especially carcinoma in situ, may cause symptoms similar to those of interstitial cystitis.

Cystoscopy with hydrodistention causes mucosal hemorrhages, called *glomerulations*, in patients with interstitial cystitis, although there are false-positive cystoscopies. In addition to glomerulations (Fig. 4-3), linear cracking and Hunner's ulcer may also be noted. Because significant bladder distention is needed to perform this test and this is very painful in women with interstitial cystitis, general or spinal anesthesia is usually necessary.

Cystoscopy for the diagnosis of intersitital cystitis is performed as follows: The bladder is passively distended to a pressure of 60 to 80 cmH$_2$O. This may require compression of the urethra by upward digital compression of the anterior vaginal wall against the urethroscope to prevent leakage. Although the risk is low, it is possible to rupture the bladder in interstitial cystitis patients during this distention. Findings during this first filling are usually normal, although occasionally increased trabeculation or Hunner's ulcer may be noted. As soon as maximal capacity is reached, the volume is noted. Distention is maintained for 3 to 5 minutes and then the irrigant is drained. If videocystoscopy is performed and the bladder is visualized during this emptying phase, diffuse bleeding from the mucosa is noted that causes the terminal portion of drained irrigant to be blood-tinged (see Fig. 4-3). The bladder is refilled and examination reveals splotchy, submucosal hemorrhages (glomerulations) throughout the bladder of the patient with interstitial cystitis. Bladder biopsies are useful but not essential unless other abnormalities are seen. In such cases biopsies must be done to rule out carcinoma in situ or cancer. Up to 1% of women diagnosed with interstitial cystitis may actually have carcinoma in situ. It is important that any infection has been cleared for several weeks before cystoscopy, not only because of infection concerns, but also because current or recent infection may cause cystoscopic findings similar to those of interstitial cystitis. Postprocedure pain may be decreased by instillation of a dilute solution of local anesthetic after completing cystoscopy (for example, 30 mL of 0.25% bupivacaine).

The potassium sensitivity test has been proposed as an office screening test for interstitial cystitis. This test evaluates pain and urgency after intravesical instillation of 40 mL of potassium chloride (0.4 mEq/mL) compared to symptoms with 40 mL of water. It is reportedly positive in 70% to 90% of patients with interstitial cystitis. As many as 85% of women evaluated by gynecologists for chronic pelvic pain may have positive intravesical potassium sensitivity tests.[13] It is probably appropriate to diagnose interstitial cystitis in women with characteristic symptoms and a positive potassium sensitivity test. Pain caused by a positive potassium sensitivity test should be alleviated by intravesical instillation of 20 to 30 mL of 1% lidocaine or 0.5% bupivacaine. Figure 4-4 shows a questionnaire that may expedite the identification of patients likely to have interstitial cystitis.

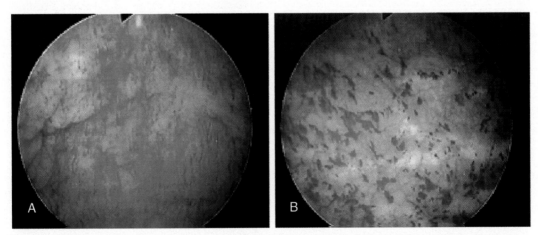

**Figure 4-3 Glomerulations with cystoscopic hydrodistention in a patient with interstitial cystitis.** *A,* Mucosal hemorrhages during emptying phase after hydrodistention. *B,* Glomerulations after refilling the bladder.

Ambulatory Office Practice

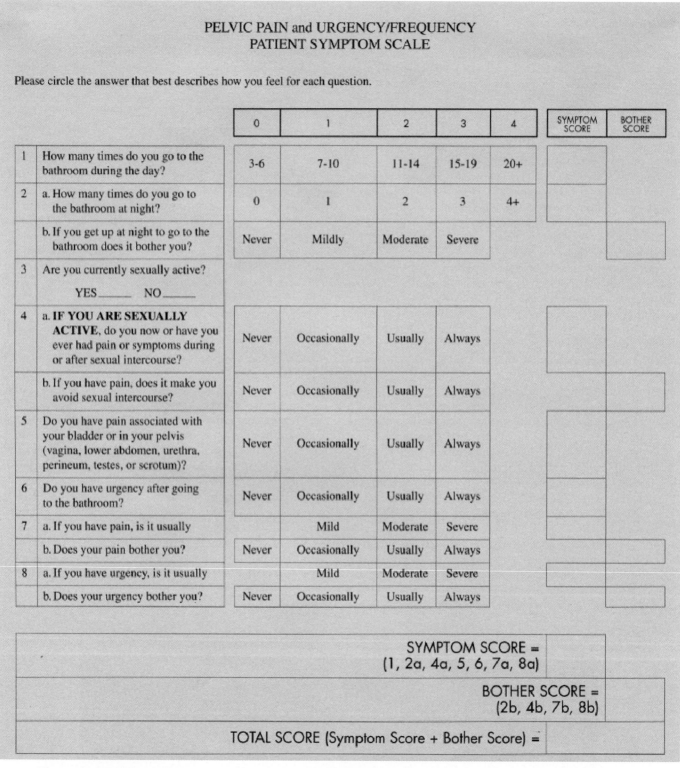

## PELVIC PAIN and URGENCY/FREQUENCY PATIENT SYMPTOM SCALE

Please circle the answer that best describes how you feel for each question.

| | | 0 | 1 | 2 | 3 | 4 | SYMPTOM SCORE | BOTHER SCORE |
|---|---|---|---|---|---|---|---|---|
| 1 | How many times do you go to the bathroom during the day? | 3-6 | 7-10 | 11-14 | 15-19 | 20+ | | |
| 2 | a. How many times do you go to the bathroom at night? | 0 | 1 | 2 | 3 | 4+ | | |
| | b. If you get up at night to go to the bathroom does it bother you? | Never | Mildly | Moderate | Severe | | | |
| 3 | Are you currently sexually active? YES_____ NO_____ | | | | | | | |
| 4 | a. **IF YOU ARE SEXUALLY ACTIVE**, do you now or have you ever had pain or symptoms during or after sexual intercourse? | Never | Occasionally | Usually | Always | | | |
| | b. If you have pain, does it make you avoid sexual intercourse? | Never | Occasionally | Usually | Always | | | |
| 5 | Do you have pain associated with your bladder or in your pelvis (vagina, lower abdomen, urethra, perineum, testes, or scrotum)? | Never | Occasionally | Usually | Always | | | |
| 6 | Do you have urgency after going to the bathroom? | Never | Occasionally | Usually | Always | | | |
| 7 | a. If you have pain, is it usually | | Mild | Moderate | Severe | | | |
| | b. Does your pain bother you? | Never | Occasionally | Usually | Always | | | |
| 8 | a. If you have urgency, is it usually | | Mild | Moderate | Severe | | | |
| | b. Does your urgency bother you? | Never | Occasionally | Usually | Always | | | |

SYMPTOM SCORE =
(1, 2a, 4a, 5, 6, 7a, 8a)

BOTHER SCORE =
(2b, 4b, 7b, 8b)

TOTAL SCORE (Symptom Score + Bother Score) =

**Figure 4-4    The PUF questionnaire: a screening questionnaire that may be useful in identifying patients with interstitial cystitis.**

## Endometriosis

Endometriosis is the presence of ectopic endometrial glands and stroma (i.e., endometrium located outside of the endometrial cavity). Classically the woman with endometriosis presents with one or more of the following triad: an adnexal mass (endometrioma), infertility, or pelvic pain. Estimates are that 5% to 40% of women with endometriosis have chronic pelvic pain. Endometriosis-associated pain almost always starts as menstrual pain, then progresses to include more and more of the luteal phase, and in many women progresses to constant pain with premenstrual and menstrual exacerbation. Most women with endometriosis-associated pelvic pain have severe dysmenorrhea as a component of their pain symptoms. Dyspareunia is present in at least 40%. The clinical diagnosis of endometriosis based on the history and physical examination is accurate in about 85% of women with chronic pelvic pain, but for absolute confirmation of the diagnosis there must be histological confirmation of ectopic endometrium. A solely visual diagnosis at the time of laparoscopy has a significant false-positive rate.

## Pelvic Inflammatory Disease

From 15% to 30% of all women with acute PID subsequently develop chronic pelvic pain. PID is most common among teenagers and women younger than age 25, which is about a decade younger than the mean age of women with chronic pelvic pain. Chronic pelvic pain secondary to prior PID is usually related to coitus and physical activity and is acyclic, although sometimes there may be premenstrual or menstrual exacerbation. The diagnosis is based on past history of PID and on operative findings consistent with prior PID, such as adnexal adhesions, tubo-ovarian complexes, tubal agglutination and phimosis, and hydrosalpinges. Little is known about the actual mechanisms by which chronic pelvic pain results from PID. Some evidence suggests it is related to the severity of adnexal adhesions and damage.

Antibiotic treatment is often empirically tried in women with suspected chronic pelvic inflammatory disease or sub-clinical, chronic pelvic infection. There is scant evidence that any pathogenic microorganisms persist in the uterus or tubes after PID, and there is no published evidence of efficacy of empiric antibiotic treatment of chronic pelvic pain when there is no suggestion of active, acute infection.

Although not a common diagnosis in the United States, tuberculous PID must be remembered as a potential diagnosis in patients with chronic pelvic pain, especially as the incidence of tuberculosis has increased in association with human immuno-deficiency virus infection/acquired immunodeficiency syndrome. As many as 25% of women with pulmonary tuberculosis have pelvic tuberculosis, and about 25% of women with pelvic tuber-culosis will have chronic pelvic pain.

## Pelvic Congestion Syndrome

Although not a common cause of chronic pelvic pain, pelvic congestion syndrome may be more common than generally recognized. Pain associated with pelvic congestion is typically worst premenstrually and although menstrual pain may be present, menses are not usually the time of most severe pain. Pain is usually dull and aching, similar in quality to the leg pain produced by leg varicosities. It is usually not constant and may be brought on by simple acts such as walking or changing posture. Occasional acute, severe exacerbations of sharp pain may occur. Backache is common, characteristically sacral in position, and made worse by standing. Deep dyspareunia is present in three fourths of women with pelvic congestion syndrome. Postcoital aching pain, lasting in some cases up to 24 hours, is present in 65% of cases.

Abdominal palpation at the ovarian point, which lies at the junction of the upper and middle thirds of a line drawn from the anterior superior iliac spine to the pubic symphysis (Fig. 4-5) reproduces the pelvic pain in 80% of women with pelvic congestion syndrome. Diffuse pelvic tenderness, particularly at the adnexae, is characteristic at bimanual pelvic examination.

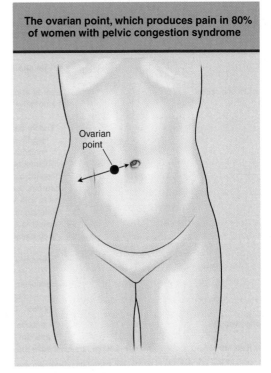

The ovarian point, which produces pain in 80% of women with pelvic congestion syndrome

Ovarian point

**Figure 4-5   The ovarian point, which reproduces pain in 80% of women with pelvic congestion syndrome.**

The diagnosis is confirmed by pelvic venography showing venous stasis, dilation, and plexus formation of the ovarian or uterine vessels. Venography can be performed by transuterine injection of the myometrium (Fig. 4-6) or by retrograde injec-tion of the ovarian veins.

## Adhesions

Adhesions are aberrant fibrous tissues that abnormally attach anatomic structures to one another. Immediately following a peritoneal wound, a cascade of events is unleashed that ulti-mately determines whether or not adhesions develop. In women

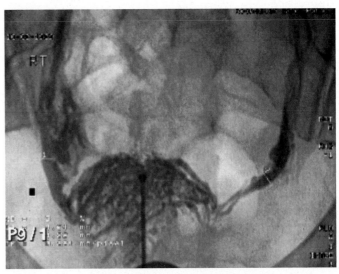

**Figure 4-6   Example of a positive transuterine pelvic venogram.**

the major causes of adhesions are surgery, PID, appendicitis, endometriosis, inflammatory bowel disease, and neoplasia. Post-mortem studies reveal that 67% of all patients develop adhesions postoperatively.

It is generally accepted that adhesions can cause intestinal obstruction and infertility, but their role as a cause of chronic pelvic pain is not clear. There is an association between adhesions and chronic pelvic pain, because intra-abdominal and pelvic adhesions are found more often in women with chronic pelvic pain than in women without pain, but this association does not prove causation. Laparoscopic conscious pain mapping has demonstrated that at least one third of patients with adhesions have focal, dramatic tenderness of some of their adhesions.[10] This suggests that adhesions cause pain in some, but not all, women with pelvic adhesions.

Pelvic pain due to adhesions is usually consistent in its location and may be exacerbated by sudden movements, intercourse, or certain physical activities. A history of PID, endometriosis, perforated appendix, prior abdominopelvic surgery, or inflammatory bowel disease makes adhesive disease a more likely diagnosis. A history of at least one of these is present in only 50% of women with adhesions, however.

Although nonsurgical methods such as computed tomography, magnetic resonance imaging, or ultrasound may suggest the presence of adhesions, presently the only definitive way to diagnose them is by surgical visualization. Laparoscopy, not laparotomy, is the gold standard for diagnosing pelvic adhesive disease.

### Chronic Pain Syndrome

Some chronic pain sufferers seem to maintain a good level of physical and psychological function despite significant pain, whereas others develop a set of emotional and behavioral characteristics that is called *chronic pelvic pain syndrome* (Table 4-11). The recognition of chronic pelvic pain syndrome can be critical to the successful treatment of chronic pelvic pain. In general, surgical and medical treatment are less successful in women with chronic pain syndrome compared to those without chronic pain syndrome.[14]

### Depression

The etiologic relationship between depression and chronic pain is complex and confusing. Regardless, depression is one of the major findings that leads to a diagnosis of chronic pain syndrome and it is a major predictor of pain severity and response to treatment. It is important to seek evidence of depression in women with chronic pelvic pain.

## TREATMENT

Two primary approaches to the treatment of chronic pelvic pain are used:

1. Treatment of pain (pain-specific treatment)
2. Treatment of specific diseases responsible for chronic pelvic pain (disease-specific treatment)

Randomized clinical trials have been conducted to evaluate treatment of several of the common diagnoses associated with chronic pelvic pain, such as endometriosis, IBS, and interstitial cystitis. Pain-specific treatment of chronic pelvic pain is not as well studied.

### Disease-Specific Treatment

#### Endometriosis

Endometriosis may be treated surgically, medically, or with combined surgical and medical therapy. Laparoscopic surgical treatment by destruction of endometriotic lesions and lysis of adhesions relieves pain in a substantial percentage of patients. One published randomized, clinical trial of laparoscopic treatment showed that at 6 months, 63% of patients had significant relief of pain (the placebo effect was 23%).[15] This study showed a number needed to treat of 2.5, meaning that to obtain pain relief at 6 months in two women it is necessary to surgically treat five women.

Neurolytic procedures, particularly uterosacral ligament transections and presacral neurectomy, are sometimes performed to treat endometriosis-associated pelvic pain. Controlled clinical trials suggest that presacral neurectomy (excision of the superior hypogastric plexus) gives a small improvement in pain relief over that obtained with excision of endometriosis alone, with a number needed to treat for presacral neurectomy of 4.8 (meaning five patients would need to have a presacral neurectomy performed, in addition to excision of endometriosis, to have one patient who is better because of the presacral neurectomy).[16,17] However, transection of the uterosacral ligaments showed no efficacy in the treatment of endometriosis-associated pelvic pain over that obtained with only surgical excision of lesions in randomized clinical trials.[18,19] Transection of the uterosacral ligaments may have efficacy for the treatment of primary, central dysmenorrhea in women without endometriosis, with a number needed to treat of 2.2.[20]

Although hysterectomy and bilateral salpingo-oophorectomy are thought to be curative for endometriosis, no clinical trials of hysterectomy or salpingo-oophorectomy for endometriosis-associated pelvic pain have been reported. It is probably important that all endometriosis be resected or destroyed at the time of hysterectomy and bilateral salpingo-oophorectomy to minimize the potential of recurrence.

The mainstay of medical treatment of endometriosis-associated pelvic pain is hormonal, usually with oral contraceptives, danazol, progestins, or gonadotropin-releasing hormone (GnRH) agonists. Danazol and GnRH agonists are approved by

---

**Table 4-11**
**Criteria for Chronic Pelvic Pain Syndrome**

Chronic pelvic pain (usually pain of 6 or more months' duration)
Pain out of proportion to pathology
Altered physical activities at home or work (e.g., stopping running or playing tennis, stopping working)
At least one vegetative sign of depression, usually early-morning awakening not caused by pain
Significantly altered emotional roles within the family or identification of the patient's illness as the most significant problem the family faces. Examples of alterations of emotional roles are:
  Family decision making
  Supervision and discipline of children
  Nurturing of children and partner

the Food and Drug Administration (FDA) for endometriosis treatment. The GnRH agonists available in the United States are nafarelin, goserelin, and leuprolide. They work at the hypothalamic-pituitary level to shut down luteinizing hormone and follicle-stimulating hormone production and release. This down-regulation leads to a dramatic decline in estradiol levels. GnRH agonists have been evaluated in several placebo-controlled, randomized clinical trials, as well as numerous trials comparing them to danazol. Placebo-controlled trials suggest that the number needed to treat for GnRH agonists for endometriosis-associated pelvic pain is 2.0 to 2.5.[21,22] Comparative trials suggest that danazol and GnRH agonists have similar efficacies, whereas oral contraceptives and progestins may be somewhat less effective. The only placebo-controlled trial of medroxy-progesterone acetate, a commonly prescribed progestin, used a high dose, 100 mg/day. Lower doses and other progestins are probably effective. Side effects observed with medical therapy include breakthrough bleeding, mood changes, depression, hot flushes, weight gain, and irritability. Danazol may also cause androgenic side effects. Loss of bone density is a concern with GnRH agonists.

To minimize loss of bone density, GnRH agonist treatment may be given for less than 6 months[23] or add-back treatment with estrogen and/or progestins may be used. Add-back regimens evaluated with clinical trials include conjugated equine estrogen (0.625 mg or 1.25 mg) plus norethindrone acetate (2.5 mg or 5 mg) or norethindrone acetate alone.[24] All of the add-back regimens significantly decreased the loss of bone density (they also decreased hot flashes), but they slightly increased the likelihood of breakthrough bleeding and pain symptoms.

Preliminary results with mifepristone, an antiprogesterone, suggest that it induces amenorrhea and improves endometriosis-associated pelvic pain when given at 50 to 100 mg daily. It may be possible to achieve similar results with lower doses, but this remains to be adequately studied.

### Interstitial Cystitis

Dimethylsulfoxide (DMSO) was the first FDA-approved drug indicated for interstitial cystitis. Intravesical treatments with DMSO are usually repeated four to eight times at 1- to 2-week intervals. In addition to subjective evidence of decreased symptoms, objective evidence of significantly increased bladder capacity (<100 mL increase) has also been demonstrated. The number needed to treat for DMSO therapy of interstitial cystitis-associated pelvic pain is estimated at 3.6.[25] Unfortunately, DMSO treatments result only in remission of disease, not cure. At least 30% to 60% of patients relapse within the first year after successful treatment. Other intravesical therapies for interstitial cystitis have been less extensively studied and none other than DMSO has FDA approval for treatment of interstitial cystitis.

The other FDA-approved treatment of interstitial cystitis is oral pentosan polysulfate sodium, a polyanionic analog of heparin. One randomized clinical trial showed decreased pelvic pain in 45% of treated patients, compared to 18% with placebo, giving a number needed to treat of 3.7.[26] The dosage of sodium pentosan polysulfate is 100 mg orally three times a day.

Intravesical capsaicin therapy, in a small, placebo-controlled, randomized clinical trial of 36 patients showed significant improvements in frequency and nocturia, but no improvement in pain levels.[27] A small placebo-controlled trial of intravesical bacillus Calmetté-Guerin showed a response rate of 60%, compared to 27% in the placebo group, with a mean decrease of pain in 81%.[28] Amitriptyline also has shown efficacy in a clinical trial, but anticholinergic side effects hinder its use.[29]

Oral cyclosporine, L-arginine, nifedipine, and hydroxyzine have been used to treat interstitial cystitis but have not been substantiated as effective in randomized clinical trials.

The primary surgical treatment of interstitial cystitis for more than 50 years has been hydrodistention of the bladder. This procedure can be performed at the time of diagnostic cystoscopy if general or spinal anesthesia is used—hydrodistention is too painful to be done without anesthesia. Observational studies suggest that about 50% of patients have a successful response to hydrodistention. Remission generally lasts for 6 to 10 months, with a gradual recurrence of symptoms in almost all patients. Retreatment with hydrodistention has a greatly diminished success rate.

Neurolytic surgery via laser destruction of the vesicoureteric plexus has been reported to show some degree of success, but only in uncontrolled studies with limited follow-up. Further confirmation is essential before this procedure is widely used. Nd:YAG laser treatment has also been used, but data are limited regarding its efficacy.

Approximately 5% of patients have unresponsive, intractable, incapacitating symptoms. Such patients usually have small-capacity bladders (<400 mL), void 18 to 20 times per day, and have severe, uncontrolled pain. Augmentation cystoplasty or cystectomy-urethrectomy-continent diversion have been the most successful and acceptable radical surgical treatments.

### Irritable Bowel Syndrome

Dietary interventions constitute the initial approach to IBS. Lactose, fructose, and sorbitol can contribute to symptoms and should be eliminated from the diet, at least on a trial basis. Caffeinated products, carbonated beverages, and gas-producing foods (such as broccoli, cabbage, Brussels sprouts, asparagus, cauliflower, and beans) may contribute to bloating and should be avoided if possible. Smoking and chewing gum lead to more swallowed air and may also increase gas and bloating. Excessive alcohol consumption may lead to increased rectal urgency. Fiber supplementation is often useful for both diarrhea and constipation symptoms.

Pharmacologic treatment is not specific to the disease but rather is directed to relief of symptoms. Patients may be divided into one of three major symptom categories, depending on which symptoms are dominant. The three symptom categories are abdominal pain, gas, and bloating; constipation predominant; and diarrhea predominant. Unfortunately many patients do not fall clearly into one of these three groups but have overlapping symptoms. The severity of the symptoms also influences the choice of pharmacologic treatment.

With predominantly abdominal pain, gas, and bloating symptoms, a trial of an antispasmodic is suggested if there is no evidence of small bowel obstruction. Commonly used antispasmodics are dicyclomine (Bentyl), hyoscyamine (Levsin), Donnatal, and Librax. None has been shown to be consistently efficacious. Because many patients have these symptoms postprandially, it is best to give these medications 30 minutes before meals. Beano (a D-galactosidase) or a simethicone preparation (Gas X, Phazyme) also can be tried.

If constipation is the predominant symptom, a trial of increased roughage and psyllium is prescribed. Many patients have increased gas with increased fiber, and about 15% cannot tolerate fiber therapy. It is recommended, therefore, that fiber be increased gradually and be taken with a meal (usually breakfast). Sometimes tap water enemas during the initiation of fiber supplements are helpful. If necessary, a stool softener or osmotic laxative also can be used temporarily. An insufficient dose of fiber is a frequent cause of failure. Chronic use of stimulant laxatives should be discouraged. There may be a role for prokinetic agents in constipation, but data from clinical trials have been inconsistent. Cisapride, one of the most studied agents, is no longer readily available, because its use has been restricted in the United States. Tegaserod is FDA-approved for constipation-predominant IBS, but its approval is for 12 weeks of treatment.

In diarrhea-predominant patients, over-the-counter loperamide is a commonly used agent. An advantage of loperamide over many other antidiarrheal agents is that it does not cross the blood-brain barrier. Ondansetron, a serotonin receptor antagonist that slows colonic transit time may be useful in the treatment of diarrhea-predominant IBS, but studies have shown inconsistent results. Ondansetron is not approved by the FDA for this indication.

Peppermint oil is the major constituent of several over-the-counter remedies for IBS. It is a safe and inexpensive treatment, but clinical trials have shown inconsistent efficacy.

Psychotherapy with cognitive/behavioral therapy (including stress management), dynamic psychotherapy, hypnosis, and relaxation therapy may be helpful and may improve clinical response over medical treatment only. Factors that predict a good response to psychotherapy include diarrhea and pain as the predominant symptoms, the association of overt psychiatric symptoms, intermittent pain exacerbated by stress, short duration of bowel complaints, and few sites of abdominal pain. Patients with constant abdominal pain do poorly with psychotherapy or hypnotherapy. A recent review of controlled trials of psychological treatments for IBS found that 8 out of 14 studies reported that psychological therapy was significantly superior to control treatment in reducing the primary symptoms of IBS.[30]

### Adhesions

The traditional treatment of abdominopelvic adhesions is surgical adhesiolysis. The only randomized trial of adhesiolysis for chronic pelvic pain failed to show any significant improvement after lysis of adhesions by laparotomy, compared to a control group that did not undergo adhesiolysis.[31] Only when a subgroup analysis of 15 women with severe, stage IV adhesions was done could any detectable improvement in pain be attributed to adhesiolysis. A randomized trial of laparoscopic adhesiolysis for abdominal pain (in men and women) also failed to show any significant difference between surgically treated versus nontreated patients.[32]

A problem with studies of surgical adhesiolysis is that there are no effective methods for preventing recurrence of adhesions. The current adhesion barriers, oxidized regenerated cellulose (Interceed, Johnson & Johnson Medical, Arlington, Tex.), Gore-Tex surgical membrane (W.L. Gore., Flagstaff, Ariz.), and hyaluronic acid-methylcellulose (Seprafilm, Genzyme, Cambridge, Mass.), are only somewhat effective and at best prevent up to 50% of adhesion recurrence. Crystalloid fluids, such as Ringer's solution, are easy to use, but are not effective. Colloid fluid such as Dextran 70 can cause rapid fluid shifts and anaphylactic reactions.

Adhesions will likely remain a cause for some cases of chronic pelvic pain until a method to prevent adhesions is found.

## Pain-Specific Treatment

The fundamental steps involved in nociception provide a framework that helps explain the difference between pain-specific treatment and disease-specific treatment (Fig. 4-7). In general, disease-specific treatment attempts to remove the noxious stimulus and prevent transduction (the conversion of a noxious stimulus into a biochemical event that activates a nociceptor). Pain-specific treatment is directed not to the noxious stimulus but rather to the fundamental processes involved in nociception (i.e., transduction, transmission, modulation, or perception). Pain-specific treatment can be a crucial component of therapy because disease-specific treatment often gives inadequate pain relief. Pain-specific treatment may be pharmacological, psychological, physical, or neuroablative.

### Pharmacologic Treatment

The mosaic of neural elements and chemical mediators involved in pain perception make it possible to decrease pain with medications with different pharmacologic profiles and mechanisms. Oral analgesics are particularly important in the treatment of pain, yet optimization of analgesic medications is sometimes overlooked in the initial treatment of chronic pelvic pain. Optimization of analgesia is usually best accomplished with a scheduled regimen, not an as-needed regimen. However, a scheduled regimen also presents some hazards. For example, with nonsteroidal anti-inflammatory drugs (NSAIDs) it may lead to gastric irritation or renal damage and with opioids it may lead to constipation, sedation, habituation, addiction, or diminished analgesic potency.

#### Peripheral-Acting Analgesics

Aspirin is a prototype peripheral-acting analgesic. It interferes with transduction by acting to inhibit prostaglandin synthesis, which decreases inflammation and the activation of nociceptors, and by blocking the action of bradykinin on pain receptors. The NSAIDs generally work via the same mechanisms, although potencies may vary significantly. The potential of side effects with NSAIDs is significant and their chronic use requires careful observation, especially for gastric or intestinal ulceration with gastrointestinal bleeding and less commonly for nephropathy. NSAIDs also inhibit platelet function and may lead to significant bleeding. They promote retention of salt and water and may cause edema in some patients. Certain individuals have intolerance to NSAIDs and display a "hypersensitivity reaction" to them that can manifest as vasomotor rhinitis, angioneurotic edema, urticaria, bronchial asthma, laryngeal edema, bronchoconstriction, or hypotension and shock. A history of hypersensitivity reaction to aspirin is an absolute contraindication to

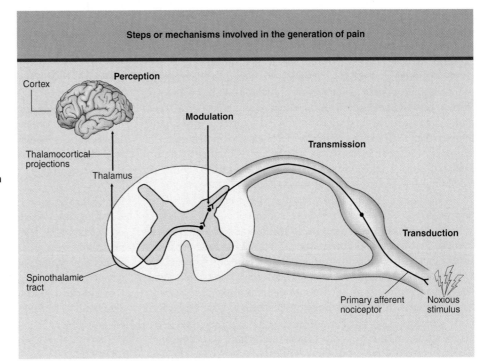

**Figure 4-7  Steps or mechanisms involved in the generation of pain.**

the use of any NSAID. Such hypersensitivity reactions do not appear to occur with acetaminophen.

### Opioid Analgesics

Although still controversial, the use of opioid analgesics to treat chronic pain is common in pain centers. Chronic dose opioid therapy provides improved quality of life and daily function in many patients who have failed other treatments.[33]

Some of the a priori bias of physicians against opioid treatment of chronic pelvic pain stems from a lack of understanding of the difference between tolerance, dependence, and addiction. Tolerance is the diminution of effectiveness over time from the same dose of drug. Physical dependence is the appearance of an abstinence syndrome if the drug is withdrawn. The initial symptoms of the abstinence syndrome are yawning, diaphoresis, lacrimation, coryza, and tachycardia, followed by peak symptoms at 72 hours of abdominal cramps, nausea, and vomiting. Withdrawal symptoms can be minimized by tapering opioids prior to discontinuation and by avoiding the use of antagonists. The term *addiction* should probably be replaced by the term *psychological dependence*. Psychological dependence represents a mental illness manifest by aberrant behaviors, consisting of drug craving, efforts to secure its supply, interference with physical health or psychological function, and recidivism after detoxification. Although tolerance and physical dependence are significant problems with opioid treatment, psychological dependence or addiction is the only complication that leads to unacceptable and illegal behavior by the patient. Greater than 90% of pain patients on chronic opioid maintenance never manifest addictive behavior.[34] Clinical experience suggests that a prior history of addiction to legal or illegal substances is a major risk factor and that patients with such histories are not good candidates for opioid treatment of chronic pelvic pain. The diagnosis and treat-

ment of addiction can be difficult; it is best diagnosed and managed by an expert on treatment of substance abuse.

After all traditional attempts at pain control have failed, opioid maintenance therapy for chronic pelvic pain should be considered.[33] Before opioid treatment is initiated there should be documentation that the patient has failed nonnarcotic treatment and has entered knowingly into a trial of opioid maintenance. A written or documented verbal contract or agreement should be made with the patient that includes at least the following particulars:

- The treating doctor is the sole provider of opioids
- The patient is seen by this physician before having her opioid prescription refilled
- Lost medications or prescriptions will not be refilled
- The patient agrees she will actively participate in strategies to develop alternative pain therapies.

Some physicians have advocated inclusion of random urine drug testing as a condition of opioid maintenance therapy.

Combining opioid treatment with central-acting and peripheral-acting medications may optimize efficacy with lower opioid doses, but use of commercially available formulations of opioids with acetaminophen, aspirin, or ibuprofen can lead to overdosage of the nonopioid drug. All medications are best given on a scheduled, not an as-needed, basis. Titration of the selected opioid should be done over several weeks with the goals of improvement in physical and social function and at least partial analgesia. Failure to achieve these goals at relatively low doses in the nontolerant patient should cause the clinician to question the feasibility of opioid maintenance therapy.

It is important to assess the extent of pain relief provided by the opioid medication and determine its role in restoring function and improving quality of life. When improved function and reasonable analgesia are achieved, close and regular follow-up is essential in chronic pelvic pain patients on opioid maintenance therapy. Most patients should be seen and drugs prescribed monthly. If doses escalate during opioid maintenance, hospitalization is recommended to evaluate the medication requirements and, if possible, return medications to their baseline level. If inappropriate use occurs, such as using the medication to treat depression or anxiety, drug diversion, or hoarding, this should be pursued and managed firmly. Use of the medication for symptoms other than those for which it is prescribed (e.g., use for headaches in addition to pelvic pain) may lead to increased tolerance and dose escalation, and should be discouraged. If control cannot be maintained, treatment with opioids should be discontinued.

Table 4-12 summarizes most of the opioids available in the United States as oral formulations and gives doses that are equivalent to 10 mg of morphine administered intramuscularly. Side effects are common with opioid therapy. Opioids may cause drowsiness, difficulty in mentation, decreased physical activity, mood changes, respiratory depression, nausea, vomiting, dizziness, pruritus, constipation, increased biliary tract pressure, urine retention, miosis, depression, and (rarely) convulsions. Considering this long list of untoward effects, as well as the risks or tolerance and addiction, it is again worth stating that opioid treatment should be initiated only after other treatments have been insufficient, the patient has been carefully counseled, and assurance of close follow-up is possible.

### Antidepressants

Antidepressants, particularly tricyclic antidepressants (TCAs), have been used to treat a number of chronic pain syndromes, including arthritis, diabetic neuropathy, headache, back pain, and cancer pain. TCAs may result in improved pain levels at doses much lower than those typically used for the treatment of depression. Pain levels generally are decreased by 20% to 50% in chronic pain syndromes, although it is not clear that TCAs are effective in all pain syndromes. There are no randomized, clinical trials of TCAs for treatment of chronic pelvic pain. One open-label study suggested that nortriptyline at 100 mg/day was effective, but the dropout rate due to side effects was 50%.[35] Depression is common in women with chronic pelvic pain; when it is diagnosed, it should be treated with an appropriate antidepressant in most cases.

### Combination Drug Therapy

Combination drug therapy uses medications with different sites or mechanisms of action to improve the treatment of pain. For example, combining a central-acting opioid analgesic and a peripheral-acting NSAID often gives better pain relief than either analgesic alone. Similarly, combining two medications that are central-acting but with different mechanisms, such as a TCA and an opioid analgesic, might result in better pain relief than monotherapy. Combination drug therapy may improve pain relief, but it also increases adverse effects and potential drug interactions.

### Psychological Treatment

Ideally psychological evaluation and treatment would be part of the care of every patient with chronic pelvic pain. Patients with chronic pain develop psychological changes that maintain or increase the distress of their pain regardless of the degree of physical trauma or disease. Combining psychotherapy (usually cognitive/behavioral therapy) with traditional surgical or medical treatment results in better outcomes than those obtained with surgical or medical treatment alone.[36–40] Unfortunately, many women are unable to afford or reluctant to accept referral to a psychologist or psychiatrist for evaluation and treatment.

### Other Treatments

Other treatments, especially alternative or complementary treatments, are used by women with chronic pelvic pain. Most patients use alternative treatments as adjuncts to conventional therapy, not as replacements. Thus the name *complementary medicine* may be better terminology. Most complementary treatments are not well-studied for chronic pain, let alone for chronic pelvic pain.

*Relaxation therapy* is a commonly used technique to aid in treatment of chronic pain and especially for acute exacerbation of pain. Music therapy is also used by many women. There appear to be no randomized clinical trials of efficacy.

*Transcutaneous electrical nerve stimulation* (TENS) has been extensively used by physical medicine and pain physicians and by physical therapists with seemingly good results. About three fourths of patients treated with TENS for chronic pain show improvement, although the degree of pain relief is not great. One might expect similar or better results with *acupuncture*, but not as much has been published.

*Bodywork* of a less traditional nature than physical therapy, such as *massage therapy*, *chiropractic manipulation*, and *reflexology*, is often used but there is no published research sufficient to reach a valid conclusion on such approaches as yet.

**Table 4-12**
**Some of the Opioids Available in the United States***

| Generic Name | Proprietary Name(s) | Mean Duration (hrs) | Equianalgesic Dose (mg) |
|---|---|---|---|
| Butorphanol | Stadol | 3–6 | 2–3 (intranasal) (agonist-antagonist) |
| Codeine | | 4–6 | 200 (oral) |
| Fentanyl | Duragesic | 72 | 25–100 µg/hr (transdermal) |
| Hydrocodone | Hycodan, Vicodin, Lortab, Lorcet, others | 4–5 | 5–10 (oral) |
| Hydromorphone | Dilaudid | 4–5 | 6–7.5 (oral) |
| Methadone | Dolophine | 4–6 | 20 (oral) |
| Morphine | MSIR MS Contin | 4–7 | 30–60 (oral) |
| Oxycodone | Percodan, Tylox, Percocet* Oxycontin | 4–6 | 5–10 (oral) |
| Pentazocine | Talwin | 4–7 | 180 (oral) |
| Propoxyphene | Darvon, Darvocet* | 4–6 | 180–240 (oral) |

*Equianalgesic doses to 10 mg of morphine administered intramuscularly are given.

*Magnetic therapy* and *magnetic field therapy* have shown results in animal studies that suggest they decrease pain levels. No significant clinical studies have been published. There is also insufficient clinical evidence to reach a conclusion about the efficacy of *hypnosis* in the treatment of chronic pain.

*Spiritual or religious treatments* such as intercessionary prayer, healing, divine intercession, and meditation are important aspects of health care for many people, but have not been extensively studied with scientific techniques for pain treatment.

*General comfort measures* should always be included in the treatment of chronic pelvic pain. Examples are heat packs, hot baths or whirlpools, ice packs, back rubs, enhanced empathy and attentive listening by clinicians, and compassionate interactions between doctor and patient.

## PITFALLS AND CONTROVERSIES

There is still not a widely accepted definition of chronic pelvic pain. This hinders the applicability of published research, because it makes it difficult to know whether a particular investigation or treatment is applicable to one's specific patient. It is crucial that all research on chronic pelvic pain clearly define the population being studied.[41] It would be quite helpful if a consensus definition were available.

The role of laparoscopy in the evaluation of chronic pelvic pain is another area of controversy. Unfortunately many gynecologists, and thus their patients, consider laparoscopy the definitive diagnostic test in the evaluation of chronic pelvic pain. In reality, laparoscopy is important in diagnosing endometriosis and adhesions, but is not essential in the diagnosis of almost all other clinical conditions associated with chronic pelvic pain. A review of Table 4-3 will confirm that most of the other diagnoses can be made with less invasive laboratory and imaging tests. Yet it remains common for many women to undergo numerous laparoscopic evaluations in spite of prior negative or minimal prior laparoscopic findings. Although there is optimism that conscious laparoscopic pain mapping may improve the usefulness of laparoscopy, this is not sufficiently substantiated to recommend it in routine gynecologic practice.

The concept of pain as a diagnosis, not necessarily a symptom, and the use of therapies directed at pain rather than only at specific diagnoses, is another controversial subject. The current understanding of chronic pain would suggest that pain often represents a diagnosis, but this concept is not well studied or substantiated in chronic pelvic pain. As a corollary, the use of opioids in chronic pelvic pain is not well established.

Finally, a major pitfall for gynecologists is to assume that all or most chronic pelvic pain is due to the reproductive tract. Clearly, this is not the case, with gastrointestinal and urologic disorders both notably more frequent with chronic pelvic pain. Although a gynecologist may choose to only treat gynecologic disorders in women with chronic pelvic pain, it is essential that the gynecologist properly evaluate each patient for nongynecologic diseases before assuming that gynecologic disorders, such as mild endometriosis, are the cause of the patient's pain. There are numerous examples of women with other disorders, such as interstitial cystitis, being treated repeatedly for insignificant or asymptomatic endometriosis, because a thorough evaluation was not done for nongynecologic diseases.

## REFERENCES

1. Zondervan K, Barlow DH: Epidemiology of chronic pelvic pain. Baillieres Best Pract Res Clin Obstet Gynaecol 2000;14:403–414. **(III, B)**
2. Lippman SA, Warner M, Samuels S, et al: Uterine fibroids and gynecologic pain symptoms in a population-based study. Fertil Steril 2003;80:1488–1494. **(III, B)**
3. Mathias SD, Kuppermann M, Liberman RF, et al: Chronic pelvic pain: prevalence, health-related quality of life, and economic correlates. Obstet Gynecol 1996;87:321–327. **(III, B)**
4. Ness RB, Soper DE, Holley RL, et al: Effectiveness of inpatient and outpatient treatment strategies for women with pelvic inflammatory disease: results from the Pelvic Inflammatory Disease Evaluation and Clinical Health (PEACH) randomized trial. Am J Obstet Gynecol 2002;186:929–937. **(Ib, A)**
5. Carlson KJ, Miller BA, Fowler FJ II: The Maine Women's Health Study: I. Outcomes of hysterectomy. Obstet Gynecol 1994;83:556–565. **(III, B)**
6. Kjerulff KH, Rhodes JC, Langenberg PW, Harvey LA: Patient satisfaction with results of hysterectomy. Am J Obstet Gynecol 2000;183:1440–1447. **(III, B)**
7. Almeida EC, Nogueira AA, Candido dos Reis FJ, Rosa e Silva JC: Cesarean section as a cause of chronic pelvic pain. Int J Gynaecol Obstet 2002;79:101–104. **(III, B)**
8. IASP Subcommittee on Taxonomy: Pain terms: a list with definitions and notes on usage. Pain 1979;6:249. **(IV, C)**
9. Zondervan KT, Yudkin PL, Vessey MP, et al: Chronic pelvic pain in the community—symptoms, investigations, and diagnoses. Am J Obstet Gynecol 2001;184:1149–1155. **(III, B)**
10. Howard FM, El Minawi AM, Sanchez RA: Conscious pain mapping by laparoscopy in women with chronic pelvic pain. Obstet Gynecol 2000;96:934–939. **(III, B)**
11. Demco LA: Effect on negative laparoscopy rate in chronic pelvic pain patients using patient assisted laparoscopy. JSLS 1997;1:319–321. **(III, B)**
12. Zondervan KT, Yudkin PL, Vessey MP, et al: Chronic pelvic pain in the community—symptoms, investigations, and diagnoses. Am J Obstet Gynecol 2001;184:1149–1155. **(III, B)**
13. Parsons CL, Bullen M, Kahn BS, et al: Gynecologic presentation of interstitial cystitis as detected by intravesical potassium sensitivity. Obstet Gynecol 2001;98:127–132. **(III, B)**
14. Steege JF, Stout AL: Resolution of chronic pelvic pain after laparoscopic lysis of adhesions. Am J Obstet Gynecol 1991;165:278–281. **(III, B)**
15. Sutton CJ, Ewen SP, Whitelaw N, Haines P: Prospective, randomized, double-blind, controlled trial of laser laparoscopy in the treatment of pelvic pain associated with minimal, mild, and moderate endometriosis. Fertil Steril 1994;62:696–700. **(Ib, A)**
16. Zullo F, Palomba S, Zupi E, et al: Effectiveness of presacral neurectomy in women with severe dysmenorrhea caused by endometriosis who were treated with laparoscopic conservative surgery: a 1-year prospective randomized double-blind controlled trial. Am J Obstet Gynecol 2003;189:5–10. **(Ib, A)**
17. Candiani GB, Fedele L, Vercellini P, et al: Presacral neurectomy for the treatment of pelvic pain associated with endometriosis: a controlled study. Am J Obstet Gynecol 1992;167:100–103. **(Ib, A)**
18. Vercellini P, Aimi G, Busacca M, et al: Laparoscopic uterosacral ligament resection for dysmenorrhea associated with endometriosis: results of a randomized, controlled trial. Fertil Steril 2003;80:310–319. **(Ib, A)**
19. Sutton C, Pouley AS, Jones KD, et al: A prospective, randomized, double-blind controlled trial of laparoscopic uterine nerve ablation in the treatment of pelvic pain associated with endometriosis. Gynaecol Endoscopy 2001;10:217–222. **(Ib, A)**
20. Lichten MM, Bombard J: Surgical treatment of primary dysmenorrhea with laparoscopic uterine nerve ablation. J Reprod Med 1987;32:37–41. **(IIb, B)**
21. Ling FW: Randomized controlled trial of depot leuprolide in patients with chronic pelvic pain and clinically suspected endometriosis. Pelvic Pain Study Group. Obstet Gynecol 1999;93:51–58. **(Ib, A)**

22. Adamson GD, Kwei L, Edgren RA: Pain of endometriosis: effects of nafarelin and danazol therapy. Int J FertilMenopausal Stud 1994; 39:215–217. **(Ib, A)**

23. Hornstein MD, Yuzpe AA, Burry KA, et al: Prospective randomized double-blind trial of 3 versus 6 months of nafarelin therapy for endometriosis associated pelvic pain. Fertil Steril 1995;63:955–962. **(Ib, A)**

24. Hornstein MD, Surrey ES, Weisberg GW, Casino LA: Leuprolide acetate depot and hormonal add-back in endometriosis: a 12-month study. Lupron Add-Back Study Group. Obstet Gynecol 1998; 91:16–24. **(Ib, A)**

25. Perez-Marrero R, Emerson LE, Feltis JT: A controlled study of dimethyl sulfoxide in interstitial cystitis. J Urol 1988;140:36–39. **(IIb, B)**

26. Parsons CL, Benson G, Childs SJ, et al: A quantitatively controlled method to study prospectively interstitial cystitis and demonstrate the efficacy of pentosanpolysulfate. J Urol 1993;150:845–848. **(Ib, A)**

27. Lazzeri M, Beneforti P, Benaim G, et al: Intravesical capsaicin for treatment of severe bladder pain: a randomized placebo controlled study. J Urol 1996;156:947–952. **(Ib, A)**

28. Peters K, Diokno A, Steinert B, et al: The efficacy of intravesical Tice strain bacillus Calmetté-Guerin in the treatment of interstitial cystitis: a double-blind, prospective, placebo controlled trial. J Urol 1997; 157:2090–2094. **(Ib, A)**

29. van Ophoven A, Pokupic S, Heinecke A, Hertle L: A prospective, randomized, placebo controlled, double-blind study of amitriptyline for the treatment of interstitial cystitis. J Urol 2004;172:533–536. **(Ib, A)**

30. Talley NJ, Owen BK, Boyce P, Paterson K: Psychological treatments for irritable bowel syndrome: a critique of controlled treatment trials. Am J Gastroenterol 1996;91:277–283. **(Ia, A)**

31. Peters AA, Trimbos-Kemper GC, Admiraal C, et al: A randomized clinical trial on the benefit of adhesiolysis in patients with intra-peritoneal adhesions and chronic pelvic pain. Br J Obstet Gynaecol 1992;99:59–62. **(Ib, A)**

32. Swank DJ, Swank-Bordewijk SC, Hop WC, et al: Laparoscopic adhesiolysis in patients with chronic abdominal pain: a blinded randomised controlled multi-centre trial. Lancet 2003;361:1247–1251. **(Ib, A)**

33. Portenoy RK: Opioid therapy for chronic nonmalignant pain: a review of the critical issues. J Pain Symptom Manage 1996;11:203–217. **(IV, C)**

34. Joranson DE, Ryan KM, Gilson AM, Dahl JL: Trends in medical use and abuse of opioid analgesics. JAMA 2000;283:1710–1714. **(III, B)**

35. Walker EA, Roy-Byrne PP, Katon WJ, Jemelka R: An open trial of nortriptyline in women with chronic pelvic pain. Int J Psychiatry Med 1991;21:245–252. **(III, B)**

36. Guthrie E, Creed F, Dawson D, Tomenson B: A randomised controlled trial of psychotherapy in patients with refractory irritable bowel syndrome. Br J Psychiatry 1993;163:315–321. **(Ib, A)**

37. Guthrie E, Creed F, Dawson D, Tomenson B: A controlled trial of psychological treatment for the irritable bowel syndrome. Gastroenterol 1991;100:450–457. **(IIa, B)**

38. Svedlund J, Sjodin I, Ottosson JO, Dotevall G: Controlled study of psychotherapy in irritable bowel syndrome. Lancet 1983;2:589–592. **(IIa, B)**

39. Farquhar CM, Rogers V, Franks S, et al: A randomized controlled trial of medroxyprogesterone acetate and psychotherapy for the treatment of pelvic congestion. Br J Obstet Gynaecol 1989;96:1153–1162. **(Ib, A)**

40. Peters AA, van Dorst E, Jellis B, et al: A randomized clinical trial to compare two different approaches in women with chronic pelvic pain. Obstet Gynecol 1991;77:740–744. **(Ib, A)**

41. Williams RE, Hartmann KE, Steege JF: Documenting the current definitions of chronic pelvic pain: implications for research. Obstet Gynecol 2004;103:686–691. **(III, B)**

# Female Sexual Dysfunction

## Gloria Bachmann, MD, and Nidhi Gupta, MD

### KEY POINTS

- Female sexual dysfunction occurs in approximately 40% of the adult population and is especially prevalent among teens and women over 65 years of age.
- Women expect physicians to ask questions directed to their sexual health. Reluctance to discuss sexual matters often results from patient anxiety and embarrassment to bring up the topic; many women will discuss the topic only after direct clinician query.
- Using the PLISSIT model of sexual inquiry is an efficient way to address sexual concerns and problems in a busy practice.
- The use of hormonal therapy should be considered in appropriate postmenopausal women, especially surgically menopausal women, since urogenital atrophy and loss of sexual desire are common problems in this age group.
- Regardless of how advanced in age a woman is, sexual history taking should be a part of the annual examination and counseling and treatment should be offered if the woman reports distress from a sexual dysfunction.

## EPIDEMIOLOGY, RISK FACTORS, AND PATHOGENESIS

Sexuality is an intimate and integral portion of a woman's life, reflecting both her physical health and emotional well-being. A neglected medical topic for many years, the emergence of effective pharmacologic interventions, especially for male sexual dysfunction, has infused the field with renewed research and clinical interest. Sexual function, however is a difficult area to objectively analyze because it is influenced by emotional, biologic, and psychosocial factors, which makes the clinical diagnosis, treatment, and study of female sexual dysfunction (FSD) more challenging than other medical problems, such as diabetes mellitus, in which there is an objective clinical value to diagnose the condition and prove efficacy of the intervention.

FSD affects the entire spectrum of ages, races, and socio-economic backgrounds and is influenced—to differing degrees—by biological, physical, and psychosocial factors. Since many conditions and personal experiences adversely affect sexual health, it is not surprising that the prevalence of FSD is high (Table 5-1). The National Health and Social Life study evaluated 1749 women aged 18 to 59 by personal interview technique. From this study, a 43% overall prevalence of female sexual dysfunction was reported, with 22% reporting low sexual desire, 14% reporting arousal difficulties, and 7% reporting sexual pain[1] (Fig. 5-1). Data from a study of 1480 women

showed even higher percentages of various FSDs. In this group of women aged 18 to 87 years, hypoactive sexual desire was reported by 87%, followed by 83% with orgasmic disorders, 75% with insufficient vaginal lubrication, 71% with dyspareunia, 69% with body image concerns, 67% with unmet sexual needs, and 63% with inadequate information on sexual issues.[2] A recent on-line Web-based survey of 3807 women confirmed these high rates of FSD.[3] Of these respondents, who were 88% Caucasian, 5% black, 3% Hispanic, and 1.4% Asian, the most common sexual complaint was low sexual desire (77%). Other prevalent complaints included low sexual arousal (62%), inability to achieve orgasm or difficulty achieving orgasm (56%), and vaginal dryness (46%). Forty percent of the respondents reported that they did not seek help from a physician for these complaints. Of the group who did not seek professional assistance, 54% reported that they would like to, and 33% were not sure whether they would pursue help.[3]

Data suggest that FSD is increased in women who are younger, unmarried, have lower levels of education and social status, are African American, and have a history of sexual abuse or coercion. As expected, the more sexual dysfunctions a woman notes, the more adversely they impact her quality of life. Some classes of medications such as antidepressants and oral contraceptives as well as medical conditions such as diabetes, high blood pressure, multiple sclerosis, endocrine disorders, spinal cord injury, and mastectomy interfere with sexual wellness. Gynecologic conditions such as vaginitis, pregnancy, lactation, and menopause also increase sexual problems in women. Often ignored by women and their clinicians, psychological and social stressors such as depression, anxiety, rape, interpersonal conflicts with partner, and sexual identity disorders commonly lead to sexual dysfunction.

A major contributor to FSD, especially in the aging population, is poor vascular integrity that can lead to adverse anatomic and physiologic changes. Arterial insufficiency from atherosclerosis of the iliohypogastric/pudendal arterial bed may result in decreased blood flow to the clitoris or vagina that can have a major impact on sexual wellness.[4] This vascular insufficiency over time leads to loss of corporal smooth muscle and replacement by fibrous connective tissue in clitoral cavernosal arteries, ultimately leading to vaginal dryness and dyspareunia.[5] Traumatic injury from pelvic fractures, blunt trauma, surgical disruption, and chronic perineal pressure from bicycle riding can also lead to disruption of the iliohypogastric/pudendal arterial bed and result in diminished vaginal and clitoral blood flow and complaints of sexual dysfunction.[6] Verification of this phenomenon was demonstrated in rabbit studies. When the pelvic nerves of an atherosclerotic female rabbit were stimulated, the increase in clitoral and vaginal blood flow was less than in a

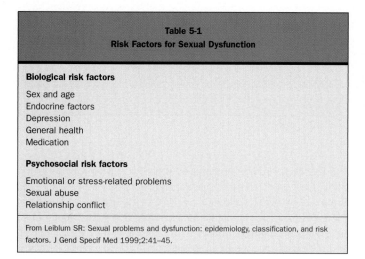

**Table 5-1**
**Risk Factors for Sexual Dysfunction**

**Biological risk factors**

Sex and age
Endocrine factors
Depression
General health
Medication

**Psychosocial risk factors**

Emotional or stress-related problems
Sexual abuse
Relationship conflict

From Leiblum SR: Sexual problems and dysfunction: epidemiology, classification, and risk factors. J Gend Specif Med 1999;2:41–45.

normal control.[5] Postmenopausal women with atrophic changes in vaginal and clitoral vasculature frequently report diminished vaginal lubrication and arousal (Table 5-2).

At the neurogenic level, nitric oxide, phosphodiesterase V, and vasoactive intestinal peptide are considered to play a significant role in sexual response. Autonomic innervation of the vagina originates from the hypogastric and sacral plexus, which gives rise to uterovaginal nerves. The uterovaginal nerves contain both parasympathetic and sympathetic nervous system fibers. The pudendal nerve provides somatic sensory innervation to the vulvar/clitoral region, whereas the autonomic innervation to the clitoris is from the sympathetic (T1–L3) and parasympathetic (S2–S4) fibers.

Sympathetic nervous system activation can impair genital blood flow in women with spinal cord injury or diseases of the

central or peripheral nervous system, such as multiple sclerosis, parkinsonism, temporal lobe epilepsy, and spinal cord injuries. In females with multiple sclerosis there is demyelination of the central nervous system pathways. Because of this disruption of pudendal somatosensory afferents in women with multiple sclerosis, orgasmic dysfunction may be reported.[7] Women with complete upper motor neuron injuries affecting sacral spinal segments are unable to achieve psychogenic lubrication. However, when incomplete injuries occur, women usually retain their capacity for psychogenic lubrication, especially if there is sensory preservation at the T11 to L2 dermatomes.[8] Women with spinal cord injuries also report more difficulty achieving orgasm than women with an intact spinal cord.[9]

Both estrogen and testosterone play a role in female sexual response. Other conditions, including endocrine dysfunctions, especially those of the hypothalamic/pituitary axis; diabetes mellitus; hypo- and hyperthyroidism; surgical or medical castration; premature ovarian failure; natural menopause; certain commonly used medications like antihypertensives, psychotropics, antidepressants, and the birth control pill, also can lead to FSD through a primary or secondary effect on the gonadal hormones. Use of oral contraceptives, gonadotropin-releasing hormone (GnRH) agonists, and tamoxifen may also result in decreased desire and libido, vaginal dryness, and lack of sexual arousal. Studies on women with hyperprolactinemia resulting from the use of antipsychotic medication report higher rates of sexual dysfunction than in unaffected women. The level of depression or dose of medication is not as strong a predictor of sexual problems as the level of prolactin. This implies that hyperprolactinemia is the main cause of sexual dysfunction in females taking antipsychotic medication.[10] Clinicians should avoid prescribing antipsychotics that raise the prolactin level, or if no alternative drugs are available, then monitoring prolactin

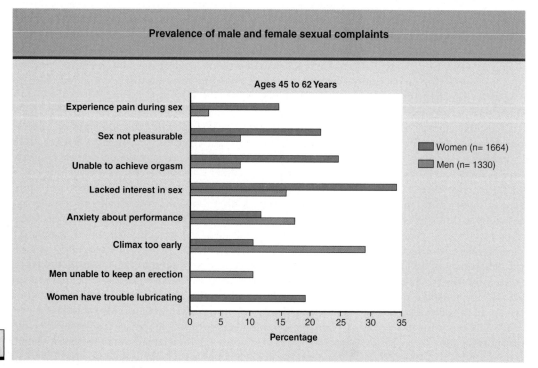

**Figure 5-1 Prevalence of male and female sexual complaints.** Data from National Health and Social Life Survey, subjects aged 46 to 62 years. (From Laumann EO, Gagnon JH, Michael RT, Michaels S: The Social Organization of Sexuality: Sexual Practices in the United States. Chicago, University of Chicago Press, 1994.)

**Table 5-2**
**Common Drugs That Affect Sexuality in Women**

**Decreased desire**

Antilipid medications
Antipsychotics
Barbiturates
Benzodiazepines
β-Blockers
Clonidine
Danazol
Digoxin
Fluoxetine
Gonadotropin-releasing hormone agonists
H$_2$-blockers and antireflux agents
Indomethacin
Ketoconazole
Lithium
Phenytoin
Spironolactone
Tricyclic antidepressants

**Diminished arousal**

Alcohol
Anticholinergics
Antihistaminics
Antihypertensives
Benzodiazepines
Selective serotonin reuptake inhibitors
Monoamine oxidase inhibitors
Tricyclic antidepressants

**Orgasmic dysfunction**

Methyldopa
Amphetamines and related anorexia drugs
Antipsychotics
Benzodiazepines
Selective serotonin reuptake inhibitors
Narcotics
Trazodone
Tricyclic antidepressants—also associated with painful orgasm

Adapted from Weiner DN, Rosen RC: Medications and their impact. In Sipski ML, Alexander CJ (eds): Sexual Function in People with Disability and Chronic Illness. Gaithersburg, Md, Aspen Publishers, 1997, pp 856–1118.

receptor antagonist also has been reported to reverse SSRI-induced sexual dysfunction.[12]

During pregnancy and the postpartum period women experience profound physical changes, fluctuating hormone levels, and other coexisting conditions that influence their sexual health. In recently delivered women, postpartum depression and sexual dysfunction are a concern. Treatment may require psychotherapy or pharmacologic intervention.

On the other end of the reproductive spectrum, the prevalence of diminished sexual desire and libido, dyspareunia, and decreased sexual activity and arousal is increased in the menopausal and postmenopausal periods of a woman's life. During menopause, the natural depletion of oocytes and ovarian follicles lead to a decline in serum estrogen levels to a fraction of reproductive-aged levels, causing loss of vaginal moisture and dyspareunia. Declining androgen levels commencing in the fourth decade of a woman's life can also lead to sexual problems. Therefore, in addition to estrogen, androgens are an important contributor to sexual wellness. A recent double-blind, randomized controlled study compared the effects of oral esterified estrogens with and without methyltestosterone on endocrine profiles and dimensions of sexual function in postmenopausal women experiencing hypoactive sexual desire.[13] The concentration of bioavailable testosterone was significantly increased and sex hormone–binding globulin (SHBG) decreased after treatment with combination estrogen/androgen therapy as compared with estrogen alone. As anticipated, mean changes in sexual interest or desire as rated on the Sexual Interest Questionnaire increased from baseline with combination treatment and were significantly greater than those achieved by esterified estrogens alone. Increased circulating level of unbound testosterone and suppression of SHBG by exogenous testosterone appears to be the reason for the improved sexual functioning in women on combination therapy.

Psychiatric illnesses, both long term and acute, such as affective and anxiety disorders, anorexia nervosa, depression, obsessive-compulsive disorder, schizophrenia, and bipolar disease can cause female sexual dysfunction. Interpersonal conflicts not psychiatrically related in a sexual relationship may also lead to changes in sexual interest and response. Religious beliefs and history of rape or other forms of abuse are some of the most common reasons causing FSD in subsets of younger women.

Even short-term emotional problems can lead to sexual problems. The National Health and Social Life Survey (NHSLS) data reported that deteriorating social position and worsening economic status, leading to a high level of stress, can negatively affect sexual functioning.[1]

In addition to the anatomic alterations that result from surgical procedures and radiologic treatments such as hysterectomy, vulvectomy, radiation therapy, bladder suspension, cystocele/rectocele repair, and mastectomy, emotional issues also may have a negative impact on a woman's sexual wellness.[14] For example, women who undergo treatment for cervical cancer often experience decreased lubrication and genital swelling owing to damage to peripheral nerves and vasculature during surgery. Disruption of the vasculature due to any pelvic surgery or radiotherapy may have an adverse impact on sexual function. Superimposed on these effects are the psychological issues that

levels in these women is advisable. Another class of pharmacologic interventions that may contribute to sexual dysfunction is the selective serotonin receptor reuptake inhibitor (SSRI). Some evidence suggests that activation of the 5-hydroxytryptamine 2 (5-HT$_2$) receptor produces vasoconstriction of the genital vasculature as compared with stimulation of the 5-HT1A receptor, which facilitates sexual functioning.[11] Serotonin produces vasodilation by acting on 5-HT$_1$ receptors to stimulate release of nitric oxide and also by activating 5-HT$_3$ receptors. The role of 5-HT$_3$ receptors in female sexual response is currently not definitively known.

In affected individuals, buspirone, a 5-HT1A agonist may be useful in reversing SSRI-induced sexual dysfunction. Another intervention, nefazodone, a 5-HT$_2$ antagonist, causes up-regulation of 5-HT1A receptors. It has been reported to cause fewer sexual side effects than traditional SSRIs. Cyproheptadine acts as a histamine and serotonin (5-HT$_2$) antagonist and has been reported to reduce antidepressant-induced sexual dysfunction. Mirtazapine, an α$_2$-adrenergic, 5-HT$_2$, and 5-HT$_3$

have to be dealt with afterward, including loss or diminution of female identity.[14] Sometimes all that is addressed is the vaginal shortening, reduced vaginal elasticity, and vaginal bleeding that may occur with coitus. Additionally, clinicians could address the anatomic and emotional changes that may occur. Alterations in level of sexual functioning after major surgery can often be predicted by a number of factors that are present prior to surgery. The level of sexual wellness presurgery appears to be the most important one. Treating and counseling women for anxiety, depression, type of surgery, alterations in physical appearance, and changes in sexual function that may result will reduce the number of sexual complaints arising from psychological issues postoperatively. However, it is important to note that after hysterectomy, women often report greater sexual pleasure.

## CLINICAL FEATURES OF SEXUAL RESPONSE

Masters and Johnson in 1966 first characterized the female sexual response as four successive phases: excitement, plateau, orgasm, and resolution.[15] In 1979, Kaplan proposed the aspect of "desire" and the three-phase model consisting of desire, arousal, and orgasm. (Fig. 5-2). Kaplan's three-phase model is the basis of classifications of female sexual dysfunction in the Diagnostic and Statistical Manual of Mental Disorders IV (DSM-IV) and also the World Health Organization International Classification of Diseases 10 (ICD-10). Later, Basson proposed an intimacy-based female sex response cycle[16] (Fig. 5-3). According to her, the female sexual response is a circular, more complex model than the linear sequence of desire, arousal, orgasm, and resolution and the key to female sexual response is emotional intimacy and sexual stimuli.

A major barrier to the development of clinical research in the area of sexual function has been the absence of a well-defined, broadly accepted diagnostic framework and classification for female sexual dysfunction. The International Consensus Development Conference on Female Sexual Dysfunction in 1998 developed a classification system that has four major

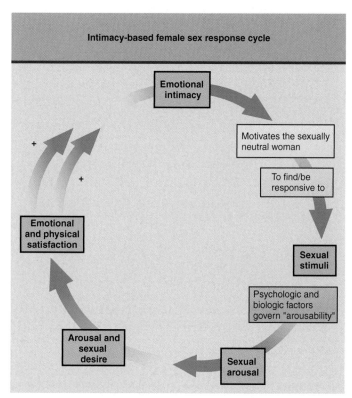

**Figure 5-3   Intimacy-based female sex response cycle.** (From Basson R: Female sexual response: the role of drugs in the management of sexual dysfunction. Obstet Gynecol 2001;98:350–353.)

categories of dysfunction: desire, arousal, and orgasmic and sexual pain disorders. According to this international panel of sex researchers, therapists, and clinicians, DSM-IV categorizes only psychiatric-related sexual disorders. This group proposed that the classification of sexual dysfunctions be based on both physiological and psychological problems. Definitions of several disorders were altered to include this premise. This consensus classification defines four types of dysfunction and five subtypes. A new category of sexual pain disorder, including noncoital sexual pain, also was added. The DSM-IV requirement that a woman must experience personal distress for a diagnosis of sexual dysfunction was retained.[15]

In 1998, the American Foundation of Urologic Disease Consensus panel also published an updated FSD definition and classification system.[15] Each classification is further subtyped as lifelong or acquired, generalized or situational, and of organic, psychogenic, mixed, or unknown etiology. This classification from the International Consensus Panel is as follows:

I.   Hypoactive sexual desire disorder
     This is defined as persistent or recurring deficiency (or absence) of sexual fantasies/thoughts and/or receptivity to sexual activity, which causes personal distress. It is the most common female problem. Loss of desire may result from psychological/emotional factors, physiologic problems such as hormonal deficiencies, physical illnesses, medications, medical and surgical interventions, stress, fatigue, very restrictive upbringing, and negative or traumatic sexual experiences. In postmenopausal

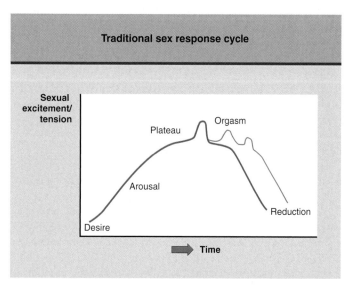

**Figure 5-2   Traditional sex response cycle.** (From Kaplan HS: The New Sex Therapy: Active Treatment of Sexual Dysfunctions. New York, Brunner/Mazel, 1974.)

women, especially those who are surgically menopausal, low testosterone levels are associated with loss of sexual desire. (Fig. 5-4).

A subtype of hypoactive sexual desire is sexual aversion disorder, defined as the persistent or recurring phobic aversion to and avoidance of sexual contact with a sexual partner, which causes personal distress. Sexual aversion disorder is generally a psychologically or emotionally based problem that can result from a variety of causes such as physical abuse, sexual abuse, or other childhood trauma.

II. Sexual arousal disorder

This is defined as persistent or recurring inability to attain, or maintain, sufficient sexual excitement, causing personal distress. It may be experienced as lack of subjective excitement or lack of genital (lubrication/swelling) or other somatic response. Disorders of arousal include lack of or reduced vaginal secretions, decreased clitoral and labial sensation, decreased clitoral and labial engorgement, and lack of vaginal smooth muscle relaxation. Causes can be psychologic and medical/physiologic and from prior pelvic trauma, pelvic surgery, medications (e.g., SSRIs), and neural and peripheral vascular diseases.

III. Orgasmic disorder

This is defined as persistent or recurrent difficulty, delay, or absence of orgasmic potential after sufficient sexual stimulation and arousal, which causes personal distress. Primary disorder occurs when the female has never experienced orgasm through any means of stimulation,

and secondary disorder occurs when the female has previously experienced orgasm but is currently non-orgasmic. Medications, chronic illnesses, trauma to the nerves associated with pelvic surgery and spinal cord injury, medical conditions affecting the nerve supply of the pelvis (such as multiple sclerosis, diabetic neuropathy), hormonal imbalance, relationship difficulties, emotional trauma, or sexual abuse are associated with orgasmic failure.

IV. Sexual pain disorders

These are classified as dyspareunia, vaginismus, and noncoital sexual pain disorders.

A. Dyspareunia

Dyspareunia is recurrent or persistent genital pain associated with genital touching, entry attempt, deep thrusting, or pain immediately after intercourse. Sites of pain include the vaginal opening, areas on the vestibule, the entire vulva, and the pelvis. Inadequate lubrication is a common cause in the postmenopausal female. Inadequate arousal, pelvic infections, endometriosis, vulvodynia, uterine prolapse, vaginal atrophy, scars, and tumors can cause dyspareunia in women across the adult life cycle.

B. Vaginismus

Vaginismus is recurrent or persistent involuntary spasm of the outer third of the vagina that interferes with vaginal penetration and causes personal distress. Vaginismus may result from vaginal scarring, previous trauma, surgeries, childbirth, or chronic vaginal infection.

C. Noncoital sexual pain disorder

Noncoital sexual pain disorder is recurrent or persistent genital pain induced by noncoital sexual stimulation. This new category recognizes that sexual pain can occur in situations other than penile penetration.

## DIAGNOSIS

Sexual assessment is an integral part of the general medical evaluation and should be taken in a quiet atmosphere in which the patient is seated comfortably and assured privacy and confidentiality. Clinicians who are cognizant of their own sexual beliefs are most comfortable with this part of the medical history and are more likely to take a sexual history. Full evaluation of FSD, in addition to history, must include a physical examination, pelvic examination, and in selected cases a hormonal profile (follicle-stimulating hormone, luteinizing hormone, testosterone, and estradiol levels).

Because many women are reluctant to talk about sexual issues, especially if they have a specific problem, a useful way to commence sexual inquiry is with basic, nonthreatening questions such as "Are you sexually active?" and "Is sex satisfying?" Providing information such as, "Many of my patients who stop hormonal therapy complain of pain with sex soon afterward. Has this happened to you?" also is helpful. In some practices, a preconsultation questionnaire including sexual questions has proved useful; however, many women are reluctant to put sexual problems down on paper (Fig. 5-5).

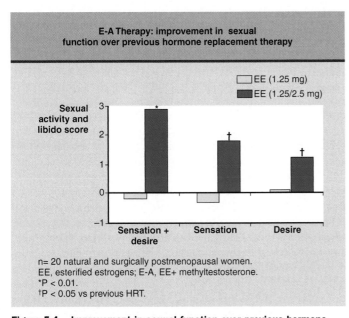

**E-A Therapy: improvement in sexual function over previous hormone replacement therapy**

EE (1.25 mg)
EE (1.25/2.5 mg)

n= 20 natural and surgically postmenopausal women.
EE, esterified estrogens; E-A, EE+ methyltestosterone.
*$P < 0.01$.
†$P < 0.05$ vs previous HRT.

**Figure 5-4 Improvement in sexual function over previous hormone replacement therapy (HRT) with estrogen-androgen replacement therapy.** (From Sarrel P, Dobay B, Wiita B: Estrogen and estrogen-androgen replacement in postmenopausal women dissatisfied with estrogen-only therapy: sexual behavior and neuroendocrine responses. J Reprod Med 1998;43:847–856. Reproduced with permission from the Journal of Reproductive Medicine, permission conveyed through the Copyright Clearance Center, Inc.)

## Ambulatory Office Practice

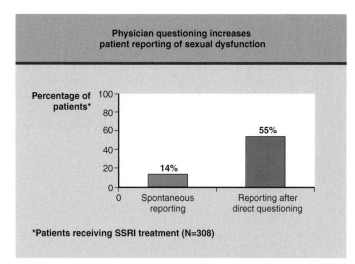

**Physician questioning increases patient reporting of sexual dysfunction**

Percentage of patients*

*Patients receiving SSRI treatment (N=308)

**Figure 5-5** **Physician questioning increases patient reporting of sexual dysfunction.** (From Montejo AI, Llorca G, Izquierdo JA, et al: [Sexual dysfunction secondary to SSRIs: a comparative analysis in 308 patients.] Actas Luso Esp Neurol Psiquiatr Cienc Afines 1996;24:311–321.)

The PLISSIT model for assessment and treatment of sexual health is a useful tool that gives basic structure to sexual inquiry and treatment.[17] PLISSIT stands for permission (to engage in sexual exchange), limited information (education to clarify myths and misconceptions), specific suggestions (addressing the problem of the patient with options for intervention and treatment), and intensive therapy (referring the patient with complex problems who will need long-term care to a professional who deals with FSD).

Permission assists many women who need a clinician to tell them it is OK to experience sexual pleasure without guilt. Limited information is educating and giving information, clarifying misunderstandings and myths about sexuality. Specific suggestions are detailed suggestions relating to a particular concern such as sensate focus training for arousal disorders. Intensive therapy by a qualified sex therapist is helpful for women who do not respond to the first three measures.

Currently, there are no useful, easy to use and interpret, objective measures that a clinician can use in the office setting to measure sexual dysfunction and response to intervention. Measurements that have been used in the research setting include changes in pelvic hemodynamics, measurement of vaginal smooth muscle relaxation, and genital vibratory perception thresholds. Clitoral, labial, urethral, vaginal, and uterine blood velocity (peak systolic velocity) and venous pooling (end-diastolic velocity) are assessed using duplex Doppler ultrasound. The most used and validated estimate of vaginal blood flow is photoplethysmography. Vaginal photoplethysmography measures vasoengorgement, vaginal blood volume, and vaginal pulse amplitude (VPA). However, the data are difficult to interpret when patient movement occurs during the study and so this instrument is not suitable during stimulation or orgasm. As well, photoplethysmography provides relative rather than absolute units of measurement and does not provide anatomic information. Measurements by this tool have not correlated significantly with subjective arousal reports in women.

Other methods for assessment of female genital vasocongestion are labial temperature, clitoral blood flow measures, Doppler ultrasound, and magnetic resonance imaging. Sommers et al described a new device for measuring vaginal and labial blood flow during sexual arousal and orgasm. The device assesses transcutaneous oxygen partial pressure by measuring the amount of electrical power needed to maintain a set temperature. Advantages of this device over the photoplethysmograph are that it is relatively free from movement artifacts and can be calibrated in terms of absolute blood flow.[18]

Vaginal pressure-volume changes and clitoral and labial vibratory thresholds are recorded both at baseline and after sexual stimulation. Results of vibratory testing may support a diagnosis of vascular, hormonal, or neurologic dysfunction as a cause of the FSD.[19]

Vaginal pH, which is the only test that can be routinely done in a physician's office, is an indirect measurement for the assessment of vaginal flora and the support of urogenital atrophy.

Currently, FSDs are mainly diagnosed and interventions assessed for efficacy by clinician inquiry. Questionnaires, some validated and others not, have proliferated in recent years, spurred in large part by the development of new treatments for male sexual dysfunctions. These are most useful in research settings. Recently, a variety of brief, self-report measures that show a high degree of reliability and validity and are sensitive to treatment interventions, have been used for the multidimensional assessment of female sexual function.[20] Self-administered questionnaires, daily diary records, and event log measures of sexual behavior are geared mainly for use in clinical trials on female sexual dysfunction, especially since they are easier to administer and score than clinical measures.

A commonly used questionnaire is the Female Sexual Function Index (FSFI). This self-report questionnaire assesses sexual function in six domains: desire, arousal, lubrication, orgasm, satisfaction, and pain. The use of this questionnaire for clinical trials in female sexual dysfunction has been validated, and it is currently being used in a number of clinical trials. It is easy to administer, is very sensitive, and has a high degree of internal consistency and test-retest reliability.[21]

The Brief Sexual Function Index for Women (BSFI-W) is a self-report instrument that assesses current levels of female sexual functioning and satisfaction such as sexual thought/desires, arousal, frequency of activity, receptivity/initiation, pleasure/orgasm, relationship satisfaction, and sexual problems.[20] The Sexual Function Questionnaire (SFQ), which has been validated by large-scale clinical trials, assesses sexual function in seven domains: desire, physical arousal-sensation, lubrication, enjoyment, orgasm, pain, and partner satisfaction.[22] This questionnaire has demonstrated strong internal consistency and test-retest reliability, making it valuable in evaluating and diagnosing various types of FSD. It is sensitive to treatment interventions, making it valuable in determining their efficacy in clinical trials.

### Daily Diaries and Event Logs

These tools are used to assess variables such as intercourse frequency, successful attempts at intercourse, and medication use and to obtain frequency data in clinical trials.[23] Diaries require the subject to record sexual activity on a daily basis, whereas event logs are completed only on days when sexual activity occurs. However, they are not suitable for subjective assessment of female sexual response, are restricted in the scope of measurement, and are susceptible to various forms of response bias or error, since they are completed at home.

## Structured Interviews

The Derogatis Sexual Function Interview is a structured interview that has been validated by large-scale clinical trials for the assessment of male and female sexual dysfunction.[24] The advantages of this interview are breadth of the assessment and the clinical validation.

## Personal Distress and Quality of Life

The Female Sexual Distress Scale is a 12-item scale that has shown a high degree of test-retest reliability and internal consistency.[25] It is highly recommended for clinical trials in FSD, since it assesses the subjective distress associated with sexual dysfunction.

## TREATMENT

The treatment options for FSD are limited. However, new interventions are gradually evolving as more clinical and basic science research is being directed to this problem.

## Estrogen

Estrogen (with or without progestogen) therapy is indicated in postmenopausal women (either spontaneous or surgical) who complain of symptoms of urogenital atrophy, dryness, burning, urinary frequency, urgency, and dyspareunia. Diminished sex response, difficulty reaching orgasm, and decreased sexual activity may also be improved with estrogen therapy but usually because of elimination of vasomotor symptoms and not directly from an effect on sexual motivation. Estrogen depletion leads to decreased pelvic blood flow and sensory perception, ultimately leading to dyspareunia. Estrogen therapy improves clitoral sensitivity, increases genital blood flow, improves vaginal cytology, improves lubrication, and decreases pain with intercourse. In women with contraindications to systemic hormone therapy or who need treatment only for urogenital atrophy, local therapy such as with an estrogen cream, ring, or tablet might be considered. Vaginal estrogens have a profound local estrogenic effect on the urogenital tissue with minimal systemic absorption.

## Testosterone

Androgens play a major role in sexual motivation behaviors and sexual desire (Table 5-3). A randomized, double blind, placebo-controlled cross-over trial of transdermal testosterone patches in doses of 150 and 300 µg combined with oral estrogen in 75 women after total abdominal hysterectomy with bilateral oophorectomy found a positive effect on sexual motivational activities. Serum free testosterone levels were substantially increased at both treatment doses. Sexual function measures of sexual desire, orgasm pleasure, and general well-being improved significantly above baseline with 300 µg testosterone.[26]

Methyltestosterone (1.25 or 2.5 mg) used orally in combination with esterified estrogens (0.625 and 1.25 mg) is available as hormonal therapy for menopausal women with vasomotor symptoms. In a study of postmenopausal women who were

| Table 5-3 Sexual Complaints Associated with Androgen Decline | | |
|---|---|---|
| | Patients (%) | |
| | Testosterone <10 ng/mL (n=11) | Testosterone >30 ng/mL (n=11) |
| Decreased desire | 100 | 80 |
| Decreased orgasm | 100 | 45* |
| Dyspareunia | 55 | 63 |
| Sexual avoidance | 80 | 36 |
| Sexual aversion | 15 | — |
| The symptoms are global | 100 | 45* |

*P < 0.05.
From Kaplan HS, Owett T: The female androgen deficiency syndrome. J Sex Marital Ther 1993;19:3–24.

dissatisfied with estrogen alone, improvement was seen in sexual function in women who were switched to estrogen plus androgen as compared with estrogen alone (see Fig. 5-4).[27] With androgen creams increased clitoral sensitivity, decreased vaginal dryness, and increased libido have been reported.[27] Side effects that are dose dependent are similar to those seen with the oral preparation, such as acne, weight gain, voice deepening, clitoral enlargement, increased facial hair, and androgenic alopecia. A decrease in high-density lipoprotein cholesterol and in triglycerides may also occur when high systemic levels of androgens are used. Dehydroepiandrosterone (DHEA) is a precursor to testosterone and is produced in both the ovary and the adrenal gland in women. In cases of adrenal insufficiency, oral DHEA brings testosterone levels into the normal range.[28] Data are not available on DHEA use and FSD.

## Tibolone

Tibolone is a synthetic steroid compound used outside the United States in women who are naturally or surgically menopausal. It has estrogenic, progestagenic, and androgenic effects. The effect of tibolone on women with sexual dysfunction is still inconclusive.

## Sildenafil

Sildenafil is a potent phosphodiesterase type V (PDE-5) inhibitor that causes the accumulation of cyclic 3′,5′ guanosine monophosphate leading to smooth muscle relaxation. Nitric oxide and phosphodiesterase type V (the enzyme responsible for cyclic 3′,5′-guanosine monophosphate degradation and nitric oxide production) have been identified in human clitoral and cavernosal smooth muscle.[29]

After the enormous success of sildenafil citrate in male erectile disorder, the impact on FSD was studied. Although an organ bath study reported that sildenafil causes a dose-dependent relaxation of female rabbit clitoral corpus cavernosum, which would indicate a positive effect on arousal, this consistent positive result has not been observed in women.[30]

In one open-label, nonrandomized sildenafil study of 33 postmenopausal women, no significant improvement in sexual function was found.[31] The most commonly reported side effects were clitoral discomfort and hypersensitivity, reported in 21% of women. In a double-blind, placebo-controlled, cross-over trial of 53 premenopausal women aged 22 to 28 years with arousal disorder, both sildenafil 25 mg and 50 mg significantly improved sexual function from baseline.[32] Women taking sildenafil reported significantly increased arousal, orgasm, enjoyment, satisfaction, and frequency of intercourse and frequency of sexual fantasies. There was no difference between the two doses. The investigators found that 70.5% women in this study wanted to continue treatment with sildenafil. Another randomized, double-blind, cross-over, placebo-controlled trial of sildenafil was performed in premenopausal women with multiple sclerosis who had an active sexual relationship, normal estrogen and androgen levels, and no significant medical or recent psychiatric study.[33] Sildenafil increased lubrication and sensation in these women with MS and FSD, but there was no improvement in the capacity to reach orgasm, overall enjoyment, or quality of life. The starting dose of sildenafil was 50 mg and was increased or decreased depending on the response.

Potential future treatments for FSD include the following:

1. L-Arginine: an amino acid precursor that leads to the formation of NO, which mediates the relaxation of vascular and nonvascular smooth muscle, leading to vascular dilation.
2. Prostaglandin $E_1$: a prostaglandin $E_1$ intravaginal application is under investigation for treatment of female sexual dysfunction.
3. Phentolamine: functions as a nonspecific α-adrenergic blocker leading to vascular smooth muscle relaxation and increased vaginal blood flow. A pilot study to analyze the effects of oral phentolamine on postmenopausal women with sexual arousal difficulties have shown improvement in vaginal lubrication and other measures of sexual arousal.[34]
4. Apomorphine: a short-acting dopamine agonist reported to improve sexual function.

### Mechanical Devices

The U.S. Food and Drug Administration (FDA) approved a device known as the EROS clitoral therapy device (EROS-CTD) for the treatment of female sexual arousal disorder.[35] It is designed to treat women who experience reduced sensation, lubrication, and ability to achieve orgasm. Available by prescription, it consists of a small, soft, plastic vacuum pump that is placed over clitoris. With gentle suction to the region, blood flow is increased, aiding in sexual arousal. No adverse effects have been reported from this battery-operated device. EROS may be particularly effective in postmenopausal women, but clinical data are needed to confirm this assumption.

### Dietary Supplements

Dietary supplements such as ginseng, gingko biloba, B vitamins, calcium, and folic acid have no clinical data to support claims that they are useful in the treatment of FSD.

### Pelvic Exercises

Pelvic floor exercises (Kegel exercises) are prescribed to strengthen the pubococcygeal muscles and increase blood flow to the pelvis. No objective data document improved sexual and orgasmic responses in women doing these exercises.

### Vaginal Dilators

Vaginal dilators are most often used to treat vaginismus. At the commencement of treatment, the smallest dilators are placed in the vagina for 15 minutes twice daily. As the woman becomes comfortable with that size, she gradually replaces it with the next one with an increased diameter.

### Lubricants

Lubricants can be used in conditions of vaginal dryness and dyspareunia. They are best used during coital activity, as their maximal effects are temporary.

## RESEARCH

The Center for Drug Evaluation and Research, a branch of FDA, issued a guidance document in May 2000 that outlines FDA recommendations for conduct of clinical trials in FSD.[36] According to this document, the definition of FSD should include a measure of personal distress that reflects a degree of psychological dissatisfaction with sexual functioning in the affected woman. Appropriate study populations are defined and include premenopausal women and naturally and surgically postmenopausal women taking hormone-containing products for menopausal symptoms. To demonstrate efficacy in clinical trials and to minimize recall bias, it is recommended that subjects record sexual events or encounters on a daily basis during the pretreatment period of 4 to 8 weeks and then during the intervention. According to this document, to find the lowest effective dose for FSD, two adequate, well-controlled, phase III trials should be carried out for about 6 months. This document recognizes the value of questionnaires and self-report measures, which should be validated separately before their use in clinical trials. To demonstrate efficacy in a treatment, women with the following conditions should be excluded from clinical trials: women with significant relationship difficulties or sexual dysfunction in the partner, women using medications that affect sexual function, and women having medical illnesses that affect sexual function. End points for clinical trials should be based on the number of successful and satisfactory sexual events or encounters over time, the determination of which should be by the woman participating in the trial, as opposed to her partner. These events or encounters can be sexual intercourse (with or without orgasm), oral sex resulting in orgasm, or manual stimulation by self or partner resulting in orgasm, and they should be recorded in daily records or event logs.

## PITFALLS AND CONTROVERSIES

Sexuality is an important component of a woman's life and has a significant impact on her quality of life. Research on the cause and treatment of female sexual dysfunction has lagged far behind many other conditions that affect women. Available pharmacologic interventions are increasing as research in this area becomes widespread. Drugs under investigation include gonadal hormones and vasodilators. To understand the impact of drugs, there is a great need to study and understand the myriad of factors that contribute to a woman's psychological experience of sexual satisfaction.

Inquiry about sexual symptoms should be routine, even though the only treatment at times may be acknowledging and validating the sexual complaint. Patients expect the physician to raise questions related to sexual well-being. Along these lines, more efforts should be made to emphasize training in human sexuality during medical school and residency training. For the field to progress, the use of standardized clinical trial tools must be adopted so that data sets can be compared. Of great importance is the need for large-scale, randomized, placebo-controlled, double-blind trials to determine long-term efficacy and side effects of pharmacologic interventions used to treat FSD.

## REFERENCES

1. Laumann E, Paik A, Rosen R: Sexual dysfunction in the United States: prevalence and predictors. JAMA 1999;281:537–544. **(III, B)**

2. Nusbaum MR, Gamble G, Skinner B, Heiman J: The high prevalence of sexual concerns among women seeking routine gynecological care. Fam Pract 2000;49:229–232. **(III, B)**

3. Berman L, Berman J, Felder S, et al: Seeking help for sexual function complaints: what gynecologists need to know about the female patient's experience. Fertil Steril 2003;79:572–576. **(III, B)**

4. Myers LS, Morokof PJ: Physiological and subjective sexual arousal in pre- and postmenopausal women taking replacement therapy. Psychophysiology 1986;23:283–292. **(IIb, B)**

5. Park K, Goldstein I, Andry C, et al: Vasculogenic female sexual dysfunction: the hemodynamic basis for vaginal engorgement insufficiency and clitoral erectile insufficiency. Int J Impot Res 1997;9:26–27. **(IIa, B)**

6. Berman JR, Berman L, Werbin TJ, Goldstein I: Female sexual dysfunction: anatomy, physiology, evaluation and treatment options. Curr Opin Urol 1999;9:563–568. **(IV, C)**

7. Yang CC, Bowen JR, Kraft GH, et al: Cortical evoked potentials of the dorsal nerve of the clitoris and female sexual dysfunction in multiple sclerosis. J Urol 2000;164:2010–2013. **(III, B)**

8. Tarcan T, Park K, Goldstein I, et al: Histomorphometric analysis of age-related structural changes in human clitoral cavernosal tissue. J Urol 1999;161:940–943. **(III, B)**

9. Sipski ML, Alexander CJ, Rosen RC: Sexual response in women with spinal cord injuries: implications for our understanding of the able-bodied. J Sex Marital Ther 1999;25:11–22. **(III, B)**

10. Smith SM, O'Keane V, Muray R: Sexual dysfunction in patients taking conventional antipsychotic medication. Br J Psychiatry 2002;181:49–55. **(IIa, B)**

11. Meston CM, Frohlich PF: The neurobiology of sexual function. Arch Gen Psychiatry 2000;57:1012–1030. **(IV, C)**

12. Gelenberg AJ, Laukes C, McGahuey C, et al: Mirtazapine substitution in SSRI-induced sexual dysfunction. J Clin Psychiatry 2000;61:356–360. **(IIb, B)**

13. Lobo RA, Rosen RC, Yang H-M: Comparative effects of oral esterified estrogens with and without methyltestosterone on endocrine profiles and dimensions of sexual function in postmenopausal women with hypoactive sexual desire. Fertil Steril 2003;79:1342–1352. **(Ib, A)**

14. Bergmark K, Avall-Lundqvist E, Dickman PW: Vaginal changes and sexuality in women with a history of cervical cancer. N Engl J Med 1999;340:1383–1389. **(III, B)**

15. Basson R, Berman J, Burnett A, et al: Report of the International Consensus Development conference on female sexual dysfunction: definitions and classifications. J Urol 2000;163:888. **(IV, C)**

16. Basson R: Female sexual response: the role of drugs in the management of sexual dysfunction. Obstet Gynecol 2001;98:350–353. **(IV, C)**

17. Annon JS: Behavioral Treatment of Sexual Problems. San Francisco, Harper & Row, 1976. **(IV, C)**

18. Sommers F, Caspers H, Esders K, et al: Measurement of vaginal and minor labial oxygen tension for the evaluation of female sexual function. J Urol 2001;165:1181–1184. **(IIb, B)**

19. Berman JR, Berman L, Goldstein I: Female sexual dysfunction: incidence, path physiology, evaluation, and treatment options, Urology 1999;54:385–391. **(IV, C)**

20. Taylor JE, Rosen RC, Leiblum SR: Self-report assessment for female sexual function: psychometric evaluation of the Brief Index of Sexual Functioning for Women (BISF-W). Arch Sex Behav 1994;23:627–643. **(III, B)**

21. Rosen RC, Brown C, Helman J, et al: The Female Sexual Function Index (FSFI): a multidimensional self-report instrument for the assessment of female sexual function. J Sex Marital Ther 2000;26:191–208. **(III, B)**

22. Quirk FH, Heiman J, Rosen R, et al: Development of a sexual function questionnaire for clinical trials of female sexual dysfunction. J Womens Health Gend Based Med 2002;11:277–289. **(III, B)**

23. Rosen RC: Assessment of female sexual dysfunction: review of validated methods. Fertil Steril 2002;77:S89–S93. **(IV, C)**

24. Derogatis LR: The Derogatis Interview for Sexual Functioning (DISF/DISF-R): an introductory report. J Sex Marital Ther 1997;23:291–296. **(III, B)**

25. Derogates LR, Burnett A, Heiman J, et al: Development and continuing validation of the Female Sexual Distress Scale (FSDS). Presented at 4th annual Female Sexual Function Forum. Boston, Mass, Oct 29, 2001. **(III, B)**

26. Shifren JL, Braunstein GD, Simon JA, et al: Transdermal testosterone treatment in women with impaired sexual function after oophorectomy. N Engl J Med 2000;343:682–688. **(Ib, A)**

27. Sarrel P, Dobay B, Wiita B: Estrogen and estrogen-androgen replacement in postmenopausal women dissatisfied with estrogen-only therapy. J Reprod Med 2000;43:847–856. **(IIb, B)**

28. Arlt W, Callies F, Van Vlijmen JC, et al: Dehydroepiandrosterone replacement in women with adrenal insufficiency. N Engl J Med 1999;341:1013–1020. **(Ib, A)**

29. Berman JR, Adhikari SP, Goldstein I: Anatomy and physiology of female sexual function and dysfunction: classification, evaluation, and treatment options. Eur Urol 2000;38:20–29. **(IV, C)**

30. Vemulapalli S, Kurowski S: Sildenafil relaxes rabbit clitoral corpus cavernosum. Life Sci 2000;67:23–29. **(IIb, B)**

31. Kaplan SA, Reis RB, Kown IJ, et al: Safety and efficacy of sildenafil in postmenopausal women with sexual dysfunction. Urology 1999;53:481–486. **(IIb, B)**

32. Caruso S, Intelisano G, Lupo L, Agnello C: Premenopausal women affected by sexual arousal disorder treated with sildenafil: a double-blind, cross-over, placebo-controlled study. Br J Obstet Gynecol 2001;108:623–628. **(Ib, A)**

33. Wiseman OJ, Dasgupta R, Fowler CJ: A randomized double-blind, cross-over, placebo-controlled trial of sildenafil in neurogenic female sexual dysfunction. BJU Int 2003;91:89. **(Ib, A)**

34. Rosen RC, Phillips NA, Gendrano NC III, et al: Oral phentolamine and female sexual arousal disorder: a pilot study. J Sex Marital Ther 1999;25:137–144. **(IIb, B)**

35. Josefson D: FDA approves device for female sexual dysfunction. BMJ 2000;320:1427. **(IV, C)**

36. Center for Drug Evaluation and Research: Female sexual dysfunction: clinical development of drug products for treatment. Rockville, Md, U.S. Department of Health and Human Services, May 2000. **(IV, C)**

# Chapter 6

# Alternative Medicine

Jennifer S. Gell, MD

**KEY POINTS**

- Complementary and alternative medicines are commonly used to treat disorders throughout reproductive age.
- Complementary medicines must be used carefully and thoughtfully owing to herb-drug and herb-herb interactions.
- Chasteberry is used to treat premenstrual syndrome.
- Evening primrose oil may diminish cyclic mastalgia symptoms.
- Phytoestrogens, black cohosh, wild yam, and dong quai are proposed to improve menopausal symptoms.

Complementary and alternative medicine (CAM) is becoming widely practiced within the United States. By conservative estimates, Americans spend approximately $27 billion per year on complementary and alternative medication. A therapy is called complementary when it is used in addition to conventional treatment, and alternative when it replaces conventional treatment. Women especially are turning more often to CAM therapies to treat common ailments. While many herbal therapies offer therapeutic benefits, they are not without risk. It is important for women and their health care providers to have information regarding common herbal therapies, their potential risks, and possible interactions with both conventional and alternative treatment modalities.

## COMMONLY USED THERAPIES

### St. John's Wort (*Hypericum perforatum*)

St. John's wort is a flowering plant found in Europe, Asia, Africa, Australia, and North and South America. The yellow flowers were traditionally gathered for the feast of St. John the Baptist. The leaves and flowers of this plant contain hypericin, pseudohypericin, hyperforin, flavonoids, and other components. Hypericin and hyperforin appear to be the active components. St. John's wort is most often made from the flower and based in an ethanolic extract standardized to 0.3% hypericin. Recently, it has been questioned whether hypericin is the main active ingredient, since it does not cross the blood-brain barrier. Hyperforin actually may be the key component. Hyperforin, however, is less stable, and its concentration may vary considerably in St. John's wort. Importantly, significant differences in concentrations exist depending on when and how St. John's wort is harvested.

St. John's wort is commonly used for treatment of depression. St. John's wort appears to act similarly to selective serotonin reuptake inhibitors (SSRIs) in that it decreases the rate of reuptake of monoamine neurotransmitters such as serotonin.[1]

Multiple studies have been performed evaluating *Hypericum* extracts for treatment of depression. A German group looked at an extract of *Hypericum* as compared to placebo for treatment of mild-to-moderate depression.[2] The treatment group showed an improvement in depression scores as compared with the placebo group, with no adverse effects in either group. Other groups have evaluated *Hypericum* as compared with SSRIs in the treatment of mild-to-moderate depression. In an evaluation of the LI 160 extract of *Hypericum* as compared with sertraline, clinical response was noted in 47% of patients receiving *Hypericum* and 40% of patients receiving sertraline.[3] In a study investigating the use of *Hypericum* extract as compared with fluoxetine,[4] both treatment groups demonstrated improvement in multiple depression scoring systems. Several meta-analyses similarly suggest that in patients with mild-to-moderate depression, St. John's wort has similar efficacy to low-dose tricyclic antidepressants but may be better tolerated.[5,6]

St John's wort, however, does not appear to significantly improve moderate to severe depression. In a randomized, placebo-controlled study evaluating the use of LI 160 as compared with sertraline and placebo for the treatment of moderate-to-severe depression, no difference in depression scores was detected, although a higher rate of full response was noted in the patents with a lower initial depression score.[7,8] Although St. John's wort may not treat moderate-to-severe depression as evaluated by depression scoring scales, most patients using St. John's wort have mild-to-moderate symptoms and therefore may experience some improvement in mood (Figs. 6-1 and 6-2).

Researchers have evaluated St. John's wort in premenstrual syndrome (PMS). Women with PMS note the appearance of symptoms late in the luteal phase with resolution after menses. Mood disorders are frequently reported also. A pilot study was performed evaluating the use of daily *Hypericum* extract for the treatment of PMS.[9] Women completed a daily symptom ratings calendar for one cycle before starting daily *Hypericum* tablets standardized to 900 μg hypericin. Symptoms were rated daily and then scored after one and two cycles of treatment. Overall premenstrual scores decreased by 51% between baseline and completion of the trial, suggesting that *Hypericum* may be useful as a treatment for PMS.

The recommended daily dose is 2 to 4 g St. John's wort or 0.2 to 1 mg hypericin. Adverse effects include photosensitivity, rash, nausea, fatigue, and restlessness.[10] Although well tolerated, St. John's wort appears to have significant drug-herb interactions. St. John's wort induces cytochrome P-450 enzymes and increases the metabolism of protease inhibitors, oral contraceptives, warfarin, digoxin, and theophyline.[11] St. John's wort decreases cyclosporine levels, resulting in organ transplantation

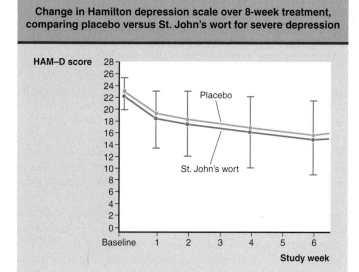

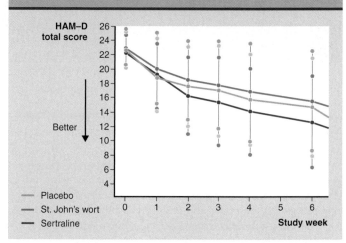

**Figure 6-1   Change in Hamilton Depression Scale (HAM-D) score over 8-week treatment period comparing placebo with St. John's wort for severe depression.** (From Shelton RC, Keller MB, Gelenber A, et al: Effectiveness of St. John's wort in major depression: a randomized controlled trial. JAMA 2001;285:1978–1986.)

**Figure 6-2   Change in Hamilton Depression Scale (HAM-D) score over 6-week treatment period comparing placebo with St. John's wort or sertraline for severe depression.** (From Hypericum Depression Trial Study Group: Effect of *Hypericum perforatum* [St. John's wort] in major depressive disorder: a randomized controlled trial. JAMA 2002;287:1807–1814.)

rejection.[12] Finally, St. John's wort should not be used during pregnancy or lactation.

### Chasteberry (*Vitex agnus-castus*)

Chasteberry is commonly used for the treatment of PMS symptoms. The active part of the chaste tree is the fruit. The active constituents of chasteberries are iridoid glycosides, flavonoids, and the diterpenes. The active iridoids are aucubin and agnoside, and many chasteberry extracts are standardized to contain 6% agnoside. Chasteberries also contain several essential fatty acids including oleic acid, linolenic acid, palmitic acid, and stearic acid.[13]

The mechanism of action of chasteberry seems to be through indirect effects on neurotransmitters and hormones. Chasteberry extracts may have agonistic activity at the pituitary dopamine (D2) receptors. At high doses, chasteberry may suppress prolactin release.[14] Chasteberry also appears to selectively bind to the β-estrogen receptor (β-ER). The isolated ligand for the β-ER appears to be linoleic acid.[15] Linoleic acid has been shown to stimulate mRNA β-ER expression in a breast cancer cell line.

Chasteberry has been evaluated for the treatment of PMS. In one large, nonrandomized trial, over 1600 German women used chasteberry extract for treatment of PMS.[16] After 3 months of treatment, 81% of women reported feeling much better than at the start of treatment. Another group investigated *Vitex agnus-castus* extract Ze 440 in 50 women with PMS.[17] These women took one tablet daily containing 20 mg native extract for three menstrual cycles. The 43% of the women who continued the study responded with a reduction of at least 50% on the Moos menstrual distress questionnaire. Symptoms gradually recurred after cessation of treatment; however, a difference from baseline did persist for up to three additional cycles. No difference

was seen between women taking or not taking oral contraceptives. However, this group was also not compared with a placebo group. More recently, a prospective, randomized, placebo-controlled study evaluated daily treatment of chasteberry fruit extract Ze 440 in 170 women with PMS.[18] Women rated six symptoms using a visual analog scale. After 3 months of treatment, women receiving chasteberry extract noted a greater than 50% improvement in their symptoms.

Chasteberry extracts are generally well tolerated. Some patients complain of gastrointestinal (GI) upset, headache, nausea, itching, and rash. Some patients also complain of fatigue. Women may note irregular bleeding when chasteberry is first started. Chasteberry should be avoided during pregnancy, since it may have uterine stimulating properties. In addition, it should be avoided during lactation because it appears to be a dopamine agonist and may inhibit prolactin release.

### Evening Primrose Oil (*Oenothera biennis*)

Evening primrose oil is obtained from the seed of *Oenothera biennis*. It contains 2% to 16% γ-linolenic acid, 65% to 88% linoleic acid, and vitamin E. Evening primrose oil has been suggested as a treatment option for women with cyclic mastalgia. The hypothesis is that women with cyclic mastalgia have an altered proportion of fatty acid esters as compared with unaffected women. Therefore, one therapeutic option is supplemental fatty acid intake. Australian data suggest evening primrose oil at a dose of 1000 mg three times daily improves cyclic mastalgia.[19] In addition, a cohort of 66 Australian women treated with gamolenic acid demonstrated a marked reduction in cyclic mastalgia after 6 months of treatment.[20]

Evening primrose oil is generally well tolerated orally, but nausea, indigestion, and headache have been reported. Usually these side effects are easily tolerated and do not result in discontinuation of therapy. Evening primrose oil may have anticoagulant effects owing to its γ-linolenic acid component. Therefore, evening primrose oil may theoretically increase anticoagulant or antiplatelet effects of other drugs such as aspirin, nonsteroidal anti-inflammatory drugs, clopidogrel, heparin, warfarin, and enoxaparin. Caution should be used with concomitant use of other herbal products with coumarin activity such as dong quai. Finally, evening primrose oil should not be used in schizophrenic patients being treated with phenothiazine drugs because this combination has been reported to cause seizures.[13]

### Ginkgo

Ginkgo is derived from the leaf of *Ginkgo biloba*. *Ginkgo biloba*, which is also known as the maidenhair or fossil tree, is the oldest living species of tree. Ginkgo leaf and its extracts contain several active constituents including flavonoids, terpenoids, and organic acids. The terpenoids include ginkgolides A, B, C, M, and J, and bilobalide. The major flavonoids are kaempferol, quercetin, and isohamnetine derivatives. Ginkgo leaf flavonoids have antioxidant and free radical scavenging effects as seen by their ability to inhibit the expression of inducible nitric oxide synthase.[13] Ginkgolide B competitively inhibits platelet activating factor (PAF) in laboratory animals. PAF inhibition decreases platelet aggregation and protects against hypoxia-induced neuronal injury as well as decreasing free radical production.[21] This effect on platelet aggregation may also increase the risk of spontaneous bleeding. One case has been reported of excessive bleeding requiring transfusion after laparoscopy.[22] Gingko extracts should be used cautiously in patients taking other anticoagulant or antiplatelet drugs. Ginkgo extracts also contain ginkgotoxin, a neurotoxin. Ginkgotoxin is more concentrated in gingko seed than in gingko leaf; therefore, it is unlikely to be at high enough concentration to cause toxicity.[23] However, there are reports of patients having seizures who were previously well controlled on antiseizure medications.[24] Therefore, patients with seizure disorders or taking other medications known to lower seizure threshold should avoid using ginkgo extracts. Other side effects of oral ginkgo supplements include GI upset, headache, dizziness, constipation, and allergic skin reactions.

While gingko leaf is most commonly used for dementia, ginkgo has been used to treat sexual dysfunction caused by SSRIs. In one open trial, ginkgo extracts improved sexual response in women taking SSRI antidepressants.[25] A more recent placebo-controlled, randomized trial did not demonstrate a difference after 8 weeks of therapy between placebo and ginkgo groups. In fact, both treatment arms showed improvement in sexual function.[26] Ginkgo should be used cautiously in patients with infertility, since it might interfere with oocyte fertilization.[27]

### Dong Quai

Dong quai, which is extracted from the root of *Angelica sinesis*, is a Chinese herb often used to treat gynecologic conditions such as menstrual disorders and menopausal symptoms. The primary active ingredients are coumarin derivatives including psoralen, osthol, and bergapten. Osthol appears to inhibit platelet aggregation. Psoralen and bergapten are photosensitizing, which

may result in phototoxicity with external application of dong quai. Bergapten and other dong quai constituents have been shown to be carcinogenic; however, what concentration or duration of use is unsafe is unknown.[13] Because of the coumarin derivatives, there is a theoretical risk of bleeding. Therefore, dong quai should be used cautiously or not at all in patients taking other anticoagulants or antiplatelet drugs.

It has been suggested that dong quai has estrogenic effects resulting in improvement in menopausal symptoms. A randomized, placebo-controlled study evaluated the effects of dong quai 4.5 g/day as compared with placebo for treatment of hot flashes (hot flushes) and menopausal side effects. Patients were evaluated at 6, 12, and 24 weeks. Both dong quai and placebo decreased hot flashes with no differences noted in endometrial thickness, vaginal maturation index, or Kupperman index.[28] The Kupperman index classifies 11 menopausal symptoms including vasomotor symptoms, nervousness, insomnia, melancholia, paresthesias, formication, fatigue, headache, palpitation, arthralgia, and vertigo. Therefore, dong quai does not alleviate menopausal symptoms. When investigators in Houston evaluated the estrogenicity of dong quai through its ability to proliferate MCF-7 breast cancer cells in vitro,[29] dong quai significantly stimulated the human breast cell cancer line. Dong quai did not, however, activate either the α- or β-ER and did not increase uterine weight in treated mice. At this time, dong quai should be used cautiously or not at all in patients with known breast cancer.

### Phytoestrogens

Phytoestrogens are one of the main alternatives women use for estrogen replacement therapy. Phytoestrogens are diphenolic compounds found in grains, legumes, and grasses. Because they possess a phenolic ring, they are able to bind to estrogen receptors specifically, binding with greater affinity to β-ER than to α-ER. Even though these compounds bind to the estrogen receptor, they are much weaker than human estrogens. Phytoestrogens are classified into three groups: isoflavones, lignans, and coumestans. Isoflavones are plant sterol molecules found in soy and legumes (Fig. 6-3). Lignans are a constituent of the plant cell wall and are found in grains and the husks of seeds such as flaxseed. Coumestans are found in sprouts such as alfalfa and red clover.[30]

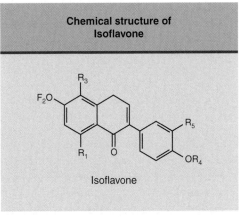

**Chemical structure of Isoflavone**

Isoflavone

**Figure 6-3   Chemical structure of isoflavone.**

Soybeans, which contain 1 to 2 mg of isoflavone per gram of soy protein, are the richest food source of isoflavones. The amount of phytoestrogen in a soy product depends on how it is processed. Soy milk and soy flour contain less phytoestrogen than do soybeans. Some soy capsules and powders have no remaining active phytoestrogen after being processed with an alcohol extract. Soybeans contain three different types of isoflavones: genistein, daidzein, and glycitein. Red clover extracts also contain genistein and daidzein in addition to their methylated precursors, formononetin and biochanin (Fig. 6-4).

Genistein has 1/400 to 1/1000 the potency of 17β-estradiol and binds with greater affinity to β-ER than to α-ER. Genistein may act as either an estrogen or antiestrogen depending on the tissue type and amount of endogenous circulating estrogens.

Hot flashes and night sweats are the most bothersome symptoms of menopause. The severity of symptoms, however, differs among national groups. Only 10% to 25% of Asian women report hot flashes as compared with 70% to 80% of American women. Since Asian women have a much greater dietary intake of soy, there has been interest in evaluating the efficacy of phytoestrogens for treating menopausal symptoms (Fig. 6-5; Table 6-1).

An early study evaluated the effects of a short-term, phytoestrogen-rich diet on menopausal symptoms. Women were randomized to either a diet rich in phytoestrogens or to a regular diet with instructions to avoid specific soy products and flax seed. The phytoestrogen-rich diet included 80 g of

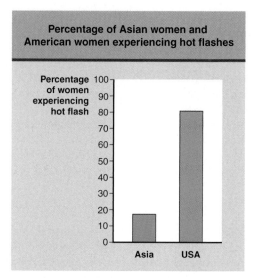

Figure 6-5    Percentage of Asian women and American women experiencing hot flashes.

tofu daily (containing approximately 75 mg/g daidzein and 200 mg/g genistein), one teaspoon of miso (40 mg/g daidzein and 35 mg/g genistein), and two teaspoons of ground flax seed (4 mg/g lignans). Throughout the study period, women recorded the frequency and severity of their menopausal symptoms. Symptoms improved in both groups with a significantly greater improvement in vaginal dryness and hot flashes in the phytoestrogen group as compared with the control group.[31] However, another investigator found no significant difference between frequency of hot flashes or night sweats in women randomized to diets containing either isoflavone-rich soy protein (80.4 mg/day) or isoflavone-poor soy protein (4.4 mg/day) or a control diet containing whey protein. Albertazzi performed a double-blind, placebo-controlled trial in which 104 women were randomized to either 60 g of isolated soy protein daily consisting of 76 mg of isoflavone or to 60 g of casein as a placebo. Women recorded both the number and severity of hot flushes and night sweats during the 12-week study period. Women in the isoflavone group demonstrated a 45% decrease in hot flashes as compared with a 30% decrease reported by women in the placebo group.[32] Albertazzi then evaluated the change in serum levels of isoflavones after 60 g/day soy supplementation. Marked

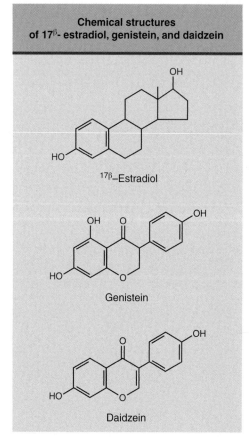

Figure 6-4    Chemical structures of 17β-estradiol, genistein, and daidzein.

| | Amount (cup) | Isoflavone (mg) | Calories (kcal) | Fat (g) |
|---|---|---|---|---|
| **Table 6-1** Isoflavone Content of Soy Products | | | | |
| Low-fat tofu | ½ | 35 | 60 | 2 |
| Regular tofu | ½ | 35 | 110 | 6 |
| Soy milk | 1 | 30 | 130–150 | 4 |
| Low-fat soy milk | 1 | 20 | 105 | 2 |
| Soy nuts | ¼ | 60 | 195 | 9 |

From Bieber EJ, Gell JS: Complementary and alternative medicine in the perimenopause and menopause. In Yuan CS, Bieber EJ (eds): Textbook of Complementary and Alternative Medicine. New York, Parthenon, 2003, pp 319–332.

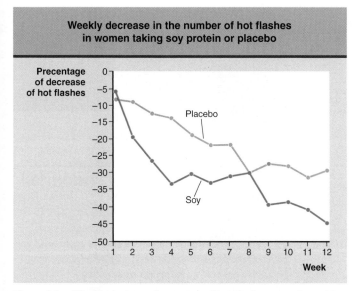

**Figure 6-6    Weekly decrease in number of hot flashes experienced by women taking soy protein or placebo.** (From Albertazzi P, Pansini F, Bonaccorsi G, et.al: The effect of dietary soy supplementation on hot flush. Obstet Gynecol 1998;91:6–11.)

increases were seen in genistein, daidzein, and equol; however, these marked increases did not correlate with decreased vasomotor symptoms[33] (Figs. 6-6 and 6-7).

A review of the literature on phytoestrogens and menopausal symptoms was performed. Trials were eligible if they were placebo controlled, reported hot flash frequency, and lasted at least 4 weeks. Neither the soy food nor the soy extract trials demonstrated improvement in menopausal symptoms. Reasons for no benefit may be inadequate amount of soy

ingested for a response or poor bioavailability of phytoestrogen preparations.[34]

Another source of isoflavones is red clover. Unlike soy, red clover is not a dietary staple and if ingested at all may be consumed in small quantities as a flavoring. Standardized extracts of red clover have been developed to treat menopausal symptoms. A randomized controlled trial evaluated the use of Promensil (82 mg of total isoflavones per day) with Rimostil (57 mg of total isoflavones per day) to placebo. After 12 weeks of therapy, all three groups showed a similar decrease in daily hot flashes. Women taking Promensil reported a more rapid reduction of hot flashes as compared with placebo; Rimostil did not appear to have this effect[35] (Fig. 6-8).

Since isoflavones have estrogenic effects, one concern with long-term use is their ability to stimulate the endometrium. Wilcox found an increase in the maturation index in women supplementing their diet with soy flour, red clover sprouts, and linseed. However, other studies have not demonstrated any increase in vaginal maturation index with increasing isoflavone supplementation. No difference has been seen in endometrial thickness after treatment with either placebo or soy supplementation. Finally, endometrial histology has not been reported to change after ingestion of an isoflavone-enriched diet.[36]

A final concern is the use of phytoestrogens in women with breast cancer. Many newly menopausal women are diagnosed with breast cancer and are advised to avoid the use of estrogen therapy, turning instead to soy products as an alternative treatment for hot flashes. Patients beginning tamoxifen therapy may experience significant worsening of vasomotor symptoms. One trial enrolled 177 breast cancer survivors in a randomized, double-blind, crossover trial in which they consumed 150 mg/day of soy (equivalent to approximately three glasses of soy milk). Soy was no more effective than placebo in diminishing hot flashes. Unfortunately, minimal clinical safety data exist

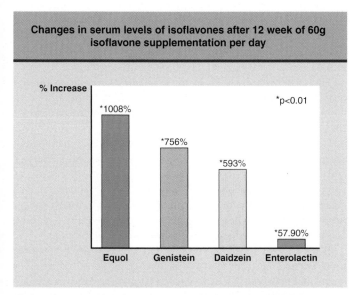

**Figure 6-7    Change in serum level of isoflavone after 12 weeks of isoflavone supplementation 60 g/day in women with moderate to severe hot flashes.** (From Albertazzi P, Pansini F, Bottazzi M, et al: Dietary soy supplementation and phytoestrogen levels. Obstet Gynecol 1999;94:229–231.)

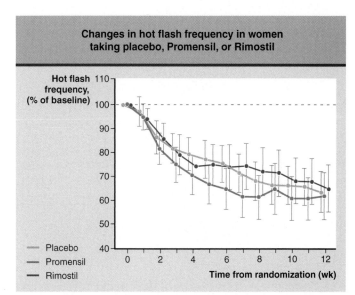

**Figure 6-8    Change in hot flash frequency over 12-week treatment period comparing placebo, Promensil, and Rimostil.** (From Tice JA, Ettinger B, Ensrud K, et al: Phytoestrogen supplements for the treatment of hot flashes—the isoflavone clover extract [ICE] study: a randomized controlled trial. JAMA 2003;290:207–214.)

regarding the use of phytoestrogens and risk of recurrence of breast cancer.[37]

### Wild Yam (*Dioscorea villosa*)

Wild yam root and tubers are known to contain diosgenin, a steroid precursor used in early commercial production of steroid hormones. For this reason, wild yam extracts have been used topically to treat menopausal symptoms. However, conversion of diosgenin to estrogen, progesterone, or any other steroid does not occur in the human body. Diosgenin may enhance estradiol binding to estrogen receptors and may stimulate growth of mammary tissue.[13] A double-blind, placebo-controlled, crossover study evaluated the effects of wild yam cream on menopausal symptoms.[38] Women were treated with either active or placebo cream for 12 weeks in random order and instructed to keep a diary of symptoms. Hormone assays were performed on both serum and saliva samples. Both study groups showed minimal improvement on flushing severity and number with no significant difference between wild yam extract and placebo. After 3 months of therapy, there was no change in FSH, estradiol, or serum or salivary progesterone. Therefore, while wild yam extract appears to be well tolerated without significant side effects, it also does not appear to be beneficial for the treatment of menopausal symptoms (Fig. 6-9).

### Black Cohosh (*Cimicifuga racemosa* Rhizome)

Black cohosh is a herb native to Eastern North America and traditionally has been used by Native Americans to treat

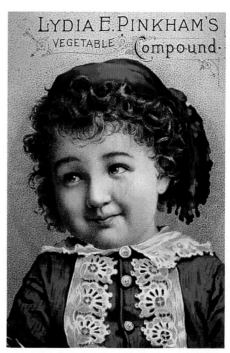

Figure 6-10    Label from Lydia Pinkham's Vegetable Compound.

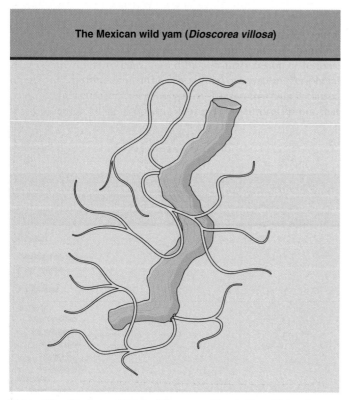

**The Mexican wild yam (*Dioscorea villosa*)**

Figure 6-9    **Mexican wild yam (*Dioscorea villosa*).** (From Bieber EJ, Gell JS: Complementary and alternative medicine in the perimenopause and menopause. In Yuan CS, Bieber EJ [eds]: Textbook of Complementary and Alternative Medicine. New York, Parthenon, 2003, pp 319–332.)

gynecologic conditions including menopause. Black cohosh was commercially available during the 19th century as Lydia Pinkham's Vegetable Compound (Fig. 6-10) and during the early 20th century as Huntington's 11, and currently is available as Remifemin.

The primary active constituents are flavonoids and triterpenes such as 27-deoxyactein.[13] Remifemin is standardized to contain 1 mg of 27-deoxyactein per 20 mg tablet. The estrogenic activity remains unclear. Black cohosh did not demonstrate estrogenic activity in a study utilizing several different assay systems.[39] Another study evaluated the effects of 17β-estradiol as compared with *Cimicifuga racemosa* extract BNO 1055 on ovariectomized rats.[40] While estradiol-treated rats demonstrated increased uterine weight and expression of progesterone receptor, no such effects were seen in the *Cimicifuga racemosa*–treated rats. In an additional study, black cohosh did not appear to induce the growth of a human breast cancer cell line or activate the α- or β-ER.[29]

Clinically, black cohosh has been used to treat menopausal symptoms. German investigators reported decreased frequency and severity of hot flashes in women taking black cohosh as compared with placebo.[41] In another trial evaluating black cohosh as treatment for menopausal symptoms in breast cancer survivors most of whom were on tamoxifen therapy,[42] placebo and black cohosh reduced hot flashes to the same extent.

Black cohosh appears to be safe and well tolerated; however, there are no long-term safety data. Therefore, the recommended length of treatment is not to exceed 6 months. Side effects are limited but include GI upset, bradycardia, headache, and nausea. Black cohosh may also cause uterine contractility and should not be used during pregnancy. Black cohosh should not be confused with blue cohosh, which has potent vasoconstrictive constituents.[13]

**Table 6-2**
**Possible Interactions Between Conventional Medicines and Botanicals**

| Herb | Relevant Pharmacologic Effects | Perioperative Concerns | Preoperative Discontinuation |
|---|---|---|---|
| Gingko | Inhibits platelet-activation factor | Potential to increase risk of bleeding especially in combination with other anticoagulants or antiplatelet drugs | At least 36 hours before surgery |
| St. John's wort | Decreases rate of uptake of monoamine neurotransmitters such as serotonin | Induction of cytochrome P-450 enzymes affecting cyclosporine, warfarin, steroids, digoxin | At least 5 days before surgery |
| Evening primrose oil | May have anticoagulant effects owing to its γ-linolenic component | May increase anticoagulant or antiplatelet effects of other drugs | No data |
| Dong quai | Primary active ingredients are coumarin derivatives | May increase anticoagulant or antiplatelet effects of other drugs | No data |

## HERBAL MEDICINES AND PREOPERATIVE CARE

With the ever-increasing use of herbal products, presurgical patients are also likely to be ingesting herbal medications. In a recent survey, 32% of patients in an ambulatory surgical setting admitted to using herbal medications; however, more than 70% did not report herbal medications during a perioperative evaluation. Because of potential interactions with conventional medications causing increased risk during surgical care, health care professionals should specifically ask about use of botanical products[43] (Table 6-2).

## REFERENCES

1. Perovic S, Muller WEG: Pharmacological profile of hypericum extract: effect of serotonin uptake by postsynaptic receptors. Arztl Forsch 1995;45:1145–1148. **(IIb, B)**
2. Kalb R, Trautmann-Sponsel RD, Kieser M: Efficacy and tolerability of hypericum extract WS 5572 versus placebo in mildly to moderately depressed patients: a randomized double-blind multicenter trial. Pharmacopsychiatry 2001;34:96–103. **(Ib, A)**
3. Brenner R, Axbel V, Madhusoodanan S, et al: Comparison of an extract of hypericum (LI 160) and sertraline in the treatment of depression: a double-blind, randomized pilot study. Clin Ther 2000;22:411–419. **(Ib, A)**
4. Behnke K, Jensen GS, Graubaum HG, et al: *Hypericum perforatum* versus fluoxetine in the treatment of mild to moderate depression. Adv Ther 2002;19:43–52. **(IIa, B)**
5. Linde K, Ramirez G, Mulrow CD, et al: St. John's wort for depression. BMJ 1996;313:253–258. **(Ia, A)**
6. Gaster B, Holroyd J: St. John's wort for depression: a systematic review. Arch Intern Med 2000;160:152–156. **(Ia, A)**
7. Shelton RC, Keller MB, Gelenber A, et al: Effectiveness of St. John's wort in major depression: a randomized controlled trial. JAMA 2001;285:1978–1986. **(Ib, A)**
8. Hypericum Depression Trial Study Group: Effect of *Hypericum perforatum* (St. John's wort) in major depressive disorder: a randomized controlled trial. JAMA 2002;287:1807–1814. **(Ib, A)**
9. Stevinson C, Ernst E: A pilot study of *Hypericum perforatum* for the treatment of premenstrual syndrome. BJOG 2000;107:870–876. **(IIa, B)**
10. Ernst E, Rand JI, Barnes J, et al: Adverse effects profile of herbal anti-depressant St. John's wort. Eur J Clin Pharmacol 1998;54:589–594. **(III, B)**
11. Baede-van Dijk PA, van Galen E, Lekkerkerker JF: Drug interactions of *Hypericum perforatum* are potentially hazardous. Ned Tijdschr Geneesk 2000;144:811–812. **(III, B)**
12. Ernst E: St. John's wort supplements endanger the success of organ transplantation. Arch Surg 2002;137:316–319. **(III, B)**
13. Available at http://www.naturaldatabase.com. Accessed 3/26/05. **(III, B)**
14. Jarry H, Leonhardt S, Gorkow C, et al: In vitro prolactin but not LH and FSH release is inhibited by compounds in extracts of *Agnus castus*: direct evidence for a dopaminergic principle by the dopamine receptor assay. Exp Clin Endocrinol 1994;102:448–454. **(III, B)**
15. Liu J, Burdette JE, Sun Y, et al: Isolation of linoleic acid as an estrogenic compound from the fruits of *Vitex agnus-castus* L. (chaste-berry). Phytomedicine 2004;11:18–23. **(III, B)**
16. Loch EG, Selle H, Boblitz N: Treatment of premenstrual syndrome with a phytopharmaceutical formulation containing *Vitex agnus castus*. J Womens Health Gend Based Med 2000;9:315–320. **(IIa, B)**
17. Berger D, Schaffner W, Schrader E, et al: Efficacy of *Vitex agnus castus* L. extract Ze 440 in patients with pre-menstrual syndrome (PMS). Arch Gynecol Obstet 2000;264:150–153. **(IIa, B)**
18. Schellenberg R: Treatment for the premenstrual syndrome with agnus castus fruit extract: prospective, randomized, placebo controlled study. BMJ 2001;322:134–137. **(Ib, A)**
19. Wetzig NR: Mastalgia: a 3 year Australian study. Aust N Z J Surg 1994;64:329–331. **(III, B)**
20. Cheung KL: Management of cyclical mastalgia in oriental women: pioneer experiment of using gamolenic acid (Efamast) in Asia. Aust N Z J Surg 1999;69:492–494. **(III, B)**
21. Brautigam MR, Blommaert FA, Verleye G, et al: Treatment of age-related memory complaints with *Gingko biloba* extract: a randomized double blind placebo-controlled study. Phytomedicine 1998;5:425–434. **(Ib, A)**
22. Fessenden JM, Wittenborn W, Clarke L: *Gingko biloba*: a case report of herbal medicine and bleeding postoperatively from a laparoscopic cholecystectomy. Am Surg 2001;67:33–35. **(III, B)**
23. Arenz A, Kelin M, Flehe K, et al: Occurrence of neurotoxic 4'-O-methylpyridoxine in ginkgo biloba leaves, ginkgo medications and Japanese ginkgo food. Planta Med 1996;62:548–551. **(III, B)**
24. Granger AS: Ginkgo biloba precipitating epileptic seizures. Age Aging 2001;30:523–525. **(III, B)**
25. Cohen AJ, Bartlik B: *Ginkgo biloba* for antidepressant-induced sexual dysfunction. J Sex Marital Ther 1998;24:139–143. **(III, B)**
26. Kang BJ, Lee SJ, Kim MD, et al: A placebo-controlled, double-blind trial of *Ginkgo biloba* for antidepressant-induced sexual dysfunction. Hum Psychopharmacol 2002;17:279–284. **(Ib, A)**
27. Ondrizek RR, Chan PJ, Patton WC, et al: An alternative medicine study of herbal effects on the penetration of zona-free hamster oocytes and the integrity of sperm deoxyribonucleic acid. Fertil Steril 1999;71:517–522. **(III, B)**
28. Hirata JD, Swierz LM, Zell B, et al: Does dong quai have estrogenic effects in postmenopausal women? A double-blind placebo-controlled trial. Fertil Steril 1997;68:981–986. **(Ib, A)**
29. Amato P, Christophe S, Mellon PL: Estrogenic activity of herbs commonly used as remedies for menopausal symptoms. Menopause 2002;9:145–150. **(III, B)**

30. Mackey R, Eden J: Phytoestrogens and the menopause. Climacteric 1998;1:302–308. **(III, B)**

31. Brzezinski A, Adlercruetz H, Shaoul R, et al: Short-term effects of phytoestrogen-rich diet on postmenopausal women. Menopause 1997; 2:89–94. **(Ib, A)**

32. Albertazzi P, Pansini F, Bonaccorsi G, et.al: The effect of dietary soy supplementation on hot flush. Obstet Gynecol 1998;91:6–11. **(Ib, A)**

33. Albertazzi P, Pansini F, Bottazzi M, et al: Dietary soy supplementation and phytoestrogen levels. Obstet Gynecol 1999;94:229–231. **(III, B)**

34. Kronenber G, Fugh-Berman A: Complementary and alternative medicine for menopausal symptoms: a review of randomized, controlled trials. Ann Intern Med 2002;137:805–813. **(Ia, A)**

35. Tice, JA, Ettinger B, Ensrud K, et al: Phytoestrogen supplements for the treatment of hot flashes—the isoflavone clover extract (ICE) study: a randomized controlled trial. JAMA 2003;290:207–214. **(Ib, A)**

36. Wilcox G, Wahlquist ML, Burger HG, Medley G: Oestrogenic effects of plant foods in postmenopausal women. BMJ 1990;301:905–906. **(III, B)**

37. Quella SK, Loprinzi CL, Barton DL et al: Evaluation of soy phytoestrogens for the treatment of hot flashes in breast cancer survivors: a North Central Cancer Treatment Group trial. J Clin Oncol 2000; 18:1068--1074. **(Ib, A)**

38. Komesaroff PA, Black CV, Cable V, et al: Effects of wild yam extract on menopausal symptoms, lipids and sex hormones in healthy menopausal women. Climacteric 2001;4:144–150. **(Ib, A)**

39. Lupu R, Mehmi I, Atlas E, et al: Black cohosh, a menopausal remedy, does not have estrogenic activity and does not promote breast cancer cell growth. Int J Oncol 2003;23:1407–1412. **(III, B)**

40. Seidlova-Wuttke D, Hesse O, Jarry H, et al: Evidence for selective estrogen receptor modulator activity in a black cohosh (*Cimicifuga racemosa*) extract: comparison with estradiol-17β. Eur J Endocrinol 2003;149:351–362. **(III, B)**

41. Stoll W: Phytopharmaceutical influences on atrophic vaginal epithelium: double-blind study on *Cimicifuga v* an estrogen preparation. Therapeutickon 1987;1:23–32. **(Ia, A)**

42. Jacobson JS, Troxel AB, Klaus EJ, et al: Randomized trial of black cohosh for the treatment of hot flashes among women with a history of breast cancer. J Clin Oncol 2001;19:2739–2745. **(Ia, A)**

43. Ang-Lee MK, Moss J, Yuan CS: Herbal medicines and perioperative care. JAMA 2001;286:208–216. **(III, B)**

# Domestic Violence

Judy C. Chang, MD, MPH

## KEY POINTS

- Intimate partner violence is prevalent among women in the United States.
- Intimate partner violence is associated with significant morbidity and mortality.
- Obstetricians and gynecologists have unique opportunities and responsibilities to address intimate partner violence.
- Asking about intimate partner violence in a supportive, nonjudgmental manner may increase awareness of the problem and offer a message of caring and support.
- Interventions for intimate partner violence should emphasize validation, information/resources, options, and autonomy.

## EPIDEMIOLOGY AND RISK FACTORS

Authors in the health care and social science literature have used many different terms to represent violence against women perpetrated by her partner. These include *domestic violence, spouse abuse, wife battering, battered women, partner abuse, wife abuse, partner violence,* and *women abuse.* Recognition of these variations and the resulting inconsistencies in prevalence and incidence estimations prompted the Centers for Disease Control and Prevention to develop and publish *Intimate Partner Violence Surveillance: Uniform Definitions and Recommended Data Elements.* An *intimate partner* includes current spouses, common-law spouses, nonmarital dating partners or boyfriends/ girlfriends, former marital partners, former nonmarital partners, opposite-sex partners, and same-sex partners. *Violence* includes physical violence, sexual violence, threats of physical/sexual violence, and psychological/emotional abuse.[1]

A recent report describing the findings of the National Violence Against Women Survey estimated that 1.5 million women experience physical or sexual violence from a current or former intimate partner each year in the United States. This same study revealed that approximately 25% to 30% of women in the United States experience intimate partner violence.[2] Of women seen in emergency departments (EDs) and in community clinics, 15% to 30% have a history of intimate partner violence.[3-5] Between 42% and 52% of female victims of intimate partner violence sustained an injury,[2,6] and 41% required medical care as a result of a physical assault by their intimate partner.[6]

National reports from the U.S. Department of Justice repeatedly find that intimate partner violence affects women of various ages, races, cultures, and socioeconomic levels. These reports find higher incidence rates of intimate partner violence among women in the reproductive-age group, particularly those between ages 19 and 29, compared to other age groups. Other characteristics associated with a higher incidence of intimate partner violence include lower socioeconomic and education status.[7-9] However, these reports relied on violent crime data and report univariate rates without comparing to nonvictims and without controlling for other factors. Reviews of studies that included less severe forms of intimate partner violence and compared factors between assaulted and nonassaulted groups show no consistent factors to predict a woman's risk for experiencing intimate partner violence.[10]

Among pregnant women who present for medical care, between 14% and 46% report a past history of intimate partner violence.[11-14] Prevalence rates of intimate partner violence that occur during pregnancy vary from 0.9% to 20.1%, with most estimates between 4% and 8%,[15-18] similar to prevalence rates for routinely screened conditions such as preeclampsia[19] and gestational diabetes.[20] Although most women who report experiencing violence during the pregnancy also experienced violence before the pregnancy, between 12.5% and 28.9% report that the violence first began during the pregnancy.[21-24]

Several studies examining homicide data reveal that between 30% and 66.9% of women who are killed are killed by a current or former intimate partner.[8,25-27] Of the women killed by their partner, two thirds reported physical assault prior to murder and 83% were threatened by the man who eventually killed them.[26] In one study, half of the couples in which murder occurred had a separation event (e.g., divorce, break-up, separation) preceding the murder. In another study, 44% of intimate partner violence murder victims had presented to an ED within 2 years of their murder.[28] Estimates of the cost of care for women suffering from partner abuse are generally higher than for the nonabused population. One study calculated $1.8 billion per year for direct medical care of injuries.[29] Another study found that female victims of violence were twice as likely to use outpatient health care services as were nonvictims, with 2.5 times the health care costs.[30] Another study examining female enrollees in a single large health plan showed that victims of intimate partner violence had significantly higher mental health service use and cost the health plan 92% more than a random sample of general female enrollees.[31] Additional factors that could also affect cost include days of work missed, utilization of police and/or ambulance services, and costs of care for children exposed to violence.

## CLINICAL FEATURES

Despite studies (Table 7-1) showing that between 41% and 51% of women who experience intimate partner violence suffer physical injury from their attacks,[2,6,8] only 28% of those who

**Table 7-1**
**Health Conditions Associated with Intimate Partner Violence**

| General and Mental Health Associations | Reproductive Health Associations |
| --- | --- |
| · Death | · Sexually transmitted infections |
| · Major and minor injuries | · HIV/AIDS |
| · Gastrointestinal disorders | · Delayed or lack of prenatal care |
| · Chronic pain disorders | · Low birthweight babies |
| · Depression | · Pelvic pain |
| · Anxiety disorders | · Unplanned/unwanted pregnancies |
| · Post-traumatic stress disorder | · Lack of reproductive control |
| · Suicide | |
| · Alcohol and substance abuse | |

were injured sought medical care.[2] Findings from the National Violence Against Women Survey revealed that the majority of women experiencing an injury from intimate partner violence described relatively minor injuries such as bruises, scratches, or welts. However, 11% suffered broken bones or dislocated joints, 8.8% reported lacerations or knife wounds, and 8.8% described head and spinal cord injuries.[2]

Because injuries are often absent or no longer apparent when a victim of intimate partner violence presents for care, more attention has been placed on other clinical signs of intimate partner violence. Studies have demonstrated associations between partner violence and other medical problems, including gastrointestinal disorders,[32] depression,[33] anxiety, chronic pain syndromes,[34] increased substance abuse, and suicidal ideation.[35]

The Commonwealth Fund's 1993 National Survey of Women's Health found that women who have experienced partner violence were more likely to report having gynecologic problems, sexually transmitted diseases, and pelvic pain.[36] Other studies have indicated an association between intimate partner violence and unintended pregnancies,[37,38] elective pregnancy terminations,[39,40] and delayed entry into prenatal care.[41] In one study surveying more than 1400 women, 23% of the women who reported intimate partner violence described experiencing either sexual assault or rape from their partner.[42] Additionally, one qualitative study revealed that abusive partners often controlled access to and use of contraception.[37] Two studies examining the prevalence of intimate partner violence among women seeking services from abortion clinics found that 30% to 39% report a history of intimate partner violence.[39,40] Additionally, women who experienced physical intimate partner violence were 1.8 times more likely (95% confidence interval [CI], 1.5–2.1) to have delayed entry into prenatal care compared to those who had not experienced violence.[41]

Studies examining associations between intimate partner violence and pregnancy outcomes have not shown consistent results. According to a review of published studies on pregnancy outcomes and intimate partner violence, only mean birthweight and low birthweight achieved statistical significance in more than one study.[43] Recent studies examining causes of maternal death, however, have shown that homicides represent between 13% and 25% of deaths in pregnant or recently pregnant women.[44–46] A statewide analysis in Maryland between 1993 and 1998 revealed that homicide was the leading cause of all

pregnancy-associated deaths (20.2%) with cardiovascular disorders representing the second most common cause of maternal death (19.4%).[46] Women who experienced intimate partner violence during pregnancy had three times higher odds of suffering a life-threatening attack compared to intimate partner violence victims who did not report experiencing abuse during pregnancy.[47] This study also suggested that intimate partner violence that occurs during pregnancy may represent a more severe and potentially dangerous type of partner abuse.

## DIAGNOSIS

In recognition of intimate partner violence as a public health problem, various advocacy groups and medical organizations have called for health care facilities and providers to develop and implement routine screening and intervention for violence. The Family Violence Prevention Fund released clinical guidelines that recommend screening "all women over the age of 14, whether or not symptoms or signs are present and whether or not the provider suspects abuse has occurred."[48] Medical organizations such as the American Medical Association,[49,50] American College of Obstetricians and Gynecologists,[51] the American College of Emergency Room Physicians,[52] the American Academy of Family Physicians,[53] and the American Nurses' Association[54] advocate similar recommendations for routine screening. Additionally, since 1992, the Joint Commission on Accreditation of Healthcare Organizations has required hospital departments and clinics to provide interventions for identified victims of intimate partner violence.[55]

Compared to other medical specialists, obstetrician/ gynecologists have an increased opportunity to identify and provide intervention for women at risk for intimate partner violence. A study in 1995 estimated that approximately 72% of women in the United States aged 15 to 44 received at least one reproductive health visit during that year.[56] Obstetrician/ gynecologists provide the majority of women's reproductive health services to women of all ages, as well as the majority of nonreproductive health care to women between ages 18 and 44.[57] According to a National Vital Statistics Report in 2000, the mean number of care visits received in pregnancy in 1995 was 12.3,[58] representing numerous opportunities for an obstetrician/ gynecologist to develop patient trust, address the issue of intimate partner violence, and, if needed, offer resources and intervention. Additionally, pregnancy is often regarded as an opportunity to address and intervene for a number of behavioral health issues, such as smoking,[59–64] substance abuse,[65] and depression.[66,67] Studies also suggest that pregnant patients may be more motivated to consider and initiate certain health behavioral changes.[62–65]

The majority of studies exploring how health providers address the topic of intimate partner violence focus on how often they ask. These studies show that rates of routine screening for intimate partner violence by health care providers range between 1% and 40%, with increased rates of screening among patients when the provider suspects abuse.[5,12,68–71] Among the reasons physicians cite for their reluctance to broach the subject with their patients are lack of training regarding how to address the issue, uncertainty in their ability to help, and frustration with their perception of the patient's lack of change or

### Table 7-2
### Barriers to Provider Screening and Patient Disclosure of Violence

| Provider Barriers to Screening | Patient Barriers to Disclosure |
|---|---|
| • Concern about offending patients or belief that asking invades family privacy<br>• Personal discomfort about discussing topic, lack of experience with abused patients, or concern about misdiagnosis<br>• Feeling powerless to help<br>• Frustration with patients who return to abuser<br>• Concern that identification may compromise the victim's ability to get/keep health insurance<br>• Fear for their own personal safety<br>• Cultural differences between patients and clinicians<br>• Reluctance to become involved with justice system<br>• Belief that abuse is not a medical problem<br>• Lack of awareness about violence against women<br>• Inadequate provider training<br>• Shortage of time during patient visits<br>• Underestimation of the prevalence of violence among their female patients<br>• Lack of 24-hour access to social worker<br>• Marginalization of practitioners who take leadership roles in dealing with family violence | • Fear of escalating violence<br>• Feelings of shame and embarrassment<br>• Fear of losing custody of their children<br>• Concern about confidentiality<br>• Fear of police involvement<br>• Sense of family duty or responsibilities<br>• Lack of access or partner preventing access to health care<br>• Denial of abuse<br>• Thinking abuse was controllable<br>• Feeling that physician could not help and that it was not part of the physician's job<br>• Negative physician attitude or negative past experience with a physician |

response[70-72] (Table 7-2). Compared to other medical specialties, such as family practice and internal medicine, obstetrician/gynecologists are most likely to perform routine screening for intimate partner violence,[71] and they are more likely to do so during the first prenatal visit.[68]

Female participants in many studies reported that they think providers should routinely ask about violence and provide information on community and legal resources.[73-76] One study by Rodriguez and colleagues suggested that if asked directly whether they have been abused, women who experience intimate partner violence will disclose.[77] However, several other studies found that many women experiencing current partner violence will deny their abuse even when asked.[76,78,79] Studies exploring patients' perceived barriers to disclosure of partner abuse showed that fear of escalating violence,[73,76,78,79] feelings of shame and embarrassment,[73,75,76,78] fear of losing the children, concern about confidentiality,[76,79] and fear of police involvement[76] were common reasons for denying the abuse (see Table 7-2).

## TREATMENT

### Asking About Intimate Partner Violence May Itself Be an Intervention

Multiple qualitative studies suggest that just the act of asking about intimate partner violence in a nonjudgmental and com-

passionate manner is helpful to women experiencing intimate partner violence.[78,80–82] Gerbert and colleagues interviewed women who had experienced intimate partner violence and who had helpful encounters with health care providers. The women described that providers were most helpful by validating and helping them recognize that the violence was a problem they did not deserve.[83,84] Chang and colleagues found that just asking about intimate partner violence not only helps women recognize the abuse, but also begins to decrease her isolation. This also allows the patient to feel that her provider cares about the situation.[82] As a result of these findings, experts have begun to recommend that health care providers view asking about intimate partner violence not merely as a screening tool, but also as potentially therapeutic in and of itself.[80,82,83,85–87]

### How to Ask About Intimate Partner Violence
The American College of Obstetricians and Gynecologists (ACOG) recommends asking all patients about intimate partner violence. They suggest that for women who are not pregnant, these inquiries occur at routine gynecologic visits, family planning visits, and preconception visits. Pregnant women can be asked at the first prenatal visit, at least once per trimester, and at the postpartum checkup.[51] Several screening tools have been developed to assist clinicians in assessing for intimate partner violence.[4,88–92] One of the most common assessment tools is the Abuse Assessment Screen, developed by the Nursing Research Consortium on Violence for use with pregnant patients (Table 7-3).[90] The ACOG has adapted this screening tool into three recommended questions preceded by an explanatory statement (Table 7-4).[93]

Some studies suggest that the style of asking about intimate partner violence may make a difference. Chang and colleagues found that while women identified positive consequences with

### Table 7-3
### Abuse Assessment Screen

1. Have you ever been emotionally or physically abused by your partner or someone important to you? (yes/no)
2. Within the last year, have you been hit, slapped, kicked, or otherwise physically hurt by someone? (yes/no)
   a. If yes, by whom? (husband/ex-husband/boyfriend/stranger/other/multiple)
   b. Number of times?
3. Since you've been pregnant, have you been hit, slapped, kicked, or otherwise physically hurt by someone? (yes/no)
   a. If yes, by whom? (husband/ex-husband/boyfriend/stranger/other/multiple)
   b. Number of times?
   c. Mark the area of injury on the body map.
   d. Score the most severe incident to the following scale:
      1 = Threats of abuse including use of a weapon
      2 = Slapping, pushing; no injuries and/or no lasting pain
      3 = Punching, kicking, bruises, cuts, and/or continuing pain
      4 = Beaten up, severe contusions, burns, broken bones
      5 = Head, internal, and/or permanent injury
      6 = Use of weapon, wound from weapon
4. Within the past year, has anyone forced you to have sexual activities? (yes/no)
   a. If yes, who? (husband/ex-husband/boyfriend/stranger/other/multiple)
   b. Number of times?
5. Are you afraid of your partner or anyone you listed?

**Table 7-4**
**ACOG Recommended Screening Questions for Intimate Partner Violence**

1. Within the past year—or since you have been pregnant—have you been hit, slapped, kicked, or otherwise physically hurt by someone?
2. Are you in a relationship with a person who threatens or physically hurts you?
3. Has anyone forced you to have sexual activities that made you feel uncomfortable?

some methods of inquiry, other styles of discussing intimate partner violence resulted in negative consequences, such as feeling judged by the provider, increased anxiety about the unknown, and disappointment in the provider's response.[82] Hamberger and colleagues surveyed 115 battered women to identify desirable and undesirable physician behaviors and practices. They found that battered women valued assessment for violence as a part of their complete medical history as long as it did not create "an atmosphere of interrogation."[94] In focus groups, immigrant Latino and Asian women who were victims of intimate partner violence described feeling that open communication about intimate partner violence was facilitated by compassionate and supportive provider behavior, provider initiation of discussion of intimate partner violence, and a continued relationship with the same provider.[95] Generally, health providers should address intimate partner violence in a nonjudgmental, sensitive manner, taking care to ensure the patient's safety, confidentiality, and dignity. Women should be asked about intimate partner violence without others present, particularly her partner. Professional interpreters should be used for women who do not speak English.

**What to Do When a Woman Says "Yes"**
No good studies have tested responses to a woman's disclosure of violence to determine the best response. However, the general feeling among female survivors, advocates, and health care providers who care for abused women is that one needs to include the following in one's response:

- Validation—Acknowledge the woman's disclosure and emphasize to her that she did not deserve the abuse or violence. Emphasize that she did not do or say anything "wrong." She is not the one with a problem in the relationship—the perpetrator has the problem.
- Support—Express a willingness to support her. Offer an invitation to use the health care setting as a resource and a source of support and safety.
- Information—Provide referral information and/or hotline numbers to community domestic violence programs. Ask if she can take the information safely. Write the numbers down without labeling them if she is afraid to take anything. The National Domestic Violence Hotline is a 24-hour toll-free resource that will help women locate and contact shelters and other support services in their own community. Other national organizations such as the Family Violence Prevention Fund and the National Coalition Against Domestic Violence will also provide links to local resources (Table 7-5).

- Safety planning—Ask if she is currently safe and/or if she needs shelter. If she intends to return to the batterer, ask if she has a plan for what to do/how to escape if the violence occurs again (Table 7-6). Suggest having money hidden or put somewhere else to have if she needs to leave quickly; having copies of birth certificates, immunizations, Social Security numbers, and other important documents that she could keep somewhere else or quickly take; having a hidden spare car key; making a list of hotline numbers; developing a code with friends, family, and/or neighbors to get help in an emergency. McFarlane and colleagues found increased safety behaviors (e.g., hiding money, removing weapons from the home, and establishing a coded method of calling for help from friends and family) among pregnant victims of intimate partner violence who underwent a brief intervention focused on safety planning.[96]
- Danger assessment—In various studies, Campbell and colleagues have examined potential risk factors associated with increased risk of homicide[97] (Table 7-7). From this work, these investigators have developed a danger assessment tool to aid in counseling women regarding their lethality risk in their intimate partner violence situation[98] (Fig. 7-1). Although currently no outcome data is available regarding the benefits or risks of using this instrument, the objective regarding its use is to increase women's awareness of their danger and individualize their safety counseling.
- Documentation—Although this is still a somewhat controversial issue, both victims advocates and legal counselors working on behalf of victims of intimate partner violence

**Table 7-5**
**National Domestic Violence Organizations and Resources**

**Family Violence Prevention Fund**

Main office
383 Rhode Island St., Suite #304
San Francisco, CA 94103-5133

Phone: (415) 252-8900
Fax: (415) 252-8991
TTY: (800) 595-4889

Washington, DC, office
1522 K St., NW #550
Washington, DC 20005

Boston office
67 Newbury St., Mezzanine Level
Boston, MA 02116

Email: info@endabuse.org
Website: http://endabuse.org/

**National Coalition Against Domestic Violence**

P.O. Box 18749
Denver, CO 80218

Phone: (303)-839-1852
Fax: (303)-831-9251

Email: mainoffice@ncadv.org
Website: http://ncadv.org/

**Table 7-6**
**Safety Planning**

**Making safety plans**

If you are being abused, making a safety plan now will help you when you have to act quickly in the future. If you make a decision to permanently leave your partner, planning ahead for your safety is very important.

The following ideas are ways that other women have planned for their safety. Some of these ideas may work for you. You may come up with additional ideas for yourself. You know your own situation better than anyone else, so plan what will work best for you.

**Planning for an episode of violence**

· Know which doors, windows, stairwells, elevators, or fire escapes you can use if you have to leave quickly. Practice using them so that they feel familiar to you.
· Know how to reach the police and your local women's shelter.
· Keep emergency items like bus/cab fare, house and car keys, a list of important phone numbers, change for telephone calls, and an extra coat or sweater in a safe place where you can get to them quickly. You may want to keep them with a trusted neighbor.
· Every day, think about where you can go immediately if you have to leave. Is a neighbor home today? A relative? A friend?
· If you can, remove weapons from your home.
· If you have children, teach them a signal (like a code word) that means they should call the police or go for help. You may want to have a code for a neighbor (like putting on a particular light) that means you want them to call the police.
· Something to think about: When you cannot get away and your partner becomes violent, which room is the safest for you to get to? Is there a room that has a phone and a lock on the door? Can you stay out of rooms with easy weapons, such as the kitchen?
· Check yourself and your children for injuries and go to the hospital, if necessary.
· Try not to leave without your children. But if you have to leave your children with the abuser, call the police immediately after you escape.
· If you need to get an emergency protection order (PFA), call your local women's shelter or the police for instructions in your area. **To access your local shelter, call 1-800-799-SAFE**
· Is there anything else that might help with planning for your safety?

**Safety planning for when you permanently leave the relationship**

Often, violence gets worse immediately before and after a woman leaves her abuser. Although you do not have control over your partner's violence, you can take steps to increase the chances of your safety. Even if you hope to be able to stay in your own home, you may need to leave temporarily until the abuser is forced to leave.

· Secretly make preparations. Who can you trust to keep extra house/car/office keys, clothes, money, children's favorite toy/blanket, and copies of important papers (e.g., identification, birth certificates for yourself and your children, Social Security cards, school and vaccination records, money, checkbook or savings account and ATM cards, driver's license and car registration, welfare and medical assistance cards, and divorce papers)?
· Make a list of important phone numbers—like family, friends, minister, and women's shelter.
· Where can you stay for a while right after you leave? Can you stay with a family member or friend? Will you need a shelter? Make arrangements ahead if you can.
· Open a savings account in your own name.
· To help make an escape plan, call a hotline at a women's shelter from a phone outside your home. **To access your local shelter, call 1-800-799-SAFE**.
· Rehearse your plan with someone you trust.
· After you leave the relationship, change your daily patterns. Do your grocery shopping at different stores and at different times than you used to. If you use the bus, try to alter the time or route. If you drive, change the roads you use. If you routinely go to a laundromat, bank, hair appointment, etc., change something about how you accomplish your task.
· Do you need to change the locks and install security lights or a security system?
  Do you need to get an unlisted phone number?
· Build a support network. It takes courage and incredible energy to make the changes you have started by leaving your abuser. There will be times when you feel sad and like you need to return to the abusive situation. Make a plan about who you can call. Think of a way to remind yourself that you are courageous and you deserve to live without violence in your home. If reading helps you, know what books or magazines will help you stay on track with your changes. You can also attend workshops or support groups.
· The use of drugs or alcohol can be very unsafe. Illegal drugs or alcohol can also be very hard on your body. They can affect your relationship with your children and could cause problems in legal actions with your batterer. Drugs and alcohol can also reduce your awareness and ability to act quickly to protect you and your children when you are in danger. If you use drugs or alcohol, make a plan to use them safely.
· Is there anything else that might help with planning for your safety?

From the Office Reference Manual for Recognition and Referral of Victims of Domestic Violence publlished by The Domestic Violence Resource Center of Magee-Womens Hospital, University of Pittsburgh Medical Center. Copyright 2003.

emphasize that documentation by a medical provider can help a woman in her legal case.[99,100] However, there have been past concerns regarding confidentiality breaches and some cases of insurance denial. Many clinical settings use the screening/documentation form developed by the Family Violence Prevention Fund (Fig. 7-2).

Studies in which women described bad experiences with health care providers included situations during which clinicians ignored or minimized the intimate partner violence, made excuses for the batterer, or blamed the woman.[73,78,79,81,94] Women described feeling criticized and blamed when they are asked questions such as "What did you do to deserve this?" and "Why don't you just leave?"[78]

Experts recommend offering women various options for dealing with the intimate partner violence.[101] Although a natural inclination would be to recommend that a woman leave her violent relationship, many women experiencing intimate partner violence are either unwilling or unable to do so. A few homicide studies also suggest that leaving the batterer can still be dangerous. In Moracco's study of femicide in North Carolina, half of women killed by their partners had some form of separation event (e.g., divorce, break-up, separation) immediately before the murder.[26]

**Danger assessment tool**

### Danger Assessment
From: Jacquelyn C. Campbell, PhD, RN, FAAN
*Copyright 2004 Johns Hopkins University, School of Nursing*

Several risk factors have been associated with increased risk of homicides (murders) of women and men in violent relationships. We cannot predict what will happen in your case, but we would like you to be aware of the danger of homicide in situations of abuse and for you to see how many of the risk factors apply to your situation.

Using your calendar, please mark the approximate dates during the past year when you were abused by your partner or ex-partner. Write on that date how bad the incident was according to the following scale:

1. Slapping, pushing; no injuries and/or lasting pain
2. Punching, kicking; bruises, cuts, and/or continuing pain
3. "Beating up"; severe contusions, burns, broken bones, miscarriage
4. Threat to use weapon; head injury, internal injury, permanent injury, miscarriage
5. Use of weapon; wounds from weapon

(If **any** of the descriptions for the higher number apply, use the higher number.)

Mark **Yes** or **No** for each of the following.
("He" refers to your husband, partner, ex-partner, or whoever is currently physically hurting you.)

| Yes | No | |
|---|---|---|
| ____ | ____ | 1. Has the physical violence increased in severity or frequency over the past year? |
| ____ | ____ | 2. Does he own a gun? |
| ____ | ____ | 3. Have you left him after living together during the past year? |
| | | 3a. (If have never lived with him, check here ____) |
| ____ | ____ | 4. Is he unemployed? |
| ____ | ____ | 5. Has he ever used a weapon against you or threatened you with a lethal weapon? |
| | | 5a. (If yes, was the weapon a gun?____) |
| ____ | ____ | 6. Does he threaten to kill you? |
| ____ | ____ | 7. Has he avoided being arrested for domestic violence? |
| ____ | ____ | 8. Do you have a child that is not his? |
| ____ | ____ | 9. Has he ever forced you to have sex when you did not wish to do so? |
| ____ | ____ | 10. Does he ever try to choke you? |
| ____ | ____ | 11. Does he use illegal drugs? By drugs, I mean "uppers" or amphetamines, speed, angel dust, cocaine, "crack", street drugs or mixtures. |
| ____ | ____ | 12. Is he an alcoholic or problem drinker? |
| ____ | ____ | 13. Does he control most or all of your daily activities? (For instance: does he tell you who you can be friends with, when you can see your family, how much money you can use, or when you can take the car?) |
| | | (If he tries, but you do not let him, check here: ____) |
| ____ | ____ | 14. Is he violently and constantly jealous of you? |
| | | (For instance, does he say, "If I can't have you, no one can.") |
| ____ | ____ | 15. Have you ever been beaten by him while you were pregnant? |
| | | (If you have never been pregnant by him, check here: ____) |
| ____ | ____ | 16. Has he ever threatened or tried to commit suicide? |
| ____ | ____ | 17. Does he threaten to harm your children? |
| ____ | ____ | 18. Do you believe he is capable of killing you? |
| ____ | ____ | 19. Does he follow or spy on you, leave threatening notes or messages on answering machine, destroy your property, or call you when you don't want him to? |
| ____ | ____ | 20. Have you ever threatened or tried to commit suicide? |
| | | TOTAL "Yes" Answers |

**Thank you. Please talk to a nurse, advocate, or counselor about what the Danger Assessment means in terms of your situation.**

**Figure 7-1 Danger assessment tool.** (From Jacquelyn C. Campbell, PhD, RN, FAAN. Copyright 2004 Johns Hopkins University, School of Nursing. http://www.dangerassessment.org/WebApplication1/)

## Domestic violence screening/documentation form

**DV Screen**
- ☐ DV +(Positive)
- ☐ DV? (Suspected)

Date _____ Patient ID#_____
Patient Name _____
Provider Name _____
Patient Pregnant      ☐ Yes     ☐ No

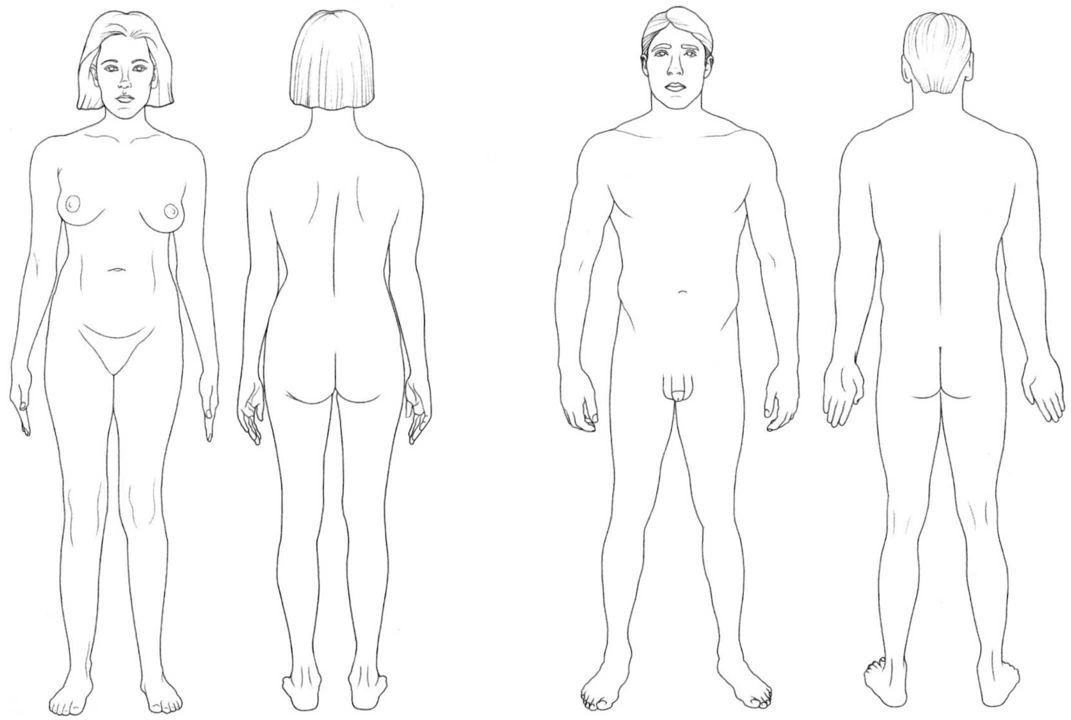

**Assess Patient Safety**

| Yes | No | | |
|-----|-----|-----|---|
| ____ | ____ | 1. | Is abuser here now? |
| ____ | ____ | 2. | Is patient afraid of her partner? |
| ____ | ____ | 3. | Is patient afraid to go home? |
| ____ | ____ | 4. | Has physical violence increased in the severity? |
| ____ | ____ | 5. | Has partner physically abused children? |
| ____ | ____ | 6. | Have children witnessed violence in the home? |
| ____ | ____ | 7. | Threats of homicide? By whom:_____ |
| ____ | ____ | 8. | Threats of suicide? By whom: _____ |
| ____ | ____ | 9. | Is there a gun in the house? |
| ____ | ____ | 10. | Alcohol or substance abuse? |
| ____ | ____ | 11. | Was safety plan discussed? |

**Referrals**

____ Hotline number given
____ Legal referral made
____ Shelter number given
____ In-house referral made
    Describe:_____
____ Other referrals made
    Describe:_____

**Reporting**

____ Law enforcement report made
____ Child protective Services report made
____ Adult Protective Services report made

**Photographs**

☐ Yes  ☐ No  Consent to be photographed?
☐ Yes  ☐ No  Photographs taken?

**Figure 7-2  Domestic violence screening/documentation form.** (From Preventing domestic violence: Clinical guidelines on routine screening, October 1999. Produced by The Family Violence Prevention Fund, 383 Rhode Island St., Suite 304, San Francisco, CA 94103–5133. www.endabuse.org.)

**Table 7-7**
**Intimate Partner Violence Risk Factors Associated with Homicide**

**Risk factors**

Abuser unemployed, not seeking job
Abuser access to gun
Victim had a child by a previous partner in the home
Abuser is controlling
Separation after living together
History of abuser threatening victim with weapon
History of abuser threatening to kill victim
History of forced sex

**Incident-level risk factors**

Abuser used gun
Trigger: jealousy—victim left for another relationship
Trigger: victim left abuser for other reasons

### What to Do When a Woman Says "No"

Women who have experienced intimate partner violence often describe experiences of denying the violence to others because of fear and denial. So denial of violence, even in highly suspicious cases, can be expected. The women also describe that this denial is not because they do not want help—often they do want help but are confused and afraid to ask for it.[101] Easy, anonymous access to information on intimate partner violence and to resources through posters, flyers, brochures, and information booklets would allow any woman—regardless of disclosure—to obtain help.

## PITFALLS AND CONTROVERSIES

Few states have mandatory reporting laws for intimate partner violence. These laws have generated controversy because there is uncertainty regarding whether they help or harm victims of intimate partner violence.[102–104] Although not explicit to intimate partner violence, many states require physicians to report to law enforcement specific injuries (e.g., gunshot or stab wounds) that may have resulted from a criminal act. If possible, the victim should be informed of the reporting laws and her rights as a crime victim before the report is made.

Little information exists regarding outcomes and consequences of health care screening and counseling for intimate partner violence.[105,106] Three recent reviews on interventions and screening for intimate partner violence[105–107] highlight the lack of measurable evidence showing effectiveness of these practices. Two reviews focused on intimate partner violence screening and interventions in health care settings. Ramsay and colleagues examined 20 papers, of which 9 addressed screening for intimate partner violence and 6 addressed interventions for intimate partner violence. The screening and intervention papers were included if they were conducted in a health care setting, had a comparison group, and measured a quantifiable outcome. Of the screening studies, only one was a randomized, controlled trial, with most of the remaining studies comparing women who underwent intimate partner violence screening with historical controls.[105] All six intervention studies were felt to be poor in quality, and most focused on referral rates and

service utilization as outcomes.[105] Nelson and colleagues selected studies that focused on studies that tested screening instruments for intimate partner violence and the effectiveness of health care interventions for victims of intimate partner violence. Of the 14 studies on screening instruments, 4 were rated to be good in quality and all involved the comparison of one screening instrument with another. The two intervention studies and the other screening studies were deemed to be fair or poor in quality.[106] All three reviews illustrated the dearth of studies examining health and safety outcomes for women experiencing intimate partner violence.

These reviews highlight the challenges of defining measurable outcomes for intimate partner violence screening and intervention programs and protocols. Nelson and colleagues admit that the definition of outcomes should not focus merely on violence incidents but should be broadened to include "improved quality of life, mental health, social support, self-esteem, and productivity." Currently, however, measures specific to women experiencing intimate partner violence do not exist.

Despite these reviews and the lack of large randomized, controlled trials in intimate partner violence, our knowledge and understanding regarding intimate partner violence should not merely depend on quantitative studies. A large body of well-done qualitative studies are available that examine how health care providers can help women experiencing intimate partner violence. Multiple qualitative studies suggest that although a single clinical encounter may not be associated with direct health and safety outcomes, there may be important intermediate cognitive and emotional changes, such as increased awareness of intimate partner violence as a problem, realizing the existence of options, and feeling that change is possible.[82–84,108] Several experts have found that seeking help for and finding safety from intimate partner violence may occur in stages or steps.[109–113] Thus a health care provider's inquiry about and offering interventions for intimate partner violence could contribute to changes in a patient's attitude, thoughts, and feelings that may facilitate future help-seeking actions.

## REFERENCES

1. Saltzman LE, Fanslow J, McMahon P, Shelley G: Intimate Partner Violence Surveillance: Uniform Definitions and Recommended Data Elements, Version 1.0. Atlanta: National Center for Injury Prevention and Control, Centers for Disease Control and Prevention, 1999. **(IV, C)**
2. Tjaden P, Thoennes N: Extent, Nature, and Consequences of Intimate Partner Violence. NCJ Publ. 181867. Washington, DC: National Institute of Justice/Centers for Disease Control and Prevention, 2000. **(III, B)**
3. Abbott J, Johnson R, Koziol-McLain J, Lowenstein SR: Domestic violence against women: incidence and prevalence in an emergency department population. JAMA 1995;273:1763–1767. **(III, B)**
4. Feldhaus KM, Koziol-McLain J, Amsbury HL, et al: Accuracy of 3 brief screening questions for detecting partner violence in the emergency department. JAMA 1997;277:1357–1361. **(IIb, B)**
5. Hamberger LK, Saunders DG, Hovey M: Prevalence of domestic violence in community practice and rate of physician inquiry. Fam Med 1992;24:283–287. **(III, B)**
6. Craven D: Female Victims of Violent Crime. NCJ Publ.162602. Washington, DC: Bureau of Justice Statistics, U.S. Department of Justice, 1996. **(III, B)**

7. Zawitz MW: Violence Between Intimates. NCJ Publ. 149259. Washington, DC: Bureau of Justice Statistics, 1994. **(III, B)**

8. Greenfeld LA, Rand MR, Craven D, et al: Violence by Intimates: Analysis of Data on Crimes by Current or Former Spouses, Boyfriends and Girlfriends. NCJ Publ. 167237. Washington, DC: Bureau of Justice Statistics, U.S. Department of Justice, 1998. **(III, B)**

9. Bachman R, Saltzman LE: Violence against Women: Estimate from the Redesigned Survey. Washington, DC: U.S. Department of Justice, 1995. **(III, B)**

10. Hotaling GT, Sugarman DB: A risk marker analysis of assaulted wives. J Fam Violence 1990;5:1–13. **(III, B)**

11. Canterino JC, VanHorn LG, Harrigan JT, et al: Domestic abuse in pregnancy: a comparison of a self-completed domestic abuse questionnaire with a directed interview. Am J Obstet Gynecol 1999; 181:1049–1051. **(IIb, B)**

12. McGrath ME, Hogan JW, Peipert JF: A prevalence survey of abuse and screening for abuse in urgent care patients. Obstet Gynecol 1998; 91:511–514. **(III, B)**

13. Norton LB, Peipert JF, Zierler S, et al: Battering in pregnancy: an assessment of two screening methods. Obstet Gynecol 1995; 85:321–325. **(IIb, B)**

14. Sequin RE: Domestic violence in pregnancy: a survey of obstetrical patients at the UAMS Department of Obstetrics and Gynecology Clinics. J Arkansas Med Soc 1998;95:187–189. **(III, B)**

15. Gazmararian JA, Petersen R, Spitz AM, et al: Violence and reproductive health: current knowledge and future research directions. Matern Child Health J 2000;4(2):79–84. **(III, B)**

16. Gazmararian JA, Lazorick S, Spitz A, et al: Prevalence of violence against pregnant women. JAMA 1996;275:1915–1920. **(III, B)**

17. Cokkinides VE, Coker AL: Experiencing physical violence during pregnancy: prevalence and correlates. Fam Community Health 1998; 20:19–37. **(III, B)**

18. Martin SL, English KT, Andersen Clark K, et al: Violence and substance use among North Carolina pregnant women. Am J Public Health 1996;86:991–998. **(III, B)**

19. Sibai BM, Ewell M, Levine RJ, et al: Risk factors associated with preeclampsia in healthy nulliparous women. Am J Obstet Gynecol 1997;177:1003–1010. **(III, B)**

20. Coustan D: Gestational diabetes. In National Institutes of Diabetes and Digestive and Kidney Diseases: Diabetes in America, 2nd ed. NIH Publication No. 95-1468. Bethesda, Md.: National Institutes of Diabetes and Digestive and Kidney Diseases, 1995. **(III, B)**

21. Martin SL, Mackie L, Kupper LL, et al: Physical abuse of women before, during, and after pregnancy. JAMA 2001;285:1581–1584. **(III, B)**

22. Helton AS, McFarlane J, Anderson ET: Battered and pregnant: a prevalence study. Am J Public Health 1987;77:1337–1339. **(III, B)**

23. Ballard TJ, Saltzman LE, Gazmararian JA, et al: Violence during pregnancy: measurement issues. Am J Public Health 1998;88:274–276. **(IV, C)**

24. Stewart DE, Cecutti A: Physical abuse in pregnancy. Can Med Assoc J 1993;149:1257–1263. **(III, B)**

25. Kellermann AL, Mercy JA: Men, women, and murder: gender-specific differences in rates of fatal violence and victimization. J Trauma 1992; 33:1–5. **(III, B)**

26. Moracco KE, Runyan CW, Butts J: Femicide in North Carolina, 1991–1993, a statewide study of patterns and precursors. Homicide Stud 1998;4:422–446. **(III, B)**

27. Center VP: When Men Murder Women: An Analysis of the 1997 Homicide Data. Violence Policy Center, 2000 [fulltext online]. Available at: http://www.vpc.org/studies/dv2cont.htm. Accessed 20 October 2003. **(III, B)**

28. Wadman MC, Muelleman RL: Domestic violence homicides: ED use before victimization. Am J Emerg Med 1999;17:689–691. **(III, B)**

29. Miller TR, Cohen MA, Rossman SB: Victim costs of violent crime and resulting injuries. Health Aff (Millwood) 1993;12(4):186–197. **(III, B)**

30. Koss MP, Koss PG, Woodruff WJ: Deleterious effects of criminal victimization on women's health and medical utilization. Arch Intern Med 1991;151:342–347. **(III, B)**

31. Wisner CL, Gilmer TP, Saltzman LE, Zink TM: Intimate partner violence against women: do victims cost health plans more? J Fam Pract 1999;48:439–443. **(III, B)**

32. Drossman DA, Talley NJ, Lesserman J, et al: Sexual and physical abuse and gastrointestinal illness: review and recommendations. Ann Intern Med 1995;123:782–794. **(III, B)**

33. Scholle Rost K, Golding J: Physical abuse among depressed women. J Gen Intern Med 1998;13:607–613. **(III, B)**

34. Walling MK, O'Hara MW, Reiter RC, et al: Abuse history and chronic pain in women: II. A multivariate analysis of abuse and psychological morbidity. Obstet Gynecol 1994;84:200–206. **(III, B)**

35. McCauley J, Kern DE, Kolodner K, et al: Relation of low-severity violence to women's health. J Gen Intern Med 1998;13:687–691. **(III, B)**

36. The Commonwealth Fund Survey of Women's Health. New York: The Commonwealth Fund, 1993. **(IV, C)**

37. Campbell JC, Pugh LC, Campbell D, Visscher M: The influence of abuse on pregnancy intention. Womens Health Issues 1995;5:214–223. **(III, B)**

38. Goodwin MM, Gazmararian JA, Johnson CH, et al: Pregnancy intendedness and physical abuse around the time of pregnancy: findings from the Pregnancy Risk Assessment Monitoring System, 1996–1997. Matern Child Health J 2000;4:85–92. **(III, B)**

39. Glander SS, Moore ML, Michielutte R, Parsons LH: The prevalence of domestic violence among women seeking abortion. Obstet Gynecol 1998;91:1002–1006. **(III, B)**

40. Evins G, Chescheir N: Prevalence of domestic violence among women seeking abortion services. Womens Health Issues 1996;6:204–210. **(III, B)**

41. Dietz PM, Gazmararian JA, Goodwin MM, et al: Delayed entry into prenatal care: effect of physical violence. Obstet Gynecol 1997; 90:221–224. **(III, B)**

42. Coker AL, Smith PH, McKeown RE, King MJ: Frequency and correlates of intimate partner violence by type: physical, sexual, and psychological battering. Am J Public Health 2000;90:553–559. **(III, B)**

43. Petersen R, Gazmararian JA, Spitz AM, et al: Violence and adverse pregnancy outcomes: a review of the literature and directions for future research. Am J Prev Med 1997;13:366–373. **(III, B)**

44. Dannenberg AL, Carter DM, Lawson HW, et al: Homicide and other injuries as causes of maternal death in New York City, 1987 through 1991. Am J Obstet Gynecol 1995;172:1557–1564. **(III, B)**

45. Parsons LH, Harper MA: Violent maternal deaths in North Carolina. Obstet Gynecol 1999;94:990–993. **(III, B)**

46. Horon IL, Cheng D: Enhanced surveillance for pregnancy-associated mortality—Maryland, 1993–1998. JAMA 2001;285:1455–1459. **(III, B)**

47. McFarlane J, Campbell JC, Sharps P, Watson K: Abuse during pregnancy and femicide: urgent implications for women's health. Obstet Gynecol 2002;100:27–36. **(III, B)**

48. Lee D, James L, Sawires P: Preventing Domestic Violence: Clinical Guidelines on Routine Screening. San Francisco: The Family Violence Prevention Fund, 1999. **(IV, C)**

49. American Medical Association: Physicians and domestic violence: ethical considerations. JAMA 1992;267:3190–3193. **(IV, C)**

50. Flitcraft AH, Hadley SM, Hendricks-Matthews MK, et al: American Medical Association diagnostic and treatment guidelines on domestic violence. Arch Fam Med 1992;1:39–47. **(IV, C)**

51. Horan D, Himes C: Violence against women: screening tools. American College of Obstetricians and Gynecologists [website]. 20 July 1999. Available at: http://www.acog.org/from_home/departments/dept_notice.cfm?reçno=17&bulletin=585. Accessed 20 October 2003. **(IV, C)**

52. Emergency Medicine and Domestic Violence. American College of Emergency Physicians [website]. Available at: http://www.acep.org/policy/po400163.htm. Accessed 20 October 2003. **(IV, C)**

53. Age Charts for Periodic Health Examination. Kansas City, MO: American Academy of Family Physicians, Commission on Public Health and Scientific Affairs, 1993. **(IV, C)**

54. Position Statement on Physical Violence Against Women. Washington, DC: American Nurses Association, 1991. **(IV, C)**

55. Accreditation Manual for Hospitals. Chicago: Joint Commission on Accreditation of Healthcare Organizations, 1992. **(IV, C)**

56. Abma J, Chandra A, Mosher W, et al: Fertility, Family Planning and Women's Health: New Data from the 1995 National Survey of Family Growth. National Center of Health Statistics. Vital Health Stat 1997; 23:19. **(III, B)**

57. Scholle SH, Chang JC, Harman J, McNeil M: Trends in women's health services by type of physician seen: data from the 1985 and 1997–98 NAMCS. Womens Health Issues 2002;12:165–177. **(III, B)**

58. Martin JA, Hamilton BE, Ventura SJ, et al: Births: Final Data for 2000. Hyattsville, Md.: National Center for Health Statistics, 2002. **(III, B)**

59. O'Campo P, Davis MV, Gielen AC: Smoking cessation interventions for pregnant women: review and future directions. Semin Perinatol 1995;19:279–285. **(III, B)**

60. Mullen PD, Pollak KI, Titus JP, et al: Prenatal smoking cessation counseling by Texas obstetricians. Birth 1998;25:25–31. **(III, B)**

61. Todd SJ, LaSala KB, Neil-Urban S: An integrated approach to prenatal smoking cessation interventions. MCN Am J Matern Child Nurs 2001;26:185–190. **(III, B)**

62. Stotts AL, DiClemente CC, Carbonari JP, Mullen PD: Postpartum return to smoking: staging a "suspended" behavior. Health Psychol 2000;19:324–332. **(III, B)**

63. Curry SJ, McBride C, Grothaus L, et al: Motivation for smoking cessation among pregnant women. Psychol Addict Behav 2001;15: 126–132. **(III, B)**

64. O'Campo P, Faden RR, Brown H, Gielen AC: The impact of pregnancy on women's prenatal and postpartum smoking behavior. Am J Prev Med 1992;8:8–13. **(III, B)**

65. Corse SJ, Smith M: Reducing substance abuse during pregnancy. Discriminating among levels of response in a prenatal setting. J Subst Abuse Treat 1998;15:457–467. **(III, B)**

66. Josefsson A, Berg G, Nordin C, Sydsjo G: Prevalence of depressive symptoms in late pregnancy and postpartum. Acta Obstet Gynecol Scand 2001;80:251–255. **(III, B)**

67. Evans J, Heron J, Francomb H, et al: Cohort study of depressed mood during pregnancy and after childbirth. BMJ 2001;323:257–260. **(III, B)**

68. Horan DL, Chapin J, Klein L, et al: Domestic violence screening practices of obstetrician-gynecologists. Obstet Gynecol 1998; 92:785–789. **(III, B)**

69. Parsons LH, Zaccaro D, Wells B, Stovall TG: Methods of and attitudes toward screening obstetrics and gynecology patients for domestic violence. Am J Obstet Gynecol 1995;173:381–387. **(III, B)**

70. Sugg NK, Thompson RS, Thompson DC, et al: Domestic violence and primary care: attitudes, practices, and beliefs. Arch Fam Med 1999; 8:301–306. **(III, B)**

71. Rodriguez MA, Bauer HM, McLoughlin E, Grumbach K: Screening and intervention for intimate partner abuse: practices and attitudes of primary care physicians. JAMA 1999;282:468–474. **(III, B)**

72. McGrath ME, Bettacchi A, Duffy SJ, et al: Violence against women: provider barriers to intervention in emergency departments. Acad Emerg Med 1997;4:297–300. **(III, B)**

73. Caralis PV, Musialowski R: Women's experiences with domestic violence and their attitudes and expectations regarding medical care of abuse victims. South Med J 1997;90:1075–1080. **(III, B)**

74. Friedman LS, Samet JH, Roberts MS, et al: Inquiry about victimization experiences: a survey of patient preferences and physician practices. Arch Intern Med 1992;152:1186–1190. **(III, B)**

75. McNutt L-A, Carlson BE, Gagen D, Winterbauer N: Reproductive violence screening in primary care: perspectives and experiences of patients and battered women. JAMWA 1999;54:85–90. **(III, B)**

76. Rodriguez MA, Quiroga SS, Bauer HM: Breaking the silence: battered women's perspectives on medical care. Arch Fam Med 1996; 5:153–158. **(III, B)**

77. Rodriguez MA, Sheldon WR, Bauer HM, Perez-Stable EJ: The factors associated with disclosure of intimate partner abuse to clinicians. J Fam Pract 2001;50:338–344. **(III, B)**

78. Gerbert B, Johnston K, Caspers N, et al: Experiences of battered women in health care settings: a qualitative study. Women Health 1996;24:1–17. **(III, B)**

79. McCauley J, Yurk R, Jenckes MW, Ford DE: Inside "Pandora's Box": abused women's experiences with clinicians and health services. J Gen Intern Med 1998;13:549–555. **(III, B)**

80. Hathaway JE, Willis G, Zimmer B: Listening to survivors' voices: addressing partner abuse in the health care setting. Violence Against Women 2002;8:687–719. **(III, B)**

81. Bacchus L: Women's perceptions and experiences of routine enquiry for domestic violence in a maternity service. Br J Obstet Gynaecol 2002;109:9–16. **(III, B)**

82. Chang JC, Decker M, Moracco KE, et al: What happens when health care providers ask about intimate partner violence? A description of consequences from the perspectives of female survivors. JAMA 2003;58:76–81. **(III, B)**

83. Gerbert B, Caspers N, Bronstone A, et al: A qualitative analysis of how physicians with expertise in domestic violence approach the identification of victims. Ann Intern Med 1999;131:578–584. **(III, B)**

84. Gerbert B, Caspers N, Milliken N, et al: Interventions that help victims of domestic violence. A qualitative analysis of physicians' experiences. J Fam Pract 2000;49:889–895. **(III, B)**

85. Ferris LE, Norton PG, Dunn EV, et al: Guidelines for managing domestic abuse when male and female partners are patients of the same physician. The Delphi Panel and the Consulting Group. JAMA 1997;278:851–857. **(IV, C)**

86. Rittmayer J, Roux G: Relinquishing the need to "fix it": medical intervention with domestic abuse. Qual Health Res 1999;9:166–181. **(III, B)**

87. Titus K: When physicians ask, women tell about domestic abuse and violence. JAMA 1996;275:1863–1865. **(III, B)**

88. Brown JB, Lent B, Schmidt G, Sas G: Application of the Woman Abuse Screening Tool (WAST) and WAST—short in the family practice setting. J Fam Pract 2000;49:896–903. **(IIb, B)**

89. Brown JBL, Brett PJ, Sas G, Pederson LL: Development of the Woman Abuse Screening Tool for use in family practice. Fam Med 1996;28:422–428. **(IIb, B)**

90. McFarlane J, Parker B, Soeken K, Bullock L: Assessing for abuse during pregnancy: severity and frequency of injuries and associated entry into prenatal care. JAMA 1992;267:3176–3178. **(III, B)**

91. McFarlane J, Hughes RB, Nosek MA, et al: Abuse assessment screen-disability (AAS-D): measuring frequency, type, and perpetrator of abuse toward women with physical disabilities. J Womens Health Gend Based Med 2001;10:861–866. **(III, B)**

92. Sherin KM, Sinacore JM, Li XQ, et al: HITS: a short domestic violence screening tool for use in a family practice setting. Fam Med 1998;30:508–512. **(IIb, B)**

93. America College of Obstetricians and Gynecologists: Screening Tools—Domestic Violence. Available at: http://www.acog.org/departments/dept_notice.cfm?recno=17&bulletin=585. Accessed 9 May 2005. **(IV, C)**

94. Hamberger LK, Ambuel B, Marbella A, Donze J: Physician interaction with battered women: the women's perspective. Arch Fam Med 1998;7:575–582. **(III, B)**

95. Rodriguez MA, Bauer HM, Flores-Ortiz Y, Szkupinski-Quiroga S: Factors affecting patient–physician communication for abused Latina and Asian Immigrant women. J Fam Pract 1998;47:309–311. **(III, B)**

96. McFarlane J, Parker B, Soeken K, et al: Safety behaviors of abused women after an intervention during pregnancy. J Obstet Gynecol Neonatal Nurs 1998;27:64–69. **(Ib, A)**

97. Campbell JC, Webster D, Koziol-McLain J, et al: Risk factors for femicide in abusive relationships: results from a multisite case control study. Am J Public Health 2003;93:1089–1097. **(III, B)**

98. Campbell JC: Danger Assessment. Available at: http://www.dangerassessment.org/WebApplication1/. Accessed 10 May 2005.

99. Easley M: Domestic violence. Ann Emerg Med 1996;27:762–763. **(IV, C)**

100. Buel SM, Harvard JD: Family violence: practical recommendations for physicians and the medical community. Womens Health Issues 1995;5:158–172. **(IV, C)**

101. Chang JC, Cluss PA, Ranieri L, et al: Health care interventions for intimate partner violence: what women want. Womens Health Issues 2005;15:21–30. **(III, B)**

102. Rodriguez MAC, Mooney DR, Bauer HM: Patient attitudes about mandatory reporting of domestic violence: implications for health care professionals. West J Med 1998;169:337–341. **(III, B)**

103. Hyman A, Chez RA: Mandatory reporting of domestic violence by health care providers: a misguided approach. Womens Health Issues 1995;5:208–213. **(IV, C)**

104. Hyman AS, Lo B: Laws mandating reporting of domestic violence: do they promote patient well-being? JAMA 1995;273:1781–1787. **(IV, C)**

105. Ramsay J, Richardson J, Carter YH, et al: Should health professionals screen women for domestic violence? Systematic review. BMJ 2002; 325:314–326. **(Ib, A)**

106. Nelson HD, Nygren P, McInerney Y, Klein J: Screening women and elderly adults for family and intimate partner violence: a review of the evidence for the u.s. preventive services task force. Ann Intern Med 2004;140:387–396. **(Ib, A)**

107. Wathen CN, MacMillan HL: Interventions for violence against women: scientific review. JAMA 2003;289:589–600. **(Ib, A)**

108. Gerbert B, Abercrombie P, Caspers N, et al: How health care providers help battered women: the survivor's perspective. Women Health 1999;29:115–135. **(III, B)**

109. Frasier PY, Slatt L, Kowlowitz V, Glowa P: Using the stages of change model to counsel victims of intimate partner violence. Patient Educ Couns 2001;43:211–217. **(IV, C)**

110. Kramer A: Domestic violence: how to ask and how to listen. Nurs Clin North Am 2002;37:189–210. **(IV, C)**

111. Landenburger K: A process of entrapment in and recovery from an abusive relationship. Issues Ment Health Nurs 1989;10:209–227. **(III, B)**

112. Landenburger KM: The dynamics of leaving and recovering from an abusive relationship. J Obstet Gynecol Neonatal Nurs 1998; 27:700–706. **(III, B)**

113. Nicolaidis C: The Voices of Survivors documentary: using patient narrative to educate physicians about domestic violence. J Gen Intern Med 2002;17:117–124. **(III, B)**

# Chapter 8

# Abnormal Uterine Bleeding

## Randall B. Barnes, MD

### KEY POINTS

- The distinction between ovulatory and anovulatory abnormal uterine bleeding is critical because causes and therapies are distinct.
- The diagnosis of menorrhagia is usually subjective, with the only objective indicator readily available to the physician being a low hemoglobin.
- Uterine fibroids, endometrial polyps, and adenomyosis are common anatomic abnormalities causing menorrhagia.
- Nonanatomic causes of menorrhagia include bleeding disorders, hypothyroidism, and essential menorrhagia.
- Evaluation of the uterine cavity by means of saline infusion sonography, TSH level, and coagulation studies is the core workup in patients with menorrhagia.
- Medical therapy is usually effective in patients with menorrhagia.
- Any cause of normoestrogenic anovulation can present as dysfunctional uterine bleeding.
- In anovulatory patients with dysfunctional uterine bleeding, prolactin, TSH, and FSH should be measured.
- In anovulatory patients and patients with menorrhagia over the age of 40 years, endometrial biopsy should be considered to rule out hyperplasia.
- Medical therapy is the first-line therapy for dysfunctional uterine bleeding.

Abnormal uterine bleeding is a common and vexing problem. In England, about 30 per 1000 female patients per year consult with their general practitioners for evaluation of abnormal uterine bleeding. About 20% of referrals from general practitioners to gynecologists are for abnormal uterine bleeding; and of those referred, about half undergo hysterectomy.[1] About 11% of hysterectomies performed in the United States are for abnormal bleeding.[2] Abnormal uterine bleeding has significant economic impact, with work loss estimated to be almost U.S.$1700 annually for women with menorrhagia.[3]

## CLINICAL FEATURES

### Definitions and Scope

Uterine bleeding associated with early pregnancy may be due to threatened abortion, incomplete abortion, or ectopic pregnancy. This chapter is concerned only with abnormal uterine bleeding in nonpregnant, reproductive-aged women. The critical distinction to be made in the evaluation and treatment of abnormal uterine bleeding is whether it is associated with ovulation or anovulation. In this chapter, abnormal uterine bleeding associated with anovulation is referred to as dysfunctional uterine bleeding. However, the term *dysfunctional uterine bleeding* sometimes also is used for essential menorrhagia, which is menorrhagia without evidence of an anatomic or other cause.[4] Menorrhagia is heavy menses in ovulatory women, whereas metrorrhagia is irregular bleeding during an ovulatory cycle (Table 8-1). The distinction between ovulatory and anovulatory bleeding is critical because causes and therapies are distinct.

### Menometrorrhagia

The diagnosis of menorrhagia is usually made by the patient. Menstrual bleeding lasting longer than 7 days or associated with clotting is common in menorrhagia. The average menstrual blood loss is about 40 mL per cycle; any loss greater than 80 mL is associated with an increased risk of anemia and is considered menorrhagia.[5,6] Menstrual blood loss can most accurately be quantified by the alkaline hematin method, in which catamenial receptors are soaked in 5% sodium hydroxide to convert the blood to alkaline hematin and optical density is measured. Weighing of total menstrual fluid also has been described as being sufficient for the diagnosis of menorrhagia. A pictorial blood loss assessment chart has been developed that provides a semiquantitative measurement of menstrual blood loss and may be better suited to clinical practice.[4] However, all these methods are inconvenient and cumbersome, and the diagnosis of menorrhagia is usually subjective, with the only objective indicator readily available to the physician being a low hemoglobin.

Metrorrhagia may be physiologic when it presents as midcycle spotting, which is probably the result of falling estradiol levels during the time of the luteinizing hormone surge. All intrauterine devices (IUDs), except those containing progestins, increase the prevalence of menorrhagia. Depending on the type used, menorrhagia occurs in 25% to 50% of IUD users after 1 year.[6]

Uterine leiomyomata, particularly those that distort the uterine cavity, endometrial polyps, and adenomyosis all have been associated with menometrorrhagia. Both polyps and myomas are more common in women with abnormal uterine bleeding than in asymptomatic women. In a study using sonohysterography in 80 women with abnormal uterine bleeding and 100 asymptomatic, age-matched controls, endometrial polyps (32% vs 10%), intracavitary myomas (21% vs 1%), and intramural myomas (57% vs 13%) were all significantly more common in women with abnormal uterine bleeding.[7] In studies of women undergoing hysteroscopy for menorrhagia, 10% to 15% had submucosal myomas and 15% to 30% had endometrial polyps.[8]

Adenomyosis is the benign invasion of endometrial glands and stroma into the myometrium. Most cases (90%) occur in

**Table 8-1**
**Causes of Abnormal Uterine Bleeding**

**Menometrorrhagia**

Anatomic
    Leiomyomata
    Endometrial polyp
    Adenomyosis
IUD
Bleeding disorder
    von Willebrand's disease
    Platelet disorders
    Warfarin therapy
Hypothyroidism or hyperthyroidism
Essential menorrhagia

**Dysfunctional uterine bleeding**

Physiologic
    Perimenarcheal and perimenopausal anovulation
Hypothalamic dysfunction
    Stress
    Exercise
    Weight loss
Hyperprolactinemia
Premature ovarian failure
Androgen excess
    Polycystic ovary syndrome
    Late onset 21-hydroxylase deficiency
Hypothyroidism or hyperthyroidism
Consequences of chronic anovulation
    Endometrial hyperplasia
    Endometrial cancer

multiparous women, and about 80% of women with adenomyosis are 40 to 50 years old.[9] The most frequent symptoms are menorrhagia, dysmenorrhea, and metrorrhagia. Classically the uterus is diffusely enlarged and tender to palpation. The role of adenomyosis in the pathogenesis of menometrorrhagia is perplexing, in part because it frequently occurs in asymptomatic women.[9] Adenomyosis has been found in 54% of uteri examined at autopsy.[10] In a prospective study of patients undergoing hysterectomy, there was no difference in duration of menstrual bleeding or presence of dysmenorrhea in the 28 patients found to have adenomyosis and the 157 without adenomyosis or endometriosis.[11]

On the other hand, adenomyosis often is associated with abnormal uterine bleeding. Adenomyosis was found in hysteroscopic biopsy specimens in 37% of 90 menorrhagic women. However, if the uterine cavity was normal, the number of patients who had significant adenomyosis increased to 66%.[8] Adenomyosis was found in 20 of 43 women with an enlarged uterus without evidence of leiomyomata on ultrasound who had hysterectomy for persistent menorrhagia.[12] Ultimately, the role of adenomyosis in abnormal uterine bleeding may prove to be quantitative, with more extensive disease and greater depth of myometrial invasion more likely to cause abnormal bleeding.[9]

Hyperthyroidism rarely causes menometrorrhagia. Polymenorrhea or hypermenorrhea was noted in only 8% of 214 reproductive-aged women with hyperthyroidism.[13] Hypothyroidism causes a range of menstrual abnormalities from amenorrhea to menometrorrhagia. In a study of 171 reproductive-aged women with hypothyrodism, 23% had menstrual abnor-

malities. Menorrhagia accounted for about one third of the abnormalities.[14] Early hypothyroidism has been found in 22% of women with menorrhagia[15] and overt hypothyroidism in 2% of women with menorrhagia evaluated for endometrial ablation.[8]

Bleeding disorders should always be considered in women with menorrhagia without an anatomic cause. In particular, bleeding disorders should be considered in adolescents admitted to the hospital with acute menorrhagia. A primary coagulation disorder has been reported in 19% to 28% of such patients, with 50% of patients hospitalized with excessive bleeding at menarche having clotting disorders.[16,17] Of the 18 adolescents described in the two reports, 11 had thrombocytopenia due to idiopathic thrombocytopenia purpura (n = 8) or to leukemia, thalassemia major, or Fanconi's anemia (one each), and 5 had von Willebrand's disease.

In adults with objectively proved menorrhagia, inherited bleeding disorders have been found in 13% to 20%.[18–20] The prevalence is somewhat less, about 11%, in women who have menorrhagia without objective verification.[21] The majority of patients had von Willebrand's disease, but deficiencies of factor VII, X, and XI and platelet dysfunction also were found. Inherited bleeding disorders were more likely in women with a history of menorrhagia since menarche or with a history of excessive bleeding after tooth extraction, surgery, or childbirth.[19] Menorrhagia has been demonstrated objectively in 5 of 11 women of reproductive age undergoing treatment with oral anticoagulants.[22]

There is debate about whether tubal sterilization increases a woman's risk of increased menstrual and intermenstrual bleeding, often referred to as the post-tubal-sterilization syndrome. A study of more than 9500 women who underwent tubal sterilization and 573 whose partners underwent vasectomy found no increased risk of abnormal bleeding in the tubal sterilization group. The women who underwent sterilization had significantly fewer days of bleeding and significantly lesser amounts of bleeding and dysmenorrhea.[23]

Essential menorrhagia is probably the most common cause of menorrhagia. About 50% of cases of objectively proved menorrhagia have no pathologic cause at hysterectomy.[4] Essential menorrhagia has been reported to occur in about 10% of western European women.[6] Pathogenic mechanisms include increased production of prostaglandins $E_2$ and $F_2\alpha$ and prostacyclin by the endometrium and myometrium, increased myometrial concentrations of prostaglandin receptors, and elevated fibrinolytic activity in the endometrium.[4]

## Dysfunctional Uterine Bleeding

Any cause of anovulation with normal estrogen levels can present as dysfunctional uterine bleeding (see Table 8-1). Typically patients have irregular, unpredictable bleeding without symptoms of ovulation such as breast tenderness, mood changes, or dysmenorrhea. Anovulatory cycles are considered physiologic in the first year after menarche and in the perimenopause and do not require hormonal evaluation.[24] However, the cause of anovulatory cycles at other times in a woman's reproductive life should be investigated. Dysfunctional bleeding may occur during the transition to premature ovarian failure, just as it does at the time of physiologic menopause. Dysfunctional uterine bleeding is a common symptom of androgen excess. In women with

| Table 8-2 |
| --- |
| Evaluation of Abnormal Uterine Bleeding |

**All patients**

Pregnancy test if sexually active
CBC
TSH
Platelet count, PT, PTT, and platelet function analysis if coagulation disorder
  suspected

**Ovulatory vs anovulatory**

Serum progesterone
Endometrial biopsy
Basal body temperature

**Ovulatory bleeding (menometrorrhagia)**

Saline infusion sonography
Endometrial biopsy (if over 40 years old)

**Anovulatory bleeding (dysfunctional uterine bleeding)**

Prolactin, FSH
If androgen excess present: testosterone, free testosterone,
  17-hydroxyprogesterone
If anovulatory for more than 1 year: consider endometrial biopsy
If unresponsive to medical therapy: rule out anatomic defect

The long-term consequence of chronic anovulation is endometrial hyperplasia and carcinoma. Chronically anovulatory women have a threefold increased risk of endometrial cancer.[25] Endometrial hyperplasia occurs in about 5% and endometrial cancer in about 0.5% of premenopausal women who undergo sampling for abnormal uterine bleeding. Risk factors include age of 45 years or older, weight of 90 kg or greater, a history of infertility, family history of cancer of the colon, and nulliparity.[26]

## DIAGNOSIS

### Menometrorrhagia

Menometrorrhagia is often difficult to distinguish from dysfunctional uterine bleeding. Ovulation should be confirmed in uncertain cases by an ovulatory serum progesterone level or finding secretory endometrium on biopsy. Basal body temperature charting is useful to time the preceding tests during the midportion of the temperature rise (Table 8-2).

The patient with menometrorrhagia should be evaluated for the presence of an anatomic abnormality. Oftentimes, this is easily accomplished by palpating a fibroid uterus on physical examination. However, symptomatic submucosal fibroids or endometrial polyps can be present in a normal-size uterus (Fig. 8-1). Therefore, all patients with menometrorrhagia should undergo imaging of the uterine cavity. Transvaginal ultrasound with saline infusion of the uterine cavity (saline infusion sonography [SIS] or sonohysterography) is the best initial choice among current options. A large meta-analysis found a sensitivity of 0.95 and a specificity of 0.88 for SIS compared with the gold standard of either hysteroscopy or hysterectomy, and only about 7% of uterine cavity abnormalities were missed by SIS.[27] SIS can be performed successfully in 95% of premenopausal women and is as accurate as diagnostic hysteroscopy.[27] SIS is more reliable than magnetic resonance imaging (MRI) in detecting endometrial polyps, is equivalent to MRI in detecting submucosal

dysfunctional bleeding and evidence of hirsutism or acne, the most likely diagnosis is polycystic ovary syndrome.

If there is no evidence of hyperprolactinemia, hypothyroidism, premature ovarian failure, or androgen excess, dysfunctional uterine bleeding is characterized as hypothalamic dysfunction. The patient may be anovulatory as a result of stress, weight loss, or exercise or the cause may be idiopathic. These patients can be reassured that, as long as they continue to withdraw to a progestin challenge, there is no serious cause for their anovulation.

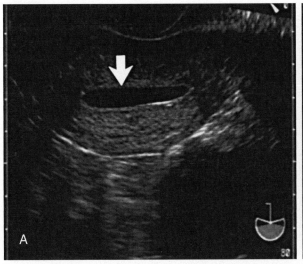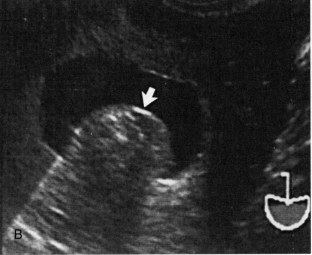

**Figure 8-1   Images from saline-infused sonograms from two different patients.** *A,* Normal study, with saline filling the uterine cavity *(arrow).* The borders are regular, and no masses protrude into the cavity. *B,* In this magnified view, a myoma protrudes into the cavity from the posterior uterine wall. (From Bayer SR: Clinical management of abnormal uterine bleeding. In Gershenson DM, DeCherney AH, Curry SL, Brubaker L [eds]: Operative Gynecology, 2nd ed. Philadelphia, W.B. Saunders, 2001, p 478.)

fibroids, and can provide information regarding intramural extension.[28] SIS also is easier to perform and better accepted by patients than hysteroscopy or MRI.[27]

Preoperative diagnosis of adenomyosis may be difficult to make. The physical finding of a diffusely enlarged, tender uterus is not always present. Transvaginal ultrasound is about 80% sensitive in detecting adenomyosis, with a 26% false-positive rate.[12] The most reliable preoperative method for detecting adenomyosis is MRI.[29] Based on histopathologic diagnosis, MRI correctly revealed adenomyosis in 88% of cases versus 53% of cases uncovered by transvaginal ultrasonography. MRI correctly distinguished between leiomyomata and adenomyosis in 92 of 93 patients with an enlarged uterus.

Thyroid-stimulating hormone (TSH) should be measured in all patients with menometrorrhagia as a screening test for both hypothyroidism and hyperthyroidism.

In patients with an otherwise normal evaluation, consider testing for bleeding disorders before making the diagnosis of essential menorrhagia. As mentioned above, the mostly likely bleeding disorders are thrombocytopenia from various causes and von Willebrand's disease. Menorrhagia since menarche, bleeding following surgical or dental procedures, and postpartum hemorrhage are predictive of von Willebrand's disease in adult women with menorrhagia.[30] If there is suspicion of a clotting disorder, a prothrombin time, partial thromboplastin time, platelet count, and platelet function analysis should be performed.[30] The ristocetin cofactor assay of von Willebrand's factor function may be the best single screening test for von Willebrand's disease.[31] Consultation with a hematologist is helpful if there is concern that a bleeding disorder may be the cause of menorrhagia.

### Dysfunctional Uterine Bleeding

Prolactin, follicle-stimulating hormone (FSH), and TSH should be measured in all patients with anovulation whether they have amenorrhea, oligomenorrhea, or dysfunctional uterine bleeding to rule out hyperprolactinemia, hypothyroidism, and premature ovarian failure. The diagnosis of polycystic ovary syndrome is clinical and is based on a history of anovulation, symptoms or signs of androgen excess, and the finding of polycystic ovaries on ultrasound. Laboratory confimation is made by finding elevated total or free testosterone levels.[32] Late-onset or nonclassic 21-hydroxylase deficiency is an uncommon cause of androgen excess, occurring in less than 5% of hyperandrogenic women. It can be reliably ruled out by a 17-hydroxyprogesterone of less than 2 ng/mL.[33]

Endometrial biopsy should be considered for all patients with abnormal uterine bleeding and a risk factor for endometrial cancer, particularly those 45 years of age or older and those who weigh 90 kg or more. Some authors recommend that an endometrial biopsy be done in a patient of any age with a history of anovulatory bleeding of more than 1 year's duration because there have been reports of endometrial cancer in patients as young as 15 years of age.[24,34] The Pipelle endometrial sampling device is superior to other biopsy techniques. It is an office procedure that is easily performed and well tolerated. It has a sensitivity of 91% for the diagnosis of premenopausal endometrial carcinoma, sensitivity of 81% for the diagnosis of atypical endometrial hyperplasia, and specificity for both of greater than 98%.[35] Although an endometrial thickness of 5 mm or greater

on transvaginal ultrasound detects 96% of endometrial cancer in postmenopausal women, there are no data concerning its role in the diagnosis of endometrial cancer in premenopausal women.[36]

## TREATMENT

### Menometrorrhagia

The two general approaches to treatment of menometrorrhagia are surgical and medical therapy (Table 8-3). Hysteroscopic resection of a submucosal myoma or polyp in patients with menometrorrhagia has become standard practice (see Chapter 38). About 80% of women with menometrorrhagia treated with resection of endometrial polyps report the return to a normal pattern of menstrual bleeding, with a mean follow-up of 5 years.[37] After hysteroscopic resection of a submucosal myoma, the 3-year probability of recurrence of myomas and menorrhagia is 34% and 30%, respectively.[38]

As a general rule in patients with menometrorrhagia without obvious uterine myomas and no intracavitary lesions, medical treatments should be attempted before surgical therapy. If

---

**Table 8-3**
**Treatment of Abnormal Uterine Bleeding**

**Menometrorrhagia**

Anatomic defect
  Endometrial polyp or submucosal myoma
    Hysteroscopic resection
  Other uterine myoma
    More children desired: myomectomy
    No more children desired: hysterectomy
  Adenomyosis
    More children desired: medical therapy (see essential menorrhagia)
    No more children desired: hysterectomy
Bleeding disorders
  Consultation with hematologist
  Oral contraceptive pill
  Intranasal desmopressin
  Tranexamic acid
  Endometrial ablation
Hypothyroidism
  Thyroid replacement therapy
Essential menorrhagia
  Oral contraceptive pill
  NSAIDs
  Combination of oral contraceptive pill and NSAID
  Levonorgestrel IUD
  Failure of above treatments and more children desired: GnRH agonist and add-back therapy; danazol
  Failure of above treatments and no more children desired: endometrial ablation

**Dysfunctional uterine bleeding**

Hyperprolactinemia
  Carbergoline
  Bromocriptine
Hypothyroidism
  Thyroid replacement therapy
Other causes of anovulation
  Oral contraceptive pill
  Cyclic progestins
  Failure of above treatments and more children desired: levonorgestrel IUD; GnRH agonist and add-back therapy
  Failure of above treatments and no more children desired: hysterectomy

hypothyroidism is present, patients respond very quickly to thyroid hormone replacement therapy, with a rapid decline in menstrual blood loss.[39,40] Medical therapies for von Willebrand's disease include the oral contraceptive pill, intranasal desmopressin, and antifibrinolytics such as tranexamic acid. Endometrial ablation also may be effective.[31,41]

Medical therapies for menorrhagia include the oral contraceptive pill, oral progestins, progestin-containing IUDs, nonsteroidal anti-inflammatory drugs (NSAIDs), danazol, tranexamic acid, and gonadotropin-releasing hormone (GnRH) agonists. The oral contraceptive pill is probably the first line of therapy for treating menorrhagia, and its efficacy is supported by wide clinical experience.[4] However, few objective data support this common clinical practice. A recent review found a single randomized trial of the oral contraceptive pill in menorrhagia. The oral contraceptive pill reduced menstrual blood loss by 43% and did not differ in efficacy from danazol, mefenamic acid, or naproxen.[42]

An oral progestin given only during the luteal phase is not effective in the treatment of menorrhagia. However, when started on cycle day 5 and continued for 21 days, norethindrone acetate 5 mg three times a day resulted in an 87% reduction in menstrual blood loss compared with baseline. Oral norethindrone acetate was less efficacious than the levonorgestrel-releasing IUD and had a lower proportion of patient acceptability.[43]

The levonorgestrel-releasing IUD reduces menstrual blood loss by 96% after 12 months in patients with essential menorrhagia and to a significantly greater degree than an NSAID or tranexamic acid.[44] After an initial randomized treatment period of 6 months, 64% of women scheduled for hysterectomy because of menorrhagia postponed surgery and continued treatment with the levonorgestrel-releasing IUD compared with 14% undergoing other medical treatments ($P < 0.001$).[45] In a randomized trial in women with menorrhagia, the levonorgestrel IUD was as effective as endometrial resection as determined by hemoglobin concentrations after 6 months of therapy and by rates of satisfaction with treatment.[46] However, women with menorrhagia who underwent endometrial resection had a significantly greater reduction in menstrual blood loss, higher rates of amenorrhea, and fewer progestogenic side effects.[47] Five-year follow-up of 236 women with menorrhagia randomized to either the levonorgestrel IUD or hysterectomy found similar improvement in health-related quality of life in the two groups. Although 42% of women randomized to the IUD eventually had a hysterectomy, the costs in the IUD group remained substantially lower than in the hysterectomy group.[48]

The levonorgestrel IUD also is effective in treating menorrhagia in women with adenomyosis diagnosed by transvaginal ultrasound. Treatment resulted in resolution of menorrhagia in all 24 patients and a significant increase in hemoglobin at 3, 6, and 12 months of therapy.[49] In contrast, the levonorgestrel IUD is relatively ineffective in treating menorrhagia in women with leiomyomas and a uterine volume equivalent to 8 to 12 weeks of pregnancy but without intracavitary abnormalities, with 14 of 19 women having persistent menorrhagia after 12 months of therapy.[50]

Randomized trials have shown that NSAIDs reduce menstrual blood loss by 20% to 50% in women with objectively verified menorrhagia and are well tolerated when given for about 5 days.[51] Mefenamic acid 500 mg three times a day is the most studied drug. However, both ibuprofen 400 mg three times a day and naproxen 250 mg four times a day are efficacious. Limited data do not suggest a difference in efficacy among the NSAIDs.

Danazol 200 mg daily for 3 months reduces menstrual blood loss by 80%.[52] Small clinical trials have found that danazol is more effective than the oral contraceptive pill or mefenamic acid in treating menorrhagia.[53] Its usefulness is limited by daily administration and the need for adequate contraception owing the risk of masculization of a female fetus exposed to danazol between 8 and 18 weeks' gestation. Other androgenic side effects of danazol include weight gain, acne, hirsutism, and hoarseness. Thus, danazol is effective but rarely used to treat menorrhagia because of side effect and safety concerns.

Tranexamic acid is a plasminogen activator inhibitor approved in the United States for treatment of acute episodes of bleeding in hemophilia. It reduces menstrual blood loss by 50% in women with objectively proved essential menorrhagia.[54] The usual dose is 1 g four times a day during days 1 through 5 of the menstrual cycle. Tranexamic acid is more effective than NSAIDs but has not been compared with hormonal treatments for menorrhagia. The major concern about use of tranexamic acid is the risk of thrombosis. Long-term studies in Sweden show that the rate of thrombosis in women treated with tranexamic acid is comparable with the rate in untreated women. However, there have been at least three cases of intracranial arterial thrombosis in women using antithrombolytics for menorrhagia.[6]

GnRH agonists have been investigated in patients with essential menorrhagia and adenomyosis. There are case reports of pregnancy following GnRH agonist therapy of severe adenomyosis.[55,56] A GnRH agonist given with cyclic hormone replacement therapy reduced menstrual blood loss by 43% in women with objectively proved essential menorrhagia.[57] Because of their expense, GnRH agonists should be reserved for use in women with essential menorrhagia or adenomyosis who are unresponsive to other medical therapy and who wish to preserve childbearing.

Surgical therapy of essential menorrhagia is discussed in detail in Section 6 of this text but is briefly considered here, particularly in comparison to medical therapy. Hysterectomy and endometrial ablation are the two general categories of surgical treatment for essential menorrhagia. First-generation endometrial ablation techniques include endometrial resection, rollerball, and laser ablation. Second-generation ablative techniques include inflatable balloons inserted into the endometrial cavity through which heated water is circulated, hot water instillation systems, endometrial cryoablation, and intrauterine diode laser fiber arrays.[58] The goal of these second-generation techniques is to achieve effectiveness similar to that of first-generation techniques but with greater patient safety and ease of operator use. Most second-generation techniques give similar results. Generally, there is about a 30% to 50% prevalence of amenorrhea and 80% to 90% satisfaction rate 6 months after second-generation treatments.[58]

After 6 months to 2 years of treatment or follow-up, both hysterectomy and endometrial ablation are superior to oral medical therapy with regard to control of bleeding, patient satisfaction, and side effects as determined in randomized trials.[58–60]

## Ambulatory Office Practice

As noted previously, the levonorgestrel IUD is somewhat less effective than endometrial ablation or hysterectomy but remains a reasonable alternative.

When surgical techniques are compared, patient satisfaction rates are slightly but significantly higher after hysterectomy than after first-generation endometrial ablation techniques. Within 5 years of ablation, about 15% of women will have a second ablation and about 20% will undergo hysterectomy.[58]

If deep adenomyosis is present, hysterectomy, not ablation, is probably a more appropriate therapy. Adenomyosis is a frequent finding in hysterectomy specimens from patients whose ablation treatment has failed.[61,62]

### Dysfunctional Uterine Bleeding

When dysfunctional uterine bleeding is due to hyperprolactinemia, a dopamine agonist, such as cabergoline or bromocriptine, is effective in restoring ovulatory function. Carbergoline is more effective and better tolerated than bromocriptine, but only bromocriptine is approved for ovulation induction in women desiring pregnancy.[63] The oral contraceptive pill may also be used to control abnormal bleeding in hyperprolactinemic patients, although there is some concern that it could result in growth of a prolactin-secreting microadenoma.[64] Patients with dysfunctional uterine bleeding and hypothyroidism respond quickly to thyroid hormone replacement therapy, as noted above.

In other patients with dysfunctional uterine bleeding, periodic progestin administration is probably effective in restoring a normal bleeding pattern (see Table 8-3). A progestin, such as medroxyprogesterone acetate, is given by mouth 5 mg daily for the first 14 days of each month. There are some objective data that either cyclic medroxyprogesterone acetate or norethindrone acetate given for 14 days of each month results in a significant decrease in blood loss and duration of bleeding in women with dysfunctional uterine bleeding.[65] The oral contraceptive pill is often used and widely accepted as effective treatment in patients with dysfunctional uterine bleeding, although objective data are scarce. A randomized, double-blind, multicenter trial found a triphasic norgestimate-ethinyl estradiol oral contraceptive pill superior to placebo in treating anovulatory dysfunctional uterine bleeding. Subjects treated with the oral contraceptive pill were nearly twice as likely to note improvement in their bleeding pattern than were women treated with placebo (87% vs 45%), and 47% of treated subjects developed regular bleeding patterns in the relatively brief three study cycles.[66]

Metformin, usually in dosages of 1500 to 1700 mg/day, results in ovulation in 50% or more of women with polycystic ovary syndrome.[67] However, it has not been investigated as a treatment for dysfunctional uterine bleeding in this disorder.

The levonorgestrel IUD is a reasonable next option in women who do not respond to therapy with progestins or the oral contraceptive pill, although there are no data on its efficacy in this subgroup. As with essential dysmenorrhea, the last resort of medical therapy in women desiring more children is a GnRH agonist with add-back therapy.

Occasionally, patients with dysfunctional uterine bleeding have acute episodes of extremely heavy bleeding that require immediate therapy. An effective outpatient therapy is to give any low-dose oral contraceptive pill, one or two pills twice daily for 5 to 7 days. Patients usually stop bleeding within 12 to 24 hours, but therapy should be continued for the full 7 days. Upon completion of therapy, the patient will have a self-limited episode of bleeding, which may be heavy. Five days after discontinuing the initial dosage, the birth control pill can be restarted, one tablet daily as for contraception.[68] In patients with significant anemia, the withdrawal bleed may be postponed by continuing the oral contraceptive until the hemoglobin is adequate to allow it. In women requiring inpatient observation and therapy, intravenous Premarin, 25 mg every 3 to 4 hours for up to three doses, is effective in the treatment of dysfunctional uterine bleeding.[69] After the acute episode of bleeding is treated, it is important to give the patient chronic intermittent progestin therapy or the oral contraceptive pill to prevent further episodes.

Endometrial ablation is not the ideal therapy for patients with dysfunctional uterine bleeding, because chronic anovulation and unopposed ovarian estrogen production continue despite ablation. Since the endometrium may not be completely destroyed by endometrial ablation, there is continued need for progestin therapy to prevent endometrial carcinoma in the residual islands. Endometrial carcinoma has been reported in a variety of circumstances following endometrial ablation, including in two perimenopausal patients 3 and 5 years after endometrial ablation for dysfunctional uterine bleeding.[70,71] In the author's opinion, hysterectomy may be a more appropriate surgical choice for patients who cannot tolerate or do not respond to medical therapy for dysfunctional uterine bleeding.

## REFERENCES

1. Coulter A, Bradlow J, Agass M, et al: Outcomes of referrals to gynaecology outpatient clinics for menstrual problems: an audit of general practice records. Br J Obstet Gynaecol 1991;98:789–796. **(IIa, B)**
2. Farquhar CM, Steiner CA: Hysterectomy rates in the United States 1990–1997. Obstet Gynecol 2002;99:229–234. **(IIa, B)**
3. Cote I, Jacobs P, Cumming D: Work loss associated with increased menstrual loss in the United States. Obstet Gynecol 2002;100:683–687. **(IIa, B)**
4. Oehler MK, Rees MC: Menorrhagia: an update. Acta Obstet Gynecol Scand 2003;82:405–422. **(IV, C)**
5. Hallberg L, Hogdahl AM, Nilsson L, Rybo G: Menstrual blood loss—a population study: variation at different ages and attempts to define normality. Acta Obstet Gynecol Scand 1966;45:320–351. **(IIa, B)**
6. Van Eijkeren MA, Christiaens GC, Sixma JJ, Haspels AA: Menorrhagia: a review. Obstet Gynecol Surv 1989;44:421–429. **(IV, C)**
7. Clevenger-Hoeft M, Syrop CH, Stovall DW, Van Voorhis BJ: Sonohysterography in premenopausal women with and without abnormal bleeding. Obstet Gynecol 1999;94:516–520. **(IIa, B)**
8. McCausland AM: Hysteroscopic myometrial biopsy: its use in diagnosing adenomyosis and its clinical application. Am J Obstet Gynecol 1992;166(6 Pt 1):1619–1626. **(IIa, B)**
9. Ferenczy A: Pathophysiology of adenomyosis. Hum Reprod Update 1998;4:312–322. **(IV, C)**
10. Emge LA: The elusive adenomyosis of the uterus: its historical past and its present state of recognition. Am J Obstet Gynecol 1962; 83:1541–1563. **(IV, C)**
11. Kilkku P, Erkkola R, Gronroos M: Non-specificity of symptoms related to adenomyosis: a prospective comparative survey. Acta Obstet Gynecol Scand 1984;63:229–231. **(IIa, B)**

12. Fedele L, Bianchi S, Dorta M, et al: Transvaginal ultrasonography in the diagnosis of diffuse adenomyosis. Fertil Steril 1992;58:94–97. **(IIa, B)**

13. Krassas GE, Pontikides N, Kaltsas T, et al: Menstrual disturbances in thyrotoxicosis. Clin Endocrinol (Oxf) 1994;40:641–644. **(IIa, B)**

14. Krassas GE, Pontikides N, Kaltsas T, et al: Disturbances of menstruation in hypothyroidism. Clin Endocrinol (Oxf) 1999;50:655–659. **(IIa, B)**

15. Wilansky DL, Greisman B: Early hypothyroidism in patients with menorrhagia. Am J Obstet Gynecol 1989;160:673–677. **(III, B)**

16. Claessens EA, Cowell CA: Acute adolescent menorrhagia. Am J Obstet Gynecol 1981;139:277–280. **(III, B)**

17. Oral E, Cagdas A, Gezer A, et al: Hematological abnormalities in adolescent menorrhagia. Arch Gynecol Obstet 2002;266:72–74. **(III, B)**

18. Edlund M, Blomback M, von Schoultz B, Andersson O: On the value of menorrhagia as a predictor for coagulation disorders. Am J Hematol 1996;53:234–238. **(III, B)**

19. Kadir RA, Economides DL, Sabin CA, et al: Frequency of inherited bleeding disorders in women with menorrhagia. Lancet 1998; 351:485–489. **(III, B)**

20. Woo YL, White B, Corbally R, et al: von Willebrand's disease: an important cause of dysfunctional uterine bleeding. Blood Coagul Fibrinolysis 2002;13:89–93. **(IIa, B)**

21. Dilley A, Drews C, Miller C, et al: von Willebrand disease and other inherited bleeding disorders in women with diagnosed menorrhagia. Obstet Gynecol 2001;97:630–636. **(IIa, B)**

22. van Eijkeren MA, Christiaens GC, Haspels AA, Sixma JJ: Measured menstrual blood loss in women with a bleeding disorder or using oral anticoagulant therapy. Am J Obstet Gynecol 1990;162:1261–1263. **(IIa, B)**

23. Peterson HB, Jeng G, Folger SG, et al: The risk of menstrual abnormalities after tubal sterilization: U.S. Collaborative Review of Sterilization Working Group. N Engl J Med 2000;343:1681–1687. **(IIa, B)**

24. Bayer SR, DeCherney AH: Clinical manifestations and treatment of dysfunctional uterine bleeding. JAMA 1993;269:1823–1828. **(IV, C)**

25. Coulam CB, Annegers JF, Kranz JS: Chronic anovulation syndrome and associated neoplasia. Obstet Gynecol 1983;61:403–407. **(IIb, B)**

26. Farquhar CM, Lethaby A, Sowter M, et al: An evaluation of risk factors for endometrial hyperplasia in premenopausal women with abnormal menstrual bleeding. Am J Obstet Gynecol 1999;181:525–529. **(IIa, B)**

27. de Kroon CD, de Bock GH, Dieben SW, Jansen FW: Saline contrast hysterosonography in abnormal uterine bleeding: a systematic review and meta-analysis. BJOG 2003;110:938–947. **(Ia, A)**

28. Dueholm M, Lundorf E, Hansen ES, et al: Evaluation of the uterine cavity with magnetic resonance imaging, transvaginal sonography, hysterosonographic examination, and diagnostic hysteroscopy. Fertil Steril 2001;76:350–357. **(IIa, B)**

29. Togashi K, Ozasa H, Konishi I, et al: Enlarged uterus: differentiation between adenomyosis and leiomyoma with MR imaging. Radiology 1989;171:531–534. **(IIa, B)**

30. Kouides PA: Menorrhagia from a haematologist's point of view. 1. Initial evaluation. Haemophilia 2002;8:330–338. **(IV, C)**

31. Committee Opinion No. 263, December 2001: von Willebrand's disease in gynecologic practice. Obstet Gynecol 2001;98:1185–1186. **(IV, C)**

32. Revised 2003 consensus on diagnostic criteria and long-term health risks related to polycystic ovary syndrome (PCOS). Hum Reprod 2004;19:41–47. **(IV, C)**

33. Azziz R, Hincapie LA, Knochenhauer ES, et al: Screening for 21-hydroxylase-deficient nonclassic adrenal hyperplasia among hyperandrogenic women: a prospective study. Fertil Steril 1999;72:915–925. **(IIa, B)**

34. Farhi DC, Nosanchuk J, Silverberg SG: Endometrial adenocarcinoma in women under 25 years of age. Obstet Gynecol 1986;68:741–745. **(III, B)**

35. Dijkhuizen FP, Mol BW, Brolmann HA, Heintz AP: The accuracy of endometrial sampling in the diagnosis of patients with endometrial carcinoma and hyperplasia: a meta-analysis. Cancer 2000;89:1765–1772. **(Ia, A)**

36. Smith-Bindman R, Kerlikowske K, Feldstein VA, et al: Endovaginal ultrasound to exclude endometrial cancer and other endometrial abnormalities. JAMA 1998;280:1510–1517. **(IV, C)**

37. Cravello L, Stolla V, Bretelle F, et al: Hysteroscopic resection of endometrial polyps: a study of 195 cases. Eur J Obstet Gynecol Reprod Biol 2000;93:131–134. **(III, B)**

38. Vercellini P, Zaina B, Yaylayan L, et al: Hysteroscopic myomectomy: long-term effects on menstrual pattern and fertility. Obstet Gynecol 1999;94:341–347. **(III, B)**

39. Higham JM, Shaw RW: The effect of thyroxine replacement on menstrual blood loss in a hypothyroid patient. Br J Obstet Gynaecol 1992;99:695–696. **(III, B)**

40. Scott JC Jr, Mussey E: Menstrual patterns in myxedema. Am J Obstet Gynecol 1964;90:161–165. **(III, B)**

41. Siegel JE, Kouides PA: Menorrhagia from a haematologist's point of view. 2. Management. Haemophilia 2002;8:339–347. **(IV, C)**

42. Iyer V, Farquhar C, Jepson R: Oral contraceptive pills for heavy menstrual bleeding. Cochrane Database Syst Rev 2000:CD000154. **(Ib, A)**

43. Lethaby A, Irvine G, Cameron I: Cyclical progestogens for heavy menstrual bleeding. Cochrane Database Syst Rev 2000:CD001016. **(Ib, A)**

44. Milsom I, Andersson K, Andersch B, Rybo G: A comparison of flurbiprofen, tranexamic acid, and a levonorgestrel-releasing intrauterine contraceptive device in the treatment of idiopathic menorrhagia. Am J Obstet Gynecol 1991;164:879–883. **(IIa, B)**

45. Lahteenmaki P, Haukkamaa M, Puolakka J, et al: Open randomised study of use of levonorgestrel releasing intrauterine system as alternative to hysterectomy. BMJ 1998;316:1122–1126. **(Ib, A)**

46. Crosignani PG, Vercellini P, Mosconi P, et al: Levonorgestrel-releasing intrauterine device versus hysteroscopic endometrial resection in the treatment of dysfunctional uterine bleeding. Obstet Gynecol 1997; 90:257–263. **(Ib, A)**

47. Lethaby AE, Cooke I, Rees M: Progesterone/progestogen releasing intrauterine systems versus either placebo or any other medication for heavy menstrual bleeding. Cochrane Database Syst Rev 2000:CD002126. **(Ib, A)**

48. Hurskainen R, Teperi J, Rissanen P, et al: Clinical outcomes and costs with the levonorgestrel-releasing intrauterine system or hysterectomy for treatment of menorrhagia: randomized trial 5-year follow-up. JAMA 2004;291:1456–1463. **(Ib, A)**

49. Fedele L, Bianchi S, Raffaelli R, et al: Treatment of adenomyosis-associated menorrhagia with a levonorgestrel-releasing intrauterine device. Fertil Steril 1997;68:426–429. **(IIb, B)**

50. Mercorio F, De Simone R, Di Spiezio Sardo A, et al: The effect of a levonorgestrel-releasing intrauterine device in the treatment of myoma-related menorrhagia. Contraception 2003;67:277–280. **(IIb, B)**

51. Lethaby A, Augood C, Duckitt K: Nonsteroidal anti-inflammatory drugs for heavy menstrual bleeding. Cochrane Database Syst Rev 2002:CD000400. **(Ia, A)**

52. Chimbira TH, Anderson AB, Naish C, et al: Reduction of menstrual blood loss by danazol in unexplained menorrhagia: lack of effect of placebo. Br J Obstet Gynaecol 1980;87:1152–1158. **(Ib, A)**

53. Beaumont H, Augood C, Duckitt K, Lethaby A: Danazol for heavy menstrual bleeding. Cochrane Database Syst Rev 2002:CD001017. **(Ia, A)**

54. Lethaby A, Farquhar C, Cooke I: Antifibrinolytics for heavy menstrual bleeding. Cochrane Database Syst Rev 2000:CD000249. **(Ia, A)**

55. Hirata JD, Moghissi KS, Ginsburg KA: Pregnancy after medical therapy of adenomyosis with a gonadotropin-releasing hormone agonist. Fertil Steril 1993;59:444–445. **(III, B)**

56. Nelson JR, Corson SL: Long-term management of adenomyosis with a gonadotropin-releasing hormone agonist: a case report. Fertil Steril 1993;59:441–443. **(III, B)**

57. Thomas EJ, Okuda KJ, Thomas NM: The combination of a depot gonadotrophin releasing hormone agonist and cyclical hormone replacement therapy for dysfunctional uterine bleeding. Br J Obstet Gynaecol 1991;98:1155–1159. **(IIb, B)**

58. Sowter MC: New surgical treatments for menorrhagia. Lancet 2003;361:1456–1458. **(IV, C)**

59. Learman LA, Summitt RL Jr, Varner RE, et al: Hysterectomy versus expanded medical treatment for abnormal uterine bleeding: clinical outcomes in the medicine or surgery trial. Obstet Gynecol 2004;103 (5 Pt 1):824–833. **(Ib, A)**

60. Marjoribanks J, Lethaby A, Farquhar C: Surgery versus medical therapy for heavy menstrual bleeding. Cochrane Database Syst Rev 2003:CD003855. **(Ia, A)**

61. Daniell JF, Kurtz BR, Ke RW: Hysteroscopic endometrial ablation using the rollerball electrode. Obstet Gynecol 1992;80(3 Pt 1):329–332. **(III, B)**

62. Derman SG, Rehnstrom J, Neuwirth RS: The long-term effectiveness of hysteroscopic treatment of menorrhagia and leiomyomas. Obstet Gynecol 1991;77:591–594. **(III, B)**

63. Webster J, Piscitelli G, Polli A, et al: A comparison of cabergoline and bromocriptine in the treatment of hyperprolactinemic amenorrhea. Cabergoline Comparative Study Group. N Engl J Med 1994; 331:904–909. **(Ib, A)**

64. Schlechte JA: Clinical Practice: prolactinoma. N Engl J Med 2003; 349:2035–2041. **(IV, C)**

65. Hickey M, Higham J, Fraser IS: Progestogens versus oestrogens and progestogens for irregular uterine bleeding associated with anovulation. Cochrane Database Syst Rev 2000:CD001895. **(IIa, B)**

66. Davis A, Godwin A, Lippman J, et al: Triphasic norgestimate-ethinyl estradiol for treating dysfunctional uterine bleeding. Obstet Gynecol 2000;96:913–920. **(Ib, A)**

67. Costello MF, Eden JA: A systematic review of the reproductive system effects of metformin in patients with polycystic ovary syndrome. Fertil Steril 2003;79:1–13. **(IV, C)**

68. Dysfunctional uterine bleeding. In Speroff L, Glass R, Kase N (eds): Clinical Gynecologic Endocrinology and Infertility, 6th ed. Baltimore, Md, Lippincott Williams & Wilkins, 1999:pp 575–594. **(IV, C)**

69. DeVore GR, Owens O, Kase N: Use of intravenous Premarin in the treatment of dysfunctional uterine bleeding—a double-blind randomized control study. Obstet Gynecol 1982;59:285–291. **(Ib, A)**

70. Copperman AB, DeCherney AH, Olive DL: A case of endometrial cancer following endometrial ablation for dysfunctional uterine bleeding. Obstet Gynecol 1993;82(4 Pt 2 Suppl):640–642. **(III, B)**

71. Valle RF, Baggish MS: Endometrial carcinoma after endometrial ablation: high-risk factors predicting its occurrence. Am J Obstet Gynecol 1998;179(3 Pt 1):569–572. **(III, B)**

# Chapter 9

# Preventive Health

Alice W. Chuang, MD, and Frank W. Ling, MD

## KEY POINTS

- Preventive medicine involves a spectrum of interventions, including primary, secondary, and tertiary prevention.
- Screening tests should not be utilized or interpreted in the same way as diagnostic tests.
- A basic knowledge of epidemiology is important for understanding preventive health care and implementing preventive evaluations and interventions.
- Many different preventive recommendations or guidelines are offered by various professional medical, research, and epidemiologic societies.
- Important preventive health topics include tobacco use, alcohol misuse, unintentional injury, seat belt use, depression, hyperlipidemia, hypertension, and obesity. Physicians can make a difference in these areas with appropriate screening and counseling.
- As health care resources become more scarce and practitioners become busier, it is important to use only those interventions that have been proven to change outcomes.

## INTRODUCTION

The advent of health care maintenance organizations and the concept of primary care physicians as gatekeepers have brought preventive medicine to the forefront as the key to better use of health care resources. The purpose of preventive medicine is to detect disease before its onset or in its early stages in order to implement early treatment. Preventive counseling can empower a patient to take appropriate measures to eliminate risks and to adopt healthful behaviors to prevent disease.

Although many diseases present clear potential for prevention, many interventions have not been proved to prevent disease. It is paramount that clinicians know which tests, types of counseling, and treatments actually work as demonstrated by rigorous research. Unfortunately, screening of the asymptomatic individual is time consuming and is often unwelcomed by the patient and not reimbursed by third-party payers.

While screening for disease seems only beneficial, there are potential harms. There certainly is harm if screening is performed incorrectly. But even when performed correctly, screening has downfalls. Screening inevitably produces a certain number of false-positive results. Subsequent testing, particularly if invasive, can increase morbidity and mortality. The patient can experience anxiety and stress induced by the diagnostic limbo created by a positive screening test. Patients who are incorrectly screened can be mislabeled. False-negative screens, on the other hand, can give a false sense of security.

Additionally, clinicians need to be knowledgeable about the appropriate interpretation of screening tests. The possible outcomes of screening should be reviewed with patients before the test and then more specifically reviewed after test results are returned. The imprecise role of screening for diagnosis should be clarified for patients.

Preventive medicine is inherently different from the classical curative model of the physician's role.[1] Historically, patients come to physicians with complaints. Preventive medicine requires the physician to be proactive—the instigator of questions, screening, and treatment. A physician's skills as an educator are paramount for a successful preventive practice. The physician must be able to assess a nondiseased patient's risks, offer applicable screening for diseases, determine the most appropriate preventive interventions, counsel the patient about these interventions, and then educate the patient about the potential results and necessary follow-up plans. The physician has to be able to motivate the unmotivated patient and to change patient behavior and compliance—and to be able to do all of this in the setting of a busy ambulatory practice!

## DEFINITIONS

*Primary prevention* is preventing the onset of disease. It should be applied to all patients. Common examples include obesity counseling and immunizations. *Secondary prevention* is diagnosing disease in its asymptomatic state. It is often applied to a more narrow population, perhaps those at risk for a specific disease. For instance, the Papanicolaou (Pap) smear is a screening test for early dysplastic changes that can be treated, preventing progression to cervical cancer. *Tertiary prevention* is preventing serious sequelae from previously diagnosed disease. An example is anticoagulation in patients with known coagulopathy in order to prevent deep vein thrombosis and subsequent pulmonary embolus.

To evaluate a screening test, it is important to be familiar with some basic epidemiologic concepts and link them to important clinical questions. *Sensitivity* is the proportion of the population with disease who have a positive test. (What percentage of people who actually have the disease will test positive?) *Specificity* is the proportion of the population *without* disease who have a negative test. (What percentage of people who do *not* have the disease will test negative?) *Positive predictive value* is the proportion of the population with a positive test who have the disease. (What is the chance that you have the disease if your test is positive?) *Negative predictive value* is the proportion of the population with a negative test who do *not* have the disease.

# Ambulatory Office Practice

(What is the chance that you really do *not* have the disease if your test is negative?)

Additional concepts that are important to be familiar with include the following. *Incidence* is the number of new cases of disease in a certain period of time. *Prevalence* is the total number of existing cases. This is a particularly important concept because a disease with low prevalence decreases positive predictive value, highlighting the point that certain screening tests are inappropriate in certain populations. *Reliability* is a test's ability to produce the same result time after time. *Validity* is the ability of a test to measure what it claims to measure.

In general very few tests have good sensitivity and good specificity. Most involve trade-offs between the two. Experts have tried to develop different measures of validity to help clinicians understand and gauge which tests are appropriate. One example is diagnostic accuracy, which is defined as the sum of true positives and true negatives divided by the number of all those tested.[2] Others suggest that the definition of a "good" screening test is one in which the sum of the sensitivity and specificity is greater than or equal to 1.5. A "very good" test has a sum of at least 1.8.

A good screening test is sensitive but often not specific. Screening tests should be designed to detect a significant majority of those affected, sometimes at the cost of falsely detecting some who are not. Screening protocols, constructed with a series of tests, correct for this by further evaluating those who are screen positive. These tests usually proceed in a stepwise fashion, becoming progressively more invasive, more diagnostically accurate, and more expensive in order to maximally utilize resources. It is possible also to screen by performing two tests simultaneously, thus often improving sensitivity.

Though many health care dollars are spent researching and implementing screening strategies, screening is only appropriate if the following criteria are met.[3] (1) The disease being screened for is a significant public health problem. What is the burden of disease compared with the burden of prevention? What are the long-term outcomes of this disease? What is the severity of the disease? What is the prevalence of the disease? (2) The disease can be detected in the asymptomatic state. In other words, there is a definable period prior to the onset of disease that can be identified. Various methods of screening include questionnaires and history-taking, laboratory results, and physical examination findings. (3) The disease can be treated in the early stages. There is no point to screen for disease if no intervention will improve outcomes.

To make the situation even more confusing, many governing bodies offer different recommendations colored by their organizational biases and based on different data. Sometimes their recommendations even conflict! Examples of such organizations are the American Cancer Society (ACS), the American College of Obstetricians and Gynecologists (ACOG), the World Health Organization (WHO), the Centers for Disease Control and Prevention (CDC), the American Academy of Family Physicians (AAFP), the American Heart Association (AHA), the National Institutes of Health (NIH), the American College of Physicians (ACP), the American Medical Association (AMA), the United States Preventive Services Task Force (USPSTF), and the American College of Preventive Medicine (ACPM).

The best strategy is to examine all the data with a critical eye; however, in light of the plethora of literature, not to mention clinical responsibilities, this is impossible for most practitioners. All these organizations strive to summarize the data, but their conclusions can differ. USPSTF and its Canadian equivalent, the Canadian Task Force, adhere to rigorous standards in their evaluation of preventive care data. Their recommendations offer solid guidelines based on objective review of the best data available.

## TOPICS FOR PREVENTIVE MEDICINE

The following discussion does not address preventive issues that are discussed elsewhere in this text, such as osteoporosis, cancer prevention, preventive health in pregnancy, domestic violence, screening in the pediatric patient, preconceptional screening, contraception screening, and sexually transmitted infection screening. The following discussions occur in no particular order.

### Skin Cancer

Skin cancer is the most common cancer in the United States. There are three major types: melanoma, basal cell carcinoma, and squamous cell carcinoma. Basal cell carcinoma is the most common; melanoma is the most lethal, accounting for 75% of deaths from skin cancer. The incidence of melanoma is increasing from 5.7/100,000 in 1973 to 17.7/100,000 in 2000. The overall mortality also is increasing from 1.6/100,000 to 2.4/100,000 in the same time period. Melanoma is the sixth most common cancer-causing death, with 44,000 new cases diagnosed in 1999. The 5-year survival from melanoma is 89.6%, increased from previous years.[4]

It is important to distinguish between melanoma and non-melanoma (basal cell and squamous cell) skin cancers. Basal cell and squamous cell carcinoma treatments are almost always curative. Most screening protocols are directed at melanoma because of its increased morbidity and mortality.

A successful screening program with early treatment has the potential in theory to prevent some of the morbidity associated with advanced skin cancer treatments including disfigurement, anxiety, and complications of treatment. Screening techniques that have been studied in this area include full-body skin examination, questionnaires identifying risk, and education about sun avoidance, including wearing sun block and staying out of the sun during times of highest ultraviolet ray exposure. The morbidity associated with these techniques is limited to inconvenience to the patient, embarrassment from full-body skin examination, possible skin reactions from sun block, and misdiagnosis.

The official recommendation of USPSTF is that the evidence is insufficient to recommend for or against performing full-body examination for early detection of skin cancer.[5] The benefit is unproved even in patients at high risk for melanoma, including fair-skinned men and women older than 65 years of age, individuals with atypical moles, and those with more than 50 moles. Of course, suspicious lesions, specifically those with asymmetry, variable coloring, irregular borders, or a diameter greater than 6 mm should be sampled for biopsy.

No randomized-controlled trials have examined whether skin cancer screening of the general population results in a difference in skin-cancer deaths. In populations that were self-selected secondary to interest in free screening or that had lesions requiring examination, dermatologic specialists were able to identify cancerous lesions with greater sensitivity and specificity than were general practitioners. These results cannot be extrapolated to a general population for screening. General screening does not seem to increase the detection rate compared with partial examination or lesion-focused examination.[6]

One case-control study examined the effect of self-examination on morbidity and mortality from melanoma.[7] Berwick and colleagues studied 650 Caucasians with primary melanoma and matched them to 549 Caucasians from the general population. They followed both groups for 5 years and queried them about whether they performed skin examinations of any kind. They found that self–skin examination was associated with a decreased incidence of melanoma (OR 0.66, 95% CI 0.44–0.99) in the control group and a decreased incidence of lethal melanoma (OR 0.37, 95% CI 0.16–0.84) in those who already had the diagnosis.

It is important to remember that self-examination is not the same intervention as routine screening by a primary care physician. Self-examination usually occurs at more frequent intervals and thus can detect changes in lesions more effectively. However, one benefit of physician total-body examination is increased self-skin examination. Screening has been shown to increase biopsies.

USPSTF also has concluded that the evidence is insufficient to recommend routine counseling to change behaviors as a means to prevent long-term morbidity and mortality associated with skin cancer.[8] These behaviors include wearing sunscreen with UVA and UVB protection, avoiding tanning beds, avoiding sun from 10 AM to 4 PM, wearing protective clothing and accessories, and self-examining of the skin. Intense exposure, fair complexion, severe sunburn, and intermittent (as opposed to chronic) sun exposure all have been shown to increase risk for melanoma.

Wearing sunscreen decreases squamous cell carcinoma, but the results concerning preventing melanoma are mixed. Several descriptive studies show increased melanoma in those using sunscreen. Perhaps those using sunscreen are more likely to be at risk for other reasons and spend more hours in the sun when wearing sunscreen. The effect of tanning beds on melanoma incidence is mixed as well. There is no decreased vitamin D level in those using sunscreen.[9] One study has shown that youths are more likely to use sunscreen if their parents do. Thus, one benefit of changing adult behavior is to potentially alter the behavior of their children[10] (Table 9-1).

## Physical Activity

All evidence points to the benefits of physical activity in preventing many common chronic illnesses: obesity, hypertension, osteoporosis, cardiovascular disease, diabetes, and depression to name a few. This benefit is seen at even modest increases in activity or moderate activity for 30 minutes on most days of the week, with a dose-response effect. Despite these commonly known benefits, only 20% to 30% of adults achieve this activity level, with no appreciable change from 1990 to 1998.[11] At this writing, tobacco is the number one preventable cause of death, but obesity is predicted to soon surpass it. Epidemiologists who

| Table 9-1 | |
|---|---|
| **Skin Cancer Screening Recommendations** | |
| **Organization** | **Recommendation** |
| **U.S. Preventive Services Task Force** | **Insufficient evidence for or against routine screening examination** |
| Canadian Task Force | No routine screening. Regular total-body skin examination in high-risk individuals |
| American Cancer Society | Monthly skin self-examination. Total-body skin examination every 3 years between ages 20 and 39, every year after age 40 |
| National Institutes of Health. American Academy of Dermatology | Annual total-body skin examination |
| American College of Preventive Medicine. American Academy of Family Physicians. American College of Obstetricians and Gynecologists | No routine screening. Interval total-body skin examination in high-risk individuals |

study obesity have found that most obese people do not eat significantly more than nonobese people but are much less active. A sedentary lifestyle is more and more common in U.S. culture. Watching television is an independent risk factor for obesity.[12]

USPSTF states that the evidence is insufficient to recommend for or against routine counseling for increased physical activity.[13] Many organizations recommend this routine counseling, but it is based on the obvious benefit of exercise rather than the true impact counseling might have. Although it is clear patients would be healthier if they exercised more, it is unclear whether clinicians can have a meaningful impact on their activity levels.

Possible interventions include brief counseling, written exercise prescriptions, specific physical activity goal setting, mail or phone follow-up, and individualized exercise regimens. Trials that compare physical activity counseling with routine primary care have mixed results in both the short term (<6 months) and the long term (>6 months), with a majority finding no difference. There are six controlled trials comparing intervention versus usual care or no intervention and two trials comparing two or more different interventions. All these trials demonstrate mixed results.[14] One trial showed that patients who received a written prescription in addition to advice about exercise were more active at 6-week follow-up.[15] Another trial comparing increasingly intensive counseling ranging from 18 minutes over 2 years to 9 hours over 2 years did not show a difference in physical activity up to 24 months later.[16]

Adverse effects of physical activity counseling potentially include increased injury to deconditioned patients attempting exercise. Presently, there is no convincing evidence to support this, and in fact there is evidence to demonstrate decreased falls in elderly community-dwelling patients after participating in exercise programs[17] (Table 9-2).

## Dietary Activity

Many dietary habits are associated with diseases including coronary arterial disease, osteoporosis, obesity, diabetes, and

# Ambulatory Office Practice

| Table 9-2 | |
|---|---|
| **Physical Activity Counseling Recommendations** | |
| **Organization** | **Recommendation** |
| **U.S. Preventive Services Task Force** Canadian Task Force | **Insufficient evidence for or against routine counseling** |
| Department of Health and Human Services Centers for Disease Control and Prevention American Academy of Family Physicians American Heart Association American College of Obstetricians and Gynecologists | Routine counseling for increased physical activity |

| Table 9-3 | |
|---|---|
| **Healthy Diet Counseling Recommendations** | |
| **Organization** | **Recommendation** |
| **U.S. Preventive Services Task Force** | **Insufficient evidence for or against routine counseling** |
| American College of Preventive Medicine American Academy of Family Physicians American College of Obstetricians and Gynecologists National Institutes of Health | Counsel all patients at average risk for disease |
| American Dietetic Association Joint National Committee on Prevention, Detection, Evaluation and Treatment of High Blood Pressure | Screen in all patients at risk for nutrition-related illness, and counsel appropriately |

some neoplasia. The evidence is convincing that a diet low in saturated fat and cholesterol and high in fruits, vegetables, and whole-grain products helps prevent and treat these diseases as well as the associated morbidity and mortality. The Dietary Guidelines for Americans recommend daily consumption of 2 to 4 servings of fruit or fruit juice, 3 to 5 servings of vegetables or vegetable juices, 2 to 3 servings of protein, 2 to 3 servings of dairy products, and 6 to 11 servings of grains. They also recommend limiting total daily fat intake to less than 30% of total calories, total cholesterol to less than 300 mg/day, and total saturated fat intake to less than 10% of total calories.[18] Fewer than 20% of Americans follow these guidelines.

USPSTF performed a large meta-analysis to determine if counseling in patients results in dietary changes. They examined randomized-controlled trials performed in patients without chronic disease, though some had risk factors for chronic disease. They included only trials involving counseling as the intervention with dietary change as the endpoint and compared net change in consumption. For various nutrients, they determined standards for "small," "medium," and "large" net effects, and they standardized definitions for "low," "medium," and "high" intensity counseling. Low intensity was defined as one counseling session lasting 30 minutes or less. This is similar to what most primary care providers can achieve in a single office visit. High intensity was defined as six or more counseling sessions of 30 minutes or more. Medium intensity included all interventions that fell in between. When these studies were examined in this systematic way, overall counseling did produce dietary change with regard to fruit and vegetable intake, fiber intake, and fat intake. Low intensity counseling produced minimal positive change in diet; more intense counseling was associated with greater changes. Larger changes were also produced in those with risk factors for disease and those who were counseled in a research clinic versus a primary care setting. Goal setting, involving family and social support, dietary assessment, individualized and personalized interventions, and group counseling, also seemed to increase dietary change. There are no studies to prove that these specific interventions ultimately produced change in disease status.[19]

USPSTF states that there is insufficient evidence to promote or discourage routine dietary counseling.[20] There is good evidence that medium to high intensity counseling should be offered to patients at risk for chronic disease associated with diet deficiencies. If counseling is to be offered, a validated dietary survey can be used for assessment of dietary deficiencies, keeping in mind that patients are notorious at underreporting unhealthful behaviors. There seem to be no significant adverse effects of this type of counseling (Table 9-3).

## Tobacco

Smoking is the most reversible cause of disease in the United States, responsible for one in five deaths. The burden of disease is oppressive, with smoking being linked to not only oropharyngeal and pulmonary neoplasia but also pancreatic, renal, and cervical neoplasia. Smoking promotes atherosclerosis and increases the risk for myocardial infarction, ischemic stroke, and other vascular disease. Smoking is a key factor in the development of chronic obstructive pulmonary disease. It exacerbates asthma and can lead to pneumonia.

The effects extend beyond smokers to those in their environment. Fetuses carried by pregnant smokers are at risk for decreased birth weight, perinatal death, and preterm delivery and potentially for sudden infant death syndrome. Passive smoking in children increases the incidence of upper respiratory infections and otitis and exacerbates asthma. In adults, passive smoking can be linked to 3000 deaths per year from lung cancer! Cigarettes are responsible for 25% of deaths from residential fires.[21] Despite the well-known dangers of smoking, millions of people continue to smoke, and 2000 adolescents daily become regular smokers. However, it is encouraging to note that 50% of ever-smokers have successfully quit.

The evidence for the benefit of smoking cessation is compelling. After 1 year of smoking cessation, the risk of myocardial infarction or myocardial death is halved. After 5 years of smoking cessation, the risk for oropharyngeal neoplasia is halved. After 10 years of abstinence, the risk for lung cancer is halved. After 15 years of abstinence, the risks for myocardial infarction and stroke are almost equivalent to those of nonsmokers. A pregnant smoker who has quit by as late as her 30th week of gestation can increase her infant's birth weight relative to infants of women who smoke during their entire pregnancy.[21]

USPSTF makes it clear that screening for and education about tobacco use is beneficial.[22] They make a strong recommendation for screening adults. Benefits can be inferred in light of the evidence for strong association with cardiovascular disease, pulmonary disease, and neoplasia. Short counseling sessions (3 minutes) as well as pharmacotherapy increase rates of smoking cessation with an effect lasting at least a year. More intensive counseling, setting a goal "stop date," and scheduling follow-up visits to address smoking cessation are associated with a longer lasting effect. The highest relapse rate is in the first 2 weeks; intense follow-up should be directed at this clinical window.[21]

The recommendation for pregnant women is similar but emphasizes that slightly lengthier counseling, 5 to 15 minutes, is necessary as is distribution of literature specifically addressing smoking in pregnancy and fetal effects. There is direct evidence of increased abstinence rates and increased birth weight with these interventions.[21] The evidence is insufficient to support routine screening in children and adolescents.

There are several Food and Drug Administration (FDA)-approved pharmacotherapies for smoking cessation. Nicotine substitution or replacement methods include gum and patch, which are available over the counter, and prescription inhaler and nasal spray. All have been shown to be safe and effective, with an 18% to 31% abstinence rate as compared with 10% to 17% in those who do not use these products.[21,23] The nicotine patch is effective regardless of the level of smoker. The nicotine gum, specifically the 4 mg dose, is more effective for treating heavy smokers. The inhaler and nasal spray have not been studied extensively. Combinations of the above methods are more effective than single therapy alone. If these therapies are used while a person is still smoking, there is a risk for nicotine toxicity.

Other therapies that have demonstrated increased cessation rates when compared with placebo include sustained-release bupropion, clonidine, and nortriptyline. Bupropion is the only one of the three having FDA approval for this indication.

The safety and efficacy of these interventions in pregnant individuals, adolescents, and children are not well studied; therefore, specific recommendations cannot be made (Table 9-4).

## Alcohol

USPSTF defines alcohol misuse by defining a range of alcohol consumption and consequences. "Risky" or "hazardous" drinking means drinking more than seven drinks per week or more than three per occasion for women, and more than 14 per week or more than four per occasion for men. "Harmful" drinking is drinking to the point of causing physical, social, or psychological consequences, but not to the point of meeting the criteria for true alcohol dependence. Patients who meet the criteria for alcohol dependence, as defined by the *Diagnostic and Statistical Manual of Mental Disorders*, 4th edition, should be referred for treatment.[24] This discussion is limited to discovering alcohol misuse prior to the development of alcohol dependence in the primary care setting.

Excessive alcohol use can cause neurologic, hepatic, pancreatic, and cardiac insult. It increases risk for various neoplasms including those of the liver, breast, digestive tract, and oropharynx and is responsible for both intentional and unintentional injury. Alcoholism is also at the root of many social problems including divorce, unemployment, decreased productivity, increased risky behavior, and domestic violence. It is responsible for the fetal effects of mental and growth retardation in the pregnant patient. Moderate levels of alcohol consumption, defined as two or fewer drinks per day for men and one or fewer drinks per day for women, are associated with health benefits. No drinks are considered safe for pregnant patients.

The USPSTF recommends that all patients be screened for alcohol abuse via standardized methods and counseled if found to be misusing alcohol.[24] Pregnant women should be counseled to discontinue alcohol use. All patients should be cautioned against driving while consuming alcohol. Practical screening tests include the Alcohol Use Disorders Identification Test (AUDIT), with a sensitivity of 51% to 97% and specificity of 78% to 96%, and the CAGE (*c*ut back, *a*nnoyed by criticism, *g*uilty, *e*ye-opener) questionnaire, with a sensitivity of 43% to 94% and specificity of 70% to 97%.[24] The TWEAK [*t*olerance, *w*orried, *e*ye-opener, *a*mnesia, *k* (for cut down)] and T-ACE (*t*olerance, *a*ngry or *a*nnoyed, *c*ut down, *e*ye-opener) are designed for pregnant patients, who are at risk at lower levels of alcohol consumption. Laboratory data are not effective for screening for alcohol abuse.[25]

Multiple studies have demonstrated the benefit of counseling to decrease alcohol abuse. A meta-analysis of 12 controlled studies examined the effect of counseling in those who were screened and found to have risky or harmful levels of alcohol consumption.[26] The counseling was stratified as "very brief" (one 5-minute session or less), "brief" (one 15-minute session or less), or "brief multicontact" (initial 15-minute session with follow-up contacts). The brief, multicontact sessions decreased weekly drinking, decreased risk from drinking, and had a questionable effect on binge drinking. Shorter counseling produced less significant results. One study with extensive follow-up showed decreased mortality in heavy drinkers. Studies in pregnant women show that many women reduce alcohol consumption during pregnancy, but this reduction has not been linked with counseling or interventions[25] (Table 9-5).

## Drug Abuse

Drug abuse and drug use are a source of not only medical morbidity and mortality but also severe social consequences, including criminal activity and violence. In the United States, marijuana accounts for the most drug use and abuse, with more than 5 million Americans using it at least weekly. Other major drugs used include illicit drugs, such as cocaine and heroin, legal but unprescribed drugs such as barbiturates and amphetamines, and inhalants such as gasoline and glue.

| Table 9-4 Tobacco Counseling Recommendations | |
|---|---|
| **Organization** | **Recommendation** |
| **U.S. Preventive Services Task Force** American Academy of Family Physicians Centers for Disease Control and Prevention American College of Preventive Medicine American Academy of Family Physicians American College of Obstetricians and Gynecologists | **Screen all patients for tobacco use, and counsel for tobacco cessation** |

## Ambulatory Office Practice

**Table 9-5**
**Alcohol Misuse Screening and Counseling**

| Organization | Recommendation |
|---|---|
| U.S. Preventive Services Task Force<br>American Medical Association<br>American Academy of Family Physicians<br>Canadian Task Force<br>American College of Obstetricians and<br>Gynecologists | Screen in all patients, including pregnant women, using standardized tools; counsel those misusing alcohol |

Morbidity and mortality can stem from both acute and chronic effects, and occasional and regular use. Cocaine is associated with acute cardiac compromise from arrhythmia or infarction. Infectious complications can result from use of all intravenously injected drugs including the spread of human immunodeficiency virus (HIV). Chronic use or abuse of many substances decreases work productivity and increases insomnia. Drug use in pregnancy clearly has effects on the fetus including abruption, low birth weight, preterm delivery, and withdrawal in the neonate. Drug use is involved in a significant portion of motor vehicle accidents and other recreational injury.

Screening can be performed by taking a detailed history, including type of drug used, amount, duration, and frequency, as well as noting any social disruption caused by drug use. There are no validated screening questionnaires for drug use. Other screening might involve obtaining objective laboratory data. Drug screens are sensitive but depend on the timing of the drug use and the timing of the laboratory test. Marijuana can be detected up to 14 days after use, but cocaine, opiates, amphetamines, and barbiturates can be detected only 2 to 4 days after use. These limits can be manipulated if the patient alters the urine sample or purposely uses diuretics. Positive tests are of course not indicative of drug abuse but only of recent drug use. Patient consent should be obtained prior to drug testing, and results should be reviewed with patients.

USPSTF recommends taking a substance abuse history. There is insufficient evidence to recommend for or against laboratory screening.[27] Clinicians should note signs or symptoms of drug abuse or addiction. Drug use should be discouraged and drug abuse should be addressed with intensive therapy or other appropriate treatment plans. There is little evidence that treating the asymptomatic drug user or abuser impacts outcome. These

**Table 9-6**
**Drug Abuse Counseling Recommendations**

| Organization | Recommendation |
|---|---|
| U.S. Preventive Services Task Force | Insufficient evidence for or against standardized screening; take history of drug use, and follow with appropriate counseling or treatment |
| American Medical Association<br>American Academy of Family Physicians<br>American College of Obstetricians and<br>Gynecologists | Routine in-depth substance abuse history |

recommendations are based on the potential for preventing addiction and the subsequent medical and social consequences. The asymptomatic user is commonly less motivated to make lifestyle changes (Table 9-6).

### Household and Recreational Injuries

Unintentional injuries, half of which are household and recreational injuries, are the fifth leading cause of death in the United States. The most common types of accidents in order of frequency are motor vehicle accidents, falls, and poisonings. Others include fires, drowning, strangulation, aspiration, firearm injury, and injury resulting from use of recreational vehicles including bicycles, motorcycles, boats, and all-terrain vehicles.[28]

The prevention of injuries in children is not discussed here, but an important risk factor for injuries in adolescents and young adults is substance abuse. Alcohol abuse has been implicated in 25% to 40% of fatal unintentional injuries in this age group and provides another reason for alcohol abuse screening and counseling. Drug abuse contributes to the incidence of overdose. Cigarette smoking is a common cause of residential fires.

Many recreational injuries are preventable by use of common sense. Swimming lessons, flotation devices, and close supervision of beginners all are associated with decreased fatal swimming or boating accidents. Careful handling of firearms and careful supervision of young firearm handlers can prevent some of these injuries. Again, it is unclear whether physician counseling can change recreational behavior.[28] It is hypothesized that this type of counseling may induce an adolescent to increase risk-taking behavior and thus may cause additional morbidity and mortality, but this hypothesis is not supported by any data.

In the elderly, the most common cause of household injury is falls. The elderly population is at risk secondary to decreased muscle strength, decreased balance and flexibility, and possible mild impairment secondary to multiple medication use and poor vision. Those with osteoporosis, syncope, or dementia are more likely to be injured after a fall. Possible interventions to minimize these risks include exercise, mobility therapy, careful monitoring of medications, close monitoring of bone density, protection against hard surfaces, and correction of environmental obstacles such as slippery floors and poor lighting. These have had variable success in preventing falls. Exercise programs, which target improved balance, have been associated with fewer falls. External hip protectors have been shown to decrease injury from falls but are not FDA approved for this purpose.

The most effective measures to decrease unintentional injury are passive. Examples are childproof packaging on poisonous household materials and smoke detection devices. Some measures must be instituted at a community or legislative level rather than a clinical level. Individual behavior modification with regard to recreational behavior or household routine has been shown to be ineffective; thus, physician counseling is ineffective. A more promising approach is to counsel specifically with regard to substance abuse to prevent injury. In the elderly, interventions that decrease falls include home health visits or visits with medical educators, assessment of home environment, assessment of risk factors for falls, medication review, and exercise.

USPSTF recommends periodic counseling of children, adolescents, those using alcohol or illicit drugs, and elderly patients based on the risk for recreational and household

**Table 9-7**
**Injury Prevention Counseling Recommendations**

| Organization | Recommendation |
|---|---|
| U.S. Preventive Services Task Force | Counsel all patients periodically on household and recreational hazards, particularly those patients using alcohol or drugs |
| American Academy of Pediatrics American Academy of Family Physicians American Medical Association | Provide age-specific counseling |
| American College of Obstetricians and Gynecologists | Provide routine counseling on safety helmets, recreational hazards, and firearms |

injury.[28] Counseling should be individualized. Though not supported by the data to date, it might be justified owing to the emotional devastation caused by an unintentional death secondary to injury. Keep in mind that patients underreport the level of safety measures taken at home[29] (Table 9-7).

## Motor Vehicle Accidents

The two most important risk factors for a motor vehicle accident are failure to wear a seat belt and alcohol use. Interventions for alcohol abuse are described earlier in this chapter, and the evidence overwhelmingly shows that alcohol intoxication is associated not only with increased motor vehicle accidents but also with increased mortality, increased serious injury, longer hospitalization, and increased neurologic impairment following motor vehicle accidents.[30]

The evidence is clear that seat belts, when used appropriately, decrease injury and death associated with motor vehicle collision by up to 50%. Use of seat belts also decreases the severity of injury, the likelihood of hospital admission, and the cost of hospitalization.[31] Seat belt laws increase the use of seat belts. In model year 1998, driver- and passenger-side air bags became a requirement for passenger vehicles. These have further reduced injury and mortality.

Most studies examining the effectiveness of physician seat belt counseling involve counseling the parent of a pediatric patient. Studies in pregnant women who were counseled several times during their prenatal care showed increased proper car seat use, suggesting that counseling can potentially change behavior with regard to safety restraints. Most studies looking at personal seat belt use found some improvement in self-reported seat belt use, although in some studies this increase was not sustained. One study suggests that a brief reminder by physicians increases seat belt use,[32] but this study was neither controlled nor randomized. It is important to remember that self-reported seat belt use is not necessarily correlated with true seat belt use.

USPSTF recommends that clinicians remind patients to wear seat belts and inform them that air bags are effective in further reducing motor vehicle injuries.[33] Doctors should not neglect to remind patients that driving under the influence of alcohol or recreational drugs is dangerous. The appropriate interval for counseling is undetermined. Counseling is most important for

high-risk groups including adolescents, young adults, and those with substance use or abuse problems. This recommendation is not based on direct evidence that counseling will change outcomes but on the potential benefit of changing patient behavior with regard to motor vehicle safety and on the low morbidity and mortality associated with counseling (Table 9-8).

## Suicide and Depression

Depression is common and has a prevalence of 5% to 8% in the primary care setting. Detection and subsequent treatment can decrease not only associated morbidity but also the irreversible endpoint of suicide. Risk factors for depression include a family history of mental illness, unemployment, and chronic illness. Risk factors for suicide include mental illness, substance abuse, living alone, recent grieving, access to firearms, personal or family history of suicide attempt or suicide completion, divorce, separation, or unemployment. Women are more likely to be depressed and more likely to attempt suicide. Men over the age of 65 years are the most common suicide completers.

USPSTF recommends screening for depression in care settings where accurate diagnosis, treatment, and follow-up are feasible.[34] The evidence is insufficient to recommend for or against suicide risk screening.[35] There are many standardized tools for depression screening. Asking the two questions, "Over the past 2 weeks, have you felt down, depressed, or hopeless?" and "Over the past 2 weeks, have you felt little interest or pleasure in doing things?" may be as effective as some more elaborate screening tools.[36] Most depression screening tools have good sensitivity and fair specificity. The obvious potential adverse effect is misdiagnosis and associated stigma. Positive screening should be followed by more specific diagnostic evaluation.

Fourteen randomized-controlled trials, comparing outcomes in patients who were screened for depression and those who were not screened, were examined in a meta-analysis.[37] Some studies examined the effect of feedback of screening results to practitioners. Detection rates of depression increased when feedback, either positive or negative screening results, was given to practitioners, but treatment rates did not change. Other studies examined outcomes when usual care was compared with a screening and treatment protocol; patients who were screened demonstrated clinical improvement. This result suggests that clinics which can follow positive screening with more specific diagnosis and appropriate treatment can change outcomes in depression.

**Table 9-8**
**Seat Belt Counseling Recommendations**

| Organization | Recommendation |
|---|---|
| U.S. Preventive Services Task Force American Medical Association American College of Physicians American Academy of Family Physicians American Academy of Pediatrics American College of Obstetricians and Gynecologists Canadian Task Force National Highway Traffic Safety Administration | Counsel all patients to use passive restraints |

| Table 9-9 Depression Screening and Suicide Screening Recommendations | |
| --- | --- |
| Organization | Recommendation |
| U.S. Preventive Services Task Force | Screen for depression in all adults in settings that have systems in place for appropriate follow-up; insufficient evidence for or against routine suicide screening |
| Canadian Task Force | Exclude depression screening as part of routine health examination, but maintain high degree of suspicion; insufficient evidence for or against routine suicide screening |
| American College of Obstetricians and Gynecologists | Be aware of symptoms; inquire about social stressors and family history of depression at routine examination |
| American Medical Assocation | Screen for depression in adolescents at risk |

Studies on suicide are difficult to perform because it is a relatively rare event. All subjects who succeed in committing suicide are not available to compare with those who survive. Information on those who attempt suicide and fail cannot necessarily be extrapolated to those who attempt and succeed. Though it seems intuitively reasonable that identifying a patient who will attempt suicide allows for timely intervention, there is no solid evidence that intervention is effective. Treatment of psychiatric disease and substance abuse may potentially prevent suicide. Removal of firearms may prevent suicide. Neither of these interventions has been clearly demonstrated to reduce suicide rates (Table 9-9).

### Anemia

Anemia is defined by the World Health Organization as hemoglobin of less than 13 g/dL in men and less than 12 g/dL in menstruating women as determined by venous blood sampling. The prevalence in reproductive age women is below 2%, and the burden of disease is minimal. Severe anemia can certainly cause decreased activity, decreased exercise tolerance, fatigue, and cardiorespiratory difficulty, but mild anemia or asymptomatic anemia is associated with little morbidity and mortality. Additionally, iron supplementation in the mildly anemic produces little significant change in symptoms or sense of well-being, despite improvement by laboratory evidence.

USPSTF recommends screening for anemia in pregnant women and high-risk infants. There is insufficient evidence to recommend for or against screening in asymptomatic adults.[38] Militating against screening are the cost of the test, the adverse effects of iron therapy, and the low prevalence of the disease. For anyone who is found to be anemic, the type of anemia should be determined and the patient treated appropriately. Routine iron supplementation in nonanemic pregnant or nonpregnant adults is not supported.

### Lipid Disorders

There is little debate that an abnormal lipid profile signifies increased risk for coronary heart disease, the leading cause of morbidity, mortality, and disability in the United States. The lifetime risk of coronary heart disease is 49% for men by the age of 40 years and 32% for women. USPSTF recommends routine screening for men aged 35 and older and women aged 45 and older. Abnormal results should be treated. Men aged 20 to 35 and women aged 20 to 45 should be screened if they have risk factors for coronary heart disease, specifically diabetes, a family history consistent with familial hyperlipidemia, multiple other coronary risk factors, or a family history of cardiovascular disease at a young age. There is no recommendation for adults younger than age 20. All patients should be counseled about a diet low in saturated fat and high in fiber.[39]

The screening tests of choice are total cholesterol and high-density lipoprotein (HDL) cholesterol.[40] These tests are reliable, have acceptable variability, and can be performed on nonfasting venous blood. Two measurements should be made on two separate occasions to ensure accuracy. The addition of triglycerides and low-density lipoprotein (LDL) cholesterol necessitates a fasting sample. In general, patients are open to screening for lipid disorders, and the test is feasible and convenient for most physicians. Other possibilities for screening include sequential protocols based on stratified risk assessment and varying levels and ratios of the different cholesterol measurements. These are more time consuming and require more physician counseling time.

The evidence is clear that dietary manipulation can decrease total cholesterol and improve the lipid profile on average from 2% to 6% to 10% to 20%.[41] These changes translate to decreased cardiac risk, but studies have not linked dietary changes to decreased cardiac events. Medications such as HMG-CoA inhibitors and gemfibrozil, when taken for 5 to 7 years, improve the lipid profile; a meta-analysis of the main drug therapy trials also demonstrates a 30% decrease in cardiac events in patients with moderate to high cholesterol levels[42] and a 20% reduction in strokes in patients with known coronary heart disease.[43] These benefits should be weighed against the side effects of these medications including but not limited to myopathy and liver enzyme abnormalities. It is unclear whether drug therapy has any effect on overall mortality after the first 5 to 7 years of therapy, particularly in the lower risk patient (Table 9-10).

### Thyroid Disorders

Subclinical thyroid disease affects 3% to 5% of adults, with increasing prevalence in older individuals, females, and white individuals. In women over age 75 years, it is estimated to be 17.4%. It is defined as an abnormal thyroid stimulating hormone (TSH) level with normal thyroid hormones in an asymptomatic individual. The population at risk for thyroid disease includes elderly and postpartum patients, those with Down syndrome, and those who have a history of high-level radiation exposure.

Subclinical hyperthyroidism is much less common than subclinical hypothyroidism. Both entities, if untreated, can lead to overt disease or at least some of the same morbidity associated with overt disease. Subclinical hyperthyroidism is associated in some studies with atrial fibrillation, osteoporosis, and dementia; untreated hyperthyroidism is associated with those findings as well as congestive heart failure. Subclinical hypothyroidism is associated in some studies with dyslipidemia and atherosclerosis; untreated hypothyroidism can lead to fatigue, weight gain, heart failure, and elevated lipid levels.[44] It is important to note that

| Table 9-10 Cholesterol Screening Recommendations | |
|---|---|
| **Organization** | **Recommendation** |
| **U.S. Preventive Services Task Force** | **Screen routinely in men at least 35 years of age and in women at least 45 years of age; screen in men 20–35 years of age and in men and women 20–45 years of age if they have coronary risk factors** |
| American Heart Association | Screen all adults over age 20 every 5 years |
| American College of Obstetricians and Gynecologists | Screen all women over age 45 every 5 years |
| American College of Physicians American Academy of Family Physicians | Screen men aged 35–65 and women aged 45–65 periodically |
| American Diabetes Association | Screen in all patients with diabetes annually |

the associations with subclinical disease are merely that, associations, often not reaching statistical significance, often not studied with appropriate controls, and often not measured by true clinical outcomes but by physiologic endpoints or laboratory data.

It would seem reasonable to screen patients to prevent this morbidity and mortality; however, it is estimated that only a small number of cases of subclinical thyroid disease discovered by mass screening progress to true thyroid disease with clinically relevant outcomes. There are no controlled studies examining whether screening, and thus early detection, of thyroid disease changes long-term morbidity and mortality.[44] Screening does *not* mean testing a patient who comes in with complaints consistent with thyroid disease. In a referral population tested in a specialty clinic, the sensitivity and specificity of TSH are 92% and 98%, respectively.[44] When used for confirmatory reasons, TSH is very useful. In a primary care population, however, the positive predictive value of the same TSH test ranges from 0.06 to 0.24.[45]

This potential benefit has to be balanced with the adverse effects associated with treatment and the possibility of false-positive results. Overtreatment of hypothyroidism has been associated with a small risk of atrial fibrillation. Thus, USPSTF can make no recommendation for or against routine screening[46] (Table 9-11).

## Diabetes

Various tests are used to help diagnose diabetes in the symptomatic or high-risk patient. The American Diabetes Association recommends using the fasting plasma glucose at a cut-off of greater than 126 mg/dL. Compared with hemoglobin $A_1C$, random glucose testing, and the 2-hour glucose load test, fasting plasma glucose is faster, easier, more reproducible, more convenient, more reliable, and less expensive. It also correlates with development of microvascular complications. An abnormal test must be corroborated by a second abnormal screen on a separate day.

Studies show that lifestyle interventions in patients with impaired glucose tolerance by various criteria can prevent

development of diabetes.[47] We know these patients are at higher risk of developing diabetes in the future. However, diabetes is preceded by an asymptomatic phase whose length has yet to be determined. It is estimated that up to a third of individuals with laboratory criteria for diabetes have not yet received a diagnosis.[48] There are no randomized-controlled trials studying screening for diabetes or the effectiveness of intervention during the asymptomatic phase.

A wealth of research demonstrates that treatment for diabetes decreases microvascular and macrovascular complications that can develop 10 to 15 years after clinical diagnosis. These include retinopathy, nephropathy, cardiovascular disease, stroke, and amputation. Possible treatments include blood pressure control, glycemic control, angiotensin-converting enzyme (ACE) inhibitors, foot-care programs, aspirin, and dyslipidemia treatment. Do these interventions work better if started in the asymptomatic phase?

One way to tackle this question is to see whether these treatments improve outcomes differently in diabetic and nondiabetic patients. Because the risk for cardiovascular disease in the asymptomatic diabetic patient is significant, there is interest in interventions geared toward cardiovascular risk reduction. There is evidence that treatment of hypertension and dyslipidemia in diabetics decreases cardiovascular risk more than in nondiabetics. On the other hand, foot-care programs, diet and activity counseling, and smoking cessation do not offer added benefit or effectiveness in the diabetic patient.[49]

USPSTF does not recommend for or against routine screening for diabetes or any form of glucose intolerance. USPSTF does, however, recommend screening for diabetes in patients with hypertension or dyslipidemia.[50] Potential harms of screening include the anxiety and stress caused by labeling with the diagnosis of diabetes and the stigma attached when applying for insurance policies. Risk associated with treatment includes hypoglycemia and side effects of medications (Table 9-12).

| Table 9-11 Thyroid Disease Screening Recommendations | |
|---|---|
| **Organization** | **Recommendation** |
| **U.S. Preventive Services Task Force** | **Insufficient evidence for or against routine screening** |
| American Thyroid Association | Measure thyroid function every 5 years after age 35 years |
| Canadian Task Force | Use clinical suspicion to determine appropriate screening, particularly in the perimenopausal and postmenopausal woman |
| American College of Physicians | Screen in women > 50 years of age with one or more symptoms |
| American Association of Clinical Endocrinologists American Academy of Family Physicians | Screen in all women > 50 years of age |
| American College of Obstetricians and Gynecologists | Use clinical suspicion to determine appropriate screening, particularly in the postpartum period |

| Table 9-12 Diabetes Screening Recommendations | |
| --- | --- |
| **Organization** | **Recommendation** |
| **U.S. Preventive Services Task Force** | **Insufficient evidence for or against routine screening** |
| American Diabetic Association | Consider screening with fasting plasma glucose at 45 years of age, or younger in the high-risk patient |
| American College of Obstetricians and Gynecologists | Screen routinely every 3 years in women aged 45 and older |
| American Heart Association | Consider screening with fasting plasma glucose at age 20 years and older based on risk |

## Hypertension

Hypertension is systolic blood pressure 140 mm Hg or higher and diastolic blood pressure 90 mm Hg or higher on two occasions at least 1 week apart. Complications of untreated hypertension include congestive heart failure, myocardial infarction, chronic renal failure, retinopathy, stroke, and aortic aneurysm. The risks of these endpoints depend on the level of blood pressure elevation as well as various risk factors such as concomitant dyslipidemia, smoking, diabetes, age, and sex.

Hypertension can be treated with a wide variety of interventions including the lifestyle changes of decreasing sodium intake, adding potassium to the diet, decreasing alcohol intake, increasing exercise, reducing weight, and managing stress. Though these lifestyle changes have been shown to lower blood pressure, no trials have demonstrated a decrease in cardiovascular events as a result. Antihypertensive medications decrease cardiovascular events, stroke, myocardial infarction, and congestive heart failure, some more significantly than others. Though no studies directly measure the benefit of screening, most patients are found by screening in the asymptomatic state.[51]

USPSTF strongly recommends blood pressure screening for adults aged 18 and older. The evidence is insufficient to recommend for or against screening those younger than age 18.[52] There are no studies evaluating whether all patients should be screened or only those with risk factors. Possible harms from screening include the risks of the various treatments. Studies evaluating quality of life and well-being showed mixed results with regard to absenteeism from work but found no psychological burden caused by the diagnosis of hypertension (Table 9-13).

## Obesity

Obesity is the accumulation of an excessive amount of a body fat and is most universally defined as a body mass index (BMI) greater than 30, with the precursor of obesity, overweight, defined as a BMI of 25 to 29.9. Morbid obesity is defined as BMI greater than 35. Other methods of measuring body fat include skinfold measurements, which are notoriously unreliable owing to high inter- and intra-observer variability. Waist-to-hip ratio has been used to measure obesity and more specifically to link it to cardiovascular outcomes and those diseases associated with visceral adiposity. Other less practical, more invasive, and more accurate measurement tools include hydrostatic weighing and

bioelectric impedance. BMI calculation is simple, is linked most broadly with various outcomes, and is the most appropriate screening tool, with a 0.7 to 0.8 correlation with true body fat content.

Obesity is linked to a host of diseases including cardiovascular disease, hyperlipidemias, diabetes, disorders of glucose metabolism, many types of neoplasia including endometrial, breast, ovarian, and colon cancer, and sleep apnea. Much morbidity and mortality is associated with obesity including perioperative and postoperative complications and pregnancy-related complications. There are social and cultural stigmas against obesity, causing difficulties with quality of life secondary to physical limitations and potential discrimination in professional and social settings. Obesity will soon become the leading preventable cause of death, surpassing tobacco use, in the United States.

The reasons to screen for obesity are many. First, the yield of screening should be high, secondary to its high prevalence. It is important to prevent those who are not obese from becoming obese, and to prevent morbidity and mortality in those who already are obese by helping them lose weight. There are no randomized-controlled trials examining mass screening for obesity and its implications for long-term outcomes, but there is evidence that addressing obesity at preventive health care visits can improve weight loss. Weight loss, specifically lower BMI, is associated with lower overall morbidity and mortality.[53]

USPSTF recommends that all patients be screened by means of BMI for obesity or overweight. Those who are obese should undergo intensive counseling and behavior modification to initiate and sustain weight loss.[54] Fair-to-good evidence shows that those with a BMI greater than 30, with the help of intense counseling including behavioral modification, diet, and exercise, can sustain weight loss in the range of 3 to 5 kg over the course of a year. Intense counseling is defined as counseling at intervals greater than monthly. The ideal setting for this counseling is not clear. Randomized-controlled trials demonstrate that counseling that stresses diet modification, specifically caloric restriction, produces weight loss. Counseling that stresses increased physical activity also produces weight loss. Counseling that includes elements of both types produces even greater weight loss.[53] Behavioral modification was also an important component of this counseling. The 5-A framework (assess, advise, agree, assist, and arrange) has been used for behavior modification with

| Table 9-13 Hypertension Screening Recommendations | |
| --- | --- |
| **Organization** | **Recommendation** |
| **U.S. Preventive Services Task Force** | **Screen in all adults 18 years of age and older** |
| American Heart Association | Screen at least once every 2 years in adults over age 20 |
| American Academy of Family Physicians | Screen periodically in adults over age 21 |
| American College of Obstetricians and Gynecologists | Screen annually in adults over age 13 |

regard to tobacco use and may be useful in this scenario. Long-term success depends on continued counseling. There are no identified harms in weight loss counseling except possible embarrassment about obesity. Counseling that is less intense, defined as containing fewer components or occurring less than or equal to once a month, has not been effective. It is unclear whether counseling in those who are overweight but not obese is beneficial.

Another aspect of obesity screening and treatment includes pharmacotherapy. Only two medications are FDA-approved for the long-term treatment of obesity: sibutramine, which is a centrally acting appetite suppressant, and orlistat, a lipase inhibitor that prevents absorption of fat in the gastrointestinal tract. They should be used in patients with a BMI greater than 30 or with a BMI greater than 27 with risk factors. Multiple randomized-controlled trials have shown significant weight loss in the short term with these therapies when compared with placebo, with average weight loss of 5% to 10% of body weight.[53] Those who continued to use these medications had more successful weight loss maintenance up to 2 years when compared with those who took placebo. Obviously, the possible side effects of these medications must be considered. Orlistat can cause headache, oily discharge, flatus, diarrhea, or fecal urgency. Sibutramine can cause headache, insomnia, gastro-intestinal upset, agitation, constipation, and other symptoms. Other medications that have been studied include metformin, phentermine, fluoxetine, and diethylpropion. These treatments did not show consistent benefit and are not approved for long-term use. They are best used in the context of a regimented diet and exercise plan.

Surgical intervention is a consideration for patients with BMI greater than 40 or BMI greater than 35 with risk factors. There are several options, both laparoscopic and open, but all induce a malabsorptive state by bypassing portions of the gastrointestinal tract or restricting gastric storage capacity and thus oral intake. The quality of evidence is limited by ethical concerns and the lack of blinded subjects, but randomized trials demonstrated significant weight loss on the order of 30 to 50 kg, with an average of 20 kg of weight loss maintenance after 8 years. Again, the risks of these surgical procedures must be weighed against the benefit of weight loss for these patients (Table 9-14).

## CONCLUSION

Preventive care is an area that is wide open for more research to clarify the issues that can determine a patient's future health or illness. As health care resources become more and more scarce and as practitioners become more and more busy, it is important to use only those interventions that have been proven to change outcomes.

## REFERENCES

1. Kern DE, Roberts JC: Preventive medicine in ambulatory practice. In Barker LR, Burton JR, Zieve PD (eds): Principles of Ambulatory Medicine, 4th ed. Baltimore, Md, Williams & Wilkins, 1995. (IV, C)
2. Grimes DA, Schulz KF: Uses and abuses of screening tests. Lancet 2002;359:881–884. (IV, C)
3. Ling FW, Peterson H: Cancer screening. In Ling FW, Duff P (eds): Obstetrics and Gynecology: Principles for Practice. New York, McGraw-Hill, 2001, pp 576–580. (IV, C)
4. Ries LAG, Eisner MP, Kosary CL, et al (eds): SEER Cancer Statistics Review, 1975–2000. Bethesda, Md, National Cancer Institute. Available at http://seer.cancer/gov/csr/1975_2000/. Accessed 4/10/04. (III, B)
5. U.S. Preventive Services Task Force: Screening for skin cancer: recommendations and rationale. Am J Prev Med 2001;20(Suppl 3): 44–46. (IV, C)
6. Helfand M, Mahon SM, Eden KB, et al: Screening for skin cancer. Am J Prev Med 2001;20(Suppl 3):47–58. (III, B)
7. Berwick M, Begg CB, Fine JA, et al: Screening for cutaneous melanoma by skin self-examination. J Natl Cancer Inst 1996;88:17–23. (IIb, B)
8. U.S. Preventive Services Task Force: Counseling to Prevent Skin Cancer: Recommendations and Rationale. Rockville, Md, Agency for Healthcare Research and Quality, Oct 2003. Available at http://www.ahrq.gov/clinic/3rduspstf/skcacoun/skcarr.htm. Accessed 3/12/04. (IV, C)
9. Helfand M, Krages KP: Counseling to Prevent Skin Cancer: A Summary of the Evidence for the U.S. Preventive Services Task Force. Rockville, Md, Agency for Healthcare Research and Quality, Jun 2003. Available at http://www.ahrq.gov/clinic/3rduspstf/skcacoun/skcounsum.htm. Accessed 3/12/04. (Ia, A)
10. Cokkinides VE, Weinstock MA, Cardinez CJ, et al: Sun-safe practices in U.S. youth and their parents, role of caregiver on youth sunscreen use. Am J Prev Med 2004;26:147–151. (IIb, B)
11. Centers for Disease Control and Prevention: Physical activity trends—United States, 1990–1998. Morbid Mortal Wkly Rep 2001;50:166–169. (III, B)
12. Shaw J: The deadliest sin. Harvard Magazine Mar–Apr 2004:36–43. (IV, C)
13. U.S. Preventive Services Task Force: Behavioral Counseling in Primary Care to Promote Physical Activity: Recommendations and Rationale. Rockville, Md, Agency for Healthcare Research and Quality, Jul 2002. Available at http://www.ahrq.gov/clinic/3rduspstf/physactivity/physactrr.htm. Accessed 3/20/04. (IV, C)
14. Eden KB, Orleans CT, Mulrow CD, et al: Does counseling by clinicians improve physical activity? Summary of the evidence for the U.S. Preventive Services Task Force. Ann Intern Med 2002;137:208–215. (Ia, A)
15. Swinburn BA, Walter LG, Arroll B, et al: The green prescription study: a randomized controlled trial of written exercise advice provided by general practitioners. Am J Public Health 1998;88:288–291. (Ib, A)
16. Writing Group for the Activity Counseling Trial Research Group: Effects of physical activity counseling in primary care—The activity counseling trial: a randomized controlled trial. JAMA 2001;286:677–687. (Ib, A)
17. Province MA, Hadley EC, Hornbrook MC, et al: The effects of exercise on falls in elderly patients: a preplanned meta-analysis of the FICSIT trials. JAMA 1995;273:1341–1347. (Ia, A)

| Table 9-14 | |
| :-- | :-- |
| **Obesity Screening Recommendations** | |
| **Organization** | **Recommendation** |
| **U.S. Preventive Services Task Force**<br>American Academy of Family Physicians<br>American Diabetes Association<br>American College of Preventive Medicine<br>American College of Obstetricians and Gynecologists | Take periodic height and weight measurements in all patients; offer intensive counseling for weight loss in those who are overweight or obese |
| Canadian Task Force | Insufficient evidence to recommend for or against periodic body mass index measurements |

18. U.S. Department of Agriculture, U.S. Department of Health and Human Services, Dietary Guidelines Advisory Committee, Center for Nutrition and Policy and Promotion: Nutrition and Your Health: Dietary Guidelines for Americans. Home and Garden Bulletin No. 232, 2000. Available at http://198.102.218.57/dietaryguidelines/dga2000/document/build.htm#pyramid. Accessed 4/12/04. **(IV, C)**

19. Pignone MP, Ammerman A, Fernandez L, et al: Counseling to Promote a Healthy Diet in Adults: A Summary of the Evidence for the U.S. Preventive Services Task Force. Rockville, Md, Agency for Healthcare Research and Quality. Available at http://www.ahrq.gov/clinic/3rduspstf/diet/dietsum.htm. Accessed 3/23/04. **(Ia, A)**

20. U.S. Preventive Services Task Force: Behavioral Counseling in Primary Care to Promote a Healthy Diet: Recommendations and Rationale. Rockville, Md, Agency for Healthcare Research and Quality, Dec 2002. Available at http://www.ahrq.gov/clinic/3rdustpstf/dietrr.htm. Accessed 3/23/04. **(IV, C)**

21. U.S. Preventive Services Task Force: Counseling to Preventive Tobacco Use. In Guide to Clinical Preventive Services, 2nd ed. Rockville, Md, Agency for Healthcare Research and Quality, 1996, pp 597–609. Available at http://hstat.nlm.nih.gov/hq/Hquest/db/local.gcps.cps/screen/Browse/s/49188/cmd/HF/action/GetText?IHR=CH54. Accessed 2/25/04. **(IV, C)**

22. U.S. Preventive Services Task Force: Counseling to Prevent Tobacco Use and Tobacco-Related Diseases: Recommendation Statement. Rockville, Md, Agency for Healthcare Research and Quality, Nov 2003. Available at http://www.ahrq.gov/clinic/3rduspstf/tobaccoun/tobcounrs.htm. Accessed 4/11/04. **(IV, C)**

23. Fiore MC, Hatsukami DK, Baker TB: Effective tobacco dependence treatment. JAMA 2002;288:1768–1771. **(IV, C)**

24. U.S. Preventive Services Task Force: Screening and Behavioral Counseling Interventions in Primary Care to Reduce Alcohol Misuse: Recommendation Statement. Rockville, Md, Agency for Healthcare Research and Quality, Apr 2004. Available at http://www.ahrp.gov/clinic/3rduspstf/alcohol/alcomisrs.htm. Accessed 4/12/04. **(IV, C)**

25. U.S. Preventive Services Task Force: Screening for problem drinking. In Guide to Clinical Preventive Services, 2nd ed. Rockville, Md, Agency for Healthcare Research and Quality, 1996, pp 567–582. Available at http://hstat.nlm.nih.gov/hq/Hquest/db/local.gcps.cps/screen/Browse/s/49891/cmd/HF/action/GetText?IHR=CH52. Accessed 2/22/04. **(IV, C)**

26. Whitlock EP, Polen MR, Green CA, et al: Behavioral counseling interventions in primary care to reduce risk/harmful alcohol use by adults. Ann Intern Med 2004;140:558–569. **(Ia, A)**

27. U.S. Preventive Services Task Force: Screening for drug abuse. In Guide to Preventive Services, 2nd ed. Rockville, Md, Agency for Healthcare Research and Quality, 1996, pp 583–594. Available at http://hstat.nlm.nih.gov/hq/Hquest/db/local.gcps.cps/screen/Browse/s/51553/cmd/HF/action/GetText?IHR=CH53. Accessed 3/3/04. **(IV, C)**

28. U.S. Preventive Services Task Force: Counseling to prevent household and recreational injuries. In Guide to Preventive Services, 2nd ed. Rockville, Md, Agency for Healthcare Research and Quality, 1996, pp 659–685. Available at http://hstat.nlm.nih.gov/hq/Hquest/db/local.gcps.cps/screen/Browse/s/51553/cmd/HF/action/GetText?IHR=CH58. Accessed 3/3/04. **(IV, C)**

29. Chen LH, Gielen AC, McDonald EM: Validity of self reported home safety practices. Inj Prev 2004;9:73–75. **(Ib, A)**

30. Kraus JF, Morgenstern H, Fife D, et al: Blood alcohol tests, prevalence of involvement, and outcomes following brain injury. Am J Public Health 1989;79:294–299. **(IIb, B)**

31. Marine WM, Kerwin EM, Moore EE, et al: Mandatory seatbelts: epidemiologic, financial, and medical rationale from the Colorado matched pairs study. J Trauma 1994;36:96–100. **(IIb, B)**

32. Kelly RB: Effect of a brief physician intervention on seat belt use. J Fam Pract 1987;24:630–632. **(IIb, B)**

33. U.S. Preventive Services Task Force: Counseling to prevent motor vehicle injuries. In Guide to Preventive Services, 2nd ed. Rockville, Md, Agency for Healthcare Research and Quality, 1996, pp 659–685. Available at http://hstat.nlm.nih.gov/hq/Hquest/db/local.gcps.cps/screen/Browse/s/51553/cmd/HF/action/GetText?IHR=CH57. Accessed 3/3/04. **(IV, C)**

34. U.S. Preventive Services Task Force: Screening for Depression: Recommendations and Rationale. Rockville, Md, Agency for Healthcare Research and Quality, May 2002. Available at http://www.ahrq.gov/clinic/3rduspstf/depressrr.htm. Accessed 3/17/04. **(IV, C)**

35. U.S. Preventive Services Task Force: Screening for Suicide Risk. In Guide to Preventive Services, 2nd ed. Rockville, Md, Agency for Healthcare Research and Quality, 1996, pp 547–554. Available at http://hstat.nlm.nih.gov/hq/Hquest/db/local.gcps.cps/screen/Browse/s/53589/cmd/HF/action/GetText?IHR=CH50. Accessed 3/3/04. **(IV, C)**

36. Whooley MA, Avins AL, Miranda J, et al: Case-finding instruments for depression: two questions are as good as many. J Gen Intern Med 1997;12:439–445. **(IIb, B)**

37. Pignone MP, Gaynes BN, Rushton JL, et al: Screening for depression in adults: summary of the evidence for the U.S. Preventive Services Task Force. Ann Intern Med 2002;136:765–776. **(Ia, A)**

38. U.S. Preventive Services Task Force: Screening for iron deficiency anemia—including iron prophylaxis. In Guide to Preventive Services, 2nd ed. Rockville, Md, Agency for Healthcare Research and Quality, 1996, pp 231–247. Available at http://hstat.nlm.nih.gov/hq/Hquest/db/local.gcps.cps/screen/Browse/s/54796/cmd/HF/action/GetText?IHR=CH22. Accessed 3/23/04. **(IV, C)**

39. U.S. Preventive Services Task Force: Screening adults for lipid disorders: recommendations and rationale. Am J Prev Med 2001;20(3 Suppl):73–76. **(IV, C)**

40. Screening Adults for Lipid Disorders: What's New from the USPSTF? AHRQ Publication No. APPIP 01-0011. Rockville, Md, Agency for Healthcare Research and Quality, Mar 2001. Available at http://www.ahrq.gov/clinic/prev/lipidwh.htm. Accessed 3/18/04. **(IV, C)**

41. Pignone MP, Phillips CJ, Atkins D, et al: Screening and treating adults for lipid disorders: a summary of the evidence. Am J Prev Med 2001;20(Suppl 3):77–89. **(Ia, A)**

42. Pignone MP, Phillips CJ, Mulrow CD: Use of lipid lowering drugs for primary prevention of coronary heart disease: a meta-analysis of randomized trials. BMJ 2000;321:983–986. **(Ia, A)**

43. Hebert PR, Gaziano JM, Chan KS, Hennekens CH: Cholesterol lowering with statin drugs, risk of stroke and total mortality: an overview of randomized trials. JAMA 1997;278:313–321. **(Ia, A)**

44. Helfand M: Screening for subclinical thyroid dysfunction in nonpregnant adults: a summary of the evidence for the U.S. Preventive Services Task Force. Ann Intern Med 2004;140:128–141. **(Ia, A)**

45. Attia J, Margetts P, Guyatt G: Diagnosis of thyroid disease in hospitalized patients. Arch Intern Med 1999;159:658–665. **(III, B)**

46. U.S. Preventive Services Task Force: Screening for Thyroid Disease: Recommendation Statement. Rockville, Md, Agency for Healthcare Research and Quality, Jan 2004. Available at http://www.ahrq.gov/clinic/3rduspstf/thyroid/thyrrs.htm. Accessed 3/21/04. **(IV, C)**

47. Tuomilehto J, Lindstrom J, Eriksson JG, et al: Prevention of type 2 diabetes mellitus by changes in lifestyle among subjects with impaired glucose tolerance. N Engl J Med 2001;344:1343–1350. **(Ia, A)**

48. Harris R, Donahue K Rathore S, et al: Screening for Type 2 Diabetes Mellitus in Adults: Review of the Evidence. Rockville, Md, Agency for Healthcare Research and Quality, 2003. Available at http://www.ahrq.gov/clinic/3rduspstf/diabscr/diabrev.htm. Accessed 3/31/04. **(Ia, A)**

49. Harris MI, Flegal KM, Cowie CC, et al: Prevalence of diabetes, impaired fasting glucose, and impaired glucose tolerance in U.S. adults: the Third National Health and Nutrition Examination Survey, 1988–1994. Diabetes Care 1998;21:518–524. **(III, B)**

50. U.S. Preventive Services Task Force: Screening for Type 2 Diabetes Mellitus in Adults: Recommendations and Rationale. Rockville, Md, Agency for Healthcare Research and Quality, Feb 2003. Available at http://www.ahrq.gov/clinic/3rduspstf/diabscr/diabetrr.htm. Accessed 3/31/04. **(IV, C)**

51. Sheridan S, Pignone M, Donahue K: Screening for high blood pressure: review of the evidence for the U.S. Preventive Services Task Force. Am J Prev Med 2003;25:151–158. (Ia, A)

52. U.S. Preventive Services Task Force: Screening for High Blood Pressure: Recommendations and Rationale. Rockville, Md, Agency for Healthcare Research and Quality, July 2003. Available at http://www.ahrq.gov/clinic/3rduspstf/hibloodrr.htm. Accessed 3/9/04. (IV, C)

53. McTigue K, Harris R, Hemphill B, et al: Screening and interventions for obesity in adults: summary of the evidence for the U.S. Preventive Services Task Force. Ann Intern Med 2003;139:933–949. (Ia, A)

54. U.S. Preventive Services Task Force: Screening for Obesity in Adults: Recommendations and Rationale. Rockville, Md, Agency for Healthcare Research and Quality, November 2003. Available at http://www.ahrq.gov/clinic/3rduspstf/obesity/obesrr.htm. Accessed 2/29/04. (IV, C)

# Chapter 10

# Preconception Counseling

Marion S. Verp, MD

## KEY POINTS

- Preconception counseling and anticipation of genetic or medical problems is superior to postconception discovery and management.
- Genetic counseling and screening can be initiated before conception.
- Folic acid begun before conception reduces the risk for a child with a neural tube defect and should be prescribed for every woman anticipating pregnancy.

Most physicians would agree that preventive care and anticipation of potential medical problems is likely to result in a superior outcome as compared to secondary intervention. Unfortunately, almost half of all pregnancies are "unintended." Therefore, by the time of the first prenatal visit, the opportunity for prevention of harm to the mother and the fetus may have been lost. For example, pregnancy may be contraindicated by a maternal medical condition, required medications, or use of illicit substances. In many cases, recognition by the care provider of the possibility of conception would allow modification of the medication schedule, recommendation to postpone pregnancy until a chronic disease is in remission, or advice to change the patient's lifestyle before undertaking a pregnancy. Knowing that a pregnancy may adversely affect her own health or that she is at high risk for an abnormal fetus may result in a woman's firmer commitment to reliable contraception. Optimally, then, physicians seeing reproductive-age women would briefly explore with them their desire for pregnancy in the near future and their personal and family medical histories. Those patients expressing an interest in conception should have an appointment scheduled for fuller exploration of these issues.

In the case of a familial disorder, addressing potential problems before conception will allow adequate time to explore all of the reproductive options, possibilities for prenatal diagnosis, and the patient's feelings about intervention in an abnormal pregnancy. These issues can be much more calmly and thoughtfully dealt with when the pregnancy is anticipated rather than a fact.

## GENETIC HISTORY

The most important part of a genetic evaluation is asking the right questions. Many patients are ignorant of which disorders are genetic and therefore will not volunteer any information when asked if there is a genetic disease in the family. Therefore, one must be specific and ask the patient her age, ethnic background, outcome of all prior pregnancies, as well as information on chronic illness or death of a child, sibling, or parent. An initial screening questionnaire may be useful, but the information must be reviewed verbally with the patient to ensure that she has understood the questions. The health of the prospective parents, their parents and grandparents, aunts and uncles, siblings, nieces, and nephews should all be queried. Consanguinity (descent from a common ancestor) should be routinely sought. Details regarding prior pregnancy losses and anomalous fetuses or infants should be explored and relevant medical records obtained if possible. The records should be studied to verify the diagnosis, to determine how the diagnosis of a genetic condition was made, and whether other diagnoses were appropriately excluded. Consideration of whether the condition is sporadic or familial, alternative patterns of inheritance, and the risk to the consultant's offspring are all relevant. In many cases the latter issues are complex and referral to a genetic specialist is appropriate (Table 10-1). Sufficient time to obtain old records and to evaluate the level of risk and the patient's options is available if counseling is initiated prior to conception.

## PARENTAL AGE

A common concern for the preconception patient is the effect of her and her partner's age on the health of their offspring. Risk for chromosome abnormalities in offspring increases with maternal age[1] (Table 10-2). Many gynecologists are familiar with the risks associated with advancing maternal age and are comfortable advising their patients of these risks and the routine ways of addressing them (i.e., first-trimester or second-trimester screening or diagnosis). Educational brochures from the American College of Obstetricians and Gynecologists are available for patients to read and consider.

Advanced paternal age (45 years or older) does not increase the risk for chromosome abnormalities but does confer increased risk for a child with a new dominant mutation (e.g., neurofibromatosis, achondroplasia) and for cardiac defects.[2] Although elevated severalfold compared to that of younger men, the risk for a new dominant mutation in the child of a father older than age 40 is still less than 1%. Because a new dominant mutation can be for any of a variety of disorders, prenatal diagnosis cannot exclude the possibility of a new mutation. However, we advise pregnant partners of men older than age 45 to have a detailed ultrasound examination at 18 to 20 weeks' gestation because a skeletal disorder will occasionally be detected. Because cardiac detects are also more common in the offspring of older men, we may also suggest a fetal echocardiogram.

### Table 10-1
### Indications for Considering Genetic Referral

Personal or family history of child (or fetus) with congenital anomaly,
 chromosome abnormality, genetic disorder, early neonatal death
Multiple pregnancy losses
Advanced maternal age
Personal or family history of individual(s) with mental retardation
Personal or family history of genetic disorder
Couple both heterozygous for the same genetic condition
Potential exposure to teratogen

### Table 10-2
### Risk of Having a Live-Born Child with Down Syndrome or Other Chromosomal Abnormality

| Maternal Age | Risk of Down Syndrome | Total Risk for All Chromosomal Abnormality* |
|---|---|---|
| 20 | 1/1667 | 1/526 |
| 21 | 1/1667 | 1/526 |
| 22 | 1/1429 | 1/500 |
| 23 | 1/1429 | 1/500 |
| 24 | 1/1250 | 1/476 |
| 25 | 1/1250 | 1/476 |
| 26 | 1/1176 | 1/476 |
| 27 | 1/1111 | 1/455 |
| 28 | 1/1053 | 1/435 |
| 29 | 1/1000 | 1/417 |
| 30 | 1/952 | 1/384 |
| 31 | 1/909 | 1/384 |
| 32 | 1/769 | 1/322 |
| 33 | 1/625 | 1/317 |
| 34 | 1/500 | 1/260 |
| 35 | 1/385 | 1/204 |
| 36 | 1/294 | 1/164 |
| 37 | 1/227 | 1/130 |
| 38 | 1/175 | 1/103 |
| 39 | 1/137 | 1/82 |
| 40 | 1/106 | 1/65 |
| 41 | 1/82 | 1/51 |
| 42 | 1/64 | 1/40 |
| 43 | 1/50 | 1/32 |
| 44 | 1/38 | 1/25 |
| 45 | 1/30 | 1/20 |
| 46 | 1/23 | 1/15 |
| 47 | 1/18 | 1/12 |
| 48 | 1/14 | 1/10 |
| 49 | 1/11 | 1/7 |

Because sample size for some intervals is relatively small, 95% confidence limits are sometimes relatively large. Nonetheless, these figures are suitable for genetic counseling.
*47,XXX excluded for ages 20–32 (data not available).
Data from Hook EB: Rates of chromosome abnormalities at different maternal ages. Obstet Gynecol 1981;58:282; and Hook EB, Cross PK, Schreinemachers DM: Chromosomal abnormality rates at amniocentesis and in live-born infants. JAMA 1983;249:2034.

## GENETIC DISORDERS

In couples with a history of a prior chromosomally abnormal fetus or liveborn, or with a history of a chromosomal rearrangement in one of the parents, we advise formal genetic counseling to confirm the diagnosis, assess risk, and consider reproductive options. In many cases the additional risk based on this history is not great, yet the anxiety level in the potential parents can be enormous.

Families that have had a child with an X-linked recessive, autosomal dominant, or autosomal recessive genetic syndrome are frequently at high risk for recurrence. In addition, if one of the parents has an autosomal dominant genetic disorder (e.g., achondroplasia or neurofibromatosis), each fetus is at 50% risk for inheriting the mutant parental allele. If the father has an X-linked disorder, none of his sons will inherit the gene, but all of his daughters will inherit the gene and eventually be at high risk for affected offspring. Pregnancy may also exacerbate certain maternal genetic conditions (e.g., Marfan syndrome), with implications for maternal life and health. Therefore, identifying the high-risk patient, obtaining records to confirm the diagnosis, and counseling or referring the patient to the appropriate medical specialist before conception is crucial.

Multifactorial conditions, including isolated structural defects, usually recur in 2% to 5% of siblings or offspring. Some of these conditions (e.g., neural tube defects [NTDs]) can be detected during pregnancy; others, such as pyloric stenosis, will not be apparent prenatally. In families that have previously had a child or fetus with an NTD the opportunity exists to decrease the risk of recurrence by starting high-dose (4 mg/day) folic acid supplementation before conception and continuing through the period of embryogenesis.

### Ethnic and Racial Background

Ethnic background is important to ascertain because members of different ethnic and racial groups are at increased risk for specific disorders. Because almost all of these disorders are autosomal recessive in inheritance, prospective parents can be screened for the appropriate conditions once their ethnic/racial backgrounds are known. If both parents are heterozygous (carriers) for the same condition, options are available prior to conception (e.g., adoption, donor gametes, preimplantation diagnosis) that will not be available once a pregnancy is in progress. Although it is not possible to describe in detail each disorder for which screening is available, following is an example of the kind of information we provide verbally and in take-home pamphlets to our patients, prior to their deciding on screening.

#### African Background

Sickle cell disease (which includes SS disease, SC disease, and sickle cell–thalassemia disease) occurs in 1 in 500 African Americans. Children and adults with sickle cell disease have painful crises, which may occur frequently or rarely. They are also at risk for poor growth and for childhood death due to infections. Strokes or kidney failure may occur at a young age. Carrier frequency is 1 in 12.

### Ashkenazi Jewish Background

Several conditions are more common in the Ashkenazi Jewish population. If one member of the couple is Jewish and the other is not, the Jewish parent can be tested first. If he or she is positive for a trait, the non-Jewish parent can then be tested. For some of these conditions, testing a non-Jewish individual is less reliable.

Tay-Sachs disease causes mental and physical deterioration of the child, with death usually by age 5. The carrier frequency is 1 in 30, and 1 in 3600 Jewish children are affected. The Tay-Sachs gene is also more common among French Canadians from eastern Quebec and Cajuns in southern Louisiana. Canavan disease causes symptoms similar to Tay-Sachs disease. One in 40 Ashkenazi Jews carries this trait, and 1 in 6400 children is affected.

Familial dysautonomia is a neurologic disorder. Children with familial dysautonomia have trouble regulating their temperature, blood pressure, and digestive systems. About half of affected individuals live to age 30. The carrier frequency is 1 in 30, and 1 in 3700 children is affected.

Niemann-Pick disease type A causes an enlarged liver and spleen, poor growth, and progressive physical and mental deterioration, with death by age 4. The carrier rate is 1 in 90, with 1 in 32,000 Jewish children affected.

Children with Fanconi anemia type C have anemia, short stature, learning disabilities, or mental retardation. Birth defects of the limbs, heart, or kidneys may also be present. The risk for leukemia and early death is increased. The carrier rate is 1 in 89 Jewish individuals, and 1 in 31,000 Jewish children is affected.

Bloom syndrome results in poor growth and poor resistance to infection. There is a high rate of cancer, from which individuals usually die before age 30. One in 100 Jewish individuals carries this trait, and 1 in 46,000 children is affected.

Gaucher disease type 1 can be very mild or severe. Children and adults may have nosebleeds, anemia, an enlarged liver and spleen, bone pain, and easily broken bones. Because the severity is so variable, decisions about testing are difficult. The carrier frequency is 1 in 12, and 1 in 600 children is affected.

Mucolipidosis IV is a disorder of motor and mental retardation beginning in the first year of life. The carrier frequency is 1 in 100.

### Northern European Background

Cystic fibrosis (CF) is common among whites, particularly those of northern European origin. The disease causes lung infections, difficulty breathing, and problems with bowel function, weight gain, and growth. Children frequently need to be hospitalized, have physical therapy, and take several medications. The average life span is 30 years. One in 2500 white newborns has cystic fibrosis, and 1 in 25 whites carries the CF trait. CF is also found in the Ashkenazi Jewish population.

### Mediterranean Background (also Southeast Asian, African)

Beta-thalassemia causes severe anemia in children, requiring frequent blood transfusion. Children may grow poorly, have bone deformities or fractures, and develop heart failure from their disease. Carrier frequency varies with ethnic group.

| Table 10-3 Heterozygote Screening | |
|---|---|
| **Disorder** | **Screening Test** |
| Alpha-thalassemia | MCV |
| Beta-thalassemia | MCV |
| Sickle cell anemia | Hemoglobin electrophoresis |
| Cystic fibrosis | Mutation analysis |
| Tay-Sachs | Hexosaminidase assay and mutation analysis |
| Canavan | Mutation analysis |
| Familial dysautonomia | Mutation analysis |
| Gaucher type 1 | Mutation analysis |
| Fanconi anemia type C | Mutation analysis |
| Bloom syndrome | Mutation analysis |
| Niemann-Pick type A | Mutation analysis |
| Mucolipidosis IV | Mutation analysis |

MCV, mean corpuscular volume.

### Southeast Asian Background

Alpha-thalassemia is a blood disease that results in severe anemia and, in some forms, death of the fetus or newborn. Carrier frequency varies but may be as high as 1 in 20.

Carrier testing for some of the conditions described is possible using routine blood tests. However, for other conditions specialized testing is needed to determine whether an individual is a carrier (Table 10-3). Carrier tests cannot entirely eliminate the possibility of being a carrier, but a negative test makes the chance very low.

If the patient is interested in carrier testing, this may be arranged through the primary care provider, alternatively, a genetic counseling appointment can be made to discuss the most appropriate testing, the accuracy of test results, which laboratories do the testing, and the cost.

## CONSANGUINITY

Consanguinity is occasionally the reason couples will present for preconception counseling. If one of the members of the couple is the result of a consanguineous union or has a close relative who is, there is no concern as long as the individual in question is phenotypically normal and does not have a genetic disorder. However, if the couple itself is consanguineous, the exact degree of relatedness must be sought. Offspring of first-cousin unions have a twofold increase in risk for perinatal and childhood death, malformation, or mental retardation, as compared to the general population risk.[3] This assumes that both parents are phenotypically normal and there is no family history of a recessive disorder. If the family does have an autosomal recessive disorder, or if the ethnic background warrants, heterozygote testing should be offered to the couple.

## Ambulatory Office Practice

As the degree of relatedness decreases, the likelihood of carrying identical mutant genes decreases sharply. Therefore the risk to offspring of second and third cousins is not increased as compared to the general population.[3] Obviously if a known genetic disorder exists in the family, specific counseling should be offered.

# MEDICAL ISSUES

## Nutritional Status

As part of the preconception counseling process, a complete medical history should be obtained. This must include information on the patient's nutritional status (i.e., whether she has an eating disorder or unusual diet, whether she is underweight or overweight, and whether she takes dietary supplements or weight loss products). A history of bulimia or anorexia should be explored to determine the patient's current eating practices.

Underweight women are at increased risk for preterm delivery and a low-birth-weight infant or fetus with intrauterine growth restriction (IUGR).[4] Overweight women have an increased likelihood of developing hypertension, preeclampsia, gestational diabetes, thrombophlebitis, preterm or post-term delivery, abnormal labor, and delivery by cesarean section with increased postoperative complications.[5] Offspring of obese women are at greater risk of late fetal demise, macrosomia, birth trauma, and congenital malformations (e.g., spina bifida).[5,6] In addition, obese women (body mass index > 27) have a greater risk of anovulatory infertility.

Women deficient in iron have an increased chance of preterm delivery and low-birth-weight infants. Pica, or the ingestion of nonfood substances, can result in lead poisoning or iron deficiency. Vegetarian diets may be satisfactory for pregnancy as long as there is adequate protein intake.

Ocean fish (e.g., shark, king mackerel, swordfish) are known to be contaminated with methyl mercury; however, the level of contamination varies with type of fish and geographic origin. Women with high ingestion of heavily contaminated fish have had children with microcephaly, cerebral atrophy, mental retardation, and seizures.[7] On the other hand, ingestion of fish with a lower mercury concentration has not been demonstrated to cause these defects.[8] Nonetheless, the U.S. Food and Drug Administration (FDA) and the Environmental Protection Agency (EPA) have recommended that pregnant women avoid eating any shark, swordfish, king mackerel, or tilefish and that they limit other small ocean fish, canned tuna, and shellfish to less than 12 ounces per week, with no more than one serving of any one type of fish per week. Local freshwater fish will also vary in their level of contamination. The EPA can be contacted to obtain advice on specific locales.[9]

Supplementation with 0.4 mg of folic acid/day in low-risk women (4 mg/day in women who have previously had a child with an NTD) has been shown to substantially reduce the risk for an open NTD when started at least 1 month prior to conception and continued through the first trimester.[10] Because so many pregnancies are unplanned, folic acid supplementation should be recommended to all women of childbearing age. Although the FDA has mandated folic acid fortification of food, intake is inadequate in most women to meet the required dose without further supplementation. Multivitamins containing folic acid have also been associated with decreased risk for neuroblastoma, genitourinary anomalies, and facial clefts.[11,12] Low maternal levels of zinc, most likely to be found in women who exercise strenuously or who are vegans, have been associated with occurrence of NTD.[13] Therefore, a multivitamin containing folic acid and zinc should be recommended to all potentially pregnant women. Additional folic acid supplementation must be prescribed to women at high risk for NTD.

Oversupplementation with vitamin A (retinol) has been reported to be associated with a variety of congenital anomalies, including cardiac, central nervous system, and urinary tract defects, as well as IUGR. Although these reports have been contested,[14] it is safest for patients not to take supplements with more than 10,000 IU retinol/day. Most prenatal vitamin supplements are currently formulated to have 8000 IU or less. The beta-carotene form of vitamin A has not been associated with birth defects, even when ingested in large doses.

## Chronic Medical Conditions

Pregnancy may have a deleterious effect on some chronic medical conditions; conversely, medical conditions and medications can affect the outcome of pregnancy. Therefore, before conception, each woman should be queried as to the medical conditions she has been or is currently being treated for and all of the medications and over-the-counter substances she is ingesting. The primary care provider may not be familiar with the effect of the disorder, or drug, on pregnancy and may elect to refer the patient to a specialist who can assess whether a disease is in good control, help plan the timing of a pregnancy, and consider the potential teratogenicity of required medications and the alternatives (Table 10-4).

There are, however, a few disorders that are sufficiently common to warrant familiarity of the primary physician caring for the preconception patient. For example, carbohydrate intolerance affects 1.5 million women of reproductive age in the United States. Although maternal and fetal mortality associated with diabetes in pregnancy has decreased, congenital malformations still occur 2 to 3 times more commonly in offspring of diabetics than in offspring of women with normal carbohydrate metabolism.[15] Cardiac, renal, and neural tube defects are especially common. Although they occur infrequently, holoprosencephaly and sacral agenesis are much more common among offspring of diabetic than nondiabetic mothers.

| Table 10-4 |
| --- |
| **Medications Contraindicated During Pregnancy** |
| ACE inhibitors and angiotensin II receptor antagonists |
| Alkylating agents |
| Amiodarone |
| Androgens |
| Diphenylhydantoin |
| Etretinate |
| Isotretinoin |
| Leflunomide |
| Tetracycline |
| Trimethoprim |
| Valproic acid |
| Warfarin |

Poorly controlled diabetics have a higher pregnancy loss rate and a higher fetal malformation rate than do well-controlled diabetics.[15] However, because most embryologic development occurs before 10 weeks' gestational age, good control must be achieved before conception and must be continued through the phase of organogenesis to impact the morbidity and mortality rates. Control starting after the first prenatal visit, although it may have other beneficial effects on maternal health and fetal growth, is usually too late to reduce the risk of malformation. Other complications in diabetic women and their fetuses are maternal hypertension and preeclampsia, increased need for cesarean section, macrosomia and associated birth trauma, and IUGR; complications in the neonate include hypoglycemia, respiratory distress syndrome, hypocalcemia, polycythemia, and hyperbilirubinemia. If the maternal diabetes is of long standing, diabetic nephropathy may be present, increasing the likelihood of preterm birth, hypertensive complications, and the need for maternal dialysis or transplantation in the near future, while her child is very young.[16] Progression of diabetic retinopathy, again requiring aggressive treatment and possible permanent morbidity, is more common in pregnant women with poor control than in pregnant women with good control.[17]

Ideally, the patient's renal, cardiac, and retinal function would be assessed prior to conception. Glycosylated hemoglobin levels can be used to assess the level of control for the previous 3 months. Tight control may require changing from an oral hypoglycemic agent to several injections of insulin each day. The patient will have to manage her disease intensively, measuring her blood sugar frequently at home, and plan for frequent medical visits both in the early and late stages of pregnancy. Discussing these issues before conception allows the patient the opportunity to think about whether she is prepared to make this commitment to preconception control and prenatal care. If not, she may want to consider a very effective method of contraception or sterilization.

Hypertension, likewise, is a common disorder in the general population. Although this condition can usually be satisfactorily managed without complication during pregnancy, women with hypertension are at increased risk for cerebrovascular accident, renal failure, preeclampsia, gestational diabetes, placental abruption, IUGR, fetal demise, and preterm delivery.[18] The most severe complications occur in women over age 30 with evidence of end-organ disease (long-standing hypertension). Also, certain antihypertensive agents (e.g., angiotensin-converting enzyme inhibitors or angiotensin II receptor antagonists) are contraindicated in pregnancy for their fetopathic effect.[19] Atenolol has been associated with IUGR.[20] Hypertensive women should have their retinal, renal, and cardiac functions assessed prior to conception. If the patient requires an antihypertensive drug to maintain normal blood pressure, and the medication she is taking is not teratogenic, she should continue the medication during pregnancy. Alternatively, if the hypertension is mild and not complicated by renal disease or diabetes mellitus, a trial off medication with close monitoring is also reasonable.

An uncommon (1 in 14,000 women) disorder, but one that is extremely important to recognize prior to conception, is phenylketonuria (PKU). Women with PKU will report having been on a special diet throughout childhood and requiring multiple physician visits to monitor phenylketone levels. Women who have adhered to this diet throughout childhood are usually of normal intelligence. However, many have stopped their phenylalanine-free diet on reaching adolescence. Although this may not be causing them any physical or mental harm, their phenylalanine levels will be very high on a normal diet. This in turn will have a teratogenic effect on their offspring (i.e., microcephaly, mental retardation, cardiac anomalies, and IUGR).[21] Therefore such women must be identified and aggressively treated with a phenylalanine-restricted diet prior to conception.

Seizure disorders are the most common neurologic problem in women who present for preconception counseling. Seizure frequency is unchanged or decreased in about half of pregnant women, and the other 50% report an increase in seizure frequency. Many women will have been on anticonvulsant medications for many years, and some will have a history of no recent seizures. In the latter case, it would be appropriate to arrange a consultation for the patient with her neurologist to see if a trial off anticonvulsants is reasonable. The usual guideline is that if no seizures have occurred for the preceding 2 years, and the seizure history does not include tonic-clonic seizures, then a trial off medication is warranted.[22] Even if such a trial proves successful, however, a patient with a history of idiopathic seizures must be advised of her twofold increased risk for a child with a nonspecific birth defect.[23] The latter is true even if no anticonvulsant medication is taken during the pregnancy. The explanation for this empirical finding is that some individuals may have genetic syndromes characterized both by seizures and by increased risk for dysmorphogenesis.

Additionally, the patient who must continue her anticonvulsant medication during pregnancy should be advised that many anticonvulsants are known to have teratogenic effects. Both valproic acid and carbamazepine are associated with an increased risk for NTDs. Diphenylhydantoin is associated with a pattern of dysmorphogenesis that includes growth restriction, microcephaly, mental retardation, and hypoplastic fingernails and toenails. Other anticonvulsants are also associated with similar dysmorphism. Some of the newer anticonvulsants (e.g., topiramate, gabapentin, lamotrigine) may ultimately prove safer, but only a minimal amount of data is currently available.[23] Folic acid may reduce the risk for a birth defect, and women taking valproic acid or carbamazepine are advised to take a dose of 4 mg/day starting before conception and continuing through the stage of neural tube closure (4 weeks' postconception). Anticonvulsant levels should be monitored serially throughout pregnancy to assure that they are at a therapeutic level. The required dose is likely to change during pregnancy, given the increased volume of distribution, decreased plasma protein levels, and change in liver metabolism and gastrointestinal absorption. Most important is the ability to manage the disorder with single rather than multiple drug therapy, the latter resulting in a higher malformation rate.

Once pregnancy occurs, maternal serum alpha-fetoprotein screening, amniocentesis, or detailed ultrasound examination at the appropriate gestational ages are available for screening and diagnosis of fetal NTDs. Ultrasound may also detect some cases with anticonvulsant-associated facial clefts or cardiac defects.

Patients may be receiving chronic anticoagulation for a number of reasons, including a history of antiphospholipid syndrome, thromboembolism, or prosthetic heart valve. First-trimester exposure to Coumadin (warfarin sodium), an oral anticoagulant, is associated with fetal nasal hypoplasia. Second-trimester exposure infrequently results in optic nerve or cerebral damage.[24] Therefore, the safest option is for the patient to change to a form of heparin (regular or low molecular weight), which does not cross the placenta, prior to conception. Because heparin must be injected daily, this will obviously be a more difficult therapy for the patient, and requires discussion in the preconception period.

### Infections

The preconception period is ideal for screening for infectious disease and immunizing when appropriate. High-risk patients should be screened for tuberculosis. A rubella titer should be drawn. If no antibodies are present, the patient should be immunized and advised not to conceive for the next 3 months. The same is true for varicella in women who have no history of the infection. Patients without a history of hepatitis B can be immunized also if they fall into a high-risk group (e.g., health care worker, household contact, multiple sexual partners). Women with exposure to outdoor cats or raw meat should take precautions to avoid exposure to *Toxoplasma* unless they have a positive antibody titer. Childcare workers are at increased risk for cytomegalovirus and parvovirus. If they do not have antibodies they need to adopt appropriate precautions (e.g., wearing gloves when handling wet diapers). Testing for human immunodeficiency virus (HIV) and syphilis can be offered, as well as screening for other sexually transmitted diseases.

### Environmental Exposures

Other issues that should be raised in the course of pre-conception counseling include the patient's use of caffeine, tobacco, alcohol, and illicit drugs. Consumption of more than 2 cups of regular strength coffee (250 mg) a day has been associated with a slight decrease in fertility; more than 4 cups per day has been associated with pregnancy loss.[25] Causality, however, may be questioned on the grounds that women who drink such high levels of coffee in early pregnancy don't have the usual aversion and nausea commonly present in a healthy first-trimester pregnancy.

Approximately 15% of women smoke during pregnancy despite the known association with preterm delivery and low birth weight, placental abruption, placenta previa, and, more recently reported, facial clefting and clubfeet.[26] The odds ratio of delivering a small for gestational age infant in a smoker is 2.07 (95% confidence interval [CI], 1.69 to 2.53), with a direct dose–response association between number of cigarettes smoked and risk of growth restriction.[27] Because pregnancy is a powerful inducement to change, attempts to stop smoking in preparation for gestation may be more successful than at other times in a woman's life. Suggestions by the physician regarding use of nicotine replacement or other pharmacointerventions may be more positively received by the patient interested in her offspring's welfare. Because secondhand smoke exposure has also been associated with full-term low-birth-weight infants, the male partner should be encouraged to participate in these efforts. Cigarette smoking is associated with accelerated attrition of oocytes, decreased fertility, and earlier menopause, an issue for the older patient attempting pregnancy.[28]

| | Table 10-5 <br> The T-ACE Questionnaire |
|---|---|
| T | How many drinks does it take to make you feel "high" (can you hold)? (*Tolerance:* a positive response consists of two or more drinks) |
| A | Have people *annoyed* you by criticizing your drinking? |
| C | Have you ever felt you ought to *cut down* on your drinking? |
| E | Have you ever had a drink first thing in the morning to steady your nerves or to get rid of a hangover (*eye-opener*)? |

Scoring: 2 points for the first question and 1 point each for the other three questions. A score of ≥ 2 is high risk.

Alcohol is a known teratogen and the leading preventable cause of mental retardation. There is a dose–response relationship between alcohol and congenital abnormalities and although low levels of exposure are not associated with the fetal alcohol syndrome, it cannot be assumed that even low-level exposure is without long-term subtle behavioral effects on the developing fetal brain. The preconception interview can include a few questions to screen for heavy alcohol use (e.g., the T-ACE questionnaire; Table 10-5).[29] Infertility secondary to anovulation is more common in women who consume alcohol, and heavy alcohol use by the male reduces spermatogenesis.[30]

Use of cocaine, heroin, or other illicit substances is known to confer increased risk for low birth weight and other obstetric complications. Referral to a detoxification program before conception would be beneficial to mother and child.

Domestic violence during pregnancy has been reported in at least 4% to 8% of women, most of whom are already suffering abuse prior to pregnancy. In fact, 59% of women abused prior to pregnancy have reported continuation of violence during pregnancy.[31] Counseling and resources should be made available to women in this situation.

Because there is data from animal studies indicating that hyperthermia during organogenesis is teratogenic, particularly for NTDs, use of hot tubs in very early pregnancy has been a concern. A study done by Milunsky and colleagues[32] showed that women who used a hot tub in the first 8 weeks of pregnancy had a 2.9 relative risk (95% CI, 1.4 to 6.3) of a child with an NTD. Although most women will not stay in a hot tub long enough to become hyperthermic, caution would suggest limiting exposure in the periconception period.

Although most workplaces are safe for pregnant women, an occupational history should be taken. If there is concern regarding exposure to excess physical stress, organic solvents, lead, mercury, or pesticides, which may be associated with pregnancy loss or teratogenesis, further investigation of the level of exposure, whether the patient is retaining toxic substances in her blood, and the need for a more protected work environment should be explored.

## REFERENCES

1. Hook EB, Cross PK, Schreinemachers DM: Chromosomal abnormality rates at amniocentesis and in live-born infants. JAMA 1983; 249:2034–2038. (IIb, B)

2. Olshan AF, Schnitzer PG, Baird PA: Paternal age and the risk of congenital heart defects. Teratology 1994;50:80–84. **(IIa, B)**

3. Bennett RL, Motulsky AG, Bittles A, et al: Genetic counseling and screening of consanguineous couples and their offspring: recommendations of the National Society of Genetic Counselors. J Genet Couns 2002;11:97–119. **(IV, C)**

4. Ehrenberg HM, Dierker L, Milluzzi C, Mercer BM: Low maternal weight, failure to thrive in pregnancy, and adverse pregnancy outcomes. Am J Obstet Gynecol 2003;189:1726–1730. **(IIb, B)**

5. Rosenberg TJ, Garbers S, Chavkin W, Chiasson, MA: Prepregnancy weight and adverse perinatal outcomes in an ethnically diverse population. Obstet Gynecol 2003;102:1022–1027. **(IIb, B)**

6. Watkins ML, Rasmussen SA, Honein MA, et al: Maternal obesity and risk for birth defects. Pediatrics 2003;111:1152–1158. **(IIa, B)**

7. Harada M: Congenital Minamata disease: intrauterine mercury poisoning. Teratol 1978;18:285–288. **(III, B)**

8. Myers GJ, Davidson PW, Cox C, et al: Prenatal methylmercury exposure from ocean fish consumption in the Seychelles child development study. Lancet 2003;361:1686–1692. **(IIb, B)**

9. http://www.epa.gov/waterscience/fishadvice/advice.html or 1-800-723-3366. **(IV, C)**

10. Centers for Disease Control and Prevention: Recommendations for use of folic acid to reduce number of spina bifida cases and other neural tube defects. JAMA 1993;269:1233–1238. **(Ib, A, IIa, B)**

11. Olshan AF, Smith JC, Bondy ML, et al: Maternal vitamin use and reduced risk of neuroblastoma. Epidemiol 2002;13:575–580. **(IIa, B)**

12. Hernandez-Diza S, Werler MM, Alexander MW, Mitchell AA: Folic acid antagonists during pregnancy and the risk of birth defects. New Eng J Med 2000;343:1608–1614. **(IIa, B)**

13. Groenen PM, Peer PG, Wevers RA, et al: Maternal myo-inositol, glucose, and zinc status is associated with the risk of offspring with spina bifida. Am J Obstet Gynecol 2003;189:1713–1719. **(IIa, B)**

14. Mastroiacovo P, Mazzone T, Addis A, et al: High vitamin A intake in early pregnancy and major malformations: a multicenter prospective controlled study. Teratol 1999; 59:7–11. **(IIa, B)**

15. Green MF, Hare JW, Cloherty JP, et al: First-trimester hemoglobin A$_1$ and risk for major malformation and spontaneous abortion in diabetic pregnancy. Teratol 1989;39:225–231. **(IIb, B)**

16. Gordan M, Landon M, Samuels P, et al: Perinatal outcome and long-term follow-up associated with modern management of diabetic nephropathy. Obstet Gynecol 1996;87:401–409. **(IIb, B)**

17. Chew EY, Mills JL, Metzger BE, et al: Metabolic control and progression of retinopathy. Diabetes Care 1995;18:631–637. **(IIb, B)**

18. Rey E, Couturier A: The prognosis of pregnancy in women with chronic hypertension. Am J Obstet Gynecol 1994;171:410–416. **(IIb, B)**

19. Barr M II: Teratogen update: angiotensin-converting enzyme inhibitors. Teratol 1994;50:399–409. **(IV, C)**

20. Tabacova S, Kimmel CA, Wall K: Atenolol developmental toxicity: animal-to-animal comparisons. Birth Defects Res 2003;67:181–192. **(III, B)**

21. Rouse B, Azen C, Koch R, et al: Maternal phenylketonuria collaborative study (MPKUCS) offspring: facial anomalies, malformations, and early neurological sequelae. Am J Med Gen 1997;69:89–85. **(IIb, B)**

22. Delgado-Escueta AV, Janz D: Consensus guidelines: preconception counseling management, and care of the pregnant woman with epilepsy. Neurol 1992;42(Suppl 5):149–160. **(IV, C)**

23. Pennell PB: The importance of monotherapy in pregnancy. Neurol 2003;60(Suppl 4):S31–S38. **(IIb, B)**

24. Van Driel D, Wesseling J, Sauer PJJ, et al: Teratogen update: fetal effects after in utero exposure to coumarins. Overview of cases, follow-up findings, and pathogenesis. Teratol 2002;66:127–140. **(IIa, B)**

25. Christian MS, Brent RL: Teratogen update: evaluation of the reproductive and developmental risks of caffeine. Teratol 2001;64:51–78. **(IIa, B)**

26. Shepard TH, Brent RL, Friedman JM, et al: Update on new developments in the study of human teratogens. Teratol 2002;65:153–161. **(IIa, B)**

27. Horta BL, Victora CG, Menezes AM, Barros HR: Low birthweight, preterm births and intrauterine growth retardation in relation to maternal smoking. Paediatr Perinat Epidemiol 1997;11:140–151. **(IIa, B)**

28. Cramer DW, Barbieri RL, Xu H, Reichardt JK: Determinants of basal follicle-stimulating hormone levels in premenopausal women. J Clin Endocrinol Metab 1994;79:1105–1109. **(IIb, B)**

29. Sokol RJ, Martier SS, Ager JW: The T-ACE questions: practical prenatal detection of risk-drinking. Am J Obstet Gynecol 1989;160:863–868. **(IIb, B)**

30. Nagy F, Pendergrass PB, Bowen DC, Yeager JC: A comparative study of cytological and physiological parameters of semen obtained from alcoholics and non-alchoholics. Alcohol Alcoholism 1986;21:17–23. **(IIb, B)**

31. Martin SL, Mackie L, Kupper LL, et al: Physical abuse of women before, during, and after pregnancy. JAMA 2001;285:1581–1584. **(III, B)**

32. Milunsky A, Ulcickas M, Rothman K: Maternal heat exposure and neural tube defects. JAMA 1992;268:882–885. **(IIa, B)**

# Chapter 11

# Cervical Cancer Screening*

## Herschel W. Lawson, MD

This chapter presents principles of cervical cancer screening and follow-up of abnormal Papanicolaou (Pap) test results that result in the histologic diagnosis of premalignant changes of the cervix. More detailed information about diagnostic follow-up of abnormal cervical cancer screening results by colposcopy and clinical features of cervical intraepithelial neoplasia and invasive cancer are discussed in Chapters 12 and 43, respectively. Issues related specifically to diagnosis and management of invasive cancer of the cervix are covered in Section 7.

In 1957, the United States Commission on Chronic Illness defined health screening as "the presumptive identification of unrecognized disease or defect by the application of tests, examinations or other procedures that can be applied rapidly."[1] Thus, health screening is the use of methods to detect unrecognized health risks or diseases in order to permit timely intervention.

Screening tests are usually applied on a large scale. They are used to distinguish apparently unaffected people from those who may have or may develop a disease. A screening test is not intended to be diagnostic. Screening procedures are generally easier to perform and cheaper than diagnostic procedures. Their results require confirmation through definitive diagnostic tests, or sometimes direct treatment is offered on the basis of a positive test. Even if the screening test is harmless, it can cause anxiety and the subsequent investigations and treatment may be hazardous. Ensuring the safety of screening is also important because large numbers of individuals will be screened, creating a potential for greater numbers to be harmed by the screening process.[2]

Screening comprises three elements:

1. It is a preliminary process of selection to identify individuals at sufficiently high risk of a specific disorder to warrant further investigation or direct action.
2. It is offered to a largely healthy population not seeking attention for symptoms of the disease for which the screening is being conducted.
3. It is meant to benefit the individuals being screened.

These principles imply an ethical approach to participants in the screening process. In clinical practice, the special nature of the patient/provider relationship has resulted in the need to create a core of ethical principles to govern this relationship. An important distinction between screening and episodic care for medical diagnosis and treatment is that the screening encounter is not initiated by the subject but by the provider. This is true whether screening is offered in an organized way by governmental public health units or opportunistically by providers in a variety of ambulatory care settings. When a patient consults a health provider for diagnosis of, and hopefully relief of symptoms, or for treatment of an established condition, the provider exercises skills only to the extent that knowledge is currently available. In screening, however, those who participate are not patients in the sense that they are ill, and in the majority of situations, do not become patients in the traditional sense. The screener promotes the test based on evidence that as a result of screening, the overall health of the community will be better. This does not mean that the condition of every individual screened will be better, although in general, this should be so.[3] There is also an ethical responsibility of the provider community to (1) minimize the potential harms and anxiety that affect certain individuals being screened, (2) ensure that quality control of the screening tests is maintained and the effectiveness of proven, beneficial programs is continually monitored, and (3) guarantee that assurance is available that a useful course of management is available for all individuals identified as being truly test-positive.

Equity of access to screening services is another important consideration. Ideally, all who stand to gain from screening should have access to the procedure. Those who organize the service have an obligation to ensure that those who have not heard of the test/ procedure but who stand to benefit from it are adequately informed and are encouraged or invited to be screened. An additional issue concerns the extent to which the offer of screening in a community could divert resources from other important health care programs. This is of particular importance in low resource settings in which limited resources

---

*All material in this chapter is in the public domain, with the exception of any borrowed figures or tables.

## EPIDEMIOLOGY, PATHOGENESIS, AND RISK FACTORS FOR CERVICAL INTRAEPITHELIAL NEOPLASIA

Persistence of DNA from a high-risk type of HPV is significantly associated with development of high-grade cervical intraepithelial neoplasia (CIN) or dysplasia and invasive cervical cancer.[4,5] CIN III and invasive cancer are most commonly found at the junction between the squamous and glandular cells of the uterine cervix, which is called the *squamocolumnar junction* (SCJ). This cervical *transformation zone*, an active area of squamous metaplasia, is especially vulnerable to HPV-induced cellular transformation (Fig. 11-1).

After infection with HPV, one of two clinical pathways may occur: (1) transient viral expression followed by clinical clearance, or (2) viral persistence. Most infections remain undetectable or produce transient cytologic changes that are missed by infrequent screening. Some infections cause detectable cytologic changes diagnostic of HPV infection, including a low-grade squamous intraepithelial lesion (LSIL) or high-grade squamous intraepithelial lesion (HSIL), or induce the shedding of cells that demonstrate only some, but not all, features of an HPV infection (e.g., atypical squamous cells of undetermined significance, or ASC-US). CIN is a tissue-based classification; i.e., it is based on reviewing the histopathology of biopsy specimens. The designation of CIN I, II, or III is based on the thickness of the epithelium showing abnormal cells, the degree of mitotic activity, and nuclear atypia[6] (Fig. 11-2). Since more than one naming system is used, it is important to note that CIN I and II correspond to mild and moderate dysplasia, respectively; CIN III is analogous to severe dysplasia, and this category includes carcinoma in situ. Pathologists often disagree about the interpretation of samples at the lower end of the cytologic and histologic spectra (ASC-US and CIN I, respectively).[7] The disparity between the high rate of infection with HPV and the relatively low risk of cervical cancer reflects the fact that many women become infected with HPV but most infections spontaneously regress over time. Attempts to understand why the virus persists in some women have focused on variants of high-risk HPV types and cofactors such as smoking, other infectious agents (chlamydia, herpes, bacterial vaginosis), parity, use of oral contraceptives, and host immune factors. In the end, any important role played by HPV variants and cofactors is likely to be due to promotion of viral persistence because it is the most important factor in determining whether an HPV infection has the potential to progress to a precancerous lesion or cancer. The incidence of invasive cervical cancer reaches a plateau in women approximately 15 years later than the peak incidence of CIN III, suggesting a slow progression from CIN III to invasive carcinoma in most instances.[8] This prolonged period from development of CIN III to invasion probably reflects the long period of time required for the accumulation of mutations following viral integration and down-regulation of the apoptotic functions of certain tumor suppressor oncogenes (p53 tumor suppressor gene, or p53, and the retinoblastoma protein, or pRb). Inhibition of p53 and pRb leads to an increased cell proliferation rate and to genomic instability. The infected cell acquires more and more DNA damage that cannot be repaired, leading eventually to oncogenic transformation.

## NATURAL HISTORY OF HUMAN PAPILLOMAVIRUS

It is now clear that the natural history of cervical neoplasia and HPV are intimately related. The natural history of HPV begins with infection followed by a variable period of time during which disease expression is absent. Over time there may be an active growth phase and a finally a host-containment phase (Fig. 11-3). Most HPV infections do not result in signs or symptoms of disease.[4,9,10] If HPV infection is not controlled,

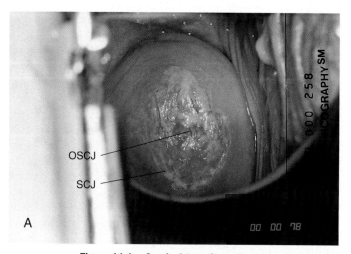
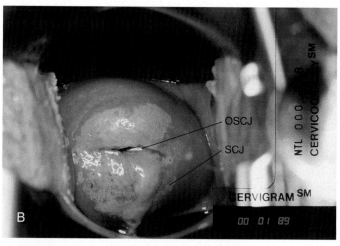

**Figure 11-1    Cervical transformation zone seen on cervigrams showing visual inspection with acetic acid (VIA).**
The transformation zone lies between the new squamocolumnar junction (SCJ) and the original squamocolumnar junction (OSCJ). The new squamocolumnar junction is defined by the leading edge of squamous cells as they abut the columnar epithelium. *A,* Small, flat, dull acetowhite lesion. *B,* Large, thick, shiny acetowhite lesion. Both are examples of high-grade squamous intraepithelial lesions (HSILs). (Courtesy of K. Dahlquist and J. Sellors, MD.)

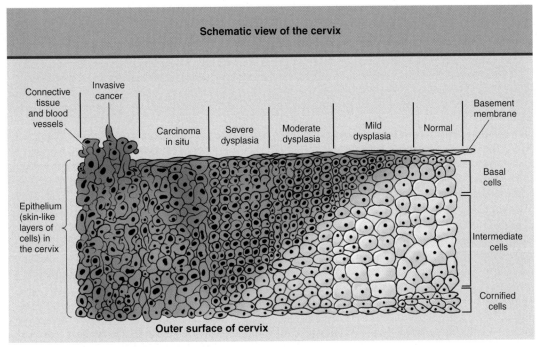

**Figure 11-2   Schematic development of cervical cancer from normal and precursor lesions.** (Courtesy of V. Hanson, MD.)

owing to host, viral, or environmental factors, an active growth phase will be expressed as one or more morphologic changes such as abnormalities of cervical cytology, cutaneous warts, CIN, or invasive cervical cancer. For the majority of patients, a phase of host containment begins following immune recognition of HPV presence. A successful immune response results in viral control or clearance. A minority of individuals do not develop adequate host control and are at risk for persistence of HPV. The persistence of high-risk HPV infection is a necessary step for the development of cervical cancer precursor lesions and

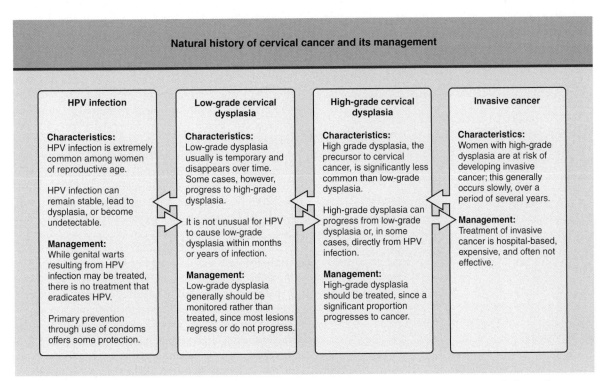

**Figure 11-3   Natural history of cervical cancer and program implications.** (From Sherris J, Herdman C: Preventing cervical cancer in low-resource settings. Outlook 2000;18:3. Used with permission of Program for Appropriate Technology in Health [PATH], Seattle, Wash.)

invasive cancer.[11] In summary, the basic segments of the natural history of transient HPV infection include viral entry, viral replication, productive viral infection, and host containment. The viral life cycle is depicted in Fig. 11-4.

HPV first enters the basal cells in the stratum germinativum of the epithelium.[12] The virus is most often transmitted by skin-to-skin contact and enters through sites of microtrauma, most commonly found in women at the introitus and perineum during or following sexual relations. Areas with increased vulnerability to HPV infection are the epithelial layers of immature squamous metaplasia located in the transformation zone of the cervix and anal verge.

HPV is a small, double-stranded DNA virus encased in a protein capsid. To enter the host cell, it must shed its protein capsid, injecting naked DNA into the cytoplasm of the cell. From the cytoplasm, the DNA travels to the cell nucleus. The viral genome usually exists in an episomal (circular) configuration that can be divided into three regions: the long control region (LCR), the early region (E), and the late region (L)[12] (Fig. 11-5). The LCR is responsible for regulation of viral replication and controls transcription of some sequences in the early region. The early region encodes mainly for proteins that are important in viral replication, occurring "early" in the viral life cycle. The late region encodes for viral structural proteins that are necessary for capsid production, which occurs "late" in the viral life cycle.[12] The early region has eight different regions that encode for proteins that play vital roles in the HPV life cycle. Two regions, designated E6 and E7, are crucial in the process of oncogenesis in high-risk types of HPV. The E6 protein binds to p53 and accelerates its destruction. The E7 protein binds to pRb, inhibiting its function.[13] The actions of the E6 and E7 proteins lead to cellular transformation.[12] Low-risk HPV types have a much lower capacity to induce malignant transformation in vitro

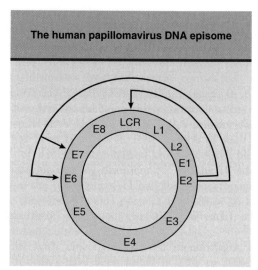

**Figure 11-5    Human papillomavirus (HPV) DNA.** Most HPV exists in episomal (circular) DNA. The important genomic sites are called open reading frames (ORFs). In the episomal state, E2 regulates both the long control region (LCR), which is responsible for regulation of viral transcription, and E6 and E7, the two sites most often responsible for malignant transformation. (From Cox JT: Clinical Proceedings, Association of Reproductive Health Professionals, September 2003, p 5, with permission.)

than high-risk HPV types because of functional differences between their E6 and E7 proteins.[12] For example, the E6 proteins of low-risk HPV types bind to the protein product of p53 poorly, and thus are less able to transform infected cells.[12] The two late regions, L1 and L2, encode for proteins involved in construction of the capsid of the infective HPV genome. In benign lesions associated with HPV, viral DNA exists as a circular extrachromosomal DNA in the nucleus. However, in cancerous cells and in some precancerous lesions associated with HPV, the viral DNA is integrated into the host genome. Generally, the integration of the viral DNA deletes or disrupts the E2 region, resulting in loss of normal E2 down-regulation of E6 and E7, which leads to increased expression of these two regions.

At some point, daughter cells of the infected basal cells may begin to carry transcriptionally active episomal HPV DNA. As these cells differentiate and mature, HPV replicates, making 50 to 100 replicated copies per cell. Activation of the L1 region of the HPV genome in the upper epithelial layers envelopes each episomal DNA in a protein capsid, recreating the infective unit. HPV induction of cytoplasmic proteins in some of the infected epithelial cells results in the hallmark cell of HPV infection, the koilocyte described by Koss in 1956.[14] Although described, it was not recognized as significant until 20 years later when Meisels and colleagues reported the changes in mild dysplasia.[15] Koilocytes are large, polygonal squamous cells with a wrinkled nucleus and a large perinuclear cavity[13] (Fig. 11-6). Shedding of the dead, surface squamous cells as part of the natural process of the cell cycle releases HPV virions to infect other cells or transmit the virus to another individual. In productive infection, viral replication is associated with proliferation of all layers except the basal layer.[12] In high-grade CIN, however, viral

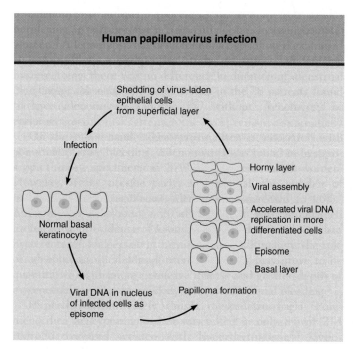

**Figure 11-4    The viral life cycle.** (From Cox JT: Clinical Proceedings, Association of Reproductive Health Professionals, September 2003, p 5, with permission.)

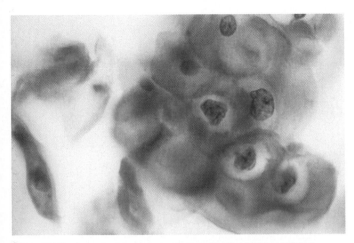

**Figure 11-6    Low-grade squamous intraepithelial lesions (LSILs).** Classic koilocytes, as seen here, have a large cytoplasmic cavity with a sharply defined inner edge and are frequently binucleate. (Courtesy of ES Cibas, MD)

replication is associated with proliferation of the cells in the basal layer and with an increased number of mitoses, some of which are abnormal.[12] The exact factors that determine the transition from productive infection to persistent infection associated with high-grade lesions are unknown, but a complex interplay of host, viral, and environmental factors is most likely important.

Recognition of the presence of HPV by the immune system results in a T-cell response. T cells are the primary effectors of the cellular immune response, which is known to be of prime importance in limiting HPV infection.[10] The humoral immune system may also be involved with fighting HPV infection and preventing reinfection with the same HPV type. Antibodies against the viral capsid have been detected in individuals with cutaneous or urogenital warts.[16–18] In most cases, genital HPV infection appears to be transient. In one study of college women, the median duration of HPV detection by sensitive molecular tests was 8 months; this may be an underestimate because it was not possible to document when these infections began.[19] Other studies have documented a longer duration of detection of HPV that is type-specific, with a mean duration of 13.4 months for low-risk types and 16.3 months for high-risk types.[20] Ninety percent of HPV infections will be cleared or suppressed below the limits of detection by host defenses within 1 to 2 years.[4] Viral persistence is necessary for HPV-induced oncogenesis to occur. Persistent infection with high-risk HPV types correlates with age and high viral load and is associated with increased risk of CIN.[19, 21,22] In a 2-year study, CIN lesions were 11 times more likely to develop in women with HPV type 16 or 18 infection at baseline than in women without HPV infection at baseline.[23]

## CERVICAL CANCER SCREENING

Screening for cervical neoplasia to date primarily involves assessment of the cervical epithelium; the future of such screening may involve detection of high-risk HPV types.[24] More than 90% of lower genital tract neoplasia in women originates at the squamocolumnar junction of the cervix, where columnar and nonkeratinizing squamous epithelia meet.[25] Under the influence of various factors, a variety of intraepithelial changes take place before invasive cancer develops, and these changes are confined to the squamous epithelium above the basement membrane— "cervical intraepithelial neoplasia" (see Fig. 11-2). Because the cervical transformation zone is large in adolescence and during a woman's first pregnancy, early age at first sexual activity and at first pregnancy have been suggested as risk factors for cervical cancer. Given the progression of cytologic lesions of the cervix in some women, it is important to monitor those with persistent cytologic abnormalities to detect and treat high-grade intraepithelial lesions if they are detected. Screening and monitoring are done by the Pap test or possibly by HPV DNA testing.

For more than 50 years, the Pap test has been the primary screening tool for cervical disease. It is a cytologic screening test of a direct scraping or brushing of the uterine cervix and lower endocervical canal. In a conventional Pap test, the sample tissue is smeared onto a slide and fixed and stained. The slide is viewed under a microscope and a cytotechnologist or cytopathologist interprets the observed cellular changes. As noted earlier, this is a screening test and is not meant to be explicitly diagnostic. Patient preparation and appropriate provider technique help optimize collection of cellular material. In the conventional dry slide methodology, a single slide combining endocervical and ectocervical samples, or two separate slides for individual components, should be used. The most important consideration is rapid fixation of the samples to avoid air-drying artifacts. If liquid-based preparations are used, rapid immersion in liquid media is equally important.

In the past two decades, many refinements to techniques for collecting cervical cytology samples have been developed. In the 1980s, newer devices to enhance collection of exfoliated cells, such as nylon endocervical brushes and "broom" devices were created. These devices were responsible for improved collection of cellular material and of dysplastic cells from the transformation zone than was formerly possible with cotton swabs or the wooden Ayres spatula[26,27] (Figs. 11-7 and 11-8). In the 1990s, efforts to improve sampling turned to the development of liquid-based cytology methods and computer-based reading systems. In 1996, the first of two liquid-based systems currently available in the United States was approved by the U.S. Food and Drug Administration (FDA). The ThinPrep 2000 system was considered to be more effective in detecting LSILs and more severe lesions and to provide a better specimen than the conventional Pap test preparation[28] (Fig. 11-9). The basis of the liquid-based system is collection of a cervical cytology specimen using one of the new improved sampling devices and then suspending the sample in an alcohol-based preservative solution. Almost all the cells are transferred to the liquid preservative, with blood, mucus, and inflammatory cells generally filtered out or lysed. In the laboratory, a technician subsamples the cells, which are then deposited by an automatic device on to a slide. This technique thus removes much of the noncervical obscuring material from the sample, allowing for staining and screening of a uniform single-layer sample. The remaining sample can be stored for further testing if indicated (such as for HPV DNA testing). Even though the sampling may be improved, there still is no convincing evidence that thin-layer technology reduces morbidity or mortality from cervical cancer or its precursors.

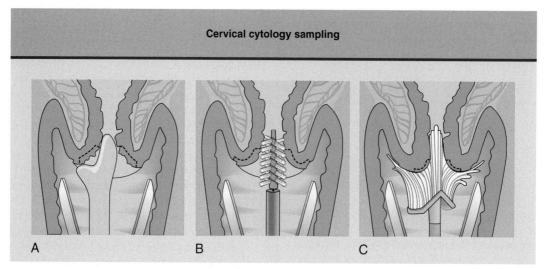

**Figure 11-7**    **Direct cervical cytology sampling using wooden Ayres spatula (A), Cytobrush (B), Cervex-Brush (C).**
(From ThinPrep Pap Test Quick Reference Guide. Courtesy of Cytyc Corporation and Affiliates.)

Moreover, increased detection of LSIL may not be of great importance as the majority serve as a proxy for the presence of an acute HPV infection, and in most women, HPV infections are cleared without consequence in less than 24 months. It is important to remember that little reduction in the burden of cervical cancer morbidity or mortality will be achieved without recruiting and screening women who are rarely or never screened.

In addition to new sampling devices and the liquid-based collection systems, automated computer-based technologies have been developed that use digitally scanned images and neural intelligence to facilitate primary cervical cancer screening and the Clinical Laboratory Improvement Amendments

(CLIA)–mandated 10% rescreening of cervical cytology tests that have negative results. The rationale for such systems involves the notion that false-negative readings may be secondary to human error and fatigue. While there is great potential benefit

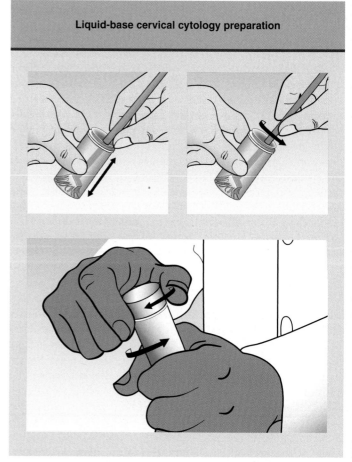

**Figure 11-9    Preparation of specimen for liquid-based cytologic applications.** (From ThinPrep Pap Test Quick Reference Guide. Courtesy of Cytyc Corporation and Affiliates.)

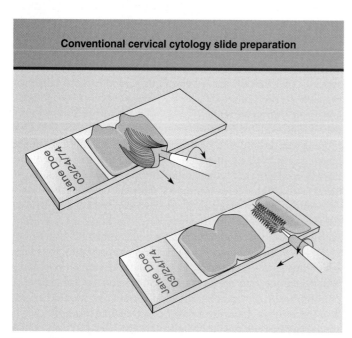

**Figure 11-8    Applying specimen to slide in conventional cervical cytologic testing.** (From ThinPrep Pap Test Quick Reference Guide. Courtesy of Cytyc Corporation and Affiliates.)

of computerized screening devices to assist in identification of potentially abnormal cells or samples, using such devices will not compensate for specimens that are inadequately prepared or not representative of the cervical transformation zone, or result in interpretation errors when cytotechnologists and cytopathologists conduct secondary screenings.

One measure of screening effectiveness is knowing the population covered by the screening test. In the United States, where cervical cancer screening is entirely opportunistic (i.e., there is no organized system for inviting women to be screened at certain intervals as in some European countries), the only measure of coverage is based on self-reports by women enrolled in either the Behavioral Risk Factor Surveillance System (BRFSS), or the National Health Interview Survey (NHIS), both administered by the Centers for Disease Control and Prevention (CDC). BRFSS and NHIS show that more than 85% of women in the United States have had a previous cervical cancer screening test, and that approximately 80% have had one in the past 2 to 3 years.[29,30] Some variations exist by age, race/ethnicity, and availability of insurance coverage. Only one national program exists in the United States that covers women who are either uninsured or underinsured—the National Breast and Cervical Cancer Early Detection Program (NBCCEDP), administered by the CDC. This program was developed as a result of the U.S. Congress passing the Breast and Cervical Cancer Mortality Prevention Act in 1990.[31]

This comprehensive women's health initiative is implemented through cooperative agreements with qualifying health agencies, including state and U.S. territorial health departments and American Indian and Alaska Native tribes and tribal organizations. In addition to providing screening, participating programs conduct activities in a number of other critical areas: diagnostic tests; surveillance, tracking, and follow-up; case management; public education and outreach; professional education and training; quality assurance of screening tests; coalition and partnership development; and program evaluation. NBCCEDP-sponsored programs have initiated outreach efforts to serve women in high-priority groups, including older women, racial/ethnic minorities, foreign born women, women with disabilities, lesbians, and women living in rural or other hard-to-reach areas.

During the time period 1991 to 2003, 1.4 million women received approximately 2.5 million Pap tests through NBCCEDP-sponsored programs. During this time period, 14,000 women were found to have histologically confirmed CIN II or greater for a rate of 5.8 per 1000 Pap tests, and 929 women were diagnosed with invasive cervical cancer for a rate of 0.3 cervical cancers per 1000 Pap tests. Approximately 50% of the women served were members of racial and ethnic minorities. Tables 11-1 to 11-4 show more detailed NBCCEDP information on Pap test results and final diagnoses for the time period 1995 to 2002.[32,33]

In recent years, a large number of studies have updated information about cervical cancer screening and have been the basis for updating screening guidelines and recommendations by several U.S. professional organizations and government agencies from 2001 to 2004.[34,35] They are derived from clinical-based studies of cervical cytology and from mathematical modeling in situations where clinical data are not available. Issues covered

| Table 11-1 Characteristics of Women Receiving First Pap Tests in NBCCEDP | | |
|---|---|---|
| Characteristic | Number of Women (N = 750,591) | Percent Distribution |
| **Age (yr)** | | |
| 18–29 | 41,919 | 5.6 |
| 30–39 | 74,783 | 10.0 |
| 40–49 | 259,830 | 34.6 |
| 50–64 | 327,841 | 43.7 |
| ≥65 | 46,218 | 6.2 |
| **Race/ethnicity** | | |
| White, non-Hispanic | 403,670 | 53.8 |
| Black, non-Hispanic | 108,404 | 14.4 |
| Asian/Pacific Islander | 33,309 | 4.4 |
| American Indian/Alaskan Native | 36,302 | 4.8 |
| Hispanic | 145,172 | 19.3 |
| Other, unknown | 23,734 | 3.2 |
| **Pap test before program (by self-report)** | | |
| Yes | 569,525 | 75.9 |
| No | 66,402 | 8.9 |
| Unknown | 114,664 | 15.3 |

NBCCEDP, National Breast and Cervical Cancer Early Detection Program, U.S. Centers for Disease Control and Prevention.

are age to initiate screening, frequency of rescreening and intervals between screening, and age to stop screening. Also covered is use of new screening technologies such as liquid-based cytology preparations and HPV DNA testing, as well as screening in special situations such as among postmenopausal women, pregnant women, women posthysterectomy, and immunocompromised women. While there are some differences in the recommendations of these groups, they all address the fact that certain high-risk HPV types are necessary in the chain of events leading up to the diagnosis of cervical cancer, that screening should begin for a woman by age 21, that a Pap test should be performed at least every 3 years, if prior tests were normal, and that screening may end by age 65 to 70 years depending on health status and confirmation that cervical screening tests in the prior 5 to 10 years were negative for malignant change. Less consistent are recommendations for use of liquid-based screening technologies and HPV testing because of concerns about test specificity and false-positive results. Included here is a summary of pertinent studies relating to these subjects, and a table comparing the various new U.S. professional organization screening recommendations[34,35] (Table 11-5).

## When to Initiate Screening

The natural history of cervical cancer is important in determining when to initiate screening, how often to screen, when to discontinue screening, and when to recommend treatment or follow-up evaluation (see Fig.11-3). Cervical cancer most often develops in women after age 40 years, and high-grade CIN generally is detectable 10 to 15 years before cancer develops, with a peak high-grade CIN rate at about age 35. Therefore, where program resources are limited, screening initially should focus on women in their thirties and forties.

### Table 11-2
### Distribution of Pap Test Results by Age Group and Screening Round

| | | | Age (yr) | | | |
|---|---|---|---|---|---|---|
| | All[†] | 18–29 | 30–39 | 40–49 | 50–64 | ≥65 |
| **First round** | | | | | | |
| Total Pap tests (N) | 750,591 | 41,919 | 74,783 | 259,830 | 327,841 | 46,218 |
| Results (%) | | | | | | |
| Normal | 79.9 | 66.8 | 74.6 | 78.8 | 82.2 | 85.4 |
| Infection/reaction | 12.8 | 13.9 | 15.0 | 13.6 | 12.0 | 9.9 |
| ASCUS | 4.1 | 7.9 | 5.5 | 4.6 | 3.4 | 2.7 |
| LSIL | 1.1 | 7.9 | 2.4 | 1.1 | 0.6 | 0.4 |
| HSIL | 0.6 | 2.4 | 1.3 | 0.6 | 0.4 | 0.3 |
| SqCa | 0.1 | <0.1 | <0.1 | <0.1 | 0.1 | 0.1 |
| Other | 0.7 | 0.4 | 0.4 | 0.6 | 0.9 | 0.6 |
| Unsatisfactory | 0.6 | 0.8 | 0.8 | 0.6 | 0.6 | 0.5 |
| Total abnormal tests* | 1.8 | 10.3 | 3.7 | 1.7 | 1.0 | 0.8 |
| **Subsequent rounds** | | | | | | |
| Total Pap tests (N) | 373,851 | 12,610 | 28,303 | 111,539 | 201,330 | 20,069 |
| Results (%) | | | | | | |
| Normal | 78.6 | 71.3 (71.2) | 73.2 | 77.1 | 81.0 | 83.4 |
| Infection/reaction | 13.7 | 14.4 | 17.0 | 14.4 | 12.7 | 11.4 |
| ASCUS | 5.0 | 7.6 | 6.1 | 5.6 | 4.2 | 3.5 |
| LSIL | 1.2 | 4.8 (4.7) | 1.9 | 1.3 | 0.7 | 0.5 |
| HSIL | 0.3 | 1.0 | 0.6 | 0.3 | 0.2 | 0.1 |
| SqCa | <0.1 | 0.0 | <0.1 | <0.1 | <0.1 | <0.1 |
| Other | 0.6 | 0.3 | 0.4 | 0.6 | 0.7 | 0.5 |
| Unsatisfactory | 0.5 | 0.7 | 0.8 | 0.6 | 0.5 | 0.4 |
| Total abnormal tests* | 1.5 | 5.7 | 2.5 | 1.7 | 0.9 | 0.7 |

ASCUS, atypical squamous cells of undetermined significance; HSIL, high-grade intraepithelial lesion; LSIL, low-grade intraepithelial lesion; SqCa, squamous cell cancer.

*Includes LSIL, HSIL, and SqCa.

[†]All Pap test results are age-adjusted to 2000 NBCCEDP population. *P* value for trend <0.001 for higher percentage of total abnormal results with greater age.

### Table 11-3
### Rates of Biopsy-confirmed Cervical Intraepithelial Neoplasia and Invasive Cancer

| | | | Age (yr) | | | |
|---|---|---|---|---|---|---|
| | All[‡] | 18–29 | 30–39 | 40–49 | 50–64 | ≥65 |
| **First round*** | | | | | | |
| CIN/invasive (n) | 9557 | 2853 | 1835 | 2748 | 1968 | 153 |
| CIN I | 5.1 | 37.2 | 10.9 | 4.8 | 2.4 | 0.8 |
| CIN II | 2.0 | 16.3 | 5.0 | 1.8 | 0.8 | 0.5 |
| CIN III/CIS | 3.5 | 14.4 | 8.2 | 3.5 | 2.1 | 1.5 |
| Invasive | 0.6 | 0.2 | 0.4 | 0.5 | 0.6 | 0.5 |
| CIN II or worse[†] | 6.0 | 30.9 | 13.7 | 5.8 | 3.6 | 2.5 |
| **Subsequent rounds*** | | | | | | |
| CIN/invasive (n) | 3180 | 424 | 487 | 1077 | 1126 | 66 |
| CIN I | 5.6 | 20.7 | 9.5 | 6.2 | 3.6 | 1.5 |
| CIN II | 1.6 | 6.8 | 3.6 | 1.6 | 0.8 | 0.6 |
| CIN III/CIS | 1.7 | 6.1 | 4.1 | 1.7 | 1.0 | 0.9 |
| Invasive | 0.1 | 0.0 | 0.1 | 0.2 | 0.1 | 0.2 |
| CIN II or worse[†] | 3.4 | 12.9 | 7.7 | 3.5 | 2.0 | 1.7 |

CIN, cervical intraepithelial neoplasia; CIS, carcinoma in situ.

*Rates calculated as number of CINs or invasive cancers diagnosed per 1000 Pap tests; includes in the denominator 2726 Pap tests in first round and 1040 (1038) in subsequent rounds with abnormal findings for which work-ups were incomplete.

[†]CIN II or higher includes CIN II, CIN III, CIS, or invasive cancer; *P* value for trend <0.001 for CIN II or worse with age.

[‡]Rates are age-adjusted to 2000 NBCCEDP population.

**Table 11-4**
**Age-adjusted Pap Test Results and Rates of Biopsy-confirmed Cervical Intraepithelial Neoplasia**

| | | | Race/Ethnicity | | | |
| --- | --- | --- | --- | --- | --- | --- |
| | All[§] | White | Black | Asian/ Pacific Islander | American Indian/ Alaskan Native | Hispanic |
| **First round** | | | | | | |
| Total Pap tests* (N) | 750,591 | 403,607 | 108,404 | 33,309 | 36,302 | 145,172 |
| Pap test results (% of total Pap tests) | | | | | | |
| LSIL | 1.1 | 1.2 | 1.1 | 0.7 | 1.0 | 1.1 |
| HSIL | 0.6 | 0.6 | 0.6 | 0.4 | 0.4 | 0.6 |
| SqCa | 0.1 | <0.1 | <0.1 | <0.1 | <0.1 | <0.1 |
| Percentage of all Pap tests abnormal[†] | 1.8 | 1.9 | 1.8 | 1.2 | 1.4 | 1.8 |
| Biopsy-detection rate (per 1000 Pap tests) | | | | | | |
| CIN II | 2.0 | 2.5 | 1.8 | 1.0 | 1.1 | 1.7 |
| CIN III/CIS | 3.5 | 4.0 | 2.9 | 2.5 | 1.7 | 3.2 |
| Invasive | 0.6 | 0.6 | 0.5 | 0.7 | 0.3 | 0.6 |
| Rate of CIN II or worse[‡] | 6.0 | 7.1 | 5.2 | 4.1 | 3.2 | 5.4 |
| **Subsequent rounds** | | | | | | |
| Total Pap tests* (N) | 373,851 | 213,489 | 46,129 | 13,573 | 28,487 | 64,351 |
| Pap test results (% of total Pap tests) | | | | | | |
| LSIL | 1.2 | 1.2 | 1.2 | 0.9 | 0.9 | 1.2 |
| HSIL | 0.3 | 0.3 | 0.4 | 0.4 | 0.2 | 0.3 |
| SqCa | <0.1 | <0.1 | <0.1 | <0.1 | <0.1 | <0.1 |
| % of all Pap tests abnormal[†] | 1.5 | 1.6 | 1.6 | 1.3 | 1.1 | 1.5 |
| Biopsy-detection rate (per 1000 Pap tests) | | | | | | |
| CIN II | 1.6 | 1.9 | 1.6 | 0.8 | 0.6 | 1.2 |
| CIN III/CIS | 1.7 | 1.9 | 1.6 | 1.6 | 1.1 | 1.6 |
| Invasive | 0.1 | 0.1 | 0.2 | 0.1 | 0.1 | 0.1 |
| Rate of CIN II or worse[‡] | 3.4 | 3.9 | 3.3 | 2.5 | 1.7 | 3.0 |

ASCUS, atypical squamous cells of undetermined significance; HSIL, high-grade intraepithelial lesion; LSIL, low-grade intraepithelial lesion; SqCa, squamous cell cancer, CIN, cervical intraepithelial neoplasia; CIS, carcinoma in situ.

*Total number of Pap tests includes 31,556 (31,542) of other/unknown race.

[†]Includes LSIL, HSIL, and SqCa.

[‡]Includes CIN II, III, CIS, or invasive cancer.

[§]All percentages and rates are age-adjusted to the 2000 NBCCEDP population.

The incidence of invasive cervical carcinoma is low under the age of 20 but begins to climb from 20 to 24 years. In a cohort study from British Columbia, Canada, the incidence of carcinoma in situ at the ages of 20 to 24 was approximately 16 per 100,000.[36–38] This led to a National Workshop in Canada which recommended that screening begin at the age of 20.[37] Similar conclusions were derived by American Cancer Society in 2002, with the recommendation to begin screening no later than age 21.[38]

Other groups have taken a different view. In Europe, age to start screening varies widely, with Finland inviting women to their organized program from age 30.[39] Sasieni et al conducted a study designed to evaluate frequency of rescreening and recommended that women not be screened under the age of 25.[40] For developing countries, given the low incidence of cervical cancer below the age of 35 and with an objective of maximizing use of resources, it is generally recommended that screening start at age 35.[41]

**How Often to Screen**

In most instances, cervical cancer develops slowly from precursor lesions; therefore, screening can take place relatively infrequently (less than annually) and still have a considerable impact on morbidity and mortality. Screening every 3 years has almost as great an impact as screening every year or every 2 years (Table 11-6). Even screening every 10 years or once in a lifetime can have significant impact.[41,42] The emphasis of screening programs, therefore, should be on coverage of risk-appropriate women rather than on frequency.

Determining the frequency of screening is helped by knowledge about the natural history of the condition being screened for, including the duration of the asymptomatic or latent phase. Screening too frequently will result in a low number of cases per screen and thus a low predictive value for the test. The reason is that the prevalence of asymptomatic disease will be low in the population when the screening frequency is high. On the other hand, infrequent or no screening will leave much of the disease uncontrolled.[43]

The goal of screening programs is to maximally reduce incidence and mortality from disease given available resources. The optimal screening interval is one that provides the most favorable degree of disease control and cost of screening. The design of a screening program defines two key parameters for achieving these objectives: the target population and the screening interval. Adherence to these parameters is crucial in maintaining the effectiveness of the program, measuring

Ambulatory Office Practice

| | Table 11-5 Recommendations for Cervical Cancer Screening, United States, 2003 | | | |
|---|---|---|---|---|
| | **Organization** | | | |
| | *American Cancer Society (ACS), Nov/Dec 2002* | *American College of Obstetricians and Gynecologists (ACOG), Aug 2003* | *American Society for Colposcopists and Cervical Pathologists (ASCCP), Apr 2002* | *U.S. Preventive Task Force (USPSTF), Jan 2003* |
| When to start cervical cancer screening | Age 21 or within 3 years of start of sexual activity | Age 21 or within 3 years of start of sexual activity | N/A | Age 21 or within 3 years of start of sexual activity |
| Interval | Annually with conventional or every 2 years with liquid-based cytology; ≥ age 30, women with 3 negative may be screened every 2–3 yr  HPV negative, Pap negative: every 3 years | Every year for women <30 or every 2–3 years for women ≥30 (except women with HIV, immunosuppression or DES exposure)  HPV negative, Pap negative: every 3 years | N/A | At least every 3 years |
| Thin Prep | Recommend | Option | N/A | Insufficient evidence |
| HPV testing with ASCUS | N/A | Option | Recommend/preferred | Insufficient evidence |
| HPV testing >30 | Guidelines out before FDA approval—preliminary recommend | Option | Guidelines out before FDA approval | Insufficient evidence |
| Posthysterectomy | Discontinue if for benign reasons | Discontinue except in special circumstances | N/A | Discontinue |
| When to stop cervical cancer screening | Age 70 or 3 or more negative tests within 10-yr period | It depends | N/A | >65 |

cost-effectiveness, and maximizing population coverage. Deviation from the recommended screening intervals or target populations may reduce program effectiveness either by using excessive resources as with annual rescreening for cervical cancer or by allowing the disease to "escape" the interval during which early intervention can lead to treatment of precursor lesions or cure of early-stage invasive disease. Modeling can facilitate decisions on the optimal frequency of screening.

An early evaluation of the British Columbia data using a Markov-Chain model supported a prolonged natural history of carcinoma in situ (an average sojourn time of at least 9 years) and concluded that women with a negative cytologic test should be rescreened every 5 years.[44] Nevertheless, the International Agency for Research on Cancer (IARC) report in 1986, based

on the best available data of the time, recommended cervical cancer screening every 3 years. This was based on a sojourn time of 5 to 8 years and predicted a cumulative reduction in incidence of approximately 90%[42] (see Table 11-6). Contrary to this recommendation, the cervical cancer screening program in Finland, utilizing screening every 5 years, achieved the level of success that the IARC model suggested would require triennial screening. As validation of the Finnish report, a reevaluation of British Columbia data using the Miscan model developed in Rotterdam showed that although the median duration for progression from carcinoma in situ to invasive cancer in the IARC study was about 5 to 8 years, this was calculated by including women with screen-detected (prevalent) cancers, whose prognosis is excellent and who are affected by the lead time gained by screening.[45] Adjusting for screen-detected cancers lengthened the median sojourn time from CIS to invasive cancer to 15 years. The implication is that screening every 5 rather than 3 years will yield a 90% reduction in invasive cancer incidence and mortality.[45]

While Table 11-6 shows the expected impact on the cumulative incidence of invasive cancer of the cervix in optimally screened populations, it is important to emphasize that even in optimal circumstances, based on the presence of highly effective cytology screening programs, no realistic screening schedule will result in complete elimination of invasive cervical cancer. In most countries, including the United States, this failure to attain optimally reduced morbidity and mortality may involve any of the essential components of a program, occurring at the level of the woman, her provider, or the laboratory reviewing her Pap test.[46] Another reason may be the variability of the natural

| | Table 11-6 Percentage Reduction in Cumulative Rate of Invasive Cervical Cancer over Age Range of 35 to 64 with Different Frequencies of Screening | |
|---|---|---|
| Frequency of Screening (yr) | Percent Reduction in Cumulative Rate* | No. of Tests |
| 1 | 93 | 30 |
| 2 | 93 | 15 |
| 3 | 91 | 10 |
| 5 | 84 | 6 |
| 10 | 64 | 3 |

*Assuming that a screen occurs at age 35 and that a previous screen had been performed. Data from IARC, 1986.

history in different women. Models are based on averages of transition probabilities, each with a different distribution or range of time periods during which some lesions progress from one state to the next, while others regress to normal. Still others remain stable for long periods of time. Some lesions may progress so rapidly that they cannot be detected in a curable stage even with annual screening, and it seems unlikely that the majority of such lesions would be detected by more frequent screening. This does not mean that there are different types of cancers of the cervix, as suggested many years ago, but that the fast-growing lesions represent one extreme of the distribution of progression or sojourn times.[47]

Celentano et al conducted a case-control study that included 153 women with invasive cancer, 153 case-nominated controls, and 392 randomly selected controls.[48] Cases were much less likely to have been screened within 2 to 3 years than controls (Odds ratio [OR] 8.3, 95% confidence interval [CI] 3.4–19.9 compared with case-nominated controls, OR 4.6, 2.0–10.5 compared with randomly selected controls). Moreover, some degree of protection was seen among screened women for 4 to 6 years (OR 4.3, 1.5–12.7, and 3.6, 1.4–9.6, respectively) after adjusting for a number of confounding variables.

Herbert et al studied the incidence of cervical cancer in a region of the United Kingdom after the introduction of the UK computerized invitation and recall system.[49] The incidence of invasive cancer was significantly higher in those not screened in the previous 5 years than among those screened (relative risk [RR] 2.6, 95% CI 1.6–4.3].RRs were even higher when screen-detected cancers were excluded. Based on their results, the authors concluded that a 5-year screening interval was too long.

Goldie et al modeled the natural history of cervical cancer using published data on transition and regression rates, and data from a study in South Africa.[50] They concluded that in developing countries, it would be more cost-effective if resources were available to screen three times in a lifetime, and that these tests should occur every 5 years from age 35 or 40, rather than every 10 years from age 35, as had been modeled by the IARC study.[39]

Miller et al conducted a case-control study within a U.S. health maintenance organization (Kaiser Permanente) between 1983 and 1995 of cases of invasive cancer diagnosed, and 934 controls, matched for length of membership in the HMO and race.[51] The ORs for different interval lengths between screens with 1-year interval as the referent are given in Table 11-7. The authors emphasized the low absolute risk of an abnormal cervical cancer screening test within 3 years of a prior negative test.

Sawaya et al studied the prevalence of biopsy-proved cervical neoplasia among 938,576 women less than 65 years of age in the NBCCEDP.[52] The prevalence of all grades of CIN was highest in women below age 30 and higher in those with no previous negative cytology tests than in those with one or more tests. No invasive cervical cancers were detected in women with three or more previous negative tests. Using a Markov model and various rates of progression and regression from the literature, they estimated that for women aged 30 to 64 with three or more consecutive negative tests, extending the rescreening interval to every 3 years would result in an average excess risk of cancer of approximately 3 per 100,000.

Sasieni et al conducted a case-control study based on the screening histories of 1305 women aged 20 to 69 with stage 1B cancer of the cervix and 2532 age-matched controls from the records of the National Health Service in the UK.[40] The odds of cervical cancer occurrence increased with time from the last negative test, reaching 1.0 (no protection) at 3 years for women aged 20 to 39, approached 1.0 at 6 years for women aged 40 to 54, and remained approximately 0.5 at 6 years for women aged 55 to 69. The authors estimated the proportion of cancer of the cervix that could be prevented by using different schedules of rescreening, and based on their results, these proportions varied by age. For women aged 20 to 39, 30% could have been prevented by 5-year screening, 61% by triennial screening, and 76% by annual screening. The respective percentages for women aged 40 to 54 were 73%, 84%, and 88%, and for women aged 55 to 69, 83%, 87%, and 87%. The authors recommended triennial screening for women aged 25 to 49, a 5-year screening interval for women aged 50 to 64, and for women aged 65 or more, to only screen those who had not been screened since age 50. These

| Table 11-7 Odds Ratios of Invasive Cancer by Screening Intervals | | | | |
|---|---|---|---|---|
| **Interval\*** | | | | |
| 2 yr | 3 yr | 3–5 yr | 5–10 yr | >10 yr |
| **Unadjusted** | | | | |
| 1.72 (1.12–2.64) | 2.06 (1.21–3.50) | 3.16 (1.93–5.18) | 4.73 (3.03–7.38) | 8.86 (5.29–14.8) |
| **Adjusted†** | | | | |
| 2.06 (1.30–3.92) | 2.24 (1.28–3.92) | 3.37 (1.97–5.76) | 5.72 (3.48–9.41) | 11.80 (6.70–20.8) |
| **Subsample with at least one previous negative Pap test (unadjusted)** | | | | |
| 2.15 (1.12–4.1) | 3.60 (1.50–8.68) | 4.28 (1.80–10.3) | 4.15 (1.80–9.55) | 6.90 (2.76–17.2) |

\*Referent group is annual screening (95% confidence intervals in parentheses).
†Adjusted for ever having abnormal cervical cytology before the last negative Pap test, and for having at least one negative Pap test less than 36 months before last negative test.

conclusions differed from those of the IARC Working Group on Cervical Cancer Screening, which recommended against different screening frequencies for different age groups.[41]

### When to Discontinue Screening

With the age-specific incidence of cervical cancer in all countries showing relatively high rates of invasive cancer in older women, there is a consensus that women over the age of 60 years who have never been screened or have not been screened for many years should be encouraged to have at least two tests over a period of a few years, and only if both are negative should they cease screening.[37,39]

Cecchini et al reviewed data for women aged 60 to 70 from the Florence screening program and the Tuscany Cancer Registry.[53] Only 5 of 242 women with invasive cervical cancer had two or more negative Pap tests between 50 and 60 years of age. However, of 11,342 women aged 58 to 60 with a negative test during 1980 to 1987 and followed to December 1990, only one invasive cancer was diagnosed, compared with the nearly 14 cases expected from age-specific incidence data from the cancer registry (OR 0.07, 95% CI 0.002–0.39). The authors recommended reconsideration of continuing screening after 60 to 64 years of age.

In North America, it is generally recommended that women actively screened and consistently negative could end screening at 70 years of age.[37,38] In Europe, guidelines recommend 64 as the upper age limit of the population to be actively invited for screening.[54]

It has been suggested that women without cytologic abnormalities who have been actively screened could end screening at even younger ages (e.g. 50 to 55).[39] No population-based studies to date have specifically addressed this issue.

## DIAGNOSIS

Exfoliative cytology is currently the most common means of screening for preinvasive disease. Other methods include screening colposcopy, visual inspection with acetic acid (VIA), visual inspection with Lugol's iodine (VILI), HPV DNA testing, and still largely experimental methods such as real-time imaging technology and tumor markers.

A recent revision of the Bethesda system (Table 11-8) of cervical cytologic classification includes prior terms used for high- and low-grade cervical cytology changes—low-grade squamous intraepithelial lesion (LSIL) and high-grade squamous intraepithelial lesion (HSIL). However, it subdivides the equivocal level of abnormalities—atypical squamous cells (ASC)—into two subcategories, namely, atypical squamous cells of undetermined significance (ASC-US), which lack certain expected cellular elements to more specifically categorize the test, and atypical squamous cells that cannot rule out a high-grade lesion (ASC-H), recognizing that some cytology specimens contain high-risk elements that may suggest a more serious endpoint (HSIL) and require immediate follow-up.[55] Management of abnormal Pap test results has been the subject of intense interest to researchers, providers, and the public. As noted earlier, a screening test result is of little value if there is no system of appropriate follow-up and management of abnormal results.

---

**Table 11-8**
**The Bethesda System 2001 (Abridged)**

**Satisfactory for evaluation**

A satisfactory squamous component must be present (see text)
Note presence/absence of endocervical/transformation zone component
Obscuring elements (inflammation, blood, drying artifact, other) may be mentioned if 50–75% of epithelial cells are obscured

**Unsatisfactory for evaluation**

Specimen rejected/not processed because (specify reason). Reasons may include
· Lack of patient identification
· Unacceptable specimen (e.g., slide broken beyond repair)

Specimen processed and examined but unsatisfactory for evaluation of an epithelial abnormality because (specify reason). Reasons may include
· Insufficient squamous component (see text)
· Obscuring elements cover more than 75% of epithelial cells

**General categorization (optional)**

Negative intraepithelial lesion or malignancy
Epithelial cell abnormality
Other

**Interpretation/Results**

*Negative for intraepithelial lesion or malignancy*
Organisms
  *Trichomonas vaginalis*
  Fungal organisms morphologically consistent with *Candida* species
  Shift in flora suggestive of bacterial vaginosis
  Bacteria morphologically consistent with *Actinomyces* species
  Cellular changes consistent with herpes simplex virus
Other non-neoplastic findings (Optional to report; list not comprehensive)
Reactive cellular changes associated with inflammation (includes typical repair), irradiation, intrauterine contraceptive device (IUD)
  Glandular cells status posthysterectomy
  Atrophy
*Epithelial cell abnormalities*
Squamous cell
Atypical squamous cells (ASC)
  of undetermined significance (ASC-US)
  cannot exclude HSIL (ASC-H)
Low-grade squamous intraepithelial lesion (LSIL)
  encompassing: human papillomavirus (HPV)/mild dysplasia/cervical intraepithelial neoplasia (CIN) 1
High-grade squamous intraepithelial lesion (HSIL)
  encompassing: moderate and severe dysplasia, carcinoma in situ; CIN 2 and CIN 3
Squamous cell carcinoma
Glandular cell
  Atypical glandular cells (AGC) (specify endocervical, endometrial, or not otherwise specified)
  Atypical glandular cells, favor neoplastic (specify endocervical or not otherwise specified)
Endocervical adenocarcinoma in situ (AIS)
Adenocarcinoma
Other (list not comprehensive)
  Endometrial cells in a woman ≥40 years of age

**Automated review and ancillary testing (include as appropriate)**

**Educational notes and suggestions (optional)**

---

In 2002, the American Society of Colposcopy and Cyto-pathology (ASCCP) published results of a consensus conference held in September 2001 that dealt with management and follow-up of abnormal Pap test results closely following the newly updated Bethesda system classification of cervical cytology results[56] (Figs. 11-10 through 11-14). The process included an evidence-based review of pertinent published literature that was graded to assure that decisions could be based upon results of the most rigorous studies possible. A draft of the recommendations was then published on the ASCCP Web site (www.asccp.org), and all interested parties were invited to participate in a Web-based forum of the draft to recommend changes and additions to be most consistent with the science and clinical applications of the time. A revised draft document was developed and this document was discussed by those invited to participate in the 2001 consensus conference for final review and recommendations.

Atypical squamous cells (ASC) on Pap tests are associated with a risk of detecting high-grade CIN in 5% to 17% of cases.[56] The ASC-US/LSIL Triage Study (ALTS) confirmed that using HPV DNA testing was helpful in differentiating those women with ASC-US Pap test results at risk of having underlying high-grade histologic disease from those having little or no risk.[7,55] Women with negative tests for high-risk HPV types would be immediately excluded from further investigation, while those with positive results would be immediately referred for colposcopy and directed cervical biopsy if indicated. Alternatives to HPV testing include repeat Pap testing at 6-month intervals for up to 2 years, or immediate colposcopy. While all

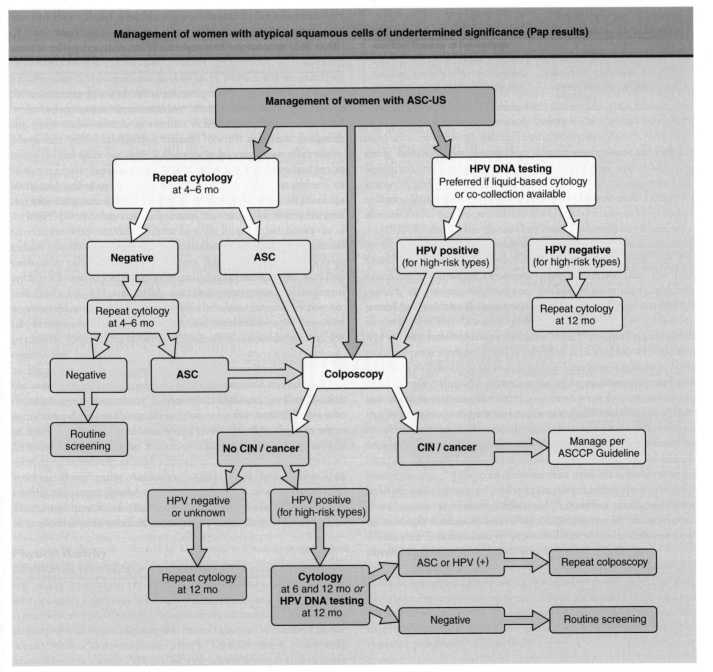

**Figure 11-10** Algorithm for management of atypical squamous cells of undetermined significance (ASC-US). (Reprinted from The Journal of Lower Genital Tract Disease Vol. 6 Issue 2, with the permission of ASCCP © American Society for Colposcopy and Cervical Pathology 2002.)

## Ambulatory Office Practice

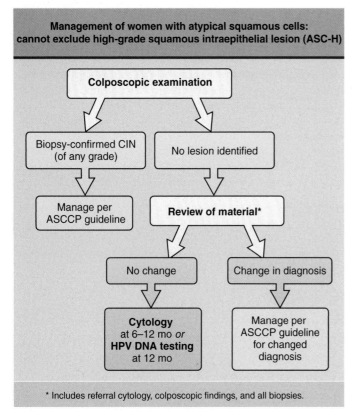

**Management of women with atypical squamous cells: cannot exclude high-grade squamous intraepithelial lesion (ASC-H)**

Colposcopic examination

→ Biopsy-confirmed CIN (of any grade)
→ No lesion identified

Biopsy-confirmed CIN (of any grade) → Manage per ASCCP guideline

No lesion identified → Review of material*

Review of material* → No change
Review of material* → Change in diagnosis

No change → Cytology at 6–12 mo *or* HPV DNA testing at 12 mo

Change in diagnosis → Manage per ASCCP guideline for changed diagnosis

\* Includes referral cytology, colposcopic findings, and all biopsies.

**Figure 11-11    Algorithm for management of ASC-H.** (Reprinted from *The Journal of Lower Genital Tract Disease* Vol. 6 Issue 2, with the permission of ASCCP © American Society for Colposcopy and Cervical Pathology 2002.)

three are considered to be of equal value in the follow-up process, reflex HPV testing using the Digene Hybrid Capture II test is recommended if the Pap test sample is obtained by means of a liquid-based system.[56]

In traditional cytology-based cervical cancer screening programs, it is usual to attempt to acquire a histologic diagnosis of the preinvasive lesion from either a colposcopically directed biopsy or an excisional procedure. In addition, some studies have shown cervicography to be as useful as colposcopy as a secondary means of assessing patients with abnormal Pap test results; however, the procedure has not gained wide acceptance for this use (Figs. 11-15 through 11-18).

If a woman has an LSIL, HSIL, or ASC-H Pap report, it is recommended that she undergo immediate colposcopy with endocervical assessment. The LSIL report is often equated with the presence of active HPV DNA in the cells demonstrated by the presence of koilocytes. As noted earlier, these vacuoles are now known to represent the presence of viral activity within the cell. In the ALTS trial, more than 70% of women with LSIL results were positive for HPV types.[57]

While immediate colposcopy is currently recommended for LSIL Pap results, it should be kept in mind that not all LSIL reports are due to high-risk HPV types. Any genital-tract HPV type can cause changes consistent with LSIL. Moreover, these changes may be transient, since the sample is likely being collected during an active HPV viral infection; most will clear spontaneously, leaving no persistent viral infection or residual

cervical cytologic changes. For reports of HSIL and ASC-H, the potential for identifying CIN II or CIN III is considerably higher than with LSIL results. Moreover, the interrater reliability for detecting HSIL and high-grade CIN is better than for detecting either ASC-US or LSIL. For ASC-H, cellular elements are absent that would otherwise allow the reviewer to report the test as HSIL, but the level of suspicion is high enough to warrant the slide being classified separately from other ASC slides. The histologic diagnosis of CIN based on colposcopically directed biopsies is similarly complicated. Not only might a large proportion of CIN lesions regress spontaneously, but analysis of data from the ALTS trial showed that 43% of biopsies originally classified as CIN I were reclassified downward in 40% of cases and upgraded to CIN II/III in 13% of cases.[7]

Whereas histologically confirmed CIN I lesions are associated with a low risk of progression to invasive cervical cancer, histologically confirmed CIN II lesions are associated with a risk of advancement to cancer of 20% and CIN III lesions with a risk of advancement to cancer of 30%.[58–60] Therefore, except in special circumstances as noted below, treatment needs to be initiated promptly for high-grade disease once histologic confirmation is available.

During pregnancy, regression of CIN II/III is reported to be minimal, however post partum; spontaneous regression is higher.[61] When a pregnant woman is found to have an LSIL or HSIL Pap result, immediate colposcopy is indicated; however, invasive evaluation of the endocervical canal is not. Although colposcopic examination in early pregnancy may be unsatisfactory, as the pregnancy progresses, repeat colposcopy will likely be satisfactory, since the transformation zone of the cervix may be more easily visualized. Biopsies of pregnant women should be reserved for situations in which there is high suspicion that invasive cancer is present. In certain circumstances, when there is a very high suspicion of invasive cancer, it is appropriate to consider performing a cold-knife conization of the cervix for definitive diagnosis.

Among postmenopausal women, special consideration needs to be given for most abnormal Pap test reports. If the result is ASC-US or LSIL and the woman has cytologic or clinical evidence of atrophic changes, a short course of intravaginal estrogen cream is indicated before repeating the test 1 week after completion of treatment. If the result is ASC-US or LSIL and no atrophy is present, it is satisfactory to repeat Pap tests at 6- and 12-month intervals or to perform an HPV DNA test at 12 months and refer for colposcopy if the Pap test result is ASC-US or greater or if the HPV test is positive.

For adolescents with LSIL, it is appropriate to postpone immediate colposcopy and biopsy in favor of a repeat Pap test at 6 and 12 months, using a threshold of ASC-US for colposcopy referral or performing an HPV-DNA test at 12 months and referring those adolescent women positive for high-risk HPV DNA for colposcopy. When biopsy-confirmed CIN II or III is not found in a young woman with confirmed HSIL cytology reports, observation with cytology and colposcopy at 4- to 6-month intervals is acceptable if colposcopic findings are satisfactory, endocervical sampling is negative, and the patient understands and accepts the risk of occult disease.[56] If progression is observed or HSIL Pap tests persist, consideration for invasive diagnostic excision (LEEP or cold-knife conization) is recommended.

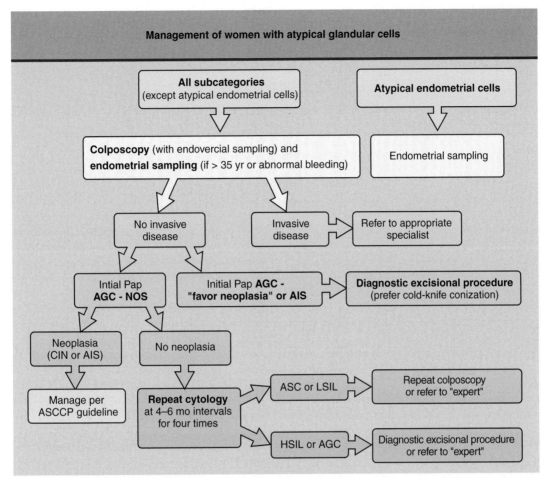

**Figure 11-12    Algorithm for management of atypical glandular cells (AGC).** (Reprinted from The Journal of Lower Genital Tract Disease Vol. 6 Issue 2, with the permission of ASCCP © American Society for Colposcopy and Cervical Pathology 2002.)

Immunosuppressed women have a higher incidence of persistent HPV infections and in turn higher incidence of all grades of abnormal Pap test results and cervical neoplasia.[62] Among HIV-positive women treated for histologically confirmed CIN II and III there is a high rate of recurrence and persistence of disease, with treatment failure rates approaching 25%.[63] For invasive cervical cancer, there is no clear picture about increased incidence among HIV-seropositive women; however, Selik and Rabkin in 1998 reported a relative risk of 5.5 for cervical cancer in HIV-positive women compared with seronegative women.[64] In 2000, Frisch et al, using data from the U.S. Cancer Match Registry for the period 1978 to 1996, showed an RR of 5.4 for invasive cervical cancer among HIV-positive women compared with the general U.S. population.[65] Careful adherence to CDC recommendations for cervical cancer screening of HIV-positive women is highly recommended.[66] Referral for colposcopy is recommended for all immunosuppressed women with ASC-US or abnormal Pap test results. This includes all women infected with HIV, regardless of CD4 count, HIV viral load, or antiretroviral therapy.[56]

The 2001 Bethesda system classified cervical glandular cell abnormalities less severe than adenocarcinoma into three categories: atypical glandular cells—either endocervical, endometrial, or "glandular cells" not otherwise specified (AGC

NOS); atypical glandular cells—either endocervical or "glandular cells" favoring neoplasia ("AGC neoplasia" category); and endocervical adenocarcinoma in situ (AIS).[55] The AGC category is associated with higher risk for cervical neoplasia than ASC or LSIL is. A number of studies show that 9% to 54% of women with AGC have at least biopsy-confirmed CIN.[67-72] These studies also suggest that there is a higher risk of high-grade lesions among women with "AGC favor neoplasia" than among women with AGC NOS. Biopsy-confirmed CIN II or III, AIS, or invasive cancer has been identified in 9% to 41% of women with AGC NOS compared with 27% to 96% of women with "AGC favor neoplasia." The cytologic interpretation of AIS is associated with a high risk of either AIS—48% to 69%—or invasive cervical adenocarcinoma—38%.[73,74]

AIS is the only well-characterized preinvasive glandular lesion of the uterine cervix and is uncommon relative to squamous counterparts. The Surveillance Epidemiology and End Results (SEER) program from the U.S. National Cancer Institute during the time period 1973 to 1995 reported an estimated 121,793 cases of carcinoma in situ of the cervix.[75] Of these, only 1% were adenocarcinoma in situ. Although terminology has been proposed for intraepithelial glandular lesions with lesser degrees of nuclear atypia and mitotic activity than AIS, because of the rarity of biopsy-documented non-AIS preinvasive glandular

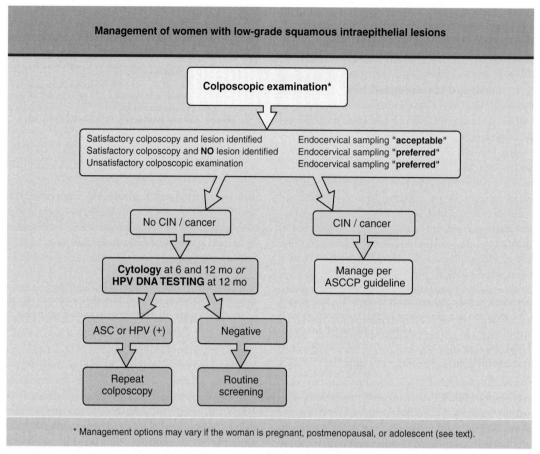

**Management of women with low-grade squamous intraepithelial lesions**

**Colposcopic examination***

Satisfactory colposcopy and lesion identified  Endocervical sampling **"acceptable"**
Satisfactory colposcopy and **NO** lesion identified  Endocervical sampling **"preferred"**
Unsatisfactory colposcopic examination  Endocervical sampling **"preferred"**

No CIN / cancer    CIN / cancer

**Cytology** at 6 and 12 mo *or*    Manage per
**HPV DNA TESTING** at 12 mo    ASCCP guideline

ASC or HPV (+)    Negative

Repeat    Routine
colposcopy    screening

* Management options may vary if the woman is pregnant, postmenopausal, or adolescent (see text).

**Figure 11-13    Algorithm for management of low-grade squamous intraepithelial lesions (LSIL).** (Reprinted from The Journal of Lower Genital Tract Disease Vol. 6 Issue 2, with the permission of ASCCP © American Society for Colposcopy and Cervical Pathology 2002.)

lesions, their utility has not been established.[56,76–78] AIS coexists with preinvasive squamous lesions or invasive squamous cell carcinoma in nearly two-thirds of cases, and risk factors for AIS are similar to those for preinvasive squamous lesions.[79,80] Because no natural history studies for AIS have been published owing to its relative rarity, the evidence that AIS is the precursor lesion for invasive endocervical adenocarcinoma remains circumstantial.[56] Like high-grade squamous intraepithelial neoplasia, AIS is associated to a high degree with persistence of high-risk HPV types.[81,82]

The value of traditional follow-up of AGC and AIS with repeat cytology, colposcopy, and endocervical sampling is limited. The sensitivity of all these modalities to detect either AIS or adenocarcinoma is low. Many cases of biopsy-confirmed AIS have no associated observed colposcopic abnormalities, and even combinations of cytologic testing and colposcopy can miss AIS and small endocervical adenocarcinomas localized in the endocervical canal. Nevertheless, colposcopy with endocervical sampling is recommended for women with all subcategories of AGC except those with atypical endometrial cells, who should initially be evaluated with endometrial sampling.[56] This should be done along with colposcopy in women older than age 35 with AGC, and among women under age 35 with AGC who have unexplained vaginal bleeding. Absence of sufficient data so far does not allow assessment of HPV DNA testing in management

of women with either AGC or AIS. Further follow-up depends on outcome of initial evaluation. If invasive disease is not identified, women with "AGC favor neoplasia" or endocervical AIS should undergo a diagnostic excision procedure. The preferred procedure is cold-knife conization. If invasive disease is not identified among women with AGC NOS, they should be followed using a program of repeat cervical cytology at 4- to 6-month intervals until four consecutive "negative for intraepithelial lesion or malignancy" results are obtained, after which they may return to routine screening. The ASCCP guidelines state that if a result of either ASC or LSIL is obtained on any of the follow-up Pap tests, acceptable options include repeat colposcopic examination or referral to a clinician experienced in the management of complex cytologic situations.[56]

## TREATMENT

Whatever technique is employed to treat histologically confirmed preinvasive CIN, it must be effective in eradicating the lesion, as well as safe and associated with minimal patient morbidity. Two categories of treatment are available—destructive/ablative procedures and excisional procedures.

Techniques involving destruction or ablation of the abnormal transformation zone can be used only when strict criteria are available to ensure that for all practical purposes the presence of

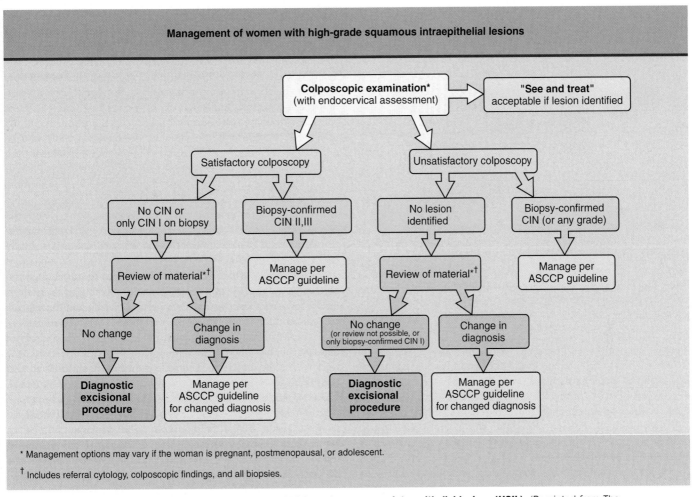

**Management of women with high-grade squamous intraepithelial lesions**

**Colposcopic examination*** (with endocervical assessment) → **"See and treat"** acceptable if lesion identified

Satisfactory colposcopy → Unsatisfactory colposcopy

No CIN or only CIN I on biopsy | Biopsy-confirmed CIN II,III | No lesion identified | Biopsy-confirmed CIN (or any grade)

Review of material*† | Manage per ASCCP guideline | Review of material*† | Manage per ASCCP guideline

No change | Change in diagnosis | No change (or review not possible, or only biopsy-confirmed CIN I) | Change in diagnosis

**Diagnostic excisional procedure** | Manage per ASCCP guideline for changed diagnosis | **Diagnostic excisional procedure** | Manage per ASCCP guideline for changed diagnosis

* Management options may vary if the woman is pregnant, postmenopausal, or adolescent.

† Includes referral cytology, colposcopic findings, and all biopsies.

**Figure 11-14    Algorithm for management of high-grade squamous intraepithelial lesions (HSIL).** (Reprinted from The Journal of Lower Genital Tract Disease Vol. 6 Issue 2, with the permission of ASCCP © American Society for Colposcopy and Cervical Pathology 2002.)

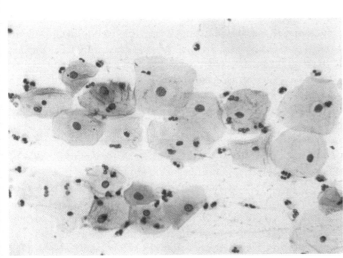

**Figure 11-15    Superficial and intermediate squamous cells.** The mature squamous epithelium of the ectocervix in women of reproductive age is composed throughout most of its thickness by superficial and intermediate cells. (Courtesy of ES Cibas, MD.)

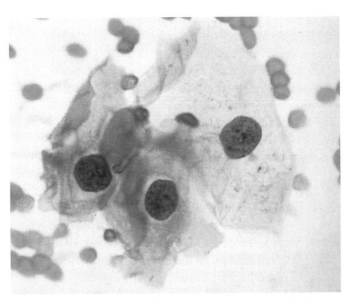

**Figure 11-16    "Nonkoilocytic" low-grade squamous intraepithelial lesions (LSIL).** Nuclei are significantly enlarged and show mild hyperchromasia and nuclear contour irregularity. No definite koilocytes are seen. (Courtesy of ES Cibas, MD.)

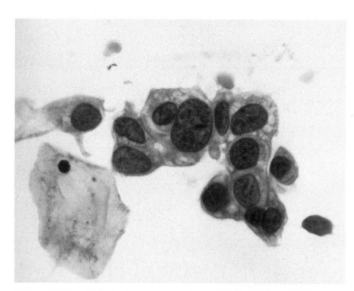

**Figure 11-17    High-grade squamous intraepithelial lesions (HSIL).**
These squamous cells have scant cytoplasm and markedly hyperchromatic nuclei with highly irregular nuclear contours. (Courtesy of ES Cibas, MD.)

invasive cervical cancer has been excluded. Except where so-called "see and treat" modalities are used in developing countries, it is essential that treatment be preceded by a biopsy result that is concordant with other screening and diagnostic tests. The most common techniques are cryotherapy, $CO_2$ laser vaporization, and electrocautery. The last technique, although effective, is not used with great frequency. The level of tissue destruction is estimated to be approximately 3 to 7 mm based on information that crypt involvement by CIN extends on average to a depth of 3 mm.[83] All three have estimated success rates of about 90%.[84] Cure rates depend on size of lesion, endocervical gland involvement, and status of lesion margins.[85,86] Currently, cryotherapy is the most frequently used method of ablative treatment. The

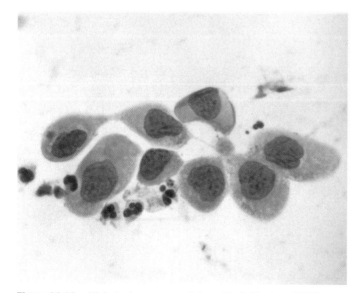

**Figure 11-18    High-grade squamous intraepithelial lesions (HSIL).**
Cells with a moderate amount of cytoplasm, formerly called "moderate dysplasia" or "CIN II," are included in the HSIL category. (Courtesy of ES Cibas, MD.)

equipment is relatively inexpensive; it requires nitrous oxide gas (−89°C) or carbon dioxide gas (−65°C), which achieve the temperatures necessary (−20°C to −30°C) for effective cellular destruction and are readily available in many locations; the technique can be learned and applied with minimal instruction; it can be performed in most any ambulatory health care setting; and the discomforts and side effects are mild and complications rare. Cryotherapy instruments designed with probes specifically intended for treatment of cervical lesions facilitate the ease with which the technique can be applied. Cryotherapy destroys the surface epithelium of the cervix by crystallizing the intracellular water, resulting in eventual destruction of the cell. The most effective technique seems to be a freeze-thaw-freeze method in which an ice ball is achieved 5 mm beyond the edge of the probe. The time required for the procedure depends on the pressure of the gas; the higher the gas pressure, the more rapidly the ice ball forms.

$CO_2$ laser vaporization, on the other hand, requires considerable outlays for the equipment, electric power source, training in the form of a laser course or a preceptorship, and experience to become adept at applying the technique correctly and safely. The operator must be familiar with the physics of the procedure and thoroughly understand the safety precautions. For these reasons, in recent years, less attention has been paid to this technique as a means of cervical ablation therapy. However, laser vaporization is particularly suited for treating large lesions that the cryo-probe cannot adequately cover, for treating an irregular cervix with a "fish mouth" appearance and deep clefts, for treating disease extending to the vagina, and for treating lesions with extensive glandular involvement to reach the deepest gland clefts.

Excisional methods include the loop electrode excision procedure (LEEP), $CO_2$ laser excision, cold-knife conization, and total hysterectomy and trachelectomy (removal of the cervical stump). Traditionally, cold-knife conization of the cervix has been the gold standard for obtaining an adequate tissue specimen to assure maximal opportunity to eliminate the presence of preinvasive disease, and also for obtaining the best specimen for histologic review. Prior to the availability of colposcopy, conization was the standard method of evaluating an abnormal Pap test result. It can be either diagnostic or therapeutic. Today, the disadvantages of this procedure are that it requires hospitalization, anesthesia, and considerable training; is expensive; and is associated with a moderate amount of both short- and long-term morbidity. Nevertheless, the procedure is indicated when the limits of the lesion cannot be visualized with colposcopy or the SCJ is not seen, if endocervical curettage is histologically CIN II or III, if there is a lack of correlation between various study results, and if either microinvasion or more advanced disease cannot be ruled out.

In many western countries, LEEP is currently the most popular technique. In some centers, extended uses of the procedure have replaced cold-knife conization. The advantages of this procedure are that, although it depends on the availability of an electrosurgical unit and a source of electricity, it can be performed in an ambulatory setting with local anesthesia and requires less intensive training to master the technique and apply it effectively and safely. This electrosurgical unit produces a constant low voltage flow of energy with the ability to blend

**Loop electrode excision procedure**

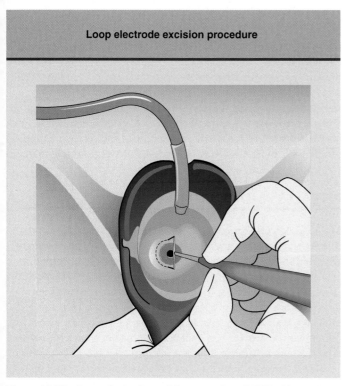

**Figure 11-19    Loop electrode excision procedure (LEEP).** (Used with permission of Cooper Companies, Lake Forest, Ca.)

and mold both cutting and coagulation characteristics of current. It should be used primarily for management of CIN II and III lesions. It must be performed after a comprehensive colposcopic examination and is intended to remove the entire transformation zone with an adequate margin of normal squamous epithelium surrounding the abnormal area and with minimal artifactual damage to the excised specimen.[87] Descriptions of the technique can be found in modern textbooks of operative gynecology, but basically it is important to assess the size of the transformation zone, location of the squamocolumnar junction, size of the lesion in question, and amount of tissue necessary to excise. The tissue effect of electricity depends on the concentration of electrons, the power, and the water content of the tissue. Low power settings may cause extensive thermal damage to the tissue. Higher power settings when a small wire loop is used will result in an electrosurgical effect with little thermal damage. The actual cutting is the result of a steam envelope developing at the interface between the wire

loop and the water-laden tissue. This envelope is then pushed through the tissue, separating it from surrounding structures.

To obtain a specimen with clear margins, an appropriate-sized wire loop should be selected and the depth gauge set to achieve the best specimen possible. It is important to use a grounding pad on the patient's thigh and nonconductive instruments in the vagina, to have a vacuum source to exhaust any smoke created from the procedure, and to use local anesthesia with epinephrine. Performing colposcopy prior to the procedure may help delineate the lesion and determine endocervical involvement. The electrosurgical generator should use a blend of cutting and coagulation current and should be set to 35 to 55 watts. Using a continuous motion, beginning either on the posterior lip or the lateral aspect of the cervix, allowing for a margin of normal tissue, the operator moves the loop electrode perpendicularly to the limit of the depth guide and then either upward or transversely to a point on either the anterior lip or the opposite side of the cervix, allowing for a margin of normal tissue, and then draws the loop out of the cervix toward herself or himself (Figs. 11-19 and 11-20). Although removing the specimen in one piece is encouraged, it is satisfactory to remove the specimen in two parts depending on its size. After the specimen is removed, the base should be coagulated using a ball electrode at 50 watts of power. Application of Monsel's solution for additional chemical coagulation is optional.

A meta-analysis of 28 trials of various treatments for CIN showed that while there was no considerable difference overall between ablative and excisional techniques, LEEP behaved as an ideal method for treating CIN because it produced the least morbidity and the most favorable surgical specimen for histologic assessment.[84]

The effectiveness of LEEP was analyzed by Flannelly et al in studies in 1997 and 2001.[88,89] Women less than 50 years of age with clear margins in excised specimens had a 92% chance of normal Pap tests on subsequent examinations, while those without clear margins had an 86% chance of normal Pap tests. Among women over 50 years of age who had margin involvement, only 57% had normal Pap tests on follow-up examination. Although the latter group comprised only a small proportion of those treated, this group appears to be at higher risk of recurrence and possibly should be more intensely followed by cytology and colposcopy than the younger age cohort. Other studies confirm the low failure rate of LEEP. The finding overall of CIN in specimen margins did not translate to a high risk of recurrence at 1 year posttreatment.[88] Moreover, the finding of microinvasive carcinoma in the excised specimen did not seem

**Wire loop for loop electrode excision procedure**

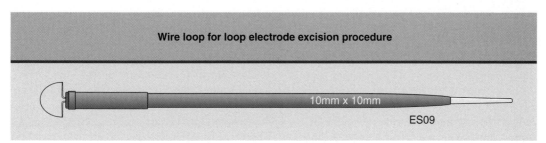

**Figure 11-20    Example of wire used in loop electrode excision procedure (LEEP).** (Used with permission of Cooper Companies, Lake Forest, Ca.)

to increase the efficacy of an excisional technique over that of a destructive procedure.[88]

Laser excisional conization can be used similarly to LEEP or cold-knife conization with equivalent therapeutic effectiveness. Local anesthetic with epinephrine should be injected directly into the cervical stroma to assist with hemostasis during and after the procedure. The laser beam is adjusted to a watt size of 0.2 to 0.5 mm in diameter and set at 20 to 30 watts to outline the peripheral margins of the area to be removed. The incision is deepened circumferentially by passing the laser beam across tissue, and traction instruments are used on the cone specimen to facilitate visualization of the underlying stroma as the procedure extends deep enough to remove all abnormal tissue. Once appropriate depth is reached, the tissue at the endocervical margin can be sharply removed with laser, scissors, or scalpel. Deep or large cone defects are at greater risk of bleeding and postoperative discharge, but only rarely is additional hemostatic medication necessary.[90]

Hysterectomy and trachelectomy are not currently considered as primary treatment for CIN. The risk of significant morbidity with these procedures is higher than with the other described modalities of treatment. Nevertheless, there are some indications for which hysterectomy is a valid treatment option for CIN: (1) conization specimen margins positive for CIN, especially in women who have completed childbearing or who are expected to adhere poorly to follow-up recommendations; (2) presence of coexisting gynecologic conditions requiring hysterectomy; and (3) request by patient with CIN III or carcinoma in situ who cannot be persuaded otherwise based on informed decision making (cancer phobia).

## CLINICAL COURSE AND PROGRESSION

Inherent in the above discussions about the natural history of HPV infection and cervical neoplasia is that HPV infections and low-grade cervical neoplasia regress to a high degree without intervention, and although there is no actual treatment for HPV infections, the various methods of treating CIN result in cures in approximately 90% of cases. The most important issues are to screen women for cervical cancer, to follow up abnormal results adequately and in a timely manner, to apply therapy appropriately, and to insure long-term follow-up. Along with appropriate follow-up is the need for culturally appropriate patient education and reassurance to enhance adherence to a program of continued surveillance if necessary. Overall, an estimated 93% of cervical cancers can be prevented by screening and appropriate management of abnormal results. The most difficult task may be encouraging, recruiting, and inviting those women who for a variety of reasons do not come in for screening.

For cryotherapy, grade of lesion is of great importance to recurrence of disease; CIN III has the greatest chance of failure. Size of lesion is most important. Large lesions are associated with recurrence or progression rates of 42%, whereas there is only a 7% rate of recurrence when lesions are 1 cm or less.[91] Moreover, finding a positive endocervical curettage specimen can ultimately reduce the usefulness of this technique at the time of colposcopy as it is associated with recurrence or progression rates of 27% versus 9% among women without positive endocervical curettage.[83]

Laser therapy has highly varied results. In properly selected patients, cure rates of 95% or higher can be achieved. Probably the most important lesson learned over time is that treating the entire transformation zone rather than just localized lesions is necessary to effect appropriate levels of cure.[92,93]

LEEP is effective in reducing the proportion of recurrences if performed correctly. In a review of several studies including almost 2500 women, only 97, or 4%, of lesions recurred following treatment.[94] For cold-knife conization of the cervix, recurrence of disease is most closely associated with having positive margins or gland involvement.[86]

## PITFALLS AND CONTROVERSIES

Most controversy in cervical cancer screening currently relates to new technologies and the frequency with which women are screened in largely opportunistic clinical settings. Information is available on a variety of technologies such as aided visualization (VIA, VILI), cervicography, computer-assisted screening devices, optical probe devices, self-collected vaginal samples for HPV DNA testing, and spectroscopy/electronic detection devices but not enough to provide satisfactory evidence of their efficacy and effectiveness in clinical practice settings.

Much current interest on new technologies focuses on how liquid-based testing and HPV-DNA testing enhance the accuracy of cervical cancer screening. For evaluating and comparing the utility of the technologies, several points need to be emphasized.[37] For the most part, data on sensitivity of testing are derived from research settings with optimized testing conditions. The same results may not be achievable in actual practice. Certain research designs by their nature may over- or underestimate test sensitivity. Test sensitivity must be distinguished from program sensitivity. Test sensitivity is the probability that a single test performed at a specified time will detect the presence of underlying disease. Program sensitivity is the probability that tests repeated at specified intervals will detect underlying disease over a period of time. Repeat screening at regular intervals therefore compensates somewhat for limitations in the sensitivity of a technique. For any test, sensitivity for detection of disease can be improved by lowering the test threshold for a "positive" result but only with concomitant loss in specificity, resulting in more false-positive results. When screening a population for a disease of very low prevalence, even a small percentage change in specificity affects a large number of women because the vast majority of women screened do not have disease. For example, if disease prevalence is 10% and test specificity 95%, then a 5% decrement of specificity for 50 million screening tests represents an increase of approximately 2.5 million women (from 2.2 million to 4.5 million) who will receive a "false-positive" result and may in turn have unnecessary diagnostic tests performed with potentially harmful effects.[37] With regard to liquid-based testing, the reader is directed to the literature on the subject most of which has come from studies supported by industry. Taken as a whole, the available evidence supports the conclusion that LBP is an acceptable option for cervical cancer screening, that LBP is somewhat more sensitive but less specific for high-grade lesions, and that it may increase the number of ASC-US referrals and possibly the proportion of samples lacking an endocervical component. Any decision for its use should be based on looking at all the evidence as well as the additional costs involved and determining whether the end result is in the interest of all patients served. A similar decision should be made about HPV-DNA testing for all currently recommended uses.

Since the mid-1990s there has been interest in the use of HPV DNA testing as a cervical cancer screening tool based on the premise that standardized molecular testing of exfoliated cervical cells for the causative agent of cervical cancer could demonstrate acceptable diagnostic performance while being more reproducible and more easily adapted for clinical practice than conventional cytology. Several studies have assessed the relative utility of both a cytology test and HPV DNA testing compared with the cytology test alone as a primary cervical cancer screening tool. Most of these studies indicate that women with a concurrent normal cytology test and a negative HPV-DNA result have little risk of a high-grade lesion being found on colposcopy relative to those for whom the only screening information is a normal conventional cytology result. On the other hand, a positive high-risk HPV result is not an absolute indicator that high-grade lesions exist or will develop; the prognostic value of a positive test result, especially in the absence of a cytologic abnormality, has not been fully evaluated in prospective studies. While definitive evidence of efficacy is still needed from long-term follow-up studies with CIN II/III as an outcome and from randomized controlled trials, evidence supports consideration of the use of HPV DNA testing (high-risk HPV types only) as an adjunct to cervical cytology with a screening interval no more frequent than every 3 years if both tests are negative. More frequent screening would not significantly improve sensitivity but would likely result in overevaluation and possible overtreatment of many women with transient HPV infections.[95]

Prevailing management paradigms, medicolegal issues, economic factors, and societal expectations all are factors in determining the balance between sensitivity and specificity for screening programs. Risk perception, understanding, and acceptability vary among individual patients, care providers, and policy makers.[96–99] In recent years, the public has been bombarded with direct-to-consumer advertising for all categories of goods and services including many drugs, medical treatment modalities, and screening tests. Vast improvement in public health education is necessary to enable individuals to understand these complex issues well enough to make informed decisions about the effectiveness of new technologies and the impact they might have on their individual needs and health status.

Lengthening the cervical cancer screening interval remains a controversial issue in the United States. While the evidence supports the conclusion that conventional cytology can be safely performed at 2- to 3-year intervals, many women and providers in the United States may be more comfortable with annual screening. A key factor is the limited sensitivity of the conventional Pap test. A significant proportion of false-negative conventional cytology results are due to inadequate sampling; improvement in the ability to obtain an adequate sample would increase the sensitivity and effectiveness of cytology, either conventional or liquid-based. Some improved sensitivity and cost-effectiveness of screening may be realized by utilizing new technologies but at longer intervals. If the new technologies are

used as frequently as annually, they would greatly increase the number of women referred for colposcopy unnecessarily, increasing health care costs and potential harms to patients, with little or no benefit. The greatest gain in reducing cervical cancer incidence and mortality would be achieved by increasing screening rates among women who have not been screened or who have not been screened regularly. Missed opportunities for screening abound, particularly among unscreened older women, foreign-born women, women of low income or low education, and women who are uninsured or underinsured. Clinicians, hospitals, health plans, and public health officials should seek to identify and screen these women and to ensure continued screening at regular intervals.

## REFERENCES

1. Commission on Chronic Illness (eds): Chronic Illness in the United States, Vol. 1. Cambridge, Mass, Harvard University Press, 1957. **(IV, C)**

2. Wilson JMG, Junger G (eds): Principles and Practice of Screening for Disease. Public Health Paper No. 34. Geneva, World Health Organization, 1968. **(IV, C)**

3. Hakama M, Chamberlain J, Day NE, et al: Evaluation of screening programmes for gynaecological cancer. Br J Cancer 1985;52:669–673. **(III, B)**

4. Moscicki AB, Shiboski S, Broering J, et al: The natural history of human papillomavirus infection as measured by repeated DNA testing in adolescent and young women. J Pediatr 1998;132:277–284. **(IIb, B)**

5. Nobbenhuis MAE, Walboomers JMM, Helmerhorst TJM, et al: Relation of human papillomavirus status to cervical lesions and consequences for cervical-cancer screening: a prospective study. Lancet 1999;354:20–25. **(IIb, B)**

6. Eifel PJ, Verek JS, Thigpen JT: Cancer of the cervix, vagina, and vulva. In DeVita VT Jr, Hellman S, Rosenberg SA (eds): Cancer: Principles and Practice of Oncology, 6th ed. Philadelphia, Lippincott Williams & Wilkins, 2001. **(III, B)**

7. Stoler MH, Schiffman M: Atypical Squamous Cells of Undetermined Significance-Low-grade Squamous Intraepithelial Lesion Triage Study (ALTS) Group: Interobserver reproducibility of cervical cytologic and histologic interpretations: realistic estimates from the ASCUS-LSIL Triage Study. JAMA 2001;285:1500–1505. **(Ib, A)**

8. Kivlahan C, Ingram E: Papanicolaou smears without endocervical cells: are they inadequate? Acta Cytol 1986;30:258. **(III, B)**

9. Hildesheim A, Schiffman MH, Gravitt PE, et al: Persistence of type-specific human papillomavirus infection among cytologically normal women. J Infect Dis 1994;169:235–240. **(IIb, B)**

10. Oguchi M, Komura J, Tagami H, et al: Ultrastructural studies of spontaneously regressing plane warts: macrophages attack verruca-epidermal cells. Arch Dermatol Res 1981;270:403–411. **(III, B)**

11. Bosch FX, Lorincz A, Munoz N, et al: The causal relation between human papillomavirus and cervical cancer. J Clin Pathol 2002;55:244–265. **(IIa, B)**

12. Burd EM: Human papillomavirus and cervical cancer. Clin Microbiol Rev 2003;16:1–17. **(IIa, B)**

13. Bonnez W, Reichman RC: Papillomaviruses: In Mandell GL, Bennett JE, Dolin R (eds): Principles and Practice of Infectious Disease, 5th ed. Philadelphia, Churchill Livingstone, 2000. **(IIb, B)**

14. Koss L, Durfee G: Unusual patterns of squamous epithelium of the uterine cervix: cytologic and pathologic study of koilocytotic atypia. Ann NY Acad Sci 1956;63:1235–1240. **(III, B)**

15. Meisels A, Fortin R, Roy M: Condylomatous lesions of the cervix. 2. Cytologic, colposcopic and histopathologic study. Acta Ctyol 1977; 21:379–390. **(IIb, B)**

16. Kienzler JL, Lemoine MT, Orth G, et al: Humoral and cell-mediated immunity to human papillomavirus type 1 (HPV-1) in human warts. Br J Dermatol 1983;108:665–672. **(IIa, B)**

17. Bonnez W, DaRin C, Rose RC, et al: Use of human papillomavirus type 11 virions in an ELISA to detect specific antibodies in humans with condylomata acuminata. J Gen Virol 1991;72:1343–1347. **(IIa, B)**

18. Bonnez W, Kashima HK, Leventhal B, et al: Antibody response to human papillomavirus (HPV) type 11 in children with juvenile-onset recurrent respiratory papillomatosis. Virology 1992;188:384–387. **(III, B)**

19. Ho GY, Bierman R, Beardsley L, et al: Natural history of cervicovaginal papillomavirus infection in young women. N Engl J Med 1998; 338: 423–428. **(III, B)**

20. Richardson H, Kelsall G, Tellier P, et al: The natural history of type-specific human papillomavirus infections in female university students. Cancer Epidemiol Biomarkers Prev 2003;12:485–490. **(III, B)**

21. Brown DR, Rawlings K, Handy V, et al: Human papillomavirus detection by hybrid capture in paired cervicovaginal lavage and cervical biopsy specimens. J Med Virol 1996;48:210–214. **(IIa, B)**

22. Londesborough P, Ho L, Terry G, et al: Human papillomavirus genotype as a predictor of persistence and development of high-grade lesions in women with minor cervical abnormalities. Int J Cancer 1996; 69: 364–368. **(IIb, B)**

23. Koutsky LA, Holmes KK, Critchlow CW, et al: A cohort study of the risk of cervical intraepithelial neoplasia grade 2 or 3 in relation to papillomavirus infection. N Engl J Med 1992;327:1272–1278. **(IIb, B)**

24. Cuzick J, Szarewski A, Cubie H, et al: Management of women who test positive for high-risk types of human papillomavirus: the HART study. Lancet 2003;362:1871–1876. **(IIa, B)**

25. Histology of the normal cervix. Available at: http://www.ASCCP.org/edu/practice/cervix/histology.shtml. Accessed 8/15/05. **(III, B)**

26. Hutchinson M, Fertitta L, Goldbaum B, et al: Cervex-Brush and Cytobrush: comparison of their ability to sample abnormal cells for cervical smears. J Reprod Med 1991;36:581–586. **(III, B)**

27. Martin-Hirsch P, Lilford R, Jarvis G, et al: Efficacy of cervical-smear collection devices: a systematic review and meat-analysis. Lancet 1999;354:1763–1770. **(Ib, A)**

28. Gutman S: FDA clarifies labeling of liquid-based systems (recent letters to the editors, Acta Cytologica). Available at: http://www.aqch.com/letters/recentletters.htm. Accessed 4/4/05. **(III, B)**

29. Blackman DK, Bennett EM, Miller DS: Trends in self-reported use of mammograms (1989–1997) and Papanicolaou tests (1991–1997)—Behavioral Risk Factor Surveillance System. MMWR CDC Surveill Summ 1999;48:1–22. **(IIa, B)**

30. Swan J, Breen N, Coates RJ, et al: Progress in cancer screening practices in the United States: results from the 2000 National Health Interview Survey. Cancer 2003;97:1528–1540. **(IIa, B)**

31. Henson RM, Wyatt SW, Lee NC: The National Breast and Cervical Cancer Early Detection Program: a comprehensive public health response to two major health issues for women. J Public Health Manag Pract 1996;2:36–47. **(III, B)**

32. Benard VB, Eheman CR, Lawson HW, et al: Cervical screening in the National Breast and Cervical Cancer Early Detection Program, 1995–2001. Obstet Gynecol 2004;103:564–571. **(IIb, B)**

33. Lawson HW, Lee NC, Thames SF, et al: Cervical cancer screening among low-income women: results of a national screening program, 1991–1995. Obstet Gynecol 1998;92:745–752. **(IIb, B)**

34. U.S. Preventive Services Task Force: Screening for Cervical Cancer: Guide to Preventive Clinical Services. Rockville, Md, AHRQ Publications Clearinghouse, 2003. **(Ia, A)**

35. American College of Obstetricians and Gynecologists: ACOG Practice Bulletin No. 45: Clinical management guidelines for obstetrician-gynecologists: cervical cytology screening. Obstet Gynecol 2003;102: 417–427. **(III, B)**

36. Miller AB, Anderson G, Brisson J, et al: Report of a National Workshop on Screening for Cancer of the Cervix. CMAJ 1991;145:1301–1325. **(IV, C)**

37. Miller AB, Knight J, Narod S: The natural history of cancer of the cervix, and the implications for screening policy In Miller AB, Chamberlain J, Day NE, et al (eds): Cancer Screening, 1991. Cambridge, Cambridge University Press, pp 144–152. **(III, B)**

38. Saslow D, Runowicz CD, Solomon D, et al: American Cancer Society guideline for the early detection of cervical neoplasia and cancer. CA Cancer J Clin 2002;52:342–362. **(Ib, A)**

39. Miller AB: The (in)efficiency of cervical screening in Europe. Eur J Cancer 2002;38:321–326. **(III, B)**

40. Sasieni P, Adams J, Cuzick J: Benefit of cervical screening at different ages: evidence from the UK audit of screening histories. Br J Cancer 2003;89:88–93. **(IIb, B)**

41. Miller AB: Cervical Cancer Screening Programmes: Managerial Guidelines. Geneva, World Health Organization, 1992. **(IV, C)**

42. IARC Working Group on Evaluation of Cervical Cancer Screening Programmes: Screening for squamous cervical cancer: duration of low risk after negative results of cervical cytology and its implication for screening policies. BMJ 1986;293:659–664. **(III, B)**

43. Cole P, Morrison AS: Basic issues in population screening for cancer. J Natl Cancer Inst 1980;64:1263–1272. **(III, B)**

44. Yu SZ, Miller AB, Sherman GJ: Optimising the age, number of tests, and the test interval for cervical screening in Canada. J Epidemiol Community Health 1982;36:1–10. **(IIb, B)**

45. van Oortmarssen GJ, Habbema JD: Duration of preclinical cervical cancer and reduction in incidence of invasive cancer following negative pap smears. Int J Epidemiol 1995;24:3007. **(IIb, B)**

46. Miller AB: Failures of cervical cancer screening. Am J Public Health 1995;85:761–762. **(III, B)**

47. Ashley DJ: Evidence for the existence of two forms of cervical carcinoma. J Obstet Gynaecol Br Commonw 1966;73:382–389. **(IV, C)**

48. Celentano DD, Klassen AC, Weisman CS, et al: Duration of relative protection of screening for cervical cancer. Prev Med 1989;18:411–422. **(III, B)**

49. Herbert A, Stein K, Bryant TN, et al: Relation between the incidence of invasive cervical cancer and the screening interval: is a five year interval too long? J Med Screen 1996;3:140–145. **(III, B)**

50. Goldie SJ, Kuhn L, Denny L, et al: Policy analysis of cervical cancer screening strategies in low-resource settings: clinical benefits and cost-effectiveness. JAMA 2001;285:3107–3115. **(IIb, B)**

51. Miller MG, Sung HY, Sawaya GF, et al: Screening interval and risk of invasive squamous cell cervical cancer. Obstet Gynecol 2003;101: 29–37. **(IIb, B)**

52. Sawaya GF, McConnell KJ, Kulasingam SL, et al: Risk of cervical cancer associated with extending the interval between cervical-cancer screenings. N Engl J Med 2003;349:1501–1509. **(IIb, B)**

53. Cecchini S, Iossa A, Ciatto S: Upper age limit for cervical cancer screening. Eur J Cancer 1996;32A:180. **(III, B)**

54. Coleman D, Day N, Douglas G, et al: European Guidelines for Quality Assurance in Cervical Cancer Screening: Europe against cancer programme. Eur J Cancer 1993;29A(Suppl 4):S1–S38. **(III, B)**

55. Solomon D, Davey D, Kurman R, et al: The 2001 Bethesda system: terminology for reporting results of cervical cytology. JAMA 2002; 287:2114–2119. **(III, B)**

56. Wright TC Jr, Cox JT, Massad LS, et al: 2001 Consensus guidelines for the management of women with cervical cytological abnormalities. For the 2001 ASCCP-Sponsored Consensus Conference. JAMA 2002; 287:2120–2129. **(Ia, A)**

57. Koutsky LA, for the Atypical Squamous Cells of Undetermined Significance/Low-Grade Squamous Intraepithelial Lesions Triage Study (ALTS) Group: Human papillomavirus testing for triage of women with cytologic evidence of low-grade squamous intraepithelial lesions: baseline data from a randomized trial. JNCI 2000;92:397–402. **(Ib, A)**

58. Mitchell MF, Tortolero-Luna G, Wright T, et al: Cervical human papillomavirus infection and intraepithelial neoplasia: a review. J Natl Cancer Inst Monogr 1996;21:17–25. **(III, B)**

59. Melnikow J, Nuovo J, Willan A, et al: Natural history of cervical squamous intraepithelial lesions: a meta-analysis. Obstet Gynecol 1998;92:727–735. **(IIb, B)**

60. Jones RW: The natural history of lower genital tract precancer: historical perspective. In MacLean A, Singer A, Critchley H (eds): Lower Genital Tract Neoplasia. London, RCOG Press, 2004, pp 69–81. **(IIb, B)**

61. Yost NP, Santoso JT, McIntire DD, Iliya FA: Postpartum regression rates of antepartum cervical intraepithelial neoplasia II and III lesions. Obstet Gynecol 1999;93:359–362. **(IIb, B)**

62. Massad LS, Riester KA, Anastos KM, et al: Prevalence and predictors of squamous cell abnormalities in Papanicolaou smears from women infected with HIV-1. Women's Interagency HIV Study Group. J Acquir Immune Defic Syndr 1999;21:33–41. **(IIb, B)**

63. Holcomb K, Matthews RP, Chapman JE, et al: The efficacy of cervical conization in the treatment of cervical intraepithelial neoplasia in HIV-positive women. Gynecol Oncol 1999;74:428–431. **(IIb, B)**

64. Selik RM, Rabkin CS: Cancer death rates associated with human immunodeficiency virus infection in the United States. J Natl Cancer Inst 1998;90:1300–1302. **(IIb, B)**

65. Frisch M, Biggar R, Goedert J: Human papillomavirus-associated cancers in patients with human immunodeficiency virus infection and acquired immunodeficiency syndrome. J Natl Cancer Inst 2000;92:1500–1510. **(II, B)**

66. Centers for Disease Control and Prevention: Sexually transmitted diseases treatment guidelines 2002. MMWR 2002;51(RR-6):53–57. **(Ia, A)**

67. Jones BA, Novis DA: Follow-up of abnormal gynecologic cytology: a college of American Pathologists Q-probes study of 16,132 cases from 306 laboratories. Arch Pathol Lab Med 2000;124:665–671. **(IIb, B)**

68. Ronnett BM, Manos MM, Ransley JE, et al: Atypical glandular cells of undetermined significance (AGUS): cytopathologic features, histopathologic results, and human papillomavirus DNA detection. Hum Pathol 1999;30:816–825. **(III, B)**

69. Duska LR, Flynn CF, Chen A, et al: Clinical evaluation of atypical glandular cells of undetermined significance on cervical cytology. Obstet Gynecol 1998;91:278–282. **(IIb, B)**

70. Zweizig S, Noller K, Reale F, et al: Neoplasia associated with atypical glandular cells of undetermined significance on cervical cytology. Gynecol Oncol 1997;65:314–318. **(IIb, B)**

71. Goff BA, Atanasoff P, Brown E, et al: Endocervical glandular atypia in Papanicolaou smears. Obstet Gynecol 1992;79:101–104. **(III, B)**

72. Taylor R, Guerrieri J, Nash J, et al: Atypical cervical cytology: colposcopic follow-up using the Bethesda system. J Reprod Med 1993;38:443–447. **(III, B)**

73. Laverty C, Farnsworth A, Thurloe J, et al: The reliability of a cytological prediction of cervical adenocarcinoma in situ. Aust N Z J Obstet Gynecol 1988;28:307–312. **(IIb, B)**

74. Lee K, Manna E, St John T: Atypical endocervical glandular cells: accuracy of cytologic diagnosis. Diagn Cytopathol 1995;71:894–897. **(III, B)**

75. Ries LAG, Eisner MP, Kosary et al: SEER Cancer Statistics Review, 1975–2002. Bethesda, Md, National Cancer Institute, 2004. Available at: http://seer.cancer.gov/csr/1975–2002. Accessed 8/16/05. **(IIb, B)**

76. Bousfield L, Pacey F, Young Q, et al: Expanded cytologic criteria for the diagnosis of adenocarcinoma in situ of the cervix and related lesions. Acta Cytol 1980;24:283–296. **(III, B)**

77. Ayer B, Pacey F, Greenberg M, Bousfield L: The cytologic diagnosis of adenocarcinoma in situ of the cervix uteri and related lesions. 1. Adenocarcinoma in situ. Acta Cytol 1987;31:397–411. **(III, B)**

78. Gloor E, Hurlimann J: Cervical intraepithelial glandular neoplasia (adenocarcinoma in situ and glandular dysplasia): a correlative study of 23 cases with histologic grading, histochemical analysis of mucins, and immunohistochemical determination of the affinity for four lectins. Cancer 1986;58:1272–1280. **(IIb, B)**

79. Denehy TR, Gregori CA, Breen JL: Endocervical curettage, cone margins, and residual adenocarcinoma in situ of the cervix. Obstet Gynecol 1997;90:1–6. **(IIb, B)**

80. Ursin G, Pike MC, Preston-Martin S, et al: Sexual, reproductive, and other risk factors for adenocarcinoma of the cervix: results from a population-based case-control study. Cancer Causes Control 1996; 7:391–401. **(IIa, B)**

81. Tase T, Okagaki T, Clark BA, et al: Human papillomavirus DNA in adenocarcinoma in situ, microinvasive adenocarcinoma of the uterine cervix, and coexisting cervical squamous intraepithelial neoplasia. Int J Gynecol Pathol 1989;8:8–17. **(IIb, B)**

82. Duggan MA, Benoit JL, McGregor SE, et al: Adenocarcinoma in situ of the endocervix: human papillomavirus determination by dot blot hybridization and polymerase chain reaction amplification. Int J Gynecol Pathol 1994;13:143–149. **(IIa, B)**

83. Anderson MC, Hartley RB: Cervical crypt involvement by intraepithelial neoplasia. Am J Obstet Gynecol 1980;55:546–550. **(IIb, B)**

84. Martin-Hirsch PL, Paraskevaidis E, Kitchener H: Surgery for cervical intraepithelial neoplasia. Cochrane Database of Systematic Reviews 2000; 2:CD001318. **(Ia, B)**

85. Mitchell MF, Tortolero-Luna G, Cook E, et al: A randomized clinical trial of cryotherapy, laser vaporization, and loop electrosurgical excision for treatment of squamous intraepithelial lesions of the cervix. Obstet Gynecol 1998;92:737. **(Ib, A)**

86. Demopoulos RI, Horowitz LF, Vamvakas EC: Endocervical gland involvement by cervical intraepithelial neoplasia grade III: predictive value for residual and/or recurrent disease. Cancer 1991;68:1932. **(IIa, B)**

87. Prendiville W: Treatment of grade 3 cervical intraepithelial neoplasia. In Prendiville W, Ritter J, Tatt S, Twiggs L (eds): Colposcopy Management Options. London, WB Saunders, 2003. **(III, B)**

88. Flannelly G, Bolger B, Fawzi H, et al: Follow up after LLETZ: could schedules be modified according to risk of recurrence?. BJOG 2001; 108:1025–1030. **(III, B)**

89. Flannelly G, Langhan H, Jandial L, et al: A study of treatment failures following large loop excision of the transformation zone for the treatment of cervical intraepithelial neoplasia. BJOG 1997;104:718–722. **(III, B)**

90. Burke L: The use of the carbon dioxide laser in the therapy of cervical inraepithelial neoplasia. Am J Obstet Gynecol 1982;144:377-80. **(III, B)**

91. Townsend DE: Cryosurgery for CIN. Obstet Gynecol Surv 1979; 34:828. **(III, B)**

92. Larsson G, Gullberg B, Grundsell H: A comparison of complications of laser and cold knife conization. Obstet Gynecol 1983;62:213–217. **(III, C)**

93. Baggish M, Dorsey J, Adelson M: A ten-year experience treating cervical intraepithelial neoplasia with $CO_2$ laser. Am J Obstet Gynecol 1989;161:60–68. **(IIb, C)**

94. Hatch K, Hacker N: Intraepithelial disease of the cervix, vagina and vulva. In Berek J, Adashi E, Hillard P (eds): Novak's Gynecology, 12th ed. Baltimore, Md, Williams & Wilkins, 1996, pp 447–474. **(IIa, B)**

95. Goldie SJ, Kim JJ, Wright TC: Cost-effectiveness of human papillomavirus DNA testing for cervical cancer screening in women aged 30 years or more. Obstet Gynecol 2004;103:619–631. **(IIb, B)**

96. Dominitz JA, Provenzale D: Patient preferences and quality of life associated with colorectal cancer screening. Am J Gastroenterol 1997; 92:2171–2178. **(IIb, B)**

97. Lawrence VA, Gafni A, Kroenke K: Evidence-based vs emotion-based medical decision-making: routine preoperative HIV testing vs universal precautions. J Clin Epidemiol 1993;46:1233–1236. **(IIa, B)**

98. Ward J: Population-based mammographic screening: does "informed choice" require any less than full disclosure to individuals of benefits, harms, limitations, and consequences? Aust N Z J Public Health 1999; 23:301–304. **(IIb, B)**

99. Marteau TM, Senior V, Sasieni P: Women's understanding of a "normal smear test result": experimental questionnaire based study. BMJ 2001; 322:526–528. **(IIb, B)**

# Chapter 12

# Colposcopy

## Lisa Flowers, MD

## KEY POINTS

- Human papillomavirus (HPV) infection in young women is generally transient, and the majority of women with HPV infection will not develop squamous intraepithelial lesions (SIL).
- Risk factors for development of SIL and progression of low-grade squamous intraepithelial lesions (LSIL) to high-grade squamous intraepithelial lesions (HSIL) are persistence of HPV infection and presence of high-risk oncogenic subtypes.
- Additional risk factors for progression to high-grade squamous intraepithelial lesions (HSIL) are cigarette smoking, multiple pregnancies, multiple sexual partners, long-term contraceptive use, and immunosuppression.
- The role of colposcopy is to locate and describe cervical abnormalities detected by cytologic screening in order to rule out invasive disease.
- Consistent and frequent use of colposcopic assessment systems such as Reid colposcopic index (RCI) and Rubin and Barbo during colposcopy assist in characterizing and identifying the most abnormal lesions for focused sampling and confirmation of the most severe disease.
- For colposcopy to be satisfactory or adequate, the entire lesion, squamocolumnar junction (SCJ), and transformation zone (TZ) must be visualized.
- Important colposcopic features to assess are color, margin, surface contour, vessels, and iodine coloration of the lesion.
- The role of colposcopy in pregnancy is to rule out invasive disease.
- Cervical sampling is generally not needed in pregnancy unless concern for microinvasive disease is present.
- Indications for conization are an unsatisfactory colposcopy, microinvasive disease, positive endocervical curettage, discrepancy between Pap test and biopsy, and adenocarcinoma in situ.
- Colposcopic findings of concern for microinvasive disease are atypical vessels, spontaneous areas of bleeding (lakes and pools), and ulcerations.
- A short course of intravaginal estrogen can assist with the atrophic cervix and vagina in evaluation of the postmenopausal patient.
- In the diethylstilbestrol (DES) patient, complete evaluation of the lower genital tract, particularly palpation of the upper vagina, is necessary to ensure no evidence of cancer.

Since the early 1900s colposcopy has been the clinician's instrument for identifying cellular abnormalities detected by the Papanicolaou (Pap) test or for evaluating gross lesions suspicious for cancer. The main purpose of colposcopy is to identify the most abnormal lesions within the lower genital tract for directed sampling and confirmation of grade of disease. Of the approximately 50 million Pap tests performed each year in the United States, 10% will show some cytologic abnormality and 5% will reveal a LSIL or higher.[1] These cellular abnormalities will require evaluation with colposcopy, and the ability to accurately detect disease will depend on the experience and expertise of the colposcopist.

## ACCURACY OF COLPOSCOPY

Several studies have evaluated the efficacy and accuracy of colposcopy as a tool for identification of dysplasia and invasive disease of the cervix. Clearly, the ability to accurately grade the level of disease in the lower genital tract is dependent on the experience of the examiner, and there is variation in sensitivity and specificity among studies. However, in a meta-analysis by Mitchell et al[2] of over 80 articles, the sensitivity of diagnostic colposcopy ranged between 87% and 99% with a positive predictive value of 53% to 96%. Its specificity was variable at 23% to 87%. In general, colposcopy is a predictive tool for the determination of disease, and even in pregnancy, when most biopsies are not performed until after delivery, the colposcopic impression is typically within one grade of level of disease as compared with pathologic results from biopsy specimens taken after delivery.

## INDICATIONS FOR COLPOSCOPY

The Pap smear is the primary screening test for referral of patients to colposcopy. Abnormalities detected by the cytopathologist suggesting premalignant or malignant changes on the cervix or lower genital tract are based on certain morphologic cellular characteristics distinguishing LSIL from HSIL.

There are several indications for referral to colposcopy:

1. Cellular abnormalities suggesting LSIL on a Pap test
2. Cellular abnormalities suggesting HSIL on a Pap test
3. Cellular abnormalities suggesting atypical squamous cells of high-grade disease (ASC-H) on a Pap test
4. Cellular abnormalities suggesting atypical squamous cells of undetermined significance (ASC-US) on two consecutive occasions within a 1-year time period
5. Atypical squamous cells of undetermined significance (ASC-US) with concurrent high-risk HPV
6. Glandular abnormalities such as atypical glandular cells (AGCs) or adenocarcinoma in situ (AIS)

145

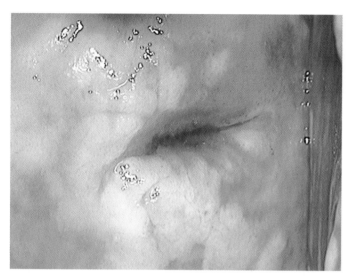

**Figure 12-1** Several areas representative of leukoplakia with elevated white plaques present prior to application of 3% to 5% acetic acid. This finding may be secondary to intraepithelial neoplasia, cancer, trauma, or infection.

7. Any Pap test or suspicious cervical lesion seen on pelvic examination suggestive of invasive cancer
8. Repetitive unsatisfactory Pap tests
9. Persistent clinical impression of cervicitis and bloody vaginal discharge with no evidence of cervical infection (negative cervical cultures)
10. Evidence of HPV infection (condyloma) in other areas of the lower genital tract such as the vagina and vulva
11. History of DES exposure with no prior evaluation

These indications justify a thorough colposcopic assessment of the lower genital tract, with particular focus on the cervix. Components of the colposcopic evaluation allow for proper management and treatment in the follow-up period. The colposcopic report should include the indication for colposcopy, whether the examination was satisfactory or adequate, description of all lesions seen, and impression of level of disease.

## COLPOSCOPIC PROCEDURE

During the colposcopic examination, the patient is placed in a modified lithotomy position and the external genitalia are completely evaluated for any physical evidence of HPV infection (condyloma) or abnormally pigmented (e.g., hyperpigmented areas) areas requiring biopsy. The vaginal speculum is placed into the vagina until the cervix is located and in complete view of the colposcopist. The vagina and cervix are inspected for suspicious lesions or leukoplakia (white patches suggestive of keratinization due to dysplasia, cancer, or trauma; Fig. 12-1). The colposcope is a microscope using illuminated magnification to allow for visualization of lesions with 6- to 40-fold magnification. The Pap test may be repeated if indicated and normal saline applied to allow for visualization of the subepithelial capillary network. Typically a green filter is used to accentuate vessels by deepening the red color to identify any abnormal vascular patterns (Figs. 12-2A and 12-2B).

Next, 3% to 5% acetic acid is applied to the cervix and vagina to assist with visualization of dysplastic lesions. When acetic acid is applied to the epithelium of the cervix, it rapidly penetrates the tissue, creating a hyperosmotic environment that causes transient contraction of the cytoplasmic volume, thus increasing the nuclear cytoplasmic ratio in cervical cells. An additional effect is interaction of acetic acid with the nucleoproteins, causing precipitation of these nucleoproteins. Dysplastic cells have a higher nuclear density and contain more nucleoprotein compared with normal cells. The elevated nucleoprotein level obscures the underlying vessels, and when light is reflected from the colposcope, the epithelium appears white, thus, acetowhite epithelium (Fig. 12-3). In normal squamous

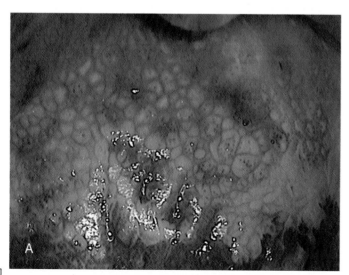

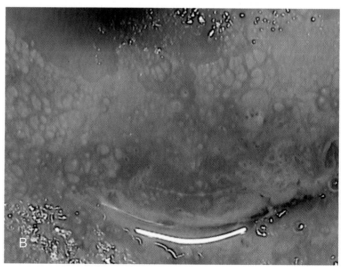

**Figure 12-2** *A* and *B*, The green filter accentuates coarse mosaic tiles bordered by vessels within the field of acetowhite epithelium.

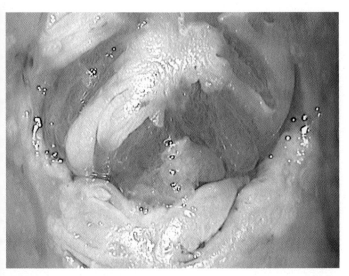

**Figure 12-3** After application of 3% to 5% acetic acid to the cervical epithelium, a dense white color change occurs in areas suspicious for intraepithelial neoplasia.

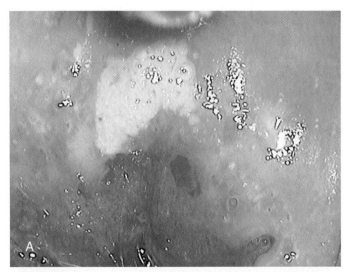

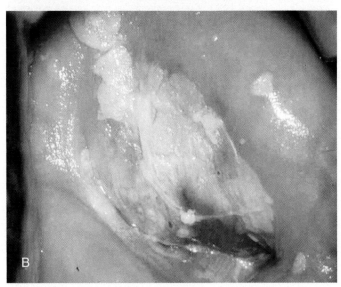

**Figure 12-4** **Acetowhite cervical lesions.** *A,* Transient appearance of an acetowhite lesion characteristic of a low-grade lesion on the anterior lip of the cervix at 12 o'clock. *B,* Dense acetowhite lesion with internal borders entering the os consistent with a high-grade squamous intraepithelial lesion. The squamocolumnar junction cannot be completely visualized; therefore, this is an unsatisfactory colposcopy. Biopsy of the lesion revealed a CIN II lesion.

epithelial cells acetic acid produces little precipitation, and the pink color from the underlying stroma with its network of subepithelial vessels is predominantly seen. Therefore, in low-grade lesions the onset of white is delayed and transient, since the nuclear to cytoplasmic ratio (N/C) is not so pronounced as in high-grade disease in which the acetowhite effect occurs rapidly (Figs. 12-4A and 12-4B). Acetowhitening of the epithelium can occur in other instances in which the N/C ratio is increased such as metaplasia, healing regenerating epithelium, and presence of viruses. The effect is reversible and typically lasts for 50 to 60 seconds.

Another diagnostic tool is Lugol's solution or Schiller's test. Lugol's solution is $\frac{1}{4}$ iodine to $\frac{3}{4}$ water, and it stains normal squamous epithelium brown secondary to the large amount of glycogen in the cytoplasm of normal cells. In abnormal epithelium, application of Lugol's will demonstrate various levels of staining based on the amount of glycogen and the severity of disease (Figs. 12-5A and 12-5B).

## Satisfactory or Adequate Colposcopy

The term satisfactory or adequate colposcopy indicates to the clinician that the area most at risk for disease—the present SCJ or TZ—and the margin of any visible abnormal lesion were completely visualized by the colposcopist. The SCJ is the junction of the squamous epithelium and columnar (glandular) epithelium usually located near the external cervical os (opening of the cervix; Fig. 12-6). Visualization of the SCJ may require use of an endocervical speculum to evaluate the endocervical canal for the presence of neoplasia. The transformation zone is the area undergoing active metaplastic change and the likely region for abnormal colposcopic findings. It lies between the original SCJ and the "new" or present SCJ.

If the examination is determined to be unsatisfactory for either reason, a diagnostic excisional procedure (conization) of the cervix may have to be performed to ensure that the transformation zone, endocervical canal, and any associated lesion within those areas have been investigated (Figs. 12-7A and 12-7B).

*Conization* is an excisional technique to remove a cone-shaped or cylinder-shaped piece of cervix to obtain a specimen from the transformation zone and endocervical canal for histologic evaluation. Types include laser conization, cold-knife conization, and loop electrosurgical conization.

Other indications for conization are

- Microinvasive disease
- Positive endocervical curettage
- Discrepancy of two grades between the Pap test and biopsy (e.g., a discrepancy of two grades would be an HSIL Pap test, with no evidence of disease found on the cervical and endocervical biopsies.
- Adenocarcinoma in situ

147

Ambulatory Office Practice

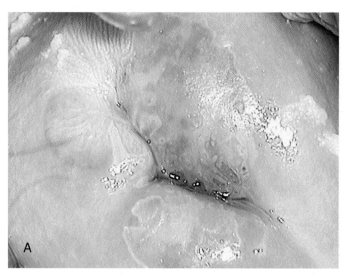

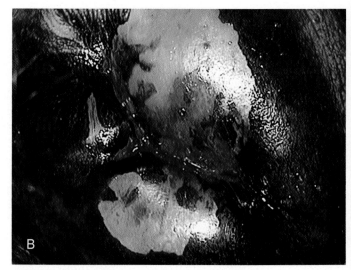

**Figure 12-5   Aceteowhite lesion with varying grades of dysplasia ranging from CIN I to CIN II.** *A,* An area of fine mosaic tile at 1 o'clock near opening of the os. *B,* Same lesion after application of Lugol's solution demonstrating the borders and extent of the lesion.

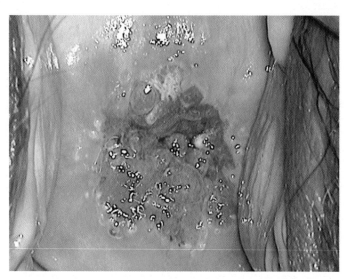

**Figure 12-6   The current, or new, squamocolumnar junction is where the squamous and columnar cells meet on the surface of the cervix at the time of colposcopy.** The entire SCJ is seen, with a small area of CIN I at 12 o'clock.

In the case of microinvasive disease or adenocarcinoma in situ, cold-knife conization is the preferred procedure to preserve tissue for optimal histologic review.

### Colposcopy of the Normal Transformation Zone

The normal transformation zone is bordered by the original squamous epithelium and columnar epithelium. The original squamous epithelium has a smooth surface with lacy or branching vessels giving a pink color to its surface. It retains its pink color after application of acetic acid and acquires a brown color after iodine application secondary to the abundant glycogen content. The columnar epithelium is made up of a single layer of mucus-secreting tall columnar cells that line the endocervical canal and appear grapelike under colposcopic visualization. The

original SCJ is the border between the SCJ present at birth and the current transformation zone. The new SCJ demarcates the border between the squamous epithelium and the endocervical columnar cells at the time of colposcopy.

Within the new and original SCJ lies mature squamous metaplasia, the region on the cervix that was previously covered with columnar epithelium that has undergone metaplastic transformation secondary to hormonal influences and acidity of the vagina. It is characterized by the presence of nabothian cysts, gland openings, and branching vessels. It is similar in appearance to the original squamous epithelium and at times cannot be differentiated from it. Immature squamous metaplasia can be confused with abnormal epithelium by its reaction to acetic acid with acetowhiteness similar to CIN. Cells of immature squamous metaplasia lack glycogen and so can exhibit less staining with Lugol's solution similarly to low-grade CIN.

### Colposcopy of the Abnormal Transformation Zone

The colposcopist uses physical characteristics of lesions revealed during colposcopy to differentiate low-grade lesions from high-grade lesions at risk for progression to malignancy. The epithelial and vascular changes present prior to or after acetic acid and Lugol's solution may be used with various colposcopic grading systems to objectively identify the grade of disease and the lesions most appropriate for biopsy. Examples of such abnormal colposcopic findings are leukoplakia, acetowhite epithelium, internal borders, punctation, mosaic, atypical vessels, and ulceration.

*Leukoplakia* is the presence of areas of reflecting white epithelium prior to acetic acid application. The increased keratinization causing leukoplakia may be secondary to SIL, cancer, or trauma. Samples for biopsy are taken from areas of leukoplakia in addition to other abnormal lesions found during the colposcopic procedure to rule out disease. As previously mentioned, acetowhite epithelium may reveal SIL depending on its characteristics such as its color, margins, and surface contour. Another feature is the *internal border*, the presence of an internal line of demarcation separating a high-grade acetowhite lesion

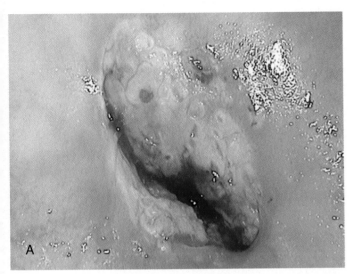

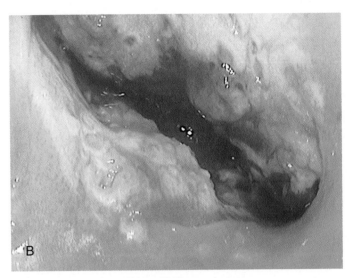

**Figure 12-7** *A and B,* **High-grade squamous intraepithelial lesion with dense acetowhite epithelium and coarse mosaic pattern extending into the canal.** Biopsy confirmed CIN III disease. The full extent of the lesion and the SCJ were not visualized; therefore, the examination is unsatisfactory.

from a low-grade lesion. In general when an internal border or margin is seen, the HSIL is centrally located closer to the SCJ. *Punctations* are vessels seen infiltrating the epithelium perpendicular to the basement membrane and when coarse in appearance are generally indicative of a high-grade lesion. If bridges are created between the vessels infiltrating the epithelium, a *mosaic* pattern is expressed with vessels running horizontal to the basement membrane. The coarse appearance of these vascular patterns and the increased intercapillary distance between the vessels further support the presence of a high-grade lesion. Finally, signs suspicious for microinvasive disease are atypical vessels and ulcerations or lakes and pools of blood. *Atypical vessels* appear as isolated, nonbranching vessels, irregular with loss of pattern. Various descriptions for atypical vessels are corkscrew and spaghetti loops. Associated with atypical vessels may be areas of spontaneous pooling of blood and ulceration. These features are highly suggestive of cancer.

## COLPOSCOPIC ASSESSMENT SYSTEMS

Several classification systems of colposcopy have been created to assist clinicians in objectively grading changes seen in the abnormal transformation zone. Two commonly used systems are the Reid colposcopic index (RCI), and the Rubin and Barbo colposcopic assessment system.[3-6] These colposcopic assessment systems integrate physical traits seen with the colposcope to objectively grade the level of disease.

### Reid's Colposcopic Index
In RCI, a numeric value is given to a lesion based on several key features: margin, color, vascular patterns, and iodine staining (Table 12-1).[7] All of the colposcopic signs are determined after the application of 3% to 5% acetic acid except for the iodine staining as the last step. The numerical value places the lesion in a low-grade (CIN I) or a high-grade (CIN II/III) category.

| Table 12-1 Reid's Colposcopic Index | | | |
|---|---|---|---|
| **Colposcopic Sign** | **0 Points** | **1 Point** | **2 Points** |
| Margin | Flocculated or feathered edges Indistinct margins | Smooth, straight lines Sharp peripheral margins | Rolling, peeling edges Internal border between lesions of different grade |
| Color | Shiny or snow white Transparent Indistinct acetowhite epithelium | Shiny, gray-white | Dull white Oyster gray |
| Vessels | Uniform, fine caliber Fine mosaic or punctations | Absence of blood vessels after acetic acid | Coarse punctation and mosaicism Large intercapillary distance Dilated individual vessels |
| Iodine staining | Positive iodine uptake producing brown color Low grade by other criteria (<2/6) | Partial variegated iodine uptake Tortoise shell color | Mustard yellow color in uptake High grade by other criteria (>3/6) |
| **Colposcopic score** | 0–2 = HPV or CIN I | 3–4 = CIN I or CIN II | 5–8 = CIN II or CIN III |

CIN, cervical intraepithelial neoplasia; HPV, human papillomavirus.

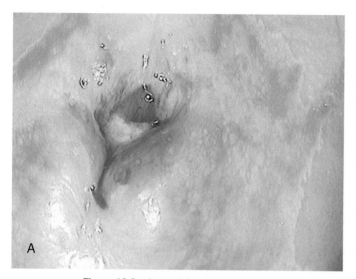
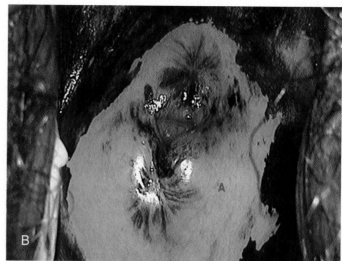

**Figure 12-8    Large, high-grade dense acetowhite lesion with mosaic pattern entering the canal.** *A,* Biopsy confirmed CIN III disease. *B,* Lugol's solution applied to the cervix, with lack of staining in areas of disease.

These features are more than 90% accurate in predicting pathologic findings and assist the colposcopist in identifying and properly sampling the most severe lesion.[3–8]

In using Reid's colposcopic index for the case represented in Figs. 12-8A and 12-8B, the RCI score would be 2 points for margin, 1 point for color, 2 points for vessels, and 2 points for iodine staining for a total of 7 points, placing the lesion in the high-grade disease category. This patient also has an unsatisfactory or inadequate colposcopy and requires a conization.

### Rubin and Barbo System

The Rubin and Barbo assessment method uses descriptors to categorize severity of disease and focuses on presence of microinvasive disease. The key components of the Rubin and Barbo assessment include color, vessels, border, and surface pattern (Table 12-2).

Use of the Rubin and Barbo system (Figs. 12-9A and 12-9B) demonstrates a dense acetowhite lesion with rolling, peeling edges and internal borders suggestive of microinvasive disease.

## LOW-GRADE SQUAMOUS INTRAEPITHELIAL LESIONS

More than 70% of LSIL lesions resolve spontaneously or remain the same without change over time. In a meta-analysis of studies examining the natural history of LSIL, 47% of lesions regress to normal within 2 years, 21% progressed to HSIL (CIN II/III), and 0.15% progressed to cancer.[9] Thus, most low-grade lesions remain stable or resolve, and treatment should be delayed unless progression to high-grade disease occurs. This category contains lesions with histologic features of CIN I disease or koilocytosis indicating HPV infection. The rationale for combining HPV

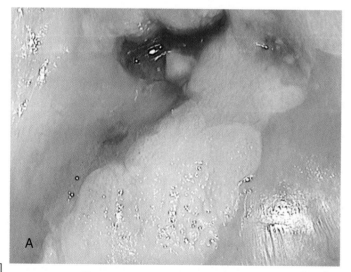
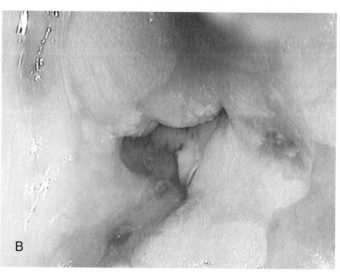

**Figure 12-9    Large, high-grade lesion.** *A and B,* Several elevated dense acetowhite areas with internal borders and peeling edges noted on entry into the os. Biopsy revealed microinvasive disease.

| | Table 12-2 | | | |
|---|---|---|---|---|
| | **Rubin and Barbo Colposcopic Assessment System** | | | |
| **Grade** | **Color** | **Vessels** | **Border** | **Surface** |
| Normal | Pink<br>Translucent | Fine<br>Lacy<br>Normal branching | Normal T-zone<br>Geographic | Flat |
| Grade I<br>HPV/mild dysplasia<br>CIN I<br>LSIL | White<br>Shiny white<br>Snow white | None<br>Fine punctation<br>Fine mosaic | Diffuse<br>Feathery<br>Flocculated<br>Geographic | Flat<br>Micropapillary<br>Macropapillary |
| Grade II<br>Moderate dysplasia<br>CIN II<br>HSIL | White<br>Shiny gray | None<br>Punctation<br>Mosaic | Demarcated | Flat<br>Slightly raised |
| Grade III<br>Severe dysplasia<br>CIS<br>CIN III<br>HSIL | Whitest<br>Dull white<br>Oyster white | None<br>Coarse punctation<br>Coarse mosaic<br>Dilated<br>Intercapillary distance | Sharp<br>Clearly<br>Demarcated<br>Straight<br>Internal border | Raised |
| Microinvasion<br>Frank invasion | Red<br>Yellow<br>Dull gray | Atypical<br>Irregular<br>Bizarre | Clearly<br>Demarcated<br>Peeling<br>Rolling edges | |

CIN, cervical intraepithelial neoplasia; CIS, carcinoma in situ; HPV, human papillomavirus; HSIL, high-grade squamous intraepithelial lesion; LSIL, low-grade squamous intraepithelial lesion.

koilocytotic changes with CIN I disease is based on the rate of progression to CIN III disease (14% for HPV koilocytotic changes and 16% for CIN I) and both demonstrate a mixture of low-risk and oncogenic HPV subtypes.[10] Though HPV subtypes 6 and 11 are frequently associated with low-grade disease; as many as 86.1% of women with low-grade disease have oncogenic HPV subtypes as demonstrated by the ASCUS/LSIL triage study (ALTS).[11] HPV 16 is the most common oncogenic subtype detected, but 18, 45, 56, 31, 33, and 35 also have been found. It is common for multiple HPV subtypes to be found in LSIL lesions (as seen in the ALTS trial) with over 58% of LSIL cases having multiple HPV subtypes. Certain factors determine whether HPV infection will translate to LSIL disease. Such factors are longevity of the HPV infection, young age, and the presence of oncogenic HPV subtypes. Typically, the presence of HPV infection, especially in young populations, is indicative of sexual activity.[12] The younger the onset of sexual activity in the presence of an immature transformation zone, the greater the risk of development of LSIL. The rate of squamous metaplastic maturation appears critical for LSIL development. As women approach their 30s, detection of HPV infection declines from the initial peak in late adolescence. This decrease appears to be due to a reduction in new sexual partners and to cell-mediated immune response to HPV. In summary, infection with oncogenic HPV subtypes and persistence of HPV infection for more than a year are strong risk factors for progression from LSIL to HSIL.[12]

## Colposcopic Features of Low-grade Disease
Colposcopic features of low-grade disease include the following:

- Color: transient, shiny, snowy acetowhite lesion or translucent, faint acetowhite lesion
- Margin: geographic, feathery, flocculated lesion with indistinct borders
- Surface contour: flat satellite lesions or exophytic condyloma
- Vessels: no vessels seen or fine punctuations and mosaic pattern, normal intercapillary distance (50 to 250 μm)
- Iodine: partial uptake or poor uptake with pale yellow iodine staining for condylomatous lesions

An example of a low-grade lesion is shown in Figure 12-10.

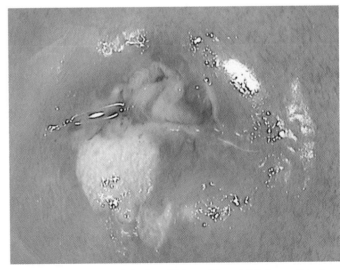

**Figure 12-10** Low-grade lesions (flat condylomata) between 6 and 7 o'clock.

# HIGH-GRADE SQUAMOUS INTRAEPITHELIAL LESIONS

The main purpose for colposcopy is to identify lesions most likely to progress to cancer, in particular high-grade disease. To have the highest impact in preventing cervical cancer, clinicians should focus on screening women from age 20 to 39 years, when the rate of CIN III is highest.[13] The average rate of progression from LSIL to HSIL is approximately 10% to 20% following an LSIL Pap smear. Duggan et al[14] in a longitudinal study demonstrated that 18.6% of 342 women with a cytologic diagnosis of LSIL progressed to CIN II or III. However, in patients with high-grade disease the potential for progression if untreated is significant.[15] A natural history study of 894 women with CIN II over 50 to 78 months revealed regression, persistence, and progression rates of 54%, 16%, and 30%, respectively.[16] In a limited series of patients untreated for CIS, the reported progression rate was 12% to 70%. The diagnosis of HSIL includes CIN II, CIN III, and carcinoma in situ. The rationale for combining CIN II and CIN III is based on similarities on cellular morphology, HPV subtypes associated with invasive cancer, aneuploidy, and malignant potential. However, many authors believe that CIN II and III should not be grouped together and point out the potential for CIN III to develop de novo.[15] The theory that cervical dysplasia progresses stepwise from CIN I to II and finally to III has been questioned by studies demonstrating women with CIN III and no evidence of current or previous history of CIN I.[17] In addition, HSIL is monoclonal, similarly to invasive cancer, while 32% of LSIL is polyclonal.[18] However, at present there is sufficient reason to consider CIN II as having malignant potential to justify the same management guidelines as CIN III.

Risk factors for progression to high-grade disease are

- Oncogenic HPV types
- Cigarette smoking
- Multiple pregnancies
- Multiple sexual partners
- Long-term contraceptive use
- Immunosuppression

Persistent infection with oncogenic HPV subtypes, in particular HPV 16, has consistently played a role in the progression to HSIL. In patients with normal cytology who demonstrated continual positive HPV 16 infection for a duration of 2 years versus transient infection, 44% of these women developed CIN at the end of the studies, and those with persistent positivity had more severe lesions.[19] In a study by Moscicki et al, clearance rate for HPV over 5 years was 92%. Those whose disease persisted harbored HPV 16 subtype.[12] The potential to advance to high-grade disease within a 2-year period in cytologically normal women stresses the importance of persistent HPV 16 in determining risk for HSIL.[19]

Several studies confirm that cigarette smoking is directly related to progression to high-grade disease, and its effect is increased by time of exposure and years of smoking.[20-23] In addition, size and degree of dysplasia correlates with the amount of cigarette smoking by the individual. Oral contraceptive pills, cigarette smoking, and HPV 16 subtype had little or essentially no relationship to CIN I disease, in contrast to high-grade disease.

Women in an immunodeficient state, in particular HIV-infected women, are at greater risk for developing CIN than HIV-negative women. Various studies give the estimated prevalence of CIN to be 20% to 77% in HIV-positive women.[24-26] In a meta-analysis of examining risk of CIN in HIV-positive versus HIV-negative women, the relative risk of CIN in HIV-positive women was five times as high as in HIV-negative women.[27] The higher prevalence of HPV may be the role of HIV as a cofactor in the increased replication, persistence, or reactivation of acquired HPV infection.[28]

Additional risk factors such as low socioeconomic status and sexual behavior of the male partner need to be taken into consideration.[29]

## Colposcopic Features of High-grade Disease

Interobserver and intraobserver agreement in diagnosis of high-grade disease is more accurate than in diagnosis of low-grade disease.[30] Most attribute this disagreement to the abnormal vascular patterns seen in high-grade lesions that assist in differentiating these lesions from low-grade lesions. Most severe lesions are found near the SCJ, and particular attention must be placed on sampling and visualizing disease entering the endocervical canal.

Typical colposcopic features of high-grade disease are the following:

- Color: persistent dull, oyster white dense acetowhite lesion
- Margin: sharp, demarcated, smooth borders, rolling and peeling edges, with or without internal border within a lower grade lesion (lesion within a lesion)
- Surface contour: raised and elevated lesion
- Vessels: coarse punctations or mosaic pattern, wide intercapillary distance between vessels, mosaic lesion with central punctation or umbilication
- Iodine: lacks staining, mustard yellow color

Typically in colposcopy the most severe lesion is sampled to avoid patient discomfort. However, complex lesions may require more samples to assure accurate diagnosis. An example of a lesion demonstrating high-grade features is shown in Figure 12-11.

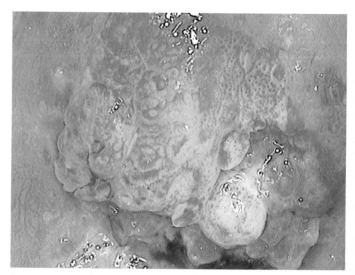

**Figure 12-11    High-grade intraepithelial lesion with a combination of coarse mosaic pattern and punctations.**

# CANCER

Atypical vessels, areas of ulceration and spontaneous bleeding and dull yellow or reddish tone may indirectly suggest colposcopic evidence of stromal invasion. The borders are frequently peeling or rolled, with lakes and pools, and easily friable. If the lesion is visible, immediate biopsy is warranted. Several studies have revealed the inaccuracy of detection of occult invasive squamous cell carcinoma by colposcopy in as many as 50% of cases.[31,32] Other abnormal colposcopic findings seen with microinvasion are thick, elevated acetowhite epithelium, coarse mosaic pattern and punctation, and keratosis. The deeper the invasion, the greater the frequency of atypical vessels seen in the majority of patients with 3 to 5 mm of invasion having atypical vessels detected on colposcopy.[33] An example of typical features of microinvasive disease is shown in Figure 12-12.

## Colposcopic Features of Cancer

Colposcopic features of cancer include the following:

- Color: red or dull gray and yellow necrotic appearance
- Margin: sharp, demarcated, with rolling and peeling edges
- Surface contour: raised, polypoid, nodular, exophytic lesion, ulcerative
- Vessels: corkscrew- and comma-shaped vessels, bizarre shapes with abrupt changes in size
- Iodine: lacks staining

Diagnostic conization may be necessary for sufficient histologic confirmation of depth of invasion or invasive disease. Figures 12-13A and 12-13B are reflective of lesions of concern for cancer.

# COLPOSCOPY IN PREGNANCY

The goal of cervical screening during pregnancy is to identify invasive disease. Colposcopy can be challenging secondary to all the normal physiologic changes of pregnancy and requires great expertise in localizing disease. The pregnant state does not

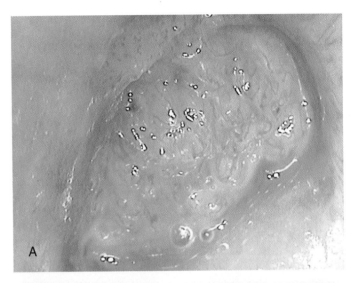

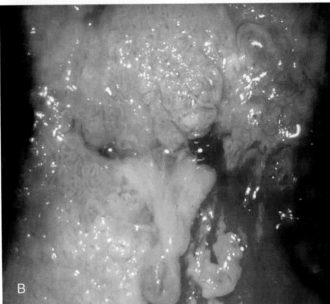

**Figure 12-13    Colposcopic appearance of invasive cancer.**
*A,* Endocervical mass with bizarre vessels suspicious for cancer and confirmed by biopsy. *B,* Large, irregular, papillary acetowhite lesion with lakes and pools and atypical vessels consistent with cancer. Biopsy revealed invasive cancer.

accelerate cervical neoplasia, and there is no difference in survival between pregnant and nonpregnant women with cervical cancer. The incidence of SIL found during pregnancy is 1% to 2% with greater than 85% of the cytologic abnormalities being LSIL and approximately 14% HSIL. Detection of histologic CIN in all pregnant patients can range between 0.19% and 0.53%.[4,35] Invasive cancer presents in 1/3000 pregnancies, with more than 70% presenting in stage I and IIA and a typical mean age of 32 years.[36] Some of the physiologic changes are softening of the cervix, increased vascularity and mucus production, hypertrophy of the fibromuscular stroma, and eversion of the endocervical canal, all due to the high estrogen state. In addition, the cellular changes such as immature metaplasia, decidualization, basal cell hyperplasia, and the Arias-Stella reaction can make

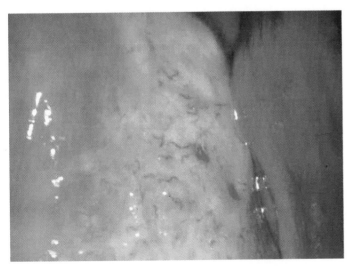

**Figure 12-12    Dense acetowhite lesion with atypical vessels suspicious for microinvasive disease.**

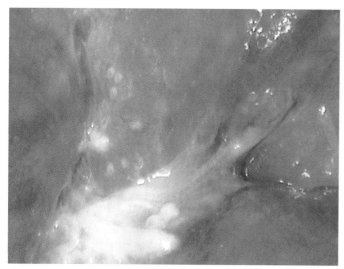

**Figure 12-14** Thick tenuous mucus in the os of a pregnant woman with squamous metaplasia at 12 o'clock.

accurate cytologic assessment difficult. Colposcopic evaluation is limited by extensive immature squamous metaplasia, increased vascularity causing upgrading of cervical lesions, and thick endocervical mucus (Fig. 12-14). However, it allows conservative management of cytologic abnormalities of the cervix with delay of treatment until after delivery. Views differ about whether sampling is necessary during pregnancy in absence of concern for microinvasive disease.[37–40] Most investigators agree on performing a biopsy if there are colposcopic signs suggestive of microinvasion (atypical vessels), a gross lesion on the cervix, or a large, high-grade lesion covering most of the ectocervix (Fig. 12-15). If a biopsy is necessary, the most severe lesion should be sampled with Monsel's solution in hand to apply to the biopsy site. Though there are few risks for infection and hemorrhage from biopsy, most colposcopists wait until the second trimester

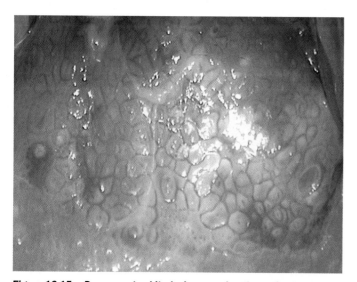

**Figure 12-15** **Dense acetowhite lesion covering the entire posterior lip of the cervix in a pregnant patient.** Note the coarse mosaic and punctations on the inferior border. Biopsy confirmed microinvasive disease.

to sample the cervix.[41] Generally by 20 weeks' gestation the SCJ is easily seen as a result of eversion of the endocervical canal, and most colposcopies will be satisfactory.

Once cytologic, colposcopic, and if needed histologic evaluation is complete and no evidence of microinvasive or invasive disease is noted, then follow-up with colposcopy or cytology every 8 weeks can be done with repeat colposcopy with sampling after delivery. Diagnostic cone biopsy is reserved for cases in which microinvasive or invasive disease is suspected from histologic evaluation of a simple biopsy or a cytologic test suspicious for cancer with inconclusive colposcopy or colposcopic-directed biopsy or adenocarcinoma in situ is found. A wedge biopsy may be performed instead of standard conization to decrease morbidity. Owing to the risk of preterm labor, premature rupture of membranes, and excessive bleeding, endocervical curettage is not recommended.[37] Low-grade disease may be followed with only repeat colposcopy postpartum, while high-grade disease should be followed with repeat colposcopy with or without cytology every 8 to 12 weeks.[41] There is a high regression rate for cervical dysplasia after delivery, with rates of 74% for CIN II and 54% for CIN III.[42] The regression rate of LSIL to normal can be as high as 65%. Postpartum colposcopic evaluation of cytologic abnormalities found during pregnancy should take place 8 to 12 weeks after delivery. Treatment and follow-up are determined by cytologic, colposcopic, and histologic confirmation of disease.

Nonetheless, the diagnosis of microinvasive disease may require wedge or cone biopsy to exclude invasive disease. Conization during pregnancy is associated with significant morbidity consisting of hemorrhage, preterm labor, and maternal chorioamnionitis.[43] Additionally in as many as 50% of cone biopsies performed during pregnancy, there may be residual CIN disease.[44] Therefore, clear indications are needed. Vaginal delivery in the presence of only microinvasive disease is appropriate.

Several factors direct care in the case of invasive cancer during pregnancy. Important variables are stage of disease, gestational age of the fetus, and the patient's desire to continue the pregnancy. If the cancer is detected at an early stage and beyond 20 weeks' gestation, the option of delaying treatment until there is fetal viability is reasonable.[45] When the cancer is further advanced or found in the first trimester of pregnancy, consideration of immediate treatment needs to be discussed with the patient. If pregnancy is continued, preferred treatment for early-stage disease is a cesarean section for delivery and radical hysterectomy with node dissection.[46]

## POSTMENOPAUSAL CERVIX

Postmenopausal squamous epithelium is pale because of the loss of stromal blood supply, and the cervix may appear red owing to the thin epithelium and easy visualization of the subepithelial capillaries. On application of acetic acid, a distinct area of whitening may not be apparent, since atrophy may complicate the ability to identify the most severe area (Fig. 12-16). Because it is devoid of glycogen, Lugol's solution will stain the cervix and vagina a pale yellow color. In certain cases, Lugol's solution can help identify areas most likely to be CIN versus atrophy. Another challenge in the postmenopausal patient requiring colposcopy is

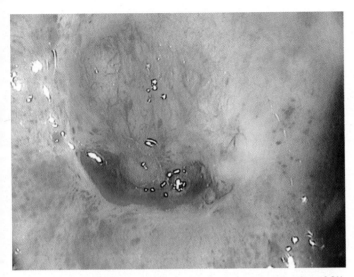

**Figure 12-16    Atrophic postmenopausal cervix after application of 3% to 5% acetic acid.** Nabothian cyst at 11 o'clock with prominent vessels. No distinct lesion was identified, and only endocervical curettage (ECC) was performed. The ECC result was negative.

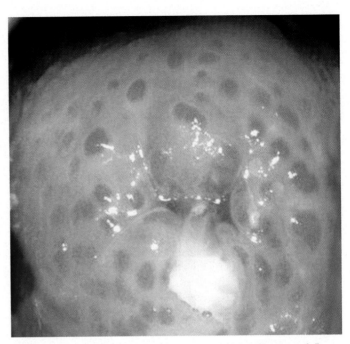

**Figure 12-17    Trichomonas infection with the "strawberry cervix" seen after application of acetic acid.** Colposcopy was delayed until treatment was completed.

the location of the SCJ in the endocervical canal. The external os may be stenotic and difficult to enter with an endocervical speculum. A short course of intravaginal estrogen may be necessary to soften the cervix and increase the glycogen content to allow for better visualization.

## COLPOSCOPIC CHALLENGES

Despite the various colposcopic assessment systems, particular cases provide a challenge to the colposcopist. As previously mentioned, atrophy of the epithelium can make identifying the most severe lesion difficult in the postmenopausal patient not on hormone replacement. The presence of infection may result in a higher grading than the histologic diagnosis. When active infection is suspected, colposcopy should be delayed until the infection is treated (Fig. 12-17). Differentiating between normal changes and real disease such as the acetowhite of squamous metaplasia versus the acetowhite of CIN I is a dilemma. Radiation can cause dramatic changes such as bizarre-appearing blood vessels and pale areas, making colposcopy challenging to the most experience colposcopist. Women exposed to DES in utero have cervical structural changes and vaginal epithelial abnormalities. Vaginal changes appear to be dependent on total dose of exposure, and close colposcopic evaluation of the cervix and vagina is necessary. A potential risk from DES exposure is the development of clear cell adenocarcinoma of the vagina and cervix.[47] After an extensive colposcopic evaluation has been performed, the upper vagina should be palpated to ensure no evidence of cancer. Common changes are the cervical collar, hypoplastic cervix, coxcomb cervix, pseudopolyp, shortened fornix, and vaginal strictures.[48] These changes should be documented and suspicious areas sampled. However, aggressive treatment in the absence of cancer should be avoided, since many of these changes will disappear over time.

## MANAGEMENT AFTER COLPOSCOPY

Colposcopy allows for identification of the most severe lesion for proper sampling. In general, agreement within one grade of disease among the initial Pap test, colposcopic impression, and histologic grade is preferred. However, the colposcopic impression and histologic diagnosis are the gold standard and ultimately determine management and treatment of disease. In instances of discrepancy between the Pap test and the gold standard, a full review of the slides and possibly a repeat colposcopy are performed. Patients with CIN I or no evidence of disease by colposcopy or histology may be followed with Pap tests per the ASCCP Consensus Guidelines.[49] Patients with biopsy-confirmed high-grade disease (CIN II/III) may require excisional or ablative therapy depending on the severity of grade, volume of disease, extension of disease into the endocervical canal or the rest of the lower genital tract, glandular involvement, HIV status, and patient compliance and desire for fertility. Types of ablative therapy are cryosurgery, diathermy, cold (Semm) coagulation, and carbon dioxide laser. Advantages of these procedures are preservation of cervical tissue, anatomy, and function, allowing for future follow-up with cytology and colposcopy and lack of interference with fertility. The disadvantage is lack of histologic evaluation for confirmation of biopsy results. This may be an issue in the case of an inexperienced colposcopist when the most severe lesion is not sampled or disease in the endocervical canal is missed. In this circumstance, invasive and glandular abnormalities may be missed and lead to inappropriate treatment. Therefore, the following critical criteria must be adhered to ensure a good outcome:

- Visualization of the squamocolumnar junction
- Visualization of the entire lesion or lesions

- No evidence of glandular pathology
- Negative endocervical curettage
- Patient compliance

If there is any doubt, excisional treatment should be considered in the form of LEEP (loop electrosurgical excision procedure), LLETZ (large loop excision of transformation zone), or conization. LEEP utilizes a fine loop wire attached to a high-frequency electrical generator that allows precise removal of abnormal tissue from the cervix. This is a common outpatient procedure for cervical disease and has a success rate of over 95%. The procedure allows for minimal tissue to be excised and sufficient material for diagnosis. The disadvantage is the cautery effect, which can create a heat artifact causing some difficulty in evaluating the margin of the specimen.

The key issue in the management of patients with cervical disease is proper counseling about the potential for recurrence and critical need for consistent follow-up. With regular cytologic follow-up and appropriate referral for colposcopy, the risk of future invasive disease is minimal.

## KEY TERMS

**Abnormal transformation zone:** areas on the cervix or vagina that may contain columnar epithelium and squamous metaplasia and that often contain intraepithelial neoplasia with an abnormal colposcopic pattern.

**Acetic acid (3% to 5%):** a contrast solution to enhance the detection of cervical neoplasia during colposcopic examination.

**Acetowhite epithelium:** used to describe epithelium that initially looks normal but appears white after the application of acetic acid. Suggestive of intraepithelial neoplasia or human papillomavirus (HPV) infection, in which case the term subclinical papilloma infection (SPI) is used.

**AGC (atypical glandular cell of undetermined significance):** term used in the Bethesda cytologic classification to indicate abnormal glandular cells that are not sufficiently abnormal to allow a definite diagnosis of neoplasia.

**ASC-US (atypical squamous cells of undetermined significance):** term used in the Bethesda cytologic classification to indicate abnormal squamous cells that are not sufficiently abnormal to allow a definite diagnosis of neoplasia.

**Bethesda classification:** a cytologic classification developed in the United States in 1988, which defines two levels of squamous neoplasia (low-grade or high-grade squamous intraepithelial neoplasia).

**Carcinoma in situ:** a morphologic alteration of the epithelium that usually precedes, occasionally gives rise to, and is usually present in the vicinity of invasive carcinoma. The full thickness of the epithelium is replaced with neoplastic cells.

**Cervical intraepithelial neoplasia (CIN):** a premalignant change in the cervical epithelium that can progress to cervical carcinoma. The degree of change from mild to severe is described as CIN I, II, or III.

**Colposcope:** an instrument used to magnify and examine the epithelium of the transformation zone to identify abnormal areas in the lower genital tract that warrant biopsy. It is a stereoscopic binocular field microscope with a long focal length and powerful light source. Lower magnification yields a wider view and a greater depth of field for observation. Higher magnification can reveal small features such as abnormal blood vessel patterns.

**Colposcopy:** examination of the cervix, vagina, and occasionally the vulva with the colposcope after the application of a 3% to 5% acetic acid solution; in addition, utilized to obtain directed biopsies of suspected lesions representing neoplasia.

**Cone biopsy, conization:** an excisional technique to remove a cone-shaped or cylinder-shaped piece of cervix for diagnosis or treatment of intraepithelial neoplasia.

**Cold knife cone:** Using a scalpel as the tool for conization of the cervix for diagnostic purposes.

**Cryotherapy:** freezing of the cervix to abate abnormal epithelium.

**Diagnostic excisional procedure:** obtaining a specimen from the transformation zone and endocervical canal for histologic evaluation, which includes laser conization, cold-knife conization, LEEP, and loop electrosurgical conization.

**Dysplasia:** describes varying degrees of cervical intraepithelial neoplasia. It may be mild, involving approximately one third of the epithelium (CIN I); moderate, involving approximately two thirds of the epithelium (CIN II); or severe, involving full thickness of the epithelium (CIN III).

**Endocervical curettage (ECC):** a biopsy procedure used to obtain endocervical tissue for histologic diagnosis.

**Endocervical sampling:** use of an endocervical curette or a cytobrush to obtain a specimen for histologic evaluation; or of a cytobrush for cytologic evaluation.

**Endocervical assessment:** method of evaluating the endocervical canal for the presence of neoplasia by means of colposcopy or endocervical sampling.

**Endocervical curette:** obtains a histologic sample by scraping the endocervical canal. The distal end of the basket is sharp and acts as a blade for curettage. A cytobrush may be rapidly spun in the endocervical canal to provide a specimen.

**Endocervical speculum:** may be necessary to obtain a satisfactory colposcopy that includes visualization of the entire squamocolumnar junction.

**Endometrial sampling:** endometrial biopsy, "dilation and curettage," or hysteroscopy used to obtain a specimen for histologic evaluation.

**Human papillomavirus (HPV):** a subgroup of papillomaviruses, which are small DNA tumor viruses that are classified by their DNA sequences.

**Koilocytosis:** a cellular change associated with papillomavirus infection, which includes perinuclear cavitation and nuclear atypia.

**Leukoplakia:** an area that appears white to the naked eye even before the application of 3% acetic acid.

**Loop electrosurgical excision procedure (LEEP):** a procedure that utilizes a fine loop wire attached to a high-frequency electrical generator that allows precise removal of abnormal tissue from the cervix.

**Lugol's solution:** an iodine based contrast solution that is mainly used when examining the vagina but may also be used in cervical colposcopy. It is less irritating and equally effective when diluted to half strength with water or saline.

**Monsel's solution:** the most common hemostatic agent used for lower genital tract biopsy or excision. It works best in a toothpaste consistency. Silver nitrate sticks and gel foam also may be used.

**Mosaic pattern:** the rosette appearance of capillary vessels in an abnormal transformation zone.

**Native squamous epithelium:** the normal original squamous epithelium found in the vagina and on the portio of the cervix.

**Normal transformation zone:** area of columnar epithelium and squamous metaplasia that has a normal colposcopic pattern.

**Punctation:** the stippled appearance of capillary vessels in an abnormal transformation zone.

**Radiation dysplasia:** abnormal cytologic smear from patients who have been treated by ionizing radiation for lower genital tract malignancies. These patients have increased risk of recurrent disease.

**Satisfactory colposcopy:** a colposcopic examination in which the entire transformation zone, including the squamocolumnar junction, is adequately visualized plus the margin of any visible lesion. If this area is not visualized, the colposcopy is termed unsatisfactory.

**Squamocolumnar junction (SJC):** the junction of the squamous epithelium and columnar (glandular) epithelium, usually located near the external cervical os.

**Squamous intraepithelial lesion (SIL):** abnormal squamous cells according to the Bethesda classification. Low-grade (LSIL) corresponds to koilocytosis and CIN I. High-grade (HSIL) corresponds to CIN II and III.

**Squamous metaplasia:** a physiologic process by which squamous tissue replaces columnar tissue.

**Subclinical papilloma infection (SPI):** colposcopically evident papillomavirus infection not clinically visible. Area looks normal to the naked eye but colposcopically appears white after acetic acid application.

## REFERENCES

1. Kurman RJ, Henson DE, Herbst AL, et al: Interim guidelines for management of abnormal cervical cytology. JAMA 1994;271:1886–1869. **(IV, C)**
2. Mitchell MF, Schottenfeld D, Zortolero-Luna G, et al: Colposcopy for the diagnosis of squamous intraepithelial lesions: a meta-analysis. Obstet Gynecol 1988;91:626–631. **(IIa, B)**
3. Reid R, Stanttope CR, Herschman BR, et al: Genital warts and cervical cancer. 4. A colposcopic index for differentiating subclinical papillomaviral infection from cervical intraepithelial neoplasia. Am J Obstet Gynecol 1984;149:815–823. **(IV, C)**
4. Reid R, Herschman BR, Crum CP, et al: Genital warts and cervical cancer. 5. The tissue basis of colposcopic change. Am J Obstet Gynecol 1984;149:293–303. **(IV, C)**
5. Reid R, Scaizi P: Genital warts and cervical cancer. 7. An improved colposcopic index for differentiating benign papillomaviral infections from high-grade cervical intraepithelial neoplasia. Am J Obstet Gynecol 1985;153:611–618. **(IV, C)**
6. Rubin M: Follow-up of an abnormal Pap test and colposcopy. In Wallis LA (ed): Textbook of Women's Health. New York, Little, Brown, 1997, p 901. **(IV, C)**
7. Apgar BS, Brotzman GL, Spitzer M, et al: Colposcopy: Principles and Practice Textbook and Atlas. Philadelphia, WB Saunders, 2002.
8. Hopman EH, Voorhorst FJ, Kenemans P, et al: Observer agreement on interpreting colposcopic images of CIN. Gynecol Oncol 1995; 58:206–209. **(III, B)**
9. Melnikow J, Nuovo J, Willan AR, et al: Natural history of cervical squamous intraepithelial lesions: a meta-analysis. Obstet Gynecol 1998; 92:727–735. **(IIa, B)**
10. Kurman RJ, Malkasian GD, Sedlis A, et al: From Papanicolaou to Bethesda: the rationale for a new cervical cytology classification. Obstet Gynecol 1991;77:779–782. **(IV, C)**
11. ALTS Group: Human papillomavirus testing for triage of women with cytologic evidence of low-grade squamous intraepithelial lesions: baseline data from randomized trial. J Natl Cancer Inst 2000; 92:397–402.
12. Moscicki AB, Shiboski S, Broering J, et al: The natural history of human papillomavirus infection as measured by repeated DNA testing in adolescent and young women. J Pediatr 1998;132:277–284. **(IIb, B)**
13. Herbert A, Smith JAE: Cervical intraepithelial neoplasia grade III (CIN III) and invasive cervical carcinoma: the yawning gap revisited and the treatment of risk. Cytopathol 1999;10:161–170. **(III, B)**
14. Duggan MA, McGregor SE, Stuart GC, et al: The natural history of CIN I lesions. Eur J Gynaecol Oncol 1998;19:338–344. **(IIa, B)**
15. Kiviat N: Natural history of cervical neoplasia: overview and update. Am J Obstet Gynecol 1996;175:1099–1104. **(III, B)**
16. Nasiell K, Roger V, Nasiell M: Behavior of mild cervical dysplasia during long-term follow-up. Obstet Gynecol 1986;67:665–669. **(IIa, B)**
17. Cuzick J, Szarewski A, Terry G, et al: Human papillomavirus testing in primary cervical screening. Lancet 1995;345:1533–1536. **(IIa, B)**
18. Park TW, Richart RM, Sun XW, Wright TC: Association between human papillomavirus type and clonal status of cervical squamous intraepithelial lesions. J Natl Cancer Inst 1996;88:317–318. **(IIb, B)**
19. Moscicki AB, Palefsky J, Gonzales J, Schoolnik GK: Human papillomavirus in sexually active adolescent females: prevalence and risk factors. Pediatr Res 1990;28:507–513. **(IIb, B)**
20. Daly SF, Doyle M, English J, et al: Can the number of cigarettes smoked predict high-grade cervical intraepithelial neoplasia among women with mildly abnormal cervical smears? Am J Obstet Gynecol 1998;179:399–402. **(IIa, B)**
21. Brisson J, Morin C, Fortier M, et al: Risk factors for cervical intraepithelial neoplasia: differences between low and high-grade lesions. Am J Epidemiol 1994;140:700–710. **(IIa, B)**
22. Ho GY, Kadish AS, Burk RD, et al: HPV 16 and cigarette smoking as risk factors for high-grade cervical intraepithelial neoplasia, Int J Cancer 1998;78:281–285. **(IIa, B)**
23. Roteli-Martins CM, Panetta K, Alves VA, et al: Cigarette smoking and high-risk HPV DNA as predisposing factors for high-grade cervical intraepithelial neoplasia (CIN) in young Brazilian women. Acta Obstet Gynecol Scand 1998;77:678–682. **(IIa, B)**
24. Schrager LK, Friedland GH, Maude D, et al: Cervical and vaginal squamous cell abnormalities in women infected with human immunodeficiency virus. J Acquir Immune Defic Syndr 1989;2:570–575. **(III, B)**
25. Schafer A, Friedmann W, Mielke M, et al: The increased frequency of cervical dysplasia-neoplasia in women infected with the human immunodeficiency virus is related to the degree of immunosuppression. Am J Obstet Gynecol 1991;164:593–599. **(III, B)**
26. Vermund SH, Kelley KF, Klein RS, et al: High risk of human papillomavirus infection and squamous intraepithelial lesions among women with symptomatic human immunodeficiency virus infection. Am J Obstet Gynecol 1992;165:392–400. **(IIb, B)**
27. Mandelbatt JS, Fahs M, Garibaldi K, et al: Association between HIV infection and cervical neoplasia: implications for clinical care of women at risk for conditions. AIDS 1992;6:173–178. **(IIa, B)**
28. Klein RS, Ho GYF, Vermund SH, et al: Risk factors for squamous intraepithelial lesions on Pap smear in women at risk for human immunodeficiency virus infection. J Infect Dis 1994;170:1404–1409. **(IIb, B)**
29. Giuliano AR, Papenfuss M, Schneider A, et al: Risk factors for high-risk type papillomavirus infection among Mexican-American women. Cancer Epidemiol Biomarkers Prev 1999;8:615–620. **(IIa, B)**
30. Ismail SM, Colclough AB, Dinnen JS, et al: Observer variation in histopathological diagnosis and grading of cervical intraepithelial neoplasia. BMJ 1989;298:707–710. **(III, B)**

31. Parakevaidis E, Kitchener HC, Miller ID, et al: A population-based study of microinvasive disease of the cervix—a colposcopic and cytologic analysis. Gynecol Oncol 1992;45:9–12. **(III, B)**

32. Hopman EH, Kenemans P, Helmerhorst TJM: Positive predictive rate of colposcopic examination of the cervix uteri: an overview of literature. Obstet Gynecol Surv 1998;53:97–106. **(III, B)**

33. Liu WM, Chao KC, Wang KI, et al: Colposcopic assessment in microinvasive carcinoma of the cervix. Chin Med J 1989;43:171–176. **(IV, C)**

34. Lurain JR, Gallup DG: Management of abnormal Papanicolaou smears in pregnancy. Obstet Gynecol 1979;53:484–488. **(IV, C)**

35. Yoonessi M, Wieckowska W, Mariniello D, et al: Cervical intraepithelial neoplasia in pregnancy. Int J Gynaecol Obstet 1982;20:111–118. **(III, B)**

36. Nevin J, Soeters R, Dehaeck K, et al: Cervical carcinoma associated with pregnancy. Obstet Gynecol Surv 1995;50:228–239. **(III, B)**

37. Ostergard DR: The effect of pregnancy on the cervical squamocolumnar junction in patients with abnormal cervical cytology. Am J Obstet Gynecol 1979;134:759–760. **(IV, C)**

38. McDonnell JM, Mylotte MJ, Gustafson RC, et al: Colposcopy in pregnancy: a twelve year review. BJOG 1981;88:414–420. **(III, B)**

39. Benedet JL, Selke PA, Nickerson KG: Colposcopic evaluation of abnormal Papanicolaou smears in pregnancy. Am J Obstet Gynecol 1987;157:932–937. **(III, B)**

40. Apgar BS, Zoschnick LB: Triage of the abnormal Papanicolaou smear in pregnancy. Prim Care Clin North Am 1998;24:483–503. **(III, B)**

41. Economos K, Veridiano NP, Delke I, et al: Abnormal cervical cytology in pregnancy: a 17-year experience. Obstet Gynecol 1993;81:915–918. **(III, B)**

42. Kiguchi K, Bibbo M, Hasegawa T, et al: Dysplasia during pregnancy: a cytologic follow-up study. J Reprod Med 1981;26:66–72. **(III, B)**

43. Hannigan EV, Whitehouse HH, Atkinson WD, et al: Cone biopsy during pregnancy. Obstet Gynecol 1982;60:450–455. **(III, B)**

44. Larsson G, Grunsdell H, Gullberg B, et al: Outcome of pregnancy after conization. Acta Obstet Gynecol Scand 1982;61:461–466. **(III, B)**

45. Greer BE, Goff BA, Koh WJ, et al: Cancer in the pregnant patient. In Hoskins WJ, Perez CA, Young RC (eds): Principles and Practice of Gynecologic Oncology, 2nd ed. Philadelphia, Lippincott-Raven, 1997, p 463.

46. Hacker NF, Berek JS, Lagasse LD, et al: Carcinoma of the cervix associated with pregnancy. Obstet Gynecol 1982;59:735–746. **(III, B)**

47. Herbst AL, Ulfelder H, Poskancer DC: Adenocarcinoma of the vagina: association of maternal stilbestrol therapy with tumor appearance in young women. N Engl J Med 1971;284–878. **(III, B)**

48. Jefferies JA, Robboy SJ, O'Brien PC, et al: Structural anomalies of the cervix and vagina in women enrolled in the diethylstilbestrol adenosis (DESAD) project. Am J Obstet Gynecol 1984;148:59–66. **(IIa, B)**

49. Wright TC, Cox JT, Massad LS, et al: 2001 Consensus guidelines for the management of women with cervical intraepithelial neoplasia. Am J Obstet Gynecol 2003;189:295–304. **(Ia, A)**

# Chapter 13 Endometriosis

David B. Redwine, MD

Endometriosis is estimated to affect approximately 10% of women, making it one of the most common diseases affecting humankind. Asymptomatic disease that has not been diagnosed may increase the prevalence even higher. For example, up to 40% of parous and apparently asymptomatic women undergoing laparoscopic tubal sterilization have been found to be affected. The ubiquitous nature of endometriosis has not necessarily led to a clear understanding of the disease. Historically, controversy has accompanied all facets of the definition, origin, diagnosis, and treatment of the disease, although modern insights are finally leading to a more accurate distillation of opinion.

## DEFINITION

Endometriosis is tissue somewhat resembling eutopic endometrium that is found outside the uterus. Although for many decades it had been believed that endometriosis was identical to endometrium, this notion is incorrect.[1] The most common and most specific symptom of endometriosis is pelvic pain, which can be of several types.

## EPIDEMIOLOGY

The true epidemiology of endometriosis has been mischaracterized by early misleading observations, which have been repeated by rote for decades. These notions have been magnified by errors of visual diagnosis at surgery.

Sampson in the 1920s noticed that 56% of married women with surgically diagnosed chocolate cysts of the ovaries had conceived. Because at that time the "normal" fertility rate among married couples was thought to be 100%, the notion was advanced that endometriosis caused infertility. The inverse side of this unfounded conclusion was that pregnancy might protect against the disease. Because none of the 23 patients in this original study was menopausal or teenaged, the notion arose that endometriosis did not occur in these age groups. As a result, this one seminal paper[2] sowed several bad seeds: that infertility was a prime symptom, that pregnancy protected against the disease, that it did not occur in teenage women, and that menopause could cure the disease. Modern clinicians will recognize these notions existing today but may not realize that of the 23 patients with chocolate cysts described by Sampson, most of the cysts were corpora lutea, not endometriotic. Some of the most widely held notions surrounding endometriosis have therefore come from women who apparently did not even have the disease. This combination of errors guaranteed the confusion that surrounds the disease today. Indeed, in retrospect, it seems simplistic to conclude that the correct theory of origin or important modern treatment principles should arise from one of the first publications on the disease.

Early onset of menses, heavy menstrual flows, müllerian outflow tract anomalies, a positive family history, and nulliparity have been positively associated with endometriosis in past studies, whereas exercise, cigarette smoking, and pregnancy have negative associations. It is unclear whether any of these associations represents a truth or is simply a result of selection bias stemming from the particular criteria used to assemble study subjects. As one example, it is clear that most women with endometriosis do not have müllerian outflow obstruction defects, which could theoretically impede the outflow of menses and predispose to reflux menstruation, thus facilitating the establishment of disease. Alleged loose epidemiologic associations do not automatically lead to helpful insights or useful therapies.

To know the true epidemiology of endometriosis requires a more perfect knowledge of the disease. Such knowledge would include, among other things, the cardinal symptoms of the disease, the age groups affected, more accurate diagnosis in the office and at surgery, and a comprehensive understanding of how endometriosis behaves in the pelvis and how it responds to treatment. Even better epidemiologic understanding may follow more complete understanding of the molecular genetic basis of endometriosis, a subject finally attracting overdue attention.[3] Currently there is no noninvasive test that is 100% accurate in diagnosing all stages of endometriosis, so the true prevalence of the disease could be known only by performing diagnostic surgery on asymptomatic women, which is not feasible from a research standpoint. Thus the fundamental misunderstandings of endometriosis have persisted for decades. Even observational papers that have sought to accurately characterize clinical aspects of the disease have turned out to be misleading.

## PATHOGENESIS

### Classical Teaching: Sampson's Theory of Reflux Menstruation

There has been a dramatic shift in opinion of the origin of endometriosis as a consequence of modern research. Sampson's theory of reflux menstruation, once the most widely accepted theory of origin of the disease, is now in the slow process of being discarded. This theory should not be used as the basis for research or clinical treatment, because it appears to be invalid.

Supporters of this theory allege the following: During menses viable particles of normal endometrium travel in a retrograde direction against the normal peristaltic action of the fallopian tubes and are regurgitated out the tubal fimbriated ends. After these endometrial particles enter the peritoneal cavity they are attacked and destroyed by some as-yet unidentified immunologic process that has not been investigated. Women destined to develop endometriosis were felt to have a defective immune system that does not attack these particles, allowing them to continue to exist and to attach to peritoneal surfaces where they proliferate, invade, and become the disease called endometriosis. The ovaries are the most frequently involved sites of occurrence of the disease because these organs are the pelvic surfaces closest to the tubal ostia and are the first to receive the regurgitated endometrial tissue fragments. Otherwise, the distribution of pelvic disease results from a combination of several factors: the effect of gravity and the clockwise circulation of peritoneal fluid down the descending colon and sigmoid, across the pelvis from left to right, and up the ascending colon. Although billions of endometrial tissue particles or individual cells have been refluxed in probably tens or hundreds of millions of women over the years, the important initial steps of attachment, proliferation, and invasion of refluxed endometrial cells all occur sequentially in less than 24 hours. This is why it has been and will always be impossible to obtain the important photomicrographic proofs of attachment, proliferation and invasion. Such rapid attachment, proliferation, and invasion is also why studies on "invisible" microscopic endometriosis[4] have not found these important initiating steps.

Because reflux menstruation can't explain all sites of occurrence of disease, endometriosis may have multiple other pathogenetic origins.

### Modern Thinking

A more modern theory of the origin of endometriosis would embrace current knowledge of the disease, including the following known proven facts, which directly oppose the precepts of the theory of reflux menstruation, as well as those of vascular or lymphatic spread:

- Endometriosis is not identical to endometrium, but differs in dozens of fundamental and profound ways.[1] Endo-

metriosis therefore cannot be an autotransplant as predicted by Sampson's theory, because autotransplants remain similar or identical to the eutopic tissue of origin.

- The initial attachment of refluxed endometrium to the peritoneum and secondary proliferation and invasion of these cells hasn't been demonstrated by photomicrography in biopsies taken from human females. Regardless of how short a time attachment, proliferation, and invasion may span, the billions of instances of this occurrence guarantee that such evidence should exist by now. Because such photographic proof would be simple to obtain, the lack of such photographs is the most concrete evidence against the theory of reflux menstruation.

- The most common site of involvement is the cul-de-sac, not the ovaries, as originally suggested by Sampson, but endometriosis can occur in remote locations outside the peritoneal cavity, as well as in males.

- Endometriosis seems to be positionally static, sometimes locally invasive with surrounding fibromuscular metaplasia, but there is no evidence of progressive geographic spread throughout the pelvis with advancing age, as Sampson's theory would predict. Most untreated women do not have surgically proven progression of disease. The age-related evolution in color appearance of endometriosis may spuriously give the impression of disease spread if early, subtle disease was not recognized.

- Endometriosis occurs in consistent patterns in the pelvis, intestines, and diaphragm, not in a random distribution.

- The cure rate by conservative excision is greater than 50% per surgery, not 0% as predicted by Sampson's theory. Cure is more difficult in teenagers and in women with widespread disease.

- If recurrent endometriosis is found after excision, it is virtually always superficial, with fewer areas of pelvic or intestinal involvement.

- Endometriosis is only very rarely associated with müllerian defects, which would theoretically facilitate reflux menstruation.

- Pulmonary endometriosis is extremely rare, as are coexisting cardiac atrioventricular septal defects. Hematogenous spread of endometriosis would require a high prevalence of either or both of these pathologic entities, so hematogenous spread through the uterine veins can be ruled out as a major origin of disease.

- Lymphatic endometriosis is extremely rare, effectively ruling out lymphatic spread of disease.

In the vacuum left after discarding reflux menstruation, hematogenous spread, and lymphatic spread as theories of origin of endometriosis, coelomic metaplasia of embryologically patterned mesenchyme and epithelium or embryologically patterned rests emerges as the leading candidate for the origin of endometriosis. At the moment of conception, polygenic, environmental, and chance factors combine to result in embryologically patterned tracts of tissue being laid down between 6 and 8 weeks of embryogenesis. These tracts of tissue generally follow the pathways of normal organogenesis of the female pelvic organs across the posterior coelomic cavity, but can be found elsewhere in the body, depending on defects of differentiation and migration that may occur in the tiny volume of the embryo. Incomplete dedifferentiation of the müllerian tract in males sets the stage for later occurrence of disease in the bladder or prostate of elderly males undergoing estrogen therapy for palliation of symptoms due to metastatic prostate cancer. In females, these embryologically patterned tracts either already contain endometriosis or consist of substrate, which may undergo metaplasia into endometriosis and the associated fibromuscular metaplasia, which can be seen when the disease involves parenchymal structures such as the uterosacral ligaments, intestine, or bladder. These tracts are most commonly found within the posterior pelvic peritoneum because that is the main migratory pathway of organogenesis, but undifferentiated substrate may extend more deeply. It is possible that when ovarian production of estrogen begins at pubarche, these tracts exhibit varying degrees of biologic response, depending on the potentialities imparted during embryogenesis.

Early endometriosis in teenagers can be colorless because capillaries are not prominent. Individual glands, however, are readily visible to the trained surgeon's eye, appearing like specks of tapioca. The glandular elements of endometriosis secrete a paracrine substance that may cause an inflammatory response in surrounding tissue and destabilize adjacent capillaries, resulting in local fibrosis and occasional hemorrhage. Underlying fibromuscular metaplasia may occur either as a result of this paracrine secretion or because of hormonal stimulation of mesenchymal substrate. With the passage of time, surrounding fibrosis may give a whitish or yellowish appearance to the disease, and fibromuscular metaplasia will result in whitish nodularity. Because glands do not bleed and not all endometriotic lesions are well-vascularized, hemorrhage is not a consistent histologic or morphologic feature of endometriosis, even in the presence of advanced angiogenesis or invasive disease. Blood is not a product of the glands and stroma of endometriosis, but comes from blood vessels, so it is somewhat incorrect to say that endometriosis bleeds. In some older patients with more biologically active disease or leakage of chocolate fluid from endometrioma cysts, a dark, hemorrhagic component may seem more apparent, although a fibrotic component may still prevail. This age-related evolution in color appearance of the disease is largely due to reactive changes surrounding areas of active endometriosis. These changes, such as fibrosis, hemorrhage, and fibromuscular metaplasia, are sequelae of endometriosis. Older patients do not have more areas of pelvic involvement, and most untreated patients do not have progression of disease between surgical investigations. Most women will have developed their lifetime load of endometriosis by their early twenties, with ongoing fibromuscular metaplasia or enlargement of ovarian endometrioma cysts occurring in a minority.

This modern theory of origin predicts exactly what is seen after surgical excision. If all embryologically patterned tracts of tissue have changed into endometriosis, as has usually occurred by the mid-twenties, removal of these tracts can cure the disease. If some tracts have not undergone metaplasia, as might be the case in teenagers, these tracts might escape excision because there is no distinguishing characteristic that would allow the surgeon to identify them for removal. In such cases, a certain rate of recurrence might be expected, especially in women who had undergone excision as teenagers, although the amount of disease at reoperation is typically less than that found at the initial surgery. After excision in some patients, müllerian-directed epithelial growth factors associated with tissue healing may allow metaplastic formation of superficial deposits of endometriosis around the margins of an excised area or, rarely, in the center of an excised area.

## SYMPTOMS

The symptoms associated with endometriosis are pain and infertility, pain being the more common and more specific symptom. Although endometriosis may be the most common cause of pelvic pain seen by gynecologists, not all pain or infertility in women with endometriosis is necessarily due to the disease. Less common causes of pelvic pain include other diseases of the uterus, tubes, or ovaries; intestinal diseases; urologic processes; muscular syndromes of the pelvis or abdominal wall; and pelvic or abdominal adhesions. Given the widespread distribution of estrogen and progesterone receptors throughout the body, some of these other nongynecologic causes of pain may also exhibit aggravation before or during menses. Accurate diagnosis of pain specifically due to endometriosis and prediction of the patient's prognosis after treatment are both made more difficult by this lack of exact correlation of symptoms with the disease. Nonetheless, women with endometriosis can exhibit consistent patterns of symptoms highly suggestive of the disease because the sites of disease can produce characteristic symptoms.

### Dysmenorrhea
*Dysmenorrhea* refers to painful menses and is often the first symptom of endometriosis. A common history in women with endometriosis is the memory of severe pain with menses from an early age, frequently from menarche or even before. The term immediately brings to mind uterine cramping as the prototypical characteristic of dysmenorrhea. However, clinicians must be cautious about blaming the uterus for all pain during menses. Pain during menses could be due either to uterine cramps or to simultaneous occurrence of menstrually timed aggravation of nonuterine pain, including endometriosis. Dysmenorrhea is therefore a common but somewhat nonspecific symptom associated with endometriosis. Both endometriosis pain and uterine pain can radiate into the sacral region, whereas uterine pain can radiate up to the umbilicus and into the upper anterior thighs.

### Nonmenstrual Pelvic Pain
Menstrual pain can worsen in severity and duration over several years and may eventually begin to occur in the luteal phase of the ovarian hormonal cycle, before menses begins. The pain may cause absence from school for up to several days each month, and sport or social activity may be curtailed due to the pain. The pain frequently is trivialized by family and friends as "just cramps" even though it is not necessarily directly associated with menses, and the patient is encouraged to "just deal with it" as part of being a woman. The patient may be seen as somewhat of a malingerer, especially if seen by a physician who finds nothing apparently wrong on abdominal examination or diagnostic imaging scan. This trivialization of the patient's pain by family, friends, and medical practitioners leads to a delay in diagnosis of 10 to 15 years in many cases.

# General Gynecology

By late teenage years, the patient may be aware of a sharp character of the pain and may use adjectives such as "stinging," "burning," or "knifelike" to describe the pain. When describing her pain, the patient may clench a fist as if holding an invisible knife and stab at her pelvis or make a twisting thrust of the unseen blade toward the interviewer. The pain can eventually begin around the time of ovulation, in which case it may be diagnosed as simple ovulation pain, and may increase in severity as the menstrual flow approaches. During menses, the pain can be greatly aggravated; some patients may also be able to discriminate the occurrence of uterine cramping on top of pain that began before the flow. The pain may abate after menses, although some patients may still be aware of pain at a lower level even during the "good" times of the monthly cycle.

## Dyspareunia, Dyschezia
Endometriosis is most commonly found in the cul-de-sac, medial broad ligaments, and uterosacral ligaments (Table 13-1), where it can cause specific and consistent symptoms. These common areas of involvement are located immediately adjacent to both the end of the vagina and the rectum. Accordingly, any physical stimulation to these diseased areas can be painful. Endometriosis of the cul-de-sac and uterosacral ligaments will frequently be associated with dyspareunia and painful bowel movements during menses because these actions will mechanically impact on the disease.

Obliteration of the cul-de-sac occurs when the rectum is adherent across the posterior cervix or lower uterine segment with simultaneous adherence to the uterosacral ligaments. This signifies invasive disease of the uterosacral ligaments, cul-de-sac, and usually the anterior wall of the rectum. Sacral back pain, rectal pain, rectal pain with flatus or intercourse, rectal pain with sitting, and painful bowel movements throughout the month are

characteristic symptoms of obliteration of the cul-de-sac. Many patients describe rectal pain with vaginal intercourse. Because intestinal endometriosis rarely penetrates to the mucosa, cyclic rectal bleeding is an uncommon sign, even with significant bowel wall involvement.

## Lateral Pelvic Pain
Endometrioma cysts of the ovaries can cause chronic ipsilateral pain and fullness due to swelling of the cyst. Intermittent sharper exacerbations of pain may occur, with leakage of cyst contents. Such leakage can cause pain that can last for several days and can initially mimic an acute abdominal emergency. Superficial endometriosis of the ovarian cortex appears to be asymptomatic. Periovarian adhesions due to endometriosis can contribute to lateral pain because an ovarian cyst of any type can increase in size and place traction on such adhesions. This pulls on the peritoneum where the adhesion inserts and can result in pain.

Pain caused by invasive disease of a uterosacral ligament can occasionally radiate into the back or upper posterior thigh. Endometriosis of the pelvic sidewalls or lateral to the sigmoid colon or cecum near either pelvic brim can also cause ipsilateral pain. Endometriosis invading from the peritoneum to involve the sciatic or obturator nerve can cause pain or motor dysfunction in the distribution of those nerves, especially during menses.

Constriction of a ureter occurring due to entrapping fibrosis extending from a large uterosacral ligament nodule can cause both ipsilateral low pelvic pain as well as ipsilateral renal or ureteral colic. Actual invasion of the ureter by endometriosis is rare. When the constriction occurs slowly over the course of several years, ureteric symptoms may be absent, even when the ipsilateral kidney is destroyed by ureteral obstruction. When an endometrioma cyst compresses a ureter or when the ureter is constricted by surrounding fibrosis or invaded by endometriosis, cyclic stricture of the ureter may occur, especially in the luteal or menstrual phase of the cycle. This can produce cyclic symptoms of ureteral obstruction such as flank pain and backache.

## Lower Back Pain
Endometriosis of the uterosacral ligaments may radiate pain into the lower back, especially if invasive disease or obliteration of the cul-de-sac is present. Uterine pain can also radiate to this area.

## Bladder Pain, Frequency, Dysuria
Superficial lesions of the bladder peritoneum are usually asymptomatic. Lesions invading the muscularis may cause symptoms of dysuria and urgency throughout the month, with some perimenstrual aggravation of pain. Because the bladder mucosa is rarely involved, hematuria is rare. Occasionally, frequency and urgency seem to be the result of irritation of the pelvic plexus by invasive disease of the uterosacral ligaments. Interstitial cystitis can cause bladder pain, and this can worsen during menses also, contributing some confusion to the case of a woman with bladder pain.

## Irregular Vaginal Bleeding
Although it is said that irregular or heavy menses may occur with increased frequency among women with endometriosis, this

| Table 13-1 Sites of Pelvic Involvement in 2115 Patients with Biopsy-proven Endometriosis* | |
| --- | --- |
| **Pelvic Site** | **Number (Frequency) of Involvement** |
| Cul-de-sac | 1521 (71.9%) |
| Left broad ligament | 1038 (49.1%) |
| Left uterosacral ligament | 878 (41.5%) |
| Right broad ligament | 871 (41.2%) |
| Right uterosacral ligament | 795 (37.6%) |
| Bladder | 600 (28.4%) |
| Left ovary | 233 (11.0%) |
| Right ovary | 209 (9.9%) |
| Left fallopian tube | 134 (6.3%) |
| Right fallopian tube | 90 (4.3% |
| Left round ligament | 49 (2.3%) |
| Right round ligament | 27 (1.3%) |

*Treated at the Endometriosis Treatment Program at St. Charles Medical Center, Bend, OR. 476 patients with obliteration of the cul-de-sac or Stage IV disease have been excluded because most patients do not have such disease and most clinicians will not commonly encounter such disease.

is a very nonspecific multifactorial symptom that contributes little or nothing to the diagnosis. Vaginal endometriosis occurs in the posterior fornix, and this can bleed perimenstrually or after hysterectomy. Vaginal endometriosis represents extension of invasive endometriosis of a uterosacral ligament or of a rectal nodule associated with obliteration of the cul-de-sac.

## Partial Bowel Obstruction

Symptoms of partial bowel obstruction during menses occur almost exclusively with nodular disease of the ileum. With progression of the nodularity and ileal distortion, partial obstructive symptoms are possible throughout the month. Symptoms of partial obstruction due to colonic endometriosis are rare due to the larger diameter of the large intestine. Complete bowel obstruction due to endometriosis almost never occurs.

## Irritable Bowel Syndrome

Nodular disease of the large or small bowel may be associated with alternating constipation and diarrhea, bloating, or intestinal cramping. Peritoneal endometriosis without bowel involvement can also cause irritable bowel symptoms, apparently because the bowel can be irritated by laying against these endometriotic areas or irritated by the increased volume of reactive peritoneal fluid that can be associated with endometriosis.

## Perimenstrual Chest and Shoulder Pain

Diaphragmatic endometriosis is rare and occurs most frequently on the right hemidiaphragm. Ipsilateral chest and shoulder pain during or just before menses is a common symptom. This pain can sometimes radiate into the neck or down the arm and can be described as resembling a muscular ache. Some patients may progress to suffer symptoms all month long, with severe menstrual aggravation of pain. Occasionally a patient may need to sleep in a sitting position to relieve the pain.

## Abdominal Wall Pain

Umbilical endometriosis presents as a small darkly hemorrhagic nodule located usually in the inferior midline of the umbilicus. Pain and swelling may occur during menses, occasionally associated with a slight bloody discharge from the umbilicus.

Scar endometriosis occurs most commonly after cesarean sections, but can also be found after hysterectomy. A rare and specialized form of scar endometriosis has occurred after prenatal diagnostic amniocentesis. Scar endometriosis manifests as a slowly growing lump, which may enlarge slightly and become more painful during menses.

Inguinal endometriosis arises from nodular endometriosis of the round ligament as it traverses the inguinal canal, causing a tender lump most commonly found overlying the right pubic ramus, which may be more painful and slightly larger during menses. This lesion is one of the earliest types reported, probably because it was so obvious on examination and presented an easy surgical target.

## Nonpelvic Pain

With increasingly deranged differentiation and migration of müllerian tract derivatives during embryogenesis, endometriosis can be found outside the abdominal cavity, with pain as a result. Endometriosis has been reported to involve the posterior thigh, posterior knee, left neck, brain, cauda equina, thorax, and liver in females and the bladder and prostate in elderly males undergoing estrogen therapy for palliation of metastatic prostate cancer.

## Asymptomatic Endometriosis

Apparently asymptomatic endometriosis may be diagnosed during pelvic surgery done for other reasons, such as tubal sterilizations. After removal of such "asymptomatic" disease, some previously "asymptomatic" patients may realize for the first time in their lives that they were, in fact, symptomatic. The visual appearance of endometriosis does not guarantee whether the disease is symptomatic or not. Disease with a subtle morphology may hurt, whereas disease with a spectacular morphology may not.

## Infertility

Fecundity is decreased in women with endometriosis compared to age-matched women without endometriosis. Although fertility may be lower because of endometriosis, it is not eliminated. Even women with untreated severe disease may become pregnant, although success takes longer. When a patient has unsuccessfully attempted pregnancy for 2 years or more, this may indicate some other cause of infertility besides endometriosis, especially if superficial disease is present. Therefore, in women with long-standing infertility, treatment directed at endometriosis will be less successful because this group of women will be more likely to have some other cause of infertility. Important among the other causes of infertility among women with endometriosis is the age-related decline in fertility of both females and males.

Many women with infertility due to endometriosis also suffer from pain. Rarely will a patient present only with the symptom of infertility. After successful treatment of their disease, however, some of these "pain-free" infertile women will realize that they actually were having pain as well; the pain was thought to be low-level or "normal."

# DIAGNOSIS

Because endometriosis is the most common cause of pelvic pain in reproductive-age women, it should always lead the list of differential diagnoses. A presumptive diagnosis of endometriosis can be made in most patients on the basis of a characteristic history of pain and characteristic findings on pelvic examination. Abdominal examination is rarely helpful, although occasionally a large ovarian cyst will be palpated, or nonspecific direct tenderness in the lower quadrants will be present. Leakage of an ovarian endometrioma can be associated with symptoms of an acute abdomen initially, with clearing of the pain spontaneously over several days.

## Pelvic Examination

The pelvic examination is important both for the diagnosis of endometriosis as well as for prediction of the likelihood of pain relief following surgical treatment. Given the ubiquitous nature of the disease, gynecologists in training must first become expert in mastering the pelvic examination as it relates to endometriosis, then later worry about the examination as it relates to less common entities such as pelvic infection, ovarian cysts, pelvic adhesions, uterine retroversion, and uterine enlargement.

# General Gynecology

The external genital examination will rarely yield any useful information contributing to the diagnosis of endometriosis, although rare cases of endometriosis of an episiotomy scar will be manifest as a tender lump, which is occasionally discolored by underlying hemorrhage and which is more obvious with menses.

Speculum examination of the cervix may reveal hemorrhagic spots less than 3 mm in diameter located within the squamous epithelium. Occasionally there may be a droplet of blood on the epithelial surface adjacent to the spot (Fig. 13-1). This may be cervical endometriosis, although biopsy is the only way to be sure. The speculum should also be directed posteriorly to examine the posterior vaginal fornix. Often, cases of nodular endometriosis of the uterosacral ligaments or cul-de-sac that are invading the vagina are missed because the speculum is used only to examine the cervix, and the posterior blade hides the lesion. Endometriosis of the posterior fornix may have several morphologies, including subtle epithelial piling (see Fig. 13-1), small bluish cysts, and red hemorrhagic fleshy lesions.

Manual pelvic examination for endometriosis should focus on four specific areas: the uterus, the left and right uterosacral ligaments, and the cul-de-sac. Although endometriosis uncommonly involves the uterus, the uterus may still be an important cause of pain unrelated to endometriosis. During bimanual palpation of the uterus, the size, shape, position, and consistency should of course be noted. However, one of the most important things the examiner can do is to gently squeeze the uterus between the fingers of the external and internal hands to see what degree of tenderness might be present and whether this reproduces any component of the patient's pain. When the uterus is retroverted, it is almost impossible to determine if it might be a source of pain because only its posterior wall can be palpated through the cul-de-sac. Any tenderness ascribed to the uterus when uterine retroversion is present could be caused either by the uterus or by cul-de-sac endometriosis.

After examining the uterus, ovarian enlargement and tenderness should be sought. Normal ovaries are not always palpable. Enlarged ovaries are easier to detect but not always discretely because the adhesive process associated with advanced cases of endometriosis may cause the uterus and enlarged ovaries to move as one indistinct mass.

The examiner's attention should now shift to the most important part of the examination: gentle palpation of the cul-de-sac and uterosacral ligaments. These are among the areas most commonly involved by disease, and these areas can be easily reached by most physicians during examination, although the length of the examining physician's fingers becomes an important limiting factor. The external examining hand will not be helpful in detecting positive findings in these commonly involved areas because the external hand cannot press deeply enough to reach the posterior pelvis. Also, discomfort associated with attempting this deep palpatory maneuver with the external hand will mask positive findings. Therefore, the cul-de-sac and both uterosacral ligaments should be examined only with the examiner's internal fingers, without any use of the external examining hand. Each of these three areas should be gently palpated or stroked while watching the patient's face. A normal pelvic examination should not provoke pain. If the patient's face winces, or if she arches her back or pushes away from the end

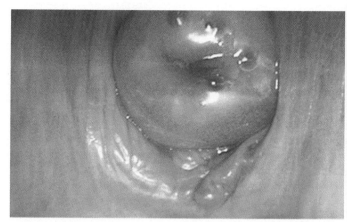

**Figure 13-1 Endometriosis of the vagina occurs in the posterior fornix and represents extension of nodular disease of a uterosacral ligament or a rectal nodule.** Such disease can be easily seen if the speculum is directed toward the fornix. Some lesions are hemorrhagic. Other lesions, such as this one, may be manifest as epithelial piling without hemorrhage. Notice the superficial cervical endometriosis, which appears to be asymptomatic.

of the table, these are positive findings suggestive of endometriosis. Extremely rarely the anterior vaginal wall may have nodularity and tenderness, which is an indication of invasive disease of the trigone region of the bladder. Nodularity in any of these areas should be noted, and the patient should be asked if palpation of each particular site reproduces any symptoms. This clinical pain mapping is helpful because nodularity, tenderness on examination, and reproduction of symptoms by examination are findings predictive of a better prognosis following surgical removal of endometriosis in these areas.[5]

Some patients cannot describe their pain succinctly and may have equivocal or no findings on pelvic examination. These patients may have some other reason for pain besides endometriosis and the prognosis for pain relief following treatment for endometriosis is low.

## Diagnostic Tests

The morphological manifestations of endometriosis are most frequently rather two-dimensional with little invasion or three-dimensional volume. Ultrasound, magnetic resonance imaging (MRI) or computed tomography scans are therefore negative in most cases but may be helpful in obese patients, who are difficult to examine, or if a uterine component of pain is present. If a patient has uterine symptoms, an abnormal uterine scan, and has completed her child-bearing, hysterectomy may be a rational treatment option.

Because intestinal endometriosis rarely penetrates from the seromuscular layer through to the mucosa, intestinal barium studies and colonoscopy are notoriously negative in all but the most advanced cases. Advanced cases of obliteration of the cul-de-sac with involvement of the anterior rectal wall may be suggested by MRI or rectal ultrasound, but symptoms and pelvic examination will have already suggested the presence of such disease even if scans are not performed. When lesser degrees of nodularity and tenderness are found on pelvic examination, imaging scans will usually be negative.

Endometriosis of the urinary tract will not always be found on scans either. Like intestinal endometriosis, bladder disease beginning on the peritoneum rarely penetrates through to the mucosa, so cystoscopy is rarely positive. Constriction of one or both ureters may be identified by imaging tests in patients with suggestive symptoms, with silent loss of renal function identified in extreme cases.

Ovarian enlargement may be undetectable by pelvic examination in some patients, either due to obesity interfering with the accuracy of the examination or because ovarian size is still below the threshold of clinical detection by the individual examiner. Imaging scans can arrive at an accurate assessment of solid and cystic portions of the ovary, the diameter of a cyst, the thickness of the wall of the cyst, and the consistency of the fluid contents. Ovaries involved by endometrioma cysts are frequently described as "complex" on scans because they have a solid component, which can represent normal ovarian tissue, and a cystic component, which is thick walled and filled with hyper-echogenic fluid representing old thick bloody ("chocolate") fluid. Hemorrhagic corpora lutea may have a similar imaging signature. Although peritoneal fluid volume can be increased with endo-metriosis, frank ascites is uncommon. Findings suggestive of ovarian malignancy include thick-walled septations of cysts, internal or external excrescences, and associated ascites.

In the uncommon instance when diagnostic imaging is positive or extremely suggestive of endometriosis, the patient's symptoms and findings on pelvic examination are frequently flagrant, and the correct diagnosis of endometriosis will be obvious at surgery. When imaging is negative but disease exists, the findings will also be obvious to the trained surgeon's eye. Surgical investigation is thus more accurate than any scan. Positive scans focus attention on their findings, and other areas of disease not identified by scanning can be overlooked during surgery. For example, an ovarian endometrioma cyst will be easily identified on imaging scans, and the surgeon may focus only on its removal during surgery, leaving other areas of endometriosis behind. Negative scans do not guarantee absence of pathology and should not be used to ignore a patient's complaints. The patient's pain is the most important factor in the decision to treat, and the pelvic examination is usually more helpful than any scan.

The CA 125 level may be elevated or normal with endo-metriosis. This test may also be elevated or normal with a variety of other gynecologic pathologies, including adhesions, adenomyosis, leiomyomata, ovarian cancer, or unknown causes. For these reasons, the CA 125 test lacks the sensitivity and specificity that would make it a useful test for diagnosing endometriosis.

## Surgical Diagnosis

Surgery is the most accurate measure of the sites of and extent of involvement and is most commonly done by laparoscopy. The visual appearances possible with endometriosis are protean, the spectrum ranging from the extremely subtle to the spectacular. All visual manifestations may be present in a single patient. Errors of diagnosis can be made at either end of this morpho-logic spectrum. Invisible microscopic endometriosis has not been proven to be a concern in diagnosis, treatment, prognosis, or recurrence.[5] The incidence of unanticipated endometriosis existing in apparently visually normal peritoneum is directly

| Table 13-2 |  |
| :-- | :-- |
| Incidence of Unanticipated Endometriosis in Visually Normal Peritoneum, According to Distance of Observation |  |
| **Distance** | **Incidence of Unanticipated Endometriosis** |
| Approximately 5 cm at laparotomy | 25% |
| 5 cm at laparoscopy | 13% |
| 4 cm at laparoscopy | 6% |
| 2 cm at laparoscopy | 2% |
| 1 cm at laparoscopy | 0% |

From Redwine DB: Invisible microscopic endometriosis: a review. Gynecol Obstet Invest 2003;55:63–67.

related to magnification used during surgical inspection and can be effectively reduced to almost zero with near-contact laparoscopy (Table 13-2).

There is a premium on accurate identification of early forms of the disease, because failure to identify extant disease will give the spurious impression of the development of new disease or of progressive geographic spread if previously unidentified subtle disease has become more obvious by the time surgery is done.[6]

Women in the teenage years may have disease that is extremely subtle and colorless, sometimes with adjacent clear papules, which appear to be localized collections of glandular secretions either on or just beneath the peritoneal surface (Figs. 13-2 and 13-3). Close examination with the tip of the laparoscope within 1 cm of the pelvic surfaces will disclose individual gland/stroma complexes of endometriosis without surrounding hemorrhage or fibrosis. These findings may be missed if only panoramic viewing of the pelvis is performed. In some patients the disease is stable in appearance over the patient's

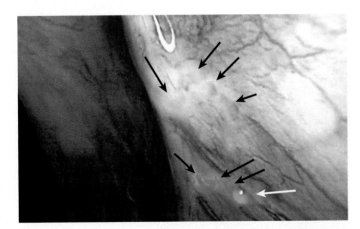

**Figure 13-2 Subtle endometriosis of the right uterosacral ligament in a young woman.** Individual gland/stroma complexes of endometriosis are seen *(black arrows)*. These colorless, clear, macular lesions secrete a paracrine substance, which may remain trapped beneath the peritoneal surface, although occasionally clear papules *(white arrow)* may be present, which appear to be extrusion of secretions trapped under a monolayer of peritoneum.

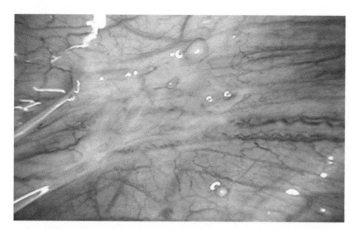

**Figure 13-3   With the passage of time, these subtle lesions of the left broad ligament are associated with increased clear papular change, faint whitish fibrosis, and beginning angiogenesis but no hemorrhagic change.**

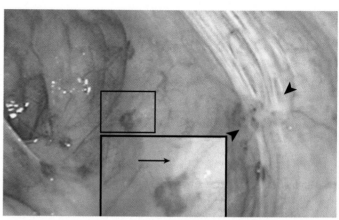

**Figure 13-5   With the passage of time, further hemorrhage and fibrosis may occur.** A hemorrhagic area of the right cul-de-sac *(small box)* is seen on magnification to lie adjacent to a clear macule of endometriosis *(large box)* and may contain a gland/stroma complex of endometriosis obscured beneath the hemorrhage. The base of the right uterosacral ligament demonstrates thickening of whitish fibrosis and entrapment of old dark blood between the arrowheads.

symptomatic lifetime; in others, the predetermined biologic potential of the disease will result in reactive sequelae, which can change the morphology of the disease over time.

With the passage of time, the paracrine secretions of endometriosis may cause superficial peritoneal fibrosis surrounding the lesions, with a resultant whitish coloration. If the paracrine secretions destabilize adjacent capillaries, a hemorrhagic appearance may be associated with the disease, resulting in either a reddish or blackish hue adjacent to the disease (Figs. 13-4 and 13-5). Occasionally the paracrine secretions can stimulate angiogenesis, and some lesions may be associated with adjacent or overlying obvious (Fig. 13-6) or subtle (Fig. 13-7) neovascularity. Particularly active lesions will continue to incite reactive fibrosis, and the scarring over the active lesion will become thicker as well as whitish or yellowish and will obscure visualization of the gland/stroma complexes, which may formerly have been

visible. This is the well-known morphology of "burned-in" endometriosis (Fig. 13-8). This formerly was termed *burned-out* endometriosis, a term that erroneously implied to several generations of gynecologists that no active disease was present, when actually very active disease has simply been buried under thick, reactive fibrosis. Classic "black powderburn" lesions tend to be most common in women after age 30. Biopsy of such lesions may simply return old hemorrhage, because the endometriosis responsible for provoking the bleeding may be some distance away. With further passage of time, pelvic areas predestined to undergo fibromuscular metaplasia will do so, leading to an increased volume of disease.

The uterus can occasionally be involved by endometriosis (Fig. 13-9), and this represents a clinical problem of diagnosis

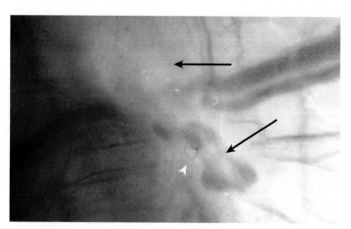

**Figure 13-4   Subtle lesions of endometriosis *(black arrows)* of the right bladder peritoneum with adjacent dark hemorrhage.** Faint whitish fibrosis is forming within the peritoneum, slightly obscuring the retroperitoneal vascular pattern. Angiogenesis is beginning, evidenced by a tiny capillary loop *(white arrowhead)*.

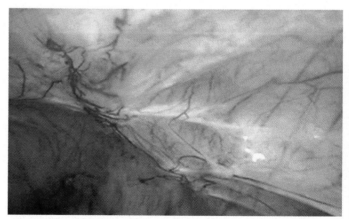

**Figure 13-6   This endometriosis of the cul-de-sac exhibits thicker fibrosis and advanced angiogenesis, which some lesions display over time.** The individual gland/stroma complexes of endometriosis are now largely hidden beneath the increasing fibromuscular metaplasia.

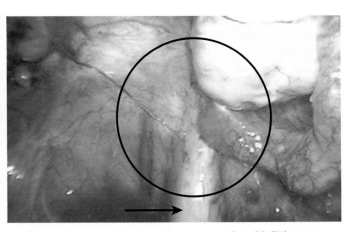

**Figure 13-7 Advanced invasive disease can exist with little or no hemorrhagic changes.** This patient has partial obliteration of the cul-de-sac, with the rectum *(arrow)* tented up to the right uterosacral ligament. The right ovary and fimbriated end of the tube are also adherent to and obscure this area *(circle)*. Invasive disease of the uterosacral ligament and anterior rectal wall is present without any hemorrhagic change, although mild neovascularity overlies the entire region.

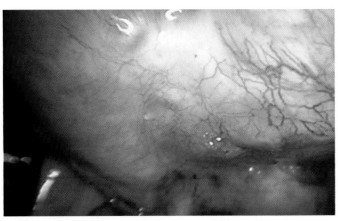

**Figure 13-9 The uterus is infrequently involved by endometriosis, most commonly on its posterior surface.** The disease can be manifest as subserosal collections of dark blood associated with unseen gland/stroma complexes, sometimes with impressive neovascular changes.

that is distinctly different from peritoneal disease. Whereas normal peritoneum is transparent and underlying disease can be separated from identifiable normal surrounding structures, the uterus is opaque. Endometriosis on the serosa may be isolated or may signify the underlying presence of invasive disease of the myometrium, which cannot be easily distinguished or separated from normal uterine tissue.

Fibromuscular metaplasia is most common in parenchymal structures, such as the uterosacral ligaments (Fig. 13-10) or the muscularis of the bladder or bowel (Figs. 13-11 and 13-12), in which case the morphology at surgery will be nodular and the histologic picture will be adenomyotic. The age-related evolution in color appearance of endometriosis can give the spurious impression that new disease is appearing.

Not all peritoneal epithelial changes are due to endometriosis. Laser vaporization can leave behind flecks of carbon as well as treatment granulomas, which overlie incompletely treated endometriosis (Fig. 13-13). Carbon deposits can induce a foreign body giant cell reaction, which can be a new source of pain. Carbon may mimic old hemorrhage associated with endometriosis, but its chief contribution to the diagnosis of endometriosis is the possibility that incompletely treated endometriosis lies beneath it. Laser vaporization can also cause superficial adhesions overlying incompletely treated endometriosis (Figs. 13-14 and 13-15).

All pelvic and intestinal areas involved by endometriosis can be visualized by a laparoscope inserted through an umbilical port. Occasionally atraumatic graspers may be helpful in

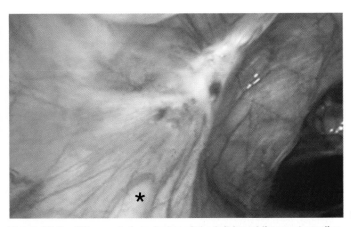

**Figure 13-8 This powderburn lesion of the left broad ligament overlies the path of the left ureter *(asterisk)*.** Black hemorrhagic changes are present both in the center of the dense yellow-white fibrosis as well as at its edge. The most active disease is buried in the center of the yellowish fibrotic nodule. When the fibrosis eventually completely obscures the hemorrhagic component, the malapropism "burned out" disease might be applied, instead of the correct term of "burned in" disease.

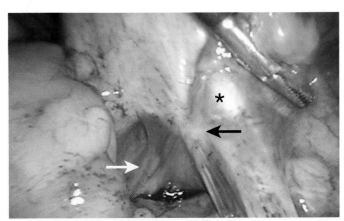

**Figure 13-10 The right uterosacral ligament *(black arrow)* is involved by invasive endometriosis manifest as a yellowish nodule with no associated hemorrhage.** The normal rectum *(white arrow)* is slightly tethered to this nodule, which will histologically show fibromuscular tissue surrounding gland/stroma complexes of endometriosis. A small right ovarian cyst *(asterisk)* is also adherent to this region.

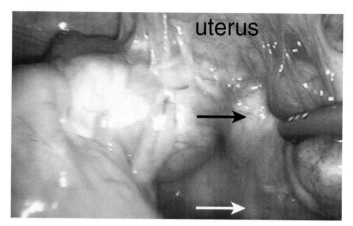

**Figure 13-11    Obliteration of the cul-de-sac.** The normal rectum *(white arrow)* can be seen to lead to a portion of the rectum which is rounded in appearance *(black arrow)* and adherent to both uterosacral ligaments. The ovaries are also adherent to their ipsilateral uterosacral ligaments. When the wall of the rectum is rounded, the muscularis is involved by significant endometriosis and some type of rectal surgery will be necessary to ensure complete removal of all invasive disease.

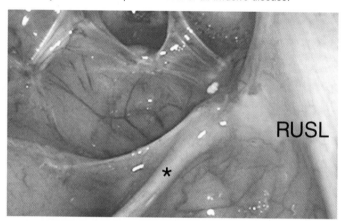

**Figure 13-12    The normal rectum *(asterisk)* leads into a small rectal nodule which is fused with a retroperitoneal nodule extending from the adjacent right uterosacral ligament (RUSL).** Nearby, areas of active endometriosis in the cul-de-sac are associated with peritoneal scarring and retraction.

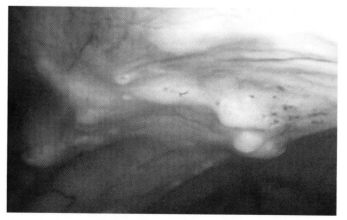

**Figure 13-13    Laser vaporization can leave behind abnormalities that can be confused with endometriosis.** Discrete flecks of carbon are usually easily distinguished from hemorrhage because of their dark black color with sharp borders. The white papular lesions are composed of a combination of incompletely treated endometriosis and foreign body giant cell reaction.

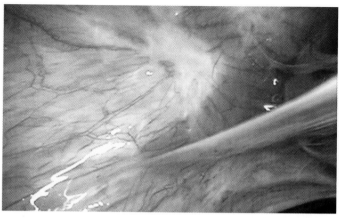

**Figure 13-14    This patient underwent laser vaporization of endometriosis performed by an experienced surgeon.** At second-look laparoscopy, persistent superficial endometriosis was present, as well as filmy adhesions induced by laser therapy.

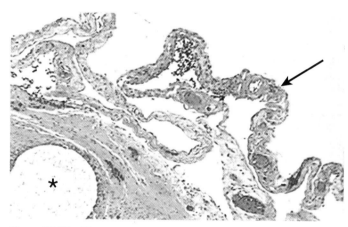

**Figure 13-15    Photomicroscopy of the lesion seen in Figure 13-14.** Superficial filmy adhesions with slight vascularity *(arrow)* were present over untreated superficial endometriosis *(asterisk).*

examining the ileum or redundant sigmoid colon loops, because even large nodules can be initially hidden (Fig. 13-16). Disease of the ileum can be superficial, in which case it is distributed linearly along the antimesenteric aspect of the ileal wall, or invasive and nodular (Fig. 13-17), in which case symptoms of obstruction may be present. Endometriosis of the appendix is often manifest as a white fibrotic area, which may curl the appendix upon itself so that it cannot be straightened out (Fig. 13-18). Disease of the cecum is rare and is frequently located near the base of the appendix (Fig. 13-19).

Symptomatic endometriosis of the diaphragm usually involves the posterior diaphragm and is not always visible with a laparoscope inserted through an umbilical port but is always visible through a second small-diameter laparoscope inserted beneath the right costal margin (Fig. 13-20).

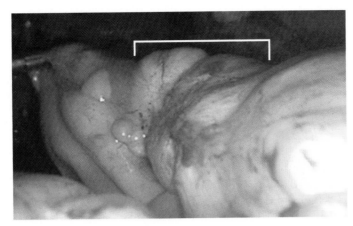

**Figure 13-16    A large nodule of endometriosis of the sigmoid colon (within the *white bracket*) is displayed by suspending the bowel with an atraumatic grasper.** This lesion was not visible when the sigmoid was in its normal position and appears slightly smaller due to foreshortening caused by the position of the bowel in the frame.

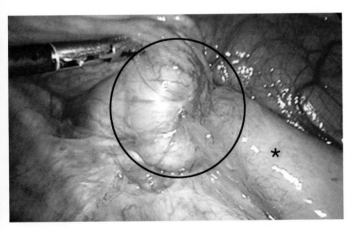

**Figure 13-17    A large obstructing nodule of ileal endometriosis is seen (within the *black circle*).** The graspers at the upper left of the frame are in the vicinity of the ileocecal valve. The last portion of the normal distal ileum is marked by an asterisk. This patient lost 25 pounds in 4 months due to symptoms of intestinal obstruction and was treated by segmental resection and anastomosis.

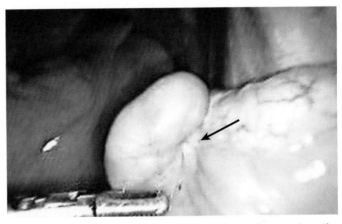

**Figure 13-18    Endometriosis of the appendix is usually asymptomatic and frequently subtle.** It is almost always manifest as whitish fibrosis *(arrow)*, which curls the appendix toward the fibrosis. Hemorrhagic change or neovascularity is rarely present.

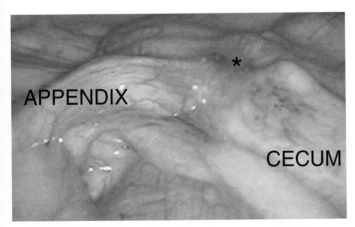

**Figure 13-19    The center of a cecal nodule of endometriosis is marked by the asterisk.** There is slight nodularity of the bowel wall with some puckering and surrounding minimal neovascularity.

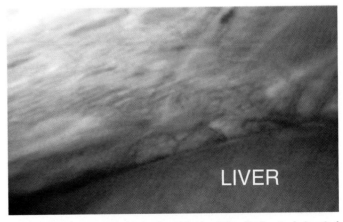

**Figure 13-20    Symptomatic endometriosis of the diaphragm is located along the posterior edge of the diaphragm and cannot always be seen with a laparoscope inserted through an umbilical port.** This view was obtained through a 5-mm laparoscope inserted beneath the right costal margin and passed over the liver.

Quantifying the extent of endometriosis at surgery is problematic. The revised American Fertility Society (now called the American Society for Reproductive Medicine) classification system[7] of endometriosis is commonly used, but this system has limitations for measuring disease extent for the following reasons: Most of the available points score for adhesions rather than endometriosis. Of the endometriosis component of this system, most of the points are awarded the ovaries, which are not the most common site of involvement. The peritoneal surfaces of the posterior pelvis are the most common sites of involvement, but peritoneal disease is accorded only 10 points (4 points for superficial disease and 6 points for deep disease). No points are allowed for intestinal disease or disease in distant sites. Multiple manifestations of disease may produce the same point total, and there are over 100,000 possible combinations in which points can be scored.

Pelvic mapping of individual pelvic or intestinal sites of involvement is a more accurate measure of disease extent and is easier to apply than measuring the diameter of each implant and adding the results to obtain a total additive diameter of the implants.

## TREATMENT

Because fecundity is not improved by medical therapy in women with endometriosis-associated infertility and no medical therapy eradicates endometriosis, the only indication for medical treatment of endometriosis is for temporary relief of pain symptoms. Medical therapy is contraindicated in women with endometriosis-associated infertility. These patients are better served by advanced reproductive technology techniques or by surgery. Traditional medical therapies have aimed at producing states of pseudopregnancy or pseudomenopause, with resultant amenorrhea. These hormonal states induced by medical treatment were originally thought to physically eradicate endometriosis because for decades it had been erroneously thought that pregnancy and menopause physically eradicate the disease.

### Pseudopregnancy Therapy

Because some early studies identified a relatively high percentage of nulliparous women among endometriosis patients, it was concluded that pregnancy protected against the occurrence of the disease and could, in fact, cure endometriosis by a cytocidal toxic effect called *necrobiosis*. When oral contraceptive steroids were developed in the early 1960s, they were adopted as treatment for endometriosis because the estrogen/progestin mix within the birth control pills was thought to mimic the alleged beneficial effects of pregnancy. The hormone levels in early oral contraceptives (OCs) were very high compared to those of the modern era, and the dosage formulations that helped popularize OC therapy of endometriosis are no longer available. With newer, lower-dose formulations come fewer side effects, but possibly a decrease in efficacy for preventing or treating functional ovarian cysts.

Although the hormonal dosage in OCs has been reduced substantially over the years, symptom reduction during treatment is still observed in some women. There are many combinations of estrogens and progestins in OCs, and new OCs are brought to market as others are dropped. It is impossible to mention a dose formulation that will be effective in reducing symptoms for all women for all time, but general guidelines can be followed. A monophasic low-dose ($<50\,\mu g$ of estrogen) pill with a non-varying hormone level may be preferable because endometriosis or troublesome breakthrough bleeding might be stimulated by changing hormone levels. A pill with less than $20\,\mu g$ of estrogen may be associated with a higher incidence of breakthrough bleeding. Continuous therapy for 3 to 6 months without a withdrawal bleed may be preferable to cyclic therapy resulting in a menstrual flow every 28 days. Although presence of a menstrual flow probably has nothing to do with initiation of endometriosis, dysmenorrhea, whatever its cause, may be lessened during this induced amenorrhea. Newer contraceptive skin patches are available that contain similar hormones delivered by some OCs, but these have not been studied specifically for treatment of endometriosis symptoms. However, one would expect efficacy similar to OCs.

Medroxyprogesterone acetate (MPA) 30 mg orally for 90 days to mimic the high progesterone state existing in pregnancy resulted in decreased pain and a decrease in nodularity and tenderness on examination in many patients during therapy. Norethynodrel, a progestin, given orally at dosages of 30 mg daily for 6 months was reported to relieve pain in most patients during therapy and to be associated with a culdoscopically confirmed cure rate of almost 80%. The long-term outcome after cessation of therapy is unknown.

### Pseudomenopausal Treatment

Symptomatic postmenopausal endometriosis occurs less commonly than premenopausal symptomatic disease. The historical notions that either natural or surgical menopause physically eradicates endometriosis are clearly incorrect, although endometriosis certainly may be less symptomatic during estrogen deficiency of any origin. Accordingly, medications that decrease or suspend the production of estrogen by the ovaries have been developed.

Danazol was the first medicine approved in America for treatment of endometriosis. Although it is an androgen with masculinizing side effects, it was originally thought to produce primarily a pseudomenopausal state. It was later found to produce a chronic anovulatory state, similar to OCs, by reducing the midcycle luteinizing hormone (LH) surge. The recommended dose of 600 to 800 mg orally daily for 6 months is associated with a high prevalence of androgenic side effects, some irreversible, including acne, hirsutism, clitoral hypertrophy, temporal hair loss, or deepening of the voice and is equivalent to MPA given in a dose of 100 mg orally daily for 6 months.[8]

Gonadotropin-releasing hormone (GnRH) agonists are currently the most widely prescribed medicines for treating the symptoms of endometriosis. GnRH is secreted in a pulsatile fashion by the hypothalamus and binds to cells in the anterior pituitary gland to stimulate production of the pituitary gonadotropins LH and follicle-stimulating hormone (FSH), both responsible for normal ovarian function. The half-life of endogenous GnRH is 3.5 minutes. If the normal hypothalamic pulsatile release of GnRH is replaced by a release that is too high or too low, the pituitary gland will eventually stop producing LH and FSH in normal quantities. To capitalize on this biologic effect,

GnRH agonists bind to receptor sites on cells in the pituitary gland and, because of their long half-life of 3 to 8 hours, mimic a pulsatile GnRH signal which is too rapid and sustained, resulting in an initial increase and then a cessation of pituitary gonadotropin output. Ovarian function correspondingly increases temporarily, then subsides to menopausal status during treatment if suppression has occurred. The resultant clinical effect may be one of initial worsening of estrogen-dependent symptoms (because ovarian production of estrogen increases), followed by amenorrhea associated with improvement or absence of estrogen-dependent symptoms. Estrogen-dependent pain caused by adenomyosis, uterine fibroids, primary dysmenorrhea, ovulation pain, endometriosis, or unknown factors may all be relieved by such ovarian suppression. It is generally agreed that ovarian suppression of estrogen production by GnRH agonists is more profound than occurs with OC or danazol therapy. GnRH agonists can be given by nasal spray, injection, or pellet insertion.

Temporary improvement of symptoms on GnRH agonist therapy can be associated with an overall worsening of disease extent, as shown by reoperation 12 months after cessation of treatment[9] as well as a return of pain to baseline levels 9 months after cessation of therapy.[10] The efficacy of GnRH agonists is similar to danazol, whether the agonist is given by the intranasal[11] or the subcutaneous[12] route.

With nasal spray therapy, absorption across the nasal mucosa can be erratic, and the twice-daily dosing increases the likelihood of patient noncompliance. For these reasons, and because subcutaneous administration of some forms of GnRH agonists was found to be more efficacious than nasal administration,[13] intranasal therapy has largely been replaced by systemic therapy, either by injection of depot forms of GnRH agonists or by insertion of pellets of goserelin.

Gonadotropin-releasing hormone agonist therapy is associated with a significant rate of estrogen-deficiency side effects, including vasomotor symptoms, atrophic vaginitis, arthralgias, decreased libido, and weight gain. Loss of bone mineral density (BMD) appears during the first 3 months of treatment[14]; it remains controversial whether this is associated with irreversible loss of bone mineral content.[15]

Because cessation of GnRH agonist therapy is followed quickly by return of symptoms, longer durations of treatment with GnRH agonists (for 6 to 24 months) have been studied. "Add-back" estrogen therapy can be given to ameliorate hypoestrogenic side effects, including loss of BMD, with the target window of serum estradiol being between 30 and 50 pg/mL. Above this window, endometriosis may be stimulated to remain symptomatic. Below this window, bone loss may be substantial. Estrogen-only add-back therapy can increase pain due to endometriosis, so other add-back schemes have been studied.

Add-back therapy with norethindrone 5 mg daily without oral conjugated equine estrogens, 0.625 mg daily, preserved BMD without provoking symptoms.[16] MPA[17] and levonorgestrel have also been used effectively as add-back therapies. Add-back therapies have challenged the historical concept of "pseudomenopausal" therapy of endometriosis by GnRH agonists because such treatments have created a hybrid class of therapy.

Gonadotropin-releasing hormone agonist therapy is expensive, does not eradicate endometriosis, and long-term treatment is associated with symptoms in many women despite add-back therapy. These concerns may limit the use of such treatment in some patients.

Gestrinone (ethylnorgestrienone) is an antiprogestin that causes a decrease in serum estradiol as well as in the concentrations of estrogen and progesterone receptors on cell surfaces. Approved for use in Europe, it has androgenic side effects, including clitoromegaly, deepening of the voice, and hirsutism, all of which may be irreversible. It is taken orally one to three times per week to deliver a total weekly dose of 2.5 to 10 mg.

## Efficacy of Medical Therapy

### Infertility

Medical therapy directed against treatment of endometriosis alone does not improve fertility in women with endometriosis-associated infertility[18] and has actually been associated with a reduction of fertility in these women. This may be due either to some direct negative effect of the medications or to the fact that the natural age-related decline in fertility is manifest following 6 months or more of treatment and eventual resumption of ovarian function. Medical therapy is therefore contraindicated for the symptom of infertility associated with endometriosis. However, medical therapy as an adjunct to assisted reproductive techniques appears to be helpful. In women with infertility associated with advanced stages of endometriosis, an extended course of a GnRH agonist given before ovulation induction and intrauterine insemination was found to improve fecundity over a shorter course of GnRH agonist.[19]

### Pain

Both high-dose (50 mg/day) oral MPA and placebo given for 3 months were associated with improvement of symptoms and surgical findings at reoperation.[20]

Oral contraceptives given for 12 months appear equivalent for treating pain to GnRH agonists given for 4 months followed by OCs for another 8 months.[21] Low-dose OCs (0.02 mg of ethinyl estradiol plus 0.15 mg desogestrel) given for 6 months have an equivalent effect to the GnRH agonist goserelin given for 6 months, with the return of pain in most patients by 6 months after discontinuation of medication.[22]

Oral danazol and injections of the GnRH agonists leuprolide depot[23] or triptorelin depot[24] had equivalent effects on laparoscopic assessment of extent of endometriosis, pain, and tenderness, although reduction of the serum estradiol level was more pronounced with the GnRH agonist and the free androgenic index and liver enzymes were elevated by danazol treatment.

In women with rectovaginal disease, a levonorgestrel-releasing intrauterine system used for 12 months was associated with reduction of both symptoms and size of lesions.[25]

### Future Medical Treatments

With the advance of research, new therapies are being developed that depart radically from the traditional historical categories of pseudopregnancy or pseudomenopausal therapy. These new therapies may allow more effective symptom control. These include aromatase inhibitors and medications to block angiogenesis. Also being studied are GnRH antagonists, which have similar actions as GnRH agonists, although without the

# General Gynecology

initial stimulation of ovarian estrogen production. Selective progesterone modulators, RU486, and tumor necrosis factor-$\alpha$ inhibitors are also being studied. It will be important to judge whether these medications are advanced on the basis of the response of symptoms rather than eradication of endometriosis.

## Ablative Surgical Treatment

Some surgical treatments do not require extensive tissue dissection and can be applied quickly, potentially by any surgeon. These include thermal ablation performed by laser vaporization, monopolar or bipolar electrocoagulation, argon beam coagulation, endocoagulation, and harmonic scalpel coagulation. The many variables affecting each of these treatments reduce their efficacy, one of the most important being the depth of destruction possible with each energy system. Although depth of tissue destruction may depend in part on the technique used by a particular surgeon, it is generally agreed that all thermal ablation techniques have the potential of incomplete treatment because of inadequate depth of tissue destruction. For example, the carbon dioxide ($CO_2$) laser may vaporize only 100 microns in one short burst, whereas endometriosis may invade several centimeters beneath the visible surface. Deeper tissue destruction is possible with the laser in continuous mode. In some cases, the laser beam may be passed across the tissue too swiftly to allow any chance of eradication of even superficial disease. With monopolar electrocoagulation, the maximal depth of destruction may be only 1 or 2 mm, and the zone of desiccated tissue that builds up around the active electrode serves as an insulator that retards further flow of electrons, thus effectively limiting severely the depth of destruction by electrocoagulation. Bipolar electrocoagulation can be associated with a higher sustained temperature than monopolar coagulation because the close approximation of the bipolar paddles can allow continued electron flow and heat generation even when the tissue between the paddles is desiccated. Also, when the tissue between the paddles is desiccated, electrons will begin to pass through tissue alongside the paddles. This gives a much larger and possibly more dangerous electrosurgical "footprint" than monopolar coagulation. The details of electrocoagulation, such as the type of electrosurgical generator, power settings, type of active electrode, manner of use, and visual endpoint of adequate destruction, have not been adequately described in the literature. This lack of detailed instructional information makes its clinical use inconsistent.

With any thermal ablation technique, all important endpoints depend on the opinion of the surgeon. What is being destroyed, the depth of invasion of the pathology, and how completely it has been destroyed are all controlled only by the surgeon's opinion. The visual endpoint of adequate thermal destruction is ill-defined, other than for laser vaporization of superficial endometriosis, in which case normal yellow retroperitoneal fat is exposed. With all thermal ablation techniques, disease that may be deeply invasive will be treated identically to superficial disease, because the surgeon remains unaware of the difference. Thus, thermal ablation techniques effectively transform all endometriosis into superficial disease in the surgeon's eye. Unintentional damage to underlying structures is another danger of thermal ablation techniques, and the surgeon's understandable hesitancy to burn an underlying vital structure is yet another contributing factor resulting in treatment that is too superficial and possibly incomplete.

## Surgical Excision

Many experts in endometriosis treat the disease by surgical excision, which may allow complete removal of superficial or invasive disease. Excision is the only form of treatment with cure of disease documented among reoperated patients. Conservative excision can usually be performed entirely laparoscopically, although laparotomy may be necessary for extreme cases with profound pelvic distortion, diaphragmatic involvement, or multiple areas of intestinal involvement. Excision may be performed with scissors, electrosurgery, $CO_2$ or fiber lasers, or harmonic scalpel. Small-diameter (3 mm) monopolar scissors are a versatile tool, allowing multiple operations with one instrument, thus decreasing instrument changes (Table 13-3).

In addition to appropriate instrumentation, the surgeon must have a strategy that will allow the case to progress. Fortunately, endometriosis exhibits recurring patterns of pelvic involvement, which can be treated virtually the same way every time. Thus, a surgeon will need to learn only five or six separate techniques to manage most of the cases that will be seen.

In severe cases, the ovaries may be involved by endometriosis, with bilateral endometrioma cysts, which often are adherent to the uterosacral ligaments and/or pelvic sidewalls (see Fig. 13-10 and 13-11) and may obscure the posterior pelvis completely (Fig. 13-21). The size of these cysts may impede all other endometriosis surgery, so it is most advantageous to begin by puncturing and draining such cysts for decompression.

Endometrioma cysts of an ovary are best treated by cystectomy, because only drainage and burning the cyst wall is associated with a high rate of persistence. The ovary involved by an endometrioma cyst is frequently adherent either to the pelvic sidewall peritoneum, the ipsilateral uterosacral ligament, or both. The cyst wall is typically thick and fibrous, which helps the cystectomy process. After cortical incision to expose the cyst wall (Fig. 13-22), ovarian cystectomy is most typically performed using two atraumatic graspers, one to pull on the cyst wall, the other to provide countertraction on the normal ovarian cortex. Cystectomy will proceed fairly smoothly in most cases

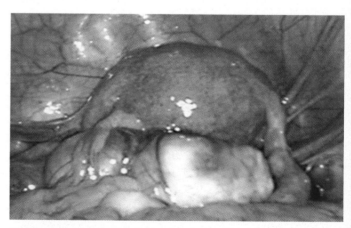

**Figure 13-21** Enlarged, adherent ovaries may call attention only to themselves but can hide impressive pathology. Complete obliteration of the cul-de-sac was hidden beneath these ovaries.

**Table 13-3**
**Range of Functions Possible with Different Surgical Techniques for Endometriosis in Typical Use**

| Function | Surgical Technique | | | Excision | | |
|---|---|---|---|---|---|---|
| | Laser Vaporization | Argon Beam Coagulation | Electro-coagulation | CO$_2$ Laser | Fiber Laser | Scissors* |
| Palpation | — | — | + | — | + | + |
| Grasp, retract | — | — | + | — | + | + |
| Blunt dissect | — | — | — | — | + | + |
| Sharp dissect | — | — | — | — | — | + |
| Cut tissue | + | — | — | + | + | + |
| Cut suture† | — | — | — | — | + | + |
| **Hemostasis** | | | | | | |
| Vessels ≥3mm | — | — | — | — | — | + |
| Smaller vessels | ± | ± | + | ± | ± | + |
| Capillary bleeding | + | + | + | + | + | + |
| **Disease eradication** | | | | | | |
| Superficial | + | + | + | + | + | + |
| Deep | — | — | — | + | + | + |
| All intestinal | — | — | — | + | + | + |
| Angiolysis | + | — | — | + | + | + |
| Ureterolysis | + | — | — | + | + | + |
| **Adhesiolysis** | | | | | | |
| Dense, confluent | + | — | — | + | + | + |
| Filmy | + | + | + | + | + | + |

*Monopolar electrosurgical scissors
†Suture can be cut with the CO$_2$ laser, but this is not recommended unless a backstop for the laser beam is used.

until the process encounters the area where the ovary is adherent to the uterosacral ligament. At this point, the cyst wall, ovarian cortex, and uterosacral ligament are all fused tightly together. It is helpful to approach this problem from the exterior of the ovary by simply amputating the small fused area from the rest of the ovary. The cystectomy process can be completed more easily, and the area of ovary that is still fused to the uterosacral ligament can be removed separately with disease of the ligament. When the ovary is adherent to the peritoneum of the ovarian fossa, this peritoneum is commonly involved by endometriosis, frequently with impressive retroperitoneal fibrosis. This peritoneum can also be removed.

When surgery is performed on or around the ovaries, postoperative adhesions may form, especially if adhesions were already present. To reduce the chance of dense periovarian adhesions from forming, temporary ovarian suspension may be helpful.[26] The ovary can be suspended (Fig. 13-23) from the ipsilateral round ligament with 3-0 or 4-0 absorbable sutures

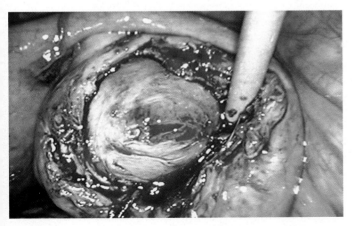

**Figure 13-22    Enlarged ovary incised to expose the underlying ovarian cyst.**

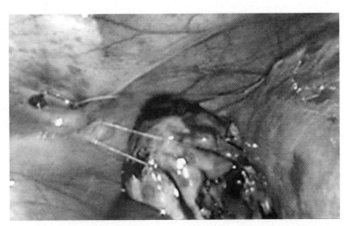

**Figure 13-23    The left ovary has undergone ovariolysis and cystectomy.** It has been suspended from the left round ligament with 3-0 Vicryl suture to avoid re-adherence to the raw surgical site on the left pelvic sidewall.

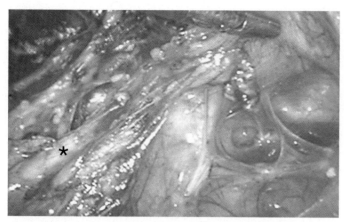

**Figure 13-24** The left ureter *(asterisk)* has been freed from retroperitoneal fibrosis related to endometriosis. The diseased peritoneum has been dissected bluntly and with electrosurgery from the ureter and is being held by the graspers.

or with nylon sutures that pass through the abdominal wall and can be removed 1 week postoperatively. An additional advantage of ovarian suspension is that it keeps the ovaries out of the surgical field during the rest of the case.

Invasive endometriosis of a uterosacral ligament can be excised by first creating a releasing incision in relatively normal peritoneum lateral and parallel to the ligament. The ligament can be bluntly undermined laterally and then separated from the posterior cervix by transection above the invasive disease. The ligament can then be isolated medially by a peritoneal incision

alongside it. The cut edge of the ligament adjacent to the cervix can then be grasped and the ligament shaved off the pelvic floor, with the line of excision occurring in soft, normal tissue.

When endometriosis is more biologically active, the peritoneum may be thickened and yellow, thus obscuring the active disease. Furthermore, retroperitoneal scarring associated with invasive disease may involve retroperitoneal structures, including the ureter and pelvic vessels. Dissection once again begins through normal peritoneum, but quickly involves ureterolysis (Fig. 13-24) or angiolysis, because all retroperitoneal fibrosis must be removed for complete excision of the disease.

Superficial peritoneal involvement can be identified by easy movement of the peritoneum containing the lesions over an underlying positionally static structure (Fig. 13-25). This is treated by grasping the abnormal peritoneum and tenting it up and away from underlying vital structures. An incision is created in normal peritoneum adjacent to the abnormality, and the abnormal peritoneum can be dissected away from the underlying normal tissue with blunt dissection or shaving with laser or electrosurgery.

Invasive disease of the bladder may require partial-thickness or full-thickness cystectomy. When the ureter is stenotic due to restrictive fibrosis or invasion by endometriosis, the origin of the ureteral pathology is always the ipsilateral uterosacral ligament. Treatment may require difficult ureterolysis followed by segmental ureteral resection and anastomosis. Simply relieving the obstruction by segmental resection/anastomosis and leaving the offending uterosacral ligament disease behind will guarantee continuation of symptoms and invite re-occlusion of the bypassing ureter.

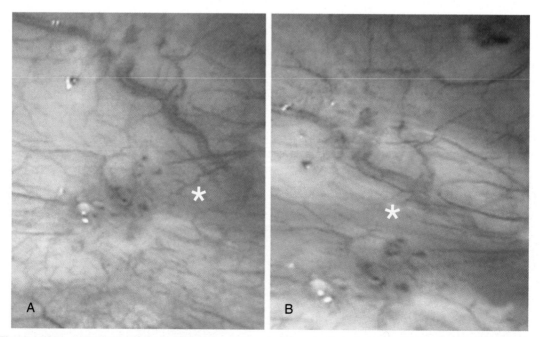

**Figure 13-25** Superficial disease of the bladder. *A,* An asterisk marks the edge of a rather large retroperitoneal venous structure, which will remain unchanged in position by peritoneal traction. Areas of endometriosis are located in the center and top of the frame. *B,* When the peritoneum is pulled downward with a grasper, the areas of endometriosis and small peritoneal vessels are seen to move freely over the large retroperitoneal vein, as noted by the relative change of position with respect to the asterisk.

The rectosigmoid colon is the intestinal site most commonly involved by endometriosis (Table 13-4). As the number of intestinal sites of involvement increases, the likelihood of a full-thickness or segmental bowel resection increases. In its most severe form intestinal involvement presents as obliteration of the cul-de-sac. Obliteration of the cul-de-sac represents invasive disease of the uterosacral ligaments, cul-de-sac, posterior cervix, and usually the anterior rectal wall as well. When the wall of the rectum is rounded at its adherence to the posterior cervix, the muscularis is involved by significant endometriosis. Obliteration of the cul-de-sac is most efficiently treated by en bloc resection, which does not always require a segmental bowel resection to be done. The ileum, appendix, and cecum are less commonly involved by endometriosis. Intestinal disease can be treated by partial thickness, full-thickness, or segmental bowel resection as required. This can be done laparoscopically or by laparotomy. Disease of the appendix is treated by appendectomy.

Symptomatic diaphragmatic endometriosis penetrates the full thickness of this rather thin muscle and is usually concentrated along the posterior diaphragm near the posterior chest wall. The best treatment results are obtained by laparotomy with full-thickness resection of the affected areas of the diaphragm followed by repair with permanent suture.

Umbilical endometriosis is treated by local excision. Endometriosis of a surgical scar occurs most commonly following cesarean section. Scar endometriosis of a low transverse incision is commonly located near the end of the incision, more frequently on the right side. The endometriosis always involves the fascia and rarely communicates with the uterus or peritoneal cavity. The subcutaneous fat is sometimes minimally involved. Excision of fibrosis at all levels is curative in most cases. It is necessary in all cases to remove the portion of fascia involved by fibrosis because not all lesions will appear to be hemorrhagic. It is usually possible to close the fascia primarily without creating fascial relaxing incisions. Closure can be facilitated by flexing the operating table to reduce stretching of the abdominal wall.

Uterine cramps, either during menses or away from menses, may not be due to endometriosis. Uterine cramping is a uterine symptom that may not respond to endometriosis surgery alone. In women with uterine cramping that severely affects their lifestyle, a presacral neurectomy (Fig. 13-26) will enhance the pain relief beyond excision of endometriosis only.[27] Transection or resection of normal uterosacral ligaments does not add to the pain relief of excision of endometriosis only.[28]

Surgery for endometriosis does not treat symptoms not due to endometriosis. Although persistent or recurrent pain following thermal ablation is frequently due to incompletely treated disease, pain following excision is usually due to something other than endometriosis because most patients will have been cured of their disease. A second excisional surgery will be less successful at pain relief than the first excisional surgery.

### Efficacy of Surgical Treatment

The efficacy of a surgical technique is most accurately assessed by comparing disease extent before surgical treatment and at later reoperation. There has been no systematic, biopsy-controlled study in reoperated patients to assess the efficacy of any of the thermal ablation techniques. Aggressive excision at laparotomy[29] or laparoscopy,[30,31] however, is associated with a cure rate of more than 50%, even in patients with disease resistant to other forms of therapy. Excision of endometriosis is associated with impressive and long-lasting symptom reduction and quality of life improvement. Excision has been shown by a randomized, controlled trial to be more effective than placebo surgery in relieving pain due to endometriosis.[31]

Thermal ablation techniques have looked toward symptom reduction, rather than disease reduction, as a measure of efficacy. In a randomized, controlled trial, laser vaporization of peritoneal endometriosis was found to reduce pain compared to placebo surgery by 6 months after treatment.[32] Electrocoagulation or resection has been found to improve fecundity in endometriosis-associated infertility in early-stage disease in a randomized, controlled trial,[33] although an Italian study did not confirm this.[34] After surgical treatment of endometriosis, ovulation augmentation with clomiphene citrate combined with intrauterine insemination has been shown to improve fertility.[35]

Ovarian cystectomy is superior to cyst puncture, drainage and coagulation of endometriotic cysts for both pain relief and pregnancy rates.[36]

### Efficacy of Combined Medical/Surgical Treatment

Intrauterine devices containing progestins may reduce dysmenorrhea after conservative surgical treatment of endometriosis.[25,37] A 3-month course of nasal GnRH agonist has not been found to contribute to pain relief after excision of endometriosis in patients with Stage III or IV disease.[38]

In women who have undergone excision of ovarian endometrioma cysts, postoperative use of OCs is associated with a slightly higher rate of new cyst formation compared to untreated patients.[39]

## CLINICAL COURSE AND PROGRESSION

The clinical course of endometriosis is highly variable. Some women seem destined to have only scattered superficial disease, whereas others are destined to have widespread invasive disease. Many will have both superficial and invasive disease in different pelvic areas. Disease at either end of the clinical spectrum may or may not cause symptoms, and symptoms can worsen even if the disease does not. The age-related evolution in color

| Table 13-4 Frequency of Involvement of Intestinal Sites among 2589 Patients with Biopsy-proven Endometriosis* | |
|---|---|
| **Site** | **Number of Patients** |
| Rectal nodule | 342 |
| Sigmoid | 445 |
| Ileum | 116 |
| Appendix | 79 |
| Cecum | 41 |
| Total patients with intestinal involvement | 732[†] |

*Treated at the Endometriosis Treatment Program at St. Charles Medical Center, Bend, OR.
[†]Total of sites of involvment exceeds number of patients with intestinal involvement because 213 patients had more than one site of intestinal involvement.

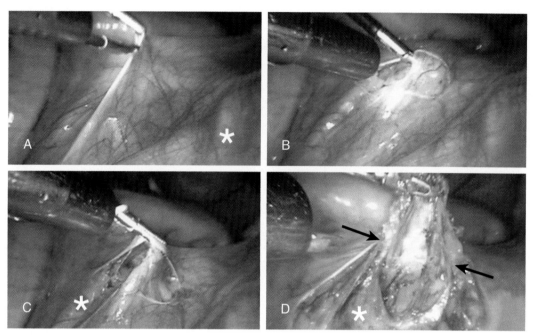

**Figure 13-26  Surgical steps in laparoscopic presacral neurectomy.** *A,* The peritoneum overlying the sacral promontory is elevated and the pleat of tissue created is being cut with electrosurgery. The right ureter is marked by an asterisk. *B,* A transverse peritoneal incision is created between the edge of the sigmoid mesentery on the left and the right common iliac vessels on the right. Blunt dissection at the left angle of this incision allows the periosteum to be exposed and the presacral plexus to be isolated. *C,* The edge of the sigmoid mesentery is marked by the asterisk. The left common iliac vein is seen as a bluish structure beneath the mesenteric vessels at the left margin of the peritoneal incision. The presacral plexus is being elevated by graspers and will be transected adjacent to the superior cut peritoneal edge. *D,* After proximal transection of the presacral plexus, it is dissected bluntly off of the underlying periosteum and from small presacral vessels. The left common iliac vein *(asterisk)* is seen. The presacral plexus will then be transected distally along a line between the two arrowheads.

appearance of endometriosis will cause the spurious impression of appearance of new disease if early, subtle forms of the disease were not correctly diagnosed at initial surgery. Actually, endometriosis appears to usually be geographically static and nonspreading by any type of measurement of pelvic involvement. Local fibromuscular hyperplasia of involved parenchymal structures associated with invasive disease or enlargement of endometriotic cysts represent the chief modes of "progression" of endometriosis, although such local proliferation does not indicate more widespread geographic involvement of more pelvic areas. This positionally static nature of endometriosis is what leads to its potential curability by excisional surgery. At the same time, the positionally static nature of the disease can contribute to a picture of success following any therapy because if it is assumed that endometriosis is progressively spreading, then lack of spread during or after treatment can be attributed to the "success" of treatment rather than simply a consequence of the natural history of the disease.

## PITFALLS AND CONTROVERSIES

Historic pitfalls surrounding endometriosis persist almost unchanged today compared to previous eras. "New" discoveries about the disease have frequently already been discovered, only to be forgotten by succeeding generations of clinicians. There

are many important examples of this phenomenon. Retroperitoneal "adenomyotic" disease was one of the first manifestations described in the literature almost a century ago, only to be rediscovered in Europe at the millennium's end. By 1940 it was apparent that peritoneal endometriosis was more common and more clinically important than ovarian disease, but it is still thought by some that the ovaries are the most commonly involved pelvic site. Subtle endometriosis and even colorless lesions were known by the mid-20th century. In the same era, clinicians were amazed by the apparent increase in prevalence of endometriosis, attributing it to better diagnosis of subtle lesions and looking for it in age groups where it was unexpected, such as teenagers. By the 1950s, it appeared that endometriosis could be cured by conservative excisional surgery, which has once again been proven to be true.

A randomized, controlled trial is considered the "gold standard" of evidence of therapeutic efficacy. Randomized, controlled trials on endometriosis therapy have frequently been conducted with inherent fundamental errors, such as inadequate identification of disease at initial surgery or reoperation, assessing the response of symptoms rather than the response of the disease, or basing some portion of the study in part on the assumed correctness of the theory of reflux menstruation. The result of this is that errors of understanding and clinical management have become even more firmly entrenched.

# REFERENCES

1. Redwine DB: Was Sampson wrong? Fertil Steril 2002;78:686–693. **(IV, C)**

2. Sampson JA: Perforating hemorrhagic chocolate cysts of the ovary. Arch Surg 1921;3:245–323. **(IV, C)**

3. http://www.well.ox.ac.uk/`krinaz/genepi_endo.htm **(IV, C)**

4. Redwine DB: "Invisible" microscopic endometriosis: a review. Gynecol Obstet Invest 2003;55:63–67. **(IV, C)**

5. Redwine DB, Wright J: Laparoscopic treatment of obliteration of the cul de sac in endometriosis: long term followup. Fertil Steril 2001; 76:358–365. **(IIa, B)**

6. Redwine DB: Age related evolution in color appearance of endometriosis. Fertil Steril 1987;48:1062–1063. **(III, B)**

7. American Fertility Society: Revised American Fertility Society classification of endometriosis, 1985. Fertil Steril 1985;43:351–352. **(IV, C)**

8. Telimaa S, Puolakka J, Ronnberg L, et al: Placebo-controlled comparison of danazol and high-dose medroxyprogesterone acetate in the treatment of endometriosis. Gynecol Endocrinol 1987;1:13–23. **(Ib, A)**

9. Lemay A, Quesnel G: Potential new treatment of endometriosis: reversible inhibition of pituitary–ovarian function by chronic intranasal administration of a luteinizing hormone-releasing hormone LH-RH agonist. Fertil Steril 1982;38:376–379. **(III, B)**

10. Hornstein MD, Yuzpe AA, Burry KA, et al: Prospective randomized double-blind trial of 3 versus 6 months of nafarelin therapy for endometriosis associated pelvic pain. Fertil Steril 1995;63:955–962. **(Ib, A)**

11. Henzol MR, Corson SL, Moghissi K, et al: Administration of nasal nafarelin as compared with oral danazol for endometriosis. A multicenter double-blind comparative clinical trial. N Engl J Med 1988; 318:485–489. **(Ib, A)**

12. Shaw RW: An open randomized comparative study of the effect of goserelin depot and danazol in the treatment of endometriosis. Fertil Steril 1992;58:265–272. **(Ib, A)**

13. Donnez J, Nisolle-Pochet M, Clerckx-Braun F, et al: Administration of nasal Buserelin as compared with subcutaneous Buserelin implant for endometriosis. Fertil Steril 1989;52:27–30. **(Ib, A)**

14. Orwoll ES, Yuzpe AA, Burry KA, et al: Nafarelin therapy in endometriosis: long-term effects on BMD. Am J Obstet Gynecol 1994; 171:1221–1225. **(III, B)**

15. Dawood MY, Lewis V, Ramos J: Cortical and trabecular bone mineral content in women with endometriosis: effect of gonadotropin-releasing hormone agonist and danazol. Fertil Steril 1989;52:21–26. **(Ib, A)**

16. Hornstein MD, Surrey EX, Weisberg GW, et al: Leuprolide acetate depot and hormonal add-back in endometriosis: a 12-month study. Obstet Gynecol 1998;91:16–24. **(Ib, A)**

17. Carr BR, Breslau NA, Peng N, et al: Effect of gonadotropin-releasing hormone agonist and medroxyprogesterone acetate on calcium metabolism: a prospective, randomized, double-blind, placebo-controlled, crossover trial. Fertil Steril 2003;80:1216–1223. **(Ib, A)**

18. Hughes E, Fedorkow D, Collins J, et al: Ovulation suppression for endometriosis. Cochrane Database Syst Rev 2003, Vol. 3. CD000155. **(Ia, A)**

19. Kim CH, Cho YK, Mok JE: Simplified ultralong protocol of gonadotrophin-releasing hormone agonist for ovulation induction with intrauterine insemination in patients with endometriosis. Hum Reprod 1996;11:398–402. **(Ib, A)**

20. Harrison RF, Barry-Kinsella C: Efficacy of medroxyprogesterone treatment in infertile women with endometriosis: a prospective, randomized, placebo-controlled study. Fertil Steril 2000;74:24–30. **(Ib, A)**

21. Parazzini F, Di Cintio E, Chatenoud L, et al: Estroprogestin vs. gonadotrophin agonists plus estroprogestin in the treatment of endometriosis-related pelvic pain: a randomized trial. Gruppo Italiano per lo Studio dell'Endometriosi. Eur J Obstet Gynecol Reprod Biol 2000;88:11–14. **(Ib, A)**

22. Vercellini P, Trespidi L, Colombo A, et al: A gonadotropin-releasing hormone agonist versus a low-dose oral contraceptive for pelvic pain associated with endometriosis. Fertil Steril 1993;60:75–79. **(Ib, A)**

23. Wheeler JM, Knittle JD, Miller JD: Depot leuprolide versus danazol in treatment of women with symptomatic endometriosis. I. Efficacy results. Am J Obstet Gynecol 1992;167:1367–1371. **(Ib, A)**

24. Cirkel U, Ochs H, Schneider HP: A randomized, comparative trial of triptorelin depot D-Trp6-LHRH and danazol in the treatment of endometriosis. Eur J Obstet Gynecol Reprod Biol 1995;59:61–69. **(Ib, A)**

25. Fedele L, Bianchi S, Zanconato G, et al: Use of a levonorgestrel-releasing intrauterine device in the treatment of rectovaginal endometriosis. Fertil Steril 2001;75:485–488. **(IIa, B)**

26. Ouahba J, Madelenat P, Poncelet C: Transient abdominal ovariopexy for adhesion prevention in patients who underwent surgery for severe pelvic endometriosis. Fertil Steril 2004;82:1407–1411. **(III, B)**

27. Zullo F, Palomba S, Zupi E, et al: Effectiveness of presacral neurectomy in women with severe dysmenorrhea caused by endometriosis who were treated with laparoscopic conservative surgery: a 1-year prospective randomized double-blind controlled trial. Am J Obstet Gynecol 2003;189:5–10. **(Ib, A)**

28. Vercellini P, Aimi G, Busacca M, et al: Laparoscopic uterosacral ligament resection for dysmenorrhea associated with endometriosis: results of a randomized, controlled trial. Fertil Steril 2003;80:310–319. **(Ib, A)**

29. Wheeler JM, Malinak LR: Recurrent endometriosis. Contrib Gynecol Obstet 1987;16:13– 21. **(IIa, B)**

30. Redwine DB: Conservative laparoscopic excision of endometriosis by sharp dissection: life table analysis of reoperation and persistent or recurrent disease. Fertil Steril 1991;56:628–634. **(IIb, B)**

31. Abbott J, Hawe J, Hunter D, et al: Laparoscopic excision of endometriosis: A randomized, placebo-controlled trial. Fertil Steril 2004; 82:828–884. **(Ib, A)**

32. Sutton CJ, Ewen SP, Whitelaw N, et al: Prospective, randomized, double-blind, controlled trial of laser laparoscopy in the treatment of pelvic pain associated with minimal, mild, and moderate endometriosis. Fertil Steril 1994;62:696–700. **(Ib, A)**

33. Marcoux S, Maheux R, Berube S: Laparoscopic surgery in infertile women with minimal or mild endometriosis. Canadian Collaborative Group on Endometriosis. N Engl J Med 1997;337:217–222. **(Ib, A)**

34. Parazzini F, Gruppo Italiano per lo Studio dell'Endometriosi: Ablation of lesions or no treatment in minimal–mild endometriosis in infertile women: a randomized trial. Hum Reprod 1999;14:1332–1334. **(Ib, A)**

35. Deaton JL, Gibson M, Blackmer KM, et al: A randomized, controlled trial of clomiphene citrate and intrauterine insemination in couples with unexplained infertility or surgically corrected endometriosis. Fertil Steril 1990;54:1083–1088. **(Ib, A)**

36. Beretta P, Franchi M, Ghezzi F, et al: Randomized clinical trial of two laparoscopic treatments of endometriomas: cystectomy versus drainage and coagulation. Fertil Steril 1998;70:1176–1180. **(Ib, A)**

37. Vercellini P, Frontino G, De Giorgi O, et al: Comparison of a levonorgestrel-releasing intrauterine device versus expectant management after conservative surgery for symptomatic endometriosis: a pilot study. Fertil Steril 2003;80:305–309. **(IIb, B)**

38. Parazzini F, Fedele L, Busacca M, et al: Postsurgical medical treatment of advanced endometriosis: results of a randomized clinical trial. Am J Obstet Gynecol 1994;171:1205–1207. **(Ib, A)**

39. Muzii L, Marana R, Caruana P, et al: Postoperative administration of monophasic combined oral contraceptives after laparoscopic treatment of ovarian endometriomas: a prospective, randomized trial. Am J Obstet Gynecol 2000;183:588–592. **(Ib, A)**

# Chapter 14

# Uterine Leiomyomas

Rahi Victory, MD, Walter Romano, MD, John Bennett, MD, and Michael P. Diamond, MD

## KEY POINTS

- Fibroids occur commonly in reproductive-age women and can cause significant morbidity.
- Risk factors include primarily age and African American race, but incidence may also be affected by menstrual history, endogenous and exogenous hormone exposure, infertility history, and cigarette smoking.
- Symptoms differ widely but may include menorrhagia, pelvic pain and pressure, infertility, and pregnancy-related complications.
- Diagnosis can be made by radiographs, transabdominal and transvaginal ultrasound, magnetic resonance imaging, and hysteroscopy.
- Treatment includes both medical therapy, primarily in the form of gonadotropin-releasing hormone agonists, and surgical therapy using either endoscopic or open laparotomy approaches for myomectomy or hysterectomy.
- Significant controversy exists regarding many aspects of the impact, diagnosis, and management of uterine leiomyomas.

Uterine leiomyomas (leiomyomata or fibroids) are benign smooth muscle tumors of the human uterus that represent one of the most common gynecologic problems in women of reproductive age. While most leiomyomas are asymptomatic, they can result in debilitating symptoms having a significant impact on quality of life. They are the primary indication for the nearly 600,000 hysterectomies performed each year in the United States, and for 37,000 myomectomies performed annually.[1]

Risk factors for the development of myomas, complications and symptoms related to fibroids, and reproductive outcomes related to these benign tumors are areas of controversy. Patients are frequently confused or unaware of the range of options available for treatment of myomas. This chapter reviews the epidemiology, symptomatology, diagnosis, medical therapy, and surgical treatment of fibroids. Controversies still existing in the literature are also reviewed as are suggested future directions for research and current principles for counseling patients with fibroids.

## EPIDEMIOLOGY

The exact incidence of leiomyomas in reproductive age women is difficult to ascertain for several reasons. Primarily, the majority of fibroids are asymptomatic, resulting in low clinical detection rates.[2,3] Cadaveric studies are also hampered by the fact that many fibroids regress in size with age. Furthermore, different diagnostic methodologies have highly variable sensitivities for the detection of uterine leiomyomas.. In a comprehensive review of patients in the United States conducted by Schwartz, incidence rates varied from 2.0 to 12.8 per 1000 women per year.[1]

Age plays a significant role in the detection of fibroids, with increasing incidence rates as women approach the perimenopause, followed by fibroid regression in the postmenopausal years.[4] Marshall et al demonstrated that in 95,061 patients followed in the Nurses Health Study, the baseline incidence was 4.3 per 1000 women-years in women between 25 and 29 years of age, 9.0 between 30 and 34 years of age, 14.7 between 35 and 39, and 22.5 between 40 and 44, demonstrating a linear increase in incidence with increasing age.[5] Thus, in the group aged 40 to 44 years, there was a 5.2 fold increase in fibroid incidence compared with women aged 25 to 29 years. With declining hormonal stimulation in the postmenopausal years, incidence rates decline.[2,6]

Racial disparities also play a significant role in the epidemiology of leiomyomas. Multiple studies have demonstrated significant differences between patients of African American descent and white patients. Shwartz demonstrated that when adjusting for age, standardized rates of incidence were 2 to 3 times higher in black vs. white patients.[1] Faerstein et al demonstrated that even when controlling for age at menarche, oral contraceptive use, body size, smoking, hypertension, diabetes, and history of pelvic inflammatory disease, black patients had an adjusted odds ratio of 9.4 compared with white control cases.[7] More recently, Baird et al examined a random selection of patients without any specific gynecologic complaints from an urban, prepaid health plan.[8] This study demonstrated that both premenopausal and postmenopausal black patients had a higher rate of diagnosis of fibroids prior to the study (45% vs. 21% and 74% vs. 42%, respectively). In women with no previous history of fibroids, 59% of black women were newly diagnosed by ultrasound to have fibroids versus 43% of white women. When controlling for body mass index (BMI) and parity, black women had an odds ratio of 2.7 for the presence of leiomyoma (95% CI, 2.3 to 3.2; $P < 0.001$). Black women were also found to have a higher incidence of multiple fibroid tumors (74% vs. 31%). Although there were no racial differences in fibroid size in women with a previous history of fibroids, black women with newly diagnosed fibroids were more likely to have larger leiomyomas than white women. These differences also manifest in different management strategies, with black women being more likely to undergo hysterectomy for fibroids and at a younger age than white patients. Marshall et al demonstrated that age standardized rates (per 1000 woman-years) for fibroid incidence were lowest for Asian women, followed by white women, then Hispanic women, and substantially increased for black women (10.4, 12.5, 14.5, 37.9 per 1000 woman-years, respectively).[5]

## RISK FACTORS

While age and race are, epidemiologically, the most significant risk factors for the development of uterine fibroids, many other factors have been analyzed for their potential contribution to the development of these tumors. Although the impact and prevalence of these risk factors vary among specific populations, their pathophysiologic associations may be categorized according to hormonal and nonhormonal mechanisms.

### Menstrual Factors

Multiple studies have demonstrated increased fibroid growth in response to estrogenic stimuli, with a correspondingly significant reduction in growth when gonadotropin-releasing hormone (GnRH) analogs are used to induce a hypoestrogenic state.[9] Thus, prolonged estrogen exposure should increase the incidence of leiomyomas. This theory is supported by data that indicate an increased risk of fibroid incidence in patients with early menarche.[10–13] Although these studies are not consistent with regard to populations examined, both Marshall and Faerstein demonstrated significant increases in fibroid incidence in women with menarche occurring below 11 years of age.[7,10] However, while both studies demonstrated increased risks, Faerstein demonstrated nearly twice the risk found in Marshall's study with an adjusted odds ratio of 2.4 (95% CI 1.1, 5.6) versus Marshall's adjusted odds ratio of 1.35 (95% CI 1.19, 1.53). In contrast, most studies demonstrate either significant decreases or trends toward decreased fibroid incidence in women in whom menarche occurred after 13 years of age.[1] Against referent menarchal ages of 12 or 13, patients with menarche occurring after age 13 had reductions in fibroid incidence ranging from 17% to 60%. These reductions were greatest in women who experienced menarche at age 16 or greater.[9,13] More recently, Wise et al examined a cohort of 22,895 African American women. For women with menarche after the age of 12 to 13, the risk progressively decreased with increasing menarchal age, resulting in a 30% reduction among women with menarche after age 15.[14]

Menstrual patterns also may have an effect on the risk of fibroids. Chen et al assessed risk factors for fibroids in women undergoing tubal sterilization, in a population of reproductive age women (Table 14-1).[15] White women with heavy menstrual flow and cycle duration longer than 6 days had significantly increased risk of uterine leiomyoma, with odds ratios of 1.4 and 1.5, respectively. However, there were no significant menstrual-related associations for African American women. Cycle regularity, dysmenorrhea, prolonged cycle length, and intermenstrual bleeding had no significant association with leiomyoma. While Faerstein found no significant association between fibroids and cycle interval, cycle duration, or menstrual irregularity, patients with menstrual flow longer than 6 days demonstrated a trend

toward increased fibroid incidence, with an odds ratio of 1.4 (95% CI 0.9, 2.1) when controlled for confounding variables.[7]

### Gravidity and Parity

Women with a history of pregnancy and childbearing appear to have a reduced risk of fibroids. The risk with at least one live-born child is reduced by 20% to 50%.[1] The majority of studies have demonstrated that increasing parity corresponds with lower fibroid incidence, with reductions of up to 70% to 80% for women with greater than four deliveries.[6,10,13,16] In contrast, Faerstein found no difference in risk of fibroids when controlling for parity in a multivariate model that accounted for all relevant confounding variables.[7] Interestingly, Chen et al found a substantial risk reduction of up to 70% in white women with two or more live children; however, in women of African American descent, there was no relationship between parity and fibroid incidence.[15] Wise also demonstrated no significant impact of parity on fibroid incidence in African American women.[14] Thus, while it would appear that the risk of fibroids decreases with increasing parity, there is some suggestion that other factors, such as race, likely account for a greater degree of the variance in fibroid incidence. Moreover, it is possible that women with fibroids have a greater incidence of infertility (see later discussion) and thus fewer pregnancies.[9]

Until recently, there was no evidence that age at first delivery has a significant impact on the incidence of fibroids. In the cohort study by Wise, multivariate analyses demonstrated that African American women with progressively greater age at first delivery had significantly lower risks of uterine leiomyomas compared with women whose first delivery occurred before 20 years of age.[14] No such relationship has been demonstrated among white women. In contrast, there is some controversy about the significance of age at last delivery and its impact on fibroid risk. Women who deliver prior to the age of 35 are at significantly increased risk of developing or having fibroids compared with women who were older than age 35 at their last delivery.[6,13] In contrast, Faerstein demonstrated no significant increase in risk of fibroids in women greater than 35 years of age compared with women less than 25 years of age when controlled for covariates.[7] Similarly, Chen et al demonstrated no increase in risk of fibroids based on age at last delivery compared with a reference group of women less than 24 years of age whether they were white or African American.[15]

### Infertility

Discussions of the impact of a diagnosis of infertility on the risk of fibroids are marred by heterogeneity in definitions of infertility, prior infertility investigations, and prior exposure to infertility-related treatments, as well as difficulty in ascertaining whether the fibroids caused the infertility or whether the infertility caused the fibroids. However, most studies suggest an association between infertility and the risk of developing fibroids. Biologically, the substantial proportion of oligomenorrheic women who constitute most infertile populations would be at risk of unopposed estrogen states with consequent impact on leiomyoma growth and development. However, to date no epidemiologic studies have specifically examined this relationship. Marshall et al demonstrated a 35% increase in fibroid risk in nulliparous patients with a prior history of infertility compared

**Table 14-1**

**Risk of Uterine Fibroids Relative to Menstrual Cycle Abnormalities in White and African American Women**

| Menstrual Cycle Characteristic | White Women | | | | | | African American Women | | | | | |
|---|---|---|---|---|---|---|---|---|---|---|---|---|
| | Cases (n=247) | | Controls (n=988) | | Odds Ratio* | 95% Confidence Interval | Cases (n=70) | | Controls (n=280) | | Odds Ratio* | 95% Confidence Interval |
| | No. | Percent | No. | Percent | | | No. | Percent | No. | Percent | | |
| **Heavy flow** | | | | | | | | | | | | |
| No | 131 | 53.5 | 591 | 60.0 | 1.0† | | 38 | 54.3 | 177 | 63.2 | 1.0† | |
| Yes | 114 | 46.5 | 394 | 40.0 | 1.4 | 1.01, 1.8 | 32 | 45.7 | 103 | 36.8 | 1.4 | 0.8, 2.5 |
| **Irregular cycles** | | | | | | | | | | | | |
| No | 218 | 89 | 844 | 85.7 | 1.0† | | 65 | 92.9 | 254 | 90.7 | 1.0† | |
| Yes | 27 | 11 | 141 | 14.3 | 0.7 | 0.4, 1.1 | 5 | 7.1 | 26 | 9.3 | 0.7 | 0.3, 2.1 |
| **Duration of bleeding (days)** | | | | | | | | | | | | |
| 1–5 | 150 | 61.7 | 660 | 68.3 | 1.0† | | 61 | 87.1 | 239 | 86.3 | 1.0† | |
| ≥6 | 93 | 38.3 | 306 | 31.7 | 1.5 | 1.1, 2.0 | 9 | 12.9 | 38 | 13.7 | 0.8 | 0.3, 1.8 |
| Median duration (days) | 5.0 | | 5.0 | | | | 5.0 | | 5.0 | | | |
| p for trend | 0.08 | | | | | | 0.83 | | | | | |
| **Severe pain** | | | | | | | | | | | | |
| No | 160 | 65.6 | 695 | 70.7 | 1.0† | | 45 | 64.3 | 190 | 68.1 | 1.0† | |
| Yes | 84 | 34.4 | 288 | 29.3 | 1.3 | 0.9, 1.8 | 25 | 35.7 | 89 | 31.9 | 1.2 | 0.7, 2.2 |
| **Cycle length** | | | | | | | | | | | | |
| ≤30 | 204 | 82.6 | 827 | 83.7 | 1.0† | | 63 | 90.0 | 256 | 91.4 | 1.0 | |
| >30 | 24 | 9.7 | 61 | 6.2 | 0.7 | 1.0, 2.9 | 3 | 4.3 | 3 | 1.1 | 4.8 | 0.9, 25.9 |
| Unknown | 19 | 7.7 | 100 | 10.1 | 0.8 | 0.4, 1.3 | 4 | 5.7 | 21 | 7.5 | 0.8 | 0.3, 2.8 |
| Median length (days) | 28.0 | | 28.0 | | | | 28.0 | | 28.0 | | | |
| p for trend | 0.37 | | | | | | 0.06 | | | | | |
| **Spotting between cycles** | | | | | | | | | | | | |
| No | 223 | 91.0 | 928 | 94.2 | 1.0† | | 61 | 87.1 | 253 | 90.4 | 1.0† | |
| Yes | 22 | 9.0 | 57 | 5.8 | 1.3 | 0.7, 2.2 | 9 | 12.9 | 27 | 9.6 | 1.4 | 0.6, 3.3 |

*Adjusted for age at sterilization and number of living children (continuous variables), using unconditional logistic regression.

†=Referent.

Reproduced with permission from Chen CR, Buck GM, Courey NG, et al: Risk factors for uterine fibroids among women undergoing tubal sterilization. Am J Epidemiol 2001;153:20–26.

with nulliparous patients with no history of infertility, while Faerstein found no increased risk in general, but a nearly 2.5-fold increase in risk in patients diagnosed with infertility prior to age 25.[7,10]

## Hormone Exposure

Animal studies have demonstrated hormonal responsiveness of leiomyomas to estrogens and progestins. Based on these studies, it is plausible that exogenous estrogen and progestin exposure would influence the risk of uterine leiomyoma. Studies examining the relationship between combined oral contraceptives (OCs) and fibroids have yielded conflicting results, with some showing increased risks and others showing no risk or risk reductions of up to 31% in women using oral contraceptives for more than 10 years. In African Americans, the evidence appears to suggest that OC users are at increased risk of fibroid growth, especially when OCs are initiated during adolescence.[14]

Although one study demonstrated a strong correlation between depot medroxyprogesterone acetate injectable contraception and decreased fibroid incidence, the majority of clinical studies demonstrate a significant role of progestins in stimulation of fibroid growth. At least three randomized, controlled trials of GnRH analog suppression plus progestin add-back therapy demonstrated that progestin add-back nullified the

suppressive effects of GnRH therapy, with at least one study showing an increase in fibroid growth in the progestin add-back group.[17]

It is well established that fibroids regress in the post-menopause period. Thus, persistent hormonal stimulation may negate the natural tendency of leiomyomas to decrease in volume and incidence following menopause. Studies of postmenopausal hormone replacement therapy suggest either no growth or a minimal increase in fibroid growth and symptomatology.[18–21] The studies examining this relationship have been conducted in small population samples with limited statistical power. Reed et al studied the effect of HRT use on having a first diagnosis of fibroids.[22] HRT use for more than 5 years resulted in a 4-fold increase in incidence of first diagnosis of uterine leiomyomas in peri- and postmenopausal women with a BMI less than 24 kg/m$^2$.

BMI itself has been investigated as an independent risk factor for fibroid growth. Increasing BMI appears to substantially increase risk of fibroid development and growth.[6,7,13,23] Increasing BMI appears to lead to increased risks. Faerstein demonstrated a 2.3-fold increase in risk only for women with BMI greater than 25.4 kg/m$^2$.[7] However, others have not shown a significant increase in risk related to BMI.[11,12,15,24] Wise demonstrated that BMI had an impact on the relationship of parity to fibroid risk.[14] Parous women with a BMI less than 27 kg/m$^2$ had a 40% reduction in risk compared with nulliparous women, whereas this risk reduction was reduced to only 20% in parous women with a BMI greater than 27 kg/m$^2$.

Cigarette smoking has consistently been shown to reduce the risk of fibroids. Most studies demonstrate a 20% to 50% reduction in fibroid risk when controlled for confounders, including BMI.[6,12,13,25] In contrast, Chen et al demonstrated that increased risk was present only in white smokers with a daily habit of more than 1 pack per day use.[15] Ex-smokers had no increased risk. Wise et al similarly demonstrated no significant change in risk among African American women based on smoking status.[14] Although, theoretically, smoking contributes to lower estrogen levels with consequent decreases in fibroid growth, this relationship has not been proved.[26] Derangements in estrogen metabolism, however, may contribute to the risk reductions observed. Furthermore, the association between decreased fibroid incidence and smoking may in part be due to the strong correlation between smoking and decreased BMI.

## Summary

In summary, many factors have a potential contribution to fibroid risk. The preponderance of risk is likely associated with age and race. Increasing age contributes to increasing fibroid incidence until the menopause at which time significant fibroid regression occurs almost universally. Menarchal age also appears to significantly affect fibroid risk. African American women are at significantly increased risk of leiomyomas. The significance of the contributions of age and race may outweigh the effect of other variables and explain the frequent discrepancy in findings between the various epidemiologic studies cited. Hormone-related risk factors appear to increase risk, but there is significant controversy among studies about the degree and nature of these risks. Furthermore, prospective large-scale studies are necessary to determine the actual contribution and significance of risk factors for leiomyomas.

## PATHOGENESIS

A variety of mechanisms have been proposed for the initiation of tumorigenesis necessary for fibroid formation. Hypotheses include genetic predisposition, menstrual cycle–related mitotic dysregulation, myometrial cell phenotype transformation in response to ischemia, and an inherent myometrial predisposition to fibroid formation. Despite the abundance of theories and evidentiary support, a specific common cause has yet to be identified in fibroid formation.

### Genetic Etiology

Fibroid tumors appear to develop from a single progenitor cell, causing them to be monoclonal. Initially, this evidence was derived from analyzing the two different alleles of the X-linked glucose-6-phosphate dehydrogenase (G6PD) enzyme in fibroid tumors.[27] Townsend demonstrated that each tumor had only one of the two alleles, with either only type A or type B G6PD isoenzymes present in any given tumor. Moreover, within the same uterus, different fibroids could have different alleles, establishing the individual origin of each tumor. More recently, these data have been supported by studies using methylation

sensitive restriction endonuclease enzymes that have demonstrated monoclonal origins based on analysis of the androgen receptor allele and the phosphoglycerokinase gene.[28,29]

### Specific Gene Defects

Further evidence for a genetic basis for leiomyomas derives from the presence of common genetic abnormalities. While the majority of fibroids are chromosomally normal, approximately 40% have chromosomal abnormalities.[30] Gross et al classified these abnormalities into six cytogenetic subgroups: t(12;14) chromosomal translocation, trisomy 12, rearrangements of the short arm of chromosome 6, rearrangements of the long arm of chromosome 10, and chromosome 3 and 7 deletions.[30]

To date, the chromosomal anomaly most commonly identified is the t(12;14)(q14-q15;q23-q24) translocation, which is evident in approximately 20% of all leiomyomas.[30] The q14-q15 region on chromosome 12 is significant because of its anomalous presence in other mesenchymal tumors. Rearrangements of the 12q14-q15 region have been found in gynecologic related neoplasms, including endometrial polyps and breast fibroadenomas, as well as in salivary gland adenomas, angiomyxomas, hemangiopericytomas, pulmonary chondroid hamartomas, and salivary gland adenomas. This region is of particular interest because it codes for a high mobility group protein (HMGIC) that binds to DNA, inducing transcription-related conformational changes.[31] The HMGIC (and HMGIY; see later discussion) proteins are both expressed highly in tumor cells and during embryogenesis.[31] Although their precise role is not understood, it is believed that both function as proliferation factors in tissues of mesenchymal origin. Molecular analyses revealed that normal endometrium had no expression of the HMGIC protein, while chromosomally aberrant leiomyomas had high levels of HMGIC protein expression.[31] The 14q23-24 region is also of interest because of its specificity for uterine leiomyomas and its proximity to the estrogen receptor beta gene (ERβ). Interaction between these two loci may factor in the development of uterine fibroids. However, to date there is no evidence to indicate up-regulation of ERβ transcription in uterine leiomyomas.[32] Recently the RAD51L1 gene has been implicated in 14q23-24 rearrangements, with a purported function in cell cycle regulation. However, its specific role in leiomyoma genesis has yet to be determined.[26]

Rearrangements of the short arm of chromosome 6 (6p21) have been found in less than 5% of leiomyomas.[26] This region is of interest because it codes for HMGIY, a protein with similar properties to the HMGIC gene. This protein has been demonstrated in other common neoplasias including lipomas, hamartomas, and endometrial polyps.[33-37] Expression is increased in fibroids with 6p21 abnormalities compared with normal endometrium, but unlike HMGIC, HMGIY expression is also present in normal endometrium and chromosomally normal leiomyomas.[38] Thus, its exact function in the genesis of leiomyomas is not known.

Deletional abnormalities of chromosome 7, del(7)(q22q32) for example, have been found in 17% of chromosomally abnormal fibroids.[39] These aberrations are often present in mosaic cell lines in fibroids. Their presence has been noted in other neoplasms such as lipomas and endometrial polyps although they are most commonly found in leiomyomas. The specific region of 7q22 has been implicated as the region affected by deletions; however, this region codes for a variety of genes with cell growth and development functions. No specific deletion of any of these genes has elucidated the pathogenesis of fibroids.

Trisomy 12 cell lines are thought to play a role by increasing HMGIC expression.[40] Aberrations in chromosomes 10 and 3 also have been noted in leiomyomas, but putative genes and their role in fibroid pathogenesis remain to be identified.[41]

### Heritability

As discussed earlier, ethnicity plays a significant role in the predilection for developing uterine leiomyomas. Women of African American descent have a 2- to 10-fold increase in the incidence of uterine fibroids compared with white women, supporting a genetic predisposition to fibroids based on differing racial DNA profiles. These data may be used to help isolate specific genes responsible for these differences. However, to date, there has been no identification of a racially specific gene or alteration of gene expression leading to increased fibroid formation.

Two studies of fibroid incidence in twins validate a heritable genetic hypothesis for fibroids. The Australian twin registry demonstrated a greater than 2-fold twin-pair correlation for hysterectomy in monozygotic versus dizygotic twins.[42] Fibroids represent the most common indication for hysterectomy; thus supporting a genetic link for fibroids. However, this study did not specifically assess the number of uterine leiomyomas, leaving other genetic variables as potential contributors to the increased hysterectomy incidence among monozygotic twins. More recently, a Finnish twin cohort study analyzed hospitalization for fibroids and determined that there was a higher incidence of hospitalization among monozygotic compared with dizygotic twins.[43] However, ultrasonographic assessment demonstrated no significant increase in risk based on zygosity. The authors concluded that other risk factors may contribute as much to the incidence of fibroids as genetic predisposition.

Family history of fibroids has been reported, first by Winkler and Hoffman in 1938, who demonstrated a 4.2-fold increase in fibroids among first-degree relatives.[44] Two further studies demonstrated similar findings in first-degree relatives and sisters of affected individuals in a Russian population, with one study demonstrating an increase from a baseline of 2.45% to 26.1% in sisters of affected patients and to 19.7% in daughters of affected patients.[45,46] Schwartz et al examined familial aggregation patterns in a study of 638 women.[47] All patients were between the ages of 18 and 59 years and had either operative or ultrasonographic evidence of leiomyomas. These patients were matched to 617 controls. The odds ratio for leiomyomas was 2.5 in patients with a positive family history, increasing to 5.7 in patients with a family history of fibroids and a positive diagnosis prior to 45 years of age.

Further evidence of genetic associations can be derived from analysis of heritable conditions that predispose to fibroid development. For example, Reed syndrome is an inherited autosomal dominant trait that causes a significant increase in both uterine and cutaneous leiomyomas. The gene responsible codes for a tumor suppressor gene, and mutations in the gene decrease tumor suppressor function.[26]

### Summary

In summary, molecular, genomic, and epidemiologic evidence all support a genetic hypothesis in the genesis of some uterine leiomyomas. Although no specific genetic defects have been clearly linked to the initiating mechanism in fibroid development, further studies are warranted to determine whether specific genetic derangements contribute to the formation of fibroids. Since the majority of fibroids remain chromosomally normal, other factors also must play a crucial role in the pathogenesis of leiomyomas.

### Hormonal Etiology

It has long been believed that uterine leiomyomas are estrogen-dependent tumors. More recent evidence suggests a plausible causative role for progesterone as well.[48] Despite a substantial number of studies evaluating the role of sex hormones in fibroid etiology, growth, and development, controversy exists and many questions remain.

### Estrogen

Extensive effort has been devoted to the study of estrogen receptors and uterine leiomyomas. Although some controversy exists over the presence of increased estrogen receptors in leiomyomas, most studies indicate that fibroids have a higher concentration of estrogen receptors than does normal myometrium.[26] While myometrial estrogen receptor concentrations vary during the normal menstrual cycle, Sadan et al demonstrated that fibroid estrogen receptor concentrations remain elevated throughout the menstrual cycle, regardless of fibroid volume.[49] Others have demonstrated that estrogen receptor alpha and beta both are present in leiomyomas and that both may be up-regulated when compared with normal myometrium.[32,50] The finding of ERβ up-regulation in myomas is significant because of the proximity of the gene locus to the region of chromosome 14 involved in the t(12;14) chromosomal translocation commonly found in uterine leiomyomas.

Several authors have demonstrated increased concentrations of estrogen within leiomyomas.[51,52] Yamamoto et al showed that there was a decreased conversion of estradiol to its bioactively weaker metabolite of estrone in leiomyomas as compared with normal endometrium.[53] Potential causes may be related to reduced activity of 17β-hydroxysteroid dehydrogenase, or to increased levels of aromatase enzyme.[52] Via either pathway, precursors would be converted to increased levels of estrogenic compounds, with potential stimulatory effects on myometrial and hence leiomyomatous cells. These effects are thought to occur in an autocrine or intracrine manner, suggesting a local effect. This theory is supported by multiple studies that fail to demonstrate any substantial difference in serum levels of estradiol in patients with leiomyomas as compared with normal controls.[54–56] Estrogenic activity may also be increased by modification of the estradiol molecule. Leihr et al demonstrated higher concentrations of $C_4$ hydroxylated estradiol metabolites in myomas, the likely result of increased estradiol 4-hydroxylase activity.[57] The 4-hydroxylated estradiol molecule has a greater affinity for the estradiol receptor than estradiol does, thus presenting another source of locally produced growth stimulants.

To date, no evidence proves a direct role of estrogen in fibroid pathogenesis. However, estrogen has been shown to up-regulate numerous other factors with potential effects on fibroid growth including epidermal growth factor, insulin-like growth factor, gap junction proteins, and the progesterone receptor.[48] By exerting an influence on the concentration of these factors it is likely that estrogen plays a significant role in the genesis of leiomyomas.

### Progesterone

Progesterone receptors are also found in increased concentration in leiomyomas.[58] Although it is controversial, it appears that fibroid progesterone receptors have also been found in increased concentrations throughout the menstrual cycle.[49] These findings are particularly noteworthy because during the normal menstrual cycle estrogen (normally) would stimulate an increase of progesterone receptors, yet in fibroids, this regulatory system is abolished and receptor concentration is maintained at an elevated level. Both progesterone receptor A and progesterone receptor B are expressed in fibroids with progesterone receptor A levels higher than those of the type B receptor in both leiomyomatous and normal myometrial tissues.[59]

In contrast to estrogen, progesterone levels do not appear to be elevated within myomas as compared with surrounding normal endometrium.[60] However, increased progesterone levels have been shown to increase mitotic indices in fibroids, potentiating growth both during cyclic hormonal changes in the menstrual cycle and when administered exogenously.[61,62] Kawaguchi et al examined menstrual cycle–dependent mitotic rates in uterine leiomyomas in 181 women.[62] They found that the mitotic count was highest, at 12.7 per high-powered field, in the progesterone-dominant secretory phase, achieving a middle value of 8.3 per high-powered field during menses and down to a low of 3.8 per high-powered field during the estrogen-dominant proliferative phase. Kawaguchi subsequently analyzed the effect of progesterone and estrogen on fibroid myocytes in culture.[63] Cells cultured in progesterone and estrogen-enriched media had more active growth and development than those cultured in an estrogen-only medium. Serum progesterone levels also are not increased in women with leiomyomas. Unless exogenously administered, the impact of progesterone appears limited to autocrine and intracrine mechanisms, where, at a molecular level, it appears to exert a significant influence on the growth and development of fibroids.

### Growth Factors

Both estrogen and progesterone appear to interact through a variety of growth factors in leiomyomas to induce and stimulate growth. Epidermal growth factor (EGF) and its receptor (EGF-R) can be found in both normal myometrium and leiomyoma cells. Maruo et al demonstrated that estrogen increases the local production of EGF in leiomyoma cell cultures, while progesterone synergistically increases EGF-R levels.[64] Several authors have demonstrated the importance of this growth factor in regulation of fibroid growth.[65–68] Transforming growth factor β3 (TGFβ3) mRNA levels are up to 5-fold higher in myomas compared with normal myometrium.[69] This factor likely contributes to increasing mitogenic potential of leiomyoma cells while also increasing extracellular matrix deposition. TGFβ3 is of significant importance, not only because of the functional potential of the product, but also because of its proximity to the

t(12;14) breakpoint on chromosome 14, downstream of the ERβ gene. Other factors with potential contributions not yet clearly elucidated include platelet-derived growth factor, vascular endothelial growth factor, insulin-like growth factor I, basic fibroblast growth factor, and prolactin.[26]

Recent studies have also focused on the potential influence of alterations of the growth cycle in fibroids.[62,70–72] During normal menses, myocytes undergo growth arrest and potentially undergo apoptosis. However, leiomyomatous cells have increased rates of cellular proliferation with a decreased apoptotic rate compared with normal endometrium. This combination could easily explain the growth of leiomyomas as cells replicate more rapidly without dying as frequently.

Thus, within the peptide and hormone milieu of the endometrium and myometrium, significant interaction appears to occur—between genetic elements, sex steroids, and growth factors—to initiate and then stimulate the growth and development of fibroids. With further research, specific pathways demonstrating the interaction of these factors and potential initiating events or catalysts may be identified. Identification of these pathways is essential to management of both symptoms and manifestations of uterine leiomyomas.

## CLINICAL MANIFESTATIONS

The high prevalence of fibroids has led most authorities to attribute multiple clinical manifestations to the presence of these tumors. Despite the high prevalence of these tumors and the frequency with which they necessitate medical or surgical intervention, the majority of women remain asymptomatic. Most studies of fibroid symptomatology rely on paired comparisons before and after intervention strategies.[73] These studies do not accurately reflect the incidence of clinical presentations of fibroids, since the patients are selected because of one or more complications related to their leiomyomas. Moreover, because both medical and surgical strategies have significant physical and psychological impact, combined with the inevitable placebo effect, these studies cannot be relied upon to explain the true clinical nature of uterine leiomyomas.

While controversy exists about the exact role of fibroids in the generation of specific symptomatology, it is important for the practicing gynecologist to be familiar with the classic manifestations of these tumors, as they may play a role in a variety of symptoms as diverse as pelvic pain and constipation. To classify the wide range of presentations potentially attributable to fibroids, we recommend a modification of Stewart's classification system,[74] dividing presentations into one of four subgroups: abnormal uterine bleeding, pelvic pain or pressure including affected organ system dysfunction, reproductive dysfunction such as infertility and miscarriage, and pregnancy-related complications.

### Abnormal Uterine Bleeding

Abnormal uterine bleeding (AUB) is the most frequently cited symptom in women with fibroids.[75] While menorrhagia is the most common type of abnormal bleeding experienced, patients may have metrorrhagia or menometrorrhagia. Buttram and Reiter reviewed nine studies citing an incidence of menorrhagia between 17% and 62%.[2] Bettocchi et al examined women with

AUB who underwent hysterectomy within 2 months of having a diagnostic dilation and curettage procedure.[76] Hysterectomy confirmed that in 40% of these women myomas were the source of their AUB. In the Ontario Uterine Fibroid Embolization Trial (OUFET), 74% of 538 women undergoing bilateral uterine artery embolization (UAE) had four or fewer myomas.[77] Overall, 17% of women with myomas came in with menorrhagia and 63% with a combination of menorrhagia and pain. Chen et al reported that white women with menorrhagia had a 40% increased incidence of leiomyomas, whereas African American women had no increase in risk.[15]

Thirty percent of women in the OUFET trial reported having menses that lasted more than 7 days. The median pad count was 9 per day. Rybo et al demonstrated that fibroids were four times more common in women with excessive menstrual loss of greater than 200 mL.[78] Chen reported that in white women with fibroids, nearly 40% had a duration of menses equal to or greater than 6 days, while only 13% of African American women experienced prolonged menses.[15] Both African American and white women experienced an approximately 10% incidence of intermenstrual bleeding.

The mechanism of menorrhagia in women with fibroids has not been clearly delineated. Myoma location may be important in determining the severity of bleeding associated with fibroids (Fig. 14-1). Submucosal myomas may increase the likelihood of menorrhagia either by local effects on endometrium adjacent to the fibroid or by alteration of endometrium directly over the fibroid surface. However, no hysteroscopic or microscopic evidence supports this hypothesis.[73] Vascular changes have been suggested as a potential mechanism of fibroid-induced menorrhagia.[79] Myometrium adjacent to myomas undergoes venous compression leading to formation of venous lakes in the myometrium that may influence bleeding patterns. Numerous growth factors as well as local hormone and prostaglandin influences may play roles in the development of menorrhagia. These may include elevated levels of 6-keto prostaglandin $F_{1\alpha}$ ($PGF_{1\alpha}$) and prostacyclin.[80] Others have suggested impaired endometrial hemostasis as a mechanism for altered bleeding in patients with fibroids.[81]

It is unclear how often leiomyomas can cause menstrual loss significant enough to cause anemia. In a small study of 61 women with AUB and moderate-to-severe anemia, 38% of patients had a submucosal myoma.[82] Little evidence directly correlates the presence of myomas and the incidence of iron deficiency anemia, even though they are often cited as a common cause of iron deficiency anemia in reproductive-age women.

Fibroids are also commonly associated with dysmenorrhea. In the OUFET trial, 60% of patients had dysmenorrhea.[77] In contrast, Lippman et al demonstrated no increased risk of dysmenorrhea in fibroid affected women compared with patients without fibroids.[83] However, when evaluating pain symptoms by fibroid location, these authors demonstrated a nearly 3-fold increase (29% vs. 11%) in moderate-to-severe dysmenorrhea in women with submucosal fibroids versus women without myomas. The elevated levels of prostaglandins $PGF_{1\alpha}$ and $PGF_{2\alpha}$ demonstrated in leiomyomatous uteri have also been associated with dysmenorrhea. Thus, it is biologically plausible that fibroids contribute to the development of dysmenorrhea.

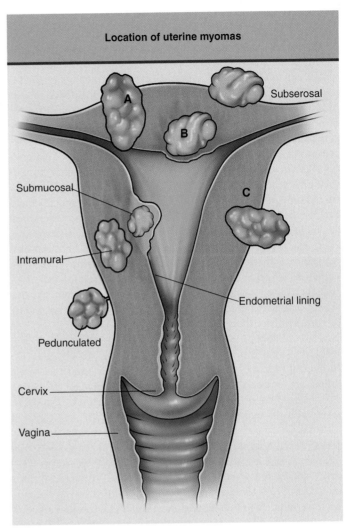

**Location of uterine myomas**

Subserosal

Submucosal

Intramural

Pedunculated

Cervix

Vagina

C

Endometrial lining

**Figure 14-1    Locations of uterine myomas.** Submucosal fibroids intrude into or are contained in the uterine cavity; intramural fibroids are contained within the wall of the uterus, and subserosal ones create the characteristic irregular feel of the myomatous uterus. Most myomas are of mixed type, however, as illustrated by A, B, and C. (From Stewart EA: Uterine fibroids. Lancet 2001;357:293–298. Reprinted with permission from Elsevier.)

## Pelvic Pain and Pressure

Pelvic pain and pressure are the second most frequently reported symptoms. The presence of pain may be related to compression of organs or nerves, to ureteric compression from large, broad ligament or cervical fibroids, or to compression from torsion of pedunculated fibroids. Pain may also be related to prolapsed leiomyomas that undergo ischemic or necrotic changes.[3] Kjerulff et al recorded 41% of white and 59% of African American patients complaining of severe pelvic pain.[84] Chen et al found an approximately 35% incidence of severe pain in both races.[15] The study by Lippman et al, which evaluated 635 women who had a pelvic ultrasound and were subsequently followed for reproductive outcome, demonstrated a trend toward increased risks of dyspareunia and noncyclic pelvic pain in women found to have fibroids.[83] These authors also found an increased risk of dyspareunia and noncyclic pelvic pain when myomas were located in the fundal portion of the uterus. Other authors have also found that fibroid location influences the severity and location of pain.[75]

Pelvic pressure symptoms can occur in women with a myomatous uterus. Few data exist on the relative contribution of fibroids to the development of these symptoms in unselected populations. The OUFET trial reported an 8% incidence of only bulk or pressure-related symptoms prior to study enrollment.[77] However, nearly 86% of patients complained of bulk and pressure symptoms and 57% complained of urinary urgency/frequency symptoms as components of their clinical presentation. Anterior fibroids can cause bladder dysfunction, whereas posterior fibroids may affect bowel function. Such symptoms are dependent on the volume of the leiomyomas. Bladder dynamics can be significantly altered by changes in bladder capacity, urethrovesical angle changes, and incomplete bladder emptying. Although rare, complete ureteric obstruction has been reported.[85] Symptoms related to urinary changes must be investigated for alternative explanations prior to surgical management of leiomyomas.[2,3,86] Although rare, bowel complications can be significant. In one report, a patient experienced a large bowel obstruction secondary to compressive effects of a uterine leiomyoma.[87]

### Infertility

In clinical practice, leiomyomas are frequently used to explain otherwise unexplained infertility. Indeed, between 27% and 40% of women with myomas experience infertility.[2] However, some authors suggest that myomas are rarely the sole cause of infertility, accounting for a true fibroid related incidence of only 1% to 2%.[2] Other authors rarely suggest that more than 10% of infertility cases are attributable to the presence of leiomyomas.[88] Pritts conducted a meta-analysis (Table 14-2) to answer three questions: (1) Is there a higher incidence of infertility in patients with fibroids? (2) Does fibroid location affect the incidence of infertility? (3) Does myomectomy enhance fertility?[89] Women

with subserosal and intramural fibroids did not have a higher risk of infertility, although a subanalysis of almost 4000 patients showed a strong trend toward a significant reduction in implantation rates. Women with submucosal fibroids had significantly reduced fertility. The presence of submucosal fibroids resulted in a 68% reduction in implantation and a 73% reduction in clinical pregnancy. It is important to note that this meta-analysis demonstrated no significant increase in infertility when all women with fibroids were pooled, regardless of leiomyoma location. Most authors support the concept that fibroids affect fertility with decreasing significance from submucosal to intramural to subserosal anatomic locations.[90] In contrast, in a study by Bulletti et al, 11% of patients with myomas and infertility went on to conceive, while 27% of patients with infertility without myomas achieved conception, a highly significant difference between groups ($P < 0.001$).[91]

The potential for myomas to affect fertility also appears clear from studies examining the positive benefits of myomectomy on fertility rates. Bulletti's study demonstrated that women with myomectomy had an even higher pregnancy rate of 42% than the 11% rate found in untreated controls.[91] Interestingly, the pregnancy rate in the myomectomized group was nearly twice that of the no-myoma infertility group!

In keeping with the findings from the previously mentioned studies, patients who experience infertility and subsequently undergo in vitro fertilization (IVF) therapy also appear to have adverse effects if fibroids are present. In an analysis of seven separate studies of the effects of myomas on in vitro fertilization therapy, Donnez and Jadoul found that patients with uterine cavity–distorting myomas had a 9% pregnancy rate compared with 29.1% for patients with myomas without cavity distortion, and 25.1% for patients without myomas.[92] When conducting a meta-analysis of the results of these studies, these authors demonstrated a 9% pregnancy rate for women with endometrial

| | No. of Studies with Infertile Controls | No. | Relative Risk | 95% CI |
|---|---|---|---|---|
| **Table 14-2** **Relative Risks and Confidence Interval (CI) of Pregnancy, Implantation, and Delivery Rate in Women with Fibroids, Compared with Infertile Controls** | | | | |
| Mixed subserosal, intramural, and submucosal pregnancy rates | 8 | 3616 | 1.021 | 0.885–1.171 |
| Mixed subserosal, intramural, and submucosal implantation rates | 5 | 3724 | 0.746 | 0.625–0.888* |
| Mixed subserosal, intramural, and submucosal delivery rates | 5 | 1490 | 0.833 | 0.682–1.010 |
| Subserosal and intramural pregnancy rates | 7 | 1507 | 0.963 | 0.822–1.122 |
| Subserosal and intramural implantation rates | 6 | 3906 | 0.862 | 0.726–1.022 |
| Subserosal and intramural delivery rates | 4 | 588 | 0.979 | 0.795–1.194 |
| Subserosal pregnancy rates | 1 | 359 | 1.108 | 0.065–1.720 |
| Subserosal delivery rates | 1 | 359 | 1.094 | 0.580–1.858 |
| Intramural pregnancy rates | 3 | 614 | 0.944 | 0.727–1.201 |
| Intramural implantation rates | 1 | 321 | 0.813 | 0.600–1.088 |
| Intramural delivery rates | 2 | 649 | 1.005 | 0.734–1.341 |
| Submucosal pregnancy rates | 2 | 510 | 0.321 | 0.130–0.697* |
| Submucosal implantation rates | 1 | 541 | 0.277 | 0.096–0.720* |

*Denotes statistical significance.
Modified with permission from Pritts EA: Fibroids and infertility: a systematic review of the evidence. Obstet Gynecol Surv 2001;56:483–491.

cavity–distorting myomas, 33.5% pregnancy rate for women with myomas not distorting the endometrial cavity, and 40% pregnancy rate for women without myomas. However, as with many meta-analyses, not all the studies independently demonstrated a significant effect of myomas on infertility therapy. Additional, recent studies appear to support a detrimental role of myomas on fertility therapy and assisted reproductive technologies. Hart et al conducted a prospective study of the effects of intramural myomas smaller than 5 cm on patients undergoing IVF therapy.[93] They found that, when controlled for age and number of embryos transferred, women with intramural fibroids had a 54% reduction in ongoing pregnancy rates, although biochemical pregnancy and implantation rates were not significantly different between groups in their models. It is becoming progressively more apparent that fibroids causing endometrial distortion or having extension into the endometrial cavity likely have a negative impact on the success of infertility therapy. The results appear to substantiate severe reductions in IVF success and mandate careful investigation and consideration of surgical intervention prior to assisted reproductive technology therapies.

To date two studies have examined the relationship between IVF and myomas that do not distort the endometrial cavity. Oliveira et al examined 245 women undergoing IVF and intracytoplasmic sperm injection (ICSI) with subserosal or intramural myomas determined by transvaginal ultrasound and compared these patients against 245 matched controls with no evidence of myomas.[94] In women with myomas less than 4 cm, there was no difference in outcome with regard to pregnancy, implantation, and abortion rates. However, women with myomas greater than 4 cm had a 30% pregnancy rate compared with a 52% pregnancy rate in women with myomas smaller than 4 cm. The number and location of the myomas had no impact on results. Check et al examined 61 women with exclusively intramural myomas, finding no difference in IVF outcomes, including positive β–human chorionic gonadotropin (β-hCG) levels, chemical pregnancies, clinical pregnancies, ectopic pregnancies, abortions, or live births.[95] Ng and Ho also confirmed these findings, demonstrating no difference in implantation rates (13.8% vs. 14.4%) or ongoing pregnancy rates (19.5% vs. 21.5%).[96] Thus, it would appear that the presence of intramural leiomyomas that have no impact on endometrial cavity architecture does not lead to any significant decrease in assisted reproductive technology success. These data are consistent with the proposed mechanisms for leiomyoma interference with implantation (Table 14-3).[97] Most of these hypotheses require fibroid proximity to the endometrium for a deleterious effect. The lack of such proximity and consequent endometrial distortion may significantly decrease the impact of these tumors on infertility therapy.

## Pregnancy and Pregnancy Outcomes

Between 1% and 4% of pregnancies are affected by the presence of fibroids.[88] The majority of these do not significantly change during pregnancy and frequently remain asymptomatic.[98] Some leiomyomas may shrink during pregnancy. Leiomyomas that increase in volume during pregnancy rarely grow by more than 25%.[99] Up to 10% of women with myomas experience some type of antepartum, intrapartum, or postpartum complication. Complications attributed to leiomyomas include recurrent

| Table 14-3 |
| Pathophysiologic Mechanisms of Fibroid-related Infertility |

- Potential effects on implantation and sperm transport as well as uterine contractility and perfusion
- Changes in the myometrial microvasculature consisting of abnormalities within tight junctions between endothelial cells
- Aberrant local expression of growth factors involved with angiogenesis

Adapted from Surrey ES: Impact of intramural leiomyomata on in-vitro fertilization-embryo transfer cycle outcome. Curr Opin Obstet Gynecol 2003;15:239–242.

miscarriage, antepartum and postpartum hemorrhage, placental disturbances including placental insufficiency and placental abruption, increased risk of preterm labor and delivery, increased cesarean section rate, and acute ischemic changes and fibroid degeneration secondary to decreased perfusion or torsion.

Fibroids appear to increase the risk of spontaneous first-trimester miscarriage. Benson et al assessed leiomyoma presence in the first trimester by transvaginal ultrasonography usually prior to 7 weeks of gestational age.[100] They compared 143 patients with leiomyomas with 715 control patients without myomas. The results of this study are presented in Table 14-4. Overall, patients with myomas had a 14% spontaneous loss rate versus 7.4% for patients without myomas. Patients with a single myoma had a small but significantly higher spontaneous loss rate, with only a 0.4% increase compared with patients without myomas. However, patients with multiple myomas had a 3-fold increase in spontaneous miscarriage rates and a 16% decrease in live-birth rates. There was no correlation between fibroid size or location and loss rates. Interestingly, only one patient had a submucosal fibroid and therefore the authors could not determine the impact of these specifically located myomas on miscarriage rate. Others, however, have reported high loss figures if implantation occurs over a submucosal fibroid. Li et al observed a 17% incidence of second-trimester miscarriage in affected patients with intramural and subserosal fibroids.[101] The pathophysiologic mechanisms may involve abnormal calcium

| Table 14-4 |
| Pregnancy Outcome Based on Number of Fibroids |

| No. of Fibroids | No. of Patients | Liveborn Rate (%) | Spontaneous Pregnancy Loss Rate (%) |
| --- | --- | --- | --- |
| No fibroids, normal uterus | 715 | 92.4 | 7.6 |
| Single fibroid | 88 | 92.0 | 8.0 |
| Multiple fibroids | 55 | 76.4 | 23.6 |
| Two | 25 | 76.0 | 24.0 |
| Three | 8 | 87.5 | 12.5 |
| Four or more | 22 | 72.7 | 27.3 |

$P < 0.05$ (Fisher's exact test) for comparison of loss rates with single vs. multiple fibroids.
Reproduced with permission from Benson CB, Chow JS, Chang-Lee W, et al: Outcome of pregnancies in women with uterine leiomyomas identified by sonography in the first trimester. J Clin Ultrasound 2001;29:261–264.

**Table 14-5**
**Association Between Uterine Leiomyomas and Pregnancy Complications**

| Pregnancy Complication | Percent Leiomyoma (n=2065) | Percent No Leiomyoma (n=4243) | Multivariate-adjusted* | |
|---|---|---|---|---|
| | | | OR | 95% CI |
| Any complication[†] | 40.44 | 24.86 | 1.87 | 1.59, 2.20 |
| First-trimester bleeding[†] | 1.84 | 0.80 | 1.82 | 1.05, 3.20 |
| Placenta previa | 0.87 | 0.49 | 1.76 | 0.76, 4.05 |
| Abruptio placentae | 1.84 | 0.60 | 3.87 | 1.63, 9.17 |
| Oligohydramnios | 1.07 | 0.66 | 1.80 | 0.80, 4.07 |
| Polyhydramnios | 0.68 | 0.40 | 2.44 | 1.02, 5.84 |
| Preeclampsia | 0.15 | 0.19 | 1.50 | 0.29, 7.87 |
| Other complications | 25.91 | 12.61 | 2.62 | 2.15, 3.20 |
| Anemia | 1.26 | 2.10 | 0.68 | 0.38, 1.19 |
| PROM | 4.55 | 2.50 | 1.79 | 1.20, 2.69 |

CI, confidence interval; OR, odds ratio; PROM, premature rupture of membranes.

*Adjusted for maternal age (<25, 25–34, ≥35 yr) and maternal weight gain (<25, 25–39, ≥40 lb).

[†]Data collected only for years 1989–1993 (n=1538 women with uterine leiomyomas, 3189 women without uterine leiomyomas).

Reproduced with permission from Coronado GD, Marshall LM, Schwartz SM: Complications in pregnancy, labor, and delivery with uterine leiomyomas: a population-based study. Obstet Gynecol 2000;95:764–769.

metabolism and consequent irregularities in myometrial contractions.[88]

In one of the largest studies of fibroid-related pregnancy complications, Coronado et al examined 2065 women from Washington State with hospital discharge records indicating the presence of leiomyomas.[102] These authors were able to assess a wide range of pregnancy complications while controlling for confounding variables including maternal age, race, ethnicity, marital status, residence, smoking status, parity, prior cesarean delivery, maternal weight gain, hypertension, and diabetes (Table 14-5). They reported significantly increased antepartum risks, with an odds ratio of 1.87 (CI 1.59, 2.20) for risk of

any complication. Specifically, first-trimester bleeding, placental abruption, polyhydramnios, and premature rupture of the membranes were all significantly increased, with odds ratios ranging from 1.79 for premature rupture of the membranes to an astounding 3.87 for placental abruption.

Labor- and delivery-related complications were also significantly increased in these patients (Table 14-6). Patients with leiomyomas had increased labor dysfunction, an increased incidence of breech presentation, and a greater than 6-fold increase in risk of cesarean section. Adverse birth outcomes were also increased, with leiomyomas being associated with higher risks of Apgar scores below 7 at 5 minutes, malformations, birth

**Table 14-6**
**Association Between Uterine Leiomyomas and Labor and Delivery Complications**

| Labor and Delivery Complication | Percent Leiomyoma (n=2065) | Percent No Leiomyoma (n=4243) | Multivariate-adjusted* | |
|---|---|---|---|---|
| | | | OR | 95% CI |
| Labor complications | 50.61 | 30.73 | 1.90 | 1.65, 2.18 |
| Dysfunctional labor[†] | 4.12 | 1.65 | 1.85 | 1.26, 2.72 |
| Prolonged labor | 3.58 | 1.84 | 1.17 | 0.80, 1.71 |
| Excessive bleeding[†] | 0.82 | 0.71 | 1.58 | 0.76, 3.29 |
| Delivery complications | | | | |
| Breech presentation | 12.59 | 3.04 | 3.98 | 3.07, 5.16 |
| Precipitous labor[†] | 0.58 | 1.89 | 0.41 | 0.21, 0.81 |
| Cesarean delivery | 58.31 | 17.51 | 6.39 | 5.46, 7.50 |

CI, confidence interval; OR, odds ratio.

*Adjusted for maternal age (<25, 25–34, ≥35 yr), maternal parity (nulliparous, primiparous, multiparous) and previous cesarean delivery (yes/no).

[†] Data collected only for years 1989–1993 (n=1538 women with uterine leiomyomas, 3189 women without uterine leiomyomas).

Reproduced with permission from Coronado GD, Marshall LM, Schwartz SM: Complications in pregnancy, labor, and delivery with uterine leiomyomas: a population-based study. Obstet Gynecol 2000;95:764–769.

weight less than 2500 g, and delivery prior to 38 weeks of gestational age.

Interestingly, a recent study found no increase in risk of miscarriage in women with myomas undergoing genetic amniocentesis compared with women with myomas who did not undergo the diagnostic procedure.[103] The exact mechanism of action for causation of these various pregnancy-related complications is not well understood. Leiomyoma location, abnormal uterine distensibility, abnormal uterine contractility, and abnormal maternal-fetal vascularization may all play a part.

Perhaps the most common complication of myomas in pregnancy is hemorrhagic infarction, frequently termed "red degeneration."[104] This syndrome occurs more frequently in enlarged myomas with volumes greater than 200 mL, usually during the second trimester. The syndrome is thought to occur as a result of vascular insufficiency, ischemia, and edema. Typically, affected patients have pain but also may have fever, contractions, nausea, vomiting, and mild leukocytosis. Diagnostic ultrasound can demonstrate changes of cystic spaces or a coarse heterogeneous pattern in up to 70% of patients. Treatment is optimally managed by anti-inflammatory agents, which have been shown to reduce duration of hospital stay and readmission.[105]

## DIAGNOSIS

Diagnosis of uterine leiomyomas begins with careful history-taking and physical examination. A bulky, large, irregular, or firm uterus is suggestive of the presence of leiomyomas. A careful clinical examination to determine uterine size in the presence of myomas is highly correlated with ultrasonographic findings of uterine length and subsequent pathologic specimens.[106] However, clinical examination has a limited capacity to differentiate submucosal, intramural, and subserosal myomas. Anatomic location often dictates management, and therefore in clinical practice diagnostic radiology frequently is employed to determine the precise location of uterine leiomyomas. Many different imaging modalities are available, including hysterosalpingography, sonography, sonohysterography, CT scan, magnetic resonance imaging, and hysteroscopy. The practical benefits and disadvantages of each are reviewed briefly.

### Hysterosalpingography

Hysterosalpingography (HSG) is a common method of assessing tubal patency. It frequently is used in the evaluation of infertile patients who are at increased risk for the presence of myomas. Myomas can be detected by hysterosalpingography if they are present within the uterine cavity or significantly distort the uterine cavity. There is an associated false-positive rate. For example, a submucosal myoma may be identified when myomas are actually intramural with extension into the endometrium, since the radiograph can distinguish only endometrial cavity distortion rather than precise fibroid location. In one study, almost 25% of hysterosalpingogram reports were incorrect when followed-up with sonohysterograms.[107] There was high false-positive detection of polyps and myomas by HSG that were not found on subsequent investigation with hysteroscopy. While technically simple, the procedure is invasive and frequently causes discomfort. Patients with a previous history of pelvic inflammatory disease are at risk of recurrence following HSG.[108] Pretest β-hCG levels to rule out pregnancy and premedication with analgesics, nonsteroidal anti-inflammatory drugs, and antibiotics where indicated may reduce some of the associated complications. Although a viable option for diagnosis of tubal occlusion secondary to uterine myomas, HSG is not optimal in the evaluation of uteri affected by leiomyomas because of its inefficacy in providing information on myomas that do not involve the uterine cavity.

### Ultrasonography

The most common imaging modality used in the detection and diagnosis of leiomyomas is the two-dimensional ultrasound. Both transabdominal and transvaginal approaches are frequently used. Transabdominal images provide a wider field of view and are obviously less invasive; however, they cannot detect myomas smaller than 1 cm. Transvaginal approaches allow for detailed high-resolution images, giving precise location information and detection for even 4- to 5-mm myomas. However, this modality may have decreased sensitivity in detecting pedunculated, subserosal myomas or those high in the abdominal cavity, since they may remain outside the field of view.[109] Ultrasonographic appearances of fibroids can vary widely depending on location, size, ratio of fibrous to smooth muscle tissue, and degree of calcification.[110] Fibroids that have undergone degenerative changes may also demonstrate cystic, hypoechoic, or fluid-filled areas consistent with regions of necrosis. Typically myomas present as large, well-defined, echogenic, rounded lesions in the uterus.

Transabdominal ultrasound is less accurate in the identification of myomas that extend into the broad ligament.[111] Furthermore, because of the significant variation in ultrasonographic appearance, it has poor sensitivity in the differentiation of sarcomatous myomas from benign leiomyomas. While transvaginal ultrasonography (TVUS) improves on the detection of myomas over transabdominal scanning, it is still limited in discerning pedunculated from sessile myomas and detecting the degree to which myomas extend into the endometrial cavity. Fedele et al reported 100% sensitivity in detection of submucosal myomas with transvaginal sonography when compared with hysterectomy specimens.[112] One study demonstrated that TVUS was as sensitive in detecting the presence of myomas as magnetic resonance imaging (MRI), but that MRI detected twice as many myomas as TVUS.[113] However, detection of intracavitary abnormalities is significantly reduced in comparison with hysteroscopic diagnoses, with 63% sensitivity.[114]

Three-dimensional ultrasonography has recently been incorporated into gynecologic practice. This modality provides more detailed information on the uterine cavity and uterine anatomy and may reduce the required skill necessary for accurate determination of fibroid location.[109,115] To date there is little data on its efficacy in improving on traditional, two-dimensional ultrasound; however, it may improve volumetric assessment.[116] Newer studies have examined the use of three-dimensional ultrasound in conjunction with saline infusion hysterography. While some authors have demonstrated improvements in the detection of intracavitary abnormalities using this technique, considerable controversy exists.[117] Pretorius et al suggest that it may assist in reducing hysteroscopy for potentially inoperable myomas.[118]

# General Gynecology

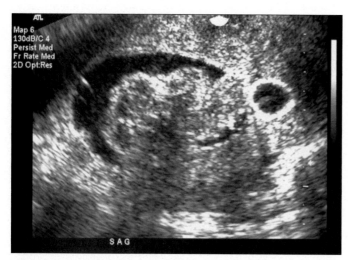

**Figure 14-2    Sonohysterogram demonstrating a large, submucosal fibroid growing cephalad into the endometrial canal.** The myoma interferes with the majority of the endometrial canal. (Courtesy of W. Romano, St. Joseph's Health Care Center, London, Ontario, Canada.)

**Figure 14-4    Sonohysterogram demonstrating two anterior, submucosal fibroids and one small endometrial polyp.** (Courtesy of W. Romano, St. Joseph's Health Care Center, London, Ontario, Canada.)

Hysterosonography is taking on a more significant role in the diagnosis of myomas. This technique allows clearer visualization of endometrial cavity contours. Polyps, as well as pedunculated and sessile fibroids, can all be more clearly delineated. Furthermore, this allows for specific determination of the extent of myoma presence within the uterine cavity when they are located submucosally or in the intramural regions (Figs. 14-2 to 14-5). With the use of sonographic contrast media, tubal patency also can be determined. Complications such as infection are extremely rare although precautions are recommended in patients with a prior history of pelvic inflammatory disease. The sensitivity for the detection of intrauterine abnormalities using hysterosonography compared with hysteroscopy is 88% with a

specificity of 95%.[114] The majority of studies examining the utility of hysterosonography in pre- and postmenopausal patients have revealed sensitivities of 88% to 100% and specificities of 76% to 96%. It has been suggested that up to 72% of hysteroscopic procedures could be avoided by use of sonohysterography and only 4% of intracavitary lesions would be missed.[119]

## Magnetic Resonance Imaging

MRI is possibly the most useful technique for the diagnosis of uterine fibroids because of its accuracy in the detection and localization of uterine fibroids.[120] It also may provide advantages to patients undergoing fertility preserving therapy, such as myomectomy or uterine artery embolization, or when endovaginal

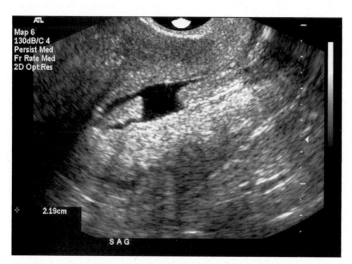

**Figure 14-3    Sonohysterogram demonstrating two endometrial polyps/ fibroids.** The first polyp is fundal, and the second arises from a point near the internal cervical os and grows cephalad. Doppler flow (not shown) demonstrated significant vascularization of the neoplasms. (Courtesy of W. Romano, St. Joseph's Health Care Center, London, Ontario, Canada.)

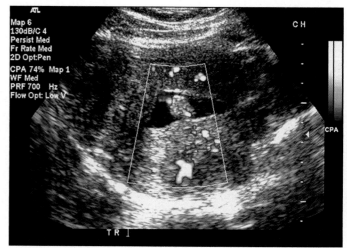

**Figure 14-5    Sonohysterogram demonstrating a large submucosal uterine leiomyoma and a concurrent endometrial polyp.** Doppler flow demonstrates significant arterial vascularization and blood flow to both neoplasms. (Courtesy of W. Romano, St. Joseph's Health Care Center, London, Ontario, Canada.)

ultrasound has been equivocal or nondiagnostic.[121] Fibroids generally appear as homogenous, dark (i.e., low intensity), well-circumscribed masses (Figs. 14-6 and 14-7). Endometrial polyps often can be distinguished from myomas on the basis of the myometrial origin of myomas visible on MR scans. Fibroids as small as 0.5 cm can be detected using this imaging modality. When myomas grow beyond 3 cm they often have inhomogeneous architecture because of various degrees of degenerative, hemorrhagic, and necrotic changes within the tumor.[120] Specialized coils have been developed specifically for pelvic MR images that increase signal intensity. Several adjunctive techniques may also be useful in enhancing images, including the use of glucagon for restriction of bowel activity, rectal air insufflation, and oral contrast media.[111] In addition to localization of myomas, MR angiograms can help in detection of collateral ovarian blood supply to uterine myomas. This is particularly useful information for patients considering undergoing uterine artery embolization (UAE), since fibroids with ovarian blood supply may not respond adequately to UAE procedures.

Despite the high resolution of MRI for uterine fibroids, its utility is limited in determining pathologic differences in degenerating fibroids or in distinguishing benign leiomyomas from their malignant counterparts, leiomyosarcomas. Additionally, despite its proven efficacy, the substantial costs associated with MRI have generally limited its use in routine evaluation of uterine leiomyomas.[109]

## Hysteroscopy

Hysteroscopic evaluation of myomas is the gold standard for evaluation of intrauterine extension of fibroids. This technique is particularly useful in women with submucosal fibroids and polyps amenable to surgical intervention at the time of hysteroscopic evaluation. Hysteroscopic evaluation allows for accurate

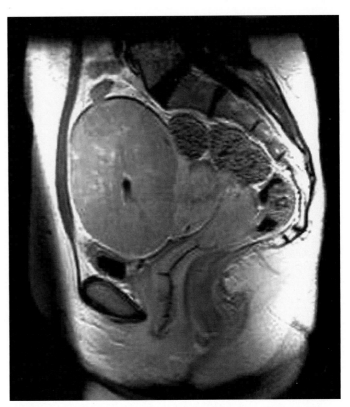

**Figure 14-7    T1-weighted MR image in sagittal view after gadolinium injection.** The MRI demonstrates a massive subserosal uterine myoma with central necrosis and cavitation. (Courtesy of J. Bennett, St. Joseph's Health Care Center, London, Ontario, Canada.)

localization of submucosal fibroids and for clear delineation of pedunculated and sessile myomas and polyps. This technique also provides visualization of the extent of endometrial distortion caused by intramural myomas and the extent to which tubal ostia may be occluded by adjacent myomas. The advantages of this technique include direct visualization, potentially simultaneous therapeutic intervention, out-patient or office setting use, and minimal complications. The disadvantages include inability to detect intramyometrial extension, need for significant analgesia/sedation or anesthetic, and potential for rare but significant complications associated with operative hysteroscopy (see Chapters 38 and 39).

de Vries et al reviewed the evidence comparing saline infusion sonography (SIS) with hysteroscopy for the evaluation of endometrial abnormalities.[119] Although SIS had between 88% and 100% sensitivity, these values were still lower, in general, than the reference category of hysteroscopy.

## MANAGEMENT

Because the vast majority of uterine myomas are asymptomatic, in most cases no therapeutic intervention is necessary. Patients experiencing complications related to the presence of leiomyomas generally have several options for management: medical therapy, embolotherapy, and surgical therapy. The choice depends on many factors including severity of symptomatology, desire for future fertility, comorbid conditions, and access to physicians with appropriate surgical knowledge, skill, and equipment.

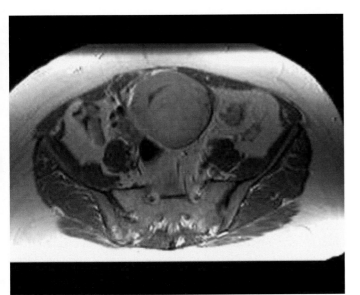

**Figure 14-6    T1-weighted MR image in axial view after gadolinium injection.** The MRI depicts a large uterine leiomyoma, with compression of the posterior myometrium and distortion of the endometrial canal. (Courtesy of W. Romano, St. Joseph's Health Care Center, London, Ontario, Canada.)

Implicit in consideration of management options is ruling out the potential for malignancy within a myomatous mass. The incidence of uterine leiomyosarcomas is 1.7 per 100,000 women, with an incidental finding of leiomyosarcoma in asymptomatic uterine fibroids of 1 in 2000.[86,122] Schwartz et al analyzed six studies evaluating typical clinical presentations of patients with leiomyosarcoma. The majority of patients were near 45 to 50 years of age and had an enlarged uterus (>6 week size).[123] The authors found that 95% of leiomyosarcomas present as the largest or only uterine mass. The importance of correctly diagnosing uterine myomas is highlighted by reports of inadvertent treatment of leiomyosarcomas with GnRH agonist therapy.[124]

## Medical Management

Medical management of leiomyomas is a rapidly expanding field aimed at reducing the symptoms associated with fibroids without the risks and complications of surgical intervention. Medical therapy involves manipulation of factors that contribute to fibroid growth by either reducing the concentration of growth factors, using competitive antagonists against hormones, interfering with growth factor receptor function, altering uterine blood flow, or altering endometrial properties. To date, many different agents have been used but generally may be categorized into six primary modalities: endometrial suppression drugs, GnRH agonist therapy, antisteroid therapy, androgen therapy, leiomyoma receptor growth factor antagonists, and most recently uterine blood flow–altering drugs.

### Oral and Injectable Contraceptives

Oral contraceptives have long been used in the control of abnormal uterine bleeding by reducing endometrial growth. They are frequently used in clinical practice to control fibroid-related menorrhagia despite the lack of evidence supporting their efficacy. In theory, reducing endometrial growth should reduce bleeding; however, there is no practical or theoretical evidence to support a decrease in bulk- or pain-related symptoms. Although no direct evidence links fibroid growth and progestins, medroxyprogesterone acetate may actually stimulate growth of uterine leiomyomas.[125] In fact, the data regarding OCs suggest an increase in the incidence of leiomyomas if initiated prior to the age of 16 years.[10] Because of the relative safety of OCs and the contraceptive benefits, their use may provide a reasonable first-line approach to the control of fibroid-related menorrhagia in patients over age 16. However, in patients with bulk-related symptoms, no evidence supports the use of oral contraceptives and other agents with proven efficacy in reducing leiomyoma volume should be considered.

### Levonorgestrel Intrauterine Systems

In contrast to OC use, fibroid-related menorrhagia and fibroid volume may be reduced in patients using levonorgestrel intra-uterine contraceptive systems (LN-IUS). The endometrial suppressive effects of this device are well documented, but its efficacy in the treatment of myomas is only recently being evaluated. Traditionally, intrauterine devices have been contra-indicated in patients with fibroids because of the frequency of endometrial cavity distortion leading to decreased contraceptive efficacy. However, one study demonstrated a decreased incidence of leiomyoma development in patients using the LN-IUS for more than 5 years, with decreased uterine surgery and hyster-ectomy rates as well.[126] A study conducted in a small population of women demonstrated decreased myoma volume within 6 to 18 months of LN-IUS use. Although the LN-IUS controls fibroid-related menorrhagia by progestin-induced endometrial suppression, it is believed to exert its effect on fibroid volume by increasing the concentration of insulin-like growth factor-binding protein-1, thereby reducing a potential leiomyoma-related growth factor.[127]

### Nonsteroidal Anti-Inflammatory Drugs

Nonsteroidal anti-inflammatory drugs (NSAIDs) that can significantly reduce abnormal uterine bleeding do not appear to reduce fibroid-induced menorrhagia. In two studies, no benefit was shown in patients undergoing therapy with either naproxen or ibuprofen if myomas were present.[128,129] Moreover, there is likely no alteration in fibroid volume and growth, resulting in no significant benefit in the use of these agents in fibroid-affected patients.

### Gonadotropin-releasing Hormone Agonists

GnRH agonists are the most common form of medical therapy employed in the treatment of leiomyoma-related symptomatology. These agents are thought to exert their influence by inducing a hypoestrogenic state unfavorable to fibroid and endometrial growth. Thus, use of these agents can potentially reduce both bleeding- and bulk-related symptoms. While there are many different agents, most studies have examined the use of leuprolide acetate. The route of administration can signifi-cantly influence the efficacy of these agents. Friedman et al demonstrated that intranasal administration of leuprolide acetate resulted in no reduction in uterine volume compared with a 53% reduction when it was administered subcutaneously, with a concurrently higher level of mean serum estradiol concen-trations in patients undergoing intranasal administration.[130]

The majority of studies indicate that fibroid and uterine volume can effectively be reduced on average by 50% with the use of these agents.[131] However, individual leiomyomas have a high degree of heterogeneity in their response to GnRH agonists, with response rates varying from 0% to 100% after 3 to 6 months of continuous therapy.[132] Response is usually seen within 1 to 2 months of therapy and maximal response after 12 weeks. The greatest proportion of shrinkage occurs after the first month and subsequently progressively declines.[133] Reductions of up to 38% have been demonstrated in the surface area of submucosal myomas at 8 weeks of therapy.[134] Uterine volume can similarly be decreased on average by 25% to 80% with maximal reductions achieved after 12 weeks of therapy.[135] The reduction in uterine volume extends to reductions in the intrauterine cavity. Two studies used hysterography to demonstrate reductions in the volume of the endometrial cavity. The first study demonstrated a reduction of 35% at 8 weeks,[136] while the second demonstrated that prolonged use resulted in a 40% decrease at 24 weeks.[137] The efficacy of GnRH agonists appears to be dependent on circu-lating levels of estrogen. Thus, women with obesity or without a significant suppressive response to GnRH agonist administration have reductions in amenorrhea and volume decrease.[138] Up to 10% of myomas will have no response to therapy (Table 14-7).

**Table 14-7**

**Factors Contributing to Failure of GnRH Agonist Therapy for Treatment of Leiomyomas**

- Leiomyoma histopathologic subtype
- Extracellular matrix composition
- Steroid and growth factor receptor content
- Intracrine production of steroid hormones and growth factors
- Paracrine-mediated growth stimulation
- Fibroid location and number

Gutmann et al demonstrated a 5-fold increased degree of hyalinization in myomas that were unresponsive to leuprolide acetate in a small study of 12 patients with surgical histopathologic evaluation following short-term administration of depot leuprolide.[139] Pedunculated fibroids may have an attenuated response as compared with myomas contained within the uterus.

Lemay et al reviewed data on symptom improvement following GnRH agonist use[134] (Table 14-8). Even patients without significant myoma shrinkage experience up to 92% improvement in symptoms following GnRH agonist therapy. Additionally, there can be improvements in hematocrit, hemoglobin, and iron indices. These improvements provide not only symptomatic benefit, but can make potential surgery safer by reducing the impact of blood loss and the need for transfusion and allowing for preoperative autologous blood donation.

### Preoperative

The use of GnRH agonists preoperatively for uterine leiomyomas may be one of the most effective strategies for improving outcomes. There are preoperative, intraoperative, and postoperative benefits. Preoperative GnRH agonist use is the subject of a meta-analysis of 21 randomized controlled trials.[140] Preoperative hemoglobin was significantly increased by 1.3 g/dL and hematocrit by 3.1%, uterine size decreased by 159 mL and 2.2 gestational weeks, and fibroid volume decreased by 12 mL.

**Table 14-8**

**Beneficial Effects of GnRH Agonist Treatment on Clinical Symptoms of Myomas**

| Symptom | Improvement (%) |
|---|---|
| Dysmenorrhea | 95–100 |
| Abnormal bleeding | 93–100 |
| Pelvic pain | 85–95 |
| Pelvic pressure | 75–93 |
| Urinary frequency | 50–94 |
| Dyspareunia | 69–80 |
| Constipation | 66–78 |
| Abdominal bloating | 69–75 |

Reproduced with permission from Lemay A, Maheux R: GnRH agonists in the management of uterine leiomyoma. Infert Reprod Med Clin North Am 1996;7:33–55.

### Intraoperative

Intraoperative benefits included a 58 mL reduction in blood loss at hysterectomy and a 68 mL reduction in blood loss at myomectomy. Although these values are statistically significant, their clinical relevance is questionable. Despite the reduction in blood loss, the rate of blood transfusion did not significantly differ between groups. The odds ratio for vaginal hysterectomy was substantially increased in patients undergoing GnRH agonist treatment, with a nearly 5-fold increase in vaginal hysterectomy rate in treatment patients, although the largest trial with a placebo-controlled group demonstrated no difference in surgical approach. These differences may be attributable to other patient factors including previous pelvic surgery, history consistent with adhesions, and physician skill and preference. However, physicians found an 8% reduction in risk of difficult surgery in pretreated patients. For patients undergoing abdominal hysterectomy, the choice of Pfannenstiel incision was more common, with an OR of 0.36 for vertical incisions, a significant clinical value in light of the increase in wound complications associated with vertical incisions. Patients also benefited from a decreased duration of operating time and a 1.1 day reduction in hospital stay. However, in a study of 426 patients undergoing laparoscopic myomectomy, patients who had received GnRH therapy prior to surgery had a higher risk of conversion to open laparotomy.[141]

### Postoperative

Overall, postoperative complications did not differ in groups undergoing myomectomy, but there was a 38% reduction in risk of postoperative complications with hysterectomy including blood loss and pyrexia. Compared with no treatment, postoperative hemoglobin and hematocrit values appear to be elevated, but these results were not evident in placebo-controlled trials. Of interest is the finding of a 4-fold increase in risk of myoma recurrence 6 months postoperatively in patients who had received treatment. It has been hypothesized that this is due to shrinkage of small myomas that subsequently become undetectable at surgery but then undergo regrowth postoperatively.

### Complications

Several complications are associated with the administration of GnRH agonists for uterine myomas. The most important is the rapid regeneration of myomas and regrowth of the uterus within 6 months of cessation of treatment.[132] Often these increases occur within weeks of treatment cessation. Friedman et al demonstrated that within 3 months of cessation fibroids exhibited regrowth to 88% of their original size.[142] This may be due, in part, to a rapid return of ovarian steroidogenesis following treatment cessation, or it may involve the return of uterine blood flow to pretreatment levels. Matta et al demonstrated that pretreatment uterine artery resistive indices were 0.52, peaked at 0.92 at 4 months of treatment, and were 0.59 at 6 weeks posttreatment.[143] Shaw found that blood flow was strongly correlated with uterine and fibroid volume, with increasing resistive indices seen with decreased fibroid and uterine volumes.[144] Others have found that the relationship of uterine blood flow to fibroid growth may even be predictive of GnRH agonist treatment success.[133]

Although two thirds of women are amenorrheic during GnRH agonist therapy, menses often return within 4 to 10 weeks after cessation of treatment. Patients with a history of menorrhagia are at risk for recurrence. Symptoms may reappear following myoma regrowth, but some studies support a prolonged benefit after cessation of therapy. Up to 65% of patients remain symptom free after therapy, and two thirds of patients may continue to avoid operative intervention 8 to 12 months after the completion of therapy.[145] Some patients derive enough resolution of their symptoms to avoid subsequent hysterectomy.[146]

### Hypoestrogenic Side Effects

In general, administration of GnRH agonists results in profound pituitary suppression of gonadotropin release and a consequent state of hypoestrogenemia. Hypoestrogenemia results in menopausal-like symptoms. Several studies have examined the side effects of GnRH agonist treatment and described their incidence compared with patients receiving placebo and a Cochrane review also evaluated odds ratios for four adverse outcomes (Table 14-9).[131,132,140,147,148] These side effects may in general be classified as physiologic changes, physical changes, and nonphysiologic effects. Hot flashes (hot flushes) occur with the highest frequency and are the most debilitating, often resulting in intolerance and treatment discontinuation. Combined with the accompanying diaphoretic episodes, these symptoms limit the utility of these drugs in the long-term treatment of fibroids.

While physiologic changes are particularly distressing to the patient, physicians frequently focus on the bone loss that occurs with prolonged GnRH agonist therapy. Because of the hypoestrogenic state, bone remodeling is altered and new bone formation decreased. Initially, concerns were derived from studies of young women undergoing long-term GnRH agonist treatment for the suppression of pelvic endometriosis. In these women, after 6 months of therapy, 5% to 6% of the trabecular

bone in the lumbar spine was lost. Although most patients regained the lost bone following treatment cessation, the age-dependent decrease in new bone deposition resulted in concern about prolonged GnRH use. More recent studies in patients with fibroids have demonstrated smaller decreases, with a maximal bone loss of 3%.[134] It is postulated that the diminished loss results from treatment of perimenopausal women with increased body mass index as compared with patients undergoing therapy for endometriosis. However, treatment for longer than 6 months often is discouraged owing to concern about potential bone loss.

Other rare but significant complications include fibroid degeneration, which results in episodes of pain, fever, and bleeding. Frequently these patients come to the emergency room for acute pelvic pain management. Some patients also undergo degenerative vascular changes resulting in massive hemorrhage necessitating emergent management.

Thus, while GnRH agonist treatment affords considerable efficacy in reduction of both fibroid volume and related symptomatology, the effect is limited to continuation of drug administration. Absence of suppression results in myoma regrowth and a return of symptoms in a substantial proportion of treated patients. Short-term treatment carries a significant degree of morbidity, and long-term therapy is contraindicated because of concerns regarding bone loss. Although some patients continue to benefit following cessation of GnRH administration, the adverse effects and cost of this drug reduce its efficacy as a long-term treatment strategy.

### Add-back Therapy

Concerns regarding side effects and decreased efficacy of GnRH agonist therapy led several investigators to consider hormonal add-back regimens to ameliorate the side effects induced by short- and long-term GnRH agonist use. Following an initial 3-month treatment period, patients are started on regimens including progestin only or estrogen and progestin. Theoretically, this would allow for long-term suppressive therapy while minimizing potential side effects, risks, and complications and would be particularly beneficial in temporizing symptomatic perimenopausal patients.

**Progestin Only.** Studies of progesterone add-back have been disappointing. If initiated simultaneously with the GnRH agonist, hot flashes are reduced, but fibroids do not shrink significantly compared with pretreatment levels. In a randomized controlled trial, when norethindrone was initiated after 3 months of GnRH agonist therapy, bone mineral density decreased by 3% but then stabilized over the ensuing year of therapy.[149] However, fibroids regained 92% of their original volume with progesterone add-back therapy. Other authors have demonstrated a maximum of 20% reduction in fibroid volume with progesterone add-back therapy. Thus, while these regimens improve the side effect profile of GnRH agonists, they significantly impede the therapeutic efficacy, limiting their usefulness.

**Estrogen and Progestin.** Friedman initially tested a combined regimen in a small population of five patients with fibroids treated with leuprolide for 3 months, followed by initiation of a cyclic regimen of 0.625 mg of conjugated equine estrogen and 5 mg of medroxyprogesterone acetate daily for 24 months.[150] The initial leuprolide-only phase resulted in a 50% volume

### Table 14-9
**Adverse Effects of GnRH Agonist Therapy for Treatment of Fibroids**

| Adverse Effect | Incidence (%) | OR | 95% CI |
|---|---|---|---|
| **Physiologic changes** | | | |
| Hot flashes | 80–100 | 6.5 | 4.6, 9.2 |
| Diaphoresis | 45–63 | 8.3 | 4.5, 15.3 |
| **Physical changes** | | | |
| Breast changes | 11–47 | 7.7 | 2.4, 24.9 |
| Vaginitis/vaginal dryness | 5–29 | 4.0 | 2.1, 7.6 |
| Bone loss | 3–6 | | |
| **Other changes** | | | |
| Depression | 11–23 | | |
| Decreased libido | 3–34 | | |
| Emotional lability | 8–32 | | |
| Sleep disturbance | 10–45 | | |
| Nausea | 10–19 | | |
| Arthralgia | 8–14 | | |
| Headache | 20–26 | | |
| **Fibroid changes** | | | |
| Hyaline degeneration | 1–2 | | |
| Submucosal vascular disruption | <1 | | |

CI, confidence interval; OR, odds ratio.
Data from references 131, 132, 140, 147, and 148.

reduction in fibroids that was maintained during the course of add-back therapy, with no detrimental effects on bone mineral density.

Subsequently, Friedman evaluated a combined regimen in a randomized controlled trial of 51 premenopausal women.[149] Patients had a 25% reduction in uterine volume with add-back therapy at 1 year, although there was a significant decrease in bone mineral density that remained at study completion.

On the basis of results of add-back therapy trials, it is evident that patients amenable to GnRH agonist treatment would benefit from some estrogen-progesterone combined therapy in either continuous or cyclic regimens. These patients may experience some diminution of symptoms but are at risk for decreased efficacy and potential bone loss. Alternative therapies for the prevention of bone loss, including bisphosphonates, may reduce the complication of bone loss and in combination with add-back therapy provide a rational option for symptomatic women nearing menopause, unwilling or unable to undergo surgery, or wishing to preserve fertility.

### Alternative Forms of Medical Therapy

The complications and side effects of GnRH agonists have led to the development of several alternatives in the medical management of uterine myomas.

#### Antiprogesterones

Antiprogesterones such as RU 486 have been used in the treatment of leiomyomas. Two studies have demonstrated that even at low doses there is a reduction in fibroid volume of 25% to 50% at 12 weeks.[151] This effect may be mediated through alteration of uterine blood flow, to an even greater degree than that seen with GnRH agonists. Although these studies were promising, numbers were small and firm conclusions cannot be drawn about the safety and efficacy of long-term use without further analysis.

Selective progesterone receptor modulators (SPRMs) represent a relatively new class of drugs with both agonist and antagonist activities at progesterone, glucocorticoid, and androgen receptors.[152] Although their use in the treatment of uterine myomas is currently investigational only, initial results appear to show promise in both control of symptoms and reduction in myoma volume.[153]

#### Androgens

Androgens used in the treatment of uterine fibroids include danazol and gestrinone. Danazol provides reversible pituitary suppression by binding to multiple steroid receptors and indirectly suppressing LH and FSH production. Danazol has been compared with the GnRH agonist buserelin in a prospective trial of 164 women.[154] Patients receiving danazol had a 57% reduction in fibroid volume at 6 months, compared with 76% in patients receiving buserelin. De Leo examined the effects of danazol following GnRH agonist discontinuation and found that fibroid volume had a 30% lower rebound compared with volume in control patients.[155] Others have found that minimal dosages of danazol may alleviate symptoms despite a lack of efficacy in reducing fibroid volume.[156] Currently, danazol is not indicated for long-term use and must be considered in light of its potential androgenic side effects and the rare consequence of virilization.

Gestrinone, a synthetic derivative of nortestosterone, was used in a prospective trial for the treatment of fibroids in 100 patients.[157] While 73% of patients had a significant reduction in fibroid volume similar to that observed with GnRH agonist therapy, 20% to 100% of patients suffered androgenic side effects, including acne, hirsutism, and weight gain. These changes reversed with treatment cessation, and only 4% of patients discontinued therapy because of side effects. This may be a viable option in patients who wish to minimize fibroid regrowth and are willing to accept the potential hyperandrogenic consequences of therapy.

#### Aromatase Inhibitors

The incorporation of aromatase inhibitors into ovulation induction, pioneered by Mitwally et al, has stimulated renewed interest in the use of these agents in the treatment of uterine myomas.[158] At present there are only case reports of the use of the newer orally administered aromatase inhibitors for the treatment of uterine leiomyomas[159]; however, concerns have been raised regarding the significance of potential long-term estrogen suppression resulting from chronic administration.[160]

#### Other Antiestrogens

Many compounds with antiestrogenic activity have been used to reduce fibroid volume, including clomiphene citrate, tamoxifen, and raloxifene. The side effects, potential risks, and lack of large prospective studies currently limit the use of the majority of these drugs. Selective estrogen receptor modulators have had some limited success.[161] Further studies may reveal new antiestrogens with growth-inhibiting efficacy for leiomyomas, but at present no data supports the use of these agents in clinical practice.

### Embolotherapy

The fact that reduced uterine blood flow corresponds with significant decreases in fibroid and uterine volume contributed to the development of uterine artery embolization. This technique was first described in 16 patients in Paris.[162] Using coils, microspheres, and most recently a transvaginal clamp, the uterine arteries or those feeding the myoma are selectively occluded. Patients are treated using conscious sedation and are monitored either overnight or as outpatients.

Fibroids are particularly well-suited to this treatment because of the hypervascular peripheral supply and the hypovascular central core. This pattern allows for central infarction and necrosis of the myoma when the external blood supply is compromised. Uterine artery embolization (UAE) techniques take advantage of this pathophysiologic finding to induce irreversible necrosis and consequent fibroid volume reduction. Patients should be preoperatively evaluated by a gynecologist, and diagnostic testing for the number, size, and location of fibroids is indicated. Using either a unilateral or a bilateral femoral approach, the vascular bed supplying individual fibroids or the uterine arteries is embolized (Fig. 14-8). Selective embolization of fibroid vascular beds may result in decreased complications and decreased postoperative pain. Radiographic exposure is significant but not excessive. In one study, patients received an average of 44 angiographic exposures, with a mean ovarian exposure of 22 cGy and a mean fluoroscopy time of 22 minutes.[163]

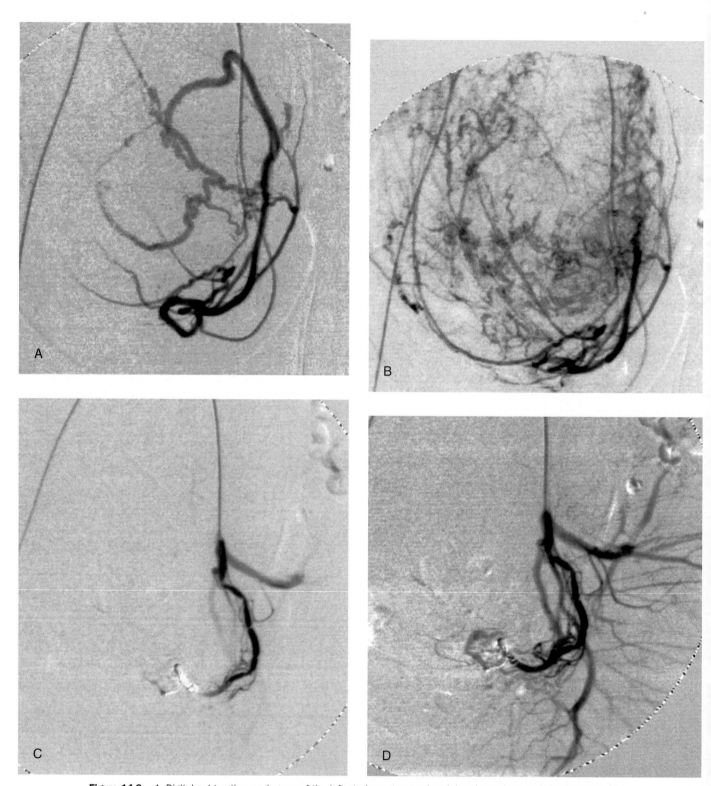

**Figure 14-8** *A,* Digital subtraction angiogram of the left uterine artery and peripheral supply to a uterine myoma. The image depicts early dye infusion prior to uterine artery embolization. *B,* Digital subtraction angiogram taken prior to uterine artery embolization. The image depicts continued spread of dye, highlighting the typical observed pattern of hypervascularity in uterine leiomyomas. *C,* Digital subtraction angiogram taken immediately after uterine artery embolization. Note the massive reduction in peripheral and central blood supply to the myoma. *D,* Digital subtraction angiogram taken after uterine artery embolization. This image demonstrates the complete and persistent occlusion of arterial flow to the myoma, with consequent redistribution of blood flow to peripheral blood vessels. (Courtesy of J. Bennett, St. Joseph's Health Care Center, London, Ontario, Canada.)

Results indicate that fibroid volume reduction, symptomatic improvement, and patient satisfaction all are high. Up to 85% of patients report significant reductions in menorrhagia and bulk-related symptoms following embolization procedures.[164] On average, up to 50% of fibroid volume can be reduced within 6 months of therapy. Similarly to GnRH agonist therapy, the majority of shrinkage occurs over the first few months of therapy, although some further volume reductions can be seen between 6 and 12 months after the procedure.

The OUFET trial recently reported on findings in a large population of women undergoing uterine artery embolization.[77] Five hundred thirty-eight patients underwent bilateral uterine artery embolization with polyvinyl alcohol particles. The study was composed of 65% white women, with a mean age of 43 years, 50% of whom were nulliparous, and 30% of whom were desirous of retaining their fertility potential. The majority of patients had 2 to 4 fibroids (44%), and 60% of all fibroids were intramural. At 3 months postembolization, the mean reduction in fibroid volume was 23% for fibroids less than 200 cm$^3$ pretreatment, 38% for fibroids 201 to 400 cm$^3$, and 49% for fibroids greater than 401 cm$^3$, with reductions in uterine volume of 11% to 44% depending on pretreatment uterine volume.

Effects on symptoms were dramatic, with 83% of women reporting improvement in menorrhagia, mean reductions of over 2 days in menstrual duration, and a 50% reduction in pad count on the heaviest day of menstrual flow. Interestingly, 7% of patients reported worsening of menorrhagia following the procedure. Dysmenorrhea was reduced in 77%, bulk in 84%, and urinary urgency in 86% of patients.

The effect of UAE on future pregnancy is not well understood. Theoretically, the consequent restriction of uterine blood flow through the uterine arteries could result in utero-placental insufficiency. Goldberg et al reported that, based on the first 50 reported cases of pregnancy following embolization, patients were at increased risk for malpresentation (17%), fetus small for gestational age (7%), premature delivery (28%), cesarean delivery (58%), and postpartum hemorrhage (13%).[165] Although these figures are increased compared with unaffected patients, no data indicate that risks following embolization are significantly greater than those experienced by other patients with similarly sized fibroids. However, Chen et al reported a greater than 40% risk of miscarriage following UAE and suggested that the procedure be limited to patients who do not desire fertility.[166] Patients must be counseled that data regarding safety in pregnancy is lacking and there are both theoretical concerns and some early evidence that patients are at risk of increased complications. Early consultation with an obstetrician and close follow-up should be considered mandatory.

Although this procedure appears safe and efficacious, several complications exist. Overall, complications occur in less than 0.5% of patients. The most important concern following embolization is potential infection, with these patients at risk for hysterectomy. However, there is no consensus on the use of antibiotic prophylaxis for this procedure. Infection-related death has been reported following embolization, so careful consideration of the risks and benefits of antibiotic use should be made for each patient.[167] Fibroids with intracavitary exposure may be at increased risk of infective complications.[168] Because of the inflammation and necrosis that occurs in the process of fibroid ischemia, leukocytosis and febrile morbidity are common. Thus, markers of infection are frequently present even under sterile conditions. Sudden increases in temperature greater than 38.5°C associated with increasing pain, foul discharge, or hypotension are of particularly concern and mandate formal evaluation for possible infection. MRI may be helpful in delineating infection.

Other authors have raised concerns regarding diminished ovarian reserve observed in patients following uterine artery embolization. Smaller occlusive particles may embolize into the ovarian blood supply and cause occlusion or restriction of blood flow, resulting in decreased ovarian function. Patients over age 45 years may be at increased risk of premature ovarian failure following embolization. In one study, 43% of women over age 45 subsequently had ovarian failure.[169] While selective arterial embolization and larger particle sizes should resolve some of these concerns, women over age 45 should be warned of the potential complication of diminished ovarian function and the attendant menopausal symptoms.

Additional complications may include pain, which commonly is severe over the initial 24 hours following embolization and may last up to 2 weeks. Pain can be well controlled with patient-controlled narcotic analgesic pumps and liberal use of anti-inflammatory agents. Prolonged pain in conjunction with fever should raise concerns about a possible septic uterus. Rare complications, including transcervical passage of necrotic submucosal fibroids, bowel necrosis, uterine infarction, and infection of other pelvic organs including the appendix, have been reported. Although these complications are rare, they can result in significant morbidity and mortality if diagnosis and acute intervention are delayed.

Up to 16.5% of procedures will fail owing to early treatment-related factors such as inability to catheterize, arterial dissection, incorrect diagnosis, and excessive myoma size.[170] Patients with submucosal or extremely large myomas may be at increased risk of treatment failure. Approximately 10% of patients with embolization had regrowth or recurrence of myomas at 2 years of follow-up.[170] Thus, while this therapy provides highly efficacious short-term results, long-term safety and efficacy have not been fully evaluated. Patients must be informed of the potential risks of both early and delayed procedure failure prior to embolization.

Surgical intervention following embolization occurs in 4% to 5% of patients.[171] The majority of these patients subsequently undergo hysterectomy. Many patients requiring surgery were treated for submucosal myomas. Most failures occur within 6 months of treatment and are secondary to menorrhagia or prolapse of pedunculated or submucosal myomas. Laparotomy may be complicated by the presence of bowel adhesions to the serosal surface overlying myomas.

## Surgical Management

For many women, the lack of prolonged efficacy, desire for fertility, concern regarding potential pregnancy-related complications and attendant side effects result in unacceptable compromises when undergoing medical treatment. Patients with extremely large myomas may find that medical treatment lacks sufficient efficacy in controlling pressure-related symptoms. In these cases, surgery is a viable and potentially curative option.

## Hysterectomy

Ultimately, hysterectomy provides a permanent cure for fibroid-related symptoms. Whether conducted vaginally, abdominally, or laparoscopically, removal of the uterus resolves bleeding-, pressure-, and pain-related symptomatology. Vaginal hysterectomy should be the primary approach where possible, as it has the lowest morbidity and cost and a relatively rapid recovery time compared with abdominal hysterectomy. For a subtotal hysterectomy, the laparoscopic approach provides significant benefits in terms of recovery. Enlarged uteri may be amenable to vaginal hysterectomy with pretreatment using either GnRH analogs or UAE. Asymptomatic women with myomas should not undergo hysterectomy, as the risk of malignant transformation is 0.3% to 1%, a value less than the risk of morbidity associated with the surgical morbidity of hysterectomy.

In symptomatic women, hysterectomy provides significant relief of symptoms and resolution of anemia. The risk of fibroid growth posthysterectomy is exceedingly low and has only been reported as a metastatic process.[172] The Maine Women's Health study demonstrated that in women with myomas, the most significant factor correlated with positive outcome at 1 year of follow-up was hysterectomy.[173] Satisfaction rates following hysterectomy approximate 90%.[174] Although highly efficacious in the treatment of myomas, hysterectomy has a 3% to 6% morbidity rate. It has been estimated that 1 to 2 per 1000 women undergoing hysterectomy will die of procedural complications.[175] Compared with UAE, patients undergoing hysterectomy had fewer emergency room visits, a decreased rate of minor and moderate complications, but a 5% to 10% incidence of severe complications including deep venous thrombosis, wound infection, need for blood transfusion, and intraperitoneal abscess.[176]

Several studies have examined differences in the route of hysterectomy in women with myomatous uteri. In a randomized, controlled clinical trial comparing total abdominal hysterectomy, vaginal hysterectomy, and laparoscopically assisted vaginal hysterectomy for myomas greater than 6 cm in size, febrile morbidity was increased significantly in women with abdominal hysterectomy.[177] Operative outcomes from this study are shown in Table 14-10. Blood loss was highest with laparoscopically assisted vaginal hysterectomy, followed by total abdominal hysterectomy, with vaginal hysterectomy showing the least blood loss. Although hospital stays were significantly different, there was little clinical difference in the observed values. The interval from surgery to return to work, however, was significantly longer for abdominal hysterectomies compared with the laparoscopically assisted vaginal hysterectomy or vaginal hysterectomy. Vaginal hysterectomy elicits the least amount of inflammatory reaction as measured by C-reactive protein and interleukin 6 levels, compared with abdominal hysterectomy and total laparoscopic hysterectomy.[178] There does not appear to be any difference in satisfaction or complication rates for total abdominal hysterectomy versus supracervical abdominal hysterectomy.[179]

With delayed child-bearing becoming more common, and medical options available for temporization of fibroid symptoms, the role of hysterectomy in the treatment of fibroids is becoming smaller. However, for women with considerable symptomatology, no desire for future fertility, and acceptance of the potential morbidity associated with hysterectomy, it is the only curative procedure available. Adjunctive use of GnRH agonist or UAE may facilitate the vaginal approach to the myomatous uterus. When vaginal hysterectomy is not possible, total laparoscopic and laparoscopically assisted hysterectomy may provide significant benefits in terms of recovery but carry operator-dependent risks of morbidity that patients must consider prior to electing the route of hysterectomy.

For patients who want to preserve fertility or do not want to have uterine extirpation, four alternative forms of surgical therapy are available: hysteroscopic resection (see Chapters 38 and 39), laparoscopic or hand-assisted laparoscopic myomectomy (see Chapter 37), myomectomy via laparotomy, and myolysis.

**Table 14-10**
**Comparison of Operative Events Among Women in the Study Groups**

|  | LAVH (n) | Mean Value | TAH (n) | Mean Value | TVH (n) | Mean Value | P Value |
|---|---|---|---|---|---|---|---|
| Operation time (min) with second procedure | 13 | 119 ± 20 | 8 | 117 ± 32 | 3 | 93 ± 15 | 0.12* |
| Without second procedure | 17 | 109 ± 22 | 22 | 98 ± 16 | 27 | 74 ± 23 | <0.001* |
| Blood loss (mL) | 30 | 343 ± 218 | 30 | 293 ± 182 | 30 | 215 ± 134 | 0.04 |
| Hospital stay (days) | 30 | 4.7 | 30 | 5 | 30 | 4.7 | 0.003* |
| Postoperative tenderness scores after 24 h | 30 | 4 | 30 | 6 | 30 | 3 | <0.001* |
| Return to work (days) | 30 | 30 ± 16 | 30 | 41 ± 10 | 30 | 29 ± 11 | <0.001* |
| Days of antibiotics used | 30 | 1.3 | 30 | 1.7 | 30 | 1.3 | <0.001* |
| Pathology ultrasound correlation (%) | 30 | 93.3 | 30 | 100 | 30 | 93.3 | 0.54† |
| Uterine weight (g) | 30 | 748 ± 255 | 30 | 1020 ± 383 | 30 | 835 ± 330 | 0.02* |

LAVH, laparoscopically assisted vaginal hysterectomy; TAH, abdominal hysterectomy; TVH, vaginal hysterectomy.
*Based on Kruskal-Wallis test.
†Fisher's exact test.
From Hwang JL, Seow KM, Tsai YL, et al: Comparative study of vaginal, laparoscopically assisted vaginal and abdominal hysterectomies for uterine myoma larger than 6 cm in diameter or uterus weighing at least 450 g: a prospective randomized study. Acta Obstet Gynecol Scand 2002;81:1132–1138, with permission.

## Abdominal Myomectomy

For women wishing to preserve the uterus, indications for abdominal myomectomy are similar to those for laparoscopic myomectomy, although because of the increased access provided by laparotomy, multiple fibroids and those that are either large or located in technically challenging locations can generally be resected. Preoperative and intraoperative adjuvant treatments are equally applicable; however, abdominal myomectomy permits minimization of blood loss by temporary mechanical obstruction of the uterine arteries with instruments such as the Bonny clamp.[180] Technically, abdominal and laparoscopic myomectomy procedures are similar, absent the need for laparoscopic instrumentation. Abdominal procedures may be conducted through a Pfannenstiel skin incision, although larger myomas may necessitate vertical skin incisions, with the attendant increase in wound-related morbidity. Uterine incisions should be minimized, since laparotomy often allows for removal of multiple myomas through a single uterine incision.[181] Careful attention to minimization of blood loss, avoidance of tissue trauma, and complete closure of the myoma cavity are the guiding principles of abdominal myomectomy procedures.

Efficacy rates are high with rare cases requiring hysterectomy for intractable bleeding.[182] Buttram and Reiter reviewed five studies and demonstrated an 81% rate of symptom resolution following myomectomy procedures.[2] Recently, Campo et al compared fertility outcomes of patients undergoing both abdominal and laparoscopic myomectomies, in a retrospective cohort evaluation.[183] There was a nonsignificant reduction of nearly 70% in pregnancy loss following abdominal myomectomy and a highly significant 75% reduction in pregnancy loss following laparoscopic myomectomy. Nearly 58% of patients with abdominal myomectomy were able to conceive versus 64% of patients with laparoscopic myomectomy. Eighty percent of patients gave birth successfully, with a cesarean section rate of 50%. Interestingly, these authors noted a 14-fold increase in chance of conception in patients who underwent laparoscopic versus abdominal myomectomy. In their evaluation of 46 separate studies on fertility following myomectomy, Donnez and Jadoul found that pregnancy rates for laparoscopic and abdominal myomectomy patients were 49% and 48%, respectively.[92]

Compared with hysterectomy, abdominal myomectomy demonstrates decreased morbidity.[184] Other sources of morbidity including fever, infection, blood loss, and visceral injury do not significantly differ from those of laparoscopic myomectomy. Adhesion formation rates after abdominal myomectomy may be as high as 90% compared with a lower rate for laparoscopic myomectomy. Leiomyoma recurrence rates following abdominal myomectomy are generally between 15% and 30%. In a randomized, controlled trial comparing abdominal and laparoscopic myomectomy procedures, recurrence rates were 23% and 27%, respectively, with no significant difference detected between the two groups.[185] In Fauconnier's review, excluding studies using ultrasound for diagnosis, recurrence rates were between 5.7% and 11.1%.[186] Inclusion of ultrasound significantly increases the rate of recurrence up to 50%, but many of these myomas may remain asymptomatic. The mean time to recurrence of myomas is 5.6 to 7.6 years following abdominal myomectomy procedures. Studies using life table analysis demonstrated a cumulative risk of 10% at 5 years after abdominal myomectomy. Hysterectomy rates are similar for both abdominal and laparoscopic approaches, varying in studies from 4.3% to 16.8% for patients who previously underwent myomectomy. These values represent nearly one of every three patients who have recurrence. Predictors of recurrence include uterine size less than 12 weeks of gestational age, history of endometriosis, history of menorrhagia, and parity of one or more.[187]

## Laparoscopic Myolysis

In patients with fibroids not amenable to myomectomy, some authors advocate the use of laparoscopic myolysis. Acceptable candidates for this procedure include those with exceptionally large myomas, multiple myomas, or symptoms of pain or pressure. Myomas are coagulated with laser sources, diathermy, or electrical coagulation, usually starting with the central core followed by application to the entire myoma. Noselle et al treated 48 patients by laparoscopic Nd:YAg laser myolysis and followed patients with ultrasonographic assessment.[188] The authors found that myoma volume progressively decreased by a mean of 4% at 6 weeks postoperatively to a mean reduction of 41% after 6 months. Bipolar myoma coagulation has even higher efficacy with 80% to 90% reduction in uterine and fibroid volume at 6 months and almost universal patient satisfaction levels.[189]

Intraoperative complication rates are low and usually involve hemorrhagic areas within or around the coagulated myoma. Myoma regrowth following myolysis has not been reported. Most studies indicate a 3% to 6% rate of subsequent hysterectomy for persistent symptoms, in accord with reoperation rates following other surgical modalities of leiomyoma management. Although pregnancy has been reported following use of myolytic therapy, complications including uterine rupture also have been noted.[190] Because of its unknown effect on pregnancy, this procedure is not currently recommended for patients wishing to conceive following therapy.

## Alternative Therapies

In an attempt to reduce the complications associated with operative myomectomies, some authors have investigated the utility of performing hysteroscopic global endometrial ablation techniques for the treatment of fibroid-related menorrhagia. In a study of 22 women undergoing hydrothermal endometrial ablation for submucosal fibroids, 54% of patients were amenorrheic, 235 were oligomenorrheic, 14% were eumenorrheic, and only 4.5% (one patient) continued to have menorrhagia, necessitating hysterectomy, after a mean follow-up period of 15.4 months.[191] These results show significant promise, but the modality is unacceptable for patients wishing to conserve fertility. For physicians lacking technical proficiency in hysteroscopic resection techniques, the global ablative technique may be a reliable and effective means of controlling fibroid-related symptoms in selected patients.

# CONTROVERSIES

Epidemiologic studies on fibroids often conflict. Differences in patient populations, diagnostic techniques, and lack of control of confounding variables riddle many of the studies. Although race and hormonal-related factors appear to have significant impact on the incidence of myomas, precise estimates of risk are difficult to ascertain. Moreover, causality or pathophysiologic associations have not been clearly delineated between risk factors and the genesis of uterine leiomyomas.

The effect of myomas on reproductive outcome also requires further investigation. Increasing evidence suggests that submucosal and some intramural fibroids can impair fertility as well has have adverse effects on women undergoing infertility treatment. However, these findings have not been confirmed in large, prospective studies, and the impact of subserosal myomas and smaller intramural fibroids on fertility outcomes is not clear. Moreover, the data regarding fibroids and pregnancy outcomes are mainly derived from retrospective case control studies with limited statistical power. Thus, the value of preconceptional myomectomy in patients with pregnancy loss and even those without symptoms needs further evaluation. Currently, the American College of Obstetricians and Gynecologists recommends that if patients with mild symptoms or reproductive failure undergo therapy, it should be conducted as close to the time of conception as possible owing to the relatively high rate of myoma recurrence over time.[192] Similarly, the association of myomas with recurrent miscarriage has not been assessed prospectively. The authors have reviewed the existing evidence, which indicates that resection of myomas is associated with a reduced miscarriage rate, and agree with Manyonda et al who conclude that from a pragmatic standpoint excision of myomas in patients with recurrent miscarriage not attributable to other factors is a reasonable therapeutic option.[193]

The role of medical therapy in the treatment of myomas is also riddled with numerous unanswered questions. While GnRH agonists have an obvious salutary effect on symptoms and myoma shrinkage, the severity and complexity of associated side effects limits their long-term use. Moreover, little evidence indicates that these agents are useful in patients wishing to subsequently conceive. The utility of preoperative GnRH agonists has not been fully evaluated, since some trials demonstrate potentially increased risks of surgical complexity, longer operative times, and higher recurrence rates in patients pretreated. These potential complications must be weighed against the observed benefits of decreased blood loss and results of some studies that demonstrate reduced operating times. A large, multicenter, randomized, controlled trial assessing the impact of preoperative GnRH analogs on intraoperative and postoperative outcomes would resolve these questions.

The optimal invasive approach is dependent on patient-specific factors. Laparoscopic myomectomy is associated with some improved short-term benefits, but long-term recurrence rates are likely higher than those found with abdominal myomectomy. Uterine artery embolization also has resulted in significant improvements in fibroid symptomatology, but the effects on pregnancy are not well understood. Thus, no single procedure can be considered the gold standard, because patients not wishing to undergo repeat surgical procedures, those who desire to conceive, and those who need rapid relief of symptoms without significant morbidity may each benefit from different procedures. Until the specific benefits, morbidities, and long-term patient and reproductive outcomes have been assessed the authors recommend that physicians review all options with

patients and decide on a course of therapy only after extensive consideration of the risks and benefits of each strategy for each patient.

The quandaries of myoma management are best summarized by Myers et al, who undertook a review of 1084 separate studies on the surgical and nonsurgical management of uterine leiomyomas with outcomes data.[194] Despite the large number of studies evaluated, these authors were unable to conduct any meta-analyses because of the "inconsistency in reporting of severity of symptoms, uterine anatomy, and response to therapy." Two issues thus are paramount in establishing evidence-based guidelines for myoma management: (1) research on myomas must use standardized classification systems, symptom measurement scales, and outcome measures and their respective assessment tools; and (2) greater collaboration between centers is necessary to enable the initiation of adequately powered, large-scale, prospective, randomized controlled trials. Until such circumstances arise, physicians must rely on careful analysis of the current body of evidence and use clinical judgment and skill in the counseling and guidance of patients.

## REFERENCES

1. Schwartz SM: Epidemiology of uterine leiomyomata. Clin Obstet Gynecol 2001;44:316–326. **(IV, C)**
2. Buttram VC, Reiter RC: Uterine leiomyomata: etiology, symptomatology and management. Fertil Steril 1981;36:433–445. **(IV, C)**
3. Lumsden MA, Wallace EM: Clinical presentation of uterine fibroids. Baillieres Clin Obstet Gynaecol 1998;12:177–195. **(IV, C)**
4. Cramer SF, Patel A: The frequency of uterine leiomyomas. Am J Clin Pathol 1990;94:435–438. **(IIb, B)**
5. Marshall LM, Speigelman D, Barbieri R, et al: Variation in the incidence of uterine leiomyoma among premenopausal women by age and race. Obstet Gynecol 1997;90:967–973. **(IIb, B)**
6. Ross RK, Pike M, Vessey MP, et al: Risk factors for uterine fibroids: reduced risk associated with oral contraceptives. BMJ 1986; 293:359–362. **(III, B)**
7. Faerstein E, Szklo M, Rosenshein NB: Risk factors for uterine leiomyoma: a practice-based case control study. 1. African-American heritage, reproductive history, body size, and smoking. Am J Epidemiol 2001;153:1–10. **(III, B)**
8. Baird DD, Dunson DB, Hill MC, et al: high cumulative incidence of uterine leiomyoma in black and white women: ultrasound evidence. Am J Obstet Gynecol 2003;188:100–107. **(IIb, B)**
9. Walker CL: Role of hormonal and reproductive factors in the etiology and treatment of uterine leiomyoma. Rec Prog Horm Res 2002; 57:277–294. **(IV, C)**
10. Marshall LM, Spiegelman, Goldman MB, et al: A prospective study of reproductive factors and oral contraceptive use in relation to the risk of uterine leiomyomata. Fertil Steril 1998;70:432–439. **(IIb, B)**
11. Samadi AR, Lee NC, Flanders WD, et al: Risk factors for self reported uterine fibroids: a case control study. Am J Public Health 1996; 86:858–862. **(III, B)**
12. Romieu I, Walker AM, Jick S: Determinants of uterine fibroids. Post Market Surveil 1991;5:119–133. **(IV, C)**
13. Lumbiganon P, Rugpao S, Phandhu-Fung S, et al: Protective effect of depot-medroxyprogesterone acetate on surgically treated uterine leiomyomas: a multicenter case-control study. BJOG 1995;103: 909–914. **(IIb, B)**
14. Wise LA, Palmer JR, Harlow BL, et al: Reproductive factors, hormonal contraception, and risk of uterine leiomyomata in African-American women: a prospective study. Am J Epidemiol 2004;159:113–123. **(IIb, B)**

15. Chen CR, Buck GM, Courey NG, et al: Risk factors for uterine fibroids among women undergoing tubal sterilization. Am J Epidemiol 2001;153:20–26. **(III, B)**

16. Parazzini F, Negri E, La Vecchia C, et al: Reproductive factors and risk of uterine fibroids. Epidemiology 1996;7:440–442. **(III, B)**

17. Rein MS, Barbieri RL, Friedman AJ: Progesterone: a critical role in the pathogenesis of uterine myomas. Am J Obstet Gynecol 1995; 172:14–18. **(IV, C)**

18. Sener AB, Seckin NC, Ozmen S, et al: The effects of hormone replacement therapy on uterine fibroids in postmenopausal women. Fertil Steril 1996;65:354–357. **(Ib, A)**

19. Yang CH, Lee JN, Hsu SC, et al: Effect of hormone replacement therapy on uterine fibroids in postmenopausal women—a 3-year study. Maturitas 2002;43:35–39. **(III, B)**

20. Fedele L, Bianchi S, Raffaelli R, et al: A randomized study of the effects of tibolone and transdermal estrogen replacement therapy in postmenopausal women with uterine myomas. Eur J Obstet Gynecol Reproid Biol 2000;88:91–94. **(Ib, A)**

21. de Aloysio D, Altieri P, Penacchioni P, et al: Bleeding patterns in recent postmenopausal outpatients with uterine myomas: comparison between two regimens of HRT. Maturitas 1998;29:261–264. **(Ib, A)**

22. Reed SD, Cushing-Haugen KL, Daling JR, et al: Postmenopausal estrogen and progestogen therapy and the risk of uterine leiomyomas. Menopause 2004;11:214–222. **(III, B)**

23. Marshall LM, Spiegelman D, Manson JE, et al: Risk of uterine leiomyomata among premenopausal women in relation to body size and cigarette smoking. Epidemiol 1998;9:511–517. **(IIb, B)**

24. Parazzini F, LaVecchia C, Negri E, et al: Epidemiologic characteristics of women with uterine fibroids: case-control study. Obstet Gynecol 1988;72:853–857. **(III, B)**

25. Parazzini F, Negri E, La Vecchia C, et al: Uterine myomas and smoking: results from an Italian study. J Reprod Med 1996;41:316–320. **(III, B)**

26. Flake GP, Andersen J, Dixon D: Etiology and pathogenesis of uterine leiomyomas: a review. Environ Health Perspect 2003;111:1037–1054. **(IV, C)**

27. Townsend DE, Sparkes RS, Baluda MC, et al: Unicellular histogenesis of uterine leiomyomas as determined by electrophoresis of glucose-6-phosphate dehydrogenase. Am J Obstet Gynecol 1970;107:1168–1173. **(III, B)**

28. Mashal RD, Fejzo MLS, Friedman AJ, et al: Analysis of androgen receptor DNA reveals the independent clonal origins of uterine leiomyomata and the secondary nature of cytogenetic aberrations in the development of leiomyomata. Genes Chromosomes Cancer 1994;11:1–6. **(IIb, B)**

29. Hashimoto K, Azuma C, Kamiura S, et al: Clonal determination of uterine leiomyomas by analyzing differential inactivation of the X-chromosone-linked phosphoglycerokinase gene. Gynecol Obstet Invest 1995;40:204–208. **(IIb, B)**

30. Gross KL, Morton CC: Genetics and the development of fibroids. Clin Obstet Gynecol 2001;44:335–349. **(IV, C)**

31. Gattas GJ, Quade BJ, Nowak RA, et al: HMGIC expression in human adult and fetal tissues and in uterine leiomyomata. Genes Chromosomes Cancer 1999;25:316–322. **(IIb, B)**

32. Pedeutour F, Quade BJ, Weremowicz S, et al: Localization and expression of the human estrogen receptor beta gene in uterine leiomyomata. Genes Chromosomes Cancer 1998;23:361–366. **(IIb, B)**

33. Kazmierczak B, Dal Cin P, Wanschura S, et al: HMGIY is the target of 6p21.3 rearrangements in various benign mesenchymal tumors. Genes Chromosomes Cancer 1998;23:279–285. **(IIb, B)**

34. Tallini G, Dal Cin P, Rhoden KJ, et al: Expression of HMGI-C and HMGI(Y) in ordinary lipoma and atypical lipomatous tumors: immunohistochemical reactivity correlates with karyotypic alterations. Am J Pathol 1997;151:37–43. **(III, B)**

35. Xiao S, Lux M, Reeves R, et al: HMGI(Y) activation by chromosome 6p21 rearrangements in multilineage mesenchymal cells from pulmonary hamartoma. Am J Pathol 1997;150:901–910. **(Comment)**

36. Dal Cin P, Wanschura S, Christiaens MR, et al: Hamartoma of the breast with involvement of 6p21 and rearrangement of HMGIY. Genes Chromosomes Cancer 1997;20:90–92. **(III, B)**

37. Dal Cin P, Van Den Berghe H, et al: Involvement of 6p in an endometrial polyp. Cancer Genet Cytogenet 1991;51:279–280. **(III, B)**

38. Somberger KS, Weremowicz S, Williams AJ, et al: Expression of HMGIY in three uterine leiomyomata with complex rearrrangements of chromosome 6. Cancer Genet Cytogenet 1999;114:9–16. **(III, B)**

39. Ligon AH, Morton CC: Genetics of uterine leiomyomata. Genes Chromosomes Cancer 2000;28:235–245. **(III, B)**

40. Vanni R, Van Roy N, Lecca U, et al: Uterine leiomyoma cytogenetics. 3. Interphase cytogenetic analysis of karyotypically normal uterine leiomyoma excludes possibility of undetected trisomy 12. Cancer Genet Cytogenet 1992;62:40–42. **(III, B)**

41. Ligon AH, Morton CC: Leiomyomata: heritability and cytogenetic studies. Genes Chromosomes Cancer 2000;28:235–245. **(IV, C)**

42. Treloar SA, Martin NG, Dennerstein L, et al: Pathways to hysterectomy: insights from longitudinal twin research. Am J Obstet Gynecol 1992;167:82–88. **(IIb, B)**

43. Luoto R, Kaprio J, Rutanen EM, et al: Heritability and risk factors of uterine fibroids—the Finnish Twin Cohort study. Maturitas 2000; 37:15–26. **(IIb, B)**

44. Winkler VDH, Hoffmann W: Regarding the question of inheritance of uterine myoma. Deutsche-Medizinische Wochenschrift 1938; 68:235–257. **(IV, C)**

45. Kurbanova M, Koroleva AG, Sergeev AS: Genetic-epidemiological analysis of uterine myoma: estimate of risk to relatives. Genetika 1989;25:1896–1898. **(IV, C)**

46. Vikhlyaeva EM, Khodzhaeva ZS, Fantschenko ND: Familial predisposition to uterine leiomyomas. Int J Gynecol Obstet 1995; 51:127–131. **(IIb, B)**

47. Schwartz SM, Voigt L, Tickman E, et al: Familial aggregation of uterine leiomyomata. Am J Epidemiol 2000;151:S10. **(III, B)**

48. Rein MS, Barbieri RL, Friedman AJ: Progesterone: a critical role in the pathogenesis of uterine myomas. Am J Obstet Gynecol 1995; 172:14–18. **(IV, C)**

49. Sadan O, van Iddekinge B, van Gelderen CJ, et al: Oestrogen and progesterone receptor concentrations in leiomyoma and normal myometrium. Ann Clin Biochem 1987;24:263–267. **(III, B)**

50. Benassayag C, Leroy MJ, Rigourd V, et al: Estrogen receptors (ERalpha/ERbeta) in normal and pathological growth of the human myometrium: pregnancy and leiomyoma. Am J Physiol 1999; 276:E1112–1118. **(III, B)**

51. Folkerd EJ, Newton CJ, Davidson K, et al: Aromatase activity in uterine leiomyomata. J Steroid Biochem 1984;20:1195–1200. **(IIb, B)**

52. Sumitani H, Shozu M, Segawa T, et al: In situ estrogen synthesized by aromatase P450 in uterine leiomyoma cells promotes cell growth probably via an autocrine/intracrine mechanism. Endocrinol 2000; 141:3852–3861. **(IIb, B)**

53. Yamamoto T, Takamori K, Okada H: Estrogen biosynthesis in leiomyoma and myometrium of the uterus. Horm Metab Res 1984; 16:678–679. **(III, B)**

54. Spellacy WN, Le Maire WJ, Buhi WC, et al: Plasma growth hormone and estradiol levels in women with uterine myomas. Obstet Gynecol 1972;40:829–834. **(III, B)**

55. Maheux R, Lemay-Turcot L, Lemay A: Daily follicle-stimulating hormone, luteinizing hormone, estradiol, and progesterone in ten women harboring uterine leiomyomas. Fertil Steril 1986;46:205–208. **(IIb, B)**

56. Dawood MY, Khan-Dawood FS: Plasma insulin-like growth factor-I, CA-125, estrogen, and progesterone in women with leiomyomas. Fertil Steril 1994;61:617–621. **(IIa, B)**

57. Liehr JG, Ricci MJ, Jefcoate CR, et al; 4-hydroxylation of estradiol by human uterine myometrium and myoma microsomes: implications for the mechanism of uterine tumorigenesis. Proc Natl Acad Sci USA 1995;92:9220–9224. **(III, B)**

58. Brandon DD, Bethea CL, Strawn EY, et al: Progesterone receptor messenger ribonucleic acid and protein are overexpressed in human uterine leiomyomas. Am J Obstet Gynecol 1993;169:78–85. **(III, B)**

59. Viville B, Charnock-Jones DS, Sharkey AM, et al: Distribution of the A and B forms of the progesterone receptor messenger ribonucleic

acid and protein in uterine leiomyomata and adjacent myometrium. Hum Reprod 1997;12:815–822. **(III, B)**

60. Otubu JA, Buttram VC, Besche NF, et al: Unconjugated steroids in leiomyomas and tumor-bearing myometrium. Am J Obstet Gynecol 1982;143:130–133. **(III, B)**

61. Tiltman AJ: The effect of progestins on the mitotic activity of uterine fibromyomas. Int J Gynecol Pathol 1985;4:89–96. **(III, B)**

62. Kawaguchi D, Fujii S, Konishi I, et al: Mitotic activity in uterine leiomyomas during the menstrual cycle. Am J Obstet Gynecol 1989; 160:637–641. **(III, B)**

63. Kawaguchi K, Fujii S, Konishi I, et al: Ultrastructural study of cultured smooth muscle cells from uterine leiomyoma and myometrium under the influence of sex steroids. Gynecol Oncol 1985;21:32–41. **(III, B)**

64. Maruo T, Matsuo H, Samoto T, et al: Effects of progesterone on uterine leiomyoma growth and apoptosis. Steroids 2000;65:585–592. **(III, B)**

65. Hofmann GE, Rao CV, Barrows GH, et al: Binding sites for epidermal growth factor in human uterine tissues and leiomyoma. J Clin Endocrinol Metab 1984;58:880–884. **(III, B)**

66. Nelson KG, Takahashi T, Bossert NL, et al: Epidermal growth factor replaces estrogen in the stimulation of female genital-tract growth and differentiation. Proc Natl Acad Sci U S A 1991;88:21–25. **(III, B)**

67. Yeh J, Rein M, Nowak R: Presence of messenger ribonucleic acid for epidermal growth factor (EGF) and EGF receptor demonstrable in monolayer cell cultures of myometrial and leiomyoma. Fertil Steril 1991;56:997–1000. **(III, B)**

68. Rossi MJ, Chegini N, Masterson BJ: Presence of epidermal growth factor, platelet-derived growth factor (PDGF), and their receptors in human myometrial tissue and smooth muscle cells: their action in smooth muscle cells in vitro. Endocrinol 1992;130:1716–1727. **(III, B)**

69. Lyons RM, Moses HL: Transforming growth factors and the regulation of cell proliferation. Eur J Biochem 1990;187:467–473. **(IV, C)**

70. Matsuo H, Maruo T, Samoto T: Increased expression of Bcl-2 protein in human uterine leiomyoma and its up-regulation by progesterone. J Clin Endocrinol Metab 1997;82:293–299. **(III, B)**

71. Valenti MT, Azzarello G, Vinante O, et al: Differentiation, proliferation and apoptosis levels in human leiomyoma and leiomyosarcoma. J Cancer Res Clin Oncol 1998;124:93–105. **(III, B)**

72. Vu K, Greenspan DL, Wu T-C, et al: Cellular proliferation, estrogen receptor, progesterone receptor, and bcl-2 expression in GnRH agonist-treated uterine leiomyomas. Hum Pathol 1998;29:359–363. **(III, B)**

73. Lumsden MA, Wallace EM: Clinical presentation of uterine fibroids. Baillieres Clin Obstet Gynecol 1998;12:177–195. **(IV, C)**

74. Stewart EA: Uterine fibroids. Lancet 2001;357:293–298. **(IV, C)**

75. Stovall DW: Clinical symptomatology of uterine leiomyomas. Clin Obstet Gynecol 2001;44:364–371. **(IIb, B)**

76. Bettocchi S, Ceci O, Vicino M, et al: Diagnostic inadequacy of dilation and curettage. Fertil Steril 2001;75:803–805. **(III, B)**

77. Pron G, Bennett J, Common A, et al: The Ontario Uterine Fibroid Embolization Trial. 2. Uterine fibroid reduction and symptom relief after uterine artery embolization for fibroids. Fertil Steril 2003; 79:120–127. **(IIb, B)**

78. Rybo G, Leman J, Tibbin R: Epidemiology of Menstrual Blood Loss: Mechanisms of Menstrual Bleeding, New York, Raven Press, 1985, pp 181–193. **(III, B)**

79. Farrer-Brown G, Bobbeilby JOW, Tarbit NH: Venous changes in the endometrium of myomatous uteri. Obstet Gynecol 1971;38:743–751. **(III, B)**

80. Yamaguchi M, Mori N: Prostaglandin production by human myometrium, uterine cervix and leiomyoma. Prostaglandins Leukot Med 1987;29:107–112. **(III, B)**

81. Anderson J: Factors in fibroid growth. Baillieres Clin Obstet Gynecol 1998;12:233–238. **(IV, C)**

82. Vercellini P, Vendola N, Ragni G, et al: Abnormal uterine bleeding associated with iron deficiency anemia: etiology and role of hysteroscopy. J Reprod Med 1993;38:502–504. **(IV, C)**

83. Lippman SA, Warner M, Samuels S, et al: Uterine fibroids and gynecologic pain symptoms in a population-based study. Fertil Steril 2003;80:1488–1494. **(IIb, B)**

84. Kjerulff KH, Langenberg P, Seidman JD, et al: uterine leiomyomas: racial differences in severity, symptoms, and age at diagnosis. J Reprod Med 1994;41:483–490. **(IIb, B)**

85. Hara T, Tsuchida M, Takai K, et al: Ureteral obstruction in a transplanted kidney secondary to a subserous myoma uteri. Transplant 2003;75:1915–1916. **(III, B)**

86. Reiter RC, Wagner PL, Gambone JC: Routine hysterectomy for large asymptomatic uterine leiomyomata: a reappraisal. Obstet Gynecol 1992;79:481–484. **(III, B)**

87. Chaparala RPC, Fawole AS, Ambrose NS, et al: Large bowel obstruction due to a benign uterine leiomyoma. Gut 2004;53:386. **(III, B)**

88. Bajekal N, Li TC: Fibroids, infertility and pregnancy wastage. Hum Reprod Update 2000;6:614–620. **(IV, C)**

89. Pritts EA: Fibroids and infertility: a systematic review of the evidence. Obstet Gynecol Surv 2001;56:483–491. **(IV, C)**

90. Ubaldi F, Tournaye H, Camus M, et al: Fetility after hysteroscopic myomectomy. Hum Reprod Update 1995;1:81–90. **(IV, C)**

91. Bulletti C, De Ziegler D, Polli V, et al: The role of leiomyomas in infertility. J Am Assoc Gynecol Laparosc 1999;6:441–445. **(III, B)**

92. Donnez J, Jadoul P: What are the implications of myomas on fertility? A need for a debate? Hum Reprod 2002;17:1424–1430. **(IV, C)**

93. Hart R, Khalaf Y, Yeong CT, et al: A prospective controlled study of the effect of intramural uterine fibroids on the outcome of assisted conception. Hum Reprod 2001;16:2411–2417. **(IIa, B)**

94. Oliveira FG, Abdelmassih VG, Diamond MP, et al: Impact of sub-serosal and intramural uterine fibroids that do not distort the endometrial cavity on the outcome of in vitro fertilization-intracytoplasmic sperm injection. Fertil Steril 2004;81:582–587. **(IIa, B)**

95. Check JH, Choe JK, Lee G, et al: The effect on IVF outcome of small intramural fibroids not compressing the uterine cavity as determined by a prospective matched control study. Hum Reprod 2002; 17:1244–1248. **(IIa, B)**

96. Ng EHY, Ho PC: Doppler ultrasound examination of uterine arteries on the day of oocyte retrieval in patients with uterine fibroids undergoing IVF. Hum Reprod 2002;17:765–770. **(IIb, B)**

97. Surrey ES: Impact of intramural leiomyomata on in-vitro fertilization-embryo transfer cycle outcome. Curr Opin Obstet Gynecol 2003; 15:239–242. **(IV, C)**

98. Muram D, Gillieson M, Walters JH: Myomas of the uterus in pregnancy: ultrasonographic follow-up. Am J Obstet Gynecol 1980;138:16–19. **(IV, C)**

99. Myers ER, Barber M, Couchman GM, et al: Management of uterine fibroids. Evidence Report/Technology Assessment. Rockville, Md, Agency for Health Care Research and Quality, 2001. Available at http://www.ahcpr.gov/clinic/epcix.htm. Accessed 4/15/05. **(IV, C)**

100. Benson CB, Chow JS, Chang-Lee W, et al: Outcome of pregnancies in women with uterine leiomyomas identified by sonography in the first trimester. J Clin Ultrasound 2001;29:261–264. **(III, B)**

101. Li TC, Mortimer R, Cooke ID: Myomectomy: a retrospective study to examine reproductive performance before and after surgery. Hum Reprod 1999;14:1735–1740. **(III, B)**

102. Coronado GD, Marshall LM, Schwartz SM: Complications in pregnancy, labor, and delivery with uterine leiomyomas: a population-based study. Obstet Gynecol 2000;95:764–769. **(III, B)**

103. Salvador E, Bienstock J, Blakemore KJ, et al: Leiomyomata uteri, genetic amniocentesis, and the risk of second-trimester spontaneous abortion. Am J Obstet Gynecol 2002;186:913–915. **(IIa, B)**

104. Lanouette JM, Diamond MP: Pregnancy in women with myoma uteri. Infert Reprod Med Clin North Am 1996;7:19–32. **(IV, C)**

105. Katz V, Dotters DJ, Droegemueller W: Complications of uterine leiomyomas in pregnancy. Obstet Gynecol 1989;73:593–596. **(III, B)**

106. Cantuaria GHC, Angioli R, Frost L, et al: Comparison of bimanual examination with ultrasound examination before hysterectomy for uterine leiomyoma. Obstet Gynecol 1998;92:109–112. **(III, B)**

107. Goldberg JM, Falcone T, Attaran M: Sonohysterographic evaluation of uterine abnormalities noted on hysterosalpingography. Hum Reprod 1997;12:2151–2153. **(III, B)**

108. Pittaway DE, Winfield AC, Maxson W, et al: Prevention of acute pelvic inflammatory disease after hysterosalpingography: efficacy of doxycycline prophylaxis. Am J Obstet Gynecol 1983;147:623–626. **(III, B)**

109. Hurley V: Imaging techniques for fibroid detection. Baillieres Clin Obstet Gynecol 1998;12:213–224. **(IV, C)**

110. Karasick S, Lev-Toaff AS, Toaff ME: Imaging of uterine leiomyomas. Am J Roentgenol 1992;158:799–805. **(IV, C)**

111. Mayer DP, Shipilov V: Ultrasonography and magnetic resonance imaging of uterine fibroids. Obstet Gynecol Clin North Am 1995; 22:667–725. **(IV, C)**

112. Fedele L, Bianchi S, Dorta M, et al: Transvaginal sonography versus hysteroscopy in the diagnosis of uterine submucous myomas. Obstet Gynecol 1991;77:745–748. **(III, B)**

113. Dueholm M, Lundorf E, Hansen ES, et al: Accuracy of magnetic resonance imaging and transvaginal ultrasonography in the diagnosis, mapping, and measurement of uterine myomas. Am J Obstet Gynecol 2002;186:409–415. **(IIb, B)**

114. de Vries LD, Dijkhuizen FP, Mol BW, et al: Comparison of transvaginal sonography, saline infusion sonography, and hysteroscopy in premenopausal women with abnormal uterine bleeding. J Clin Ultrasound 2000;28:217–223. **(IIb, B)**

115. Sylvestre C, Child TJ, Tulandi T, et al: A prospective study to evaluate the efficacy of two- and three-dimensional sonohysterography in women with intrauterine lesions. Fertil Steril 2003;79:1222–1225. **(IIb, B)**

116. Brunner M, Obruca A, Bauer P, et al: Clinical application of volume estimation based on three dimensional ultrasonography. Ultrasound Obstet Gynecol 1995;6:359–361. **(III, B)**

117. Jurkovic D: Three-dimensional ultrasound in gynecology: a critical evaluation. Ultrasound Obstet Gynecol 2002;19:109–117. **(IV, C)**

118. Pretorius DH, Becker E, Lev-Toaff AS: Impact of sonohysterography on the management of women with uterine myomas. Ultrasound Obstet Gynecol 2001;18(Suppl):2. **(IV, C)**

119. de Vries LD, Paul HLF, Dijkhuizen J, et al: Comparison of transvaginal sonography, saline infusion sonography, and hysteroscopy in premenopausal women with abnormal uterine bleeding. J Clin Ultrasound 2000;28:217–223. **(IIb, B)**

120. Hricak H, Tscholakoff D, Heinrichs L, et al: Uterine leiomyomas: correlation of MR, histopathological findings, and symptoms. Radiology 1986;158:385–391. **(III, B)**

121. Ascher SM, Jha RC, Reinhold C: Benign myometrial conditions: leiomyomas and adenomyosis. Top Magn Reson Imaging 2003; 14:281–304. **(IV, C)**

122. Lefebvre G, Vilos GA, Allaire C, et al: SOGC Clinical practice guidelines: the management of uterine leiomyomas. J Obstet Gynaecol Can 2003;25:396–405. **(III, B)**

123. Schwartz LB, Diamond MP, Schwartz PE: Leiomyosarcomas: clinical presentation. Am J Obstet Gynecol 1993;168:180–183. **(III, B)**

124. Meyer WR, Mayer AR, Diamond MP, et al: Unsuspected leiomyosarcoma: treatment with a gonadotropin-releasing hormone analogue. Obstet Gynecol 1990;75:529–532. **(III, B)**

125. Carr BR, Marshburn PB, Weatherall PT, et al: An evaluation of the effect of gonadotropin-releasing hormone analogs and medroxyprogesterone acetate on uterine leiomyomata volume by magnetic resonance imaging: a prospective, randomized, double blind, placebo-controlled, crossover trial. J Clin Endocrinol Metab 1993;76:1217–1223. **(Ib, A)**

126. Sivin I, Stern J: Health during prolonged use of levonorgestrel 20 mcg/d and the copper TCu 380Ag intrauterine contraceptive devices: a multicenter study. International Committee for Contraception Research. Fertil Steril 1994;61:70–77. **(Ib, A)**

127. Pekonen F, Nyman T, Lahteenmaki P, et al: Intrauterine progestin induces continuous insulin-like growth factor-binding protein-1 production in the human endometrium. J Clin Endocrinol Metab 1992;75:660–664. **(IIb, B)**

128. Makarainen L, Ylikorkala O: Primary and myoma-associated menorrhagia: role of prostaglandins and effects of ibuprofen. BJOG 1986;93:974–978. **(Ib, A)**

129. Ylikorkala O, Pekonen F: Naproxen reduces idiopathic but not fibromyoma-induced menorrhagia. Obstet Gynecol 1986;68:10–12. **(IIa, B)**

130. Friedman AJ, Barbieri RL, Benacerraf BR, et al: Treatment of leiomyomata with intranasal or subcutaneous leuprolide, a gonadotropin-releasing hormone agonist. Fertil Steril 1987;48:560–564. **(Ib, A)**

131. Friedman AJ, Hoffman DI, Comite F, et al: Treatment of leiomyomata uteri with leuprolide acetate depot: a double-blind, placebo-controlled, multicenter study. Obstet Gynecol 1991;77:720–725. **(Ib, A)**

132. Chavez NF, Stewart EA: Medical treatment of uterine fibroids. Clin Obstet Gynecol 2001;44:372–384. **(IV, C)**

133. Shaw RW: Gonadotropin hormone-releasing hormone analogue treatment of fibroids. Baillieres Clin Obstet Gynecol 1998;12:245–268. **(IV, C)**

134. Lemay A, Maheux R: GnRH agonists in the management of uterine leiomyoma. Infert Reprod Med Clin North Am 1996;7:33–55. **(IV, C)**

135. Farquhar C, Arroll B, Ekeroma A, et al: An evidence based guideline for the management of uterine fibroids. Aust N Z J Obstet Gynaecol 2001;41:125–140. **(IV, C)**

136. Donnez J, Schrurs B, Gillerot S, et al: Treatment of uterine fibroids with implants of gonadotropin-releasing hormone agonist: assessment by hysterography. Fertil Steril 1989;51:947–950. **(III, B)**

137. Watanabe Y, Nakamura G: Effects of two different doses of leuprolide acetate depot on uterine cavity area in patients with uterine leiomyomata. Fertil Steril 1995;63:487–490. **(Ib, A)**

138. Friedman AJ, Daly M, Juneau-Norcross MJ, et al: Predictors of uterine volume reduction in women with myomas treated with a gonadotropin-releasing hormone agonist. Fertil Steril 1992;8:413–415. **(III, B)**

139. Gutmann JN, Thornton KL, Diamond MP, et al: Evaluation of leuprolide acetate treatment on histopathology of uterine myomata. Fertil 1994;61:662–626. **(III, B)**

140. Lethaby A, Vollenhoven B, Sowter M: Efficacy of pre-operative gonadotrophin hormone releasing analogues for women with uterine fibroids undergoing hysterectomy or myomectomy: a systematic review. BJOG 2002;109:1097–1108. **(IV, C)**

141. Dubuisson JB, Fauconnier A, Fourchotte V, et al: Laparoscopic myomectomy: predicting the risk of conversion to an open procedure. Human Reprod 2001;16:1726–1731. **(IIb, B)**

142. Friedman AJ, Harrison-Atlas D, Barbieri RL, et al: A randomized, placebo-controlled, double-blind study evaluating the efficacy of leuprolide acetate depot in the treatment of uterine leiomyomata. Fertil Steril 1989;51:251–256. **(Ib, A)**

143. Matta WHM, Stabile I, Shaw RW, et al: Doppler assessment of uterine blood flow changes in patients with fibroids receiving the gonadotropin releasing hormone agonist buserelin. Fertil Steril 1988;46:1083–1085. **(III, B)**

144. Shaw RW: Blood flow changes in the uterus induced by treatment with GnRH analogues. Hum Reprod 1996;11:27–32. **(IV, C)**

145. Serra GB, Panetta V, Colosimo M, et al: Efficacy of leuprorelin acetate depot in symptomatic fibromatous uteri: the Italian multicenter trial. Clin Ther 1992;14:57–73. **(IIb, B)**

146. West CP, Lumsden MA, Baird JT: Goserelin in the treatment of fibroids. BJOG 1992;99(Suppl):27–30. **(IV, C)**

147. Cirkel U, Ochs H, Scheiner HPG, et al: Experience with leuprolin acetate depot in the treatment of fibroids: a German multicenter study. Clin Ther 1992;14(Suppl A):37–50. **(IIb, B)**

148. Lumsden MA, West CP, Thomas E, et al: Treatment with the gonadotropin-releasing hormone agonist goserelin before hysterectomy for uterine fibroids. BJOG 1994;101:438. **(Ib, A)**

149. Friedman AJ, Daly M, Juneau-Norcross M, et al: A prospective, randomized trial of gonadotropin-releasing hormone agonist plus estrogen-progestin or progestin "add-back" regimens for women with leiomyomata uteri. J Clin Endocrinol Metab 1993;76:1439–1445. **(Ib, A)**

150. Friedman AJ: Treatment of leiomyomata uteri with short-term leuprolide followed by leuprolide plus estrogen-progestin hormone replacement therapy for 2 years: a pilot study. Fertil Steril 1989;51:526–528. **(III, B)**

151. Murphy AA: RU 486 in the treatment of leiomyomata uteri. Infert Reprod Med Clin North Am 1996;7:57–68. **(IV, C)**

152. DeManno D, Elger W, Garg R, et al: Asoprisnol (J867): a selective progesterone receptor modulator for gynecological therapy. Steroids 2003;68:1019–1032. **(IV, C)**

153. Chwalisz K, Lamar Parker R, Williamson S, et al: Treatment of uterine leiomyomas with the novel selective progesterone receptor modulator (SPRM) J867. J Soc Gynecol Invest 2003;10 [abstract 636].

154. Ueki M, Okamoto Y, Tsurunaga T, et al: Endocrinological and histological changes after treatment of uterine leiomyomas with danazol or buserelin. J Obstet Gynecol 1995;21:1–7. **(IIa, B)**

155. De Leo V, Morgante G, Lanzetta D, et al: Danazol administration after gonadotropin-releasing hormone analogue reduces rebound of uterine myomas. Hum Reprod 1997;12:357–360. **(III, B)**

156. Takebayashi T, Fujino Y, Umesaki N, et al: Danazol suspension injected into the uterine cervix of patients with adenomyomas and myoma. Gynecol Obstet Invest 1995;39:207–211. **(III, B)**

157. Coutinho EM, Goncalves MT: Long-term treatment of leiomyomas with gestrinone. Fertil Steril 1989;51:939–946. **(Ib, A)**

158. Mitwally MF, Casper RF: Use of an aromatase inhibitor for induction of ovulation in patients with an inadequate response to clomiphene citrate. Fertil Steril 2001;75:305–309. **(IIb, B)**

159. Shozu M, Murakami K, Segawa T, et al: Successful treatment of a symptomatic uterine leiomyoma in a perimenopausal woman with a nonsteroidal aromatase inhibitor. Fertil Steril 2003;79:628–631. **(III, B)**

160. Eldar-Geva T, Healy DL: Other medical management of uterine fibroids. Baillieres Clin Obstet Gynaecol 1998;12:269–288. **(IV, C)**

161. Jirecek S, Lee A, Pavo I, et al: Raloxifene prevents the growth of uterine leiomyomas in premenopausal women. Fertil Steril 2004; 81:132–136. **(Ib, A)**

162. Ravina JH, Herbreteau D, Ciraru-Vigneron N, et al: Arterial occlusion to treat uterine myomata. Lancet 1995;346:671–672. **(IIb, B)**

163. Nickolic B, Spies JB, Lundsten MJ, et al: Patient radiation dose associated with uterine artery embolization. Radiology 2002; 214:121–125. **(IIb, B)**

164. Walker WJ, Pelage JP, Sutton C: Fibroid embolization. Clin Radiol 2002;57:325–331. **(IV, C)**

165. Goldberg J, Pereira L, Berghella V: Pregnancy after uterine artery embolization. Obstet Gynecol 2002;100:869–872. **(IV, C)**

166. Chen YJ, Wang PH, Yuan CC, et al: Pregnancy following treatment of symptomatic myomas with laparoscopic bipolar coagulation of uterine vessels. Hum Reprod 2003;18:1077–1081. **(IIb, B)**

167. Vashisht A, Studd J, Carey A, et al: Fatal septicaemia after fibroid embolization. Lancet 1999;354:307–308. **(III, B)**

168. Pelage JP, Le Dref O, Soyer P, et al: Fibroid-related menorrhagia: treatment with superselective embolization of the uterine arteries and mid term follow-up. Radiology 2000;215:428–431. **(IIb, B)**

169. Chrisman HB, Saker MB, Ryu R, et al: The impact of uterine fibroid embolization on resumption of menses and ovarian function. J Vasc Interv Radiol 2000;11:699–703. **(IIb, B)**

170. Marret H, Alonso AM, Cottier JP, et al: Leiomyoma recurrence after uterine artery embolization. J Vasc Interv Radiol 2003;14:1395–1399. **(IIb, B)**

171. Al-Fozan H, Tulandi T: Factors affecting early surgical intervention after uterine artery embolization. Obstet Gynecol Surv 2002; 57:810–815. **(IV, C)**

172. Heinig J, Neff A, Cirkel U, et al: Recurrent leiomyomatosis peritonealis disseminata after hysterectomy and bilateral salpingo-oophorectomy during combined hormone replacement therapy. Eur J Obstet Gynecol Reprod Biol 2003;111:216–218. **(III, B)**

173. Carlson KJ, Miller BA, Fowler FJ: The Maine Women's Health Study: 1. Outcomes of hysterectomy. Obstet Gynecol 1994;83:556–565. **(IIb, B)**

174. Dwyer N, Hutton J, Stirrat GM: Randomised controlled trial comparing endometrial resection with abdominal hysterectomy for the surgical treatment of menorrhagia. BJOG 1993;100:237–243. **(Ib, A)**

175. Manyonda I, Sinthamoneya E, Belli AM: Controversies and challenges in the modern management of uterine fibroids. BJOG 2004; 111:95–102. **(IV, C)**

176. Pinto I, Chimeno P, Romo A, et al: Uterine fibroids: uterine artery embolization versus abdominal hysterectomy for treatment—a prospective, randomized, and controlled clinical trial. Radiol 2003; 226:425–431. **(Ib, A)**

177. Hwang JL, Seow KM, Tsai YL, et al: Comparative study of vaginal, laparoscopically assisted vaginal and abdominal hysterectomies for uterine myoma larger than 6 cm in diameter or uterus weighing at least 450 g: a prospective randomized study. Acta Obstet Gynecol Scand 2002;81:1132–1138. **(Ib, A)**

178. Ribeiro SC, Ribeiro RM, Santos NC, et al: A randomized study of total abdominal, vaginal and laparoscopic hysterectomy. Int J Gynecol Obstet 2003;83:37–43. **(Ib, A)**

179. Learman LA, Summitt RL Jr, Varner RE, et al: A randomized comparison of total or supracervical hysterectomy: surgical complications and clinical outcomes. Obstet Gynecol 2003;102:453–462. **(Ib, A)**

180. Vollenhoven BJ, Lawrence AS, Healy DL: Uterine fibroids: a clinical review. BJOG 1990;97:285–298. **(IV, C)**

181. Wallach EE: Myomectomy. In Thompson JD, Rock JA (eds): TeLinde's Operative Gynecology, 7th ed. Philadelphia, JB Lippincott, 1992, p 647. **(IV, C)**

182. LaMorte AL, Lalwani S, Diamond MP: Morbidity associated with abdominal myomectomy. Obstet Gynecol 1993;82:897. **(III, B)**

183. Campo S, Campo V, Gambadauro P: Reproductive outcome before and after laparoscopic or abdominal myomectomy for subserous or intramural myomas. Eur J Obstet Gynecol Reprod Biol 2003; 110:215–219. **(IIa, B)**

184. Iverson RE, Chelmow D, Strohbehn K, et al: Relative morbidity of abdominal hysterectomy and myomectomy for management of uterine leiomyomas. Obstet Gynecol 1996;88:415–419. **(III, B)**

185. Rossetti A, Sizzi O, Soronna L, et al: Long-term results of laparoscopic myomectomy: recurrence rate in comparison with abdominal myomectomy. Hum Reprod 2001;16:770–774. **(Ib, A)**

186. Fauconnier A, Chapron C, Babaki-Fard, et al: Recurrence of leiomyomata after myomectomy. Hum Reprod Update 2000;6:595–602. **(IV, C)**

187. Stewart EA, Faur EA, Wise LA, et al: Predictors of subsequent surgery for uterine leiomyomata after abdominal myomectomy. Obstet Gynecol 2002;99:426–432. **(IIb, B)**

188. Nisolle M, Smets M, Gillerot S, et al: Laparoscopic myolysis with the Nd:YAg laser. J Gynecol Surg 1993;9:95–99. **(III, B)**

189. Phillips DR, Nathanson HG, Milim SJ, et al: Experience with laparoscopic leiomyoma coagulation and concomitant operative hysteroscopy. J Am Assoc Gynecol Laparosc 1997;4:425–433. **(IIb, B)**

190. Vilos G, Daly L, Tse B: Pregnancy outcome after laparoscopic myolysis. J Am Assoc Gynecol Laparosc 1998;5:289–292. **(III, B)**

191. Glasser MH, Zimmerman JD: The hydrothermablator system for management of menorrhagia in women with submucous myomas: 12- to 20-month follow-up. J Am Assoc Gynecol Laparosc 2003; 10:521–527. **(IIb, B)**

192. Surgical alternatives to hysterectomy in the management of leiomyomas. ACOG practice Bulletin No. 16. Int J Gynaecol Obstet 2001;73:285–294. **(IV, C)**

193. Manyonda I, Sinthamoney E, Belli AM: Controversies and challenges in the modern management of uterine fibroids. BJOG 2004; 111:95–102. **(IV, C)**

194. Myers ER, Barber MD, Gustilo-Ashby T, et al: Management of uterine leiomyomata: what do we really know? Obstet Gynecol 2002; 100:8–17. **(IV, C)**

## KEY POINTS

- An ectopic gestation can implant on any surface outside the normal endometrium; however, 95% of ectopic pregnancies occur within the fallopian tube.
- While the incidence of ectopic pregnancy in the United States has plateaued over the last several years, the incidence among minority populations has almost doubled.
- The most common risk factors associated with the development of an ectopic gestation are previous ectopic pregnancy, previous tubal surgery including tubal sterilization, current use of an IUD, and a history of proven pelvic inflammatory disease.
- The patient with an unruptured ectopic pregnancy may be asymptomatic or may appear almost identical to the patient with a threatened abortion.
- Serial quantitative hCG measurements combined with transvaginal ultrasound are the primary modes for excluding a viable intrauterine pregnancy and thus making the diagnosis of ectopic gestation.
- Treatment of the unruptured ectopic pregnancy has moved from surgical toward nonsurgical management over the last two decades, while surgery continues to be the only treatment for the patient with a ruptured ectopic pregnancy.
- Following resolution, the patient continues to have an increased likelihood of a subsequent ectopic pregnancy and an overall decreased risk of a subsequently viable pregnancy.

A pregnancy can occur in either an intrauterine or an extrauterine location. While intrauterine pregnancies can be abnormal (incomplete or missed abortion), an extrauterine (ectopic pregnancy) pregnancy is always abnormal. An ectopic pregnancy occurs when the fertilized ovum implants in a location other than on the normal endometrium lining the endometrial cavity. Ectopic pregnancy appears to be confined to humans, since it has rarely been reported in other mammalian species. The most common site for an ectopic pregnancy is the ampullary segment of the fallopian tube; however, it may occur in other locations (Table 15-1).

## EPIDEMIOLOGY

Ectopic pregnancies are a common occurrence among reproductive-aged women, and the rates have been increasing over the last 30 years. The overall ectopic pregnancy rate is approximately 16 per 1000 pregnancies. Among women aged 35 to 44 years, the rate averages approximately 27 per 1000 preg-

nancies. Minority populations have a much higher rate of ectopic pregnancies. The rate for ectopic pregnancies is approximately 21 per 1000 among minorities versus 13 per 1000 in the white population. Women with ectopic pregnancies also have a significant risk for maternal mortality. Teenage women have the highest mortality rates with African American women having a risk five times greater than that of whites. The mortality rate associated with ectopic pregnancies accounts for approximately 15% of the annual maternal deaths in the United States.[1]

Once a woman has had one ectopic pregnancy, she has a 7- to 13-fold increased risk for a subsequent ectopic pregnancy. After an ectopic pregnancy, the following pregnancy has a 50% to 80% chance of being intrauterine and a 10% to 25% chance of again being ectopic, with the remainder of the patients becoming infertile.[2]

## ETIOLOGY AND RISK FACTORS

It is felt that the majority of ectopic pregnancies develop from an underlying tubal factor. The fallopian tubes can become damaged as a result of prior infection, inflammation, or surgery. Table 15-2 provides a listing of the known risks factors for ectopic pregnancy development. Associated risk factors include salpingitis, tubal sterilization, prior reconstructive tubal surgery, partial salpingectomy or congenital anomalies associated with the fallopian tubes. Changing levels of estrogen and progesterone as women age may account for the increased rates of ectopic pregnancies in women over age 35. While the etiology is uncertain, it may be secondary to the effects of estrogen on smooth muscle contractility and progesterone on smooth muscle relaxation.

Many risk factors are associated with development of an ectopic pregnancy; however, a few have been found to significantly increase a woman's risk. Women with a history of proved pelvic inflammatory disease (PID), a prior ectopic pregnancy, current use of an intrauterine contraceptive device (IUD), and previous tubal surgery as a treatment for infertility all have an increased risk for development of an ectopic pregnancy.

One of the major risk factors associated with development of an ectopic pregnancy is a history of a PID. Additional PID episodes may increase the inflammatory response within the pelvis, and subsequently the damage to the fallopian tube and tubal obstruction worsens. Although chlamydia infections may manifest only mild symptoms, there can be significant damage to the fallopian tubes. This may result in many cases being untreated or inadequately treated in the outpatient setting. Women with antichlamydial titers of 1:64 or greater are three times more likely to have an ectopic pregnancy than women with negative titers.[3] With each episode of PID, the rate of tubal obstruction is increased and the first pregnancy after an episode

**Table 15-1**
**Ectopic Pregnancy Locations**

| Type of Ectopic Pregnancy | Location |
| --- | --- |
| Tubal pregnancy | A pregnancy occurring in the fallopian tube Most commonly found in the ampullary region |
| Interstitial pregnancy | A pregnancy that implants in the interstitial portion of the fallopian tube |
| Abdominal pregnancy | Primary: The first and only implantation occurs on a peritoneal surface Secondary: The first implantation begins in the tubal lumen; the pregnancy is later aborted and then reimplants on a peritoneal surface |
| Cervical pregnancy | The developing ovum implants within the cervical canal |
| Ligamentous pregnancy | A pregnancy that occurs when a primary ectopic pregnancy erodes into the broad ligament and secondarily implants and develops between the leaves of the broad ligament |
| Heterotopic pregnancy | Concurrent intrauterine and ectopic pregnancies |
| Ovarian pregnancy | A pregnancy that develops within the ovarian cortex |

of PID has a higher rate for an ectopic gestation at 6% versus 0.9% in the control group of women without prior PID.[4,5]

The type of contraception that a woman is using affects her risk for development of an ectopic pregnancy. IUDs are effective at preventing intra- and extrauterine pregnancies. However, if a woman does conceive with an IUD in place, she is six to ten times more likely to have an ectopic pregnancy than is a woman using no contraception method. The use of other contraceptive methods has also been evaluated. Women have many options such as combined oral contraceptives, progesterone-only hormonal preparations, as well as condom and diaphragm use. Of these, the only method shown to increase the rate for ectopic pregnancies was progesterone-only, by 4% to 10%. Levonorgestrel (Norplant) has shown a 30% increase in the risk of ectopic pregnancy.[6,7] However, this form of birth control is no longer marketed in the United States.

**Table 15-2**
**Risk Factors for Ectopic Pregnancy**

- History of documented pelvic inflammatory disease/salpingitis
- Tubal sterilization
- Prior reconstructive tubal surgery
- Congenital anamolies of the fallopian tube
- Advanced maternal age
- Prior ectopic pregnancy
- Current use of an intrauterine contraceptive device
- Progestin-only contraceptive method
- Smoking
- Prior pelvic surgery
- Conception with an associated reproductive technology

Tubal sterilization is the most popular form of birth control throughout the world. However, tubal sterilization is not without risks and is associated with the development of future ectopic pregnancies. The use of bipolar electrocautery as the sterilization method is associated with a higher incidence of tubal pregnancies.[8] However, failures resulting in an ectopic pregnancy can occur with all types of sterilization procedures and can occur for many years following the procedure. Because tubal sterilization is such a popular method of sterilization, there is also a high incidence of regret associated with the procedure. As a result, many women are now opting to undergo reversal of the sterilization procedure. Not only do these women have an increase in the risk of developing an ectopic pregnancy secondary to their prior sterilization procedure, but they also are at risk because of the subsequent reanastomosis. The risks vary according to the method of sterilization used, the site of the prior tubal occlusion, the residual tube length after reanastomosis, coexisting disease, and surgical technique. The ectopic pregnancy risks associated with a tube that was cauterized are significantly higher than for a tube that was occluded using the Pomeroy or tubal banding techniques.[9]

Surgical sterilization is not the only tubal surgery that can increase a woman's risk for ectopic pregnancy. Tubal surgery can be performed to relieve an obstruction, lyse adhesions, or treat an existing ectopic pregnancy. Surgery on the tube is felt to place a woman at increased risk for an ectopic pregnancy, but it is unclear whether the increased risk is due to the surgery itself or from the underlying problem that existed prior to the surgery.

Patients who have had prior abdominal surgery are at an increased risk for developing an ectopic pregnancy. Surgery or conditions that result in the development of abdominal/pelvic adhesive disease are felt to place a patient at increased risk for ectopic pregnancy. Spontaneous and elective abortions are not believed to play a significant role in the development of future ectopic pregnancies so long as complications from the procedure do not occur.

The increasing number of women undergoing treatment for infertility is affecting the number of ectopic pregnancies. The majority of women undergoing treatment for infertility are older, and women of increased age are known to be at a greater risk of ectopic pregnancy. Women seeking treatment for infertility also are undergoing sterilization reversal, ovulation induction, and in vitro fertilization. Women undergoing ovulation induction with clomiphene citrate and gonadotropins have been found to be at a greater risk of ectopic pregnancy, even women with normal hysterosalpingography. The increased rate of an ectopic pregnancy with these techniques is between 1.1% and 4.6%.[2] In vitro fertilization is thought to place a woman at greater risk for ectopic pregnancy, owing to either the procedure itself or the underlying pathology resulting in infertility.

Tubal pathology resulting from salpingitis isthmica nodosa (SIN) is felt to place a woman at a greater risk for ectopic pregnancy. SIN is diverticulum of the fallopian tube as the endothelial tissue extends outward into the myosalpinx. It is not known whether the SIN causes ectopic pregnancies or whether its presence in the fallopian tubes of a woman with an ectopic pregnancy is coincidental.

Endometriosis and leiomyomata are two common conditions affecting women of reproductive age. Both conditions can result in obstruction of the fallopian tubes. However, neither is commonly associated with the development of an ectopic pregnancy.

Smoking is one of the few truly modifiable risk factors associated with the development of an ectopic pregnancy. Women who smoke cigarettes have a two-fold risk for developing an ectopic pregnancy when compared with women who do not smoke. Coste et al suggest that this relationship with smoking may be dose dependent. Women who smoked more than 20 cigarettes per day had a risk 2.5 times greater than nonsmokers; while women smoking between 1 and 10 cigarettes a day had a relative risk of 1.3 for ectopic pregnancy.[10]

## PATHOGENESIS

An ectopic pregnancy is the attempted implantation and development of the fertilized ovum in an extrauterine location. The presence of chorionic villi is pathognomonic for an ectopic pregnancy. The chorionic villi are usually located within the lumen of the fallopian tube; however, they can be found elsewhere in the abdomen. When the ectopic pregnancy is located within the fallopian tube, the tube characteristically exhibits an irregular dilatation and bluish discoloration secondary to the surrounding hematosalpinx.

Patients with an ectopic pregnancy often have associated bleeding. The bleeding is usually extraluminal; however, it can remain confined to the fallopian tube, forming a hematosalpinx. The presence of hemoperitoneum can cause a varying degree of peritoneal irritation and subsequent pain. The hemoperitoneum is usually confined to the cul-de-sac unless rupture of the ectopic pregnancy and fallopian tube has occurred. Ectopic pregnancies can progress to the point of expulsion of the pregnancy out the fimbriated end of the fallopian tube, to rupture of the tube, or to natural involution of the pregnancy. The most common time for rupture of the ectopic pregnancy occurs around the sixth to eighth week of gestation, but is variable.

Histologically, the fallopian tubes may exhibit evidence of chronic salpingitis and/or SIN. The associated inflammation can result in the development of adhesive disease associated with the tubes. Women who have ectopic pregnancies have been found to demonstrate evidence of prior salpingitis.[11]

Histologic findings in the endometrium include the Arias-Sella reaction, which is characterized by localized hyperplasia of endometrial glands that are hypersecretory. The cells have enlarged nuclei that are hyperchromatic and irregular. The Arias-Sella reaction is a nonspecific finding that can be seen in patients with intrauterine pregnancies.

## CLINICAL FEATURES AND DIAGNOSIS

Because ectopic pregnancies are associated with a significant degree of morbidity and mortality, clinicians should have a high degree of suspicion for an ectopic pregnancy. Patients' presentations may range from asymptomatic to experiencing an acute abdomen with hemodynamic instability. The majority of patients with an unruptured ectopic gestation demonstrate vaginal spotting, bleeding, or lower abdominal cramping. While the patient's history and physical examination findings are important, the symptoms and physical examination findings in a patient with an ectopic pregnancy are sometimes indistinguishable from the patient with an early viable intrauterine pregnancy or threatened abortion. Therefore, the degree of suspicion must be high, especially in areas of high prevalence. Because the goal is to make the diagnosis prior to rupture of the ectopic pregnancy, other diagnostic modalities than the physical examination must be utilized. If the diagnosis is made prior to rupture, morbidity can be reduced and future fertility maximized. Once rupture of the pregnancy has occurred, the goal shifts to stabilizing the patient and achieving hemostasis (Fig. 15-1).

### History

The patient's history is an important component in raising the clinician's awareness of the possibility of an ectopic pregnancy. Many patients will not exhibit clinical symptoms; however, when they do occur they usually involve one or all three of a classic triad. The classic triad consists of amenorrhea, irregular vaginal bleeding, and abdominal pain. This triad is present approximately 50% of the time and increases along with an increasing rate of rupture of the ectopic pregnancy. Abdominal pain is the most common symptom at presentation in the patient with a ruptured ectopic pregnancy and may result after the development of a hemoperitoneum. The severity of the pain can vary widely among patients, and no particular type of abdominal pain is pathognomonic. The pain can occur on only one side or bilaterally. It may be located in the upper or lower abdomen and characterized by being dull, sharp, or crampy in nature. The pain may be constant or intermittent. It can remain localized but more commonly radiates to the shoulders if a hemoperitoneum exists. Patients may also present with syncope or shock.

In addition to the preceding symptoms, patients should be questioned regarding a history of abnormal menses, prior pregnancy outcomes, history of infertility as well as current contraceptive use, specifically regarding progestin-only preparations or an IUD.

### Physical Examination

The physical examination, like the history, is an important component in recognizing and diagnosing an ectopic pregnancy. The clinician should be mindful of the patient's vital signs to evaluate for hemodynamic instability and examine the abdomen and pelvis to evaluate for rupture of the ectopic pregnancy.

Prior to rupture of the ectopic pregnancy, the patient often exhibits nonspecific symptoms. The vital signs are most often normal and the abdomen may be nontender or only mildly tender to palpation. The abdominal examination is usually nonspecific, and cervical motion tenderness may or may not exist. An adnexal mass may be present; however, this could represent a functional corpus luteum cyst. As the ectopic pregnancy ruptures and the patient subsequently develops intra-abdominal bleeding, the physical examination findings change as well. The first change usually is the development of tachycardia and, with increasing hemodynamic instability, hypotension. The abdomen becomes distended, and peritoneal signs with tenderness and rebound become evident. At this point patients usually have cervical motion tenderness.

Because the patient's history and physical examination generally do not provide the complete diagnosis, clinicians must be prepared to initiate the appropriate work-up to diagnose

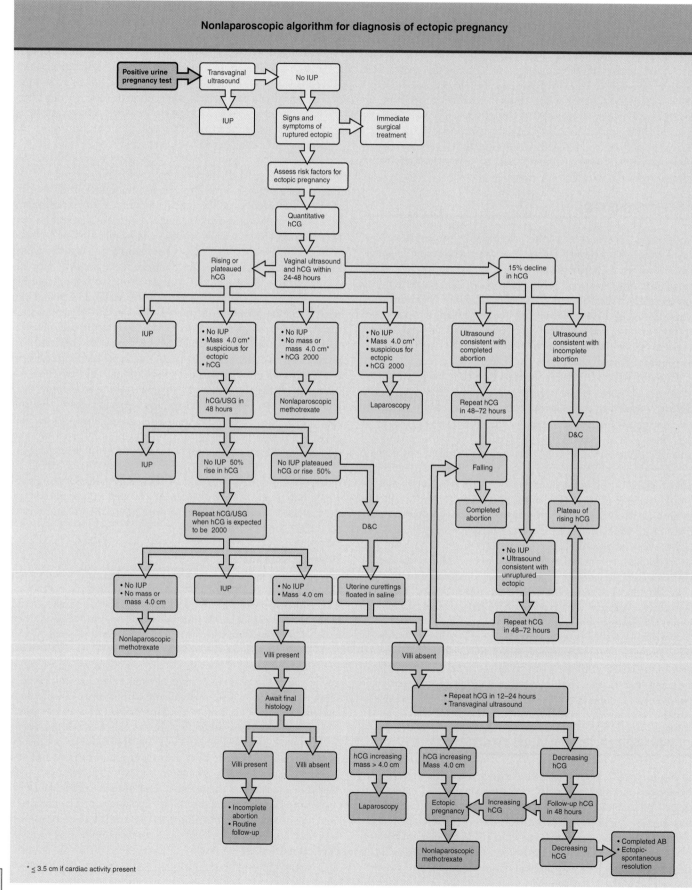

**Figure 15-1    Nonlaparoscopic algorithm for diagnosis of ectopic pregnancy.**

the ectopic pregnancy. A combination of diagnostic modalities generally is required including measurement of human chorionic gonadotropin (hCG) levels, transvaginal ultrasound, and possibly endometrial curettage and laparoscopy.

## Laboratory Tests

### Serial Quantitative hCG Measurements

The history and physical examination are important components of diagnosing an ectopic pregnancy; however, the most important test is the quantitative β-subunit measurement of hCG. The enzyme-linked immunoassay (ELISA) hCG is positive with virtually all ectopic pregnancies because of its sensitivity to 25 mIU/mL. Once a positive pregnancy has been identified, the goal is to determine whether it is intra- or extrauterine.

#### Reference Standards

There are three reference standards for β-hCG measurements. The World Health Organization (WHO) introduced the First International Standard (1st IS) in the 1930s. Testing for hCG and its subunits have improved over the years. The Second International Standard (2nd IS), introduced in 1964, has varying amounts of hCG α and β subunits. A purified preparation of β-hCG is now available. Originally referred to as the First International Reference Preparation (1st IRP), the test standard is now referred to as the Third International Standard (3rd IS). Although each standard has its own scale, as a general rule, the 2nd IS is about one-half of the 3rd IS. For example, if a level is reported as 500 mIU/mL (2nd IS), it is equivalent to a level of 1000 mIU/mL (3rd IS). The assay standard used must be known in order to correctly interpret hCG results. In several recent articles, attention has been drawn to a problem known as phantom hCG, in which the presence of heterophile antibodies or proteolytic enzymes cause a false-positive hCG result. Because the antibodies are large glycoproteins, significant quantities of the antibody are not excreted in the urine. Thus, in the patient with hCG levels of less than 1000 mIU/mL, a confirmatory positive urine pregnancy test should be obtained prior to instituting treatment.

A single measurement of the hCG level is not helpful in and of itself, especially when the level is below the discriminatory zone for ultrasound visualization. There is a wide range of variability of hCG levels for both intrauterine and ectopic pregnancies, and the location of the pregnancy for a given patient cannot be determined using a single hCG measurement. The single hCG is useful if the test is negative, which essentially excludes the diagnosis of pregnancy. Also, if the hCG level is greater than the discriminatory zone for ultrasonography, the results can be used to aid in the diagnosis of an ectopic pregnancy. If the hCG level is elevated above the discriminatory zone and the ultrasound was inconclusive, the physician would still need to follow serial hCG measurements to differentiate between an ectopic pregnancy and a completed abortion. Thus, in almost all instances, serial hCG measurements are required. The doubling time associated with serum hCG is an important parameter for following an early pregnancy and differentiating a normal from an abnormal pregnancy. A patient's hCG level correlates closely with gestational age early in pregnancy. Within the first 6 weeks of pregnancy, the patient's hCG level increases exponentially.

Kadar and Romero reported that in early gestations the hCG doubles approximately every 1.98 days (95% CL).[12] These hCG levels are useful for diagnosing pregnancy, identifying an abnormal pregnancy at risk for an early abortion or ectopic gestation, and following the resolution of a treated ectopic pregnancy.

Serial measurements of hCG are useful in differentiating a viable intrauterine pregnancy from an ectopic pregnancy. With a viable intrauterine pregnancy, the hCG typically exhibits at least a 66% increase over a 48-hour period (85% CL). However, approximately 15% of viable pregnancies will have less than a 66% increase and the same number of ectopic pregnancies will have more than a 66% increase. Thus, to confirm pregnancy nonviability, an increase of less than 50% over 48 hours should be used in patients with hCG less than 2000 mIU/mL. Patients with a normal intrauterine pregnancy have at least a 50% rise in the hCG level over 48 hours unless the starting level is above 2000 mIU/mL when the rate of rise is more unpredictable. When measurements are repeated in less than 48 hours between samplings, there is even more overlap between normal and abnormal, and so from a clinical perspective the values are not as useful. When serial hCG measurements are followed, the clinical pattern of an hCG that has plateaued (doubling time of >7 days) is the most predictive for an ectopic pregnancy.[13] For falling levels, a 50% decrease in less than 1.4 days is rarely associated with an ectopic pregnancy, whereas a less than 50% decrease over more than 7 days is most predictive of ectopic pregnancy.

If the physician is initially suspicious that a patient has an ectopic pregnancy, an initial ultrasound is obtained. However, if the ultrasound evaluation is indeterminate for either an intrauterine or an ectopic pregnancy, serial hCG levels are obtained. As long as the hCG levels continue to rise appropriately (>50% over 48 hours) and the patient is relatively asymptomatic, the physician could follow the patient until the hCG level reaches the transvaginal discriminatory level of 2000 mIU/mL. At this point a repeat vaginal ultrasound should be obtained. If the levels do not rise appropriately, either an ectopic or nonviable intrauterine pregnancy is present. The location of the pregnancy at this point would have to be found surgically; first, with dilation and curettage (D&C), and possibly with laparoscopy depending on the clinical situation.

### Serum Progesterone Measurement

Initial progesterone analysis helps differentiate viable from nonviable gestations. In studies by Stovall et al, if the initial progesterone level was 25 ng/mL or greater, the diagnosis of ectopic pregnancy could virtually be excluded with approximately 98% certainty. If the progesterone level was less than 5.0 ng/mL, the diagnosis of a nonviable pregnancy, either intrauterine or ectopic, could be guaranteed with almost 100% sensitivity.[14] The risk of a normal pregnancy with a serum progesterone level below 5.0 ng/mL is approximately 1/1500. For this reason, serum progesterone is not included in the diagnostic algorithm presented here (see Fig. 15-1). The difficulty with progesterone interpretation is when a patient's level is between 5 ng/mL and 25 ng/mL. In this case, the clinician must continue to use hCG, ultrasound, and clinical history for diagnosis.

### Other Markers

Other maternal serum markers such as estradiol, creatine kinase, pregnancy-associated plasma protein C, relaxin, CA-125, material serum α-fetoprotein, and C-reactive protein have all been analyzed with regard to ectopic pregnancy. Their clinical reliability has been mixed, and they are not currently used clinically in the management of ectopic pregnancies.

### Ultrasonography

Ultrasound evaluation of the patient is an important tool in diagnosis. Transvaginal ultrasound is superior to transabdominal ultrasound in visualization of pelvic structures, and an intrauterine gestational sac can be visualized as much as 1 week earlier with transvaginal imaging. However, both have clinical relevance in the complete evaluation of a patient with an expected ectopic pregnancy. Figure 15-2 demonstrates a right tubal ectopic pregnancy as visualized on ultrasound.

The ultrasound results obtained should be correlated with the patient's β-hCG level, which is termed the discriminatory zone. The discriminatory zone is the hCG level above which the ultrasonographer should be able to visualize normal intrauterine pregnancies. With abdominal ultrasonography viable intrauterine pregnancies should be seen above hCG levels of 6500 mIU/mL as opposed to 1500 to 2000 mIU/mL transvaginally. If the hCG is 6500 mIU/mL or greater for an abdominal ultrasound and 2000 mIU/mL or greater for a vaginal ultrasound and a pregnancy is not visualized, it is either a failed intrauterine pregnancy or an ectopic pregnancy. The difficulty with utilizing the discriminatory zone for analysis is that there is no discriminatory zone associated with an ectopic pregnancy. An ectopic pregnancy can exist with either a high or low hCG level. A word of caution is warranted, even in those patients with an hCG titer above the discriminatory zone for an intrauterine pregnancy. In the stable patient, the hCG titer and ultrasound should be repeated prior to instituting treatment. In other words, unless cardiac activity is seen in the ectopic pregnancy or the clinical situation dictates more immediate management, the ultrasound and hCG findings are confirmed by repeat testing.

With ultrasound, early findings indicative of an intrauterine pregnancy are the presence of a small, fluid-filled space and the gestational sac with a surrounding echogenic ring. The gestational sac typically has an eccentric uterine location. The gestational sac can be visualized at 4 weeks postconception vaginally versus 5 weeks abdominally. In an intrauterine pregnancy, the sac grows followed by the presence of a yolk sac and subsequently an embryo with cardiac activity.

A normal gestational sac is often confused with a pseudosac. The pseudosac is probably due to bleeding from the decidua into the endometrial cavity. Investigators have wondered whether the presence of pseudosac is indicative of an ectopic pregnancy; in a recent study of 77 patients it was felt that the presence of the pseudosac could not be used reliably. Ahmed et al found that the presence of the pseudosac was not indicative of an ectopic pregnancy because an intrauterine pregnancy failure could not be differentiated from an ectopic pregnancy using ultrasonography.[15]

It has long been believed that the presence of a double decidual sac sign (DDSS) is the best method to determine if a sac present is a true gestational sac or a pseudosac. The DDSS is thought to be a layer of decidua surrounding the chorionic sac. Its presence is felt to be indicative of an intrauterine pregnancy, and the clinician's confidence can increase when the yolk sac has been seen on ultrasound. The yolk sac is usually visible with abdominal ultrasound when the gestational sac reaches a size of 2.0 cm and 0.6 to 0.8 mm vaginally. When cardiac activity is seen within the uterine cavity, definitive evidence of an intrauterine pregnancy exists.

When a gestational sac with fetal pole and cardiac activity is present within the adnexa, the clinician can be relatively confident that an ectopic pregnancy exists. However, ultrasonography of the adnexa is not particularly sensitive in diagnosing ectopic pregnancies.

If, after ultrasonography is used to aid in diagnosis, the uterus is found to be empty and the hCG level is below the discriminatory zone, the clinician must consider the differential diagnosis of: an early normal intrauterine pregnancy, an abnormal intrauterine gestation, miscarriage, ectopic pregnancy, and even the nonpregnant state.

In this situation, further diagnostic tests such as a follow-up laboratory studies, repeat ultrasounds, D&C, and laparoscopy can all be useful.

### Dilation and Curettage

D&C should be performed once the pregnancy has been determined to be nonviable or its exact location cannot be verified ultrasonographically. Care must be taken to not perform D&C in the presence of a viable intrauterine pregnancy; therefore, D&C should be performed when the ultrasound is inconclusive above the level of the discriminatory zone and hCG levels have plateaued or are rising suboptimally. The physician can immediately examine the specimen removed at the time of the endometrial curettage. The specimen can be placed in normal saline and examined. Chorionic villi exhibit a lacy, frond-like appearance and float on the saline. This technique has sensitivity and specificity of greater than 95%. The specimen also should be examined by a pathologist for the presence of chorionic villi and a serum hCG level obtained.

If the follow-up hCG levels decrease by 15% or more in the initial 12-hour period after the D&C, a completed abortion is suspected. However, if the follow-up hCG levels plateau or rise, the diagnosis of an ectopic pregnancy has been made.[14]

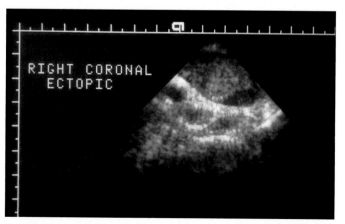

**Figure 15-2    Right tubal ectopic pregnancy, visualized by ultrasound.**

## Culdocentesis

The practice of culdocentesis has declined in popularity for the diagnosis of ectopic pregnancies with the advent of transvaginal ultrasonography and serial hCG measurements. In culdocentesis the posterior fornix of the vagina is visualized by means of a speculum. The posterior cul-de-sac is then entered with a spinal needle and the contents are aspirated with a syringe. With a positive test—the presence of nonclotting blood—a ruptured ectopic pregnancy may exist. If serous fluid is aspirated, the test is thought to be negative. Culdocentesis is considered non-diagnostic if clotted blood or no fluid is aspirated. The problem associated with culdocentesis is that the majority of patients with an ectopic pregnancy will have a positive test, yet the majority of these patients will not have a ruptured ectopic pregnancy.

Historically, if the culdocentesis results were positive, surgery was performed for a presumed diagnosis of ruptured tubal pregnancy. However, the results of culdocentesis do not always correlate with the status of the pregnancy. Although approximately 70% to 90% of patients with an ectopic pregnancy have a hemoperitoneum demonstrated by culdocentesis, only 50% of patients have a ruptured tube. Furthermore, approximately 6% of women with positive culdocentesis results do not have an ectopic gestation at the time of laparotomy. Non-diagnostic fluid occurs in 10% to 20% of patients with ectopic pregnancy and therefore is not definitive.

## Laparoscopy

The gold standard for diagnosing an ectopic pregnancy has long been laparoscopy. Laparoscopy allows for visualization of the pelvis, fallopian tubes, and ovaries (Fig. 15-3). Disadvantages of laparoscopy are that the patient has to undergo a surgical procedure with its inherent risks, including anesthesia, and that small ectopic pregnancies may be missed. Since many ectopic pregnancies occur in normal fallopian tubes, if surgery can be avoided, the fallopian tube has been spared, which may increase a patient's future fertility. A distinct advantage of laparoscopy is that diagnosis and treatment can occur in the same setting.

At the time of laparoscopy, with the presence of a tubal ectopic pregnancy, the tubal architecture is usually distorted. If the patient has experienced prior PID or tubal damage resulting in adhesive disease, the assessment of the fallopian tubes may be compromised.

## Diagnostic Algorithm: A Combination of Assessment Techniques

This diagnostic algorithm (see Fig. 15-1) was found to be 100% accurate in a randomized clinical trial.[14,16] Serial hCG levels are used to assess the viability of a pregnancy, correlate the given transvaginal ultrasound findings, and determine whether the hCG titer increases or falls following suction curettage in those patients who require curettage before beginning medical therapy for an ectopic pregnancy.

Transvaginal ultrasound is an important diagnostic tool in the algorithm. If the patient is found to have an intrauterine sac or pregnancy, ectopic pregnancy can be excluded with a reasonable degree of certainty. If the patient's hCG is greater than the discriminatory level and no intrauterine gestational sac is visualized, the patient is considered to have an ectopic pregnancy. If cardiac activity is found in an extrauterine location, most specifically the adnexa, the diagnosis of ectopic pregnancy is confirmed. With the sensitivity of ultrasound, masses greater than 1 cm can be identified. When the size of the ectopic pregnancy reaches 3.5 to 4.0 cm, depending on the presence of fetal cardiac activity, surgical treatment becomes the preferred method of treatment.

Endometrial curettage is used to distinguish between a non-viable intrauterine pregnancy and an ectopic pregnancy. Suction curettage is performed when a patient experiences an inappropriate rise in the hCG level of less than 50% over 48 hours and an hCG level of 2000 or greater with an indeterminate ultrasound. With D&C the clinician can avoid using methotrexate for medical management in patients with an abnormal intrauterine gestation that can effectively be diagnosed via uterine evacuation. The only real drawback to curettage is the presence of a heterotopic gestation or missing an extremely early nonviable intrauterine gestation.

## TREATMENT

Medical and surgical options exist for the treatment of ectopic pregnancy. Both methods are effective, and the individual patient's clinical scenario including the site and size of the ectopic pregnancy should determine her treatment.

### Surgical Treatment

Surgical treatment has been the gold standard for treatment of ectopic pregnancy. Experts are unsure which operative treatment is best, and the surgical options range from salpingo-oophorectomy, salpingectomy, segmental resection, and salpingostomy. Salpingo-oophorectomy was once considered appropriate because it was theorized that this technique would eliminate transperitoneal migration of the ovum or zygote, which was thought to predispose to recurrent ectopic pregnancy. Ovary removal results in all ovulations occurring on the side with the remaining normal fallopian tube. Subsequent studies have not confirmed that ipsilateral oophorectomy increases the likelihood of conceiving an intrauterine pregnancy; therefore, this practice is not recommended.

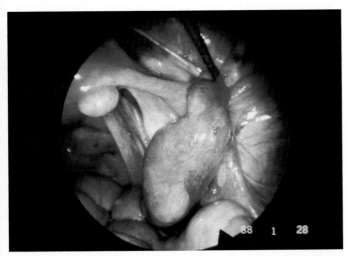

**Figure 15-3   Right tubal ectopic pregnancy, visualized by laparoscopy.**

# General Gynecology

The most widely accepted method for surgical treatment in a patient who has not experienced rupture of the ectopic pregnancy and who desires future fertility is salpingostomy. The fallopian tube is opened along the antimesenteric border, and the products of conception are removed (see Chapter 37). A fine incision should be utilized and carried out with the needle tip bovine cautery, scalpel, scissors, or laser. The surgery can be done either through a laparotomy or laparoscopically. When patients undergoing salpingectomy and salpingostomy were followed, no difference was found in future fertility rates.[17] The patients who had a history of infertility were more likely to have an ectopic pregnancy following salpingostomy. Therefore, consideration should be given in this patient group to salpingectomy in order to reduce their risk for ectopic pregnancy. However, the status of the contralateral tube must be considered when this decision is made.

There is also debate over whether the patient requiring surgery should be treated with a laparotomy or laparoscopically. The primary treatments of salpingectomy, salpingostomy, and segmental resection can be accomplished via both techniques. The hemodynamic stability of the patient and the comfort level of the surgeon are the primary factors that determine the surgical approach. Typically, laparotomy is indicated if the patient becomes hemodynamically unstable. Rupture of the ectopic pregnancy does not necessitate laparotomy. Laparotomy is typically chosen if the patient has an abdominal or ovarian pregnancy.

Studies have shown that laparoscopy and laparotomy are both safe and effective treatment measures. However, laparoscopy is more economical secondary to reduced costs and shorter hospitalizations. Laparoscopically treated patients also have a shorter time for recovery and convalescence and reduced postoperative pain requirements. It has also been concluded that laparoscopy results in the formation of fewer adhesions postoperatively and less blood loss. For these reasons, many physicians consider laparoscopy the preferred method of surgical treatment for ectopic pregnancies.[18] Future pregnancy rates are similar in patients treated by both laparotomy and laparoscopy.

## Medical Treatment

The most popular current medical treatment for ectopic pregnancy is methotrexate although other agents such as potassium chloride (KCl), hyperosmolar glucose, prostaglandins, and RU-486 have been studied. The routes of treatment vary from systemic administration—intravenous, intramuscular, and oral—to local administration—laparoscopically guided direct injections, transvaginal ultrasound directed injections, and retrograde fallopian tube treatments.

### Methotrexate

Methotrexate is the most popular form of medical treatment for women with unruptured ectopic pregnancies. Methotrexate is a folic acid analog and functions by inhibiting dihydrofolate reductase. With the synthesis of folate disrupted, the synthesis of DNA is prevented. Methotrexate is also used for the treatment of gestational trophoblastic disease. The most common side effects are leukopenia, thrombocytopenia, bone marrow aplasia, ulcerative stomatitis, diarrhea, and hemorrhagic enteritis. Other less common side effects include alopecia, dermatitis, elevated

liver function tests, and pneumonitis. These side effects are more common at the higher therapeutic doses associated with chemotherapy and are not associated with the lower dosing regimens necessary to treat ectopic pregnancies. A patient who requires multiple doses for treatment of ectopic pregnancy is more prone to develop the minor side effects. The incidence of these side effects can be reduced with the administration of citrovorum factor.

Stovall et al studied the use of multidose (Table 15-3) intramuscular methotrexate (1 mg/kg/day) followed by citrovorum factor (0.1 mg/kg/day). One hundred patients received injections on alternate days with a success rate of 96%.[19,20] This treatment regimen was continued until the hCG level began to decline by at least 15% between two consecutive hCG levels. Citrovorum factor was given on the day following the methotrexate injection even if the patient required no further methotrexate injections. Once the treatment was discontinued, the patient's hCG levels were measured until they became negative. A second treatment course of methotrexate was given only if the patient's hCG levels plateaued or began to rise. In this study 96 patients were treated effectively. Seventeen received one methotrexate/citrovorum injection while 19 patients received four doses. Four of 100 patients ultimately required surgical management secondary to rupture. Each of these four patients differed with respect to ectopic pregnancy size, hCG level, and time of rupture. Five patients had ectopic pregnancies with cardiac activity, and four of the five (80%) were treated successfully.

In an effort to reduce the side effects associated with methotrexate, a single-dose protocol was devised. Initially, 31 patients were treated with a single dose of methotrexate (50 mg/m$^2$). Citrovorum factor was eliminated. Approximately 97% of the treated patients (29/30) were treated successfully.

| Table 15-3 Multidose Methotrexate-Citrovorum Protocol for Unruptured Ectopic Pregnancy | |
|---|---|
| **Day** | **Therapy** |
| 1 | CBC, SGOT, BUN, creatinine, β-hCG, blood type and Rh, MTX |
| 2 | CF, β-hCG |
| 3 | MTX, β-hCG |
| 4 | CF, β-hCG |
| 5 | MTX, β-hCG |
| 6 | CF, β-hCG |
| 7 | MTX, β-hCG |
| 8 | CF, β-hCG, CBC, SGOT, BUN, creatinine |
| >8 | Weekly β-hCG until <10 mIU/mL |

BUN, blood urea nitrogen; CBC, complete blood count with differential and platelet count; CF, intramuscular citrovorum factor 0.1 mg/kg; hCG, human chorionic gonadotropin; MTX, intramuscular methotrexate 1.0 mg/kg; SGOT, serum glutamic–oxaloacetic transaminase. Notes: (1) Methotrexate/citrovorum is given until there is a 15% decline in two consecutive hCG titers; (2) any time methotrexate is given, citrovorum is given on the following day; (3) patients with a hematocrit <35% are given oral iron therapy; (4) patients are told to refrain from alcohol, folic acid–containing vitamins, and sexual intercourse during the treatment period; (5) oral or barrier contraceptives are used until the hysterosalpingogram is completed; (6) hysterosalpingogram is requested on days 6–9 after the second menstrual cycle.

**Table 15-4**
**Single-Dose Methotrexate Protocol for Ectopic Pregnancy**

| Day | Therapy |
|-----|---------|
| 0 | D&C, hCG |
| 1 | CBC, SGOT, BUN, creatinine, blood type and Rh, methotrexate 50 mg/m$^2$ IM |
| 4 | hCG |
| 7 | hCG |

BUN, blood urea nitrogen; CBC, complete blood count; D&C, dilation and curettage; hCG, human chorionic gonadotropin; SGOT, serum glutamic–oxaloacetic transaminase.
Notes: (1) Treatment is never begun based on a single hCG titer unless cardiac activity is visualized on transvaginal scan in the ectopic pregnancy. (2) If <15% decline in hCG level between days 4 and 7, give second dose of methotrexate 50 mg/m$^2$ on day 7. (3) If >15% decline in hCG level between days 4 and 7, follow weekly until hCG<10 mIU/mL. (4) In patients not requiring D&C (hCG>2000 mIU/mL and no gestational sac on transvaginal ultrasonography), days 0 and 1 are combined.

**Table 15-6**
**Initiation of Methotrexate: Physician Checklist**

- Obtain hCG level
- Perform transvaginal ultrasound within 48 hours
- Perform endometrial curettage if hCG level <2000 mIU/mL
- Obtain normal liver function (SGOT), normal renal function (BUN, creatinine), and normal CBC (WBC >2000/mL and platelet count >100,000)
- Administer Rh$_o$(D) immune globulin if patient is Rh-negative
- Identify unruptured ectopic pregnancy <3.5 cm
- Obtain informed consent
- Prescribe FeSO$_4$ 325 mg PO bid if hematocrit <30%
- Schedule follow-up appointment on days 4, 6, and 7

BUN, blood urea nitrogen; CBC, complete blood count; hCG, human chorionic gonadotropin; SGOT, serum glutamic–oxaloacetic transaminase; WBC, white blood cell.

Currently, 600 patients have been treated with this protocol with an overall success rate of 93% (Table 15-4). A major advantage of this treatment regimen is that no patients experienced methotrexate-related side effects. In addition, the single-dose treatment protocol is less expensive than the multidose protocol, has increased patient acceptance/compliance secondary to decreased patient monitoring during therapy, with similar treatment results and prospects for future fertility.

Most clinicians who oppose the use of methotrexate do so owing to the potential side effects. The majority of patients who experience side effects were treated with the intravenous form of the medication, with higher doses or for longer period of time. When the single-dose regimen was utilized, the incidence of side effects was less than 1%, while the failure rate was similar to that of conservative forms of laparoscopic surgery.

### Treatment Initiation

Before methotrexate therapy can be initiated, the physician must confirm that the patient is a good candidate for therapy (Table 15-5), that the pretreatment check-in has been completed (Table 15-6), and that the patient has been given the appropriate instructions (Table 15-7). This is essential to maximize the safety of the therapy and decrease the chance that a patient with an early intrauterine or nonviable intrauterine gestation will receive methotrexate. Good candidates for therapy are patients who (1) have a rising or plateaued hCG level after salpingostomy; (2) who have a rising or plateaued hCG level at least 12 to 24 hours following a diagnostic D&C; and (3) who are without an intrauterine gestational sac or fluid collection by transvaginal ultrasound, have an abnormally rising hCG level below 2000, have an ectopic mass of 3.5 cm or less with fetal cardiac activity or 4.0 cm and less without fetal cardiac activity.

### Follow-up

Once methotrexate has been administered, the patient is sent home for follow-up as an outpatient. During the initial treatment phase, the frequency of follow-up is determined based on whether the multidose (see Table 15-3) or the single-dose (see Table 15-4) protocol is being followed. Serial hCG measurements, usually weekly, are obtained until negative. Following the initial treatment, patients are instructed to monitor their pain and to call in if there is any increase in pain. If the pain is prolonged or severe, the hematocrit is evaluated and a transvaginal ultrasound should be obtained. If a drop of greater than 3% to 4% occurs in the hematocrit or if the patient becomes unstable, the physician should suspect a tubal rupture. Transvaginal ultrasound may be helpful if an increase in abdominal free fluid is noted; however, a small amount of physiologic fluid may be present within the pelvis. Although there is no scientific base for doing so, the authors ask patients to refrain from becoming pregnant for 2 months after methotrexate treatment is completed.

**Table 15-5**
**Candidates for Methotrexate Treatment of Ectopic Pregnancy**

- An hCG level is present and plateaued or rising after salpingostomy or salpingectomy
- A rising or plateaued hCG level is present at least 12–24 hours after suction curettage (needed if hCG is <2000 mIU/mL)
- No intrauterine gestational sac or fluid collection is detected by transvaginal ultrasound,* hCG level is >2000 mIU/mL, and an ectopic pregnancy mass ≤3.5 cm is demonstrated with cardiac activity or ≤4.0 cm without cardiac activity

*The ultrasound finding must be interpreted with caution because most unruptured ectopic pregnancies will be accompanied by fluid in the cul-de-sac.

**Table 15-7**
**Initiation of Methotrexate: Patient Instruction**

- Refrain from alcohol use, multivitamins containing folic acid, and sexual intercourse until hCG level is negative
- Call your physician if you experience prolonged or heavy vaginal bleeding, or if pain is prolonged or severe (lower abdomen and pelvic pain is normal during the first 10–14 days of treatment).
- Use oral contraception or barrier contraceptive methods
- Know that ~5% of women experience unsuccessful methotrexate treatment and require surgery

## Other Modalities

The primary alternative treatment modality—salpingocentesis—includes the injection of various substances into the ectopic pregnancy either transvaginally utilizing ultrasound guidance, transcervically via tubal cannulization, or laparoscopically. Agents such as KCl, methotrexate, prostaglandins, and hyperosmolar glucose are used.[21] The advantages of this treatment are that it is a one-time, localized treatment that can avoid most of the systemic side effects associated with methotrexate.

## CLINICAL COURSE, PROGRESSION, AND ECTOPIC PREGNANCY TYPES

### Spontaneous Resolution

Not all ectopic pregnancies require medical or surgical management. Some resolve by resorption or by a tubal abortion. Some investigators feel that expectant management may be appropriate for the management of early ectopic pregnancies. Following serum hCG levels until resorption or tubal abortion occurs has been advocated. Some authors feel that expectant management is the best way to preserve future fertility; however, this is controversial. Falling hCG levels are the most reliable indicator of success, but the physician should be mindful that rupture can occur even with a falling or low $\beta$-hCG level. Expectant management should be attempted only in extremely compliant patients.[22]

### Persistent Ectopic Pregnancy

A persistent ectopic pregnancy is present when a patient has already undergone a conservative form of surgery such as salpingostomy or fimbrial expression and viable trophoblastic tissue remains. The persistent trophoblastic tissue is usually located in the medial segment of the fallopian tube; however, it can be located on the peritoneal surface as well.[23]

The incidence of persistent ectopic pregnancies is increasing as the incidence of tubal conservation surgery is increasing. The persistent ectopic pregnancy is suspected and later diagnosed as the $\beta$-hCG levels remain elevated following conservative surgery.

The risk factors for development of a persistent ectopic pregnancy vary from the type of initial surgical procedure, initial hCG level, duration of amenorrhea, and size of the ectopic pregnancy.

The treatment of a persistent ectopic pregnancy is similar to the treatment of the initial ectopic pregnancy; either medical or surgical. Methotrexate can be used as a medical treatment for patients who are hemodynamically stable. Many feel that methotrexate is the treatment of choice, since the trophoblastic tissue may have been spread to multiple locations during the initial surgical procedure. If follow-up surgery is indicated, repeat salpingostomy can be performed; however, salpingectomy is more commonly performed.

### Chronic Ectopic Pregnancy

Chronic ectopic pregnancy occurs as a result of expectant medical management or occasionally following salpingostomy. In the course of the treatment, if the ectopic pregnancy does not completely resorb, chorionic villi will still be present. Because of the persistent chorionic villi, the patient may develop bleeding into the wall of the fallopian tube. As a result, the tube distends slowly and does not rupture. Patients usually have symptoms of pain and vaginal bleeding. On examination the majority of patients have a pelvic mass. The treatment for a chronic ectopic pregnancy is surgery with removal of the affected fallopian tube.

### Nontubal Ectopic Pregnancies
#### Cervical Pregnancy

The rates associated with a cervical pregnancy have been reported to range from 1 in 2400 to 1 in 50,000 in the United States. The differential diagnosis initially must include cervical cancer, presence of a cervical fibroid, trophoblastic tumor, and abnormalities of placental location such as a placenta previa or low-lying placenta. Patients are at risk of developing a cervical pregnancy if they have undergone a prior elective abortion, developed Asherman's syndrome, had a prior cesarean delivery, been exposed to diethylstilbestrol, developed leiomyomata, or undergone in vitro fertilization.[24]

Clinical criteria that should alert the physician to the possibility of a cervical pregnancy include smaller size of the surrounding uterus than of the distended cervix, the presence of a closed internal os, no chorionic tissue found on curettage of the endometrial cavity, and dilation of the external os sooner than would be expected in the presence of a spontaneous miscarriage.

Utilization of ultrasound is useful in diagnosis of a cervical pregnancy. Ultrasound diagnostic criteria of a cervical pregnancy (Table 15-8) consist of the presence of an echo-free uterine cavity, decidual transformation of the endometrium, a diffuse uterine wall structure in an hourglass shape, enlargement and ballooning of the cervical canal, a closed internal cervical os with a gestational sac and placental tissue within the cervical canal (Fig. 15-4).

When a cervical pregnancy is diagnosed, the patient can be treated medically with methotrexate or surgically. If surgical treatment is to be performed, the patient should give consent for a D&C with the possibility of blood transfusion and even hysterectomy. Typed and cross-matched blood should be available prior to initiation of the procedure. If bleeding does occur at the time of diagnosis or treatment, it may range from light to heavy. Attempts to control the bleeding can be accomplished through various techniques such as uterine packing, lateral cervical suture placement in an attempt to ligate the lateral cervical vessels, placement of a cerclage, or insertion of a 30-mL Foley catheter into the cervix for tamponade. If these measures

| Table 15-8 |
| :-- |
| **Ultrasound Criteria for Diagnosis of Cervical Pregnancy** |

- Echo-free uterine cavity or the presence of a pseudogestational sac only
- Decidual transformation of the endometrium with dense echo structure
- Diffuse uterine wall structure
- Hourglass uterine shape
- Ballooned cervical canal
- Gestational sac in the endocervix
- Placental tissue in the cervical canal
- Closed internal os

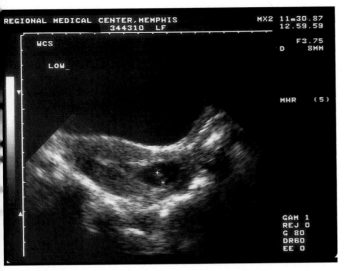

**Figure 15-4  Cervical pregnancy, visualized by ultrasound.**

are unsuccessful, embolization of the bleeding vessels can be attempted. If the patient requires laparotomy, the uterine arteries can be ligated. If all these methods are unsuccessful, the patient requires hysterectomy.

### Ovarian Pregnancy

The most common site for a nontubal ectopic pregnancy is the ovary. Ovarian pregnancy represents 0.5% to 1.0% of all ectopic pregnancies, and the incidence varies from 1 in 7000 to 1 in 40000.[25] The primary difference between a tubal ectopic pregnancy and an ovarian pregnancy is that an ovarian pregnancy is not associated with PID or infertility. The primary risk factor associated with the development of an ovarian pregnancy is concurrent use of an IUD. Patients with an ovarian ectopic pregnancy have similar symptoms to those of other ectopic pregnancies.

Ovarian pregnancy may be misdiagnosed as a ruptured corpus luteum cyst, and ultrasonography may aid in the diagnosis. The primary criteria for diagnosis of an ovarian pregnancy (Table 15-9) are that the fallopian tube on the affected side must be intact, the fetal sac must replace the position of the ovary, and the ovary must remain attached to the uterus by the ovarian ligament. Finally, ovarian tissue must be located within the wall of the gestational sac.

Historically, the treatment for an ovarian pregnancy was oophorectomy; however, the current trend is to perform an ovarian cystectomy. If medical treatment is an option, methotrexate therapy could also be attempted.

| Table 15-9 |
|---|
| **Spiegelberg's Criteria for Diagnosis of Ovarian Pregnancy** |
| • The fallopian tube on the affected side must be intact |
| • The fetal sac must occupy the position of the ovary |
| • The ovary must be connected to the uterus by the ovarian ligament |
| • Ovarian tissue must be located in the sac wall |

| Table 15-10 |
|---|
| **Studdiford's Criteria for Diagnosis of Primary Abdominal Pregnancy** |
| • Presence of a pregnancy related exclusively to the peritoneal surface and early enough to eliminate the possibility of secondary implantation after primary tubal nidation |
| • Presence of normal tubes and ovaries with no evidence of recent or past pregnancy |
| • No evidence of uteroplacental fistula |

### Abdominal Pregnancy

Abdominal pregnancies occur with a frequency of approximately 1 in 372 to 1 in 9714 live births in the United States.[26] Abdominal pregnancies are classified as either primary or secondary, with secondary being the most common.

A primary abdominal pregnancy (Table 15-10) occurs in the presence of normal fallopian tubes and ovaries without evidence of a prior pregnancy. With a primary pregnancy there is also no evidence of uteroplacental fistula. A primary pregnancy must be related exclusively to the peritoneal surface. Secondary abdominal pregnancies usually develop as a result of a tubal abortion, tubal rupture, or uterine rupture with intra-abdominal implantation.

Abdominal pregnancies carry a significant risk of maternal morbidity and mortality. The risk of mortality associated with an abdominal pregnancy is approximately eight times greater than for ectopic pregnancy and 90 times greater than for intrauterine gestation. Few abdominal pregnancies are carried to term. If they are, these pregnancies are associated with significant perinatal morbidity, mortality, and congenital anomalies.

Patients with an abdominal pregnancy in the first and second trimesters often have symptoms similar to those of a tubal ectopic pregnancy. Ultrasound is helpful in establishing the diagnosis (Fig. 15-5). As a patient achieves an advanced gestational age, she may have vague complaints. She may feel misplaced fetal movements in the upper abdomen or extremely painful fetal movements. On physical examination, the patient

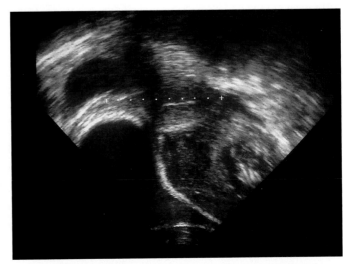

**Figure 15-5  Abdominal pregnancy, visualized by ultrasound.**

215

will often have persistent abnormal fetal lies, abdominal tenderness, a displaced cervix, easily palpated fetal parts, and a uterus that is palpated separately from the fetus. If there are no uterine contractions with pitocin infusion, the diagnosis is often suspected.

Once an abdominal pregnancy is suspected, the patient should be treated with surgery. The placenta should be removed only if its vascular supply can be identified and ligated. Many patients require abdominal packing, which is left in place and removed after 24 to 48 hours. If the vascular supply to the placenta is not identifiable, it should be left in place and the umbilical cord ligated at the base. The involution of the placenta can be followed with serial ultrasound images and serial β-hCG levels. Patients should be monitored for the development of a bowel obstruction, fistula formation, and sepsis as the placental tissue degenerates. In this situation, methotrexate is contraindicated, since it leads to rapid tissue necrosis, subsequently causing a high rate of complications such as sepsis and death.[27]

### Interstitial Pregnancy

Interstitial pregnancies present later than typical ectopic pregnancies and represent 1% of all ectopic pregnancies. These pregnancies are associated with a higher rate of maternal mortality than are typical ectopic pregnancies secondary to the increased rate of uterine rupture. The treatment is to attempt to achieve hemostasis and perform a cornual resection either through laparotomy or laparoscopy.

### Interligamentous Pregnancy

The development of an interligamentous pregnancy is a rare occurrence in the development of ectopic gestations, but there have been reported cases of live births from an interligamentous pregnancy. It is believed that an interligamentous pregnancy develops as the trophoblastic tissue penetrates the tubal serosa into the mesosalpinx with further implantation between the leaves of the broad ligament. It can also occur if a fistula is present between the uterine cavity and the retroperitoneal space of the broad ligament. Complications arise as the placenta can be firmly adherent to the adjacent pelvic organs and side walls. As is the case with an abdominal pregnancy, the placenta should be removed if possible; however, if the placenta cannot be removed with good hemostasis, it should be left in place and allowed to resorb.

## Heterotopic Pregnancy

A heterotopic pregnancy is the presence of both an intrauterine and an ectopic pregnancy. Patients having undergone ovulation induction with clomiphene citrate and gonadotropins, or in vitro fertilization, are at a greater risk for a heterotopic pregnancy. The ectopic pregnancy may be missed as the ultrasonographer focuses on the intrauterine gestation. Serial β-hCG levels are usually not useful secondary to the normal intrauterine gestation causing a normal doubling time.

The treatment for a heterotopic pregnancy is surgical management of the ectopic pregnancy with expectant management of the intrauterine gestation. Heterotopic pregnancies have been successfully treated with KCl and hyperosmolar glucose solutions injected directly into the ectopic pregnancy either laparoscopically or transvaginally.[21]

## Multiple Ectopic Pregnancies

Multiple ectopic pregnancies occur rarely, with approximately 250 case reports for twin ectopic gestations.[28] The majority of multiple ectopic pregnancies are twin tubal pregnancies; however, there have been reports of ovarian, interstitial, and abdominal pregnancies. Management of multiple ectopic pregnancies is similar to that of single ectopic pregnancies and depends on patient stability and location of the pregnancies.

## Pregnancy After Hysterectomy

Hysterectomy is expected to eliminate the risk of an ectopic pregnancy; however, the situation has been reported.[29] A patient undergoing hysterectomy could have a luteal-phase pregnancy at the time of the initial surgery and subsequently have an ectopic pregnancy within the remaining fallopian tube. Additionally, in a patient with a vaginal wall defect or supracervical hysterectomy, sperm could gain intra-abdominal access to the peritoneal cavity and fertilize an egg, resulting in an ectopic pregnancy.

## REFERENCES

1. National Center for Health Statistics: Annual Summary of Births, Marriages, Divorces and Deaths: United States, 1989. Hyattsville, Md, U.S. Department of Health and Human Services, Public Health Service, 1990, Vol 38, p 23. **(IIb, B)**
2. Chow WH, Daling JR, Cates W Jr, et al: Epidemiology of ectopic pregnancy. Epidemiol Rev 1987;9:70–94. **(IIb, B)**
3. Chow JM, Yonekura ML, Richwald GA, et al: The association between *Chlamydia trachomatis* and ectopic pregnancy: a matched-pair, case-control study. JAMA 1990;263:3164–3167. **(IIb, B)**
4. Westrom L, Bengtsson LPH, Mardh P-A: Incidence, trends, and risks of ectopic pregnancy in a population of women. BMJ 1981;282:15–18. **(IIb, B)**
5. Westrom L: Influence of sexually transmitted diseases on sterility and ectopic pregnancy. Acta Eur Fertil 1985;16:21–24. **(IIb, B)**
6. Liukko P, Erkkola R, Laakso L: Ectopic pregnancies during low-dose progestogens for oral contraception. Contraception 1977;16:575–580. **(IIb, B)**
7. Shoupe D, Mishell DR Jr, Bopp BL, et al: The significance of bleeding patterns in Norplant implant users. Obstet Gynecol 1991;77:256–260. **(IIb, B)**
8. Cheng MC, Wong YM, Rochat RW, et al: Sterilization failures in Singapore: an examination of ligation techniques and failure rates. Stud Fam Plann 1977;8:109–115. **(IIb, B)**
9. Hulka JF, Halme J: Sterilization reversal: results of 101 attempts. Am J Obstet Gynecol 1988;159:767–774. **(IIb, B)**
10. Coste J, Job-Spira N, Fernandez H: Increased risk of ectopic pregnancy with maternal cigarette smoking. Am J Public Health 1991;81:199–201. **(IIb, B)**
11. Westrom L: Effect of acute pelvic inflammatory disease on fertility. Am J Obstet Gynecol 1975;121:707–713. **(IIb, B)**
12. Kadar N, Romero R: Further observations on serial human chorionic gonadotropin patterns in ectopic pregnancies and spontaneous abortions. Fertil Steril 1988;50:367–370. **(IIb, B)**
13. Kadar N, Caldwell BV, Romero R: A method of screening for ectopic pregnancy and its indications. Obstet Gynecol 1981;58:162–165. **(IIb, B)**
14. Stovall TG, Ling FW, Carson SA, et al: Serum progesterone and uterine curettage in differential diagnosis of ectopic pregnancy. Fertil Steril 1992;57:456–458. **(Ib, A)**
15. Ahmed A, Tom BDM, Calabrese P: Ectopic pregnancy diagnosis and the pseudo-sac. Fertil Steril 2004;81:1225–1228. **(IIb, B)**

16. Stovall TG, Ling FW: Ectopic pregnancy: diagnostic and therapeutic algorithms minimizing surgical intervention. J Reprod Med 1993; 38:807–810. **(Ib, A)**

17. Ory SJ, Nnadi E, Herrmann R, et al: Fertility after ectopic pregnancy. Fertil Steril 1993;60:231–235. **(IIb, B)**

18. Brumstead J, Kessler C, Gibson C, et al: A comparison of laparoscopy and laparotomy for the treatment of ectopic pregnancy. Obstet Gynecol 1988;71:889–892. **(Ib, A)**

19. Stovall TG, Ling FW, Buster JE: Outpatient chemotherapy of unruptured ectopic pregnancy. Fertil Steril 1989;51:435–438. **(IIb, B)**

20. Stovall TG, Ling FW, Gray LA: Single-dose methotrexate for treatment of ectopic pregnancy. Obstet Gynecol 1991;77:754–757. **(IIb, B)**

21. Strohmer H, Obruca A, Lehner R, et al: Successful treatment of a heterotopic pregnancy by sonographically guided instillation of hyperosmolar glucose. Fertil Steril 1998;69:149–151. **(III, B)**

22. Makinen JI, Kivijarvi AK, Irjala KMA: Success of non-surgical management of ectopic pregnancy. Lancet 1990;335:1099. **(III, B)**

23. Seifer DB, Gutmann JN, Grant WD, et al: Comparison of persistent ectopic pregnancy after laparoscopic linear salpingostomy. Obstet Gynecol 1990;76:1121–1125. **(III, B)**

24. Parente JT, Ou CS, Levy J, et al: Cervical pregnancy analysis: a review and report of five cases. Obstet Gynecol 1983;62:79–82. **(III, B)**

25. Grimes HG, Nosal RA, Gallagher JC: Ovarian pregnancy: a series of 24 cases. Obstet Gynecol 1983;61:174–180. **(III, B)**

26. Atrash HK, Friede A, Hogue CJR: Abdominal pregnancy in the United States: frequency and maternal mortality. Obstet Gynecol 1987; 69:333. **(IIb, B)**

27. Martin JN Jr, Sessums JK, Martin RW, et al: Abdominal pregnancy: current concepts of management. Obstet Gynecol 1988;71:549–557. **(IIb, B)**

28. Olsen ME: Bilateral twin ectopic gestations with intraligamentous and interstitial components: a case report. J Reprod Med 1994;39:118–120. **(IIb, B)**

29. Jackson P, Barrowclough IW, France JT, et al: A successful pregnancy following total hysterectomy. Br J Obstet Gynaecol 1980;87:353–355. **(III, B)**

## NORMAL VULVA

The vulva is a convergence of the integumentary, genital, and urinary systems. The vulvar boundaries are the genitocrural folds laterally, the vestibule medially, the mons pubis anteriorly, and the perineal posterior border. The major vulvar areas include the labia majora, labia minora, clitoris, vestibule, and hymen. The external border of the vestibule is Hart's line, which is a subtle skin demarcation on the inner labia minora.

### Anatomic Variants

There are many anatomic variants of the normal vulva, including labial asymmetry (Fig. 16-1). One of the most commonly misinterpreted normal vulvar variants is vestibular papillae (Fig. 16-2), which is estimated to exist in 44% of premenopausal women and 8% of postmenopausal women.[1] These symmetric flesh-colored or pink projections are asymptomatic. They may be mistaken for condylomata accuminata, but the regularity and symmetry of the papillae help distinguish them from human papilloma virus (HPV)–related changes.

Over time, an individual's vulvar appearance may change. In menopause, atrophy may produce thinning of the labia minora.

Unlike skin on other surfaces, the vulva is exposed to constant moisture and pressure due to its anatomic position and its covering by restrictive, occlusive clothing.

Distinctions between normal and abnormal changes in the vulva are sometimes difficult to discern. Accurate diagnosis requires an understanding of the complex interaction of skin occlusion from clothing, anatomic variance, and physiologic processes of the vulva.

## EVALUATION OF VULVAR DISEASE

### Prevalence

Vulvar disorders are common complaints in gynecology, primary care, and dermatology practices. Because patients present to a variety of practitioners, the prevalence of many vulvar diseases is unknown. Most reports on the prevalence of vulvar disorders are based on information derived from genital dermatology clinics, but these numbers may not adequately represent the prevalence in the general population.

### Classification Guidelines

Benign vulvar disorders fall into the following main categories: infectious, inflammatory, neoplastic, and neuropathic etiologies. Much of our knowledge about treatment of vulvar diseases is supported by Level III evidence. Few randomized trials are available to shape our therapeutic decisions. Some of the challenges in developing a consensus for treatment exist in regard to terminology. Because a number of different health care providers treat vulvar disease and each discipline has its own categorization to identify vulvar disorders, a multidisciplinary approach to the study of vulvar disease, vulvology, has been proposed.[2] The International Society for the Study of Vulvovaginal Disease (ISSVD) has established classification guidelines. This terminology is reviewed and updated periodically. ISSVD terminology for vulvar nonneoplastic disease includes the categories found in Table 16-1.[3,4]

### Patient History

A systematic, detailed approach to the evaluation of vulvar complaints is optimal. The clinician should begin with an extensive exploration of the chief complaint. Patients may not be exact in their description of the problem. The nature and timing of symptoms should be as accurate as possible, and the quality of discomfort should be delineated, with distinctions made between itching, burning, sharp pain, and dull ache. The interview should also focus on any inciting events or topical product use. Patients should be questioned about hygiene practices, including bubble baths and douching. Currently, douching is not recommended for routine hygiene, but the practice continues.[5]

Patients should provide a detailed list of any over-the-counter products or prescription medications used in the genital region. According to one observational study conducted in Finland, 76% of women complaining of chronic vulvovaginal symptoms were confident in their own self-diagnosis and used at least one over-the-counter preparation for self-treatment without consulting a health care provider.[6] Physicians surveyed in the same study estimate adverse events related to patient self-medication in 74% to 95% of patients seen in follow-up. Level III evidence indicates that the most commonly noted problems with self-treatment are misdiagnosis and delay in receiving adequate therapy.[6]

A detailed problem list, including a history of systemic dermatologic disorders, should be compiled. Any disorder of the

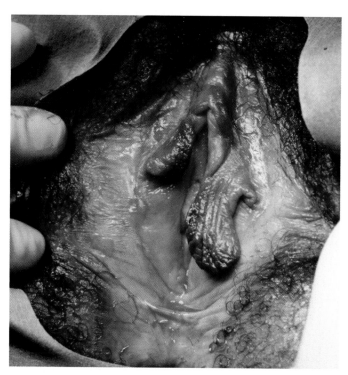

**Figure 16-1    Asymmetry of the labia minora is a common normal vulvar variant.**

| Table 16-1 |
| :---: |
| **Classification of Noninvasive Epithelial Disorders of the Vulva** |

**Non-neoplastic epithelial disorders of skin and mucosa**

Lichen sclerosus
Squamous cell hyperplasia (formerly hyperplastic dystrophy)
Other dermatoses

**Vulvar intraepithelial neoplasia**

VIN I Mild dysplasia
VIN II Moderate dysplasia
VIN III Severe dysplasia
VIN III Carcinoma in situ

**Nonsquamous intraepithelial neoplasia**

Paget disease
Melanoma in situ

From Ridley CM, Frankman O, Jones IS, et al: New nomenclature for vulvar disease: International Society for the Study of Vulvar Disease. Hum Pathol 1989;20:495–496.

skin can affect the vulva. Disorders of mucous membranes, such as lichen planus, can also be found in the vulva and vagina. One case series of 37 female patients with lichen planus indicated that vulvar involvement is present in 19 (51%) of the patients treated for extragenital lichen planus.[7]

Acquisition of the past medical history should also include any history of a self-limited disorder that could predispose a patient to long-term sequelae as well as chronic disorders or trauma that may increase the likelihood of vulvar disease (Table 16-2). For example, chronic postherpetic neuralgia can develop in patients with a history of genital herpes. Patients with diabetes may have more severe candidal infection of the vulva. Patients with a history of neurologic trauma or generalized chronic pain disorders may be at increased risk for vulvar pain syndromes. Level III

evidence compiled from a survey of patients with vulvodynia revealed that 55% of 300 women also had other chronic health conditions.[8] These disorders included pain syndromes such as chronic fatigue, endometriosis, fibromyalgia, interstitial cystitis, irritable bowel syndrome, depression, low back pain, and migraine headaches. Due to the complexity of disorders associated with vulvar disease, interdisciplinary collaboration may be essential for diagnosis and treatment.

**Physical Examination**

The physical examination should begin with a clinical inspection of the skin on the entire body. Inspection of the mouth and vagina may be helpful because some conditions can lead to erosions of the mucous membranes. Other body surfaces including the trunk and extremities may have easily recognized lesions that may also be found on the vulva but with an altered appearance.

*Lesion Characteristics*

A vulvologist is akin to an art historian in some key ways. Both use the power of recognition for identification. Lesion characteristics

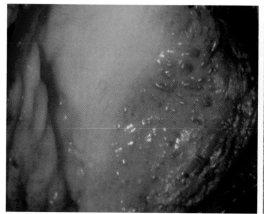
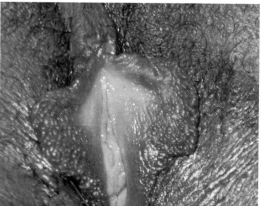

**Figure 16-2    Vulvar papillae may be found on the labia minora.** The symmetric distribution and frondlike individual projections help distinguish them from HPV lesions.

| |
|---|
| **Table 16-2**<br>**Pertinent Medical History** |

**Chronic medical disorders**

Allergies
Autoimmune disorders
Chronic fatigue syndrome
Diabetes
Fibromyalgia
Irritable bowel syndrome
Lumbosacral vertebral disk disease
Systemic dermatologic disorders
Thyroid disease

**Infections**

Sexually transmitted infections, including HIV, HPV, and HSV
Shingles

**Genitourinary conditions**

Gynecologic history
   Contraception
   Endometriosis
   Menopause
   Sexual practices
   Genital tract dysplasia
Urologic history
   Interstitial cystitis
   Incontinence
Obstetrical history
   Breastfeeding history
   Episiotomy
   Vulvovaginal laceration

**History of trauma**

Sexual abuse
Back injury
Straddle injury

**Surgical history**

Laser of the vagina/vulva
Vulvar excision

**Psychological history**

Domestic violence/abuse
Depression

help support the diagnosis. Types of lesions include the macule, papule, plaque, vesicle, ulcer, nodule, and tumor. Lesions may be flesh colored, erythematous, hyperpigmented, hypopigmented, or variegated. Categorizing the vulvar appearance into these descriptions facilitates the diagnostic process. The presence of one or multiple lesions can define the disorder. On inspection of the vulva, the absence of lesions may also give clues to neuropathic origins of disease.

Physical examination of the external genitalia should focus on important vulvar landmarks. Distortion of the normal vulvar anatomy gives clues to the diagnosis. For example, patients who present with labial thinning may have symptoms related to vulvovaginal atrophy. Lichen planus or lichen sclerosus may present with labial agglutination or clitoral phimosis.

Mapping of pain symptoms may be helpful. Some conditions such as vestibulodynia may present with pain confined to the vulvar vestibule. Several techniques are used to map vulvar pain.

A cotton-tipped applicator can be used to delineate point tenderness. Although this is the most common technique for assessing vulvar pain, this method is subjective and it is not quantified or always reproducible. A vulvar algesiometer, a noninvasive tool for the measurement of vulvar pain, has been implemented in some studies in an attempt to quantify vulvar pain.[9]

### Associated Signs

Vaginal discharge may be obtained and examined for pH and wet preparation. A maturation index can confirm the diagnosis of vulvovaginal atrophy. Scrapings of the vulvar skin can also be examined microscopically for fungal infection. If the patient has had recurring symptoms, a vaginal culture may reveal resistant fungal organisms. A bacterial culture can reveal *Streptococcus agalactiae* overgrowth. Herpes simplex virus (HSV) cultures should be obtained in any patient who presents with vulvar vesicles or ulcers. Serologic tests such as those for HSV antibody, human immunodeficiency virus antibody, and antinuclear antibodies can support the vulvar diagnosis.

### Diagnosis

Ultimately a biopsy confirms the diagnosis of most vulvar disorders. A magnified view of the vulva with either a magnifying lens or a colposcope can target the biopsy site, and a dermatopathologist may be consulted to confirm histopathologic diagnoses. Specialized testing, including direct immunoflouresence studies of vulvar biopsies, requires special handling of the tissue.

### Treatment Options

Topical corticosteroids are the mainstay of therapy for many vulvar disorders. Steroids reduce inflammation, but the local immunosuppressive effect of steroids on the skin may worsen a pre-existing vulvar infection. Bacterial, viral, or fungal infections should be excluded before initiating treatment. Topical steroids are categorized into seven classes based on potency, and many steroid options exist within each class. Class I steroids are in the ultrapotent category. Class VII steroids are the mildest topical steroid preparations. A practitioner usually uses a few steroids in each general potency group (Fig. 16-3).

Topical steroids exist in a variety of preparations, including creams, lotions, and ointments. In general creams and lotions are easier to apply; however, they contain more allergens and preservatives than ointments and so stinging may occur on skin contact. Ointment-based steroids are more occlusive; therefore, they have a longer-lasting, more potent effect on the skin.

### Steroid Side Effects

It is important to remember that the stronger the steroid, the more likely it is to produce side effects. Systemic absorption of ultrapotent steroids such as 0.05% clobetasol propionate can be significant, with the risk of hypothalamic-pituitary axis suppression. Aseptic necrosis of the femoral head has been reported. Additionally, long-term use may result in skin atrophy and striae. Steroid rebound dermatitis can occur when long-term high-potency steroid use is discontinued; therefore, this class of steroids should be used with caution. Limits should be set on the amount and duration of use. The potent steroid should be tapered to a milder class or discontinued as soon as a response is obtained.

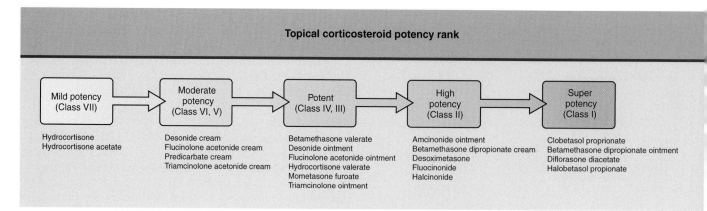

**Topical corticosteroid potency rank**

| Mild potency (Class VII) | → | Moderate potency (Class VI, V) | → | Potent (Class IV, III) | → | High potency (Class II) | → | Super potency (Class I) |

Hydrocortisone
Hydrocortisone acetate

Desonide cream
Flucinolone acetonide cream
Predicarbate cream
Triamcinolone acetonide cream

Betamethasone valerate
Desonide ointment
Flucinolone acetonide ointment
Hydrocortisone valerate
Mometasone furoate
Triamcinolone ointment

Amcinonide ointment
Betamethasone dipropionate cream
Desoximetasone
Fluocinonide
Halcinonide

Clobetasol proprionate
Betamethasone dipropionate ointment
Diflorasone diacetate
Halobetasol propionate

**Figure 16-3 Topical corticosteroid potency rankings.**

### Immune Modulators

A new class of topical preparations is now available for use in vulvar conditions. Tacrolimus and pimecrolimus are nonsteroidal drugs that reduce inflammation by inhibiting T-lymphocyte activation. This class of drugs is currently only approved by the Food and Drug Administration for atopic dermatitis, but it has been used for treatment of other vulvar disorders.

Other immunmodulators include imiquimod cream, which augments the immune response. Primarily used in the treatment of HPV, it is applied three times per week, and a response should be noted within 16 weeks. The side effects of imiquimod include skin irritation, which may prohibit its use in some patients. Case reports suggest that imiquimod may be used in vulvar intraepithelial neoplasia. One report even noted utility in recurrent Paget's disease, once an associated malignancy has been excluded.

## VULVAR DISORDERS

### Infection

Vulvar infections include a wide variety of disorders. These disorders will be reviewed in detail in Chapter 18 and include vulvar candidiasis.

### Candida

Vulvar candidiasis can have a variety of presentations. Vulvar pruritus, erythema with satellite papules, fissures, or vaginal discharge are common signs and symptoms. In the acute setting, *Candida albicans* accounts for the majority of fungal infections. Chronic or recurrent infections may be associated with the more resistant non-*albicans* species. Cyclic vulvovaginitis, a recurring entity characterized by intermittent postovulatory vulvar discomfort and a sensation of labial swelling, has been linked to infection and hypersensitivity to fungus. In a retrospective review of 40 cases of cyclic vulvitis, 61.5% of patients had positive fungal cultures.[10] Only 54% of the positive cultures revealed *C. albicans*. *Candida glabrata* was the most common non-*albicans* species isolated. Fungal cultures may be useful because non-*albicans* candidiasis may be more difficult to diagnose and treat. In general, cultures for bacteria have limited value because a wide variety of organisms are considered part of the normal flora.

### Human Papillomavirus

Human papillomavirus may present with vulvovaginal condylomata acuminata. The verrucoid appearance of these lesions aids in identification of the disorder. If vulvar intraepithelial neoplasia or squamous cell carcinoma is suspected, a biopsy should be performed.

### Herpes Simplex Virus

Herpes simplex virus should be included in the differential diagnosis of anyone who presents with vulvar vesicles or ulcers. HSV-1 or -2 can be confirmed by viral culture. Direct fluorescent antibody testing can yield results in the same day. Serologic testing for HSV proves a history of the infection but is not site specific. Serum antibody testing is mainly useful in ruling out a history of infection with a negative result. HSV vesicles can be found on the vulva or on other body surfaces (Figs. 16-4 and 16-5).

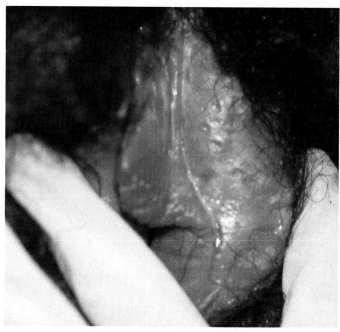

**Figure 16-4 Vulvar herpes simplex virus.** The initial vesicular lesions have ruptured to reveal round coalescent erosions.

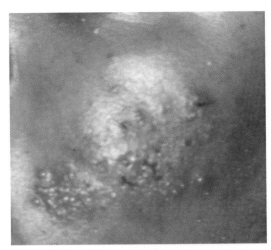

Figure 16-5    Facial herpes simplex virus.

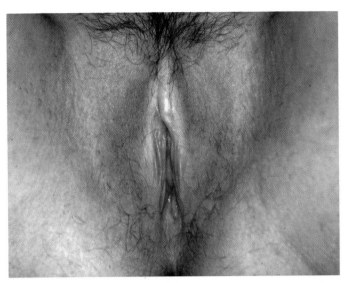

**Figure 16-6    Vulvar lichen sclerosus.** Skin pallor may be noted on the labia in a keyhole distribution or may be noted around the labial and anal areas in a figure-of-eight distribution.

## Benign Dermatoses

Nonmalignant vulvar dermatoses can be subdivided into three categories: non-neoplastic epithelial disorders, tumors, and intra-epithelial neoplasias. Clinically these lesions can be categorized by appearance based on color, pattern, and location (Table 16-3; Figs. 16-6 through 16-18).

## Non-neoplastic Epithelial Disorders

Any disorder that can involve the skin can exist in the vulva. Given the moist environment of the vulva, lesions may appear altered compared to other skin. An example is psoriasis, which usually presents as erythematous plaques with silvery white scales, but on the vulva often appears as red plaques without scales (Fig. 16-19). Depending on the pigmentation of the affected individual, lesions may also vary. Vulvar disorders in individuals with dark skin may have a different appearance than the same types of lesions in a woman with less pigmented skin.

### Contact Dermatitis

Contact dermatitis is an inflammatory skin reaction to an irritant or allergen. The skin barrier of the vulva is more susceptible to irritation than skin in other anatomic sites due to constant moisture, occlusion, and frictional forces. Vulvar irritants may

| Table 16-3 Characterization of Vulvar Lesions by Appearance | | |
|---|---|---|
| **Lesion Characteristics** | **Examples** | **Illustrations** |
| **Color** | | |
| White lesions | Lichen sclerosus (LS), squamous hyperplasia, vulvar intraepithelial neoplasia (VIN), vitiligo | LS (Fig. 16-6) |
| Red lesions | Vestibulodynia, vulvar candidiasis, lichen planus (LP), VIN | Candidiasis (Fig. 16-7) |
| Brown lesions | VIN, nevi, acanthosis nigricans | VIN (Fig. 16-8) |
| **Pattern** | | |
| Macule | Vitiligo, melanosis, HPV, VIN | Melanosis (Fig. 16-9) |
| Papule | Skin tag, nevus, molluscum contagiosum, seborrheic keratosis | Seborrheic keratosis (Fig. 16-10) |
| Plaque | Eczema, Paget's disease, psoriasis, HPV, VIN | Paget's disease (Fig. 16-11) |
| Verrucae | HPV, verrucous xanthoma | HPV (Fig. 16-12) |
| Vesicles | HSV, varicella | Varicella (Fig. 16-13) |
| Cyst | Bartholin cyst, Skene's duct cyst, keratinous cysts | Skene's duct cyst (Fig. 16-14) |
| Ulcer | Behçet's disease, HSV, Crohn's disease, LGV, syphilis, chancroid | HSV (Fig. 16-15) |
| Tumor | Fibroma, hemangioma, lipoma, VIN | Lipoma (Fig. 16-16) |
| **Location** | | |
| Vulvodynia subsets | Vestibulodynia | (Fig. 16-17) |
| | Pudendal neuralgia, generalized vulvodynia | (Fig. 16-18) |

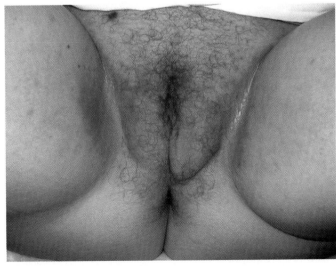

**Figure 16-7    Vulvar candidiasis.** Erythematous patches on the vulva and intertriginous areas may be surrounded by satellite papular lesions.

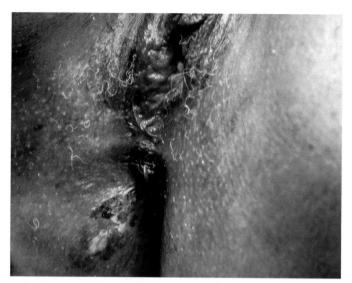

**Figure 16-8    Vulvar intraepithelial neoplasia.** Vulvar intraepithelial lesions may be hyperpigmented and eroded.

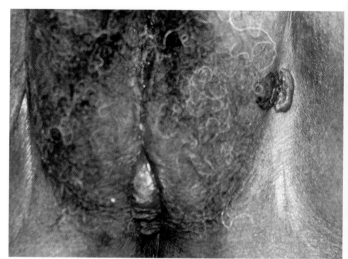

**Figure 16-10    Seborrheic keratosis.** These hyperpigmented lesions vary in size and may be single or multiple. The oily, "stuck on" appearance helps distinguish this lesion from other dermatoses.

range from caustic agents such as 5-fluorouracil to more typical irritants such as perfumed soaps and detergents.[11] Vulvar exposures and hygiene practices such as overzealous cleansing, piercing of genitalia, and wearing constrictive, synthetic undergarments and clothing can exacerbate the condition.

Allergic contact dermatitis is an immune-mediated response to an allergen in a previously exposed and sensitized individual.[12] Both irritant and allergic contact dermatitis may present with vulvar erythema, edema, itching, stinging, or burning sensations (Fig. 16-20).

History is an important key to identifying the type of dermatitis and the causative agent. Patch testing may be helpful

in distinguishing an allergen. According to Level III evidence compiled from a vulvar clinic in 2000, 20% to 30% of patients had dermatitis, with 26% associated with positive patch tests.[13] Treatment should focus on identifying and eliminating the causative agent. Short-term use of anti-inflammatory agents such as a midpotency to ultrapotency topical corticosteroid may be useful in controlling pruritus. Contact dermatitis is usually self-limited if the inciting factors are removed.

### Lichen Simplex Chronicus

Lichen simplex chronicus is one of the most common vulvar dermatoses. Lichen simplex chronicus is the vulvar manifestation of a chronic dermatitis. The hallmark of lichen simplex chronicus

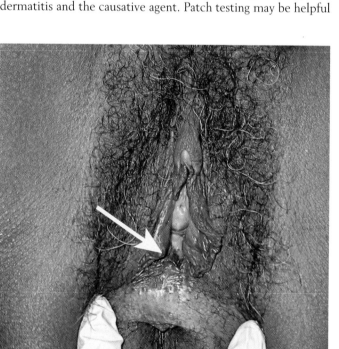

**Figure 16-9    Vulvar melanosis.** This benign change is more commonly seen on the labia minora of postmenopausal women.

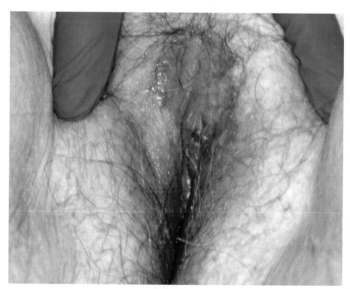

**Figure 16-11    Paget's disease of the vulva.** This plaque has a velvet-like appearance. Affected patients typically present with chronic pruritus that may be misdiagnosed as candidiasis.

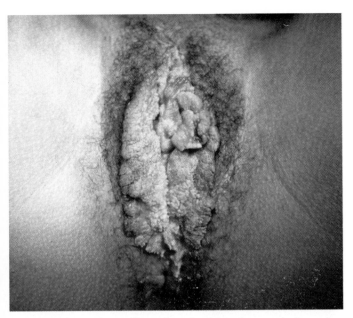

**Figure 16-12    Human papillomavirus.** Condylomata accuminata can be single or confluent verrucoid lesions.

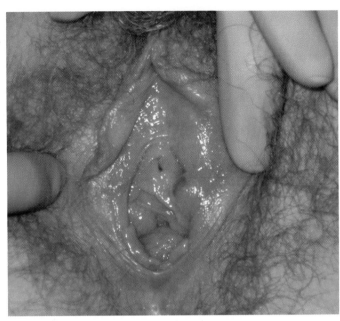

**Figure 16-14    Skene's gland cyst.**

is pruritus. Patients may complain of intense itching with temporary relief with scratching. Indeed the itch-scratch cycle is the perpetuating force with lichen simplex chronicus.

A careful history regarding vulvar hygiene is an important key to resolution of symptoms. Patients must be interviewed about the use of topical agents because seemingly benign things such as soaps, feminine hygiene products, and bubble bath may be the inciting irritants. Clinical evaluation should be performed to assess for infection and other dermatoses. In addition to lichen simplex chronicus, the differential diagnosis for these patients includes any dermatosis that may present with pruritus, including lichen sclerosus, atopic dermatitis, and psoriasis. Inspection of the skin may reveal lichenification or thickening of the labia minora and the labia majora (Fig. 16-21). Within the thickened whitish or grayish plaques, normal skin markings may be accentuated (Fig. 16-22). If a patient scratches excessively,

linear excoriations may be found (Fig. 16-23). Vulvar biopsy may be indicated to confirm the diagnosis. Hyperkeratosis and acanthosis may also be noted.

Tests to ascertain inciting factors include cutaneous and vaginal swabs with microscopic evaluation for fungal infection. If a longstanding history of lichen simplex chronicus is present, further evaluation is warranted. Culture for non-*albicans* candidiasis should be obtained. If perianal pruritus is also noted, parasitic examination of the stool for pinworms should be considered. Level III evidence supports patch testing to identify allergens if there is a history of prolonged use of topical irritants or topical treatments. In one case series, 48% of women diagnosed with lichen simplex chronicus tested positive for allergens, and 27% of these allergens were found to be relevant to the pathology.[13] Although rare, corticosteroid allergy has been reported.[14]

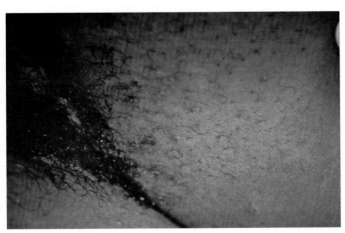

**Figure 16-13    Vulvar vesicles.** Vesicles on the vulva are fragile and easily rupture. This patient was diagnosed with varicella.

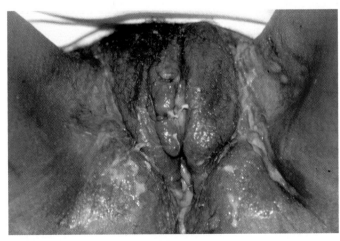

**Figure 16-15    Hidradenitis suppurativa.** This condition may present with ulceration, sinus tracts, and abscess formation.

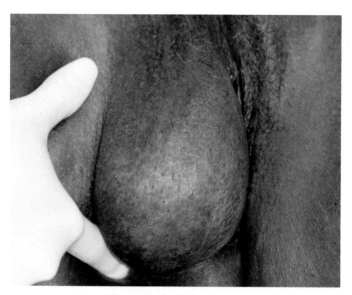

**Figure 16-16    Vulvar lipoma.**

Identification of the etiologic factor, avoidance of skin irritants, and cessation of the itch-scratch cycle are the simplified keys to resolution of this dermatosis. Breaking the itch-scratch cycle is the challenge. Often a medium- to high-potency topical corticosteroid must be applied to the affected skin. Oral antihistamines may be used to treat intense pruritic symptoms. The sedative properties of some antihistamines may be preferable for suppression of nocturnal exacerbations. In extreme cases, a short course of oral corticosteroids may be indicated.

### Lichen Sclerosus

Lichen sclerosus is a chronic dermatosis that may present with vulvar pruritus. Lichen sclerosus was previously considered a disorder of hypoestrogenic girls and women. Currently, many

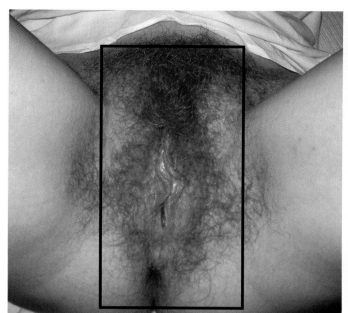

**Figure 16-18    Generalized vulvodynia and pudendal neuralgia present with a wide distribution of vulvar pain.**

cases of lichen sclerosus are first identified in women of reproductive age. The pathogenesis of lichen sclerosus is unknown. Reports of multiple members of a family being affected suggest a genetic link. Patients with lichen sclerosus may also have hypothyroidism, indicating a possible autoimmune association.[15]

Examination reveals a pale parchment-like appearing of the labia (Fig. 16-24). Labial agglutination may also be present in longstanding dermatoses. Lichen sclerosus may increase the fragility of the vulvar skin; therefore, fissures and ecchymosis may develop (Fig. 16-25). Lichen sclerosus can also present with white plaques on other body surfaces (Fig. 16-26).

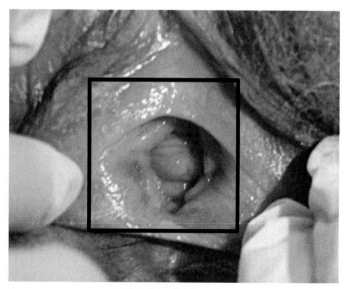

**Figure 16-17    Vestibulodynia.** Patients have point tenderness confined to the vulvar vestibule. The inner border of the vestibule is the hymen/hymenal tags. The outer border is Hart's line, a demarcation on the medial labia minora.

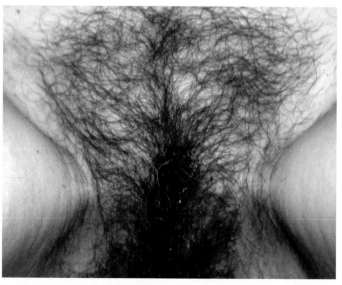

**Figure 16-19    Vulvar psoriasis.** Psoriasis on the vulva has a bright red appearance. Due to the moist environment of the vulva, it lacks the silvery scale that is typical of psoriasis on other skin surfaces.

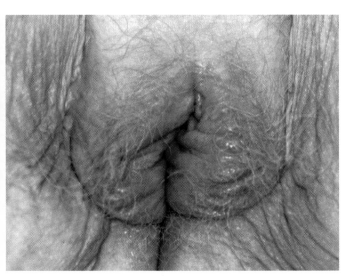

**Figure 16-20** **Dermatitis.** Erythema and pruritus are common manifestations of dermatitis.

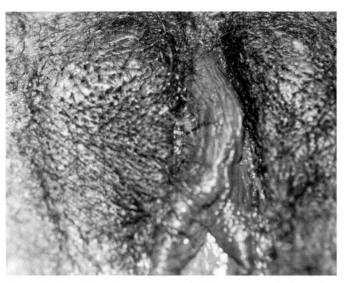

**Figure 16-22** **Lichen simplex chronicus.** Edematous changes may produce exaggerated skin markings.

Treatment protocols for lichen sclerosus have evolved over time. Initially this condition was treated with testosterone preparations. A randomized, controlled study of testosterone versus a petrolatum base (placebo) revealed that the hormone is no more potent in treatment of lichen sclerosus than the petrolatum ointment in which it is prepared.[16] In a study of 79 women with lichen sclerosus, each patient was randomized into a topical therapy group of testosterone (2%), progesterone (2%), clobetasol propionate (0.05%), or a cream-based preparation. After 3 months of treatment, remission was noted in 20% of the testosterone-treated group, 10% in the progesterone-treated group, 75% in the clobetasol propionate group, and 10.5% in the group treated with the cream-based preparation. Histologic improvement of the lichen sclerosus was found only in the clobetasol propionate–treated group.[17] Ultrapotent topical corticosteroids such as 0.05% clobetasol propionate are now standard therapy for lichen sclerosus. Improvement of symptoms is usually noted within the first month of use. Daily treatment should be limited given potential side effects of long-term ultrapotent steroid use. Small case series also suggest the utility of tacrolimus and pimecrolimus for the treatment of lichen sclerosus.[18–20] Surgical excision is not advocated because lichen sclerosus can recur in the surrounding vulvar skin.

If left untreated, lichen sclerosus can be a progressive disorder. Loss of normal vulvar architecture may occur due to scarring. Introital narrowing and dyspareunia may result.

Lichen sclerosus can be associated with vulvar carcinoma. In a cohort study of 20 months' duration, squamous cell carcinoma resulted in 3 of 211 patients with lichen sclerosus.[21] Lichen sclerosus has been found in skin adjacent to squamous cell carcinoma at the time of excision. A retrospective review of

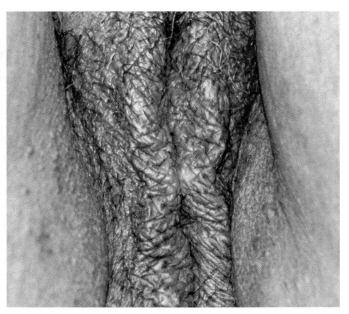

**Figure 16-21** **Lichen simplex chronicus.** Patients with this chronic condition may have hyperpigmented, lichenified skin.

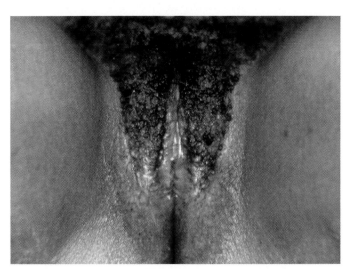

**Figure 16-23** **Linear excoriations.** Patients with chronic dermatitis may develop linear erosions from persistent scratching.

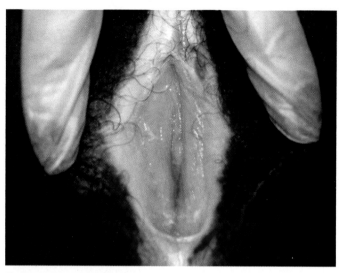

**Figure 16-24   Lichen sclerosus.** The pallor of lichen sclerosus presents a striking contrast in a dark-skinned patient.

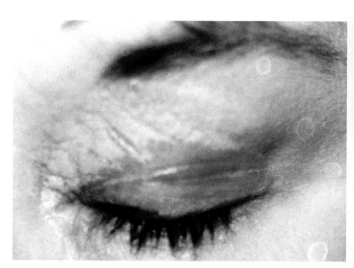

**Figure 16-26   Lichen sclerosus on the eyelid.** Lichen sclerosus can affect other skin surfaces.

72 cases of non-HPV-related squamous cell carcinoma found 25 cases associated with lichen sclerosus.[22] Because vulvar carcinoma arises in only a small fraction of the many women affected by the dermatosis, lichen sclerosus is not a direct precursor for the disease. Other contributing factors remain undetermined. Regular evaluation of the skin should be performed to detect malignant changes. A biopsy should be performed on hyperkeratotic or ulcerated lesions when malignancy is suspected.

### Lichen Planus

Vulvar lichen planus is an uncommon but chronic, debilitating condition that is often misdiagnosed initially.[23] The etiology of lichen planus is unknown, but a cell-mediated autoimmune reaction is suspected. The difficulty in diagnosis of lichen planus

may be related to the variable symptoms, appearance, and anatomic sites of presentation. Patients with vulvar lichen planus complain of burning, irritation, or itching. The three types of vulvar lichen planus are hypertrophic, papular, and erosive disease. The hypertrophic form may reveal subtle thickening on examination; itching may be reported by the patient. The papular form reveals raised lesions that may be pruritic or asymptomatic. The erosive form reveals denuded surfaces with ill-demarcated borders on exam and usually presents with complaints of a burning sensation (Fig. 16-27). Pain with urination may be reported if the urine irritates eroded vulvar skin.

Erosive lichen planus can also affect mucous membranes. Vaginal erosions may yield an inflammatory vaginal discharge. This discharge may be characterized by an alkaline pH, lack of maturation (parabasal cells on wet prep), replacement of lactobacilli with cocci, and many inflammatory cells (mainly eosinophils).[24] Extragenital lesions may include oral lichen planus, which may appear as erosion or a reticulate pattern known as *Wickham's striae*. Violaceous papules may also be

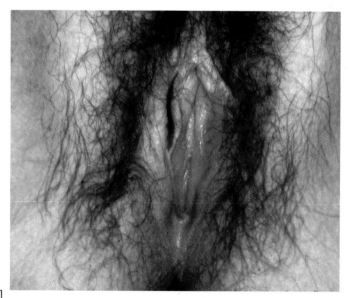

**Figure 16-25   Lichen sclerosus.** Skin fragility may lead to fissures, tears, petechiae, and ecchymosis.

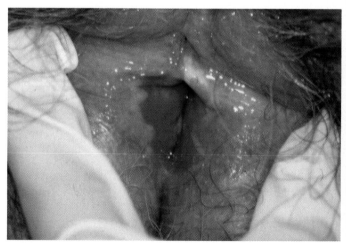

**Figure 16-27   Erosive vulvar lichen planus.**

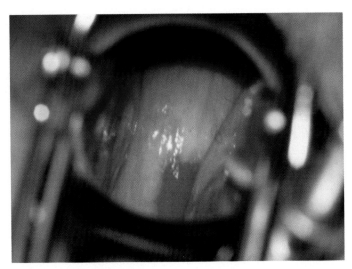

**Figure 16-28    Vaginal erosive lichen planus.** This lesion developed after hysterectomy along the vaginal vault scar.

found on the extremities and trunk. Lichen planus may exhibit the koebner response; it tends to develop at sites of friction or scars. It may even develop at the vaginal cuff suture line after hysterectomy (Fig. 16-28).

Treatment usually consists of mid-potency to high-potency topical steroids. An ointment may produce less burning than a cream preparation when applied to eroded skin. Initial therapy for an advanced case may consist of clobetasol propionate applied sparingly once or twice per day for the first month. The patient should be reevaluated monthly until the condition improves. The topical steroid should be tapered, either by decreasing the frequency of application or by decreasing the potency of the preparation. One case series reports 81% subjective improvement in patients with vulvovaginal lesions treated with 25 mg intravaginal hydrocortisone suppositories.[25] Foam steroid preparations can also be used in the vagina. Severe cases of lichen planus may be treated with a short course of oral steroids. Small case series suggest that tacrolimus may be beneficial in the treatment of recalcitrant vulvar lichen planus.[26,27] If untreated, the hypertrophic and papular types of lichen planus may be self-limited, but the erosive form has a progressive course. Distortion of labial architecture, with loss of the labia minora and midline labial agglutination can be seen. Narrowing of the introitus with scarring and shortening of the vagina may result in dyspareunia.

## Vulvodynia

Although the symptom of vulvar pain has always existed, the identification of the disorder is still undergoing classification. The recognition of vulvar pain in the literature has certainly lagged behind the existence of the disorder, but as awareness of vulvodynia increases, new light has been shed on the disorder.

Vulvar pain can be divided into identifiable disorders, neuropathic disease, or idiopathic causes (Fig. 16-29).

*Vulvodynia*, defined as chronic vulvar pain existing in the absence of an underlying recognizable disease,[28] has long been considered a clinical entity. The chronicity of the disorder usually is at least 3 months' duration. In 1976, this disorder was initially recognized as the *burning vulva syndrome*. Debate over vulvodynia as a symptom versus a disease continues.

Various terminology has evolved to characterize this entity, including recently defining the distinct terms *dysesthetic vulvodynia* and *vestibulitis*. In 2003, at the 17th World Congress, the ISSVD updated the terminology.[28] *Vulvodynia* remains the preferred term, with subsets of generalized, localized, or mixed groups. Further subclassification of these groups includes spontaneous or provoked pain with reference to anatomic sites (Fig. 16-30).

*Vestibulitis*, a subset of vulvodynia, was originally defined as a triad of severe pain on vestibular touch or attempted vaginal entry, tenderness to pressure localized within the vulvar vestibule, and physical findings confined to vestibular erythema of various degrees.[29] The popular term *vestibulitis* has been deemed a misnomer by the ISSVD because local inflammation, as implied by its suffix, has not been the defining histologic picture. The term has been officially replaced by the term *provoked vestibulodynia*. Modifications to terminology may continue as new information about the disorder is discovered. Pain rather than pruritus is the hallmark of this entity.

Early studies of vulvodynia described the disease as an entity of non-Hispanic white women. Interestingly, in a population-based cross-sectional survey conducted in the Boston area of 3358 women age 18 to 64, Hispanic women were at greatest risk of unexplained chronic vulvar pain. African American and white women had similar risk of unexplained vulvar pain, but Hispanic women were 80% more likely than white women to report chronic vulvar pain.[30] Although the exact incidence of vulvodynia is unknown, this study estimated the lifetime cumulative incidence at 16% in women age 18 to 64. Researchers extrapolated these figures to estimate that approximately 14 million U.S. women may experience vulvodynia.[30]

Several etiologies of vulvodynia have been postulated, including embryologic abnormalities, increased urinary oxalate

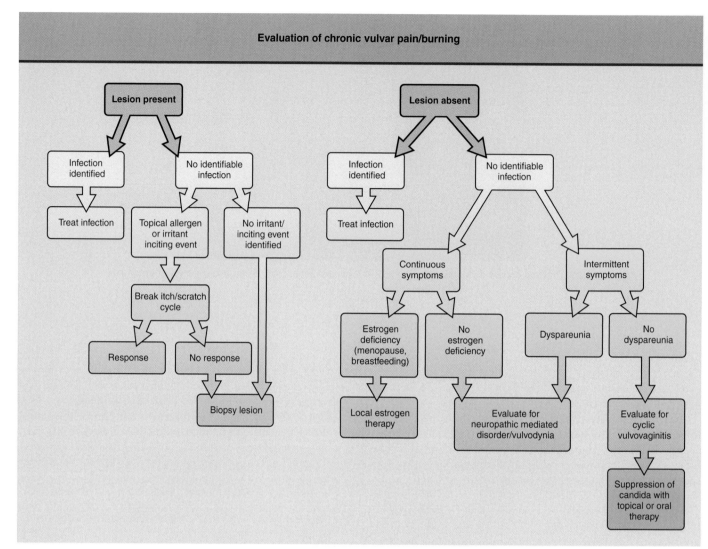

**Figure 16-29** Evaluation of chronic vulvar pain and burning.

levels, genetic or immune factors, hormonal factors, inflammation, infection, and neuropathic changes.[31] The etiology of the disorder may be multifactoiral; no one cause has been isolated. Other causes of vulvar burning or pain should be excluded, including monilial infection, postherpetic neuralgia, dermatitis, vulvovaginal atrophy, lichen sclerosus, erosive lichen planus, and other dermatoses. Early researchers postulated a link between HPV and vulvodynia, but this association has been discredited by a number of studies. Biopsy has limited usefulness, except to exclude other causes. The histopathologic characteristics described in the literature are varied. Inflammation of the vestibule may exist,[32–34] but there is controversy over whether it is definitive.[35] Proliferation of intraepithelial nerve fibers has been noted in patients with vestibulodynia,[36,37] but the significance of this finding is also unclear.

Patients with generalized unprovoked vulvar pain should be assessed for pudendal neuralgia and other disorders in the complex regional pain syndrome. Tricyclic antidepressant therapy has been a widely used pharmacologic approach to treatment.[38] The use of tricyclic antidepressants is based originally on their use in the treatment of postherpetic neuralgia. In both entities, an inciting event may lead to allodynia. Unlike postherpetic neuralgia, the inciting event in vulvodynia is often unknown. Other pharmacologic therapeutic regimens include the use of gabapentin, topical lidocaine ointment and vulvar injections of steroids and anesthetic agents. Nonpharmacologic agents include physical therapy with rehabilitation of the pelvic floor musculature and biofeedback exercises. Less information is available about acupuncture, dietary restrictions, vitamin supplementation, and other alternative therapies. Surgical excision of the vestibule with advancement of vaginal mucosa should only be considered when conservative options have been exhausted. Treatment options must be individualized because varied responses are reported and few prospective trials have been performed to validate the effectiveness of most therapeutic protocols.

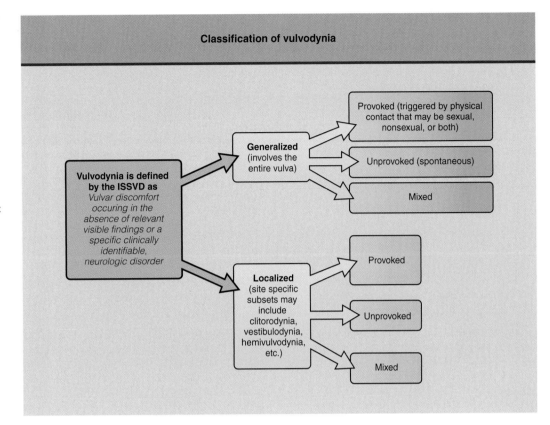

**Figure 16-30 Classification of vulvodynia.** (Adapted from Moyal-Barracco M, Lynch P [eds]: 2003 ISSVD Terminology and Classification of Vulvodynia. J Reprod Med 2004;49:48.)

# REFERENCES

1. Moyal-Barracco M, Leibowitch M, Orth G: Vestibular papillae of the vulva. Lack of evidence for human papillomavirus etiology. Arch Dermatol 1990;126:1594–1598. **(III, B)**

2. Micheletti L, Preti M, Bogliatto F, et al: Vulvology: a proposal for a multidisciplinary subspecialty. J Reprod Med 2002;47:715–717. **(IV, C)**

3. Ridley CM, Frankman O, Jones IS, et al: New nomenclature for vulvar disease: International Society for the Study of Vulvar Disease (letter). Hum Pathol 1989;20:495–496. **(IV, C)**

4. Wilkinson EJ, Kneale B, Lynch PJ: Report of the ISSVD terminology committee. J Reprod Med 1986;31:973–974. **(IV, C)**

5. Martino JL, Vermund SH: Vaginal douching: evidence for risks or benefits to women's health. Epidemiol Rev 2002;24:109–124. **(IV, C)**

6. Sihvo S, Ahonen R, Mikander H, et al: Self medication with vaginal antifungal drugs: physicians' experience and women's utilization patterns. Family Pract 2000;17:145–149. **(III, B)**

7. Lewis FM, Shah M, Harrington CI: Vulval involvement in lichen planus: a study of 37 women. Br J Dermatol 1996;135:89–91. **(III, B)**

8. Sadownik LA: Clinical profile of vulvodynia patients: a prospective study of 300 patients. J Reprod Med 2000;45:679–684. **(III, B)**

9. Eva LJ, Reid W, MacLean A, et al: Assessment of response to treatment in vulvar vestibulitis syndrome by means of the vulvar algesiometer. Am J Obstet Gynecol 1999;181:99–102. **(III, B)**

10. Handa V, Stice C: Fungal culture findings in cyclic vulvitis. Obstet Gynecol 2000;96:301–303. **(III, B)**

11. Margesson LJ: Contact dermatitis of the vulva. Dermatol Ther 2004; 17:20–27. **(IV, C)**

12. Crone AM, Stewart EJ, Wojnarowska F, et al: Aetiological factors in vulvar dermatitis. J Eur Acad Dermatol Venereol 2000;14:181–186. **(IV, C)**

13. Virgili A, Corazza M, Bacilieri S, et al: Contact sensitivity in vulval lichen simplex chronicus. Contact Dermatitis 1997;37:296–297. **(IV, C)**

14. Chow ETY: Multiple corticosteroid allergies. Aus J Dermatol 2001; 42:62–63. **(III, B)**

15. Meyrick-Thomas RH, Ridley CM, MacGibbon DH, et al: Lichen sclerosus et atrophicus and autoimmunity: a study of 350 women. Br J Dermatol 1988;108:41. **(III, B)**

16. Sideri M, Origoni M, Spinaci L, et al: Topical testosterone in the treatment of vulvar lichen sclerosus. Int J Gynaecol Obstet 1994;46:53–56. **(Ib, A)**

17. Bracco GL, Carli P, Sonni L, et al: Clinical and histologic effects of topical treatments of vulval lichen sclerosus, a critical evaluation. J Reprod Med 1993;38:37–40. **(Ib, A)**

18. Goldstein A, Marinoff S, Chistopher K: Pimecrolimus for the treatment of vulvar lichen sclerosus. J Reprod Med 2004;49:778–780. **(III, B)**

19. Kunstfeld R, Reinhard K, Stingl G, et al: Successful treatment of vulvar lichen sclerosus with topical tacrolimus. Arch Dermatol 2003; 139:850–852. **(III, B)**

20. Bohm M, Frieling U, Luger T, et al: Successful treatment of anogenital lichen sclerosus with topical tacrolimus. Arch Dermatol 2003; 139:922–924. **(III, B)**

21. Carli P, Cattaneo A, De Magnis A, et al: Squamous cell carcinoma arising in vulvar lichen sclerosus: a longitudinal cohort study. Eur J Cancer Prev 1995;4:491–495. **(IIb, B)**

22. Carli P, De Magnis A, Mannone F, et al: Vulvar carcinoma associated with lichen sclerosus, experience at the Florence Italy vulvar clinic. J Reprod Med 2003;48:313–317. **(III, B)**

23. Edwards L: Vulvar lichen planus. Arch Dermatol 1989;125:1677–1680. **(III, B)**

24. Edwards L, Friedrich E: Desquamative vaginitis: lichen planus in disguise. Obstet Gynecol 1988;71:832–836. **(III, B)**

25. Anderson M, Kutzner S, Kaufman R: Treatment of vulvovaginal lichen planus with vaginal hydrocortisone suppositories. Obstet Gynecol 2002;100:359–362. **(III, B)**

26. Byrd J, Davis M, Rogers R: Recalcitrant symptomatic vulvar lichen planus, response to topical tacrolimus. Arch Dermatol 2004;140:715–720. **(III, B)**

27. Jensen J, Bird M, LeClair C: Patient satisfaction after the treatment of vulvovaginal erosive lichen planus with topical clobetasol and tacrolimus: a survey study. Am J Obstet Gynecol 2004;190:1759–1765. **(III, B)**

28. Moyal-Barracco M, Lynch P: 2003 ISSVD terminology and classification of vulvodynia. J Reprod Med 2004;49:772–777. **(IV, C)**

29. Friedrich EG: Vulvar vestibulitis syndrome. J Reprod Med 1987; 32:110–114. **(III, B)**

30. Harlow B, Stewart S: A population-based assessment of chronic unexplained vulvar pain: Have we underestimated the prevalence of vulvodynia? JAMA 2003;58:82–88. **(III, B)**

31. Haefner H, Collins M, Davis G, et al: The vulvodynia guideline. J Lower Genital Tract Disease 2005;9:40–51. **(IV, C)**

32. Pyka RE, Wilkinson EJ, Friedrich EG, et al: The histopathology of vulvar vestibulitis syndrome. Int J Gynecol Pathol 1988;7:249–257. **(III, B)**

33. Chadha S, Gianotten WL, Drogendijk AC: Histopathologic features of vulvar vestibulitis. Int J Gynecol Pathol 1998;17:7–11. **(III, B)**

34. Prayson R, Stoler M, Hart W: Vulvar vestibulitis, a histopathologic study of 36 cases, including human papillomavirus in situ hybridization analysis. Am J Surg Pathol 1995;19:154–160. **(III, B)**

35. Lundquist E, Hofer P, Olofsson J: Is vulvar vestibulitis an inflammatory condition? A comparison of histological findings in affected and healthy women. Acta Derm Venereol 1997;77:319–322. **(III, B)**

36. Westrom LV, Willen R: Vestibular nerve fiber proliferation in vulvar vestibulitis syndrome. Obstet Gynecol 1998;91:572–576. **(III, B)**

37. Bohm-Starke N, Hilliges M, Falconer C: Increased intraepithelial innervation in women with vulvar vestibulitis syndrome. Gynecol Obstet Invest 1998;46:256–260. **(III, B)**

38. Edwards L: New concepts in vulvodynia. Am J Obstet Gynecol 2003; 189:S24–S30. **(IV, C)**

# Chapter 17

# Preoperative Evaluation and Postoperative Management

Daniel L. Clarke-Pearson, MD, Monique A. Spillman, MD, PhD, Christopher V. Lutman, MD, and Paula S. Lee, MD, MPH

## KEY POINTS

- Multimodality postoperative pain management usually is optimized by a combination of opioids and nonsteroidal anti-inflammatory drugs (NSAIDs).
- Perioperative antibiotic prophylaxis is effective in reducing postoperative infection in most major abdominal and vaginal procedures.
- The use of low-dose heparin, low-molecular-weight heparins, and external pneumatic compression significantly reduces venous thromboembolic complications in moderate- and high-risk surgery patients.
- Red blood cell transfusion should not be dictated by a single hemoglobin value but rather by the patient's risk of developing complications of inadequate oxygenation.
- Obese patients are at high risk for postoperative complications including obesity hypoventilation syndrome, prolonged mechanical ventilation, aspiration, wound infection and dehiscence, and venous thromboembolism.
- Perioperative care of patients with coronary artery disease is based on maximizing delivery of oxygen to the myocardium as well as decreasing myocardial oxygen utilization.

The successful outcome of gynecologic surgery is based on thorough evaluation, careful preoperative preparation, and attentive postoperative care. Approaches to the general perioperative management of patients undergoing major gynecologic surgery with specific medical problems that could complicate the surgical outcome are discussed in this chapter.

## MEDICAL HISTORY AND PHYSICAL EXAMINATION

Gynecologic surgery should be undertaken only after obtaining a thorough understanding of a patient's medical history and performing a complete physical examination.

The detailed medical history will identify any medical illnesses that might be aggravated by surgery or anesthesia. Coronary artery disease and pulmonary diseases are the most common sources of postoperative complications.

Medications currently being taken (including nonprescription drugs) as well as those discontinued within the month prior to surgery should be recorded. In addition, the use of "alternative therapies," herbs, and vitamins should be elicited. Specific instructions must be given to the patient regarding the need to discontinue any medications prior to surgery (e.g., aspirin, antiplatelet agents) as well as those medications that should be continued (e.g., cardiac or antihypertensive medications).

The patient should be questioned regarding known allergies to medications (e.g., sulfa and penicillin), foods, or environmental agents. A history of sensitivity to shellfish may be the only clue of iodine sensitivity, which can be fatal if intravenous (IV) contrast is used without corticosteroid preparation.

Previous surgical procedures and the patient's course following those surgical procedures should be reviewed to identify previous complications that might be avoided. The patient should be asked about specific complications, such as excessive bleeding, wound infection, deep vein thrombosis, peritonitis, and bowel obstruction. A history of pelvic surgery should alert the gynecologist to the possibility of distorted surgical anatomy and possible preexisting injury to adjacent organ systems such as small bowel adhesions or ureteral stenosis from previous periureteral scarring. In such cases it may be prudent to identify any preexisting abnormality by performing an intravenous pyelogram (IVP) or computed tomography (CT) scan. Many patients may not be entirely clear about the extent of the previous surgical procedure or the details of intraoperative findings. Operative notes from previous operations can be obtained and reviewed.

Family history may identify familial traits that might complicate planned surgery. A family history of excessive intraoperative or postoperative bleeding, venous thromboembolism, malignant hyperthermia, and other potentially inherited conditions should be sought.

A review of systems should be detailed to identify any coexisting medical or surgical conditions. Inquiry about gastrointestinal and urologic function is particularly important prior to undertaking pelvic surgery, since many gynecologic diseases also involve adjacent nongynecologic viscera.

Although many women undergoing gynecologic surgical procedures are otherwise healthy, with disease identified only on pelvic examination, other major organ systems should not be neglected in the physical examination. Identification of abnormalities such as a heart murmur or pulmonary compromise should lead the surgeon to obtain additional testing and consultation in order to minimize intraoperative and postoperative complications.

## Laboratory Evaluation

The selection of appropriate preoperative laboratory studies depends on the extent of the anticipated surgical procedure and the patient's medical status.

For patients undergoing general anesthesia, a blood count including hematocrit, white cell count, and platelet count should be obtained routinely. (For low-risk laparoscopy procedures even a hematocrit may be unnecessary.)

Serum chemistries and liver function testing results are rarely abnormal in the asymptomatic patient who has no significant medical history and who is not taking medications.

Coagulation studies are of little value unless the patient has a significant medical history.[1]

In women under 50 years of age, chest radiography and electrocardiography are of low yield in identifying asymptomatic cardiopulmonary disease and thus are not necessary.[2,3]

Radiographic evaluation of adjacent organ systems should be undertaken in individual cases as follows:

- Intravenous pyelography is helpful to delineate ureteral patency and course, especially in the presence of a pelvic mass, gynecologic cancer, or congenital müllerian anomaly. However, an IVP is not of value in the evaluation of most patients undergoing pelvic surgery.[4]
- A barium enema or upper gastrointestinal series with small bowel assessment may be of value in evaluating some patients before pelvic surgery. Because of the proximity of the female genital tract to the lower gastrointestinal tract, the rectum and sigmoid colon may be involved with benign (endometriosis or pelvic inflammatory disease) or malignant gynecologic conditions. Conversely, a pelvic mass could have a gastrointestinal origin such as a diverticular abscess or Crohn's disease. Clearly, any patient with gastrointestinal symptoms should be further evaluated.
- Other imaging studies, including ultrasound, CT scanning, or magnetic resonance imaging (MRI), may be useful in selected patients.

## PREOPERATIVE DISCUSSION AND INFORMED CONSENT

The goals of the preoperative discussion are to detail issues relevant to the surgery, its expected outcome, and risks and is the basis for obtaining signed informed consent.[5] Informed consent is an educational process for the patient and her family and fulfills the physician's need to convey information in understandable terms. The following items (Table 17-1) should be discussed, and after each item, the patient and family should be invited to ask questions.

1. A discussion of the nature and the extent of the disease process should include an explanation in lay terms of the significance of the disease. Printed materials, computer-based learning programs, and videotapes may assist in this process.
2. The goals of surgery should be discussed in detail. Some gynecologic surgical procedures are performed purely for diagnostic purposes (e.g., dilation and curettage, cold knife conization, diagnostic laparoscopy) although most are aimed at correcting a specific disease process. The extent

| **Table 17-1** |
| --- |
| **Key Topics of Preoperative Informed Consent Discussion** |

1. Nature and extent of the disease process
2. Extent of the actual operation proposed and the potential modifications of the operation, depending on intraoperative findings
3. Anticipated benefits of the operation, with a conservative estimate of successful outcome
4. Risks and potential complications of the surgery
5. Alternative methods of therapy and the risks and results of those alternative methods of therapy
6. Likely results if the patient is not treated

of the surgery should be outlined, including which organs will be removed. Most patients like to be informed about the type of surgical incision and the estimated duration of anesthesia.

3. The expected outcome of the surgical procedure should be explained. If the procedure is being performed for diagnostic purposes, the outcome will depend on surgical or pathologic findings that are not known before surgery. When treating anatomic deformity or disease, the expected success of the operation should be discussed, as well as the potential for failure (i.e., failure of tubal sterilization or the possibility that stress urinary incontinence may not be alleviated). When treating cancer, the possibility of finding more advanced disease and the potential need for adjunctive therapy (e.g., postoperative radiation therapy or chemotherapy) should be mentioned. Other issues of importance to the patient include loss of fertility or loss of ovarian function. These issues should be raised by the physician to ensure that the patient adequately understands the pathophysiology that may result from the surgery and to allow her to express her feelings regarding these emotionally charged issues. Unanticipated findings at the time of surgery should also be mentioned. For example, if the ovaries are unexpectedly found to be diseased, the best surgical judgment may be to remove them.
4. The risks and potential complications of the surgical procedure should be discussed with the patient, including the most frequent complications of the particular surgical procedure. For most major gynecologic surgery, the risks include intraoperative and postoperative hemorrhage, postoperative infection, venous thrombosis, injury to adjacent viscera, and wound complications. If the patient has a preexisting medical problem, additional risks should be reviewed.
5. The usual postoperative course should be discussed in enough detail to allow the patient to understand what to expect in the days following surgery. Information regarding the need for a suprapubic catheter or prolonged central venous monitoring helps the patient accept her postoperative course and avoids surprises that may be disconcerting. The expected duration of the recovery period, both in and out of the hospital, should be outlined.
6. Alternative methods of therapy should be discussed including medical management or other surgical approaches. The patient should also have an understanding of the outcome of the disease if nothing is done.

## PERIOPERATIVE PAIN MANAGEMENT

Current therapeutic strategies for perioperative pain control are largely dependent on opioid analgesics and NSAIDs. Multimodal therapy is recommended in postoperative surgical patients to reduce opioid consumption by coadministration of NSAIDs. This may reduce the side effects of opioid use such as respiratory depression, central nervous system depression and sedation, nausea, vomiting, diminished gastrointestinal motility, and pruritus.

Nonselective NSAIDs inhibit both cyclooxygenase (COX)-1 and COX-2. Potential adverse effects associated with the use of NSAIDs include an increased risk of renal compromise, gastrointestinal side effects, hypersensitivity reactions, and bleeding. The anti-inflammatory and analgesic effects are produced by COX-2 inhibition, whereas gastrointestinal toxicity and platelet dysfunction are caused by COX-1 inhibition. With the development of COX-2 selective inhibitors, several randomized control studies involving both minor and major abdominal surgeries have shown a benefit of preoperative COX-2 selective inhibitor use to reduce acute postoperative pain and perioperative opioid use.[6-8] However, the use of IV NSAIDs such as ketorolac, which has an analgesic potency comparable to morphine, may be more effective than the orally administered COX-2 selective inhibitors.[9] Rofecoxib has been withdrawn from the marketplace after concerns about myocardial risk.

The use of patient-controlled analgesia (PCA) devices shortens the time between the onset of pain and the administration of pain medication, provides more continuous access to analgesics, and allows for an overall steadier state of pain control. Anesthetics and narcotics administered either in the epidural space or intrathecally have greater efficacy than is provided by IV PCA techniques. Epidural analgesia has been shown to be associated with improved pulmonary function postoperatively, a lower incidence of pulmonary complications, a decrease in postoperative venous thromboembolic events, fewer gastrointestinal side effects, a lower incidence of central nervous system depression, and shorter convalescence.[10] Severe respiratory depression is the most serious potential complication, occurring in less than 1% of patients.

## ANTIMICROBIAL PROPHYLAXIS

Gynecologic procedures often involve breaching of the reproductive and gastrointestinal tracts. These locations harbor endogenous flora that are capable of causing polymicrobial infections in the postoperative period. Despite advances in aseptic technique and drug development, bacterial contamination of the operative site and postoperative infections are an inevitable part of the practice of gynecologic surgery.

Infections in the skin or pelvis that result from gynecologic surgery (i.e., parametritis, cuff cellulitis, pelvic abscess) are typically polymicrobial. These infections are complex and often involve gram-negative rods, gram-positive cocci, and anaerobes. Antibiotic prophylaxis should be sufficiently broad as to cover these potential pathogens.[11]

As the number and virulence of bacteria increase within a surgical site, the risk for postoperative infection increases. Excessive tissue injury and foreign material, such as suture and drains, may further increase the risk for infection. Antibiotic prophylaxis is given to the gynecologic surgery patient with the belief that antibiotics can enhance the immune mechanisms in the host tissues that would resist such infections by killing bacteria that inoculate the surgical site at the time of surgery.[12]

The timing of antimicrobial prophylaxis is important. There is a relatively narrow window of opportunity for affecting outcomes.[13] In the United States, it is customary to give antimicrobial prophylaxis shortly before or during the induction of anesthesia. Data have revealed that a delay of 3 or more hours between the time of bacterial inoculation (i.e., skin incision) and administration of antibiotics may result in ineffective prophylaxis. Evidence indicates that for prophylaxis, one dose of antibiotic is appropriate. When the surgical procedure is longer than one to two times the half-life of the drug or blood loss is greater than 1.5 L, the data suggest that additional intraoperative doses of antibiotics maintain adequate levels of drug in serum and tissues. There are no data to support the continuation of prophylactic antimicrobial agents into the postoperative period for routine gynecologic procedures.

The cephalosporins have emerged as the most important class of antimicrobial agents for antimicrobial prophylaxis. These drugs have a broad spectrum and relatively low incidence of adverse reactions. Cefazolin (1 g) appears to be most widely used by gynecologic surgeons in the United States because of its relatively low cost and long half-life. Other cephalosporins, such as cefoxitin, cefotaxime, and cefotetan, are also widely used for prophylaxis. These agents appear to have a broader spectrum of activity against anaerobic bacteria. Most data do not indicate a clinically relevant distinction between cefazolin and the other agents; however, data have emerged from randomized controlled trials indicating that cefotetan and cefotaxime are superior to cefazolin in women undergoing abdominal hysterectomy.[14]

Women undergoing gynecologic surgery who are given antimicrobial prophylaxis may have adverse reactions to this treatment. A single dose of broad-spectrum antibiotic can result in pseudomembranous colitis, caused by *Clostridium difficile*. Diarrhea may develop in as many as 15% of hospitalized patients treated with β-lactam antibiotics. In patients receiving clindamycin, the rate of diarrhea is nearly 30%. These gastrointestinal complications from antibiotics may cause serious morbidity in the surgical patient, and the surgeon should be familiar with recognizing and managing these problems.[15] Anaphylaxis is the greatest life-threatening complication from antibiotic use.

Anaphylactic reactions to penicillins occur in 0.2% courses of treatment. The fatality rate is 0.0001%. Data indicate that it is generally safe to administer cephalosporins to women who report a history of adverse reactions to penicillins. The incidence of adverse reactions (i.e., skin flushing, itching) in women with a history of penicillin allergy who are given cephalosporins is 1% to 10%. The incidence of anaphylaxis in this setting is less than 0.02%.[16]

Not all gynecologic surgery patients need to receive prophylactic antibiotics. The surgeon should choose agents to cover procedures based on available data, thereby avoiding the potential for adverse reactions and minimizing the frivolous use of antibiotics, which may contribute to increased rates of antimicrobial resistance. In patients reporting adverse reactions to

**Table 17-2**
**Antimicrobial Prophylaxis for Gynecologic Surgical Procedures**

| Procedure | Drug |
| --- | --- |
| Hysterectomy (vaginal/abdominal) | 1–2 g IV cefazolin, 2 g IV cefoxitin, 1–2 g IV cefotetan, 1 g IV cefotaxime |
| Hysterosalpingogram | 100 mg doxycycline PO bid for 5 days |
| Abortion/dilation and curettage | 100 mg doxycycline PO 1 hour before procedure, then 200 mg PO after the procedure |
| Cervical conization | No clear recommendations; doxycycline suggested by some authors |
| Colporrhaphy | No clear recommendations; cephalosporins suggested by some authors |
| Laparoscopy (clean) | None |
| Laparotomy (clean) | None |
| Hysterosocopy | None |

the above agents, the surgeon should choose other drugs or combinations that will provide adequate prophylactic coverage. For example, metronidazole and levofloxacin or clindamycin and gentamycin are two alternative broad-spectrum prophylactic regimens in hysterectomy patients that cover anaerobes, gram-positive cocci and gram-negative rods.[17] Some commonly used regimens are listed in Table 17-2.

### Spontaneous Bacterial Endocarditis Prophylaxis

Often, the gynecologic surgeon encounters the issue of endocarditis prophylaxis. Most commonly, a woman will report a history of a murmur or mitral valve prolapse to the surgeon during the preoperative interview. Data clearly indicate that surgeons and dentists in the United States overtreat these women with prophylactic antibiotics meant to prevent endocarditis. The majority of patients who report these cardiac issues are at no increased risk for endocarditis. For example, most patients with mitral valve prolapse or benign murmurs do not require endocarditis prophylaxis at the time of gynecologic surgery. A thorough history and physical examination, coupled with a preoperative echocardiogram and consultation with a cardiologist, will provide detailed assessment of endocarditis risk in these patients.

The American Heart Association (AHA) has published guidelines for physicians and dentists to use in selecting patients and procedures for endocarditis prophylaxis. If the surgeon is uncertain, consultation with a cardiologist is most appropriate. If it appears that the patient would benefit from endocarditis prophylaxis, based on the cardiac lesion and the procedure she will undergo, then the risk is stratified as high or moderate. High-risk patients receive ampicillin or vancomycin *plus* gentamycin in a multidose regimen; moderate-risk patients receive amoxicillin or ampicillin or vancomycin in a single-dose regimen. Low-risk patients require no prophylaxis regardless of the procedure.

Antibiotics administered to prevent surgical site infection are not sufficient for endocarditis prophylaxis; however, some experts feel that antibiotics given for endocarditis prophylaxis

may provide adequate coverage against postoperative infections. This claim may be suspect, however, in the gynecologic surgery patient. Some regimens (e.g., single-dose oral amoxicillin) prescribed for endocarditis prophylaxis in some patients may not provide adequate coverage for flora (gram-negative rods and anaerobes) found in the reproductive or gastrointestinal tracts. The reader is referred to the AHA guidelines for detailed dosing and schedule information on the topic of endocarditis prophylaxis[18] (Table 17-3).

### Bowel Preparation

The structures of the female genital tract lie in close proximity to the small bowel, large bowel, and vermiform appendix. Pathologic conditions such as endometriosis, pelvic inflammatory disease, adnexal cysts, leiomyomata, inflammatory bowel disease, cancer, and prior surgery often give rise to adhesions between genital and gastrointestinal structures. Given the anatomic proximity of these structures and the frequency of involvement between them, the gynecologic surgeon must have an understanding of the available data regarding preoperative bowel preparation.

General surgeons, gynecologists, and gynecologic oncologists often point to numerous potential benefits of mechanical bowel preparation before abdominal or pelvic operations. These include removal of feces, facilitation of intraoperative palpation, ease of packing for pelvic surgery, lowering of the bacterial load, and reduction in spillage or contamination. These are reasonable benefits; however, mechanical bowel preparation is potentially harmful to patients. Patient discomfort, noncompliance, electrolyte abnormalities, and dehydration before major surgery are frequently reported.[19]

Mechanical bowel preparation prior to pelvic surgery can be completed with the use of several commercially available products. Magnesium citrate, polyethylene glycol, and sodium phosphate are each effective in mechanically cleansing the bowel. Effective mechanical cleansing of the gastrointestinal tract can be achieved by combining the agent of choice with a clear liquid diet for 24 hours prior to surgery. Although numerous options for mechanical bowel preparation exist, a randomized trial comparing polyethylene glycol and sodium phosphate found that sodium phosphate was more effective, less expensive, and better tolerated.[20]

**Table 17-3**
**Antimicrobial Prophylaxis for Endocarditis**

| Patient Description | Drug |
| --- | --- |
| Patients at "high risk" for endocarditis | Ampicillin plus gentamicin |
| Patients at "high risk" for endocarditis and allergic to penicillins | Vancomycin plus gentamicin |
| Patients at "moderate risk" for endocarditis | Amoxicillin or ampicillin |
| Patients at "moderate risk" for endocarditis and allergic to penicillins | Vancomycin |
| Patients at "negligible risk" for endocarditis (e.g., mitral valve prolapse without regurgitation) | No antibiotics needed |

Despite dogma, prospective studies have failed to prove the benefit of mechanical bowel preparation. The available prospective data have not shown a decreased risk of wound or abdominal infections.[21] The incidence of anastomotic breakdown was not lowered in patients undergoing preoperative mechanical bowel preparation. These reports have not typically controlled for surgical indications, actual procedures, or other associated comorbidities, so the astute pelvic surgeon will exercise caution interpreting these data. Until these data mature and more randomized, controlled studies are available, it appears prudent to recommend mechanical bowel preparation for patients undergoing pelvic surgery at risk for gastrointestinal complications.

The role for perioperative antibiotics in patients undergoing abdominal or pelvic operations anticipated to involve the gastrointestinal tract remains controversial. A variety of perioperative antibiotic regimens have been proposed and defended. The use of oral, parenteral, and combination prophylaxis is described widely in the literature. The typical oral regimen involves the preoperative administration of neomycin, erythromycin, or metronidazole. Various doses and combinations exist in the literature. The lack of solid data and the increased incidence of preoperative gastrointestinal distress (e.g., nausea and vomiting) seen in patients treated with these preoperative oral antibiotics raise questions about their utility and advisability.

Perioperative parenteral antibiotics are used widely in patients undergoing abdominal operations. A single dose of a broad-spectrum agent (i.e., one that covers anaerobes, gram-positive cocci, and gram-negative rods) given 30 to 60 minutes prior to the operation will provide adequate antibacterial prophylaxis for patients undergoing gastrointestinal operations. Parenteral antibiotics appear to be an adequate substitute for preoperative oral antibiotics. If a lengthy operation is encountered (greater than twice the half-life of the antibiotic) or if blood loss (greater than 1 L) is encountered, the surgeon should consider ordering one or two additional doses of parenteral antibiotics during or after the operation.[22]

## POSTOPERATIVE COMPLICATIONS

### Thromboembolism and Pulmonary Embolism

#### Risk Factors

Deep venous thrombosis (DVT) and pulmonary embolism, although largely preventable, are significant postoperative complications. The magnitude of this problem is relevant to the gynecologist, since 40% of all deaths following gynecologic surgery are directly attributed to pulmonary emboli[23] and they are the most frequent cause of postoperative death in patients with uterine or cervical carcinoma.[24]

The causal factors of DVT were first proposed by Virchow in 1858 and include a hypercoagulable state, venous stasis, and vessel endothelial injury. Risk factors include major surgery; advanced age; nonwhite race; malignancy; history of DVT, lower extremity edema, or venous stasis changes; presence of varicose veins; being overweight; a history of radiation therapy; and hypercoagulable states, such as factor V Leiden; pregnancy; and use of oral contraceptives, estrogens, or tamoxifen. Intraoperative factors associated with postoperative DVT include increased anesthesia time, increased blood loss, and the need for

| Table 17-4 |
| :-- |
| **Thromboembolism Risk Stratification** |

| |
| :-- |
| **Low risk** |
| Minor surgery |
| No other risk factors* |
| **Moderate risk** |
| Age >40 years and major surgery |
| Other risk factors* and major surgery |
| **High risk** |
| Age >60 years and major surgery |
| Cancer |
| History of DVT or PE |
| Thrombophilia |
| **Highest risk** |
| Age >60 and cancer or history of venous thromboembolism |

DVT, deep venous thrombosis; PE, pulmonary embolism.
*Risk factors: obesity; varicose veins; history of DVT or PE; current estrogen, tamoxifen, or oral contraceptive use.

transfusion in the operating room. It is important to recognize these risk factors (Table 17-4) to provide the appropriate level of DVT prophylaxis.[25,26]

#### Thromboembolism Prophylaxis

A number of prophylactic methods have been shown to significantly reduce the incidence of DVT, and a few studies have demonstrated a reduction in fatal pulmonary emboli. The ideal prophylactic method would be effective, free of significant side effects, well accepted by the patient and nursing staff, widely applicable to most patients, and inexpensive.

##### Low-Dose Heparin

The use of small doses of subcutaneously administered heparin for the prevention of DVT and pulmonary embolism is the most widely studied of all prophylactic methods. More than 25 controlled trials have demonstrated that heparin given subcutaneously 2 hours preoperatively and every 8 to 12 hours postoperatively is effective in reducing the incidence of DVT. The value of low-dose heparin in preventing fatal pulmonary emboli was established by a randomized, controlled, multicenter international trial that demonstrated a significant reduction in fatal postoperative pulmonary emboli in general surgery patients receiving low-dose heparin every 8 hours postoperatively.[27] Trials of low-dose heparin in gynecologic surgery patients have shown a significant reduction in postoperative DVT.

Although low-dose heparin is considered to have no measurable effect on coagulation, most large series have noted an increase in the bleeding complication rate, especially a higher incidence of wound hematoma.[28] Although relatively rare, thrombocytopenia is associated with low-dose heparin use and has been found in 6% of patients after gynecologic surgery.[28] If patients remain on low-dose heparin for greater than 4 days it is reasonable to check the platelet count to assess the possibility of occurrence of heparin-induced thrombocytopenia.

# General Gynecology

## Low-Molecular-Weight Heparins

Low-molecular-weight heparins (LMWHs) are fragments of heparin that vary in size from 4500 to 6500 Da. When compared with unfractionated heparin, LMWHs have more anti-Xa and less antithrombin activity, leading to less effect on partial thromboplastin time and possibly to fewer bleeding complications.[29] An increased half-life of 4 hours leads to increased bioavailability when compared with unfractionated heparin. The increase in half-life of LMWHs also allows the convenience of once a day dosing.

Randomized controlled trials have compared LMWH with unfractionated heparin in patients undergoing gynecologic surgery. In all studies, there was a similar incidence of DVT. Bleeding complications[30] were also similar. A meta-analysis of general and gynecologic surgery patients from 32 trials likewise indicated that daily LMWH administration is as effective as unfractionated heparin in DVT prophylaxis with no difference in hemorrhagic complications.

## Mechanical Methods

Stasis in leg veins has been clearly demonstrated while the patient is undergoing surgery and continues postoperatively for varying lengths of time. Stasis occurring in the capacitance veins of the calf during surgery, plus the hypercoagulable state induced by surgery, are the prime factors contributing to the development of acute postoperative DVT. Prospective studies of the natural history of postoperative DVT have shown that the calf veins are the predominant site of thrombi and that most thrombi develop within 24 hours of surgery.[31]

Although probably of only modest benefit, reduction of stasis by short preoperative hospital stays and early postoperative ambulation should be encouraged for all patients. Elevation of the foot of the bed, raising the calf above heart level, allows gravity to drain the calf veins and should further reduce stasis.

**Elastic Stocking.** Controlled studies of graduated pressure stockings are limited but suggest modest benefit when they are carefully fitted.[32] Poorly fitted stockings may be hazardous to some patients, who develop a tourniquet effect at the knee or midthigh.[24] Variations in human anatomy do not allow perfect fit of all patients to available stocking sizes. The simplicity of elastic stockings and the absence of significant side effects are probably the two most important reasons that they are often included in routine postoperative care.

**External Pneumatic Compression.** The largest body of literature dealing with the reduction of postoperative venous stasis deals with intermittent external compression of the leg by pneumatically inflated sleeves placed around the calf or leg during intraoperative and postoperative periods. Various pneumatic compression devices and leg sleeve designs are available, and the current literature does not demonstrate superiority of one system over another. Calf compression during and after gynecologic surgery significantly reduces the incidence of DVT on a level similar to that of low-dose heparin. In addition to increasing venous flow and pulsatile emptying of the calf veins, external pneumatic compression also appears to augment endogenous fibrinolysis, which may result in lysis of very early thrombi before they become clinically significant.[33]

The duration of postoperative external pneumatic compression differs in various trials. External pneumatic compression may be effective when used in the operating room and for the first 24 hours postoperatively[33,34] in patients with benign conditions who will ambulate on the first postoperative day.

External pneumatic compression used in patients undergoing major surgery for gynecologic malignancy reduces the incidence of postoperative venous thromboembolic complications by nearly threefold,[35] but only if calf compression is applied intraoperatively and for the first 5 postoperative days.[36] Patients with gynecologic malignancies may remain at risk because of stasis and hypercoagulable states for a longer period than general surgical patients and therefore appear to benefit from longer use of external pneumatic compression.

External pneumatic leg compression has no significant side effects or risks and is considered slightly more cost-effective than pharmacologic methods of prophylaxis.[37]

## Management of Postoperative Deep Venous Thrombosis

Because pulmonary embolism is the leading cause of death following gynecologic surgical procedures, identification of high-risk patients and the use of prophylactic DVT regimens are an essential part of management.[23,24,38] In addition, the early recognition of DVT and pulmonary embolism and immediate treatment are critical. Most pulmonary emboli arise from the deep venous system of the leg although following gynecologic surgery, the pelvic veins are a known source of fatal pulmonary emboli as well.

The signs and symptoms of DVT of the lower extremities include pain, edema, erythema, and prominent vascular pattern of the superficial veins. These signs and symptoms are relatively nonspecific; 50% to 80% of patients with these symptoms will not actually have DVT.[39] Conversely, approximately 80% of patients with symptomatic pulmonary emboli have no signs or symptoms of thrombosis in the lower extremities.[40] Because of the lack of specificity when signs and symptoms are recognized, additional diagnostic tests should be performed to establish the diagnosis of DVT.

### Doppler Ultrasound

B-mode duplex Doppler imaging is currently the most common technique for the diagnosis of symptomatic DVT, especially when it arises in the proximal lower extremity. With duplex Doppler imaging, the femoral vein can be visualized and clots may be seen directly.[41] Compression of the vein with the ultrasound probe tip allows assessment of venous collapsibility; the presence of a thrombus diminishes vein wall collapsibility. Doppler imaging is less accurate when evaluating the calf venous system and pelvic veins.

### Venography

Although venography has been the "gold standard" for diagnosis of DVT, other diagnostic studies are accurate when performed by a skilled technologist and, in most patients, may replace the need for routine contrast venography. Venography is moderately uncomfortable, requires the injection of a contrast material that may cause allergic reaction or renal injury, and may result in phlebitis in approximately 5% of patients.[42]

### Magnetic Resonance Venography

Magnetic resonance venography (MRV) has a sensitivity and specificity comparable to venography. In addition, MRV may detect thrombi in pelvic veins that are not imaged by venography.[43] The primary drawbacks to MRV are the time involved in examining the lower extremity and pelvis and the expense of this technology.

The treatment of postoperative DVT requires the immediate institution of anticoagulant therapy. Treatment may be with either unfractionated heparin or LMWHs, followed by 6 months of oral anticoagulant therapy with warfarin.

### Unfractionated Heparin

After DVT is diagnosed, unfractionated heparin should be initiated to prevent proximal propagation of the thrombus and allow physiologic thrombolytic pathways to dissolve the clot. After an initial bolus of 5000 units intravenously, continuous infusion of 30,000 units per day should be implemented and dosage adjusted to maintain activated partial thromboplastin time (APTT) level at a therapeutic level 1.5 to 2.5 times the control value. Patients having subtherapeutic APTT levels in the first 24 hours have a risk of recurrent thromboembolism 15 times the risk of patients with appropriate levels. Patients, therefore, should be managed aggressively using IV heparin to achieve prompt anticoagulation. Oral anticoagulant (warfarin) should be started on the first day of heparin infusion. The international normalized ratio (INR) should be monitored daily until a therapeutic level is achieved (INR 2.0 to 3.0). The change in INR resulting from warfarin administration often precedes the anticoagulant effect by approximately 2 days, during which time low protein C levels are associated with a transient hypercoagulable state. Therefore, heparin should be administered until the INR has been maintained in a therapeutic range for at least 2 days, confirming proper warfarin dose. IV heparin may be discontinued in 5 days if an adequate INR level has been established.

### Low-Molecular-Weight Heparin

LMWHs are effective in the treatment of venous thromboembolism and have a cost-effective advantage over IV heparin because they can be administered in the outpatient setting. The dosages used in treatment of thromboembolism are unique and weight adjusted according to each LMWH preparation. Because LMWHs have a minimal effect on APTT, serial laboratory monitoring of PTT levels is not necessary. Similarly, monitoring of anti-Xa activity (except in difficult cases) has not been shown to be of significant benefit in a dose adjustment of LMWH. The increased bioavailability associated with LMWH allows for twice-a-day dosing, potentially making outpatient management for a subset of patients an option. A meta-analysis involving more than 1000 patients from 19 trials suggests that LMWH is more effective, safer, and less costly than unfractionated heparin in preventing recurrent thromboembolism.

### Management of Pulmonary Embolism

Many signs and symptoms of pulmonary embolism are associated with other, more commonly occurring pulmonary complications following surgery. The classic findings of pleuritic chest pain, hemoptysis, shortness of breath, tachycardia, and tachypnea should alert the physician to the possibility of a pulmonary embolism. Many times, however, the signs are more subtle and may be suggested only by persistent tachycardia or a slight elevation in the respiratory rate. Patients suspected of pulmonary embolism should be evaluated initially by chest radiography, electrocardiography, and arterial blood gas assessment. Any evidence of abnormality should be further evaluated by ventilation-perfusion lung scan or a spiral CT scan of the chest. Unfortunately, a high percentage of lung scans may be interpreted as "indeterminate." In this setting, careful clinical evaluation and judgment are required to decide whether pulmonary arteriography should be obtained to document or exclude the presence of a pulmonary embolism.

#### Treatment

1. Immediate anticoagulant therapy, identical to that for the treatment of DVT, should be initiated.
2. Respiratory support, including oxygen and bronchodilators and an intensive care setting, may be necessary.
3. Although massive pulmonary emboli are usually quickly fatal, pulmonary embolectomy has been performed successfully on rare occasions.
4. Pulmonary artery catheterization with the administration of thrombolytic agents bears further evaluation and may be important in patients with massive pulmonary embolism.
5. Vena cava interruption may be necessary in situations in which anticoagulant therapy is ineffective in the prevention of repeat thrombosis and repeat embolization from the lower extremities or pelvis. A vena cava umbrella or filter may be inserted percutaneously above the level of the thrombosis and caudad to the renal veins.
6. In most cases, however, anticoagulant therapy is sufficient to prevent repeat thrombosis and embolism and to allow the patient's endogenous thrombolytic mechanisms to lyse the pulmonary embolus.

## BLOOD COMPONENT THERAPY

Most hematologic problems observed in the postoperative period are related to perioperative bleeding and blood component replacement. Adherence to proper indications for blood component therapy is necessary to avoid potential adverse effects and costs of transfusion. Adverse effects include most commonly nonhemolytic transfusion reactions, rarely hemolytic reactions from incompatible blood, and exposure to infectious diseases including bacterial contamination.

Red blood cell transfusions should not be dictated by a single hemoglobin value but rather by the patient's risk of developing complications due to inadequate oxygenation. Red blood cell transfusion is rarely indicated in hemoglobin concentrations greater than 10 g/dL and is almost always indicated when it is less than 6 g/dL. The determination of whether intermediate hemoglobin concentrations (6 to 10 g/dL) require transfusion should be dependent on clinical assessment. Autologous blood donation has been advocated as a safer alternative for the patient; however, preoperative autologous blood donation is not cost-effective, especially in low-transfusion-risk operations.[44] Furthermore, having preoperative autologous blood may lead to more liberal blood transfusion, iatrogenic anemia, volume overload, and other risks such as hemolytic reactions due to clerical errors and bacterial contamination.[45] The National Heart, Lung, and Blood Institute Expert Panel does not recommend collection of autologous blood for procedures with a likelihood of transfusion less than 10%, such as uncomplicated abdominal and vaginal hysterectomies.[46]

Replacement of platelets and clotting factors in patients with massive transfusion and microvascular bleeding is dependent on clinical and surgical assessments. Guidelines are provided by the American Society of Anesthesiologists task force.[47] Platelet transfusion is rarely indicated for counts greater than 100,000/μL and usually indicated for counts <50,000/μL. With intermediate platelet counts of 50,000/μL to 100,000/μL, transfusion should be based on the risk of bleeding. Fresh-frozen plasma therapy is indicated in massively transfused patients with microvascular bleeding or hemorrhage if the prothrombin or APTT values exceed 1.5 times the normal values. Cryoprecipitate transfusions are recommended for prophylaxis in nonbleeding perioperative patients with fibrinogen deficiencies or von Willebrand's disease refractory to desmopressin, bleeding patients with von Willebrand's disease, and correction of microvascular bleeding in massively transfused patients with fibrinogen concentrations less than 80 to 100 mg/dL.

## MANAGEMENT OF MEDICAL DISORDERS

### Inherited Disorders of Coagulation and Menorrhagia

Menorrhagia is a common gynecologic complaint in reproductive aged women. A specific cause for menorrhagia is identified in less than 50% of affected women.[48] Many of these women are referred for surgical intervention and require a thorough preoperative evaluation for possible inherited disorders of coagulation, such as factor VIII (hemophilia) and factor IX (Christmas disease) deficiencies and von Willebrand's disease. Von Willebrand's disease is a common hereditary bleeding disorder with prevalence in the general population of 0.8% to 1.3%,[49] but in women with menorrhagia, its prevalence is 10% to 18%.[49] Identified women can be treated effectively with desmopressin nasal spray, thus improving quality of life and preventing unnecessary surgical intervention. In addition, unanticipated and excessive bleeding during surgery can be avoided with prophylactic treatment.

A careful medical history identifying a long history of menorrhagia; bleeding after dental procedures, operations, or childbirth; easy bruising; and mucosal bleeding may predict an increased risk of a bleeding disorder. However, women with von Willebrand's disease may present only with easy bruising.[50] In the absence of a genetic diagnosis, the diagnosis of von Willebrand's disease is difficult and involves a combination of clinical and laboratory assessments including von Willebrand factor antigen and von Willebrand factor (vWF) functional activity or ristocetin cofactor assay. Physiologic fluctuations occur with vWF levels, requiring repeated testing and consultation or referral to a hematologist. Nevertheless, it is recommended that women with menorrhagia without obvious uterine or endometrial abnormalities should be routinely screened for inherited bleeding disorders, especially von Willebrand's disease, before undergoing invasive procedures.

### Diabetes

#### Preoperative Assessment and Optimization of Management

According to the American Diabetes Association, 9.3 million American women, or 8.7% of all women older than 20 years have diabetes.[51] The risk is increased 2.4 fold in African American, Hispanic, Native American, and Asian/Pacific Islander women. Prevalence rates of diabetes are 4.7% in non-Hispanic white women, 12.6% of non-Hispanic African American women, and 11.3% in Mexican American women.[52]

In older classification systems, diabetes was classified as childhood or adult-onset diabetes. These classifications have been supplanted by the terminology of insulin-dependent diabetes mellitus (IDDM, type 1) and non-insulin-dependent diabetes mellitus (NIDDM, type 2) with the recognition that either type can occur in any age group. From a practical point of view, patients with NIDDM are managed with oral hypoglycemic agents and those with IDDM require insulin.

Preoperative assessment of patients with diabetes requires knowledge of the patient's routine glucose management regimen, including finger-stick testing regimens and medications.[53] The presence of symptoms of hyperglycemia and hypoglycemia should be documented. Complications of diabetes should also be noted, including nephropathy, neuropathy, and retinopathy. A serum HgbA1$_c$ level should be obtained for independent assessment of long-term blood sugar control in known diabetic patients.

The current recommendations for making a diagnosis of diabetes include the following[54]: (1) random nonfasting blood glucose greater than 200 mg/dL with symptoms of diabetes (polyuria, polydipsia, unexplained weight loss), or (2) fasting plasma glucose greater than 126 mg/dL, or (3) 2-hour post-75 g glucose load with a serum glucose greater than 200 mg/dL. To confirm the diagnosis, one of the above criteria must be verified on a subsequent day. It is imperative that diabetes be controlled before proceeding to the operating room. Referral to internal medicine or endocrine physicians and dietitians is appropriate prior to elective gynecologic surgery.

Diabetic patients are at higher risk of other comorbidities, including coronary heart disease and silent cardiac ischemia, which are discussed in other sections of this chapter.

#### Perioperative and Postoperative Management

Ideally, surgery on the diabetic patient should be accomplished early in the operative day. Type 2 diet-controlled diabetics can safely receive IV fluids that do not contain dextrose, and they should be provided a sliding scale insulin regimen for postoperative management. Type 2 diabetics on oral hypoglycemic regimens should not take their oral hypoglycemic medicines on the morning of surgery. Postoperatively, a sliding scale insulin regimen can be instituted until oral intake is sufficient to resume hypoglycemic medicines.

Type 1 diabetics who require insulin need special consideration. The general heuristic procedure is that one third to one half of the morning NPH insulin should be taken on the day of surgery. The patient will require dextrose-containing IV fluids. For particularly long or complex surgeries, intraoperative assessment of blood glucose levels and administration of subcutaneous or IV insulin may be instituted by the anesthesiologist.

Postoperatively, the hormonal regulation of blood glucose is altered. Insulin production is decreased, and ACTH and glucagon production are increased. The countervailing hormones drive blood sugar levels higher. Insulin must be provided in the postoperative setting to obtain control of blood glucose with a goal of 120 to 200 mg/dL. In the DIGAMI study,[55] tight control of blood glucose contributed to a decreased overall mortality in post–myocardial infarction patients. Elevated postoperative insulin levels contribute to increased risk of infection and delayed wound healing.

At a minimum, blood glucose levels should be obtained every 6 hours in the patient without significant oral intake. Initially, sliding scale insulin may be administered. If sliding scale subcutaneous insulin does not achieve adequate blood glucose control, or if the patient will be receiving corticosteroids, an IV insulin drip should be considered.

For patients with IDDM and elevated blood glucose postoperatively, close monitoring of urine for ketones must be instituted to avoid diabetic ketoacidosis (DKA). If ketones are detected, assessment of serum electrolytes is warranted. The first signs and symptoms of impending DKA may be a drop in serum bicarbonate level and increased respiratory rate. The diagnosis of DKA mandates a search for the predisposing factor, including occult infections of the operative site, wound, urinary tract, respiratory tract, or blood.

Once oral intake has been reliably established, the patient may be gradually switched to the preoperative regimen. Caution must be used in restarting metformin in the setting of significant renal insufficiency, hepatic impairment, or congestive heart failure. Metformin may increase the risk of lactic acidosis. In addition, metformin should be held for 24 to 48 hours before and after the patient has received a CT scan to reduce the likelihood of renal insufficiency developing after contrast dye load.

## Obesity

### Incidence and Definition

Obesity is the new scourge of the American public. Centers for Disease Control and Prevention (CDC) statistics from the year 2000 indicate that 30% of U.S. adults greater than 20 years old are obese—an astounding 59 million adults! If these statistics are expanded to include overweight as well as obese persons, 64% of the U.S. adult population is facing a significant medical problem.[56]

Obesity is defined by the body mass index (BMI). BMI is calculated by dividing the weight in kilograms by the height in centimeters squared. Alternatively, the body weight in pounds is multiplied by 704 and then divided by the height in inches squared. Current American Gastroenterology Association Guidelines[57] use BMI to define classes of obesity. A BMI of 25 to 29.9 is defined as overweight; BMI 30 to 34.9, class I obesity; BMI 35 to 39.9, class II obesity; and BMI over 40 is extreme class III obesity. In practical terms, a 5 ft. 4 in. American woman who is 30 pounds overweight will have a BMI greater than 30, placing her in obesity class I.

### Preoperative Planning

A gynecologic surgeon with an obese patient faces obstacles in both surgical performance and postoperative care. Preoperative imaging may be complicated by lack of a size-appropriate CT or MRI scanner and limitations of ultrasound probe depth penetration. Vaginal ultrasound may offer more detailed infor-

mation than abdominal ultrasound. Obese patients may have multiple medical comorbidities, including diabetes, coronary heart disease, obesity hypoventilation syndrome, and hypertension. Preoperative clearance in consultation with internal medicine, endocrine, and anesthesia colleagues is imperative to optimize preoperative function and postoperative control.

The most important decisions facing the gynecologic surgeon are the timing of the operation and the possibility of referral to a more experienced consultant. Decision to proceed to the operating room should be accompanied by extensive discussion. Part of the preoperative counseling of an obese patient must include the increased risk of operative injury to adjacent structures, wound dehiscence or infection with prolonged wound healing,[58] severe sepsis syndrome, skin ulcers, venous thromboembolism, and increased risk of medical and anesthetic complications, including prolonged intubation. A study of abdominal and vaginal hysterectomy in obese and normal-weight patients found that the obese patients required a longer operating time for both procedures and had greater blood loss during vaginal hysterectomy but otherwise tolerated the procedure as well as the normal-weight patients.[59] Similar results were found with radical hysterectomy for cervical cancer in obese versus normal-weight women, where outcomes were the same but operating time and blood loss were increased in the obese patients.[60] The surgeon should plan ahead with requests for a weight-appropriate operating room bed, extra-long or bariatric surgical instruments, deep retractors, extra assistants, and possibly panniculectomy.[61,62]

Intubation may be exceedingly difficult in the morbidly obese patient.[63] These patients have a decreased functional residual capacity, decreased expiratory reserve volume, decreased compliance of the chest wall, and chronic abnormalities of room air blood gases. The lack of normal anatomic markers, redundant neck folds, small oropharynx, and a poor Mallampati class[64] also increase the risk of failed intubation. Experienced anesthesiologists with availability of fiberoptic intubation or other advanced techniques may increase the safety of the anesthetic induction. Consideration may be given to awake intubation.

### Postoperative Complications and Management

Control of the airway continues as the critical element in the immediate postoperative period.[63] Extubation may not be prudent or possible at the end of the case. If the initial intubation was difficult, tracheal edema may have developed, enveloping the endotracheal tube. Alternatively, the patient may not have the physical capacity to compensate for excess chest wall weight. Many obese patients suffer from the obesity hypoventilation syndrome (OHS), which increases their baseline hypercarbia and may delay extubation. Transfer to a surgical intensive care unit with mechanical ventilation and serial arterial blood sampling will aid in timing of extubation. Postoperative reduction in vital capacity is related more to the degree of obesity than to the site of surgery.[65]

Extubation may also be delayed by intraoperative anesthetic agents that suppress respiratory drive.[66] For this reason, preoperative placement of a regional anesthesia modality such as an epidural may lessen the amount of IV anesthetic agents used and assist with postoperative extubation. Analgesic and anesthetic

241

agents that are fat soluble will continue to slowly release from fat stores for a period time after the operation is finished. Even after extubation, ventilation of the obese patient during sleep may be aided by the use of noninvasive positive pressure ventilation units, particularly if the patient has a history of sleep apnea and uses a continuous positive airway pressure (CPAP) machine at home. Respiratory therapists can be of assistance in patient instruction and management of CPAP machinery in addition to other respiratory toilet.

Postextubation management must heed the higher risk of aspiration[67] in the obese patient. These patients have increased gastric residual volumes, a higher rate of gastroesophageal reflux disease (GERD), and increased intra-abdominal pressure from mass effect. Neutralization of the stomach contents with a proton pump inhibitor can minimize the chemical burn potential of aspirated stomach contents. Gastrointestinal motility agents such as metoclopramide may decrease residual volume by increasing intestinal transit.

Venous access poses another problem.[63] Extreme obesity obliterates anatomic landmarks and makes insertion of peripheral lines, as well as central lines, problematic. Adjunctive visualization technology such as Doppler ultrasound or fluoroscopy increases the accuracy and safety of line placement. Arterial line placement facilitates monitoring of pressures and blood gas parameters. Ideally, central venous lines and arterial lines should be placed intraoperatively by the anesthesia team to insure adequate access in the postoperative period. The intraoperative placement of central lines should be verified for position postoperatively by chest radiography in the post-anesthesia care unit.

Medication administration must take into account total body weight as well as ideal body weight.[63] Certain medications are dosed on ideal body weight (corticosteroids, penicillin, cephalosporins, β-blockers). Others are dosed on total body weight (heparin), and still others based on a calculated "dosing weight" (aminoglycosides, fluoroquinolones, vancomycin). An inpatient pharmacist should be consulted for assistance with proper dosing and monitoring of pharmacotherapy.

## Cardiac Complications

The risk of perioperative cardiac complications such as myocardial infarction in patients with no prior history of coronary artery disease is less than 1%. In contrast, the risk of perioperative infarction is doubled in patients with known or suspected coronary disease. When these complications occur, subsequent cardiac mortality is high. The goal of perioperative cardiac evaluation is to lower perioperative morbidity and mortality by identifying high-risk patients and performing tests that may modify perioperative management and improve long-term benefit.

The history and physical examination of the patient remain the key factors of preoperative risk assessment. A number of risk indices have been developed on the basis of multivariate analysis. The largest and most current scheme of clinical risk assessment for noncardiac surgery is the revised cardiac risk index.[68] The risk of major cardiac events (myocardial infarction, cardiac arrest, pulmonary edema, and complete heart block) range from 0.5% to 9.1% based on the number of risk factors (Table 17-5). Risk factors include high-risk surgical procedures

**Table 17-5**
**Major Cardiac Event Rates by Revised Cardiac Risk Index**

| Class | Events/Patients (No.) | Event Rate (95% CI), (%) |
|---|---|---|
| I (0 risk factors) | 2/488 | 0.4 (0.05–1.5) |
| II (1 risk factor) | 5/567 | 0.9 (0.3–2.1) |
| III (2 risk factors) | 17/258 | 6.6 (3.9–10.3) |
| IV (≥3 risk factors) | 12/109 | 11.0 (5.8–18.4) |

From Lee T, Marcantonio E, Mangione C, et al: Derivation and prospective validation of a simple index for prediction of cardiac risk of major noncardiac surgery. Circulation 1999; 100:1043–1049.

(intraperitoneal, intrathoracic, or suprainguinal vascular reconstruction), history of ischemic heart disease (excluding prior revascularization), history of congestive heart failure, history of transient ischemic attack or stroke, preoperative insulin therapy, and preoperative serum creatinine levels greater than 2.0 mg/dL.

The American College of Cardiology/American Heart Association Practice Guidelines stratify risk assessment into three major categories: (1) clinical predictors, (2) functional capacity, and (3) surgery-specific risk. Clinical predictors of increased perioperative cardiac risk are major, intermediate, and minor factors (Table 17-6). Poor functional capacity is the inability to perform activities that require at least four metabolic equivalents, such as climbing a flight of stairs or walking up a hill. Patients with poor functional capacity have higher perioperative risks, and self-reported exercise tolerance can be used to predict perioperative risk.[69] Surgery-specific risk is subclassified as high risk (emergency major surgery, aortic or vascular procedures, and prolonged surgeries associated with large fluid shifts or blood loss), intermediate risk (other intraperitoneal procedures), and low risk (endoscopies, breast surgery, and superficial procedures). The updated Guidelines[70] present a detailed algorithm that incorporates these factors to guide clinicians to proceed directly to surgery, obtain noninvasive testing, consider coronary angiography, or consider delay of surgery and risk factor modification (Fig. 17-1).

Preoperative testing should be used discriminately in intermediate-risk patients. Controversy exists concerning the accuracy of these tests to provide prognostic information beyond that which is obtained from clinical risk stratification for nonvascular procedures. Stress tests such as exercise electrocardiography, dipyridamole-thallium scintigraphy, and dobutamine echocardiography may provide information on ischemic threshold, maximal tolerated heart rate, and localization and amount of threatened myocardium. Echocardiography can be performed to assess left ventricular dysfunction in patients with current or poorly controlled heart failure, and in valvular heart disease. Coronary angiography should only be considered in patients who have an indication for angiography independent of the planned surgery, such as patients with acute coronary syndromes, unstable angina, angina refractory to medical therapy, or high-risk results on noninvasive testing.

Although the pathophysiologic mechanisms are complex, the causes of myocardial ischemia and infarction are related to

## Table 17-6
### Clinical Predictors of Increased Perioperative Cardiovascular Risk (Myocardial Infarction, Heart Failure, and Death)

**Major**

Unstable coronary syndromes
    Acute or recent myocardial infarction (MI)*
    Unstable or severe angina
Decompensated heart failure
Significant arrhythmia
    High-grade atrioventricular block
    Symptomatic ventricular arrhythmias in the presence of underlying heart
       disease
    Supraventricular arrhythmias with uncontrolled ventricular rate
Severe valvular disease

**Intermediate**

Mild angina
Previous myocardial infarction (>1 month before planned surgery)
Compensated or prior heart failure
Diabetes mellitus
Renal insufficiency

**Minor**

Advanced age
Abnormal electrocardiogram (ECG; left ventricular hypertrophy, left bundle
    branch block, ST-T abnormalities)
Rhythm other than sinus
Low functional capacity
History of stroke
Uncontrolled systemic hypertension

*Recent MI defined as >7 days but ≤30 days; acute MI is within 7 days. If a recent stress test does not indicate residual myocardium at risk, the likelihood of reinfarction after noncardiac surgery is low. It appears reasonable to wait 4 to 6 weeks after MI to perform elective surgery.

From American College of Cardiology/American Heart Association: Guideline update for perioperative cardiovascular evaluation for noncardiac surgery. Executive Summary. Circulation 2002;105:1257–1267.

increases in myocardial oxygen demand coupled with decreased myocardial oxygen supply, alterations in coagulation that may precipitate thrombosis, and changes in vascular tone and endothelial function.[71] Postoperative ischemic events peak on the second and third postoperative days, whereas tachycardia is maximal during days 1 and 2. Conditions leading to decreased myocardial oxygen supply include hypotension, anemia, and hypoxia. Myocardial oxygen consumption may be increased by hypothermia, tachycardia, and hypertension, which occur with stress responses to intubation and emergence from anesthesia, pain, and shifts in intravascular volume.

Perioperative care of patients with coronary artery disease is based on maximizing delivery of oxygen to the myocardium as well as decreasing myocardial oxygen utilization. Patients benefit from maintenance of normothermia, supplemental oxygen, correction of anemia, and effective pain management. In high-risk patients, close hemodynamic monitoring is integral to perioperative management and may require surveillance in an intensive care setting postoperatively. The value of pulmonary artery catheters in high-risk surgical patients is controversial. A randomized, controlled trial of patients undergoing urgent or elective major noncardiac surgery found neither benefit nor harm with pulmonary artery catheters.[72] In this randomized trial, pulmonary catheter use did not decrease perioperative

morbidity or mortality and should no longer be recommended as a risk-reduction strategy in high-risk surgical patients.

Diagnosis of perioperative myocardial infarction includes clinical symptoms, postoperative electrocardiographic changes, and elevation of myocardium-specific enzymes. Electro-cardiograms obtained at baseline, immediately after surgery, and on the first 2 days postoperatively appear to be cost effective in patients with known or suspected coronary artery disease undergoing high-risk procedures.[73] Measurement of cardiac enzymes should be reserved for patients at high risk and those with clinical, electrocardiographic, or hemodynamic evidence of cardiovascular dysfunction.

A meta-analysis of six prospective randomized studies has shown that β-blocker therapy reduces the incidence of peri-operative cardiac complications in patients undergoing non-cardiac surgery.[74] The authors suggest a clinical algorithm that recommends perioperative β-blocker therapy for patients with at least one major or two minor risk factors as defined by the revised cardiac risk index.[68] The timing and optimal duration of β-blocker therapy are uncertain. Current evidence suggests initiating therapy at least 1 week prior to surgery and continuing throughout the hospitalization. For patients receiving β-blockade therapy prior to surgery, therapy should be continued immediately in the perioperative period.

### Pulmonary Complications
#### Preoperative Predictors and Testing

Postoperative pulmonary complications occur in 2% to 80% of cases, depending on the exact definition utilized and the study population.[75] Pulmonary complications can include atelectasis, infection, prolonged mechanical ventilation, bronchospasm, exacerbation of chronic lung disease, pulmonary edema, and pulmonary embolism.[75,76] A previous history of chronic obstructive pulmonary disease (COPD) places the patient at the highest risk of postoperative pulmonary complications, with a relative risk (RR) of 2.7 to 6.0. A previous history of asthma does not significantly raise postoperative pulmonary complication risks unless the patient's peak flow is less than 80% of predicted values. Tobacco smoking in the 2 months prior to surgery increases the odds ratio of pulmonary complications to 2.3.

Many clinical studies using multivariate regression analyses have attempted to define patient risk factors that are strong predictors of postoperative pulmonary complications. Definite risk factors for postoperative pulmonary complications include the following[77]: upper abdominal, thoracic, or abdominal aortic aneurysm surgery; surgical procedure time greater than 3 hours; poor functional status; ASA (American Society of Anesthesiologists) class greater than 2; previous COPD; smoking within 2 months of surgery; and use of pancuronium as an anesthesia agent. Probable risk factors for postoperative complications include general (as opposed to regional) anesthesia, $PaCO_2$ greater than 45 mm Hg, and emergency surgery. Possible risk factors are upper respiratory infection, an abnormal preoperative chest radiograph, and age greater than 70 years.

Patients with COPD must have their pulmonary function maximized preoperatively with regimens that may include inhaled agents such as ipratropium bromide and albuterol as well as systemic and inhaled corticosteroids. Smoking cessation should be urged, possibly with a nicotine replacement regimen.

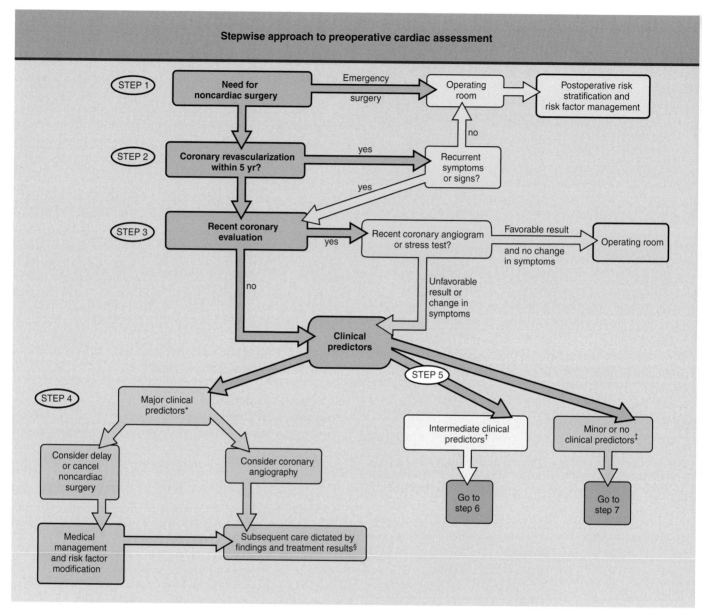

**Figure 17-1    Stepwise approach to preoperative cardiac assessment.** CHF, congestive heart failure; ECG, electrocardiogram; MET, metabolic equivalent; MI, myocardial infarction. *Major clinical predictors: unstable coronary syndromes; decompensated CHF; significant arrhythmias; severe vascular disease. †Intermediate clinical predictors: mild angina pectoris; prior MI; compensated or prior CHF; diabetes mellitus; renal insufficiency. ‡Minor clinical predictors: advanced age; abnormal ECG; rhythm other than sinus; low functional capacity; history of stroke; uncontrolled systemic hypertension. §Subsequent care may include cancellation or delay of surgery, coronary revascularization followed by noncardiac surgery, or intensified care.

Routine treatment with antibiotics is not necessary; however, the presence of purulent sputum should initiate antibiotic treatment.

The optimal tests to assess preoperative pulmonary function and surgical risk are controversial. A chest radiograph is indicated for all patients older than 60 years and for those patients in whom metastatic malignancy is a concern. Obtaining pulmonary function tests preoperatively remains controversial. Pulmonary function tests are indicated in smokers in whom COPD has not yet been diagnosed. Often, a careful physical examination can reveal as much about pulmonary function as formal spirometry.

Auscultation for adventitious respiratory sounds and assessment of the ratio of inspiration time to expiration time may give clues to the need for more formal testing.

### Postoperative Complications

The most common complication facing postoperative gynecologic surgery patients is atelectasis. Large vertical midline incisions are associated with the most pulmonary dysfunction owing to decreased vital capacity and decreased functional residual capacity. Lower abdominal and laparoscopy incisions produce much less pulmonary dysfunction. A second predisposing factor

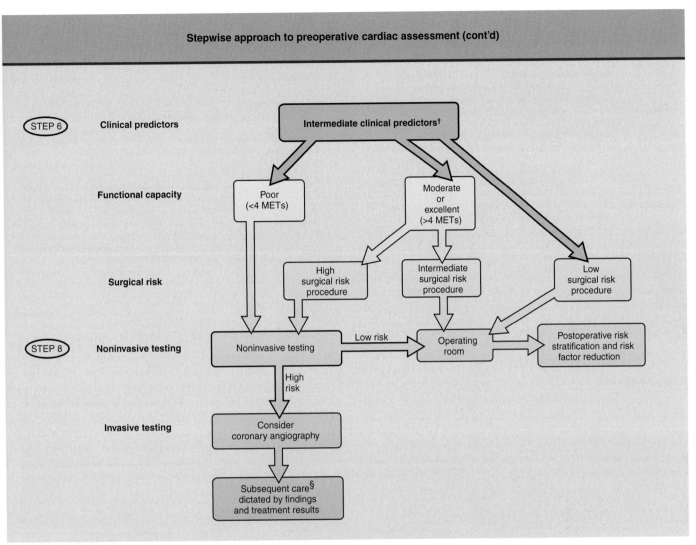

**Figure 17-1, cont'd. Stepwise approach to preoperative cardiac assessment.** CHF, congestive heart failure; ECG, electrocardiogram; MET, metabolic equivalent; MI, myocardial infarction. *Major clinical predictors: unstable coronary syndromes; decompensated CHF; significant arrhythmias; severe vascular disease. †Intermediate clinical predictors: mild angina pectoris; prior MI; compensated or prior CHF; diabetes mellitus; renal insufficiency. ‡Minor clinical predictors: advanced age; abnormal ECG; rhythm other than sinus; low functional capacity; history of stroke; uncontrolled systemic hypertension. §Subsequent care may include cancellation or delay of surgery, coronary revascularization followed by noncardiac surgery, or intensified care. *(Continued)*

is the use of narcotic analgesia with subsequent respiratory depression. The routine use of deep breathing and coughing techniques with incentive spirometry promotes pulmonary toilet. Patients should ideally be instructed in the use of an incentive spirometer preoperatively to optimize postoperative efforts. In high-risk patients (morbidly obese or with preexisting pulmonary disease), aggressive chest physiotherapy and respiratory therapy should be ordered. Adequate pain control postoperatively is important, since movement-evoked pain may significantly affect pulmonary function after hysterectomy.[78]

Pulmonary edema commonly occurs after gynecologic procedures in older women. Strict assessment of intake and output in the critical 24 to 48 hours after surgery should allow for volume assessment. Decrease in pulse oximetry, continued oxygen requirement, and crackles on physical examination are clues to the presence of pulmonary edema. A chest radiograph may show bilateral diffuse edema with the presence of Kerley B lines. Treatment is appropriate fluid management and administration of a diuretic agent.

Pneumonia may result from aspiration or nocosomially acquired infection. The risk of aspiration is greatest around the time of intubation and extubation. However, in patients who are morbidly obese or have Dobbhoff feeding tubes, GERD, postoperative emesis, or indwelling nasogastric suctioning tubes, the risk of aspiration pneumonia rises. On the chest radiograph, the most common side of aspiration pneumonia is the right owing to the more vertical orientation of the right mainstem bronchus. The primary insult to the lung is a chemical pneumonitis for which observation and supportive treatment are appropriate. In rare cases, the chemical pneumonitis will progress to full

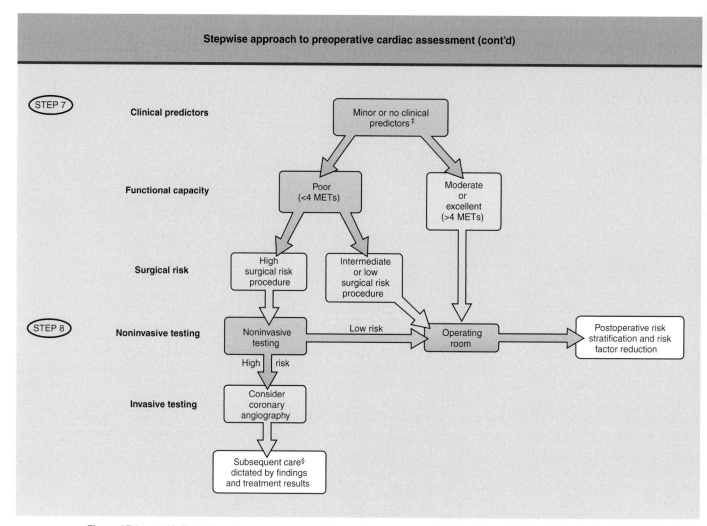

**Figure 17-1, cont'd. Stepwise approach to preoperative cardiac assessment.** CHF, congestive heart failure; ECG, electrocardiogram; MET, metabolic equivalent; MI, myocardial infarction. *Major clinical predictors: unstable coronary syndromes; decompensated CHF; significant arrhythmias; severe vascular disease. †Intermediate clinical predictors: mild angina pectoris; prior MI; compensated or prior CHF; diabetes mellitus; renal insufficiency. ‡Minor clinical predictors: advanced age; abnormal ECG; rhythm other than sinus; low functional capacity; history of stroke; uncontrolled systemic hypertension. §Subsequent care may include cancellation or delay of surgery, coronary revascularization followed by noncardiac surgery, or intensified care. (From American College of Cardiology/American Heart Association: Guideline update for perioperative cardiovascular evaluation for noncardiac surgery. Executive summary. Circulation 2002;105:1257–1267.)

adult respiratory distress syndrome (ARDS), which will require mechanical ventilation and transfer to an intensive care unit. When a secondary infection of aspiration pneumonitis is suspected, broad-spectrum antibiotic coverage should be initiated. Organisms acquired in nosocomial pneumonia infections are aerobic gram-negative species and *Staphylococcus aureus*. These are common in intensive care units, and prolonged intubation increases the risk of colonization and subsequent pneumonia.

Pulmonary embolus is one of the most feared complications of gynecologic surgery. Recognition and treatment of pulmonary emboli are covered in the preceding thromboembolism sections.

## REFERENCES

1. Rohrer M, Michelotti M, Nahrwold D: A prospective evaluation of the efficacy of preoperative coagulation testing. Ann Surg 1989; 208:554–557. **(IIa, B)**
2. Lamers R, van Engelshoven J, Pfaff A: Once again, the routine preoperative thorax photo. Ned Tijdschr Geneeskd 1989;133. **(IIa, B)**
3. Loder R: Routine preoperative chest radiography. Anesthesiology 1987; 66. **(IIa, B)**
4. Piscitelli J, Simel D, Addison W: Who should have intravenous pyelograms before hysterectomy for benign disease? Obstet Gynecol 1987;69:541–545. **(IIb, B)**
5. Easley H, Hammond C: Informed consent in obstetrics and gynecology. Postgrad Obstet Gynecol 1986;10:1–12. **(III, C)**

6. Karamanlioglu B, Turan A, Memis D, Ture M: Preoperative oral rofecoxib reduces postoperative pain and tramadol consumption in patients after abdominal hysterectomy. Anesth Analg 2004; 98:1039–1043. **(Ib, A)**

7. Meyer R: Rofecoxib reduces perioperative morphine consumption for abdominal hysterectomy and laparoscopic gastric banding. Anaesth Intensive Care 2002;30:389–390. **(Ib, A)**

8. Sinatra R, Shen Q, Halaszynski T, et al: Preoperative rofecoxib oral suspension as an analgesic adjunct after lower abdominal surgery: the effects on effort dependent pain and pulmonary function. Anesth Analg 2004;98:135–140. **(Ib, A)**

9. Ng A, Temple A, Smith G, Emembolu J: Early analgesic effects of parecoxib versus ketorolac following laparoscopic sterilization: a randomized controlled trial. Br J Anaesth 2004;92:846–849. **(Ib, A)**

10. Rawal N: Epidural and spinal agents for postoperative analgesia. Surg Clin North Am 1999;79:313–344. **(IIa, B)**

11. Dellinger E, Gross P, Barrett T, et al: Quality standard for antimicrobial prophylaxis in surgical procedures. Infectious Diseases Society of America. Clin Infect Dis 1994;18:422–427. **(III, B)**

12. Tanos V, Rojansky N: Prophylactic antibiotics in abdominal hysterectomy. J Am Coll Surg 1994;179:593–600. **(IIb, B)**

13. Burke JF: Preoperative antibiotic. Surg Clin North Am 1963; 43:665–676. **(IIb, B)**

14. Hemsell D, Johnson E, Hemsell P, et al: Cefazolin is inferior to cefotetan as single-dose prophylaxis for women undergoing elective total abdominal hysterectomy. Clin Infect Dis 1995;20:677–684. **(Ib, A)**

15. McFarland L, Surawicz C, Greenberg R, et al: Prevention of beta-lactam-associated diarrhea by *Saccharomyces boulardii* compared with placebo. Am J Gastroenterol 1995;90:439–448. **(Ib, A)**

16. Idsoe O, Guthe T, Willcox R, de Weck A: Nature and extent of penicillin side-reactions, with particular reference to fatalities from anaphylactic shock. Bull World Health Organ 1968;38:159–188. **(III, B)**

17. Hemsell D: Prophylactic antibiotics in gynecologic and obstetric surgery. Rev Infect Dis 1991;13(Suppl 10):S821–841. **(III, B)**

18. Dajani A, Taubert K, Wilson W, et al: Prevention of bacterial endocarditis: recommendations by the American Heart Association. JAMA 1997;277:1799. **(IIb, B)**

19. Nichols R, Smith J, Garcia R, et al: Current practices of preoperative bowel preparation among North American colorectal surgeons. Clin Infec Dis 1997;24:606–619. **(IV, C)**

20. Zmora O, Pikarsky A, Wexner S: Bowel preparation for colorectal surgery. Dis Colon Rectum 2001;44:1537–2549. **(IV, C)**

21. Zmora O, Mahajna A, Bar-Zakai B, et al: Colon and rectal surgery without mechanical bowel preparation: a randomized prospective trial. Ann Surg 2003;237:363–367. **(1b, A)**

22. American College of Obstetricians and Gynecologists (ACOG): ACOG Practice Bulletin No. 23. Antibiotic prophylaxis for gynecologic procedures. In Compendium of Selected Publications. Washington, DC, ACOG, 2005, pp 294–302. **(IV, C)**

23. Jeffcoate T, Tindall V: Venous thrombosis and embolism in obstetrics and gynecology. Aust N Z J Obstet Gynaecol 1965;5:119–130. **(III, B)**

24. Clarke-Pearson D, Jelovsek F, Creasman W: Thromboembolism complicating surgery for cervical and uterine malignancy: incidence, risk factors, and prophylaxis. Obstet Gynecol 1983;61:87–94. **(IIb, B)**

25. Clayton J, Anderson J, McNicol G: Preoperative prediction of postoperative deep vein thrombosis. BMJ 1976;2:910–912. **(IIb, B)**

26. Clarke-Pearson D, DeLong E, Synan I, et al: Variables associated with postoperative deep venous thrombosis: a prospective study of 411 gynecology patients and creation of a prognostic model. Obstet Gynecol 1987;69:146–150. **(IIa, B)**

27. Kakkar V: Prevention of fatal postoperative pulmonary embolism by low dose heparin: an international multicenter trial. Lancet 1975; 2:145–151. **(Ib, A)**

28. Clarke-Pearson D, DeLong E, Synan I, Creasman W: Complications of low-dose heparin prophylaxis in gynecologic oncology surgery. Obstet Gynecol 1984;64:689–694. **(Ib, A)**

29. Tapson V, Hull R: Management of venous thromboembolic disease: the impact of low-molecular-weight heparin. Chest 1995;16:281–294. **(Ia, A)**

30. Haas S: Recommendations for prophylaxis of venous thrombo-embolism: International Consensus and the American College of Chest Physicians Fifth Consensus Conference on antithrombotic therapy. Curr Opin Pulm Med 2000;6:314–320. **(IV, C)**

31. Clarke-Pearson D, Synan I, Coleman R, et al: The natural history of postoperative venous thromboembolism in gynecologic oncology: a prospective study of 283 patients. Am J Obstet Gynecol 1984; 148:1051–1054. **(Ib, A)**

32. Scurr J, Ibrahim S, Faber R, Le Quesne L: The efficacy of graduated compression stocking in the prevention of deep vein thrombosis. Br J Surg 1977;64:371–373. **(Ib, A)**

33. Salzman E, Ploet J, Bettlemann M, et al: Intraoperative external pneumatic calf compression to afford long-term prophylaxis against deep vein thrombosis in urological patients. Surgery 1980;87:239–242. **(Ib, A)**

34. Nicolaides A, Fernandes E, Fernandes J, Pollock A: Intermittent sequential pneumatic compression of the legs in the prevention of venous stasis and postoperative deep venous thrombosis. Surgery 1980;87:69–76. **(Ib, A)**

35. Clarke-Pearson D, Synan I, Hinshaw W, et al: Prevention of postoperative venous thromboembolism by external pneumatic calf compression in patients with gynecologic malignancy. Obstet Gynecol 1984;63:92–98. **(Ib, A)**

36. Clarke-Pearson D, Creasman W, Coleman R, et al: Perioperative external pneumatic calf compression as thromboembolism prophylaxis in gynecologic oncology: report of a randomized controlled trial. Gynecol Oncol 1984;18:226–232. **(Ib, A)**

37. Maxwell G, Myers E, Clarke-Pearson D: Cost-effectiveness of deep venous thrombosis prophylaxis in gynecologic oncology surgery. Obstet Gynecol 2000;95:206–214. **(Ia, A)**

38. Creasman W, Weed JJ: Radical hysterectomy. In Schaefer G, Grager E (eds): Complications in Obstetrics and Gynecology Surgery. Hagerstown, Md, Harper and Row, 1981, pp 389–398. **(IV, C)**

39. Haegger K: Problems of acute deep vein thrombosis. Angiolology 1969; 20:219–222. **(IIb, B)**

40. Palko P, Namson E, Fedonik S: The early detection of deep venous thrombosis using $^{135}$I-tagged fibrinogen. Can J Surg 1964;7:215–220. **(IIb, B)**

41. Lensing A, Pradoni P, Bandjes D, et al: Detection of deep-vein thrombosis by real-time B-mode ultrasonography. N Engl J Med 1989;320:342–348. **(IIb, B)**

42. Athanasoulis C: Phlebography for the Diagnosis of Deep Leg Vein Thrombosis, Prophylactic Therapy of Deep Venous Thrombosis and Pulmonary Embolism. DHEW Publication No. 76-886. Washington, DC, National Institutes of Health, 1975, pp 62–76. **(IV, C)**

43. Montgomery K, Potter H, Helfet D: Magnetic resonance venography to evaluate the deep venous system of the pelvis in patients who have acetabular fracture. J Bone Joint Surg 1995;77:1639–1649. **(IIb, B)**

44. Etchason J, Petz L, Keeler E, et al: The cost effectiveness of pre-operative autologous blood donations. N Engl J Med 1995;332: 719–724. **(Ib, A)**

45. Kanter M, van Maanen D, Anders K, et al: Preoperative autologous blood donations before elective hysterectomy. JAMA 1996;276:798–801. **(Ib, A)**

46. National Heart, Lung, and Blood Institute Expert Panel on the Use of Autologous Blood: Transfusion alert: use of autologous blood. Transfusion 1995;35:701–711. **(Ia, A)**

47. American Society of Anesthesiologists: Practice guidelines for blood component therapy. Anesthesiology 1996;84:732–747. **(IV, C)**

48. Rees M: Menorrhagia. BMJ 1987;294:759–762. **(IV, C)**

49. Shankar M, Lee C, Sabin C, et al: Von Willebrand disease in women with menorrhagia: a systematic review. BJOG 2004;111:737–740. **(Ia, A)**

50. Kadir R, Economides D, Sabin C, et al: Frequency of inherited bleeding disorders in women with menorrhagia. Lancet 1998;351:485–489. **(IIa, B)**

51. American Diabetes Association. National diabetes factsheet. Available at http://www.diabetes.org/diabetes-statistics/national-diabetes-fact-sheet.jsp. Accessed 9/6/04.

52. American Heart Association. Women and cardiovascular diseases. Statistics (revised). Updated 2005. Available at http://www.americanheart.org/downloadable/heart/1109000876764FS10WM05 REV.DOC. Accessed 9/17/05. **(IV, C)**

53. Khan NA, Ghali WA: Perioperative management of diabetes mellitus. In Rose BD (ed): Up to Date. Vol 12.2. Wellesley, Mass, Up to Date, 2004. **(IV, C)**

54. American Diabetes Association. Diagnosis and classification of diabetes mellitus. Available at http://www.guideline.gov/summary/summary.aspx?doc_id=6575&nbr=004135&string=diabetes. Accessed 9/6/04.

55. Malmberg K, Ryden L, Efendic S, et al. Randomized trial of insulin-glucose infusion followed by subcutaneous insulin treatment in diabetic patients with acute myocardial infarction (DIGAMI study): effects on mortality at 1 year. J Am Coll Cardiol 1995;26:57–65. **(Ib, A)**

56. Centers for Disease Control and Prevention. Overweight and obesity. Frequently asked questions. Available at http://www.cdc.gov/nccdphp/dnpa/obesity/faq.htm. Accessed 9/5/04. **(IV, C)**

57. Klein S, Wadden T, Sugerman H: AGA technical review on obesity. Gastroenterology 2002;123:882–932. **(IV, C)**

58. Gallup D, Gallup D, Nolan T, et al: Use of a subcutaneous closed drainage system and antibiotics in obese gynecologic patients. Am J Obstet Gynecol 1996;175:358–361. **(Ib, A)**

59. Rasmussen K, Neumann G, Ljungstrom B, et al: The influence of body mass index on the prevalence of complications after vaginal and abdominal hysterectomy. Acta Obstet Gynecol Scand 2004;83:85–88. **(Ib, A)**

60. Soisson A, Soper J, Berchuck A, et al: Radical hysterectomy in obese women. Obstet Gynecol 1992;80:940–943. **(IIa, B)**

61. Hopkins M, Shriner A, Parker M, Scott L: Panniculectomy at the time of gynecologic surgery in morbidly obese patients. Am J Obstet Gynecol 2000;182:1502–1505. **(IIa, B)**

62. Pearl M, Valea F, Disilvestro P, Chalas E: Panniculectomy in morbidly obese gynecologic oncology patients. Int J Surg Invest 2000;2:59–64. **(IIa, B)**

63. Savel R, Gropper M, Maceva J, Lazzaro R: Management of the critically ill bariatric patient. 1. In Rose BD (ed): Up to Date. Vol 12.2. Wellesley, Mass, Up to Date, 2004.**(IV, C)**

64. Mallampati S, Gatt S, Gugino L, et al: A clinical sign to predict difficult tracheal intubation: a prospective study. Can Anaesth Soc J 1985;32:429–434. **(Ib, A)**

65. Von Ungern-Sternberg B, Regli A, Schneider M, et al: Effect of obesity and site of surgery on perioperative lung volumes. Br J Anaesth 2004;92:202–207. **(IIa, B)**

66. Vasilev SA: Perioperative and Supportive Care in Gynecologic Oncology. New York, Wiley-Liss, 2000. **(IV, C)**

67. Savel R, Gropper M, Maceva J, Lazzaro R: Management of the critically ill bariatric patient. 2. In Rose BD (ed): Up to Date. Vol 12.2. Wellesley, Mass, Up to Date, 2004.**(IV, C)**

68. Lee T, Marcantonio E, Mangione C, et al: Derivation and prospective validation of a simple index for prediction of cardiac risk of major noncardiac surgery. Circulation 1999;100:1043–1049. **(Ib, A)**

69. Reilly D, McNeely M, Doerner D, Greenberg D: Self-reported exercise tolerance and the risk of serious perioperative complications. Arch Intern Med 1999;159:2185–2192. **(III, B)**

70. American College of Cardiology/American Heart Association: Guideline update for perioperative cardiovascular evaluation for noncardiac surgery. Executive summary. Circulation 2002;105:1257–1267. **(IV, C)**

71. Mangano D: Perioperative cardiac morbidity. Anesthesiology 1990;72:153–184. **(Ib, A)**

72. Sandham JD, Hull RD, Brant RF, et al: A randomized, controlled trial of the use of pulmonary-artery catheters in high-risk surgical patients. N Engl J Med 2003;348:5–14. **(Ib, A)**

73. Charlson ME, MacKenzie C, Ales K, et al: Surveillance for postoperative myocardial infarction after noncardiac operations. Surg Gynecol Obstet 1988;167:404–414. **(Ib, A)**

74. Auerbach AD, Goldman L: β-Blockers and reduction of cardiac events in noncardiac surgery: scientific review. JAMA 2002;287:1435–1444. **(Ia, A)**

75. Conde MS, Im SS: Overview of the management of postoperative pulmonary complications. 1. In Rose BD (ed): Up to Date. Vol 12.2. Wellesley, Mass, Up to Date, 2004. **(IV, C)**

76. Smetana GW: Evaluation of preoperative pulmonary risk. In Rose BD (ed): Up to Date. Vol 12.2. Wellesley, Mass, Up to Date, 2004.

77. Smetana GW: Preoperative pulmonary Eevaluation. N Engl J Med 1999;340:937–944. **(Ib, A)**

78. Gilron I, Tod D, Goldstein D, et al: The relationship between movement-evoked versus spontaneous pain and peak expiratory flow after abdominal hysterectomy. Anesth Analg 2002;95:1702–1707. **(Ib, A)**

# Chapter 18

# Vulvovaginal Infections

Sebastian Faro, MD, PhD

## KEY POINTS

- Infection of the vulva is common; the two categories are skin flora and sexually transmitted disease.
- Erythematous lesions do not always indicate infection.
- Lesions that persist should be studied histologically.

## INTRODUCTION

The vulva and vagina constitute two distinct ecologic niches. The vulva is covered by a thick and fairly resistant dermis and is subjected to a variety of environmental substances like soaps, creams, and ointments, as well as trauma, such as scratching or the placing into the vagina of a variety of instruments either for the introduction of medications or for pleasure. The vulva is inhabited by a microbial flora that, for the most part, maintains a commensal relationship with the host. Infections of the vulva and vulvar organs occur following breaks in the dermis, which allow resistant bacteria to gain entrance to the deeper tissue and cause infection. Infection can also occur following introduction of exogenous bacteria into the deeper tissues or glands of the vulva. An intact dermis and resident microflora limit the use of topical agents that can alter the normal flora and eliminate trauma that results in breaks in the skin, which can prevent vulvar infections.

Vaginal infections and alterations in the resident or endogenous microflora occur at alarming rates. Our understanding of factors and conditions that result in the development of vaginitis, vaginosis, or significant alterations in the vaginal environment are poorly understood. The basis of most alterations of the endogenous microflora, excluding the introduction of bacteria into the vaginal ecosystem, is recognition that the vaginal microflora is a complex biosphere and consists of a variety of gram-negative and gram-positive bacteria including aerobic, facultative, and obligate anaerobic bacteria. A healthy vaginal ecosystem is achieved through a variety of biologic activities that maintain *Lactobacillus* as the dominant bacterium and suppress the numerous nonpathogenic and pathogenic bacteria.

Infection occurring anywhere in the body is caused primarily by the host's endogenous bacteria or pathogens that constitute part of the normal microflora. Normally, the pathogens that reside on the skin do not cause infection unless the dermis is broken (microscopic or macroscopic disruption) and bacteria gain entrance to the deeper tissues. The deeper tissues, in contrast to the dry dermis, provide nutrients that allow the bacteria to grow. Infection occurs when bacteria invade a sterile site, adhere to cells and invade host cells, or enter the bloodstream. Subsequently the bacteria reproduce and spread to adjacent cells or distant organs. Thus, the development of infection is an orderly process that can be divided into the following steps:

1. Establishment of an initial inoculum that overwhelms the local host defenses
2. Invasion and adherence to host cells
3. Reproduction of bacteria
4. Migration to adjacent tissues or entrance into the blood stream or distant organs
5. Ability to overcome host defenses

## SOFT TISSUE INFECTIONS

Soft tissue infections of the vulva and vagina are frequently minor but under certain circumstances, such as in the diabetic patient, trauma to the vulva, and minor infections that go unnoticed, they can become associated with major morbidity and mortality. Usually, infections of the vulva are secondary to trauma of the skin, for example, scratching or nicking of the skin during depilation (especially shaving). Infection spreads from the dermis to the deeper tissues and can involve the fascia and muscle.

### Pyoderma

The most common bacteria to cause pyoderma are coagulase-positive staphylococci or hemolytic streptococci. *Staphylococcus epidermidis*, *Staphylococcus hominis*, and *Staphylococcus haemolyticus* are commonly found in areas where there are apocrine glands (e.g., axillae, vulva, inguinal and perianal areas).[1,2] Although these bacteria frequently cause vulvar pyoderma, folliculitis, furuncles, and carbuncles because of the vulva's close proximity to the vagina and rectum, other bacteria endogenous to these two areas should be considered possible causes of infection. Pyoderma is a pyogenic infection of the skin, the hair follicle and its associated glands, or the deeper dermis.

*Pyoderma* is a nonspecific term used to denote a localized purulent skin infection caused by *Staphylococcus aureus* or group A streptococci (*Streptococcus pyogenes*). Infection caused by either of these bacteria is indistinguishable on clinical presentation. However, infection caused by *S. aureus* is characterized by its rapid progression to deeper tissues, resulting in cellulitis.[3] Identification of the bacterium can be only established by obtaining a specimen for Gram staining, culture, and identification.

Antibiotic sensitivities should be obtained on the bacterial isolate. Because of the possibility that bacteria from the vagina and rectum can also cause infection of the vulvar skin, two specimens should be obtained for culture and placed in an anaerobic and aerobic transport system. Gram's stain can differentiate between *Staphylococcus* and *Streptococcus*, but it cannot identify the species. Cases of impetigo have been reported where both *S. aureus* and *S. pyogenes* skin and soft tissue have been reported as coinfecting bacteria.[4,5] If the Gram stain reveals a mixture of gram-positive and gram-negative bacteria, the infection should be considered polymicrobial, and the presence of obligate anaerobic bacteria should be considered when treatment is administered.

## Erysipelas

Erysipelas is an infection involving the skin but not the subcutaneous tissue found in patients with cellulitis. In addition to *S. aureus* and *S. pyogenes*, *Streptococcus agalactiae* solely or in combination with *S. aureus* can cause skin infections of the vulva. Erysipelas and cellulitis usually arise secondary to trauma of the tissue (e.g., abrasions secondary to scratching). The initial lesion is the development of an erythematous area associated with pain. There also may be central necrosis as the disease process progresses. Patients with erysipelas or cellulitis can develop systemic disease (i.e., bacteremia and sepsis); therefore, administration of antibiotic therapy should not be delayed.

## Folliculitis

Folliculitis is an infection that originates in a hair follicle from bacteria that reside permanently or transiently on skin appendages (Fig. 18-1). The bacterium most commonly associated with folliculitis is *S. aureus*. Other bacteria from the vagina and rectum can cause folliculitis. In patients with recurrent infection, specimens should be obtained from the lesion and cultured for aerobic, facultative, and obligate anaerobic bacteria. Folliculitis typically presents as a central pustule in a hair follicle surrounded by a narrow erythematous base. If folliculitis is widely distributed over the patient's body, the possibility of

"hot-tub folliculitis" or "swimmer's itch" is considered. "Hot-tub folliculitis" is associated with bathing in poorly chlorinated water at 98.6°F to 104°F, and is caused by *Pseudomonas aeruginosa*.[6] This is a rare infection contracted from recreational or therapeutic use of improperly chlorinated hot tubs, whirlpools, and swimming pools. Clinically the disease presents with painful, papulopustular skin lesions, low-grade fever, and malaise. The infection usually is self-limiting, but it has been associated with serious disseminated disease (e.g., bacteremia and septic shock).

Folliculitis can advance to a subcutaneous abscess that is referred to as a furuncle or "boil." This is usually self-limiting, drains spontaneously, and resolves without requiring antibiotic or surgical intervention (Figs. 18-2 and 18-3). However, if a group of furuncles coalesce, a large, painful, swollen, erythematous, indurated mass with a large central pustule develops. The central pustule is typically a solid core of coagulated pus. Resolution of a carbuncle is accomplished by the administration of antibiotic therapy, especially if the patient is febrile, and surgical incision to remove the central core and drain any pus that may be behind the central core. The abscess cavity should be thoroughly irrigated with either an antibiotic solution (bacitracin 50,000 units plus kanamycin 1 g in 1 L of normal saline). All necrotic tissue should be débrided, and the abscess cavity should be packed with iodoform gauze. The packing should be removed in 24 to 48 hours and the defect allowed to close spontaneously. Antibiotic therapy should be continued until the lesion has healed.

## Hidradenitis Suppurativa

Hidradenitis suppurativa (also known as Verneuil's disease, acne inverse, and pyoderma fistulans) is a chronic inflammatory disease involving the axillae, inguinal area, vulva, and anogenital area. It can also occur in the breast, under the breast, and in sacral areas. Women are affected more frequently than men, by approximately three to one.[7] The etiology is unknown; however, it is a complex disease that has genetic, hormonal, inflammatory, and infection components.[8,9] The disease process appears to be initiated by occlusion of a hair follicle, resulting in blockage of apocrine gland contents. Bacteria trapped below the occlusion infect the apocrine gland, which results in an intense inflammatory response and the development of an abscess. Bacterial involvement is a secondary feature of hidradenitis, and antibiotic therapy appears to be effective only in early and mild disease. Once the disease has become well established and is chronic, antimicrobial therapy is ineffective.

The infection component of hidradenitis suppurativa appears to be polymicrobial, involving at least two bacteria, with *S. aureus* playing a major role[10–12] (Table 18-1).

### Treatment

Various treatment modalities have been described. However, the mainstay of treatment is surgical excision of the entire lesion and the tracts that develop as the disease progresses. When administered early in the disease process, antibiotic therapy appears to be beneficial if one or two lesions are present. Prior to institution of antibiotic therapy, a specimen should be obtained from the lesion via aspiration or swab. Specimens should be obtained for the isolation of facultative and obligate anaerobic

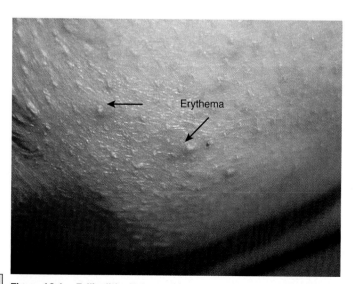

**Figure 18-1  Folliculitis.** Note pustules surrounded by erythematous base.

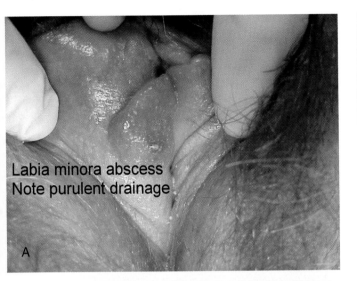

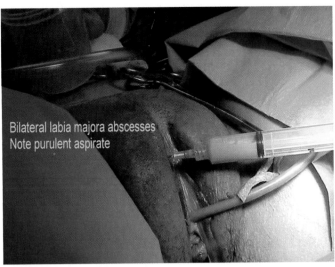

Figure 18-3   **Bilateral labia majora abscesses.** Note purulent aspirate.

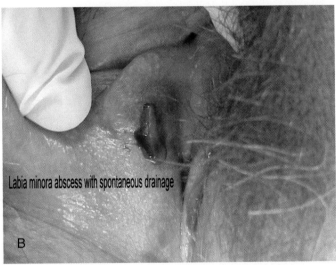

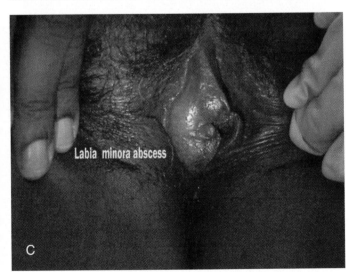

Figure 18-2   *A,* Labia minora abscess (*right*). Note necrotic center, surrounding erythema, and swelling. *B,* Purulent drainage. *C,* Totally intact abscess on the labia minora.

bacteria. Although the infection may be caused by a single bacterium (e.g., *S. aureus*), it is also likely that the infectious component is polymicrobial. Therefore, empirical administration of antibiotics should provide broad antibacterial coverage, for example, metronidazole plus a quinolone or clindamycin plus a quinolone; a cephalosporin may be substituted for a quinolone. However, if metronidazole is used with a quinolone, such as levofloxacin, the latter would be preferred to a first-generation cephalosporin in an attempt to provide better coverage against *S. aureus*. A specimen for culture should be obtained because if community-acquired *S. aureus* is present, it is likely to be methicillin resistant (MRSA) and may be resistant to the quinolones. Therefore, the sensitivity pattern of the isolate is important to direct the appropriate administration of antibiotic therapy. However, when the disease progresses to the stage where multiple lesions are present and chronically recurring, antibiotic therapy neither arrests the disease nor results in resolution of the disease process. Antibiotic therapy should be instituted prior to performing surgery on these patients in order to provide adequate levels of antibiotic in the tissue surrounding the involved areas.

Oral isotretinoin (Accutane) demonstrated a positive effect in 50% of patients tested.[13] Acitretin administered in a dose of 25 mg twice a day also seems to be effective, but studies are

| Table 18-1 Bacteria Involved in Hidradenitis Suppurativa | |
| --- | --- |
| **Gram-Positive Organisms** | **Gram-Negative Organisms** |
| *Staphylococcus aureus* | *Acinetobacter* |
| *Staphylococcus epidermidis* | *Pseudomonas aeruginosa* |
| *Staphylococcus hominis* | *Bacteroides* |
| *Streptococcus milleri* | *Fusobacterium* |
| *Streptococcus pyogenes* | *Prevotella* |
| *Propionibacterium acnes* | |
| *Peptostreptococcus* | |
| *Corynebacterium* | |
| *Lactobacillus* | |

limited.[14,15] Administration of isotretinoin is recommended for patients several weeks prior to surgery and should be continued for several weeks after surgery.[16]

Infliximab and etanercept are immunosuppressive agents that block tumor necrosis factor alpha (TNF-α) and have been used to treat inflammatory diseases such as Crohn's disease, psoriasis, and rheumatoid arthritis.[17] Infliximab is a monoclonal antibody with an affinity for TNF-α. It is hypothesized that TNF-α induces proinflammatory cytokines that may play a role in a number of inflammatory conditions, such as hidradenitis suppurativa. Infliximab was administered for the treatment of hidradenitis in a small number of patients, who responded favorably.[18] It is plausible that immunosuppressive agents such as infliximab and etanercept may be useful in the treatment of hidradenitis.

The surgical approach for hidradenitis has included laser ablation, curettage, skinning techniques followed by skin grafts, simple drainage, simple excision with primary closure, simple excision with secondary closure, radical excision with primary closure, radical excision with secondary closure, and radical excision of the lesions and skin grafts. The surgical approach appears to have the best effect on the natural history of severe hidradenitis suppurativa.[19] In a study of 82 patients treated with radical surgical excision, the recurrence rates 3 to 72 months following surgery were as follows: axillary 3%, perianal 0%, inguinoperineal 37%, and submammary 50%.[20] In a study of 106 patients with chronic hidradenitis suppurativa treated with wide surgical excision, 2.5% of the patients experienced a recurrence.[21] In this study, 17.8% of the patients experienced minor complications (e.g., superficial suture dehiscence, post-operative bleeding, and hematoma formation), and 3.7% of the patients developed a wound infection.[21] Prior to institution of any therapy, the patient should be informed that hidradenitis suppurativa is a chronic condition and recurrences are likely to occur. All excised specimens should be submitted for histologic analysis because of the possibility of squamous cell carcinoma and verrucous carcinoma arising in areas of hidradenitis suppurativa, especially anogenital hidradenitis suppurativa.[22,23]

## BARTHOLIN'S GLAND ABSCESS

A Bartholin abscess can be differentiated from a Bartholin cyst by the clinical characteristics listed in Table 18-2 and illustrated in Figures 18-4 and 18-5. For a patient with a Bartholin cyst, specimens should be obtained from the endocervix to identify the presence of *Chlamydia trachomatis* and *Neisseria gonorrhoeae*.

For a Bartholin abscess, the surface of both the skin and the vagina should be cleansed with betadine prior to performing marsupialization of the abscess, an incision, drainage, or placement of a Word catheter. A needle should then be inserted at the center of the gland along the vermilion border. A portion of the aspirated pus should be placed into each of the following: one vial containing appropriate transport medium for the isolation of obligate anaerobic bacteria, one vial for the isolation of facultative anaerobic bacteria, and one vial for the detection of *C. trachomatis*; the remaining pus should be sent for Gram staining.

If a Word catheter is to be used, a stab incision with a No. 15 scalpel blade is made. The purulent contents of the abscess

| Table 18-2 |
|---|
| **Differentiation Between Bartholin Abscess and Bartholin Cyst** |

| Bartholin Abscess | Bartholin Cyst |
|---|---|
| Gland is enlarged | Gland is enlarged |
| Erythema is present in skin overlying and surrounding the gland | No erythema |
| Skin overlying the gland typically feels warm to the touch | No increase in temperature |
| Fever is present, especially if there is tachycardia | No fever |
| An advancing cellulitis can be present | No cellulitis |
| WBC count is elevated | No elevation in WBC count |
| Bacteria and WBCs are present in fluid (pus) contained within Bartholin's gland | No bacteria or WBCs present in fluid (serous fluid contained within the cyst) |

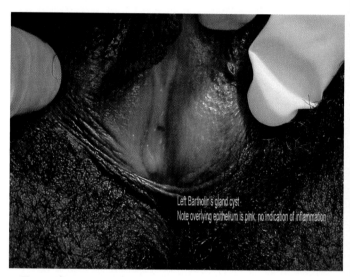

**Figure 18-4  Bartholin cyst.** The tissue overlying the gland is pink.

should be completely drained and the gland irrigated with sterile saline until the effluent is clear. The Word catheter is placed into the gland through the stab incision and the balloon is distended with saline. The balloon should not be distended with air because it will not remain distended and the catheter will fall out. The catheter should be left in place until it falls out spontaneously, which usually occurs after 3 to 6 weeks. The patient should also be placed on an antibiotic regimen that provides activity against *C. trachomatis*, *N. gonorrhoeae*, and gram-positive and gram-negative facultative and obligate anaerobic bacteria, for example, metronidazole 500 mg every 8 hours plus levofloxacin 500 mg every 24 hours orally for 7 to 10 days. The patient should be reevaluated within 3 weeks and again at 6 weeks. The patient should be directed to monitor her temperature, and if she develops an oral temperature above 100.4°F, shaking, chills, nausea, or flu-like symptoms, she should call her physician and be evaluated.

## VULVOVAGINAL CANDIDIASIS

Vulvovaginal candidiasis is probably the most common condition of altered vaginal microflora that occurs in the reproductive-age

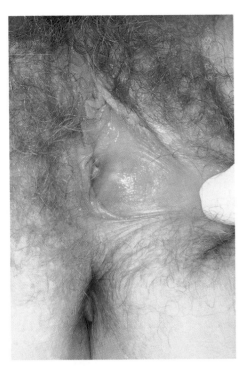

**Figure 18-5    Bartholin abscess.** Note erythema of the tissue overlying Bartholin's gland.

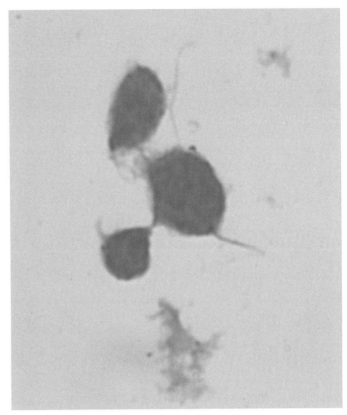

**Figure 18-6    Gram's stain of *Trichomonas vaginalis*.** Note flagella.

group. Approximately 75% of women in the reproductive-age group will experience at least one episode, with up to 50% of these women experiencing a subsequent episode and 5% evolving to recurrent and chronic vulvovaginal candidiasis.[24-28] *Candida* can be isolated from the lower genital tract in approximately 15% to 20% of asymptomatic women with a healthy vaginal ecosystem and microflora.[29-31] Typically the colony counts are extremely low and rarely detected on wet preparation microscopic examination of the vaginal discharge, but the organism is detected on culture of the vaginal discharge. Thus, women with vaginal *Candida* can be grouped into the following categories: (1) asymptomatic individuals with a healthy vaginal ecosystem and *Candida* as part of the endogenous vaginal microflora (i.e., symptomatic carriers); (2) individuals who have infrequent episodes of symptomatic vaginal candidiasis; (3) individuals with recurrent episodes of vaginal candidiasis, less than four episodes per year; (4) individuals with chronic recurrent vulvovaginal candidiasis, more than four episodes per year; (5) individuals with chronic persistent vulvovaginal candidiasis; and (6) individuals with chronic persistent vulvovaginal candidiasis, usually caused by *Candida glabrata*.

Yeasts occupy an interesting position in the schema of vaginitis. Approximately 20% of women will be colonized by yeast that can be considered part of their endogenous healthy vaginal microflora. Therefore, when these women are in an asymptomatic state and lactobacilli are the dominant microbe, a healthy vaginal microflora and ecosystem exist; when these women develop symptomatic vulvovaginal candidiasis, what is the endpoint of treatment? Should the endpoint be eradication of the fungus or resolution of the signs and symptoms of vulvovaginal candidiasis? When evaluating a patient for vulvovaginal candidiasis, the physician should perform the standard pelvic

examination and determine the presence of typical signs of vulvovaginal candidiasis. In addition, the pH of the vagina should be determined because if yeasts are present and the pH is equal to or greater than 5, additional causes of vaginitis or vaginosis should be sought, for example, trichomoniasis (Figs. 18-6 and 18-7). If white blood cells are present (>5/hpf), specimens should be obtained from the endocervix to determine whether *C. trachomatis* or *N. gonorrhoeae* is present. If the patient's

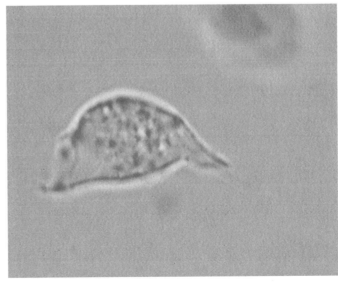

**Figure 18-7    Microscopic photograph of wet preparation of *Trichomonas vaginalis*.**

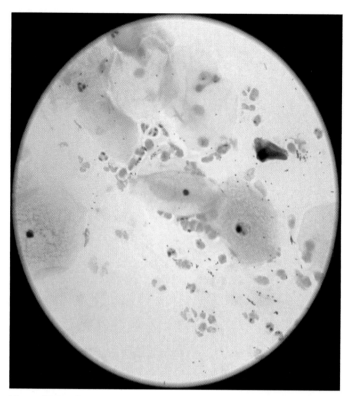

**Figure 18-8    Gram's stain of vaginal discharge.** Note estrogenized squamous epithelial cells, relative absence of bacteria, and numerous white blood cells. The pH of the vaginal fluid was 5.8. Further evaluation revealed no detectable pathogen or cervical infection.

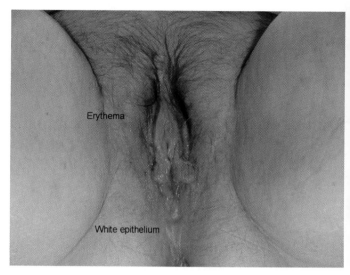

Erythema

White epithelium

**Figure 18-9    Vulvar candidiasis.**

uterus is tender to palpation, consideration should be given to the possible presence of upper genital tract infection, that is, endometritis or salpingitis (Fig. 18-8). A vaginal specimen should be obtained and cultured for the presence of yeast. The specific species should be identified because this information can be of assistance in determining appropriate antifungal therapy should the initial treatment fail.

### Diagnosis and Management

The clinical presentation of vulvovaginal candidiasis initially is itching, which can be severe and results in scratching that leaves excoriations on the vulva and introitus. The involved tissue becomes inflamed and can develop a rich erythematous color (Fig. 18-9). The discharge is typically white, unless there is a concomitant infection or abnormality present within the vaginal microflora. The consistency can range from liquid to thick and pasty, and the latter is often referred to as a cottage cheese–like discharge. The patient may also complain of burning and pain following sexual intercourse and urination. Risk factors for vulvovaginal candidiasis include a variety of diseases as well as therapeutic agents and practices[32,33] (Table 18-3).

Establishing a diagnosis of vulvovaginal candidiasis is often difficult even when the patient has all the yeast vaginitis symptoms. Handa and Stice compared potassium hydroxide (KOH) preparations with culturing and found that KOH preparations were positive in 40.5% and fungal cultures were positive in 61.5% of 30 women.[34] Vaginal culture for yeast should be performed when the examiner finds that the signs and

symptoms are suggestive of yeasts but the wet preparation of the discharge, including a KOH preparation, is negative.[31]

The physician should obtain two specimens of the vaginal discharge with a cotton or Dacron-tipped swab, one for culture and one for microscopic examination. The specimens for microscopic examination should be placed in a tube containing 2 to 3 mL of normal saline. Once immersed in saline, the swab should be agitated briskly for several seconds. Then the swab is removed and lightly touched to a glass slide to release one to two drops of the diluted discharge onto the surface of the glass slide. The diluted vaginal discharge is covered with a glass coverslip and examined microscopically under 40× magnification (Fig. 18-10). A second slide is prepared, and the diluted discharge is mixed with 10% KOH. The KOH will dissolve the squamous epithelial cells and white blood cells but not the hyphae or yeast cells. The yeast cell wall is made up of chitin, which is resistant to strong alkali. Culture is necessary to identify the species of yeasts (Table 18-4), since nonalbicans species tend to be resistant to the azole antifungal agents.

| Table 18-3 |
| Risk Factors for Development of Vulvovaginal Candidiasis |

| |
| --- |
| Pregnancy |
| Poorly controlled diabetes mellitus |
| Cushing's disease |
| Addison's disease |
| Hypothyroidism |
| Hyperthyroidism |
| Cancer |
| HIV/AIDS |
| Vaginal trauma |
| Oral contraceptive use |
| Antibiotic use |
| Immunosuppressive therapy |
| Frequent sexual intercourse |
| Wearing of tight clothing |
| IUD use |
| Ingestion of large amounts of sugar-containing foods |

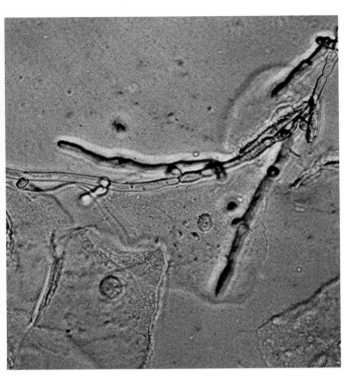

**Figure 18-10   Wet preparation of yeasts, squamous epithelial cells, and bacteria.** This is a hyphal form of *Candida albicans*.

---

**Table 18-5**
**Antifungal Agents for Treatment of Vulvovaginal Candidiasis**

**Intravaginal agents (no prescription required)**

Clotrimazole cream 1%—one applicatorful daily for 7 days
Clotrimazole vaginal inserts 100 mg—one insert daily for 7 days
Clotrimazole vaginal inserts 200 mg—one insert daily for 3 days
Clotrimazole 100 mg, 1% cream combination—one vaginal insert daily and
   cream; 7-day therapy
Butaconazole nitrate 2% cream—3-day therapy
Butaconazole nitrate 2% emulsion—one-time treatment
Clotrimazole 100 mg—7-day therapy
Clotrimazole 1% cream—7-day therapy
Clotrimazole 100 mg, 1% cream combination—one vaginal insert daily and
   cream; 7-day therapy
Clotrimazole 500 mg vaginal tablet—1-day therapy
Miconazole nitrate 2%—7-day therapy
Miconazole nitrate 200 mg, 2% cream combination suppositories and cream—
   7-day therapy
Miconazole nitrate 100 mg suppositories—7-day therapy
Miconazole nitrate 1% cream—7-day therapy
Miconazole nitrate 100 mg, 2% suppositories and cream combination—7-day
   therapy
Miconazole nitrate 2% cream—7-day therapy
Monistat nitrate 2% cream—7-day therapy
Tioconazole 6.5% ointment—1-day therapy

**Intravaginal preparations (prescription required)**

Terconazole 0.8% cream—3-day therapy
Terconazole 80 mg suppositories—3-day therapy
Terconazole 0.4% cream—3-day therapy

**Oral preparations (prescription required)**

Fluconazole 150 mg tablets—1-time therapy
Fluconazole 100 mg tablets—2 tablets day 1, 1 tablet days 2–5
Ketoconazole 100 mg tablets—2 tablets daily for 7 days

---

Individuals who experience either their first yeast infection or who have an infrequent recurrent yeast infection can be treated with various antifungal agents (Table 18-5). Patients who have recurrent vulvovaginal candidiasis—four or more episodes within a 12-month period—should probably be placed on suppressive therapy once the acute episode has been resolved. It is in these patients where identification of the yeasts becomes important because the nonalbicans species tend to be resistant to over-the-counter preparations. The nonalbicans species probably account for up to 20% of recurrent cases of vulvovaginal candidiasis, with *C. glabrata* responsible for 95% of the cases. Approaches to the treatment of acute recurrent vulvovaginal candidiasis are listed in Table 18-6.

## NECROTIZING INFECTION

Necrotizing fasciitis is a relatively infrequent infection that affects the subcutaneous tissue and fascia, can result in systemic toxicity, and has a mortality of 30%.[35,36] Necrotizing infections in the obstetric and gynecologic patient basically occur in one of three areas: the abdominal incision; the perineum following episiotomy repair, following trauma, or following the development of folliculitis commonly seen in the diabetic patient; or in the uterus following the development of postpartum endometritis. The development of a necrotizing infection is not predictable because any surgical incision or traumatic wound,

---

**Table 18-4**
**Species of *Candida* Isolated from Lower Genital Tract in Women with Yeast-Caused Vaginitis**

| Species | Frequency | Response to Azoles |
|---|---|---|
| C. albicans | 80%–90% | Sensitive |
| C. glabrata | 5%–10% | Resistant |
| C. krusei | <1% | Tends to be resistant |
| C. lusitaniae | <1% | Tends to be resistant |
| C. parapsilosis | <1% | Tends to be resistant |
| C. pseudotropicalis | <1% | Tends to be resistant |
| C. tropicalis | <1% | Tends to be resistant |

---

**Table 18-6**
**Recommendations for Treatment of Acute Recurrent Vulvovaginal Candidiasis**

1. Tioconazole 6.5% cream once a week for 3 weeks*
2. Terconazole 0.4% cream daily for 14 days†
3. Fluconazole 150 mg orally once then repeated in 3 days†
4. Boric acid 600 mg capsule twice daily for 2–3 weeks†
5. Boric acid 600 mg tampon for 8 hours, then a 600 mg suppository at
   bedtime for 14 days*

*Author's regimen; no data.
†Centers for Disease Central and Prevention: Sexually transmitted diseases treatment
   guidelines 2002. MMWR 2002;51:47.
†Sobel JD, Chaim W, Nagappan V, Leaman D: Treatment of vaginitis caused by *Candida
   glabrata*: use of topical boric acid and flucytosine. Am J Obstet Gynecol
   2003;189:1297–1300.

no matter how minor, can progress to a necrotizing infection without warning. Successful management of necrotizing fasciitis depends on early recognition and knowledge of the bacteria most likely involved in the infectious process.[37,38]

Infections such as folliculitis, furunculosis, and carbuncles of the vulva, and the infected episiotomy have the potential to evolve into necrotizing fasciitis, especially in immunocompromised patients (e.g., diabetics). In fact, any event that causes a break in the skin and allows bacteria to enter the subcutaneous fatty tissue has the potential to develop into necrotizing fasciitis. Minor infections that have the potential to develop into necrotizing fasciitis are usually those in which the area has been traumatized—by squeezing, pricking with a pin, or scratching. The patient at greatest risk for developing necrotizing fasciitis of the vulva and perineum is the diabetic, especially the insulin-dependent diabetic. Individuals who do not have an impaired immune system and maintain good tissue perfusion resulting in high oxygen concentrations in the tissue are less likely to develop necrotizing fasciitis following tissue trauma.

Necrotizing fasciitis is an infection that typically begins in the subcutaneous tissue and progresses to the fascia, which results in destruction of the fatty subcutaneous tissue as well as the fascia. The skin may be spared; however, if the process remains unchecked, necrosis of the skin occurs. The hallmark of necrotizing fasciitis is the initial development of severe pain at the site of infection. Typically the patient states that the pain is severe, even when gentle pressure is applied to the area.

The bacteriology of necrotizing fasciitis of the vulva commonly involves *S. aureus*, *S. pyogenes* (group A *Streptococcus*), *Escherichia coli*, *Peptostreptococcus*, *Prevotella*, and *Bacteroides* as well as many other bacteria.[38] These bacteria are derived from the patient's skin, vagina, and rectum. Involvement is not unexpected, since the vulva and perineum are constantly exposed to these bacteria. In the study reported by Brook and Frazier,[38] the clinical signs and symptoms of necrotizing fasciitis were reviewed over a 17-year period; although they were collected from a variety of cases, the findings are applicable to necrotizing fasciitis of the vulva and perineum (Table 18-7).

| Table 18-7 Clinical Findings Associated with Necrotizing Fasciitis | |
|---|---|
| **Finding** | **Percentage of Patients** |
| Necrosis | 100 |
| Fever | 86 |
| Tachycardia | 80 |
| Leukocytosis | 78 |
| Edema | 77 |
| Foul odor | 70 |
| Gas and crepitation | 39 |
| Hypotension | 33 |
| Hyperglycemia | 27 |
| Local anesthesia | 24 |
| Disorientation | 23 |
| Anemia | 10 |

Brook I, Frazier EH: Clinical and microbiological features of nectrotizing faciitis. J Clin Microbiol 1995;33:2382–2387.

## Diagnosis and Management

If a patient is suspected of having necrotizing fasciitis of the vulva and perineum or of any site, it is imperative that the diagnosis be established promptly and therapy initiated immediately. If the diagnosis is in question, a computed tomography (CT) scan can often facilitate in making the diagnosis. Broad-spectrum antibiotic therapy should be administered intravenously immediately, for example, clindamycin 900 mg every 8 hours, ampicillin 2 g every 6 hours, and gentamicin 5 mg/kg of body weight every 24 hours. Gentamicin should be calculated on ideal body weight for patients over 91 kg (200 lb) and should be adjusted for individuals with renal impairment. The patient should be taken to surgery immediately following establishment of the diagnosis, because if imaging studies cannot be performed immediately, surgical exploration of the infected site should not be delayed. The infected area should be thoroughly explored and all necrotic tissue removed. The excision of necrotic tissue should involve all necrotic tissue as well as adjacent tissue and continue until healthy tissue that bleeds briskly is encountered. The débridement should involve all necrotic subcutaneous tissue, fascia, muscle, and skin. Failure to remove all necrotic tissue will necessitate a return to the operating room. Hyperbaric oxygen therapy following débridement has been beneficial in some cases.

## SUMMARY

Infections of the vulva and perineum should not be taken lightly, and the diagnosis should be established early and appropriate antibiotic therapy instituted. The bacteria most likely to be involved are *S. aureus* methicillin-sensitive (MSSA) as well as methicillin-resistant (MRSA), coagulase-negative staphylococci, *S. agalactiae* (GBS), *S. pyogenes* (GAS), other streptococci, facultative gram-negative anaerobic bacteria (e.g., *E. coli*), and obligate anaerobic bacteria originating from the vagina and rectum. The MRSA community-acquired strains have been changing their resistance patterns; some are sensitive to clindamycin, quinolones, minocycline, trimethoprim/sulfamethoxazole, and rifampin, whereas others are resistant to clindamycin and still others to the quinolones. A culture specimen from the infected site (e.g., an aspirate, tissue, or swab), should always be obtained. This is necessary in the event that the initial, empirically chosen antibiotic regime is not effective. Finally, in the event of an abscess, the area should be incised, loculations broken, and the area completely drained and thoroughly irrigated. In the presence of necrotizing fasciitis, the immediate administration of broad-spectrum antibiotics is required with thorough surgical débridement of all necrotic tissue.

## REFERENCES

1. Kloos WE: Ecology of the human skin. In Märdh PA, Schleifer KH (eds): Coagulase-negative Staphylococci. Stockholm, Almquist and Wiksell International, 1986, pp 37–50 (**IIa, B**)
2. Kloos WE, Musselwhite MS: Distribution and persistence of *Staphylococcus* and *Micrococcus* species and other aerobic bacteria on human skin. Appl Microbiol 1975;30:381–385. (**III, B**)
3. Waldvogel FA: *Staphylococcus aureus* (including staphylococcal toxic shock). In Mandell GL, Bennett JE, Dolin R (eds): Principles and

Practice of Infectious Diseases. Philadelphia, Churchill Livingstone, 2000, p 2079. **(III, B)**

4. Feingold DS: Staphylococcal and streptococcal pyodermas. Semin Dermatol 1993;12:331–335. **(III, B)**

5. Bisno AL, Stevens DL: Streptococcal infections of the skin and soft tissues. N Engl J Med 1996;34:229–234. **(IIb, B)**

6. Fowler JF Jr, Stage GC III: Hot tub (*Pseudomonas*) folliculitis. J Ky Med Assoc 1990;88(2):66–68. **(III, B)**

7. Jemec GB, Heidenheim M, Nielsen NH: The prevalence of hidradenitis suppurativa and its potential precursor lesions. J Am Acad Dermatol 1996;35:191–194. **(III, B)**

8. Slade DE, Powell BW, Mortimer PS: Hidradenitis suppurativa: pathogenesis and management. Br J Plast Surg 2003;56:451–461. **(III, B)**

9. Von Der Werth JM, Williams HC, Raeburn JA: The clinical genetics of hidradenitis suppurativa revisited. Br J Dermatol 2000;142:947–953. **(III, B)**

10. Brook I, Frazier EH: Aerobic and anaerobic microbiology of axillary hidradenitis suppurativa. J Med Microbiol 1999;48:103–105. **(III, B)**

11. Lapins J, Jarstrand C, Emtestam L: Coagulase-negative staphylococci are the most common bacteria found in cultures from the deep portions of hidradenitis suppurativa lesions, as obtained by carbon dioxide laser surgery. Br J Dermatol 1999;140:90–95. **(III, B)**

12. Jemec GB, Faber M, Gutschik E, Wendelboe P: The bacteriology of hidradenitis suppurativa. Dermatology 1996;193:203–206. **(III, B)**

13. Dicken CH, Powell ST, Spear KL: Evaluation of isotretinoin treatment of hidradenitis suppurativa. J Am Acad Dermatol 1984;11:500–502. **(IIb, B)**

14. Chow ET, Mortimer PS: Successful treatment of hidradenitis suppurativa and retroauricular acne with etretinate. Br J Dermatol 1992;126:415. **(IIb, B)**

15. Jemec GB, Gniadecka M: Sebum excretion in hidradenitis suppurativa. Dermatology 1997;194:325–328. **(III, B)**

16. Boer J, van Gemert MJ: Long-term results of isotretinoin in the treatment of 68 patients with hidradenitis suppurativa. J Am Acad Dermatol 1999;40:73–76. **(IIb, B)**

17. Agnholt J, Dahlerup JF, Kaltoft K: The effect of etanercept and infliximab on the production of tumor necrosis factor alpha, interferon-gamma and GM-CSF in in vivo activated intestinal T lymphocyte cultures. Cytokine 2003;23:76–85. **(IIb, B)**

18. Sullivan TP, Welsh E, Kerdel FA, et al: Infliximab for hidradenitis suppurativa. Br J Dermatol 2003;149:1046–1049. **(IIb, B)**

19. Banerjee AK: Surgical treatment of hidradenitis suppurativa. Br J Surg 1992;79:863–866. **(III, B)**

20. Harrison BJ, Mudge M, Hughes LE: Recurrence after surgical treatment of hidradenitis suppurativa. BMJ (Clinical research ed) 1987; 294:487–489. **(III, B)**

21. Rompel R, Petres J: Long-term results of wide surgical excision in 106 patients with hidradenitis suppurativa. Dermatol Surg 2000; 26:638–643. **(III, B)**

22. Cosman BC, O'Grady TC, Pekarske S: Verrucous carcinoma arising in hidradenitis suppurativa. Int J Colorectal Dis 2000;15:342–346. **(III, B)**

23. Manolitsas T, Biankin S, Jaworski R, Wain G: Vulvar squamous cell carcinoma arising in chronic hidradenitis suppurativa. Gynecol Oncol 1999;75:285–288. **(III, B)**

24. Hurley R, De Louvois J: *Candida* vaginitis. Postgrad Med J 1979; 55:645–647. **(III, B)**

25. Sobel JD: Pathogenesis of *Candida* vulvovaginitis. Curr Top Med Mycol 1989;3:86–108. **(IIb, B)**

26. Geiger AM, Foxman B: Risk factors in vulvovaginal candidiasis: a case-control study among university students. Epidemiology 1996;7:182–187. **(III, B)**

27. Sobel JD: Candidal vulvovaginitis. Clin Obstet Gynecol 1993; 36:153–165. **(Ib, A)**

28. Faro S: Systemic vs. topical therapy for the treatment of vulvovaginal candidiasis. Infect Dis Obstet Gynecol 1993;1:202–208. **(III, B)**

29. Odds FC: *Candida* and Candidosis. London, Balliere-Tindall, 1988, pp 104–110. **(III, B)**

30. Fleury FJ: Adult vaginitis. Clin Obstet Gynecol 1981;24:407–438. **(III, B)**

31. Sobel JD, Faro S, Force RW, et al: Vulvovaginal candidiasis: epidemiologic, diagnostic, and therapeutic considerations. Am J Obstet Gynecol 1998;178:203–211. **(III, B)**

32. Sobel JD: Candidal vulvovaginitis. Clin Obstet Gynecol 1993; 36:153–165. **(IIb, B)**

33. Scudamore JA, Tooley PJ, Allcorn RJ: The treatment of acute and chronic vaginal candidosis. Br J Clin Pract 1992;46:260–263. **(IIb, B)**

34. Handa VL, Stice CW: Fungal culture findings in cyclic vulvitis. Obstet Gynecol 2000;96:301–303. **(III, B)**

35. Giuliano A, Lewis F Jr, Hadley K, Blaisdell FW: Bacteriology of necrotizing fasciitis. Am J Surg 1977;134:52–7. **(III, B)**

36. Pessa ME, Howard RJ: Necrotizing fasciitis. Surg Gynecol Obstet 1985;161:357–361. **(III, B)**

37. Sudarsky LA, Laschinger JC, Coppa GF, Spencer FC: Improved results from a standardized approach in treating patients with necrotizing fasciitis. Ann Surg 1987;206:661–665. **(IIb, B)**

38. Brook I, Frazier EH: Clinical and microbiological features of necrotizing fasciitis. J Clin Microbiol 1995;33:2382–2387. **(III, B)**

# Chapter 19

# Sexually Transmitted Diseases

## Richard L. Sweet, MD

**KEY POINTS**

- Sexually transmitted diseases (STDs) are associated with significant social, health and economic burdens.
- Increased resistance of *Neisseria gonorrhoeae* to quinolones antibiotics has limited options for treatment of gonorrhea.
- *Chlamydia trachomatis* is the most common treatable bacterial STD in the United States.
- After a decade of decline, in 2001 rates of primary and secondary syphilis began to rise.
- More than 25% of females in the United States have been infected with genital herpes simplex virus 2.
- *Trichomonas vaginalis* infects approximately 5 million people annually in the United States.
- 500,000 to 1 million new cases of human papillomavirus (HPV)-induced genital warts occur annually in the United States.

Despite many advances in the diagnosis and treatment of STDs, the epidemic of STDs continues unabated.[1-3] Moreover, STDs are associated with significant social, health, and economic burdens both in the United States and worldwide.[1,2,4]

In the developing countries of the world, STDs (excluding HIV/AIDS) are the second leading cause of lost healthy life among women aged 15 to 44 years. The World Health Organization (WHO) estimated in 1995 that 333 million new cases of the four curable STDs occurred in the 15- to 49-year-old age group worldwide annually: gonorrhea 62.6 million, syphilis 12.2 million, chlamydia 89.1 million, and trichomoniasis 167.2 million.[5]

The Institute of Medicine (IOM) in their report, "The Hidden Epidemic: Confronting Sexually Transmitted Diseases," estimated that as of 1993, 12 million new cases of STDs occur annually in the United States.[1] As a result, the United States had the highest rates of curable STDs among countries in the developed world.[1] In fact, the Centers for Disease Control and Prevention (CDC) noted in 1995 that five of the ten most frequently reported infections in the United States were STDs (Table 19-1).[6] In its report, the IOM noted that the economic impact of this "hidden epidemic" was substantial, with an estimated total cost for a selected group of major STDs and related syndromes (excluding HIV) of $10 billion in 1994.[1] This estimate did not include bacterial vaginosis and trichomoniasis and thus is an underestimate. The estimated annual cost of sexually transmitted HIV infection was nearly $7 billion, leading to a total annual cost of STDs in the United States of $17 billion.[1] In 1998, the American Social Health Association (ASHA)

estimated that 15 million new STD cases occur in the United States each year (see Table 19-1).[2] More recently, Weinstock et al estimated that approximately 18.9 million new STD cases occurred in the United States in 2000.[3]

Of particular concern is the incidence and prevalence of STDs among adolescents and young adults (15- to 24-year-olds). Berman and Hein reported that sexually active adolescents have the highest rates of STDs of any age group.[7] An estimated 3 million adolescents acquire an STD annually in the United States.[8] In 2000, of the approximately 18.9 million new cases of STD, 9.1 million (48%) occurred among persons aged 15 to 24.[3] The estimated economic burden of the nine million new cases of STDs that occurred among 15- to 24-year-olds in 2000 was $6.5 billion.[4]

Clinicians should be aware of several important recent trends in STDs. First is expansion of the scope of STDs from the classic five venereal diseases of gonorrhea, syphilis, chancroid, lymphogranuloma venereum, and granuloma inguinale to include over 30 microorganisms. The spectrum of sexually transmitted infections (STIs) has expanded to include diseases such as vaginitis, mucopurulent cervicitis, pelvic inflammatory disease, infertility, perinatal infections, hepatitis, enteric infections, arthritis syndromes, nongonococcal urethritis, epididymitis, genital tract oncogenesis, and severe immunosuppression (e.g., AIDS).

Secondly, there has been a changing emphasis in the field of STDs. As noted by Cates, there has been a progression in focus from the traditional STDs, such as syphilis and gonorrhea, to the STIs caused by *Chlamydia trachomatis*, herpes simplex virus (HSV), HPV, and most recently to HIV infection and AIDS.[9,10]

Thirdly, the traditional STDs—syphilis, gonorrhea and chlamydia—were caused by bacteria. Consequently, they were relatively easily cured with antimicrobial therapy. The newer STDs tend to be of viral etiology and thus associated with incurable or fatal conditions. Examples include chronic recurrent HSV, HPV-associated genital tract cancer, and HIV and AIDS.

Fourthly, there exists an epidemiologic synergy among STDs. STDs and STIs are historically, behaviorally, and biologically related. Initially, the ulcerative STDs (e.g., syphilis, HSV, chancroid) were shown to be associated with an increased risk of acquiring and transmitting HIV. More recently, STDs associated with cervicitis and vaginal discharge (e.g., gonorrhea, chlamydia, trichomoniasis, and bacterial vaginosis) have also been implicated in increasing the risk for transmission and acquisition of HIV. Further, the immunosuppression seen with HIV infection may worsen the clinical findings of other STDs and cause them to be more difficult to treat.

Lastly, with the exception of HIV/AIDS, the burden of STDs is greater among women than men, and women are more likely

Gynecologic Infectious Disease

**Table 19-1**
**Most Commonly Reported Notifiable Diseases in the United States, 1995**

1. Chlamydia*
2. Gonorrhea*
3. AIDS*
4. Salmonellosis
5. Hepatitis A
6. Shigellosis
7. Tuberculosis
8. Syphilis (primary and secondary)*
9. Lyme disease
10. Hepatitis B*

*Sexually transmitted disease.
Data from Centers for Disease Control: MMWR 1996;45:883–884.

to develop serious long-term consequences of STDs and STIs. Among these are (1) infertility and ectopic pregnancy secondary to damaged fallopian tubes with *Neisseria gonorrhoeae* and *C. trachomatis;* (2) complications of pregnancy, including spontaneous abortion, stillbirth, chorioamnionitis, preterm birth, and low birth weight; (3) congenital or vertically transmitted neonatal infections; and (4) an increased risk for genital cancer with HPV.

This chapter focuses on specific STDs with emphasis on the most common and those having a substantial impact on the health of women.

## GONORRHEA

### Epidemiology, Risk Factors, and Pathogenesis

Gonorrhea, which is caused by the gram-negative diplococcus *N. gonorrhoeae,* is the second most common reported communicable disease (after chlamydia) in the United States, with over 350,000 cases reported in 2002.[11] Because of an assumed 50% under-reporting, it is estimated that approximately 700,000 cases of *N. gonorrhoeae* actually occurred in 2002 in the United States. Following a 74% decrease in reported cases of gonorrhea from 1975 through 1997, an 8.9% increase occurred in 1998. Since then the number of reported cases and the rate of gonorrhea have essentially plateaued.[11] In 2002, the reported gonorrhea rate among women (125.3 cases per 100,000) was similar to that among men (124.2 cases per 100,000). For women, the highest rates of gonorrhea have been reported in non-Hispanic black women aged 15 to 19 years (3307.7 cases per 100,000).[1] The CDC reported that in 2000, 60% of reported gonorrhea cases were in the age group 15 to 24 years.[12]

Humans are the only natural host for *N. gonorrhoeae.* Because of its predilection for columnar or pseudostratified epithelium, mucous membranes that are lined by columnar, cuboidal, or noncornified squamous epithelial cells are most susceptible to infection with *N. gonorrhoeae* in adults. Thus gonococcal infection is most commonly found in the urogenital tract.

Over the past 30 years there has been a phenomenal expansion in our understanding of the pathogenic mechanisms of the gonococcus.[13] Initially, Kellogg et al demonstrated differences in the virulence of *N. gonorrhoeae,* associated with specific colony types.[14] Of the Kellogg colony types, only types 1 and 2 (now called P+), which contain pili, are capable of producing infection, while types 3 and 4, which do not contain pili (now called P colonies), fail to cause infection.[14] The pili appear to facilitate attachment of gonococci to epithelial surfaces.[14] Other gonococcal surface structures in addition to pili are associated with pathogenesis. These surface structures and functions are determined by proteins present in the outer membrane of the gonococcus, including porin protein (Por), opacity-associated proteins (Opa), and reduction modifiable protein (RmP).

Additional gonococcal virulence factors include (1) lipopolysaccharides,[15] (2) IgA,[13] and (3) iron-repressible proteins that are involved in uptake of iron—an essential requirement for growth of gonococci.[5]

Like other infections, the initial step in gonococcal infection is adherence of *N. gonorrhoeae* to mucosal cells lining the genitourinary tract. This process of adherence is mediated by pili and other surface proteins.[16] This step is followed by the process of pinocytosis by which the organism is transported into epithelial cells and then into submucosal tissues.[17] Attachment of *N. gonorrhoeae* also results in the release of the endotoxin, gonococcal lipopolysaccharide, which damages the ciliated and nonciliated cells of the fallopian tube epithelium.[15]

Race and age are important determinants and risk factors for gonorrhea.[11] Rates of gonorrhea among non-Hispanic blacks (570 cases per 100,000) are higher than for any other racial/ethnic group in the United States.[11] Hook and Handsfield[18] reported that 77% of reported cases of gonorrhea in the United States in 1995 were among persons aged 15 to 29 years with the highest rates occurring in the 15- to 19-year-old age group. If only sexually active females are considered, the incidence of gonorrhea is twice as high in adolescents than in women aged 20 to 24 years.[18] Additional risk factors for gonorrhea include low socioeconomic status, early onset of sexual activity, unmarried marital status, a past history of gonorrhea, illicit drug use, and prostitution.[4]

Transmission of gonorrhea is almost entirely by sexual contact. The female is at greater risk of infection than the male. While it is estimated that a male having a single sexual encounter with a gonorrhea-infected female will become infected 20% to 25% of the time, the risk of transmission from male to female is estimated at 50% to 90%.[19] A short incubation time of 3 to 5 days occurs.

Among nonpregnant women, *N. gonorrhoeae* is an important cause of urethritis, cervicitis, and pelvic inflammatory disease (PID).[19] Pharyngeal gonorrhea and disseminated gonorrhea occur in men and women. Infection with *N. gonorrhoeae* in pregnancy is also a major concern. Gonorrheal ophthalmia neonatorum has long been recognized as a major consequence of maternal infection. More recently, an association between maternal gonococcal infection and disseminated gonococcal infection, amniotic infection syndrome, and perinatal complications such as premature rupture of membranes (PROM), chorioamnionitis, prematurity, intrauterine growth retardation, neonatal sepsis, and postpartum endometritis has been recognized.

### Clinical Features

*N. gonorrhoeae* infects both males and females. In adults, the gonococcus attaches to nonsquamous epithelium-lined mucosal membranes, and thus the primary involvement site is the genito-urinary tract. In males, the infection is usually acute symptomatic urethritis. Female infection is often asymptomatic, and the primary site of involvement is the endocervical canal and the transition zone of the cervix. However, women with endocervical gonorrhea may be symptomatic and most commonly have a vaginal discharge, dysuria, and abnormal uterine bleeding.[18] Urethral colonization occurs in the majority of women with endocervical gonorrhea, and infection of the paraurethral (Skene's) glands, Bartholin's glands, and anorectum also occur.

Uncomplicated anogenital gonorrhea in women may involve the endocervix, urethra, Skene's glands, Bartholin's glands, or anus. The most commonly infected site is the endocervix. Gonococcal infection of the vagina is rare except in prepubertal and postmenopausal patients. Urethral colonization is present in 70% to 90% of women infected with *N. gonorrhoeae*.[20]

It is now recognized that although the majority of women harboring *N. gonorrhoeae* are asymptomatic, a large number of women with anogenital gonorrhea are symptomatic. Common symptoms include vaginal discharge, dysuria, intermenstrual bleeding, menorrhagia, and pelvic discomfort. The incubation period for urogenital gonorrhea in women is unclear, but those who develop symptomatic gonococcal infection do so within 10 days. In 15% to 20% of women with uncomplicated ano-genital gonorrhea, upper genital tract infection (PID) occurs.[21] Gonococcal-associated PID tends to occur at the end of or just after menstruation.

The cervix infected with *N. gonorrhoeae* can appear healthy or reveal an inflamed cervical canal with ectopy and a muco-purulent exudate (Fig. 19-1). The area of ectopy is edematous, erythematous, and friable. In general, these signs of gonococcal cervicitis are indistinguishable from other causes of cervicitis, and thus an absolute diagnosis of gonococcal cervicitis requires confirmatory laboratory tests. Gonococcal infection of the urethra, Skene's glands, or Bartholin's glands may be associated with mucopurulent exudate that can be expressed from these structures. If routine screening for *N. gonorrhoeae* is not employed during pelvic examinations, the presence of lower genital tract complaints or signs such as abnormal bleeding, discharge, dysuria, mucopurulent endocervicitis, or pelvic dis-comfort should suggest that cultures be obtained to determine whether the gonococcus is present.

Non-lower-tract gonococcal disease may result from direct or contiguous spread and by bloodstream dissemination. Direct or contiguous spread occurs for PID, anorectal infection, perihepatitis (Fitz-Hugh-Curtis syndrome), conjunctivitis, and pharyngeal gonococcal infection.

Acute PID is a local complication and the most common com-plication of gonorrhea in women, occurring in an estimated 10% to 20% of untreated cases.[21] Bartholin's gland abscess is the next most frequent complication of gonococcal infection in women.

Disseminated gonococcal infection (DGI), the most common systemic complication of gonorrhea, occurs when gonococcal bacteremia produces extragenital manifestations of gonococcal infection. The prevalence of DGI among total gonorrhea cases ranges from 0.1% to 0.3%, with females predominating over males by about 4:1.[22] The majority of women with DGI develop symptoms either during pregnancy, especially in the third trimester, or within 7 days from the onset of menstruation.

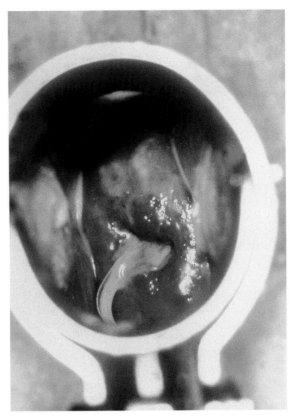

**Figure 19-1   Gonococcal mucopurulent endocervicitis.** (Reprinted with permission from Sweet RL, Gibbs RS: Atlas of Infectious Diseases of the Female Genital Tract. Philadelphia, Lippincott Williams & Wilkins, 2004.)

Patients are considered to have proven DGI if they have positive cultures from blood, joint fluid, skin lesions, or other-wise sterile sources.[2] This group makes up less than 50% of DGI cases.[23] DGI is defined when *N. gonorrhoeae* can be cultured from the primary site in the lower genital tract or pharynx or in a sexual partner. Patients with a clinical syndrome consistent with DGI and an appropriate clinical response to treatment but in whom all culture sites are negative are considered to have possible DGI.[18]

Disseminated gonococcal infection manifests two stages: an early bacteremia stage and a late stage. The bacteremia stage is characterized by chills, fever, typical skin lesions, and asymmetric joint involvement. Blood cultures are positive for *N. gonorrhoeae* in half of cultures during the bacteremia stage. The bacteremia stage is associated with a dermatitis that is characterized by a variety of skin lesions due to gonococcal emboli and occurs in 50% to 75% of cases.[24] These lesions appear initially as small vesicles that become pustules and develop a hemorrhagic base. The center becomes necrotic. These lesions occur on any body region but are most frequently present on the volar aspects of the upper extremities, the hands, and the digits. These skin lesions resolve spontaneously without residual scarring.

Joint symptoms are frequently present during the early stage, with arthritis developing in 30% to 40% of cases.[18,24] Asymmetric joint involvement is the usual pattern, most often affecting the knee, elbow, wrist, ankle, and metacarpophalangeal joints. The arthritis is migratory (i.e., one joint heals as another becomes affected). In two thirds of patients, tenosynovitis is present.[24] The most frequent sites are the dorsal tendons of the hands, wrists, and ankles.

The late stage of disseminated gonococcal infection is characterized by frank arthritis with permanent joint damage, endocarditis, meningitis, pericarditis, osteomyelitis, and perihepatitis.[18,24] With arthritis, the knees, ankles, and wrist joints are the sites most commonly involved.

While the problem of gonococcal ophthalmia neonatorum has been addressed for over 100 years, the effects of gonorrheal infection on both mother and fetus were not fully appreciated until 30 years ago. Studies have demonstrated an association between untreated maternal endocervical gonorrhea and perinatal complications, including an increased incidence of PROM, preterm delivery, chorioamnionitis, neonatal sepsis, and maternal postpartum sepsis.[21-24]

## Diagnosis

The laboratory diagnosis of infection with *N. gonorrhoeae* requires identification of the organism at infected sites. Methods available include Gram's stain, cultures, immunochemical detection, and molecular diagnostic techniques.

In men with urethral discharge and dysuria, the Gram stain of the urethral exudate is considered diagnostic for *N. gonorrhoeae* when gram-negative diplococci are seen within or closely associated with polymorphonuclear leukocytes. However, the majority of women with gonorrhea (pregnant and nonpregnant) are asymptomatic. Thus, the diagnosis depends on sampling of potential infected sites. The major site of primary infection in women is the endocervix. Unfortunately, microscopic examination of a gram-stained specimen from the endocervix in asymptomatic women produces a diagnosis of gonorrhea in only 60% of women compared with 95% of men.[18]

In women the diagnosis of *N. gonorrhoeae* infection requires isolation of the organism by culture or use of nucleic acid amplification tests (NAATs). Ideally, all sexually active women should be screened at every opportunity (i.e., annual routine pelvic examination, any visit for a gynecologic complaint). Obviously, this would be a major logistic and economic burden, especially in patient populations with low rates (<1%) of gonorrhea. At a minimum, certain at-risk patient groups should be routinely screened. These include partners of men with gonorrhea or urethritis, women with symptoms and signs referred to the lower genital tract, patients with known other STDs, patients with multiple sexual partners, and patients with PID.

Clinical isolation is best performed using selective media for *N. gonorrhoeae*, such as Thayer-Martin medium containing the antibiotics that inhibit the growth of contaminating organisms present in the same body sites as the gonococcus. Proper collection, handling, and processing of culture specimens are crucial to obtaining accurate results. *N. gonorrhoeae* does not tolerate drying and thus requires immediate inoculation on an appropriate medium and placement in an incubator. When culture facilities are not readily available, a holding or transport medium should be used.

The diagnosis of *N. gonorrhoeae* infection is made by identification of the organism with a typical growth on selective media, a positive oxidase reaction, and a gram-negative diplococcal

morphology on gram staining of the isolated colonies. Fermentation reactions may be also performed. They take advantage of the ability of the gonococcus to ferment glucose but not sucrose or maltose.

Reliable nonculture assays for detection of gonorrhea have recently become available and have gained increasing acceptance.[18] Hook and Handsfield suggested that utilization of these new nonculture assays will continue to increase owing to their satisfactory performance and extensive promotion by manufactures and because specimens used by those assays for gonorrhea can also often be used to test for *C. trachomatis*.[18] The first widely accepted technique was the nonamplified DNA probe test (e.g., Gen-Probe PACE 2). Currently nonamplified DNA probes are the most commonly used nonculture method for diagnosis of gonorrhea in the United States.[13] Nonamplified DNA probes have sensitivity ranging from 89% to 97% and specificity of 99%. Thus, they compare favorably to culture with selective media.

More recently, NAATs have been introduced for detection of *N. gonorrhoeae*. These techniques include ligase chain reaction (LCR), polymerase chain reaction (PCR), and transcription-mediated amplification (RMA). NAATs have excellent sensitivity and specificity.[25]

## Treatment

The choice of antimicrobial agents for the treatment of gonococcal infection is largely dependent on in vitro resistance patterns to *N. gonorrhoeae*. Additional factors that influence the choice of antimicrobial agents include maximizing compliance with single-dose (observed) therapy and the probability that patients infected with *N. gonorrhoeae* are coinfected with other STDs (especially *C. trachomatis*).[18]

While most *N. gonorrhoeae* is sensitive to a large number of antimicrobial agents including penicillins, tetracyclines, macrolides, cephalosporins, erythromycin, aminoglycosides, and quinolones, increasing resistant strains have appeared.[26] These resistant strains include penicillinase-producing *N. gonorrhoeae* (PPNG), as well as high-level chromosomal resistance to penicillin; plasmid-mediated resistance to tetracycline; chromosomally mediated resistance to cephalosporins, tetracycline, spectinomycin, and aminoglycosides; and most recently fluoroquinolone resistance. The prevalence of fluoroquinolone-resistant *N. gonorrhoeae* in Asian countries is high (China 86.9%, Japan 64%, and the Philippines 54.3%).[27] Of concern is the rapid increase in fluoroquinolone-resistant strains in the United States, with 12% in Hawaii, 19% in California, and 14% in Massachusetts in 2003.[28] The recommended treatment regimens for uncomplicated gonorrhea of cervix and urethra are listed in Table 19-2.

Among women with gonorrhea, 10% to 30% are coinfected with chlamydia.[18] Thus, CDC recommends that women treated for gonorrhea should also be presumptively treated for chlamydial infection. Azithromycin 1 g orally in a single dose or doxycycline 100 mg orally twice a day for 7 days are the preferred regimens in nonpregnant women, while in pregnancy an erythromycin regimen or amoxicillin should be used (see chlamydia treatment).

Pregnant or lactating women should not be treated with quinolones.[26] In pregnant women *N. gonorrhoeae* should be

## Table 19-2
### CDC–recommended Treatment of Uncomplicated Gonococcal Infections of the Cervix, Urethra, and Rectum in Adults, 2002

**Recommended regimen**

Cefixime 400mg orally in a single dose
*or*
Ceftriaxone 125 mg IM in a single dose
*or*
Ciprofloxacin 500 mg orally in a single dose
*or*
Ofloxacin 400 mg orally in a single dose
*Plus*
Azithromycin 1 g orally in a single dose
*or*
Doxycycline 100 mg orally twice a day for 7 days

**Alternative regimens**

1. Spectinomycin 2g IM in a single dose
2. Single dose of cephalosporins such as ceftizoxime 500 mg IM, cefotaxime 500 mg IM, cefotetan 1 g IM, and cefoxitin 2 g IM with probenecid 1 g orally
3. Single dose of other quinolones such as enoxacin 400 mg orally, lomefloxacin 400 mg orally, and norfloxacin 800 mg orally

treated with a recommended or alternative cephalosporin.[26] When cephalosporins can not be tolerated, spectinomycin 2 g should be administered intramuscularly (IM). Either erythromycin or amoxicillin is the recommended treatment for presumptive chlamydial infection in pregnancy.

Test of cure is no longer recommended for individuals with uncomplicated gonorrhea who received any CDC-recommended regimen for uncomplicated gonorrhea.[29] Persons with persistent

## Table 19-3
### CDC–recommended Treatment for Disseminated Gonococcal Infection, 2002

**Recommended initial regimen**

Ceftriaxone 1 g IM or IV every 24 hours

**Alternative initial regimens**

Cefotaxime 1 g IV every 8 hours
*or*
Ceftizoxime 1 g IV every 8 hours
*or*
For persons allergic to β-lactam drugs
Ciprofloxacin 500 mg IV every 12 hours
*or*
Ofloxacin 400 mg IV every 12 hours
*or*
Spectinomycin 2 g IM every 12 hours
All regimens should be continued for 24 to 48 hours after improvement begins, at which time therapy may be switched to one of the following regimens to complete a full week of therapy:
Cefixime 400 mg orally twice a day
*or*
Ciprofloxacin 500 mg orally twice a day*
*or*
Ofloxacin 400 mg orally twice a day*

*Ciprofloxacin and ofloxacin are contraindicated in pregnant or lactating women.

symptoms should be retested, and any *N. gonorrhoeae* recovered should be tested for antimicrobial susceptibility. Because patients infected with gonorrhea are at high risk for reinfection, repeat screening 1 to 2 months after treatment is appropriate.

In addition, sexual partners of patients with gonorrhea should be examined, tested, and treated (prior to culture results). Treatment should be with one of the CDC regimens for uncomplicated gonorrhea, preferably with treatment for coexistent chlamydial infection.

Ceftriaxone is the drug of choice for DGI. Patients allergic to penicillins and cephalosporins can be treated with spectinomycin 2 g IM every 12 hours. The current CDC recommendations and alternative drugs are listed in Table 19-3.

## CHLAMYDIA

*Chlamydia trachomatis* is the most common bacterial sexually transmitted organism in the United States, with an estimated 4 million new cases occurring each year at an estimated cost of $2.4 billion.[30] In addition, chlamydial infection is the most commonly reported infectious disease in the United States, and in 2002 834,555 cases of genital chlamydial infection were reported to the CDC.[31] Washington et al estimated that over three fourths of the health care costs associated with chlamydial infection are for women.[32] Of most concern is the recognition that the health consequences of chlamydial infection are greatest for women. This is primarily due to the increased risk of women infected with *C. trachomatis* for PID and its sequelae of tubal factor infertility, ectopic pregnancy, and chronic pelvic pain.[30] Additionally, pregnant women infected with *C. trachomatis* but untreated are at increased risk for adverse pregnancy outcome including preterm delivery, PROM, and low-birth-weight infants.[31] Infants born to mothers with untreated chlamydial infection of the cervix are at increased risk for neonatal conjunctivitis and pneumonia.[32] Moreover, women infected with *C. trachomatis* appear to be at increased risk for acquisition of HIV infection.[33]

During the past 20 years, the spectrum of diseases caused by *C. trachomatis* has expanded dramatically, and an increasing number of infections have been attributed to *C. trachomatis* (Table 19-4).[30]

*C. trachomatis* is a high-prevalence agent associated with a wide variety of complications. Unfortunately, the majority (50% to 70%) of chlamydial infections of the lower genital tract in women are asymptomatic and can progress to the upper genital tract to produce serious complications such as PID, tubal factor infertility, and ectopic pregnancy.[30] Other long-term consequences of chlamydial infection include neonatal conjunctivitis and chlamydial pneumonia of the newborn; and association with fetal wastage, PROM, preterm labor and delivery, and postpartum endometritis also has been suggested.

There are four recognized species within the genus *Chlamydia*: *C. trachomatis, C. psittaci, C. pneumoniae,* and *C. pecorum. C. psittaci* is the causative agent of psittacosis, a common pathogen in avian species and lower mammals. *C. pneumoniae* (TWAR) is a recently identified species that causes acute respiratory tract infection.[34] The clinical syndromes associated with *C. pneumoniae* infection include bronchitis, pneumonia, otitis, pharyngitis, and sinusitis.[34] *C. pneumoniae*

# Gynecologic Infectious Disease

| **Table 19-4** <br> **Clinical Spectrum of *Chlamydia trachomatis* Infection** | | |
|---|---|---|
| **Men** | **Women** | **Infants** |
| Urethritis | Bartholinitis | Conjunctivitis |
| Postgonococcal urethritis | Mucopurulent cervicitis | Pneumonia |
| Epididymitis | Endometritis | Asymptomatic pharyngeal carriage |
| Prostatis | Salpingitis | Asymptomatic gastrointestinal tract carriage |
| Conjunctivitis | Perihepatitis | Otitis media |
| Pharyngitis | Urethritis | |
| Lymphogranuloma venereum | Lymphogranuloma venereum | |
| Reiter's syndrome | Conjunctivitis | |
| Sterility | Pharyngitis | |
| | Tubal factor infertility | |
| | Ectopic pregnancy | |
| | Postpartum endometritis* | |
| | Preterm labor and delivery* | |
| | Premature rupture of membranes* | |
| | Reactive arthritis | |
| | Stillbirth* | |
| *Relationship not firmly established. | | |

may play a role in coronary artery disease.[35] *C. pecorum* is a recently recognized species that causes disease in the reproductive tract of sheep, cattle, and swine.[36]

Although all chlamydiae share a common genus-specific antigen (chlamydial lipopolysaccharide), *C. trachomatis* may be further differentiated on a serologic basis. There are currently 15 recognized serotypes (Table 19-5). The *C. trachomatis* serotypes are responsible for three major groups of infections. Three of these serotypes (L1, L2, L3) represent the agents causing lymphogranuloma venereum. Serotypes A, B, Ba, and C are the agents responsible for endemic blinding trachoma. The remaining serotypes of *C. trachomatis* (D, E, F, G, H, I, J, K) are the oculogenital and sexually transmitted strains that cause inclusion conjunctivitis, newborn pneumonia, urethritis, cervicitis, epididymitis, salpingitis, acute urethral syndrome, and perinatal infections.

The chlamydial organism exists in two forms: (1) the elementary body, which is the infectious particle and capable of entering uninfected cells; and (2) the reticulate body, which multiplies by binary fission within the host cell to produce the inclusions that are identified in properly stained cells.[37] The reticulate bodies condense and reorganize to form new elementary bodies, and at the end of the 48- to 72-hour growth cycles, the cell bursts with release of elementary bodies.

*C. trachomatis* is an obligatory intracellular bacterium.[37] It is an extremely well-adapted human parasite that depends on the host cell for nutrients and energy.[37] Although chlamydiae are

capable of limited metabolic activities, they do not possess an enzyme system capable of generating ATP and have been considered energy parasites.

## Epidemiology, Risk Factors, and Pathogenesis

For the oculogenital serotypes, the primary method of transmission is sexual. Schachter has stated that *C. trachomatis* is probably the most common sexually transmitted bacterial pathogen in Western industrialized society.[37] *C. trachomatis* appears to be more difficult to transmit than *N. gonorrhoeae*.[38] Lycke et al studied partners of men with chlamydial or gonococcal urethritis and noted that female partners were infected 45% and 80% of the time, respectively.[38] Male-to-female and female-to-male transmission of chlamydia are equally efficient.[38]

Chlamydiae cause between one third and one half of nongonococcal urethritis in men.[39] Double infections with gonococci are common in both men and women, and between 20% and 40% of men and between 30% and 50% of women with lower genital gonorrheal infection have concomitant chlamydial infection.[38] Epididymitis is an important complication of chlamydial infection of the male urethra, and *C. trachomatis* is the major cause of epididymitis in men under the age of 35. Rectal and pharyngeal infections also occur in both sexes.[40] Reiter's syndrome is a systemic clinical syndrome associated with chlamydial infection in men.

A number of clinical conditions in the female have been attributed to *C. trachomatis* (see Table 19-4).[40] These include mucopurulent endocervicitis, endometritis, salpingitis, acute urethral syndrome, urethritis, and perinatal infections. The anatomic site within the female genital tract most commonly infected with *C. trachomatis* is the cervix. No specific symptoms are associated with the cervical infections, and so many of the chlamydial infections of the cervix are clinically inapparent. This is unfortunate because mucopurulent cervicitis (the female equivalent of nongonococcal urethritis) caused by *C. trachomatis* predisposes to acute PID in nonpregnant women and to maternal and infant infections during pregnancy. In addition,

| **Table 19-5** <br> **Taxonomy and Association of Chlamydia with Human Disease** | | |
|---|---|---|
| **Species** | **Serotype** | **Disease** |
| *Chlamydia psittaci* | Many | Psittacosis |
| *Chlamydia pneumoniae* | TWAR | Acute upper and lower respiratory tract infections |
| *Chlamydia trachomatis* | A, B, Ba, C | Hyperendemic blinding trachoma |
| | D, E, F, G, H, I, J, K | Inclusion conjunctivitis, nongonococcal urethritis, proctitis, epididymitis, cervicitis, endometritis, salpingitis, pneumonia of newborn |
| | L1, L2, L3 | Lymphogranuloma venereum |
| *Relationship not firmly established. | | |

asymptomatic chlamydial cervicitis is a major reservoir for sexual transmission of C. trachomatis.

In 1996 chlamydia became a notifiable disease, and by 2002 over 834,000 cases of genital chlamydia infection were reported to the CDC (296.55 cases per 100,000) making chlamydia the most frequently reported infection in the United States.[31] The annual incidence of new chlamydia infections in the United States is estimated to be over 4 million cases.[37] Of the reported U.S. cases, over 75% were in women.[31] These reported rates for women are an overestimate of the female-to-male ratio of chlamydial infection because women are more likely to be screened. Chlamydial infections are present through all strata of society, but the highest rates occur in the young and the poor. As noted by Stamm, in areas where intensive chlamydia control programs have been instituted, dramatic decreases in the prevalence of chlamydia have occurred.[40] Such has been reported in Sweden where the number of cases of chlamydial infection decreased greater than 50% from 1987 to 1994[29] and in selected areas of the United States (e.g., Pacific Northwest and Wisconsin) where similar results have been reported.[39]

While 3% to 5% of sexually active women in the United States carry chlamydia in their cervix, high-risk populations can be readily identified. A number of patient characteristics have been found to be predictors of chlamydial genital infections.[40-42] These include young age (<25 years), socioeconomic status, nonwhite race, number of sexual partners, new partner, douching, and use of nonbarrier methods of contraception.

The majority of women with chlamydial disease remain untreated because their infection is either asymptomatic or relatively inapparent. In general, one half to two thirds of chlamydial infections of the cervix are asymptomatic.[40,43] Untreated, the infection can persist for several years and subject those infected to the risks of spread of C. trachomatis to the upper genital tract, with subsequent infertility and ectopic pregnancy.[44]

Over 1 million women acquire PID each year in the United States. Both medically and economically PID is the most important genital disease caused by C. trachomatis. Studies in the United States suggest that 20% to 50% of these cases are associated with C. trachomatis.[45] Thus, 200,000 to 500,000 cases of chlamydia-associated PID occur annually in the United States and are estimated to require 50,000 to 100,000 hospitalizations each year. In addition, these women are exposed to a significantly increased risk for infertility and ectopic pregnancy.

The infant born to a woman with a chlamydial infection of the cervix is at 60% to 70% risk of acquiring the infection via vertical transmission during passage through the birth canal.[45] Approximately 25% to 50% of exposed infants will develop chlamydial conjunctivitis in the first 2 weeks of life, and 10% to 20% of the infants will develop chlamydial pneumonia within 3 to 4 months of birth.

## Clinical Features

The majority (up to 85% to 90%) of chlamydial infections are asymptomatic.[40,45] Although the majority of infected women are asymptomatic, an estimated one third will have signs of infection at the time of examination.[40] In women, the most common findings on examination are the presence of mucopurulent endocervical discharge and hypertrophic cervical ectopy

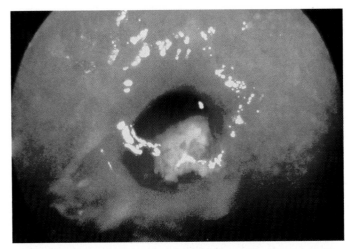

**Figure 19-2  Chlamydial mucopurulent endocervicitis.** (Reprinted with permission from Sweet RL, Gibbs RS: Atlas of Infectious Diseases of the Female Genital Tract. Philadelphia, Lippincott Williams & Wilkins, 2004.)

(Fig. 19-2). A broad spectrum of clinical presentations has been described for chlamydial infection in women. These include bartholinitis, endocervicitis, endometritis, PID, perihepatitis, acute urethral syndrome, urethritis, and reactive arthritis (Reiter's syndrome).[40,45]

### Endocervicitis

The anatomic site within the female genital tract most commonly infected with C. trachomatis is the cervix. C. trachomatis is a major cause of mucopurulent cervicitis (MPC). The infected cervix may range from clinically normal to a severely eroded cervix with a hypertrophic cervical erosion and a mucopurulent endocervical discharge. Hypertrophic cervicitis is the term applied to the presence of cervical ectopy that is edematous, congested, and friable.

A diagnosis of mucopurulent cervicitis is suggested by demonstrating (1) yellow or green mucopus on a swab of endocervical secretions ("positive swab test"); (2) more than 10 PMNs per oil immersion field of a Gram stain of the endocervix; or (3) friability, erythema, or edema within a zone of cervical ectopy.[40]

The acute urethral syndrome, which is defined as acute dysuria and frequent urination in women with pyuria but whose voided urine is sterile or contains less than 10 microorganisms/mL[32] is a common and perplexing problem for the clinician. Based on studies in STD clinics of cultures for C. trachomatis from the cervix and urethra, 25% of positive women harbor the organism only in their urethra[46]; an additional 50% harbor the organism in both cervix and urethra. Stamm and coworkers identified a causative role for C. trachomatis in up to 25% of women with the acute urethral syndrome.[47] Several findings on history are suggestive of C. trachomatis as the causative agent in women with symptoms of acute urethral syndrome.[47] These include a recent change in sexual partner, the use of oral contraceptives, and a longer duration of presenting symptoms—approximately 7 to 10 days—as compared with 4 days for women with acute cystitis or bacteriuria. In addition, women with chlamydia are less likely to give a history of recurrent urinary tract infections, in contradistinction to women with acute cystitis or bladder bacteriuria.

Multiple investigations have demonstrated that endometritis in nonpregnant women is another manifestation of genital chlamydial infection.[48] Histologic endometritis based on the presence of plasma cells and infiltration of the superficial epithelium by PMN leukocytes has been detected in nearly one half of patients with chlamydial mucopurulent cervicitis.[40] The presence of histologic endometritis has been associated with both cultural and immunohistologic detection of C. trachomatis.[48] In addition, histologic endometritis can be detected in nearly all patients with chlamydial salpingitis.[40]

The most serious complication of chlamydial infection in women is acute PID. As reviewed by Cates et al[49] and Sweet,[50] microbiologic and serologic studies have firmly established C. trachomatis as an important sexually transmitted organism that leads to acute PID.

Initial evidence that C. trachomatis is an important etiologic agent in acute salpingitis came from European investigations (predominantly Scandinavian).[45] Of major importance was the report by Mardh et al of a 30% isolation of C. trachomatis from the fallopian tubes of women with acute salpingitis in whom isolation attempts were performed on material aspirated from the involved fallopian tubes visualized by laparoscopy.[51]

In the mid 1980s studies in the United States that utilized appropriate methodology for obtaining chlamydial specimens (i.e., tubal biopsy, tubal aspirate, swab of endosalpinx, endometrial biopsy, with or without protected endometrial aspirate) confirmed that C. trachomatis is a major etiologic agent for acute PID in the United States.[52-54] Currently it is estimated that C. trachomatis is responsible for 20% to 40% of clinically apparent acute PID in the United States.[30,32,50]

Cates and Wasserheit have estimated that clinically apparent PID (symptomatic or visually confirmed) accounts for less than half of the total cases of PID.[30] The remaining cases are due to unrecognized ("silent" or "atypical") PID. Thus, chronic, subacute, or latent upper genital tract infection is present in a large number of women.[55] Neither the magnitude of nor an accepted definition of these unrecognized infections has been established. Unfortunately, unrecognized PID appears to be as likely as recognized PID to result in progressive scarring of the fallopian tubes, resulting in tubal factor infertility and ectopic pregnancy.[56] Further support for the role of C. trachomatis in the etiology and pathogenesis of acute PID arises from a large number of studies demonstrating a statistically significant association for tubal factor infertility and ectopic pregnancy with previous systemic chlamydial infection identified by the presence of antibody against C. trachomatis.[45]

Acute perihepatitis (Fitz-Hugh-Curtis syndrome) is a localized fibrinous inflammation affecting the anterior surface of the liver and the adjacent parietal peritoneum. Most commonly, this entity is associated with acute PID. However, the symptoms of PID are often moderate or even absent in this syndrome. The clinical picture is often characterized by an acute onset of severe right upper quadrant abdominal pain resembling that of acute cholecystitis. Several investigations have demonstrated a putative role for C. trachomatis in the Fitz-Hugh-Curtis syndrome.[57,58]

Infection with C. trachomatis in pregnant women is a major concern. The prevalence of chlamydial infection of the cervix in pregnant women has been reported to range from 2% to 37%, with the general estimate for the United States being 5%.[45] In general, the higher prevalence rates occur in studies conducted among indigent patients in urban inner city areas and among adolescents.[52] While it is well documented that infants born through an infected birth canal are likely to become infected with C. trachomatis and develop inclusion conjunctivitis or pneumonia, the effect of maternal chlamydial infection on pregnancy outcome and perinatal complications such as preterm labor and delivery, PROM, and postpartum endometritis has also been demonstrated.

An association between C. trachomatis and postpartum infection was initially described in the ophthalmology literature.[53,54] Subsequently in a prospective investigation, Wager et al from Seattle suggested that pregnant women in whom C. trachomatis was recovered at their initial prenatal visit were at significant increased risk for developing late-onset endometritis following a vaginal delivery.[59] Subsequent studies have both confirmed[60] and not confirmed[61] a putative role for C. trachomatis in postpartum endometritis.

Several studies have demonstrated that patients with chlamydial cervicitis who undergo pregnancy termination are at high risk for postabortion endometritis.[62] Approximately 10% to 35% of women who have cervical C. trachomatis at the time of elective abortion develop postabortal pelvic infection compared with 2% to 10% of chlamydia negatives.

## Diagnosis

Until recently, the "gold standard" for the diagnosis of C. trachomatis was cell culture. However, methodologic difficulties, including cold-chain transport of specimens, delay in obtaining results (7 days), expense, need for substantial technical expertise, and relative insensitivity, led to the development of non–culture based testing for C. trachomatis.[45] Antigen and nucleic acid detection methods were introduced during the 1980s into clinical practice for diagnosing genital chlamydia infection and rapidly became the most widely available diagnostic tests for detection of C. trachomatis. More recently, nucleic acid amplification technology was introduced into clinical practice for detection of C. trachomatis.[45]

Because chlamydiae are obligatory intracellular parasites, culture cannot be performed on artificial media but requires a susceptible tissue culture cell line. Culture has the advantage that it preserves organisms for further studies including antimicrobial susceptibility testing and genotyping. Moreover, because it detects only viable chlamydial elementary bodies and is unlikely to be contaminated, culture remains the standard for medicolegal matters such as sexual abuse in adults or children.

Nonculture, non-nucleic acid amplification testing is based on direct visualization of chlamydia by staining with fluorescein-labeled specific antibodies (direct immunofluorescence; DFA), immunohistochemical detection of antigen (enzyme-linked immunoassay [EIA] and rapid tests), and detection of hybridization to a DNA probe.[63] The advantages of these nonculture, non-nucleic acid amplification techniques include (1) laboratories lacking the expertise or facilities to perform culture can make these tests widely available, (2) specimen transport is less rigorous, and (3) the technology is standardized.[63] Multiple investigations have compared these tests favorably to culture.[63]

As a result, most laboratories in North America and Western Europe use antigen detection tests (DFA and EIA) or nucleic acid hybridization tests (DNA probe).[63]

However, these tests have reduced sensitivities and specificities compared with culture and even more so when compared with NAATs.[63] In addition, use of nonculture, non-nucleic acid amplification techniques in populations with a low prevalence of infection is problematic as the proportion of false positives will rise as the prevalence of infection decreases.

In general, direct fluorescent monoclonal antibody staining in the hands of an experienced technician has sensitivity of 80% to 85% and specificity greater than 99% compared with cell culture.[40,63] The EIA method has a sensitivity that is generally in the range of 60% to 80% compared with culture.[63] Its specificity, with use of antibody-blocking reagents is greater than 99%.[63] Rapid, office-based direct EIA kits have been developed for detection of C. trachomatis. The results are read visually, usually in about 30 minutes. In general, the rapid tests have proved to be less sensitive and specific than laboratory-performed EIAs or the PACE 2 DNA probe.[63]

DNA probes are commercially available for detection of C. trachomatis. This DNA probe uses the technique of nucleic acid hybridization to identify C. trachomatis DNA directly from urogenital swab specimens.

An important advantage of the DNA probe is that it can be used in conjunction with a probe for detection of N. gonorrhoeae as a single-swab specimen.[63] In addition, DNA probe does not require cold-chain transportation or that specimens remain stable in storage; minimal technical expertise is required, and testing procedures can be automated, leading to decreased costs. Black noted that the DNA probe is probably the most commonly used test for detecting C. trachomatis in public health laboratories in the United States.[63] However, DNA probe is less sensitive than NAATs, and CDC recommends that positive results in a low prevalence population be confirmed.[52]

The most important recent advance in the diagnosis of chlamydial infections of the genital tract has been development of tests utilizing NAATs.[40,63] Nucleic acid amplification testing is extremely sensitive (detects as little as a single gene copy) and highly specific.[63] As a result, these tests can be utilized for non-invasive (urine or vaginal swab) specimen procurement to screen asymptomatic men and women for chlamydial infection.[40,63] The two most widely used nucleic acid amplification tests are PCR and LCR, which target nucleotide sequences on the plasmid of C. trachomatis, which are present in multiple copies within each elementary body. A third methodology, transcription-mediated amplification (TMA) is now available; this test amplifies chlamydial ribosomal RNA. The lower limit of detection for these tests is in the range of 1 to 10 elementary bodies (Ebs). In comparison, EIA requires 10,000 Ebs, DNA probe 1000 Ebs, and culture 10 to 100 Ebs. Thus NAATs are the most sensitive.

Nucleic acid amplification technologies detect DNA or RNA targets and do not require the presence of viable or intact organisms for a positive test.[63] This has major implications when considering "test of cure." It has been suggested that a culture-negative, nucleic acid–positive state following appropriate treatment lasts up to 3 weeks after which both culture and NAAT will be negative.

## Table 19-6
### CDC–recommended Treatment for Chlamydial Infection of the Lower Genital Tract, 2002

**Recommended regimen**

Azithromycin 1 g orally in a single dose
or
Doxycycline 100 mg orally twice a day for 7 days

**Alternative regimens**

Erythromycin base 500 mg orally four times a day for 7 days
or
Erythromycin ethylsuccinate 800 mg orally four times a day for 7 days
or
Ofloxacin 300 mg orally twice a day for 7 days

## Treatment

CDC-recommended treatment for chlamydial infection of the lower genital tract in nonpregnant patients is provided in Table 19-6.[64] Either doxycycline 100 mg orally twice a day for 7 days or azithromycin 1 g orally as a single dose are the suggested treatments of choice. The fluoroquinolones, ofloxacin and levofloxacin, and erythromycin base or erythromycin ethylsuccinate are alternative regimens.

An antichlamydial agent, usually doxycycline or clindamycin in the parenteral regimens and doxycycline or ofloxacin in the oral regimens,[64] is part of a combination therapy approach to the treatment of acute PID.

CDC recommendations for the treatment of chlamydial genital tract infection during pregnancy is provided in Table 19-7.[64] Since doxycycline and fluoroquinolones are contraindicated for pregnant women, erythromycin base and amoxicillin are the recommended regimens for treatment of chlamydial infection during pregnancy. Crombleholme et al were the first group to demonstrate the efficacy of amoxicillin in preventing vertical transmission of C. trachomatis.[65] In addition amoxicillin was well tolerated. Subsequent randomized, prospective trials comparing amoxicillin and erythromycin for the treatment of chlamydial infection in pregnancy demonstrated treatment success in 85% to 99% of amoxicillin-treated patients compared with 72% to 88% of erythromycin-treated cases. At the time

## Table 19-7
### CDC–recommended Treatment of Chlamydial Genital Tract Infection During Pregnancy, 2002

**Recommended regimen for pregnant women**

Erythromycin base 500 mg orally four times a day for 7 days
or
Amoxicillin 500 mg orally three times a day for 7 days

**Alternative regimens for pregnant women**

Erythromycin base 250 mg orally four times a day for 14 days
or
Erythromycin ethylsuccinate 400 mg orally four times a day for 14 days
or
Azithromycin 1 g orally in a single dose

267

# Gynecologic Infectious Disease

when the current CDC guidelines for treatment of chlamydial infection were published, the safety and efficacy of azithromycin in pregnant and lactating women had not been established.[48] Thus, azithromycin was suggested as an alternative regimen for pregnant women.[48] Other alternatives include erythromycin ethylsuccinate and the option of reducing the dose of erythromycin base or ethylsuccinate by half but doubling the length of therapy for patients not able to tolerate the larger dose of erythromycin.[48] Erythromycin estolate is contraindicated in pregnancy because it is associated with drug-induced hepatotoxicity.[48]

## SYPHILIS

Syphilis is a chronic systemic infectious process caused by the spirochete *Treponema pallidum*. In the late 1980s syphilis reemerged in epidemic form in the United States with significant increases in the incidences of primary and secondary syphilis and especially of syphilis in pregnancy and of congenital syphilis.[66,67] Starting in 1991 syphilis rates sharply declined in the United States.[68] However, in 2001, the number of reported cases of syphilis began to increase again.[69]

That syphilis in pregnant women caused infection of the fetus, with resultant stillbirths, premature births, congenital abnormalities, and active disease at birth has been known for several centuries. Because of this significant morbidity, great emphasis has been placed on routine screening of all pregnant women for the presence of syphilis.

### Epidemiology, Risk Factors, and Pathogenesis

Acquisition, with the exception of congenital syphilis, is generally through sexual contact. *T. pallidum* enters the body through breaks in mucosal surfaces or abraded areas of the skin. Subsequently, the chancre (the primary lesion) appears at the site of entry of the spirochetes. The chancre, if untreated, resolves within 3 to 6 weeks and is followed by a secondary stage. Secondary syphilis is a systemic disease with dermatologic manifestations, lymphadenopathy, and spirochetemia and lasts 2 to 6 weeks. This stage is also self-limiting, and with resolution of the secondary stage, the patient enters the latent phase in which there are no clinical manifestations of disease. Individuals with primary, secondary, or early latent (up to 1 year) syphilis have replicating treponemal organisms and are capable of transmitting syphilis to susceptible hosts. Without therapy, approximately one third of patients develop tertiary syphilis, with progressive damage to the central nervous system (CNS), cardiovascular system, musculoskeletal system, or other parenchyma.

The incidence of primary and secondary syphilis (best indicator of incidence trends) peaked in 1947 at 76 cases per 100,000 population.[70] Following the introduction of penicillin into clinical practice, the incidence of primary and secondary syphilis fell dramatically, reaching a nadir of 4 cases per 100,000 by the late 1950s. Beginning in 1959 this trend reversed with a 3-fold increased incidence by 1965. From 1965 through 1982 there was steady but slow increase in the incidence of reported cases of primary and secondary syphilis that peaked in 1982 at 14.6 cases per 100,000 persons. Much of this increase was due to increased rates among homosexual and bisexual men.[71] From 1982 until 1985 there was a 22% decrease in reported cases of primary and secondary syphilis. In large part this decrease occurred among white homosexual and bisexual men[67] probably as a result of changes in sexual behavior as a result of the AIDS epidemic.

Commencing in 1985 the United States experienced the most recent epidemic of syphilis.[68] From 1985 to 1990 the incidence of primary and secondary syphilis rose sharply, reaching a peak in 1990 of 23.5 cases and 17.3 cases per 100,000 in men and women, respectively.[69,70] Much of the increase occurred among African American men and women. This increased spread of syphilis has been linked to increased use of illicit drugs, especially "crack cocaine," and high-risk sexual behavior associated with drug use. In 1991 the rates of primary and secondary syphilis again fell dramatically.

During 2002, a total of 6862 primary and secondary syphilis cases were reported (2.4 cases per 100,000 population), an increase from the 6103 cases reported in 2001.[72] While the rate in men increased by 27%, in women it decreased by 21%.[72] A total of 412 cases of congenital syphilis were reported in 2002 (10.2 per 100,000 live births). This is a sharp decline from the peak of 107.3 per 100,000 in 1991. This decline is related to the reduction in the rate of primary and secondary syphilis among women over that period of time.

### Clinical Features

The probability of acquiring syphilis from an infectious partner during a sexual encounter is approximately 50%. Following exposure to syphilis, there is an incubation period ranging from 10 to 90 days before the primary lesion, the chancre, appears at the point of entry. The chancre is a painless, ulcerated lesion with a raised border and an indurated base (Fig. 19-3). Most commonly, the "hard" chancre of syphilis appears in the genital area. In men, the lesion is easily apparent, and syphilis is often diagnosed in its primary stage in men. Although chancres on the female external genitalia are easily recognized, more commonly the lesion is on the cervix or in the vagina and not recognized. Thus, the chancre often escapes detection in women, and it is unusual to diagnose the primary stage of syphilis in females. Usually only a single chancre is present, but multiple chancres occur in up to 30% of cases.[73] Painless inguinal lymphadenopathy is frequently present. The primary chancre, even without treatment, heals spontaneously in 3 to 6 weeks.

Following resolution of the primary stage, the patient enters the secondary or spirochetemia (bacteremia) stage. Syphilis always disseminates. Thus, any organ can potentially be infected especially the CNS. While the secondary stage of syphilis is characterized by involvement of all major organ systems by *T. pallidum*, it presents most commonly with skin and mucous membrane lesions. These clinical manifestations of secondary syphilis include a generalized maculopapular rash that begins on the trunk and proximal extremities and spreads to the entire body especially the palms and soles; there are mucous patches, condyloma latum, and generalized lymphadenopathy.

During the secondary stage of syphilis, the CNS is invaded by spirochetes in 40% of cases.[74] Although abnormal levels of protein and cell counts in the cerebrospinal fluid (CSF) are common and headache or meningismus may develop, frank "aseptic" meningitis is uncommon (1% to 2% of cases).[73] Even

The clinical spectrum in congenital syphilis includes still-births, neonatal death, clinical apparent congenital syphilis during the early months of life (early congenital syphilis), and development of the classic stigmata of late congenital syphilis.[76] While the most severe effects on pregnancy outcome occur with primary or secondary syphilis, at present pregnant women with syphilis are usually asymptomatic in the latent stage and have had the disease for more than 1 year. Consequently, most infants (approximately two thirds) with early congenital syphilis are asymptomatic at birth and do not develop evidence of active disease for 3 to 8 weeks. Chancres do not occur unless the disease is acquired at the time of passage through the birth canal. The characteristic manifestations of early congenital syphilis (onset <2 years of age) include a maculopapular rash that may progress to desquamation or vesiculae and bullae formation, snuffles (a flu-like syndrome associated with a nasal discharge), mucous patches in the oral pharyngeal cavity, hepatosplenomegaly, jaundice, lymphadenopathy, Parrot's pseudoparalysis due to osteochondritis, chorioretinitis, and iritis.[76]

Untreated or incompletely treated early congenital syphilis will progress to the classic manifestations of late congenital syphilis. These include Hutchinson's teeth, mulberry molars, interstitial keratitis, eighth nerve deafness, saddle nose, rhagades, saber shins, and neurologic manifestations (mental retardation, hydrocephalus, general paresis, optic nerve atrophy, and Clutton's joints). These stigmata associated with late congenital syphilis are the result of scarring induced by early lesions or reactions to persistent inflammation.[76]

### Diagnosis

The most specific and sensitive method for diagnosing syphilis is demonstration of *T. pallidum* in fresh specimens obtained from the lesions of infected individuals. Dark-field examination and direct fluorescent antibody tests are the definitive methods for diagnosing early syphilis. However, this methodology is applicable only to the lesions of primary or secondary syphilis. A specimen for dark-field examination or fluorescent antibody test should be obtained from any lesion suspected of being a chancre or manifestation of secondary syphilis.

The majority of men and nearly all women diagnosed with syphilis are in the latent stage. Thus, the diagnosis is most often based on serologic testing, which is a two-step process initially using nonspecific tests for reagin-type antibodies followed by specific antitreponemal antibody tests.[77] Nonspecific antibody tests for syphilis available today include the VDRL and the rapid plasma reagin test (RPR). These are used as screening tests. The titers of nontreponemal tests usually correlate with active disease and so results of the VDRL or RPR should be quantitated.[77] Treponema-specific tests are employed for confirming the diagnosis of syphilis in patients that have reactive VDRL or RPR tests. These tests include the *T. pallidum* immobilization (TPI) test, the fluorescent treponemal antibody absorbed (FTA-ABS) test, and the microhemagglutination assay for antibody to *T. pallidum* (MHA-TP). Because MHA-TP is less expensive and easier to perform, it has largely replaced the FTA-ABS test for confirmation of positive screening tests.

CDC recommends that all pregnant women should be screened serologically for syphilis early in pregnancy (i.e., first prenatal visit)[77] For populations that do not have optimal

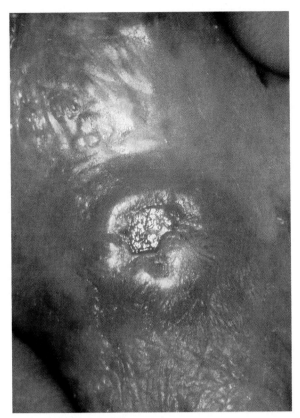

**Figure 19-3    Primary chancre of syphilis.** (Reprinted with permission from Sweet RL, Gibbs RS: Atlas of Infectious Diseases of the Female Genital Tract. Philadelphia, Lippincott Williams & Wilkins, 2004.)

without treatment these findings of secondary syphilis spontaneously clear within 2 to 6 weeks, and the latent stage of syphilis is entered, in which there is no apparent clinical disease. In the prepenicillin era about 25% of such patients had a recrudescence of secondary syphilis. These relapses usually occurred within 1 year, and thus the term early latency applies to this time period (<1 year). The mucocutaneous lesions associated with such relapses are highly contagious. The late latent stage (>1 year) is not infectious by sexual transmission, but the spirochete may still be transplacentally transmitted to the fetus.

If treatment is not provided, one third of patients progress and develop tertiary syphilis with involvement of the cardiovascular, central nervous, or musculoskeletal system, with or without involvement of various organ systems by gummas (late benign tertiary syphilis).[75] When tertiary syphilis occurs, one half of patients develop late benign syphilis (gummas), one fourth cardiovascular disease, and one fourth neurologic disease. The cardiovascular manifestations of tertiary syphilis include aortic aneurysm and aortic insufficiency. In the CNS, tertiary disease produces general paresis, tabes dorsalis, optic atrophy, and meningovascular syphilis; the Argyll-Robertson pupil (which does not react to light, but accommodates) is virtually pathognomonic. The pathogenesis of tertiary syphilis is based on the tropism of *T. pallidum* for arterioles, resulting in obliterative endarteritis with subsequent tissue destruction.[73]

# Gynecologic Infectious Disease

Table 19-8
Criteria for Performance of Cerebrospinal Fluid Examination in
Patients with Latent Syphilis to Exclude Neurosyphilis

- Neurologic or ophthalmic signs or symptoms
- Evidence of active tertiary syphilis (e.g., aortitis, gumma, and iritis)
- Treatment failure
- HIV infection with late latent syphilis or syphilis of unknown duration

prenatal care, CDC recommends that RPR-card test screening (a rapid screening test for syphilis) be performed when pregnancy is diagnosed and treatment given if the card is positive.[77] In populations with a high prevalence of syphilis or for patients at high risk, serologic testing should be performed twice during the third trimester—at 28 weeks' gestation and at delivery.[77]

Controversy has arisen over whether all patients (including pregnant women) who are asymptomatic but have a positive serologic diagnosis of syphilis should have a lumbar puncture for the detection of asymptomatic neurosyphilis. The lumbar puncture ensures proper treatment of neurosyphilis (see treatment section). Evaluation of syphilis patients with neurologic abnormalities should include CSF examination.[77] Although there is a high frequency of CSF abnormalities (elevated cell count, elevated protein concentration, reactive VDRL) in early syphilis, treatment results are good and so CSF examination is not necessary in asymptomatic early syphilis.[21] CDC recommends that all patients with latent syphilis be evaluated clinically for evidence of tertiary disease (e.g., aortitis, neurosyphilis, gummas, or iritis). Patients who demonstrate any of the criteria listed in Table 19-8 should have a prompt CSF examination.[77] With syphilis of more than 1 year's duration, CSF examination should be considered. CSF demonstrating pleocytosis, elevated protein concentrations, and a reactive VDRL is diagnostic of active neurosyphilis.

CDC emphasizes that no single test can be used to diagnose neurosyphilis.[77] The diagnosis can be made using various combinations of reactive serologic tests, abnormal CSF cell count, elevated protein, or a reactive CSF VDRL. The RPR test should not be performed on CSF. When reactive in a nonbloody tap, CSF VDRL is diagnostic of neurosyphilis. However, it may be nonreactive in the presence of neurosyphilis.

## Treatment

All patients with a history of sexual contact with a person with documented syphilis or either a positive dark-field examination or serologic evidence of syphilis with a specific treponemal test should be treated. In addition, those for whom the diagnosis cannot be ruled out with certainty or in those with previous treatment who have evidence of reinfection such as dark-field positive lesions or a 4-fold rise in titer of a quantitative nontreponemal test should receive appropriate treatment.

Parenteral penicillin G is the preferred drug for the treatment of all stages of syphilis.[77] The type of penicillin preparation used (i.e., benzathine, aqueous procaine, or aqueous crystalline), dosage, and length of treatment are dependent on the stage of syphilis and the clinical manifestations present. Parenteral penicillin G is the only therapy with documented efficacy for

treating neurosyphilis or syphilis in pregnancy. Thus, CDC recommends that patients with neurosyphilis and pregnant women with syphilis who report being allergic to penicillin should be treated with penicillin after desensitization.[77]

Table 19-9 contains CDC-recommended treatment regimens for the various stages of syphilis in nonpregnant, pregnant, and HIV-infected patients. Forty years of CDC experience

Table 19-9
CDC–recommended Treatment of Syphilis in Adults, 1998

**Primary and secondary syphilis**

Recommended regimen
  Benzathine penicillin G, 2.4 million units IM in a single dose
Penicillin allergy (nonpregnant)
  Doxycycline 100 mg orally twice a day for 2 weeks
  *or*
  Tetracycline 500 mg orally four times a day for 2 weeks

**Latent Syphilis**

Early latent syphilis (<1 year)—recommended regimens
  Benzathine penicillin G, 2.4 million units IM in a single dose
Late latent syphilis (>1 year)—recommended regimens
  Benzathine penicillin G, 7.2 million units total, administered as 3 doses of
    2.4 million units IM each, at 1-week intervals
Penicillin allergy (nonpregnant)
  Doxycycline 100 mg orally twice a day
  *or*
  Tetracycline 500 mg orally 4 times a day
  Both drugs administered for 2 weeks if duration of infection known to have
    been <1 year; otherwise administered for 4 weeks

**Tertiary syphilis (gumma and cardiovascular)**

Recommended regimen
  Benzathine penicillin G, 7.2 million units total, administered as 3 doses of
    2.4 million units IM, at 1-week intervals
Penicillin allergy
  Same as for late syphilis

**Neurosyphilis**

Recommended regimen
  Aqueous crystalline penicillin G 18–24 million units per day, administered as
    3–4 million units IV every 4 hours, for 10–14 days
Alternative regimen (if compliance assured)
  Procaine penicillin 2.4 million units IM daily, plus probenecid 500 mg orally
    four times a day, both for 10–14 days

**Syphilis during pregnancy**

Recommended regimens
  Penicillin regimen appropriate for the pregnant woman's stage of syphilis
  Some experts recommend additional therapy (e.g., a second dose of
    benzathine penicillin 2.4 million units IM) 1 week after the initial dose,
    particularly for women in the third trimester and for those who have
    secondary syphilis during pregnancy
Penicillin allergy
  A pregnant woman with a history of penicillin allergy should be treated with
    penicillin after desensitization

**Syphilis among HIV-infected patients**

Primary and secondary syphilis
  Recommended benzathine penicillin 2.4 million units IM
  Some experts recommend additional treatments such as multiple doses of
    benzathine penicillin G as in late syphilis
  Penicillin allergic patients should be desensitized and treated with penicillin
Latent syphilis (normal CSF examination)
  Benzathine penicillin G 7.2 million units as 3 weekly doses of 2.4 million
    units each

demonstrate that parenteral penicillin G is effective in achieving local cure (healing of lesions and prevention of sexual transmission) and in preventing tertiary syphilis when used for the treatment of primary and secondary syphilis.[77] Thus, for patients (nonpregnant and pregnant) who are not allergic to penicillin, the recommended regimen for primary and secondary syphilis is benzathine penicillin G 2.4 million units IM in a single dose. CDC suggests that all patients with syphilis be tested for HIV infection.[77] Patients with syphilis who have symptoms or signs suggesting neurologic or ophthalmic disease should have CSF analysis and slit-lamp examination to rule out neurosyphilis and syphilitic eye disease, respectively.[21] Lumbar puncture is recommended for patients when clinical signs or symptoms of neurologic disease are present or patients fail to respond to treatment.[77]

In nonpregnant penicillin-allergic patients with primary or secondary syphilis, treatment with doxycycline 100 mg twice a day for 2 weeks or tetracycline 500 mg four times a day for 2 weeks is suggested.

An additional alternative in nonpregnant patients allergic to penicillin, for whom compliance and follow-up can be assured, is erythromycin 500 mg orally four times a day for 2 weeks.[77] However, erythromycin is less effective than other recommendations for treatment of primary or secondary syphilis.[77] Pregnant patients who are allergic to penicillin should be desensitized and treated with penicillin.

Assessing response to treatment is based on serologic titers as well as clinical findings. With primary or secondary syphilis patients should be reexamined clinically and serologically at 6 months and 12 months after treatment.[77] HIV-infected patients should be examined more frequently at 3-month intervals. Quantitative nontreponemal titers (VDRL or RPR) should decline 4-fold by 6 months after treatment.[77] Failure to do so identifies patients at risk for treatment failure and those who should be screened for HIV infection. At a minimum, such patients require additional clinical and serologic follow-up. When follow-up cannot be assured, re-treatment is recommended. Those patients whose signs or symptoms either persist or recur or who have a 4-fold rise in titer of nontreponemal testing are either considered to be reinfected or the treatment has failed.[77] For re-treatment it is best to provide three weekly injections of benzathine penicillin G 2.4 million units IM, unless CSF examination demonstrates the presence of neurosyphilis, which requires treatment as discussed following.

For non-penicillin-allergic patients with early latent syphilis and with normal CSF examination (if performed), the recommended regimen is benzathine penicillin G 2.4 million units IM in a single dose. With late latent syphilis (duration >1 year or unknown), the recommendation is benzathine penicillin G 7.2 million units total, administered as three doses of 2.4 million units each IM, at 1-week intervals. In nonpregnant patients with latent syphilis who are allergic to penicillin, nonpenicillin therapy should be used only after CSF examination rules out neurosyphilis. Either doxycycline 100 mg orally twice a day or tetracycline 500 mg orally four times a day are recommended in such individuals. For early latent syphilis, the duration of therapy is 2 weeks, and with a duration greater than 1 year it is 4 weeks.[77] Pregnant patients allergic to penicillin should be desensitized and treated with penicillin.

Follow-up in patients with latent syphilis requires quantitative nontreponemal serologic tests to be repeated at 6 months, 12 months, and 24 months after treatment.[77] If titers increase 4-fold or if a titer initially greater than 1:32 fails to decline 4-fold within 12 to 24 months, or if the patient develops signs or symptoms of syphilis, the patient should be evaluated for neurosyphilis and re-treated appropriately depending on the findings of CSF examination.

Patients with late (tertiary) syphilis findings of gumma or cardiovascular disease (not neurosyphilis) should be treated with benzathine penicillin G 7.2 million units total, administered as 3 doses of 2.4 million units IM, at 1-week intervals. Penicillin-allergic nonpregnant patients are treated according to the regimens recommended for late latent syphilis (see Table 19-9). Pregnant penicillin-allergic patients should be desensitized and treated with penicillin (see later discussion).[77] All patients with symptomatic late syphilis should undergo CSF examination before therapy in order to exclude neurosyphilis.[77]

Patients with neurosyphilis or syphilitic eye disease who are not allergic to penicillin should be treated with 18 to 24 million units of aqueous crystalline penicillin G daily, administered as 3 to 4 million units IV every 4 hours for 10 to 14 days. For patients for whom compliance can be assured, 2.4 million units of procaine penicillin IM daily, plus probenecid 500 mg orally 4 times a day for 10 to 14 days, is an alternative.[77]

# CHANCROID

Chancroid, commonly referred to as "soft" chancre, is an acute ulcerative disease often associated with inguinal adenopathy (bubo). The causative agent of chancroid is *Haemophilus ducreyi*. This bacterium is a small, nonmotile, gram-negative rod that has a characteristic "chaining" appearance on Gram's stain that results in its "school of fish" appearance.

### Epidemiology, Risk Factors, and Pathogenesis

Chancroid is a common disease and major public health problem in many countries in the developing world. In many of these countries, chancroid is endemic and WHO estimates an annual incidence of 7 million cases.[78] Although rare in the United States, outbreaks of chancroid have been reported in urban areas.[79] In 2002 only 67 cases of chancroid were reported to CDC. Although chancroid has become an infrequent STD in the United States, in endemic areas it should be considered in the differential diagnosis of high-risk patients with a painful genital ulcer.

Sex workers are thought to be the reservoir of disease in the epidemics that have occurred in North America.[80] Major risk factors for chancroid include use of crack cocaine and exchange of sex for money or drugs.[81] The disease occurs most commonly in men, especially young, sexually active males who have a history of recent contact with sex workers.[80] Chancroid is more prevalent among lower socioeconomic groups. Uncircumcised males appear to be more susceptible to *H. ducreyi*.[80] Males are more frequently symptomatic. Asymptomatic women with lesions of chancroid are rarely seen.

The importance of chancroid is further demonstrated by the recognition that chancroid is a major cofactor in the heterosexual transmission of HIV and has been strongly associated with increased infection rates for HIV, especially in Africa.[82]

## Clinical Features

The lesions of chancroid are generally limited to genital sites. In men, they are most commonly found in the internal surface of the prepuce and the frenulum, and in women on the labia, clitoris, and fourchette.

The incubation period of chancroid is 3 to 10 days, with most from 4 to 7 days. At the site of entry, a small papule develops surrounded by a zone of erythema. Within 2 to 3 days the lesion becomes pustular or vesiculopustular and ulcerates. The classic ulcer of chancroid is superficial and shallow with a ragged edge. The chancre is surrounded by an inflammatory red halo. The base of the ulcer is covered with a necrotic exudate. The chancre of chancroid is painful and tender. In addition, it is not indurated (i.e., "soft"). Whereas only a single ulcer is present in 50% of male patients, multiple ulcers are the rule in women; Plummer et al report that women have a mean of 4.5 discrete ulcers.[83]

In approximately half of cases, a bubo develops. The bubo appears 7 to 10 days after the initial lesion and is characterized by acute, painful, tender, inflammatory inguinal adenopathy. The bubo is unilateral in about two thirds of cases and is unilocular. If untreated, the bubo will rupture, forming a large ulcer in the inguinal area. Bubo formation is less common in women.[83]

In men the usual clinical complaints relate to the ulcerative lesion or tender inguinal adenopathy. Women tend to have less specific symptoms such as dysuria, rectal bleeding, dyspareunia, or vaginal discharge.[83] The combination of a painful ulcer and tender inguinal adenopathy is suggestive of chancroid but only occurs in one third of patients. The presence of a painful ulcer in combination with suppurative inguinal adenopathy is almost pathognomonic for chancroid.

## Diagnosis

The diagnosis of chancroid is based on gram-stained smears, culture, and clinical characteristics of lesions. Gram's stain of the exudate from the lesion or an aspirate of the bubo may reveal the presence of gram-negative rods that tend to form chains ("school of fish"). However, the sensitivity of gram staining is only 50%.[84] A definitive laboratory diagnosis of chancroid depends on isolation of *H. ducreyi* from the lesion or bubo. However, the organism is fastidious, and isolation of *H. ducreyi* is not routinely performed in most general clinical microbiology laboratories. Gonococcal agar base or Mueller-Hinton agar base supplemented with 0.2% activated charcoal, 1% bovine hemoglobin, 1% CVA enrichment, and 3 mg/mL vancomycin is the preferred medium for primary isolation of *H. ducreyi*.[12] Even with use of specific media the sensitivity of culture is at best 80%.[82] PCR assays compare favorably with culture, having a sensitivity of greater than 95%.[85] However, no U.S. Food and Drug Administration (FDA)–approved PCR test is available. The CDC recommends that a probable diagnosis of chancroid may be made if the following criteria exist: (1) the individual has one or more painful genital ulcers, (2) there is no evidence of syphilis by dark-field examination of lesion or by serology performed at least 7 days after onset of ulcers, and (3) either the clinical presentation of the genital ulcer or regional lymphadenopathy is typical for chancroid and a test for HSV is negative.[86]

| Table 19-10 |
| --- |
| CDC–recommended Treatment of Chancroid, 2002 |

**Recommended regimen**

Azithromycin 1 g orally in a single dose
*or*
Ceftriaxone 250 mg IM in a single dose
*or*
Ciprofloxacin* 500 mg orally twice a day for 3 days
*or*
Erythromycin base 500 mg orally four times a day for 7 days

*Contraindicated for pregnant and lactating women.

## Treatment

Current CDC recommendations for the treatment of chancroid are presented in Table 19-10. No instance of antimicrobial resistance by *H. ducreyi* to azithromycin, ceftriaxone, or erythromycin has been reported. The fluoroquinolones are also effective treatment for chancroid. CDC suggests that all patients diagnosed with chancroid be tested for HIV infection.

Follow-up examination should occur 3 to 7 days after initiation of therapy.[82] With successful treatment, symptomatic improvement of the ulcer is present within 3 days and objective improvement within 7 days after therapy. Clinical resolution of fluctuant buboes is slower than that of ulcers and may require needle aspiration.[82]

In pregnancy, ciprofloxacin is contraindicated and the safety of azithromycin has not been established. Thus, ceftriaxone or erythromycin is the preferred regimen for pregnant and lactating women. No adverse effects of chancroid on pregnancy outcome or on the fetus have been demonstrated.[82]

## LYMPHOGRANULOMA VENEREUM

Lymphogranuloma venereum (LGV) is a sexually transmitted disease caused by *C. trachomatis* serotypes L1, L2, and L3. The disease is manifested by both generalized systemic symptoms and a wide spectrum of anogenital lesions, lymphadenopathy, and gross devastation of perineal tissue.[87] LGV is uncommon in the United States. It usually presents as inguinal adenopathy, since the painless genital ulcer stage of the disease often goes unnoticed.

### Epidemiology, Risk Factors, and Pathogenesis

Although LGV is worldwide in distribution, it most commonly occurs in tropical areas. LGV is endemic in East and West Africa, India, parts of southeastern Asia, South America, and the Caribbean.[87] In North America, Europe, Australia, and most of Asia and South America it is a sporadic disease.[87]

While LGV is no longer a reportable disease, an estimated 350 cases per year occur in the United States. The majority of acute LGV cases occur in men, with a male-to-female ratio of 5:1 or greater. As is true for other STDs, LGV is more common in urban settings, among people with numerous sexual partners, and among lower socioeconomic classes.[87] While transplacental congenital infection has not been reported, acquisition during passage through an infected birth canal can occur.[87]

## Clinical Features

LGV is primarily an infection of lymphatic tissue in which inflammation spreads from infected lymph nodes into adjacent tissue.[88] The infected lymph nodes enlarge, necrose, and form abscesses that coalesce and rupture, leading to fistula formation and sinus tracts.[88] Healing is the result of fibrosis, with resultant obstruction of lymphatic vessels, chronic edema, and enlargement of affected anatomic locations. It is believed that most of the tissue damage associated with LGV is caused by a cell-mediated "hypersensitivity" to chlamydial antigens.[88]

The clinical presentation of LGV has primary, secondary, and tertiary stages. Following an incubation time that ranges from 3 to 21 days, the primary lesion in men usually occurs on the coronal sulcus, while in females, the most common site is the posterior vaginal wall, followed by the fourchette, cervix, and vulva. This primary lesion is vesicular or papular and painless; it may ulcerate but heals within a few days without scarring. The primary lesion generally is not appreciated or recognized by patients.

The secondary stage of LGV develops 1 to 4 weeks following the primary lesion and is characterized by acute lymphadenitis with bubo formation (inguinal syndrome) with or without acute hemorrhagic proctitis (anogenitorectal syndrome). This invasive stage of LGV is often preceded by the onset of systemic symptoms such as fever, malaise, headache, and myalgia.[88] Inguinal adenopathy is the most frequent clinical manifestation of LGV. The adenopathy is unilateral in two thirds of cases and begins as firm, discrete, multiple nodes that are slightly tender. Over the next week or two, a more extensive adenitis commences as the nodes become matted together and adherent to the subcutaneous tissue and overlying skin. The skin often is discolored, and the lesion becomes painful. The horizontal group of superficial inguinal nodes is most commonly involved, but the femoral nodes may also be affected. If both groups become involved, the inguinal ligament creates a groove between the node groups, producing the "grove sign," which is considered pathognomonic for LGV. The matted mass proceeds to suppurate, and multiple draining sinuses arise from the necrotic lymph nodes. Approximately one third of inguinal buboes in LGV become fluctuant and rupture. In the anogenitorectal syndrome, proctocolitis and hyperplasia of intestinal and perirectal lymphatic tissue occur. This form of secondary LGV is found predominantly in women and homosexual men. Symptoms include anal pruritus, mucous rectal discharge, fever, rectal pain, and tenesmus.[88]

The tertiary stage involves the external genitalia and anorectal areas. It is characterized by progressive tissue destruction and extensive scarring. Especially in women, this phase of disease may be the initial clinical manifestation for which the patient seeks care. This stage may present as hypertrophic ulceration and elephantiasis. Hypertrophic lesions are more common among women, but elephantiasis occurs in both men and women. Sinuses, fistula tracts, and ultimately strictures may occur in the vulva, perineum, and rectum.

## Diagnosis

Diagnosis of LGV solely on clinical grounds is, at best, difficult. The diagnosis can be made by isolation or identification of the chlamydial organism or with the use of serology. Schachter and coworkers reported that aspiration and culture of pus from fluctuant nodes was positive in approximately 50% of cases.[89]

The Frei intradermal test was for many years the backbone of diagnostic efforts for LGV. A positive Frei is not evidence of active infection but only indicates previous LGV infection. Moreover, the Frei antigen is common to all *Chlamydia*, and thus the specificity of a positive Frei test is poor for LGV, limiting its clinical usefulness.

The most commonly used diagnostic test for LGV at present is the complement fixation test for *Chlamydia* group antibodies. This test is very sensitive, and titers greater than 1:64 are considered diagnostic. However, CF titers are present with mucosal infections due to other chlamydial subgroups, although usually at lower titers.[89] The microimmunofluorescence test of Wang and Grayston can be used for typing isolates of *Chlamydia* and thus can identify the chlamydia biovars responsible for LGV. However, this test is available only in a limited number of laboratories.

## Treatment

As recommended by CDC, doxycycline 100 mg orally twice a day for 21 days is the therapy of choice for LGV.[90] An alternative regimen is erythromycin 500 mg orally four times a day for 21 days. Although the activity of azithromycin against *C. trachomatis* suggests it would be effective in multiple doses over 2 to 3 weeks, no clinical studies have been reported.[90] In pregnant or lactating women the erythromycin regimen should be used. Sexual contacts of a person with LGV within 30 days prior to onset of symptoms should be examined, tested for urethral or cervical chlamydial infection, and treated. Fluctuant inguinal nodes should be aspirated to prevent sinus tract formation. Incision and drainage or surgical extirpation of nodes is contraindicated, as such intervention will delay healing and may further obstruct lymphatic drainage. Late sequelae such as strictures or fistulas may require surgical intervention.

# DONOVANOSIS (GRANULOMA INGUINALE)

Donovanosis (granuloma inguinale) is a chronic, progressively destructive ulcerative infection of the genital area caused by the bacterium *Calymmatobacterium granulomatis*. Previously the disease was called granuloma inguinale. The presence of Donovan bodies characterizes this infection.

## Epidemiology, Risk Factors, and Pathogenesis

Donovanosis is most common in Papua New Guinea, Southern Africa, northeast Brazil, French Guyana, and Australia among aboriginal tribes.[90] It is rare in temperate climates. Although no longer a reportable disease, an estimated fewer than 100 cases occur annually in the United States.[91]

The variable incubation time and initial subtle clinical findings have confused the epidemiology of donovanosis.[92] It is generally believed that donovanosis is an STD. However, its exact mode of transmission is still not clearly understood, and young children and very old adults also develop the infection in the absence of sexual activity.

The sexually transmitted hypothesis is supported by a variety of evidence[92] including the following: (1) most lesions occur on the genitalia, (2) the disease occurs most frequently in the

# Gynecologic Infectious Disease

sexually active age group, (3) there is almost always a history of sexual exposure before the appearance of the ulcer, (4) other STDs are present among donovanosis patients, and (5) donovanosis has been proved to exist in more than 50% of the sexual partners of patients with the disease.

## Clinical Features

Donovanosis is a low-grade chronic infection of low infectiousness, and repeated close physical contact seems to be necessary for transmission.[92] The incubation period varies from a few days to a few months. The disease has an insidious onset, and the earliest lesion presents as a painless papule or nodule that often is unnoticed by patients. Most cases (90%) involve the genitals. In women the most common sites are the labia and fourchette. The epithelium overlying the lesion subsequently ulcerates, producing an enlarging granulomatous, beefy red, velvety ulcer. If untreated, the lesions may spread to involve the inguinal regions, producing a "pseudobubo," which is a subcutaneous granulomatous process rather than adenopathy. Unless secondarily infected, the lesions of granuloma inguinale are painless.

## Diagnosis

The diagnosis of donovanosis is usually made on clinical grounds because of the characteristic granulomatous process. C. *granulomatis* is difficult to culture, and so the diagnosis is made by histologic identification of C. *granulomatis*. Donovan bodies in macrophages on the smear or biopsy specimen must be demonstrated for a certain diagnosis.

## Treatment

CDC proposes either trimethoprim-sulfamethoxazole one double strength tablet orally twice a day or doxycycline 100 mg orally twice a day given over a minimum 3-week period of time as the recommended agents for the treatment of donovanosis.[93] Alternative agents include ciprofloxacin 750 mg orally twice a day or erythromycin base 500 mg orally four times a day for a minimum 3-week course. Addition of gentamicin 1 mg/kg IV every 8 hours should be considered if lesions fail to respond in the first few days of therapy.[93] Therapy should be continued until the lesions are completely healed.

Sexual partners should be examined and treated if they had sexual contact in the 60 days preceding the onset of symptoms and have clinical signs and symptoms of the disease. In pregnancy and during lactation the erythromycin regimen is recommended and the addition of parenteral gentamicin should be given strong consideration.[93]

## HERPES SIMPLEX VIRUS (GENITAL HERPES)

Herpes simplex virus (HSV), a member of the Herpesviridae family, is a double-stranded DNA virus. Two major serotypes, HSV-1 and HSV-2, are recognized. Genital herpes is an STD caused by either HSV-1 (also associated with oral/facial lesions) or HSV-2. These viruses cause infection following entry through mucous membranes or skin, resulting in typical vesicular lesions. HSV is neurotropic with sensory nerve involvement and latency within dorsal root ganglia.[91] Following primary infection, HSV replicates at the site of entry and subsequently ascends via the axon to the dorsal root ganglion, where it persists in a latent form throughout life. Active replication and recurrent infection may or may not ensue.

## Epidemiology, Risk Factors, and Pathogenesis

There has been a dramatic increase in the prevalence of HSV infections in the United States with the CDC demonstrating a 9-fold increase in physician visits for genital herpes from 1966 to 1997.[94] An estimated 500,000 to 1 million new cases of genital HSV infections occur annually in the United States. While approximately 5 million adults in the United States have a history of genital herpes infection, large serologic studies for HSV-2 assessing type-specific HSV-2 antibodies to glycoprotein G have demonstrated an overall seroprevalence for HSV-2 infection of 21.9% with 25.6% of females seropositive.[95] Thus, an estimated 45 million Americans have been infected with HSV-2 genital herpes.

Based on clinical history, serologic testing, and HSV typing, three types of genital herpes infection have been recognized (Table 19-11). Primary infection is an initial infection with either HSV-1 or HSV-2 in the absence of evidence for prior exposure (i.e., lack of antibodies to either). Nonprimary first clinical episode is an initial episode (either clinical or subclinical) with HSV-1 and HSV-2 in an individual with serologic evidence of prior exposure to the other serotype. Recurrent genital herpes is reactivation of latent virus.

As noted previously, recent seroprevalence studies with type specific anti-HSV-2 antibody (glycoprotein G) demonstrate that the overwhelming majority of HSV-2 seropositive adults report no history of clinically diagnosed genital herpes.[94] In addition, even the majority of "severe" first clinical episodes are not true primary infections but rather recurrent infections of nonprimary first episodes. Of significant importance is the recognition that patients with past clinical or subclinical genital herpes may asymptomatically shed HSV from the genital tract on approximately 1% of days.

More recent prospective studies on the natural history of genital herpes infection report that nearly 40% of newly acquired HSV-2 infections were associated with clinically symptomatic disease.[96] This large study of 2393 sexually active HSV-2 seronegative patients demonstrated rates of new HSV-1 and HSV-2 infection of 1.6 and 5.2 cases per 100 person-years, respectively. Women were significantly more likely to have symptomatic infection. Survey studies of adult women have identified isolation of HSV from the genital tract of 0.02% to 4% of women, with the higher rates occurring in high-risk patients attending STD clinics. Among pregnant women, isolation of HSV has been reported in 0.01% to 4% of asymptomatic

| Table 19-11 |
| --- |
| **Types of Genital Herpes Simplex Infection** |

- Primary infection: initial infection with either HSV-1 or HSV-2, without evidence of prior exposure to either (i.e., antibodies)
- Nonprimary first episode: initial clinical episode with HSV-1 or HSV-2 in patient with prior exposure to the other viral serotype
- Recurrent infection: reactivation of latent virus

women; patients without symptoms account for one third to two thirds of positive cultures.[97]

It appears that there is not an increase in frequency or severity of genital herpes infections during pregnancy. A 3-fold increase in spontaneous abortion has been reported with maternal HSV infection in early pregnancy. While Brown et al reported no overall differences in mean birth weight, gestational age at birth, risk of intrauterine growth restriction (IUGR), stillbirth, or neonatal death with acquisition of HSV infection during pregnancy, primary genital herpes in the third trimester was associated with preterm birth, IUGR, and substantial risk for neonatal herpes infection.[98]

Clearly, the major impact of genital herpes infection in pregnancy is neonatal herpes infection. An estimated 700 to 1000 cases of neonatal herpes occur each year in the United States, an incidence of 1 in 3500 to 1 in 5000 births. In utero transplacental acquisition of herpes producing congenital herpes rarely occurs. However, when it does, it is associated with devastating outcomes—death in 31% and neurologic sequelae in nearly all survivors.[90] The overwhelming majority (>85%) of neonatal herpes is acquired intrapartum from an infected maternal genital tract.[99]

Risk factors associated with the transmission of HSV from mother to neonate include HSV type (HSV-2 > HSV-1), mother's clinical stage of infection, anatomic site of viral shedding, use of fetal scalp electrode, and presence and specificity of transplacental passively transferred HSV antibodies from mother to infant. Infants born to mothers with recently acquired first episodes of HSV infection were 10-fold more likely to acquire neonatal herpes as were those born to mothers with recurrent infection. With first-episode infection, whether primary or nonprimary, the rate of neonatal infection is similar, 40% and 31%, respectively. Passive transfer of maternal antibodies to HSV-2 (but not HSV-1) are protective, as demonstrated by Prober et al who reported that following exposure to HSV at vaginal delivery. 0 of 34 infants in whom antibody was present developed neonatal herpes infection 95% confidence interval, 0% to 8%).[100] Cervical shedding of HSV is associated with an increased risk of perinatal transmission.

In pregnancy, primary infection may range from asymptomatic to severe, produce transplacental or neonatal infection, and result in up to 40% or higher risk for neonatal herpes (depending on presence or absence of maternal antibody). With nonprimary first episode transmission, maternal symptoms range from asymptomatic to severe, mainly neonatal infection occurs, and the risk for neonatal infection is up to 40%. For recurrent infection, maternal symptoms range from asymptomatic to severe, only neonatal infection occurs, and the estimated risk for neonatal infection is from less than 1% to 4%.

## Diagnosis

Until recently viral culture was the best diagnostic test for confirmation of HSV infection. HSV grows rapidly (most cultures are positive at 48 to 72 hours) and is easily transported. A false-negative rate of 5% to 30% is associated with a single herpes culture. Cultures are more likely to be positive with first episodes of HSV infection and in patients with vesicles or pustules compared with ulcerative and crusted lesions. Use of specific monoclonal antibodies in immunofluorescence or immunoassay

tests have enhanced and accelerated detection of HSV in culture with resultant good sensitivity and specificity.[101]

Similarly to other infections, the laboratory diagnosis of HSV infections has been revolutionized by introduction of NAATs such as PCR. PCR has excellent sensitivity and specificity compared with viral culture for detection of HSV.

The introduction of type-specific serology has further facilitated diagnosis. Each HSV type has identifiable proteins in a characteristic protein coat. Glycoprotein G-1 is associated with HSV type 1 and glycoprotein G-2 with HSV type 2. Within several weeks of infection, type-specific antibodies to the viral proteins develop and persist.[102] Detection of HSV-2 antibodies, using glycoprotein G technology, is virtually diagnostic of genital herpes infection. Type-specific serologic assays are commercially available and can be used for patients without active lesions or who have lesions which are culture negative. Current FDA-approved type-specific assays include HerpeSelect-1 ELISA IgG and HerpeSelect-2 ELISA IgG and HerpeSelect 1/2 Immunoblot IgG. When submitting specimens, confirm that glycoprotein G–based serologic testing is available. Screening for HSV-1 and -2 infection in the general population is not indicated.[103] However, screening may be useful in counseling couples when one partner has genital HSV and the other does not know or is uncertain, especially for planning pregnancy or in pregnancy.

## Treatment

While there is no cure for HSV infection, antiviral medications are available that reduce the duration and frequency of outbreaks, reduce asymptomatic HSV shedding, and reduce transmission.[104] Acyclovir, the first effective antiviral agent for genital herpes, became available in the early 1980s. Acyclovir interferes selectively with viral thymidine kinase and inhibits viral DNA synthesis. Because of its selectivity for HSV-infected cells, acyclovir has a high margin of safety. Subsequently, two additional antiviral agents, valacyclovir and famciclovir, have become available for the treatment and suppression of HSV infection. These agents also inhibit actively replicating virus by interfering with viral DNA synthesis.

Current CDC-recommended treatment guidelines for HSV infections are listed in Table 19-12. If lesions of first-episode herpes infection are not fully healed, treatment with antiviral agents can be extended beyond 10 days. Intravenous acyclovir should be reserved for severe primary outbreaks or disseminated herpes infections. In these instances, the recommended treatment is acyclovir 5 to 10 mg/kg every 8 hours IV for 2 to 7 days or until clinical improvement followed by oral antiviral therapy to complete at least a total of 10 days of therapy.[104]

Following the first clinical episode of genital herpes, patients may choose two alternative approaches. They may take episodic therapy upon signs of recurrent outbreak, or they may select to receive continuous suppressive therapy. Episodic treatment has been shown to decrease the proportion of patients with outbreaks, reduce duration of symptoms, and shorten the duration of viral shedding.[102] On the other hand, suppressive therapy reduces the frequency of genital herpes recurrences by 70% to 80% among patients with frequent recurrences, with many patients reporting no symptomatic outbreaks.[102]

Interest has focused on the use of acyclovir prophylaxis during late pregnancy to prevent HSV recurrence at delivery.[105]

Gynecologic Infectious Disease

| Table 19-12 |
| --- |
| **CDC–recommended Regimens for Genital Herpes, 2002** |

**Recommended regimens: first clinical episode**

Acyclovir 400 mg orally three times a day for 7–10 days
Acyclovir 200 mg orally five times a day for 7–10 days
Famciclovir 250 mg orally three times a day for 7–10 days
Valacyclovir 1 g orally twice a day for 7–10 days

**Recommended regimens: episodic recurrences**

Acyclovir 400 mg orally three times a day for 5 days
Acyclovir 200 mg orally five times a day for 5 days
Acyclovir 800 mg orally twice a day for 5 days
Famciclovir 125 mg orally twice a day for 5 days
Valacyclovir 500 mg orally twice a day for 3–5 days
Valacyclovir 1 g orally once a day for 5 days

**Recommended regimens: suppression of recurrent episodes**

Acyclovir 400 mg orally twice a day
Famciclovir 250 mg orally twice a day
Valacyclovir 500 mg orally once a day*
Valacyclovir 1 g orally once a day

*Valacyclovir 500 mg once a day might be less effective than other dosing regimens in patients who have frequent (≥10 episodes per year) recurrences.

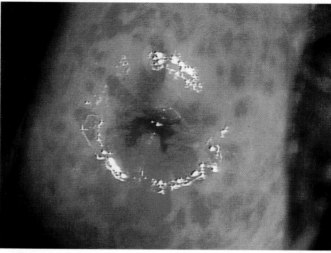

**Figure 19-4    Strawberry cervix associated with trichomoniasis.** (Reprinted with permission from Sweet RL, Gibbs RS: Atlas of Infectious Diseases of the Female Genital Tract. Philadelphia, Lippincott Williams & Wilkins, 2004.)

Acyclovir is well tolerated in pregnancy with minimal fetal drug accumulation. The Acyclovir in Pregnancy Registry assessed data from over 1200 pregnant women exposed to acyclovir and found no increases in drug-related fetal abnormalities attributed to acyclovir use.[105] However, long-term developmental outcomes were not evaluated. Although some authorities believe that insufficient data exist to recommend prophylaxis in pregnancy,[104] the American College of Obstetricians and Gynecologists suggests that use of acyclovir to suppress recurrent HSV infection in late pregnancy is acceptable.[106] Sheffield and colleagues performed a meta-analysis of acyclovir prophylaxis to prevent HSV recurrence at delivery.[107] Acyclovir prophylaxis commencing at 36 weeks' gestation was effective in reducing clinical HSV recurrence for the following: at the time of delivery (OR 0.25; 95% CI 0.15–0.40), cesarean deliveries for clinical recurrence of genital herpes (OR 0.30; 95% CI 0.13–0.67), total HSV detection at delivery (OR 0.11; 95% CI 0.04–0.31), and asymptomatic HSV shedding at delivery (OR 0.09; 95% CI 0.02–0.39).

## TRICHOMONIASIS

*Trichomonas vaginalis*, a flagellated protozoan, is the etiologic agent of trichomoniasis (Fig. 19-4). The urogenital tract is the primary site of infection, which presents with a wide spectrum of symptoms.[106] Trichomoniasis has been suggested as a putative agent for adverse pregnancy outcomes, including PROM, low-birth-weight infants, preterm delivery, and spontaneous abortion.[107] In addition, *T. vaginalis* has been identified as a predisposing factor in transmission and acquisition of HIV.[108]

### Epidemiology, Risk Factors, and Pathogenesis

At one time *T. vaginalis* was responsible for approximately 25% of cases of clinically evident vaginitis.[109] During the past decade the prevalence appears to have decreased. The prevalence of *T. vaginalis* is estimated at 3% to 5%, ranging from 2% to 3% in middle-class women to over 50% in women attending STD clinics.[109,110]

Contradictory results have been reported regarding an association between *T. vaginalis* and adverse pregnancy outcomes. Hardy et al reported that in an adolescent pregnant population with a prevalence of 34%, *T. vaginalis* was associated with low birth weight and preterm birth.[111] Despite a similar high prevalence of trichomoniasis, Mason and Brown found no association with adverse pregnancy outcome.[112] Similarly, Minkoff et al found no significant association between *T. vaginalis* and preterm labor.[7] On the other hand, the Vaginal Infection and Prematurity Study demonstrated that the presence of *T. vaginalis* in the vagina at mid pregnancy was significantly associated with preterm low birth weight (OR 1.6; 95% CI 1.3–1.9).[97] However, a recent treatment trial sponsored by NIH demonstrated that metronidazole treatment of asymptomatic women with trichomoniasis (based on culture) resulted in an increased risk of preterm birth compared with placebo.[113]

### Clinical Features

Patients with symptomatic trichomoniasis present with a copious vaginal discharge that most commonly is yellow-green and malodorous. Vulvar irritation is also frequently noted. The pH of the discharge is above 4.5. While the discharge is classically described as frothy or bubbly yellow-green, observational studies have demonstrated that frothiness was detected in only

12% to 34% of cases.[110] In addition, punctate mucosal hemorrhages of the cervix (strawberry cervix), may occur. These hemorrhages are noted by the naked eye in less than 10% of trichomoniasis cases; this finding is more commonly identified with colposcopy.[110] These data emphasize the inaccuracy of diagnosing vaginal infections on the basis of "characteristic" discharges or clinical signs and symptoms.

## Diagnosis

Most commonly, the diagnosis of trichomoniasis is made by light microscopic examination of a saline wet mount demonstrating motile organisms. In addition, a heavy polymorphonuclear infiltrate is present.[110] Unfortunately, the sensitivity of the wet mount is only 60% to 70%. Trichomoniasis also can be diagnosed on a Papanicolaou (Pap) smear, but sensitivity is low (52% to 67%), as is specificity.[110]

At present, culture is the best available method for confirming the presence of *T. vaginalis*.[110] Although culture for *T. vaginalis* is not difficult, it requires use of special media, such as Diamond or Kupferberg. The medium is incubated after inoculation, and a drop of the medium is examined daily by light microscopy for 5 to 7 days to look for motile trichomonads.

An FDA-approved DNA probe-based test for *T. vaginalis*, Affirm VP III, has sensitivity of 90% to 100% compared with culture methods.[114] Use of PCR testing for *T. vaginalis* was assessed in several recent studies that demonstrated higher sensitivity with PCR than with wet-mount microscopy, Diamond culture, modified Kupferberg culture, or Pap smear. The PCR test also was highly specific for *T. vaginalis*. Most importantly, PCR has excellent sensitivity and specificity for both symptomatic and asymptomatic women. An additional advantage of PCR testing is that patients can self-collect specimens from the distal vagina, precluding the need for a vaginal speculum examination.[115]

## Treatment

Until recently, the only treatment available in the United States for trichomoniasis was metronidazole. Tinidazole, a related 5-nitroimidazole derivative, has recently received FDA approval. An additional 5-nitroimidazole derivative, ornidazole, is available in other countries.

CDC guidelines for treatment of trichomoniasis are listed in Table 19-13.[25] Cure rates are equivalent (86% to 97%) for the single 2-g dose, and the 7-day regimens and side effects (mainly nausea) are similar.[110,116] The physician should prescribe metronidazole for the sexual partners of women with trichomoniasis.[116] Metronidazole can be used safely in pregnancy.[116]

While uncommon, relative resistance of *T. vaginalis* to metronidazole has been documented.[117] CDC recommendation for treatment failures is re-treatment with metronidazole 500 mg twice daily for 7 days. If repeated failure occurs, a single 2-g dose once daily for 3 to 5 days is suggested. If patients still have persistent trichomoniasis, CDC recommends excluding reinfection, evaluating in vitro susceptibility of the isolate, and managing in consultation with an expert.[26] Such consultation is available through CDC.

The suggested tinidazole treatment regimen for trichomoniasis is a single 2-g oral dose. Tinidazole has been reported to be effective in cases of metronidazole-resistant trichomoniasis (cure rate of 90%) when used in a dosage of 1 g orally twice a day plus 500 mg twice a day vaginally for 14 days.

## SCABIES

Scabies is a highly contagious infection caused by the itch mite *Sarcoptes scabiei*. The adult female excavates a burrow in the skin, where fertilization takes place. Following fertilization, the female emerges and excavates a new burrow, which she extends by 0.5 to 5 mm a day as she begins laying 2 to 3 eggs per day. The eggs hatch in 3 to 4 days, and the larvae emerge from the burrow and dig into adjacent skin where three moltings occur before adulthood is achieved.

### Epidemiology, Risk Factors, and Pathogenesis

Scabies is common throughout the world and appears in epidemics at 10- to 30-year intervals.[118] It is more common in men than in women and in whites than in blacks. Scabies is now considered an STD, and close and prolonged contact with an infected person is required for transmission. Unlike other STDs scabies is also spread by nonsexual contact; close person-to-person contact (e.g., crowded living conditions or sharing a bed) can be responsible.

### Clinical Features

Scabies presents with a pruritic, pleomorphic rash. It has an insidious onset and a characteristic pattern of involvement that includes wrist, finger webs, elbows, axillae, genitals, and buttocks. Patients report a gradual onset of pruritus and rash over 3 to 4 weeks after the initial infestation.[118] With repeat infestations, the onset of symptoms is relatively prompt, within hours. Much of the symptomatology of scabies is the result of the host immune response to *S. scabiei*.[118]

Pruritus is the predominant symptom and may be intense. Typically, the itching is worse at night. The physical findings include presence of the burrows, a papular erythematous rash, and persistent pruritic nodules.[26] The burrows are 5 to 10 mm long, and the organism may be seen as a tiny brown and white speck at the inner end of the burrow.

### Diagnosis

The burrow of scabies is pathognomonic. It is a short, wavy, dirty-appearing line that often crosses skin lines and is most commonly located on finger webs, volar wrists, and elbows.[118] Use of a magnifying glass is sufficient, and the burrows can be more easily seen after ink staining.[118] Most sites also contain small, erythematous, excoriated papules. Confirmation of the diagnosis is made by identifying the mite, eggs, or fecal pellets on microscopic examination. Fresh lesions should be used for obtaining mites. Skin scrapings are preferred for microscopic identification of scabies.[118]

| Table 19-13 |
| :--: |
| CDC–recommended Treatment for Trichomoniasis, 2002 |

**Recommended regimen**

Metronidazole 2 g orally in a single dose

**Alternative regimen**

Metronidazole 500 mg twice a day for 7 days

Scabies is called the great imitator because patients can have a variety of lesions. Thus, many dermatologic conditions must be considered in the differential diagnosis.[118] These include eczema, acute urticaria, impetigo, erythrasma, insect bites, neurodermatitis, and dermatitis herpetiformis. However, the history of insidious onset and the presence of nocturnal pruritus and of pleomorphic lesions and their characteristic distribution should strongly suggest scabies. Presence of itching in family members also indicates a high likelihood of scabies.

### Treatment

Successful treatment of scabies necessitates correct application of an effective scabicide to the patient, sexual contacts, and family members. The current CDC-recommended regimen for the treatment of scabies is permethrin cream 5% applied to all areas of the body from the neck down and washed off after 8 to 14 hours.[119] Alternative regimens include Lindane 1%, 1 ounce of lotion or 30 g of cream applied thinly to all areas of the body from the neck down and washed off thoroughly after 8 hours.[118] More recently, ivermectin 200 µg/kg orally, repeated in 2 weeks, has been suggested as an alternative therapy for scabies.[120]

Pregnant and lactating women should not be treated with lindane. Permethrin is recommended for the treatment of scabies in pregnant or lactating women.[119]

At the conclusion of therapy, the patient's underwear, nightclothes, sheets, and pillowcases should be decontaminated by machine washing or machine drying using the hot cycle or removed from body contact for more than 72 hours.[118]

Sexual partners and close household contacts should be treated as described previously. If no clinical improvement is noted, a single treatment after 1 week is appropriate. Clothing and bed linen used within the previous 2 days should be washed and dried by machine (hot cycle) or dry-cleaned.

## PEDICULOSIS PUBIS

*Phthirus pubis*, the crab louse, is the etiologic agent for pediculosis pubis. An estimated 3 million cases of pediculosis are treated each year in the United States. Infestation by the crab (or pubic) louse should be considered in any patient complaining of groin irritation or pruritus.

### Epidemiology, Risk Factors, and Pathogenesis

Acquisition of *P. pubis* is nearly always through sexual contact. However, it may be spread through fomites. Pediculosis pubis is more contagious than any other STD, with a 95% chance of contracting the disease with a single sexual encounter. Pediculosis pubis is most commonly encountered during adolescence and young adulthood; from ages 15 to 19, it is more common in females, while after 20, males are more commonly infected.[121]

Twenty-four hours after mating, the female begins to lay eggs at a rate of approximately four per day. The eggs are attached to a hair near its root. After an incubation time of 7 days, a nymph is hatched and proceeds through three molts over a period of 8 to 9 days. Once the louse reaches sexual maturity, its life expectancy is 3 to 4 weeks.[121]

### Clinical Features

The incubation time of pediculosis is 30 days. Patients come in with irritation or pruritus secondary to bites. The intense itching

is believed to be due to allergic sensitization. On occasion, patients may see the crab louse moving over the skin. Distribution involves the pubic, perineal, and perianal regions. With bites by a large number of lice over a short period of time, systemic manifestations such as mild fever, malaise, or irritability may occur.

### Diagnosis

Visualization of lice, larvae, and nits with use of a magnifying glass is diagnostic for pediculosis pubis. Microscopic examination reveals the typical crab-like morphology.

### Treatment

The recommended treatment regimens for pediculosis pubis include permethrin 1% cream-rinse applied to affected area and washed off after 10 minutes, pyrethrin with piperonyl butoxide applied to affected area and washed off after 10 minutes, and lindane 1% shampoo applied for 4 minutes to the affected area and then thoroughly washed off. Lindane is not recommended for pregnant or lactating women. Following either treatment, combing the infested areas with a fine-toothed comb facilitates removal of remaining lice and nits.

Re-treatment is indicated after 7 days if lice are found or eggs are observed at the hair-skin junction. Clothing or bed linen that may have been contaminated within the last 2 days should be washed and dried on the hot cycle or dry-cleaned. All sexual partners, family members, and close contacts must be treated at the same time, even if asymptomatic.

## MOLLUSCUM CONTAGIOSUM

Molluscum contagiosum is a viral skin infection of children and young adults. The molluscum contagiosum virus is a poxvirus. Characteristic small, firm, umbilicated papules occur on the extremities or trunk and, in sexually transmitted cases, in the genital area. Examination of infected cells reveals the pathognomonic molluscum bodies, which are ovoid accumulations of maturing virions.[122]

### Epidemiology, Risk Factors, and Pathogenesis

Molluscum contagiosum is transmitted by skin-to-skin contact, fomites, and autoinoculation. The incubation period averages from 2 to 3 months and ranges from one week to 6 months. There are two major forms of molluscum contagiosum.[26] The childhood disease affects the face, trunk, and limbs and is transmitted by skin contact and fomites. Disease affecting young adults is sexually transmitted and occurs in the genital area. It is usually acquired by skin contact during sexual intercourse. Prior to the onset of the AIDS epidemic, molluscum contagiosum cases had quadrupled in the United Kingdom from the early 1970s to 1980s and increased 11-fold in the United States according to surveys of private physicians between 1966 and 1983.[123,124]

### Clinical Features

Molluscum contagiosum affects normal skin rather than mucous membranes. The characteristic dome-shaped papules with central umbilication develop slowly and remain stable for long periods of time. Lesions are multiple but generally number less than 20.

Lesions are usually flesh-colored but may have a gray-white, yellow, or pink color.

The disease is usually asymptomatic, but occasionally pruritus is present. The usual life of a lesion is less than 2 months, but they can last for several years. Most commonly, the crop of molluscum contagiosum lesions tends to be self-limited and of 6- to 9-month duration.[123]

### Diagnosis

Examination reveals the characteristic smooth, light-colored papules with an umbilicated center. They are usually multiple and have the distribution noted previously for either childhood disease or sexually transmitted forms. Microscopic examination can confirm the diagnosis, if it is in doubt. The lesion can either be squeezed to express the white caseous material from its core or removed by curettage. The specimen is stained with Gram's, Wright's, or Giemsa stain. The cells will reveal the pathognomonic large intracytoplasmic molluscum bodies.[122]

### Treatment

Molluscum contagiosum is a benign and self-limited disease. While lesions often resolve spontaneously, treatment may shorten their duration and result in decreased autoinoculation or transmission. Several alternative therapies are available.[123] A small superficial incision in the top of the lesion may be made and the contents removed with a comedo extractor. Curettage of the lesion, followed by cautery, is effective. For multiple lesions, freezing with liquid nitrogen has been successful. Sexual partners should be examined and treated as well.

## CONDYLOMA ACUMINATUM (GENITAL WARTS)

Condylomata acuminata, or genital warts, are caused by human papillomavirus (HPV). HPVs are composed of double-stranded DNA and characterized by the ability to infect and transform epithelial cells.[125] Over 100 types of HPV have been described, of which 35 primarily infect the genital tract (Fig. 19-5).

The common genital HPV types are either high-risk or low-risk types based on their oncogenic potential. HPV types in the low oncogenic risk group include 6, 11, 42, 43, and 44. They are associated with genital warts, condyloma, and some cases of low-grade squamous intraepithelial lesions (LGSIL) but rarely invasive cancers. The high oncogenic risk group includes HPV types 16, 18, 31, 33, 35, and 39. These are commonly detected in women with high-grade squamous epithelial lesions (HSIL) and invasive cancers. Genital warts are the focus of this review.

### Epidemiology, Risk Factors, and Pathogenesis

An estimated 24 million Americans are infected with HPV, and between 500,000 and 1 million new cases of HPV-induced genital warts occur each year in the United States.[126] The prevalence of subclinical HPV infection, based on studies using PCR, is substantial, with recent studies demonstrating that at least 50% of sexually active women have been infected with one or more types of HPV. Clinically evident genital warts (condyloma acuminatum) continue to occur in epidemic proportions.[127] Gall suggests that there has been a 10-fold increase in HPV-related cases in STD clinics as well as private physician offices.[128] Thus, genital warts appear to be the most common viral STD. In 1995 genital warts accounted for more

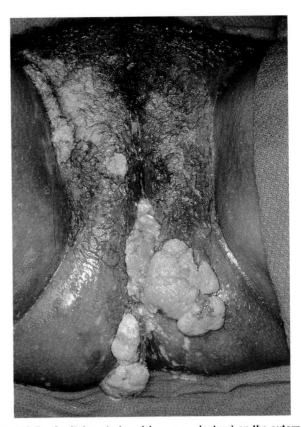

**Figure 19-5** **Genital warts (condyloma acuminatum) on the external genitalia and perineal area.** (Reprinted with permission from Sweet RL, Gibbs RS: Atlas of Infectious Diseases of the Female Genital Tract. Philadelphia, Lippincott Williams & Wilkins, 2004.)

than 240,000 initial physician office visits.[126] The Institute of Medicine estimates that the economic burden of HPV in the United States exceeded $3.8 billion in total costs in 1997 (excluding costs of HPV-related cervical cancer).[6] More recently, Insinga et al estimated the costs associated with genital warts in a private health plan; on average episodes of genital warts involved 3.1 physician visits and incurred costs of $436.[129]

Genital HPV infections are primarily transmitted through sexual contact, and the sexual transmission of HPV associated with genital warts (condyloma acuminatum) is well established.[125] The lesions occur in the urogenital and anorectal areas. The highest prevalence is in young, sexually active adolescents. An estimated 1% of sexually active men and women between 18 and 49 years of age have external genital warts.[130] The infectivity rate is about 65% among sexual contacts. The average incubation period is 2 to 3 months. Women and men are affected with equal frequency.

Risk factors associated with HPV infection include increased number of sexual partners,[26] cigarette smoking,[26] and long-term use of oral contraceptives.[26] Winer et al followed a cohort of female university students and demonstrated that in addition to smoking and oral contraceptive use, report of a new male sexual partner, especially one known for less than 8 months before sex occurred, was predictive of incident infection.[131]

A higher frequency of genital warts is associated with immunosuppressive states. An increase has been reported in female renal transplant recipients,[132] and the frequency and severity of genital warts is increased during pregnancy.[133]

# Gynecologic Infectious Disease

HPV infection in HIV-infected women has been the focus of recent interest. Of most concern has been the finding that neoplastic lesions of the cervix associated with genital HPV infection progress at an increased rate in HIV-infected women.[134]

The HPV viral genome is organized into three major regions. There are two protein-encoding regions (early and late gene regions) and a noncoding upstream regulatory region (URR).[135] The URR controls transcription of the early and late regions and thus regulates production of viral protein and infectious particles (open reading frames; ORFs), which are transcriptional units that encode for proteins and are designated E1, E2, E4, E5, E6, and E7.[135] Early region gene expression controls replication, transcription, and cellular transformation of viral DNA. In addition it plays a role in unregulated cellular proliferation. The gene products encoded by E1 and E2 ORFs are critical for viral replication. While E6 and E7 ORFs encode proteins critical for viral replication, they also encode proteins critical for host cell immortalization and transformation. The late gene region contains two ORFs (L1 and L2, which encode structural proteins critical to production of viral capsid).[135]

Acute HPV infection of the genital tract probably occurs when microtrauma allows virus to enter the skin or mucosa of the genital tract.[131] Virus enters cells at the basal layer of the epithelium and matures as it passes through the parabasal, spinous, and granular layers of epithelium.[131] It is at the granular level that viral DNA replication, late region protein synthesis, and viral particle assembly occur. Following acute HPV infection, three clinical sequelae potentially can occur.[135] First, latent viral infection occurs when the HPV genome is stabilized as a non-integrated episome and remains in host cells without causing clinical or morphologic changes in the squamous epithelium of the genital tract. Thus, with latent infection patients display no clinical evidence of infection but still harbor HPV. Second, active infection may occur, manifested by proliferation of squamous epithelial cells into benign tumors (i.e., genital warts, condyloma acuminatum). This takes place when HPV undergoes vegetative replication. Third, high-risk oncogenic types of HPV that are associated with high-grade lesions can become integrated into the host genome. Viral integration results in loss of control of proliferation by several critical oncoproteins or tumor suppressors.

In genital warts the viral DNA is an episome and not integrated into the host DNA. Major changes take place as lesions become dysplastic or invasive.[136] Viral DNA is integrated into the host genome and thus can be transferred to progeny cells. Deletion of late viral genes that encode the structural viral proteins occurs. Among the early viral genes those that play a role in abnormal growth of cells (E6, E7) continue to be expressed, whereas there is a loss of those early viral genes (E1, E2) that have a negative effect on the expression of growth-promoting genes. As a result, dysplastic and malignant lesions tend not to produce virus particles.

## Clinical Features

The American Medical Association Expert Panel on External Genital Warts developed a consensus statement regarding diagnosis, treatment, and evaluation of patients with external genital warts, as summarized by Beutner et al.[137] External genital warts are defined as visible warts occurring in the urogenital and/or anorectal regions. The morphologic appearance of external genital warts is similar whether they involve the penis, urethra, perineum, anus, rectum, vulva, or vagina. Lesions on the cervix may be flat and endophytic. External genital warts are frequently multifocal presenting with one or more lesions at a single anatomic site (e.g., vulva). Alternatively, they may be multicentric presenting with lesions on different anatomic sites.[137]

The AMA consensus group delineated four morphologic types of external genital warts: (1) condylomata acuminata that are cauliflower-shaped; (2) papular warts that are dome-shaped (usually skin-colored) 1- to 4-mm papules; (3) keratotic genital warts that have a thick horny layer and may resemble a common wart or seborrheic keratosis; and (4) flat-topped papules that appear macular to slightly raised.[137] These morphologic types are usually associated with one of the two major types of skin found in the genital area.[5] Condylomata acuminata occur generally on moist, partially keratinized and non-hair-bearing skin. Keratotic and smooth papular external genital warts occur on fully keratinized skin (hair-bearing or non-hair-bearing). Flat-topped papular warts occur on either type of skin surface.

Genital warts in women are generally located on the external genitalia and perineal regions. Exophytic genital warts (condylomata acuminata) usually present initially on the fourchette and adjacent labia and then may spread rapidly to involve other parts of the vulva. The vagina may be affected, rarely extensively. In addition, the cervix may be involved but with "flat condylomata" rather than the typical exophytic lesions. Cervical lesions are flat and endophytic condylomata that can usually be recognized only with the aid of a colposcope.

Patients with genital warts complain of lesions on their genitalia and rarely report other symptoms. Occasionally patients have itching, burning, pain, or bleeding.

## Diagnosis

Koutsky and Kiviat emphasize the importance of diagnosing two clinical manifestations of genital HPV infection: (1) genital warts that can be visualized with the naked eye, and (2) squamous intraepithelial lesions (SILs) of the cervix that can be detected by routine cytologic screening.[125]

Most condylomata are so characteristic in appearance that the diagnosis is primarily made on visual examination alone. External genital warts usually can be easily visualized with gross inspection, and such clinical is accurate and consistent with histologic diagnosis.[137] Some experts suggest that use of bright light and a hand lens, magnifying loop, or colposcope may be helpful in identifying external genital warts. In women lesions that must be differentiated from genital condylomata include epithelial papillae, small sebaceous glands, and perianal fibro-epithelial polyps. The most important infection that must be differentiated from genital warts is the condyloma latum of secondary syphilis. If lesions appear atypical or the diagnosis is uncertain, biopsy should be performed. Additional indications for biopsy include (1) progression of disease during treatment; (2) prompt or frequent recurrence; and (3) warts that are pigmented, indurated, ulcerated, or fixed to underlying tissue.[137] Histologically, condylomata acuminata are characterized by papillate epidermal hyperplasia, parakeratosis, koilocytes, occasional atypical mitotic figures, and increased numbers of dilated and tortuous capillaries.

## Treatment

The therapeutic approach for HPV infection of the genital tract is dependent on the anatomic location of disease (external genitalia/perianal, cervical, vaginal, or urethral), the clinical presentation of disease (clinical vs. subclinical), and the extent of disease. The primary goal of treatment of external genital warts (condyloma acuminatum) is to eliminate warts that cause physical or psychological symptoms or distress.[137] Elimination of genital warts may or may not decrease infectivity because internal sites (vagina or cervix) and clinically normal skin may act as reservoirs for infection.[137]

CDC issued recommendations for the treatment of HPV infection in 2002.[138] In most patients treatment will include wart-free periods of varying length. CDC notes that no evidence indicates that currently available treatment modalities eradicate or affect the natural history of HPV infection.[138] Visible genital warts that are not treated may resolve spontaneously, remain unchanged, or increase in size or number.

For external genital/perianal warts (condyloma acuminatum) the recommended therapeutic measures are listed in Table 19-14. None of the currently available treatments is superior to other treatments, and no single treatment is ideal for all patients or all warts.[138] Available treatments for visible genital warts are divided into two categories: (1) patient-applied therapies (e.g., podofilox and imiquimod) and (2) provider-administered treatments (e.g., cryotherapy, podophyllin resin, trichloroacetic acid [TCA], bichloroacetic acid [BCA], interferon, and surgery). Factors influencing choice of treatment include wart size, wart number, anatomic site, wart morphology, patient preference, cost of treatment, convenience, side effects, and provider experience.[138] Many patients require a course of therapy rather than a single treatment, and thus it is important that providers have a treatment plan or protocol for the management of genital warts.[138] CDC recommends that the treatment modality be changed if the patient has not improved substantially after three provider-administered treatments or if warts have not completely cleared following six treatments.[138]

The use of podophyllin, podofilox, and imiquimod is contraindicated in pregnancy. During pregnancy the best approach to treatment is removal of lesions by excision, electrocautery, or cryosurgery. TCA application has been used in pregnancy without adverse effects.[139] Laser therapy is another alternative for pregnant women with extensive disease.

For the treatment of vaginal exophytic warts, the recommendations include (1) cryotherapy with liquid nitrogen, (2) TCA or BCA 80% to 90%, or (3) podophyllin 10% to 25% in compound tincture of benzoin.[138] Because of concern about potential systemic absorption it is best not to use podophyllin in the vagina. Podophyllin is contraindicated in pregnancy. Podofilox is not approved for vaginal use, since the patient can not visualize the lesions for application. For urethral meatus warts either cryotherapy with liquid nitrogen or podophyllin is recommended.[138] With anal warts cryotherapy with liquid nitrogen, TCA or BCA 80% to 90%, or surgical excision is recommended.[138]

---

**Table 19-14**
**CDC-recommended Treatment for External Genital Warts, 2002**

**Recommended regimens**

Patient-applied
1. Podofilox 0.5% solution or gel: Apply podofilox-solution with a cotton swab, or podofilox gel with a finger, to visible genital warts twice a day for 3 days, followed by 4 days of no therapy. Repeat cycle as necessary for a total of four cycles.
   *or*
2. Imiquimod 5% cream: Apply with finger at bedtime, 3 times a week for up to 16 weeks

Provider-administered
1. Cryotherapy with liquid nitrogen or cryoprobe. Repeat every 1 to 2 weeks.
   *or*
2. Podophyllin resin 10%–25% in compound tincture or benzoin. Repeat weekly if necessary.
   *or*
3. TCA or BCA 80%–90%. Repeat weekly if necessary.
   *or*
4. Surgical removal by tangential scissors excision, tangential shave excision, curettage, or electrosurgery

**Alternative regimens**

1. Intralesional interferon
   *or*
2. Laser surgery

---

## REFERENCES

1. Eng TR, Butler WT (eds): The Hidden Epidemic: Confronting Sexually Transmitted Diseases. Committee on Prevention and Control of Sexually Transmitted Diseases. Washington, DC, Institute of Medicine National Academy Press, 1997. **(IV, C)**
2. Cates W and American Social Health Panel: Estimates of the incidence and prevalence of sexually transmitted diseases in the United States. Sex Transm Dis 1999;26(Suppl):S2–S7. **(Ib, A)**
3. Weinstock H, Berman S, Cates W Jr: Sexually transmitted diseases among American youth: incidence and prevalence estimates, 2000. Perspect Sexual Reprod Health 2004;36:1–10. **(Ib, A)**
4. Chesson HW, Blandford JM, Gift TL, et al: The estimated direct medical cost of sexually transmitted diseases among American youth, 2000. Perspect Sexual Reprod Health 2004;36:1–20. **(Ib, A)**
5. World Health Organization, Global Programme on AIDS: Global prevalence and incidence of selected curable sexually transmitted diseases: overview and estimates. Geneva, World Health Organization, 1996.
6. Centers for Disease Control and Prevention: MMWR 1996; 45:883–884. **(IV, C)**
7. Berman SM, Hein K: Adolescents and Sexually Transmitted Diseases. In Holmes KK, Sparling PF, Mardh P-A, et al (eds): Sexually Transmitted Diseases. New York, McGraw-Hill, 1999, pp 129–142.
8. Centers for Disease Control: 1993 Sexually transmitted diseases treatment guidelines. 1993;42:56–66. **(IV, C)**
9. Cates W Jr: Epidemiology and control of sexually transmitted diseases: strategic evaluation. Infect Dis Clin North Am 1987;1:1–23. **(IV, C)**
10. Over M, Piot P: HIV infection and sexually transmitted disease. In Jamison DT, Mosley WH, Measham AR, Bobadilla JL (eds): Disease Control Priorities in Developing Countries. New York, Oxford University Press, 1993, pp 455–527. **(IV, C)**

Gonorrhea

11. Centers for Disease Control and Prevention: Summary of notifiable diseases, United States, 2002. MMWR 2004;51:1–84. **(IV, C)**
12. Centers for Disease Control and Prevention: Sexually transmitted disease surveillance, 2000. Atlanta, CDC, 2001. **(IV, C)**
13. Meyer TF: Pathogenic Neisseriae: complexity of pathogen-host cell interplay. Clin Infect Dis 1999;28:433–441. **(IV, C)**

14. Kellogg DS Jr, Peacock WL Jr, Deacon WE, et al: *Neisseria gonorrhoeae*. 1. Virulence genetically linked to clonal variation. J Bacteriol 1963;85:1274–1279. **(IIa, B)**

15. Hook EW III, Holmes KK: Gonococcal infections. Ann Intern Med 1985;102:229–243. **(IV, C)**

16. Pierce WA, Buchanan TM: Attachment role of gonococcal pili: optimum conditions and quantification of adherence of isolated pili to human cells in vitro. J. Clin Invest 1978;61:931. **(IIa, B)**

17. Britigan BE, Cohen MS, Sparling PF: Gonococcal infections: a model of molecular pathogenesis. N Engl J Med 1985;312:1683–1694. **(III, C)**

18. Hook EW, Handsfield HH: Gonococcal infections in adults. In Holmes KK, Sparling PF, Mardh P-A, et al (eds): Sexually Transmitted Diseases. New York, McGraw-Hill, 1999, pp 451–466. **(III, C)**

19. Hooper RR: Cohort study of venereal disease. 1. The risk of gonorrhea transmission from infected women to men. Am J Epidemiol 1989; 108:136. **(IIa, B)**

20. Barlow D, Phillips I: Gonorrhea in women: diagnostic clinical and laboratory aspects. Lancet 1978;1:761. **(III, B)**

21. Sweet RL, Gibbs RS: Sexually transmitted diseases. In Infectious Diseases of the Female Genital Tract. Philadelphia, Lippincott Williams & Wilkins, 2002.

22. Suleiman SA, Grimes EM, Jones HS: Disseminated gonococcal infections. Obstet Gynecol 1983;61:48–51. **(IIa, B)**

23. Holmes KK, Counts GW, Beaty HN: Disseminated gonococcal infection. Ann Intern Med 1971;74:979–993. **(IIa, B)**

24. Devine PA: Extrapelvic manifestations of gonorrhea. Prim Care Update Ob Gyns 1998;5:233–237. **(III, B)**

25. Hook EW III, Ching SF, Stephens J, et al: Diagnosis of *Neisseria gonorrhoeae* infections in women by using the ligase chain reaction on patient-obtained vaginal swabs. J Clin Microbiol 1997;35:2129–2132. **(Ib, B)**

26. Centers for Disease Control and Prevention: 2002 Sexually transmitted diseases treatment guidelines. MMWR 2002;51(RR-6):1–77. **(IV, C)**

27. World Health Organization Western Pacific Regional Gonococcal Antimicrobial Surveillance Programme: Surveillance of antibiotic resistance in *Neisseria gonorrhoeae* in the WHO Western Pacific Region, 2001. Common Dis Intell 2002;26:541–545. **(IV, C)**

28. Centers for Disease Control and Prevention: Increases in fluoroquinolone-resistant *Neisseria gonorrhoeae*—Hawaii and California, 2001. MMWR 2002;51:1041–1044. **(IV, C)**

Chlamydia

29. Mardh P-A: Is Europe ready for STD screening? Genitourin Med 1997;73:96–98. **(III, B)**

30. Cates W Jr, Wasserheit JN: Genital chlamydial infections: epidemiology and reproductive sequelae. Am J Obstet Gynecol 1991;164:1771–1781. **(IIb, B)**

31. Centers for Disease Control and Prevention: Summary of notifiable diseases, United States, 2002. MMWR 2004;51:1–84. **(IV, C)**

32. Washington AE, Johnson RE, Sanders LL: *Chlamydia trachomatis* infections in the United States: what are they costing us? JAMA 1987; 157:2070–2072. **(IIb, B)**

33. Ghys PD, Fransen K, Diallo MO, et al: The association between cervicovaginal HIV shedding, sexually transmitted diseases and immunosuppression in female sex workers in Abidjan, Cote d'Ivoire. AIDS 1997;11:85–93. **(IIa, B)**

34. Grayston JT: Infections caused by *Chlamydia pneumoniae* strain TWAR. Clin Infect Dis 1992;15:757–763. **(IIb, B)**

35. Kuo CC, Shor A, Campbell LA, et al: Demonstration of *Chlamydia pneumoniae* in atherosclerotic lesions of coronary arteries. J Infect Dis 1993;167:841–849. **(IIa, B)**

36. Hitchcock PJ: Future directions of Chlamydial research. In Stephens RS (ed): Chlamydia: Intracellular Biology: Pathogenesis and Immunity. Washington, DC, American Society of Microbiology, 1999, pp 297–311. **(IV, C)**

37. Schachter J: Biology of *Chlamydia trachomatis*. In Holmes KK, Sparling PF, Mardh P-A, et al (eds): Sexually Transmitted Diseases. New York, McGraw-Hill, 1999, pp 391–405. **(IV, C)**

38. Lycke E, Lowhagen G-B, Hallagen G, et al: The risk of transmission of genital *Chlamydia trachomatis* infection is less frequent than that of *Neisseria gonorrhoeae* infection. Sex Transm Dis 1980;7:6–10. **(IIb, B)**

39. Katz BP: Declining prevalence of chlamydial infection among adolescent girls. Sex Transm Dis 1996;23:226–229. **(IIa, B)**

40. Stamm WE: *Chlamydia trachomatis* infections of the adult. In Holmes KK, Sparling PF, Mardh P-A, et al (eds): Sexually Transmitted Diseases. New York, McGraw-Hill, 1999, pp 407–422. **(IV, C)**

41. Oh MK, Cloud CA, Baker SL, et al: Chlamydial infection and sexual behavior in young pregnant teenagers. Sex Transm Dis 1993;20:45–50. **(III, B)**

42. Saltz GR: Chlamydia trachomatis cervical infections in female adolescents. J Pediatr 1981;98:981. **(III, B)**

43. Schachter J, Stoner E, Moncoda J: Screening for chlamydial infections in women attending Family Planning Clinics: evaluations of presumptive indicators for therapy. West J Med 1983;138:375–379. **(IIb, B)**

44. Schachter J: Chlamydia infections (3 parts). N Engl J Med 1978; 298:428–435, 490–495, 540–549. **(III, B)**

45. Sweet RL, Gibbs RS: Chlamydial infection. In Sweet RL, Gibbs RS: Infectious Diseases of the Female Genital Tract. Philadelphia, Lippincott Williams & Wilkins, 2002. **(IV, C)**

46. Brunham R: Epidemiological and clinical correlates of C. *trachomatis* and *N. gonorrhoeae* infection among women attending an STD clinic. Clin Res 1981;29:47A. **(IIa, B)**

47. Stamm WE, Wagner KF, Ansel R, et al: Causes of the acute urethral syndrome in women. N Engl J Med 1980;303:409–415. **(IIa, B)**

48. Wiesenfeld HC, Hillier SL, Krohn MA, et al: Lower genital tract infection and endometritis: insight into subclinical pelvic inflammatory disease. Obstet Gynecol 2002;100:456–463. **(IIa, B)**

49. Cates W Jr, Rolfs RT, Aral SO: Sexually transmitted diseases, pelvic inflammatory disease, and infertility: an epidemiologic update. Epidemiol Rev 1990;12:199–200. **(III, B)**

50. Sweet RL: Microbiologic etiology of acute pelvic inflammatory disease. In Sweet RL, Landers DV (eds): Pelvic Inflammatory Disease. New York, Springer-Verlag, 1996. **(IV, C)**

51. Mardh P-A, Ripa KT, Svensson L, et al: *Chlamydia trachomatis* in patients with acute salpingitis. N Engl J Med 1977;296:1377–1379. **(IIa, B)**

52. Centers for Disease Control and Prevention: Recommendations for the prevention and management of *Chlamydia trachomatis* infections. MMWR 1993;42:1–39. **(IV, C)**

53. Thygeson P, Mengert WF: The virus of inclusion conjunctivitis: further observations. Arch Ophthalmol 1936;15:377–410. **(III, B)**

54. Mordhorst CH, Dawson C: Sequelae of neonatal inclusion conjunctivitis and associated disease in parents. Am J Ophthalmol 1971;71:861–867. **(III, B)**

55. Barbacci MB, Spence MR, Kappus EW, et al: Postabortal endometritis and isolation of *Chlamydia trachomatis*. Obstet Gynecol 1986; 68:686–690. **(III, B)**

56. Patton DL, Moore DE, Spadoni LR, et al: A comparison of the fallopian tube's response to overt an silent salpingitis. Obstet Gynecol 1989;73:622–630. **(IIa, B)**

57. Muller-Schoop JW, Wang S-P, Munzinger J, et al: *Chlamydia trachomatis* as a possible cause of peritonitis and perihepatitis in young women. BMJ 1978;1:1022–1024. **(III, B)**

58. Money DM, Hawes SE, Eschenbach DA, et al: Antibodies to the chlamydia 60 kd heat-shock protein are associated with laparoscopically confirmed perihepatitis. Am J Obstet Gynecol 1997; 176:870–877. **(IIa, B)**

59. Wager GP, Martin DH, Koutsky L, et al: Puerperal infectious morbidity: relationship to route of delivery and to antepartum *Chlamydia trachomatis* infection. Am J Obstet Gynecol 1980;138:1028–1033. **(IIa, B)**

60. Plummer FA, Laga M, Brunham RC, et al: Postpartum upper genital tract infections in Nairobi, Kenya: epidemiology, etiology and risk factors. J Infect Dis 1987;156:92–97. **(IIa, B)**

61. Sweet RL, Landers DV, Walker C, Schachter J: *Chlamydia trachomatis* infection and pregnancy outcome. Am J Obstet Gynecol 1987;156:824–833. **(IIa, B)**

62. Moller BR, Ahrons S, Laurin J, et al: Pelvic infection after elective abortion associated with *Chlamydia trachomatis*. Obstet Gynecol 1982;59:210–213. **(III, B)**

63. Black CM: Current methods of laboratory diagnosis of *Chlamydia trachomatis* infections. Clin Microbiol Rev 1997;10:160–184. **(IV, C)**

64. Centers for Disease Control and Prevention: 1998 Guidelines for treatment of sexually transmitted diseases. MMWR 1998;47:53–58. **(IV, C)**

65. Quigstad E, Skaug K, Jerve F, et al: Pelvic inflammatory disease associated with *Chlamydia trachomatis* infection after therapeutic abortion. Br J Vener Dis 1983;59:189. **(III, B)**

Syphilis

66. Centers for Disease Control and Prevention: Primary and secondary syphilis—United States, 1998. MMWR 1999;48:873–878. **(IV, C)**

67. Centers for Disease Control: Continuing increase in infectious syphilis—United States. MMWR 1988;37:35–38. **(IV, C)**

68. Centers for Disease Control and Prevention: Congenital syphilis—United States, 1998. MMWR 1999;48:757–761. **(IV, C)**

69. Centers for Disease Control and Prevention: Primary and secondary syphilis—United States, 2000–2001. MMWR 2002;5143:971. **(IV, C)**

70. Aral SO, Holmes KK: Social and behavioral determinants of the epidemiology of STDs: industrialized and the developing countries. In Holmes KK, Sparling PF, Mardh P-A, et al (eds): Sexually Transmitted Diseases. New York, McGraw-Hill, 1999, pp 39–76. **(IV, C)**

71. Centers for Disease Control: Syphilis trends in the United States. MMWR 1981;31:441–444. **(IV, C)**

72. Centers for Disease Control and Prevention: Summary of notifiable diseases—United States, 2002. MMWR 2004;51:1–84. **(IV, C)**

73. Tramont EC: Syphilis in adults: from Christopher Columbus to Sir Alexander Fleming to AIDS. Clin Infect Dis 1995;21:1361–1371.

74. Chapel TA: The signs and symptoms of secondary syphilis. Sex Transm Dis 1980;7:161–164. **(III, B)**

75. Youmans JB: Syphilis and other venereal diseases. Med Clin North Am 1964;48:571–824. **(III, B)**

76. Ingall D, Sanchez PJ, Musher D: Syphilis. In Remington JS, Klein JO (eds): Infectious Diseases of the Fetus and Newborn Infant. Philadelphia, WB Saunders, 1995, pp 529–564. **(III, B)**

77. Centers for Disease Control and Prevention: 2002 Sexually transmitted diseases treatment guidelines. MMWR 2002;51(RR-6):1–77. **(IV, C)**

Chancroid

78. World Health Organization Press Release: WHO/64: Sexually transmitted diseases—three hundred and thirty-three million new, curable cases in 1995. Geneva, World Health Organization, 1995. **(IV, C)**

79. Flood JM, Safrin SK, Bolan GA, et al: Multistrain outbreak of chancroid in San Francisco, 1989–1991. J Infect Dis 1993;167:1106–1111. **(III, B)**

80. Ronald AR, Albritton W: Chancroid and *Haemophilus ducreyi*. In Holmes KK, Sparling PF, Mardh P-A, et al (eds): Sexually Transmitted Diseases. New York, McGraw-Hill, 1999, pp 515–523. **(IV, C)**

81. Dicarlo RP: Chancroid epidemiology in New Orleans men. J Infect Dis 1995;173:446–452. **(III, B)**

82. Centers for Disease Control and Prevention: 2002 Sexually transmitted diseases treatment guidelines. MMWR 2002;51(RR-6):1–77. **(IV, C)**

83. Plummer FA: Clinical and microbiologic studies of genital ulcers in Kenyan women. Sex Transm Dis 1985;12:193. **(III, B)**

84. Lockett AE: Serum-free media for the isolation of *Haemophilus ducreyi*. Lancet 1991;338:326. **(III, B)**

85. Orle KA: Simultaneous PCR detection of *Haemophilus ducreyi*, *Treponema pallidum* and herpes simplex virus types 1 and 2 from genital ulcers. J Clin Microbiol 1996;34:49–54. **(III, B)**

86. Centers for Disease Control: 1993 Sexually transmitted diseases treatment guidelines. MMWR Recomm Rep 1993;42(RR-14):20–22. **(IV, C)**

Lymphogranuloma Venereum

87. Perine PL, Stamm WR: Lymphogranuloma venereum. In Holmes KK, Sparling PF, Mardh P-A, et al (eds): Sexually Transmitted Diseases. New York, McGraw-Hill, 1999, pp 423–432. **(IV, C)**

88. Schachter J, Smith DE, Dawson CR, et al: Lymphogranuloma venereum. 1. Comparison of the Frei test, complement fixation test and isolation of the agent. J Infect Dis 1969;120:372–375. **(IIa, B)**

89. Schachter J: Chlamydial infections. N Engl J Med 1978;298:428–435, 490–495, 549–549. **(III, B)**

90. Centers for Disease Control and Prevention: 2002 Sexually transmitted diseases treatment guidelines. MMWR 2002;51(RR-6):1–77. **(IV, C)**

Donovanosis (Granuloma Inguinale)

91. O'Farrell N: Donovanosis. In Holmes KK, Sparling PF, Mardh P-A, et al (eds): Sexually Transmitted Diseases. New York, McGraw-Hill, 1999, pp 525–531. **(IV, C)**

92. In Holmes KK, Mardh P-A (eds): International Perspectives on Neglected Sexually Transmitted Diseases. Washington, DC, Hemisphere Publishing Corp., 1983, pp 205–217. **(IV, C)**

93. Centers for Disease Control and Prevention: 2002 Sexually transmitted diseases treatment guidelines. MMWR 2002;51(RR-6):1–77. **(IV, C)**

Herpes Simplex Virus (Genital Herpes)

94. Centers for Disease Control and Prevention: National Disease and Therapeutic Index (IMS American Ltd.). Available at www.cdc.gov. **(IV, C)**

95. Fleming DT, McQuillian GM, Johnson RE, et al: Herpes simplex virus type 2 in the United States, 1976 to 1994. N Engl J Med 1997; 337:1105–1111. **(III, B)**

96. Langenberg AGM, Corey L, Ashley RL, et al, for the Chiron HSV Vaccine Study Group: A prospective study of new infections with herpes simplex virus type 1 and 2. N Engl J Med 1999;341:1432–1438. **(III, B)**

97. Amstey MS, Monif GR: Genital herpes virus infection in pregnancy. Obstet Gynecol 1979;44:394. **(III, B)**

98. Brown ZA, Selke S, Zeh J, et al: The acquisition of herpes simplex virus during pregnancy. N Engl J Med 1997;337:509–515. **(IIa, B)**

99. Arvin AM, Whitley RJ: Herpes simplex virus infection. In Remington JS, Klein JV (eds): Infectious Diseases of the Fetus and Newborn Infant. Philadelphia, WB Saunders, 2001, pp 425–446. **(IV, C)**

100. Prober CG, Sullender WM, Yasukawa LL, et al: Low risk of herpes simplex virus infections in neonates exposed to the virus at the time of vaginal delivery to mothers with recurrent genital herpes simplex virus infections. N Engl J Med 1987;316:240–244. **(IIa, B)**

101. Baker DA: Herpes simplex virus infections. Curr Opin Obstet Gynecol 1992;4:676–681. **(III, B)**

102. Hollier LM, Workowski K: Treatment of sexually transmitted diseases in women. Obstet Gynecol Clin North Am 2003;30:751–775. **(III, B)**

103. Centers for Disease Control and Prevention: 2002 Sexually transmitted diseases treatment guidelines. MMWR 2002;51(RR-6):1–77. **(IV, C)**

104. Centers for Disease Control and Prevention: 2002 Sexually transmitted diseases treatment guidelines. MMWR 2002;51(RR-6):1–77. **(IV, C)**

105. Sheffield JS, Hollier LM, Hill JB, et al: Acyclovir prophylaxis to prevent herpes simplex virus recurrence at delivery: a systemic review. Obstet Gynecol 2003;102:1396–1403. **(IIa, B)**

106. Haddad J, Langer B, Astruc D, et al: Oral acyclovir and recurrent genital herpes during pregnancy. Obstet Gynecol 1993;82:102–104. **(IIa, B)**

Trichomoniasis

107. Cotch MF, Pastorek JG III, Nugent RP, et al: *Trichomonas vaginalis* associated with low birth weight and preterm delivery. The vaginal infections and preterm study group. Sex Transm Dis 1997; 24:353–360. **(IIa, B)**

108. Laga M, Manoka A, Kivuvu M, et al: Nonulcerative sexually transmitted diseases as risk factors for HIV-1 transmission in women: results from a cohort study. AIDS 1993;7:95–102. **(IIa, B)**

109. Gardner H, Dukes CD: *Haemophilus vaginalis* vaginitis: a newly defined specific infection previously classified "nonspecific" vaginitis. Am J Obstet Gynecol 1955;69:962. **(III, B)**

110. Sweet RL, Gibbs RS: Infectious vulvovaginitis. In Sweet RL, Gibbs RS: Infectious Diseases of the Female Genital Tract. Philadelphia, Lippincott Williams & Wilkins, 2002, pp 337–354. **(IV, C)**

111. Hardy PH, Nell EE, Spence MR, et al: Prevalence of six sexually transmitted disease agents among pregnant inner city adolescents and pregnancy outcome. Lancet 1984;8:333. **(IIa, B)**

112. Mason PR, Brown I: Trichomonas in pregnancy (letter). Lancet 1980; 11:1025.

113. Klebanoff MA, Carey JC, Hauth JC, et al: Failure of metronidazole to prevent preterm delivery among pregnant women with asymptomatic *Trichomonas vaginalis* infection. N Engl J Med 2001;345:487–493. **(Ib, A)**

114. Brown HL, Fuller DA, Davis TE, et al: Evaluation of the affirm ambient temperature transport system for the detection and identification of *Trichomonas vaginalis*, *Gardnerella vaginalis*, and *Candida* species from vaginal fluid specimens. J Clin Microbiol 2001; 39:3197–3199. **(Ib, A)**

115. Ryu JS, Chung HL, Min DY, et al: Diagnosis of trichomoniasis by polymerase chain reaction. Yonsei Med J 1999;40:56–60. **(Ib, A)**

116. Centers for Disease Control and Prevention: 2002 Sexually transmitted diseases treatment guidelines. MMWR 2002;51(RR-6):1–77. **(IV, C)**

117. Muller M, Lossick JG, Gorrell TE, et al: In vitro susceptibility of *Trichomonas vaginalis* to metronidazole and treatment outcome in vaginal trichomoniasis. Sex Transm Dis 1988;15:17. **(III, B)**

### Scabies

118. Platts-Mills TAE, Rein MF: Scabies. In Holmes KK, Sparling PF, Mardh P-A, et al (eds): Sexually Transmitted Diseases. New York, McGraw-Hill, 1999, pp 645–650. **(IV, C)**

119. Centers for Disease Control and Prevention: 2002 Sexually transmitted diseases treatment guidelines. MMWR 2002;51(RR-6):1–77. **(IV, C)**

120. Meinking TL, Taplin D, Hermida JL, et al: The treatment of scabies with ivermectin. N Engl J Med 1995;333:26–30. **(III, B)**

### Pediculosis Pubis

121. Oriel JD: Ectoparasites. In Holmes KK, Mardh P-A (eds): International Perspectives on Neglected Sexually Transported Diseases. Washington, DC, Hemisphere Publishing Corp., 1983:131–138. **(IV, C)**

### Molluscum Contagiosum

122. Kwitten J: Molluscum contagiosum: some new histologic observations. Mt Sinai J Med 1980;47:583–588. **(III, B)**

123. Brown ST, Nalley JF, Kraus SJ: Molluscum contagiosum. Sex Transm Dis 1981;8:227–234. **(III, B)**

124. Becker TM, Blount JH, Douglas J, et al: Trends in molluscum contagiosum in the United States, 1966–1983. Sex Transm Dis 1986; 132:88–92. **(III, B)**

### Condyloma Acuminatum (Genital Warts)

125. Koutsky LA, Kiviat NB: Genital human papillomavirus. In Holmes KK, Sparling PF, Mardh P-A, et al (eds): Sexually Transmitted Diseases. New York, McGraw-Hill, 1999, pp 347–359. **(IV, C)**

126. Centers for Disease Control and Prevention, Division of STD Prevention: Sexually transmitted disease surveillance, 1995. Atlanta, Centers for Disease Control and Prevention, U.S. Department of Health and Human Services, 1996. **(IV, C)**

127. Institute of Medicine Committee on Prevention and Control of Sexually Transmitted Diseases: The hidden epidemic: confronting sexually transmitted diseases. Washington, DC, National Academy Press, 1997. **(IV, C)**

128. Gall SA: Human papillomavirus infection. In Medd PD, Hager WD, Faro S (eds): Protocols for Infectious Diseases in Obstetrics and Gynecology. Malden, Mass, Blackwell Science, 2000, pp 380–389. **(IV, C)**

129. Insinga RP, Dasbach EJ, Myers ER: The health and economic burden of genital warts in a set of private health plans in the United States. Clin Infect Dis 2003;36:1397–1403. **(IV, C)**

130. Koutsky LA, Galloway DA, Holmes KK: Epidemiology of genital papillomavirus infection. Epidemiol Rev 1988;10:122–163. **(III, B)**

131. Winer RL, Lee S-K, Hughes JP, et al: Genital human papillomavirus infection: incidence and risk factors in a cohort of female university students. Am J Epidemiol 2003;157:218–226. **(IIa, B)**

132. Halpert R, Fruchter RG, Sedlis A, et al: Human papillomavirus and lower genital neoplasia in renal transplant patients. Obstet Gynecol 1986;68:251–258. **(III, B)**

133. Garry R, Jones R: Relationship between cervical condylomata, pregnancy and subclinical papillomavirus infection. J Reprod Med 1985; 30:393–396. **(III, B)**

134. Centers for Disease Control: 1993 Sexually transmitted diseases treatment guidelines. MMWR 1993;42:85–88. **(IV, C)**

135. Bristow RE, Montz FJ: Human papillomavirus: molecular biology and screening applications in cervical neoplasia—a primer for primary care physicians. Prim Care Update Ob Gyns 1995;5:238–246. **(III, B)**

136. Werness BA: Role of the human papillomavirus oncoproteins in transformation and carcinogenic progression. In DeVita JT (ed): Important Advances in Oncology. Philadelphia, JB Lippincott, 1991, p 3. **(IV, C)**

137. Beutner KR, Wiley DJ, Douglas JM, et al: Genital warts and their treatment. Clin Infect Dis 1999;28(Suppl):S37–56. **(III, B)**

138. Centers for Disease Control and Prevention: 2002 Sexually transmitted diseases treatment guidelines. MMWR 2002;51(RR-6):1–77. **(IV, C)**

139. Chamberlain MJ, Reynolds AL, Yeomen WB: Toxic effects of podophyllin application in pregnancy. BMJ 1972;3:391–392. **(III, B)**

# Chapter 20

# Pelvic Inflammatory Disease

## Sebastian Faro, MD, PhD

## KEY POINTS

- Clinical signs of pelvic inflammatory disease (PID) are vaginal leukorrhea, irregular uterine bleeding, breakthrough bleeding while taking oral contraceptives, vague lower abdominal pain, possible elevated body temperature.
- *Chlamydia trachomatis* tends to cause minimal symptoms (asymptomatic PID), can go undetected or result in infertility or ectopic pregnancy.
- Gonococcal or polymicrobial PID can cause significant destruction of fallopian tubes and development of pyosalpinx or tubo-ovarian abscess.
- All sexually active women should be screened for sexually transmitted infections (STIs) if they are not in a monogamous relationship, do not live with their sexual partner, have endocervical mucopus, their endocervical epithelium is hypertrophied, their cervix bleeds easily when gently touched, or a sexual partner is known to have an STI.
- A patient found to have chlamydia or gonorrhea should be treated for both STIs.
- A patient found to have trichomoniasis should be tested for other STIs.

PID has been and continues to be a devastating disease that primarily affects women in the reproductive age group. However, the disease can occur in any group if conditions permit bacteria to gain entrance to the lower or upper genitalia. The genital tract is a complex system of organs beginning with the vulva, leading to the vagina, and progressing to the cervix, uterus, fallopian tubes, and pelvic cavity. The genital tract can be viewed as a conduit leading from microbe-contaminated areas—the vulva, vagina, and cervix—to sterile areas—the uterus, fallopian tubes, pelvic cavity, and abdominal cavity.

The creation of broad-spectrum antibiotics and prevention programs caused a significant decrease in both the progression of sexually transmitted bacteria that infect the lower genital tract and the progression to PID. Educational and prevention programs have made an impact on the transmission of sexually transmitted diseases (STDs), which can lead to PID. The development of broad-spectrum antibiotics along with shorter treatment regimens has led to better compliance. Better compliance resulted in quicker eradication of the infecting bacteria, including both STDs and vaginal microflora, and reduced the progression of infection leading to PID.

## EPIDEMIOLOGY

In the United States there are an estimated 9 million cases of STDs among individuals between the ages of 15 and 24 years.[1] The estimated total costs of these STDs in the United States are between $9.3 and $15.5 billion.[2,3]

PID is actually a spectrum of infections that begins with cervicitis and can progress to endometritis, salpingitis, and tubo-ovarian abscess. The two sexually transmitted bacteria responsible for the majority of PID cases are *Chlamydia trachomatis* and *Neisseria gonorrhoeae*. Women at the greatest risk for acquiring an STD and PID are between 15 and 25 years of age.[4,5] All sexually active women are at risk for acquiring one or more STDs as well as PID if they place themselves at risk (Table 20-1). The Centers for Disease Control and Prevention (CDC) reported 80,000 cases of acute PID and approximately 40,000 cases of chronic PID in hospitals in 2002.[6] CDC estimated that there were 200,000 initial patient visits to physicians' offices for PID in 2002.[6] CDC also reported that from 1980 until 2000 the incidence of PID was declining, but there appeared to be an increase in the number of acute PID cases in 2001: in 1980 there were approximately 108,000 cases, in 2000 there were approximately 60,000 cases, in 2001 there were 70,000 cases, and in 2002 about 80,000 cases of PID.

Throughout the 1980s and early 1990s cases of PID steadily increased, and the incidence parallels the increase in the number of C. trachomatis and N. gonorrhoeae cases. However, when a decrease in the number of N. gonorrhoeae cases was seen there was a concurrent decrease in the number of PID cases. This decrease has been associated with a plateau in the number of PID cases. However, it is difficult to determine whether this plateau is real or a result of the restrictions placed on hospital admissions by the insurance industry, thus resulting in fewer individuals receiving treatment. In addition, patients are frequently given antibiotics for a variety of suspected infections, antibiotics that are also used to treat cervical chlamydial infection. However, chlamydial infection is frequently asymptomatic and, if left untreated, can progress to asymptomatic upper genital tract infection. Thus, the patient does not realize she has the infection until she attempts to become pregnant and finds out that she is infertile or has an ectopic pregnancy.

PID is a primary sequela in 10% to 40% of acute, untreated, and undiagnosed cervical chlamydial infection.[5,7] It is estimated that PID develops in 3% to 6% of acute cases of treated chlamydial cervicitis because progression of the infection occurred before treatment was initiated.[8] The cost for PID, including the sequelae of chronic pelvic pain, ectopic pregnancy, and treatment for infertility, is estimated to be $1060 to

# Gynecologic Infectious Disease

**Table 20-1**
**Risk Factors for Pelvic Inflammatory Disease Acquisition**

1. Multiple sexual partners
2. Failure to use barrier contraception
3. Illicit drug use
4. Sexual partner with an STD
5. History of STD

$3626.[9,10] However, ectopic pregnancy and infertility are unpredictable, on a per case basis, following an episode of PID because the initial episode can be asymptomatic. Ectopic pregnancy can result from damage to the lining of the fallopian tubes. In fact, 95% of ectopic pregnancies occur in the fallopian tubes, with 2.5% found in the cornua of the uterus and the remainder in the ovary, cervix, and abdominal cavity.[11] Ectopic pregnancy continues to be a significant cause of morbidity and mortality, responsible for 10% to 15% of all maternal deaths.[12] The incidence of ectopic pregnancy is 19.7 cases per 1000 pregnancies in the United States, and it is the leading cause of maternal mortality in the first trimester.[13] PID is the most common precursor to ectopic pregnancy. The bacteria that can damage the fallopian tubes, and readily do so, are C. trachomatis and N. gonorrhoeae. These bacteria typically cause asymptomatic infection that can result in significant damage to the ciliated and nonciliated epithelial cells lining the fallopian tubes. Nonfunctioning ciliated cells result, and the inflammatory response can cause adhesions within the fallopian tube (Fig. 20-1). This can all take place without the patient experiencing any significant pain. Frequently the patient may have cramping, which resembles the cramping associated with menstruation, or irregular or breakthrough bleeding. Unfortunately, the endogenous aerobic, facultative, and obligate anaerobes also can cause significant fallopian tube damage, but unlike C. trachomatis and N. gonorrhoeae, the former bacteria typically cause symptomatic infection. To prevent the sequelae of PID, the examining physician must be alert not only to the pertinent facts in the patient's history that place her at risk for PID but also to the subtle clinical signs of pelvic infection (cervicitis, endometritis, and salpingitis).

## MICROBIOLOGY

The two most common sexually transmitted bacteria that cause PID are C. trachomatis and N. gonorrhoeae, separately or together. In fact, 40% of cases of cervicitis are caused by concomitant infection with both of these bacteria.[14] Infection with either or both can be asymptomatic; therefore, these infections are typically diagnosed by the history or the pelvic examination reveals a clinical clue of infection.

Infection of the upper genital tract can occur either from the endogenous vaginal microflora secondary to infection by C. trachomatis and/or N. gonorrhoeae or via contamination from inflammatory bowel disease, for example, diverticulitis. There has been much speculation about an association between bacterial vaginosis and PID. Some investigators draw such an association because in patients who develop tubo-ovarian abscesses, obligate anaerobic bacteria are often recovered. However, other investigators report no such bacteria in patients with acute gonococcal PID.[15] That the bacteriology is qualitative and not quantitative is a common error made in many studies. The mere presence of a bacterium isolated from the lower genital tract does not mean that it is significant. Another problem is that isolating bacteria from the endometrium cannot be regarded as definitive proof that the organism is a causative agent in endometritis when instead it may be a contaminant from the lower genital tract. Other erroneous conclusions regarding the failure to recover anaerobes are that the specimens were improperly collected, were not placed in an appropriate transport medium, or were not processed appropriately by the laboratory. Not all abscesses contain obligate anaerobic bacteria. The involvement of obligate anaerobic bacteria in tubo-ovarian abscesses can originate in one of four ways: (1) bacteria ascend from the lower genital tract (a plausible hypothesis); (2) the bowel becomes inflamed because infectious exudate from the fallopian tubes covers the rectosigmoid colon and the bacteria migrate across an inflamed intact bowel; (3) a patient with diverticulitis can have an inflamed diverticulum fuse with the fallopian tube or ovary and, through pressure necrosis, a fistula forms, providing a conduit for bacteria to migrate from the large bowel to the adnexa; or (4) bacteria from the lower genital tract can be forcibly pushed into the upper genital tract during procedures, for example, hysterosalpingography, artificial insemination, chromopertubation, hysterography, and fetal reduction performed transvaginally. In fact, any procedure invading the upper genital tract via the transvaginal/cervical route can induce an upper genital tract infection if the vaginal flora is significantly altered, for example, if there is a preponderance of gram-negative bacteria.

The development of a tubo-ovarian abscess must be preceded by a break in the ovarian cortex. This usually occurs when there

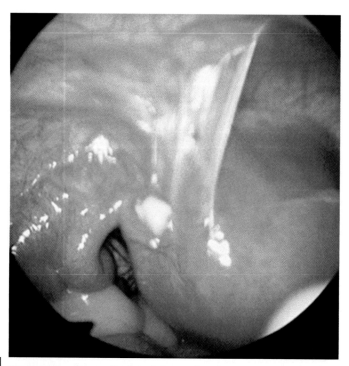

**Figure 20-1** **Filmy adhesions between the uterus and anterior abdominal wall.**

is spontaneous rupture of the ovarian cortex, for example, with ovulation or rupture of an ovarian cyst. If infected fluid is exiting the fallopian tube at the time of ovulation, an avenue for entrance of bacteria through the ruptured cortex of the ovary exists. Once bacteria enter the ovary, they can reproduce and penetrate deeper ovarian tissue, resulting in an infected ovary.

Another potential mechanism is an inflamed and infected fallopian tube densely adherent to the ovary. The pressure builds within the pyosalpinx, and via pressure necrosis the ovarian cortex is breached, which allows infected material to enter the ovary. These proposed mechanisms allow bacteria to gain entrance to sterile tissue and then grow, causing additional tissue destruction.

The progression from symptomatic or asymptomatic acute salpingitis to pyosalpinx to either hydrosalpinx or tubo-ovarian abscess depends on the bacteria involved. If the infection involves only C. trachomatis, N. gonorrhoeae, or both, the infection may not progress to abscess formation. If facultative and/or anaerobic bacteria become involved in the infection, then abscess development is more likely to occur. Infection of the cervix with either of these sexually transmitted bacteria is typically asymptomatic and if the subtle clinical presentation goes unnoticed, progression can continue. Therefore, the physician should proceed with the examination and obtain endocervical specimens for the detection of C. trachomatis and N. gonorrhoeae. Since there is no way to determine the duration of infection, the physician should consider that the infection has been in the cervix long enough to allow for ascending infection. Treatment should include coverage for upper genital tract infection.

## CLINICAL SIGNS AND SYMPTOMS

The initial infection begins with cervicitis and is usually asymptomatic but the patient may experience either postcoital bleeding or acute onset dyspareunia. Examination, in the presence of cervical infection, reveals numerous white blood cells (WBCs) in the vaginal discharge.[16,17] The infected cervix can appear inflamed, that is, the endocervical columnar epithelium becomes hypertrophied, markedly erythematous, and everted. It can be fragile and bleed easily when gently touched with a cotton-tipped applicator or when a specimen for a Papanicolaou (Pap) smear is obtained. The patient is frequently without symptoms and does not realize she is infected (has cervicitis). Untreated cervicitis can result in progression of infection to the uterus, which is known as endometritis.

Pelvic examination of a patient with cervicitis, endometritis, and salpingitis frequently reveals a purulent vaginal discharge. The discharge contains a large number of WBCs, and the morphology of the endogenous bacterial microflora can range from one dominated by large bacillary forms (consistent with lactobacilli) to one containing a variety of bacterial morphotypes. The cervix will be tender to palpation and motion. A cotton- or Dacron-tipped swab is inserted into the endocervical canal and examined for the presence of mucopus[18–20] (Fig. 20-2). Evaluation of a patient suspected of having cervicitis includes obtaining specimens from the endocervix for the isolation of C. trachomatis and N. gonorrhoeae.

The patient with endometritis may fail to realize that symptoms such as mild lower abdominal pain or cramping can

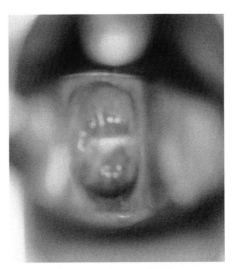

**Figure 20-2    Endocervical mucopus.**

be associated with irregular uterine bleeding or spotting. The patient taking oral contraceptive pills who has developed endometritis also can develop breakthrough bleeding. Thus, the symptoms of endometritis can be mistaken for an irregularity in estrogen and progesterone production or the presence of a submucous fibroid or endometrial polyp. The presence of endometrial cancer, however, is unlikely, since PID usually occurs in women of young reproductive age and they are unlikely to develop endometrial cancer. Patients with more advanced endometritis can have fever, purulent vaginal discharge, lower abdominal pain, or intensified cramping.

Pelvic examination can reveal the presence of an associated cervicitis, and uterine tenderness on palpation and motion. This examination should include an endometrial biopsy. The biopsy specimen should be divided as follows: (1) a portion submitted for histologic analysis; (2) a portion placed in transport medium for the processing, isolation, and identification of aerobic and facultative bacteria; (3) a portion placed in a proper transport medium for the isolation and identification of C. trachomatis and N. gonorrhoeae; and (4) a portion placed in transport medium for the processing, isolation, and identification of obligate anaerobic bacteria.

Patients with salpingitis can be completely asymptomatic, have vague symptoms, or be symptomatic. The patient can also have an elevated temperature, but less than 101°F. In a patient with salpingitis, the bimanual pelvic examination reveals the presence of pain and tenderness on palpation and motion of the adnexa.

The following laboratory tests should be obtained from the patient's venous blood work: a complete blood count, to determine whether the WBC count is elevated and whether the neutrophils are elevated; blood urea nitrogen (BUN); creatinine; and electrolytes. A C-reactive protein level or sedimentation rate should also be obtained. If a pelvic mass is suspected, a pelvic ultrasound examination should be obtained. If a mass is present, the ultrasound examination can differentiate between agglutination of the bowel (which typically appears as an amorphous mass) and the adnexa and the presence of an abscess (a uniloculated or multiloculated cystic mass). If an abscess is

# Gynecologic Infectious Disease

present, the characteristics of the abscess can be discerned, whether it is uniloculated or multiloculated, and whether the external walls are thin or thick. These characteristics may play a role in the success or failure of antibiotic therapy in the treatment of tubo-ovarian abscesses. However, there is no scientific basis for the role of the characteristics of an abscess, that is, whether the abscess is uniloculated or multiloculated or thick- or thin-walled, and whether these characteristics play a role in antibiotic treatment. Ultrasonographic examination can be helpful in determining whether there is free fluid in the pelvis. If a patient comes in with PID, free fluid in the pelvis, elevated temperature, and abdominal/pelvic rebound tenderness, a ruptured or leaking tubo-ovarian abscess should be suspected. This is a surgical emergency. A delay in administering antibiotic therapy and surgical intervention results in significant morbidity and mortality.

The patient with intact tubo-ovarian abscesses is at low risk for bacteremia and sepsis. The marked inflammation of the pelvis and abdominal peritoneum results in dilation of blood vessels, allowing for the transmigration of bacteria and resulting in bacteremia. The presence of free purulent fluid containing large numbers of bacteria, including abscessogenic combinations in the peritoneal cavity, results in the potential for abscesses to develop through the abdominal and pelvic cavities. There is also a release of endotoxins, resulting in the up-regulating of the cytokine system, which if left unchecked will lead to the release of tumor necrosis factor-$\alpha$ (TNF-$\alpha$) and then to septic shock.

Laparoscopy has become an extremely useful tool for diagnosing pelvic disease, and it is particularly useful for both diagnosing and treating PID. However, interpreting the appearance of the fallopian tubes may be difficult at times. A study by Molander and colleagues found that the accuracy of laparoscopic diagnosis of PID was 78%, the sensitivity was 27%, and the specificity was 92%.[21] These investigators found that the laparoscopic diagnosis of PID was inferior to histologically proved PID. However, laparoscopy can be used to determine the degree of infection by noting the presence or absence of edema and erythema of the uterus, tubal erythema and edema, tubal adhesions, status of tubal fimbriae, and type of fluid present in the cul-de-sac (serous, serosanguineous, bloody, or purulent). Laparoscopy without the aid of previous imaging studies may not reveal whether there is an intraloop bowel abscess or a tubo-ovarian abscess, and how complex the tubo-ovarian abscess is. In addition, the physician can determine by the presence of perihepatic adhesions whether the infection has progressed out of the pelvis. This is often referred to as the Fitz-Hugh-Curtis syndrome.[22–24] However, the presence of perihepatic adhesions is not pathognomonic of past PID. Perihepatic adhesion can result from any inflammatory process that involves the surface of the liver and the anterior abdominal wall overlying the liver.[25,26]

## MANAGEMENT

The first consideration is to determine whether the patient can be treated as an outpatient or whether hospitalization is necessary (Table 20-2). Patients with signs and symptoms of mild disease can be treated as outpatients. However, the patient must be compliant to taking the prescribed antibiotics and

| Table 20-2 |
|---|
| **Characteristics of Pelvic Inflammatory Disease to Determine Whether Patient Should Be Treated as Outpatient or Inpatient** |

| Outpatient Treatment | Inpatient Treatment |
|---|---|
| 1. Absence of nausea and vomiting | 1. Temperature ≥ 101°F |
| 2. Oral temperature < 101°F | 2. Markedly elevated WBC count |
| 3. Absence of a pelvic mass | 3. Patient has nausea or vomiting |
| 4. Compliant patient | 4. Presence of peritonitis |
| 5. No evidence of pelvic or abdominal peritonitis | 5. Presence of pelvic mass |

appear for follow-up evaluation at the specified times. The patient should also refrain from sexual intercourse and douching. The patient should be reevaluated in 72 hours. The goal of treatment is to (1) eradicate the offending bacteria, (2) prevent damage to the fallopian tubes that can result in infertility or ectopic pregnancy, and (3) prevent the formation of tubo-ovarian abscesses. Since acute early PID is most commonly, but not exclusively, caused by C. trachomatis and/or N. gonorrhoeae the antibiotic therapy should provide excellent coverage against both. In addition, since it is not possible to determine the time sequence between acquisition of the infecting bacteria, the progression from lower to upper genital tract, and possible damage to upper genital tract organs, additional antibiotic coverage for gram-negative and gram-positive facultative and obligate anaerobic bacteria should be provided.

Patients treated as outpatients should receive antibiotics that provide good activity against C. trachomatis; N. gonorrhoeae; and aerobic, facultative, and obligate anaerobic bacteria (Table 20-3). The patient must be compliant and not have nausea.

Treatment of acute uncomplicated PID in patients for whom there are uncertainties regarding compliance should be in the hospital. Intravenous antibiotic therapy should be considered in patients when there are concerns about the extent of the disease.[27] If the patient has an elevated temperature, has continued lower abdominal pain, or has a pelvic mass, she should be admitted to the hospital and reevaluated to determine whether she truly has PID. Imaging studies should be considered to determine whether a mass is present in the pelvis. The use of ultrasound to reveal the presence of a mass can have significant bearing on the management of the PID patient. The characteristics of a suspected tubo-ovarian abscess also can have significant implications with regard to medical management. A uniloculated abscess with a thin wall is more likely to respond to antibiotic therapy in contrast to the thick-walled, multiloculated abscess (Figs. 20-3 to 20-6). The latter is likely to have a decreased blood supply; therefore, antibiotics are less likely to achieve the concentrations needed to kill the offending bacteria. In addition, fluid present in the pelvis can indicate a leaking or ruptured tubo-ovarian abscess. If there was evidence of pelvic peritonitis and ileus, then the diagnosis of a leaking or ruptured abscess can be made. In this instance, antibiotic therapy alone is not indicated, and appropriate management is depicted in Table 20-4.

Intravenous antibiotics should be continued until the patient is afebrile for 72 hours, the WBC count returns to normal, peristalsis returns to the bowel, and the patient is tolerating

**Table 20-3**
**Antibiotic Choices for Treatment of PID**

| Outpatient Treatment | Inpatient Treatment |
|---|---|
| 1. Cefoxitin 2 g IM + probenecid 1 g orally *plus* doxycycline 100 mg orally twice daily for 10–14 days or tetracycline 500 mg orally four times daily for 10–14 days* *or* | 1. Cefoxitin 2 g IV every 6 hours, or cefotetan IV 2 g every 12 hours *plus* doxycycline 100 mg orally or IV every 12 hours* *or* |
| 2. Metronidazole 500 mg three times daily *plus* levofloxacin 500 mg once daily for 10–14 days[†] | 2. Clindamycin 900 mg IV every 8 hours *plus* gentamicin loading dose IV or IM (2 mg/kg body weight), followed by maintenance dose (1.5 mg/kg) every 8 hours[§] |
| 3. Ofloxacin 400 mg orally every 12 hours for 10 days[†] | 3. Ampicillin/sulbactam 3 g IV every 6 hours until signs and symptoms have resolved, followed by doxycycline 100 mg orally twice daily for 10 days[¶] |

*From Centers for Disease Control and Prevention: Pelvic Inflammatory Disease: Guidelines for Prevention and Management. MMWR Recomm Rep 1998;191:40(RR-5): 1–25.

[†] No data are available, but these combinations have been used in treatment of pelvic infections. Levofloxacin is effective in the treatment of *Chlamydia trachomatis* and *Neisseria gonorrhoeae* and gram-negative and gram-positive bacteria.

[‡] From Martens MC, Gordon S, Yarborough R, et al: Multicenter randomized trial of ofloxacin versus cefoxitin and doxycycline in outpatient treatment of pelvic inflammatory disease. South Med J 1993;86:604–610.

[§] From Hemsell DL, Little BB, Faro S, et al: Comparison of three regimens recommended by the Centers for Disease Control and Prevention for the treatment of women hospitalized with acute pelvic inflammatory disease. Clin Infect Dis 1994;19:720–727.

[¶] From Hemsell DL, Heard MC, Nobles BJ: Sublactam/ampicillin versus cefoxitin for uncomplicated acute pelvic inflammatory disease. Drugs 1988;35:39–42.

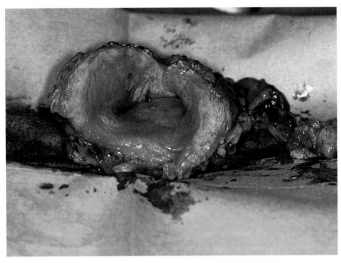

Figure 20-4    Gross specimen of uniloculated tubal abscess.

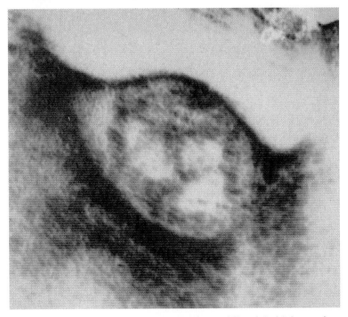

Figure 20-5    Ultrasonogram demonstrating multiloculated tubo-ovarian abscess.

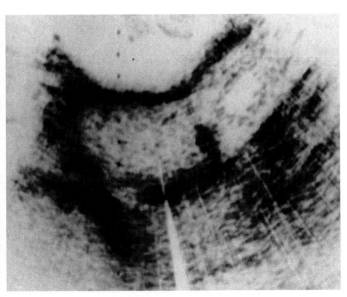

Figure 20-3    Ultrasonogram of uniloculated tubal abscess.

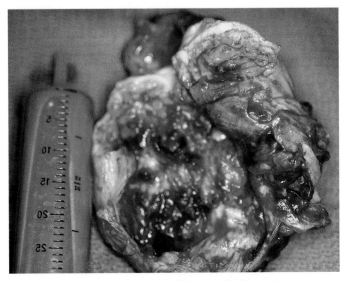

Figure 20-6    Gross specimen of multiloculated tubo-ovarian abscess.

---

**Table 20-4**
**Management of Patient with Leaking or Ruptured Tubo-ovarian Abscess**

1. Laboratory tests: CBC with differential, serum electrolytes, blood urea nitrogen, blood glucose, liver enzymes and functions

2. Imaging studies of the pelvis to reveal detail of the pelvic organs: Ultrasonography and computed tomography (CT)

3. Immediate administration of broad-spectrum antibiotics IV
   a. Metronidazole 500 mg every 8 hours *plus* ampicillin 2 g every 8 hours *plus* gentamicin 5 mg/kg body weight every 24 hours
      *or*
   b. Clindamycin 900 mg every 8 hours *plus* ampicillin 2 g every 8 hours *plus* gentamicin 5 mg/kg body weight every 8 hours
      *or*
   c. Piperacillin 3.375 g every 6 hours *plus* gentamicin 5 mg/kg body weight every 24 hours

4. Laparotomy
   a. Lower abdominal incision that can be extended to the upper abdomen
   b. Obtain specimens of infected tissue and purulent fluid for gram-staining, culture, isolation, and identification of bacteria
   c. Remove all infected tissue: typically the woman who develops PID that progresses to tubo-ovarian abscess almost always develops bilateral tubo-ovarian abscesses
   d. Patients who desire to retain child-bearing ability should not have the uterus removed

---

liquid and solid nutrition. Antibiotic therapy should then be changed to oral therapy, for example, metronidazole 500 mg every 8 hours plus levofloxacin 500 mg every 24 hours for a total of 10 days. There are no data to guide the addition of oral antibiotic therapy, but the absence of pelvic tenderness can be used as a criterion for discontinuing antibiotic therapy.

## PROGRESSION OF PELVIC INFLAMMATORY DISEASE

PID is a complex infection that ascends from the cervix to the uterus and then to the fallopian tubes. The progression is difficult to track because the initial infection and secondary infections, cervicitis and endometritis, are more often asymptomatic than not. Therefore, patients who practice high-risk sexual behavior should be suspected of having at least the initial stages of PID until proved otherwise. This is extremely important because the sequelae are devastating, and it is crucial that the patient be thoroughly evaluated. Asymptomatic, untreated, or inappropriately treated PID can result in progression of this infection.

Infection of the fallopian tubes can result in resolution without damage if antibiotic therapy is instituted early. However, women experiencing an initial episode of PID have an approximately 13% risk of becoming infertile. If the individual has a second PID episode there is a 33% chance of infertility, and the chance increases to 75% with a third episode of PID. If treatment is instituted after damage has occurred or if the infection was mild, there can be residual damage to the tube's endothelium. The damage may not be enough to leave the patient infertile but does result in a tube that does not function properly. This puts the patient at risk for ectopic pregnancy. Approximately 1.2% to 1.4% of all reported pregnancies are

ectopic.[28,29] Ectopic pregnancy continues to be the leading cause of maternal death during the first trimester of pregnancy as well as the cause of reduction in fertility.[30–32] Several factors increase an individual's risk of ectopic pregnancy (Table 20-5), with STDs that cause PID, such as *N. gonorrhoeae and C. trachomatis*, being the most common.[33–39] Even though STDs such as gonorrhea and chlamydia frequently cause PID, these bacteria tend to cause a milder form of the disease. The aerobic, facultative, and obligate anaerobic bacteria are more likely responsible for more destructive PID, for example, tubo-ovarian abscess formation.[40]

Once the fallopian tubes become infected, a substantial inflammatory response within the lumen of the tube as well as throughout the wall and involving the serosa of the tube occurs. This inflammatory reaction results in the formation of adhesions within the lumen of the fallopian tube and between the sera and adjacent organs. The inflammatory response also occurs at the fimbriae and results in agglutination. This intraluminal inflammatory response results in occlusion at the interstitial portion of the tube. The interstitial portion of the tube is embedded within the myometrium of the cornua of the uterus, thus preventing distention of this portion of the fallopian tube and allowing early occlusion of the proximal portion of that tube. The agglutination of the fimbriae results in occlusion of the distal end of the fallopian tube and, along with occlusion of the proximal end, results in a build-up of infected material within the lumen of the tube. There is a progressive build up of intraluminal fluid as the inflammatory process and infection progress. This intraluminal progressive build-up of fluid causes compression of the ciliated cells lining the lumen of the fallopian tube, which results in cessation of the ciliated movement. This malfunction of the cilia does not allow for migration of the fertilized egg, and the creation of false passages within the lumen of the fallopian tube, via the formation of adhesions, results in the fertilized egg becoming trapped within the fallopian tube. The development of a closed fallopian tube with contained infection is termed a *pyosalpinx* and is an abscess. The pyosalpinx can become symptomatic or undergo resolution and become a hydrosalpinx. A hydrosalpinx is, in essence, a nonfunctioning fallopian tube.

Infection involving the fallopian tubes can progress to the formation of a tubo-ovarian abscess. There are two theories with regard to the development of a tubo-ovarian abscess: (1) infectious fluid exits from the fallopian tube and enters the ovary via a ruptured follicle at the time of ovulation, and (2) the infected fallopian tube becomes adherent to the ovary and via pressure necrosis there is a breakdown of the fallopian tube ovarian walls and infected fluid from the fallopian tube enters

---

**Table 20-5**
**Risk Factors for Development of Ectopic Pregnancy**

1. Previous ectopic pregnancy
2. Cigarette smoking
3. Pelvic surgery
4. Use of an IUD
5. Having had an STD that results in PID

the ovary. Typically in the absence of a foreign body, for example, an intrauterine device, tubo-ovarian abscesses that develop in association with PID are bilateral (Fig. 20-7). A tubo-ovarian abscess that develops in association with a foreign body or diverticulitis is almost always unilateral.

The diagnosis of tubo-ovarian abscesses can be established with a high-degree of certainty with the assistance of either an ultrasonogram or a CT scan. Once again, the structure of the abscess will play a role in whether the abscess is likely or unlikely to respond to antibiotic therapy. In addition, the patient with peritonitis should be suspected of having a ruptured tubo-ovarian abscess. Imaging studies that reveal the presence of fluid in the pelvis or abdominal cavity, pain with rebound tenderness, or pain, elevated body temperature, and an elevated white blood cell count should be brought to the operating room for exploratory surgery. Broad-spectrum antibiotics should be administered immediately after the diagnosis is made (Table 20-6). There should be no delay in bringing the patient to surgery because a patient with a ruptured tubo-ovarian abscess is to be considered a medical and surgical emergency with a significant potential for mortality.

If imaging studies do not indicate any degree of rupture of the abscess or abscesses, consideration can be given to medical management. The anatomic characteristics of the abscesses can be used to predict the potential success or failure of antibiotic therapy. A uniloculated, thin-walled abscess is more likely to respond to antibiotic therapy. A multiloculated, thin-walled abscess is more likely to respond positively to antibiotic therapy than a thick-walled, multiloculated abscess. A thick wall implies that the blood supply to the ovary is compromised; therefore, antibiotic levels to and into the abscess will likely be below the minimum inhibitory concentration required to kill the bacteria.

Patients being treated for PID, with or without tubo-ovarian abscesses, should be monitored closely for signs of improvement or deterioration. Patients with uncomplicated PID—without a

| Table 20-6 |
| --- |
| **Author's Recommendations for Medical and Surgical Management of Patient with Tubo-ovarian Abscess** |

1. Laboratory tests
   a. CBC with differential
   b. Electrolytes
   c. BUN
   d. Creatinine
   e. Glucose
   f. Liver enzymes

2. Imaging studies
   a. Ultrasonography
   b. CT with contrast of the abdomen and pelvis

3. Antibiotic choices (IV)
   a. Clindamycin (900 mg every 8 h) *plus* ampicillin (2 g every 6 h) *plus* gentamicin (5 mg/kg of body weight every 24 h; blood trough levels should be obtained prior to the third dose and repeated with every subsequent third dose to monitor for possible toxicity)
   b. Metronidazole (500 mg every 8 h) *plus* ampicillin *plus* gentamicin
   c. Piperacillin/tazobactam (3.375 g every 6 h) + gentamicin
   d. Clindamycin or metronidazole *plus* levofloxacin (500 mg every 24 h)

4. Surgery
   a. Make a vertical lower abdominal incision that can be extended to the upper abdomen.
   b. Obtain a specimen of fluid for gram-staining and culture of aerobic, facultative, and obligate anaerobic bacteria.
   c. If the patient does not desire future pregnancy, total abdominal hysterectomy with bilateral salpingo-oopherectomy is recommended.
   d. If the patient wants to attempt future pregnancy, the uterus should remain in place and the tissue containing the abscesses be removed. If one ovary is not enlarged and is not cystic, it may be left in place and the fallopian tubes removed if infected.
   e. The abdomen and pelvis should be irrigated with copious amounts (10–15 L) of either normal saline or antibiotic solution (bacitracin 50,000 units *plus* kanamycin 1 g dissolved in 1 L normal saline).
   f. Closed drains should be placed in the pelvis, and if there was purulent fluid in the upper abdomen, drains should be placed above the liver, under the diaphragm on the left. These drains should lie along the colonic gutters and end under the diaphragm on the right and left. The drains should all be connected to suction devices (JP or Blake drains).
   g. Drains should be used to sample the fluid exiting from the abdomen and pelvis by gram-staining and culture, especially if the patient continues to have a febrile course. The drains should be removed when there is less than 30 mL exiting from each drain over a 24-hour period.

5. Medical
   a. Intravenous antibiotic therapy, as described above, should be continued until the patient becomes afebrile and remains afebrile for 48 hours, bowels sounds have returned, the WBC count has returned to normal, the patient tolerates oral liquids and solids, and the abdominal/pelvic examination does not reveal pain.
   b. After the patient has been afebrile for 48 hours, the patient can be changed to oral antibiotics
      i. Metronidazole 500 mg three times a day *plus* levofloxacin 500 mg once a day
      ii. Clindamycin 300 mg three times a day *plus* levofloxacin
      iii. Metronidazole *plus* ampicillin/clavulanic acid 875 mg twice a day
   c. Imaging studies should be repeated 2 weeks after beginning oral antibiotic therapy to determine any change in the size of the mass.
   d. The patient should monitor her oral body temperature daily, e.g., at 12, 4, and 8 PM and at bedtime. A temperature ≥ 100.4°F should be reported to her physician. The patient should also report the development of abdominal/pelvic pain.
   e. Oral antibiotic therapy should be continued until the mass has resolved or has become asymptomatic.

6. If the patient has a persistent mass that has not been significantly reduced in size (by at least 50%) or has persistent pelvic pain, laparotomy or laparoscopy should be considered.

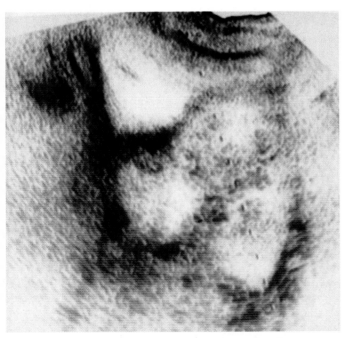

**Figure 20-7    Ultrasonogram of bilateral tubo-ovarian abscesses.**

tubo-ovarian bowel complex or abscesses—should respond to antibiotic therapy within 48 to 72 hours. They should become afebrile, WBC count and bowel function should return to normal, and their pain should be resolving. If after 48 to 72 hours of antibiotic therapy the patient's body temperature continues to be elevated, the WBC count continues to be elevated, or bowel function has not returned to normal, then the patient should be reevaluated for possible progression of PID to confirm that the initial diagnosis was correct.

In summary, a patient suspected of having PID should be treated aggressively to prevent disease progression. Patients with minimal symptoms and findings can be treated as outpatients. However, if the patient cannot be relied on to take the antibiotic therapy as prescribed, she should be hospitalized. Patients with an oral temperature of 101°F or greater, possible nausea, rebound pelvic pain, or a pelvic mass should be admitted to the hospital for treatment. Antibiotic therapy has been demonstrated to be efficacious in treating uncomplicated and suspected complicated PID.[41-43] Broad-spectrum antibiotics, that is, regimens providing activity against *C. trachomatis*, *N. gonorrhoeae*, and facultative and obligate anaerobic bacteria are efficacious in the treatment of both complicated and uncomplicated PID. When abscesses are suspected and documented by ultrasonography or CT scanning, broad-spectrum antibiotics are effective; however, there remains the question of whether a true abscess was present. If an abscess is suspected but it is not leaking or ruptured, antibiotic therapy can be administered with the expectation that the surgical approach can be held off. If there is any indication that the abscess is leaking or ruptured, then the combined approach of antibiotic and surgery should be taken.

## REFERENCES

1. Weinstock H, Berman S, Cates W Jr: Sexually transmitted diseases among American youth: incidence and prevalence estimates 2000. Perspect Sex Reprod Health 2004;36:6–10. **(IIa, B)**

2. Siegel JE: Estimates of the economic burden of STDs: review of the literature with updates. In Eng TR, Butler WT (eds): The Hidden Epidemic: Confronting Sexually Transmitted Diseases. Washington, DC, National Academy Press, 1997, pp 330–356. **(Ia, A)**

3. American Social Health Association (ASHA): Sexually Transmitted Diseases in America: How Many Cases and at What Cost? Menlo Park, CA, Kaiser Family Foundation, 1998. **(IIb, B)**

4. Washington AE, Arno PS, Brooks MA: The economic cost of pelvic inflammatory disease. JAMA 1986;255:1753–1758. **(IIb, B)**

5. Washington AE, Johnson RE, Sanders LL Jr: *Chlamydia trachomatis* infections in the United States: what are they costing us? JAMA 1987;257:2070–2072. **(IIb, B)**

6. Centers for Disease Control and Prevention: 2002 National STD Surveillance Report, STDs in Women and Infants; 2002:3. Available at http://www.cdc.gov/std/stats02/women&inf3.htm. Accesssed 4/29/05. **(IIb, B)**

7. Tait IA, Duthie SJ, Taylor-Robinson D: Silent upper genital tract chlamydial infection and disease in women. Int J STD AIDS 1997; 8:329–331. **(Ib, A)**

8. Douglas JM Jr, et al: Low rate of pelvic inflammatory disease (PID) among women with a low incidence of *Chlamydia trachomatis* (CT) infection. Int J STD AIDS 2001;12(Suppl 2):65–67. **(IIb, B)**

9. Yeh JM, Hook EW III, Goldie SJ: A refined estimate of the average lifetime cost of pelvic inflammatory disease. Sex Transm Dis 2003; 30:369–378. **(IIb, B)**

10. Rein DB, Kassler WJ, Irwin KL, Rabiee L: Direct medical cost of pelvic inflammatory disease and its sequelae: decreasing, but still substantial. Obstet Gynecol 2000:95:397–402. **(IIb, B)**

11. Hankins GD, Clark SL, Cunningham FG, Gilstrap LC: Ectopic pregnancy. In Hawkins GDV (ed): Operative Obstetrics. Norwalk, Conn, Appleton & Lange, 1995, pp 437–456. **(III, B)**

12. Ectopic pregnancy—United States, 1990–1992. MMWR 1995;44:46–48. **(IIb, B)**

13. Tenore JL: Ectopic pregnancy. Am Fam Physician 2000;61:1080–1088. **(III, B)**

14. Ness RB, Soper DE, Holley RL, et al and Clinical Health (PEACH) Study Investigators: Effectiveness of inpatient and outpatient treatment strategies for women with pelvic inflammatory disease: results from the pelvic inflammatory disease evaluation and clinical health (PEACH) randomized trial. Am J Obstet Gynecol 2002;186:929–937. **(Ia, A)**

15. Faro S, Martens M, Maccato M, et al: Vaginal flora and pelvic inflammatory disease. Am J Obstet Gynecol 1993;169:470–474. **(IIa, B)**

16. Yudin MH, Hillier SL, Wiessenfeld HC, et al: Vaginal polymorphonuclear leukocytes and bacterial vaginosis as markers for histologic endometritis among women without symptoms of pelvic inflammatory disease. Am J Obstet Gynecol 2003;188:318–323. **(IIa, B)**

17. Hakakha MM, Davis J, Korst LM, Silverman NS: Leukorrhea and bacterial vaginosis as in-office predictors of cervical infection in high-risk women. Obstet Gynecol 2002;100:808–812. **(IIa, B)**

18. Phillips RS, Hanff PA, Holmes KK, et al: *Chlamydia trachomatis* cervical infection in women seeking routine gynecologic care: criteria for selective testing. Am J Med 1989;86:515–520. **(III, B)**

19. Handsfield HH, Jasman LL, Roberts PL, et al: Criteria for selective screening for *Chlamydia trachomatis* infection in women attending family planning clinics. JAMA 1986;255:1730–1734. **(III, B)**

20. Katz BP, Caine VA, Jones RB: Diagnosis of mucopurulent cervicitis among women at risk for *Chlamydia trachomatis* infection. Sex Transm Dis 1989;16:103–136. **(IIb, B)**

21. Molander P, Finne P, Sjöberg J, et al: Observer agreement with laparoscopic diagnosis of pelvic inflammatory disease using photographs. Obstet Gynecol 2003;101:875–880. **(IIa, B)**

22. Curtis AH: A cause of adhesions in the right upper quadrant. JAMA 1930;94:1221–1222. **(IIb, B)**

23. Fitz-Hugh T: Acute gonococcic peritonitis of the right upper quadrant. JAMA 1934;102:2094–2096. **(IIb, B)**

24. Paavonen J, Saikku P, von Knorring J, et al: Association of infection with *Chlamydia trachomatis* with Fitz-Hugh-Curtis syndrome. J Infect Dis 1981;144:176. **(IIb, B)**

25. Amin-Hanjani S, Neely T, Chatwani A: Perihepatic adhesions: not necessarily pathognomonic of pelvic infection. Am J Obstet Gynecol 1992;167:115–116. **(IIb, B)**

26. Gandhi SG, Komenaka IK, Naim JH: Fitz-Hugh-Curtis syndrome after laparoscopic tubal ligation: a case report. J Reprod Med 2003; 48:302–305. **(IIb, B)**

27. Peterson HB, Walker CK, Kahn JG, et al: Pelvic inflammatory disease: key treatment issues and options. JAMA 1991;266:2605–2611. **(Ib, A)**

28. Ectopic pregnancy—United States, 1981–1983. MMWR 1986; 35:289–291. **(Ib, A)**

29. Chow WH, Daling JR, Cates W, Greenberg RS: Epidemiology of ectopic pregnancy. Epidemiol Rev 1987;9:70–94. **(IIb, B)**

30. Atrash HK, Hughes JM, Hogue CJ: Ectopic pregnancy in the United States, 1970–1983. MMWR CDC Surveill Summ 1986;35:29SS–37SS. **(IIb, B)**

31. Hughes GJ: Fertility and ectopic pregnancy. Eur J Obstet Gynecol Reprod Biol 1980;10:361–365. **(IIb, B)**

32. Sandvei R, Ulstein M, Wollen AL: Fertility following ectopic pregnancy with special reference to previous use of intra-uterine contraceptive device (IUCD). Acta Obstet Gynecol Scand 1987;66:131–135. **(IIb, B)**

33. Westrom L: Influence of sexually transmitted diseases on sterility and ectopic pregnancy. Acta Eur Fertil 1985;16:21–24. **(IIb, B)**

34. Chow JM, Yonekura ML, Richwald GA, et al: The association between *Chlamydia trachomatis* and ectopic pregnancy: a matched-pair, case-control study. JAMA 1990;263:3164–3167. **(IIb, B)**

35. Marchbanks PA, Annegers JF, Coulam CB, et al: Risk factors for ectopic pregnancy: Aa population-based study. JAMA 1988;259:1823–1827. **(IIa, B)**

36. Sherman KJ, Daling JR, Stergachis A, et al: Sexually transmitted diseases and tubal pregnancy. Sex Transm Dis 1990;17:115–121. **(IIb, B)**

37. Coste J, Job-Spira N, Fernandez H: Increased risk of ectopic pregnancy with maternal cigarette smoking. Am J Public Health 1991;81:199–201. **(IIb, B)**

38. Coste J, Laumon B, Bremond A, et al: Sexually transmitted diseases as major causes of ectopic pregnancy: results from a large case-control study in France. Fertil Steril 1994;62:289–295. **(IIa, B)**

39. Jossens MO, Schachter J, Sweet RL: Risk factors associated with pelvic inflammatory disease of differing microbial etiologies. Obstet Gynecol 1994;83:989–997. **(IIb, B)**

40. Kirshon B, Faro S, Phillips LE, Pruett K: Correlation of ultrasonography and bacteriology of the endocervix and posterior cul-de-sac of patients with severe pelvic inflammatory disease. Sex Transm Dis 1988; 15:103–107. **(IIb, B)**

41. Landers DV, Sweet RL: Tubo-ovarian abscess: contemporary approach to management. Rev Infect Dis 1983;5:876–884. **(IIb, B)**

42. Reed SD, Landers DV, Sweet RL: Antibiotic management of tuboovarian abscess: comparison of broad-spectrum beta-lactam agents versus clindamycin-containing regimens. Am J Obstet Gynecol 1991;164:1556–1561. **(IIb, B)**

43. McNeeley SG, Hendrix SL, Mazzoni MM, et al: Medically sound, cost-effective treatment for pelvic inflammatory disease and tuboovarian abscess. Am J Obstet Gynecol 1998;178:1272–1278. **(IIb, B)**

# Chapter 21

# Human Immunodeficiency Virus

Denise J. Jamieson, MD, MPH, and
Athena P. Kourtis, MD, PhD, MPH

## KEY POINTS

- Since one quarter of HIV-infected women are unaware of their serostatus, it is critical that HIV testing be offered to patients at risk.
- Although early in the HIV/AIDS epidemic concern was widespread that the gynecologic manifestations of HIV disease would be substantial, differences in gynecologic pathology between HIV-infected and -uninfected women are modest.
- Cervical dysplasia is more common and severe in HIV-infected patients. Pap tests should be performed twice in the year after diagnosis of HIV and then, if normal, annually thereafter.
- HIV-infected women have higher rates of intraepithelial neoplasia in the vagina, vulva, and perianal regions. These regions should be examined carefully during pelvic examinations. When colposcopy is performed, the entire lower genital tract should be evaluated.
- Diagnosis and treatment recommendations for bacterial vaginosis, vulvovaginal candidiasis, trichomoniasis, gonorrhea, and chlamydia do not differ with HIV status. However, topical therapies for candidiasis may be more effective if a 7-day course is prescribed.

## VIROLOGY AND LIFE CYCLE OF HIV

Human immunodeficiency virus–1 (HIV-1) is a member of the family of human retroviruses (Retroviridae) and subfamily of lentiviruses. Electron microscopy shows that the HIV virion has an icosahedral structure (Fig. 21-1) that contains an envelope formed mainly by the external glycoprotein gp120 and the transmembrane glycoprotein gp41. HIV infects CD4+ "helper" T lymphocytes, monocytes, and macrophages. Cells are infected after binding of the envelope glycoprotein gp120 to both the CD4 receptor and a chemokine coreceptor on the surface of target cells. This binding leads to a series of changes in the tertiary structure of the viral envelope that brings about virus-cell fusion.[1] After fusion of the virus with the cell membrane, the viral RNA enters the cytoplasm and reverse transcription of the viral RNA occurs by the enzyme reverse transcriptase, with production of the viral DNA copy (cDNA). cDNA is then transported to the nucleus, where integration into the host cell genome takes place through the action of the viral enzyme integrase. This provirus, which is now integrated with the nucleus of the infected cell, may remain transcriptionally inactive (latent), or it may manifest varying levels of gene expression, up to active production of virus. Productive infection of lymphocytes results in extracellular release of virions that bud through the host cell membrane. The virally encoded protease catalyzes the cleavage of a precursor to yield the mature virion. Each step in the life cycle of HIV represents a potential target for therapeutic intervention; the processes of fusion and the reverse transcriptase and protease enzymes have been subjected to pharmacologic disruption (Fig. 21-2). Integrase and other entry inhibitors are in development.

## PATHOGENESIS AND CLINICAL MANIFESTATIONS OF HIV IN WOMEN

Infection with HIV leads to a decrease in number and function of CD4+ cells through a variety of mechanisms, including direct infection and destruction of these cells and indirect acceleration of cell death through immune activation.[2] The decrease in CD4+ T lymphocytes has profound effects on both cell-mediated and humoral immunity. Without treatment, HIV infection causes generalized immunodeficiency with resultant susceptibility to opportunistic infections and neoplasms that are AIDS-defining illnesses. There is generally an inverse relationship between CD4+ cell count and the amount of virus circulating in the peripheral blood. As HIV disease progresses, the CD4+ cell count gradually declines as the amount of virus increases. The typical clinical course of an untreated HIV-infected individual will lead to AIDS and death at a mean time of approximately 10 years from primary infection (Fig. 21-3). A small proportion (<5%) of HIV-infected patients are long-term nonprogressors; the viral and host determinants that contribute to this course have not been elucidated.[3]

Overall HIV disease manifestations are similar in women and men. The most frequent AIDS-defining opportunistic processes in both men and women in the United States have so far been *Pneumocystis jirovecii* (formerly *Pneumocystis carinii*) pneumonia, *Candida* esophagitis, and wasting syndrome. With regard to malignancies, cervical cancer, Kaposi sarcoma, non-Hodgkin lymphomas, and lung cancer are more frequent in HIV-infected women compared with uninfected women. Whereas Kaposi sarcoma is less frequent in HIV-infected women than in HIV-infected men, there seem to be differences in clinical presentation, with women demonstrating a more aggressive course and a higher incidence of noncutaneous presentation and visceral involvement including, in some cases, involvement of the female genital tract.

# Gynecologic Infectious Disease

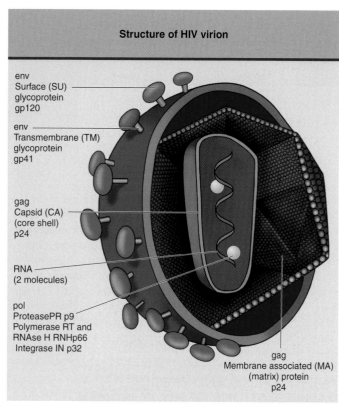

**Figure 21-1   Structure of the HIV virion.** The spikes projecting from the viral envelope represent glycoprotein gp120, which binds to the CD4 receptor on host cells. (Available at: http://www.luc.edu/depts/biology/hiv.jpg. Accessed 5/18/05.)

It was initially thought that HIV infection had a worse prognosis in women than in men; subsequent evidence, however, does not point to a difference in HIV disease-free survival or in response to antiretroviral therapy in women and in men. There may be, however, a mild sex influence on virus load levels, with women having a lower virus load than men, particularly in the initial stages of the disease when CD4+ T cell counts are higher.[4]

## EPIDEMIOLOGY AND TRANSMISSION OF HIV INFECTION

HIV is transmitted by sexual contact, percutaneous exposure to contaminated blood and blood products, and mother-to-child transmission (MTCT).[5] Risk factors for HIV infection among adults in the United States include exposure to blood products from 1978 to the spring of 1985, parenteral illicit drug use, multiple heterosexual or homosexual contacts, and a partner with one of these risk factors. Seroprevalence rates are highest among gay men and injecting drug users, but heterosexual transmission continues to rise. Youth (aged 13 to 24 years) and minority women are disproportionately affected by new infections. In developing countries, heterosexual contact is the most common mode of transmission among adults, and prevalence is similar in both sexes.

In the United States, women represent the fastest growing part of the population with newly acquired HIV infection. Whereas only 7% of all AIDS cases reported in the United

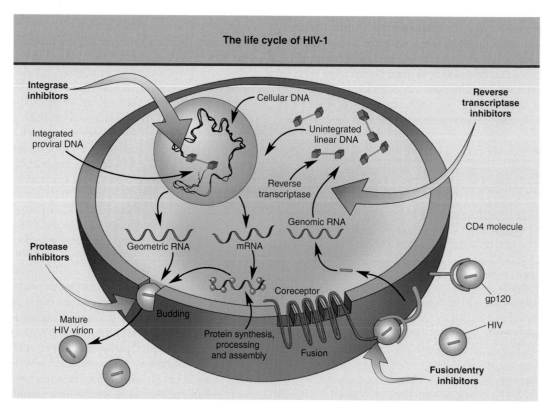

**Figure 21-2   The life cycle of HIV-1 and potential targets for antiretroviral action.** To date, fusion, reverse transcription, and protease action have been disrupted by pharmacologic agents; integrase and entry inhibitors are currently under development. (From Fauci AS: HIV and AIDS: 20 years of science. Nat Med 9:839–843.)

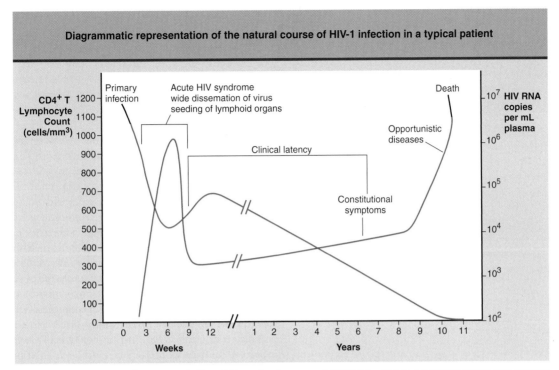

Diagrammatic representation of the natural course of HIV-1 infection in a typical patient

**Figure 21-3** **Diagrammatic representation of the natural course of HIV-1 infection in a typical patient.** The average length of time from primary HIV infection to AIDS and death is, in the absence of antiretroviral treatment, approximately 10 years. (From Pantaleo G, Graziosi C, Fauci AS: New concepts in the immunopathogenesis of human immunodeficiency virus infection. N Engl J Med 1993;327–335. Copyright 1993 Massachusetts Medical Society. All rights reserved. Adapted 2006 with permission.)

States in 1985 were in women, this proportion had reached 28% in 2003. From 1990 to 1994 AIDS cases in women increased by 89%, as compared with 29% in men. Heterosexual contact accounts for most HIV acquisition in women: 53% of women acquire HIV by contact with an HIV-infected partner and 15% by contact with a partner who is an intravenous drug user (Fig. 21-4). Minorities are disproportionately affected: approximately 80% of female AIDS cases in 2002 were in black or Hispanic women (Table 21-1). By 1995 AIDS represented the third leading cause of death among women 25 to 44 years of age in the United States and the leading cause of death in African American women of the same age.[6,7] Some evidence points to a slower decline in HIV-related mortality in women than in men after introduction of potent antiretroviral regimens. This may be related to decreased health care access or decreased utilization of protease inhibitors in women, although the evidence is inconclusive.

While the overall efficiency of HIV transmission through a single heterosexual contact is low, evidence points to increased efficiency of HIV transmission from man to woman compared with from woman to man.[8] Factors associated with increased risk of sexual transmission of HIV include concurrent sexually transmitted diseases (STDs), advanced HIV disease with low CD4+ T cell counts and high RNA virus load, acute HIV infection, absence of antiretroviral therapy, sex during menses, receptive anal intercourse, traumatic vaginal intercourse, lack of barrier contraception, lack of circumcision, and cervical ectopy.[9] Viral subtype and host genetics also play a role (Table 21-2).

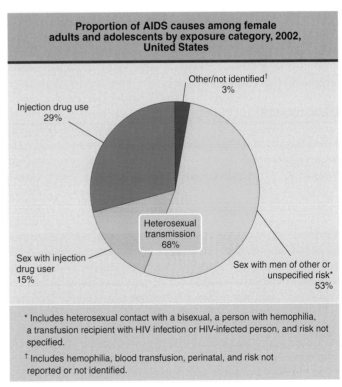

* Includes heterosexual contact with a bisexual, a person with hemophilia, a transfusion recipient with HIV infection or HIV-infected person, and risk not specified.

† Includes hemophilia, blood transfusion, perinatal, and risk not reported or not identified.

**Figure 21-4** **Proportion of AIDS cases among female adults and adolescents by exposure category in the United States in 2002.** Heterosexual transmission accounts for 68% of transmission to women. (From Centers for Disease Control and Prevention, 2005. Available at http://www.cdc.gov/hiv/graphics/images/I264/I264-2.html.)

Gynecologic Infectious Disease

**Table 21-1**
**Reported AIDS Cases and Rates among Female Adults and Adolescents by Race and Ethnicity in the United States in 2002**

| Race/Ethnicity*[†] | Number of Cases | Percentage | Rate per 100,000 Population |
|---|---|---|---|
| White, not Hispanic | 1928 | 18 | 2.2 |
| Black, not Hispanic | 7326 | 67 | 49.1 |
| Hispanic | 1556 | 14 | 11.2 |
| Asian/Pacific Islander | 68 | <1 | 1.3 |
| American Indian/ Alaska Native | 42 | <1 | 4.4 |
| **Total[†]** | **10,930** | | |

*Minorities are disproportionately affected by the epidemic.
[†] Excludes persons from U.S. dependencies, possessions, and associated nations.
[†] Includes 10 persons of unknown race.
Available at: http://www.cdc.gov/hiv/graphics/images/1264/1264-3.html. Accessed 5/17/05.

## Screening for HIV: Who Should Be Tested?

HIV counseling and testing should be offered as a routine part of gynecologic care. It is estimated that 25% of persons living with HIV are unaware that they are infected. In April 2003, the Centers for Disease Control and Prevention (CDC) announced a nationwide initiative that stressed making HIV a routine part of medical care as one of four key strategies. In a study of women in whom HIV was newly diagnosed, only 17% reported that they were tested because the test was offered or recommended by a health care provider.[10] This illustrates the need for health care providers, including gynecologists, to be proactive about offering and recommending testing.

## DIAGNOSIS

The diagnosis of HIV infection is made by detection of antibodies against HIV or direct detection of HIV or one of its components. The standard way to diagnose HIV is via a positive

**Table 21-2**
**Factors Affecting Sexual Transmission of HIV-1**

Sexually transmitted infections (ulcerative/nonulcerative)
Advanced HIV disease (low CD4+ T cell counts/high virus load)
Lack of antiretroviral therapy
Acute HIV infection
Sexual activity during menses
Receptive anal intercourse
Traumatic vaginal intercourse
Lack of barrier protection
Lack of circumcision
Cervical ectopy
?Hormonal contraception/?Pregnancy
HIV viral subtype/phenotype
Host genetics (deletions in the chemokine receptor gene CCR5)

HIV antibody test produced by an enzyme-linked immunosorbent assay (ELISA). A confirmatory test, usually a Western blot, must be performed, since occasionally false-positive ELISA results occur. Rarely an infected person may fail to make antibody. This could happen in patients with low immunoglobulin levels (sometimes the result of generalized immunodeficiency) or during the "window" period of the first 2 to 8 weeks following primary infection. Tests for the presence of virus (usually nucleic acid detection, but also HIV culture or p24 antigen) are positive and should be performed if the ELISA is negative but the clinical suspicion for HIV infection is strong.

Highly sensitive detection of proviral DNA can be accomplished using the polymerase chain reaction (PCR) technology on peripheral blood mononuclear cells isolated from whole blood. The sensitivity of PCR is greater than 95% and its specificity greater than 98%.[11] A number of assays are commercially available for the detection and quantitation of plasma HIV RNA; these assays are used for measurement of the viral load in a patient's plasma.

The absolute number and percentage of CD4 lymphocytes decline with disease progression; CD8 lymphocyte counts usually increase. Total immunoglobulin levels are usually elevated. Routine laboratory tests (complete blood count, blood chemistry profiles) are usually normal in the absence of a secondary infection or organ system disease. As disease progresses, anemia becomes common; granulocytopenia and thrombocytopenia may also occur. Mild elevation of liver enzymes is not uncommon. Serum LDH levels may be high with *P. jirovecii* infection. With brain involvement, the cerebrospinal fluid may be normal or the protein elevated and lymphocyte/mononuclear pleocytosis may be present.

## TREATMENT IN WOMEN

Specific antiretroviral therapy can prevent HIV-induced progressive immune deterioration, and prophylactic measures can prevent opportunistic infections. HIV has a high spontaneous mutation rate, and emergence of drug resistance during treatment is well recognized. Many antiretroviral drugs select for resistant mutations in the virus within weeks to months when used as monotherapy. Thus, combinations of at least three drugs and strict adherence to the dosing regimen are critical. If viral replication is not fully suppressed, the potential for emergence of resistance exists. If increasing plasma viremia is observed after treatment in a compliant patient, viral resistance is likely and the antiretroviral regimen should be changed, if possible all three drugs at the same time. Selecting a combination of drugs appropriate for an individual patient is a complex process requiring expert understanding of antiretroviral activity, cross-resistance patterns, and drug interactions; therefore, a physician with expertise in HIV treatment should be consulted whenever possible.

Four classes of drugs have been approved by the FDA for the treatment of HIV infection, and additional drugs are under development.[12] The four classes are nucleoside/nucleotide reverse transcriptase inhibitors (NRTIs/NtRTIs), nonnucleoside reverse transcriptase inhibitors (NNRTIs), protease inhibitors (PIs), and fusion inhibitors. There are currently 21 FDA-approved drugs.

NRTIs/NtRTIs are nucleoside/nucleotide analogs that block reverse transcription and production of viral DNA and thus productive infection of the cell. The first class of drugs to be developed, they vary with regard to their potency, rate of resistance development, and side effects. Zidovudine, stavudine (d4T), didanosine, lamivudine (3TC), zalcitabine (ddC), and abacavir are the best known drugs of this class. Zidovudine has moderate antiretroviral activity and a relatively long interval before development of resistance. Toxicity includes anemia, neutropenia, headache, gastrointestinal upset, myalgia, and insomnia. Stavudine has fewer side effects, the most common being peripheral neuropathy mainly seen in patients with advanced disease. Common side effects with ddI include gastrointestinal upset, pancreatitis, and peripheral neuropathy. 3TC is highly active against HIV, but resistance develops within weeks when it is used as monotherapy. Abacavir is highly active; however, approximately 10% of patients develop a hypersensitivity reaction characterized by flu-like symptoms with or without a rash. Continued treatment or rechallenge is contraindicated because the outcome may be fatal. ddC is the least potent in the class and is frequently associated with peripheral neuropathy. Emtricitabine, a newer agent in the class, is generally well tolerated; headache is an occasional side effect. Tenofovir, an agent in the NtRTI class that requires only one intracellular phosphorylation step, has a long half-life and only once daily dosing and has shown promise in preventing infection as pre- and postexposure prophylaxis in monkeys; side effects include gastrointestinal upset and headache; renal toxicity is an unusual but important side effect of this drug.[13]

NRTIs are known to induce mitochondrial dysfunction because the drugs have some affinity for mitochondrial $\gamma$-DNA polymerase. Toxicity related to mitochondrial dysfunction has been reported in patients receiving long-term treatment with NRTIs and generally resolves after discontinuation of the drug. These toxicities include neuropathy, myopathy, cardiomyopathy, pancreatitis, hepatic steatosis, and lactic acidosis; the last two are more common in women.

NNRTIs also inhibit viral DNA synthesis but act at a different site on the viral enzyme reverse transcriptase. NNRTIs have generally high-level antiretroviral potency, but resistance appears rapidly. The most common side effect is rash, which can be as severe as Stevens-Johnson syndrome. Evidence indicates that severe liver involvement with rash or systemic symptoms may be observed during the first weeks of treatment with nevirapine, particularly in women with CD4+ T lymphocyte counts greater than 250/mm$^3$.[14] Rare deaths have been reported. It is unclear whether pregnancy confers higher risk. However, in recognition of this higher risk, nevirapine is not recommended as part of an antiretroviral regimen in a woman with CD4 count greater than 250/mm$^3$ unless benefits clearly outweigh risks. Efavirenz is associated with mild central nervous system symptoms (dizziness, confusion, strange dreams), which usually resolve after the initial weeks of use. The major concern for women is its known teratogenicity (FDA pregnancy category D). Neural tube defects have been reported both in experimental animal systems and in humans inadvertently exposed to efavirenz during the first trimester of pregnancy. Women should undergo pregnancy testing before receiving efavirenz and should be counseled regarding the risk of teratogenicity. Because of

the possibility of increased failure of hormonal contraceptives related to drug interactions with certain antiretrovirals, which may include efavirenz, alternative regimens that do not contain efavirenz should be strongly considered in women at risk for unintended pregnancy.[15]

PIs inhibit viral protease during assembly of the virus and result in noninfectious particles. PIs are highly active but also induce resistance within months when used as monotherapy. Common toxicities include diarrhea (nelfinavir); nausea and perioral paresthesias (ritonavir); nephropathy and nephrolithiasis (indinavir); nausea and rash (amprenavir and fosamprenavir); nausea and diarrhea (saquinavir); hyperbilirubinemia, nausea, and diarrhea (atazanavir); nausea/vomiting (lopinavir/ritonavir); and elevation of liver enzymes, hypercholesterolemia, hypertriglyceridemia, and hyperglycemia (all). PIs are metabolized by the hepatic cytochrome P-450 enzymes, resulting in many interactions with other drugs including other antiretroviral agents, so care is needed when prescribing other medications to a patient taking a PI. Regimens combining two PIs can take advantage of the drug interaction and improve the pharmacokinetic properties of the drugs.

Enfuvirtide is the only agent in the class of fusion inhibitors. It has to be administered subcutaneously, and the most common side effects are site injection reactions, diarrhea, and nausea. Increase in rate of bacterial pneumonia in patients administered enfuvirtide has been reported.

In nonpregnant adults, initiation of antiretroviral therapy is recommended for all patients with symptomatic HIV infection. In asymptomatic infected adults, recommendations concerning when to start treatment are more controversial. The most recent recommendations are to offer therapy to nonpregnant adults with fewer than 350 CD4+ T cells per cubic millimeter or a plasma viral load exceeding 100,000 copies per milliliter and to defer therapy in otherwise asymptomatic individuals not meeting these criteria.[16] Consideration for treatment should also be given within 6 months of seroconversion. Results of therapy are evaluated through plasma HIV RNA levels, which are expected to decrease by 1.0 log$_{10}$ at 2 to 8 weeks, with no detectable virus (<50 copies/mL) at 4 to 6 months after treatment initiation. Failure of therapy at 4 to 6 months might be due to nonadherence, inadequate potency of the regimen, viral resistance, or other factors. Patients whose therapy fails in spite of a high level of adherence to the regimen should have their regimen changed. Recommended combination antiretroviral regimens include two NRTIs combined with a PI or an NNRTI; an alternative combination regimen consists of three NRTIs when the other two options cannot be used as initial therapy. In women of reproductive age, regimen selection should account for the possibility of planned or unplanned pregnancy. As part of the evaluation for initiating therapy, women should be counseled about the potential risk of efavirenz-containing regimens if pregnancy occurs. These regimens should be avoided in women who are trying to conceive or who are not using effective and consistent contraception.

## PREVENTION OF HIV TRANSMISSION

The only 100% effective method of avoiding sexual transmission of HIV is abstinence or limiting sexual contact to a monogamous partner who is not HIV-infected. Condoms, when used correctly and consistently, are highly effective in preventing transmission between sexually active couples when one partner is HIV-infected. CDC provides detailed instructions on correct condom use. Use of the spermicide nonoxynol-9, which has anti-HIV activity in vitro, was shown to increase risk of epithelial disruption and genital tract inflammation, with resultant higher risk of HIV transmission, and thus is not recommended.[17] Prompt treatment of other STDs also reduces the risk of sexual transmission of HIV. Antiretroviral prophylaxis to prevent HIV infection in people who are exposed to HIV in a circumstance that is not likely to recur (such as sexual assault or condom rupture) is now recommended[18] even though the data on the efficacy of this approach are limited. CDC recommends post-exposure prophylaxis following occupational exposure, using ZDV and 3TC, with or without a protease inhibitor, depending on the degree of risk associated with the exposure and in consultation with an infectious diseases expert.[19]

All medical equipment that can penetrate the skin should be sterile. Infected blood and secretions should be handled according to CDC recommendations.

## GYNECOLOGIC MANIFESTATIONS OF HIV

Early in the epidemic, it was widely believed that there would be large differences in the clinical manifestations of HIV/AIDS between men and women. Specifically, it was thought that many gynecologic conditions such as lower genital tract dysplasia, gynecologic cancers, menstrual irregularities, and infectious conditions such as vaginitis, cervicitis, and pelvic inflammatory disease might be more common, severe, and persistent in HIV-infected women compared with uninfected women. To address these concerns, two large cohort studies of HIV-infected and uninfected women were funded, one by CDC and the other by the National Institutes of Health (NIH).[20,21] The CDC-funded HIV Epidemiology Research Study (HERS) beginning in 1993 enrolled 871 HIV-infected women and 439 high-risk HIV-uninfected women in four cities in the United States (New York, Detroit, Providence, Baltimore). The NIH-funded Women's Interagency HIV Study (WIHS) began in 1994 and enrolled 2058 HIV-infected women and a comparison cohort of 568 HIV-uninfected women. Findings from these studies indicate that although there are subtle differences between HIV disease in men and women, the differences are much less pronounced than originally believed. In addition, the differences between HIV-infected women and well-matched high-risk HIV-uninfected women are also much less pronounced than originally thought. The most notable gynecologic difference between infected and uninfected women is the development of cervical dysplasia.

### Cervical Dysplasia

Compared with HIV-uninfected women, HIV-infected women have a markedly higher prevalence of human papillomavirus (HPV), including high-risk subtypes, and these HPV infections tend to persist longer. Furthermore, the prevalence and persistence of HPV infection among HIV-infected women increases with decreased CD4 count and increased viral load. However, the response of HPV and cervical intraepithelial neoplasia (CIN) to antiretroviral therapy remains unclear.[22] Although some studies

have shown increased clearance of HPV and regression of cervical dysplasia following immune reconstitution, others have failed to document a clinical response.[23,24]

Since HPV is more common among HIV-infected women and is the major cause of cervical dysplasia, it is not surprising that HIV-infected women have high rates of abnormal Papanicolaou (Pap) tests. In the setting of HIV infection, rates of cytologic abnormalities on Pap screening are up to 10 times greater than those observed among HIV-uninfected women. Therefore, HIV-infected women should undergo a comprehensive gynecologic examination including Pap test as part of their initial evaluation. A Pap test should also be obtained twice in the first year after diagnosis of HIV infection. If the initial Pap test results are normal, then women can begin a schedule of annual Pap tests. Pap tests are an adequate screening tool for HIV-infected women. No additional routine screening, such as colposcopy, is recommended for women with normal Pap tests.

If the results of a Pap test are abnormal, then standard diagnostic and treatment algorithms for HIV-uninfected women should be followed. As in HIV-uninfected women, the diagnosis of cervical dysplasia involves colposcope-directed biopsies. Since HIV-infected women have high rates of dysplasia, abnormal-appearing areas should be sampled liberally. Although recurrence rates are higher after treatment of cervical dysplasia among HIV-infected women, standard excisional treatment is recommended for CIN II or CIN III. Since cryotherapy has the highest rate of recurrence, it should generally be avoided. HIV-infected women may be more likely to have positive surgical margins, which may contribute to higher rates of recurrence. A randomized trial among HIV-infected women evaluated the efficacy of topical vaginal 5-fluorouracil (5-FU) maintenance therapy in preventing recurrence after standard treatment for high-grade cervical dysplasia.[25] Although this trial found a reduction in recurrence of CIN, the potential clinical role for 5-FU is still unclear. Because of limited clinical experience as well as concerns about mucosal toxicity and inflammation, this therapy is still investigational and can not be routinely recommended.

At 2 to 4 weeks following treatment for CIN, when the cervix is inflamed and ulcerated, there is a dramatic increase (as high as 10,000-fold) in the amount of HIV shed in the genital tract.[26] Therefore, abstinence should be emphasized until complete healing has occurred following treatment. Although consistent and correct condom use should always be stressed, the time after treatment of CIN may be a particularly high-risk period for sexual transmission.

### Vaginal, Vulvar, and Perianal Intraepithelial Neoplasia

Since HPV disease is multicentric in nature, it is not surprising that in addition to cervical dysplasia, HIV-infected women also have higher rates of intraepithelial neoplasia in the vagina, vulva, and perianal regions.[27] For this reason, the vaginal, vulvar, and perianal regions of HIV-infected women should be carefully examined during routine pelvic examinations. Biopsies should be taken of suspicious areas. In addition, at the time of colposcopy for cervical dysplasia, the entire lower genital tract should be evaluated. Although there is evidence that multicentric intra-epithelial neoplasia is more common in the setting of immuno-suppression, HIV-infected women should continue to be followed carefully for evidence of lower genital tract neoplasia, regardless of CD4+ count, viral load, or antiretroviral therapy.

## Gynecologic Cancers

In 1993, invasive cervical cancer was designated an AIDS-defining disorder by CDC. This was in recognition of the documented increased risk of development of cervical cancer among HIV-infected women.[28] However, HIV infection has not had a substantial impact on overall cervical cancer rates. No other gynecologic cancers have been consistently shown to be more common in HIV-infected compared with HIV-uninfected women.

## Menstrual Disorders

Although HIV-infected women frequently report menstrual disorders, these disorders are likely related to coexisting conditions rather than to HIV infection. Weight loss, substance abuse, immunosuppression, poor nutritional status, and use of certain antiretroviral agents may cause amenorrhea or other menstrual irregularities.[22] For HIV-infected women, evaluation and treatment of menstrual disorders should be similar to those in uninfected women.

## Gynecologic Surgery for HIV-Infected Women

Since women are increasingly affected by HIV infection and since gynecologic surgery is relatively common among women of reproductive age, it would be expected that a sizable number of HIV-infected women would undergo gynecologic surgical procedures such as dilation and curettage and hysterectomy. Surprisingly, however, there is little published information regarding gynecologic surgery among HIV-infected women. One retrospective review included 235 surgical procedures; 72 were major and included cesarean section, tubal sterilization, oophorectomy, and hysterectomy. They reported a higher complication rate in the HIV-infected group; major complications included postoperative fever, additional surgery, anemia requiring transfusion, and disseminated intravascular coagulation. The risk of complications was associated with immune status.[29] Another report reviewed 53 surgical procedures including nine hysterectomies. There was no difference in outcome between HIV-infected women and the uninfected women.[30] A small study from Grady Hospital in Atlanta retrospectively reviewed the hospital course of 24 HIV-infected patients who underwent hysterectomy and compared them to matched controls. Although the study was limited by small sample size, no significant differences in complication rates were found between HIV-infected and -uninfected women.[31] Since cesarean delivery is routinely recommended for HIV-infected women with viral loads higher than 1000 copies/mL, there is more published information about the obstetric surgical experience in the setting of HIV infection. Some but not all studies have found increased rates of postoperative infections, such as endometritis, wound infection, and pneumonia, among HIV-infected women compared with HIV-uninfected controls. From the limited available information, no differences in the clinical management of HIV-infected women undergoing routine gynecologic procedures can be recommended. Standard perioperative antibiotic prophylaxis should be used, and HIV-infected patients should be monitored closely for postoperative infectious complications.

Because HIV-infected women are living longer, healthier lives, increased numbers probably will undergo gynecologic surgical procedures for benign gynecologic conditions unrelated to HIV infection. In addition, since some conditions leading to gynecologic surgery, such as cervical dysplasia and cervical cancer, are more common among HIV-infected women, gynecologic surgery probably will increase among HIV-infected women as well.

## Cervicovaginal Infections

Early reports fueled concern that the prevalence and severity of lower genital tract infections such as vulvovaginal candidiasis might be increased in HIV-infected women. In 1992 CDC included vulvovaginal candidiasis among category B conditions—those for which clinical course or management is complicated by HIV infection. However, over time, it has become clear that the differences in vulvovaginal conditions such as bacterial vaginosis, vulvovaginal candidiasis, and trichomoniasis between HIV-infected and -uninfected women are less pronounced and more subtle than previously thought. In some cases, there are no meaningful clinical differences by HIV status.

The prevalence of vulvovaginitis associated with *Candida* is generally higher in HIV-infected women compared with uninfected women. Much of this difference can be attributed to immunosuppression; when HIV-uninfected women are compared with immunocompetent HIV-infected women, differences in prevalence rates are absent or modest. Increased rates of candidiasis are associated with declining CD4+ T cell count and increasing viral load among HIV-infected women. A longitudinal analysis from HERS found that vulvovaginal candidiasis occurred with higher incidence and greater persistence, but not greater severity, among HIV-infected women.[32]

In general, diagnosis and treatment of vulvovaginal candidiasis among HIV-infected women are similar to those in HIV-uninfected women. However, owing to greater persistence, topical therapies for candidiasis may be more effective if given for longer periods (e.g., 7 days). In addition, when antibiotics are given, use of prophylactic topical antifungals may be considered.

Bacterial vaginosis, a condition characterized by a shift in dominant vaginal flora, may be slightly more common among HIV-infected women compared with uninfected women, although the differences are modest. In HERS, bacterial vaginosis was more prevalent, persistent, and severe among HIV-infected women, particularly among those who were immunocompromised.[33] Diagnosis and treatment of bacterial vaginosis are the same in HIV-infected and -uninfected women.

In addition to the clinical significance of bacterial vaginosis among HIV-infected women, bacterial vaginosis may also be important among HIV-uninfected women at risk, since evidence suggests that bacterial vaginosis may be a risk factor for acquisition of HIV.

HIV infection does not appear to make a woman more likely to have incident, prevalent, or persistent trichomoniasis.[34] Diagnosis and treatment are the same as in HIV-uninfected women. Similarly, bacterial cervicitis caused by *Neisseria gonorrhoeae* or *Chlamydia trachomatis* is not more common in HIV-infected women compared with uninfected women. HIV-infected women with gonorrheal or chlamydial cervical infections should receive the same treatment as uninfected women.[35]

## Pelvic Inflammatory Disease

Despite early reports suggesting that HIV-infected women with pelvic inflammatory disease (PID) may have a more complicated clinical course than uninfected women, those differences are modest. Although not conclusive, there is some evidence that HIV-infected women are more likely to have a tubo-ovarian abscess. Overall, however, the presenting symptoms and response to standard therapy are similar. Whether the management of HIV-infected women with PID requires more aggressive treatment, such as hospitalization or parenteral antibiotics, has not been carefully evaluated. However, CDC guidelines for treatment of PID do not differ by HIV status.[35]

## CONTRACEPTION FOR HIV-INFECTED WOMEN

Preventing unintended pregnancy among HIV-infected women should be an integrated component of their gynecologic care. A wide variety of contraceptive options are appropriate for HIV-infected women.

All HIV-infected women should be counseled regarding correct and consistent condom use to decrease the risk of HIV transmission to uninfected partners. Latex male condoms are the best studied condom; they afford excellent protection when used correctly and consistently. Female condoms are also an effective barrier if intact and in place. An advantage is that they are a female-initiated method. However, cooperation and participation of the male partner are required. There are fewer data on the effectiveness of the female condom compared with the male condom, and acceptability of the female condom has been low in some populations. Although condoms provide some protection against unintended pregnancy, their effectiveness is not so high as some other methods. Therefore, some HIV-infected women may require dual protection with two different methods: a highly effective method for disease transmission prevention, such as condoms, and a highly effective method for pregnancy prevention, such as hormonal contraception.

Hormonal contraceptives can generally be prescribed according to the guidelines used for HIV-uninfected women. However, since some antiretroviral drugs may alter the bioavailability of circulating steroid levels, concomitant use of antiretroviral agents and oral contraceptives may alter the safety and effectiveness of both. It is unknown whether progesterone-only injectables are affected, since they involve much higher circulating steroid levels. For HIV-infected women taking antiretroviral therapy who desire hormonal contraception, use of an alternative or additional method of contraception is generally recommended.

In addition to concerns about the effectiveness of hormonal contraceptives, there is a theoretical concern that hormonal methods might act directly on the virus or immune system and increase HIV disease progression or severity. Limited studies suggest no such association. In addition, there is some limited evidence that hormonal contraceptives may increase genital tract shedding. Although this could have implications for sexual transmission of HIV, HIV-infected women should be advised to use condoms to protect their sexual partners from HIV and other STDs.

The World Health Organization recently revised its guidelines for the use of intrauterine devices (IUDs) in the setting of HIV. HIV-infected women can generally use IUDs. However since the risk of infection is greatest around the time of insertion, an IUD should not be inserted in a woman with AIDS unless she is clinically well on antiretroviral therapy. The appropriateness of surgical sterilization should be assessed without regard to a woman's HIV serostatus.[36]

## DISCORDANT COUPLES

Since people with HIV are living longer, healthier lives, couples may wish to have their own biologic children. This raises particularly difficult decisions for couples discordant for HIV when the man is seropositive and the woman is seronegative. Because of the risk of HIV transmission with unprotected intercourse, some authors advocate artificial insemination with semen that has been processed in an attempt to remove HIV from spermatozoa. These processing techniques generally involve semen washing and gradient centrifugation, followed by a sperm "swim-up" in which only the upper layer of medium is tested and used for insemination. After semen processing, the sample is tested for viral contamination by real-time PCR. Since the risk of sexual transmission is so low, the benefit and safety of such techniques have not been conclusively proven.[37,38]

## REFERENCES

1. Greene WC: The molecular biology of human immunodeficiency virus type 1 infection. N Engl J Med 1991;324:308–317. **(III, B)**
2. Levy JA: HIV and the Pathogenesis of AIDS, 2nd ed. Washington, DC, American Society for Microbiology, 1998. **(IV, C)**
3. Fauci AS, Lane HC: HIV disease: AIDS and related disorders. In Braunwald E, Fauci AS, Kasper DL, et al (eds): Harrison's Principles of Internal Medicine, 15th ed. McGraw-Hill, 2001, pp 1852–1913. **(III, B)**
4. Prins M, Meyer L, Hessol NA: Sex and the course of HIV infection in the pre- and highly active antiretroviral therapy eras. AIDS 2005; 19:357–370. **(IIb, B)**
5. Kourtis AP, Duerr A: Prevention of perinatal HIV transmission: a review of novel strategies. Expert Opin Investig Drugs 2003;12:1535–1544. **(IV, C)**
6. Heterosexual transmission of HIV—29 states, 1999–2002. MMWR Morb Mortal Wkly Rep 2004;53:125–129. **(III, B)**
7. Diagnoses of HIV/AIDS—32 States, 2000–2003. MMWR Morb Mortal Wkly Rep 2004;53:1106–1110. **(IV, C)**
8. Padian NS, Shiboski SC, Jewell NP: Female-to-male transmission of human immunodeficiency virus. JAMA 1991;266:1664–1667. **(III, B)**
9. Clemetson DB, Moss GB, Willerford DM, et al: Detection of HIV DNA in cervical and vaginal secretions: prevalence and correlates among women in Nairobi, Kenya. JAMA 1993;269:2860–2864. **(III, B)**
10. Advancing HIV prevention: new strategies for a changing epidemic—United States, 2003. Ann Pharmacother 2003;37:935. **(IV, C)**
11. Jongerius JM, Sjerps M, Cuijpers HT, et al: Validation of the NucliSens Extractor combined with the AmpliScreen HIV version 1.5 and HCV version 2.0 test for application in NAT minipool screening. Transfusion 2002;42:792–797. **(IIb, B)**
12. Hanna GJ, Hirsch MS: Antiretroviral therapy for HIV infection. In Bennett JE, Dolin R (eds): Mandell, Douglas, and Bennett's Principles and Practice of Infectious Diseases. Philadelphia, Elsevier Churchill Livingstone, 2005. **(IV, C)**
13. Peyriere H, Reynes J, Rouanet I, et al: Renal tubular dysfunction associated with tenofovir therapy: report of 7 cases. J Acquir Immune Defic Syndr 2004;35:269–273. **(III, B)**

14. Stern JO, Robinson PA, Love J, et al:. A comprehensive hepatic safety analysis of nevirapine in different populations of HIV infected patients. J Acquir Immune Defic Syndr 2003;34(Suppl 1):S21–S33. **(III, B)**

15. Public Health Service Task Force: Recommendations for use of anti-retroviral drugs in pregnant HIV-1-infected women for maternal health and interventions to reduce perinatal HIV-1 transmission in the United States. Available at: www.aidsinfo.nih.gov/guidelines. Accessed 9/11/05. **(IV, C)**

16. Guidelines for the use of antiretroviral agents in HIV-1-infected adults and adolescents. Available at: www.aidsinfo.nih.gov/guidelines. Accessed 9/11/05. **(IV, C)**

17. Van Damme L, Ramjee G, Alary M, et al: Effectiveness of COL-1492, a nonoxynol-9 vaginal gel, on HIV-1 transmission in female sex workers: a randomised controlled trial. Lancet 2002;360:971–977. **(Ib, A)**

18. Smith DK, Grohskopf LA, Black RJ, et al: Antiretroviral postexposure prophylaxis after sexual, injection-drug use, or other nonoccupational exposure to HIV in the United States: recommendations from the U.S. Department of Health and Human Services. MMWR Recomm Rep 2005;54(RR-2):1–20. **(IV, C)**

19. Centers for Disease Control and Prevention: Public Health Service guidelines for the management of health-care worker exposures to HIV and recommendations for postexposure prophylaxis. MMWR Recomm Rep 1998;47(RR-7):1–33. **(IV, C)**

20. Barkan SE, Melnick SL, Preston-Martin S, et al: The Women's Inter-agency HIV Study. WIHS Collaborative Study Group. Epidemiology 1998;9:117–125. **(IIb, B)**

21. Smith DK, Warren DL, Vlahov D, et al: Design and baseline participant characteristics of the Human Immunodeficiency Virus Epidemiology Research (HER) study: a prospective cohort study of human immuno-deficiency virus infection in US women. Am J Epidemiol 1997; 146:459–469. **(IIb, B)**

22. Cejtin HE: Gynecologic issues in the HIV-infected woman. Obstet Gynecol Clin North Am 2003;30:711–729. **(IV, C)**

23. Ahdieh-Grant L, Li R, Levine AM, et al: Highly active antiretroviral therapy and cervical squamous intraepithelial lesions in human immunodeficiency virus-positive women. J Natl Cancer Inst 2004; 96:1070–1076. **(IIb, B)**

24. Heard I, Palefsky JM, Kazatchkine MD: The impact of HIV antiviral therapy on human papillomavirus (HPV) infections and HPV-related diseases. Antivir Ther 2004;9:13–22. **(IIb, B)**

25. Maiman M, Watts DH, Andersen J, et al: Vaginal 5-fluorouracil for high-grade cervical dysplasia in human immunodeficiency virus infection: a randomized trial. Obstet Gynecol 1999;94:954–961. **(Ib, A)**

26. Wright TC, Jr., Subbarao S, Ellerbrock TV, et al: Human immuno-deficiency virus 1 expression in the female genital tract in association with cervical inflammation and ulceration. Am J Obstet Gynecol 2001; 184:279–285. **(IIb, B)**

27. Conley LJ, Ellerbrock TV, Bush TJ, et al: HIV-1 infection and risk of vulvovaginal and perianal condylomata acuminata and intraepithelial neoplasia: a prospective cohort study. Lancet 2002;359:108–113. **(IIb, B)**

28. Phelps RM, Smith DK, Heilig CM, et al: Cancer incidence in women with or at risk for HIV. Int J Cancer 2001;94:753–757. **(IIb, B)**

29. Grubert TA, Reindell D, Kastner R, et al: Rates of postoperative complications among human immunodeficiency virus–infected women who have undergone obstetric and gynecologic surgical procedures. Clin Infect Dis 2002;34:822–830. **(III, B)**

30. Sewell CA, Derr R, Anderson J: Operative complications in HIV-infected women undergoing gynecologic surgery. J Reprod Med 2001;46:199–204. **(III, B)**

31. Franz J, Jamieson DJ, Randall H, Spann C: Outcomes of hysterectomy in HIV-seropositive women compared to seronegative women. Infect Dis Obstet Gynecol 2005;13:167–169. **(III, B)**

32. Duerr A, Heilig CM, Meikle SF, et al: Incident and persistent vulvo-vaginal candidiasis among human immunodeficiency virus-infected women: risk factors and severity. Obstet Gynecol 2003;101:548–556. **(IIb, B)**

33. Jamieson DJ, Duerr A, Klein RS, et al: Longitudinal analysis of bacterial vaginosis: findings from the HIV epidemiology research study. Obstet Gynecol 2001;98:656–663. **(IIb, B)**

34. Cu-Uvin S, Ko H, Jamieson DJ, et al: Prevalence, incidence, and persistence or recurrence of trichomoniasis among human immuno-deficiency virus (HIV)–positive women and among HIV-negative women at high risk for HIV infection. Clin Infect Dis 2002; 34:1406–1411. **(IIb, B)**

35. Centers for Disease Control and Prevention: Sexually transmitted diseases treatment guidelines 2002. MMWR Recomm Rep 2002; 51(RR-6):1–78. **(IV, C)**

36. World Health Organization: Medical Eligibility Criteria for Contraceptive Use, 3rd ed. Geneva, World Health Organization, 2004. **(Ia, A)**

37. Duerr A, Jamieson D: Assisted reproductive technologies for HIV-discordant couples. Am J Bioeth 2003;3:45–47. **(IV, C)**

38. Jamieson DJ, Schieve L, Duerr A: Semen processing for HIV-discordant couples. Am J Obstet Gynecol 2001;185:1433–1434. **(IV, C)**

# Human Papillomaviruses

Elizabeth R. Unger, MD, PhD, Mack T. Ruffin IV, MD, MPH, and Concepcion Diaz-Arrastia, MD

## KEY POINTS

- Human papillomaviruses (HPVs) are the most common sexually transmitted infection.
- Most HPV infections are asymptomatic and transient.
- HPV is a family of more than 100 closely related viral types.
- The types found in the genital tract are divided into high risk and low risk groups based on their disease associations.
- High risk HPV types are associated with anogenital cancers, particularly cervical cancer.
- Low risk HPV types are associated with genital warts and recurrent respiratory papillomatosis.
- Treatment is not directed at HPV, rather at HPV-associated disease.
- HPV testing is recommended for triage of women with equivocal Pap smear results and may be used in combination with Pap smears for cervical cancer screening in women over age 30.

## EPIDEMIOLOGY, RISK FACTORS, AND PATHOGENESIS

HPV is the most common sexually transmitted infection. In the United States it is estimated that 80% of the sexually active population will be exposed during their lifetime. The vast majority of HPV infections are transient and asymptomatic. HPV testing is used clinically to detect HPV-associated disease. HPV infection is not treated; only HPV-associated disease is treated.

Human papillomaviruses are a family of more than 100 closely related small double-stranded DNA viruses, family Papovaviridae. HPV had been known since the turn of the 20th century to cause warts, but it was not until the advent of molecular biologic techniques that their association with cervical cancer was suspected. The genome of all papillomaviruses is episomal, about 8 kb, coding for relatively few proteins with a polycistronic message transcribed from one stand only (Fig. 22-1). The limited coding potential of the virus makes it completely dependent on the host cellular machinery for crucial steps of the viral life cycle. HPV requires a differentiating squamous epithelium to provide the appropriate cellular transcriptional and translational proteins for growth and is therefore not detectable by culture methods.

Human papillomavirus types are recognized based on their genetic sequence and are numbered in order of their discovery.

Sequence differences of more than 10% in the L1 region are recognized as another type, whereas variations of less than 2% are recognized as variants of currently numbered types. HPVs can be grouped as cutaneous or mucosal types. The cutaneous types are quite numerous and are associated with common hand and foot warts as well as a rare genetic disorder characterized by widespread warts and frequent skin cancer, erythrodermoplasia verruciformis. The cutaneous types are being investigated as risk factors for actinic keratoses, psoriasis, basal cell carcinomas, and squamous cell carcinomas. The mucosal types are those most commonly found in the anogenital region, but that may be found elsewhere, including the nail beds and oropharyngeal epithelium. The mucosal types are commonly divided into high risk and low risk groups based on their frequency of detection in malignancies. High risk types are detected in greater than 90% of cervical cancers. These types are also those most prevalent in the genital tract in the general population regardless of disease status.

The entire anogenital epithelium is exposed to HPV and may become infected during sexual contact with an infected individual. The most common site of HPV-associated neoplasia in the genital tract is the squamocolumnar junction of the cervix. Other less common sites include the squamocolumnar junction of the anus as well as the vaginal and vulvar epithelium. Most HPV infections are subclinical and do not require therapy. Detection of HPV is usually transient (median 6 to 12 months), with high risk types taking slightly longer than low risk types to clear.[1]

The mere presence of HPV DNA at the cervix does not necessarily define a woman as destined to develop cervical neoplasia. In general there is an interval of 10 or more years between HPV infection and detection of high grade squamous intraepithelial lesions or invasive cancer. Although poorly defined, additional cofactors interact with cervical HPV in the pathogenesis of cervical cancer. Some of these factors include smoking, parity, and oral contraceptive use,[2] as well as other genital tract infections, inflammation, and diet.[3] Persistent infection with high risk HPV is strongly linked to neoplastic progression. The host immune response, preceding cofactors, as well as viral factors such as viral load, type and variant types, multiple types, and integration may contribute to HPV persistence or interact in other ways to result in cervical carcinogenesis.

A variety of prospective studies have examined the issue of persistent cervical HPV infection. Ho and colleagues[4] examined the factors related to persistent squamous intraepithelial lesions among 70 women followed every 3 months for 15 months. The risk of persistent squamous intraepithelial lesions was associated

# Gynecologic Infectious Disease

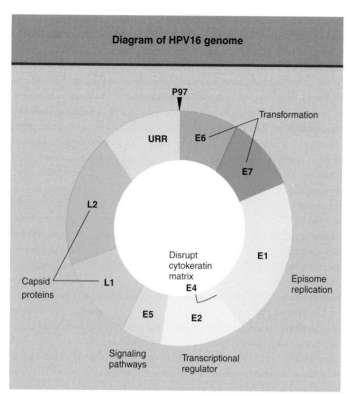

**Diagram of HPV16 genome**

**Figure 22-1    The genomes of all human papillomaviruses (HPVs) are double-stranded DNA closed circles (episomes) with similar genetic organization.** Late genes (L1 and L2) are structural proteins that make up the virus capsid. Early genes (E1, E2, E4–E7) are involved in the viral life cycle; major functions as noted on diagram. The upstream regulatory region (URR), also called the noncoding region (NCR) or long control region (LCR), contains binding sites for numerous cellular and viral transcriptional regulators. Genes are named based on relationship to bovine papillomavirus, which is why E3 is missing.

with persistent type-specific HPV infection of the cervix, with an odds ratio of 3.9 (95% CI, 1.58 to 9.65). In this study HPV persistence was defined as consecutive assessments positive for HPV. The same investigators' study of 608 college women followed every 6 months for 3 years noted a cumulative 36-month incidence of HPV infection of 43%.[1] The median duration of new infections was 8 months (95% CI, 7 to 10 months), but the accuracy of this estimate was limited by the every 6 month assessment. The risk of developing an abnormal Papanicolaou (Pap) smear increased with persistent HPV infection, particularly with high risk types (RR, 37.2; 95% CI, 14.6 to 94.8).[1]

Human papillomavirus is episomal in productive infections and in most lesions. Integration of the viral genome into host cellular DNA is found in essentially all cancers with HPV18 and most of those with HPV16. Viral integration has not been observed in all cancers, but integration clearly has implications in the perpetuation of the transformed phenotype as well as in tumor progression. HPV integration appears to be random with respect to the cellular chromosome, but nearly always occurs within the E1/E2 region of the HPV genome. Integration may be an irreversible event as a consequence of host cell genomic instability, or it may be that integration initiates a chain of events including the impairment of tumor suppressor genes

(e.g., *TP53* and *RB*), which results in genomic instability and cell immortalization.

The papillomavirus life cycle differs from that of all other virus families: infection requires the availability of epidermal or mucosal epithelial cells that are still able to proliferate.[5] In these cells, viral gene expression is largely suppressed, although the limited expression of specific "early" viral genes (such as E5, E6, and E7) results in enhanced proliferation of the infected cells and their lateral expansion.[6] Following entry into the suprabasal layers, "late" viral gene expression is initiated; the circular viral genome is then replicated, and structural proteins form. In the upper layers of the epidermis or mucosa, complete viral particles are assembled and released.

A significant role for malignant transformation can be assigned to the *E6* and *E7* genes and their respective proteins.[7] Initial observations revealed that E6 interacts with p53, and E7 interacts with RB to block the activity of these tumor suppressors. Indeed, some of the prominent functions of the E6 protein originate from its interaction with and degradation of p53 and the proapoptotic protein BAK, resulting in resistance to apoptosis and an increase in chromosomal instability.[5] E7, however, interacts with and degrades RB, which releases the transcription factor E2F from RB inhibition and up-regulates *INK4A*.[5] The resulting high E2F activity might lead to apoptosis in E7-expressing cells. Moreover, E7 stimulates the S-phase genes cyclin A and cyclin E, and seems to block the function of the cyclin-dependent kinase inhibitors *CDKN1A* (also known as *CIP1* and *p21*) and *CDKN1B*.[5]

## CLINICAL FEATURES

Human papillomavirus infection is most often asymptomatic and transient. In women, HPV infection presents clinically as warts (usually on the vulva or vaginal introitus) or is detected through cervical cancer screening as a Pap smear abnormality. HPV infection may also present as a result of a positive HPV test with or without a cytologic abnormality in women over age 30 who are screened with the "DNA-Pap" (HPV DNA test and cervical cytology).

### Genital Warts

Condylomata acuminata, or external genital warts, are generally noticed by the patient as visible cauliflower-like tan or pink papillary growths. In African American women the warts are typically hyperpigmented. They are generally painless, but may be associated with itching, burning, or redness, particularly if a secondary infection occurs. Solitary lesions do occur, but multifocal presentation is the rule. Lesions can be found anywhere on the anogenital epithelium, including the vulva, perineum, and perianal skin (Figs. 22-2 and 22-3). In men, the lesions can appear anywhere on the genitalia, including the scrotum and the pubic and perirectal areas. The lesions vary from less than 1 cm in size to massive confluences involving the entire external genitalia. These growths are benign and generally self-limited, but are treated because of cosmetic reasons or, in extreme cases, because of difficulty with ambulation. Their appearance is generally distressing to patients.

The presence of external genital warts should prompt a careful gross visual inspection, with or without magnification, of

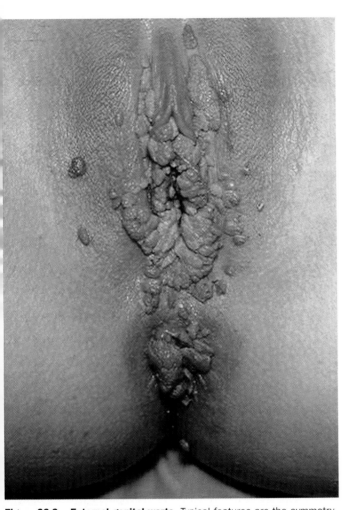

**Figure 22-2  External genital warts.** Typical features are the symmetry and multifocality of the lesions. The entire perineum is involved, including the perianal skin and mucosa.

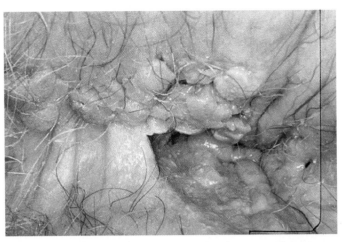

**Figure 22-3    Anal warts.** Large anal warts in a heterosexual woman with an intact immune function. She has severe psoriasis that involves the genital area.

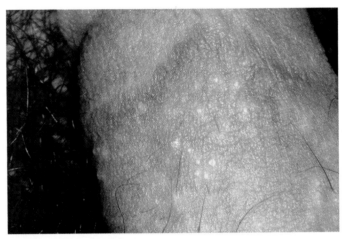

**Figure 22-4    Penile lesions.** These lesions on the penile shaft were seen only after the application of acetic acid. They were not symptomatic or apparent to the patient.

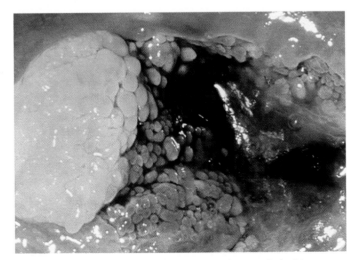

**Figure 22-5    Cervical condyloma.** This colpophotograph depicts a cervical warty lesion. Note the dense white epithelium, its location at the squamocolumnar junction, and its papillary appearance.

the entire anogenital area, as well as a Pap smear screen for coexisting HPV-associated lesions. Application of acetic acid before inspection is particularly helpful in identifying vulvar intraepithelial neoplasia and makes lesions easier to identify in men (Fig. 22-4). As with other HPV-associated diseases, condylomas can also be found in "internal" areas of the genital tract, including the vagina, cervix, and anus (Fig. 22-5). In contrast to the vulva, condylomata of the cervix are often flat (condyloma latum). Flat condylomata of the cervix are histologically indistinguishable from low-grade intraepithelial neoplasia, and the terms are interchangeable (Fig. 22-6). Condylomata of the vagina typically resemble the verrucous lesions found on the external genitalia, but may also resemble cervical warts.

Transmission generally occurs through sexual activity, and the age prevalence generally follows the age prevalence of sexual initiation and change of partners. Time from exposure to appearance of lesions varies but is on the order of several months. Transmission may occur from clinically inapparent lesions; partner tracing is not recommended. Genital warts in children are not diagnostic of sex abuse but should prompt an investigation to exclude this possibility. Testing or screening for other common sexually transmitted infections, such as *Chlamydia, Trichomonas,*

# Gynecologic Infectious Disease

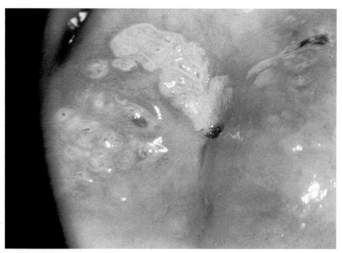

**Figure 22-6  Flat cervical wart.** This colpophotograph depicts an acetowhite lesion characteristic of flat condyloma, indistinguishable from a low-grade cervical intraepithelial lesion (LGCIN).

gonorrhea, syphilis, hepatitis, and HIV are warranted because of the common sexual routes of transmission.[8]

## Pap Smear Abnormalities

Women with Pap smear abnormalities are generally completely asymptomatic. These abnormalities come to light during routine cervical cytology performed for the purpose of cervical cancer screening. Cellular samples from the transformation zone are examined for cytologic features predicting the presence of underlying lesions that require treatment. In the United States, Bethesda terminology is used to describe cervical cytology results[9] (Table 22-1). Other than inflammatory and reactive changes

attributable to other infections such as yeast, *Trichomonas*, *Chlamydia*, or herpes, most Pap smear abnormalities are attributable to incident or persistent HPV infection. Pap smear abnormalities are very common and generally do not reflect serious disease. Because of uncertainty regarding the nature of the underlying lesion, abnormal Pap smears require further evaluation. The degree of cytologic abnormality determines the most appropriate clinical follow-up.

The ASC diagnosis (atypical squamous cells, former terminology ASCUS, atypical squamous cells of unknown significance) may prompt repeat Pap smear testing in 4 to 6 months or HPV testing.[10] The goal is to avoid missing a lesion that requires treatment, but because of limitations of sampling and cytologic sensitivity may not be diagnosed. Persistent ASC, or high risk HPV-positive ASC, as well as diagnoses of atypical squamous cells—high grade squamous intraepithelial lesion cannot be excluded, atypical glandular cells, low grade squamous intraepithelial lesion, and high grade epithelial lesion, are routinely evaluated with colposcopic examinations and directed biopsies for definitive histologic diagnosis.

## DIAGNOSIS

Human papillomavirus testing is complicated because of the nature of the virus. It cannot be cultured, and antibody methods are relatively insensitive; therefore, HPV detection requires some form of nucleic acid test. The viral life cycle is restricted to differentiating epithelium; therefore, a cellular sample collected from the site of infection is required. Further, HPV is not a single virus but a family of more than 100 closely related viral types. The types are distinguished based on differences in their DNA sequence. Assays must be designed to handle the complexity introduced by the large number of HPV types.

Human papillomavirus testing has been used to understand the epidemiology and natural history of the virus. The nature of the sample and the assay will frame the view of infection. Definitions of occult, persistent, or recurrent infection are complicated because of these issues. Based on association with disease, HPV types found in the anogenital tract are grouped into high risk and low risk types. High risk types are detected frequently in cancers, yet these are the most prevalent types in the general population. HPV testing is evaluated in terms of clinical sensitivity and specificity (ability to detect disease) or analytic sensitivity and specificity (ability to detect HPV). This section will focus on the analytic characteristics of HPV tests.

The only HPV test approved by the U.S. FDA for clinical use is Digene's Hybrid Capture 2 HPV DNA test (HC2). This test can be applied to cervical cells collected with the Digene Cervical Sampler (includes brush and media), cervical cells collected for liquid-based cytology, or with cervical biopsies collected in Digene Specimen Transport Medium. The current assay format uses liquid hybridization in a microarray platform. Samples are lysed to release nucleic acids and combined with the RNA probe mixture. The high risk probe mix includes 13 types (HPV16, 18, 31, 33, 35, 39, 45, 51, 52, 56, 58, 59, 68). The RNA probes hybridize to the DNA targets in liquid phase and are bound to the wall (i.e., captured) by antibodies specific for DNA–RNA hybrids. The same antibody linked to alkaline phosphatase is used to generate a signal after addition

| Table 22-1 The 2001 Bethesda System Terminology | |
|---|---|
| **Criteria** | **Categories** |
| Specimen adequacy | Adequate |
| | Inadequate |
| General categorization (optional) | Negative for intraepithelial lesion or malignancy |
| | Epithelial cell abnormality |
| Interpretation/Result | Negative for intraepithelial lesion or malignancy |
| | Organisms, reactive changes, atrophy, etc. |
| | Epithelial cell abnormalities |
| | Squamous cell |
| | Atypical squamous cells of undetermined significance (ASC-US) |
| | ASC cannot exclude HSIL (ASC-H) |
| | Low-grade squamous intraepithelial lesion (LSIL) |
| | High-grade squamous intraepithelial lesion (HSIL) |
| | Squamous carcinoma |
| | Glandular cell |
| | Atypical glandular cells (AGC) |
| | Atypical glandular cells, favor neoplastic |
| | Endocervical adenocarcinoma in situ (AIS) |
| | Adenocarcinoma |

From Solomon D, Davey D, Kurman R, et al: The 2001 Bethesda System: terminology for reporting results and cervical cytology. JAMA 2002;287:2114–2119.

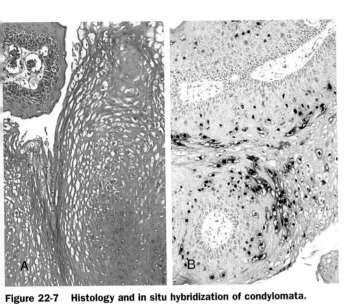

**Figure 22-7  Histology and in situ hybridization of condylomata.**
*A*, Hematoxylin and eosin-stained section demonstrating expanded epithelial layers with finger-like projections and cells with enlarged nuclei and perinuclear halos (koilocytes) that are characteristic of HPV infection. *B*, Colorimetric in situ hybridization with biotinylated probe to HPV 6/11. Dark blue/black color in scattered nuclei, particularly koilocytes, indicates presence of HPV. The uneven signal distribution within the lesion is characteristic of episomal HPV.

of chemiluminescent substrate. Cutoff for a positive result is determined by comparison of the intensity of sample to that of the 1 pg/mL control. The test has good interlaboratory comparisons and has been widely used in trials determining the clinical utility of HPV testing. The test does not control for sample cellularity and does not give type-specific results. Because the RNA probes are genetically complex and include the majority of the HPV genes, cross-hybridization with types not included as probes occurs. This could be advantageous for detection of other closely related high risk types. Occasionally large numbers of copies of low risk types will yield a positive result.

Type-specific polymerase chain reaction (PCR) assays for HPV are available and can be particularly useful in quantitative assessments of HPV. However, the large number of types that are of interest limit their usefulness in most studies. PCR assays that target sequences that are highly conserved are called *consensus assays*. These assays will generate a product for nearly all HPV types. Type-specific identification requires analysis using sequencing, restriction fragment length polymorphism assays, or hybridization. The three most widely used consensus PCR assays are PGMY09/11, GP5+/6+, and SPF.[11] All target the L1 region. They differ in the primer mix, the size of the amplified product, and the method for type identification. Results differ slightly in terms of type-specific sensitivity and specificity. Typing assays using linear arrays or strips allow for efficient detection of multiple HPV types within a sample.

Other HPV assays include serology and in situ hybridization. Serologic assays use ELISA-based detection of type-specific antibodies against L1-VLPs (virus-like particles). A positive reaction indicates past or current infection. Less than 70% of HPV-positive subjects develop detectable antibodies, and these

develop after a lagtime of several months. There is currently no gold standard for setting the threshold for positive results, and few interlaboratory comparisons are available. Competitive ELISA formats that allow titer determination are being used to follow response to HPV vaccination. The World Health Organization is developing one or more standard sera that will assist in assay standardization. In situ hybridization assays are useful for detecting virus within a morphologic context (Fig. 22-7) and can give information about integration status (Fig. 22-8). Requiring virus to be localized in abnormal cells may increase the specificity of test results, but sensitivity may be affected. The clinical utility of this format is under investigation.

In men, there is no accepted or proven method to detect HPV because the most appropriate site and method of sampling

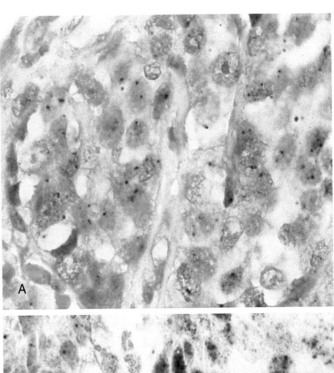

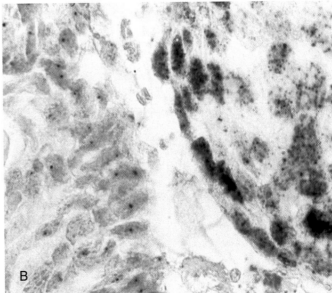

**Figure 22-8  In situ hybridization of HPV16 in cervical carcinomas.**
*A*, Dotlike signal evenly detected in most neoplastic cells is characteristic of integrated HPV. *B*, Mixed pattern of integrated HPV DNA (dot-like pattern on left) and episomal HPV DNA (uneven patchy signal on right).

Gynecologic Infectious Disease

has not been determined. A variety of anatomic sites have been studied, including urine, penile urethra, penile shaft, scrotum, and anal area. HPV testing in men has no clinical role.

## TREATMENT

It is important to recognize that treatments are not directed toward eliminating HPV infection; rather, they are directed to elimination of disease associated with HPV. There is no treatment for HPV-positive, cytology-negative women who have no genital warts. This is one reason why patient counseling can be difficult. Without careful explanation it can be quite stressful for women to learn that they have a virus associated with cervical cancer and that there is no treatment for the virus. Patients need to understand that the detection of high risk HPV in the absence of disease indicates an increased risk for disease and that regular screening must always be followed. They should be reassured about the generally transient nature of infection and the success of regular screening in preventing cancer by the detection and treatment of cancer precursors.

Human papillomavirus-associated diseases include common skin warts, genital warts, laryngeal warts (recurrent respiratory papillomatosis), cervical neoplasia, and other anogenital neoplasias (vulvar, vaginal, anal, penile). In addition, there is evidence that HPV is associated with a subset of head and neck cancers. This chapter will only address the treatment of genital warts and cervical cancer precursors, the most common HPV-associated diseases seen in gynecologic practice.

### Genital Warts

Therapeutic options for condylomata are based on removal of the lesions. A variety of chemicals can be applied topically to destroy the lesion or stimulate immune destruction. Lesions may also be removed by surgical approaches, including laser ablation, cryoablation, or excision. Regardless of the approach, a high recurrence rate, ranging from 35% to 52%, is the rule (Table 22-2), since the underlying HPV infection is not eradicated.[11,12] The choice of therapy is dictated by the size and anatomic location of the lesions, provider experience, and patient preference.[13]

### *External Genital Warts*

Based on ease of use and low toxicity, first-line therapeutic options for external genital warts include podofilox (Condylox) or imiquimod (Aldara). Both of these agents are self-administered. Patients, particularly those with keratinized warts, are advised to bathe before application to allow better penetration of the medication. Sexual contact should be avoided for 24 hours after application.

Podofilox is an antimitotic agent that is prepared as a gel or solution. Visible warts are treated twice daily for 3 consecutive days, then discontinue for 4 consecutive days. This weekly cycle can be repeated up to four times. Podofilox can be absorbed systemically and may cause bone marrow toxicity and neurotoxicity; therefore, it should be avoided in pregnancy and should not be used to treat large lesions (>10 cm$^2$). The dose should not exceed 0.5 mL per application. The clearance rate of warts with podofilox seen in multiple randomized double-blind

| | Patients with Clearance of Warts (%) | |
|---|---|---|
| Therapy | At End of Treatment | 3 Months Post-treatment |
| Cryotherapy | 70–88 | 63–92 |
| Electrocautery | 94 | 78–91 |
| Interferon | 6–90 | 18–62 |
| Laser | 31–86 | 39–86 |
| Podofilox | 32–79 | 22–73 |
| Surgery | 89–93 | 36 |
| TCA or BCA | 64–81 | 70 |
| 5-FU | 10–50 | 37 |
| Aldara | 72–84 | 72 (Females) 33 (Males) |

**Table 22-2**
**Summary of Therapeutic Response to External Genital Warts***

*References provided in text.

placebo- or vehicle-controlled trials is 45% to 91%, with a recurrence rate of 4% to 91%.[14]

Imiquimod is an immune response modifier that stimulates proinflammatory cytokines locally. It is available as a 5% cream in a predosed 250-mg sachet. Imiquimod is applied at bedtime, allowing 6 to 10 hours of overnight exposure, and is removed the following morning with soap and water. The medication is used three nonconsecutive times per week for 16 weeks or until the lesion clinically clears. As with podofilox, the wart clearance rate for imiquimod seen in multiple randomized, placebo-controlled, double-blind trials ranges from 37% to 52% after 8 to 16 weeks of therapy.[15-18] Benefits of using imiquimod over other medical therapies include a lower rate of recurrence (9% to 19%) and a greater median reduction in size of lesion.[15,19,20]

Other second-line therapies generally require administration by a health care provider and therefore multiple office visits. Trichloroacetic acid or bichloracetic acid induces a chemical burn by coagulating proteins. These strong acids are not absorbed and therefore can be used during pregnancy. Treatments are applied weekly. Podophyllin resin (10% to 25%) is another option for weekly application by a health care professional. Topical 5-fluorouracil (Efudex 5%) is a chemotherapeutic agent whose use is decreasing as other agents become available. It has toxicities, including nonhealing ulcerations of the vulva and vagina. Intralesional interferon is as effective as the other second-line therapeutics but is uncommonly used because of the high frequency of systemic side effects.

Treatment of external genital warts with surgical techniques has the advantage of providing immediate clearance of the lesions; however, high recurrence rates remain problematic. Surgical interventions include ablative and excisional procedures: cryotherapy, electrosurgery, laser, ultrasonic surgical aspiration, and cold knife excision. The recurrence rates for each method vary. The recurrence rates for cryotherapy, electrosurgery, and excisional biopsy range from 19% to 29%, in contrast to laser ablation, with recurrence rates of 60% to 77%. No randomized studies have compared one modality to the other, nor has there been a study comparing recurrence by size of lesion, which affects the recurrence rate and choice of treatment modality. For example, electrosurgery is only an option for small lesions because of to the potential for third-degree skin burn.[21]

All surgical methods require local or regional anesthesia, depending on the surface area to be treated. Because these epithelial lesions are not invasive, only superficial excision to the depth of the epithelium (1 mm) is required. However, external genital warts may have multifocal involvement, requiring treatment of extensive areas with a greater anesthetic and analgesic requirement. In general, surgical procedures require more experience and expertise than medical therapies but have the benefit of a single visit for treatment. However, convalescence from the one-day surgical treatment may extend over a month.

Cryotherapy and electrosurgery both destroy warts by thermal-induced cytolysis (freezing or burning). Overtreatment and damage to the dermis should be avoided. Local anesthesia is required for electrosurgery and may be required for cryotherapy of extensive lesions. Carbon dioxide laser destroys the warts with the benefit of low penetration of the beam; thus, underlying dermal involvement is minimized. Cold knife excision is performed by slicing the lesion off the dermis. Hemostasis is achieved with electrosurgery. Condylomata that fail to entirely clear with topical therapies alone should be considered for an excisional biopsy for both treatment and histologic diagnosis to exclude a dysplastic lesion.

Large and multifocal vulvar condylomata measuring greater than 4 cm in greatest dimension, referred to in the past as *giant condyloma of Buschke-Lowenstein*, present a management challenge, because they usually fail to respond to medical therapy. However, excision or ablation of large vulvar lesions is very painful and is associated with delayed wound healing, increased risk of scarring, and poor cosmetic result. As an alternative, a staged medical and surgical approach may be used. Topical therapy with podofilox or imiquimod can be used to reduce the size of the lesion to one that is more amenable to surgical excision with decreased morbidity.

### Cervical Warts

Cervical warts are usually flat and asymptomatic; they regress spontaneously and do not require treatment. However, a high grade intraepithelial lesion must be excluded with a biopsy. If cervical warts require treatment for progressive disease, they should be treated as high grade cervical lesions, with cryotherapy or loop electrosurgical excision procedure (LEEP).

### Vaginal and Anal Warts

Condylomata of the vagina or the anus are usually associated with vulvar or cervical condylomata. Treatment options for vaginal and anal disease are limited. Using direct visualization with a speculum as necessary, trichloroacetic acid or bichloroacetic acid may be applied. To minimize damage to adjacent tissues, the speculum should not be removed until the acid has dried and the treated tissue appears white. As with external genital warts, weekly application by a health care professional is required. Another option includes surgical removal with carbon dioxide laser or cold knife excision. Cryotherapy with a probe is not recommended due to the close proximity and potential for injury of the bladder and rectum. Topical 5-fluorouracil is not recommended because of the risk of nonhealing ulcers.

## Cervical Intraepithelial Neoplasia

Although only a small fraction of even high grade lesions are truly premalignant, therapeutic intervention of these lesions at the intraepithelial stage before they become invasive is responsible for the success of screening practices in cervical cancer prevention.

### Low-Grade Cervical Intraepithelial Neoplasia (LGCIN, CIN I)

In deciding on management of these lesions, it's important to realize that eradication of the intraepithelial lesions does not eradicate the HPV infection in the genital epithelium. It is therefore recommended to manage the patient expectantly to allow the opportunity for spontaneous clearance of the lesion. Low grade cervical epithelial neoplasia (LGCIN), also referred to as cervical intraepithelial neoplasia grade I (CIN I) or mild dysplasia, is the histologic reflection of productive HPV infection. It is characterized by a 40% to 70% rate of spontaneous regression and a 10% to 15% rate of progression to a high grade intraepithelial lesion.[22]

Expectant management may consist of a repeat evaluation in 6 to 12 months, including a repeat Pap smear alone, repeat Pap smear and colposcopic examination, or HPV DNA testing in 12 months.[23] For persistent low grade lesions, the length of observation before intervention is at the discretion of the colposcopist. A defined period of time of at least 1 year is acceptable, but indefinite observation may be appropriate in circumstances with a motivated patient in whom it is desirable to avoid instrumentation. For example, immunocompromised women such as transplant recipients, long-term corticosteroid users, or HIV-infected women, may benefit from prolonged observation to avoid multiple procedures for frequent recurring low grade lesions.[23]

The decision whether to manage CIN I expectantly or to treat the lesions must also consider the patient's preference as well as her ability to comply with follow-up. Dysplasia clinics in varied locations are notorious for no-show rates of up to 50% for any one appointment. Indications for treatment of CIN include persistent or progressive disease. Progression includes increased grade or size of lesion. Persistence or progression must be documented histologically, not only cytologically or by colposcopy. Progression by size criteria is by growth of lesion to involve additional quadrants of the cervix, or histologic progression of the grade of the dysplasia from CIN I to CIN II or III.

### High-Grade Cervical Intraepithelial Neoplasia (HGCIN, CIN II, III)

The success of Pap smear screening practices in decreasing the rates of invasive cervical carcinoma is most likely due to the treatment of HGCIN, the well established cancer precursor lesion. From 14% to 22% of HGCIN lesions progress, justifying immediate treatment of all HGCIN lesions with few exceptions.[24] Furthermore, Chang found a 20% to 30% progression of carcinoma in situ to invasive carcinoma within 5 to 10 years.[25] Before proceeding with treatment, a complete evaluation of the lesion is recommended, consisting of an adequate colposcopic examination, visualization of the entire lesion and the squamocolumnar junction, and a negative endocervical curettage. If these conditions are not met, a diagnostic conization of the cervix, which may also be therapeutic, is required.

Ablation and excision are equally efficacious treatments, with a risk of posttreatment recurrence of less than 10% for all treatment modalities: cryotherapy, laser ablation, laser conization, cold knife conization, and LEEP. Benefits of ablative procedures with cryotherapy include the broad availability of the procedure and the lack of need for anesthesia. Laser ablation of the squamocolumnar junction is also an acceptable ablative procedure.

Many colposcopists are biased toward excisional methods, in large part because these methods produce a large specimen for further pathologic evaluation, including comment on the margins of excision. Uncommonly, findings on an excision specimen upgrade the diagnosis and affect management decisions. From 4933 published LEEP specimens, 39 (0.8%) showed unsuspected microinvasive disease, 11 (0.2%) occult invasive cancers, and 14 (0.3%) adenocarcinoma in situ.

An excisional procedure is preferred over an ablative procedure for women with recurrent HGCIN or when a carcinoma is anticipated. A hysterectomy is an acceptable mode of treatment for recurrent HGCIN in a woman not interested in maintaining fertility. Hysterectomy is not an appropriate option for the primary treatment of CIN.

Cold knife conization remains the definitive treatment in select cases when the margins of excision need to be meticulously evaluated and it is felt that the submillimeter zone of cautery artifact in a LEEP specimen may compromise this evaluation. These cases include microinvasive carcinoma when a hysterectomy is not planned and adenocarcinoma in situ.

In adolescents, based on level II evidence, it is acceptable to follow a CIN II lesion with repeat Pap smear and colposcopy for 1 year, provided the examination is satisfactory and endocervical curettage is negative.

After treatment, recommended follow-up is in the form of a repeat Pap smear at 4 to 6 months, HPV testing at 12 months, or repeat Pap smear and colposcopy at 4 to 6 months.[23]

### Management of Positive Margins or Positive Endocervical Curettage Results

Many factors are to be taken into consideration in the management of patients with positive endocervical curettage results or positive conization margins. These include probability of residual cancer, which margin is positive, the degree of dysplasia at the margin or endocervical curettage, patient compliance, and fertility desires. If fertility is not an issue and a positive endocervical curettage is obtained, a repeat conization should be performed. Pap smear and colposcopy should be repeated in no later than 3 to 4 months if the patient strongly desires fertility and would prefer not to have a repeat conization, which could adversely affect obstetric outcome.

Recurrence following a conization with a negative margin is 10% compared to 26.6% if margins are positive.[26] Kobak and colleagues, in a record review of 104 patients with conization, found that 8 of 27 (29%) cases with positive margin and positive endocervical curettage had invasive cancer, whereas cancer was found in 0 of 37 cases with positive margin and benign endocervical curettage.[27] If either endocervical curettage or margin were negative, there were no cases of invasive cancer. Six of

16 patients over age 50 with positive endocervical curettage had invasive cancer (two microinvasive and four frank invasion).

The risk of recurrence of adenocarcinoma in situ is high: 40% to 70% if margins are positive and 10% to 40% with negative margins.[28,29] A repeat conization is warranted in cases of adenocarcinoma in situ with positive margins to rule out invasive disease. After confirmation of the pathology, a hysterectomy is indicated in the patient with adenocarcinoma in situ who is not interested in maintaining fertility.

### Vulvar, Vaginal, and Anal Intraepithelial Neoplasia

The entire anogenital epithelium is at risk of HPV infection. The natural history of HPV associated disease appears to be similar for the various epithelia. Similarly, low grade lesions of the vulva, vagina, and anal canal may be managed expectantly. High grade lesions share malignant potential, requiring destruction of the lesion.

## CLINICAL COURSE AND PROGRESSION

Infection with HPV is the most common sexually transmitted infection. The infection is most often without any symptoms or clinical manifestations. For most patients with intact immune function, the infection is transient. Koutsky and colleagues noted a 2-year cumulative incidence of CIN II/III from first positive HPV as 28% among college women.[30] In addition, this group noted no new cases of CIN II/III after 24 months regardless of HPV status. Moscicki and colleagues reported that most women with HPV clear it in 24 months.[31,32] A prospective study of young women with 6-month follow-up by Woodman and colleagues describes the incidence, persistence, and risk of HPV infection.[33] Among 1075 women negative for HPV and with cytologically normal cervical smears, the cumulative risk of any HPV infection over 3 years was 44%. The median duration of HPV infection by type and associated risk for developing CIN II/III are highlighted in Table 22-3. Duration was defined as one or more uninterrupted time points of HPV detection.

## PITFALLS AND CONTROVERSIES

### Human Papillomavirus Education

Despite the overwhelming prevalence of HPV and the potential consequences of an HPV infection, several studies have demonstrated an enormous lack of awareness of the disease.[34-38] In a study of 263 college-aged women, 87% replied that they had either never heard of HPV or were not sure if they had heard of HPV.[34] Another study of university students confirmed these findings, with only 38% responding that they had heard of HPV. The same study also found that 59% of participants responded that they were unaware of how HPV could be transmitted. Ramirez and colleagues quantified HPV knowledge among young women at a local university, finding a mean knowledge score at only the 68th percentile.[35] Those who had heard of HPV had received information from the following sources: health professionals (30%), class (29%), clinics (23%), friends (22%), teachers (18%), and parents and boyfriends (<8%). In contrast, adolescents' knowledge of HPV and cervical dysplasia after the diagnosis of HPV was quite high.[37] Only one published study has examined the knowledge of adults beyond college students. Adults seen in a typical family physician's office have similarly

**Table 22-3**
**Natural History of Human Papillomavirus in Young Women**

| | Median Duration (Months) [95% Confidence Interval] | Relative Risk of HSIL [95% Confidence Interval] |
|---|---|---|
| HPV 6 or 11 | 9.4 [6.1–12.0] | 3.8 [1.5–9.8] |
| HPV 16 | 10.3 [6.8–17.3] | 8.5 [3.7–19.2] |
| HPV 18 | 7.8 [6.0–12.6] | 3.3 [1.4–8.1] |
| HPV 31 | 8.6 [7.5–12.9] | 3.5 [1.0–11.8] |
| HPV 33 | 9.0 [6.1–14.0] | 0.6 [0.1–4.4] |
| HPV 52 | 13.0 [5.8–22.1] | 2.3 [0.3–17.2] |
| HPV 58 | 11.0 [7.5–18.3] | 2.9 [0.8–10.1] |
| Any HPV | 13.7 [8.0–25.4] | 7.8 [2.7–22.0] |

HPV, Human papillomavirus; HSIL, high-grade squamous intraepithelial lesion.
From Woodman CB, Collins S, Winter H, et al: Natural history of cervical human papillomavirus infection in young women: a longitudinal cohort study. Lancet 2001;357:1831–1836.

limited knowledge of HPV.[39] One tool clinicians can use to identify those with the least amount of knowledge is to ask patients how informed they are about HPV. The preferred time to receive information about HPV is before a patient becomes sexually active. However, it remains unclear whether educational intervention or knowledge changes risky behaviors.

### Psychosocial Issues Regarding Human Papillomavirus

Only one published study has examined the potential for adverse psychosexual alterations due to HPV besides an abnormal Pap smear.[40] This cross-sectional study was conducted with sexually active women aged 18 to 60. They had few sexually transmitted infections and few risk factors, yet 20% had unsuspected HPV infection. Psychosexual characteristics at baseline and at follow-up, as well as perceived changes in these characteristics by the women, did not differ between women with HPV infection and those without. Stratification by potential confounders, including the presence of a vaginal infection at the time of study enrollment, household income level, ethnic background, age, marital status, and sexual history, did not alter these results. However, there is potential for significant adverse psychosexual impact given the issues of an untreatable, sexually transmitted infection that increases a women's risk for an abnormal Pap smear. More data are needed to examine the full impact.

### Human Papillomavirus Vaccines

Because HPV infection is necessary (even though not sufficient) for cervical cancer, preventing HPV infection has the potential to eliminate cervical cancer. Phase II trials of a monovalent vaccine against HPV16[41] and a bivalent vaccine against HPV16 and HPV18[42] have been essentially 100% effective at preventing persistent infection with the types included in the vaccine. The current vaccine formulations are based on VLPs composed of L1 proteins. Vaccination has resulted in very high titers of type-specific antibodies. Phase III trials are under way and licensure can be anticipated.

Although these developments are promising, many questions must be answered before vaccine implementation. Follow-up to date has been short-term, and cancer is not the observed endpoint. Because not all viral types associated with malignancy are included in the vaccines, cervical cancer screening will not be able to be stopped. What is the most cost-effective approach to combination vaccination and screening? How long is protection maintained? What age-group should be targeted for vaccination? As a prophylactic vaccine, it should be given before exposure at the time of sexual debut. Will parents accept vaccination of their adolescent children against a sexually transmitted infection? Should both boys and girls be vaccinated? The availability of vaccine further emphasizes the need for education of the general public and health care providers about HPV.

## REFERENCES

1. Ho GY, Bierman R, Beardsley L, et al: Natural history of cervicovaginal papillomavirus infection in young women. N Engl J Med 1998; 338:423–428. **(IIb, B)**
2. Castellsague X, Munoz N: Cofactors in human papillomavirus carcinogenesis—role of parity, oral contraceptives, and tobacco smoking. J Natl Cancer Inst Monogr 2003;20–28. **(IIb, B)**
3. Castle PE, Giuliano AR: Genital tract infections, cervical inflammation, and antioxidant nutrients—assessing their roles as human papillomavirus cofactors. J Natl Cancer Inst Monogr 2003;29–34. **(IIb, B)**
4. Ho GY, Burk RD, Klein S, et al: Persistent genital human papillomavirus infection as a risk factor for persistent cervical dysplasia. J Natl Cancer Inst 1995;87:365–371. **(IIb, B)**
5. zur Hausen H: Papillomaviruses and cancer: from basic studies to clinical application. Nat Rev Cancer 2002;2:342–350. **(IIb, B)**
6. Turek LP: The structure, function, and regulation of papillomaviral genes in infection and cervical cancer. Adv Virus Res 1994;44:305–356. **(IIb, B)**
7. Flores ER, Allen-Hoffmann BL, Lee D, Lambert PF: The human papillomavirus type 16 E7 oncogene is required for the productive stage of the viral life cycle. J Virol 2000;74:6622–6631. **(IIb, B)**
8. Committee on Adolescent Health Care. Sexually transmitted diseases in adolescents. ACOG Committee Opinion No. 301. Obstet Gynecol 2004;104:891–898. **(IV, C)**
9. Solomon D, Davey D, Kurman R, et al: The 2001 Bethesda System: terminology for reporting results of cervical cytology. JAMA 2002; 287:2114–2119. **(IV, C)**
10. Wright TC Jr, Cox JT, Massad LS, et al: 2001 Consensus Guidelines for the management of women with cervical cytological abnormalities. JAMA 2002;287:2120–2129. **(IV, C)**
11. Ferenczy A, Mitao M, Nagai N, et al: Latent papillomavirus and recurring genital warts. N Engl J Med 1985;313:784–788. **(IIa, B)**
12. Zaak D, Hofstetter A, Frimberger D, Schneede P: Recurrence of condylomata acuminata of the urethra after conventional and fluorescence-controlled Nd:YAG laser treatment. Urology 2003; 61:1011–1015. **(IIa, B)**
13. Ting PT, Dytoc MT: Therapy of external anogenital warts and molluscum contagiosum: a literature review. Dermatol Ther 2004;17:68–101. **(III, B)**
14. Maw R: Critical appraisal of commonly used treatment for genital warts. Int J STD AIDS 2004;15:357–364. **(Ib, A)**
15. Beutner KR, Spruance SL, Hougham AJ, et al: Treatment of genital warts with an immune-response modifier (imiquimod). J Am Acad Dermatol 1998;38:230–239. **(Ib, A)**

16. Beutner KR, Tyring SK, Trofatter KF, Jr, et al: Imiquimod, a patient-applied immune-response modifier for treatment of external genital warts. Antimicrob Agents Chemother 1998;42:789–794. **(Ib, A)**

17. Edwards L, Ferenczy A, Eron L, et al: Self-administered topical 5% imiquimod cream for external anogenital warts. HPV Study Group. Arch Dermatol 1998;134:25–30. **(Ib, A)**

18. Sauder DN, Skinner RB, Fox TL, Owens ML: Topical imiquimod 5% cream as an effective treatment for external genital and perianal warts in different patient populations. Sex Transm Dis 2003;30:124–128. **(Ib, A)**

19. Edwards L: Imiquimod in clinical practice. Australas J Dermatol 1998;39(Suppl 1):S14–S16. **(Ib, A)**

20. Gunter J: Genital and perianal warts: new treatment opportunities for human papillomavirus infection. Am J Obstet Gynecol 2003;189(3 Suppl):S3–S11. **(Ib, A)**

21. Wiley DJ, Douglas J, Beutner K, et al: External genital warts: diagnosis, treatment, and prevention. Clin Infect Dis 2002;35(Suppl 2):S210–S224. **(III, B)**

22. Ostor AG: Natural history of cervical intraepithelial neoplasia: a critical review. Int J Gynecol Pathol 1993;12:186–192. **(IIa, B)**

23. Wright TC Jr, Cox JT, Massad LS, et al: 2001 consensus guidelines for the management of women with cervical intraepithelial neoplasia. Am J Obstet Gynecol 2003;189:295–304. **(IV, C)**

24. Mitchell MF, Tortolero-Luna G, Wright T, et al: Cervical human papillomavirus infection and intraepithelial neoplasia: a review. J Natl Cancer Inst Monogr 1996;21:17–25. **(IIa, B)**

25. Chang AR: Carcinoma in situ of the cervix and its malignant potential. A lesson from New Zealand. Cytopathol 1990;1:321–328. **(III, B)**

26. Jakus S, Edmonds P, Dunton C, King SA: Margin status and excision of cervical intraepithelial neoplasia: a review. Obstet Gynecol Surv 2000;55:520–527. **(Ib, A)**

27. Kobak WH, Roman LD, Felix JC, et al: The role of endocervical curettage at cervical conization for high-grade dysplasia. Obstet Gynecol 1995;85:197–201. **(III, B)**

28. Widrich T, Kennedy AW, Myers TM, et al: Adenocarcinoma in situ of the uterine cervix: management and outcome. Gynecol Oncol 1996;61:304–308. **(III, B)**

29. Poynor EA, Barakat RR, Hoskins WJ: Management and follow-up of patients with adenocarcinoma in situ of the uterine cervix. Gynecol Oncol 1995;57:158–164. **(III, B)**

30. Koutsky LA, Holmes KK, Critchlow CW, et al: A cohort study of the risk of cervical intraepithelial neoplasia grade 2 or 3 in relation to papillomavirus infection. N Engl J Med 1992;327:1272–1278. **(IIb, B)**

31. Moscicki AB, Hills N, Shiboski S, et al: Risks for incident human papillomavirus infection and low-grade squamous intraepithelial lesion development in young females. JAMA 2001;285:2995–3002. **(IIb, B)**

32. Moscicki AB, Shiboski S, Broering J, et al: The natural history of human papillomavirus infection as measured by repeated DNA testing in adolescent and young women. J Pediatr 1998;132:277–284. **(IIb, B)**

33. Woodman CB, Collins S, Winter H, et al: Natural history of cervical human papillomavirus infection in young women: a longitudinal cohort study. Lancet 2001;357:1831–1836. **(IIb, B)**

34. Vail-Smith K, White DM: Risk level, knowledge, and preventive behavior for human papillomaviruses among sexually active college women. J Am Coll Health 1992;40:227–230. **(IIb, B)**

35. Ramirez JE, Ramos DM, Clayton L, et al: Genital human papillomavirus infections: knowledge, perception of risk, and actual risk in a nonclinic population of young women. J Womens Health 1997;6:113–121. **(IIb, B)**

36. Yacobi E, Tennant C, Ferrante J, et al: University students' knowledge and awareness of HPV. Prev Med 1999;28:535–541. **(IIb, B)**

37. Dell DL, Chen H, Ahmad F, Stewart DE: Knowledge about human papillomavirus among adolescents. Obstet Gynecol 2000;96(5 Pt 1):653–656. **(IIb, B)**

38. Gerhardt CA, Pong K, Kollar LM, et al: Adolescents' knowledge of human papillomavirus and cervical dysplasia. J Pediatr Adolesc Gynecol 2000;13:15–20. **(IIb, B)**

39. Holcomb B, Bailey JM, Crawford K, Ruffin MT: Adults' knowledge and behaviors related to human papillomavirus infection. J Am Board Fam Pract 2004;17:16–31. **(IIb, B)**

40. Reed BD, Ruffin MT, Gorenflo DW, Zazove P: The psychosexual impact of human papillomavirus cervical infections. J Fam Pract 1999;48:110–116. **(IIb, B)**

41. Koutsky LA, Ault KA, Wheeler CM, et al: A controlled trial of a human papillomavirus type 16 vaccine. N Engl J Med 2002;347:1645–1651. **(Ia, A)**

42. Harper DM, Franco EL, Wheeler C, et al: Efficacy of a bivalent L1 virus-like particle vaccine in prevention of infection with human papillomavirus types 16 and 18 in young women: a randomised controlled trial. Lancet 2004;364:1757–1765. **(Ia, A)**

**KEY POINTS**

Sepsis should be suspected if any of these signs or symptoms are present postoperatively:

- Temperature ≥100.4°F (38°C) and tachycardia
- Elevated white blood cell count or >10% increase in immature neutrophils
- Pain adjacent to the surgical site that does not respond to narcotic analgesia
- Necrosis of skin in or adjacent to the surgical site
- Leukopenia and decreased urine output
- Hypotension, oliguria, tachypnea

Postoperative pelvic infections continue to be a significant cause of morbidity and mortality. In addition to postoperative pelvic infection, the gynecologic surgeon must be concerned with infections that are associated with the surgical procedure but occur outside of the pelvis. The key to reducing the morbidity and mortality associated with postoperative infection resides in predicting which patients are more likely to develop a postoperative infection and then applying appropriate measures preoperatively, intraoperatively, and postoperatively. The gynecologic surgeon can take measures to reduce the patient's risk for developing a postoperative infection.

## MICROBIOLOGY

Postoperative pelvic infections are most frequently caused by bacteria that make up the patient's endogenous vaginal microflora. The endogenous vaginal bacteria include gram-positive and gram-negative aerobic, facultative, and obligate anaerobic bacteria listed in Table 23-1. The status of the vaginal ecosystem, that is, whether it is in a healthy state (*Lactobacillus*-dominant) or in an altered state, appears to be of primary importance with regard to the patient's potential risk for developing a postoperative pelvic infection. When the patient's microflora is dominated by *Lactobacillus*, the species of *Lactobacillus* is important, for the species must produce a significant amount of organic acids, including lactic acid, hydrogen peroxide, and lactocin. When the ecosystem is dominated by *Lactobacillus*, the number of lactobacilli is at least $10^6$ bacteria/mL of vaginal fluid, whereas other bacteria are present in a concentration less than or equal to $10^3$ bacteria/mL of vaginal fluid. This ratio of lactobacilli to other bacteria is maintained by a vaginal pH below 4.5; the presence of hydrogen peroxide, which is toxic to those bacteria that lack catalase (i.e., obligate anaerobic bacteria); and the production of lactocin.[1–3]

When the pH of the vaginal environment begins to rise, the lactobacilli are suppressed. The bacterium that gains dominance will determine the state of the altered vaginal microflora. If *Gardnerella vaginalis* gains dominance, its growth results in either a continued decrease in the hydrogen ion concentration or a rise in pH and a reduction in the oxygen concentration. These physiologic changes in the environment cause the continued growth of *Gardnerella* and an increase in the growth of the obligate anaerobic bacteria. In addition, the facultative bacteria switch from an aerobic metabolism to an anaerobic metabolism. When this occurs, both *Gardnerella* and the obligate anaerobic bacteria dominate ($\geq 10^6$ bacteria/mL), and the facultative anaerobic bacteria are present in a concentration between $10^3$ and $10^6$ bacteria/mL of vaginal fluid. A microflora dominated by obligate anaerobic bacteria is known as *bacterial vaginosis*. Typically, bacterial vaginosis is defined as a vaginal condition in which a shift in the bacteriology of the vagina has occurred, the lactobacilli have lost dominance and the obligate anaerobes assumed dominance, and there is an absence of white blood cells (WBC). The patient's microflora can become dominated by a gram-negative facultative bacterium (e.g., *Escherichia coli*, a virulent bacterium that has been involved in pelvic infections). Patients who develop an endogenous vaginal microflora dominated by *Streptococcus agalactiae* can develop symptomatic vaginitis, but this microflora is not a risk factor for the development of a postoperative pelvic infection. However, if the patient has a significant chronic illness (e.g., insulin dependent diabetes [IDDM]) or significant immunosuppression, Group B streptococci (GBS) will place the patient at risk for infection morbidity.

The significance of an altered endogenous microflora with regard to the potential development of postoperative infection resides in two important characteristics. Infection requires that the inoculum be sufficient to overcome the host defense mechanisms. This allows the bacterium to adhere to the epithelium, invade to deeper tissues, and reproduce. The organisms that make up bacterial vaginosis contain many virulent bacteria, such as the facultative and obligate anaerobic bacteria. Many of these bacteria are gram-negative, and therefore contain lipopolysaccharide (LPS), which is responsible for initiating the pro-inflammatory response. In addition to the presence of virulent bacteria, some of these bacteria act synergistically to initiate the development of abscess formation (e.g., *E. coli* + *Bacteroides fragilis*, *E. coli* + *Prevotella bivia*, and *Enterococcus faecalis* + *P. bivia*).[4] The activity of these bacteria combinations explains why some patients who appear to have an uncomplicated hysterectomy develop a postoperative pelvic abscess. The synergistic activity of bacteria may contribute to the production of virulence factors (collagenases, proteinases, fibrinases, enzymes to break down immunoglobulins) as well as the

# Gynecologic Infectious Disease

**Table 23-1**
**Endogenous Bacteria of the Lower Genital Tract**

| Facultative anaerobes | |
| --- | --- |
| **Gram-positive** | **Gram-negative** |
| Lactobacillus | Escherichia coli |
| Corynebacterium | Enterobacter cloacae |
| Diphtheroids | Klebsiella pneumoniae |
| Enterococcus faecalis | Morganella morganii |
| α-hemolytic streptococci | Proteus mirabilis |
| Streptococcus agalactiae | Proteus vulgaris |
| Staphylococcus aureus | |
| Staphylococcus epidermidis | |

| Obligate anaerobes | |
| --- | --- |
| **Gram-positive** | **Gram-negative** |
| Eubacterium | Bacteroides fragilis |
| Peptococcus niger | Fusobacterium necrophorum |
| Peptostreptococcus anaerobius | Fusobacterium nucleatum |
| | Prevotella bivia |
| | Prevotella melaninogenica |
| | Veillonella |

Adapted from Faro S: Vaginal microflora. In Faro S (ed): Sexually Transmitted Diseases in Women. Philadelphia: Lippincott Williams & Wilkins, 2003, p. 98.

production of nutrients required by a co-colonizing bacterium. This activity allows for the growth and reproduction of the co-colonizing bacterium, thereby enabling it to achieve a population that permits it to become a co-infecting bacterium.

The endogenous microflora, not bacteria introduced from the exogenous environment, appears to be a significant factor and is the principal reason why patients who undergo hysterectomy are at risk for the development of a postoperative pelvic infection. Women with a *Lactobacillus*-dominant endogenous vaginal microflora who are undergoing a hysterectomy are at extremely low risk for the development of postoperative pelvic infection. In a study, 200 women undergoing abdominal or vaginal hysterectomy were analyzed with respect to the status of their endogenous vaginal microflora and the development of postoperative infection. The results showed that only those with bacterial vaginosis had a significant rate of infection compared to those patients who had either a *Lactobacillus*- or GBS-dominant endogenous vaginal microflora.[5]

## RISK FACTORS FOR INFECTION

For patients undergoing pelvic surgery the risk increases significantly when the vagina is entered during the course of the operation. Entry into the vagina provides a source of bacterial contamination of the pelvis. This contamination source is not limited to the pelvic peritoneum and pelvic organs; it can also allow these bacteria to colonize the abdominal incision. In cases where the vagina is not grossly entered, the presence of suture in the vaginal apex provides a conduit for bacteria to gain entrance to the pelvis. Both the grossly opened vagina and the vagina that is only penetrated by suture allows for bacteria to seed the pelvic cavity and colonize the vaginal apex as well as the

pelvic cavity continuously. Frequently, there is a collection of serum or blood at the vaginal apex, plus necrotic tissue and suture, thus providing a culture medium for the bacteria that gain entrance to this area. The suture acts as a foreign body and lowers the size of the inoculum required for infection to develop de novo. The combination of these factors allows for the reproduction of bacteria within an environment conducive to the growth of both facultative and obligate anaerobic bacteria. If the tissues at the surgical site are significantly devascularized so that the oxygen concentration and reduction potential are significantly reduced, this can result in inhibition of phagocytosis. Additionally if the area is significantly devascularized, suitable levels of antibiotic will not be achieved and both cellular and humoral host antibacterial agents will be unable to arrive at the site of bacterial colonization.

Patients with chronic illness (e.g., IDDM, severe hypertension, and immunosuppression) are at risk for postoperative infection. Patients with IDDM and severe hypertension can have peripheral vascular disease; during the operative procedure the surgical areas can experience hypoxia and are thus susceptible to infection.

Morbidly obese patients pose significant problems to the gynecologic surgeon performing a laparotomy or vaginal hysterectomy. The difficulties encountered in this instance begin with the abdominal wall; with a lower abdominal vertical incision, a significant amount of subcutaneous fatty tissue is encountered. The depth of subcutaneous fatty tissue is proportional to the amount of dead space, which allows for the collection of serum and blood. Incising the subcutaneous tissue involves cutting through lymphatic vessels and arterioles as well as venules. The pressure exerted by retraction, a decrease in blood pressure and spasm of the lymphatic vessels, arterioles, and venules results in cessation of the exiting of blood and serum. Postoperatively, the return to preoperative blood pressure and relaxation of the vessels causes the development of a seroma or hematoma. Repeated trauma to the cut surfaces of the abdominal wall occurs when the hands of surgeons and assistants brush over the exposed tissues. Bacteria can colonize the surface of the exposed tissues. Small lacerations occur in the subcutaneous fatty tissue and muscle secondary to the manipulations that occur during the operative procedure. When the abdominal incision is closed, removal of the retractors relieves the pressure from the abdominal wall and allows the serum and blood to enter the dead space of the closed incision. Bacterial colonization occurs, and this closed space with serum and/or blood serves as culture medium and an incubator. Operating in the pelvis of the morbidly obese patient is also difficult because the surgeon must operate through a thick abdominal wall. Additionally, the fatty tissue in the pelvis often hampers visualization of the operative field. There is also a significant opportunity for seepage of serum and blood around the vaginal apex. This creates a situation similar to that observed with the abdominal wound except there is a greater opportunity for bacterial colonization of the vaginal cuff. Bacteria from the vagina can gain entrance to the pelvis and cause pelvic cellulitis. If a hematoma or a seroma develop and bacteria gain entrance, an abscess can form. The microbiologic makeup of a postoperative infection that occurs in the pelvis differs from one that occurs in an abdominal surgical incision. However, the microbial pathophysiology, events that occur during the operative procedures, and host factors are probably similar.

## PREVENTION

Prevention of postoperative infection in gynecologic surgery begins with knowing the patient's past history of infection, her current status with regard to inherent risk factors, and what preventive measures were taken during the operative procedure. If the patient had surgery in the past and developed a postoperative infection, she may have an inherent defect in her immune system or a chronic subclinical infection (e.g., gingivitis) or an altered vaginal microflora. Therefore, reviewing her history may raise the need for further evaluation before performing an elective operation.

Risk factors inherent to patients fall into three categories: chronic illness (e.g., IDDM, severe chronic hypertension, immunosuppressive diseases, morbid obesity, smoking, abuse of alcohol), altered vaginal microflora syndromes, and recent antibiotic therapy.

Patients with chronic illness should be evaluated to ensure that the illness is properly managed and controlled. The diabetic patient's blood glucose should be under control weeks before the operative procedure is performed. Both severe diabetes and chronic hypertension have significant effects on the peripheral circulation. The presence of hyperglycemia in any tissue involved in the operative procedure will suppress phagocytic activity. The tissue supplied by the peripheral circulation is compromised and therefore not well perfused and oxygenated. Combine this with the mechanical effects of the operative procedure and these tissues will experience a degree of hypoxia. In addition to the hypoxia there is a decrease in antibiotic that will be perfusing this tissue. Therefore, the patient must be well oxygenated during the procedure. If the patient uses tobacco products, nicotine will also have an effect on the peripheral vascular system as well as impairing lung function. The patient should have pulmonary function studies performed to determine if there is decreased lung function. The patient should be instructed to quit smoking or using tobacco products 3 weeks before admission to the hospital for her surgery. Before surgery the patient should also be instructed in the use of incentive spirometery. The morbidly

obese patient should be evaluated for hyperglycemia, hypertension, the presence of altered vaginal microflora, and nasal carriage of *Staphylococcus aureus*, as well as have pulmonary function studies, a chest x-ray, and a consultation with a pulmonologist if the pulmonary functions are abnormal.

All patients undergoing an operative procedure involving the vagina, regardless of the degree of involvement, should have an assessment of the lower genital tract microflora to determine if it is altered. This is easily accomplished by determining the color of the discharge, the pH, and whether an odor is present, and by taking a wet preparation (Table 23-2). If microscopic examination of the vaginal discharge reveals the presence of an altered vaginal microflora or bacterial vaginosis and the presence of WBCs, the physician should evaluate the patient further for the possible existence of an associated infection (e.g., *Trichomonas vaginalis* or cervical infection with *Chlamydia trachomatis*, *Neisseria gonorrhoeae*, herpes simplex virus, or human papillomavirus). Patients with an altered vaginal microflora who are going to have elective vaginal surgery are at risk for the development of a postoperative pelvic infection. These patients are at great risk for postoperative pelvic infection even after receiving antibiotic prophylaxis before the operative procedure.[5] Although antibiotic prophylaxis has been shown to reduce the risk of postoperative infection, patients with altered vaginal microflora may derive only partial benefit from antibiotic prophylaxis.[6-9]

Antibiotic prophylaxis is recommended for patients who are not infected. Patients with an abnormal vaginal microflora should be considered to have a subclinical or clinical infection because the number of pathogenic bacteria in the vaginal microflora is in excess of $10^6$ bacteria/mL of vaginal fluid. It can be hypothesized that this amount of bacteria is too high for surgical prophylaxis to overcome.

Patients designated to receive antibiotic prophylaxis should receive a single dose within 1 hour of beginning the operative procedure. If the patient has a clinically apparent or subclinical infection she should receive therapeutic doses of antibiotic. If the operative procedure is associated with more than 1500 mL of blood loss or lasts longer than 3 hours, a second dose of antibiotic should be administered. The antibiotic should be given to noninfected patients scheduled for an operative

| | | **Table 23-2** | | | |
| | | **Assessment of the Vaginal Microflora** | | | |
| **Character of Discharge** | **Healthy** | **Bacterial Vaginosis** | **Altered Vaginal Flora** | **Trichomonas** | **Candida** |
|---|---|---|---|---|---|
| Color | White to slate-gray | Dirty gray | Gray, green-yellow, green | Dirty gray | Gray |
| Odor | No | Yes | No | Possibly | No |
| pH | <4.5 | >5 | >5 | >5 | <4.5 |
| Whiff test | Negative | Positive | Negative | Possibly negative | Positive |
| Clue cells | No | Yes | No | Maybe* | No |
| WBCs | No | No | Maybe† | Yes | Maybe† |
| Lactobacillus dominant | Yes | No | No | No | Possibly |

*Clue cells may or may not be present.
†White blood cells may or may not be present.

Gynecologic Infectious Disease

| Table 23-3 | |
|---|---|
| **Indications for Antibiotic Prophylaxis** | |
| **Procedures with a Definite Indication** | **Possible Indications (no data available)** |
| Total vaginal hysterectomy | Laparoscopic hysterectomy |
| Elective abortion | Tension-free and subobturator urethral sling |
| Abdominal hysterectomy | Retropubic urethral suspension |
| | Colposacropexy |

procedure that has been associated with a significant risk for development of a postoperative infection (Table 23-3).

Antibiotic administered prophylactically should not be given without a definite indication because of its impact on the endogenous vaginal microflora. Several investigators have demonstrated that even a single dose of antibiotic can cause changes in the endogenous microflora. Cephalosporins will select for the enterococci, even when a single dose is administered.[10]

## DIAGNOSIS AND MANAGEMENT

The clinical signs of infection are an elevated body temperature and tachycardia. These two findings should alert the physician to initiate a physical examination, including a pelvic examination, in the postoperative patient regardless of the amount of time that has elapsed since completion of the operative procedure. Additional findings indicative of infection are elevated WBC count, an increase (>10%) in immature polymorphonuclear leukocytes, an increased pulse rate that parallels the temperature, pain at the operative site that is not relieved by the prescribed analgesic, and a persistent ileus. In addition, both the patient's abdominal and vaginal incisions should be inspected.

The clinical findings that indicate that a patient may have an infection in the incisions are erythema, swelling, edema, increased temperature in the tissue surrounding the incision, pain, and drainage from the incision. The incision should be carefully inspected; if any of the above is present, the incision should be examined via ultrasonography. If a pocket of fluid is observed, it should be aspirated and Gram stain and culture of the fluid for bacteria should be performed (Table 23-4). Once the pocket of fluid has been aspirated, it should be placed into appropriate transport media for isolation of aerobic and anaerobic bacteria and mycoplasmas (*Mycoplasma* and *Ureaplasma*). The incision should then be opened and completely drained, all necrotic tissue should be débrided, and the incision packed with gauze moistened with 0.025% acetic acid. The dressing should be changed three to four times a day. If there is no evidence of infection after 48 hours of wound management, the incision can be closed. If there was documented infection or necrotic tissue, this wound management protocol should be continued until a complete layer of granulation has formed. Once this layer of tissue has formed, the incision can be closed with suture or Steri-Strips or by gradual closure. Alternatively the wound could be allowed to close by secondary intention. When initially evaluating the incision for possible infection, it is important to

ensure that the infection has not progressed to necrotizing fasciitis (as discussed in Chapter 18).

After the abdominal incision has been evaluated, the patient should be thoroughly examined. It is critical to determine if the patient has an infection outside of the pelvis. The surgical patient is at risk for developing a variety of infections because of the anesthetic, the use of peripheral lines, and an indwelling (Foley) catheter. Each of these systems must be evaluated to ensure that infection has not occurred. Once the examination is complete, an assessment of the pelvis should be performed. The vaginal discharge should be examined for the presence of pus, its origin, and the presence of erythema at the vaginal apex. The vaginal apex should be palpated to determine if the tissue is hot to the touch. A bimanual and rectal examination should also be performed to determine if a mass is present. If there is evidence of purulent fluid draining from the cuff, a needle should be inserted through the incision at this point and the fluid aspirated. Gram stain and culture for aerobic, facultative, and obligate anaerobic bacteria should be performed on the fluid.

If a mass is detected, an ultrasonogram should be obtained to determine if there is a pelvic mass and its location. If a pelvic mass is present, ultrasonography can reveal its characteristics: whether its wall is thin or thick; whether septations are present; and where free fluid is present in the pelvis. If a definitive mass is present at the vaginal cuff, it can be completely drained by gently opening the cuff. If the mass is not adjacent to the vaginal cuff, the patient should be taken to the operating room so the mass can be drained vaginally under anesthesia. Once the mass has been drained, a drain (e.g., a Foley catheter, or a mushroom or similar drain) should be attached to a suction device and should remain in place until only minimal drainage accumulates over a 24-hour period.

As soon as a diagnosis of infection is suspected, the patient should be administered intravenous broad-spectrum antibiotics (Table 23-5). If the patient received a prophylactic antibiotic, this should be considered when choosing an antibiotic regimen for treatment. Cephalosporins are the most commonly used antibiotics for prophylaxis and can select for resistant bacteria. In addition, most pelvic infections are polymicrobial; therefore, empiric antibiotic therapy should provide coverage against gram-negative and gram-positive aerobic, facultative, and obligate anaerobic bacteria. Thus, it may be prudent to initiate treatment

| Table 23-4 | | |
|---|---|---|
| **Evaluation of the Infected Wound** | | |
| **Fluid Color** | **Gram-stain Characteristics** | **Action** |
| Serous and clear | Few WBCs, no bacteria | Drain |
| Serous and cloudy | WBCs >5/hpf, no bacteria | Culture for *Mycoplasma* and *Ureaplasma* |
| Seropurulent | WBCs >5/hpf, bacteria + | Culture for aerobes and anaerobes |
| Serosanguineous | Few WBCs, no bacteria | Drain |
| Bloody | WBCs >5/hpf, bacteria +/− | Culture for aerobes, anaerobes, *Mycoplasma* and *Ureaplasma* |

**Table 23-5**
**Antibiotic Choices for Treatment of Postoperative Pelvic Infections**

Piperacillin/tazobactam 3.375 g IV q 6 hr
Ampicillin/sulbactam 3 g IV q 6 hr
Piperacillin/tazobactam or ampicillin/sulbactam + gentamicin 5 mg/kg of
    body weight q 24 hr or 2 mg/kg of body weight as a loading dose followed
    by 1.5 mg/kg of body weight q 8 hr
Metronidazole 500 mg IV q 8 hr + gentamicin + ampicillin 2 g q 6 hr
Metronidazole + levofloxacin 500 mg q 24 hr
Levofloxacin 500 mg or 750 mg q 24 hr
Clindamycin 900 mg IV q 8 hr + gentamicin + ampicillin
Clindamycin + levofloxacin
Imipenem 1 g IV q 12 hr
Invanz 1 g IV q 24 hr

with broad-spectrum penicillin or combination therapy (see Table 23-5).

When gentamicin is administered, serum levels should be obtained. If once-a-day dosing is used, a trough level should be obtained before administration of the third dose. If dosing every 8 hours is used, trough and peak serum levels should be obtained at the third dose. If the trough levels are elevated, there is an increased risk for ototoxicity and/or nephrotoxicity; peak levels will determine if a therapeutic level of gentamicin is achieved at the dose being administered.

Specimens should be obtained for culture, isolation, and identification of any bacteria. If a possible infection site is identified, a specimen should be obtained for microbiologic analysis. Venous blood should be obtained for the possible identification of bacteremia. A urine specimen should also be obtained for analysis, Gram stain, culture, identification, and sensitivity. If the surgical incision is intact, the abdominal wall should be examined via ultrasonography to determine if there is fluid collection. If there is a collection of fluid, the area should be aspirated and the fluid processed for detection and identification of bacteria (i.e., Gram stain and culture for aerobic, facultative, and obligate anaerobic bacteria). If the incision has spontaneously opened, opens easily, or is necrotic, tissue should be sent for culture of aerobic, facultative, and obligate anaerobic bacteria.

After the patient has received antibiotic therapy for 48 hours, she should show a positive response. If the patient does not demonstrate improvement (Table 23-6), consideration should be given to additional diagnostic tests and the addition of new antibiotics to broaden the range of therapy to cover the possibility of an emerging resistant bacterium. If the physical examination does not reveal anything significant and laboratory tests are not helpful, a change in antibiotic therapy may be indicated as well as more diagnostic tests (e.g., abdominal/pelvic ultrasonography and/or computed tomography [CT] scan). Choosing additional or new antibiotic therapy without microbiological data is difficult, and the antibiotic chosen often results in redundancy. The most likely bacteria to emerge as resistant to current antibiotic therapy are gram-negative facultative anaerobes (e.g., members of Enterobacteriaceae) and possibly gram-positive bacterium (e.g., *Enterococcus*). If metronidazole is being administered there is probably no need to change to another agent, such as clindamycin, because there is the possibility of

a resistant obligate anaerobic bacterium emerging within the immediate 48-hour postoperative period. If an aminoglycoside is not being administered, it should be given in place of any other antibiotic, providing coverage for possible involvement of gram-negative facultative bacteria. If gentamicin or tobramycin is being administered, it should be discontinued and amikacin initiated. Penicillin should be administered to provide activity against gram-positive bacteria and synergy with the aminoglycoside against enterococci and streptococci. Initial empiric antibiotic therapy must be broad-spectrum because the infection is frequently polymicrobial, involving gram-positive and gram-negative facultative and obligate anaerobic bacteria (Table 23-7).

The patient who continues to have an elevated body temperature but has a normal pulse rate should be considered as possibly having drug fever. Physical examination of the patient with drug fever is typically negative. It is important to perform a complete examination, including a urinalysis, urine Gram stain, urine culture, chest x-ray, CT scan of the abdomen and pelvis, complete blood count with WBC differential, and blood glucose. Once the patient's evaluation is completed and there is no focus of infection, all antibiotic therapy can be discontinued. All medication should be reviewed and consideration given to discontinuing nonessential medications. If after discontinuing antibiotic therapy and nonessential medications the patient does not become afebrile within 24 to 48 hours, re-evaluation is necessary to determine if a focus of infection (e.g., pelvic or intra-abdominal abscess, wound infection, bacteremia, or endocarditis) should be sought.

**Table 23-6**
**Clinical Findings Consistent with Ongoing Postoperative Infection**

Recent peak body temperature that is above or equal to the previous peak
    temperature
WBC count that remains elevated and has not shown a downward trend;
    WBC count dropping below the preoperative WBC count
Low blood sugar
An elevated pulse rate that continues to parallel the temperature
Persistent ileus
Level of abdominal/pelvic pain unchanged or worsening
Persistent tachypnea
Evaluation of the surgical site
    Increasing erythema
        Advancing margin of erythema (cellulites)
        Increased intensity of erythema
    Differential of pain
        Areas of intense pain, typically distant from the incision site
        Areas of anesthesia at the surgical site
    Characteristics of drainage
        Serous
        Serosanguineous
        Bloody
        Dark brownish or gray-greenish
        Frank pus
    Integrity of the incision
        Intact
        Spontaneous separation
        Necrosis

**Table 23-7**
**Antibiotic Choices for the Treatment of Postoperative Pelvic Infection**

Initial empiric choices
  Piperacillin/tazobactam 3.375 g IV q 6 hr
  Ampicillin/sulbactam 3.1 g IV q 6 hr
  Ticarcillin/clavulanic acid 3 g IV q 6 hr
  Clindamycin 900 mg IV q 8 hr + gentamicin 5 mg/kg of body weight IV q 24 hr
  Metronidazole 500 mg IV q 8 hr + gentamicin 5 mg/kg of body weight q 24 hr
  Clindamycin or metronidazole + gentamicin + ampicillin 2 g IV q 6 hr
  Clindamycin or metronidazole + levofloxacin 500 mg IV q 24 hr
  Ertapenem 1 g IV q 24 hr
  Imipenem 500 mg IV q 6 hr
  Meropenem 1 g IV q 8 hr
  Cefotetan 2 g IV q 12 hr

Alteration in antibiotic therapy for patients who fail initial therapy (after the patient has been re-evaluated and the presence of an abscess or septic pelvic vein thrombosis) is discovered
Patient is taking a penicillin: add gentamicin to increase gram-negative facultative antibacterial activity
Patient is receiving clindamycin or metronidazole + gentamicin: add ampicillin 2 g IV q 6 hr
Patient is on clindamycin or metronidazole + gentamicin + ampicillin: delete gentamicin and add amikacin 15 mg/kg. (The rationale is that it is highly unlikely that the patient has a resistant obligate anaerobic bacterium or a resistant gram-positive aerobe.)
Patient is receiving ertapenem, imipenem, or meropenem: discontinue and begin clindamycin + gentamicin + ampicillin
Patient is receiving cefoxitin or cefotetan: discontinue and begin piperacillin/tazobactam + gentamicin

## ETIOLOGY OF SEPTIC SHOCK

Failure to respond aggressively to the postoperative patient with infection leads to progressive deterioration and evolution to septic shock. Once the bacteria initiate the cytokine cascade, down-regulation of the system is prevented, thereby resulting in the production of tumor necrosis factor (TNF-$\alpha$). This cytokine cascade results in adverse effects on multiple organs. The initial response to infection is stimulation or up-regulation of the pro-inflammatory system. Once the patient enters the path to septic shock and with failure of aggressive intervention, progression to septic shock is rapid and often results in death. The mortality rate from septic shock varies from 20% to 80% and is related to the severity of the sepsis and the underlying disease.[11–13] In many cases of sepsis, the presence of microorganisms or toxins (i.e., LPS) in the blood cannot be established. This led to the establishment of the definitions listed in Table 23-8.

The patient undergoing gynecologic surgery who develops septic shock following the development of a postoperative infection may initially be a healthy individual with no particularly significant underlying illness. The patient develops an infection, which is frequently polymicrobial and involves gram-positive and gram-negative facultative and obligate anaerobic bacteria, with production and liberation of toxins that are disseminated by the bloodstream throughout the body. The patient has an exaggerated and overwhelming response to the infection and bacterial toxins occurs by release of macrophage-derived cytokines, which act on receptors of a variety of host organs. There are two classes of mediators—primary and secondary

(Table 23-9). Primary mediators—cytokines—stimulate the release of secondary mediators; together these responses have been termed the systemic inflammatory response syndrome (SIRS).

The host's initial response to infection is orderly and occurs in stages; however, if this goes unchecked, the result is severe damage to the host's organs. Stage I (pro-inflammatory response) is the release of the cytokines interleukin-1 and interleukin-6 (IL-1, IL-6) and TNF-$\alpha$, and the secondary mediators eicosanoids and platelet-releasing factor at the site of infection. This is the host's initial response to limit the infection and repair any damaged tissue. If these mediators are left unchecked or remain up-regulated, they can cause damage. If the system is to be down-regulated, the host or body initiates release of compensatory anti-inflammatory agents (i.e., IL-4, IL-10, IL-11, IL-13, soluble TNF receptors, IL-1 receptor antagonists, and TNF-$\beta$).[14–16] These anti-inflammatory compounds inhibit the expression of the major histocompatibility complex class II, impair antigen presentation, and reduce the host cell's ability to produce inflammatory cytokines. The cytokines can even down-regulate their own production.[17] Pro-inflammatory and anti-inflammatory mediators can reach high concentrations and are localized to the site of infection.

If the initial infection is severe, a systemic inflammatory response occurs (Stage II). In bacteremic or septic patients, both bacterial toxins and anti-inflammatory mediators appear in

**Table 23-8**
**Definitions for Sepsis and Septic Shock**

| Condition | Definition |
|---|---|
| Bacteremia | Positive blood cultures |
| Sepsis | Clinical evidence of infection, tachypnea (>20 breaths/min), tachycardia (>90 beats/min), hyperthermia, or hypothermia |
| Septicemia | Presence of microbes or microbial toxins in the bloodstream |
| Systemic inflammatory response syndrome | Patient reponse to disseminated infection or toxins Two or more of the following: fever (>38°C); tachypnea (>24 breaths/min); tachycardia (>90 beats/min); leukocytosis (>12,000/μL); leukopenia (<4000/μL) |
| Sepsis syndrome | Sepsis plus hypoxemia or elevated plasma lactate levels or oliguria |
| Severe sepsis | Sepsis plus one or more signs of organ dysfunction: metabolic acidosis, acute anencephalopathy, oliguria, hypoxemia, DIC, or hypotension |
| Early septic shock | Sepsis syndrome plus hypotension |
| Septic shock | Sepsis syndrome plus hypotension in the presence of adequate volume resuscitation |

Adapted from Van Amersfoort ES, Van Berkel TJ, Kuiper J: Receptors, mediators, and mechanisms involved in bacterial sepsis and septic shock. Clin Microbiol Rev 2003;16:379–414; Bone RC: Systemic inflammatory syndrome: a unifying concept of systemic inflammation. In Fein AM, Abraham EM, Balk RA, et al (eds): Sepsis and Multiorgan Failure. Baltimore, Williams and Wilkins, 1977, 3–10; and Faro S: Sepsis in obstetric and gynecologic patients. In Remington JS, Swartz MN (eds): Current Clinical Topics in Infectious Diseases. Malden, Mass, Blackwell Science, Inc., 1999; pp 60–62.

| Table 23-9<br>Components of the Systemic Inflammatory Response Syndrome | |
|---|---|
| **Primary Mediators (Cytokines)** | **Secondary Mediators** |
| Interleukin-1 (IL-1) | Platelet-activating factor |
| Interleukin-2 (IL-2) | Eicosanoids: Leukotrienes $B_4$, $C_4$, $D_4$, $E_4$<br>Thromboxane $A_2$<br>Prostaglandins $E_2$, $I_2$ |
| Interleukin-4 (IL-4) | Interferon-$\gamma$ |
| Interleukin-6 (IL-6) | Granulocyte-macrophage colony-<br>stimulating factor |
| Interleukin-8 (IL-8) | Endothelium-derived relaxing factor |
| Tumor necrosis factor-$\alpha$ (TNF-$\alpha$) | Endothelin-1 |
| | Complement fragments C3a, C5a |
| | Polymorphonuclear cells<br>Toxic oxygen radicals<br>Proteolytic enzymes |
| | Adhesion molecules<br>Endothelial-leukocyte adhesion<br>molecule 1<br>Intracellular adhesion molecule 1<br>Vascular cell adhesion molecule 1 |
| | Platelets |
| | Transforming growth factor-$\beta_1$ (TNF-$\beta_1$) |
| | Vascular permeability factor |
| | Macrophage-derived procoagulant and<br>inflammatory cytokines |
| | Bradykinin |
| | Thrombin coagulation factor |
| | Fibrin |
| | Plasmogen-activator inhibitor |
| | Myocardial depressant factor |
| | $\beta$-endorphin |
| | Heat shock protein |

the host's circulatory system. If the local infection is severe, the pro-inflammatory mediators may achieve high concentrations at the site and leak into the systemic circulation, thus initiating SIRS.[18] Initially the pro-inflammatory response acts as a normal response to infection. This results in the recruitment of neutrophils, T cells, B cells, platelets, and coagulation factors to the site of infection. If this response is left unchecked then SIRS will develop and the pro-inflammatory agents will stimulate an anti-inflammatory response.

Failure to down-regulate the pro-inflammatory response results in a massive systemic inflammatory response (Stage III). The clinical characteristics of SIRS (i.e., body temperature <36°C or >38°C; tachycardia >90 beats/min; tachypnea; a $PaCO_2$ <32 mmHg; and an elevated WBC count [<12,000/μL]) or leukopnea (<4,000/μL) develop (Table 23-10). The patient can develop edema of organs secondary to damage to endothelial cells, thereby allowing microvascular leakage.[19,20] The patient also develops sludging within the circulatory system along with increased platelet aggregation, which results in the formation of thrombi within the microcirculation and blood being diverted from tissues and organs. This results in tissue and organ ischemia,

which can result in reperfusion injury and the induction of heat shock protein.[21-24]

Once thrombosis begins activation of the coagulation system, the patient can deplete the store of coagulation factors and develop disseminated intravascular coagulation (DIC). Consumption of coagulation factors leads to bleeding. DIC can produce concurrent thrombosis that results in serious hypoperfusion of tissues, leading to gangrene, acrocyanosis, and skin necrosis. The bleeding associated with DIC leads to the development of petechiae, purpura, and ecchymosis.

Significant systemic inflammation can alter the vasodilatory and vasoconstrictive mechanisms, typically resulting in vasodilation. This causes transudation of fluids from the vascular compartment to tissues and changes blood flow. This leads to shock, organ dysfunction, and death.

Individuals who survive septic shock may, in turn, experience excessive immune suppression (Stage IV). This overcompensatory reaction results in immune suppression, "immune paralysis," or a "window of immunodeficiency."[25,26] This syndrome occurs in patients who develop shock secondary to severe burns, hemorrhage, or trauma. This may explain why gynecologic and obstetric patients who develop shock secondary to hemorrhage become infected.

The final stage in SIRS (Stage V) is referred to as immunologic dissonance and precedes multiple organ dysfunction syndrome. The presence of both SIRS and multiple organ dysfunction syndrome is the result of an overwhelming concentration of pro-inflammatory mediators. If this up-regulation cannot be reversed, the patient is at increased risk for death. Organ failure occurs in steps, the first organ to fail is the lungs, followed by the liver, then the gastrointestinal tract, and finally the kidneys.

Septicemia rates more than doubled in the United States between 1979 and 1987, resulting in approximately 250,000 deaths each year.[13,27] The proportion of infections caused by gram-negative bacteria ranges from 30% to 80%; those caused by gram-positive bacteria, from 6% to 24% of the total number of septic cases.[28] Sepsis secondary to gram-positive bacteria, especially *S. aureus* and *S. epidermidis*, rose in the 1990s and accounted for more than 50% of the cases of septicemia.[29,30] Bacterial infection is often mild or moderate but can be severe, leading to sepsis, bacteremia, or both. One key bacterial factor leading to septic shock is the endotoxin of gram-negative bacteria, LPS. The gram-negative bacterial cell wall is complex. It consists of a capsule, the outermost layer, an outer membrane that consists of LPS, a lipid bilayer, a peptidoglycan, and an inner cell membrane.[31] When LPS is contained within the bacterial cell wall, it is not toxic. However, when LPS is released (e.g., during bacterial cell multiplication) bacterial cell death or lysis disruption

| Table 23-10<br>Clinical Manifestations of Systemic Inflammatory Response Syndrome |
|---|
| Body temperature <36°C or >38°C |
| Tachycardia (90 beats/min) |
| Tachypnea (>20 breaths/min) |
| $PaCO_2$ <32 mmHg |
| WBC count <400/μL or >12,000/μL or >10% increase in immature<br>polymorphonuclear leukocytes |

# Gynecologic Infectious Disease

of the cell wall occurs, and the toxic moiety, lipid A, is exposed to immune cells and initiates an inflammatory response.[32,33] The gram-positive bacterial cell wall contains a compound similar to LPS—lipoteichoic acid (LTA)—as well as other lipid components (e.g., diglucosyldiacylglycerol, phosphatidylglycerol, diacylglycerol, and lysylphosphatidylglycerol).[34,35]

When bacteria enter the human body, two defensive systems come into action: the humoral (i.e., complement) system of antibodies and acute phase proteins and the cellular system of monocytes, macrophages, and neutrophils. Under normal physiologic conditions, the immune cells are continuously exposed to low levels of LPS from the bacteria in the gastrointestinal tract that gain entrance into the body via the portal circulation.[33] It is currently hypothesized that the continuous challenge of bacterial constituents is necessary to maintain the immune system in a ready state to infection.[36–38] Once a significant concentration of LPS or LTA is introduced into the body (i.e., infection is established), the pro-inflammatory response is triggered. If the host cannot contain the infection with or without the assistance of antimicrobial agents and the cytokine system cannot be down-regulated, the patient will progress into septic shock.

## MANAGEMENT OF SEPTIC SHOCK

Infection in the postoperative gynecologic patient should initially be considered polymicrobial (i.e., involving both gram-positive and gram-negative bacteria). Therefore, initial therapy should be with intravenous administration of broad-spectrum antibiotics (Table 23-11). Piperacillin/tazobactam, clindamycin, or metronidazole will provide excellent coverage against the obligate anaerobic bacteria. Although clindamycin does have activity against many gram-positive bacteria such as staphylococci and streptococci, gentamicin will provide slightly better activity against staphylococci and ampicillin will provide more comprehensive activity against streptococci. Gentamicin will provide broad coverage against gram-negative facultative bacteria. The combination of gentamicin and ampicillin will provide synergistic activity against enterococci and streptococci.

Patients developing, or suspected of developing, septic shock should be monitored very closely. A Foley catheter should be inserted to monitor urine output. A Swan-Ganz catheter should be placed to monitor pulmonary artery wedge pressure and cardiac output as well as to calculate oxygen delivery and utilization.[39,40] Both cardiac output and peripheral vascular resistance are important; for antibiotic therapy to be effective it must reach the site of infection and be equally distributed throughout the circulatory system. Therefore, the tissues must be adequately perfused and oxygenated. The patient's airway

must be maintained and the lungs adequately oxygenated. Volume expansion and correction of hypovolemia are critical in maintaining adequate blood pressure and, in turn, tissue perfusion. A significant decrease in blood pressure will result in poor tissue and organ perfusion, which will then be manifested by increased peripheral resistance, a decrease in kidney perfusion and urine output, and an increase in interstitial fluid or edema. If increases in fluid replacement do not result in increased urine output and cardiac output, the patient will require pressor agents. Initially, dopamine, with both alpha- and beta-adrenergic effects, is administered.[41] Doses smaller than 5 µg/kg/min are associated with increased blood flow to the kidneys and mesentery. Doses between 5 and 20 µg/kg/min primarily result in more effective myocardial contraction, increased cardiac output, and a resultant increase in myocardial oxygenation. Doses in excess of 20 µg/kg/min result in primarily alpha effects (i.e., in increased vasoconstriction and decreased tissue perfusion). Dopamine is usually administered in a dose of 2 to 5 µg/kg of body weight/min to achieve an increased blood flow (cardiac output) to the kidneys and increase urine output.[42]

Alternatives to dopamine are dobutamine and norepinephrine. Dobutamine increases cardiac output and oxygenation and improves tissue perfusion by decreasing systemic vascular resistance.[43] Dobutamine is frequently used in combination with dopamine to maintain renal perfusion and improve cardiac output. Epinephrine increases cardiac output, oxygenation, and blood pressure. However, although the patient may appear to have improved oxygenation, there is a decrease in tissue oxygenation, increased cardiac work, and greater myocardial oxygen requirements.[44,45]

If vasoconstriction becomes profound and tissue perfusion is significantly impaired, cells become hypoxic and acidotic. This leads to cell death. Arterioles cannot respond to histamine and bradykinin.[46] Immunologic complexes form and cause significant tissue injury, especially in the lung. These complexes develop within the vasculature of the lung and lead to the development of adult respiratory distress syndrome (ARDS) and within the tubules of the kidney.[47] ARDS results in a further oxygen deficit and increased tissue hypoxia. Systemic tissue hypoxia results in microscopic injury to bowel mucosa, allowing for translocation of bacteria and toxins across the bowel wall, thereby worsening septic shock.[48,49] Failure to reverse septic shock results in the development of anaerobic metabolism, which in turn leads to lactic acidosis, multiple organ dysfunction, and death.[50] Oxygen must be delivered until the concentration of lactic acid returns to normal, tissue perfusion is improved, and organ dysfunction is reversed.

Thus, the patient who develops sepsis must be regarded as on the verge of developing septic shock because this is the greatest opportunity to treat the patient and reverse the course to septic shock. The initial response of the physician is to administer broad-spectrum antibiotics and insert a Foley catheter and a Swan-Ganz catheter if there is a decrease in urine output and blood pressure. If the pulmonary wedge pressure is normal, volume replacement must be initiated; if it is decreased, dopamine should be administered. The patient should be transferred to an intensive care unit and a critical care specialist consulted.

---

**Table 23-11**
**Antibiotic Therapy for Postoperative Infection in the Septic Patient**

Piperacillin/tazobactam 3.375 g q 6 hr + gentamicin 5 mg/kg of body weight q 24 hr

Clindamycin 900 mg q 8 hr + gentamicin + ampicillin 2 g q 6 hr

Metronidazole 500 mg q 8 hr + gentamicin + ampicillin

## TREATMENT

Administering antibiotic therapy to patients having undergone gynecologic surgery and subsequently develop a pelvic infection and/or surgical site infection is based on the following principles:

- Most patients receive antibiotic prophylaxis.
- The most frequently administered antibiotic is a cephalosporin, which can select for *Enterococcus*.
- Postoperative pelvic infection is typically due to the endogenous vaginal microflora.
- Surgical site infection is due to *S. aureus* and endogenous vaginal microflora.

Therefore, the antibiotic regimen chosen for pelvic infection should provide coverage against the following:

- Gram-positive aerobic bacteria (e.g., *Streptococcus agalactiae*, *Enterococcus faecalis*)
- Gram-negative facultative anaerobic bacteria (e.g., *E. coli*, *Enterobacter* sp., *Klebsiella pneumoniae*)
- Obligate anaerobic bacteria (e.g., *Prevotella*, *Peptostreptococcus*, *Fusobacterium*, *Bacteroides*)
- Surgical-site infection, whether caused by gram-positive aerobic bacteria (e.g., *S. aureus* (MRSA), *Streptococcus* sp.) or a mixed polymicrobial infection

The initial choice of antibiotic for pelvic infection should provide broad antimicrobial coverage (Table 23-12).

Patients can initially be treated with a single agent, piperacillin/tazobactam, which provides activity against most bacteria that cause pelvic cellulitis and vaginal cuff cellulitis. If the patient does not demonstrate improvement after 48 hours of antibiotic therapy, gentamicin should be added to increase the gram-negative facultative anaerobic coverage. If the infection began within the first 24 to 48 hours postoperative, the dominant bacteria involved in the infection are gram-positive and gram-negative facultative anaerobes. If the patient continues to fail to respond, repeat the physical examination and obtain imaging studies (i.e., ultrasonography or CT scan of the abdomen and pelvis). It is important to rule out the presence of infected hematoma or abscess.

Alternatively, therapy can be initiated with either clindamycin or metronidazole, understanding that there is a significant difference between clindamycin and metronidazole. Clindamycin has activity against both obligate anaerobic bacteria and gram-positive aerobes (i.e., *S. aureus*, including some strains of MRSA, and *S. agalactiae*), whereas metronidazole only has activity against obligate anaerobes. Therefore, neither clindamycin nor metronidazole has activity against enterococci. Thus, patients treated with either of the above antibiotics and not responding should have ampicillin and gentamicin added to the regimen. The addition of ampicillin acts synergistically with gentamicin and increases activity against streptococci and enterococci. Another advantage of clindamycin and gentamicin is that this antibiotic combination provides a relatively good degree of activity against MRSA.

Surgical site infections can be divided into two categories—cellulitis and abscess. One aid in the management of surgical site infection is ultrasonography, which can delineate a collection of fluid. If fluid is present, aspiration can be performed with ultrasound guidance. A Gram stain of this fluid can assist in choosing appropriate antibiotic therapy. For example, if gram-positive cocci in chains are present, a broad-spectrum penicillin would be used; if the cocci are in clusters, clindamycin and gentamicin, which will provide coverage against MRSA, are the proper choice. If the Gram stain reveals a polymicrobial infection, piperacillin/tazobactam + gentamicin or clindamycin can be administered. If an abscess is present, the incision should be opened, the abscess drained, and any necrotic tissue present should be débrided. Aggressive management of surgical site infection can result in a speedy recovery and prevention of necrotizing fasciitis.

**Table 23-12**
**Antibiotic Choices for Treatment of Postoperative Infection**

| Antibiotic (IV) | Dose | Bacterial Coverage |
|---|---|---|
| Piperacillin/tazobactam | 3.37 g q 6 hr | Gram-positive Gram-negative Obligate anaerobes |
| Piperacillin/tazobactam + gentamicin | 5 mg/kg q 24 hr | Facultative gram-negative anaerobes |
| Clindamycin + gentamicin* | 900 mg q 8 hr | Obligate anaerobes Gram-positive aerobes |
| Metronidazole + gentamicin* | 500 mg q 8 hr | Obligate anaerobes |
| Clindamycin + gentamicin* + ampicillin | 2 g q 6 hr | Gram-positive aerobes |

*Gentamicin 5 mg/kg of body weight every 24 hours or 2 mg/kg of body weight loading dose followed by 1.5 mg/kg of body weight every 8 hours.

## REFERENCES

1. Faro S, Phillips LE, Martens MG: Perspectives on the bacteriology of postoperative obstetric-gynecologic infections. Am J Obstet Gynecol 1988;158:694–700. **(Ib, A)**
2. Aroutcheva A, Gariti D, Simon M, et al: Defense factors of vaginal lactobacilli. Am J Obstet Gynecol 2001;185:375–379. **(IIa, B)**
3. Aroutcheva A, Simoes JA, Faro S: Antimicrobial protein produced by vaginal *Lactobacillus acidophilus* that inhibits *Gardnerella vaginalis*. Infect Dis Obstet Gynecol 2001;9:33–39. **(IIa, B)**
4. Martens MG, Faro S, Riddle G: Female genital tract abscess formation in the rat. Use of pathogens including enterococci. J Reprod Med 1993; 38:719–724. **(Ib, A)**
5. Lin L, Song J, Kimber N, et al: The role of bacterial vaginosis in infection after major gynecologic surgery. Infect Dis Obstet Gynecol 1999;7:169–174. **(IIa, B)**
6. Weigelt JA, Faro S: Antimicrobial therapy for surgical prophylaxis and for intra-abdominal and gynecologic infections. Am J Surg 1998; 176:1S–3S. **(IV, C)**
7. Benigno BB, Evrard J, Faro S, et al: A comparison of piperacillin, cephalothin and cefoxitin in the prevention of postoperative infections in patients undergoing vaginal hysterectomy. Surg Gynecol Obstet 1986;163:421–427. **(Ib, A)**
8. Poindexter AN, Ritter M, Faro S, et al: Results of noncomparative studies of cefotetan in the treatment of obstetric and gynecologic infections. Am J Obstet Gynecol 1988;158:717–721. **(III, B)**

# Gynecologic Infectious Disease

9. Sweet RL, Roy S, Faro S, et al: Piperacillin and tazobactam versus clindamycin and gentamicin in the treatment of hospitalized women with pelvic infection. The piperacillin/tazobactam study group. Obstet Gynecol 1994;83:280–286. **(Ib, A)**

10. Faro S, Martens MG, Hammill HA, et al: Antibiotic prophylaxis: is there a difference? Am J Obstet Gynecol 1990;162:900–907. **(Ib, A)**

11. Bone RC: The pathogenesis of sepsis. Ann Intern Med 1991; 115:457–469. **(III, B)**

12. Bone RC: Why new definitions of sepsis and organ failure are needed. Am J Med 1993;95:348–350. **(IV, C)**

13. Parrillo JE: Mechanisms of disease: pathogenetic mechanisms of septic shock. N Engl J Med 1993;328:1471–1478. **(IIa, B)**

14. Dinarello CA, Gelfand JA, Wolff SM: Anticytokine strategies in the treatment of the systemic inflammatory response syndrome. JAMA 1993;269:1829–1835. **(IIa, B)**

15. Platzer C, Meisel CH, Vogt K, et al: Up-regulation of monocytic IL-10 by tumor necrosis factor-α and cAMP-elevating drugs. Int Immunol 1995;7:517–523. **(IIa, B)**

16. Fukushima R, Alexander JW, Gianotti L, Ogle CK: Isolated pulmonary infection acts as a source of systemic tumor necrosis factor. Crit Care Med 1994;22:114–120. **(IIa, B)**

17. Meduri GU, Kohler G, Headley S, et al: Inflammatory cytokines in the BAL of patients with ARDS: Persistent elevation over time predicts poor outcome. Chest 1995;108:1303–1314. **(IIa, B)**

18. Sauder DN, Semple J, Truscott D, et al: Stimulation of muscle protein degradation by murine and human epidermal cytokines: relationship to thermal injury. J Invest Dermatol 1986;87:711–714. **(IIa, B)**

19. Lewis RA, Austen KF, Soberman RJ: Leukotrienes and other products of the 5-lipoxygenase pathway. Biochemistry and relation to pathobiology in human disease. N Eng J Med 1990;323:645–655. **(IIa, B)**

20. Petrak RA, Balk RA, Bone RC: Prostaglandins, cyclo-oxygenase inhibitors, and thromboxane synthetase inhibitors in the pathogenesis of multiple systems organ failure. Crit Care Clin 1989;5:203–214. **(IIa, B)**

21. Conger JD, Weil JV: Abnormal vascular function following ischemia-reperfusion injury. J Invest Med 1995;43:431–442. **(IIa, B)**

22. Levi M, ten Cate H, van der Poll T, van Deventer SJ: Pathogenesis of disseminated intravascular coagulation in sepsis. JAMA 1993; 270:975–979. **(IIa, B)**

23. Gomez-Jimenez J, Salgado A, Mourelle M, et al: L-Arginine: nitric oxide pathway in endotoxemia and human septic shock. Crit Care Med 1995;23:253–258. **(IIa, B)**

24. Miyauchi T, Tomobe Y, Shiba R, et al: Involvement of endothelin in the regulation of human vascular tonus. Potent vasoconstrictor effect and existence in endothelial cells. Circulation 1990;81:1874–1880. **(IIa, B)**

25. Livingston DH, Appel SH, Wellhausen SR, et al: Depressed interferon-γ production and moncyte HLA-DR expression after severe injury. Arch Surg 1988;123:1309–1312. **(IIa, B)**

26. Mills CD, Caldwell MD, Gann DS: Evidence of a plasma-mediated "window" of immunodeficiency in rats following trauma. J Clin Immunol 1989;9:139–150. **(IIa, B)**

27. Opal SM, Cohen J: Clinical gram-positive sepsis: does it fundamentally differ from gram-negative bacterial sepsis? Crit Care Med 1999; 27:1608–1616. **(IIa, B)**

28. Glauser MP, Zanetti G, Baumgartner JD, Cohen J: Septic shock: pathogenesis. Lancet 1991;338:732–736. **(IIa, B)**

29. Bates DW, Pruess KE, Lee TH: How bad are bacteremia and sepsis? Outcomes in a cohort with suspected bacteremia. Arch Intern Med 1995;155:593–598. **(IIa, B)**

30. Geerdes HF, Ziegler D, Lode H, et al: Septicemia in 980 patients at a university hospital in Berlin: prospective studies during 4 selected years between 1979 and 1989. Clin Infect Dis 1992;15:991–1002. **(IIa, B)**

31. Van Amersfoort ES, Van Berkel TJ, Kuiper J: Receptors, mediators, and mechanisms involved in bacterial sepsis and septic shock. Clin Microbiol Rev 2003;16:379–414. **(IIa, B)**

32. Hellman J, Loiselle PM, Tehan MM, et al: Outer membrane protein A, peptidoglycan-associated lipoprotein, and murein lipoprotein are released by *Escherichia coli* bacteria into serum. Infect Immun 2000;68:2566–2572. **(IIa, B)**

33. Rietschel ET, Kirikae T, Schade FU, et al: Bacterial endotoxin: molecular relationships of structure to activity and function. FASEB J 1994; 8:217–225. **(IIa, B)**

34. Fischer W: Lipoteichoic acid and lipids in the membrane of *Staphylococcus aureus*. Med Microbiol Immunol 1994;183:61–76. **(IIa, B)**

35. Fischer W, Koch HU: Alanyl lipoteichoic acid of *Staphylococcus aureus:* functional and dynamic aspects. Biochem Soc Trans 1985;13:984–986. **(IIa, B)**

36. Takakuwa T, Endo S, Nakae H, et al: Blood cytokine and complement levels in patients with sepsis. Res Commun Chem Pathol Pharmacol 1994;84:291–300. **(IIa, B)**

37. Vogel SN, Hogan MM: Role of cytokines in endotoxins-mediated host responses, In JJ Oppenheim, EM Shevach (eds): Immunophysiology. The Role of Cells and Cytokines in Immunity and Inflammation. Oxford, UK: Oxford University Press, 1990, pp 238–258. **(III, B)**

38. Fox ES, Thomas P, Broitman SA: Comparative studies of endotoxin uptake by isolated rat Kupffer and peritoneal cells. Infect Immun 1987;55:2962–2966. **(IIa, B)**

39. Roberts JM, Laros RK II: Hemorrhagic and endotoxic shock: pathophysiologic approach to diagnosis and management. Am J Obstet Gynecol 1971;110:1041–1049. **(IIa, B)**

40. Swan HJ, Ganz W, Forrester J, et al: Catheterization of the heart in man with use of a flow-directed balloon-tipped catheter. N Engl J Med 1970;283:447–451. **(IIa, B)**

41. Porembka DT: Cardiovascular abnormalities in sepsis. New Horiz 1993; 1:324–341. **(IIb, B)**

42. Rao PS, Cavanagh D: Endotoxic shock in the primate: some effects of dopamine administration. Am J Obstet Gynecol 1982;144:61–66. **(Ib, A)**

43. Goldberg LI:. Dopamine—clinical uses of endogenous catecholamine. N Engl J Med 1974;291:707–710. **(IIa, B)**

44. Shoemaker WC, Kram HB, Appel PL, Fleming AW: The efficacy of central venous and pulmonary artery catheters and therapy based upon them in reducing mortality and morbidity. Arch Surg 1990; 125:1332–1337. **(IIa, B)**

45. Bollaert PE, Bauer P, Audibert G, et al: Effects of epinephrine on hemodynamics and oxygen metabolism in dopamine-resistant septic shock. Chest 1990;98:949–953. **(IIa, B)**

46. Hinds C, Watson D: Manipulating hemodynamics and oxygen transport in critically ill patients. N Engl J Med 1995;33:1074–1075. **(IIa, B)**

47. Altura BM, Gebrewold A, Burton RW: Failure of microscopic metarterioles to elicit vasodilator responses of acetylcholine, bradykinin, histamine, and substance P after ischemic shock, endotoxemia and trauma: possible role of endothelial cells. Microcirc Endothelium Lymphatics 1985;2:121–127. **(IIa, B)**

48. Knuppel RA, Rao PS, Cavanaugh D: Septic shock in obstetrics. Clin Obstet Gynecol 1984;27:3–10. **(III, B)**

49. Demling RH, Lalonde C, Ikegami K: Physiologic support of the septic patient. Surg Clin North Am 1994;74:637–658. **(III, B)**

50. Fiddian-Green RG, Haglund U, Gutierrez G, Shoemaker WC: Goals for the resuscitation of shock. Crit Care Med 1993;21:525–528. **(III, B)**

# Chapter 24

# The Anatomic Basis of Normal and Abnormal Pelvic Support

Robert M. Rogers, Jr., MD

## KEY POINTS

- Learn normal pelvic support anatomy by paying attention during pelvic examination of the nulliparous patient.
- Intact, fully functioning pelvic floor muscles and their innervations are more important in pelvic organ support than intact visceral support connective tissues.
- Pelvic support defects are seen as stretched and attenuated vaginal epithelium and peritoneum. What is not seen or appreciated are the breaks in the visceral connective tissues between these two layers.
- The keys to successful reparative vaginal surgery are the reconstruction of the pericervical ring and the reconstruction of the perineal body.

A directed clinical examination of the normal, nulliparous young woman teaches the clinician pelvic support anatomy. This exercise requires training and guidance as to what to observe, why, and how; and what to palpate, why, and how. This experience is further enhanced with appropriate observations during various surgeries and directed cadaver dissections. During examination of patients with existing pelvic support defects, such as high cystocele or low rectocele, often the examiner can be confused as to the specific anatomic reasons for the various observed bulges in the vagina and their associated movements on Valsalva maneuver. Even the terms *cystocele* and *rectocele* mislead the observer as to the etiology of the observed vaginal support weaknesses. We can only appreciate that which we have been trained to understand, as we process our observational and tactile input.

This chapter presents the reader with a working, hands-on overview of our present understanding of female pelvic support anatomy. This anatomy teaching is from observations from reparative vaginal surgeries and cadaver dissections by knowledgeable, anatomically minded clinicians and surgeons. This information is then correlated with clinical findings to help explain female pelvic visceral support, both normal and abnormal. This chapter explains normal vaginal support findings and anatomy, and then discusses various pelvic support defects. These include anatomic descriptions to explain the various clinical findings. Although the information offered in this chapter is basic, it should be sufficient. The goal is to give the clinician and reparative vaginal surgeon practical knowledge that can be applied

immediately in the examination room and in the operating room. However, the reader must first be forewarned. This information requires the ability to think and conceptualize in three dimensions. This must first be accomplished while reading words and sentences, and observing photographs and illustrations, on two-dimensional pages. This is challenging, even for the most experienced gynecologic anatomists and surgeons. The structural anatomy of the female pelvis is difficult to orient in one's mind. The understanding of pelvic support anatomy is even more challenging.

## EXAMINATION OF THE PATIENT WITH NORMAL PELVIC SUPPORT

Vaginal support anatomy is best learned and understood by performing focused and educated pelvic examinations on young, nulliparous patients.[1] This is most commonly performed during the patient's annual well visit, with the patient in the dorsal lithotomy position. The clinician should be professional and ask the patient for her permission to examine her after explaining the purposes of the examination. The physician will need at hand an appropriate bivalve speculum, or vaginal retractor such as a Sims' retractor, as well as a long Allis clamp or single-toothed tenaculum. Remember, these patients do not have vaginal support problems. Therefore, any feel of the tissues or movement upon patient straining or with pelvic muscular contraction gives the physician a feel for the norm. The examiner should have already been instructed about what to observe and what to palpate, with the expected findings in the nulliparous patient. The focused examination for learning pelvic support anatomy begins with observations of the vaginal area and associated movements and is followed by palpation of these organs and tissues at rest and with various movements.

### Observation of the Perineum

With the patient in the dorsal lithotomy position, the clinician should simply observe the labia, vaginal introitus, perineal body, and anus. Astute observation demands self-questioning to focus the examiner's mind to ensure that systematic observations are noted in order so as not to overlook a particular observation. This process is obviously facilitated by practice and experience. The clinician needs to establish a pattern and sequence of examination, including both observation and palpable feel of the tissues. Noting the appearance and feel of these structures gives the examiner a reference on which he/she can judge what is normal and what is not normal in all the patients examined in the office. This information on vaginal support must be correlated with patients' complaints and symptoms. The physician must adapt his/her learning to what the patients teach him/her, not to what books teach. And these observations must be correlated and integrated with newer anatomic studies and clinical reports. The learner must always question himself/herself.

## Speculum Examination

Once the external features are observed, the labia should be separated with the fingers. Note the shape and the function of the vaginal introitus. Ask the patient to squeeze your fingers. Note the action and strength of the surrounding muscles. What happens when the patient is asked to "bear down, as if having a bowel movement?" Gently insert the bivalve speculum. In what direction does the speculum travel? Is there a change in direction from the lower portion of the vagina to the upper portion? Note the cervix and surrounding vaginal fornices. Are the fornices flat or concave? Where? Describe. Ask the patient to bear down. What is the movement of the cervix? Does the cervix move down into the vagina more? Do the fornices— lateral, anterior, posterior—bulge out? What is their movement? What happens when the patient contracts her pelvic and paravaginal muscles? Place a long Allis clamp gently on the cervix. What lateral movement does the cervix show? How much? To what extent?

Slowly remove the speculum as the patient rests, as she contracts or "squeezes" her pelvic muscles, and as she bears down. What happens with the vagina? Do the vaginal walls demonstrate rugae? Where? What do they look like? What happens to the anterior vaginal wall? What happens to the lateral vaginal wall? What happens to the posterior vaginal wall? What happens as the speculum moves down toward the vaginal introitus? Do the walls demonstrate any longitudinal ridges or clefts? The bivalve speculum can be separated and the lower blade used to observe the anterior vaginal wall while retracting the posterior vaginal wall. Likewise, the posterior vaginal wall can be examined while retracting the anterior vaginal wall with the lower blade of the speculum. Pay attention and note these findings, answering these and other questions. Correlate these findings with the understood vaginal support anatomy. Why are these findings observed anatomically and physiologically?

## Palpation of Vaginal Tissues

Perform the bimanual examination and learn from palpation with the fingers through the lubricated glove. Note the tactile thickness and feel of the various areas of the vagina and surrounding viscera. Again, this is done systematically with self-directed questions. The examiner palpates the cervix, uterus, and adnexae; the four vaginal fornices; the four walls of the vagina; the lower third of the vagina underneath the urethra; laterally to feel the muscles of the levator hiatus; and posteriorly to feel the perineal body. Palpate the sidewall and the arcus tendineus fasciae pelvis, the "banjo string" traveling from the ischial spine to the pubic arch. Gently place a lubricated cotton-tipped swab in the urethra. Ask the patient to cough or bear down. How far does the cotton-tipped swab move up? Palpate the paraurethral tissues. Can you feel the pubic bone? How thick are the paraurethral tissues?

Place an Allis clamp on the cervix and gently pull while palpating posteriorly for the uterosacral ligaments. Where are they? How thick and strong are they? How far do they stretch? Be gentle. Perform a rectal examination to assess the strength of the levator ani muscles, the anal sphincter muscle, and the integrity of the perineal body. Perform this examination without and with the patient straining, and without and with the patient "squeezing" your finger. Assess the levator plate, which is easily palpable just under the posterior rectal wall. What does the anal canal feel like? How long is it? What does the rectum feel like? What is the shape of the perineal body? In what orientation are they? What happens to these areas when the patient is at rest; with contraction of the surrounding pelvic muscles; with straining? After many patients, the examiner will develop a "normal" pattern for these examinations.

## ANATOMY OF NORMAL PELVIC SUPPORT: CLINICAL CORRELATIONS

### Pericervical Ring and Levator Plate

As the "normal" findings are registered in the examiner's mind and assimilated, a discussion of the relevant pelvic support structures must be included. The uterosacral–cardinal ligament complexes on each side attach to the lateral and posterior aspects of the pericervical ring of visceral connective tissue (Fig. 24-1). This occurs at the level of the ischial spines, but slightly anterior to the interspinous diameter due to the pull of the upper portion

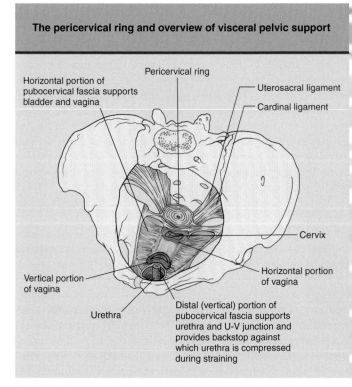

**The pericervical ring and overview of visceral pelvic support**

Horizontal portion of pubocervical fascia supports bladder and vagina

Pericervical ring

Uterosacral ligament

Cardinal ligament

Cervix

Horizontal portion of vagina

Vertical portion of vagina

Urethra

Distal (vertical) portion of pubocervical fascia supports urethra and U-V junction and provides backstop against which urethra is compressed during straining

**Figure 24-1    The pericervical ring and overview of visceral pelvic support.** The pericervical ring is formed by the cardinal–uterosacral ligament complexes and pubocervical fascia. (From Retzky SS, Rogers RM: Urinary incontinence in women. In Clinical Symposia. Summit, NJ, Ciba-Geigy, 1995;47[3], from Plate 3, p 7. Netter illustrations used with permission of Elsevier, Inc. All rights reserved.)

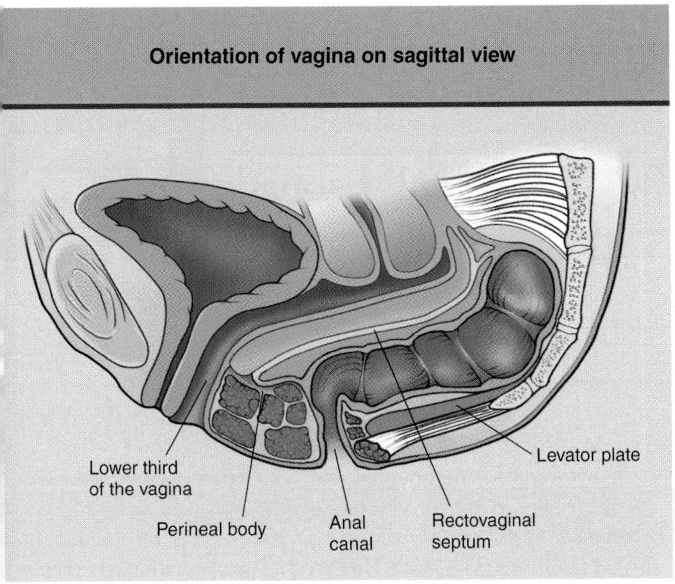

Lower third
of the vagina

Levator plate

Perineal body

Anal
canal

Rectovaginal
septum

**Figure 24-2    Orientation of the vagina.** A sagittal section through the normally oriented female pelvis. The upper portion of the vagina, the cervix, and rectum are suspended over the muscular levator plate, which dynamically contracts to entrap these pelvic organs in the pelvis on patient Valsalva straining. Note the orientation of the perineal body. (Original owned by Robert M. Rogers, Jr., MD, used with permission.)

of the cardinal ligament. The pericervical ring is located around the supravaginal portion of the cervix, which is located in the middle third of the transverse vaginal apex. Into this fuses the rectovaginal fascia posteriorly, the uterosacral ligaments posterolaterally, the cardinal ligaments laterally, and the pubocervical fascia anteriorly. The upper pelvic supports of the uterosacral–cardinal ligament complexes suspend the cervix and upper vagina over the levator plate. The active levator plate acts as a backstop against which the upper vagina and cervix are entrapped and thus prevented from prolapsing when the patient strains down[2] (Fig. 24-2). Therefore, when the patient strains, movement of the cervix down the vaginal axis is limited. In addition, the uterosacral–cardinal ligaments also secure the lateral vaginal fornices, thus giving them their upper concavity. On patient straining, the lateral fornices will flatten somewhat. However, the anterior vaginal fornix does not flatten because of the thickened attachment of the pubocervical fascia to the pericervical ring. The posterior vaginal fornix is supported by the rectovaginal fascia centrally and the uterosacral ligaments posterolaterally. Straining by the patient will allow the posterior vaginal fornix to bulge out a little. The extent must be observed and noted by the examiner.

## Anterior Vaginal Wall

Because the cardinal ligaments have a lateral attachment to the pelvic sidewall near each ischial spine[3] and because the pubocervical fascia also has lateral attachments to each arcus tendineus fasciae pelvis, which ends at the level of the ischial spine, the examiner finds limited lateral excursion of the cervix when moved with an Allis clamp (see Fig. 24-1). Also because of the lateral attachments of the pubocervical fascia mentioned, the anterior wall of the vagina exhibits an anterolateral sulcus on

each side. On straining, these sulci do not disappear but remain visible and intact while the anterior wall does move down a little. The bladder rests on the upper two thirds of the vagina, with the trigone overlying the middle third of the vagina. The urethra travels on the lower third of the anterior vaginal wall. The urethra has limited movement on Valsalva straining. Remember, the urethra is supported by a "hammock" of pubocervical fascia attached laterally to each arcus tendineus fasciae pelvis[4] (Fig. 24-3). This hammock also prevents the examiner's finger from moving around the side of the urethra to the back of the pubic bone. In addition, the distal portion of the urethra is supported by the pubourethral ligaments. The urethra also passes through the perineal membrane, an anatomic concept, which traverses between the inferior ischiopubic rami. The extent of movement in each portion of the vagina must be learned by observation. The pubocervical fascia is physiologically active and is responsible for the transverse rugations found in the well-estrogenized anterior vaginal wall (Fig. 24-4).

## Posterior Vaginal Wall

The posterior vaginal wall is supported by the rectovaginal fascia in the upper two thirds, while the lower third of the vagina is supported by its fusion with the perineal body. The rectovaginal fascia is between the rectum and just underneath the upper two thirds of the vagina, traveling from the apex of the perineal body to the iliococcygeal fascia bilaterally, and then to the uterosacral ligaments and posterior vaginal fornix. Laterally, the rectovaginal

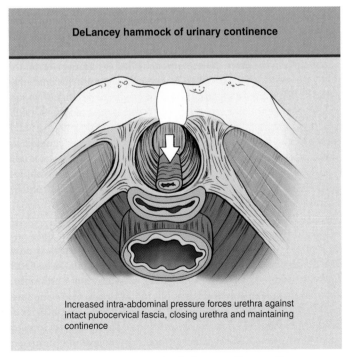

Increased intra-abdominal pressure forces urethra against intact pubocervical fascia, closing urethra and maintaining continence

**Figure 24-3    DeLancey hammock of urinary continence.** The "hammock" of pubocervical fascia underneath the urethra functions as a backstop against which the urethra is compressed on Valsalva straining. This is one of the urinary continence mechanisms in the female patient. (From Retzky SS, Rogers RM: Urinary incontinence in women. In Clinical Symposia. Summit, NJ, Ciba-Geigy, 1995, Plate 6, p 12, bottom left. Netter illustrations used with permission of Elsevier, Inc. All rights reserved.)

### The transverse rugations of the anterior vaginal wall

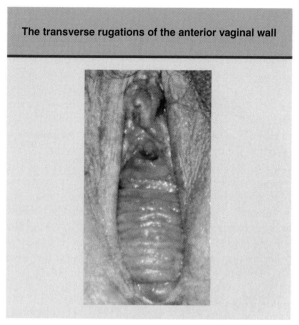

**Figure 24-4   The transverse rugations of the anterior vaginal wall.** Seen also is a bilateral paravaginal defect. (From OBG Management 2004;16[5], fig. 2, p 20; www.obgmanagement.com.)

fascia attaches to each arcus tendineus fasciae rectovaginalis, which fuses with the arcus tendineus fasciae pelvis as it travel toward the ischial spine[5] (Fig. 24-5). Therefore, posterolateral sulci also can be seen in the middle third of the posterior vaginal wall. The fibromuscular connective tissue coat surrounding the

### Lateral attachment of the rectovaginal fascia

Pubocervical fascia

Arcus tendineus fasciae pelvis

Lateral attachment of rectovaginal septum

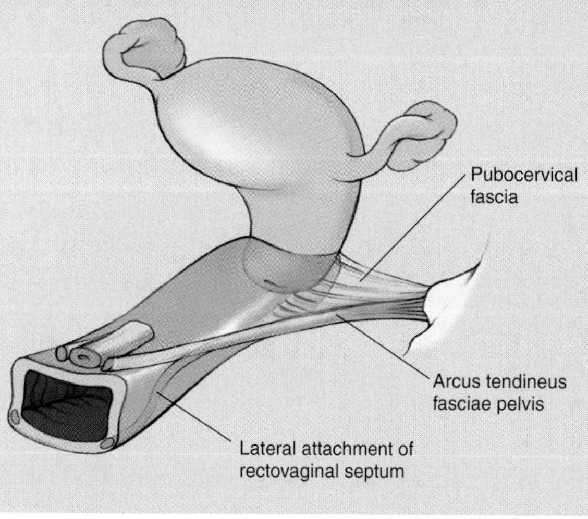

**Figure 24-5   Lateral attachment of the rectovaginal fascia.** Arcus tendineus fasciae pelvis (ATFP) of the pelvic sidewall. PCF, pubocervical fascia; RVS, rectovaginal septum, which inserts onto the arcus tendineus fasciae rectovaginalis. (From Leffler KS, Thompson JR, Cundiff GW, et al: Attachment of the rectovaginal septum to the pelvic sidewall. Am J Obstet Gynecol 2001;185:43.)

posterior vaginal wall and the rectovaginal fascia are physiologically active and are responsible for the transverse rugations found in the well-estrogenized posterior vaginal wall.

### Shape of the Vagina

In the unexamined vagina, the anterior and posterior vaginal walls rest against each other, and the lateral vaginal walls are tethered to the pelvic sidewalls by the more anterior arcus tendineus fasciae pelvis and the more posterior arcus tendineus fasciae rectovaginalis. Therefore in the resting state, the vagina in the middle third is shaped like the letter H. When the patient performs a Valsalva manuever, the anterior and posterior vaginal walls exhibit some movement, but the lateral sulci remain intact, with little movement.

### Perineal Body

The base of the perineal body is slightly concave upward because of its attachment to the rectovaginal septum, which is tethered to the hollow of the sacrum by its attachments to the uterosacral ligaments. The base is approximately 4 cm square and is almost parallel to the floor in the standing woman. The anal canal and the lower one third of the vagina fuse with the perineal body. Therefore, the apex of the pyramid-shaped perineal body is found at the junction of the lower third and middle third of the vagina. The anus, therefore, is located 1 to 2 cm above the level of the ischial tuberosities. Excursion of the perineal body by the examiner's fingers or the patient's Valsalva manuever should be approximately 1 cm and no more. The pubococcygeal muscles surround the lower third of the vagina and close off the vaginal introitus when contracted.

### Pelvic Visceral Support System

With the normal pelvic examination described and the important support structures correlated with these findings, more description is now offered to deepen the reader's understanding and appreciation in three dimensions.[2,3,6,7] The pelvic visceral support system is continuous and interdependent from the pelvic brim, along the back wall, the sidewall, and, finally, the outlet of the vagina (Fig. 24-6). Therefore, one defect in this network causes one or more defects in other areas of the network. The visceral connective tissues in the pelvis are found between the peritoneum, both visceral and parietal, and the parietal fascia covering the skeletal muscles of the pelvic basin. These visceral support tissues envelope and act as conduits for the visceral arteries, veins, nerves, lymph channels and nodes, and ureters. Visceral connective tissue is constructed of loose, meshlike collagen; some elastin; and smooth muscle. This tissue is physiologically alive, adapting to local stresses, and forms the vaginal rugae seen in the well-estrogenized vaginal epithelium.

This tissue is formed in sheets, which fuse around the contained vasculature to form sheaths (cardinal–uterosacral sheath), septa (the lateral attachments of the pubocervical fascia and rectovaginal fascia to the lateral pelvic sidewall), and even dense, direct connections with the adjacent parietal fascia (fusion of the lower third of the vagina and anal canal with the

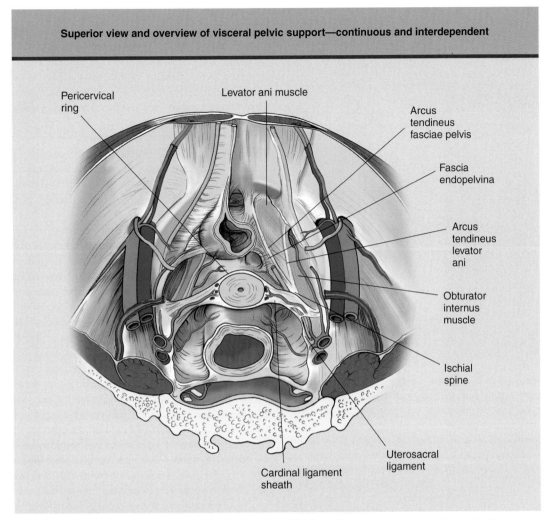

**Superior view and overview of visceral pelvic support—continuous and interdependent**

Pericervical ring

Levator ani muscle

Arcus tendineus fasciae pelvis

Fascia endopelvina

Arcus tendineus levator ani

Obturator internus muscle

Ischial spine

Uterosacral ligament

Cardinal ligament sheath

**Figure 24-6    Superior view and overview of the female pelvic visceral suspensory system, formed by the continuous and interdependent network of visceral connective tissues.** As seen after the peritoneum has been removed. (From Netter FH, Dalley AF [eds]: Netter's Atlas of Human Anatomy, 2nd ed. Novartis, 1997, Plate 341. Netter illustrations used with permission of Elsevier, Inc. All rights reserved.)

perineal body and the pubococcygeal fascia). The cardinal ligament sheath is anchored to the parietal fascia of the pelvic brim, sacrum, piriform muscle, anterior border of the greater sciatic foramen, and near the ischial spine. The sheets of visceral connective tissue coalesce and fuse around the internal iliac vessels and are led by the uterine vessels to the pericervical ring. In the standing patient, the internal iliac (hypogastric) artery and vein course in a vertical manner, along the anterior border of the greater sciatic foramen.

The visceral connective tissues also form capsules around the cervix and vagina, bladder and urethra, and the rectum and anal canal. The horizontal, lateral septa from these visceral capsules include the pubocervical fascia, rectovaginal fascia, and support pillars from the bladder and rectum. These lateral wings of visceral fascia fuse to form the medial edge of the fascia endopelvina (Fig. 24-7). The lateral edge of the fascia endopelvina inserts into the arcus tendineus fasciae pelvis, which is more horizontal in the standing patient. Remember, this travels from near the pubic arch to the ischial spine, a distance of 7.5 to 9.5 cm.[8]

## Pelvic Musculature

The pelvis is actually a basin of muscles, not bones (Fig. 24-8). There is no top to this open bowl-like form. The back wall is the sacrum centrally and the two piriform muscles laterally, one passing straight through each greater sciatic foramen to insert onto the greater trochanter of each femur. The front wall is the back of the pubic bone. The two sidewalls are bounded by the obturator internus muscles, which tail posteriorly and inferiorly to take sharp angles underneath the ischial spines and pass through the lesser sciatic foramina to insert onto the greater trochanters. The floor is formed by the levator ani and the coccygeal muscles. These latter muscles travel from the sides of the lower part of the anterior sacrum and narrow down to insert onto the ischial spines. This is also the same course as the sacrospinous ligaments, on top of which they travel. The course of direction of these is lateral and posterior. In the postmenopausal patient, the coccygeal muscles are atrophic and fibrous, appearing as part of the sacrospinous ligaments.

The levator ani muscles have an anterior portion—the pubococcygeus and puborectalis muscles—and a posterior

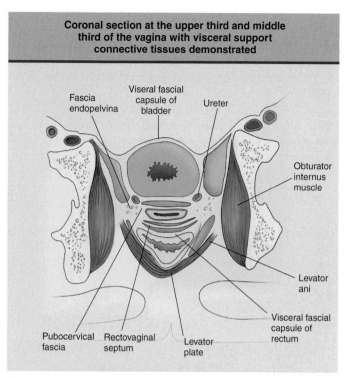

**Coronal section at the upper third and middle third of the vagina with visceral support connective tissues demonstrated**

**Figure 24-7    Frontal section through the junction of the middle third and upper third of the vagina, demonstrating the visceral suspensory connective tissues and muscular support of the pelvic floor and sidewalls.** Note the relationship of the fascia endopelvina to the fascial white line and the more medial tissue septa emanating from the capsules of the pelvic organs and the rectovaginal fascia. (Adapted from Peham HV, Amreich J: Operative Gynecology, Vol. 1. Philadelphia: Lippincott, 1934, p. 194.)

portion—the iliococcygeus muscles. The anterior portion forms the levator hiatus, through which passes the urethra, lower third of the vagina, and the anal canal. The pubococcygeus muscles produce the right angle of the rectoanal junction, which is essential for continence of solid stool. The muscles of the levator hiatus originate from the back of the pubic bone and the anterior part of the obturator internus muscles. The iliococcygeus muscles originate from the rest of the obturator internus muscles and sling down toward each other to form a common tendon between the rectoanal junction and the coccyx. This is the levator plate. This dynamic plate of tendon and muscle is responsible for entrapping the vagina and rectum horizontally at the time of downward pressures to help prevent vaginal prolapse.

### "The White Line"

The muscles of the pelvic basin are skeletal and innervated by somatic rather than visceral nerves. These nerves are derived from the lumbar and sacral plexuses. These muscles are covered by parietal fascia, which is strong, flat, and firm in contrast to the looser and more flexible visceral connective tissues. The arcus tendineus levator ani is a thickening of the parietal fascia covering each obturator internus muscle and is the origin of each portion of each levator ani muscle (see Fig. 24-8). The arcus tendineus levator ani muscle travels from the lateral aspect of the back of the pubic bone toward the ischial spine in a curvilinear course.

The arcus tendineus fasciae pelvis (*the white line*) is a thickening of the parietal fascia of the levator ani muscles and is the attachment of the pubocervical fascia and rectovaginal fascia via the fascia endopelvina (see Fig. 24-6). The arcus tendineus fasciae pelvis courses linearly from near the pubic arch to the

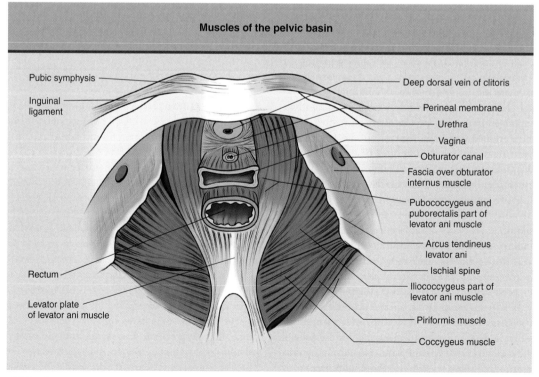

**Muscles of the pelvic basin**

**Figure 24-8    The muscles of the female pelvic basin.** (From Netter FH, Dalley AF [eds]: Netter's Atlas of Human Anatomy, 2nd ed. Novartis, 1997, Plate 333, upper illustration. Netter illustrations used with permission of Elsevier, Inc. All rights reserved.)

ischial spine. In some cases of paravaginal defects, the most common cause of anterior vaginal wall prolapse, this arcus tears away from the parietal fascia with the fascia endopelvina and attached pubocervical fascia and the rectovaginal fascia. This leaves a bare strip of muscle along the sidewall of the pelvis.

## Site-Specific Defects

Important to our present-day concepts of pelvic visceral support, the visceral connective tissues can only stretch or attenuate within a small range. Further stretching results in distinct breaks of these support tissues. Today's concepts of reparative vaginal surgeries are based on finding, diagnosing, and repairing these site-specific defects[9,10] that result in the various prolapses. The realization of this concept is difficult because the visceral connective tissues lie between the vaginal epithelium and the peritoneum, both of which can stretch endlessly. Therefore, the clinician sees redundant vagina and large protrusions of peritoneum with no intervening visceral fascia. Previously, the gynecologic surgeon assumed that the unseen visceral fascia was so attenuated that it should be plicated. Today, the gynecologic surgeon repairs the disruptions and breaks in the continuous and interdependent network of visceral supporting connective tissues.

Unfortunately, we cannot operate to repair the damaged and compromised muscles and somatic nerves, which are also crucial elements in the pelvic support system. This concept is often underplayed, underappreciated, and seldom discussed or studied. Remember, the pelvic support network of connective tissue sheaths and septa simply position the urethra and bladder, vagina and cervix, and anal canal and rectum within and over the pelvic musculature. The skeletal muscles of the pelvis are ultimately responsible for the mechanical support of the pelvic viscera. These muscles are active in reacting to the various pressure changes and other conditions presented within the pelvis. Even if the visceral support connective tissues remain intact, compromise of the pelvic musculature and its innervations can result in vaginal prolapse symptoms and signs.

## Upper Vertical Supports of Level I

The pelvic support system of visceral connective tissues is artificially described by anatomists and clinicians in distinct segments. DeLancey level I,[11] or the superior hypogastric sheath (Uhlenhuth,[3] Peham and Amreich[6]), simply describe the suspensory function of the cardinal–uterosacral sheaths (Fig. 24-9). The cardinal and uterosacral ligaments simply suspend the cervix and upper third of the vagina over the levator plate. This allows the active levator plate to counter the downward pressures generated by the patient in a Valsalva movement, such as coughing, exercising, lifting, or having a bowel movement. This flap-valve action is believed to prevent vaginal prolapse.[2] The levator plate, which occurs anatomically between the rectoanal junction and coccyx, is very strong. The levator plate and levator ani muscles should be palpated and appreciated in the young, nulliparous patient by gentle rectal examination.

## Horizontal Supports of Level II

The transition from the cardinal–uterosacral ligaments into the more horizontal supports (DeLancey level II)[11] of the pubocervical fascia and the rectovaginal fascia occurs at the level of

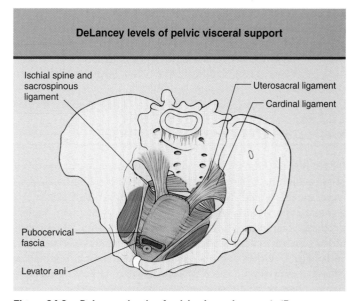

**DeLancey levels of pelvic visceral support**

Ischial spine and sacrospinous ligament

Uterosacral ligament

Cardinal ligament

Pubocervical fascia

Levator ani

**Figure 24-9    DeLancey levels of pelvic visceral support.** (From DeLancey JOL: Anatomic aspects of vaginal eversion after hysterectomy. Am J Obstet Gynecol 1992;166:1719.)

the ischial spines via the pericervical ring of visceral connective tissue (see Fig. 24-9). The pubocervical fascia is simply the thickened fibromuscular coat of visceral connective tissue surrounding the vaginal epithelium.[12,13] It is tethered to the pelvic sidewall by connective tissue septa or wings via the fascia endopelvina to the arcus tendineus fasciae pelvis. The rectovaginal septum inserts onto the pelvic sidewall in a similar manner. In cadaver dissections, the pubocervical fascia and rectovaginal fascia, along with visceral septa from the bladder and rectum, fuse and form the medial edge of a structure called the fascia endopelvina.[3] The lateral edge of the fascia endopelvina inserts onto the entire length of the arcus tendineus fasciae pelvis. Therefore, a paravaginal defect is a tearing away of the fascia endopelvina, with the attached pubocervical fascia and rectovaginal fascia, from the arcus tendineus fasciae pelvis. In some cases, the arcus and fascia endopelvina detach together from the muscular sidewall, thus leaving bare muscle tissue with no overlying parietal fascia.

## Lower Vertical Supports of Level III

The transition of the horizontal supports (DeLancey level II) to the lower vertical supports (DeLancey level III)[11] occurs at the apex of the perineal body. The perineal body is described as a pyramid with its base parallel to the floor and its apex vertically oriented (see Fig. 24-2). Fused to this is the anterior part of the anal canal and the posterior part of the lower third of the posterior vaginal wall. Also, the urethra is oriented vertically and is anchored to the pubic arch via its passage through the perineal membrane. This occurs as the middle third of the urethra follows into its distal third. The perineal membrane is more complex around the urethra and includes musculature and visceral connective tissues also.[14] In the younger patient, especially at vaginal childbirth, the structures of the perineal body can be seen—superficial transverse perineal muscles, anal sphincter muscle, rectovaginal fascia, bulbocavernosus muscle, and lower rectal layers. However, in the older, postmenopausal patient, these structures are atrophic, fibrotic, and thus obliterated and usually cannot be seen. Nevertheless, the perineal body must be reconstructed at the time of reparative vaginal surgery, with the base positioned just above the level of the ischial tuberosities.

## EXAMINATION OF THE PATIENT WITH DEFECTS OF PELVIC SUPPORT

Disruption of these visceral connective tissues along any portion of the continuous network of pelvic support, along with concomitant injury and dysfunction of the pelvic musculature and somatic innervation, leads to the various defects in vaginal support.[1] The most common causative events are vaginal childbirth, repetitive straining as with constipation and heavy lifting, and aging.[15] Other factors—genetic, environmental (such as cigarette smoking), and nutritional—also affect connective tissue integrity. These support defects include uterine/cervical prolapse, various degrees of anterior and posterior vaginal wall prolapse, vaginal apical prolapse with accompanying cul-de-sac herniation, hypermobile urethra, and perineal descent with gaping vaginal introitus.

These pelvic support defects are seen as prolapse of the vaginal walls and apex in various areas, especially with the patient straining. The examiner must have a baseline appreciation of the "normal" rugated appearance and movements of the vaginal walls in the young, nulliparous subject. The clinician must also have a three-dimensional mindset and understanding of the vaginal support structures. This allows the examiner to visualize the site-specific anatomic disruptions that are responsible for the vaginal bulges. This understanding allows the reparative vaginal surgeon to address and repair the several specific defects at the time of surgery.

Patients present with various complaints associated with pelvic floor/vaginal defects. The most common include vaginal pressure and the feeling of sitting on objects such as a "golf ball" or "tennis ball." Other complaints include urinary incontinence, urine retention, incomplete evacuation of the rectum with bowel movement, and lower back pain/pressure. With posterior vaginal wall prolapse (rectocele), some patients push on the perineal body or put a finger in the vagina to more fully empty the rectum and finish the bowel movement. The physician should listen and allow the patient to describe her symptoms. At this time, vaginal wall defects can only be appreciated and clinically diagnosed by physical examination. The office diagnoses are further confirmed and refined at the time of surgery. Physical examination with description and documentation of the findings is the standard at this time for diagnosis of pelvic support defects.[10,16] From these findings, the surgeon can then formulate a surgical plan that fits the patient and her specific vaginal defects. This is in contrast to former practices, in which all types of cystoceles were repaired by the same operation—central anterior colporrhaphy—and all types of rectoceles were repaired by posterior colporrhaphy. Most embarrassing of all, enteroceles (cul-de-sac hernias) were repaired by the plication or "purse stringing" of peritoneum and not visceral fascia!

Examination of the patient with vaginal support defects mirrors the same sequence with the same instrumentation and the same maneuvers as the examination of the normal patient without such defects. However, there is one addition. A uterine dressing forceps or straight ring forceps will assist in the evaluation of the anterior vaginal wall. In the dorsal lithotomy position, observe the perineum, labia, introitus, perineal body, and anus. What differences are seen compared to the nulliparous patient? Notice the tone, laxity, and dimensions of these structures. What is observed when the patient contracts the vaginal opening? What happens when the patient bears down? Is there descent of the perineal body and anus? Normally, the perineal body and the anus are located just above the level of the ischial tuberosities. Spread the labia. Is there gaping of the introitus? What bulges are noticeable at the introitus? Is the vagina well or poorly estrogenized? Are rugations present? Measurements in centimeters can be taken at this time.

Take the bivalve speculum and gently insert it into the depths of the vagina. What does the cervix look like? Where is it located? How far down the vaginal length does the cervix prolapse with Valsalva straining? With an Allis clamp gently placed on the cervix, how much lateral movement is allowed? Describe the vaginal fornices at rest and with the patient straining. Look at the anterior vaginal wall. Are there rugations? Where is the wall resting? What happens when the patient bears down? Are anterolateral sulci present? Do they bulge down and disappear when the patient performs a Valsalva manuever? Now place the uterine dressing forceps, curve up, or the ring forceps in the vagina with the tips placed at the level of the ischial spines. Open the forceps so that the arms rest against the pelvic side-wall and re-create the anterolateral sulci. What happens to the anterior vagina wall when the patient bears down? Describe. Does the anterior wall stay put?

Remember the forceps were originally described to correct the paravaginal defects and allow for diagnosis of a central vaginal wall defect, indicating a central defect of the visceral connective tissue underneath the bladder, as opposed to a lateral paravaginal defect. However, more importantly, the tips of the forceps also re-create the attachment of the upper edge of the pubocervical fascia with each uterosacral ligament. This action in itself significantly corrects a high cystocele. Keep this in mind when planning reparative surgery. The re-creation of the pericervical ring and its reattachment to each uterosacral ligament at the level of the ischial spines is a key element in successful repair of anterior vaginal wall prolapse (cystocele). Perform the Q-tip test. Is the urethra hypermobile?

Look at the posterior vaginal wall. Are there rugations? Where is the wall resting? What happens when the patient bears down? Are posterolateral sulci present in the middle third of the vagina? What happens when the patient bears down? Is posterior vaginal wall prolapse (rectocele) present? Anterior wall site-specific defects are usually well diagnosed and characterized in the office. In contrast, the diagnosis of posterior vaginal wall defects may be better evaluated and defined in the operating room after posterior colpotomy has been performed, and the rectovaginal septum dissected out and seen.

After the preceding observations have been made, perform the palpation portion of the examination. Place the lubricated gloved fingers in the vagina. What do the vaginal walls feel like? Can you feel the banjo string of the arcus tendineus fasciae pelvis? How do the underlying visceral connective tissues feel?

Can you feel the break of the pubocervical fascia away from the sidewall? What weaknesses in support do you notice? Can you feel the uterosacral ligaments inserting into the cervix or vaginal cuff? Place an Allis clamp on the cervix and feel again for the uterosacral ligaments. On rectovaginal examination, can you feel any distinct breaks in the rectovaginal fascia? When the patient squeezes your fingers, how strong are the levator ani muscles? How strong and functional is the levator plate? On rectal examination, move the finger laterally. Is the levator ani muscle intact and connected to the lateral pelvic sidewall? How does this examination compare to your composite "normal" patient? Describe and record in the patient's chart.

## ANATOMY OF DEFECTS IN PELVIC SUPPORT: CLINICAL CORRELATION

Our present knowledge of pelvic support anatomy allows the following correlations. Disruption of the cardinal–uterosacral ligaments from the pericervical ring is a crucial event that starts the evolution of uterine prolapse/vaginal vault prolapse. Continued disruption of the pericervical ring, especially the tearing of the pubocervical fascia away from the rectovaginal fascia, opens the apical fascial defect that results in enteroceles. An enterocele or cul-de-sac hernia is the protrusion of the cul-de-sac peritoneum, which can stretch endlessly, through the pericervical ring defect[9] (Fig. 24-10). Apical prolapse is usually a combination of both disruption of the pericervical ring (allowing the herniation) and pericervical detachment from the cardinal–uterosacral ligament complexes. As the apex is pushed distally down the vaginal length, each lateral edge of each fascia endopelvina of the pubocervical fascia and rectovaginal fascia is torn away from its sidewall insertion, thus resulting in varying degrees of severity of anterior and posterior vaginal wall prolapse.

Significant injury and compromise in function to the levator ani muscles and their somatic innervations are associated with most, if not all, pelvic support defects. This loss of real muscular support to the pelvic viscera accelerates the formation of vaginal prolapse. Without adequate muscular support, the shearing forces on the visceral connective tissues are increased, thus increasing the visceral fascial breaks. It is important to remember that reparative vaginal surgery can only attempt to repair the integrity of the network of supporting visceral connective tissues. This surgery will not rehabilitate poorly functioning muscles and nerves.

Anterior vaginal wall prolapse (cystocele) is most commonly the result of apical support defect with concomitant paravaginal defects.[17] The paravaginal defects can be a partial or complete detachment of the pubocervical fascia (via the fascia endopelvina) from each sidewall, either unilateral or bilateral, usually near the ischial spines. This is based on observations at the time of surgery and in unembalmed cadavers, especially via laparoscopic observations. The apical defects are most commonly transverse detachments of the cardinal–uterosacral ligaments from the cervix or vaginal vault apex. By observations and palpation, the detachment of the cardinal–uterosacral ligaments occurs at the points of insertion to the cervix or vaginal cuff at the level of the ischial spines. The breaks do not occur at the origin of the uterosacral ligaments to the sacrum nor at the midportion of these support tissues.[18]

The other transverse tear seen is the detachment of the pubocervical fascia away from the anterior portion of the pericervical ring, with the uterosacral ligaments still attached to the pericervical ring posterolaterally. The paravaginal defects have been observed to be a detachment of the pubocervical fascia (via the fascia endopelvina) from the arcus tendineus fasciae pelvis in most cases. Other observed cases involve the pulling away of the arcus tendineus itself from the muscle belly of the levator ani muscle. Therefore, the pelvic sidewall shows a strip of bare muscle with no overlying parietal fascia. Muscle will not hold support sutures. Many times, a "central" defect is actually the central protrusion seen anteriorly, resulting from the detachment of the cardinal–uterosacral ligaments from the middle third of the vaginal cuff or from the cervix, which is

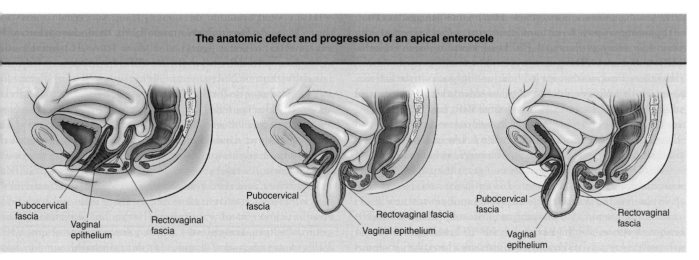

**The anatomic defect and progression of an apical enterocele**

**Figure 24-10   The anatomic defect and progresssion of an apical enterocele.** Note the separation of the pubocervical fascia of the anterior vaginal wall from the rectovaginal fascia of the posterior vaginal wall. Progression from small enterocele to complete vaginal prolapse. (From Richardson AC: The anatomic defects in rectocele and enterocele. J Pelvic Surg 1997:1:214–221.)

# Urogynecology

anatomically found in the middle third of the vaginal apex. Repair of the pericervical ring with reattachment of the uterosacral ligaments at the level of the ischial spines repairs this "central defect." By far, anterior vaginal wall prolapse is caused by detachments at the edges of the pubocervical fascia (via the fascia endopelvina) and not by tears within the pubocervical fascia.

In many cases, this same observation is true in posterior vaginal wall prolapse (rectocele) and the rectovaginal fascia. The upper edge of the rectovaginal fascia detaches from the cardinal–uterosacral ligaments, causing the posterior wall prolapse to progress, resulting in the detachment of the upper, lateral edges of the fascia endopelvina (rectovaginal fascia) from the sidewall iliococcygeus fascia. Many of these defects are found with enteroceles. Therefore, repair of the enterocele also begins the repair of the high rectocele.

Because of the disruption of the perineal body during vaginal childbirth, distal posterior vaginal wall defects can also result from detachment of the rectovaginal fascia from the perineal body. This same defect also causes perineal descent as well as disruption of the rectoanal canal. The perineal body in the multiparous, aging patient is filled with scar tissue centrally and even laterally, with thinning of the fibromuscular structures. The fibers of the superficial transverse perineal and anal sphincter muscles are rarely seen or appreciated.

The perineal body should be reconstructed at the time of reparative surgery. Reconstruct the perineal body as a pyramid with the apex 3 to 4 cm high. Then, attach the rectovaginal fascia to the perineal apex. Be sure to restore the normal diameter of the vaginal introitus by bringing the bulbocavernosus muscles into the perineal body. However, be sure to allow for a vaginal opening three fingers in diameter to facilitate comfortable penile entry during sexual intercourse.

## Goals of Reparative Vaginal Surgery

Reconstruction of the perineal body also restores the integrity of the rectoanal canal and the posterior wall of the lower third of the vagina. This brings the anus into its normal position just above the level of the ischial tuberosities. Thus, the first goals of perineal reconstruction are to correct perineal descent and to restore a more functional vaginal introitus. The second goal is to form a second backstop to assist the weakened levator plate in resisting downward Valsalva pressures that stress the restored visceral support network, just constructed during the surgery. Thus, the reconstructed pelvic outlet helps relieve the stress pressures on the upper vaginal supports, especially on the uterosacral ligaments and the reconstructed pericervical ring.

After anatomically correct reparative vaginal surgery, the lower third of the vagina should be horizontal and well supported by the perineal body in the patient in the dorsal lithotomy position. The diameter of the vagina should be three fingers. The upper two thirds of the vagina should then slope down to the ischial spines, with the apex at or slightly above the level of the ischial spines. The surgeon should be able to feel thickened visceral connective tissues underneath the vaginal epithelium with excellent peripheral attachments. This should be found anteriorly, apically, and posteriorly. At times, appropriate reinforcement of vaginal repairs with autologous, cadaveric, animal-derived tissues, or plastic meshes may be indicated. This controversial and fast-evolving clinical area of study is not addressed in this chapter. The goals of reparative vaginal surgery are to restore normal vaginal diameter and length, while also restoring more normal support and function to the bladder, urethra, vagina, rectum, and anal canal. Our understanding of pelvic support anatomy and defective vaginal support issues continues to evolve. As new knowledge and concepts appear, the clinician must integrate this knowledge into his/her understanding to better serve the many patients with pelvic floor dysfunction and prolapse.

## REFERENCES

1. Rogers RM, Richardson AC: Clinical evaluation of pelvic support defects with anatomic correlations. In Bent AE, Ostergard DR, Cundiff GW, et al (eds): Urogynecology and Pelvic Floor Dysfunction, 5th ed. Philadelphia: Lippincott Williams & Wilkins, 2003, ch. 8. (IV, C)
2. DeLancey JOL: Anatomy and biomechanics of genital prolapse. Clin Obstet Gynecol Dec 1993;36:897–909. (III, B)
3. Uhlenhuth ER, Day E, Smith R, et al: The visceral endopelvic fascia and the hypogastric sheath. Surg Gynecol Obstet 1948;86:9–28. (III, B)
4. DeLancey JOL: Structural support of the urethra as it relates to stress urinary incontinence: the hammock hypothesis. Am J Obstet Gynecol 1994;170:1713–1720. (III, B)
5. Leffler KS, Thompson JR, Cundiff GW, et al: Attachment of the rectovaginal septum to the pelvic sidewall. Am J Obstet Gynecol 2001;185:41–43. (III, B)
6. Peham HV, Amreich J: Operative Gynecology, Vol. 1. Philadelphia: Lippincott, 1934, pp 166–242. (IV, C)
7. Rogers RM: Anatomy of pelvic support. In Bent AE, Ostergard DR, Cundiff GW, et al (eds): Urogynecology and Pelvic Floor Dysfunction, 5th ed. Philadelphia, Lippincott Williams & Wilkins, 2003, ch. 2. (IV, C)
8. LaSala C, Tulikangas P: Pelvimetry and measurements of pertinent landmarks of the retropubic space in female cadavers. Poster 38, Society of Gynecologic Surgeons 29th Scientific Meeting, Anaheim, Calif, March 5–7, 2003. (III, B)
9. Richardson AC: The anatomic defects in rectocele and enterocele. J Pelvic Surg 1995;1:219. (III, B)
10. Baden W, Walker T: Surgical Repair of Vaginal Defects. Philadelphia: Lippincott, 1992. (IV, C)
11. DeLancey JOL: Anatomic aspects of vaginal eversion after hysterectomy. Am J Obstet Gynecol 1992;166:1717–1728. (III, B)
12. Weber AM, Walters MD: Anterior vaginal prolapse: review of anatomy andtechniques of surgical repair. Obstet Gynecol 1997;89:311–318. (IV, C)
13. Farrell SA, Dempsey T, Geldenhuys L: Histologic examination of "fascia" used in colporrhaphy. Obstet Gynecol 2001;98:794–798. (III, B)
14. DeLancey JOL: Structural aspects of the extrinsic continence mechanism. Obstet Gynecol 1988;72:296–301. (III, B)
15. Swift SE: Epidemiology of pelvic organ prolapse. In Bent AE, Ostergard DR, Cundiff GW, et al (eds): Urogynecology and Pelvic Floor Dysfunction, 5th ed. Philadelphia, Lippincott Williams & Wilkins, 2003, ch. 3. (IV, C)
16. Bump R, Mattiasson A, Bø K, et al: The standardization of terminology of female pelvic organ prolapse and pelvic floor dysfunction. Am J Obstet Gynecol 1996;175:10–17. (IV, C)
17. DeLancey JOL: Fascial and muscular abnormalities in women with urethral hypermobility and anterior vaginal wall prolapse. Am J Obstet Gynecol 2002;87:93–98. (III, B)
18. Buller JL, Thompson JR, Cundiff GW, et al: Uterosacral ligament: description of anatomic relationships to optimize surgical safety. Obstet Gynecol 2001;97:873–879. (III, B)

# Chapter 25

# Nonsurgical Treatment of Urinary Incontinence

## Rony A. Adam, MD, and Peggy A. Norton, MD

### KEY POINTS

- Many women with urinary incontinence may benefit from a trial of nonsurgical management.
- Pelvic floor muscle training and duloxetine are useful in the treatment of stress incontinence.
- Devices for the treatment of stress incontinence have not been well studied but show some benefit.
- Anticholinergic medications are effective at treating overactive bladder symptoms, including urge incontinence.

In women, treatment of urge urinary incontinence (overactive bladder) is primarily pharmacologic and behavioral. Although stress urinary incontinence can be treated surgically, many women choose nonsurgical options such as intravaginal devices and newer pharmacologic treatments. Both types of urinary incontinence may benefit from lifestyle interventions, physical therapy, biofeedback, bladder retraining, and behavioral modifications. Mixed urge and stress incontinence is sometimes treated as two separate entities with their respective treatments, although there is increasing evidence that both components may respond to treatments aimed at a single type of incontinence, such as anticholinergics/antimuscarinics for urge incontinence. A consensus conference on urinary incontinence was sponsored by the World Health Organization in 2001, and levels of evidence for many nonsurgical treatments were summarized by Wilson and colleagues.[1]

## GENERALIZED TREATMENTS FOR URINARY INCONTINENCE

### Lifestyle Interventions

Modest lifestyle changes are often suggested by practitioners, although much of the evidence for their use is based only on expert opinion (Table 25-1). Weight loss in morbidly obese women has been shown to decrease urinary incontinence (Level II evidence). Heavy occupational work and physical activity may be associated with urinary incontinence, but it is unknown whether cessation of these activities is beneficial or advisable (Level II evidence). Although smoking is associated with urinary incontinence, there is no data on smoking cessation in the management of incontinence. Excessive fluid intake may play a role in a minority of women, but adjustment of fluid has had conflicting results in the literature. Constipation appears to be a risk factor for urinary incontinence, but management of consti-

pation has not been studied for its effect on urinary incontinence. Other management interventions include decreasing lower extremity edema, treating pulmonary conditions such as cough, and utilizing a bedside commode for nighttime incontinence.

### Behavioral Modification

Behavior modification for urinary incontinence is a program of education, where skills are learned to improve urinary control. It emphasizes correct habits and frequency of voiding, urge suppression techniques, and in some cases scheduled voiding. Behavioral modification is often discussed in conjunction with pelvic floor muscle training (PFMT) because these muscles are an important part of urge suppression and bladder neck support during increased abdominal pressure. Despite its broad clinical use, a Cochrane review of timed (scheduled) voiding, showed insufficient quality and quantity of data to provide evidence for or against its use as a treatment for urinary incontinence.[2] This strategy continues to remain popular due to its low cost, ease of implementation, and lack of adverse effects.

Another Cochrane review determined that bladder training is better than no treatment. The reviewers cautioned, however, that such a conclusion is tenuous due to the scarcity of adequately designed studies. Regarding comparison of bladder retraining with medication for urge incontinence, the reviewers found that bladder retraining was favored over either oxybutynin or imipramine with flavoxate. Again, caution was advised in the interpretation based on the limited data found. Based on a single study reviewed for this meta-analysis, adding bladder retraining to a regimen of PFMT and biofeedback was better than PFMT or biofeedback alone when assessing patient perception of improvement and quality of life immediately after treatment. These benefits, however, were not sustained after 3 months.[3] One study found that in women with urge incontinence older than age 55, the combination of behavioral modification and oxybutynin was better at reducing incontinence episodes than either therapy alone at 8 weeks' follow-up.[4] Completion of a simple voiding diary can greatly assist in setting realistic goals for behavioral modification, and if a fluid intake/output record is kept, a better assessment of appropriate fluid management and typical voided volumes is available.

### Pelvic Floor Muscle Training

This intervention focuses on improving the strength and response of the pubococcygeal muscle to voluntary contraction. Although its role in the treatment of stress incontinence is well established, pelvic floor contraction is also a useful technique for urge suppression. In women with stress or mixed incontinence, PFMT

**Table 25-1**
**Efficacy of Lifestyle/Behavior Treatments for Urinary Incontinence**

|  | Efficacy | Effort | Evidence |
| --- | --- | --- | --- |
| **Lifestyle interventions** |  |  |  |
| Weight loss | Moderate | High | Level II |
| Active lifestyle, lifting | Assoc risk only |  | Scant II–III |
| Smoking cessation | Assoc risk only | High | Level IV |
| Fluid intake, caffeine | Moderate | Low | Scant II–III |
| Constipation | Assoc risk only | Low | Level II–III |
| Postural change (crossing legs) | Mod to high | Low | Level II |
| **Behavior modification** |  |  |  |
| Bladder retraining | Moderate | Moderate | Level I |
| Bladder retraining w/pelvic floor muscle training | Conflicting evidence | Moderate | Level I |
| Bladder retraining w/medication | Conflicting evidence | Moderate | Level I–II |
| **Pelvic floor muscle training** | Moderate | Moderate | Level I |
| "Intensive" better than "standard" | Moderate (short-term only) | Moderate | Level I |
| Adding biofeedback | No additional benefit | High | Level I |
| Adding weighted cones | No additional benefit | Moderate | Level I |

Summarized and updated from Wilson D, Hay-Smith J, Bø K: Outcomes of conservative treatment. In Cardozo L, Staskin D (eds): Textbook of Female Urology and Urogynaecology. London: Isis Medical Media, 2001, pp 325–332.

was found to be better than no treatment or sham treatment in a Cochrane review. It could not, however, be shown to be any better or worse than other conservative therapies. Adding biofeedback to PFMT shows no advantage, and the review also concludes that the role of PFMT in patients with urge incontinence remains unclear. Great heterogeneity was noted in the content of reported training programs, such as number of contractions, duration of each contraction, and number of exercise sessions per day, with no ability to determine which regimen is preferred.[5] The long-term success of PFMT depends on adherence to the exercise regimen. In a follow-up study of a randomized trial of home PFMT compared to intensive PFMT, the marked short-term benefit of intensive training did not persist after 15 years. The authors found that only 28% of subjects exercised at least once a week, 36% periodically, and 36% never, with no difference noted based on the original group assignments.[6] Obstetricians and gynecologists are in a unique position: the obstetrician sees firsthand the damage to the pelvic floor muscles during childbirth, and the gynecologist has an opportunity to teach improved muscle control every time he or she performs a digital examination of the vagina.

## URGE INCONTINENCE TREATMENTS

Although this chapter is devoted to women with incontinence, it should be noted that many women are bothered by overactive bladder symptoms without incontinence (urgency, frequency, nocturia) and may be treated for these bothersome symptoms in the absence of incontinence. Most patients with urge incontinence have some form of behavioral management included in their care, including urge suppression techniques, scheduled voiding, and fluid management. Urge suppression includes the "freeze and squeeze" technique of *not* rushing to the bathroom, contracting the pelvic floor muscles (possibly while crossing legs), and imaging the bladder contraction going away. Patients

are taught to avoid provocative situations, such as arriving home with a full bladder. A voiding diary with voided volumes recorded in a simple plastic "hat" can distinguish the patient who voids 50 to 100 mL 20 times a day from the patient who voids 400 to 600 mL 10 times a day. Both may complain of urgency, but the first will be treated with scheduled voiding and pharmacologic agents, whereas the second needs to normalize her voided volumes to a reasonable 200 to 300 mL, mostly by consuming less fluids.

Pharmacologic management of urge incontinence has good evidence for efficacy, although all of these randomized, controlled trials had significant placebo effects, probably because patients keep voiding diaries as part of these trials (Table 25-2). Newer-generation medications have sustained formulations that minimize the major side effect of dry mouth, and although all seem to have similar efficacy, the side effects seen in any individual patient may direct the medication selected. At present, differences in cognitive function in the elderly, constipation, and dry mouth are reported with several medications used to manage incontinence, but few head-to-head comparisons exist. Effects should be seen within 2 to 4 weeks of treatment, and the cost is approximately $70 to $100 per month. Generic oxybutynin 5 mg three times daily may be the cheapest option but has considerable side effects that may compromise compliance.

Extended-release oxybutynin given once daily appears to have similar efficacy as immediate-release oxybutynin, but with significantly fewer side effects.[7] Most studies show a reduction in urge incontinence episodes of approximately 70%.[7–9]

Transdermal oxybutynin is given twice a week and shows similar efficacy to oxybutynin and tolterodine, but with fewer anticholinergic side effects; the incidence of dry mouth did not differ from placebo. The primary side effect of transdermal oxybutynin is mild to moderate local skin reactions. Erythema occurs in about half the subjects, with 3% of those subjects having severe erythema and up to 17% associated pruritus.[10–12]

**Table 25-2**
**Pharmacologic Treatment of Overactive Bladder/Urge Incontinence***

| Generic/Brand Name | Dose | Citations |
|---|---|---|
| Tolterodine/Detrol LA (oral) | 2,4 mg PO once daily | Dmochowski et al., 2003,[12] Drutz et al., 1999,[14] Van Kerrebroeck et al., 2001,[15] Diokno et al., 2003[16] |
| Oxybutynin/Ditropan XL (oral) | 5, 10, 15 mg PO once daily | Anderson et al., 1999,[7] Gleason et al., 1999,[8] Appell et al., 2001,[9] Diokno et al., 2002[16] |
| Oxybutynin/Oxytrol (transdermal) | 3.9 mg/day applied twice weekly | Davila et al., 2001,[10] Dmochowski et al., 2002,[11] Dmochowski et al., 2003[12] |
| Trospium/Sanctura (oral) | 20 mg PO twice daily | Frohlich et al., 2002,[17] Halaska et al., 2003,[18] Zinner et al., 2004[19] |
| Darifenacin/Enablex (oral) | 7.5, 15 mg PO once daily | Cardozo et al., 2005,[20] Chapple et al., 2005[21] |
| Solifenacin/Vesicare (oral) | 5, 10 mg PO once daily | Cardozo et al., 2004,[22] Chapple et al., 2004,[23] Kelleher et al., 2005[24] |

*Medications available in the United States.

Tolterodine, in its immediate- and extended-release formulations, has been shown effective in the treatment of overactive bladder in numerous randomized, controlled trials.[13–15] One study compared the long-acting formulations of oxybutynin with tolterodine. Results suggest that both had similar ability to reduce the number of incontinence episodes; there was slightly more dry mouth in the oxybutynin group but no difference in discontinuation rates.[16]

Several new drugs have recently been approved by the Food and Drug Administration and appear to have similar efficacy to those already marketed[17–24] (Table 25-3). Some of these newer medications have been shown to have little effect on cognitive function. One study compared the effects of oxybutynin, tolterodine, and trospium on sleep and cognitive skills in healthy volunteers older than age 50. There was significant reduction

of rapid eye movement (REM) sleep with oxybutynin and tolterodine, but trospium showed REM sleep similar to that subjects experienced while on placebo. No differences were noted in cognitive skills or subjective reporting of sleep variables with any of the three medications tested, compared to placebo.[25] Another study showed no effect on cognitive function when darifenacin was compared to placebo in subjects age 65 or older.[26] A few older drugs have either higher side effects (propantheline bromide) or have not had efficacy established (hyoscyamine, flavoxate).

## STRESS INCONTINENCE TREATMENTS

Pharmacologic treatment of stress incontinence was previously focused on alpha stimulation of the urethral smooth muscle with ephedrine-like agents, mainly those containing phenylpropanolamine, which were removed from the market due to concerns about hemorrhagic stroke. Estrogen seemed likely to help stress incontinence due to its effects on urethral mucosal coaption and vascularity. A Cochrane review from 2003 concluded that estrogen can improve or cure incontinence, both stress and urge types,[27] but more current Level I evidence shows that oral conjugated equine estrogen with or without progestin is not useful in the treatment or the prevention of urinary incontinence—stress, urge, or mixed.[28] The role of vaginal estrogen either by cream or intravaginal device is still unclear due to lack of available studies. Duloxetine, a combined norepinephrine/serotonin reuptake inhibitor, has been shown to improve stress and mixed incontinence in multiple randomized, controlled trials (see Table 25-3). The action of the drug is unknown, but it may augment normal urethral tone without compromising voiding function. A randomized, blinded, doubly controlled trial showed that 40 mg twice a day of oral duloxetine was better than no treatment and than PFMT alone. It further showed that duloxetine and PFMT combined was better than duloxetine alone.[29] Duloxetine is approved for use in stress incontinence in Europe, but is only approved for the treatment of depression and diabetic peripheral neuropathic pain in the United States as of December 2005.

Pelvic floor muscle training has long been recognized in the treatment of stress incontinence and is based on the idea that a

**Table 25-3**
**Device/Pharmacologic Treatment for Urinary Incontinence**

| | Efficacy | Effort | Evidence |
|---|---|---|---|
| **Continence devices** | | | |
| Intravaginal (pessary-like) devices | Moderate to high | Low to moderate | Scant I–II |
| Occlusive urethral devices (not currently marketed) | Moderate | Low to moderate | Level III–IV |
| Intraurethral devices (not currently marketed) | High | Moderate | Level II–III |
| Pharmacologic treatment of overactive bladder | Moderate | Low but expensive | Level I |
| Pharmacologic treatment of stress urinary incontinence | Moderate | Low, no cost estimates | Level I |
| Pharmacologic treatment of mixed urinary incontinence | Moderate | Low | Level I |

Summarized from Wilson D, Hay-Smith J, Bø K: Outcomes of conservative treatment. In Cardozo L, Staskin D (eds): Textbook of Female Urology and Urogynaecology. London: Isis Medical Media, 2001, pp 325–342.

**Table 25-4**
**Devices for Stress Urinary Incontinence**

| Device | n | Indication | Follow-up | Outcome |
|---|---|---|---|---|
| Smith-Hodge pessary[34] | 30 | Stress incontinence | None | Cough pressure profile 24/30 patients continent |
| Randomized controlled trial of super tampon and Hodge pessary[35] | 18 | Exercise-induced stress incontinence | None | 36% pessary users continent; 58% tampon users continent |
| Bladder neck support prosthesis[36] | 77 | Stress and mixed incontinence | 12 weeks | Subjective pad test; 29% continent, 51% decreased severity by more than half; 81% combined subjective/objective some or maximum benefit |
| Bladder neck support prosthesis[37] | 70 | Stress or mixed incontinence | 4 weeks | 53/70 completed trial; significant improvement on pad tests, diaries; high subjective improvement and quality of life |
| Continence ring pessary[38] | 38 | Stress incontinence | 1 year | 6/38 continued device use long term; improved scores in pad test, voiding diary |
| Various continence pessaries[39] | 100 | Stress and mixed incontinence prolapse | 11 months | 59% patients continued use long term, with significant reduction in incontinence |
| Various continence pessaries[40] | 119 | Stress incontinence | 6 months | 89% successful device fitting; over half continued usage for 6 months |

Summarized and updated from Wilson D, Hay-Smith J, Bø K: Outcomes of conservative treatment. In Cardozo L, Staskin D (eds): Textbook of Female Urology and Urogynaecology. London: Isis Medical Media, 2001, pp. 325–347.

strong and fast contraction of the pubococcygeal muscle will press the urethra against the back of the symphysis pubis, thus creating a mechanical rise in urethral pressure. In general, patients should be assessed for their ability to perform a correct contraction; and contact with a health care provider at regular intervals may improve the effect of PFMT. One immediate benefit of PFMT may be to alert the patient to the use of a contraction before an anticipated increase in intra-abdominal pressure (the "knack"). A variety of regimens is recommended, making comparisons difficult (see Table 25-1). In most regimens, the patient is taught to perform three sets of 8 to 12 slow maximal voluntary contractions sustained for 6 to 8 seconds. These three sets should be performed three to four times a week, preferably daily, and benefit may not be appreciated until 15 to 20 weeks. Patients should expect to continue this training long term or lose its benefit.

Intravaginal devices work by creating a "backstop" at the level of the bladder neck. Devices that have been studied include a short super tampon inserted just inside the vagina, a Hodge pessary placed backward and upside down, and a variety of continence devices manufactured by companies that also manufacture pessaries for prolapse[30–36] (Table 25-4; see also Table 25-3). Additionally, there are several disposable intra-vaginal devices exist that are not currently available for use in the United States. These devices are easy to use and seem to have moderately good efficacy, especially for the woman who has predictable stress incontinence, such as with exercise or during a bad cold. Use among urogynecologic practices is variable; some specialists offer these devices to all women with stress incontinence, but others do not include intravaginal devices in their practice. The devices have not been well studied; these are low-cost, modest-volume devices whose manufacturers do not have research funds and there are no sham devices for randomized, controlled trials.

Intra-urethral devices work through occlusion of the urethra. They are removed for voiding and most cannot be reinserted.

Trials of several products have been conducted with favorable efficacy (79% of patients were completely dry) and low risk of side effects, but intra-urethral devices are less comfortable than the intravaginal devices.[37,38] These intra-urethral devices have failed to gain popularity with patients and physicians, and currently no intra-urethral device is marketed in the United States.

Occlusive extra-urethral devices or patches have been reported to significantly reduce incontinence episodes and increase quality of life.[39,40] Despite this, acceptance from physicians and patients has been poor and the devices are not currently marketed in the United States.

For more information, go to www.augs.org, the website for the American Urogynecologic Society, with sites for members and patients. For voiding diaries and bladder retraining, click on information for women, diagnostic and treatment information on overactive bladder/urge incontinence. Information on PFMT (Kegel exercises) is also available.

## REFERENCES

1. Wilson D, Hay-Smith J, Bø K: Outcomes of conservative treatment. In Cardozo L, Staskin D (eds): Textbook of Female Urology and Urogynaecology. London: ISIS Medical Media, 2001, pp 325–342 **(III, B)**

2. Ostaszkiewicz J, Johnston L, Roe B: Habit retraining for the management of urinary incontinence in adults. Cochrane Database of Systematic Reviews 2004, Vol. 2. CD002801. **(Ia, A)**

3. Wallace SA, Roe B, Williams K, Palmer M: Bladder training for urinary incontinence in adults. Cochrane Database of Systematic Reviews 2004, Vol. 1 CD001308. **(Ia, A)**

4. Burgio KL, Locher JL, Goode PS: Combined behavioral and drug therapy for urge incontinence in older women. J Am Geriatr Soc 2000 48:370–374. **(Ib, A)**

5. Hay-Smith EJ, Bo Berghmans LC, Hendriks HJ, et al: Pelvic floor muscle training for urinary incontinence in women. Cochrane Database of Systematic Reviews 2001, Vol. 1 CD001407. Last updated January 2005. **(Ia, A)**

6. Bø K, Kvarstein B, Nygaard I: Lower urinary tract symptoms and pelvic floor muscle exercise adherence after 15 years. Obstet Gynecol 2005; 105:999–1005. **(Ib, A)**

7. Anderson RU, Mobley D, Blank B, et al: Once daily controlled versus immediate release oxybutynin chloride for urge urinary incontinence. J Urol 1999;161:1809–1812. **(Ib, A)**

8. Gleason DM, Susset J, White C, et al: Evaluation of a new once-daily formulation of oxybutynin for the treatment of urinary urge incontinence. J Urol 1999;54:420–423. **(Ib, A)**

9. Appell RA, Sand P, Dmochowski R, et al: Prospective randomized controlled trial of extended-release oxybutynin chloride and tolterodine tartrate in the treatment of overactive bladder: results of the OBJECT study. Mayo Clin Proc 2001;76:358–363. **(Ib, A)**

10. Davila GW, Daugherty CA, Sanders SW: A short-term, multicenter, randomized double-blind titration study of the efficacy and anticholinergic side effects of transdermal compared to immediate release oral oxybutynin treatment of patients with urge incontinence. J Urol 2001;166:140–145. **(Ib, A)**

11. Dmochowski RR, Davila GW, Zinner NR, et al: Efficacy and safety of transdermal oxybutynin in patients with urge and mixed urinary incontinence. J Urol 2002;168:580–586. **(Ib, A)**

12. Dmochowski RR, Sand PK, Zinner NR, et al: Comparative efficacy and safety of transdermal oxybutynin and oral tolterodine versus placebo in previously treated patients with urge and mixed urinary incontinence. Urology 2003;62:237–242. **(Ib, A)**

13. Abrams P, Freeman R, Anderstrom C, Mattiasson A: Tolterodine, a new antimuscarinic agent: as effective but better tolerated than oxybutynin in patients with an overactive bladder. Br J Urol 1998;81:801–810. **(Ib, A)**

14. Drutz HP, Appell RA, Gleason D, et al: Clinical efficacy and safety of tolterodine compared to oxybutynin and placebo in patients with overactive bladder. Int Urogynecol J Pelvic Floor Dysfunct 1999; 10:283–289. **(Ib, A)**

15. Van Kerrebroeck P, Kreder K, Jonas U, et al: Tolterodine once-daily: superior efficacy and tolerability in the treatment of the overactive bladder. J Urol 2001;57:414–421. **(Ib, A)**

16. Diokno AC, Appell RA, Sand PK, et al: Prospective randomized, double-blind study of the efficacy and tolerability of the extended-release formulations of oxybutynin and tolterodine for overactive bladder: results of the OPERA trial. Mayo Clin Proc 2003;78:687–695. **(Ib, A)**

17. Frohlich G, Bulitta M, Strosser W: Trospium chloride in patients with detrusor overactivity; meta-analysis of placebo-controlled randomized double-blind multi-center clinical trials on the efficacy and safety of 20 mg trospium chloride twice daily. Int J Clin Pharmacol Ther 2002; 40:295–303. **(Ia, A)**

18. Halaska M, Ralph G, Wiedemann A, et al: Controlled double-blind multicentre clinical trial to investigate long-term tolerability and efficacy of trospium chloride in patients with detrusor instability. World J Urol 2003;20:392–399. **(Ib, A)**

19. Zinner N, Gittelman M, Harris R, et al: Trospium Study Group. Trospium chloride improves overactive bladder symptoms: a multi-center phase III trial. J Urol 2004;171:2311–2315. **(Ib, A)**

20. Cardozo L, Dixon A: Increased warning time with darifenacin: a new concept in the management of urinary urgency. J Urol 2005; 173:1214–1218. **(Ib, A)**

21. Chapple C, Steers W, Norton P, et al: A pooled analysis of three Phase III studies to investigate the efficacy tolerability and safety of darifenacin a muscarinic M3 selective receptor antagonist in the treatment of overactive bladder. BJU Int 2005;95:993–1001. **(Ib, A)**

22. Cardozo L, Lisec M, Millard R, et al: Randomized double-blind placebo controlled trial of the once daily antimuscarinic agent solifenacin succinate in patients with overactive bladder. J Urol 2004; 172:1919–1924. **(Ib, A)**

23. Chapple CR, Arano P, Bosch JL, et al: Solifenacin appears effective and well tolerated in patients with symptomatic idiopathic detrusor overactivity in a placebo- and tolterodine-controlled phase 2 dose-finding study. BJU Int 2004;93:71–77. **(Ib, A)**

24. Kelleher CJ, Cardozo L, Chapple CR, et al: Improved quality of life in patients with overactive bladder symptoms treated with solifenacin. BJU Int 2005;95:81–85. **(Ib, A)**

25. Diefenbach K, Arold G, Wollny A, et al: Effects on sleep of anticholinergics used for overactive bladder treatment in healthy volunteers aged 50 years or greater. BJU Int 2005;95:346–349. **(Ib, A)**

26. Lipton RB, Kolodner K, Wesnes K: Assessment of cognitive function of the elderly population: effects of darifenacin. J Urol 2005; 173:493–498. **(Ib, A)**

27. Moehrer B, Hextall A, Jackson S: Oestrogens for urinary incontinence in women. Cochrane Database of Systematic Reviews 2003, Vol. 2 CD001405. **(Ia, A)**

28. Hendrix SL, Cochrane BB, Nygaard IE, et al: Effects of estrogen with and without progestin on urinary incontinence. JAMA 2005; 293:935–948. **(Ib, A)**

29. Ghoniem GM, van Leeuwen JS, Elser DM, et al: Duloxetine/Pelvic Floor Muscle Training Clinical Trial Group. A randomized controlled trial of duloxetine alone, pelvic floor muscle training alone, combined treatment and no active treatment in women with stress urinary incontinence. J Urol 2005;173:1647–1653. **(Ib, A)**

30. Bhatia NN, Bergman A: Pessary test in women with urinary incontinence. Obstet Gynecol 1985;65:220–226. **(III, B)**

31. Nygaard I: Prevention of exercise incontinence with mechanical devices. J Reprod Med 1995;40:89–94. **(Ib, A)**

32. Kondo A, Yokoyama E, Koshiba K, et al: Bladder neck support prosthesis: a non-operative treatment for stress or mixed incontinence. J Urol 1997;157:824–827. **(IIb, B)**

33. Davila GW, Neal D, Horbach N, et al: A bladder-neck support prosthesis for women with stress and mixed incontinence. Obstet Gynecol 1999;93:938–942. **(IIb, B)**

34. Robert M, Mainprize TC: Long-term assessment of the incontinence ring pessary for the treatment of stress incontinence. Int Urogynecol J Pelvic Floor Dysfunct 2002;13:326–329. **(III, B)**

35. Farrell SA, Singh B, Aldakhil L: Continence pessaries in the management of urinary incontinence in women. J Obstet Gynaecol Can 2004; 26:113–117. **(III, B)**

36. Donnelly MJ, Powell-Morgan S, Olsen AL, Nygaard IE: Vaginal pessaries for the management of stress and mixed urinary incontinence. Int Urogynecol J Pelvic Floor Dysfunct 2004;15:302–307. **(IIb, B)**

37. Miller JL, Bavendam T: Treatment with the Reliance urinary control insert: one year experience. J Endourol 1996;10:287–292. **(III, B)**

38. Sand PK, Staskin D, Miller J: Effect of a urinary control insert on quality of life in incontinent women. Int Urogynecol J Pelvic Floor Dysfunct 1999;10:100–105. **(IIb, B)**

39. Eckford SD, Jackson SR, Lewis PA, Abrams P: The continence control pad—a new external urethral occlusion device in the management of stress incontinence. Br J Urol 1996;77:538–540. **(III, B)**

40. Versi E, Griffiths DJ, Harvey MA: A new external urethral occlusive device for female urinary incontinence. Obstet Gynecol 1998; 92:286–291. **(IIb, B)**

## KEY POINTS

- Multiple factors are associated with stress urinary incontinence.
- Women who have delivered a child, whether vaginally or by cesarean section, have higher rates of stress urinary incontinence.
- Nulliparous women have the lowest rates of stress urinary incontinence.
- Multichannel urodynamic testing may be useful as a diagnostic tool, but it is an imperfect test with limited reproducibility.
- Pelvic exercises rarely cure stress incontinence, but they can allow some patients to achieve a level of improvement they find acceptable.
- Treatment of stress urinary incontinence is mainly surgical; the usual methods used are retropubic suspension or midsuburethral slings.
- The selection of the type of surgery performed is based more on subjective factors such as a surgeon's taste, habits, and experience as well as by the aggressive marketing of a procedure by surgical instrument companies.

Stress urinary incontinence is defined by the International Continence Society as a symptom, a sign, and a condition. The symptom is the patient complaint of involuntary loss of urine with physical exercise. The sign is the observation of loss of urine from the urethra immediately upon increasing intra-abdominal pressure (e.g., from running, coughing, and sneezing). The condition is the social unacceptable involuntary loss of urine.

It is estimated that at least 8.5% of women suffer from some form of urinary incontinence and 37% of elderly women may have urinary incontinence.[1] It is estimated that at least 10 million adult Americans suffer from incontinence at an estimated annual cost of $10.3 million.[2] Government studies indicate that there are now 3 million adults age 85 or older who suffer from urinary incontinence; it is expected that in the next decade that number could double.[3] Urinary incontinence of a significant degree can have a major influence on a woman's life. Emotional stress is placed on a family when they must care for an incontinent member of the household. Health care workers are also psychologically affected as the hospitalized or institutionalized patient who is incontinent of both urine and feces requires more nursing time, is aesthetically unpleasant, and is more likely to spread certain pathogens. The social implications and the economic impact of incontinence are considerable given the enlarging elderly population and the prevalence of incontinence, which approaches 50% in the aged.

Incontinence refers to any involuntary loss of urine and is defined by the following:

- *Stress urinary incontinence* is involuntary leakage of urine on effort or exertion or on coughing or sneezing. The sign of stress urinary incontinence must occur at the start of coughing and end with the coughing.
- *Urge incontinence* is the strong desire to urinate. The patient may sense a degree of urgency if voiding occurs despite the desire not to void.
- *Genuine stress incontinence* is involuntary leakage of urine during increased abdominal pressure in the absence of detrusor contraction during urodynamics.
- *Functional incontinence* is involuntary leakage despite normal bladder and urethral function in patients with dementia or disorientation.
- *Total urinary incontinence* occurs when the bladder is unable to store urine because the resting urethral pressure is so low that no resistance is present for the passage of urine.

Three theories have been developed to explain the continence mechanism:

1. DeLancey's hammock hypothesis
2. Ulmsten and Petros' integral theory
3. Shafik's common sphincter mechanisms

DeLancey studied the spatial relationship and the histologic nature between the arcus tendineus fasciae pelvis, the levator ani muscles, and the fascia endopelvina.[4] A hammock-like layer on which the bladder and the urethra rest is formed by the anterior vaginal wall and the fascia endopelvina. The stability of this layer depends on the layer's intact attachment to the arcus and the levator muscles. The urethra is compressed during stress between the downward forces of intra-abdominal pressure rise and the resistance of this hammock-like supportive suburethral layer (Fig. 26-1). DeLancey believed that the stability of this layer, rather than the intra-abdominal position of the bladder neck and proximal urethra, determines urinary continence during stress. Further support for this theory was offered by the observation that operations that stabilize the pelvic fascia to the arcus tendineus fasciae pelvis have proven to be more successful and cause less voiding dysfunction than high retropubic suspension procedures.

According to the theory of Ulmsten and Petros, female stress and urge incontinence have a common etiology.[5] Laxity of the anterior vaginal wall or its supporting ligaments allows activation of stretch receptors in the bladder neck and proximal urethra, which allows an inappropriate voiding reflex that may result in detrusor instability and urgency, frequency, and nocturia. Thus,

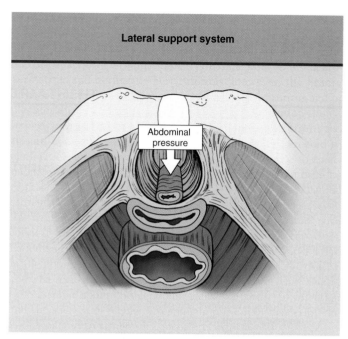

**Lateral support system**

Abdominal pressure

**Figure 26-1   The urethral support system, after the urethra and vagina have been transected just below the vaginal neck.** The arrow represents the force generated by increased abdominal pressure. (From DeLancey JOL: Structural support of the urethra as it relates to stress urinary incontinence: the hammock hypothesis. Am J Obstet Gynecol 1994;170:1713–1723. Copyright 1994, Elsevier Science.)

the anterior vaginal wall does not efficiently transmit the closure pressure that would otherwise be caused by three separate closure mechanisms. They observed three opposing muscle forces during videoradiologic studies combined with dynamic urethral pressure measurements, surface electromyography, and digital palpation. The anterior pubococcygeal muscle acts in a forward direction to lift the anterior vaginal wall to compress the urethra; two opposing muscle groups controlled by the levator ani and the longitudinal muscle of the anus move backward, which closes the bladder neck. The pelvic floor muscles, under voluntary control, lift the hammock in a cephalad direction, closing the bladder neck. This upward motion is the mechanism used in pelvic floor exercises. Thus, the overall laxity of the anterior vaginal wall or its supporting ligaments causes a dissipation of the forces, and stress incontinence occurs.

According to Shafik, the pelvic floor consists of two muscle structures, each with a different origin and innervation.[6] The puborectal muscle is considered the common pelvic organ sphincter. Contraction of the levator ani opens the bladder neck and initiates voiding and bowel evacuation. Reflex contraction of the puborectal and striated urethra muscle, mediated through the pudendal nerve, controls urinary continence.

Two of the three theories are complementary because they underline the stability of the fascia endopelvina and its intact connection to the pelvic floor muscles, which appear to be essential for adequate urethral closure during stress. The integral theory suggests a more active role for the pelvic muscles in the maintenance of continence.

This chapter reviews the most recent high-quality evidence regarding the etiology and management of urinary incontinence

in women. The data sources selected focus on the etiology or treatment of urinary incontinence in adult women and included searches in the Excerpta Medica Database (EMBASE), Medline, The Cochrane Library, and the American College of Physicians (ACP) Journal Club. Studies of treatment included only randomized, controlled trials or systematic reviews of randomized, controlled trials. Articles to determine the etiology of incontinence were found by reviewing cohort studies, case-control studies, and cross-sectional studies along with reviews of these types of studies.

Multiple factors have been found to be associated with urinary incontinence. Women who developed stress incontinence during the first pregnancy and especially those who developed stress urinary incontinence during the first 6 weeks' postpartum were found to have an increased risk of having incontinence 5 years' postpartum.[7] Increased parity was independently associated with urinary incontinence and subsequent stress incontinence surgery.[8] Women who were nulliparous had lower rates of stress incontinence than those who had either vaginal deliveries or cesarean sections.[9] Forceps delivery was associated with a higher risk of stress urinary incontinence than spontaneous vaginal delivery.[10] Vacuum delivery, vaginal laceration or episiotomy, and length of the second stage of labor were not found to be risk factors for developing stress urinary incontinence, whereas forceps delivery was an independent risk factor.[11] There appears to be an independent association between high birth weight and subsequent surgery for stress urinary incontinence.[12]

Hysterectomy in women age 60 or older was associated with a higher risk of developing urinary incontinence. This was not true for women younger than age 60.[13] After adjusting for age, parity, and educational level, a cross-sectional study demonstrated that hysterectomy was associated with urge incontinence but not stress incontinence.[14] There appears to be no association between the method of hysterectomy (abdominal or vaginal) and urge or stress incontinence.[15] The presence of a cystocele and/or the absence of the vesicourethral fold with uterine prolapse is independently associated with urinary incontinence.[16] Prolapse surgery is independently associated with urinary incontinence.[17]

Recurrent urinary tract infection appears independently associated with urge and mixed incontinence but not stress incontinence.[18] Certain medications have been independently associated with urinary incontinence, including diuretics,[19] estrogen,[20] tranquilizers, antidepressants, laxatives, and antibiotics.[20] The association between alcohol and urinary incontinence is not clear.[20] Smoking may be independently associated with urinary incontinence.[21] High caffeine intake (400 mg/day) was associated with urge incontinence.[22]

Specific diseases found to be independently associated with urinary incontinence include diabetes, stroke, elevated blood pressure, cognitive impairment, parkinsonism, arthritis, and back problems.[21,23,24]

Advancing age is associated with urge and mixed incontinence but not with stress incontinence.[25] African American women had lower rates of moderate and severe urinary incontinence but only after adjusting for educational attainment, financial assets, functional status, age, stroke, body mass index, smoking, alcohol use, and parity.[26] Increasing body mass index is associated with increasing rates of urinary incontinence.[26]

Higher level of educational achievement is associated with mild incontinence and stress incontinence.[26]

# NONPHARMACOLOGIC CONSERVATIVE MANAGEMENT

## Pelvic Floor Muscle Training

A Cochrane review that included studies of stress, urge, and mixed incontinence found that pelvic floor muscle exercises were more effective than no treatment or placebo.[27] When pelvic floor training was combined with a comprehensive clinic-based program it was found to be more effective than using a self-help booklet.[28] The combination of pelvic floor muscle training and bladder training was equally effective when administered as individual therapy or group therapy.[29] Studies that compared pelvic floor muscle training to surgery (open retropubic colposuspension, vaginal repair, or a combination) for stress urinary incontinence found no significant difference in the rates of self-reported cure or improvement, but pelvic floor training resulted in fewer self-reported cures. The surgery group had a significantly greater reduction in the number of leakage episodes.[30]

## Vaginal Cones

Therapy with vaginal cones appears to be inferior to pelvic floor muscle training.[31] Patients who have good levator tone with a substantial increase in tone with voluntary contractions may have limited benefit from vaginal cones. Small series have reported an improvement with cone therapy such that patients delayed or canceled their bladder suspension surgery. In general, cone therapy is indicated for women who are able to generate some pelvic muscle contraction.

## Vaginal Pessaries

In patients with mild to moderate cystoceles vaginal pessaries may increase urethral closure and urethral functional length. The mechanism of continence appears to be increased urethral pressure, possibly from obstruction of the urethra, or elevation of the proximal urethra into the abdominal pressure zone. A new pessary developed by Biswas (incontinence dish), with two extension arms to support the urethra has reported promising results, but more long-term studies are needed. Patients who have difficulty in using or retaining pessaries are more satisfied with definitive surgery.

## Bladder Training

Bladder training techniques involve strategies to increase the time interval voids using progressive voiding schedules. Bladder training was not significantly better than pelvic floor muscle training, but the combination of bladder training with pelvic floor muscle training was more effective than either alone.[32]

## Electrical Stimulation

The effectiveness of electrical stimulation may depend on the type of urinary incontinence. The addition of pelvic floor electrical stimulation to an extensive pelvic floor muscle training program did not significantly reduce the frequency of incontinence episodes.[32] Patients with moderate or severe incontinence with marked hypermobility of the urethra and vesicourethral descent do not respond to electrical stimulation. In general, electrical stimulation is associated with 30% to 60% improvement in stress incontinence and is most effective in patients with mild incontinence with poor pelvic muscle tone. Electrical stimulation is indicated for women who are unable to generate a pelvic muscle contraction.

## Summary

Pelvic floor exercises may be most helpful by improving the feeling that the patient can derive some benefit (positive incentive) through pelvic exercise, which improves her self-perception and sense of well-being and may minimize the patient's feeling of helplessness. These exercises rarely provide a cure for stress urinary incontinence but can achieve a level of improvement some patients find acceptable.

# PHARMACOLOGIC CONSERVATIVE THERAPY

A Cochrane review of anticholinergics for urge incontinence found anticholinergics were better than placebo in subjective cure or improvement rates.[33] In direct comparison trials, oxybutynin and tolterodine did not differ in outcomes; however, the risk of dry mouth was higher with oxybutynin than with tolterodine.[34] When extended-release oxybutynin was compared with tolterodine, there were higher mean numbers of weekly incontinence episodes with tolterodine.[30] Trospium chloride is the newest medication for urge incontinence. The effect is at least equal to the other anticholinergics, but the medication may have fewer side effects.

Magnesium hydroxide may reduce spontaneous detrusor contractions and may be effective treatment for urge incontinence. A small placebo-controlled study indicated some subjective improvement of urinary incontinence but transient diarrhea was a noted adverse effect.[35] Because of their effects on the contractile response of the urethra and bladder neck, alpha- and beta-adrenoceptor agonists have been used in the treatment of stress urinary incontinence. Likewise, ephedrine, norephedrine, and phenylpropanolamine have also been tried. However, because of the problems with hypertension from the increased vascular tone produced by these medications, their role has been diminished. Phenylpropanolamine was also found to be a risk factor in the development of hemorrhagic stroke, which has reduced the enthusiasm for alpha-adrenergic agonists.[30] Imipramine, because of its relaxing effect on the detrusor, has been used with some success. Serotonin and norepinephrine agonists have putative continence-promoting properties through parasympathetic suppression and enhancement of sympathetic and somatic activity. Dicyclomine hydrochloride is a musculotrophic/antimuscarinic agent more commonly used for the management of irritable bowel syndrome. It is a less potent agent than oxybutynin and has fewer adverse side effects. When oxybutynin is intolerable to some patients, this medication deserves consideration.

## Summary

New drug therapy that augments urethral resistance by inhibiting the reuptake of neurotransmitters, which are thought to make a key contribution to micturition may soon be available to treat stress urinary incontinence. The basis for this therapy is studies that suggest inhibition of serotonin and norepinephrine

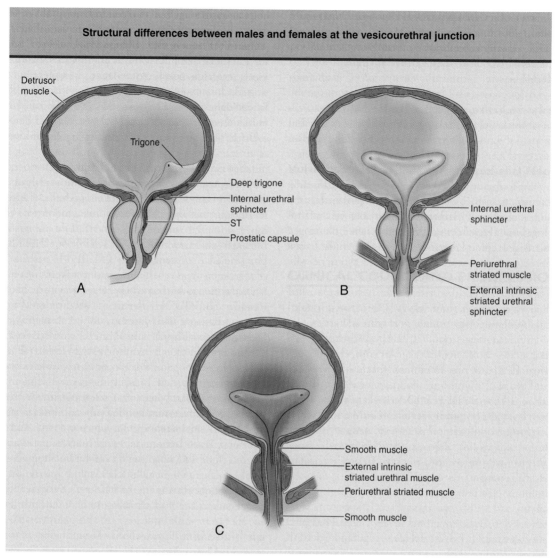

**Structural differences between males and females at the vesicourethral junction**

Figure 26-2    **Structural differences between male and female bladders at the vesicourethral junction.** *A* and *B*, Male bladder. *C*, Female bladder.

at the level of the nucleus of the pudendal nerve, which can increase signal transmission through the pudendal nerve to the urethral sphincter. This led to the development of duloxetine, a dual reuptake inhibitor, which could become the first approved medical therapy for stress urinary incontinence.

It is generally believed that the primary components that prevent stress incontinence in the female are the internal sphincter mechanism, the external urethral sphincter, and the proper anatomic support of the urethra, including the vesicourethral junction. Some researchers believe that urinary continence depends on a intact strong internal sphincter and a reactive sympathetic activity. There is a distinct structural difference between males and females at the vesicourethral junction (bladder neck). At the female bladder neck there is no comparable anatomic sphincter of smooth muscle (Fig. 26-2). Unlike the circular-oriented preprostatic smooth muscle of the

male, most of the muscle bundles in the female bladder neck extend obliquely or longitudinally into the urethral wall (see Fig. 26-1). It is doubtful that active contraction of this area plays a significant role in the maintenance of urinary incontinence in females. Due to the fact that the bladder neck and proximal urethra contain large quantities of elastin within their walls, passive elastic resistance offered by the urethral wall may be the most important single factor responsible for closure of the bladder neck and proximal urethra for maintaining continence in the female.

## ROLE OF URODYNAMICS

Despite the widespread prevalence of urinary incontinence, the diagnosis and management of urinary incontinence and voiding dysfunction is often challenging. The current role of urodynamic testing in the evaluation of stress urinary incontinence is controversial. Which women with stress urinary incontinence require urodynamic evaluation? Several studies have demonstrated that subjective symptoms alone are not predictive of stress urinary incontinence. Jensen and colleagues, in a meta-analysis of 19 articles, found the symptom of stress urinary incontinence to be 91% sensitive but only 51% specific in the diagnosis of genuine stress incontinence.[36] This usually means referral for multichannel urodynamic studies, which are expensive, not universally available, and not consistently reproducible. Rapid changes in diagnostic testing technology and further understanding of the pathophysiology of incontinence have resulted in little data and interpretation with varying degrees of consensus on its clinical applicability. This has made it difficult for the practicing clinician to decide which tests are necessary to adequately evaluate lower urinary dysfunction. Most clinicans are overwhelmed by its complexity. The criteria set developed by the American College of Obstetricians and Gynecologists does not mention cystometrography or recommend any specific urodynamic studies in the evaluation of women with stress urinary incontinence due to urethral hypermoblity.[37]

The goals of urodynamic testing should include objective observation of urinary leakage, reproduction of the patient's symptoms, correlation of the patient's symptomatology with urodynamic parameters, determination and differentiation of the etiologic factors causing urinary incontinence, and, finally, prediction and evaluation of the response to medical and surgical therapies. Little data is available to support any of these goals. Credibility is lost when the standard urodynamic results do not agree with patients who think they are cured. Nevertheless, urodynamic testing has been considered a standard in the evaluation of the incontinent female. However, studies have also shown that women who were investigated with urodynamics were more likely to receive active treatment with drugs or surgery; thus, the role of urodynamics must be further evaluated before standard use is recommended.

Clinical practice guidelines published by the Agency for Health Care Policy and Research (AHCPR) recommend considering surgery without referral for urodynamic testing for patients with symptoms of pure stress urinary loss as well as a voiding history and results of physical examination suggestive of pure hypermobility stress urinary incontinence that include the following[38]:

- Urine loss only with physical exertion (history and stress test)
- Normal voiding habits (≤ 8 episodes/day and ≤ 2 episodes/night)
- No neurologic history and no neurologic findings
- No history of anti-incontinence surgery or radical pelvic surgery
- Hypermobility of the urethra and bladder neck, pliable and compliant vaginal wall, and adequate vaginal capacity documented by physical examination
- Normal postvoid residual values
- Nonpregnant patient

Weidner and colleagues studied the predictive value of the symptom of stress urinary incontinence and the ability of other factors proposed by the AHCPR guidelines for the discrimination of patients unlikely to require urodynamic testing before surgical management.[39] They concluded that the predictive value of stress incontinence symptoms alone was not high enough to serve as the basis for surgical management. AHCPR guidelines improved the predictive value but are applicable to only a small subset of patients referred with urinary incontinence. They proposed that multichannel urodynamic testing is an imperfect diagnostic method, yet they believed that reliance on clinical assessments to determine which patients should undergo surgery was even more inaccurate and would result in some patients undergoing inappropriate surgical treatment. They concluded that their study supported routine urodynamic evaluation for most women before instigating surgical treatment with incontinence symptoms.

Urodynamists believe the basis of urodynamic testing results from the poor reliability of the patient's symptoms in accurately determining the underlying physiological or pathological state of the bladder. However, I have performed urodynamic testing on patients who give a history of stress urinary incontinence with every episode of straining, sneezing, coughing, and lifting who cannot be made to demonstrate leakage of urine in the urodynamic laboratory. This is a troubling problem. The International Continence Society has recommended that a complete urodynamic evaluation is not necessary in all patients, although some specialists believe urodynamic evaluation of the filling and voiding phases should be performed.[40] The most important aspect of a urodynamic study is that it be accurate and clinically relevant. The interpretation of the urodynamic study should never be independent of the overall clinical picture. If the results do not make sense, they are probably wrong. The generalist and the specialist should have an adequate understanding of the true value and limitations of urodynamic testing. It is beyond our scope to discuss all phases of urodynamic testing, which can be found in most textbooks on urodynamics.

Thus, the evidence to support routine urodynamic testing before any surgical treatment remains unclear. Unfortunately, this is an expensive and imperfect diagnostic test that has limited reproducibility. Physicians who perform urodynamic testing may also be reimbursed for this imperfect test more than the surgeon who performs the anti-incontinence operation. The financial incentive to recommend and perform this as a routine test before operative therapy needs further supportive evidence. Concern has been expressed that too many expensive instruments have been purchased by gynecologists and urologists who do not have the time or expertise to learn basic urodynamics or perform tests in a reproducible manner. Accurate urodynamic assessment requires a combination of appropriate equipment and technique. A retrospective study concluded that the cost and expense of running a urodynamic unit are justified when more than 200 patients are studied per year. Certainly simple office cystometry can be performed in an office setting in a cost-effective manner, providing basic information regarding voiding function and detrusor activity during bladder filling, bladder sensation, and competency of the urethral sphincter mechanism during stress. Some specialists believe that simple office cystometry should be tried first to provide the clinician with a preliminary diagnosis on which to base initial conservative therapy before further urodynamic testing is employed, if indicated.

## Summary

Many generalists believe that urodynamic studies are a necessary part of the evaluation of lower urinary tract function, but these tests are still evolving and more controlled studies are needed to clarify controversies regarding indications, techniques, and interpretation.

## SURGICAL MANAGEMENT

Controversy also continues as to the best surgical approach to treat stress urinary incontinence; it is unlikely that the necessary prospective, randomized studies with matched variables will ever be done to help resolve the matter. In the meantime, critical analysis of diagnostic methods, surgical techniques, and long-term results must continue.

Richardson's statement regarding how one chooses the surgical approach to the repair of stress urinary incontinence is enlightening:

> To determine the best approach in managing incontinent patients one must wade through a voluminous urogynecological literature inundated with contradiction, unsubstantiated opinions, speculative assertions, and modification upon modification. Adequate comparisons of results, even with ostensibly the same procedure, are generally not available.[41]

More than 200 different surgical procedures for urinary incontinence are performed, using a variety of methods. Wennberg and associates developed a conceptual approach that predicates physician decision making about clinical interventions on the presence of well-defined scientific norms (i.e., professional consensus). When consensus is lacking or ambigious, as is the case with the management of stress urinary incontinence, physician decision making is driven by subjective factors, referred to as "practice style," which incorporates physician values, attitudes, tastes, and habits.[42] To this list must be added the influence of surgical equipment companies, who actively promote a particular method before long-term studies have been done. This is why the clinical panel of the American Urological Association (AUA) recommended that at least 4 years of data on the outcomes of new technologies must be reported before those technologies are accepted, marketed, and sold to the medical community. This recommendation has gone unheeded by most companies. Eddy has described two main steps in medical decision making: The outcomes of alternative practices must be estimated first, then the desirability of the outcomes of the individual options must be compared.[43] Due to the complexity of urinary incontinence as well as its individual patient expression, the wide variation in surgical procedures offered to correct this problem is perhaps understandable. Success resides in the best understanding of a particular patient's expression, because a complete evaluation prior to surgery may still not identify the most effacious approach. Even though our present understanding of the continence mechanism and the therapeutic applications available to correct deficiencies in this mechanism is growing, therapy is not always successful.

The key to success is to define the normal anatomy of continence, understand how it becomes defective, then institute a specific surgery to correct the defect directly. Management of stress urinary incontinence has been complicated by a basic defect in knowledge, namely the anatomic basis of normal continence control. Therefore, empirical attempts to change upper urethral and bladder neck anatomy are commonly in use. Standard empirical procedures can only affect the stability, position, and mobility of the area in relation to the vesicourethral junction. Until the anatomy is understood and used as the basis for corrective surgery, the problem of deciding just what intervention to advise will continue. At present there is no definitive, ideal operation or definitive diagnostic test to separate cases on the basis of what operation to perform. Progress has been made with some very good suggestions, but for some reason surgeons do not always apply what is known.

### Summary

Among the proposed causes of stress urinary incontinence, the foremost theory is the loss of normal anatomy. Hypermobility of the urethra results in descent of this crucial area during increases in intra-abdominal pressure. The descent results in impaired pressure transmission to the urethra and ineffective compression of the suburethral hammock when discrete breaks in the fascia endopelvina and its attachment to the arcus tendineus fasciae pelvis are present.

## SURGICAL EVIDENCE

The AUA asked a select panel of seven urologists and one urogynecologist to compare the many surgical procedures for treating stress urinary incontinence on the basis of treatment outcomes.[44] The panel was charged to analyze published outcomes data on surgical procedures to treat female stress urinary incontinence and produce practice recommendations based primarily on outcomes evidence from the literature. Of the 5322 articles from the urologic, gynecologic, and general medical literature relevant to the treatment of stress urinary incontinence, 282 articles had acceptable outcome data. A meta-analysis of the data produced comparative outcome estimates for alternative surgical procedures. The panel discovered that all surgical techniques have similar outcomes for up to 48 months.

This finding is surprising when one considers the various theories and anatomic defects thought to cause incontinence. Have we reached a consensus as to what the continence mechanism is and how it should be repaired? Do we understand how each surgical anti-incontinence operation repairs the continence mechanism?

The AUA panel discovered differences in dry and cure rates that were signficant after 48 months. Slings and retropubic suspensions maintained a 82% to 84% success rate after 48 months, compared with needle suspensions, which decreased to 65% to 70% success rates.

Evaluation of anterior repairs was difficult to interpret because a sharp increase in cure/dry status at 24 to 47 months (from 68% to 85%) was followed by a marked decline after 48 months to 61%. It was believed that these results may have occurred because not all studies report outcomes at all time points studied.

Major concerns were encountered as the panel attempted to report on probability estimates for the four major procedure categories of retropubic suspensions, transvaginal suspensions, anterior repairs, and pubovaginal slings. Estimates were derived from combination cure/dry rates for the Burch procedure, Marshall-Marchetti-Krantz (MMK) procedure, and other individual retropubic suspension procedures and transvaginal suspensions, which derived combined outcomes data for Stamey, Pereyra, modified Pereyra, Gittes, and other types of individual transvaginal suspension procedures. Of interest was that no significant differences were found between individual procedures among the four groups.

## Summary

Even though the purpose of the panel was to distinguish between alternative surgical procedures and to provide estimates of the outcomes that could be expected with each, the four groups studied surgically manage the continence mechanism in different ways. Long-term outcomes data (>48 months) concluded that the surgical treatment of female stress urinary incontinence is effective despite what means was used and how the anatomic derangement of the continence mechanism was surgically corrected. Pubovaginal slings appear to closely and more directly correlate with the current theories of continence mechanism. Slings have currently evolved into the gold standard for the treatment of stress urinary incontinence caused by intrinsic sphincter deficiency and are more frequently utilized as the first-line surgical therapy for stress urinary incontinence associated with female urethral hypermobility. Slings seem to use the deranged anatomy of the continence mechanism as a basis for treatment in a more direct fashion than do other anti-incontinence procedures.

Retropubic suspensions were considered for many years the gold standard for the treatment of stress urinary incontinence. These procedures have been quite successful, yet the mechanism for their success is poorly understood. One theory is that the procedure stabilizes the proximal urethra. Thus, this assumes that urethral mobility is the cause of stress urinary incontinence. This theory differs from the original concept of retropubic procedures that were thought to be successful in treating stress urinary incontinence by placing the urethra in a high retropubic position. Furthermore, theories such as pressure transmission ratios were developed to explain why continence occurred after suspension procedures. During the 1990s procedures that neither suspend nor support the proximal urethra or bladder neck but rather place a tension-free suburethral sling under the mid-portion of the urethra were discovered to be as efficient as and less invasive than the more traditional procedures.

## CHOICE OF SURGICAL PROCEDURE

Many gynecologists seem to prefer the simplest rather than the most effective operation. Throughout the first half of the 20th century anterior colporrhaphy and the Kelly plication became the standard therapy for the treatment of female stress urinary incontinence. The purpose of this operation, described in 1914 by Kelly, was to repair the injured sphincter muscle at the vesicourethral junction. Marked variation in success of the Kelly-Kennedy plication in the literature ranges from 34% to 91%. Failure of this procedure may be the consequence of the imprecise understanding in the early 1900s of the pathophysiology of incontinence and urethral anatomy. Because it is now understood that there is no internal urethral sphincter, as

postulated by Kelly, or torn urethral sphincter, as conceived by Kennedy (see Fig. 26-2), this operation may function by being obstructive. It was also believed that this procedure could elevate the proximal urethra into the abdominal pressure zone, another theory for the cure of stress urinary incontinence, which was dismissed when the urethra was shown not to be an intra-abdominal structure. It is still confusing why this procedure works at all. Yet, Beck and McCormick[45] and Nichols[46] reported on acceptable success rates with their variations of this procedure. Beck attached the periurethral tissue to the pubic bone periosteum in a fashion similar to the abdominally performed MMK procedure. Nichols overlapped these tissues in a vest-over-trouser fashion.

Even though these investigators reported high levels of success, a considerable body of evidence does not support this approach for the treatment of stress urinary incontinence. Unfortunately there were many surgical failures, which were then subsquently treated by the sling operation. This gave rise to the unwise dictum to operate first from below and if this fails then from above. The use of anterior colporrhaphy and the Kelly-Kennedy plication as the sole operation for stress urinary incontinence appear no longer acceptable.

In 1949 Marshall, Marchetti, and Krantz collaborated on a new operation and reported on cure rates of 90% overall in patients complaining of stress urinary incontinence and 76% of patients with previously failed anti-incontinence surgery.[47] Various modifications of the MMK procedure were developed because of the occasional complication of osteitis pubis, presumably from placing sutures into the pubic bone. Further modification lead to the development of the attachment of the periurethral tissue to Cooper's ligament, the Burch procedure (Fig. 26-3). The physiological principle developed by Enhorning in 1961 was that elevation of the vesicourethral junction allows transference of abdominal pressures to the urethra.[48] Thus, many surgeons have oversuspended the urethra based on this theory. Current investigators are in conflict as to whether retropubic suspensions create urethral obstruction or simply return voiding pressures and flow conditions to normal levels. Therefore, this operation does not appear to restore the continence mechanism to normal. Until we know precisely what we are treating, we will not be able to choose the most effective, least noxious treatments for a particular patient, even though effective, non-destructive treatments do exist for particular types of stress urinary incontinence.

We really do not understand how the Burch procedure works, even though the success of the Burch procedure in the hands of many surgeons is well documented. It is a relatively simple procedure to perform, which may explain its high acceptance rate; common disadvantages include postoperative voiding dysfunction (22%) from high elevation of the vesicourethral junction and perivaginal tissues. Postoperative enterocele and vaginal prolapse (20%) are noted in the following patients:

- Women at risk for genital prolapse, including a strong history of prolapse
- Women with a history of heavy lifting or chronic constipation
- Women with coexisting genital prolapse

Burch initially fixed the paravaginal tissue to the arcus tendineus fasciae pelvis but was fearful that not enough elevation

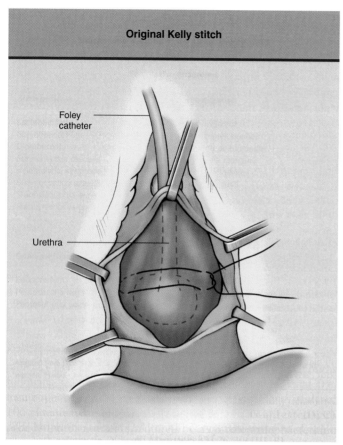

**Original Kelly stitch**

Foley
catheter

Urethra

**Figure 26-3** The original Kelly stitch, introduced to plicate a presumed internal urethral sphincter.

would be provided. Stanton modified the Burch procedure by suspending not only the vesicourethral junction, but also the entire length of the vagina to Cooper's ligament to reduce coexisting cystocele. This did cause him to report on a higher risk of enterocele because the vagina is placed in an extreme anterior position. Tanagho's modification recommended no dissection within 2 cm of the urethra as well as removing the fatty tissues from this area to stimulate fibrosis. He also avoided unnecessary tension on the sutures to Cooper's ligament by employing suture bridges to prevent hyperelevation of the urethra (Fig. 26-4).

The Burch procedure was adopted in the 20th century as the gold standard for the treatment of stress urinary incontinence by many urogynecologists, but because the Burch procedure is performed using many different techniques, it is difficult to recommend any particular type. The key to successful surgery for stress urinary incontinence is to define the normal anatomy of the continence mechanism, understand how it become defective, then institute surgery to correct the defect directly. There is no doubt that the Burch procedure is a successful operation, but is it an operation that correctly repairs the defective continence mechanism that results in incontinence? The basic goal of this procedure has always been to place the urethra in a high retropubic position, yet it has been shown that the amount of bladder neck elevation and position in relation to the pubic bone after colposuspension does not affect the cure rate. Because that

is not the normal position of the urethra, the Burch procedure must be considered an operation that distorts rather than corrects the normal anatomy of the urethra. Regrettably, surgeons who employ the Burch procedure seem to focus more on the technical merits of this operation than on the underlying pathophysiology and how best to restore the normal urethra anatomy. Yet, who can deny the long-term success rates of this operation? This questions whether it is necessary to restore normal anatomy or correct the presumed continence mechanism in the surgical management of stress urinary incontinence.

As our understanding of the pathophysiology of incontinence progressed over time, the familiar adage to the surgeon to place the urethra in a high retropubic position was questioned (Fig. 26-5). DeLancey's hammock hypothesis suggested that continence is maintained because the urethra is compressed against a hammock support layer rather than lying in a intra-abdominal position. Cadaver dissections have confirmed that the urethra is separated from the extra-abdominal area by a hammock-like supportive layer composed of fascia endopelvina and by the anterior vaginal wall, and by a distal attachment to the pubic bone. Weakening of the fascia endopelvina, anterior vaginal wall, or attachment to the pubic bone alone or in combination was believed to ultimately lead to incontinence.

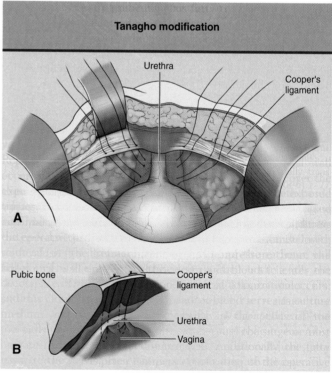

**Tanagho modification**

Urethra

Cooper's
ligament

**A**

Pubic bone

Cooper's
ligament

Urethra

Vagina

**B**

**Figure 26-4** Tanagho modification. *A,* Diaphragmatic illustration of retropubic space after mobilization of anterior wall of vagina and placement of sutures, two on either side and far lateral from midline. Distal sutures are opposite midurethra, whereas proximal sutures are at end of vesicourethral junction. Sutures are attached to Cooper's ligament. *B,* Side view of suture placement with one side tied. Anterior wall of vagina is acting as a broad sling, supporting and lifting the vesicourethral segment. Yet urethra is free in spacious retropubic space. (From Tanagho EA: Colpocystourethropexy: the way we do it. J Urol 1976;116:752. Copyright 1976, Williams & Wilkins.)

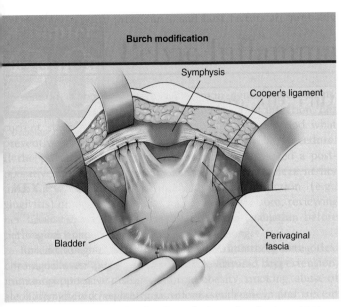

**Figure 26-5    Burch modification.** Lateral edges of vagina have been approximated to Cooper's ligament by using three interrupted sutures. (From Burch JC: Urethrovaginal fixation to Cooper's ligament for correction of stress incontinence, cystocele, and prolapse. Am J Obstet and Gynecol 1961;81:283. Copyright 1961, Mosby-Year Book.)

These findings suggest that successful correction of urinary incontinence would be best served by restoring the normal functional anatomic position of the urethra rather than by elevating the urethra to an unnatural position. Because stress urinary incontinence results when the quality and integrity of

the continence control anatomy cannot resist intra-abdominal pressures, it is logical to assume that treatment must be directed to reducing intra-abdominal pressures, restoring the continence anatomy to a functional state, or a combination of both. Hypothetically, restoring the anatomy to its normal position should produce a better clinical outcome (Fig. 26-6).

Laparoscopic colposuspension was developed to have presumed advantages over the Burch procedure: no major incisions, shorter hospital stay, and quicker return to normal activities. This is an admirable goal but due to the numerous modifications developed by individual authors and the different measures of clinical outcomes it is difficult to understand what modification results in the best outcomes. Sutures have been replaced by staples and synethetic mesh to accomplished bladder neck elevation. The evaluation of these techniques may also be difficult as a result of the difficulty and length of time required to perform this operation, the so-called "for-ever-scopy." Definitive comparative studies have not been produced. The superiority of this technique has not been demonstrated over open procedures, and long-term success of this operation is unknown. Combining these procedures demonstrates a success rate of 80% to 90% over less than 2 years. McDougall reported a success rate of 72% at 2 years, but when he studied the same patients at a mean of 45 months he found that the success rate was reduced to 30%.[49] It can be theorized that the laparoscopic technique may not duplicate the open procedure and may not offer significant fibrosis at the repair site. One of the most difficult measures in the success or failure of incontinence operations may be the judgement and skill of the operating surgeon.

In a large study by Burton in Australia women were randomized to laparoscopic Burch or standard Burch urethropexy. The results for the laparoscopic Burch procedure were initially

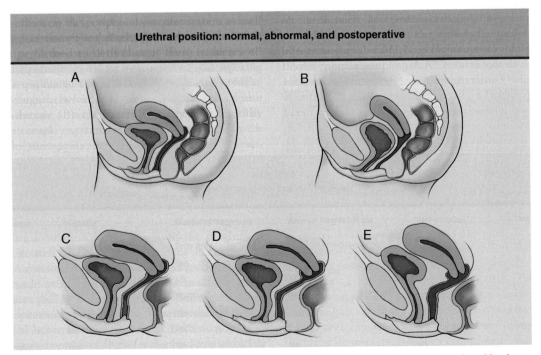

**Figure 26-6    Urethral position.** A, Normal urethral position in continent patient. B, Abnormal urethral position in incontinent patient. C–E, Abnormally high retropubic position of urethra with Marshall-Marchetti-Krantz (C), Burch (D), and needle suspension procedures (E; patient in standing position).

good at 6 weeks' evaluation, but at 6 and 12 months the laparoscopic Burch procedure had significantly poorer results than the open procedure. It is clear that more long-term data is necessary. Current available evidence suggests that laparoscopic colposuspension leads to a quicker recovery, but takes longer to perform and may be associated with more complications.

Having observed that the elevation of the vesicourethral junction was an effective means of treating urinary incontinence, Pereyra developed a vaginal approach. The aim of the procedure was to combine a high cure rate with low operative morbidity. In his original description he placed wire sutures into the peri-urethral tissues on each side of the bladder neck to the rectus fascia. These procedures were rapidly adopted because they were quicker, did not require splitting of the anterior abdominal fascia, and reduced perioperative and postoperative morbidity. The intent of needle procedures was to elevate and support the bladder neck, which achieves continence, it was presumed, like the retropubic suspensions by maintaining the bladder neck inside the sphere of abdominal pressure transmission during increased intra-abdominal pressure. There have been many modifications since the first needle suspension procedure over 40 years ago, including the Stamey, Raz, Gittes, and Muzsani modifications. Despite these modifications the long-term outcome data does not support the efficacy of needle suspension procedures, with only 67% cure/dry rate measured after 48 months. Kondo and colleagues, in a long-term study, found the Stamey procedure had a higher continence rate than Gittes (71% at 14 years vs. 31% at 6 years).[50] Clemens and collegaues found a low continence rate for the Stamey procedure (44%; mean term follow-up, 15.2 years).[51] Therefore, although needle suspension procedures may have historical significance, they currently have a limited role in the management of stress urinary incontinence because of the poor long-term results.

The newer miminally invasive suburethral slings were not studied in the AUA panel report, but their current success rates have been so remarkable that each procedure deserves mention. The first report on suburethral slings was in 1995, when Ulmstem and Petros described the transvaginal slingplasty.[52] This procedure is now known as the TVT (tension-free vaginal tape) procedure (Ethicon, Gynecare, Somerville, N.J.). The introduction of tension-free tape challenged the understanding of the continence mechanism and taught the importance of the midurethra in maintaining continence. Since 1995 the company (Data on file, Gynecare, Johnson & Johnson) believe that 750,000 TVT procedures have been performed. The procedure employs a knitted polypropylene mesh and is performed with conscious sedation with local anesthesia, with regional anesthesia, or with general anesthesia. Long-term follow-up studies (≥ 4 years) are available and indicate cure rates similar to the those for retropubic colposuspension procedures. Although few complications were noted in early reports, later reports have shown that this operation is not without risks that were infrequent with traditional procedures. Operative cystotomy has been reported in some series to occur in about 23% of cases. Twenty-eight cases of bowel injury have been reported, some leading to death; 55 cases of vascular injuries, some also leading to death; 20 urethral erosions, 20 hematomas, 60 mesh erosions, and 4 nerve injuries. Because of the number of successful TVT procedures without complications, the occasional adverse

results of this operation must be considered minimal, yet operative mortality is an unusual complication of incontinence procedures.

Another midurethral tension-free sling, the pubic bone stabilization sling involved the use of transvaginally placed bone screws (InFast, American Medical Systems, Minnetonka, Minn.) into the back of the pubic bone to support a tension-free piece of Mersilene over the midurethra. In this tension-free sling, the mesh is attached to the periurethral tissues by four sutures, which does not allow the mesh under the urethra to be placed on tension when the mesh is tied to the bone screws situated at the point where the arcus tendineus fasciae pelvis attaches to the pubic bone (Fig. 26-7). Personal communications with the company reveal that more than 150,000 of these procedures have been performed since 1997. A 4-year report on outcomes was published before the procedure was actively marketed; long-term durable results (8 years) were subsequently published in a cohort study of 105 patients with cure/dry/improved rates greater than 98%.[53] Of interest is that the pubic bone stabilization sling has been successfully used in men who have become incontinent following radical proctectomy and so is the only incontinence procedure currently used in both men and women.

Variations of this technique using bone anchors, not bone screws, with transvaginal suspension suture techniques were not reported to be as successful. Transabdominal bone anchors with sutures to suspend the urethra also reported less favorable outcomes. When transabdominal bone anchors were used to suspend a suburethral sling made of Protegen, the incidence of osteomyelitis was reported to be 480 of 60,000 cases. Although several anecdotal reports mention osteomyelitis with transvaginal bone screws, most of these have occurred with the

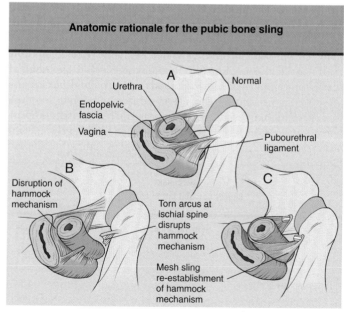

**Anatomic rationale for the pubic bone sling**

**Figure 26-7 Anatomic rationale for the sling.** *A*, Normal anatomy. *B*, Abnormal anatomy. Note the hypermobility of the urethra, caused by torn arcus from pelvis with incompetent pubourethral ligaments, paravaginal defect, and attenuated fascia endopelvina. *C*, Normal anatomy restored with pubic bone suburethral stabilization sling.

transabdominal placement of bone anchors.[54] There is only one documented case in the literature of osteomyelitis with transvaginally placed bone screws. However, the perception of such a complication became a major concern to anyone wanting to place transvaginal bone screws despite the reports of osteomyelitis occurring with other incontinence procedures, such as the retropubic procedures, the Burch procedure,[55] the MMK procedure[56] and needle suspensions.[57] Because osteomyelitis has been reported with other incontinence procedures,[58] the etiology of this condition is still unclear. Because there are no reported cases of operative cystotomy, bowel injuries, significant hemorrhage, reported deaths, or mesh erosions into the urethra with this procedure, the recommendation by some urogynecologists to avoid it because of the fear of osteomyelitis appears to be unjustified. If Eddy's description of the two main steps in medical decision making are followed, both steps would favor the pubic bone stabilization sling over the TVT procedure. The influence of surgical instrument companies must be factored into the reasons the TVT has been the most commonly used procedure performed worldwide. The rapid adoption of these minimally invasive slings may be because they have been found to be effective for both urethral hypermobility and intrinsic sphincter dysdunction; there are some reports that indicate an association with bacterial vaginosis and osteomyelitis.

Because of the reported risks with the TVT, other midurethral slings have been developed. The SPARC (American Medical Systems, Minnetonka, Minn.) passes the sling from an abdominal to vaginal approach. Initial studies appear to be promising, but no long-term studies are available. The latest suburethral sling is the transobturator sling, or TOT (American Medical Systems, Minnetonka, Minn.). This method aims to avoid the incidence of operative cystotomies and the need to use the cystoscope; however, there several cases of operative cystotomies have already been reported with this method. A small prospective randomized study comparing TVT to TOT showed that TOT was equally as efficient as TVT for the surgical management of stress urinary incontinence, with no reduction of bladder outlet obstruction at 1-year follow-up. The etiology of outlet obstruction with these procedures remains unclear. This method is being actively marketed by several companies who have developed other methods for transobturator placement of suburethral mesh; there are no studies longer than 2 years reporting on long-term outcomes.

The decision as to what type of suburethral sling procedure surgeons will use may be made on factors other than an evaluation of the outcomes of each technique. Unfortunately, this is not what patients expect or fellow colleagues expect when a patient is referred for management of stress urinary incontinence.

Pubovaginal suburethral slings (Goebel-Stockel-Frannenheim) have been in clinical use for almost a century, but because of their high complication rate, including urethral obstruction, urethral compression, detrusor instability, high postoperative residuals, and urethral and vaginal erosions, their usage is generally reserved for patients with failed surgery or a dysfunctional low-pressure urethra. The basic problem of this type of pubovaginal sling, which is not a concern with the tension-free slings, is adjusting the proper tension on the sling, which is difficult to assess and teach because the sling is attached to a high fixation point, the

rectus fascia. In a select group of patients with low urethra pressures, the pubovaginal sling may be indicated as a primary procedure.

The artifical urinary sphincter (American Medical Systems, Minnetonka, Minn.) was developed for patients with pure sphincter incompetency and normal detrusor function. It consists of four components: a pump mechanism, a cuff that encircles the bladder neck and /or urethra, a pressure-regulating balloon, and tubing connectors. Cuff placement can be abdominal or vaginal. Results of both the abdominal and transvaginal approach have been excellent, with greater than 90% attaining continence. The best results are obtained with women with total incontinence and no prolapse of the bladder base. However, only a small number (approximately 29,000) artificial urethral sphincters have been implanted worldwide, ostensibly due to the surgeon's concern regarding the technical difficulties during the crucial part of the operation, developing a space between the bladder neck and the vagina.

Glutaraldehyde cross-linked bovine collagen (GAX) is a bulking agent used effectively in patients with a fixed low-pressure urethra (Type III incontinence). GAX is injected periurethrally at the bladder neck under endoscopic control until closure of the urethra is seen through a zero-degree urethroscope. Patients must undergo a subcutaneous injection as a test for allergy before attempting periurethral injections. Small clinical studies have obtained 81% cure rates using up to two treatments. Collagen may prove to be a satifactory treatment in women who are not surgical candidates, particularly the elderly. Other bulking agents have also been used, including Teflon, cellulose, and autologous fat. Long-term success is not known.

Many surgical procedures have been described for the treatment of genuine stress incontinence in women since the early 20th century, with variable degrees of morbidity and effectiveness. The early operations were believed to share the same goal (i.e., restore the proposed normal anatomic position and mobility of the bladder neck and proximal urethra while providing adequate support). In addition, it was believed the urethra should have limited mobility without compression or obstruction. Normal anatomic position and stability of the bladder neck was thought to control continence if the urethra was placed in a high retropubic intra-abdominal position. In recent years we have learned that the urethra's normal position is not elevated to a high retropubic position, yet we have not been able to define normal urethral mobility and how it influences the continence mechanism.

Midsuburethral slings have stimulated more investigation into the mechanism of incontinence. The success of these new surgical procedures has questioned the actual mechanics of continence because these procedures do not support or suspend the proximal urethra or bladder neck. It is apparent that we really do not know why women develop incontinence and more importantly why the surgeries we perform work when they do.

Is there sufficient evidence that supports a particular surgical management of stress urinary incontinence? The answer to that question is not yet and maybe never. If we could agree on the anatomy of the continence mechanism, the physiology of the continence mechanism, and how the operations we perform relate to the anatomy and physiology of the continence. We might be able to select the appropriate operation for stress urinary incontinence by evaluating the outcomes of alternative practices and the desirability of those outcomes.

Studies that have used urodynamic criteria to assess the cure of stress urinary incontinence have also shown variable results. The evaluation of clinical evidence also presents problems in how decisions are made. For example, it is generally believed from direct comparative studies that retropubic urethropexy is more effective than needle suspensions, but not always. In at least three "same group" studies,[59–61] urethropexy had poorer results than did retropubic urethropexy. In Van Geelen's study, it was superior to retropubic urethropexy. How are these differences explained? In at least one of these studies the authors did not use permanent suture to perform the needle urethropexy that is normally described by almost all authors.[61] Early failures from retropubic surgery have long been associated with the early use of absorbable sutures. Thus, we need to be able to evaluate what role the technique, the skill, and the experience of the surgeon play in the evaluations of various procedures.

## Summary

Knowledge of various types of surgery is also mandatory so that the patient is not tailored to the surgeon's favorite or only procedure. Several other factors hamper the evaluation of any surgery for the correction of urinary incontinence: diagnostic criteria, including urodynamics (controversial); variations in patient populations, including prior incontinence surgery, age, weight, childbearing, and associated medical conditions; variations in surgical technique, operative experience, and skill; and what length of time constitutes a cure or failure.

These retropubic operations were the operation for stress urinary incontinence in the 20th century. Current evidence suggests that minimally invasive tension-free midurethral slings will be the operation for stress urinary incontinence in the 21st century.

## REFERENCES

1. Diokno AC, Wells TJ, Brink CA: Urinary incontinence in elderly women. Urodynamic Evaluation. J Am Geriatr Surg 1987;35:940–946. **(Ib, B)**
2. Palmer MA: Incontinence: the magnitude of the problem. Nurs Clin North Am 1998;1:139–157. **(III, B)**
3. Ekelund P, Rundgren A: Urinary incontinence in the elderly with implications for hospital care consumption and social disability. Arch Gerontol Geriatr 1987;6:1311–1318. **(IIb)**
4. DeLancey JOL: Structural support of the urethra as it relates to stress urinary incontinence: the hammock hypothesis. Am J Obstet Gynecol 1994;170:1713–1723. **(IIa, B)**
5. Petros PE, Ulmsten UI: An integral theory of female urinary incontinence. Experimental and clinical considerations. Acta Obstet Gynecol Scand Suppl 1990;153:7–31. **(IIa, B)**
6. Shafik A, El-Sibai O: Effect of pelvic floor muscle contraction on vesical and rectal function within dentification of puborectalis–rectovesical inhibitory reflex and levator–rectovesical excitatory reflex. World J Urol 2001;19:278–284. **(IIa, B)**
7. Viktrup L, Lose G: The risk of stress incontinence 5 years after first delivery. Am J Obstet Gynecol 2001;185:82–87. **(Ia, A)**
8. Persson J, Wolner-Hassen P, Rydstroem H: Obstetric risk factors for stress urinary incontinence: a population based study. Obstet Gynecol 2000;96:440–445. **(Ia, A)**
9. Rortveit G, Daltveit AK, Hannestand YS, Hunskaar S: Urinary incontinence after vaginal delivery or cesarean section. N Engl J Med 2003;348:900–907. **(Ia, A)**
10. Arya LA, Jackson ND, Myers DL, Verma A: Risk of new-onset urinary incontinence after forceps and vacuum delivery in primiparous women. Am J Obstet Gynecol 2001;185:1318–1324. **(Ia, A)**
11. Van Kessel K, Reed S, Newton K, et al: The second stage of labor and stress urinary incontinence. Am J Obstet Gynecol 2001;184:1571–1575. **(Ib, A)**
12. Brown JS, Sawaya G, Thom DH, Grady D: Hysterectomy and urinary incontinence: a systematic review. Lancet 2000;356:535–359. **(Ib, A)**
13. Kjerulff KH, Langenberg PW, Greenaway L, et al: Urinary incontinence and hysterectomy in a large prospective cohort study in American women. J Urol 2002;167:2088–2092. **(Ib, A)**
14. Roovers JP, van der Bom JG, Huub van der Vaart C, et al: Does mode of hysterectomy influence micturition and defecation? Acta Obstet Gynecol Scand 2001;80:945–951. **(Ib, A)**
15. Van Oyen H, Van Oyen P: Urinary incontinence in Belgium: prevalence, correlates and psychosocial consequences. Acta Clin Belg 2002; 57:207–218. **(Ib, A)**
16. Holtedahl K, Hunskaar S: Prevalence, 1-year incidence and factors associated with urinary incontinence: a population based study of women 50–74 years of age in primary care. Maturitas 1998;28:205–211. **(Ia, A)**
17. Aggazzotti G, Pesce F, Grassi D, et al: Prevalence of urinary incontinence among institutionalized patients: a cross-sectional epidemiologic study in a midsized city in northern Italy. Urol 2000;56:245–249. **(Ia, A)**
18. Moller LM, Lose G, Jorgensen T: Risk factors for lower urinary tract symptoms in women 40 to 60 years of age. Obstet Gynecol 2000; 96:446–451. **(Ia, A)**
19. Samuelsson E, Victor A, Svardsudd K: Determinants of urinary incontinence in a population of young and middle aged women. Acta Obstet Gynecol Scand 2000;79:208–215. **(Ia, A)**
20. Finkelstein MM: Medical conditions, medications, and urinary incontinence: analysis of a population-based survey. Can Fam Physician 2002; 48:96–101. **(Ib, A)**
21. Sherburn M, Guthrie JR, Dudley EC, et al: Is incontinence associated with menopause? Obstet Gynecol 2001;98:628–633. **(Ia, A)**
22. Arya LA, Myers DL, Jackson ND: Dietary caffeine intake and risk for detrusor instability: a case-control study. Obstet Gynecol 2000; 96:85–89. **(Ib, A)**
23. Schmidbauer J, Temml C, Schatzl G, et al: Risk factors for lower urinary incontinence in both sexes: analysis of a health screening project. Eur Urol 2001;39:565–570. **(Ib, A)**
24. Sampselle CM, Harlow SD, Skurnick J, et al: Urinary incontinence predictors and life impact in ethnically diverse perimenopausal women. Obstet Gynecol 2002;100:1230–1238. **(Ib, A)**
25. Fultz NH, Herzog AR, Raghunathan TE, et al: Prevalence and severity of urinary incontinence in older African American and Caucasian women. J Gerontol Biol Sci Med Sci 1999;54:M299–M303. **(Ia, A)**
26. Chiarelli P, Brown W, McElduff P: Leaking urine: prevalence and associated factors in Australian women. Neurourol Urodyn 1999; 18:567–577. **(Ia, A)**
27. Hay-Smith EJ, Bo K, Berghmans LC, et al: Pelvic floor muscle training for urinary incontinence in women (Cochrane Review). In: Cochrane Library, Issue 1. Chichester, England: John Wiley & Sons, 2003. **(Ia, A)**
28. Burgio KL, Goode PS, Locher JL, et al: Behavioral training with and without biofeedback in the treatment of urge incontinence in older women: a randomized controlled trial. JAMA 2002;288:2293–2299. **(Ia, A)**
29. Jenssen CC, Lagro-Jenssen AL, Felling AJ: The effects of physiotherapy for female urinary incontinence: individual compared with group treatment. BJU Int 2001;87:201–206. **(Ib, A)**
30. Phenylpropanolamine information page. U.S. Food and Drug Administration website. http://www.fda.gov/cder/drug/infopage/default.htm. Accessed 27 January 2004. **(IV, C)**
31. Herbison P, Plevnik S, Mantle J: Weighted vaginal cones for urinary incontinence (Cochrane Review). In: Cochrane Library, Issue 1. Chichester, England: John Wiley & Sons, 2003. **(Ib, B)**

32. Wayman JF, Fantl JA, McClish DK, Bump RC, for the Continence Program for Women Reasearch Group: Comparative efficacy of behavioral interventions in the management of female urinary incontinence. Am J Obstet Gynecol 1998;179:999–1007. **(Ib, B)**

33. Hay-Smith J, Herbison P, Ellis G, Moore K: Anticholinergic drugs verses placebo for overactive bladder syndrome in adults (Cochrane Review). In: Cochrane Library, Issue 1. Chichester, England: John Wiley & Sons, 2003. **(Ia, A)**

34. Malone-Lee J, Shaffu B, Anand C, Powell C: Tolterodine: superior tolerability than and comparable efficacy to oxybutynin in individuals 50 years old and older with overactive bladder: a randomized controlled trail. J Urol 2001;165:1452–1456. **(Ib, A)**

35. Gordon D, Groutz A, Ascher-Landsberg J, et al: Double-blind, placebo-controlled study of magnesium hydroxide for treatment of sensory urgency and detrusor instability: preliminary results. J Obstet Gynecol 1998;105:667–669. **(Ib, A)**

36. Jensen JK, Nielsen FR, Ostergard DR: The role of the patient history in the diagnosis of urinary incontinence. Obstet Gynecol 1994; 83:904–910. **(Ib, A)**

37. Thompson PK, Duff DS, Thayer PS: Stress incontinence in women under 50: does urodynamics improve surgical outcome? Int Urogynecol 2000;11:285–289. **(Ib, A)**

38. Clinical Practice Guideline No. 2. 1996 Update. Rockville, Md.: U.S. Department of Health and Human Services, Public Health Service, Agency for Health Policy and Research. HCPR Publication No. 96:682. March 1996. **(IV, C)**

39. Weidner A, Myers R, Visco G, et al: Which women with SUI require urodynamic evaluation? Am J Obstet Gynecol 2001:184:20–27. **(Ib, A)**

40. The Urodynamics Society: Standards of efficacy for evaluation of treatment outcomes in urinary incontinence: A report from the Urodynamics Society. Neurourol Urodyn 1997;16:145:1997. **(IV, C)**

41. Richardson DA: The evaluation of different surgical procedures. In Ostergard DA, Bent AE (eds): Urogynecology and Urodynamics, 3rd ed. Baltimore, Williams & Wilkins, 1991, pp 413–421. **(IV, C)**

42. Wennberg JE, Barnes BA, Zubkoff M: Professional uncertainty and the problem of supplier-induced demand. Soc Sci Med 1982;16:811–824. **(IIa, B)**

43. Eddy DM: Clinical decision making: from theory to practice. JAMA 1990;263:441–443. **(IIa, B)**

44. Leach GE, Dmochowski RR, Appell RA, et al: Female stress urinary incontinence clinical guidelines panel summary report on surgical management of female stress urinary incontinence. The American Urological Association. J Urol 1997;158:875–880. **(IV, C)**

45. Beck RP, McCormick S, Nordstrom L: A 25 year experience with 519 anterior colporrhaphy procedures. Obstet Gynecol 1991; 78:1011–1018. **(IV, C)**

46. Nichols DH: Vaginal prolapse affecting bladder function. Clin Obstet Gynecol 1985;12:449–464. **(IV, C)**

47. Marshall VF, Marchetti AA, Krantz KE: The correction of stress incontinence by simple vesicourethral suspension. Surg Gynecol Obstet 1949;88:509–518. **(IV, C)**

48. Enhorning G: Simultaneous recording of intravesical and intraurethral pressure. Acta Chir Scand 1961;276(Suppl):5–12. **(IV, C)**

49. McDougall EM, Heidorn CA, Portis AJ, Kluthe CG: Laporoscopic bladder neck suspension fails the test of time. J Urol 1999; 162:2078–2081. **(IIb, B)**

50. Kondo A, Kato K, Gotoh M, et al: The Stamey and Gittes procedures: long-term follow-up in relation to incontinence types and patient age. J Urol 1998;160(Pt. 1):756–758. **(IIb, B)**

51. Clemens JQ, Stern JA, Bushman WA, Schaeffer AJ: Long-term results of the Stamey bladder neck suspension: direct comparisan with the Marshall-Marchetti-Krantz procedure. J Urol 1998;160:372–376. **(III, B)**

52. Ulmstem U, Petros P: Intravaginal sling plasty (IVS): an ambulatory surgical procedure for treatment of female urinary incontinence. Scand J Urol Nephrol 1995;29:75–82. **(III, B)**

53. Kovac SR: A follow-up of the pubic bone suburethral stablization sling operation for recurrent urinary incontinence. The Kovac Procedure. J Pelvic Surg 1999;5:156–160. **(III, B)**

54. Wheeler JS: Osteomyelitis of the pubis: complication of a Stamey urethropexy. J Urol 1994;151:1638–1640. **(III, B)**

55. Matkov TG, Henjna MJ, Coogan CL: Osteomyelitis as a complication of vesica percutaneous bladder neck suspension. J Urol 1998;160:1427. **(III, B)**

56. Bortel DT: Candida osteomyelitis pubis following a Marshall-Marchetti procedure. Orthopedic 1993;16:1353–1355. **(III, B)**

57. Hall J, Napier-Hemy, O'Reilly PH: Case report: ostemyelitis complicating Burch colposuspension. Br J Urol 1996;77:470–471. **(III, B)**

58. Burns JR, Gregory JG: Osteomyelitis of the pubic symphysis after urologic surgery. J Urol 1977;118:803–805. **(III, B)**

59. Mundy AR: A trial comparing Stamey bladder neck suspension with colposuspension for stress urinary incontinence. Br J Urol 1983; 55:687–690.

60. Weil A, Reyes H, Bischoff P, et al: Modifications of the urethral rest and stress profiles after different types of surgery for urinary stress incontinence. Br J Obstet Gynecol 1984;91:46–55.

61. Bergman A, Koonings PP, Ballard CC: Primary stress urinary incontinence and pelvic relaxation: prospective randomized comparison of three different operations. Am J Obstet Gynecol 1990;163:2025–2026.

## KEY POINTS

- Fecal incontinence is a quality-of-life issue defined as the inability to control the elimination of rectal contents at a socially acceptable time and place.

- In women, this is frequently related to obstetric trauma to the anal sphincters, irritable bowel syndrome causing diarrhea, or neurologic diseases affecting the sphincters.

- Once medical treatment with dietary changes, bulking agents, antidiarrheals, and biofeedback has failed, surgical treatments may be considered.

- Sphincter repair offers the best likelihood for improvement in continence for patients with sphincter defects, but long-term durability of the repairs is often disappointing.

- Complex procedures such as dynamic graciloplasty, artificial neosphincters, the Secca procedure, and sacral nerve stimulation treatment are options that are still under investigation.

- Fecal diversion with ileostomy or colostomy is a final option that can provide significant improvement in quality of life.

A universally accepted definition of fecal incontinence has not been established, but most surgeons consider it to be the inability to control the elimination of rectal contents until a socially acceptable time and place. This can then be categorized into varying degrees of incontinence based on the type of material that is eliminated (gas, liquid stool, or solid stool) and the frequency with which it occurs. Incontinence can also be categorized based on the timing in the defecatory cycle as passive incontinence, urge incontinence, postdefecation leakage, or a combination of the three. A number of scoring systems have been established to try to obtain objective criteria through scoring systems for fecal incontinence,[1,2] but none of these have gained universal acceptance by those who treat the patients afflicted with this condition.[3] An example of such an incontinence scoring system can be found in Table 27-1. These systems appear to be more useful in determining the effectiveness of treatment and establishing the prevalence of incontinence within populations for the purpose of research rather than in determining the best modality of treatment for each individual patient. Some of these scales have been validated and tested for reliability,[2] but results are mixed when comparing their effectiveness head-to-head in assessing fecal incontinence.

## EPIDEMIOLOGY

The epidemiology of fecal incontinence is extremely difficult to determine due to population variability, biases (e.g., referral bias, selection bias), lack of consistency in definitions, and patient embarrassment to report symptoms or seek treatment (between 33% and less than 50% are believed to mention the condition to their physician).[4,5] Although not a life-threatening condition, fecal incontinence has significant impact on quality of life (QOL) and on the public health system as a whole. The best available data from large population-based studies and surveys shows varying degrees of fecal incontinence affecting 1% to 17% of individuals in the community[6–8] and nearly 50% of all nursing home residents.[5,9] Although fecal incontinence affects both women and men (approximately 8:1),[10] this chapter focuses on fecal incontinence in women, who have a greater incidence, likely due to increased risks from obstetric trauma. The incidence is also higher in older age groups because they more commonly suffer from associated risk factors of urinary incontinence, fecal impaction, immobility, diminished mental status, and dementia.[4,8] The economic impact of this condition has been difficult to estimate (one estimate being approximately $10,000 per year per nursing home patient), but it is believed that it is even greater than the cost of urinary incontinence, which has been shown to be $16.3 billion per year in direct health care costs alone.[4] In addition, the social and psychological impact is immense and difficult to quantify.

### Risk Factors

No controlled trials looking at the risk factors related to fecal incontinence are available. The greatest risk factors for fecal incontinence in women under age 65 are believed to be injury to the anal sphincter or pudendal nerves from obstetric trauma, irritable bowel syndrome (IBS), and neurologic diseases. Overall, however, the greatest risk factor in all women, regardless of age, is general health and physical status.[4,7,11] These risks were supported in a prospective observational survey by Chassagne and colleagues of 2602 institutionalized elderly over age 60 where the greatest independent risk factors for prolonged fecal incontinence were urinary incontinence, immobility, diminished mental status, and dementia.[7] Diseases associated with incontinence also include the following: diabetes, cerebrovascular accidents, multiple sclerosis, Parkinson's disease, spinal cord injury, and congenital abnormalities. Diarrhea, regardless of etiology, also has a strong association with incontinence, associated with 51% to 71% of cases of fecal incontinence.[7,8] Anal surgery increases the risk of fecal incontinence as well (up to 45% incidence with lateral internal sphincterotomy for anal fissure).[6,11,12]

### Obstetric Injury

The risk of developing fecal incontinence in women is highly linked with obstetric trauma. The incidence of fecal incontinence

**Table 27-1**
**Cleveland Clinic Incontinence Score**

| Frequency | Gas | Liquid Stool | Solid Stool | Pad |
|---|---|---|---|---|
| Occasionally | 1 | 4 | 7 | 1 |
| >1 per week | 2 | 5 | 8 | 2 |
| Daily | 3 | 6 | 9 | 3 |

0, perfect continence; 1–7, good continence; 8–14, moderate incontinence; 15–20, severe incontinence; 21, completely incontinent.
From Agachan F, Chen T, Pfeifer J, et al: A constipation scoring system to simplify evaluation and management of constipated patients. Dis Colon Rectum 1996;39:681–685.

to solid or liquid stool in primiparous women is 3% to 13% after vaginal delivery.[11,13] The confounding aspect of sphincter injuries at the time of vaginal delivery is that they are often occult and symptoms may not arise until long after delivery.[11,14] Therefore, the relationship between birth trauma and incontinence is not always clear. The incidence of sphincter defect based on early postpartum endoanal ultrasound has been as high as 35% in some series,[13,14] with defects being recognized by ultrasound often 7 times more frequently than by postpartum physical examination.[13] The risk of developing early fecal incontinence once an injury occurs, even if repaired, is approximately 40%.[13]

## PATHOGENESIS AND CLINICAL FEATURES

An appreciation for the pathophysiology leading to fecal incontinence can only be gained through an understanding of the normal anatomy and physiology necessary for defecation. For normal continence to occur, the rectal vault must be able to distend, an ability to sense that distention must be present, the stool must be of sufficient consistency to be held in the vault, and the complex anal sphincter mechanism must be able to hold the contents until a time when those contents can appropriately be released. Any abnormalities in these synchronized physiologic steps can lead to varying degrees of fecal incontinence.

Anatomically, the 12 to 15 cm long rectum and 2 to 5 cm long anal canal are crucial to defecatory function (Fig. 27-1). The rectum is a muscular tube with inner circular and outer longitudinal muscle that acts as a pelvic continuation of the colon and a reservoir for stool. The cephalad extent of the surgical anal canal begins at the top of the anorectal ring of musculature that includes the internal and external anal sphincters and the puborectalis muscle (the U-shaped distalmost aspect of the levator ani muscle complex). The internal sphincter is a continuation and expansion of the rectal inner circular muscle. It is the involuntary, autonomically innervated muscle responsible for 80% of the resting basal pressure of the sphincter complex.[15] The internal sphincter is responsible for maintaining continence at rest only, due to the fact that it relaxes with rectal distention (rectoanal inhibitory reflex), making the external sphincter crucial during that phase of defecation.[14] The external sphincter and puborectalis muscle are the voluntary muscles responsible for 20% of the basal resting pressure and all of the squeeze pressure of the anal canal. The external sphincter is the primary voluntary muscle bulk in women anteriorly (Fig. 27-2), and thus

can have significant sequelae in terms of continence if damaged or torn. The puborectalis muscle forms a sling around the anus that creates an anorectal angle, forming a valve while contracted at rest, thus maintaining continence (Fig. 27-3A).[14] Voluntary relaxation of this muscle straightens this angle, thus allowing stool to pass (Fig. 27-3B). Therefore, the puborectalis muscle is thought to play the key function of maintaining continence to solid stool; the internal and external anal sphincters are believed to be integral to gas and liquid stool continence. As the anal canal continues caudally; there is a transitional zone from the columnar epithelium of the rectum to cuboidal and eventually squamous epithelium of the skin at the dentate line. In addition, at this level of the canal the redundant anal mucosal folds and vascular cushions (hemorrhoids) improve the distal seal,[14] and the highly innervated anoderm (primarily from the pudendal nerve from S2-S4) provides crucial sensory input for maintaining continence. Finally, the anal canal ends as it extends from the dentate line to the anal verge, where the perianal skin becomes the nonhair-bearing anoderm, which contains many somatic sensory nerve endings.

Defecation is initiated by the peristaltic movement of feces from the sigmoid colon into the rectal vault, a capacitance organ that can hold over 500 mL of liquid in normal subjects before leaking.[15] This leads to accommodation by the internal sphincter as part of the rectoanal inhibitory reflex—also occurring intermittently during the day as part of the sampling reflex—that allows for sensation of the rectal contents to occur in the transition zone of the anal canal. Voluntary relaxation of the external sphincter and puborectalis allow for expulsion of the rectal contents when associated with an increase in abdominal pressure (Valsalva maneuver). An aberration in any of these components can lead to continence difficulties, both incontinence and constipation. This is especially true in the aged, demented, or disabled population, who have altered physiology and decreased physiologic reserve.

Alteration in stool consistency is one of the most common pathophysiologic entities leading to incontinence. This is most frequently seen in IBS with diarrhea, infectious enteritis/colitis, inflammatory bowel disease (Crohn's disease or ulcerative colitis), bile salt malabsorption, or medication abuse/misuse where the consistency of stool is so thin that it overrides the compensatory mechanisms of the external sphincter and anal cushions to seal the anal canal. This alteration in stool consistency may also be associated with a decrease in rectal compliance, especially in conditions such as inflammatory bowel disease, radiation proctitis, or malignancy, where the rectum becomes more like a nondistensible tube than a compliance vessel. Stool consistency can also lead to incontinence when severe constipation or a nonrelaxing puborectalis muscle leads to overdistention of the rectal vault and overflow incontinence.

Altered neurophysiology can also lead to incontinence, primarily due to decreased anal sensation or decreased motor function of the sphincter complex. This is frequently associated with systemic diseases such as diabetes, collagen vascular diseases, multiple sclerosis, acquired immune deficiency syndrome (AIDS), or congenital disorders such as spina bifida.[14] Altered neurophysiology is also thought to be the etiology of fecal incontinence after childbirth when no structural abnormality of the sphincter is identified. This incontinence is usually due to direct

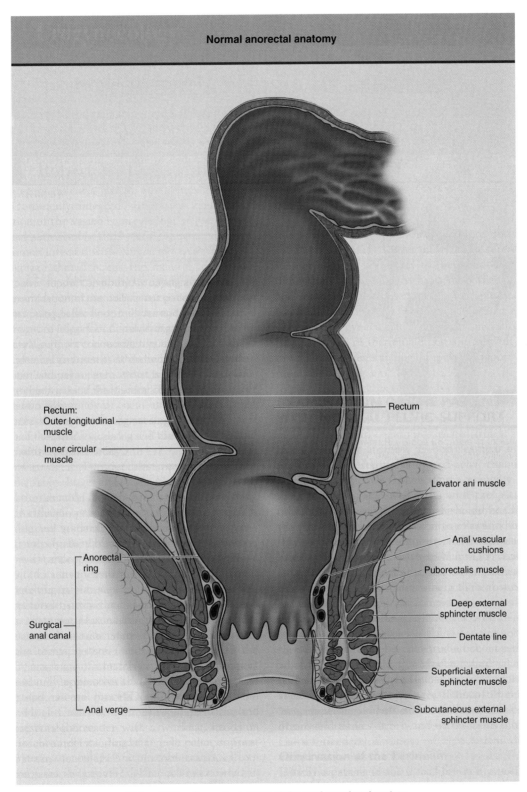

**Normal anorectal anatomy**

Rectum:
Outer longitudinal muscle

Inner circular muscle

Anorectal ring

Surgical anal canal

Anal verge

Rectum

Levator ani muscle

Anal vascular cushions

Puborectalis muscle

Deep external sphincter muscle

Dentate line

Superficial external sphincter muscle

Subcutaneous external sphincter muscle

**Figure 27-1    Normal anatomy of the anal canal and rectum.**

damage to the pudendal nerves from fetal compression, forceps trauma, or stretching of the nerves during elongation of the birth canal or with prolonged labor.[14] This damage is usually an asymmetric injury that partially recovers with time, but it can be bilateral with permanent sequelae. Similar neurologic trauma can occur over time from extensive straining at stool from

constipation leading to stretching of the pudendal nerves over the ischial spines as the perineum descends. This may be part of the etiology of the association of fecal incontinence with rectal prolapse, but this has not been clearly established.

Alteration in the structure of the anal sphincter is the most common cause of fecal incontinence in women. Trauma is

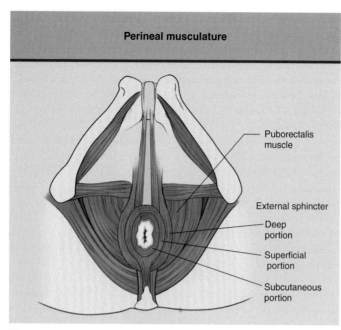

**Perineal musculature**

- Puborectalis muscle
- External sphincter
- Deep portion
- Superficial portion
- Subcutaneous portion

**Figure 27-2  Perineal musculature in the normal female.** The anal sphincter mechanism is the only substantial musculature of the perineal body in women.

usually the etiology of the change in the muscle complex; this is most frequently associated in women with childbirth, but can also occur due to anal injury or sexual trauma.[16] Muscular trauma can also occur from iatrogenic causes at the time of fistulotomy for anal fistula, sphincterotomy for anal fissure, or hemorrhoidectomy.[11] For these procedures for benign anorectal disease, the incontinence rate is believed to be up to as high as 45% (depending on the definition and follow-up period),[6,11,12] although a recent prospective study by Hyman of patients after lateral internal sphincterotomy for anal fissure showed only 1 of 35 patients postoperatively to have QOL deterioration due to fecal incontinence.[12] Other structural alterations in the sphincter complex may be due to systemic diseases such as scleroderma, inflammatory bowel disease, or AIDS.

### Obstetric Injury

The pathophysiology of birth trauma leading to fecal incontinence through sphincter or neurologic injury seems fairly intuitive, but the risk factors leading to these injuries are not always clear. Therefore, trying to identify the risk factors leading to sphincter injury is crucial to reducing the incidence of fecal incontinence in women. One survey of 475 incontinent females by Lunniss and colleagues, trying to assess potential risk factors in incontinent patients, showed that 78% of women reported a complicated delivery (episiotomy or perineal tear, forceps delivery, or vacuum extraction), with 86% of those deliveries being their first.[11] This same study also identified most of the incontinent women as having undergone pelvic surgery (58%) or anal surgery (19%) at some time in their lives before having incontinence, thus clouding the picture as to the true etiology of their incontinence. Only 40% of the women in this study could ascribe their onset of symptoms to a single event.[11] Therefore, large retrospective and some prospective case series and a few

randomized, controlled trials have looked at risk factors for fecal incontinence in relation to birth trauma.

Multiple aspects of vaginal deliveries have been noted to increase the risk of fecal incontinence. The risk seems to be greatest at the time of first delivery and decreases with subsequent deliveries in most but not all studies.[13] The foremost of the seemingly modifiable risk factors, though, is midline episiotomy or significant perineal laceration (third- or fourth-degree tears). These are usually associated with primiparity, large infant birth weight, macrosomia, prolonged labor, and forceps or vacuum extraction. Midline episiotomy has been shown to increase the sphincter injury rate by up to 9 times that of a vaginal delivery without episiotomy.[13,14] The use of mediolateral episiotomy, however, while more painful, has shown a substantially decreased risk for sphincter injury versus the midline approach in most studies.[13] Forceps deliveries have also been linked in prospective studies to an anal sphincter injury in 63% to 83% of deliveries, although a more recent analysis by de Parades and colleagues of 93 women after forceps delivery showed only 13% to have sphincter defects and 22% to be incontinent to flatus or liquid stool with limited follow-up.[17] Perineal laceration (presumably from the forceps) was the only factor in this latter study that could be linked to sphincter injury, although all episiotomies in this study were performed in the posterolateral position rather than in the midline or mediolateral. Overall, vacuum extraction and forceps deliveries have a 3 times and 7 times greater likelihood of sphincter injury, respectively. Other risks, such as prolonged active second stage of labor and the use of epidurals, have also been borne out in some studies to increase sphincter injury rates.[13]

## DIAGNOSIS

### History and Physical Examination

As with most medical conditions, the history and physical examination are the mainstays of diagnosis and can frequently divulge the etiology of fecal incontinence before any confirmatory investigations. The history should focus on the pathophysiological entities leading to incontinence and rule out any potentially confounding diseases. A detailed past medical and surgical history as well as medication review can frequently provide a source for an underlying disease or treatment/medication side effect leading to the incontinence. Queries about changes in stool consistency (diarrhea or constipation related to medications or other conditions), associated abdominal bloating or cramps (IBS or inflammatory bowel disease), perineal pain, hematochezia or purulent drainage (tumors, inflammatory bowel disease, radiation proctitis, or benign anorectal conditions such as hemorrhoids or fistula-causing disease) can elucidate other diagnoses. Consistency of the stool being leaked (gas, liquid, solid), timing of that leak (day and/or night, after bowel movements), and degree of effect on lifestyle and QOL (use of incontinence scoring systems can help standardize these questions) will help to clarify the degree of incontinence and perhaps the extent of underlying pathology. Identifying previous obstetric history, including number of children, difficult deliveries (episiotomy, perineal tear, use of forceps or vacuum, and prolonged labor) and mode of delivery, and complications of those deliveries will guide the management and anticipated need for further evaluation and possible sphincter

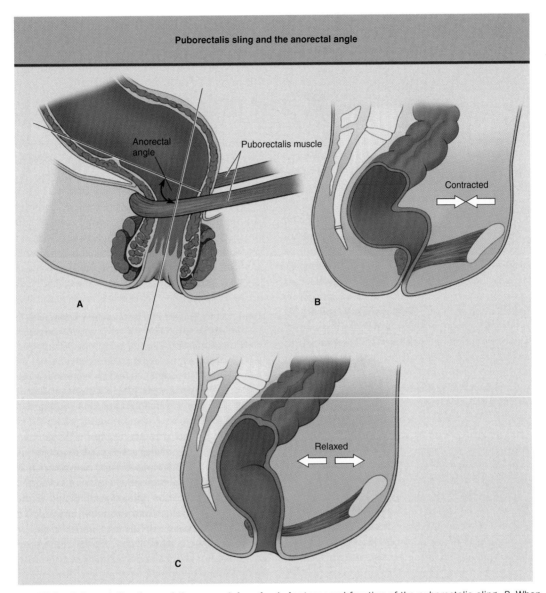

Puborectalis sling and the anorectal angle

Anorectal angle

Puborectalis muscle

A

Contracted

B

Relaxed

C

**Figure 27-3    Puborectalis sling and the anorectal angle**. *A*, Anatomy and function of the puborectalis sling. *B*, When contracted, the muscle creates the anorectal angle, which assists in maintaining continence. *C*, When relaxed, the angle changes and defecation is facilitated.

reconstruction. This should be in addition to obtaining a history about perineal or anal trauma from injury or rough sex as well as a history of past perineal operations.

After a complete physical examination looking for manifestations of diseases that can impact continence or masquerade as symptoms of incontinence, a detailed anal and perineal examination should be performed. The perineum can best be examined in the prone jackknife (Kraske), knee–chest, left lateral decubitus or, in some cases, modified lithotomy position (Fig. 27-4). Visual and digital examination should focus on the presence of mass lesions, scars, fistulae, fecal impaction, or inflammatory changes. Digital examination (including bimanual examination of the perineum) can clarify the resting sphincter tone, mobility and strength of the sphincter on voluntary squeeze, thickness of the perineum and rectovaginal septum, and presence of other pathology (e.g., rectocele). Having the patient perform a Valsalva maneuver while observing the perineum and

perianal area may show evidence of inappropriate perineal descent, rectocele, cystocele, or rectal or vaginal prolapse. The utility of these subjective examination findings has been questioned when compared to more objective studies such as ultrasound or manometry, but they are still necessary in the evaluation.[16,18]

Anoscopy, rigid or flexible sigmoidoscopy, and/or full colonoscopy with or without abdominal radiographs should be added to the investigative armamentarium when deemed appropriate. Additionally, defecography (fluoroscopic evaluation of the defecation process through voiding of barium paste) and dynamic pelvic magnetic resonance imaging are useful in select situations to confirm or identify other pathology, such as mucosal intussusception, rectal prolapse, or rectocele, that may affect continence.[18] Finally, a number of physiological tests have been shown to provide adjunctive information to the history and physical examination and may even alter the treatment plan in

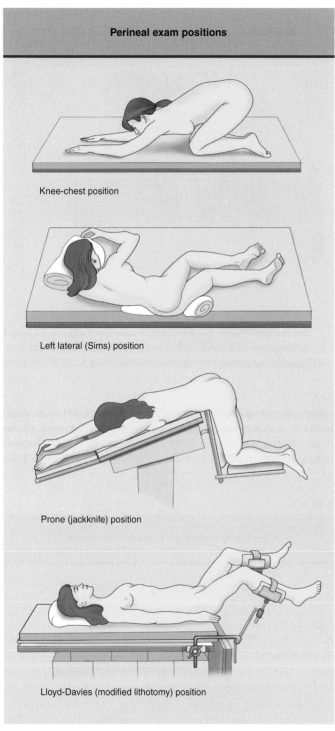

**Perineal exam positions**

Knee-chest position

Left lateral (Sims) position

Prone (jackknife) position

Lloyd-Davies (modified lithotomy) position

**Figure 27-4** **Patient positioning for examination of the anorectum and perineum.**

10% to 84% of patients with fecal incontinence.[19] These include endoanal ultrasound, anal manometry, and neurophysiology testing.

### Ultrasonography

Endoanal ultrasound has become the mainstay of fecal incontinence investigations, primarily because it is one of the few tests that can reliably, accurately, and in a minimally invasive fashion identify one of the few causes of incontinence that has shown benefit from surgical correction: the anal sphincter defect.[19] The study is performed with a rotating 360-degree 7.5- to 10-MHz ultrasound transducer with an anal cap, allowing for structural visualization and, with some instruments, three-dimensional reconstruction of the anal canal. The higher the frequency, the better the structural resolution; therefore a 10-MHz transducer is ideal for mapping the anal sphincter.[16,18] The test is best performed with the patient in prone jackknife or left lateral decubitus position, and is often facilitated by a preprocedure enema, although this is not mandatory. Normal appearance of the internal sphincter is a hypoechoic circumferential ring around the middle anal canal; the external sphincter (more difficult to interpret and identify in comparison to the internal sphincter) first appears in the upper anal canal in continuity with the horseshoe appearance of the puborectalis muscle as a hyperechoic ring that extends to the lower anal canal (Fig. 27-5A).[18] Defects are noted as unanticipated changes in the echogenicity or thickness of the sphincters (Fig. 27-5B), suggesting separation or scarring of the muscles.

Although sphincter defects may be due to injuries and may therefore be the etiology of incontinence, they may also be normal anatomic variants, which lead to false-positive results in 5% to 25% of individuals.[20] Ultrasound studies by Bollard and colleagues of 57 normal primiparous women in the first trimester showed some degree of sphincter gap in 44 (77%) of them, most in the upper anal canal.[21] These findings were substantiated in a small group of normal male and female controls, with none of the men and all of the women having some degree of anterior defect despite no previous history of trauma, surgery, or pregnancy. By limiting the definition of sphincter injury to those that had irregular borders and occurred in the lower anal canal, the authors were able to eliminate a 10% false-positive rate if an ultrasound was originally considered positive simply for showing any sphincter defect.[21] The results of this study underscore the fact that experienced technicians are necessary to provide accurate data about the anatomy of the sphincter complex. This is further underscored by studies showing variability in interobserver agreement, although significant defects are usually identified with good to very good correlation between experienced observers.[22]

The results of mapping the sphincter with ultrasound have been shown to be compatible with defects found at the time of operation,[18] and even occult defects or injuries are well-delineated with this methodology (up to 100% sensitivity with experienced technicians).[16,20] Ultrasound has also been shown to be more effective than manometry and is clearly better tolerated and at least as effective as needle electromyography (EMG) in mapping the anal sphincters.[16] It is therefore believed that ultrasound is necessary when surgical correction of a sphincter defect is planned to obtain a "road map" of the abnormal sphincter anatomy. In addition, ultrasound may provide useful information as to other pathology (such as fistula or abscess)[22] and the thickness of the perineal body, which has been found to be predictive of the presence of a pathologic sphincter defect (97% when perineal body thickness < 10 mm) but not correlated with the degree of fecal incontinence.[20] Finally, ultrasound is essential when evaluating patients with

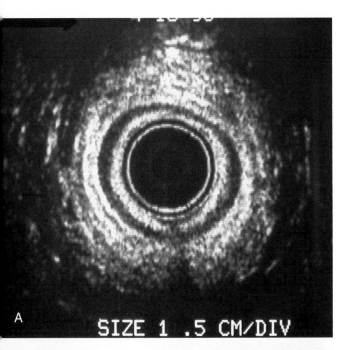

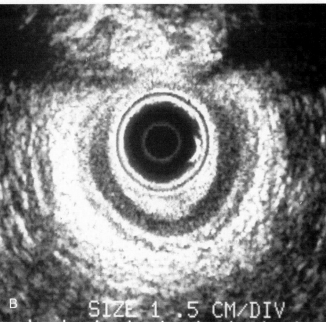

**Figure 27-5  Examples of endorectal ultrasounds.** *A*, Appearance of normal concentric ring anatomy of the internal (central hypoechoic ring) and external (outer hyperechoic ring) anal sphincters. *B*, Appearance of an abnormal endorectal ultrasound, showing an anterior defect in both internal and external anal sphincters replaced with hyperechoic scar (from obstetric trauma).

recurrent incontinence after previous sphincter repair to determine the integrity of the repair and whether other etiologies of the recurrence should be sought.

## Manometry

Anal manometry is the study of pressures within the anal canal at rest and with contraction (squeeze) as well as the determination of muscle responses to distention within the rectum

(rectoanal inhibitory reflex). At rest the pressure is indicative of the baseline tonicity of the internal and external anal sphincters, whereas squeeze pressures are indicative of external sphincter function (Fig. 27-6). The data can be used to suggest the approximate length of the anal canal (ranging from 2 to 5 cm in women)[16] and, with some instruments, the portion of the anal canal with abnormal function. It cannot, however, differentiate between muscular and neural sources of pathology in the anal canal.

The procedure is performed with any number of water-perfused catheters, solid-state transducers, or balloon-tipped catheters (Fig. 27-7). The balloon-tipped catheters are useful in determining the presence of the rectoanal inhibitory reflex as well as obtaining information about the first detected sensation of volume in the rectum (indicating ability to sense rectal filling), volume when a defecatory urge occurs (indicating normal stool volume for that patient), and the maximum tolerable volume (indicating full rectal compliance or irritability). These catheters are also used to guide biofeedback training.

The most important aspect of this testing is that it is dependent on the examiner and instrument as well as the compliance of the patient (especially for the squeeze portion of the examination and the reporting of sensory changes); therefore, the results must always be viewed in context with the clinical situation. Studies have both confirmed and refuted the reproducibility of these tests between different examiners on the same patient.[16] In addition, some studies show variability in correlating manometric results with degrees of incontinence (sensitivity, 32% to 92%; specificity, 67% to 97%, depending on the cutoffs used),[16] which is likely due to the significant variability in "normal" values detected in controls as well as the differences in "normal" values between gender and age groups.[16,18] Therefore, it is recommended that manometric techniques within laboratories be standardized and normal ranges for each laboratory be established to avoid blaming technique as the source of variability. The American Gastroenterological Association (AGA) reports that fecal incontinence is one of the indications for manometric study, despite the lack of controlled clinical trials.[16]

## Neurophysiology

The two primary means by which the integrity of the neuro-muscular function of the pelvic musculature can be tested are EMG and pudendal nerve terminal motor latencies (PNTML). Both of these tests have distinct advantages and disadvantages that make them variably useful in the assessment of fecal incontinence, and both have been used as adjuncts to the other physiological studies described in this chapter.

### Electromyography

Electromyography is used to assess external anal sphincter and puborectal muscle function, map the anal sphincter complex, and provide information on the presence of neuropathic and/or myopathic injury by measuring the electrical activity of the muscular motor units. The study requires specialized training to perform and interpret the findings.[16] It can be performed by either needle electrodes (insertion of concentric or single fibers) or anal plug (sponge or hard plug), which can indicate nerve injury and reinnervation of the muscle units by adjacent nerve

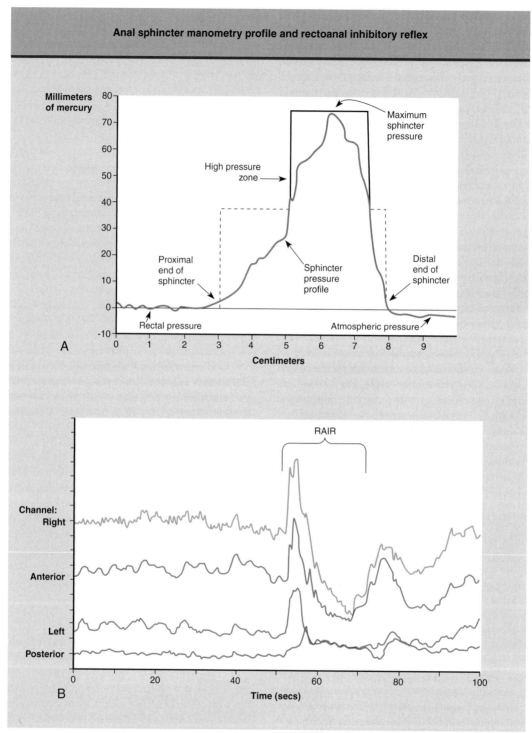

**Anal sphincter manometry profile and rectoanal inhibitory reflex**

**Figure 27-6    Normal manometric studies.** *A,* Normal manometric squeeze pressure profile of the anal canal (from an eight-channel water perfusion pressure catheter). *B,* Normal rectoanal inhibitory reflex (RAIR; from a four-channel water perfusion balloon-tipped pressure catheter).

fibers. Surface EMG electrodes are also available, but they are more useful in evaluating gross motor activity over larger areas than the needle EMG. Surface electrodes are best used for evaluating paradoxical sphincter spasm during defecation in constipated patients as well as for biofeedback training.[16,18] Of the other methods, needle EMG is more uncomfortable for the patient[18] and carries a higher risk of infection than the anal plug, but it offers the most reproducible intraobserver and interobserver results. Both needle and plug techniques are well-correlated with manometric squeeze pressures. Overall, however, EMG has not been validated by histologic evidence of nerve injury, is less sensitive than ultrasound in mapping the anal sphincter, is

**Manometric catheters and their application**

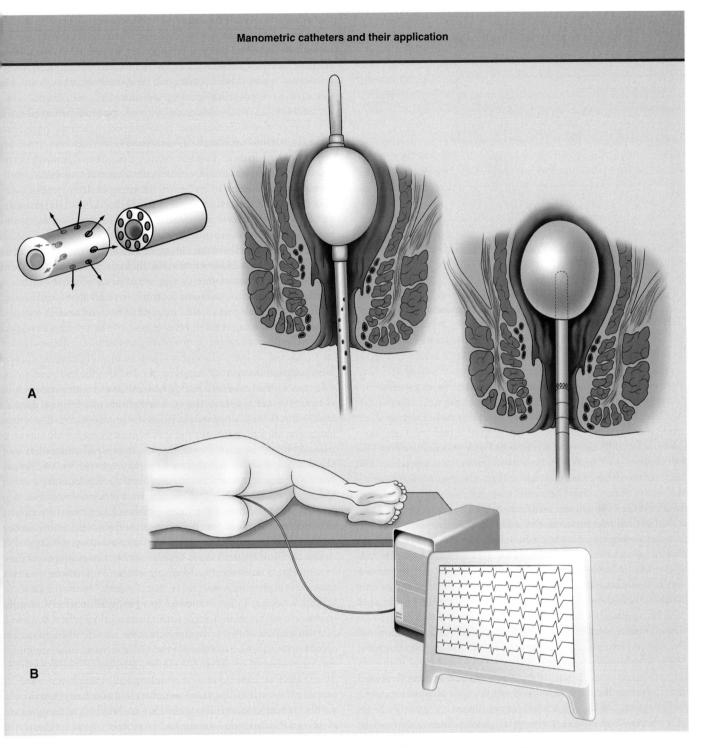

**Figure 27-7  Examples of manometric catheters (A) and their application (B).**

subject to potential sampling error, and is limited to primarily distal portions of the anal canal (although the puborectalis muscle can be examined).[16] Because of the better results and tolerability of endoanal ultrasound, the AGA has stated that "(n)eedle EMG cannot be recommended for fecally incontinent patients" while surface EMG is of "possible value" in the assessment of sphincter function in incontinence.[16]

### Pudendal Nerve Terminal Motor Latencies

The external anal sphincter is innervated by the pudendal nerve. PNTML evaluates pudendal neuropathy by measuring the time (or "latency") between stimulation of the pudendal nerve at the ischial spine and contraction of the external anal sphincter. A stimulating and recording electrode that fits on a gloved index finger was designed for this purpose (Fig. 27-8). A digital

Urogynecology

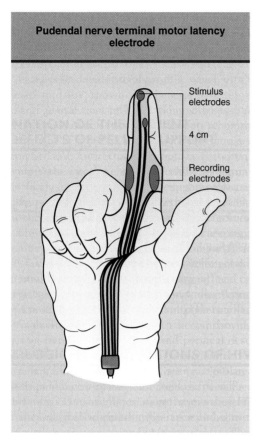

**Figure 27-8** Pudendal nerve terminal motor latencies measurement electrode.

examination is performed with the apparatus in place, and the tip of the finger electrode is placed to stimulate the nerve as it courses through Alcock's canal beneath the ischial spine (a difficult maneuver in some patients). The recording electrode is at the base of the examining finger and therefore records the motor unit potential of the external sphincter at the lower anal canal. This is tested on both sides of the pelvis to ensure that there is not a bilateral neuropathy. Because the energy used to stimulate the nerve is low (50 volts with 8 to 10 mA of current), discomfort involved in performing the test is usually minimal. Nerve conduction delay above the norm of 2.0 ± 0.2 msec is caused by demyelination of the fast-conducting fibers of the distal pudendal nerve due to aging, systemic disease (e.g., diabetes, scleroderma), and/or nerve injury or stretch (e.g., from vaginal delivery, rectal prolapse). This data is believed to best help differentiate between fecal incontinence due to nerve injury, muscle injury, or both, especially when combined with endoanal ultrasound results. Initial studies showed that patients with bilateral even more than unilateral neuropathy faired poorly after anal sphincter repair, and it was therefore believed to be a crucial preoperative test.[23] Other studies, however, have not shown PNTML results to impact surgical outcomes[24,25] or affect clinical decision making.[19] Other issues with PNTML relate to overall poor sensitivity and specificity for etiologies of incontinence, the lack of normal values for various age and gender groups, lack of data on intraobserver or interobserver reproducibility, and the fact that a normal study through a few

remaining normal distal pudendal nerve fibers could potentially camouflage a more global or proximal pudendal nerve injury.[16] It is therefore believed by some authors that this test should be abandoned in the evaluation of fecal incontinence, and the AGA has stated that "(t)he PNTML cannot be recommended for evaluation of patients with fecal incontinence," although it may be "interesting from a research point of view."[16]

## TREATMENT AND CLINICAL COURSE

Usually a complete cure for fecal incontinence cannot be attained; therefore, treatments are aimed at improving symptoms and QOL as much as possible. The treatments range from medical management through the use of bulk-forming agents and antidiarrheals to behavioral management and retraining through the use of biofeedback to multiple surgical options, including sphincter repairs, artificial and autologous neosphincters, and even fecal diversion through the creation of a stoma. Often a treatment algorithm is best followed to standardize the incontinence evaluation and avoid the pitfalls of missed diagnoses. An example of one such treatment algorithm is presented in Figure 27-9.

### Nonsurgical Treatment

The majority of patients suffering from fecal incontinence will not need surgical intervention. They often will benefit enough from nonoperative management of their disease that surgical therapies are not necessary or justified. As long as the dietary, medical, or behavioral therapies are complied with, they are effective long-term. In addition, these therapies have few side effects, avoid the potential complications associated with operative intervention, and do not preclude the potential for operative correction in the future. Therefore, most physicians will explore the use of nonsurgical treatments before more invasive means of fecal incontinence treatment.

Because incontinence is frequently related to systemic disease or medication side effects, treatment of these underlying diseases or use of alternative medications often "cures" the incontinence. Diarrhea from IBS or inflammatory bowel disease can usually be improved with pharmacologic therapies targeted to these conditions. Tumors, radiation proctitis, and benign anorectal conditions leading to incontinence will benefit from surgical therapies aimed at these conditions for those who are candidates. Medications leading to diarrhea are best discontinued, if possible, but when the medication is necessary, agents to slow motility or add bulk to the stool may be helpful. If the etiology of fecal incontinence cannot be attributed to a medication or underlying medical condition, the history, examination, and adjunctive tests can help clarify the etiology. If the incontinence symptoms are mild to moderate and are not having a substantial impact on QOL, or if the patient is not a surgical candidate, medical therapies often offer satisfactory results.

Alteration in diet is the first line of nonsurgical treatment for fecal incontinence related to alterations in stool consistency or colonic transit. This is based on increasing the dietary fiber to 25 to 30 g/day of insoluble fiber, primarily in the form of raw fruits and vegetables and whole grains. If this is not achievable through dietary means alone, bulking agents in the form of psyllium or other raw fiber can be added. This is often sufficient

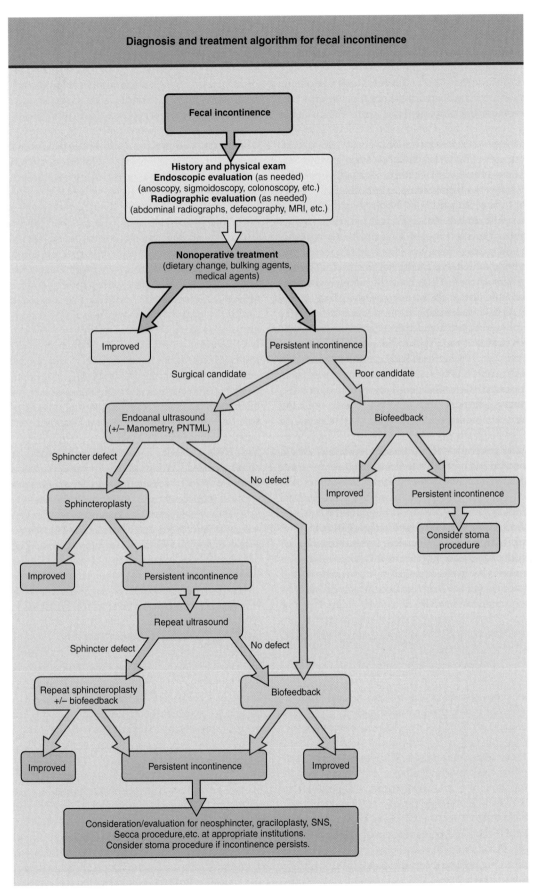

**Figure 27-9  Diagnostic and treatment algorithm for fecal incontinence.** PNTML, pudendal nerve terminal motor latencies; SNS, sacral nerve stimulation.

to increase the formed stools and thus decrease the incontinence episodes to liquid stool. A common side effect of this fiber regimen may be increased gas that requires further alteration in the diet or raw fiber until a nongas-forming regimen can be achieved. Additionally, a strict bowel movement regimen should be sought to have complete evacuation of the rectal contents each morning and thus avoid difficulty with overflow incontinence and stool leakage during the day. This may be facilitated through the use of stool softeners, laxatives (avoiding senna and cascara, which can lead to dependency), and a glycerin suppository or small enema each morning to further stimulate complete evacuation. Adherence to this regimen can lead to fewer episodes of incontinence and can be especially beneficial in the bed-bound or physically limited nursing home patient.[5]

### Medical Agents

If dietary adjustments or bulking agents are insufficient or not tenable due to patient comorbidities or limitations, pharmacotherapy may be a viable option for some patients. These agents can be especially useful when trying to alter stool consistency and thus improve bowel control and decrease stool frequency. Care must be taken to avoid constipation when using these agents, however. Loperamide (a synthetic opioid) has been shown to inhibit peristalsis, increase bowel transit time, increase anal sphincter tone, and decrease fecal urgency and stool volume. Its utility in improving incontinence episodes has been supported in a number of placebo-controlled trials. Its side effects can include paralytic ileus and central nervous system (CNS) effects on overdose. Diphenoxylate, also an opioid derivative, which is often given in combination with atropine to limit the CNS effects of the drug, has been shown to be less potent than loperamide but with a similar safety and side effect profile. This drug has also been shown to decrease stool volume and frequency in placebo-controlled trials on incontinent patients. Amitriptyline, a tricyclic antidepressant with the side effect of reducing rectal motor complexes, has been tested in incontinent patients in low doses and been shown to lead to firmer stool formation and decreased incontinence scores. This and other agents such as phenylephrine gel (applied directly to the anus to increase sphincter tone) or bile-acid binders must be examined in randomized, prospective trials before their use can be advocated in all patients with fecal incontinence.[26]

### Biofeedback

Biofeedback is a behavioral retraining technique best used in patients with pudendal neuropathy causing external anal sphincter weakness (e.g., from diabetes, pudendal stretch injury), in patients with diminished rectal sensation (from diabetes, scleroderma) leading to incontinence, or in patients with small sphincter defects who wish to avoid surgery as the initial treatment.[9] Biofeedback has also shown significant benefit when used by patients after sphincter repair.[27] Types of biofeedback include use of a balloon-tipped catheter and pressure sensors in the anal canal, use of EMG surface or anal canal electrodes, use of endoanal ultrasound, or simply use of digital self-examination. Each of the techniques focuses on training the patient to contract the anal sphincter muscles. Some of the techniques also attempt to improve the detection of rectal distention (balloon technique) and avoid inappropriate timing of the Valsalva manuever during the defecation process (EMG surface technique). They all use either visual, auditory, or sensory responses through the pressure sensors, EMG, ultrasound screen, or digital examination to provide feedback to the patient as to their progress. Given that some amount of rectal sensation and sphincter contraction must be feasible for these methods to be successful, these techniques have not been effective in patients with severe limitations such as those with spinal cord injuries. In addition, these techniques require dedication on the part of the patient as well as dedicated and well-trained therapists,[5] who are not always available in all communities and whose availability may be limited by insurance coverage.

Biofeedback techniques have been shown to be effective in 50% to 92% of selected patients, and the results are usually sustained and have been effective even when compared to sham training.[10] Primarily, there seems to be improved continence with biofeedback more often in patients with sensory deficits as compared to patients with neurologic (i.e., functional) and structural deficits, but this is based on a nonsystematic review of multiple uncontrolled studies.[28] Interestingly, the symptom improvement in these studies did not necessarily correlate to improvement in objective physiological studies or improved QOL, so the reason for the effectiveness of biofeedback remains elusive.[28] A Cochrane review of five randomized, controlled trials on biofeedback also failed to make definitive conclusions because of the variety of techniques and endpoints used in the trials.[10,28] One other well-designed randomized, controlled trial looking at various counseling and biofeedback techniques in 171 patients with and without structural sphincter defects concluded that patient–therapist interactions and patient coping strategies had a greater impact than treatment methodology or etiology of incontinence.[28] Although the reason for the effectiveness of these techniques remains unclear, they are painless, safe, and well-tolerated; and they are a useful means by which to potentially avoid the need for operative intervention.[10]

### Surgical Treatment

When dietary, medical, or biofeedback treatments are not efficacious, surgical treatments for fecal incontinence may be effective options. They include the universally accepted and performed treatment of anal sphincter repair (sphincteroplasty) in addition to more controversial procedures performed at specialized centers to create a neosphincter (graciloplasty or artificial sphincter), improve function through sacral nerve stimulation, or increase resting sphincter pressure with radiofrequency treatments (Secca). A final surgical option is stoma formation to try to improve QOL in patients with fecal incontinence.

#### Anal Sphincteroplasty

The most successful and commonly performed surgical procedure for fecal incontinence is primary repair of the anal sphincter, or anal sphincteroplasty. This procedure is for those patients with incontinence who have not responded to nonoperative measures and who have an identifiable anatomic sphincter defect on examination, ultrasound, or EMG. The majority of these patients have sphincter defects from obstetric or surgical trauma, some of which may have been identified and repaired at the time of the initial injury. The evaluation prior to sphincteroplasty, beyond a detailed history and physical examination, needs to establish the presence of a sphincter defect. Absolute contraindications to the procedure are intuitive and relate to the medical and mental fitness of the patient, active perineal or perianal infection, and the patient's eligibility for spinal or general anesthesia. Relative contraindications include radiation proctitis, malignancy, inflammatory bowel disease, or plans for subsequent vaginal deliveries. If the injury has occurred recently (<6 weeks), it is usually recommended to wait for the inflammation to decrease for at least 6 weeks, although early reoperations have shown good results in terms of postrepair continence in small case series.[13]

Sphincteroplasty at the time of acute obstetric sphincter injury (third- and fourth-degree tears) is routinely performed by most obstetricians in a direct end-to-end fashion with absorbable interrupted sutures. Fecal incontinence rates 6 to 12 months after this type of acute repair have been shown to be approximately 40% (range, 20% to 50%), depending on the definitions used.[13] This high rate of incontinence has been established by endoanal ultrasounds performed up to 12 months' postpartum, showing a persistent sphincter defect in 54% to 85% of women despite the performed repair.[18] It is unclear whether these later defects were unrecognized or whether the repairs were disrupted. Performing an overlapping repair at the time of acute injury has shown an improvement in sphincter integrity postpartum in some studies but not in others.[13] Ultimately, though, it is unclear what impact these acute repairs truly have on later continence; therefore, well-designed long-term trials need to be done before conclusions about the effectiveness of acute repair techniques can be made.

Anal sphincteroplasty for more chronic injuries is preferentially performed in the prone jackknife position via a transperineal approach, modified from that described by Parks and McPartlin in 1971.[5] Preoperative preparation for sphincteroplasty includes a full mechanical bowel preparation and appropriate broad-spectrum perioperative intravenous antibiotics (usually cefoxitin or cefotetan). Once the patient has been positioned and before preparation of the perineum, rigid proctoscopy should be performed both to evacuate any remaining stool and to reveal any previously unidentified rectal pathology. After preparation, an anterior 180-degree circumanal incision is created in the perineal body (if one still exists) approximately 1 cm distal to the dentate line (Fig. 27-10A). A flap of skin and rectal wall is elevated in the cephalad direction for 4 to 5 cm to expose the midline scar and adjacent edges of the sphincter complex (Fig. 27-10B). Lateral dissection into the ischiorectal fat provides for further identification and mobilization of the sphincters, but care must be taken to avoid injury to the pudendal nerve as it enters the sphincter complex from the posterolateral direction. Separation of the internal and external aspects of the sphincter is optional because this does not affect repair outcomes. The posterior aspect of the vagina and its adjacent perineal skin is dissected off the midline scar, and the scar is divided but not excised as it plays a crucial role in the repair (Fig. 27-10C). Once mobilization is complete, judgment is made as to whether an overlapping or abutting end-to-end repair is performed to avoid undo tension on the repair and allow the tip of the small finger or 15-mm dilator into the anus (Figs. 27-10D, 27-10E). Slow-dissolving (e.g., polydioxanone) or permanent (polypropylene) monofilament sutures are used to create a layered

horizontal mattress closure (routinely two layers three sutures deep) using the scar as suture support wherever possible. The perineal body is then closed with or without the presence of a closed suction drain. The closure frequently must be in a vertical direction, creating a T or Y configuration (Fig. 27-10F), which helps to recreate the perineal body. Postoperative care in terms of early versus late feeding, iatrogenic constipation versus early stool softeners and bulk-forming laxatives have not shown a difference in outcomes from the repair.[29] Complications are usually minor in most series and include urine retention and superficial wound infections (approximately 15%) leading to delayed healing.[30] Sitz baths and meticulous perianal hygiene is recommended to decrease wound complications, and the drain, if left in, should remain until drainage is less than 5 mL in 24 hours. The anal sphincteroplasty has also been combined with anterior levator plication or, through a posterior circumanal incision, a Parks' postanal levatorplasty with only fair long-term results.[9]

The effectiveness of sphincteroplasty alone for chronic injuries, both with overlapping and end-to-end technique, has been reported in a number of retrospective and prospective case series with a variety of clinical outcomes, incontinence scores, QOL, and physiological measures used. Most reports show 71% to 98% early improvement after anal sphincteroplasty[30] with approximately 66% of patients (52% to 83%) having excellent to good overall outcomes.[3] Factors that may lead to early poor outcomes have not been completely delineated. Diversion with a stoma at the time of initial repair has not been shown to improve outcomes,[31] although it may improve outcomes after subsequent repairs.[5] It is unclear whether the status of the pudendal nerve (specifically, PNTML duration) at the time of initial repair has an impact on the final sphincteroplasty outcomes as there are mixed results in the literature about the effect of both unilateral and bilateral PNTML delay.[3,5,19,23–25] Age has similarly shown a mixed impact on results while obesity and longer duration of incontinence before repair has been shown to have a negative impact on outcomes.[5] Reoperations for recurrent sphincter defects after prior reconstruction have not precluded good outcomes.[25,30] Finally, adjunctive measures such as the use of postsphincteroplasty biofeedback have shown improved outcomes versus sphincteroplasty alone.[3,27]

The most concerning aspect of anal sphincteroplasty is the long-term efficacy of the repair. It was originally believed that the repair had exceptional longevity. Unfortunately, recent studies have brought this into doubt. Halverson and Hull did a telephone survey at a median of 69 months postrepair of 49 of 71 patients, of whom 54% were incontinent to liquid stool and only 14% had complete continence.[32] This was in comparison to early results of the study showing 19% incontinence to liquid stool and 49% having total continence. A similar follow-up questionnaire study in 74 of 86 patients at 40 months postrepair showed a 28% complete continence rate, down from 49% at 3 months postoperatively.[31] Other studies with follow-up at 5 to 10 years showed rates of total continence of 0% to 42%, having decreased from initial total continence rates of 49% to 64%.[3] The reason for this time-dependent diminution is unclear, but it is likely related to gradual repair separation, pudendal nerve deterioration, or age effects on the pelvic floor musculature.[3] Women must be counseled before the initial sphincter repair

367

**Anal sphincteroplasty**

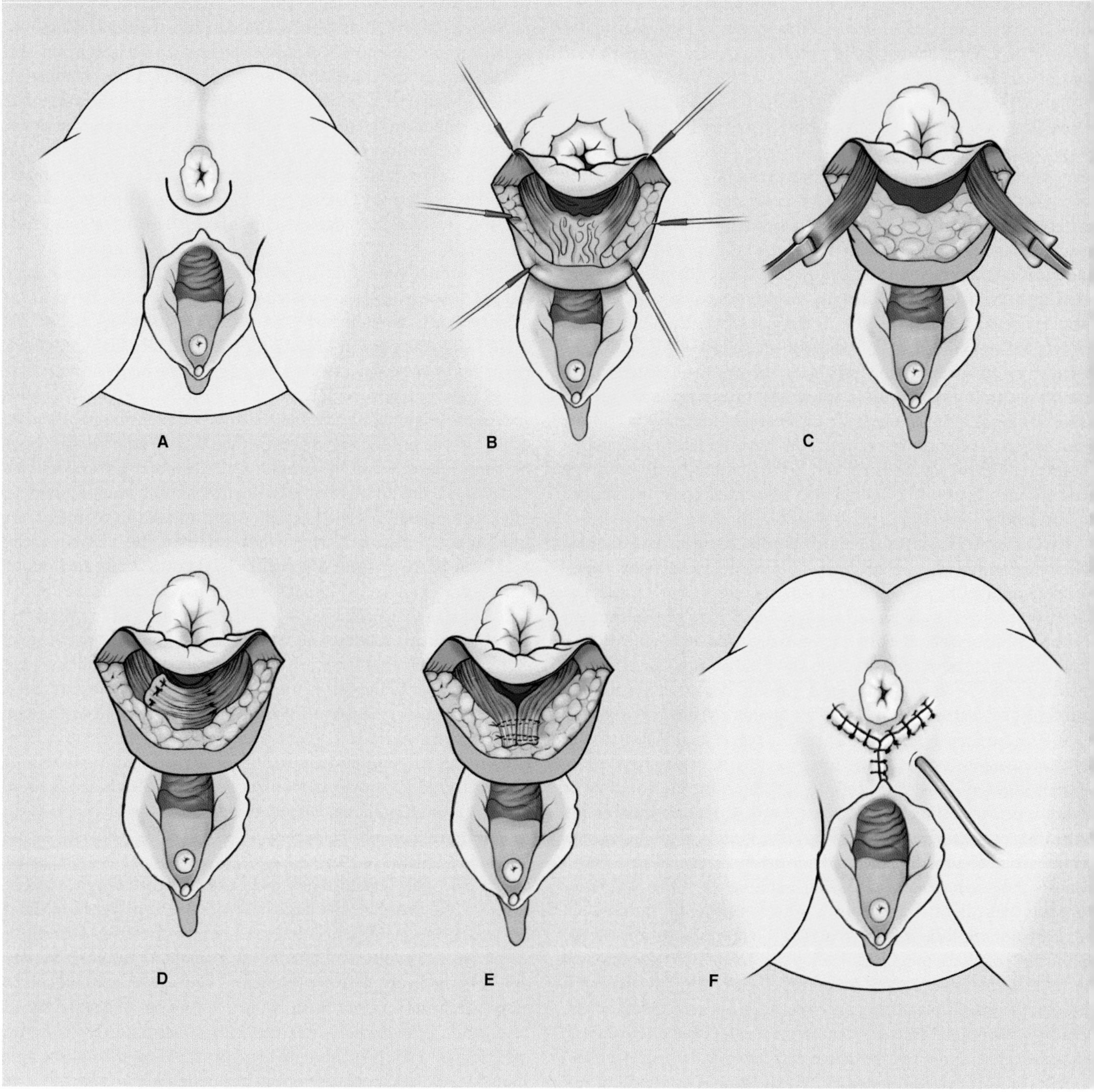

**Figure 27-10  Sphincteroplasty technique.** *A,* Anterior curvilinear incision. *B,* Flap dissection and identification of the underlying musculature and scar (facilitated by a self-retaining retractor such as the Lone Star [Lone Star Medical Systems, Stafford, Tex.]). *C,* Mobilization and central division of the anal sphincter. *D,* Creation of overlapping muscle repair. *E,* Creation of end-to-end muscle repair. *F,* Closure of the incision in a Y- or T-shape to facilitate re-creation of the perineal body.

hat reoperation or further treatments may be necessary in the future even if initial procedures are successful.

### Dynamic Gracioplasty

For patients who have failed anal sphincteroplasty, have nerve injury-related incontinence not responsive to nonoperative management, or congenital anomalies leading to fecal incontinence, attempts at creation of a new sphincter have been undertaken. Often inspired by similar attempts in the treatment of urinary incontinence, neosphincters for fecal incontinence have been created through the use of both autologous and artificial tissue. The first attempts with autologous tissue were undertaken through the use of muscles in proximity to the anal canal that could be allowed to maintain a neurovascular supply and provide some tonicity or resistance to improve continence. Initial trials were with sartorius, gluteus maximus (gluteoplasty), or gracilis (gracioplasty) muscle wraps.[33] These each involve wrapping at least a portion of the respective muscle through subcutaneous tunnels around the anal canal. Sartorius wrap results were poor due to the segmental neurovasculature, making effective wraps difficult. The initial gluteoplasties were done as early as 1902.[33] Case series for gluteoplasties developed again in the 1980s when favorable results were found in approximately 50% of patients, but because of the gluteus muscle's function in routine activities, patients had to limit those activities for almost a month after the operation, and it potentially led to long-term disability.[33] The gracioplasty also showed favorable results in initial series in the early 1950s, but these "passive" wraps had

inconsistent results because of fatiguing of the voluntary, type II, fast-twitch muscle fibers of the gracilis.[33] This prompted the addition of an implantable stimulating generator to convert these fibers into type I, slow-twitch, fatigue-resistant, involuntary muscle fibers.[3,33] This then led to the development of the stimulated or "dynamic" gracioplasty in the late 1980s.

Dynamic gracioplasty usually involves two steps. The first is the creation of the wrap by freeing the insertion of the gracilis muscle from the medial thigh through one long or two or three smaller incisions on the thigh and ligating the vessels to the distal two thirds of the muscle. The proximal neurovascular bundle from the obturator nerve and deep femoral vessels is preserved as the muscle is mobilized enough to be tunneled around the anal canal guided by one or two perianal/perineal incisions. A 360-degree wrap is then performed in any of three configurations (Fig. 27-11) to allow the new insertion to be created to the ischial tuberosity or adjacent skin.[33,34] Creation of a diverting stoma at that time is optional but does not appear to limit infectious complications and has been shown to prolong time to continence by 6 months.[34] The second step, which some surgeons perform at the time of the first operation, is placement of the pulse generator (in a lower abdominal subcutaneous pocket); this may be performed 6 to 8 weeks after the initial procedure (the generator is turned on in 6 weeks if placed at the first operation). The leads from the generator are implanted in the gracilis muscle near the main nerve trunk to facilitate conversion to slow-twitch muscle fibers. The generator is started 3 days later and is slowly increased in intensity over the course

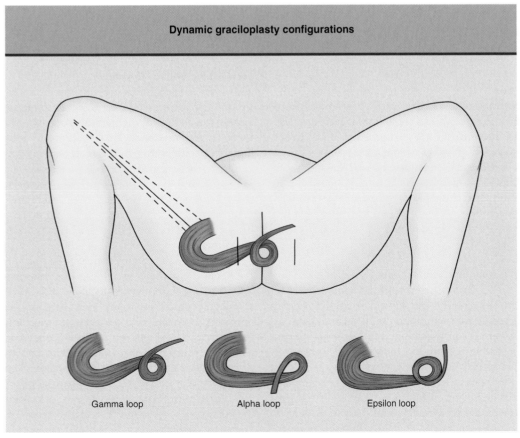

**Dynamic gracioplasty configurations**

Gamma loop

Alpha loop

Epsilon loop

**Figure 27-11   Options for gracioplasty configurations.**

of 8 weeks, eventually being left on continuously except when the patient turns it off to allow defecation. Because of the difficulty of the operation and risk for infection, it is contraindicated in patients with inflammatory bowel disease, neuromuscular disease, perianal infections, cancer, poor functional or mental status, pregnancy, or presence of a cardiac pacemaker or defibrillator.[33,34]

As with most of the technically demanding and experimental techniques for fecal incontinence, there are no randomized, controlled trials studying the use of dynamic graciloplasty.[3] Therefore, most of the outcome data come from more recent large, prospective, multicenter case series. Overall, despite varying definitions and outcomes measured, most reports show a success rate of approximately 60% (42% to 85%) and show that centers with greater experience have better outcomes with fewer complications.[3,33,34] Physiologic studies post-transposition consistently show improved sphincter tone with graciloplasty, but QOL studies have not always correlated with this improvement.[34] Mortality rates for most series have been 0, but other studies have had death rates of up to 13% (when cancer deaths are excluded), usually related to cardiopulmonary complications in small series.[33] Overall, the mortality rate is considered to be approximately 2%.[33] Morbidity rates range extensively, and many studies show substantially more complications than patients, showing that many patients have multiple complications and approximately 40% need reoperation.[33,34] In the larger series, these morbidities include major and minor infections (13% to 30%), apparatus failure (12% to 18%), chronic pain (13% to 28%), and constipation (19% to 23%).[34] Fortunately, despite the high complication rate, even patients with complications can have good outcomes after treatment.[30] Still, dynamic graciloplasty continues to be an experimental treatment best performed on highly selected, well-informed patients at high-volume centers.

### Artificial Neosphincter

Whereas the dynamic graciloplasty creates an autologous neosphincter, an artificial implantable neosphincter has also been developed to attempt to recreate the effect of an intact sphincter mechanism. The device was initially developed in the 1970s for use in the treatment of urinary incontinence but was successfully used in the late 1980s for fecal incontinence.[35] The device was then modified to a three-component mechanism (Fig. 27-12) for the treatment of fecal incontinence that includes an inflatable "sphincter" cuff implanted around the anal canal, a pressure-regulating reservoir in the retroperitoneum, and a control pump placed in the labia (or scrotum), all connected by kink-proof tubing. It functions by maintaining tonic filling of the cuff and thus closure of the anal canal until the pump is used to deflate the cuff into the reservoir and allow defecation to occur. The device is implanted after antibiotic prophylaxis through at least two perianal/perineal incisions and one lower abdominal incision (for the reservoir pocket) and then allowed to heal for 6 to 8 weeks before actually activating the system.

The indications for placement of the device have been limited due to the high cost and high complication rate associated with the device. It has primarily been reserved for patients who have congenital abnormalities, traumatic sphincter injuries or failed surgical repairs not amenable to further correction, or severe neurologic dysfunction.[35] As expected with the placement of a foreign body around the anal canal, the most common and devastating complications are infection and/or device erosion requiring explantation.[3] Other complications have included device malfunctions, chronic pain, persistent incontinence, and fecal impaction, all potentially necessitating removal or revision of the device.[3,35,36] In a review of 13 case series (there are no available randomized, controlled trials evaluating the use of the artificial neosphincter), including a multicenter trial with 112 patients, approximately 33% required explantation and 13% to 50% required surgical revision.[36] This was primarily due to an infection rate of approximately 25% (range, 4% to 38%) and an erosion rate of approximately 18% (range, 6% to 25%). Rates of postoperative fecal impaction ranged from 6% to 83% and chronic pain from 4% to 17%.[36]

Despite these potentially devastating complications, those patients that retain their devices in a functioning state have shown a statistically and clinically significant improvement in incontinence scores and QOL based on a variety of assessment tools.[35,36] Unfortunately, only one of the studies presents results on an intention-to-treat basis (showing an overall success rate in 53% of 97 patients[35]); therefore, no firm conclusions can be made as to the overall impact on continence and QOL of the artificial sphincter. Because firm conclusions cannot be drawn, it is as yet unclear whether there is a subset of incontinence patients who would more substantially benefit from the artificial neosphincter. However, as the multicenter trial by Wong and colleagues concluded:

> … there were no life-threatening complications with its use…, and it can be concluded that this procedure is a safe alternative for patients with end-stage fecal incontinence when no other medical or surgical treatment options exist.[35]

### Sacral Spinal Nerve Stimulation

Sacral nerve stimulation, or the use of an implantable device to stimulate the sacral nerves to contract the pelvic musculature, was first explored and approved by the U.S. Food and Drug Administration (FDA) in the late 1990s for use with urinary incontinence. It was noted that some of these early patients had improved fecal continence concordant with improved urinary continence; therefore trials for fecal incontinence were started in 1995.[37] The technique is still not widely available because it has not yet been approved by the FDA, but has been used in more than 1300 patients in trials for fecal incontinence.[38]

The procedure involves three steps (two diagnostic, one therapeutic) focusing on appropriate placement of electrodes into the dorsal foramina of S2–S4 that elicits the best anal sphincter contraction. The first step is performed in the operating room and involves a temporary stimulation of each of the bilateral sacral nerves to identify whether there is in fact a response from the pelvic musculature and thus confirm that the nerves are intact and adequate muscle is present. If there is an appropriate response, the second step is undertaken with continuous stimulation of the nerves (discontinued only to allow for voiding or defecation) for 2 to 3 weeks depending on the degree of incontinence. This step is initiated by attaching an external pulse generator to newly placed permanent electrodes or longer-lasting temporary percutaneous electrodes. Various settings on the pulse generator are then tested to identify which are the most effective prior to permanent implantation of the generator in the third step (with permanent electrode placement if needed). The greatest benefit of this device, therefore, is that its efficacy is confirmed prior to permanent implantation, unlike other implantable devices for incontinence.[30]

The indications for the device have broadened as more patients with varying etiologies of their incontinence have been tested. It is now felt to be indicated in any incontinent patient with an anal sphincter and any residual muscular and reflex function, and it is contraindicated in those with severe psychological or mental deficiencies or those without sphincters, with large sphincter defects, with sacral injuries/abnormalities preventing electrode placement, or with implanted cardiac pacemakers or defibrillators.[37,38] Because the indications have broadened, there has been a heterogeneous population of patients tested for a variety of endpoints. Although further controlled testing is clearly indicated to make firm conclusions about these devices, the conglomeration of preliminary studies have shown that a majority of patients have improved continence scores and QOL (most showing 75% to 100% improvement, with 41% to 75% reaching "complete" continence).[37,38] Possible complications

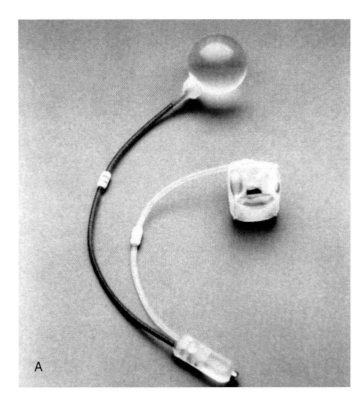

A

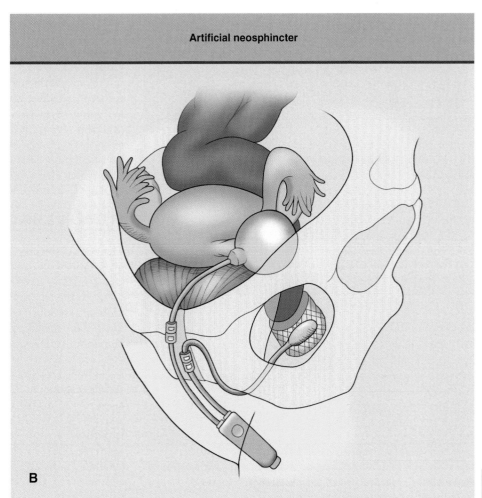

**Artificial neosphincter**

Figure 27-12   Artificial neosphincter apparatus *(A)* and appearance after implantation *(B)*.

B

(occurring in up to 50% of patients) include pain, generator or lead malfunction, or infection (no neurologic infections have been reported), lead dislocation requiring replacement, and deterioration or complete loss of effect.[37] The longevity of the results in most of these trials, however, has been excellent as long as generator and lead function has been maintained. Physiologic testing results, on the other hand, have been more inconsistent despite the subjective continence and QOL improvements.[37,38] This lack of clear change in physiology underscores the lack of understanding as to how this technique actually improves continence. Theories have included increasing the presence of

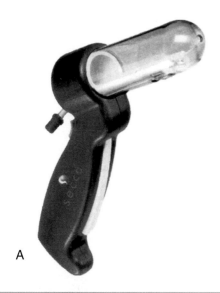

A

**Secca apparatus and application**

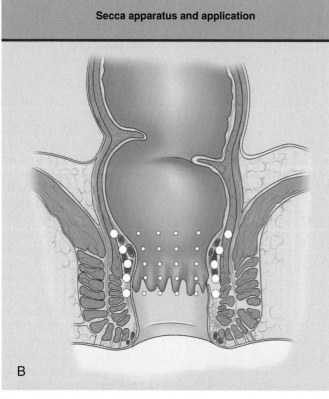

B

**Figure 27-13    Secca procedure for incontinence.** *A,* Apparatus. *B,* Radiofrequency energy application map in the anal canal.

type I, fatigue-resistant muscle fibers in the anal sphincter and increasing blood flow from autonomic nervous system effects.[38] Regardless of the mechanism, the use of sacral nerve stimulation will likely play a prominent role in the care of fecal incontinence in the future.

### Secca Procedure

Similar to the Stretta procedure for esophageal reflux disease, the Secca procedure (Curon Medical, Fremont, Calif.) uses temperature-controlled radiofrequency energy applied to the anal canal to attempt to create scarring in the internal sphincter, theoretically leading to improved anal canal apposition and resting pressures and thereby improving control.[39] The procedure is usually performed on an outpatient basis with local anesthesia, and the energy is applied through the use of a custom anoscope with needle electrodes (Fig. 27-13A) that apply the energy deep to the anal mucosa on varying levels (Fig. 27-13B). Initial data was encouraging based primarily on QOL improvement and few complications.[39] A subsequent multicenter trial by Efron and colleagues for a variety of etiologies of incontinence showed good subjective results without objective improvement in physiological measurements, thus bringing into question the true mechanism of the technique's effectiveness.[40] There were 3 complications out of 50 patients: two mucosal ulcerations and one postoperative bleed.[40] Despite the initially promising results, however, the procedure has yet to be tested on a larger scale so as to gain FDA approval or wider acceptance, likely due to the lack of data on any long-term sequelae of the procedure.

### Fecal Diversion

Creation of a colostomy or ileostomy when all other methods at improving continence have failed or are not practical is a viable means by which to relieve the social stigma of fecal incontinence and improve quality of life. Although they are not without the potential for complication and may present anesthetic and postoperative care dilemmas in the weak and frail, diverting stomas can be considered a "cure" for unremitting fecal incontinence. Performing these laparoscopically is a viable option for some patients to improve initial postoperative recovery.

## PITFALLS AND CONTROVERSIES

The first controversy in the realm of fecal incontinence is identifying a universally accepted definition and QOL indices. Other issues include developing protective strategies for preventing injury to the anal sphincters at the time of childbirth, effective methods for sphincter repair at the time of injury, and trying to identify the risk factors for fecal incontinence in women that can be altered to prevent injury. In addition, the diagnostic evaluation for fecal incontinence is far from standardized—both from a symptom/QOL standpoint as well as a physiologic and anatomic testing standpoint. Although endoanal ultrasound has provided an improved diagnostic modality, the use of manometry, EMG, and PNTML is still common despite data suggesting that the latter two are outdated and ineffectual at best. Finally, none of the listed treatment modalities have been tested in well-constructed, controlled trials with long-term follow-up to confirm their efficacy and longevity; therefore, the best treatments are left up to the surgeon and their experience with the various techniques.

# REFERENCES

1. Rockwood TH: Incontinence severity and QOL scales for fecal incontinence. Gastroenterol 2004;126:S106–S113. **(IV, C)**

2. Rockwood TH, Church JM, Fleshman JW, et al: Fecal incontinence quality of life scale. Dis Colon Rectum 2000;43:9–16. **(IIa, B)**

3. Madoff RD: Surgical treatment options for fecal incontinence. Gastroenterol 2004;126:S48–S54. **(IV, C)**

4. Miner PB: Economic and personal impact of fecal and urinary incontinence. Gastroenterol 2004;126:S175–S179. **(IV, C)**

5. Soffer EE, Hull T: Fecal incontinence: a practical approach to evaluation and treatment. Am J Gastroenterol. 2000;95:1873–1880. **(IV, C)**

6. Prather CM: Physiologic variables that predict the outcome of treatment for fecal incontinence. Gastroenterol 2004;126:S135–S140. **(IV, C)**

7. Chassagne P, Landrin I, Neveu C, et al: Fecal incontinence in the institutionalized elderly: incidence, risk factors, and prognosis. Am J Med 1999;106:185–190. **(III, B)**

8. Bliss DZ, Fischer LR, Savik K, et al: Severity of fecal incontinence in community-living elderly in a health maintenance organization. Res Nurs Health 2004;27:162–173. **(III, B)**

9. Whitehead WE, Wald A, Norton NJ: Treatment options for fecal incontinence. Dis Colon Rectum 2001;44:131–142. **(IV, C)**

10. Solomon MJ, Pager CK, Rex J, et al: Randomized, controlled trial of biofeedback with anal manometry, transanal ultrasound, or pelvic floor retraining with digital guidance alone in the treatment of mild to moderate fecal incontinence. Dis Colon Rectum 2003;46:703–710. **(Ib, A)**

11. Lunniss PJ, Gladman MA, Hetzer FH, et al: Risk factors in acquired faecal incontinence. J R Soc Med 2004;97:111–116. **(III, B)**

12. Hyman N: Incontinence after lateral internal sphincterotomy: a prospective study and quality of life assessment. Dis Colon Rectum 2004;47:35–38. **(III, B)**

13. Warshaw JS: Obstetric anal sphincter injury: incidence, risk factors, and repair. In Schoetz DJ (ed): Seminars in Colon and Rectal Surgery 2001. Philadelphia: Saunders, 2001;12:90–97. **(IV, C)**

14. Rao SSC: Pathophysiology of adult fecal incontinence. Gastroenterol 2004;126:S14–S22. **(IV, C)**

15. Bharucha AE: Outcome measures for fecal incontinence: anorectal structure and function. Gastroenterol 2004;126:S90–S98. **(IV, C)**

16. Diamant NE, Kamm MA, Wald A, et al: American Gastroenterological Association medical position statement on anorectal testing techniques. Gastroenterol 1999;116:732–760. **(IV, C)**

17. de Parades V, Etienney I, Thabut D, et al: Anal sphincter injury after forceps delivery: myth or reality? Dis Colon Rectum 2004;47:24–34. **(IIb, B)**

18. Mellgren A, Pollack J, Zetterstrom JP: Evaluation of anal incontinence. In Schoetz DJ (ed): Seminars in Colon and Rectal Surgery 2001. Philadelphia: Saunders, 2001;12:75–82. **(IV, C)**

19. Liberman H, Faria J, Ternent CA, et al: A prospective evaluation of the value of anorectal physiology in the management of fecal incontinence. Dis Colon Rectum 2001;44:1567–1574. **(IIb, B)**

20. Oberwalder M, Thaler K, Baig MK, et al: Anal ultrasound and endosonographic measurement of perineal body thickness: a new evaluation for fecal incontinence in females. Surg Endosc 2004; 18:650–654. **(III, B)**

21. Bollard RC, Gardiner A, Lindow S, et al: Normal female anal sphincter difficulties in interpretation explained. Dis Colon Rectum 2002; 45:171–175. **(III, B)**

22. Gold DM, Halligan S, Kmiot WA, et al: Intraobserver and interobserver agreement in anal endosonography. Br J Surg 1999;86:371–375. **(III, B)**

23. Gilliland R, Altomare DF, Moreira H, et al: Pudendal neuropathy is predictive of failure following anterior overlapping sphincteroplasty. Dis Colon Rectum 1998;41:1516–1522. **(III, B)**

24. Chen AS, Luchtefeld MA, Senagore AJ, et al: Pudendal nerve latency: does it predict outcome of anal sphincter repair? Dis Colon Rectum 1998;41:1005–1009. **(III, B)**

25. Ternent CA, Shashidharan M, Blatchford GJ, et al: Transanal ultrasound and anorectal physiology findings affecting continence after sphincteroplasty. Dis Colon Rectum 1997;40:462–467. **(III, B)**

26. Scarlett Y: Medical management of fecal incontinence. Gastroenterol. 2004;126:S55–S63. **(IV, C)**

27. Jensen LL, Lowry AC: Biofeedback improves functional outcome after sphincteroplasty. Dis Colon Rectum 1997;40;197–200. **(III, B)**

28. Norton C: Behavioral management of fecal incontinence in adults. Gastroenterol 2004;126:S64–S70. **(IV, C)**

29. Mahony R, Behan M, O'Herlihy C, et al: Randomized, clinical trial of bowel confinement vs. laxative use after primary repair of a third-degree obstetric anal sphincter tear. Dis Colon Rectum 2004;47:12–17. **(Ib, A)**

30. Rieger N: Surgical intervention for faecal incontinence in women: an update. Curr Opin Obstet Gynecol 2002;14:545–548. **(IV, C)**

31. Karoui S, Leroi AM, Koning E, et al: Results of sphincteroplasty in 86 patients with anal incontinence. Dis Colon Rectum 2000;43:813–820. **(III, B)**

32. Halverson AL, Hull TL: Long-term outcome of overlapping anal sphincter repair. Dis Colon Rectum 2002;45:345–348. **(III, B)**

33. Chapman AE, Geerdes B, Hewett P, et al: Systematic review of dynamic graciloplasty in the treatment of faecal incontinence. Br J Surg 2002;89:138–153. **(IV, C)**

34. Buie WD: Dynamic graciloplasty for fecal incontinence: the current status. In Schoetz DJ (ed): Seminars in Colon and Rectal Surgery 2001. Philadelphia: Saunders, 2001;12:108–114. **(IV, C)**

35. Wong WD, Congilosi SM, Spencer MP, et al: The safety and efficacy of the artificial bowel sphincter for fecal incontinence: results from a multi-center cohort study. Dis Colon Rectum 2002;45:1139–1153. **(III, B)**

36. Mundy L, Merlin TL, Maddern GJ, et al: Systematic review of safety and effectiveness of an artificial bowel sphincter for faecal incontinence. Br J Surg 2004;91:665–672. **(IV, C)**

37. Jarrett MED, Mowatt G, Glazener CMA, et al: Systematic review of sacral nerve stimulation for faecal incontinence and constipation. Br J Surg 2004;91:1559–1569. **(IV, C)**

38. Matzel KE, Stadelmaier U, Hohenberger W: Innovations in fecal incontinence: sacral nerve stimulation. Dis Colon Rectum 2004;47:1720–1728. **(IV, C)**

39. Takahashi T, Garcia-Osogobio S, Valdovinos MA, et al: Radio-frequency energy delivery to the anal canal for the treatment of fecal incontinence. Dis Colon Rectum 2002;45:915–922. **(III, B)**

40. Efron JE, Corman ML, Fleshman J, et al: Safety and effectiveness of temperature-controlled radio-frequency energy delivery to the anal canal (Secca procedure) for the treatment of fecal incontinence. Dis Colon Rectum 2003;46:1606–1616. **(III, B)**

## KEY POINTS

- Urinary incontinence is a common condition of epidemic proportions.
- History and physical examination, although a must, is not an accurate way to diagnose different types of urinary incontinence.
- Urodynamic testing is not a single test but rather a collection of various different tests that are done individually or more commonly in conjunction.
- The purpose of urodynamic testing is to objectively reproduce the patient's symptoms in a laboratory environment.

## HISTORY

History taking is at the center of all medical evaluations because it yields an appropriate diagnosis for most symptoms. Unfortunately the overlapping, nonspecific, and nonpathognomic nature of most urologic symptoms results in failure of the history to establish a correct diagnosis in a significant number of patients. It has been suggested that urologic history is only 60% accurate in establishing the correct diagnosis.[1] For example, urinary frequency and urgency are symptoms common to several different conditions, such as overactive bladder, interstitial cystitis, and urinary tract infections. Despite this shortcoming, every patient presenting with urogynecologic complaints must go through a complete history because it will guide the clinician in obtaining appropriate tests as well as help in diagnosing comorbid conditions such as diabetes insipidus. The history should include obstetric, gynecologic, medical (including review of systems and medications), surgical, and family histories (Table 28-1). It is helpful to have the patient fill out a complete medical and urogynecologic questionnaire before her consultation. This allows the patient to write down her chief complaint in her own words as well as giving her a chance to be more complete about her history. This approach allows clinicians to be more efficient and gather a larger amount of data.

Urinary incontinence is a prevalent condition, which may or may not affect a patient medically, socially, or psychologically. It is important to elucidate the most bothersome symptom during the interview process. It is important to note daytime and nighttime urinary frequency, urgency, the frequency and quantity of leakage, provoking factors, and factors that improve or worsen urine loss. It is imperative to understand which if any of these symptoms affect the patient's quality of life. This will be the guiding principle behind further investigations and treat-

ment. Table 28-2 gives examples of direct questions that might be helpful in assessing an incontinent patient.

### Voiding Diary

The voiding diary is an important part of the evaluation of urinary incontinence and could be considered the first urodynamic screening test (Fig. 28-1). The length of time a voiding diary is kept can vary significantly. A 1-week diary has been shown to be reliable in assessing urinary frequency, nocturia, and the number of incontinence episodes.[2] Ideally a patient fills out a complete diary for 1 to 2 typical days before her consultation, and the physician reviews this with her.

Urinary incontinence is often episodic and situational. It is most useful when the patient keeps the voiding diary on her most typical days (i.e., a work day, a day spent at home, and a day spent running errands). When a patient fails to complete the diary she should be given another opportunity to do so. The voiding diary can also be used to evaluate responses to treatment. During the initial visit, when the physician reviews the diary, he or she should obtain a subjective history on various voiding parameters. This is helpful in pointing out some of the subjective perceptions that are not confirmed with the diary. The voiding diary is not only a useful evaluation tool, but it can also be a very powerful treatment tool.

The voiding diary should include the following (Table 28-3):

- Type, amount, and times of fluid intake
- Time and amount of voids
- Leakage episodes
- Amount of leakage (e.g., mild, moderate, or severe)
- Events such as urgency or whether activities such as coughing or sneezing immediately precede the leakage episode

The following information should be gathered or calculated from the voiding diary:

- Average daily fluid intake and urine output
- Pattern of fluid intake (e.g., more during daytime or right before going to bed)
- Maximum and average functional bladder capacity
- Urinary frequency during daytime and after falling asleep (This should be compared with the information obtained during subjective history taking.)
- Number of leakage episodes per day and type of leakage (stress vs. urge)

The voiding diary may help the clinician to come up with a working diagnosis such as stress or urge incontinence. It may also provide more objective evidence for information obtained during history taking or may contradict the subjective history and indicate that the patient may have overestimated her

# Urogynecology

<table>
<tr><td colspan="2" align="center">**Table 28-1**<br>**Components of the Urogynecology-related History**</td></tr>
<tr><td>Obstetrical history</td><td>Number of deliveries, vaginal deliveries, birth weights, complications, including lacerations and episiotomies</td></tr>
<tr><td>Gynecologic history</td><td>Menstrual history, birth control, hormone replacement therapy, sexual history and sexually transmitted infections, results of previous Pap smears and mammograms, history of urinary tract infections</td></tr>
<tr><td>Surgical history</td><td>History of all surgical procedures and associated complications, including anesthetic complications; particular attention to pelvic surgeries and urologic surgeries and associated complications</td></tr>
<tr><td>Medical history</td><td>General medical history, with special attention to conditions that may affect urogynecologic disorder, including diabetes, neurologic conditions such as multiple sclerosis and Parkinson's disease, mental status, mobility status<br>All current medications with doses, medications that can affect urinary incontinence or lower urinary tract function, including: diuretics, beta agonists and antagonists, alpha agonists and antagonists, psychotropic medications such as antidepressants and antipsychotics<br>Current allergies</td></tr>
<tr><td>Social history</td><td>Alcohol, tobacco, and caffeine abuse</td></tr>
</table>

symptoms. The voiding diary may show that significant consumption of certain types of fluid, such as caffeinated drinks, carbonated beverages, and alcohol, coincides with the episode of urinary incontinence and/or frequency. It may establish a pattern of urine loss during certain times of the day, suggesting an associated factor, such as use of diuretics. The diary may suggest excessive fluid intake as a cofactor in urinary frequency and incontinence. Output greatly in excess of input, as indicated by the diary, is suggestive of diabetes insipidus.

The voiding diary can help guide treatment; that is, timed voiding, commonly used for the treatment of overactive bladder, requires the patient to void more frequently at the onset of treatment than her usual frequency. Usual frequency can be established based on her typical voiding pattern as recorded in her diary.

## Pad Test

The pad test is used for an objective quantification of urinary incontinence. Although its use is generally limited to research protocols, it can be used in a clinical setting in those patients in whom urinary incontinence cannot be demonstrated objectively during clinical examination or urodynamic testing. Various versions of pad tests, ranging from 20 minutes to 48 hours, have been described in the literature. The original 1-hour pad test was described by Sutherst and colleagues.[3] In this study the author demonstrated that a post-test pad weight increase of 1 g/hr or greater is considered abnormal. The International Continence Society has standardized the pad test (Fig. 28-2).[4] The pad test cannot help diagnose the type of urinary incontinence, but it may provide some estimation of the severity of urinary incontinence. Interested readers should read the review by Ryhammer and colleagues.[5]

<table>
<tr><td colspan="2" align="center">**Table 28-2**<br>**Assessment of an Incontinent Patient**</td></tr>
<tr><td>**Condition and/or Symptom**</td><td>**Helpful Questions**</td></tr>
<tr><td>Stress incontinence</td><td>Do you leak urine with strenuous activity such as coughing, sneezing, laughing, lifting, bending, pushing, pulling?<br>Do you leak with an empty or full bladder?<br>Do you leak with straining in the lying-down position?</td></tr>
<tr><td>Urinary urgency and urge incontinence</td><td>How frequently do you void during the daytime?<br>How frequently do you wake up to void after falling asleep?<br>Do you have a strong urge to void?<br>Can you make it to the bathroom with the strong urge to void?<br>Do you leak urine on your way to the bathroom?</td></tr>
<tr><td>Voiding difficulties and/or urine retention</td><td>After you empty your bladder, do you feel you emptied well?<br>Do you have any difficulty starting the stream?<br>Do you have any difficulty maintaining the stream?<br>Do you feel your stream is strong?<br>Do you have to push to void?<br>Do you have frequent bladder infections?</td></tr>
<tr><td>Severity of leakage</td><td>How often do you leak?<br>How much do you leak?<br>Do you use pads? How many pads do you go through in a typical day? How wet are these pads when you change them?</td></tr>
<tr><td>Painful bladder conditions and/or interstitial cystitis</td><td>Do you have any pain with a full bladder?<br>Does the pain get better after avoiding?<br>Do you have any suprapubic pain or pressure?<br>Do you have any urethral, vaginal, or perineal pain?<br>Do you have any pain with intercourse?<br>Do you feel a strong urge to void at once?<br>Do you void frequently during the day? After falling asleep?<br>Is there any pain or burning with urination?<br>Is there any blood in the urine?</td></tr>
<tr><td>Prolapse</td><td>Do you have any bulge or lump protruding from your vagina?<br>Do you have any pelvic pressure?<br>Do you have any difficulty voiding? Do you have any difficulty starting or maintaining the stream? Do you have postvoid fullness?<br>Do you have any difficulty emptying your bowels?<br>Do you have to push vaginally to evacuate your bowels?</td></tr>
<tr><td>Urinary tract infections and other urologic conditions</td><td>Do you have recurrent bladder infections?<br>Do you see blood in the urine?<br>Do you have a history of kidney or bladder stones?</td></tr>
<tr><td>Quality of life</td><td>Are bladder symptoms bothersome? Do they interfere with the quality of your life (e.g., not able to exercise or attend social functions)?<br>Do you have to know where all restrooms are when you go out?<br>Do you plan your day around your bladder?<br>Do you decline invitations to social functions due to concerns related to bladder control?<br>Have you declined certain jobs due to your bladder condition(s)?</td></tr>
</table>

## Frequency volume chart

| Frequency Volume Chart | | | |
|---|---|---|---|
| Day | Number | Time | Volume |
| Monday | 3 | 07:00<br>11:20<br>18:00 | 250<br>200<br>420 |
| Tuesday | 2 | 10:00<br>21:00 | 600<br>700 |
| Wednesday | 3 | 09:00<br>12:00<br>20:00 | 450<br>320<br>600 |
| Thursday | 4 | 07:20<br>11:00<br>16:00<br>21:00 | 400<br>350<br>410<br>350 |
| Friday | | | |
| Saturday | | | |

Date:_____  Name:_____

**Figure 28-1** **Typical voiding diary.** Note other information, such as amount and type of fluid intake, leakage episodes, activity, and/or urgency associated with the leakage episodes, which can also be included in such a diary. This is truly the first urodynamic test. (Courtesy of Medtronic Corporation, Minneapolis, Minn.)

| Table 28-3<br>Voiding Diary |
|---|
| Date |
| Time |
| Fluid |
| Amount intake (oz) |
| Amount voided (oz) |
| Leakage of urine (yes/no) |
| Urge preceded leak (yes/no) |
| Activity related to leak |

## PHYSICAL EXAMINATION

Physical examination, like the clinical history of the patient, is not always helpful in patients with urinary incontinence, but it may further guide the investigation and treatment. Hence, a focused physical examination is an integral part of any evaluation for urinary incontinence. The goals of physical examination should include evaluating patients for (1) future surgical candidacy, (2) physical changes due to previous pelvic and/or urinary tract surgeries, (3) the state of urethral and other pelvic organ

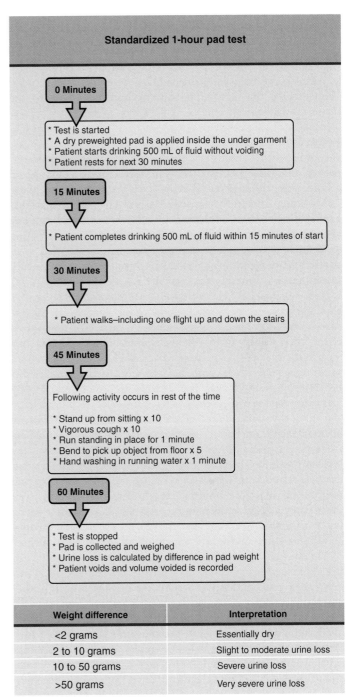

## Standardized 1-hour pad test

**0 Minutes**
* Test is started
* A dry preweighted pad is applied inside the under garment
* Patient starts drinking 500 mL of fluid without voiding
* Patient rests for next 30 minutes

**15 Minutes**
* Patient completes drinking 500 mL of fluid within 15 minutes of start

**30 Minutes**
* Patient walks–including one flight up and down the stairs

**45 Minutes**
Following activity occurs in rest of the time
* Stand up from sitting x 10
* Vigorous cough x 10
* Run standing in place for 1 minute
* Bend to pick up object from floor x 5
* Hand washing in running water x 1 minute

**60 Minutes**
* Test is stopped
* Pad is collected and weighed
* Urine loss is calculated by difference in pad weight
* Patient voids and volume voided is recorded

| Weight difference | Interpretation |
|---|---|
| <2 grams | Essentially dry |
| 2 to 10 grams | Slight to moderate urine loss |
| 10 to 50 grams | Severe urine loss |
| >50 grams | Very severe urine loss |

**Figure 28-2** **Standardized 1-hour pad test.** A figurative scheme based on the International Continence Society's recommendation for quantification of urine loss. (From Fifth Report on the Standardization of Terminology. Aachen, West Germany: International Continence Society, 1983.)

support structures, and (4) exclusion of neurologic and/or other pelvic pathologies as the cause for her urinary incontinence.

### Abdominal Examination

A general abdominal examination should be performed with attention to obesity and panus. Special attention should be devoted to previous surgical scars because they may provide important details that might not have surfaced during the interview process. The abdomen should also be inspected for incisional and inguinal hernias. The abdomen should be palpated in an attempt to reproduce any pain that the patient may have reported. Specific attention should be paid in palpation of the suprapubic area for pain, distended bladder, and midline masses. Percussion of the suprapubic area may aid in recognizing the distended bladder.

## Pelvic Examination

A complete gynecologic examination, including speculum examination, bimanual examination, and rectovaginal examination, should be performed on all incontinent patients. Gynecologic examination should begin with inspection of the external genitalia. The pelvic structures should be evaluated for any abnormality. Vaginal discharge, estrogen status, and excoriation of skin should be noted. On occasion vaginal discharge may mimic urinary incontinence. If no objective evidence for urinary incontinence is found in this patient, she should be treated for vaginal discharge. Signs suggestive of atrophic vaginitis, such as thin and friable vaginal mucosa and vulvar skin, loss of vaginal rugae, and urethral caruncle, indicate a hypoestrogenic state in the lower urinary tract. Although controversial, estrogen may have some role in the treatment of certain lower urinary tract symptoms. (This discussion is beyond the scope of this chapter, but the interested reader can review two meta-analyses by Cardozo et al[6] and Al-Badr.[7]) After a thorough examination of the vulva, the vagina should be inspected and examined. Vaginal atrophy should be noted. The anterior vaginal wall should be palpated for pain and masses. Painful urethra and bladder may suggest conditions such as urinary tract infection or interstitial cystitis. A suburethral mass with expression of pus from the urethra may suggest urethral or bladder diverticulum. The presence of a mass on the anterior vaginal wall necessitate ruling out carcinomas, Gartner's duct cyst, and other inflammatory conditions of the urethra.

Defects in pelvic organ support commonly coexist with urinary incontinence. Clinicians are expected to treat these two conditions concomitantly. Therefore, a complete examination evaluating all defects is mandatory. The choice of treatment for one condition will often guide the treatment for a coexisting condition. For example, a patient who seeks correction of prolapse via vaginal route may want to consider a vaginal procedure such as a suburethral sling to correct coexisting urodynamic stress urinary incontinence rather than an abdominal procedure such as the Burch procedure. The two halves of the vaginal speculum (Fig. 28-3) can be used sequentially to detect defects in the anterior compartment (cystocele, urethrocele), central compartment (uterine prolapse, enterocele, posthysterectomy vaginal vault prolapse), and posterior compartment (rectocele, enterocele). Prolapse is graded using a system as per personal preference. A complete speculum examination and a bimanual examination are also performed at this time, noting any vaginal scarring and/or reduction in vaginal length and/or calibration from previous surgical interventions. Any pelvic masses should be evaluated further.

## Neurologic Examination

Many neurologic conditions have a significant urologic manifestation. Neurologic conditions with significant urologic

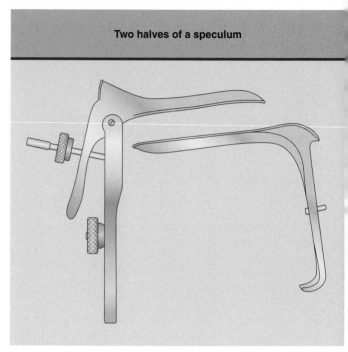

**Two halves of a speculum**

**Figure 28-3    The two halves of the speculum can be used to assess pelvic organ prolapses.** (Courtesy of Medtronic Corporation, Minneapolis, Minn.)

symptoms include multiple sclerosis, Parkinson's disease, stroke, dementia, brain tumors, and spinal cord injury of various types. The urologic manifestations of these various neurologic diseases vary depending on the location of the lesion but include urinary urgency, frequency due to detrusor hyperreflexia, and/or urinary retention due to detrusor hypoactivity. In general, lesions involving upper motor neurons cause detrusor hyperactivity (hyperreflexia) and lesions involving lower motor neurons cause hypoactive detrusor (acontractile detrusor).

Although most patients presenting with bladder symptomatology such as urinary urge incontinence and urine retention have no demonstrable nerve lesions (idiopathic), a small percentage of patients will present with urologic symptoms as their first sign of the neurologic disease. For example, 5%–10% of patients with multiple sclerosis present with urologic symptoms as their first signs of disease and up to 90% of MS patients will have urologic symptoms.[8,9] For this reason the clinician must be attuned to this possibility at all times. This requires the clinician evaluating incontinence to perform a focused neurologic examination, including evaluation of mental status and ensuring the integrity of motor, sensory, and reflex functions.

A mini-mental status examination can be performed (Table 28-4).[10] Alternatively, simple observation of the patient's orientation, speech, memory, level of consciousness, and comprehension may suffice to ensure adequate mental status.

Parasympathetic neurons originating from cord segments S2–S4 are the most important neurons involved in micturition (Fig. 28-4). There is also a significant contribution from sympathetic neurons originating from cord segments T10–L2. The rest of the neurologic examination is devoted to ensuring the integrity of these neurons. Sensory function can be evaluated with pinprick at the umbilicus (T10), labia majora (L1), labia minora (L1–L2), and all around the knee (L3–S2). Motor function can

## Table 28-4
## Mini-mental State Examination

| | Score | Points |
|---|---|---|
| **Orientation** | | |
| 1. What is the | | |
| Year? | _____ | 1 |
| Season? | _____ | 1 |
| Date? | _____ | 1 |
| Day? | _____ | 1 |
| Month? | _____ | 1 |
| 2. Where are we | | |
| State? | _____ | 1 |
| County? | _____ | 1 |
| Town/city? | _____ | 1 |
| Floor? | _____ | 1 |
| Address/name of building? | _____ | 1 |
| **Registration** | | |
| 3. Name three objects, taking one second to say each. Then ask the patient all three after you have said them. Repeat the answers until the patient learns all three. | _____ | 3 |
| **Attention and calculation** | | |
| 4. Serial sevens. Give one point for each correct answer. Stop after five answers. Alternative: Spell *world* backward. | _____ | 5 |
| **Recall** | | |
| 5. Ask for names of three objects learned in question 3. Give one point for each correct answer. | _____ | 3 |
| **Language** | | |
| 6. Point to a pencil and a watch. Have the patient name them as you point. | _____ | 2 |
| 7. Have the patient repeat "No ifs, ands, or buts." | _____ | 1 |
| 8. Have the patient follow a three-stage command: "Take the paper in your right hand. Fold the paper in half. Put the paper on the floor." | _____ | 3 |
| 9. Have the patient read and obey in the following: "Close your eyes." | _____ | 1 |
| 10. Have the patient write a sentence of his or her own choice. (The sentence should contain a subject and an object and should make sense. Ignore spelling errors when scoring.) | _____ | 1 |
| 11. Enlarge the design printed below to 1 to 5 cm per side and have the patient copy it. (Give one point if all the sides and angles are preserved and if the intersecting sides form a quadrangle.) | _____ | 1 |
| **Total** | _____ | 30 |

be evaluated with extension and flexion of the knee (L3–S1), hip (L2–L5), and ankle (L4–S1). Abduction and adduction of the ankle will also evaluate L4–S1 motor function.

Finally, testing several reflexes ensures reflex function integrity. Gently stroking the labia majora with a cotton-tipped swab and observing for contraction of the anal sphincter or pelvic floor tests for the bulbocavernosus reflex. Gently stroking the clitoris with a cotton-tipped swab and observing for the contraction of the anal sphincter or pelvic floor tests for the clitoral reflex. Presence of these two reflexes ensures the integrity of S2–S4. It should be noted that in some patients, especially in obese patients, these reflexes might be difficult to elicit; they might even be absent in some otherwise neurologically intact patients. Anal tone should also be evaluated at the time of pelvic examination. Deep tendon reflexes such as quadriceps (L3–L4), and Achilles (L5–S2) should also be evaluated. Presence of Babinski's sign will reflect an upper motor neuron lesion.

### Stress Test

As a part of a complete pelvic examination the patient is asked to perform a Valsalva maneuver or cough repetitively while leakage from the urethra is observed. Leakage that coincides with the straining is usually related to genuine stress incontinence, whereas the leakage that occurs a few seconds after the stress or persists after the stress event may be indicative of detrusor contraction. This test should be repeated after the patient has emptied her bladder, the so-called *empty supine stress test*. A positive empty supine stress test is a sensitive test for genuine stress incontinence.

### Marshall-Marchetti Test

Also known as a Bonney test, the Marshall-Marchetti test is frequently used to identify urinary leakage due to urethral hypermobility and to assess whether supporting the vesicourethral junction will prevent stress incontinence. The patient with a full bladder is asked to perform a Valsalva maneuver or cough repetitively and leakage from the urethra is observed. At this point the vesicourethral junction is supported in a high retropubic position with the examiner's index finger. The patient is asked to repeat the test and absence of leakage is considered evidence for the presence of urethral hypermobility. False-positive results may occur as a result of urethral occlusion from the examiner's fingers and render this test less sensitive and of limited use.[11]

### Q-tip Test

The Q-tip test is a very sensitive test, although nonspecific for the diagnosis of genuine stress incontinence. It is a simple, inexpensive test that may shed more light on possible pathophysiology of the patient's incontinence. While the patient is in a supine position, the urethra is prepareded with povidone-iodine solution and a well-lubricated cotton-tipped swab, preferably lubricated with lidocaine jelly, is inserted into the urethra. Once the swab is felt to be in the bladder, it is pulled back slowly until resistance is met at the vesicourethral junction. The resting angle is measured in relation to the horizontal axis (floor) using a goniometer (Fig. 28-5A). The patient is then asked to perform a Valsalva maneuver and/or cough repeatedly until maximum deflection of the swab is observed. The straining angle is then measured against the horizontal axis (Fig. 28-5B). Deflection greater than +30 degrees to the horizontal axis is considered abnormal and is called *urethral hypermobility*.

The normal resting angle is not well defined but is generally considered to be between –5 degrees and –30 degrees. Generally speaking the resting angle has little clinical significance except at the time of surgery, when it may be used to judge adequate fixation of the vesicourethral junction. During a retropubic operation such as a Burch urethropexy or bladder neck sling,

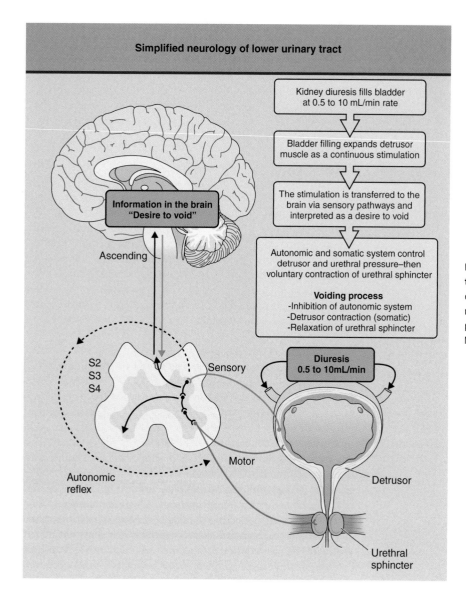

**Simplified neurology of lower urinary tract**

Kidney diuresis fills bladder at 0.5 to 10 mL/min rate

Bladder filling expands detrusor muscle as a continuous stimulation

The stimulation is transferred to the brain via sensory pathways and interpreted as a desire to void

Information in the brain "Desire to void"

Ascending

Autonomic and somatic system control detrusor and urethral pressure–then voluntary contraction of urethral sphincter

**Voiding process**
-Inhibition of autonomic system
-Detrusor contraction (somatic)
-Relaxation of urethral sphincter

**Diuresis**
0.5 to 10mL/min

S2
S3
S4

Sensory

Motor

Autonomic reflex

Detrusor

Urethral sphincter

**Figure 28-4    Simplified neurology of lower urinary tract.** Please note parasympathetic neurons originating from sacral cord segments S2–S4 are the most important neurons involved in the micturition process. (Courtesy of Medtronic Corporation, Minneapolis, Minn.)

this author routinely uses the Q-tip to fix the resting angle at 0 to –5 degrees.

As stated earlier, urethral hypermobility is not diagnostic of genuine stress incontinence but is suggestive of it.[12] Although most patients with genuine stress incontinence will have urethral hypermobility, not all with urethral hypermobility have genuine stress incontinence. Patients who demonstrate a negative Q-tip test (i.e., no urethral hypermobility) and have symptoms of stress incontinence will need a further workup to define the pathology responsible for their incontinence.[12] Many of these patients may have intrinsic urethral sphincter dysfunction and procedures such as the Burch urethropexy will have a high failure rate.

### Postvoid Residual Check

Postvoid residual check is an important part of all pelvic examinations performed in an incontinent patient. There is no universally accepted value that is considered abnormal.[13] Values ranging from 50 mL to more than 300 mL have been suggested as a clinically significant postvoid residual.[13] Postvoid residual,

including measurement, should be performed on multiple occasions. If a high value is obtained on a consistent basis, it should be viewed in context of voided volume and the potential symptomatology that the patient may have as a result of a high residual volume. For example, if two patients who voided 200 mL and 600 mL, respectively, both had residual urine measuring 150 mL, it might be considered more abnormal for the patient who only voided 200 mL. This concept is similar to the concept of ejection fraction for the heart and is based on the contractile efficiency of the bladder. We can further consider that the patient who voided 200 mL with 150 mL of residual may have symptoms such as urinary frequency and/or recurrent bladder infections. These symptoms may arise from the abnormal residual urine; their presence or absence may guide us further in deciding whether the high residual urine is clinically significant. Symptoms can guide the clinician to be more aggressive with treatment or be conservative with observation only. It is important to note that in some patients high residual urine volume could be the sole reason for incontinence in the form of overflow incontinence.

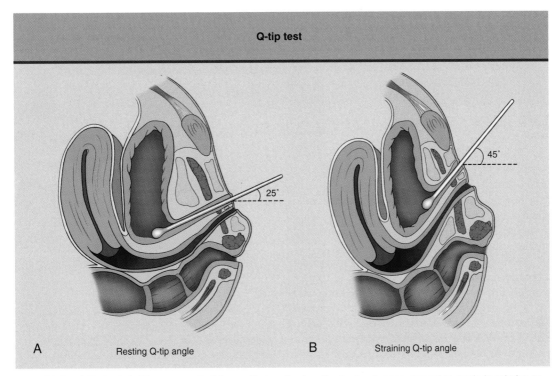

**Figure 28-5    Q-tip test.** A, Measurement of the resting urethral angle. Angle of measurement is made in relation to the horizontal axis (floor) using a goniometer. B, Measurement of the straining urethral angle. Angle greater than or equal to +30 degrees to the horizontal axis is considered abnormal and is termed urethral hypermobility. (Courtesy of Medtronic Corporation, Minneapolis, Minn.)

Many methods can be utilized to measure the postvoid residual volume. It can be estimated crudely with bimanual examination. Although it carries a small risk of urinary tract infection, transurethral catheterization is the most common method employed clinically for the accurate measurement of residual urine. Ultrasound scanning is becoming a more popular, noninvasive way to accurately and quickly measure the residual urine.[14] Residual urine can also be measured radiographically using contrast media.

## Other Laboratory Tests
### Urinalysis and Urine Culture
Urinary tract infection can mimic many bladder symptoms, particularly urinary incontinence. For this reason any patient with urinary incontinence or worsening of previously stable urinary incontinence should first have a urinalysis with or without urine culture before any extensive workup or invasive treatments. This should be viewed just as critical as getting an electrocardiogram (EKG) in a patient with complaints of chest pain. Patients with microscopic hematuria may need further workup, including urine cytology, intravenous pyelogram, and urethrocystoscopy.

## URODYNAMIC TESTING

Urodynamic testing is not a single test but rather a group of various tests that can be performed individually or in various combinations. In its simplest form it can involve insertion of a simple catheter with a measuring device; in its complex form it may involve sophisticated computerized electronics with special catheters. The purpose of urodynamic testing is to help clinicians objectively understand the function of the lower urinary tract. It objectively confirms the suspected diagnosis based on historical information about the patient in a laboratory setting. The test must be performed by, or in the presence of, the interpreter so that an accurate interpretation of data can be made as it is being collected, unlike an EKG.

The use of urodynamic testing is controversial, with more areas of disagreement than agreement. With the introduction of midurethral slings for genuine stress incontinence, the controversy surrounding urodynamic testing seems to be heating up once again. Rationalization regarding urodynamic testing remains of interest.[15] Traditional reasons for not doing urodynamic testing include complex equipment, special training, cost, patient discomfort, and a chance of lower urinary tract infection. However, most importantly, as stated by Dr. Blaivas, there will be little argument on the conclusion of many studies that suggests "neither symptoms nor response to treatment correlate very well with the specific urodynamic diagnosis."[15] Supporters of urodynamic testing have stated many benefits, including more precise diagnosis, more objective information on an otherwise very subjective clinical history of a urinary incontinent patient, and possible medicolegal issues. Despite the controversy there is little disagreement that certain groups of patients would clearly benefit from urodynamic testing. These groups of patients are listed in Table 28-5.

A closer look with specific examples gives the real flavor of this important controversy. One group of patients with lower

| Table 28-5 |
| Patients who Require Urodynamic Testing |
| · History of previous anti-incontinence surgery |
| · Mixed symptoms |
| · Failed conservative therapy after simple evaluation |
| · Patients with voiding difficulties |
| · Urine retention |
| · Surgical candidates |

urinary tract symptomatology who are not uncommonly treated empirically without urodynamic testing is patients with symptoms of overactive bladder. Overactive bladder is a collection of symptoms, including urinary frequency, urinary urgency, and/or urinary urge incontinence.[16,17] A study at a large tertiary care urogynecology center involving 4500 patients with lower urinary tract symptoms who underwent urodynamic testing showed that almost 50% of the patients with overactive bladder symptoms have no urodynamic evidence of detrusor instability. These findings suggest that it would be medically inappropriate to treat these women's symptoms if there are no objective urodynamic abnormalities. However, further evaluation of these patients results in the detection of detrusor instability by other means.[18] A second example is that of a group of patients who have cough-induced detrusor instability. One of the important reasons for performing urodynamic testing in patients with symptoms of stress urinary incontinence is to rule out cough-induced detrusor instability, which may mimic genuine stress incontinence. Treating these patients surgically can significantly worsen their condition. Less than 5% of women with symptoms of stress urinary incontinence will have cough-induced detrusor instability.

## Urodynamic Terminology
The following are commonly used terms in urodynamic testing.

### Urodynamic Setup
#### Position
The patient is generally sitting or standing (Fig. 28-6). Simple office cystometry can more easily be accomplished in a supine or lithotomy position. Changing to a more upright position is considered to be a provocative measure for the bladder and should be performed if the patient's symptoms are not reproduced.

#### Catheters
The catheters used during the test will be based on investigator's preference, experience, other equipment being used, and cost. Catheters can vary from a simple Foley catheter used for simple office cystometry to a more complex catheter containing an electronic transducer, which could be water filled or air filled (Fig. 28-7).

#### Filling Media
Various filling media can be utilized for the test. Most commonly water or physiologic saline are used. Carbon dioxide has been used as well (Fig. 28-8). The filling media is generally at room

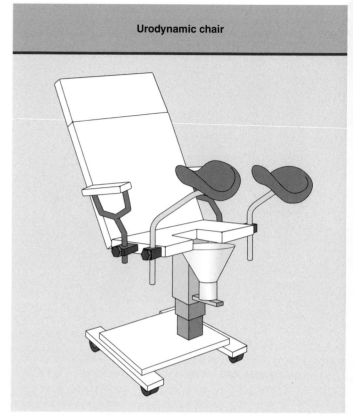

**Urodynamic chair**

**Figure 28-6** Urodynamic chair adjusted for sitting position. (Courtesy of Medtronic Corporation, Minneapolis, Minn.)

temperature or body temperature. Cold solution can be utilized as a provocative measure.

#### Filling Rate
The rate can vary. The International Continence Society has attempted to standardize this by defining a slow filling rate to be less than 10 mL/min, a medium filling rate to be between 10 mL and 100 mL/min, and a fast filling rate to be greater than 100 mL/min.[19]

### Urodynamic Measurements
Three principle pressures are simultaneously measured during the multichannel urodynamic testing: bladder, urethral, and abdominal. Single-channel urodynamic testing measures either the bladder or the urethral pressure at a time. They are depicted in the following fashion:

- **Pves**—Vesical pressure (Fig. 28-9), directly measured by a catheter in the bladder, it is a summation of pressures produced by the detrusor muscle and external pressures (i.e., abdominal) on the detrusor.
- **Pabd**—Abdominal pressure, measured by a catheter in the vagina or rectum, approximates the value of external pressures on the detrusor at rest before bladder filling. Its value should be approximately equal to Pves.
- **Pura**—Urethral pressure, directly measured by a catheter in the urethra, it is a summation of pressures produced by the urethral sphincter muscle and bladder pressures.

## Water-filled catheter set

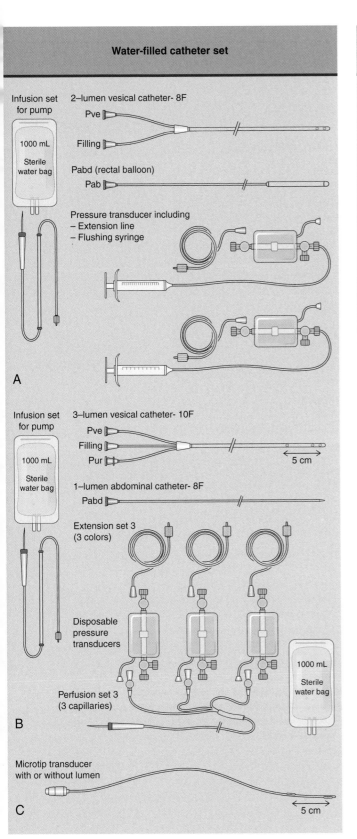

Figure 28-7 **Catheter sets.** *A,* Water-filled catheter set; note the vesicle catheter depicted has only one port for pressure measurement. *B,* Water-filled catheter set; note the vesicle catheter depicted has two ports for pressure measurement. *C,* Microtip catheter; note that a double-tip catheter is depicted. (Courtesy of Medtronic Corporation, Minneapolis, Minn.)

## Various filling media and various methods of filling bladder

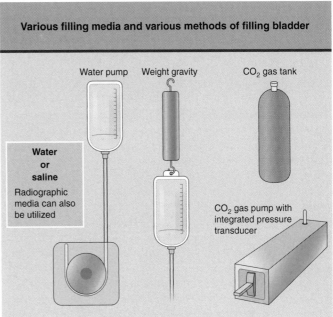

Figure 28-8 **Various filling media and various methods of filling.** The bladder can be filled utilizing gravity and a mechanical pump as shown. (Courtesy of Medtronic Corporation, Minneapolis, Minn.)

Because the sphincteric activity along the length of the urethra is not equal, the pressure measurement made along the length will vary based on the location of measurement. The urethral pressure profile (UPP) is the graph or curve created by passing the catheter and measuring pressures along the length of the urethra (Fig. 28-10).

- **Pdet**—Detrusor pressure is a measurement calculated by the following formula:

Detrusor pressure = bladder pressure − abdominal pressure

$$Pdet = Pves - Pabd$$

- **Pucp**—Urethral closure pressure is a measurement calculated by the following formula:

Urethral closure pressure = urethral pressure − bladder pressure

$$Pucp = Pura - Pves$$

Urodynamic testing evaluates the function of the bladder and urethra during two phases: storage (filling phase) and voiding. The maximum cystometric capacity is when a patient can no longer delay micturition. Functional bladder capacity is assessed from the voiding diary. VLPP (Valsalva leak point pressure) is the minimal Pves observed to cause leakage during the Valsalva maneuver in the absence of detrusor contraction. VLPP of less than 60 cm indicates severe stress incontinence and is defined as ISD (intrinsic urethral sphincter dysfunction). VLPP of 60 to 90 cm is considered to indicate moderate stress incontinence; 90 cm or greater is considered mild stress incontinence. DLPP (detrusor leak point pressure) is the true detrusor pressure that causes leakage in the absence of provocative maneuvers.

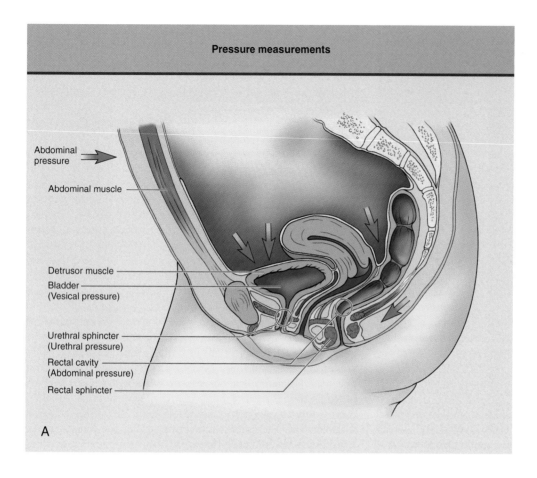

**Pressure measurements**

Abdominal pressure

Abdominal muscle

Detrusor muscle

Bladder (Vesical pressure)

Urethral sphincter (Urethral pressure)

Rectal cavity (Abdominal pressure)

Rectal sphincter

A

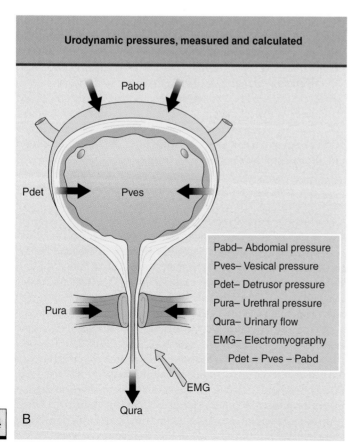

**Urodynamic pressures, measured and calculated**

Pabd

Pdet          Pves

Pura

EMG

Qura

B

Pabd– Abdomial pressure

Pves– Vesical pressure

Pdet– Detrusor pressure

Pura– Urethral pressure

Qura– Urinary flow

EMG– Electromyography

$P_{det} = P_{ves} - P_{abd}$

**Figure 28-9** **Various pressure measurements that could be made or calculated during multichannel urodynamic testing.** *A,* Measured. *B,* Measured and calculated. (Courtesy of Medtronic Corporation, Minneapolis, Minn.)

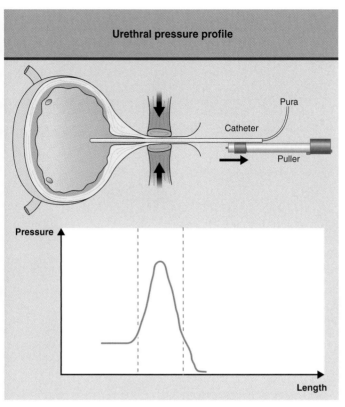

**Urethral pressure profile**

Figure 28-10  The urethral pressure profile (UPP) is the graph or curve created by passing the catheter and measuring the pressures along the length of urethra. (Courtesy of Medtronic Corporation, Minneapolis, Minn.)

### Urodynamic Sensations

The following observations could be made during the filling phase by asking patients about their sensation. The *first sensation* or first desire to void is when the patient is aware that the bladder is filling and she could void. Volume is usually equal to 150 to 250 mL (Fig. 28-11). *First urge* or normal desire to void is when patient will pass urine at the next convenient moment and could delay if she needed to. Volume is usually equal to 300 to 400 mL. *Strong desire to void* is a persistent desire to void without the fear of leakage. Volume is usually equal to 400 to 600 mL. *Urgency* is a strong desire to void with fear of leakage. Volume is usually greater than 600 mL. *Ambulatory cystometry* involves measurement of abdominal and bladder pressure during natural filling of the bladder over the course of several hours in an ambulatory format.

### Urodynamic Diagnosis

*Compliance* is the bladder volume change per detrusor pressure change (mL/cm H$_2$O). In a normal bladder capacity of 400 to 500 mL, a rise in detrusor pressure of 15 cm H$_2$O or less is considered to be normal. Decreased bladder compliance is

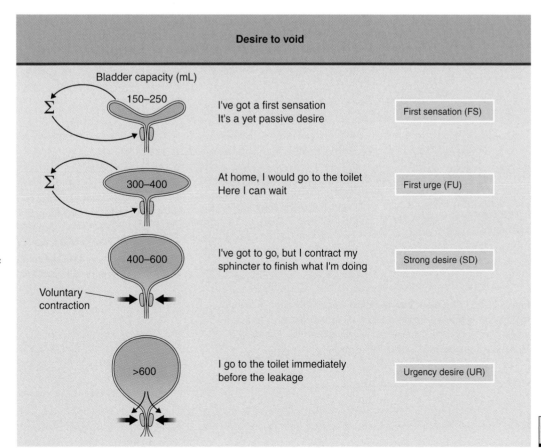

Figure 28-11  First sensation, first urge, strong desire, and urgency are the observations made during the filling phase by asking patients about their sensation. (Courtesy of Medtronic Corporation, Minneapolis, Minn.)

# Urogynecology

diagnosed when pressure rise at normal capacity exceeds 15 cm $H_2O$ (Figs. 28-12 through 28-14).

*Detrusor instability* is a urodynamic diagnosis. It is defined as the presence of spontaneous or provoked involuntary contraction during bladder filling in a patient with appropriate signs and symptoms. It is considered to be idiopathic in etiology (Fig. 28-15).

*Detrusor hyperreflexia* is the term used when there is a neurologic condition, such as multiple sclerosis, in a patient with spontaneous or provoked involuntary contraction during bladder filling, as well as appropriate signs and symptoms of the condition. Its etiology is considered to be an upper motor neuron disease (Fig. 28-16).

*Detrusor sphincter dyssynergia* is defined as lack of urethral relaxation with the bladder contraction. This could be a learned or conditioned response or may reflect upper motor neuron disease (Fig. 28-17).

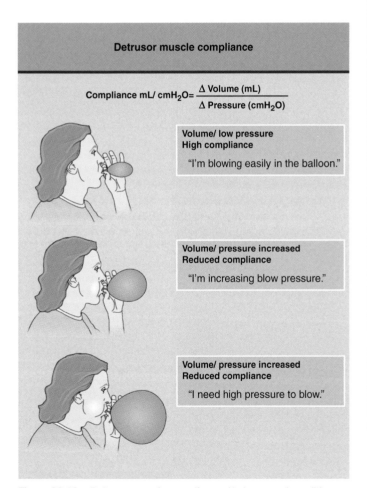

**Detrusor muscle compliance**

$$\text{Compliance mL/ cmH}_2\text{O} = \frac{\Delta \text{ Volume (mL)}}{\Delta \text{ Pressure (cmH}_2\text{O)}}$$

**Volume/ low pressure**
**High compliance**

"I'm blowing easily in the balloon."

**Volume/ pressure increased**
**Reduced compliance**

"I'm increasing blow pressure."

**Volume/ pressure increased**
**Reduced compliance**

"I need high pressure to blow."

**Figure 28-12    Detrusor muscle compliance.** Under normal condition, the bladder is a very compliant organ. A large volume change in the bladder results in a minimal rise in detrusor pressure. (Courtesy of Medtronic Corporation, Minneapolis, Minn.)

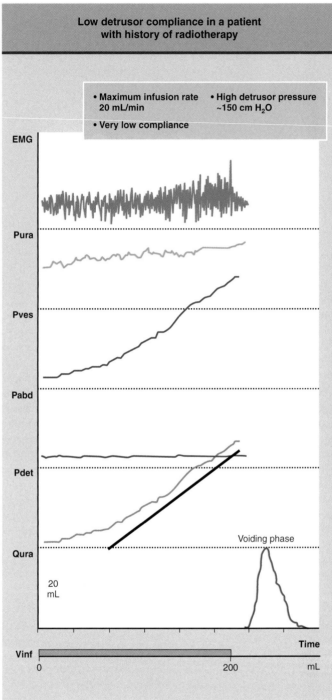

**Figure 28-13    Low detrusor compliance in a patient with a history of radiotherapy.** (Courtesy of Medtronic Corporation, Minneapolis, Minn.)

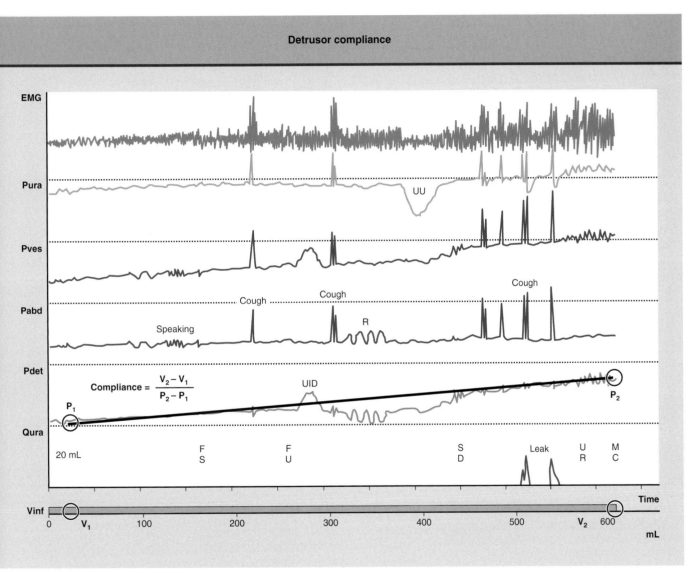

**Figure 28-14   Detrusor compliance.** Note the gradual rise in detrusor pressure. (Courtesy of Medtronic Corporation, Minneapolis, Minn.)

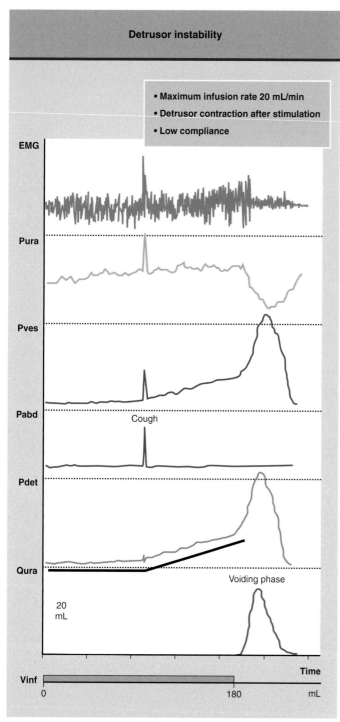

**Detrusor instability**

- Maximum infusion rate 20 mL/min
- Detrusor contraction after stimulation
- Low compliance

**Figure 28-15    Detrusor instability (DI).** Note the provoked involuntary detrusor contraction and urethral relaxation, leading to leakage. (Courtesy of Medtronic Corporation, Minneapolis, Minn.)

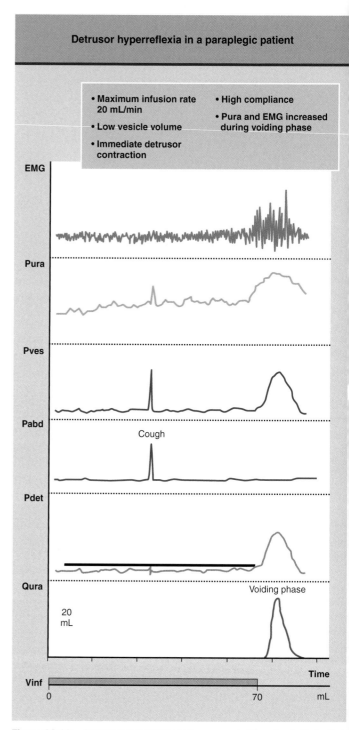

**Detrusor hyperreflexia in a paraplegic patient**

- Maximum infusion rate 20 mL/min
- Low vesicle volume
- Immediate detrusor contraction
- High compliance
- Pura and EMG increased during voiding phase

**Figure 28-16    Detrusor hyperreflexia in a paraplegic patient.** Note that the urethra remains closed during the detrusor contraction (consistent with detrusor sphincter dyssynergia). (Courtesy of Medtronic Corporation, Minneapolis, Minn.)

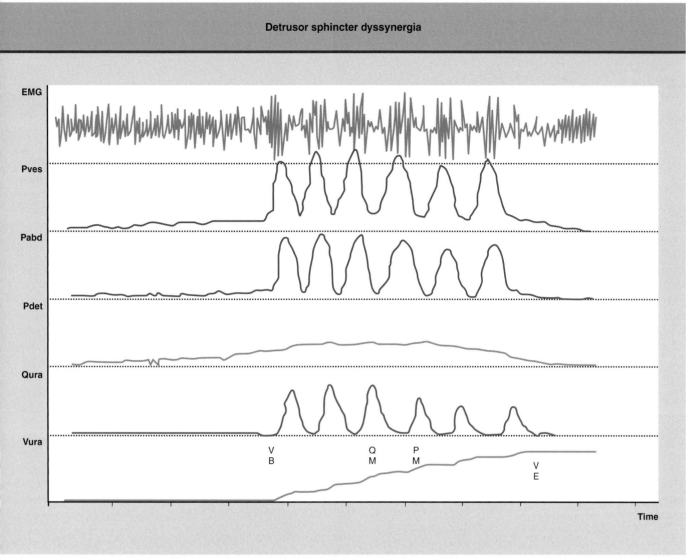

**Figure 28-17    Detrusor sphincter dyssynergia.** Note the electromyographic activity does not diminish and the urethra does not relax during the void. (Courtesy of Medtronic Corporation, Minneapolis, Minn.)

## Types of Urodynamic Tests

*"Poor man's"* or *bedside urethrocystometry* is performed with simple office equipment such as a Foley catheter and sterile water or saline (Fig. 28-18). In patients with an uncomplicated incontinence history, this test might be all that is necessary. It requires simple equipment readily available in most offices: a catheter, 60-mL syringe, graduated cylinder, and sterile saline solution. This test can be easily performed in supine lithotomy position using gynecologic stirrups. After a spontaneous void, the patient's urethra is cleansed with povidone-iodine solution and a postvoid residual is obtained and measured with a catheter. An empty supine stress test is performed at this point; if positive, the patient may need more sophisticated multichannel urodynamic testing to rule out the presence of intrinsic urethral sphincter dysfunction.[20] If negative, a 60-mL syringe without the bulb or plunger is connected to the catheter. The syringe is held at a level slightly higher than the bladder and is filled with

sterile saline solution to the 60-mL mark while pinching the catheter. Saline is then introduced into the bladder via gravity. The patient is asked to report the first sensation, first urge, and strong urge. Any rise in the meniscus during the filling is considered to be a sign of detrusor instability (the volume is noted at this point). If no change in meniscus is seen at a strong urge, the catheter is removed and a stress test is performed. Any leakage from the urethra concomitant with the stress event is considered to be positive for genuine stress incontinence. After the stress test is completed satisfactorily, a catheter can be reintroduced and more saline introduced until the maximum cystometric capacity is achieved. If no sign of detrusor instability is seen, provocative measures such as running water should also be carried out.

*Single-channel urethrocystometry* involves the measurement of urethral or bladder pressure only (Fig. 28-19). A single-channel cystometry test is performed in a fashion similar to

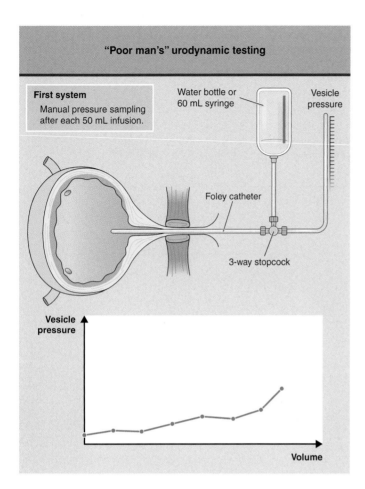

**Figure 28-18** *"Poor man's" urodynamic testing.* Note that a bladder compliance curve can be drawn by making volume and pressure measurements during each syringe fill. (Courtesy of Medtronic Corporation, Minneapolis, Minn.)

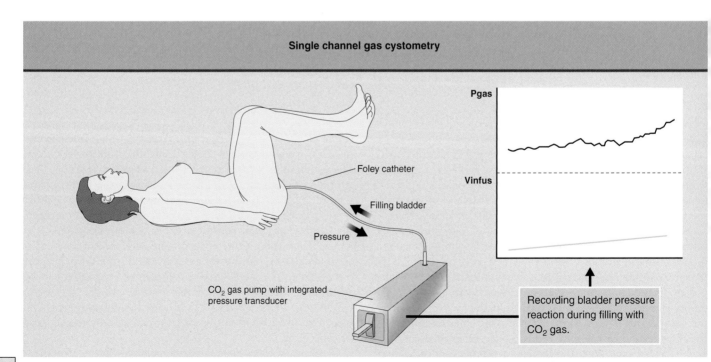

**Figure 28-19** **Single-channel cystometry shown with carbon dioxide as a filling media.** (Courtesy of Medtronic Corporation, Minneapolis, Minn.)

bedside testing with the exception that the pressure and volume measurement are made electronically. A catheter with a single pressure measuring port (see Fig. 28-7) is used to fill the bladder with saline solution or water. Various sensations are noted, as reported by the patient. An abnormal rise in bladder pressure (>15 cm H$_2$O at normal capacity) or involuntary contractions are noted along with the patient's sensation at the time. Because abdominal pressure (external pressure on detrusor) is not measured in single-channel cystometry, any rise seen in the pressure cannot be directly attributed to the detrusor muscle. This is the limiting factor of single-channel cystometry.

At bladder capacity the same catheter could be moved along the length of the urethra, either manually or by a mechanical pulley, to obtain a resting UPP. Dynamic UPP can be obtained in a similar fashion while the patient is performing various activities such as coughing or the Valsalva maneuver. Any leakage observed in the absence of a rise in bladder pressure can be diagnosed as

urodynamic stress incontinence. Leakage with a sustained rise in bladder pressure after the cough or Valsalva event may represent induced detrusor instability and require multichannel testing to confirm it.

Finally, voiding pressure studies can also be performed with single-channel testing. Because the urethral and bladder pressures cannot be measured simultaneously, it may be of limited use. Furthermore, if the bladder pressure is monitored during the test one cannot differentiate between Valsalva and/or detrusor effort during voiding.

Aside from cystometry, uroflowmetry is considered the next most important component of the multichannel testing. The patient is asked to come to the laboratory with a full bladder. As the name implies, uroflowmetry is the measurement of voided volume as a function of time (Fig. 28-20). Several measurements can be made from the uroflow including the time to initiate void, maximum and average flow rates, the time to maximum

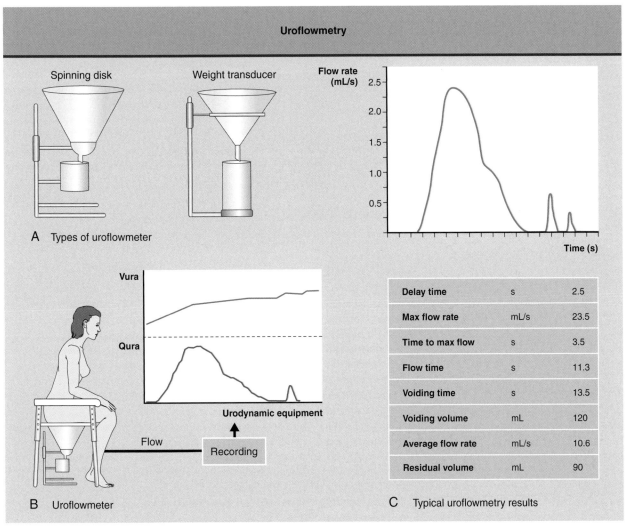

| Delay time | s | 2.5 |
|---|---|---|
| Max flow rate | mL/s | 23.5 |
| Time to max flow | s | 3.5 |
| Flow time | s | 11.3 |
| Voiding time | s | 13.5 |
| Voiding volume | mL | 120 |
| Average flow rate | mL/s | 10.6 |
| Residual volume | mL | 90 |

**Figure 28-20** **Uroflowmetry.** *A,* Types of uroflowmeter. *B,* Simple uroflowmetry: the measurement of voided volume as a function of time. *C,* Typical uroflowmetry results. (Courtesy of Medtronic Corporation, Minneapolis, Minn.)

flow rate, voided volume, the total time for void, and the pattern of uroflow curve (Fig. 28-21). It is useful to remember the rule of 20s for normal uroflow parameters in female patients. A normal uroflow curve is singleton and bell-shaped. For normal parameters the patient must void at least 200 mL of urine over 20 seconds or less, with a maximum flow rate of at least 20 mL/sec. The uroflow pattern, although not diagnostic, may provide useful information (Fig. 28-22). A pattern with a high peak, indicating very high maximum flow rate, may suggest weak urethral closure pressures, intrinsic urethral sphincter dysfunction, or hypertonic detrusor contraction. Stop-and-go (intermittent) patterns may suggest detrusor sphincter dyssynergia, bladder outlet obstruction from advanced prolapse, or Valsalva void. A pattern that is prolonged with a slow maximum flow rate may suggest hypotonic detrusor or increased urethral resistance due to partial obstruction from advanced prolapse or other causes. If the patient has abnormal uroflow parameters, she will need further studies such as the voiding pressure study, urethrocystometry, or an imaging study such as a voiding cystourethrogram to diagnose the etiology for the observed abnormality. This is particularly important in any patient who might be a surgical candidate.

Next the dual-sensor catheter is placed in the bladder, and the single-sensor catheter is placed in the vagina or rectum, electromyogram (EMG) patches and leads are placed and connected, and finally the bladder catheter is connected to a water source before beginning the next step of testing (i.e., cystometry).

*Multichannel urethrocystometry* involves the simultaneous measurement of abdominal, urethral, and bladder pressures (Fig. 28-23). Cystometry is considered to be the soul of urodynamic testing. It evaluates the pressure/volume relationship (i.e., compliance of bladder during the filling/storage phase). The sole purpose of this test is to reproduce the patient's symptoms of incontinence in the laboratory setting. Assessment of first sensation, first urge, bladder capacity, bladder compliance, involuntary detrusor activity, and urethral stability can be made. Cystometry involves placement of two catheters, a dual-sensor catheter (Fig. 28-24; see also Fig. 28-7) in the bladder and urethra to measure their respective pressures and a single-sensor catheter in either the vagina or rectum to measure abdominal pressure (one must be aware of the artifacts this may cause. Figure 28-25 shows an example of rectal artifact). In the presence of moderate to large prolapse the rectum is used to measure the abdominal pressure; in the absence of significant prolapse the vagina is used to measure the abdominal pressure. Detrusor and urethral pressures are electronically calculated and depicted in real time on the cystometrogram. During the test the bladder catheter is also used to infuse water or physiologic saline at room or body temperature in the bladder. Various

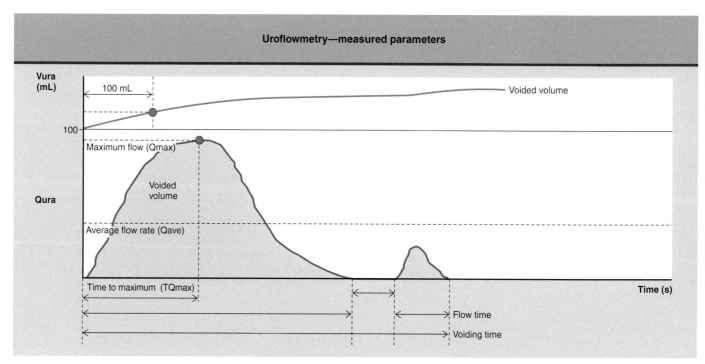

**Figure 28-21   Typical uroflowmetry curve, depicting various measured parameters.** (Courtesy of Medtronic Corporation, Minneapolis, Minn.)

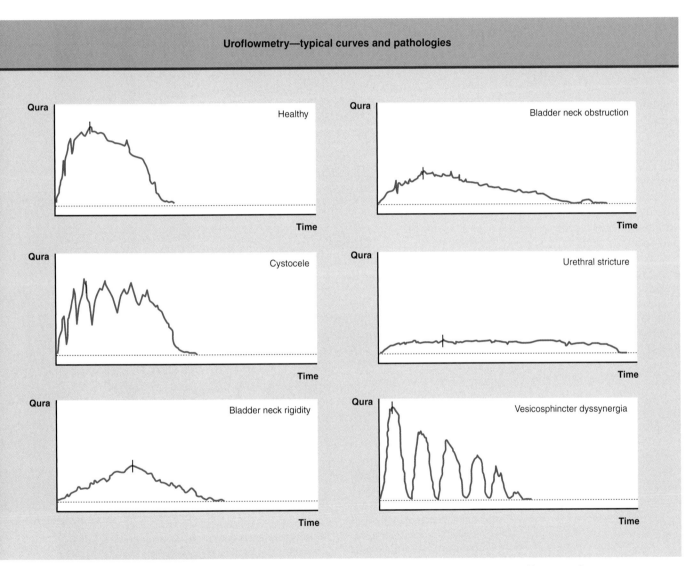

**Figure 28-22  Typical uroflowmetry curves.** Normal curve and curves in various pathologic states. (Courtesy of Medtronic Corporation, Minneapolis, Minn.)

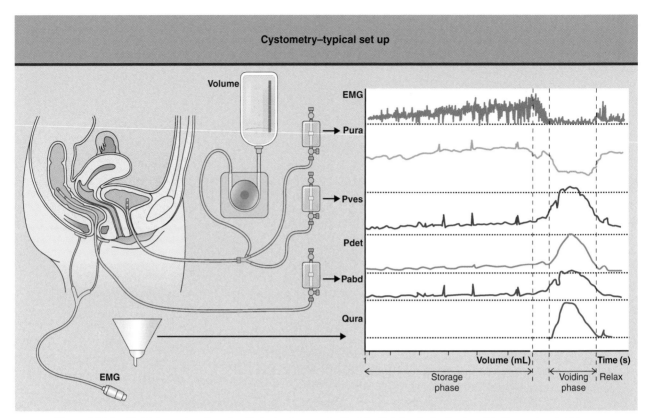

**Figure 28-23    Multichannel cystometry.** Typical set-up—note that the Pabd catheter is placed in the rectum in this case. (Courtesy of Medtronic Corporation, Minneapolis, Minn.)

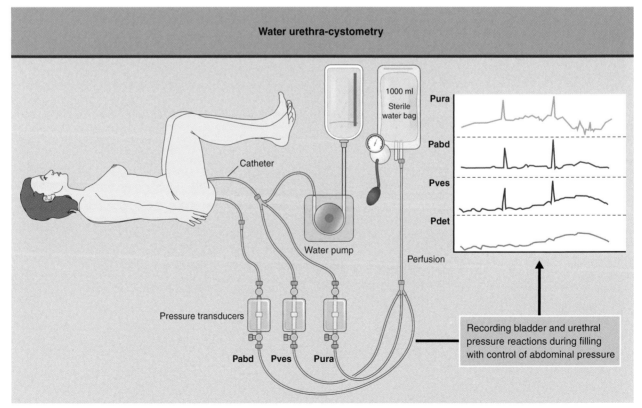

**Figure 28-24    Multichannel cystometry in a female patient in supine position with water as a filling media.** Note that the Pabd catheter is placed in the rectum and there is no EMG activity being measured in this case. (Courtesy of Medtronic Corporation, Minneapolis, Minn.)

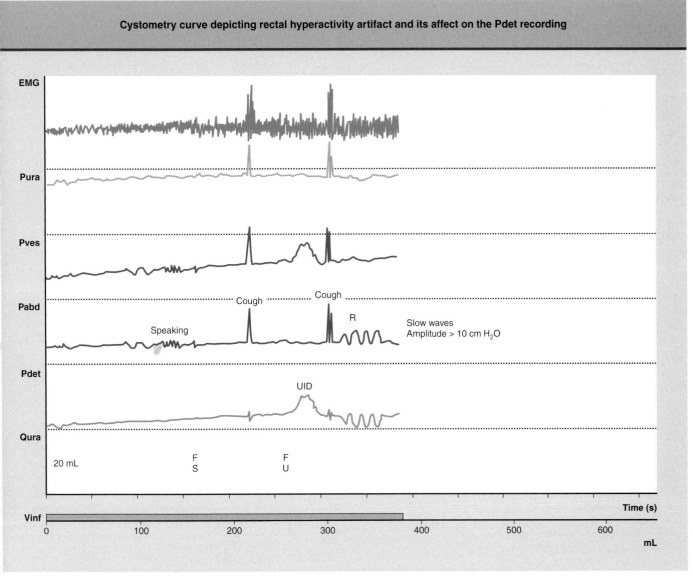

**Figure 28-25    Multichannel cystometry curve depicting rectal hyperactivity artifact and its affect on the Pdet recording.** Also note the normal reflex rise in EMG activity with increased bladder filling. (Courtesy of Medtronic Corporation, Minneapolis, Minn.)

sensations (Figs. 28-26 through 28-29) are noted as reported by the patient. Any abnormal rise in bladder pressure (>15 cm $H_2O$ at normal capacity) or involuntary contractions or involuntary urethral relaxation is noted along with the patient's sensation at the time (Figs. 28-30 and 28-31). If an involuntary contraction has not been shown during the course of the test, provocative measures such as coughing, change in position from sitting to standing, running water, or washing hands in cold water should be performed to increase the diagnostic yield of the test and to reproduce the patient's symptoms in an objective fashion.

This test is considered diagnostic only when observations made during the test correlate with the patient's symptomatology. Any observation made in the absence of proper symptoms or symptoms without urodynamic observation may represent a test artifact; or there might be another etiology behind the symptoms. In this instance the test is not diagnostic and could be considered inconclusive or unhelpful.

*Text continues on p. 401.*

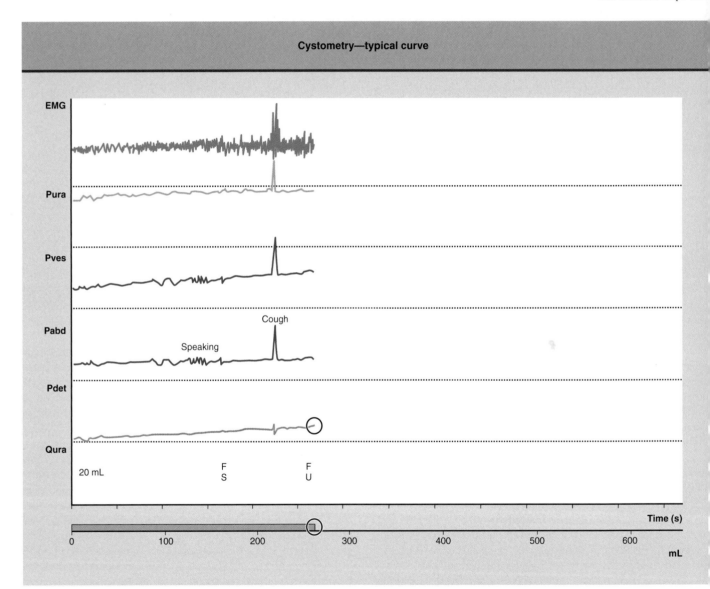

**Figure 28-26    Multichannel cystometry curve depicting first sensation and first urge.** Note the speaking and cough artifacts. (Courtesy of Medtronic Corporation, Minneapolis, Minn.)

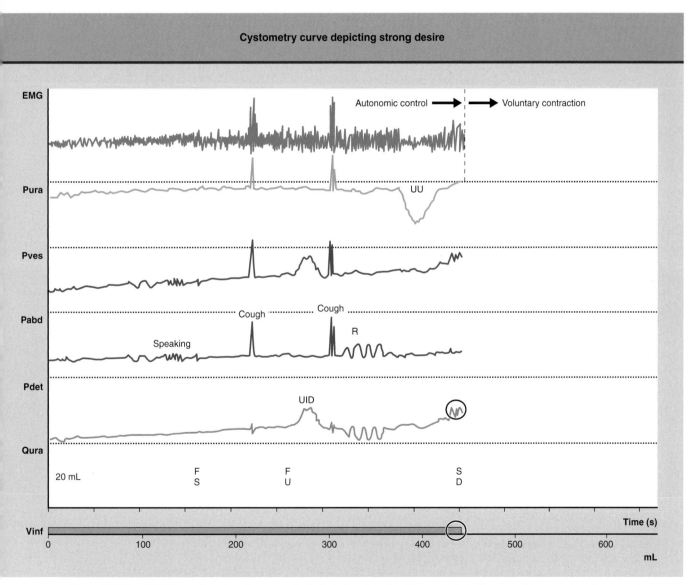

**Figure 28-27    Multichannel cystometry curve depicting strong desire.** Shown again is the normal increase in reflex EMG activity with increased bladder filling. (Courtesy of Medtronic Corporation, Minneapolis, Minn.)

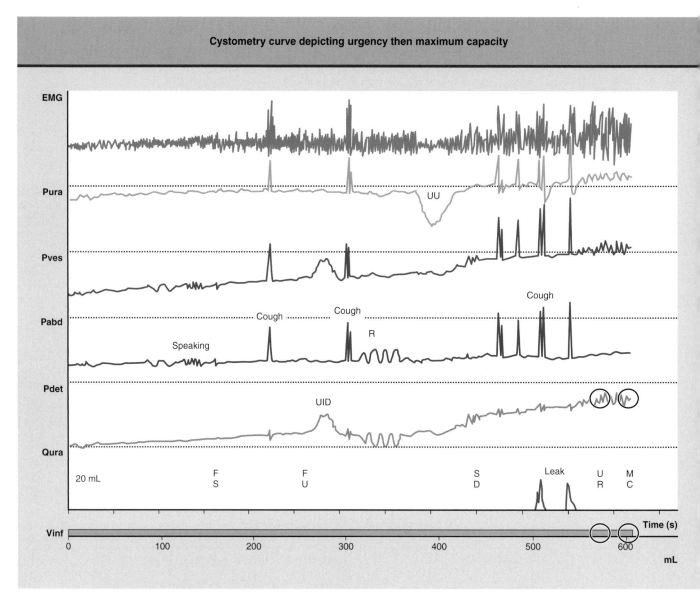

**Figure 28-28    Multichannel cystometry curve depicting urgency (UR) and then maximum capacity (MC).** (Courtesy of Medtronic Corporation, Minneapolis, Minn.)

**Typical cystometry results— storage phase**

| Events | | Pdet (cm H$_2$O) | Volume (mL) | Compliance (mL/cm H$_2$O) |
|---|---|---|---|---|
| Basic pressure | BP | 3 | 20 | — |
| First sensation | FS | 7 | 160 | 35 |
| First urge | FU | 12 | 270 | 27 |
| Strong desire | SD | 21 | 440 | 23 |
| Urgency | UR | 30 | 575 | 21 |
| Maximum cystometric capacity | MC | 32 | 610 | 20 |

**Figure 28-29    Typical cystometry results.** (Courtesy of Medtronic Corporation, Minneapolis, Minn.)

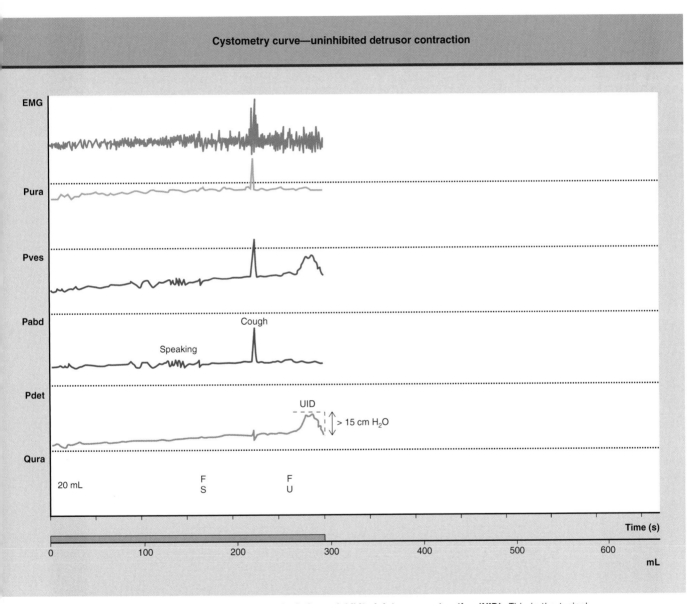

**Figure 28-30    Multichannel cystometry curve depicting uninhibited detrusor contraction (UID).** This is the typical urodynamic finding in patients with detrusor instability. Note that use of multichannel measurement allows one to assign the detrusor as the source of the increased bladder pressure during uninhibited detrusor contraction rather than the abdomen (compare uninhibited detrusor contraction curve with that for cough). (Courtesy of Medtronic Corporation, Minneapolis, Minn.)

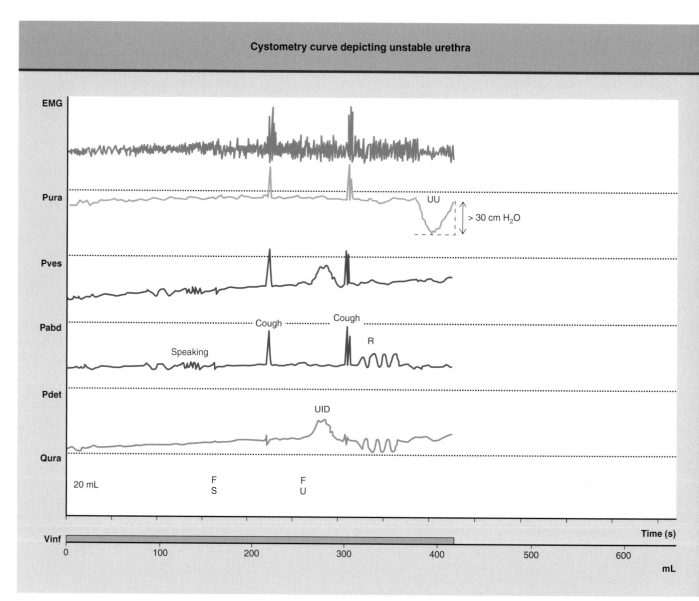

**Figure 28-31    Multichannel cystometry curve depicting unstable urethra.** Note that in some patients it could be the only sign of detrusor instability. Also note the normal reflex decrease in EMG activity during urethral relaxation. (Courtesy of Medtronic Corporation, Minneapolis, Minn.)

## Measurement of Urethral Pressure Profile

Urethral pressure profile is performed by withdrawing a urethral catheter at a constant rate by a pulley (Fig. 28-32) while making pressure measurement along the length of the urethra, generating a graph that is called the *static urethral pressure profile*. Significant data can be gathered from this profile, including maximum urethral closure pressure (MUCP), functional urethral length, and location of MUCP in relation to the bladder neck or urethral meatus (Fig. 28-33). MUCP of less than 20 cm is generally regarded as intrinsic urethral sphincter dysfunction, which carries certain therapeutic implications, discussion of which are beyond the scope of this chapter. In general intrinsic urethral sphincter dysfunction carries an implication of a higher failure rate with any therapeutic modality that is utilized. Certain modalities, such as the bladder neck sling operation, might be preferred over others such as the Burch operation. Generally two static profiles are obtained to ensure reliability and reproducibility. When these results are in close agreement, the average value of these two parameters is then utilized for the final report.

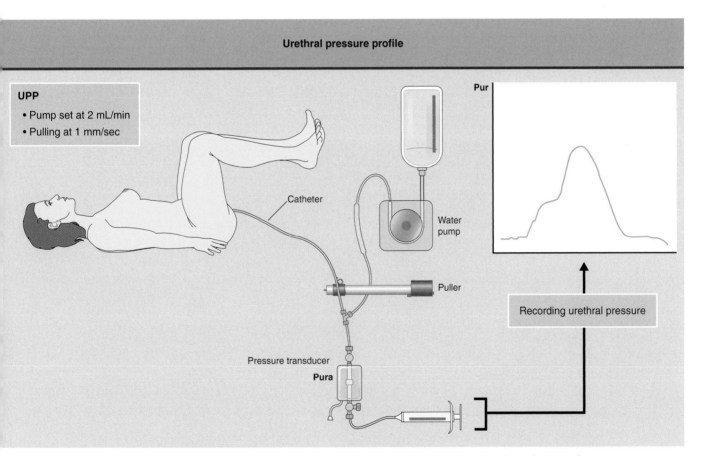

**Figure 28-32   Urethral pressure profile measurement in a single-channel setting.** Note that the catheter can be withdrawn manually or by a puller (a mechanical puller is depicted here). (Courtesy of Medtronic Corporation, Minneapolis, Minn.)

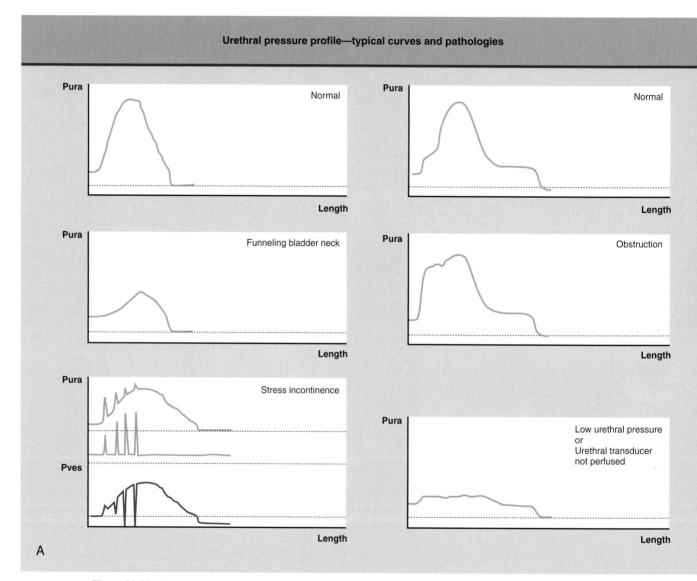

**Figure 28-33    Urethral pressure profile (UPP).** *A,* Typical UPP curves: normal curves and curves in various pathologic states.

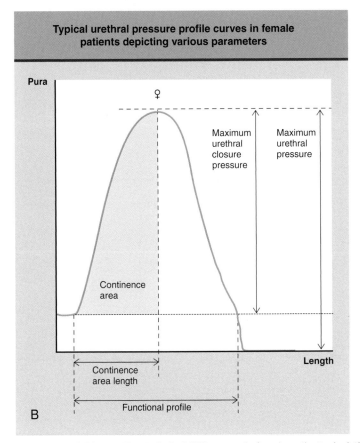

**Typical urethral pressure profile curves in female patients depicting various parameters**

Pura

♀

Maximum urethral closure pressure

Maximum urethral pressure

Continence area

Length

Continence area length

Functional profile

B

**Typical urethral pressure profile results— static profile and dynamic (stress) profile**

| Main results | |
| --- | --- |
| Volume at profile | 180 mL |
| Max urethral pressure | 72 cm H$_2$O |
| Max closure pressure | 59 cm H$_2$O |
| Closure pressure at 30% | 37 cm H$_2$O |
| Closure pressure at 70% | 41 cm H$_2$O |
| Functional length | 27 mm |
| Length of continence zone | 14 mm |
| Functional area | 795 mm*cm H$_2$O |
| Continence area | 423 mm*cm H$_2$O |

| Stress profile | | | | | |
| --- | --- | --- | --- | --- | --- |
| Cough | # | 1 | 2 | 3 | 4 |
| Percent of functional length | % | 10 | 30 | 40 | 50 |
| Transmission factor | % | 102 | 70 | 50 | 30 |

C

**Figure 28-33, cont'd** *B,* Typical UPP curves in female patients depicting various measured parameters. *C,* Typical UPP results: static profile and dynamic (stress) profile. (Courtesy of Medtronic Corporation, Minneapolis, Minn.)

After two initial static profiles are performed, two dynamic cough profiles are obtained to objectively document urodynamic stress incontinence. Dynamic cough profiles (Fig. 28-34) are performed by asking the patient to cough while the urethral catheter is passing through the functional length of the urethra; the urethral meatus is observed for leakage occurring in concert with the cough. The patient is then asked to perform a Valsalva maneuver; again the examiner observes for leakage of urine. First the patient is asked to push vigorously. If leakage is seen, she will slowly perform a Valsalva maneuver until the leakage occurs where she doesn't push any harder. In this fashion two VLPPs are documented (Figs. 28-35 and 28-36).

A *voiding pressure study* or *voiding cystometry* is a pressure flow study of the micturition act (Fig. 28-37). As the last part of multichannel testing, the patient is asked to void voluntarily around the catheter while abdominal, bladder, and urethral pressures are monitored and uroflowmetry measurements are taken (Fig. 28-38). Detrusor and urethral closure pressures are calculated in real time. This provides information on the patient's exact voiding mechanism. Normal voiding function in females includes urethral relaxation with bladder contraction (Figs. 28-39 and 28-40; see also Fig. 28-38A); Valsalva, urethral relaxation, and bladder contraction (see Fig. 28-37); Valsalva with urethral relaxation; and urethral relaxation only. By defining the exact voiding mechanism, a voiding pressure study may explain the patients' symptoms of voiding dysfunction and abnormal uroflowmetry parameters, and provide a reason for urinary retention. This component of urodynamic testing is useful in defining the etiology of postoperative voiding dysfunction, namely obstruction versus acontractile bladder. Completion of a voiding pressure study generally concludes multichannel testing.

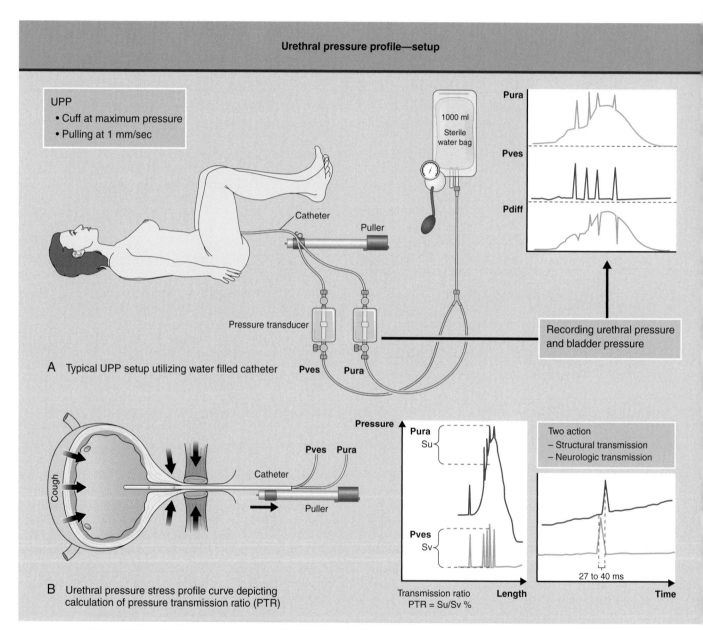

**Figure 28-34** **Urethral pressure profile (UPP).** *A,* Typical UPP setup utilizing water-filled catheter, pressurized water source, and an automatic catheter puller. Note the stress profile on the screen. *B,* Urethral pressure stress profile curve, depicting calculation of pressure transmission ratio (PTR). (Courtesy of Medtronic Corporation, Minneapolis, Minn.)

## Cystometry curve depicting cough leak point pressure measurement

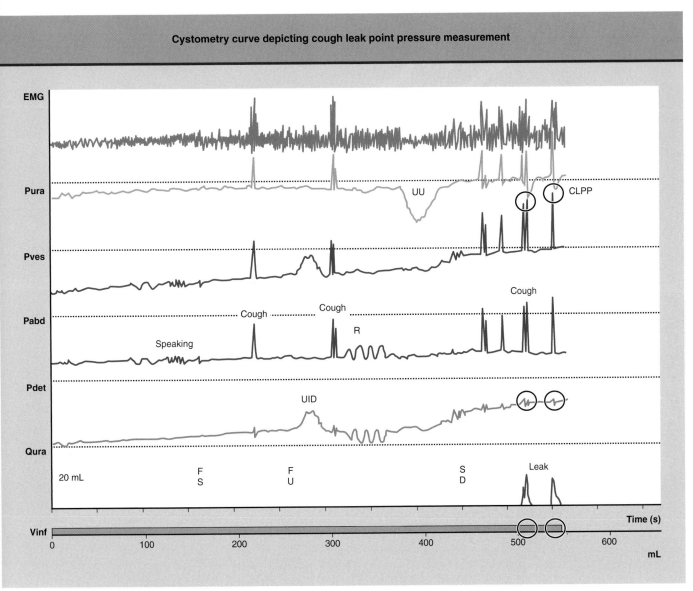

**Figure 28-35** **Multichannel cystometry curve depicting cough leak point pressure measurement.** VLPP can also be measured in a similar fashion. (Courtesy of Medtronic Corporation, Minneapolis, Minn.)

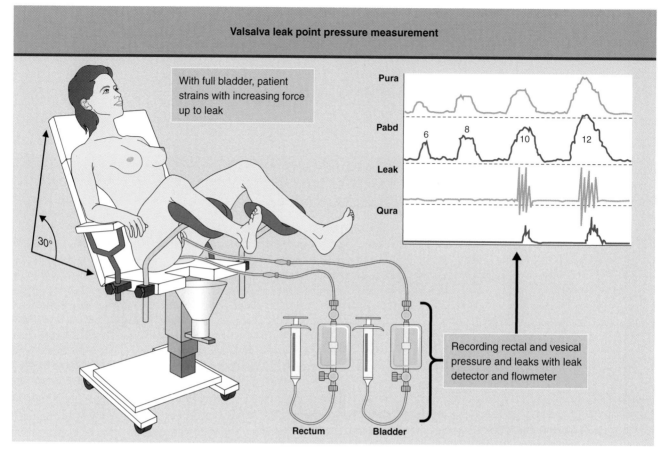

**Figure 28-36** **Multichannel cystometry curve depicting Valsalva leak point pressure measurement.** Note that patient is straining with increased force up to leak in a semisupine position. Also note that Pabd is measured through a rectal catheter and that leaks are detected with leak detector and flowmeter. (Courtesy of Medtronic Corporation, Minneapolis, Minn.)

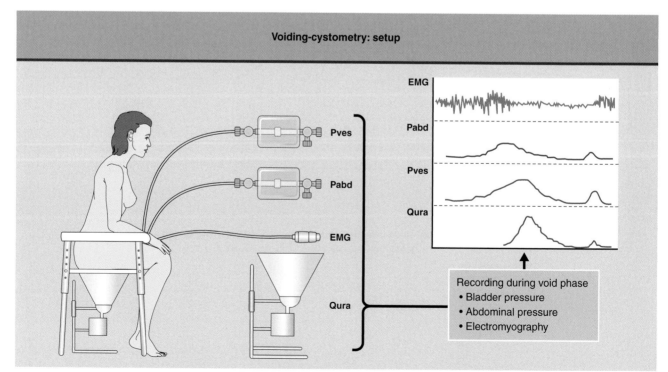

**Figure 28-37** **Typical setup for a voiding-cystometry test.** Note the recording of bladder pressure, abdominal pressure, and electromyography during the voiding phase. (Courtesy of Medtronic Corporation, Minneapolis, Minn.)

*Electromyography* is frequently performed at the time of multichannel testing (Fig. 28-41). The most common indication for EMG is to evaluate patients with a voiding dysfunction or as a therapeutic modality in the form of biofeedback treatment. EMG of the periurethral sphincter muscle is of primary interest during urodynamic testing because it can aid in diagnosis of detrusor sphincter dyssynergia. This test can be performed either directly with a needle, vaginal-surface, or urethral catheter-mounted electrodes or indirectly with an anal plug or perianal skin patch electrode. The latter is the most commonly utilized technique in clinical practice. The striated muscles of the urethral sphincter, external anal sphincter, and pelvic floor are in contracted status at baseline, as reflected by baseline EMG activity at rest. With bladder filling this baseline activity is increased further due to guarding reflex, as shown in Figures 28-19 and 28-27. At the time of voluntary void these muscles will relax, which is seen as diminished or silent EMG activity (see Fig. 28-38). In pathologic conditions causing discoordination between the detrusor and urethral sphincter, named *detrusor sphincter dyssynergia*, EMG activity will persist during a voluntary void (see Fig. 28-17).

### Video Urodynamic Testing

*Video urethrocystometry* involves the simultaneous measurement of abdominal, urethral, and bladder pressures along with the use of x-ray contrast media as a filling media. Video urodynamic testing is a combination of physiologic measurements made by a multichannel urodynamic test combined with anatomic visualization of the lower urinary tract (see Fig. 28-39). During the test, radiopaque filling media is infused in the bladder in place of water, which then is visualized by fluoroscopy. Thus, fluoroscopy provides a way of detecting leakage of x-ray contrast medium. Visualizing the lower urinary tract may make it easy to understand the complex relationship between anatomy and physiology interplaying in various pathologic conditions. Video urodynamic testing is arguably the Cadillac of urodynamic testing, although the exact indications for this particular modality are not clear.

### Ambulatory Urodynamics

As the name implies, urodynamic measurements are made in the ambulatory format, similar to Holter monitoring of the heart. Traditional urodynamic measurement is considered by many to be unnatural and embarrassing. Ambulatory testing still involves the invasiveness of catheters, but it is carried out in the patient's natural environment at a natural pace of bladder filling. Bladder and abdominal pressure are measured, and detrusor pressure is calculated. The patient wears a diaper with sensors to measure the volume leaked. The patient is also responsible for keeping a diary of symptoms and activities, as well as marking certain events on the monitor. Due to the labor-intensive nature of this type of testing, its use in daily clinical practice is limited. Other limiting factors for ambulatory testing include unknown indications for this type of testing, lack of standardization of technique, and difficulty in assessing the urethra.

### Urethral Retroresistance Pressure

Urethral retroresistance pressure (URP) is defined as the pressure required to open and to maintain an open urethral sphincter.[13] URP is not a new concept but has recently been revived, in part due to lack of correlations between current urethral assessment techniques (UPP, VLPP) and severity of illness as well as treatment outcome measurements. Some limited data is available on URP measurement utilizing the Gynecare Monitor (Gynecare, Johnson & Johnson). The Gynecare Monitor is a small, portable unit that also allows single-channel cystometry and VLPP measurements.

In Figure 28-42, Slack and colleagues recently showed a statistically significant correlation between URP and severity of incontinence as compared to current standard urodynamic measurements to assess the urethra.[21] One needs to be aware of the existence of this technique as well as the fact that the data is quite limited and in need of proof.

### Urethrocystoscopy

Cystoscopy has somewhat limited use in primary evaluation of an incontinent female patient. Some clinicians strongly believe that it should be performed in all female patients with irritative bladder symptoms, such as urinary urgency and frequency. We limit performing cystoscopy to patients with microscopic or gross hematuria, recurrent bladder infections, bladder pain with or without irritative bladder symptoms, recurrent urinary incontinence, irritative symptoms that have not responded to appropriate medical therapy, and significant nocturia. Cystoscopy can generally be performed in the office in a female patient without anesthesia with little or no discomfort. A rigid or flexible cystoscopy can be employed. Water, saline, or carbon dioxide can be utilized as distention media. Lenses measuring 0 degrees, 12 degrees, or 30 degrees can be used to inspect the urethra, bladder neck, and trigone; generally the 70-degree lens is used to evaluate the lateral, anterior, and posterior walls and the dome of the bladder. Any suspicious lesion should be biopsied and washing should be sent for cytology. Notes should be made of any ulceration or glomerulation (capillary bleeding) because they may suggest interstitial cystitis. Any other lesions, such as a cyst or raised area, should be noted. Cystoscopic bladder capacity is noted as well and we generally conduct a stress test on patients at this volume. Any bladder contraction, along with the patient's symptoms, is noted. Finally, an appropriate referral is made in the event of abnormal findings.

Figure 28-43 (see also Figs. 28-13 through 28-17 and 28-40) depicts some common urodynamic findings for readers to study.

## CONCLUSION

Urinary incontinence is a common and treatable condition that gynecologists frequently encounter This condition requires a physician to have a basic understanding of various types of incontinence and to understand that, even under the most ideal situation, history and physical examination may not accurately differentiate between various types of incontinence. When diagnosis is uncertain after clinical evaluation, as described in the history and physical examination section of this chapter, further testing may be indicated to objectively reproduce a patient's symptoms and to arrive at an accurate diagnosis. At this point the physician must decide on appropriate urodynamic testing based on the clinical situation at hand. In complex cases consultation with a urogynecologist or urologist should be considered.

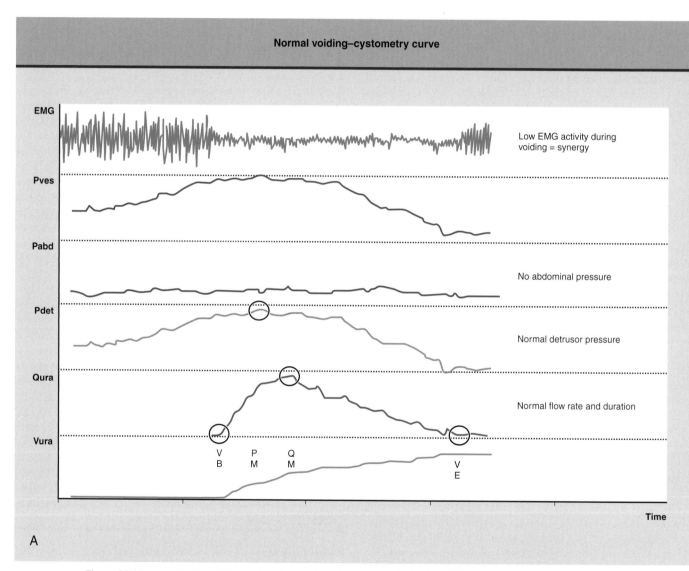

**Figure 28-38** *A,* Normal multichannel voiding–cystometry curve. Note the low EMG activity due to pelvic floor relaxation during voiding.

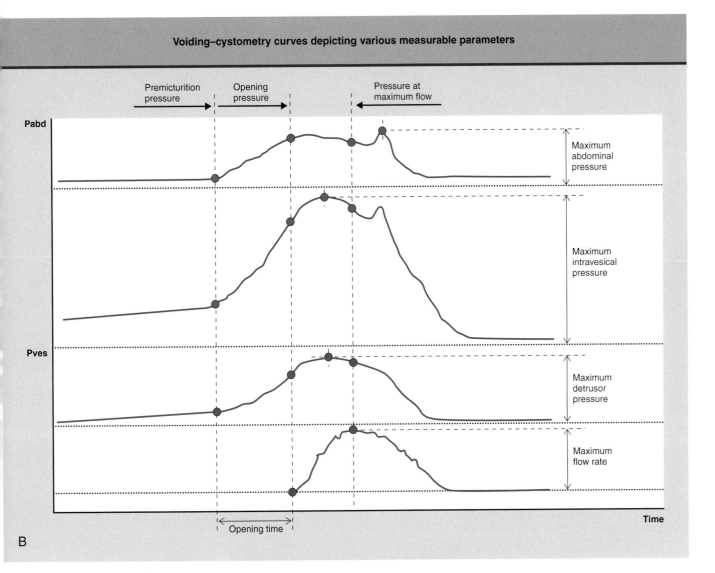

**Figure 28-38, cont'd** *B,* Voiding–cystometry curve, depicting various measurable parameters. *C,* Typical voiding cystometry results. (Courtesy of Medtronic Corporation, Minneapolis, Minn.)

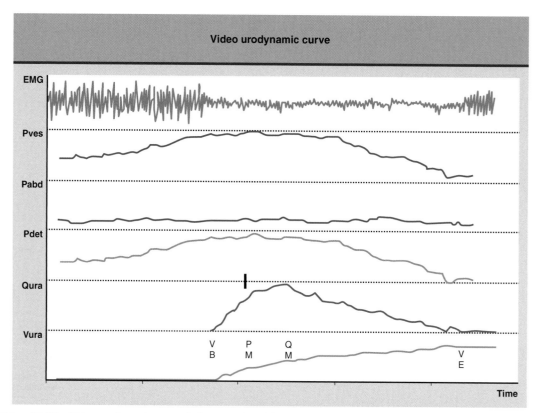

**Figure 28-39    Video urodynamic curve during normal multichannel voiding–cystometry.** Again, note the low EMG activity due to pelvic floor relaxation during voiding. (Courtesy of Medtronic Corporation, Minneapolis, Minn.)

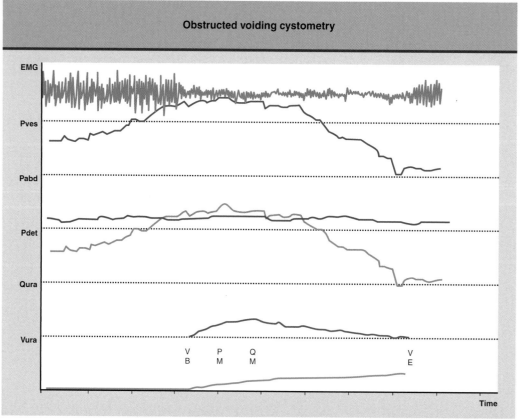

**Figure 28-40    Obstructed voiding cystometry.** Note the high detrusor pressure, low flow rate, and prolonged voiding time. (Courtesy of Medtronic Corporation, Minneapolis, Minn.)

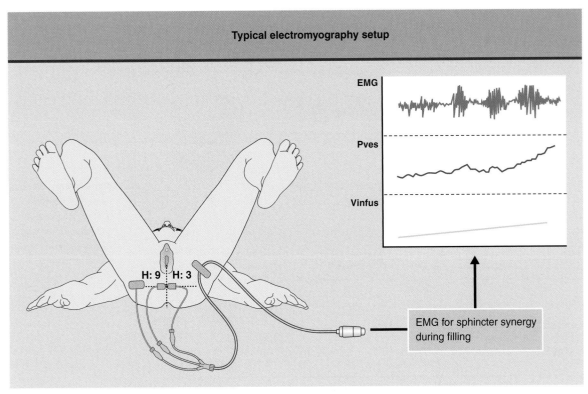

**Typical electromyography setup**

EMG for sphincter synergy during filling

**Figure 28-41** **Typical EMG setup. Note patch electrodes are being utilized in this instance.** Also note that it is easier to record anal sphincter EMG, but the best result is to record urethral sphincter with needle EMG. (Courtesy of Medtronic Corporation, Minneapolis, Minn.)

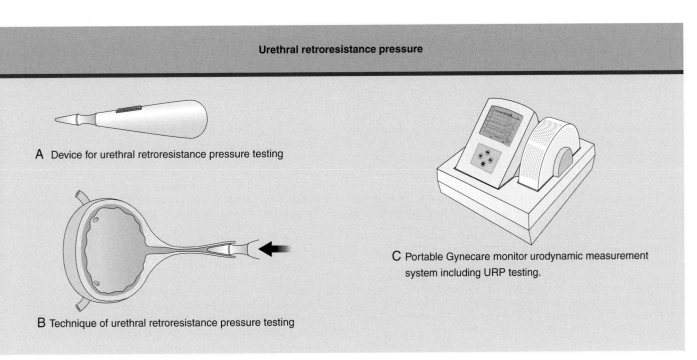

**Urethral retroresistance pressure**

A Device for urethral retroresistance pressure testing

B Technique of urethral retroresistance pressure testing

C Portable Gynecare monitor urodynamic measurement system including URP testing.

**Figure 28-42** **Urethral retroresistance pressure.** *A,* Device for urethral retroresistance pressure testing. *B,* Technique of urethral retroresistance pressure testing. *C,* Portable Gynecare MoniTorr Urodynamic Measurement System, including URP testing. (Courtesy of Gynecare Worldwide, a division of Ethicon, a Johnson & Johnson company, Bridgeport, NJ.)

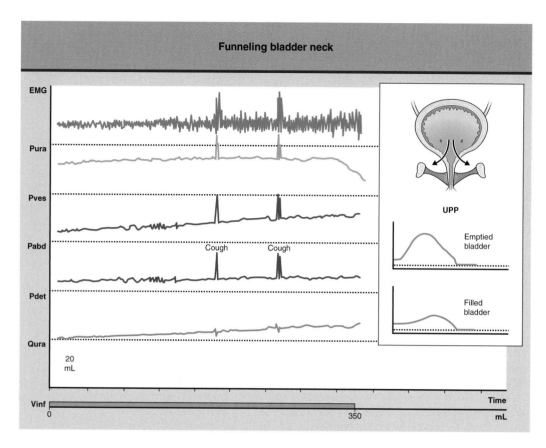

**Figure 28-43  Funneling bladder neck.** Note the decreasing urethral closure pressure at bladder capacity. (Courtesy of Medtronic Corporation, Minneapolis, Minn.)

## REFERENCES

1. Sand PK, Hill RC, Ostegard DR: The incontinence history as a predictor of detrusor instability. Obstet Gynecol 1988;71:257–260. **(IIb, B)**

2. Wyman J, Choi S, Hawkins S, et al: The urinary diary in evaluation of incontinent women: a test retest analysis. Obstet Gynecol 1988; 71:812–817. **(IIb, B)**

3. Sutherst J, Brown M, Shanner M: Assessing the severity of urinary incontinence in women by weighing perineal pads. Lancet 1981; 23:1128–1131. **(IIa, B)**

4. International Continence Society: Quantification of urine loss. In Fifth Report on the Standardization of Terminology. Aachen, West Germany: International Continence Society, 1983. **(IV, C)**

5. Ryhammer AM, Djurhuus JC, Laurberg S: Pad testing in incontinent women: a review. Int Urogynecol J Pelvic Floor Dysfunct 1999; 10:111–115. **(IV, C)**

6. Cardozo L, Lose G, McClish D, Versi E: A systematic review of the effects of estrogens for symptoms suggestive of overactive bladder. Acta Obstet Gynecol Scand 2004;83: 892–897.

7. Al-Badr A, Ross S, Soroka D, Drutz HP: What is the available evidence for hormone replacement therapy in women with stress urinary incontinence? J Obstet Gynaecol Can 2003;25:567–574.

8. Noseworthy JH, Lucchinetti C, Rodriguez M, et al: Multiple sclerosis. N Engl J Med 2000;343:938–952.

9. Awad SA, Gajewski JB, Sogbein SK, et al: Relationship between neurological and urological status in patients with multiple sclerosis. J Urol 1984;132:499–502.

10. Crum RM, Anthony JC, Bassett SS, Folstein MF: Population-based norms for the Mini-Mental State Examination by age and educational level. JAMA 1993;269:2386–2391. **(IIa, B)**

11. Bhatia NN, Berman A: Urodynamic appraisal of the Bonney test in women with stress urinary incontinence. Obstet Gynecol 1983; 62:696–699. **(IIb, B)**

12. Bergman A, McCarthy TA, Ballard CA, Yanai J: Role of the Q-tip test in evaluating stress urinary incontinence. J Repro Med 1987;32:273–275. **(IIb, B)**

13. Stevens E: Bladder ultrasound: avoiding unnecessary catheterizations. MEDSURG Nursing 2005;14:249–253.

14. Borrie MJ, Campbell K, Arcese ZA, et al: Urinary retention in patients in a geriatric rehabilitation unit: prevalence, risk factors, and validity of bladder scan evaluation. Rehab Nurs 2001;26:187–191. **(IIb, B)**

15. Blaivas JG: Editorial: urodynamics. Neurourol Urodyn 2003;22:91. **(IV, C)**

16. Kobelt G, Kirchberger I, Malone-Lee J: Quality of life aspect of the overactive bladder and the effect of the treatment with tolterodine. BJU Int 1999;83:583–590. **(IIa, B)**

17. Weber AM, Abrams P, Brubaker L, et al: The standardization of terminology for research in female pelvic floor disorders. Int Urogynecol J Pelvic Floor Dysfunct 2001;12:178–186. **(IV, C)**

18. Digesu A, Khullar V, Cardoza L, Salvatore S: Overactive bladder symptoms: do we need urodynamics? Neurourol Urodyn 2003; 22:105–108. **(IIb, B)**

19. Abrams P, Blaivas JG, Stanton SL, Andersen JT: The standardization of terminology of lower urinary tract function. The International Continence Society Committee on Standardization of Terminology. Scand J Urol Nephrol 1988;114(Suppl):5–19. **(IV, C)**

20. Lobel RW, Sand PK: The empty supine stress test as a predictor of intrinsic urethral sphincter dysfunction. Obstet Gynecol 1996; 88:128–132. **(IIb, B)**

21. Slack M, Culligan P, Tracey M, et al: Relationship of urethral retro-resistance pressure to urodynamic measurements and incontinence severity, Neurourol Urodyn 2004;23:109–114. **(Ib, A)**

# Diagnosis and Treatment of Fistulas

## Rony A. Adam, MD, and S. Robert Kovac, MD

---

### KEY POINTS

- Vesicovaginal fistulas occur most commonly following obstructed labor in developing countries.
- Although rare overall, an obstetric etiology is still common for rectovaginal fistulas in developed countries.
- In the developed world, urogenital fistulas occur rarely, but most likely following prior pelvic surgery.
- The treatment of genital fistulas is primarily surgical. The optimal timing, approach, and surgical techniques have not been established, therefore individualization is suggested.
- Further diagnostic tests to rule out inflammatory and/or neoplastic processes are required in patients that have recurrent fistulas.

---

## UROGENITAL FISTULAS

It is likely that women have suffered from urogenital fistulas since they have been giving birth. Findings of a vesicovaginal fistula have been identified in mummified remains from ancient Egypt. Since the mid-19th century, various attempts at surgical cure of urogenital fistulas as described by Marion Sims, Howard Kelly, and others have challenged gynecologic surgeons. It has long been recognized that women with vesicovaginal fistula are severely afflicted physically, socially, and emotionally owing to the constant uncontrollable dribbling of urine. While prone to litigation, patients with vesicovaginal fistulas remain among the most grateful of patients once they are cured. Although the published literature regarding urogenital fistulas is voluminous, very little scientifically validated research is available, and most of the data relies on retrospective case series and expert opinion. The various types of urogenital fistulas are listed in Table 29-1.

### Epidemiology

Genitourinary fistulas can be congenital or acquired. Congenital fistulas are rare, with only a few case reports in the literature. Most reported cases are associated with other urogenital anomalies.[1,2] Acquired fistulas may be the result of childbirth, pelvic surgery, malignancy, irradiation, infection, and an assortment of unusual presentations (Table 29-2).

In the developing world, the most common predisposing factor is obstructed childbirth, accounting for over 80% of genitourinary fistulas.[3] These difficult, often large fistulas have become exceedingly rare in developed countries owing to improvements in access to and delivery of obstetric care.

Ibrahim et al report that the mean age at diagnosis was 15 years, patients were in labor for 4 days on average, and the fetus died in 87% of cases.[4] In a rural, population-based study of parturients in Senegal, the incidence rate was 124 per 100,000 deliveries, whereas no fistulas were noted in six major cities in West Africa. It is estimated that over 33,400 new cases of obstetric fistulas occur annually in sub-Saharan Africa, with an incidence of over 120 per 100,000 births.[5] Worldwide, as many as 2 million fistulas may occur annually.[6] Risk factors include short stature, lower education and socioeconomic levels, and young maternal age.[7]

Hilton reviewed vesicovaginal fistulas in developing countries and outlined management strategies to include immediate catheter drainage as long as the tract has not yet epithelialized, perhaps even prophylactically following obstructed labor with evident vaginal sloughing. Attention to adequate vulvar skin care, nutrition, lower extremity rehabilitation, and counseling are important adjuncts in the care of fistula patients.[8] Arrowsmith et al similarly remind us of the spectrum of additional trauma sustained by the fistula patient and the need to address more than just the "hole in the bladder."[9] Surgical correction is curative in the first operation for obstetric vesicovaginal fistula in about 80% of cases. Multiple attempts may be necessary to achieve a success rate over 95% for large fistulas.[3]

The traditional tribal practice of "gishiri cutting" also is associated with formation of urogenital fistulas and is common in many parts of northern Nigeria. It involves cutting the anterior vagina with a razor or knife blade and has been noted to be the primary cause of fistula formation in 13% to 15% of cases.[10,11]

Other obstetric events and procedures have been noted to be associated with urogenital fistula formation worldwide. Cesarean section may result in formation of a vesicouterine fistula (Youssef's syndrome). Although over 700 cases have been reported in the literature, this complication is considered rare, since it represents only 1% to 4% of all genitourinary fistulas.[12,13] Vesicovaginal fistulas have also been reported following cesarean section, with or without associated hysterectomy.[14] Even more rarely reported are vesicocervical, urethrovaginal, and ureterouterine fistulas following cesarean section.[14-16] Operative vaginal delivery may result in vesicouterine fistula in the patient undergoing vaginal birth delivery after cesarean section (VBAC).[17-19] Cervical cerclage for the treatment of cervical incompetence rarely has been associated with vesicovaginal or vesicocervical fistulas.[20-22]

Nonobstetric urogenital fistulas have been reported as a consequence of gynecologic, urologic, and general surgical procedures and are the most commonly seen in developed countries with hysterectomy being the most common cause. Lee et al showed that benign hysterectomy was associated with 65% of

**Table 29-1**
**Anatomic Classification of Genitourinary Fistulas That Appear in the Literature**

- Vesicovaginal
- Urethrovaginal
- Vesicouterine
- Vesicocervical
- Ureterovaginal
- Ureterouterine
- Combination fistulas
    - Vesicoureterovaginal
    - Vesicoureterouterine
    - Vesicovaginorectal

303 genitourinary fistulas. Of 190 patients with vesicovaginal fistulas, 82% occurred following surgical treatment for benign gynecologic conditions and 11% from obstetric procedures.[23]

Harkki-Siren et al reviewed the incidence of urinary tract injuries from a Finnish national database of 62,379 hysterectomies with a vesicovaginal fistula incidence of 0.8 per 1000. Specific incidences based on the type of hysterectomy can be seen in Table 29-3.[24] In a retrospective single-institution series, Armenakas et al report on 65 patients over a 12-year period with iatrogenic bladder perforations. Obstetric and gynecologic procedures account for 62%, general surgical procedures 26%, and urologic procedures 12% of bladder perforation, excluding all endourologic procedures. Of the 40 patients from the obstetrics and gynecology service with bladder injury, there were 13 (32.5%) simple abdominal hysterectomies, 3 (7.5%) radical hysterectomies, 12 (30%) resections for pelvic mass, 10 (25%) cesarean sections, and 2 (5%) laparoscopies. Anterior vaginal repairs (done on the urology service) accounted for 6 (9%) cystotomies. All 17 cystotomies on the surgical service were sustained during colon resections. Sixty-three of the total 65 patients (97%) had their cystotomies recognized and repaired intraoperatively. With an average follow-up of 36 months, one subsequent vesicovaginal fistula occurred (1.5%).[25] Carley et al reported a 1% incidence of recognized bladder injury during

**Table 29-2**
**Associated Conditions Related to Development of Urogenital Fistulas**

**Obstetric conditions or procedures**

Prolonged, obstructed labor
Placenta percreta
Cesarean section (especially repeat cesarean section)
Cesarean hysterectomy
Operative vaginal delivery
Cervical cerclage

**Gynecologic procedures**

Hysterectomy
Suburethral slings
Anterior colporrhaphy
Periurethral bulking
Burch colposuspension
Urethral diverticulum repair
Myomectomy
Loop excision of the cervix
Voluntary interruption of pregnancy

**Pelvic conditions**

Endometriosis
Gynecologic cancer
Pelvic irradiation
Bladder stone
Infection
    Schistosomiasis
    Tuberculosis
    Lymphogranuloma venereum
Intrauterine device
Neglected pessary

| Table 29-3 Incidence of Vesicovaginal Fistula and Bladder Injury by Type of Hysterectomy, with Associated Failure Rates of Primary Repair | | | | |
|---|---|---|---|---|
| | **Failure Rate** | | | |
| | *Laparoscopic* N = 2741 | *Total Abdominal* N = 43,149 | *Subtotal Abdominal* N = 10,854 | *Vaginal* N = 5636 |
| Incidence of vesicovaginal fistula | 2.2 per 1000 | 1 per 1000 | 0 | 0.2 per 1000 |
| Incidence of bladder injury | 6.6 per 1000 | 0.2 per 1000 | 0.3 per 1000 | 0 |
| Data from Harkki-Siren P, Sjoberg J, Tiitinen A: Urinary tract injuries after hysterectomy. Obstet Gynecol 1998;92:113–118. | | | | |

hysterectomies at Parkland Hospital. Of 1722 abdominal hysterectomies, the cystotomy rate was 0.58%, of 590 vaginal hysterectomies the rate was 1.9%, and of 117 obstetric hysterectomies the rate was 5.1%.[26] A recent retrospective single-institution review of 1647 total laparoscopic hysterectomies reports 16 recognized bladder lacerations (1%) and 2 vesicovaginal fistulas (0.1%).[27]

In a review of 110 vesicovaginal fistulas following hysterectomy, Tancer reported that 92 occurred following abdominal hysterectomy, while 18 following vaginal hysterectomy. Twenty-four of these fistulas occurred despite intraoperative recognition and repair of cystotomy. In 77 of these fistulas, no risk factors such as prior cesarean section, endometriosis, recent cervical conization, or prior irradiation were identified.[28] A retrospective review of 17 urogenital fistulas following gynecologic surgery over a period of 15 years in Dublin found 12 vesicovaginal and 5 ureterovaginal fistulas. Of the vesicovaginal fistulas, three followed radical hysterectomy, one followed salpingo-oophorectomy, two followed vaginal hysterectomy, and six followed total abdominal hysterectomy. Of the ureterovaginal fistulas, three were preceded by radical hysterectomy, and one each by vaginal and total abdominal hysterectomy. It was calculated that the risk of vesicovaginal fistula is 1/605 (0.16%) of total abdominal hysterectomies, 1/571 (0.17%) vaginal hysterectomies, and 1/81 (1.2%) of radical hysterectomies.[29]

Unfortunately, not all recognized cystotomies that are repaired prevent subsequent vesicovaginal fistula formation. In their data on over 43,000 total abdominal hysterectomies, Harkki-Siren et al report failure of primary bladder repair 18% of the time.[24] Armenakas et al in their recent review of 65 iatrogenic bladder injuries that were repaired by urologists, 13 cystotomies occurred after benign abdominal hysterectomy. Of these, one vesico-vaginal fistula occurred, for a postcystotomy repair failure rate of 7.7% among total abdominal hysterectomy patients.[25]

Urethrovaginal fistulas are less common than vesicovaginal fistulas, with an incidence ratio of 1 per 8.5.[14] In the developed world, the most common predisposing event is surgery for urethral diverticulum, anterior vaginal prolapse, incontinence, radiation therapy, or trauma. Operative vaginal delivery and more rarely cesarean section also have been reported to precede urethrovaginal fistula formation.[30]

Urethrovaginal fistulas can occur from a variety of urogyneco-logic procedures such as anterior colporrhaphy,[25,31] suburethral slings,[32,33] Burch colposuspension,[14] and periurethral collagen injections.[34,35] More recently, a urethrovaginal fistula has been reported following tension-free vaginal tape.[33] It is expected that urethrovaginal fistulas may become more common with the increasing popularity of mid-urethral tapes for the treatment of stress incontinence.

Additional gynecologic procedures associated with urogenital fistulas, although with greater rarity (see Table 29-2), include myomectomy,[36] large loop excision of the cervical transformation zone for CIN,[37] and voluntary interruption of pregnancy.[38] Fistulas are noted following radiation therapy for gynecologic cancers.[39] Fistulas that form within a previously irradiated field are more prone to recurrence, and most surgeons would agree that additional pedicled flaps are needed in their surgical repair because of the microvascular compromise.[40,41]

An assortment of unusual presentations can be found in the literature associated with urogenital fistulas mostly in the form of case presentations. These include uterine artery embolization,[42,43] Behçet's syndrome,[44] infections such as schistosomiasis,[45] tuberculosis,[46,47] lymphogranuloma venereum,[48] accidental trauma,[49–51] sexual trauma,[52,53] masturbation,[54] retained foreign objects,[55,56] endometriosis,[57,58] neglected diaphragm,[59] neglected pessary,[60,61] intrauterine device,[62,63] and bladder calculus.[64]

## Pathogenesis

The precise pathophysiologic mechanism of fistula formation is elusive and poorly understood. Etiologies have been proposed based on interpretation of the epidemiologic data and risk factors previously discussed. Vascular compromise and epithelial necrosis are evident from cases of prolonged obstructed labor seen in developing countries. The pathophysiology of genital fistulas noted in developed countries, however, is more difficult to ascertain with certainty. Vascular compromise and impaired healing may be the basis of fistulas caused by infection and subsequent urethral erosion of various graft materials used for suburethral sling and tape procedures, which then result in urethrovaginal fistula formation. Similarly, vascular compromise may explain fistulas that form following periurethral collagen injection and irradiation. In posthysterectomy fistulas, it has been suggested that undiagnosed bladder injury, especially in the posterior wall, would result in vesicovaginal fistula formation, as would an inadvertently placed suture that incorporates the bladder and vagina. Direct injury with healing of the surfaces in a way to allow formation of a fistula may also explain formation of fistulas following trauma. It must be understood, however, that these explanations represent opinion rather than scientifically proved pathophysiology. A few studies have attempted to answer this question in animal models.

Meeks et al demonstrated in a rabbit model that fistula formation did not occur when absorbable sutures were placed incorporating full-thickness bladder and vaginal cuff.[65] This tends to contradict the notion that an errant suture alone is sufficient to result in fistula formation. In a laparoscopic dog model, no dogs developed a fistula after bipolar cautery injury to the bladder base, nor when absorbable sutures were placed through the bladder and vaginal cuff. Fistula formation, however, was noted in the dogs that had a monopolar cautery-induced bladder base laceration and had repair either with single-layer absorbable suture in the normal fashion or with suture that incorporated the anterior vaginal wall.[66] This suggests a possible role for microvascular compromise as an important cofactor in the pathophysiology of vesicovaginal fistula. It should be noted that these animal models of hysterectomy, because of anatomic differences, do not require any dissection of the bladder off the uterus, and in that respect may be different from humans undergoing total hysterectomy.

**Clinical Presentation**

The classic presentation of urogenital fistula is continuous urinary leakage from the vagina. This may occur in the absence of urinary urgency, Valsalva maneuvers, or changes in body position. The degree to which leakage presents depends primarily on the precise location and size of the fistula, perhaps the pliability and healing of the surrounding tissue, and the condition of the rest of the vagina. Patients have a spectrum of leakage from truly continuous to intermittent primarily at bladder capacity with attendant urinary odor. Although it is generally accepted that the larger the fistula, the worse the leakage, it is always surprising to see how much urine can leak even through a small fistula. In developed countries, a precedent gynecologic, urologic, or general surgical procedure involving the pelvis will be noted. Delivery by the operative vaginal or, more commonly, cesarean section route may precede the onset of symptoms. The vast majority of cases will present in 1 to 10 days following surgery although the authors have seen patients manifest symptoms as much as 3 months postoperatively. The increasing prevalence of multiple procedures undertaken at the same time for complex pelvic floor disorders (often by multiple surgeons) may complicate the diagnosis of subsequent fistula formation, related to multiple potential sites of injury, preexisting symptoms, and added potential postoperative urinary complications. Other factors that may potentially increase the likelihood of fistula formation are the increasing use of permanent graft materials in reconstructive and incontinence surgery placed between the lower urinary tract and the vagina, as well as the increasing complexity of laparoscopic surgery. Other potential causes of postoperative urinary leakage should be considered and ruled out, as listed in Table 29-4.

Many patients develop coexisting urinary tract infections and symptoms of frequency, urgency, and dysuria. The predominant organism is *Escherichia coli* in most cases. Urinary leakage from any genitourinary fistula may be accompanied by hematuria. Vesicouterine fistulas tend to present with cyclic hematuria, and

| Table 29-4 |
| --- |
| Differential Diagnosis of Postoperative Urinary Incontinence |

- Urogenital fistula
- Stress incontinence
- Urge incontinence
- Overflow incontinence
- Vaginal discharge/erosion of mesh

if the fistula is located above the cervix, amenorrhea may occur if all the menstrual blood is redirected into the bladder because of a closed cervical canal. Patients with coexistent mesh erosion into the urinary tract experience urgency, frequency, voiding dysfunction, and pain. If there is concurrent erosion into the vagina, coital discomfort and a vaginal discharge may occur as well.

Urine leakage for even a short period of time may result in significant irritation of the vagina, vulva, or perineum. This often occurs, despite the patient's attempt at frequent cleansing. If urine leakage persists, severe perineal dermatitis may result owing to exposure of the skin to ammonia. Phosphate crystallization may precipitate on the vagina and vulva, further irritating the area.

**Diagnosis**

Often the diagnosis of urogenital fistula is straightforward based on history and demonstrable pooling of urine in the vaginal vault; occasionally, however, the diagnosis is elusive. In all cases it is necessary to evaluate the fistula with regard to its size, precise location, degree of epithelialization, whether it is simple or complex, accessibility, and the overall health status and mobility of the surrounding tissues. In the instance of a recurrent fistula, precise knowledge of prior nonsurgical management and a detailed surgical description of prior repair attempts are mandatory for appropriate surgical planning. If no prior documentation is available to rule out upper urinary tract injury, this should be obtained by an intravenous urogram or computed tomography (CT) scan.

In the case of clinical suspicion of a urogenital fistula that cannot be verified on initial speculum examination, the physician can try concurrent Valsalva maneuvers and partial closure of the speculum to reduce the tension on the vaginal walls. If this is not helpful in visualizing vaginal leakage, then a dye test should be tried. Indigo-carmine or methylene-blue-dyed sterile water is instilled via a transurethral Foley catheter (16 French) with great care taken to avoid spilling the dye externally. Once the vagina and vulva are cleaned, a tampon is placed and the patient asked to ambulate and wait for one-half hour. The tampon is removed and inspected for presence of blue dye; if the tampon is wet with urine but not dyed then a ureterovaginal fistula is suspected and is best diagnosed by intravenous urography. On rare occasions, these office diagnostic procedures are nondiagnostic despite a compelling history. In this case, the patient is asked to take phenazopyridine (Pyridium) and wear a series of tampons at home over a longer period of time with varying degrees of physical activity. The tampons are placed individually in plastic bags and brought in to be inspected. The patient must be counseled regarding careful use of the tampons to eliminate the possibility of dye contamination during insertion or removal.

Radiologic studies are not routinely helpful in the diagnosis of urogenital fistula. However, it is often necessary to evaluate the upper urinary tract once a fistula is identified, and that is usually accomplished by an intravenous pyelogram (IVP) or contrast CT scan. Cystourethrography may be utilized to show a vesico-vaginal or urethrovaginal fistula, but it is rarely needed to make an initial diagnosis. It has been occasionally helpful in delineating a complex fistula with multiple channels and openings. Volkmer et al describe the use of Doppler ultrasound to diagnose vesico-vaginal fistulas with a sensitivity of 92%. Although this modality may be useful in the follow-up of patients undergoing conservative bladder drainage (in one of four such patients they demonstrated resolution of the fistula after 6 weeks), it too is rarely necessary to make an initial diagnosis.[67]

All patients should undergo cystourethroscopy to delineate the fistula's location and size, to determine whether it is simple or complex, and to evaluate ureteral patency and location. Although this could be done in the office, it is preferable to examine the patient under anesthesia when possible, which also allows better determination of fistula accessibility to the vaginal route of repair. If the fistula is large and does not allow adequate distention of the bladder during fluid-filled cystourethroscopy, placing a vaginal pack is helpful in allowing better visualization. When there is clinical suspicion of a vesicouterine fistula, hysterography or hysteroscopy may be helpful in making the diagnosis. If the patient is taken for examination under anesthesia and cystourethroscopy, then diagnostic hysteroscopy may help further delineate the course of such a fistula. Improved surgical planning and informed consent may be obtained when the definitive operation is done at a later time, especially in complex or recurrent cases.

Some have advocated urodynamics testing prior to repair of a urogenital fistula on clinical and medicolegal grounds.[68,69] Hilton reports abnormalities on preoperative urodynamics in most patients with urogenital fistulas. Urodynamically proved stress incontinence was noted in 75% of patients with urethral or bladder neck fistulas (n=12) and 36% with vesicovaginal fistulas (n=14), with detrusor instability, impaired bladder compliance, and voiding dysfunction noted frequently as well. Of the 24 patients who were anatomically cured in this series, 1 (4%) had stress incontinence and 9 (38%) had urgency or urge incontinence.[68] Preoperative urodynamics should be performed only if surgical management will be influenced by the results. The authors do not routinely perform urodynamics pre-operatively, since we would not usually advocate a concurrent continence procedure at the time of fistula repair even in the face of urodynamic stress incontinence. Every patient is carefully counseled regarding the variety of lower urinary tract problems that can occur or persist following such surgery, even when deemed successful.

## Prevention

Since the occurrence of a cystotomy is considered intuitively to predispose a patient to subsequent fistula formation, prevention is discussed primarily in terms of preventing a cystotomy or adequately detecting and closing one if it occurs. Careful con-sideration of the bladder, trigone, and ureteral anatomy in relation to the anterior vagina is important to maintain during a total hysterectomy (Fig. 29-1). The bladder base overlies the uterine isthmus and the cervix, the bladder trigone is positioned anterior to the upper third of the vagina, and the external cervical os is proximal to the base of the trigone (the inter-ureteric ridge). During a simple hysterectomy, mobilization of the bladder does not involve the upper third of the vagina and therefore rarely puts the trigone at risk. A subtotal (supra-cervical) hysterectomy requires no bladder mobilization and indeed resulted in no fistulas in a large series (see Table 29-3). This is not the case, however, with anterior colporrhaphy or vaginal paravaginal repair, where the anterior vaginal dissection is carried more distally and laterally.

The likelihood of cystotomy is reduced when blunt dis-section is avoided at the time of bladder mobilization during hysterectomy, especially when the vesicovaginal space is scarred from prior cesarean section. The precise direction of forces cannot be as well controlled when blunt dissection is used, as compared with sharp dissection. Gentle traction and counter-traction are helpful in dissecting the correct plane and thereby preventing bladder injury, as is utilizing an intrafascial hyster-ectomy technique. Another cause of bladder injury may be direct trauma due to retractors, which should be used with appropriate caution. In his report of urogenital fistulas, Tancer noted an absence of typical risk factors during the index surgery in 70% of cases.[28] Therefore, although it still is somewhat controversial, the authors advocate routine cystoscopy to assess for bladder and ureteral injury following hysterectomy, and certainly after surgery for pelvic prolapse or urinary incontinence.

In the event of a cystotomy, the location and size seem to be crucial to the possibility of subsequent vesicovaginal fistula formation. A small anterior bladder injury does not result in urogenital fistula formation as observed following removal of suprapubic catheters where the defect resolves spontaneously. Similarly, cumulative experience with trocar injuries from mid-urethral slings shows little or no consequence of leaving these small lateral and anterior defects to heal spontaneously, even when managed with no additional catheter drainage. Since these injuries are 0.5 cm or less in diameter, any bladder injury greater than that may benefit from primary repair. Owing to the depen-dent position of the bladder base, however, any recognized injury in this region requires suture closure and bladder drainage. Once a cystotomy is recognized, it may be repaired immediately or delayed until the hysterectomy or other surgical procedure is completed. The benefit of immediate repair is that blood and urine do not continually flow into the surgical field; however, with continued surgery and retraction there may be potential compromise to the fresh suture line, and this must be avoided. Adequate dissection of the bladder off the vagina is usually necessary to ensure tension-free closure and allow enough space for a second layer. The first layer can be accomplished with 2-0 or 3-0 absorbable suture placed in an interrupted or running fashion. There is continued controversy regarding whether this first layer can be placed through the mucosa, or should remain extramucosal. It is thought that the extramucosal technique may decrease the likelihood of subsequent fistula formation, although this has not been demonstrated. Sokol et al suggest that double layer closure is superior to single layer closure in

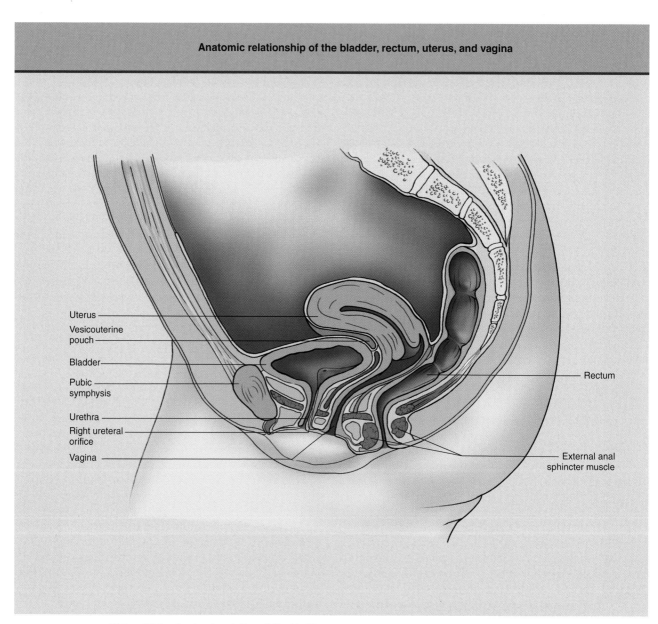

**Anatomic relationship of the bladder, rectum, uterus, and vagina**

Uterus

Vesicouterine pouch

Bladder

Pubic symphysis

Urethra

Right ureteral orifice

Vagina

Rectum

External anal sphincter muscle

**Figure 29-1    Anatomic relation of the bladder, rectum, uterus, and vagina.** See text for details.

**Repair of simple cystotomy in its nondependent portion**

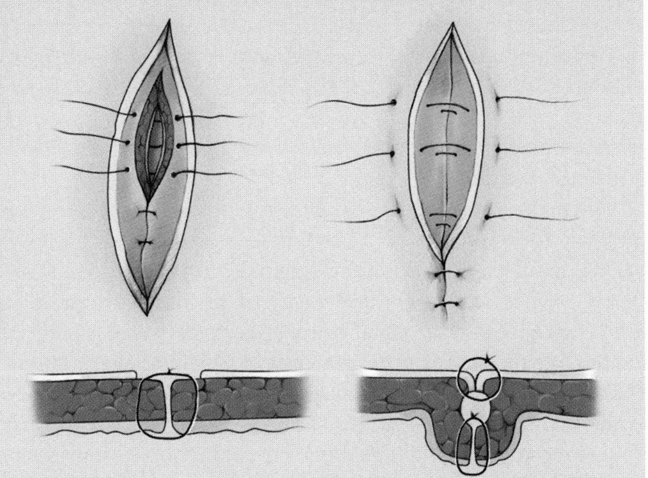

**A** The first layer incorporates the mucosal and muscularis layers

**B** The second layer imbricates over the first layer of sutures

**Figure 29-2    Simple cystotomy closure.** Two-layer bladder closure with the first layer placed full thickness through the bladder epithelium (A) and the second suture line imbricating the muscularis and serosal layer over the first to reinforce it (B).

preventing vesicovaginal fistula in an experimental laparoscopic hysterectomy model of electrocautery-induced bladder injury with laparoscopic repair in dogs.[70] The second layer placed to imbricate the first is thought to diminish tension on the suture line (Fig. 29-2). Cystoscopy is important to evaluate ureteral and bladder integrity following completion of the repair. Transurethral or suprapubic catheter drainage must prevent bladder filling to avoid stretch on the suture line. The lack of reliable postoperative catheter drainage as a cause of failure was discussed at length by Sims in his landmark paper regarding urogenital fistulas in 1852.[71] Judgment should be exercised regarding duration of drainage, based on the extent of injury, its location, the security of the closure, and any factors that may impact the normal healing process. Some advocate use of a cystogram prior to catheter removal.

## Management

### Nonsurgical Management of Urogenital Fistula

Once a urogenital fistula has been diagnosed, a trial of conservative management should be offered. This is particularly true for small fistulas that present early and have no evidence of epithelialization of the tract. Transurethral bladder drainage may help small early vesicovaginal fistulas resolve spontaneously and may be tried for 4 to 6 weeks as long as catheterization is seen to resolve the vaginal leakage. Medical management should include optimizing nutrition, correcting anemia, and improving vaginal estrogenization.[72] Some success has been reported with laser treatment of vesicovaginal fistula,[73] as well as fibrin glue and collagen.[74,75] These novel approaches have not yet been adequately studied but may be considered in selected cases. The use of various collection devices have been tried with limited success but may be offered for temporary relief of constant urinary leakage.

### Surgical Correction of Urogenital Fistula

When conservative therapy fails or the patient is not a candidate for conservative therapy, surgical repair is the only alternative to relieve the patient's condition. Prior to surgery, some advocate the need to remove any transurethral catheterization for several days to clear the urine of any infection. This may be considered as long as the patient is able to adequately prevent skin excoriation and tolerate the increased leakage.

The pelvic surgeon must determine the optimal timing, technique, and route of repair. No well-designed trials adequately address any of these dilemmas. Several general principles may apply and are discussed. Although traditionally, delayed repair for several months was the norm to allow the tissue to heal from the inciting surgery, more recently surgeons have undertaken earlier repair following surgical fistulas as long as there is no evidence of infection, inflammation, or necrosis in the tissue bed.[76–79] Obstetric and radiation injuries, however, require more time to heal prior to an attempt at fistula repair. It is generally agreed that the first attempt at cure is also the best chance of cure.

In Sims' classic article regarding the surgical treatment of vesicovaginal fistulas, he emphasized the need to excise all scar tissue within the fistula and create fresh tissue edges for reapproximation. Additional surgical principles include tension-free closure of the wound with wide mobilization of the bladder to help achieve this, careful handling of tissues, ensuring excellent hemostasis, and maintaining good bladder drainage postoperatively.[71]

Despite these original tenets, there is no consensus about whether to excise the margins of the fistula. Several series have reported success with preservation of the fistula margin, and some surgeons are concerned about making the fistulous opening larger, as occurs when the fistulous tract is trimmed.[31,80] Others have continued to report their experiences with excision of the tract.[14,81] The purported benefit is allowing fresh tissue edges to be approximated, thereby promoting healing of these surfaces and reducing failure rates. Whereas there are no adequate studies that would conclusively show superiority of either of these techniques, it is interesting to note that there is limited discussion regarding retaining the fistula collar when operating transabdominally, reserving this debate primarily for the transvaginal approach. In the case of excision, another technical dilemma is whether to permit through-and-through suture reapproximation or insist on excluding the mucosal layer from the stitch. Concern over incorporating the mucosal layer stems from the possibility that it would increase the likelihood of failure and may lead to stone formation given that this region is the most dependent portion of the bladder and is always in contact with urine. The potential benefits of a through-and-through stitch are its ease and better hemostasis at the incision site. It should also be noted that transvesical techniques used to perform complex procedures such as ureteroneocystostomy routinely make use of intravesical suture, albeit in more nondependent areas of the bladder, with no clear adverse effects. It remains for the operating surgeon to decide individually how to close the suture line.

Perhaps the most intense debate has been surrounding the route of vesicovaginal repair—transabdominal or transvaginal. There seems to be general agreement that the vaginal repair is more convenient for the patient in terms of recovery, length of hospital stay, and cosmetic issues, but little agreement regarding which is the better operation. Absolute indications for an abdominal approach include conditions that require bladder augmentation (a small capacity or poorly compliant bladder, as may occur following irradiation), a fistula involving or very close to a ureter that requires ureteral reimplantation, a combination fistula involving other intra-abdominal organs, inability to adequately expose the fistula transvaginally due to positioning, or other access problems (Table 29-5). It is also noted that the majority of vesicovaginal fistula repairs are in fact amenable to the vaginal approach.[82] Some have concluded that abdominal approaches are outright superior[83–85] while others prefer the vaginal approach as their routine.[31,78,86]

Success rates have been reported in different ways; it may be for the first surgical attempt or the ultimate rate that allows for multiple attempts. In this chapter, quoted rates are for the first attempted repair, unless otherwise stated. Through an abdominal approach the physician can do a transvesical-transperitoneal approach made popular by O'Conor[87] or a more limited transvesical repair introduced by Landes.[88] Success rates for the transvesical-transperitoneal approach have been between 68% and 100% for benign, nonirradiated fistulas.[79,84,85] A different abdominal operation for vesicovaginal fistula repair is the transvesical approach. For data pooled from three studies reporting variations of this technique, with a total of 91 fistula patients (primary and recurrent), the success rate is 100%.[83,88,89] However, a non-technique-specific series reports a 91% success rate for the transvesical approach.[14]

Vaginal repair reveals success rates of 77% to 99%.[14,23,31,90] These vaginal procedures encompass various techniques. No comparative studies are available to determine which specific vaginal procedure, if any, is superior.

Indeed with the initial success rates being comparable, there is no consensus regarding the optimal approach to repair vesicovaginal fistulas. It is clearly important that surgeons who repair these lesions be comfortable with several different approaches and individualize their techniques to the particular case at hand.

Various techniques have been described to augment fistula repairs, both for the transabdominal and transvaginal approaches. This is thought to bring additional tissue to interpose between the bladder and the vagina and with it, a healthy blood supply. Occasionally, such grafts also serve to fill in dead space, as with large fistulas where a great amount of tissue is lost. The routine use of interposition grafts has been advanced by some; however,

most surgeons use these adjuncts based on individualized clinical judgment. It is generally agreed that tissue interposition is needed in irradiation-induced fistulas or in other instances where there is local vascular compromise, such as recurrent, severely scarred or previously infected fistulas. Transabdominally the omentum or peritoneum is most often used with excellent results. Evans et al reported a 100% (10/10) success rate with such interposition grafts compared with 63% (12/19) when grafts were not used in benign vesicovaginal fistulas repaired transabdominally in a urologic residency program.[91]

Rangnekar et al report on Martius bulbocavernosus fat pad grafting to reinforce 21 obstetric urethrovaginal and vesicovaginal fistula repairs done transvaginally. Although they showed better success rates for both types of fistulas with use of the graft, because of the small sample size, statistical significance cannot be reached. Seven patients of 8 (87%) were cured of their urethrovaginal fistula, whereas all 13 patients (100%) with vesicovaginal fistulas were cured with use of the Martius graft.[92] For extremely large defects, Punekar et al reported four patients who had a myocutaneous modification of the Martius bulbocavernosus graft. The island of skin after sublabial transfer was sutured to the defect in the vaginal wall. This modified repair has been suggested for large obstetric or irradiation-induced fistulas.[93] Eilber et al report long-term results of transvaginal repair of complex or recurrent vesicovaginal fistulas with either peritoneal interposition graft for fistulas high in the vault or Martius flap or labial flap for distal defects. Cure rates were 96% of 83 patients with peritoneal graft, 97% of 34 patients with Martius fat pad graft, and 33% of three patients with a full-thickness labial flap that was rotated onto the defect and used mainly for very complex cases with multiple attempts at repair where there was insufficient vaginal epithelium to cover the fistula. Alternative flaps have been described, such as gracilis or rectus abdominis myocutaneous grafts in difficult circumstances.[94,95] In six patients who failed urethrovaginal fistula closure with Martius transposition, Bruce et al report 100% successful resolution of the fistula when treated with a pedicled, tubularized rectus abdominis muscle flap interposed suburethrally.[96]

When preparing patients for surgical correction of a urogenital fistula, detailed informed consent and discussion are very important. Patients with urogenital fistulas as complications of benign pelvic surgery have already experienced an adverse outcome that they may or may not have been prepared for. They invariably have some degree of frustration, anxiety, and suspicion. All aspects of operative risk should be discussed with the patient prior to fistula repair, including the likelihood of fistula recurrence. Even in the event of successful anatomic repair, the occurrence or persistence of lower urinary tract symptoms such as incontinence, overactive bladder, voiding dysfunction, and bladder pain should be discussed. Discussing the expected recovery course of the various available approaches and potential adverse consequences of associated procedures such as episiotomy or Schuchardt incisions, disfigurement from flaps, and discomfort from suprapubic and transurethral catheters seems to prepare patients for some of the difficulties that may lie ahead. This information should be incorporated into the decision of the route of repair, which the patient should ideally be a partner in. When ureteral reimplantation may be

| Table 29-5 |
| --- |
| Indications for Abdominal Vesicovaginal Fistula Repair |
| · Small capacity or poorly compliant bladder requiring bladder augmentation |
| · Fistula involving or very close to a ureter requiring ureteral reimplantation |
| · Combination fistula involving other intra-abdominal organs |
| · Inability to adequately expose the fistula transvaginally |

equired, the need for stenting and subsequent cystoscopic stent emoval should be discussed as well as the need for drains, the isk of ureteral stenosis, and the need for subsequent radiologic ollow-up. Patients undergoing a vaginal repair should be made ware of the possibility of conversion to an abdominal procedure, lthough this is a rare occurrence.

## Vaginal Procedures

### Vesicovaginal Fistula Repair

The patient is placed in the dorsal lithotomy position using andy-cane stirrups. Examination under anesthesia is performed vith water cystoscopy. The 30° or 70° lens is used to best visualize he fistula intravesically and identify any associated abnor- nalities. Identifying the intravesical and the vaginal openings nd assessing the tract's angle is important, since the next step s cannulation of the fistula. The fistula's proximity to the ureters s assessed, and transvaginal repair is continued if it is not too lose. Ureteral stenting may be done to continuously identify he ureters if needed. Dilation of the fistulous tract allows an 8 rench Foley catheter to be inserted and the balloon inflated. Appropriate traction allows the fistula to be brought distally for petter access and exposure. When the tissue surrounding the istula is extensively scarred, subepithelial injection of saline may pe used to facilitate dissection of the vaginal flap. Some authors dvocate the use of epinephrine to diminish surgical bleeding.

The vaginal mucosa is incised circumferentially around the istulous opening; the vaginal mucosa is then carefully dissected off the bladder to a distance that will allow tension-free multiple-layer closure, approximately 1 to 2 cm radially around he circumferential incision. All tissue must be handled delicately vith fine instruments that are of sufficient length to reach Il levels of the fistula and the dissected tissues. Excellent nemostasis is best achieved with liberal use of pressure and ubsequent suture closure, avoiding the use of electrocautery if t all possible. The fistula collar is excised and sent for pathologic evaluation. Repeat cystoscopy verifies the location of the ureters n relation to the somewhat larger fistulous opening. A supra- pubic catheter is then placed. The bladder mucosa is closed in the direction of least tension (side to side, or proximal to distal) vith interrupted 3-0 or 4-0 delayed absorbable sutures, placed pproximately 0.5 cm apart. Proximal to distal orientation is chosen if the ureters are in close proximity to the defect once the istula is excised. If extramucosal suturing is possible, it is done; however, if desired or if mucosal edge bleeding is encountered, hrough-and-through suturing is not contraindicated. A second ayer of bladder muscularis is brought together over the first uture line so it imbricates over it. This is achieved with inter- upted suture that is placed staggered in between the underlying titches on the first layer (Fig. 29-3). If the bladder peritoneum an be mobilized over the repair, it is accomplished at this point. f a Martius fat pad transposition is desired, this may be done nstead of the peritoneal layer at this time. The vaginal mucosa s then closed with interrupted suture again staggered from the econd bladder layer. At all stages of the closure, the absence of ension on each level is paramount to successful repair, as is nemostasis and verification of healthy, well-vascularized tissue or apposition.

The Latzko procedure begins in a similar fashion with a circumscribing incision and dissection of the vagina off the cervicovaginal fascia. Instead of excising the fistulous tract, it is imbricated into the bladder cavity with sequential layers of interrupted 3/0 or 4/0 delayed absorbable suture on a small tapered needle. Care should be taken to stagger the sutures so none lay atop the next layer (Fig. 29-4). Cystoscopy should be used to verify water-tight closure of the fistula and integrity of the ureters.

### Urethrovaginal Fistula Repair

The same principles of careful handling of tissues, good hemostasis, and tension-free apposition of tissues must be maintained with surgical correction of urethrovaginal fistulas. A distal fistula may be closed in a proximal to distal orientation to limit the possibility of urethral stenosis; otherwise these lesions are closed side-to-side in layers. Eversion of the fistula edges into the limited urethral lumen is not recommended, and trans- mucosally placed suture is avoided if at all possible. If there is adequate substance, the fistula is minimally excised, but often there is enough loss of urethral wall that this may be impossible without resultant stricture formation (Fig. 29-5). The authors recommend liberal use of the Martius flap to support these repairs, and a pedicled rectus muscle flap for recurrent urethro- vaginal fistula, if a previous Martius flap was employed and failed. The technique used for Martius fat pad transposition is depicted in Figure 29-6.

## Abdominal Procedures

### Retropubic Transvesical Vesicovaginal Fistula Repair

This procedure is indicated for simple posthysterectomy vesicovaginal fistula (VVF) when adequate vaginal exposure cannot be obtained or can be obtained only with a Schuchardt or episiotomy incision and the patient prefers an abdominal approach. A Cherney or midline abdominal wall incision is made, the retropubic space is entered, and a midline vertical incision is made in the bladder. The ureteral orifices are inspected and catheterized if needed. The fistula is identified and dilated to admit an 8 French pediatric Foley catheter after the position of the ureters is verified and the balloon inflated. A circumscribing incision is made 2 to 3 mm from the fistula and the vesicovaginal space dissected circumferentially 1 to 2 cm outward. The fistula is excised and the defect closed in layers with the vaginal layer first using interrupted delayed-absorbable 3-0 suture and the knots placed within the vaginal lumen. The bladder serosa and muscularis is closed next with knots placed in the vesicovaginal space. A third row incorporating bladder muscularis and mucosa is closed with 4-0 suture (Fig. 29-7). Ureteral integrity is verified. A suprapubic catheter is placed through a separate incision. The bladder incision is closed with running delayed-absorbable suture in two layers. Cystoscopy is used to verify water-tight closure and ureteral integrity prior to wound closure.

### Transvesical-Transperitoneal Vesicovaginal Repair

Cystoscopy is used to identify the pertinent anatomy and the fistula is cannulated with a stent. The bladder is vertically bisected in the midline starting at the retropubic portion and continues posteriorly in its peritoneal portion until it reaches the vesicovaginal space. This space needs to be dissected laterally and distally until the fistula is encountered, using digital traction within the bisected bladder. The fistula is identified with the aid

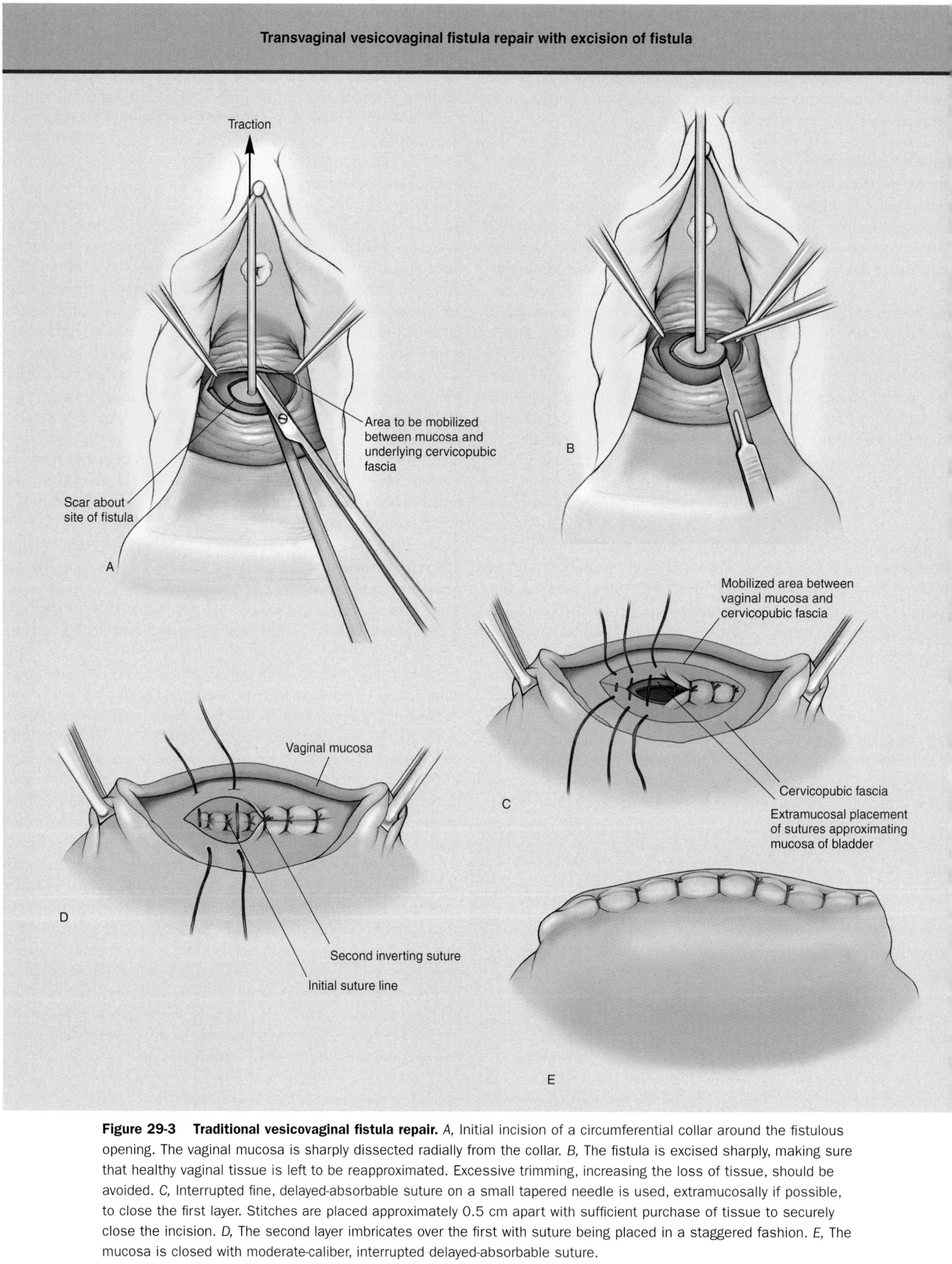

**Transvaginal vesicovaginal fistula repair with excision of fistula**

Traction

Area to be mobilized
between mucosa and
underlying cervicopubic
fascia

Scar about
site of fistula

A

B

Mobilized area between
vaginal mucosa and
cervicopubic fascia

Vaginal mucosa

Cervicopubic fascia

Extramucosal placement
of sutures approximating
mucosa of bladder

C

Second inverting suture

Initial suture line

D

E

**Figure 29-3    Traditional vesicovaginal fistula repair.** *A,* Initial incision of a circumferential collar around the fistulous opening. The vaginal mucosa is sharply dissected radially from the collar. *B,* The fistula is excised sharply, making sure that healthy vaginal tissue is left to be reapproximated. Excessive trimming, increasing the loss of tissue, should be avoided. *C,* Interrupted fine, delayed-absorbable suture on a small tapered needle is used, extramucosally if possible, to close the first layer. Stitches are placed approximately 0.5 cm apart with sufficient purchase of tissue to securely close the incision. *D,* The second layer imbricates over the first with suture being placed in a staggered fashion. *E,* The mucosa is closed with moderate-caliber, interrupted delayed-absorbable suture.

**Transvaginal vesicovaginal fistula repair by the Latzko procedure**

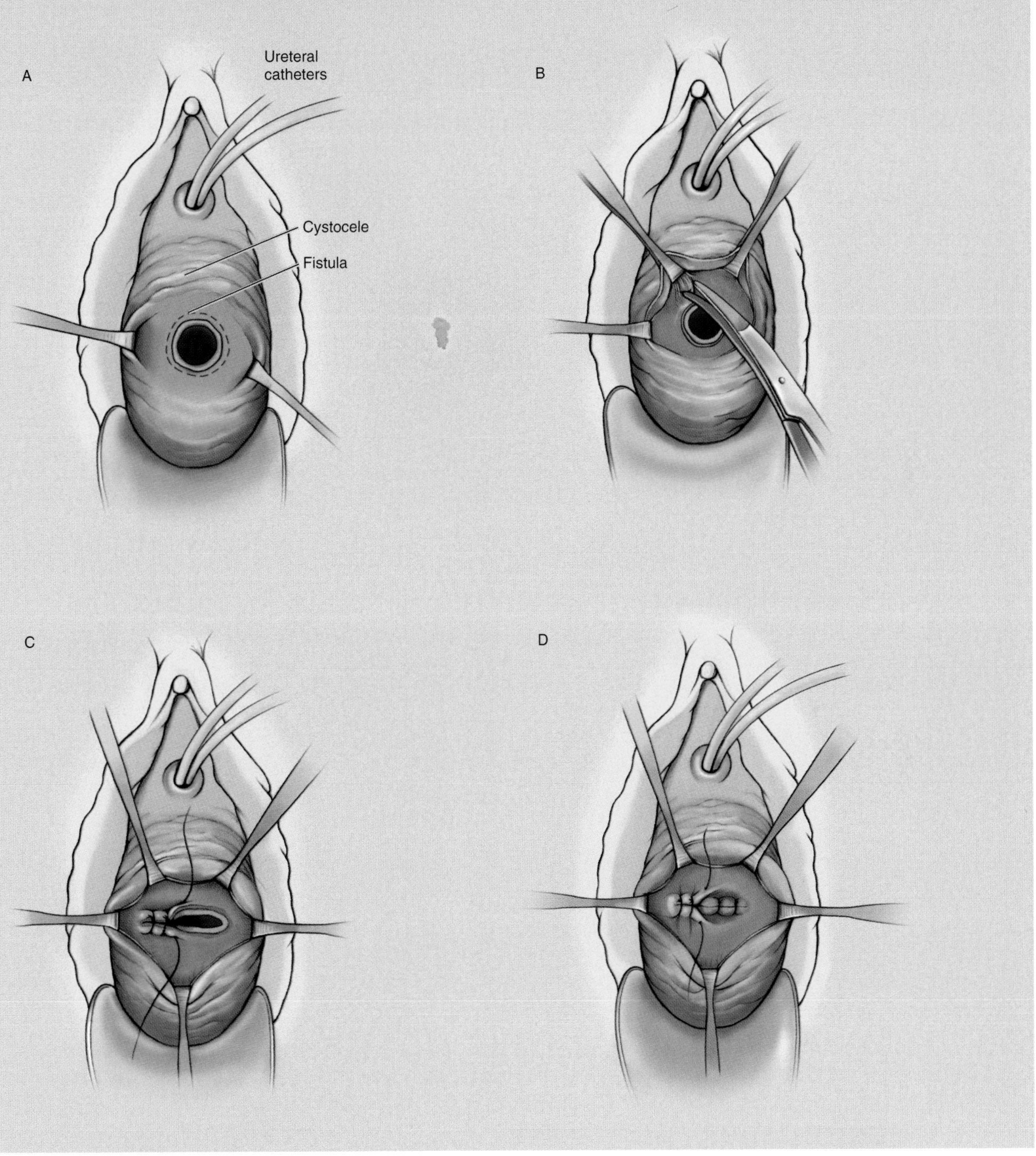

**Figure 29-4    Latzko procedure.** *A–D,* Note that the fistulous tract is left in situ and the collar of tissue is imbricated into the bladder viscus with interrupted fine, delayed-absorbable suture on a small tapered needle. The second layer further imbricates the first, and the vaginal mucosa is closed last, also with interrupted suture.

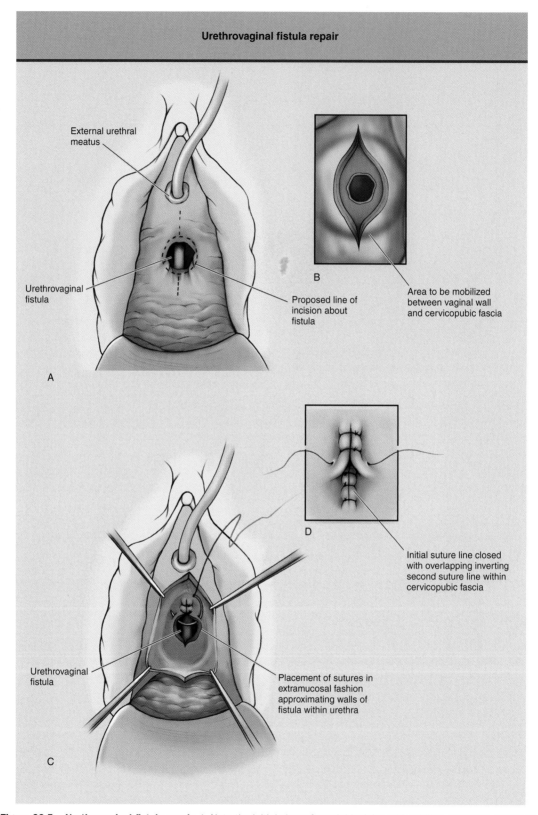

**Urethrovaginal fistula repair**

External urethral meatus

Urethrovaginal fistula

Proposed line of incision about fistula

B

Area to be mobilized between vaginal wall and cervicopubic fascia

A

D

Initial suture line closed with overlapping inverting second suture line within cervicopubic fascia

Urethrovaginal fistula

Placement of sutures in extramucosal fashion approximating walls of fistula within urethra

C

**Figure 29-5    Urethrovaginal fistula repair.** *A,* Note the initial circumferential incision with midline extension proximally and distally. *B,* Further lateral dissection exposes paraurethral tissue and allows for tension-free closure. *C,*The first layer is closed by interrupted fine, delayed-absorbable suture on a small tapered needle, avoiding intramucosal placement. *D,*The second is an interrupted imbricating layer. Martius fat pad transposition is highly recommended for these repairs.

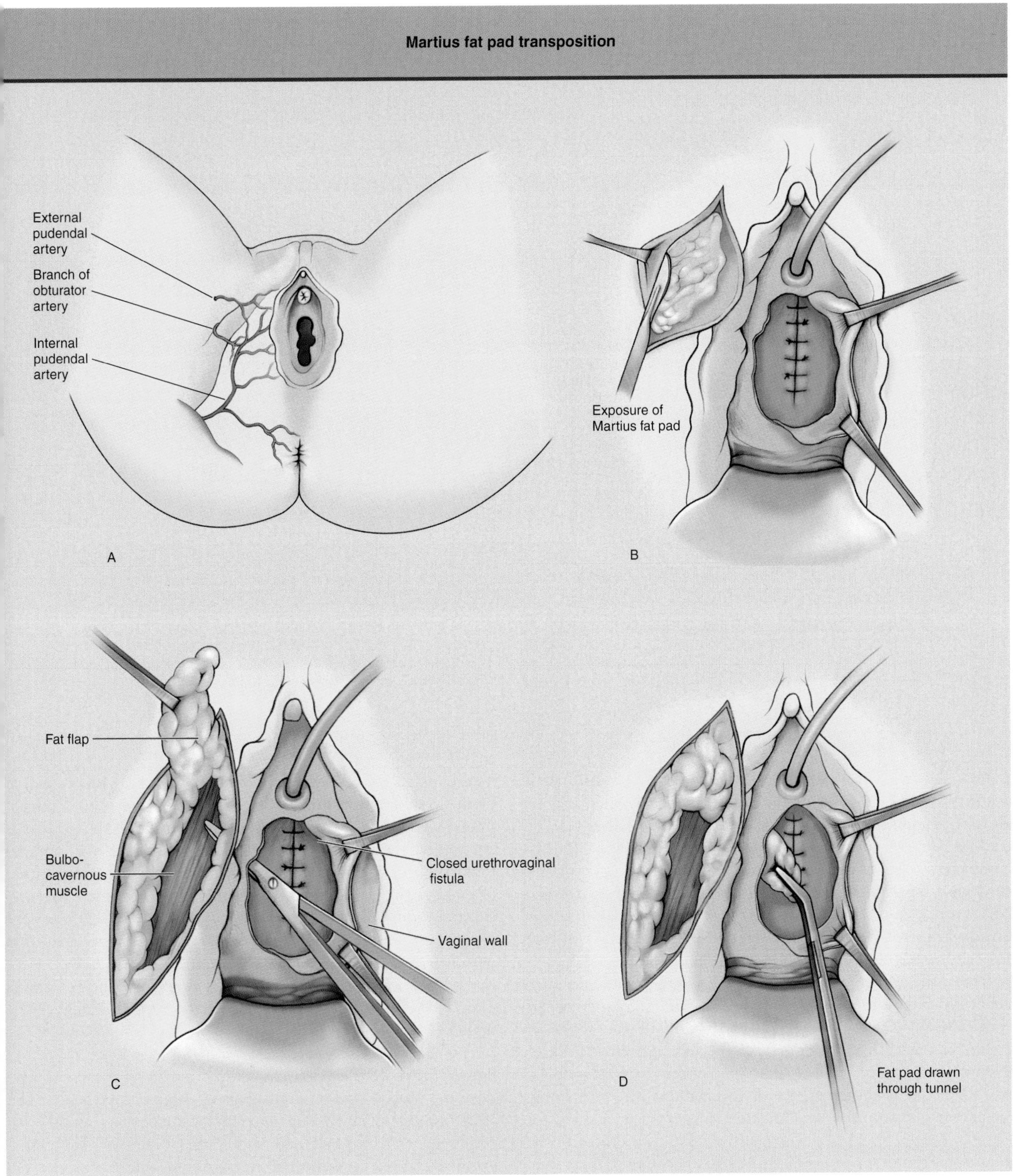

**Martius fat pad transposition**

External
pudendal
artery

Branch of
obturator
artery

Internal
pudendal
artery

A

Exposure of
Martius fat pad

B

Fat flap

Bulbo-
cavernous
muscle

Closed urethrovaginal
fistula

Vaginal wall

C

D

Fat pad drawn
through tunnel

**Figure 29-6    Martius (bulbocavernosus) fat pad transposition.** *A,* The labial fat pad is supplied anteriorly by branches of the external pudendal and obturator arteries, and posteriorly by branches of the internal pudendal artery. Although traditionally the posterior blood supply was thought to be of superior quality, the graft may be swung anteriorly or posteriorly depending on the need of the surgeon. *B,* An incision is made over the labial fat pad, and it is dissected bluntly and with electrocautery. *C,* Once it is detached, a submucosal tunnel is created and enlarged to ensure adequate blood flow to the graft. *D,* The graft is pulled through the tunnel to the area needed and sutured in place. *Continued*

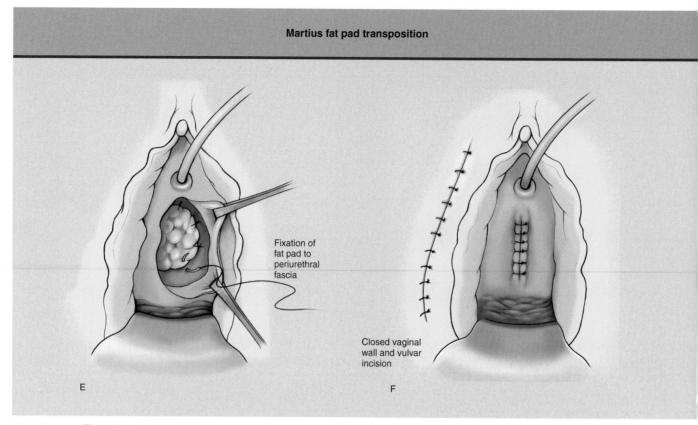

**Martius fat pad transposition**

Fixation of
fat pad to
periurethral
fascia

E

Closed vaginal
wall and vulvar
incision

F

**Figure 29-6, cont'd**  *E,* The graft is pulled through the tunnel to the area needed and sutured in place. *F,* Hemostasis of the donor site is verified, and the incisions are closed.

of the stent and is excised. Ureteral integrity is verified and continually monitored during the surgery. The vagina is closed transversely with interrupted delayed-absorbable suture with the knots within the vaginal lumen. A second layer of vagina is used to imbricate the first if sufficient tissue is found. The bladder is closed in two layers side to side (Fig. 29-8). Prior to complete closure of the bladder, a suprapubic catheter is placed through a separate stab incision. If an omental flap is deemed necessary, it is placed into the vesicovaginal space once the bladder sutures have been tied (Fig. 29-9). Cystoscopy is used to verify water-tight closure prior to wound closure.

When the fistula is adjacent to the ureteral orifice, ureteroneocystostomy must be performed at the time of fistula repair (Fig. 29-10). Once the dependent portion of the repair is complete, attention is turned to performing the ureteroneocystostomy (Fig. 29-11). The implantation site should be placed in the posterior aspect of the bladder but sufficiently distant from the repair site. A double-J stent is placed and left for 4 to 6 weeks (Fig. 29-12). The anastomosis site is drained with a Jackson-Pratt drain brought out through a separate stab incision.

### Vesicouterine Fistula Repair

A transperitoneal approach is preferred for repair of vesico-uterine fistulas. This may be done with or without hysterectomy, but should be delayed for 3 months if the inciting procedure was a cesarean section to allow for involution of the uterus. A vertical bladder incision is made and the fistula identified. If the

uterus is to be preserved, the vesicouterine space is developed sharply down to the fistula. At this point the vertical bladder incision is extended posteriorly to help with easy identification of the vesicouterine fistula. Once the planes have been appropriately dissected, layered, tension-free closure of the bladder is performed with uterine closure done separately. An omental flap may be placed and sutured into the space for interposition (Fig. 29-13). It should be kept in mind that such omental transposition will make any subsequent cesarean section more difficult. If repair is done along with a hysterectomy then it is performed in routine fashion with careful, sharp dissection of the bladder off the uterus, cervix, and vagina. The remaining vesical fistula is then excised and the defect closed in layers without tension.

### Postoperative Care

Ensuring proper bladder drainage is of utmost importance. The authors accomplish this in the early postoperative period with combined transurethral and suprapubic drainage. The transurethral catheter is removed once gross hematuria has cleared, usually a few days. This often takes longer with the transvesical-transperitoneal than with the vaginal approach. The suprapubic catheter is left for 2 to 3 weeks depending on the complexity of the repair. Some authors advocate routine evaluation with a cystogram prior to its removal, others do not.

Avoiding bladder spasms is considered important in preventing recurrence, although this has not been well studied. Some

*Text continues on p. 431.*

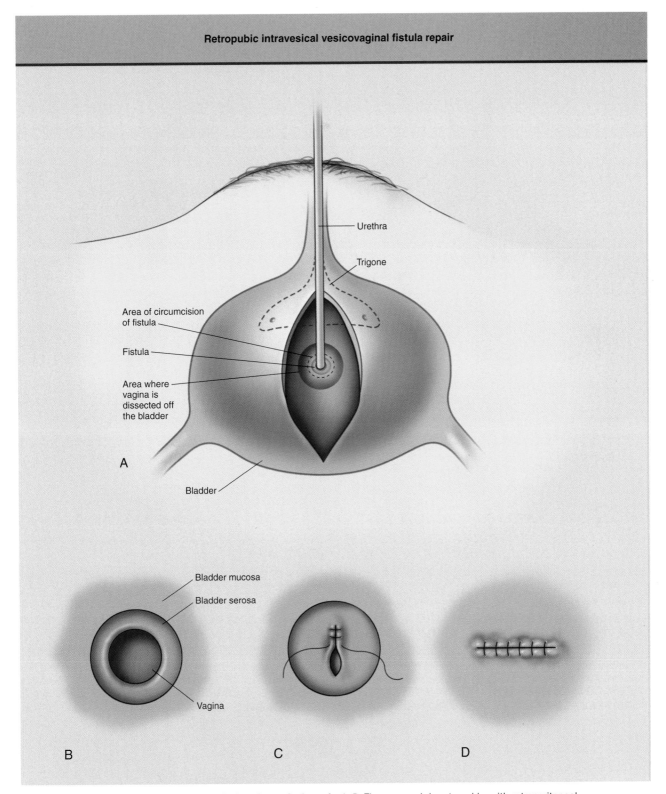

**Figure 29-7 Retropubic intravesical vesicovaginal repair.** *A–D,* The approach is retropubic, with retroperitoneal bladder incision. The fistula is identified and circumscribed, and the vesicovaginal space is dissected radially. The fistula is excised, and repair is accomplished in layers with interrupted delayed-absorbable suture on a small tapered or U-shaped needle. Staggering of the sutures is depicted for security of the closure.

**Transabdominal, transvesical closure of vesicovaginal fistula (O'Conor operation)**

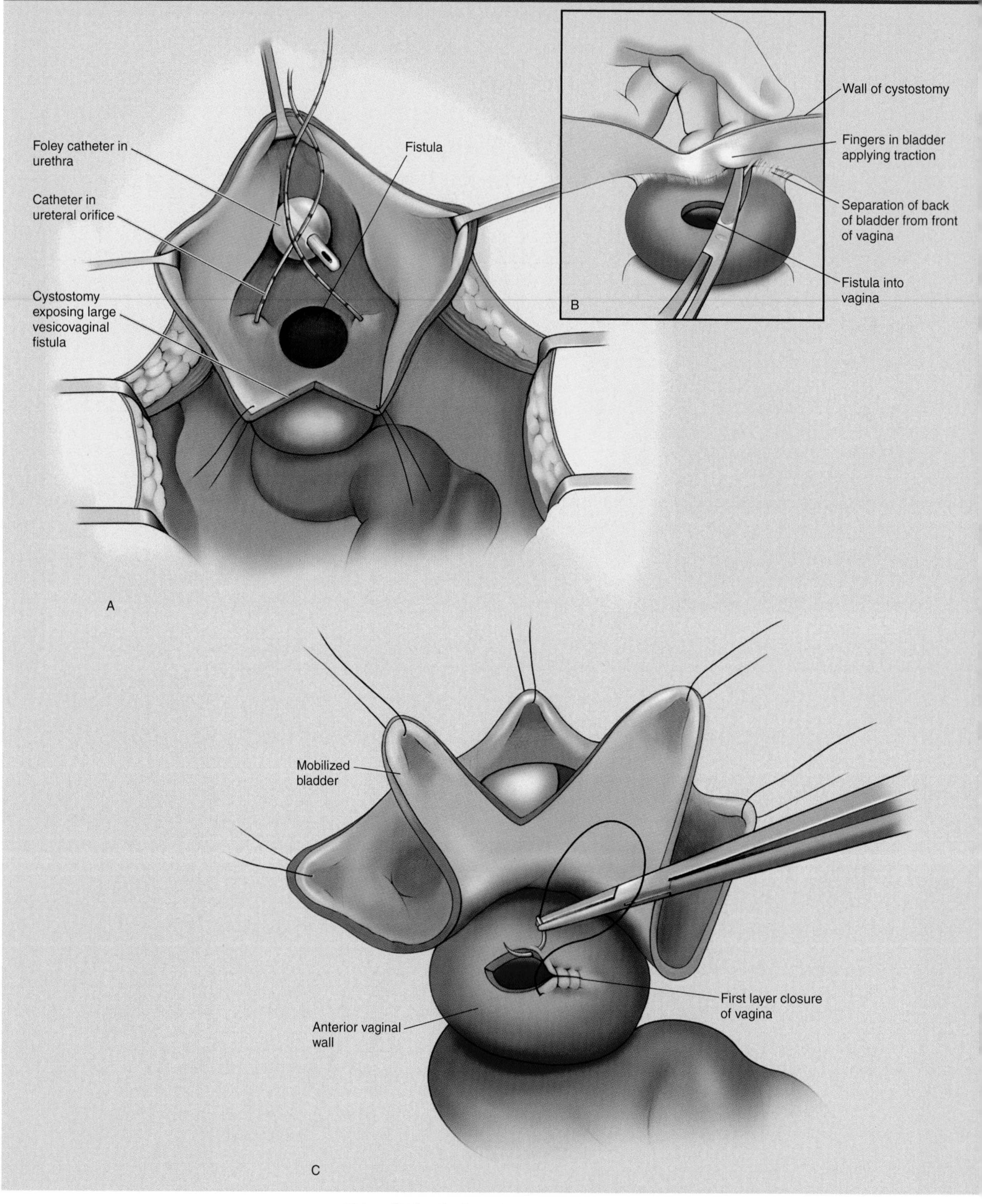

Foley catheter in urethra

Catheter in ureteral orifice

Cystostomy exposing large vesicovaginal fistula

Fistula

Wall of cystostomy

Fingers in bladder applying traction

Separation of back of bladder from front of vagina

Fistula into vagina

B

A

Mobilized bladder

Anterior vaginal wall

First layer closure of vagina

C

**Figure 29-8**   *For legend, see opposite page.*

**Transabdominal, transvesical closure of vesicovaginal fistula (O'Conor operation)**

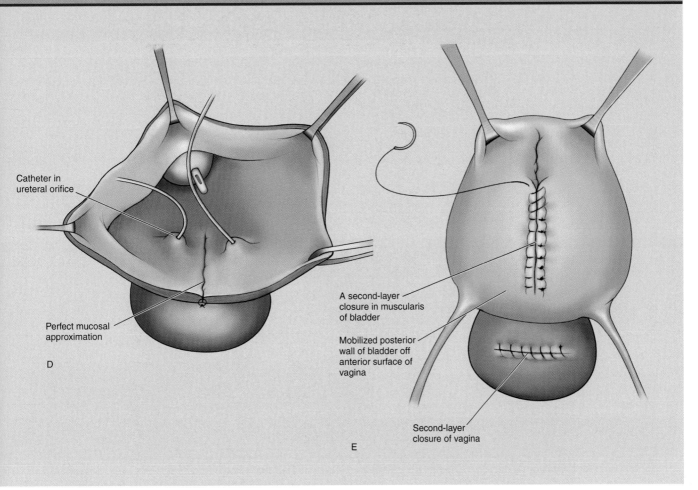

**Figure 29-8    Transperitoneal-transvesical vesicovaginal fistula repair.** *A,* The bladder is incised midline from its anterior portion back posteriorly until the fistula is reached; the fistula is excised, and the ureters are protected. *B,* Dissection is continued in the vesicovaginal space distal to the fistula to allow tension-free closure in layers. *C,* The vagina is closed with interrupted delayed absorbable suture with the knots located inside the vagina. *D,* The dependent portion of the bladder is closed with interrupted double-layer closure on the bladder and single-layer vaginal closure. *E,* The rest of the bladder incision is closed with running suture in two layers.

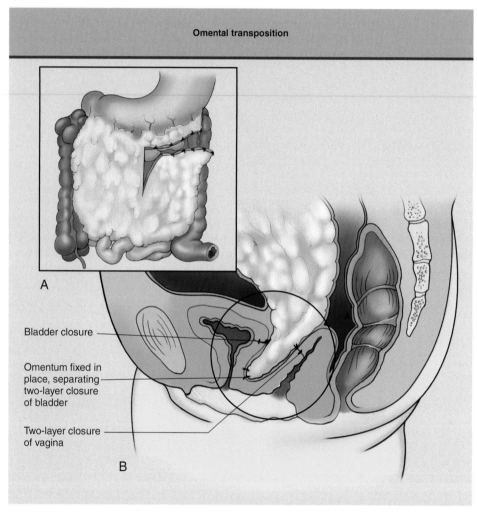

**Omental transposition**

A

Bladder closure

Omentum fixed in place, separating two-layer closure of bladder

Two-layer closure of vagina

B

**Figure 29-9    Omental transposition.** *A,* The omentum is detached by severing its vasculature on the left along the greater curvature of the stomach. *B,* This results in extra length so the flap will reach between the vagina and bladder, anchored by absorbable suture.

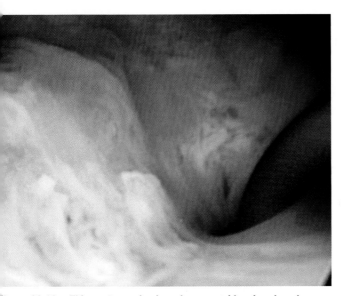

Figure 29-10    This cystoscopic view shows a guide wire placed through the fistula into the vagina, and the left ureteral orifice is seen just above it. This patient underwent a transvesical-transperitoneal fistula repair with left ureteroneocystostomy.

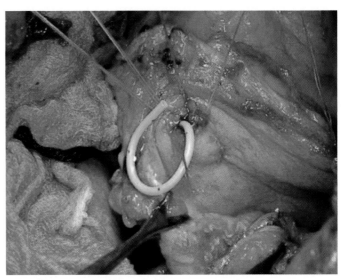

Figure 29-12    This intravesical view directed at the left dome shows the completed ureteroneocystostomy with double-J stent in place.

patients have severe pain associated with bladder spasms, and these may require belladonna and opioid (B&O) suppositories. For most patients, standard anticholinergic medication is sufficient to prevent these spasms.

Single-dose antibiotic prophylaxis is given prophylactically with a first-generation cephalosporin as in many other gynecologic surgery cases. The authors do not routinely give oral antibiotic prophylaxis even in the presence of bladder catheterization,

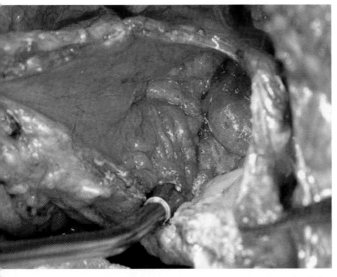

Figure 29-11    This intravesical view shows the completed repair of the most dependent portion of the bladder. The right ureteral orifice is in view near the incision line but not involved in it. The left orifice is no longer seen owing to its association with the fistula. Prior to closure of the bladder, the left ureter was identified and dissected retroperitoneally, tied off distally, then cut at the level of the cardinal ligament as close to the bladder as possible, in preparation for reimplantation.

especially with the liberal use of suprapubic catheters for these patients.

Vaginal packing rarely seems necessary following fistula surgery. Vaginal intercourse is prohibited for 2 to 3 months, to allow complete healing of the suture line. The use of vaginal estrogen cream is encouraged preoperatively and restarted 2 weeks following surgery to allow for re-epithelialization of the incision.

## RECTOVAGINAL FISTULAS

### Epidemiology and Risk Factors

Rectovaginal fistulas are uncommon, comprising less than 5% of all anorectal fistulas, but cause severe distress and discomfort to the patient and are a challenge for the operating gynecologist. They are classified on the basis of location, size, and etiology. Fistulas located between the lower third of the rectum and the lower half of the vagina are considered low, and those between the upper two thirds of the rectum and the upper vagina are considered high. Low rectovaginal fistulas are further characterized by whether they are associated with disruption of the anal sphincter or the perineum. They are, in most cases, less than one-half cm in diameter, although when they are caused by obstructive labor, they can involve loss of large areas of the rectovaginal septum.

Obstetric trauma such as perineal laceration or episiotomy, precipitous birth, forceps delivery, vacuum extraction, or unsuccessful attempts to repair 3rd or 4th degree tears may result in a low rectovaginal fistula. Prolonged labor may cause a wide area of ischemic injury of the rectovaginal septum with resulting large fistulas. Vaginal or rectal operative procedures such as hysterectomy, rectocele repair, hemorrhoidectomy, excision of rectal tumors, and low anterior resection can also result in rectovaginal fistulas. Perirectal abscesses when drained spontaneously or surgically may result in fistulas that open into

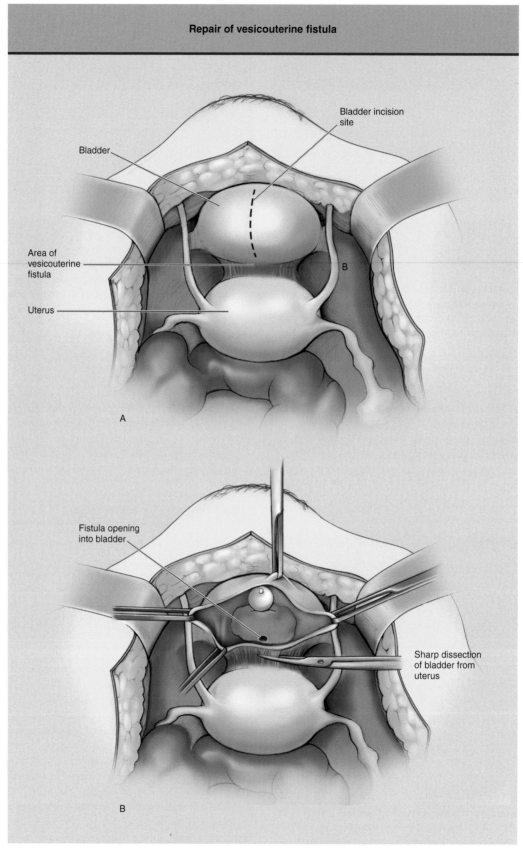

**Repair of vesicouterine fistula**

**A**

Bladder incision site

Bladder

Area of vesicouterine fistula

Uterus

B

**B**

Fistula opening into bladder

Sharp dissection of bladder from uterus

**Figure 29-13** **Vesicouterine fistula repair. Similar to the transperitoneal-transvesical approach depicted in Figure 29-8, except the fistula is located somewhat higher.** *A–C,* The bladder is incised in the midline, the fistula is identified, and the vesicouterine space is developed until the fistula is excised.

**Repair of vesicouterine fistula**

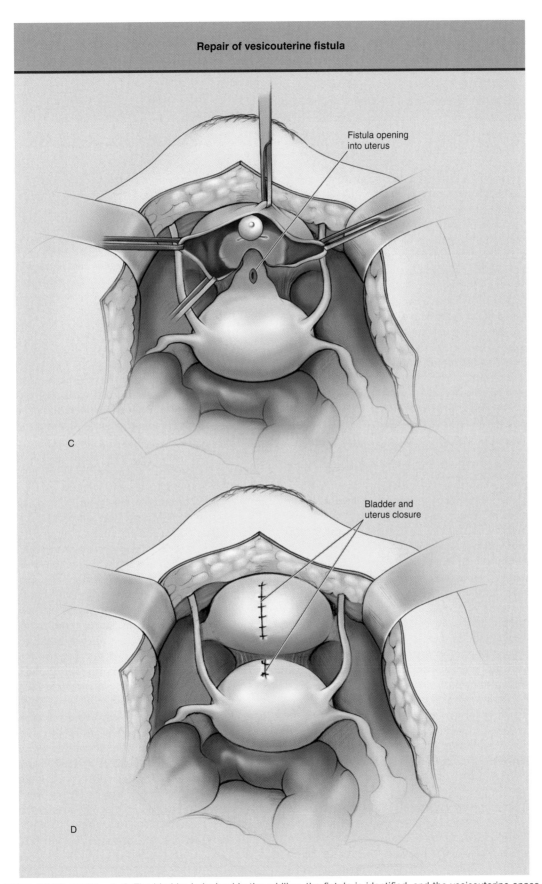

Fistula opening
into uterus

C

Bladder and
uterus closure

D

**Figure 29-13, cont'd**  *A–C,* The bladder is incised in the midline, the fistula is identified, and the vesicouterine space is developed until the fistula is excised. *D,* The uterine defect is closed with interrupted suture in one layer, and the bladder is closed in two layers similarly to the depiction in Figure 29-8.

the vagina or perineum. Traumatic penetrating or blunt trauma including forced coitus may also be responsible for development of rectovaginal fistulas.

Inflammatory bowel disease such as Crohn's or, much less commonly, ulcerative colitis is associated with rectovaginal fistula formation and should be strongly considered in any case of failed primary repair. A variety of infections including diverticulitis, Bartholin's gland abscess, lymphogranuloma venereum, tuberculosis, or human immunodeficiency virus (HIV) may be the underlying etiology.

Regressing or recurrent cervical, rectal, vaginal, or vulvar carcinoma or the neoadjuvant radiation therapy prescribed for these conditions may result in high rectovaginal fistulas. Radiation fistulas from external beam or intracavitary therapy may occur with risk being dependent on the dose and method of application. Fistulas noted in these settings must be carefully evaluated for cancer recurrence and always treated as complex fistulas, with a propensity for failure.

Obstetric injury is the most common etiology in the developing world, but many rectovaginal series in the western hemisphere also cite obstetric causes high in the list of etiologies. Although vesicovaginal fistula is the most frequent complication of obstructed labor in the developing world, rectovaginal fistulas have been seen in 17.4% of obstetric fistula patients.[9] In developed countries, rectovaginal fistulas after vaginal delivery are uncommon. A review of 20,500 vaginal deliveries in Arizona found only 25 patients (0.1%) who developed a rectovaginal fistula requiring surgical correction.[97]

## Clinical Features

Small rectovaginal fistulas may be entirely asymptomatic or intermittently so, often depending on stool consistency. When the fistulas are somewhat larger, escape of gas may be the only complaint, or a slight fecal odor can be detected in the vaginal discharge. When the fistula is large, the entire bowel content is evacuated through the vagina. Recurrent bouts of vaginitis and cystitis are common. When inflammatory bowel disease is the underlying etiology, bloody mucus and diarrhea are frequently noted.

The time from the initial insult to clinical presentation depends on the etiology of the fistula and the circumstances. Vaginal wall lacerations associated with unrecognized obstetric or operative injury typically present in the first 24 hours of the trauma. In the case of an apparently normal 4th degree laceration repair, infection or breakdown of the wound may occur within 7 to 10 days and result in formation of a rectovaginal fistula. In contrast, irradiation-induced fistulas are slowly progressive, and necrosis due to devascularization may become symptomatic a few months or even years after the original insult.

## Diagnosis

The diagnosis of simple rectovaginal fistulas usually can be accomplished by digital or anoscopic examination. In many instances merely spreading the labia and inspecting the posterior vagina and perineum may reveal the fistulous tract. A speculum can be used and rotated 90 degrees to show a more proximal fistula. The darker rectal mucosa can often be seen at the fistulous opening in contrast to the pink vaginal mucosa when the fistula is large. A pit or depression is palpable both rectally

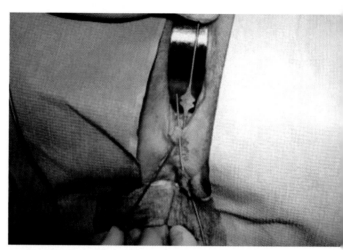

**Figure 29-14  Multiple rectovaginal and rectoperineal fistulas are identified in a patient referred for two previously failed attempts at repair.** This patient also required anal sphincteroplasty, perineorrhaphy, and reattachment of the distal rectovaginal fascia following excision of all the fistulous tracts.

and vaginally on rectovaginal or rectoperineal examination. After prior unsuccessful repair, multiple fistula tracts can often be identified by careful evaluation (Fig. 29-14). In cases in which there is difficulty in identifying the site of a small fistula despite strong clinical suspicion, filling the vagina with water and the rectum with air through a proctoscope will demonstrate bubbles rising from the fistula. If the fistula is still not demonstrated, a 20-minute ambulatory tampon test with methylene blue instilled into the rectum may help localize the fistula. If these diagnostic maneuvers are not successful, the fistula may be higher in the vagina and radiologic contrast studies are needed. This may include vaginography, barium enema, or CT scan with contrast. Proctosigmoidoscopy with biopsy should be used to exclude any underlying disease process whenever there is doubt regarding the specific etiology of a rectovaginal fistula.

Additional testing with endoanal ultrasound, anorectal manometry, and neurophysiologic studies may be useful in selected cases. It has been recommended that patients with rectovaginal fistulas secondary to obstetric injury be evaluated for occult sphincter defects, since they influence the outcome of repair as well as the type of repair used.[98] Improving and maintaining continence is just as important as healing the fistula in achieving a satisfactory outcome in the treatment of rectovaginal fistulas. The assessment for occult sphincter defects may be done by endoanal ultrasound and/or anorectal manometry. Most low rectovaginal fistulas of obstetric origin involve the anal sphincter, and success rates seem to be improved when concomitant anal sphincteroplasty is performed.[98–100] Conversely, abnormal neurophysiologic testing does not preclude surgical repair for a rectovaginal fistula with or without sphincteroplasty and is therefore not routinely used in this context.

## Management

Conservative management may be attempted in the hope of allowing spontaneous healing following a small rectovaginal istula of obstetric etiology; most, however, require surgical intervention. The timing of repair depends on the integrity and health of the surrounding tissues. All infections must be treated by appropriate drainage and antibiotics. Traditionally, postobstetric istulas required a waiting period of 3 to 6 months. However, earlier intervention is successful as long as the tissues remain oft, pliable, and adequately vascularized with no evidence of nflammation or infection. Vaginal estrogen cream and a bowel egimen including fiber supplementation to improve bowel transit and consistency may be used in preparation for surgery. t is not necessary, however, to unduly delay repair of a severely ymptomatic patient as long as the tissues appear healthy. In ontrast, attempted repair of irradiation-induced fistulas may equire up to a 1-year delay to ensure maximal resolution of issue necrosis. Rectovaginal fistulas associated with Crohn's lisease should be surgically repaired only after adequate therapy nd remission have been achieved.

The patient is carefully counseled prior to surgery regarding he route, success rate, and any associated procedures. Pre-perative standard mechanical bowel preparation is used, and prophylactic antibiotics are given intravenously 30 minutes prior o the procedure.

### Surgical Therapy

The type of surgical repair depends on the size, location, and tiology of the rectovaginal fistula as well as surgeon preference nd training. In the case of a simple low fistula, transperineal, ransvaginal, or transanal advancement flap closure may be elected. The transabdominal route of closure is often preferred or high rectovaginal fistulas. No adequately designed studies onfirm that any of the approaches is superior to the others.

Transperineal and transvaginal approaches have good success ates ranging from 85% to 100%.[101,102] In general, the trans-erineal approach is performed when the anal sphincters are nvolved and repair is necessary, or when the perineal body is leficient and a perineorrhaphy is planned. This approach may e started with a curvilinear incision along the anterior anal phincteric border with dissection continuing cephalad to the evel of the fistula and above. Alternatively, a transverse incision t the level of the posterior fourchette or dissecting off a riangular wedge of perineal skin may be used when deeper lissection is needed.

A fistulotomy involves cutting the entire bridge of perineal issue superficial to the fistula. This rarely is necessary, except when the rectoperineal fistula is very distal and superficial, hereby cutting only perineal skin.

Regardless of the incision used, the principles of repair are imilar for all transperineal approaches. Wide dissection of the ectovaginal space is achieved sharply distal, proximal, and lateral o the fistula, the fistula is excised and hemostasis achieved with uture ligature and light electrocautery as long as it is away from he incision's edge. Closure of the wound starts with the rectal nucosa using fine, delayed-absorbable suture and avoiding the owel lumen. Then the bowel serosa is imbricated on the first ayer, incorporating internal anal sphincter if it is disrupted with slightly larger caliber suture. This is followed by end-to-end epair of the external anal sphincter throughout its 4- to 5-cm ength, nearing the level of the levator ani muscle without

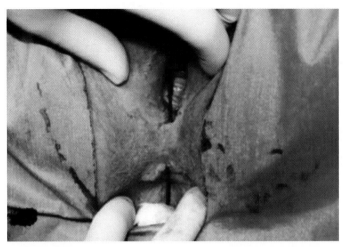

**Figure 29-15  A rectovaginal fistula involving the anal sphincters, with an attenuated perineal body.** This fistula was repaired via a transperineal approach, the rectovaginal space was dissected, and the fistula was excised.

plicating it (Figs. 29-15 and 29-16). Some authors prefer sphincteroplasty by an overlapping technique. If perineorrhaphy is needed, it is performed by plicating the posterior bulbocavernosus muscles in the usual fashion. The newly rebuilt perineal body is used to anchor the distal torn end of the rectovaginal fascia by means of proximal to distal stitches to avoid stenosis at the introitus. The vaginal mucosa is trimmed only enough to provide fresh edges for reapproximation. All stitches are interrupted to allow for careful apposition of surfaces with minimal distortion (Fig. 29-17).

A transvaginal approach is preferable for low fistulas that are proximal to the anal sphincters, or mid-vaginal fistulas, when no sphincteroplasty or perineorrhaphy is required. In all cases excision of the fistulous tract is advised with appropriate layered repair using interrupted delayed-absorbable sutures, avoiding

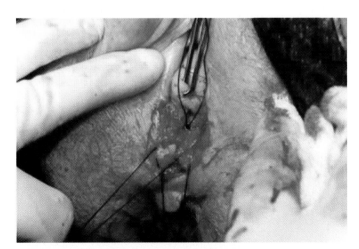

**Figure 29-16  Closure of the external anal sphincter muscle, after closure of the rectal mucosal layer, and the internal sphincter.** The authors prefer end-to-end repair including the entire 4 to 5 cm of its length. The uppermost suture in the photograph depicts the most proximal suture used; it is placed near the level of the levator ani.

**Repair of distal rectovaginal fistula involving the anal sphincter**

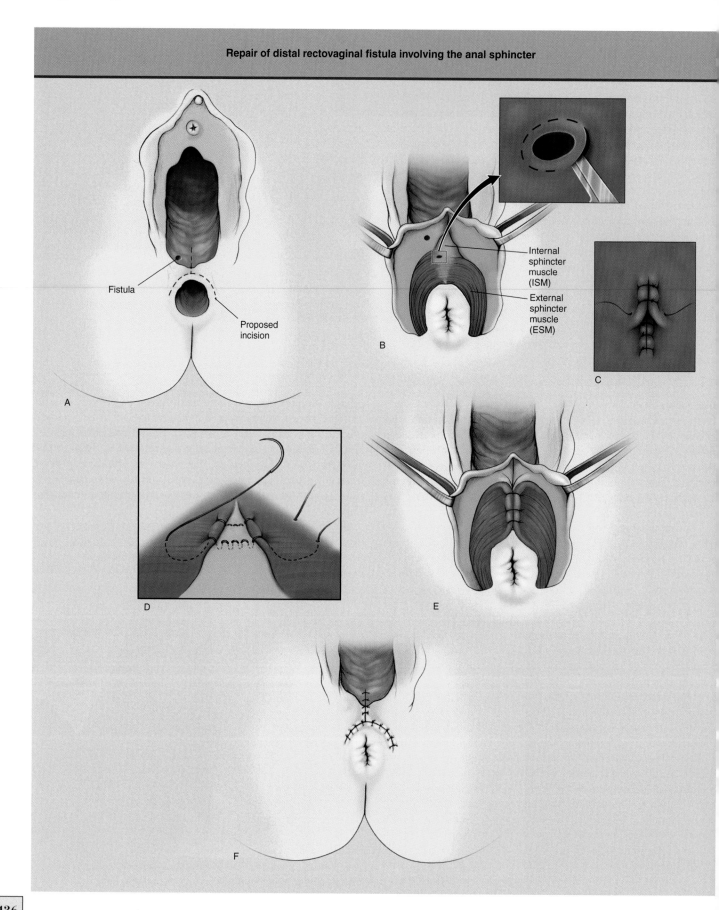

Fistula

Proposed
incision

A

Internal
sphincter
muscle
(ISM)

External
sphincter
muscle
(ESM)

B

C

D

E

F

sutures within the bowel lumen, followed by interrupted imbricating stitches (Fig. 29-18).

A Martius flap may be considered if it is a repeat repair and the tissue appears scarred, or in the case of a radiation fistula. Strong consideration for fecal diversion with colostomy should be given for patients with multiple recurrent and otherwise more complex rectovaginal fistulas.

Transanal advancement flaps are preferred by colorectal surgeons and have considerably varied success rates ranging from 41% to 100% when performed following obstetric injury.[99,103] When done in conjunction with sphincteroplasty, success rates approach about 95%.[100] Addition of a labial fat pad transposition did not appear to improve the results of transanal advancement flap repair in a report in the colorectal literature.[104]

Postoperatively, a liquid diet is recommended for several days. Pain control is administered by intravenous patient-controlled narcotics or epidural anesthesia. A Foley catheter is left in place for several days, and a low-residue diet prescribed with addition of stool softeners.

Small series of simple and recurrent rectovaginal fistulas have been treated with fibrin glue. In one report, 6 of 8 patients with recurrent rectovaginal fistulas were successfully treated.[105] This technique has not gained widespread popularity.

### Complicated Rectovaginal Fistulas

High rectovaginal fistulas and those resulting from recurrent persisting causes, radiation injury, or inflammatory bowel disease frequently require a transabdominal approach. Depending on the quality and blood supply of the tissue around the fistulous tract and the condition of the surrounding tissue, the repair may or may not require bowel resection. When the surrounding tissue is pliable without severe inflammation or scarring, the rectovaginal septum is dissected, the fistulous tract is divided and excised, and the rectal and the vaginal openings are closed primarily in layers. Interposition of an omental flap adds needed good vascularity to the area of the repair, and it will separate and support the suture lines. When the bowel is severely diseased, the involved segment has to be resected. Coloanal reconstruction with or without fashioning of a colonic reservoir pouch is preferred, often with temporary fecal diversion by a loop ileostomy.

Rectovaginal fistula associated with Crohn's disease is a difficult management problem. About 9% of the fistulas occurring in Crohn's disease are rectovaginal. The first line of treatment is medical, with surgical treatment being reserved for patients with persistent troublesome symptoms.

Irradiation-induced rectovaginal fistulas also present the surgeon with a difficult challenge. Adequate blood supply must be ensured, which is supplied by interposition of skeletal muscle with its blood and nerve supplies intact. Prior to any attempted repair, the presence of recurrent cancer must be excluded. It is important to document adequate sphincter function and absence of rectal stricture. Frequently, laparotomy is needed to expose the fistula and accomplish adequate dissection, although transvaginal repair has also reportedly been successful. The fibrotic margins of the fistulas are excised, and the vagina and bowel wall are separated. Subsequently, the freed rectal mucosa and submucosa around the fistula opening is closed transversely. Bulbocavernosus or gracilis muscle is mobilized on its vascular pedicle with preservation of nerve supply and swung to the fistula site through a subcutaneous tunnel under the labia and vaginal mucosa and sutured adjacent to the repaired fistula.[106-108] Transabdominally, an omental flap can serve as a source of a new blood supply and is often used for supporting the repair. A diverting colostomy is used to protect the surgical site. It can be reversed in 3 to 6 months.

---

**Figure 29-17** *(facing page)* **Low rectovaginal fistula involving the anal sphincter.** *A,* A transperitoneal approach is depicted that starts with an anterior perianal curvilinear incision, with midline extension. *B,* Dissection is carried up to the fistula, which is excised, and the vagina is further mobilized off the rectum proximally, medially, and laterally. Closure of the rectal defect is accomplished with interrupted delayed-absorbable suture, ensuring lack of tension on the suture line. *C,* The second layer should incorporate the internal anal sphincter and is closed with interrupted delayed absorbable suture. *D,* The external anal sphincter closure begins proximally near the levator ani incorporating internal sphincter muscle when possible. *E,* The interrupted sphincter closure stitches are tied. *F,* Perineorrhaphy, if needed, is achieved by unification of the posterior-most aspect of the bulbocavernosus muscle in the midline to rebuild an attenuated perineal body. Following vaginal mucosal trimming, closure completes the repair, ensuring that introital narrowing has not occurred.

**Repair of low rectovaginal fistula with intact perineum**

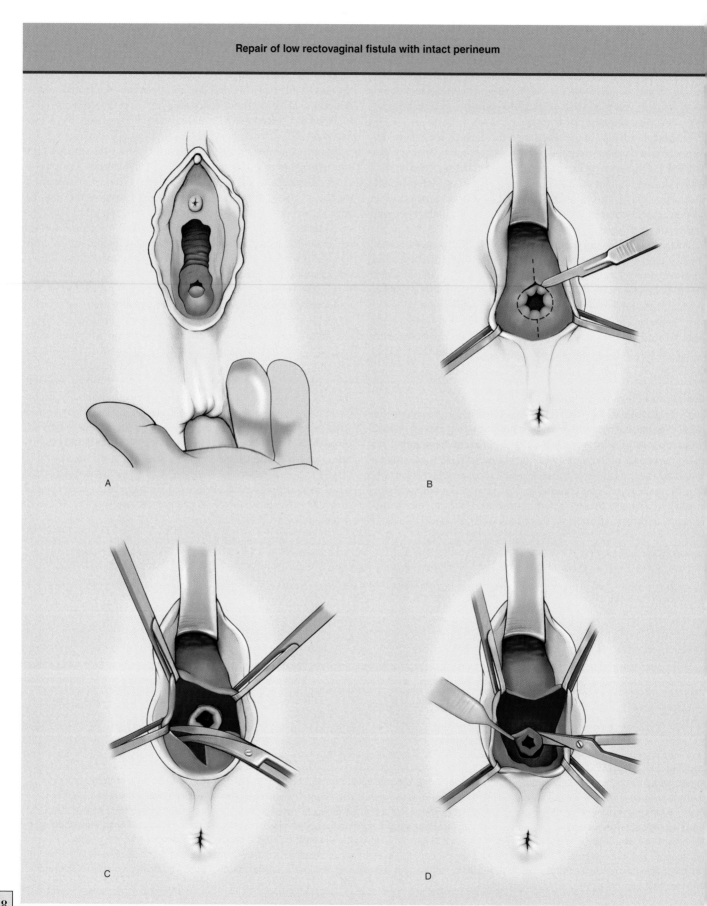

A

B

C

D

**Figure 29-18**  *For legend, see opposite page.*

**Rectovaginal fistula repair**

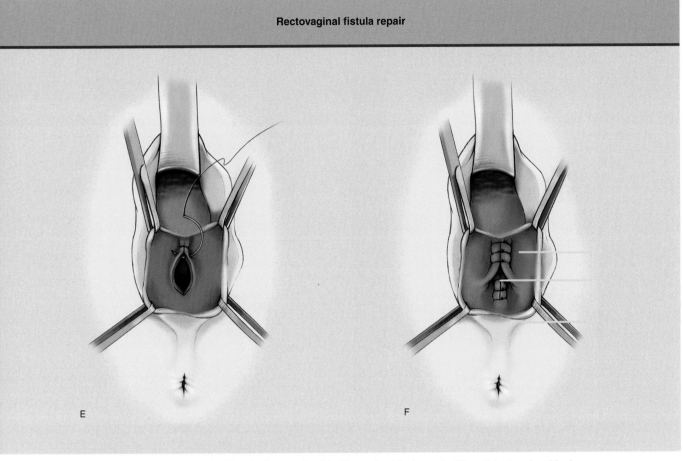

E                                                            F

**Figure 29-18   A low rectovaginal fistula, but proximal to the anal sphincter and with an intact perineal body.**
*A,* Some authors consider this a mid-vaginal fistula. Repair involves circumcision of the fistulous tract *(B),* dissection of
the vagina off the rectum *(C),* excision of the fistula *(D),* and closure of the rectal defect in two layers *(E),* followed by
vaginal mucosal closure *(F).*

# REFERENCES

1. Bai SW, Kim SH, Kwon HS, et al: Surgical outcome of female genital fistula in Korea. Yonsei Med J 2002;43:315–319. **(III, B)**

2. Asanuma H, Nakai H, Shishido S, et al: Congenital vesicovaginal fistula. Int J Urol 2000;7:195–198. **(III, B)**

3. Hilton P, Ward A: Epidemiological and surgical aspects of urogenital fistulae: a review of 25 years' experience in southeast Nigeria. Int Urogynecol J 1998;9:189–194. **(III, B)**

4. Ibrahim T, Sadiq AU, Daniel SO: Characteristics of VVF patients as seen at the specialist hospital Sokoto, Nigeria. West Afr J Med 2000; 19:59–63. **(III, B)**

5. Vangeenderhuysen C, Prual A, Ould el Joud D: Obstetric fistulae: incidence estimates for sub-Saharan Africa. Int J Gynecol Obstet 2001;73:65–66. **(III, B)**

6. Waaldijk K, Armiya'u D: The obstetric fistula: a major public health problem still unsolved. Int Urogynecol J 1993;4:126–128. **(IV, C)**

7. Ojanuga Onolemhemhen D, Ekwempu CC: An investigation of socio-medical risk factors associated with vaginal fistula in northern Nigeria. Women Health 1999;28:103–116. **(IIa, B)**

8. Hilton, P: Vesico-vaginal fistulas in developing countries. Int J Gynecol Obstet 2003;82:285–295. **(III, B)**

9. Arrowsmith S, Hamlin EC, Wall LL: Obstructed labor injury complex: obstetric fistula formation and the multifaceted morbidity of maternal birth trauma in the developing world. Obstet Gynecol Surv 1996; 51:568–574. **(III, B)**

10. Tahzib F: Vesicovaginal fistula in Nigerian children. Lancet 1985; 2(8467):1291–1293. **(III, B)**

11. Tahzib F: Epidemiological determinants of vesicovaginal fistulas. Br J Obstet Gynaecol 1983;90:387–391. **(III, B)**

12. Porcaro AB, Zicari M, Zecchini S, et al: Vesicouterine fistulas following cesarean section. Int Urol Nephrol 2002;34:335–344. **(III, B)**

13. Jozwik M, Jozwik M, Lotocki W: Actual incidence and cause of vesico-uterine fistula. Br J Urol 1998;81:341–342. **(IV, C)**

14. Flores-Carreras O, Cabrera JR, Galeano PA, et al: Fistulas of the urinary tract in gynecologic and obstetric surgery. Int Urogynecol J 2001;12:203–214. **(III, B)**

15. Hemal AK, Kumar R, Nabi G: Post-cesarean cervicovesical fistula: technique of laparoscopic repair. J Urol 2001;165:1167–1168. **(III, B)**

16. Billmeyer BR, Nygaard IE, Kreder KJ: Ureterouterine and vesi-coureterovaginal fistulas as a complication of cesarean section. J Urol 2001;165:1212–1213. **(III, B)**

17. Gil A, Sultana CJ: Vesicouterine fistula after vacuum delivery and two previous cesarean sections: a case report. J Reprod Med 2001; 46:853–855. **(III, B)**

18. Yip SK, Fung HY, Wong WS, et al: Vesico-uterine fistula—a rare complication of vacuum extraction in a patient with previous caesarean section. Br J Urol 1997;80:502–503. **(III, B)**

19. Miklos JR, Sze E, Parobeck D, et al: Vesicouterine fistula: a rare complication of vaginal birth after cesarean. Obstet Gynecol 1995; 86:638–639. **(III, B)**

20. McKay HA, Hanlon K: Vesicovaginal fistula after cervical cerclage: repair by transurethral suture cystorrhaphy. J Urol 2003;169:1086–1087. **(III, B)**

21. Kleeman SD, Vasalle B, Segal J, et al: Vesicocervical fistula following insertion of a modified McDonald suture. Br J Obstet Gynaecol 2002; 109:1408–1409. **(III, B)**

22. Golomb J, Ben-Chaim J, Goldwasser B, et al: Conservative treatment of a vesicocervical fistula resulting from Shirodkar cervical cerclage. J Urol 1993;149:833–834. **(III, B)**

23. Lee RA, Symmonds RE, Williams TJ: Current status of genitourinary fistula. Obstet Gynecol 1988;72:313–319. **(III, B)**

24. Harkki-Siren P, Sjoberg J, Tiitinen A: Urinary tract injuries after hysterectomy. Obstet Gynecol 1998;92:113–118. **(III, B)**

25. Armenakas NA, Pareek G, Fracchia JA: Iatrogeic bladder perforations: long term follow-up of 65 patients. J Am Coll Surg 2004;198:78–82. **(III, B)**

26. Carley ME, McIntire D, Carley JM, et al: Incidence, risk factors and morbidity of unintended bladder or ureter injury during hysterectomy. Int Urogynecol J 2002;13:18–21. **(II, B)**

27. Wattiez A, Soriano D, Cohen SB, et al: The learning curve of total laparoscopic hysterectomy: comparative analysis of 1647 cases. J Am Assoc Gynecol Laparosc 2002;9:339–345. **(III, B)**

28. Tancer ML: Observations on prevention and management of vesico-vaginal fistula after total hysterectomy. Surg Gynecol Obstet 1992; 175:501–506. **(III, B)**

29. Mulvey S, Foley M, Kelley DG, et al: Urinary tract fistulas following gynaecological surgery. J Obstet Gynaecol 1998;18:369–372. **(III, B)**

30. Tancer ML: A report of thirty-four instances of urethrovaginal and bladder neck fistulas. Surg Gynecol Obstet 1993;177:77–80. **(III, B)**

31. Eilber KS, Kavaler E, Rodriguez LV, et al: Ten-year experience with transvaginal vesicovaginal fistula repair using tissue interposition. J Urol 2003;169:1033–1036. **(III, B)**

32. Gerstenbluth RE, Goldman HB: Simultaneous urethral erosion of tension-free vaginal tape and woven polyester pubovaginal sling. J Urol 2003;170(2 pt 1):525–526. **(III, B)**

33. Glavind K, Larsen EH: Results and complications of tension-free vaginal tape (TVT) for surgical treatment of female stress urinary incontinence. Int Urogynecol J 2001;12:370–372. **(III, B)**

34. Pruthi RS, Petrus CD, Bundrick WS: New onset vesicovaginal fistula after transurethral collagen injection in women who underwent cystectomy and orthotopic neobladder creation: presentation and definitive treatment. J Urol 2000;164:1638–1639. **(III, B)**

35. Carlin BI, Klutke CG: Development of urethrovaginal fistula following periurethral collagen injection. J Urol 2000;164:124. **(III, B)**

36. Okafor PI, Orakwe JC, Mbonu OO: Cyclical haematuria sequel to uterine myomectomy: a case report. West African J Med 2002; 21:341–342. **(III, B)**

37. Krissi H, Levy T, Ben-Rafael Z: Fistula formation after large loop excision of the transformation zone in patients with cervical intra-epithelial neoplasia. Acta Obstet Gynecol Scand 2001;80:1137–1138. **(III, B)**

38. Lodh U, Kumar S, Arya MC, et al: Ureterouterine fistula as a complication of an elective abortion. Aust N Z J Obstet Gynaecol 1996; 36:94–95. **(III, B)**

39. Villasanta U: Complications of radiotherapy for carcinoma of the uterine cervix. Am J Obstet Gynecol 1972;114:717–726. **(III, B)**

40. Davies Q, Luesley DM: Urological problems and the treatment of gynaecological cancer. Curr Opin Obstet Gynecol 1998;10:401–403. **(III, B)**

41. Horch RE, Gitsch G, Schultze-Seemann W: Bilateral pedicled myocutaneous vertical rectus abdominis muscle flaps to close vesicovaginal and pouch-vaginal fistulas with simultaneous vaginal and perineal reconstruction in irradiated pelvic wounds. Urology 2002; 60:502–507. **(III, B)**

42. El-Shalakany AH, Nasr El-Din MH, Wafa GA, et al: Massive vault necrosis with bladder fistula after uterine artery embolization. BJOG 2003;110:215–216. **(III, B)**

43. Sultana CJ, Goldberg J, Aizenman L, et al: Vesicouterine fistula after uterine artery embolization: a case report. Am J Obstet Gynecol 2002;187:1726–1727. **(III, B)**

44. Monteiro H, Nogueira R, deCarvalho H: Behçet's syndrome and vesicovaginal fistula: an unusual complication. J Urol 1995; 153:407–408. **(III, B)**

45. Bland KG, Gelfand M: The influence of urinary bilharziasis on vesico-vaginal fistula in relation to causation and healing. Trans R Soc Trop Med Hyg 1970;64:588–592. **(III, B)**

46. Goel A, Dalela D, Gupta S, et al: Pediatric tuberculous vesicovaginal fistula. J Urol 2004;171:389–390. **(III, B)**

47. Singh A, Fazal AR, Sinha SK, et al: Tuberculous vesicovaginal fistula in a child. Br J Urol 1988;62:615. **(III, B)**

48. Ghatak DP: A study of urinary fistulae in Sokoto, Nigeria. J Indian Med Assoc 1992;90:285–287. **(III, B)**

49. Huang CR, Sun N, Wei-ping, et al: The management of old urethral injury in young girls: analysis of 44 cases. J Pediatr Surg 2003; 38:1329–1332. **(III, B)**

50. Bittard H, Bernardini S, Khenifar E, et al: Uretero-vesical rupture with vaginal fistula following pelvic fracture: value of early diagnosis and emergency surgery. J Urol (Paris) 1995;101:159–162. **(III, B)**

51. Cass AS, Luxenberg M: Management of extraperitoneal ruptures of bladder caused by external trauma. Urology 1989;33:179–183. **(III, B)**

52. Roy KK, Vaijyanath AM, Sinha A, et al: Sexual trauma—an unusual cause of a vesicovaginal fistula. Eur J Obstet Gynecol Reprod Biol 2002;101:89–90. **(III, B)**

53. Sharma SK, Madhusudnan P, Kumar A, et al: Vesicovaginal fistulas of uncommon etiology. J Urol 1987;137:280. **(III, B)**

54. Ramaiah KS, Kumar S: Vesicovaginal fistula following masturbation managed conservatively. Aust N Z J Obstet Gynaecol 1998; 38:475–476. **(III, B)**

55. Fourie T, Ramphal S: Aerosol caps and vesicovaginal fistulas. Int J Gynaecol Obstet 2001;73:275–276. **(III, B)**

56. Arikan N, Turkolmez K, Aytac S, et al: Vesicovaginal fistula associated with a vaginal foreign body. Br J Urol Int 2000;85:375–376. **(III, B)**

57. Dodero D, Corticelli A, Caporale E, et al: Endometriosis arises from implant of endometriotic cells outside the uterus: a report of active vesicouterine centrifugal fistula. Clin Exp Obstet Gynecol 2001; 28:97–99. **(III, B)**

58. Lovatsis D, Drutz HP: Persistent vesicovaginal fistula associated with endometriosis. Int Urogynecol J 2003;14:358–359. **(III, B)**

59. Staskin D, Malloy T, Carpiniello V, et al: Urological complications secondary to a contraceptive diaphragm. J Urol 1985;134:142–143. **(III, B)**

60. Grody MHT, Nyirjesy P, Chatwani A: Intravesical foreign body and vesicovaginal fistula: a rare complication of a neglected pessary. Int Urogynecol J 1999;10:407–408. **(III, B)**

61. Goldstein I, Wise GJ, Tancer ML: A vesicovaginal fistula and intra-vesical foreign body: a rare case of the neglected pessary. Am J Obstet Gynecol 1990;163:589–591. **(III, B)**

62. Szabo Z, Fiscor E, Hyiradi J, et al: Rare case of the utero-vesical fistula caused by intrauterine contraceptive device. Acta Chir Hung 1997; 36(1–4):337–339. **(III, B)**

63. Buckley P, McInerney PD, Stephenson TP: Actinomycotic vesico-uterine fistula from a wishbone pessary contraceptive device. Br J Urol 1991;68:206–207. **(III, B)**

64. Dalela D, Goel A, Shakhwar SN, et al: Vesical calculi with unrepaired vesicovaginal fistula: a clinical appraisal of an uncommon association. J Urol 2003;170(6 pt 1):2206–2208. **(III, B)**

65. Meeks GR, Sams JO, Field KW, et al: Formation of vesicovaginal fistula: the role of suture placement into the bladder during closure of the vaginal cuff after transabdominal hysterectomy. Am J Obstet Gynecol 1997;177:1298–1304. **(Ib, A)**

66. Cogan SL, Paraiso MFR, Bedaiwy MA: Formation of vesicovaginal fistulas in laparoscopic hysterectomy with electrosurgically induced cystotomy in female mongrel. Am J Obstet Gynecol 2002; 187:1510–1514. **(Ib, A)**

67. Volkmer BG, Kuefer R, Nesslauer T, et al: Colour Doppler ultrasound in vesicovaginal fistulas. Ultrasound Med Biol 2000;26:771–775. **(III, B)**

68. Hilton P: Urodynamic findings in patients with urogenital fistulae. Br J Urol 1998;81:539–542. **(III, B)**

69. Thomas K, Williams G: Medicolegal aspects of vesicovaginal fistulae. BJU Int 2000;86:354–359. **(IV, C)**

70. Sokol AI, Paraiso MFR, Cogan SL, et al: Prevention of vesicovaginal fistulas after laparoscopic hysterectomy with electrosurgical cystotomy in female mongrel dogs. Am J Obstet Gynecol 2004;190:628–633. **(Ib, A)**

71. Sims JM: On the treatment of vesico-vaginal fistula. Int Urol J 1998; 9:236–248. **(IV, C)**

72. Goh JT, Howat P, deCosta C: Oestrogen therapy in the management of vesicovaginal fistula. Aust N Z J Obstet Gynaecol 2001; 41:333–334. **(III, B)**

73. Dogra PN, Nabi G: Laser welding of vesicovaginal fistula. Int Urogynecol J 2001;12:69–70. **(III, B)**

74. Morita T, Tokue A: Successful endoscopic closure of radiation induced vesicovaginal fistula with fibrin glue and bovine collagen. J Urol 1999; 162:1689. **(III, B)**

75. Kanaoka Y, Hirai K, Ishiko O, et al: Vesicovaginal fistula treated with fibrin glue. Int J Gynecol Obstet 2001;73:147–149. **(III, B)**

76. Cruikshank SH: Early closure of posthysterectomy vesicovaginal fistulas. South Med J 1988;81:1525–1528. **(III, B)**

77. Blandy JP, Badenoch DF, Fowler CG, et al: Early repair of iatrogenic injury to the ureter or bladder after gynecological surgery. J Urol 1991;146:761–765. **(III, B)**

78. Blaivas JG, Heritz DM, Romanzi LJ: Early versus late repair of vesicovaginal fistulas: vaginal and abdominal approaches. J Urol 1995; 153:1110–1112. **(III, B)**

79. Langkilde NC, Torsten KP, Lundbeck F, et al: Surgical repair of vesicovaginal fistulae. Scand J Urol Nephrol 1999;33:100–103. **(III, B)**

80. Hadley HR: Vesicovaginal fistula. Curr Urol Rep 2002;3:401–407. **(IV, C)**

81. Akman RY, Sargin S, Ozdemir G, et al: Vesicovaginal and ureterovaginal fistulas: a review of 39 cases. Int Urol Nephrol 1999; 31:321–326. **(III, B)**

82. Carr LK, Webster GD: Abdominal repair of vesicovaginal fistula. Urology 1996;48:10–11. **(IV, C)**

83. Leng WW, Amundsen CL, McGuire EJ: Management of female genitourinary fistulas: transvesical or transvaginal approach? J Urol 1998;160:1995–1999. **(III, B)**

84. Nesrallah LJ, Srougi M, Gittes RF: The O'Conor technique: the gold standard for supratrigonal vesicovaginal fistula repair. J Urol 1999; 161:566–568. **(III, B)**

85. Mondet F, Chartier-Kastler EJ, Conort P, et al: Anatomic and functional results of transperitoneal-transvesical vesicovaginal fistula repair. Urology 2001;58:882–886. **(III, B)**

86. Miller EA, Webster GD: Current management of vesicovaginal fistulae. Curr Opin Urol 2001;11:417–421. **(IV, C)**

87. O'Conor VJ, Sokol JK: Vesicovaginal fistula from the standpoint of the urologist. J Urol 1951;66:579–585. **(III, B)**

88. Landes RR: Simple transvesical repair of vesicovaginal fistula. J Urol 1979;122:604–606. **(III, B)**

89. Gil-Vernet JM, Gil-Vernet A, Campos JA: New surgical approach for treatment of complex vesicovaginal fistula. J Urol 1989;141:513–516. **(III, B)**

90. Goodwin WE, Scardino PT: Vesicovaginal and ureterovaginal fistulas: a summary of 25 years of experience. J Urol 1980;123:370–374. **(III, B)**

91. Evans DH, Madjar S, Politano VA, et al: Interposition flaps in transabdominal vesicovaginal fistula repairs: are they really necessary? Urology 2001;57:670–674. **(III, B)**

92. Rangnekar NP, Ali NI, Kaul SA, et al: Role of the martius procedure in the management of urinary-vagina fistulas. J Am Coll Surg 2000; 191:259–263. **(IIa, B)**

93. Punekar SV, Buch DN, Soni AB, et al: Martius labial fat pad interposition and its modification in complex lower urinary fistulas. J Postgrad Med 1999;45:69–73. **(III, B)**

94. Fujiwara K, Koshima I, Tanaka K, et al: Radiation induced vesicovaginal fistula successfully repaired using gracilis myocutaneous flap. Int J Clin Oncol 2000;5:341–344. **(III, B)**

95. Viennas LK, Alonso AM, Salama V: Repair of radiation-induced vesicovaginal fistula with a rectus abdominis myocutaneous flap. Plast Reconstr Surg 1995;96:1435–1437. **(III, B)**

96. Bruce RG, El-Galley RES, Galloway NTM: Use of rectus abdominis muscle flap for the treatment of complex and refractory urethrovaginal fistulas. J Urol 2000;163:1212–1215. **(III, B)**

97. Venkatesh KS, Ramanujam PS, Larson DM, et al: Anorectal complications of vaginal delivery. Dis Colon Rectum 1989;32:1039–1041. **(III, B)**

98. Yee LF, Birnbaum EH, Read TE, et al: Use of endoanal ultrasound in patients with rectovaginal fistulas. Dis Colon Rectum 1999; 42:1057–1064. **(III, B)**

99. Tsang CB, Madoff RD, Wong WD, et al: Anal sphincter integrity and function influences outcomes in rectovaginal fistula repair. Dis Colon Rectum 1998;41:1141–1146. **(III, B)**

100. Khanduja KS, Padmanabhan A, Kerner BA, et al: Reconstruction of rectovaginal fistula with sphincter disruption by combining rectal mucosal advancement flap and anal sphincteroplasty. Dis Colon Rectum 1999;42:1432–1437. **(III, B)**

101. Tancer ML, Lasser D, Rosenblum N: Rectovaginal fistula or perineal and anal sphincter disruption, or both, after vaginal delivery. Surg Gynecol Obstet 1990;171:43–46. **(III, B)**

102. Wiskind AK, Thompson JD: Transverse transperineal repair of rectovaginal fistulas in the lower vagina. Am J Obstet Gynecol 1992; 167:694–669. **(III, B)**

103. Khanduia KS, Yamashita HJ, Wise WE, et al: Delayed repair of obstetric injuries of the anorectum and vagina: a stratified surgical approach. Dis Colon Rectum 1994;37:344–349. **(III, B)**

104. Zimmerman DDE, Gosselink MP, Briel JW, et al: The outcome of transanal advancement flap repair of rectovaginal fistulas is not improved by an additional labial fat flap transposition. Tech Colorproctol 2002:6:37–42. **(III, B)**

105. Venkatesh KS, Ramanujam P: Fibrin glue application in the treatment of recurrent anorectal fistulas. Dis Colon Rectum 1999;42:1136–1139. **(III, B)**

106. White AJ, Buchsbaum JH, Blythe JG, et al: Use of the bulbocavernosus muscle (martius procedure) for repair of radiation-induced rectovaginal fistulas. Obstet Gynecol 1982;60:114–118. **(III, B)**

107. Aartsen EJ, Sindram IS: Repair of the radiation induced rectovaginal fistulas without or with interposition of the bulbocavernosus muscle (martius procedure). Eur J Surg Oncol 1988;14:171–177. **(III, B)**

108. Rius J, Nessim A, Nogueras JJ, et al: Gracilis transposition in complicated perianal fistula and unhealed perineal wounds in Crohn's disease. Eur J Surg 2000;166:218–222. **(III, B)**

# Chapter 30

# Puberty and Precocious Puberty

Alexandra S. Carey, MD, and Pamela J. Murray, MD, MPH

## KEY POINTS

- The sequence and duration of pubertal events is relatively predictable, but there is a wide range of ages at which puberty begins.
- The decline in the age of menarche has stabilized, but there is an observable trend toward an earlier onset of puberty in American girls.
- African American girls are observed to begin puberty earlier than white girls. The significance of this trend is controversial.
- Multiple factors play a role in the timing of puberty. Genetics is still thought to have a substantial influence in the timing of normal puberty.
- It may be difficult to distinguish normal early puberty from precocious puberty.
- True precocious puberty is usually idiopathic in girls, but it is considered a diagnosis of exclusion. In boys, underlying CNS or other pathology must always be considered.
- Isolated premature pubarche is associated with an increased future risk of polycystic ovary syndrome, hyperandrogenism, and insulin resistance.

## INTRODUCTION

Puberty is a dramatic transition in a child's life, marking the change from childhood to adulthood. The changes that take place during puberty are physical, emotional, and physiological. These changes begin across a broad range of ages, with clearly recognized differences between the sexes. Although the timing of pubertal events varies, the stages of puberty occur in a predictable pattern and the overall length of pubertal development is constant (about 3 to 5 years). An understanding of normal pubertal development is required to diagnose and manage related disorders, particularly precocious puberty, delayed puberty, and other growth and maturational problems.

Precocious puberty is the onset of one or more pubertal signs, including secondary sex traits and accelerated growth, before the age that is 2 standard deviations below the mean age for the onset of puberty (Fig. 30-1).[1] In recent years the determination of when puberty is "precocious" in girls has been challenged. The mean age of the signs most associated with pubertal onset—breast development and pubic hair growth—has decreased. Complete data are still lacking on the age range of the onset of normal puberty. The majority of girls who develop signs of

puberty at an early age have no underlying disease, but determining what is "normal" early puberty versus "precocious" early puberty is not always straightforward. The diagnosis of precocious puberty is challenging and currently controversial. As appropriate, analogous states in males are presented.

The terminology used to describe precocious puberty varies, particularly when differentiating gonadotropin-releasing hormone (GnRH)–dependent, or "true," precocious puberty from other classifications of early or precocious puberty (GnRH-independent). See list of Key Terms used to describe puberty and precocious puberty. When interpreting relevant literature and communicating information, the use of specific and correct terminology is critical.

### Historical Definition

The reference standard of the normal onset and stages of puberty is based on older studies. The data collection and the resultant constructs of Tanner were revolutionary at the time. The 1969 article by Marshall and Tanner that launched "Tanner staging" included 192 white British girls from a single socioeconomic class.[2] The standard definition of precocious puberty uses Tanner staging as a clinical metric and is defined as secondary sexual development in females less than 8 years of age and secondary sexual development in males less than 9. Menarche at less than 10 is also considered precocious. This historical definition also assumes accelerated linear growth and bone maturation accompanying the changes in breasts, pubic hair, and genitals.

### Historical Trends

The factors that eventually lead to the onset of puberty are still incompletely understood. Menarche is an objective marker of puberty. Mean age of menarche has decreased over the past century. Better socioeconomic conditions and improved nutrition and general health have been associated with a secular trend toward earlier puberty. The average age of menarche has slowly decreased by 2 to 3 months per decade in industrialized European countries over the past 150 years up until the late 1970s (Fig. 30-2). In the mid-19th century the average age of menarche was 17 years in the United States, 15 years in France, and 17 years in Scandinavia.[3]

This trend to an earlier age of menarche has since abated. A decrease of about 2.5 to 4 months in age of menarche has been found over a 25-year period, which has also paralleled an increase in body mass index (BMI), although no direct relationship between menarche and BMI has been found.[4,5] African American females, on average, attain menarche earlier than white

# Pediatric and Adolescent Gynecology

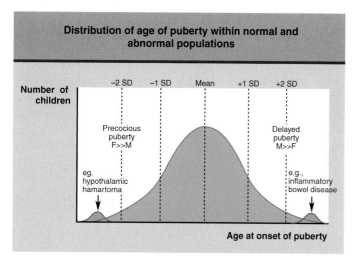

**Figure 30-1    The classic distribution of the age of onset of puberty within normal and abnormal populations.** (From Palmert MR, Boepple PA: Variation in the timing of puberty: clinical spectrum and genetic investigation. J Clin Endocrinol Metab 2001;86:2364–2368.) Copyright 2001. The Endocrine Society.

### Table 30-1
### Age of Menarche in NHE and NHANES III by Race

| | Age of Menarche (yr) | | |
| --- | --- | --- | --- |
| Study | African American Girls | White Girls | All Girls |
| NHE (1963–1970) | 12.48 | 12.8 | 12.75 |
| NHANES III (1988–1994) | 12.14 | 12.6 | 12.54 |

NHE, National Health Examination; NHANES III, National Health and Nutrition Examination Survey, cycle III (studies by National Center for Health Statistics).

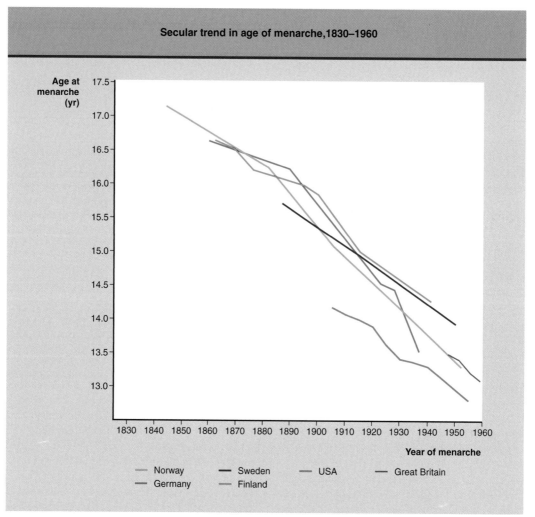

**Figure 30-2    The decreasing age of menarche over time.** (From Tanner JM: Growth at Adolescence, 2nd ed. Oxford, Blackwell Scientific, 1962, p 153.)

**Table 30-2**
**Factors Postulated to Influence Timing of Onset of Puberty**

- BMI and body composition
- Central nervous system (CNS) disease or insult
- Emotional stress or abuse
- Endocrine disorders
- Environment, e.g., geography, toxins
- Ethnicity
- Genetics, e.g., maternal history, congenital pathology
- Leptin
- Nutrition

females, but this recent trend is not consistently associated with an increase in weight in African American females (Table 30-1).

In spite of relatively stable economic conditions in the United States and a relatively constant mean age of menarche, a trend toward an earlier onset of puberty in American girls has been reported.[6] This trend toward an earlier onset of puberty raises questions regarding the interplay of known and unknown factors that contribute to pubertal timing. The factors that are thought to play a role in the timing of the onset of puberty are listed in Table 30-2.

## Current Observed Trends

The overall duration of puberty is related to its age of onset. Girls with a later onset have a slightly shorter duration of puberty and girls with an earlier onset have a longer duration.[7] Apter, from a study of a cohort of Scandinavian women, concludes that the earlier the age of menarche, the shorter the interval to regular ovulation.[8] The "earlier maturers" with menarche before 11 years have 50% of their cycles ovulatory in 6 months, "average maturers" reach this in 2 years, and "late maturers" (14+ years) take an average of 4.5 years until 50% of their cycles are ovulatory. Another contemporary trend is the correlation between earlier onset of puberty and ethnicity, with African American girls and other populations observed to start puberty at an earlier age than white American girls. This trend is likely related to genetics and lifestyle differences between these groups. The major lifestyle changes that affect growth and pubertal development are diet and exercise, with other environmental factors (food additives and topical personal care products) potentially involved but less well understood. The causes of the epidemic of childhood obesity in America contribute to earlier onset of puberty, and African American girls are more overweight and exercise less than white American girls.[9] This observation that obesity correlates with earlier onset of puberty has led to multiple hypotheses and studies regarding the role and interplay of obesity, ethnicity, genetics, and puberty.

## Contemporary Studies and Reevaluation of the Definition of Precocious Puberty

The classic definition of when puberty is early or precocious was challenged by the 1997 Herman-Giddens study through the American Academy of Pediatrics (AAP) Pediatric Research in Office Settings (PROS) Study. The PROS study was a large cross-sectional study involving 65 pediatric practices across the country with a total of 17,077 female patients included in the final study and data analysis. Only white and African American

girls were included because other races made up only 2.8% of the group. The age range was 3 to 12 years and included 9.6% African Americans and 90.4% white females, all undergoing complete physical examinations. Hispanic girls were included in both the African American and the white groups. Breast development was recorded by inspection in the majority of participants, but 39% of the sample also had their breast Tanner staging performed by inspection and palpation.[10] The study concluded that the mean age at which African American girls were exhibiting signs of puberty was 8.87 years for breast development and 8.78 years for pubic hair growth, whereas the mean age at which white American girls were starting puberty was 9.96 years for breast development and 10.51 years for pubic hair growth. Therefore, a substantial number of girls are starting puberty even earlier than these means. The study found the age of menarche to be stable compared with earlier population studies of the 1970s (National Health Examination [NHE] and others). Table 30-3 lists the significant findings from this study.

The Herman-Giddens study, with a large cohort, suggests that an earlier onset of pubertal signs is occurring but has some notable limitations. The age of menarche has not changed significantly in the past 50 years, although there is a difference between the average age of menarche in white girls and African American girls, as noted in the National Health and Nutrition Examination Study (NHANES) III study and reproduced in the PROS study. The PROS study has led to a great deal of debate on what the diagnostic guidelines should be for defining when and why precocious or early puberty occurs. The pros and cons of the PROS study are outlined in Table 30-4.

Based on the PROS study, the Lawson Wilkins Pediatric Endocrine Society proposed new guidelines for differentiating the signs of early puberty from the diagnosis of precocious puberty. The pediatric endocrine society performed a comprehensive review of the data on which the existing definitions were based and critically examined the data from the PROS study. The recommendation with the most clinical impact was that the age at which the signs of puberty would be considered precocious would be lowered to less than 6 years in African American females and less than 7 years in white females in otherwise healthy children. A summary of their findings is listed in Table 30-5.

There has been ongoing controversy over these new guidelines, and some endocrinologists have issued statements challenging

**Table 30-3**
**Significant Racial Differences in Puberty, from PROS Study**

|  | Black Girls | White Girls |
|---|---|---|
| Mean age of onset of any development | 8.11 years | 9.71 years |
| Mean age of menarche | 12.11 years | 12.88 years |
| Breast development at 7 years | 15.44% | 4.97% |
| Breast development at 8 years | 37.76% | 10.5% |
| Pubic hair growth at 7 years | 17.65% | 2.75% |
| Pubic hair growth at 8 years | 34.27% | 7.67% |

PROS, Pediatric Research in Office Settings (study by American Academy of Pediatrics).

# Pediatric and Adolescent Gynecology

| Table 30-4<br>Pros and Cons of PROS Study | |
|---|---|
| **Pro** | **Con** |
| No other large-scale studies of racially diverse girls in the United States to assess changes over time in the age of pubertal onset | A selection bias may exist in that younger females with advanced development were more likely to come in for physical examinations |
| Addresses the need for current, demographically relevant standards for assessment of the onset of pubertal changes in females | No data included on endocrine evaluations pursued in early developers as young as age 3 years<br>No information on possible pathologic conditions that may have been missed |
| Large number of subjects included and therefore may be more representative than current "norms" | Not a population-based sample, as girls were drawn only from pediatric practices over a limited period of time, making it a broad convenience, but not necessarily a representative sample |
| Impossible to assess secular trends from one generation to the next without such data | The study recognizes early pubertal signs, but it does not follow the progression through the final stages of puberty and does not include data on more advanced stages of puberty |
| Clinicians have relied on Marshall and Tanner's classic studies on pubertal changes in girls despite their limitations | Most breast examinations were by inspection without palpation. Subcutaneous fatty tissue may have been reported as breast buds |
| The trends in pubarche parallel thelarche | |

PROS, Pediatric Research in Office Settings (study by American Academy of Pediatrics).

them.[11,12] The traditional older age limits for defining precocious puberty are still used in Europe.

A subsequent study by endocrinologists (Midyett et al) contests the Lawson Wilkins guidelines. Midyett maintains that if the new guidelines are followed, there will be underdiagnosis of serious endocrine conditions.[13] This was a retrospective chart review of 223 patients referred for sexual precocity occurring between 7 and 8 years in white females and 6 and 8 years

| Table 30-5<br>Primary Conclusions of Lawson-Wilkins Pediatric Endocrine Society Regarding Precocious Puberty |
|---|
| 1. The current recommendation that breast development at less than 8 years of age is precocious is based on outdated studies. |
| 2. Stage 2 breast development and pubic hair development is being attained 1 year earlier in white females and 2 years earlier in African American females than previous studies demonstrated. |
| 3. The concern that females with moderate precocious puberty will be significantly shorter adults is overstated. The majority will have final height that is within normal limits. |
| 4. In most females with onset of puberty between 6 and 8 years, GnRH agonist therapy will not have a significant effect on adult height. |
| 5. Females with breast development or pubic hair should be evaluated if this is occurring before age 7 years in white females and before age 6 years in African American females. |

| Table 30-6<br>Findings of Midyett Chart Review[13] Regarding Precocious Puberty |
|---|
| 1. 12.3% of patients referred to Midyett et al endocrine clinic with signs of precocious puberty had underlying pathologic conditions. |
| 2. The pathologic conditions that were diagnosed did not include idiopathic precocious puberty. |
| 3. One third of the girls with two signs of precocious puberty (breast and pubic hair development) had a bone age more than three standard deviations above the mean. |
| 4. A subset of girls with isolated breast development were found to have advanced bone age. |
| 5. Although weight and body mass index (BMI) correlate positively with benign earlier sexual development, a substantial number of girls with serious endocrine conditions were obese. |
| 6. The authors conclude that all girls less than 8 years of age with secondary sexual development (one or more signs) deserve at least a bone age measurement and close longitudinal follow-up. |

in black females. The major findings of the study are listed in Table 30-6.

In view of this recent conflicting data, primary practitioners need to be cautious in their approach to the early occurring signs of puberty. The defining age of sexual precocity does not have an absolute or universally accepted answer. Therefore, the approach to early developers cannot be guided by age alone, except in the more extreme cases of girls 6 years of age or younger and boys less than 9 years old, where prompt evaluation by a pediatric endocrinologist is the standard of care.

## NORMAL PUBERTY

During puberty the central nervous system (CNS) and peripheral endocrine organs interact to initiate and sustain a reproducible series of endocrine changes. These changes occur in three endocrine axes: the adrenal glands (adrenarche), the gonads (gonadarche), and the growth hormone–insulin-like growth factor axis, "somatarche." The gonadal and growth hormone system are integrated with one another and the hypothalamic-pituitary-gonadal (HPG) axis. Adrenarche appears to be an independent process. These changes result in the acquisition of secondary sexual traits, a marked increase in growth and change in body composition, as well as psychological changes. They mark the physical and psychological transition from childhood to adulthood, with the physiologic endpoint of reproductive ability.

### Fetal, Infant, and Childhood Pubertal Endocrinology

Normal development at puberty requires a functioning hypothalamic-pituitary-gonadal axis (Fig. 30-3). GnRH is present in the hypothalamus by 14 weeks' gestation and functionally active by 20 weeks' gestation, stimulating follicle-stimulating hormone (FSH) and luteinizing hormone (LH) production. FSH and LH concentrations attain adult levels at midgestation and then fall secondary to negative feedback from pregnancy steroids. By 20 weeks' gestation the pituitary is sensitive to the negative feedback of sex steroids on FSH and LH production.

"In utero" the sex steroids and gonadotropins stimulate germ cell division and follicular development, so that by midgestation the primordial ovarian follicles reach their maximum number

## Hypothalamic-pituitary-gonadal axis

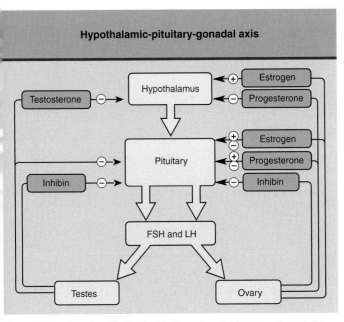

**Figure 30-3** **The hypothalamic-pituitary-gonadal (HPG) axis and the feedback effect of gonadal hormones.** (From Blair JC, Savage MO: Normal and abnormal puberty. In Besser GM, Thorner MO [eds]: Comprehensive Clinical Endocrinology, 3rd ed. Spain, Mosby, 2002, p 319.)

## Variations in oocyte number and sex hormones from early gestation to late adolescence

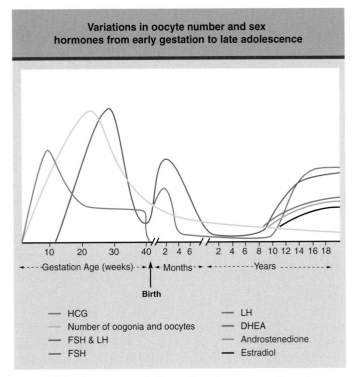

**Figure 30-4** **Serum concentrations of sex hormones and oocytes over time.** (From Speroff L, Glass RH, Kase NG [eds]: Clinical Gynecologic Endocrinology and Infertility, 6th ed. Baltimore, Lippincott Williams & Wilkins, 1999, p 382.)

and then decrease logarithmically throughout life until menopause, when they are depleted.

At birth, sex steroids, LH, and FSH are elevated but decrease postpartum. The gonadotropins and sex steroids peak in the first few months of life and then drop to low levels until puberty, although FSH levels may not be suppressed maximally until 1 to 4 years. Gonadotropin levels are lowest during mid-childhood (until 6 to 8 years). Prepubertal girls typically have lower LH to FSH ratios. Figure 30-4 depicts the changing serum concentrations of sex hormones from gestation through 18 years. The suppression of gonadotropins during childhood is dependent on a sensitive negative feedback mechanism of low level estrogen on the hypothalamus and pituitary, and there appears to be an intrinsic central inhibitory influence on GnRH.

## Hormonal Changes at Puberty

The hormonal changes that occur at puberty are due to a complex interplay of the HPG axis, with the adrenal gland functioning independently of the HPG axis. The initial pubertal changes of the hypothalamus and pituitary involve an increase in GnRH, LH, and FSH secretion in a distinctive pulsatile pattern. These hormonal changes of puberty, in general, begin 2 years before the onset of physical changes.

### GnRH and Gonadotropins

The pulsatile secretion of GnRH by the hypothalamus, released from its inhibition by the central CNS influence, is the initiator of puberty, although a decrease in the sensitivity to the negative feedback of estrogen also plays a role. GnRH is a decapeptide and is released in a pulsatile fashion. There are multiple influences on GnRH synthesis, including higher cortical centers, the limbic system, neurotransmitters, sex steroids, and gonadal peptides. GnRH binds to receptors in the anterior pituitary that synthesize

and store FSH and LH. FSH and LH are glycoproteins. Each is composed of two dissimilar peptide subunits, the alpha and beta chains. The $\alpha$ chains are similar in structure, but the $\beta$ subunit is unique and gives specificity from one hormone to the other.

GnRH gradually increases in amplitude and frequency as puberty progresses. Renewed GnRH secretion first occurs during sleep and leads to reactivation of gonadotropin synthesis and secretion. At the onset of puberty, GnRH has a priming influence on the pituitary, leading to progressive increase in LH and FSH, as well as an increase in GnRH receptors in the pituitary.

### Gonadotropins and Gonadarche

The increase in gonadotropins and sex steroids from the gonad and adrenal cortex occurs before the clinical onset of puberty. At the beginning of puberty, there is an increase in pulsatile FSH and LH secretion during sleep. As puberty progresses, this reverts to an absolute increase in daytime secretion and a relative decrease in nighttime secretion. The change is more marked for LH than for FSH, with LH levels continuing to rise as puberty progresses. The steady rise of LH secretion is marked by an increase in both pulse frequency and amplitude, especially pulse amplitude. FSH increases in amplitude but not in frequency early in puberty. A rise in FSH levels is observed before a rise in LH in females, and FSH secretion in females is greater than in males throughout puberty. Similar patterns may also be found in the reactivation of the HPG axis after suppression by disease, starvation, stress, and anorexia nervosa.

### Ovarian Maturation

FSH stimulates follicular growth of the ovary, starting at the onset of puberty. FSH stimulation and secretion lead to ovarian

447

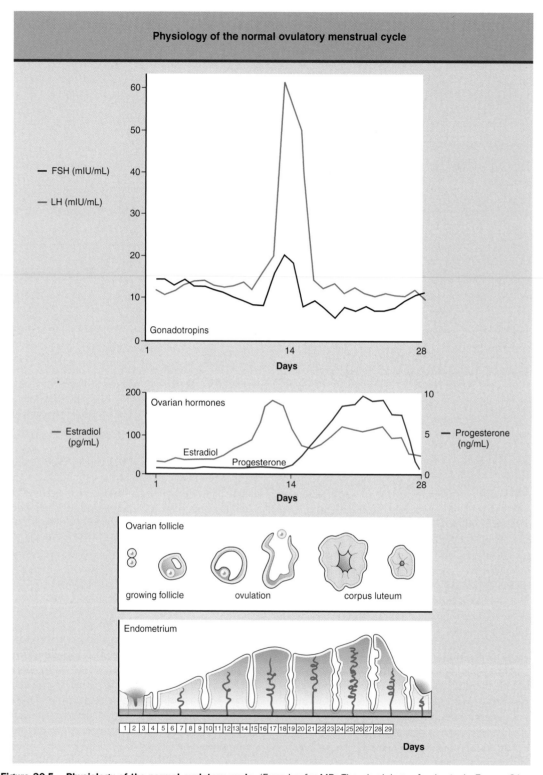

**Figure 30-5   Physiology of the normal ovulatory cycle.** (From Laufer MR: The physiology of puberty. In Emans SJ, Laufer MR, Goldstein DP [eds]: Pediatric and Adolescent Gynecology, 5th ed. Philadelphia, Lippincott-Raven, 2005, p 145.)

aromatase conversion of androgens to estrogens. Progesterone secretion increases with pubertal progression and leads to mitosis and maturation of follicular development. Mitosis leads to an increase in the layers of granulosa cells and to an increase in intercellular fluid rich in inhibin B and FSH. LH receptors increase as cell numbers increase and the ovary becomes more sensitive to LH stimulation. LH, in turn, increases the production of progesterone and androgens.

Estrogen levels rise as puberty progresses and eventually act on the hypothalamus to increase GnRH pulse amplitude. Estrogen production induces a positive feedback loop, leading to an increase in the gonadotropin surge and higher LH levels. At the same time that estrogen is enhancing the LH response, inhibin inhibits the FSH response. As LH reaches its peak levels by mid to late puberty, associated with episodic peaks of estradiol, menarche occurs. Ovulatory cycles start after a positive feedback loop is firmly established when increasing levels of estrogen trigger a midcycle LH surge. The timing at which ovulatory cycles begin to occur regularly is, on average, 2 years after menarche, but this varies considerably. The physiology of the normal ovulatory menstrual cycle is shown in Figure 30-5.

### Inhibin, Activin, and Follistatin

Inhibin, activin, and follistatin are polypeptide hormones that are synthesized in various body tissues, including the gonads, where they are secreted at their highest levels. These hormones have different local action in different tissues. Each acts to either increase (activin) or decrease (inhibin and follistatin) FSH synthesis at the pituitary level. They have been found to play a role in pubertal development, including modulation of steroid secretion in the ovary and adrenal gland. The extent of their role in puberty and reproduction is being actively investigated.[14]

### Sex Hormone–Binding Globulin

Sex hormone–binding globulin (SHBG) is a β-globulin protein that binds and transports sex steroids in plasma. Before puberty the levels of SHBG are about equal in males and females, and most estradiol and testosterone molecules are bound to SHBG reversibly. SHBG begins to decrease as pubertal age advances, and there is a consequent increase in the free or active hormones. By the end of puberty, males have one half the concentration of SHBG as females. SHBG levels may be included or implied in the battery of tests performed in obtaining a free testosterone level. Testosterone and elevated insulin levels are known to decrease SHBG levels, and estrogen increases SHBG production.

### Adrenarche

*Adrenarche* is defined endocrinologically by the increase in adrenal androgens that begins 2 years before and continues during puberty. Increased secretion of adrenal androgens occurs, including dehydroepiandrosterone (DHEA), its sulfated product (DHEAS), and androstenedione (AND). Clinically the term is also used to describe the development of pubic and axillary hair that occurs at puberty. Pubarche specifically refers to the growth of pubic hair; however, it is often used interchangeably with adrenarche to include other clinical manifestations of androgen-stimulated maturation, including acne and other skin changes, body odor, and axillary hair growth. Increases in adrenal androgen

| Table 30-7 |
| --- |
| **Chronologic Sequence of Hormonal Events of Puberty** |

**Adrenal axis**

Increase in adrenal androgens
 Dehydroepiandrosterone (DHEA)
 Dehydroepiandrosterone sulfate (DHEAS)
 Androstenedione (AND)

**Hypothalamic-Pituitary-Gonadal (HPG) axis**

Increase in GnRH frequency and amplitude
Increase in basal luteinizing hormone (LH) and follicle-stimulating hormone (FSH) concentrations
Increase in LH/FSH ratio
Increase in estradiol and testosterone
Increase in growth hormone (GH) and insulin-like growth factor 1 (IGF-1)

secretion precede the rise in gonadotropins and subsequent activation of the HPG axis, but they can overlap. Adrenarche is not under direct control of the HPG axis, and it can progress without gonadarche, as is seen in Turner's syndrome, congenital adrenal hyperplasia (CAH), and adrenal hyperandrogenism. The chronologic sequence of the hormonal events of puberty is presented in Table 30-7.

## CLINICAL SIGNS OF PUBERTY

The clinical signs of puberty occur in a generally predictable pattern in both males and females; however, there is significant variation in the onset and duration of puberty for both sexes. The first signs of puberty occur between 8 and 13 years in the majority of females and between 9.8 and 14.2 years in most males.

### Females

Usually the first sign of puberty is accelerated growth after a decrease in height velocity that precedes puberty. This is usually followed by thelarche, but either may be the cardinal sign. The sequence of pubertal events in females is listed in Table 30-8. Thelarche occurs in response to estrogen, which stimulates

| Table 30-8 |
| --- |
| **Sequence of Pubertal Development in Females** |

- Increase in growth velocity—usually the first event but can overlap with breast budding; evident by rapid change in shoe size
- Adrenarche—development of body odor and skin changes; overlaps with increase in growth velocity and thelarche
- Thelarche (or breast buds)—occurs within 1 year of the growth spurt
- Pubarche—occurs within 6 months of breast budding; the two may overlap
- Peak height velocity—occurs within 1 to 2 years of breast budding, usually at Tanner stage 2–3
- Axillary hair growth—usually occurs 1 to 2 years after pubarche
- Physiologic leukorrhea (estrogen-stimulated clear, milky vaginal discharge)— occurs 6 or more months before menarche
- Menarche—occurs within 2 years of breast budding in the majority; usually occurs within 1 year after peak height velocity, at Tanner stage 3–4
- Ovulation—can begin episodically at any time around menarche; regular ovulation can occur within 6 months of menarche and as late as 5 years after menarche, but the majority of cycles are ovulatory within 5 years of menarche

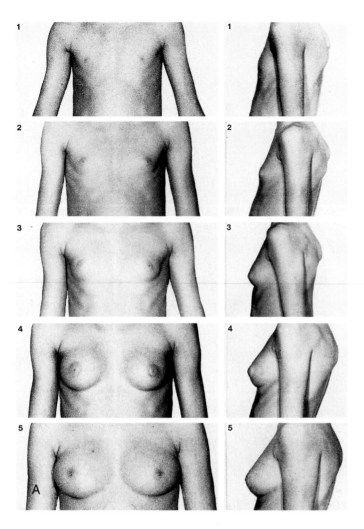

A

B

growth of the breast ductal system and the accumulation of fat. Together these produce changes in the contour of the breast. Initial breast development can be unilateral or bilateral, and this asymmetry is often more marked in premenarchal girls, often causing concern in patients and their parents. Breast tenderness in early puberty is common. There are variations in the progression of breast development. Some girls progress from Tanner stage 3 directly to Tanner stage 5 breast development, whereas others stay at Tanner stage 4 without progression to Tanner stage 5. Female Tanner staging is demonstrated in Figure 30-6.

In about 20% of girls, pubarche is the first sign of puberty, but through most of puberty the stage of breast development coincides with that of pubic hair development. Pubarche in females is dependent on adrenal androgens; however, pubic hair will not usually advance beyond Tanner stage 3 in the absence of gonadal sex steroids. Pubic hair is initially fine and sparse, and changes in quality to become coarser, curlier, and denser as puberty progresses. It expands in distribution, and should be detectable even in the presence of shaving or other hair removal techniques.

The peak height velocity usually occurs 1 to 2 years after the first appearance of breast buds, at Tanner breast stage 2–3 and precedes menarche by up to 1 year. After menarche growth rate decelerates and most girls do not grow much more than 5–6 cm thereafter. Puberty that begins earlier generally has a slightly longer duration.

Menarche is a later pubertal event, usually occurring 2 years after thelarche. This timing may vary, and menarche can occur from 1 to 5 years after thelarche, although a 5-year interval is unusual and warrants close surveillance. Menarche occurs at Tanner breast stage 3–4 in at least 75% of pubertal girls. The mean age for the onset of menstruation is 12.8 years in white American females and 12.2 in African American females.

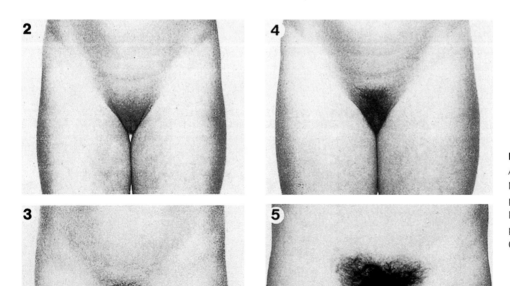

**Figure 30-6   Female Tanner stages.**
*A,* Breasts. *B,* Pubic hair. (From Marshall WA, Tanner JM: Variations in pattern of pubertal changes in girls. Arch Dis Child 1969;44:291–301. Reprinted by permission from the BMJ Publishing Group.)

The great majority of American girls (94%) have obtained menarche by 14 years. The first menstrual cycles are typically anovulatory.

### Vaginal, Uterine, and Ovarian Changes

Estrogen produces changes in vaginal contour, color, mucosa, and pH. Dulling of the vaginal mucosa occurs because of the cornification of epithelial cells. Before menarche, a clear, white vaginal discharge is noted, which is termed *leukorrhea*. Leukorrhea is desquamated epithelial cells and mucous from estrogenized mucosa. It can begin before thelarche. Unopposed estrogen exposure can cause profuse vaginal secretions with a problematic discharge that may decrease with maturity and concomitant progesterone secretion. It can be quite bothersome to the patient. As puberty progresses the vaginal pH decreases. There is also thickening of the labia majora, labia minora, and hymen. The decrease in vaginal pH allows for yeast colonization with consequent potential for infections that are microbiologically different from the typical infections of prepuberty (with gram-positive cocci and gram-negative rods) that cause vulvovaginitis.

The vagina also grows in size. The ovaries and uterus undergo substantial changes with the progression of puberty. In the years preceding puberty and as puberty progresses, the ovaries increase in size and volume and show evidence of active follicular growth and atresia. Small "cysts" are common in prepubertal ovaries (5 to 7 mm), and are usually asymptomatic. They can be an incidental finding on ultrasound. Follicular activity may be noted on ultrasound in mid to late puberty. Initially small and then larger follicular cysts appear and regress. It is common to see multiple small ovarian cysts or follicles on pelvic ultrasound during late puberty. The uterus increases in size and volume and changes shape from tubular to bulbous. These changes in the female genital tract are described in more detail in Table 30-9.

### Males

The first sign of puberty in males is testicular enlargement, with a volume of 4 mL corresponding with the onset of puberty. The

**Table 30-9**
**Changes in Gynecologic Anatomy and Physiology from Birth to Postmenarche**

| | Newborn | Early Childhood | Peripuberty (8–13 yr) | Postmenarche (>13 yr) | |
|---|---|---|---|---|---|
| Ovary | Not palpable 0.1–0.2 mL | Pelvic brim 0.7–0.9 mL | Within pelvis 2–10 mL | 1.5 × 2.5 × 4 cm 15 mL | |
| Uterine length (cm) | 2.5–4.0 | 2.0–3.0 | 3.2–5.4 | 8.0 (nulliparous) (8 × 5 × 2.5) | |
| Corpus-cervix ratio | 3:1 | 2:1 | 1:1 | 2–3:1 | |
| Vaginal length (cm) | 4 | 4–5 | 7–8.5 | 10–12 | |
| Hymen | | | | | |
|   Orifice diameter (mm) | 1–4 | 1–6 | 5–10 | 10 | |
|   Thickness | Thick | Thin | Thickening | – | |
| Clitoris | | | | | |
|   Width (mm) | 5 | 2–5 | 2–5 | ≤10 | |
|   Length (mm) | 10–15 | | | 15–20 | |
| Labia minora | Smooth | Smooth, flat | Progressive increase in size and texture | Tanner stages IV–V completed | |
| Labia majora | Hairless, prominent | Hairless, thin | Hair growth, vulval growth | Separation and differentiation of labia minora and majora | |
| Vaginal secretions | Whitish-clear, copious | Minimal | Physiologic leukorrhea | Physiologic leukorrhea may decrease | |
|   pH | 5.5–7.0 | 6.5–7.5 | 4.5–5.5 | 3.5–5.0 | |
|   Normal flora | Maternal enteric | Nonpathogenic flora including staphylococci and coliforms | Mixed vaginal flora | Lactobacilli dominant | |
| Hormonal influence | Maternal hormones | Minimal sex steroids | Low and variable levels of endogenous estrogen and androgens | High levels of endogenous cyclic hormones | |
| Maturation index of vaginal epithelium | | | | Proliferative phase* | Secretory phase† |
|   Parabasal (%) | 0 | 90–100 | 20–70 | 0 | 0 |
|   Intermediate (%) | 95 | 0–10 | 25–50 | 70 | 95 |
|   Superficial (%) | 5 | 10 | 10–20 | 30 | 5 |

*First half of cycle.
†Second half of cycle.
From Murray PM, Davis HW: Pediatric and Adolescent Gynecology. In Zitelli BJ, Davis HW (eds): Atlas of Pediatric Physical Diagnosis, 4th ed. St. Louis, Mosby, 2002, p 611.

| Table 30-10 |
| --- |
| **Sequence of Pubertal Development in Males** |

- Testicular enlargement (>2.5 mm) and thinning of scrotal skin
- Pubic hair growth—usually occurs 6 months after testicular enlargement is first noted
- Penile growth—occurs around the same time as pubic hair growth (the two may overlap); growth initially occurs in length and then in width
- Transient gynecomastia (symmetric or asymmetric)—usually seen at Tanner stage 2–3; occurs secondary to estrogen stimulation and is benign in the majority of cases
- Axillary hair growth—occurs about 1 year after pubic hair growth
- Peak height velocity—occurs at Tanner stage 3–4, at a mean age of 14 years
- Fertility—usually occurs at Tanner stage 4 but may occur earlier
- Facial and body hair, voice change—may begin at Tanner stage 3–5 but progresses for several years after puberty is complete

stimulated by androgen) and is usually seen after testicular enlargement. Pubarche in males is dependent on testicular androgens. Pubic hair is usually noted after testicular enlargement, and it is initially fine, straight, and sparse and is located at the base of the penis. It first changes in quality to become coarser and curlier and then expands in distribution, as noted in Tanner staging.

Peak height velocity occurs at a later chronologic age and Tanner stage in males than in females. It is seen, on average, at 14 years of age, when boys are between Tanner stage 3 and 4 pubertal development. Pubertal development in males progresses at a slower pace through Tanner stage 3 genital development and accelerates thereafter. The time frame from Tanner stage 2 to Tanner stage 4 in males is typically 4 years, whereas in females it is shorter. Tanner staging of genital and pubic hair development is shown in Figure 30-7.

sequence of pubertal events in males is listed in Table 30-10. The scrotum becomes darker in color and more lax. With the progression of puberty the testicular enlargement continues. At the same time, under the influence of androgens, penile growth occurs first in length and then in width. The glans develops toward the end of puberty, as adult size and shape are reached. Pubic hair usually precedes axillary hair by 1 year (both are

### Somatic Growth in Puberty
#### Clinical Events
The rate of linear growth during puberty is greater than at any other time except infancy. The pattern and rate of growth in males and females is similar until the onset of puberty. The pubertal growth spurt occurs about 2 years earlier in girls than in boys. Boys have a longer prepubertal growth period as well as

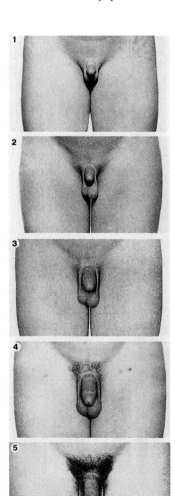

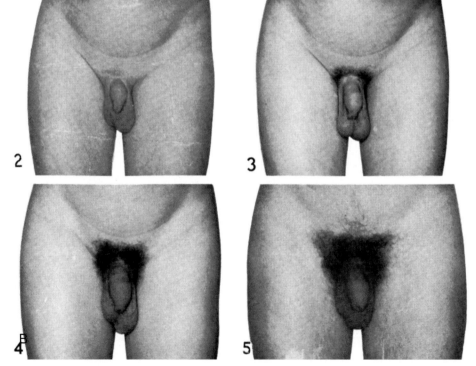

**Figure 30-7   Male Tanner stages.** A, Genitalia. B, Pubic hair. (From Marshall WA, Tanner JM: Variations in pattern of pubertal changes in boys. Arch Dis Child 1970;13–24. Reprinted by permission from the BMJ Publishing Group.)

**Relationship between growth and other changes in puberty**

## Male

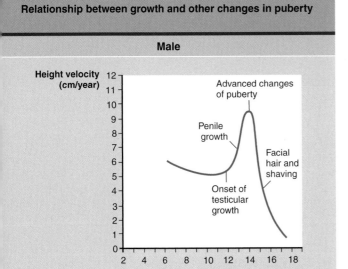

## Female

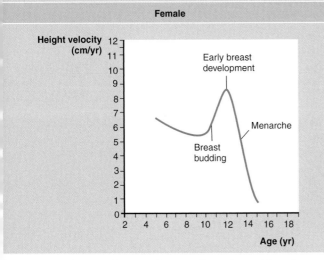

**Figure 30-8  Comparative growth curves for males and females and their relationship to other changes in puberty.** (From Blair JC, Savage MO: Normal and abnormal puberty. In Besser GM, Thorner MO [eds]: Comprehensive Clinical Endocrinology, 3rd ed. Spain, Mosby, 2002, p 326.)

a longer growth spurt and a greater peak height velocity, and thus attain taller adult heights. Figure 30-8 demonstrates the difference in growth curve and timing of pubertal changes between boys and girls.

### Hormonal Events

The major hormones that play a role in the growth spurt at puberty are estrogen, insulin-like growth factor 1 (IGF-1), and growth hormone (GH). Normal growth at puberty depends on the concerted action of all three. Other hormones are thought to also play minor roles, albeit less well defined. An increase in sex steroids, predominantly estrogen, stimulates the secretion of GH, which then stimulates IGF-1 production. Sex steroids, especially estrogen, seem to have the central role in pubertal growth for both girls and boys. The amount of estrogen required to stimulate long-bone growth is very small, which correlates

with the fact that girls achieve peak height velocity early in puberty at a time when serum estradiol levels are quite low (20 pg/mL). Estrogen at high levels, as seen toward the end of puberty, decreases GH and IGF-1 levels. Finally, the sex steroids are responsible for the termination of growth. They stimulate epiphyseal fusion and result in closure of the growth plates.

GH is secreted in pulses with a circadian pattern. For this reason, random sampling is not helpful. Before puberty, GH production is independent of the sex steroids, but during puberty its secretion is crucially dependent on the sex steroids. GH synthesis doubles during puberty, increasing in pulse amplitude, not pulse frequency. Maximal growth hormone production occurs at maximal height velocity in both sexes. Basal levels of GH are higher in girls than boys throughout puberty, reaching their maximum at Tanner stage 4. The basal level of GH secretion in boys is constant throughout puberty. By the end of puberty, GH decreases in both boys and girls regardless of continued exposure to sex steroids.

### Changes in Body Composition at Puberty

Body composition is similar between the sexes at the onset of puberty when girls and boys have the same percentage of body fat. By the end of puberty females have 2 times the body fat as males and males have 1.5 times the lean body mass and skeletal mass as females. Body proportions also change during puberty. In early puberty growth is greatest in the limbs, but at peak height velocity growth in the trunk is greater. Growth in truncal width is different between males and females—in males the maximum growth is across the shoulders (biacromial diameter) and in females the maximum growth is across the pelvis (biiliac diameter).

### Bone Density and Puberty

The major changes in bone mineral density occur during the first 3 years of life and then again during puberty, especially during peak height velocity and just after menarche in females. Estrogen is primarily responsible for the attainment of adult bone mineral density. Calcium intake has been shown to play an important role in increasing bone density in adolescent females, and supplementation is recommended in adolescent females who are ingesting suboptimal amounts of calcium (80% of the recommended daily allowance in their diet).[15] Vitamin D intake may be critical where sun exposure is limited, especially in winter. The increase in bone density during puberty ranges from 10% to 20%, which provides up to 20 years of protection against the later normal age-related loss of skeletal mass. The critical role of estrogen on bone mass accumulation is emphasized by the observation that nearly all of the bone mass in the hip and vertebral bodies is accumulated in females by late adolescence (18 years of age), mostly during the postmenarchal period. The increase in vertebral bone density is greater in African American females, as compared with white females, partly explaining why later in life osteoporosis and vertebral fractures are less common in black women than white women.[16] Deficiencies of pubertal development have been shown to adversely affect bone density in males and females, mostly due to estrogen deficiency. Children with precocious puberty have an increased bone mineral density consistent for their bone age, but treatment with GnRH analogs and antagonists reversibly decreases bone mineral density.

| Table 30-11 |
| --- |
| **Medical Conditions Associated with Early or Precocious Puberty** |

- Congenital adrenal hyperplasia (CAH)
- McCune-Albright syndrome
- Neurofibromatosis 1
- Spina bifida
- Testotoxicosis
- Tuberous sclerosis
- Williams syndrome

## Determinants of the Timing of Puberty

### Genetic

The strongest factor regulating puberty and its timing is genetic. The variance in pubertal onset can be predicted genetically 50% to 80% of the time. As discussed earlier, puberty begins with the reactivation of GnRH secretion after its suppression in mid-childhood. The mechanisms that cause this suppression and then reactivation are not clearly understood, but they help explain some of the genetic contributions to puberty. Precocious puberty is seen in several genetic disorders (Table 30-11).

The influence of genetics on puberty is demonstrated in the long-standing correlation between mothers, daughters, and sisters with timing of pubertal onset and menarche. As discussed, studies have shown that puberty varies among racial groups. It has been postulated that the genetic control of the variance in pubertal timing is linked to a complex polygenic trait or to multiple genes and that individual variation in pubertal timing involves familial, ethnic, gender, and environmental factors. Twin studies have shown a greater concordance between monozygotic than dizygotic twins in timing of skeletal maturation, age of growth spurt, age of menarche, and Tanner staging in puberty.

### General Health and Nutrition

Improved health and nutrition play an important role in the onset of puberty. Young women who have anorexia nervosa and intense exercisers with low weight and low percentage of body fat have delayed menarche or amenorrhea. This delay in menarche is more pronounced when training starts prepubertally. One theory supports that a low percentage of body fat generates less estrogen, since some estrogens are produced in adipose tissue by the aromatization of androgens. Inconsistent with a simple relationship between age of menarche and body weight is the observation that some morbidly obese girls have delayed menarche. This may be influenced by a combination of hormonal changes that are associated with extreme obesity. Variations in the timing of puberty have been observed in developing countries based on socioeconomic status, other social stressors, and demographic factors, including urban versus rural living.

Nutritional components in the diet may also play a role, although this is less well defined. It is clear that nutritional factors play a role in the age of pubertal onset through their effects on the accumulation of adipose tissue. Phytoestrogens are naturally occurring plant estrogens, and are abundant in certain food products, including soybean, clover, alfalfa, peanut, and flaxseed. Studies of phytoestrogens in the diet have demonstrated this effect of diet on puberty as well, as they have been found to interact with estrogen receptors, having either agonistic or antagonistic effects. An association between diets high in animal protein in early life compared with a diet high in vegetable protein has been associated with earlier menarche.[17] Finally, a diet high in animal fat, dairy products, refined sugars and low in complex carbohydrates, fiber, and whole-grain is associated with higher plasma sex hormones and higher urinary and fecal excretion of estrogens, as well as higher cholesterol and insulin levels.[18]

### Leptin

Leptin is a hormone produced in adipose tissue. Leptin acts on CNS neurons to regulate eating behavior and energy balance. It is thought to play a role in the stimulation and maintenance of puberty, but its exact role is still unclear. In the leptin-deficient mouse, sexual maturation and fertility are restored with leptin, and in the normal female mouse administration of leptin accelerates the onset of puberty. There seem to be sex differences in leptin concentration, with higher levels found in girls throughout life. Finally, there are low levels of leptin in athletes and patients with anorexia nervosa or delayed puberty, whereas girls with idiopathic precocious puberty have been found to have increased levels of leptin.[19] The current thinking with regard to leptin is that it plays a role in the regulation of puberty but is not the initiating hormone for the onset of puberty.

### Obesity

An association has been observed between female obesity and earlier onset of puberty, but a causal direction of this relationship has not been clearly determined. Kaplowitz et al re-evaluated the PROS population and found a positive relationship between earlier pubertal signs and obesity.[20]

A more recent longitudinal study looked at 183 white girls from age 5 to 9 years and found a significant relationship between higher percentage of body fat, greater BMI, and larger waist circumference and earlier pubertal timing in females.[21] The authors proposed factors that are thought to contribute to this positive association of obesity and earlier pubertal onset, as listed in Table 30-12.

Currently in the United States, the association of higher socioeconomic status with higher weight is no longer true. This confounds the interpretation of the association of earlier onset of puberty and obesity with the historical trend of improved socioeconomic conditions and earlier puberty.

### Biochemical Exposures

Endocrine-disrupting chemicals (EDCs) are synthetic substances such as dichlorodiphenyltrichloroethane (DDT) that can negatively influence the endocrine system.[22] Some of these compounds can act as estrogen analogs although they are structurally quite

| Table 30-12 |
| --- |
| **Factors Contributing to Earlier Puberty in Girls with Greater BMI** |

- Genetic factors
- Increased levels of estrogen from adipose tissue
- Greater stores of body fat secondary to a process of accelerated growth that starts early in development and affects both BMI and timing of puberty
- Leptin is associated with an increase in the percentage of body fat and is thought to play a permissive role in puberty

BMI, Body mass index.

different. Multiple compounds are often mixed in a suspect agent, making it challenging to sort out the effects of individual agents.

Some cosmetics also contain estrogens, and the Food and Drug Administration (FDA) does not regulate those with less than 10,000 IU of estrogen per ounce. The use of hormone-containing hair products in two case studies was associated with early puberty that regressed with discontinuation of use. The individuals using these products were African American women and girls.[23] This reinforces that sex steroids are well absorbed through the skin.

### Other Factors

One factor that is thought to play an indirect role in the timing of puberty is stress, a component of the influence of acute or chronic illness, and psychological or physical adversity. The correlation between child sexual abuse and later neurobiological consequences has been demonstrated, with adverse effects on the hypothalamic-pituitary-adrenal axis.[24]

Another factor that may play a role in pubertal timing is in utero environment, particularly low birth weight. Infants born with intrauterine growth retardation (IUGR) have been observed to be at increased risk for precocious pubarche in childhood.[25]

## PRECOCIOUS PUBERTY

Precocious puberty is, importantly, different from "early puberty" (see Key Terms). When true precocious puberty is present, there is typically substantial acceleration of linear growth and bone maturation, which can lead to early epiphyseal fusion and shorter adult height. For this reason some pediatric endocrinologists do not consider early pubertal development without growth acceleration as precocious puberty, but rather "pseudoprecocious" puberty. True precocious puberty is 20 times more common in girls than in boys.

It is prudent for primary care physicians to approach the diagnosis of precocious puberty cautiously, since it can be difficult to differentiate "normal" early developers from those with underlying disorders. Understanding the etiology and predicting the rate of progress of puberty and growth are critical in determining the urgency and aggressiveness of the workup and possible treatment options. When a girl at 6 years or less has pubertal signs or when pubertal changes are more advanced or quickly progressing, or when a boy is less than 9 years old, the approach is clear. Prompt consultation with and referral to a pediatric endocrinologist are required. In the 6- to 8-year-old female being evaluated for pubertal signs, the clinical presentation, rate of progression of changes, and level of patient and parental concern influence the clinician's approach.

The evaluation is individualized. At a minimum, a careful history and thorough physical examination, radiographic bone age, and plan for close follow-up are recommended. An initial follow-up visit provides the opportunity to review the findings and identify rapid changes. A subsequent visit 3 to 4 months later will provide documentation of progression. In addition, puberty beginning "on time" but progressing too quickly, slowly, or discordantly warrants the attention and evaluation of a pediatric endocrinologist. Continuity of care and meticulous follow-up is the way to ensure detection of slowly developing lesions of the brain, ovary, or adrenal gland or, by ongoing observation, to confirm the overall benign nature of early puberty.

| Table 30-13 |
| --- |
| Classification of Precocious Puberty |

**GnRH-dependent**

Central precocious puberty (CPP) or "true" or complete precocious puberty—always implies a hypothalamic source

**GnRH-independent**

Peripheral precocious puberty (PPP) or pseudoprecocious or incomplete precocious puberty—hormonal drive originating from exogenous, gonadal, adrenal, or other hormone-secreting tissue

Isolated precocious puberty or incomplete precocious puberty

Isolated menstruation or premature menarche

### Etiology and Pathophysiology

The typical etiologic classification scheme is given in Table 30-13 (see Key Terms for definitions). Classification by etiology helps as a general guide to the differential diagnosis, but there is overlap between categories in both etiology and presentation.

### Central Precocious Puberty

Central precocious puberty (CPP) is chronologically early pubertal development that is GnRH stimulated, as is normal puberty. In females breast development or an increase in growth appears first, and in males testicular enlargement is the first sign of puberty. Pubic hair growth follows, although all three changes can occur at the same time. There are often changes in behavior caused by sex steroid influences. The pathogenesis of CPP is not fully understood, but it has been hypothesized that it occurs secondary to suppression of or injury to the neural source of negative feedback inhibition at the level of the hypothalamus. It is much more common in females in whom it is idiopathic (95% of the time) and thought to be secondary to premature activation of the hypothalamic GnRH pulses.

Although CPP is idiopathic in the majority of cases, it is a diagnosis of exclusion, requiring a thorough investigation for other causes. Particularly, the possibility of serious CNS or peripheral endocrine pathology needs to be explored. CPP may be the only presenting sign of a hypothalamic tumor. In females below age 4, a CNS lesion is often the cause. Girls older than 4 years are more likely to have idiopathic precocious puberty. An underlying CNS pathology is highly probable in males with true precocious puberty regardless of age; they should be investigated aggressively.

### Differential Diagnosis of Central Precocious Puberty

In approaching the diagnosis of CPP all etiologic categories of precocious puberty deserve consideration. Table 30-14 illustrates the differential diagnosis of precocious puberty.

Many CNS tumors cause CPP (see Table 30-14). All these tumors are typically near the hypothalamus. Hypothalamic hamartoma, the most common CNS tumor manifesting as CPP, is a congenital malformation that contains GnRH-secreting neurons. It often presents at age 2 or less, and precocious puberty progresses quickly. The hamartoma is usually attached to or suspended from the floor of the third ventricle and is then termed *parahypothalamic*, which is more often associated with precocious puberty. The tumor can also be intrahypothalamic,

**Table 30-14**

**Differential Diagnosis of Precocious Puberty**

I. Central precocious puberty
  A. Idiopathic
  B. CNS pathology
    1. Hypothalamic hamartoma
    2. CNS tumor—craniopharyngioma, astrocytoma, glioma, optic glioma (associated with neurofibromatosis), ependymoma, suprasellar teratoma, pineal tumor—boys only
    3. Hydrocephalus
    4. Infiltrative disease (sarcoidosis, storage disease)
    5. Infectious/postinfectious—meningitis, encephalitis, brain abscess
    6. Genetic syndrome—neurofibromatosis, tuberous sclerosis, Williams syndrome
    7. Postsurgical or irradiation injury
    8. Trauma
    9. Space-occupying lesion—arachnoid cyst or suprasellar cyst
    10. Congenital defect—septo-optic dysplasia (associated with panhypopituitarism), spina bifida/myelomeningocele
    11. Skull abnormality—rickets
  C.* Excessive sex steroid exposure leading to activation of the HPG axis—androgen-secreting tumor, McCune-Albright syndrome, congenital adrenal hyperplasia (CAH), testotoxicosis, exogenous steroid use, hypothyroidism
II. Peripheral precocious puberty
  A. Gonadal tumor
    1. Ovarian tumor—granulosa cell, theca cell, mixed cell, germ cell, cystadenoma, gonadoblastoma, lipoid cell tumor, teratoma, choriocarcinoma, arrhenoblastoma, benign ovarian cyst
    2. Testicular tumor—Sertoli cell (seen in Peutz-Jeghers syndrome), Leydig cell, mixed cell, gonadoblastoma, rhabdomyosarcoma, lymphoma, neuroblastoma, leukemia
    3. β-hCG-producing tumor—germ cell tumor, hepatoblastoma, choriocarcinoma
  B. Adrenal tumor—adenoma, carcinoma
  C. Congenital adrenal hyperplasia (CAH)
  D. Hypothyroidism
  E. McCune-Albright syndome
  F. Testotoxicosis (male-limited precocious puberty)
  G. Ovarian cyst
  H. Exogenous sex steroid (oral, cutaneous intravaginal, injectable)

III. Isolated precocious puberty
  A. Premature thelarche
    1. Premature thelarche
    2. Exogenous steroid
    3. Ovarian cyst
      a. Isolated
      b. Secondary to endocrine disorder (McCune-Albright syndrome, hypothyroidism)
    4. Early central precocious puberty
  B. Premature pubarche
    1. Premature pubarche
    2. Androgen-secreting tumor
    3. CAH
    4. Exogenous steroid
IV. Isolated vaginal bleeding: first confirm that there is true blood (e.g., heme test)
  A. Vulvovaginitis
  B. Trauma
  C. Abuse
  D. Foreign body
  E. Ovarian cyst
    1. Isolated
    2. Secondary to endocrine disorder (McCune-Albright syndrome, hypothyroidism)
  F. Hypothyroidism
  G. McCune-Albright syndrome
  H. Exogenous estrogen or estrogen withdrawal
  I. Hemorrhagic cystitis
  J. Urethral prolapse
  K. Constipation
  L. Lichen sclerosis
  M. Local tumor—rhabdomyosarcoma, endodermal carcinoma, clear cell adenocarcinoma, mesonephric carcinoma
  N. Other infection—*Shigella, Streptococcus pyogenes*

*These diagnoses can overlap in all categories of precocious puberty.

Parts I and II adapted from Tomboc M, Witchel SF, Lee PA: Precocious puberty. In Sanfilippo JS, Muram D, Dewhurst J (eds): Pediatric and Adolescent Gynecology, 2nd ed. Philadelphia, WB Saunders, 2001, p 60.

which indicates that it is enveloped by the hypothalamus, causing distortion of the third ventricle. Intrahypothalamic hamartomas are more often associated with seizures and other neurologic problems than with precocious puberty. The seizures are typically gelastic seizures, which are characterized by brief stereotyped attacks of laughter, but there are often other types of seizures as well. Hypothalamic hamartomas are generally benign and do not progress over time, but they can cause growth acceleration and bone age advancement. Over recent years a greater number of cases of precocious puberty have been attributed to hypothalamic hamartoma secondary to better identification and radiographic imaging technology.

Genetic diseases that manifest as CPP are neurofibromatosis, tuberous sclerosis, Williams syndrome, McCune-Albright syndrome, and testotoxicosis. The last two disorders typically present as peripheral precocious puberty or isolated precocious puberty because the onset of puberty is due to a GnRH-independent sex steroid source, but they have the ability to trigger the HPG axis.

Other less common causes of CPP are CNS irradiation and post-traumatic damage. These patients may have simultaneous growth hormone deficiency that is masked by the exaggerated effect on growth that precocious puberty causes. Many CNS diseases, including spina bifida, are associated with earlier puberty, in contrast to most other chronic diseases that, for a variety of reasons, are often associated with delayed puberty. Finally, secondary CPP can arise from any source causing prolonged exposure to sex steroids that leads to accelerated skeletal maturation and sexual development.

## Peripheral Precocious Puberty

Peripheral precocious puberty (PPP) is the earlier onset of puberty instigated by a hormone other than GnRH. As defined in Key Terms, PPP is also referred to as pseudoprecocious and incomplete precocious puberty. It usually develops secondary to autonomous sex steroid secretion of gonadal, adrenal, or ectopic origin. It can also occur owing to an exogenous sex steroid source. Its presentation varies, and it is possible to observe some or all of the changes of CPP. Importantly, in PPP, LH and FSH levels are low or prepubertal secondary to sex steroid suppression. Finally, there is often some growth acceleration and advanced bone age, but to a lesser degree than in CPP.

### Differential Diagnosis of Peripheral Precocious Puberty

The differential diagnosis of PPP includes adrenal and gonadal tumors, genetic disorders, other endocrine disorders, and benign ovarian cysts (see Table 30-14). Androgen-secreting adrenal and gonadal tumors can all cause isolated premature pubarche, and they usually function autonomously. Androgen-producing tumors cause progressive and rapid androgen excess and usually cause virilization in females and precocious puberty in males.

Ovarian tumors are relatively uncommon but occur in about 11% of girls with precocious puberty. Granulosa cell tumors constitute 60% of ovarian tumors causing precocious puberty. Other ovarian tumor types are listed in Table 30-14. There is often a palpable abdominal mass along with an estrogen effect, since all these tumors can produce estrogen and androgens autonomously, with consequent breast and pubic hair development. Imaging studies play an important diagnostic role, including ultrasound, computed tomography (CT), and magnetic resonance imaging (MRI). Depending on the suspected lesion, different studies may offer different diagnostic information. Consultation with a pediatric radiologist is advised, and care should be taken to minimize exposure of the gonads to irradiation.

Testicular tumors in males can produce increased androgens and cause precocious puberty. The testis affected is usually larger and firmer and has an irregular consistency. These tumors are typically painless. Testicular tumors presenting as PPP are included in Table 30-14.

Human chorionic gonadotrophin (hCG)–secreting tumors are more common in males and can be associated with the 47,XXY karyotype. Germinomas occurring in the hypothalamus, pineal gland, and mediastinum can secrete hCG and thus stimulate Leydig cell secretion of testosterone in boys, independent of GnRH and LH. hCG-producing tumors can also be present in other tissues, including hepatoblastoma, hepatoma, teratoma, and chorioepithelioma. hCG induces precocious puberty in males by activating LH receptors. However, in females these tumors do not usually cause precocious puberty because LH receptor expression requires FSH stimulation.

Adrenal adenomas and carcinomas can secrete estrogens, androgens, or both. They may also secrete other adrenal hormones, such as glucocorticoids, so that Cushing's syndrome may be part of the presentation. Adrenal tumors are not usually suppressed by dexamethasone, which differentiates them from congenital adrenal hyperplasia (CAH). CAH is an endocrine disorder that occurs secondary to enzyme deficiencies in steroidogenesis. The two variants that typically present as precocious puberty or virilization in adolescents are 21-hydroxylase deficiency and 11β-hydroxylase deficiency. These are autosomal recessive disorders, although a heterozygous state has been described. In males, excessive secretion of testosterone causes precocious puberty, and in females an accumulation of adrenal androgens causes virilization and/or precocious pubarche. In females, some breast development can be seen with virilization. Late-onset CAH accounts for 1% to 5% of the cases that present as androgen excess in females.

| Table 30-15 |
| :--: |
| **Clinical Characteristics of McCune-Albright Syndrome** |

- Café-au-lait spots (irregular, large macules that do not cross the midline)
- Osteitis fibrosa or cystic bone lesions
- Endocrine abnormalities
  Precocious puberty
  Multinodular goiter and other thyroid disorders
  Pituitary gigantism
  Amenorrhea-galactorrhea
  Cushing's syndrome

McCune-Albright syndrome is a heterogeneous entity, predominantly found in females, which is diagnosed clinically and confirmed with imaging studies. The clinical characteristics of the disorder are listed in Table 30-15. When it presents as precocious puberty, it may begin with cyclic vaginal bleeding or as breast development secondary to the presence of large, hormone-secreting ovarian cysts. Precocious puberty usually occurs secondary to autonomous gonadal steroidogenesis, but it can be centrally mediated. The pathophysiology is explained by the autonomous function of tissues in which productivity is regulated by cyclic adenosine monophosphate (cAMP), as a result of a germ line mutation. A subunit of the G protein, linked to the LH receptor, becomes active, and stimulates Leydig cell production of testosterone or granulosa cell production of estradiol. Since McCune-Albright syndrome is the result of a mosaic mutation, its presentation is varied and its transmission sporadic. Precocious puberty can occur at any time from infancy to late childhood. Fertility is typically unaffected, but adult height may be compromised depending on the degree of bone age advancement.

Testotoxicosis, or familial male precocious puberty, occurs in males secondary to a germ line mutation that causes a defect in the transmembrane LH receptor, which triggers cAMP-dependent steroidogenesis. The testes secrete testosterone autonomously, usually beginning in infancy. It usually presents with virilization in preschool-aged or younger boys. There is increased testicular volume and penile and pubic hair growth. Advanced bone age and height velocity can also be seen. Testotoxicosis is inherited in an autosomal dominant pattern, but can also be inherited sporadically.

Ovarian cysts that function autonomously can occur in prepubertal females and cause precocious puberty. These follicular cysts are recurrent in nature. They are frequently associated with McCune-Albright syndrome. The ovarian cysts seen in PPP are usually unilateral, sometimes palpable on examination, and notably larger than 9 mm on ultrasound. This is in contrast to multiple, smaller cysts or follicles found in normal puberty and in GnRH-stimulated CPP. Ovarian cysts can present with early breast development or vaginal bleeding. Estradiol levels are elevated secondary to autonomous ovarian function, but GnRH and gonadotropins are prepubertal, as is bone age and height velocity. With rupture and dissolution of an estrogen-secreting cyst, there is estrogen withdrawal and bleeding.

With profound hypothyroidism, high concentrations of TSH act through the FSH and LH receptors and cause gonadal stimulation because of the similarity in structure of these

# Pediatric and Adolescent Gynecology

pituitary glycoproteins. In females, thelarche or uterine bleeding can be seen. Multiple, large cysts can occur in primary hypothyroidism. In males, macroorchidism is seen without excessive phallic or pubic hair growth. In VanWyck and Grumbach syndrome, hypothyroidism can also be associated with precocious puberty and hyperprolactinemia with secondary galactorrhea in both sexes. Notably, the symptoms of precocious puberty in hypothyroidism occur in the absence of growth acceleration. Skeletal age is typically delayed which differentiates it from true precocious puberty.

Exogenous steroid exposure is another reversible cause of early signs of puberty. The prolonged use of estrogen creams for labial adhesions can sometimes lead to premature breast development. The role of estrogens in the diet has been postulated to play a role in earlier puberty, but this has not been validated. The same is true for estrogen in cosmetics, hair products, and EDCs in the environment.

## Isolated Precocious Puberty or Incomplete Precocious Puberty

Incomplete precocious puberty is the isolated appearance of one secondary sex trait. These conditions are typically slowly progressive and benign. They must be followed closely, since they can be the presenting sign of a potentially accelerating process, such as CPP, or early evidence of a CNS or other tumor.

### Premature Thelarche

Premature thelarche is the premature onset of breast development before age 8 years. It can be unilateral or bilateral, and usually there is no darkening or widening of the areola. It is most commonly seen in girls less than 5 years old and predominantly in those less than 2. Breast buds are 2 to 4 cm. Breast tissue can be mildly tender and granular in texture, rather than smooth. Estrogen may be elevated, but gonadotropin response to GnRH is prepubertal, which differentiates it from CPP. The uterus and ovaries are prepubertal, as is the vaginal mucosa. Height velocity is typically normal, bone age is not substantially advanced, and there is no compromise in final adult height.

It is usually transient, but 10% of cases progress to CPP, especially when the age of onset is over 2 years. Evaluation includes careful questions about sources of exogenous estrogen, including pills, patches, or other medications in the household. Initial evaluation includes a bone age and plan for follow-up. Often no intervention is needed. It has been postulated that premature thelarche is caused by a derangement in the maturation of the HPG axis with higher than normal FSH secretion and increased sensitivity peripherally to sex hormones. It is crucial to keep in mind that patients with isolated premature thelarche cannot be differentiated at presentation from those with progressive precocious puberty, and therefore they require close and regular follow-up. These patients may not need referral to a pediatric endocrinologist unless there is advanced radiologic bone age or other signs of more rapidly advancing puberty.

### Premature Pubarche (or Premature Adrenarche)

Premature pubarche is defined as the onset of pubic hair growth before 8 years in girls and 9 years in boys without any other signs of puberty. It is more frequent in girls and it is usually slowly progressive. Premature pubarche is often used interchangeably with premature adrenarche, which includes other signs of increased androgens: body odor, acne, skin changes, axillary hair, and penile or clitoral enlargement. Pubic hair growth is typically limited to the labia majora or base of the penis and there is only slight, if any, penile or clitoral enlargement. Hormonal changes associated with adrenarche are also found including a slight increase in DHEA, DHEAS, and AND. These are relatively weak androgens, but they are peripherally converted to testosterone. There is no corresponding activation of the HPG axis, and the gonadotropin response to GnRH is prepubertal. There is minimal or no breast or testicular development, but there may be modest accelerated growth and bone age. Prolonged exposure of the CNS to androgens infrequently activates the HPG axis and leads to CPP.

Premature pubarche was originally thought to be a benign condition, but the differential diagnosis includes some of the causes of PPP, including CAH and androgen-secreting tumors of the adrenals or gonads. Recent studies suggest that individuals with isolated premature pubarche have an increased risk of later endocrine pathology. This encompasses the spectrum of hyperandrogenism, including functional ovarian hyperandrogenism, polycystic ovary syndrome (PCOS), and an increased risk of insulin resistance. Ovarian hyperandrogenism is characterized by signs and symptoms of androgen excess and by an exaggerated ovarian 17-hydroxyprogesterone (17-OHP) response to GnRH agonist challenge. A study by Ibanez et al found that girls with premature pubarche are at increased risk for anovulation from late adolescence onward.[26]

Certain populations appear to be at higher risk for premature pubarche and subsequent endocrine problems, including African American, Caribbean, South American, Native American, and Mediterranean populations and babies born with low birth weight. Hyperandrogenism is seen in a greater proportion of African American and Caribbean Hispanic girls with premature pubarche.[27] A link between fetal growth and adrenarche has been suggested with prenatal growth restriction associated with more pronounced adrenarche.[28]

Thus, premature pubarche in certain cases may be a precursor of insulin resistance, PCOS, and related endocrine abnormalities. The primary care provider's or gynecologist's approach to diagnostic evaluation of these patients, before consultation with a pediatric endocrinologist, includes history, physical examination, bone age, and baseline laboratory testing if the bone age is advanced. A diagnostic flowchart is depicted in Figure 30-9. These patients need to be observed closely in future years and may need referral to pediatric endocrinology and reproductive endocrinology in the future.

### Premature Menarche

Premature menarche in isolation is a rare presentation of precocious puberty that may indicate PPP or isolated precocious puberty. In the prepubertal setting, the new onset of vaginal bleeding is worrisome to the patient and family. It is helpful to determine first whether there is truly blood, and if so, the source of the blood. Many conditions, including those arising from the urethra, skin, and rectum can present with "vaginal bleeding." See Table 30-14 for the differential diagnosis.

True "vaginal" or menstrual bleeding occurs secondary to estrogen stimulation. There are typically other signs of estrogen stimulation, such as breast development and vaginal epithelia

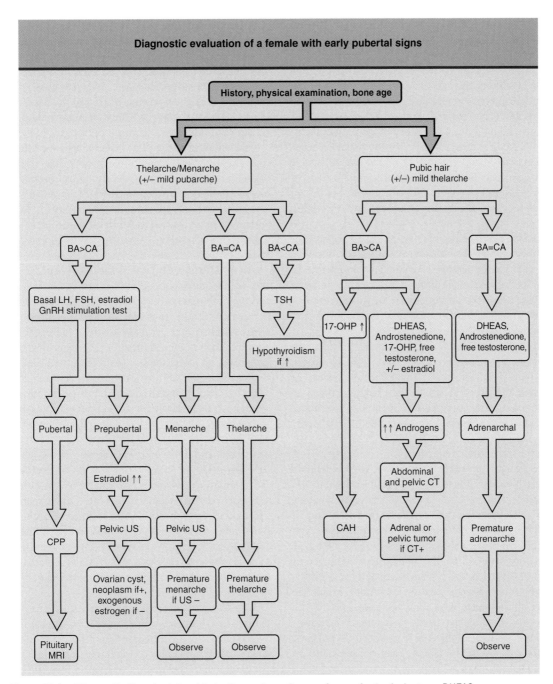

**Figure 30-9** **Diagnostic flowchart for girls in the workup of precocious puberty.** Androgens, DHEAS, androstenedione, testosterone; BA, bone age; CA, chronologic age; CAH, congenital adrenal hyperplasia (nonclassical form); CPP, central precocious puberty; CT, computed tomography; DHEAS, dehydroepiandrosterone sulfate; GnRH, gonadotropin-releasing hormone; LH, luteinizing hormone; MRI, magnetic resonance imaging; 17OHP, 17α-hydroxyprogesterone; US, ultrasonography. (Adapted from Root A: Precocious puberty. Pediatr Rev 2000;21:16.)

changes. Less common causes of isolated vaginal bleeding, which are associated with precocious puberty, include ovarian cysts, McCune-Albright syndrome (polyostotic fibrous dysplasia), hypothyroidism, and exogenous estrogen exposure. Ovarian cysts usually occur in isolation but can be associated with McCune-Albright syndrome or hypothyroidism. Following "premature menarche," growth and fertility are usually unimpaired. Most cases of premature menarche require at least one consultation with a pediatric endocrinologist. However, vaginal bleeding

secondary to ovarian cysts can be followed by the primary care provider, with serial ultrasound evaluations every 3 months, and referral if the problem persists.

## Diagnosis and Evaluation of Precocious Puberty

The initial evaluation of the signs of precocious puberty should take into account the possibility of CNS pathology or hormone-secreting tumors. These warrant immediate referral and evaluation by pediatric subspecialists, possibly including endocrinologists, neurosurgeons, oncologists, and general surgeons among others.

### History

A detailed history includes the age of onset of symptoms and progression of pubertal development and overall growth, and an in-depth review of any other potentially involved systems.

Past medical history includes any history of past CNS infection, trauma, irradiation, seizures, headaches, or visual changes. Other helpful questions include history of recent weight loss or excessive weight gain, recent history of more rapid or slower growth, changes in energy level or fatigue, recent history of exogenous steroid use, and finally any other symptoms related to hypothyroidism.

Family history should include history of early puberty or pubertal signs especially in the otherwise well child between 6 and 8 years of age. Family history is particularly important in constitutional early puberty, male-limited precocious puberty, CAH, and other inherited conditions, including neuro-fibromatosis (autosomal dominant, variable penetrance) and tuberous sclerosis (autosomal dominant).

In taking the history, consider that the sequence of development for CPP is similar to normal puberty, but it begins earlier. Therefore, it is helpful to ask about the expected events of normal puberty and the order in which they have occurred so far. Abrupt onset and rapid progression suggest a hormone-secreting lesion. If there is premature thelarche, ask whether neonatal breast development has persisted or regressed and then recurred. The latter indicates a new process.

If vaginal bleeding is the presenting complaint, elicit a detailed description of the bleeding. Bleeding is typically irregular and heavy with ovarian tumors or cysts and with early, anovulatory menstrual cycles. The bleeding may originate from the skin or mucosa, or a different orifice. Factitious bleeding may occur, and "blood" can be confirmed with a simple office test for blood.

Growth charts are central to the diagnosis of precocious puberty. Accelerated growth and advanced skeletal age differentiate CPP from more benign forms. The more rapid the growth rate, the more concerning and the more likely the condition is to be CPP, whereas the growth rate is steady or slow in GnRH-independent categories of precocious puberty. Increased appetite and emotional lability may be seen with an increased estrogen effect.

Questions about urinary symptoms, bowel symptoms, and abdominal pain are critical components of the history. It is important to question the parent or guardian and the child alone about the possibility of sexual abuse in the setting of prepubertal vaginal bleeding. It is common to find that vulvovaginal complaints, including bleeding and discharge, have been treated by providers without an examination of the child. This is not an acceptable practice, and findings need to be evaluated firsthand by a provider.

### Physical Examination

Normal growth parameters, such as height, weight, and BMI, along with percentiles for height, weight, and BMI, are crucial in assessing a child with early onset of puberty. Look at the patient's growth chart and document changes in height, clothes, shoe and hand size as reported by patients and their families. In younger children, an increase in head circumference can indicate hydrocephalus or other CNS anomalies.

Vital signs can pinpoint particular sources of pathology. An elevated blood pressure may be seen in certain forms of CAH and heart-rate alterations are observed in a variety of illnesses such as a decreased resting heart rate in hypothyroidism. Vital signs change through each stage of puberty and adult values are substantially different from prepubertal values.

Examination of the skin offers diagnostic clues. Skin changes to evaluate include acne, oiliness, odor, hair (pubic, axillary, and other), and café-au-lait marks. In neurofibromatosis café-au-lait marks are brown with smooth edges ("coast of California") and typically multiple in number (6 or more). In contrast, café-au-lait spots in McCune-Albright syndrome are larger in size with irregular borders ("coast of Maine"), and fewer in number (1 or 2).

An eye examination is critical to visualize the optic discs and to evaluate visual fields in assessing for CNS pathology and possible mass effect. With any suspicion of abnormalities in the region of the pituitary or hypothalamus, a sophisticated electronic mapping of visual fields is required. In addition to a comprehensive eye examination, a neurologic examination is important to assess for any CNS abnormalities.

A thorough examination of the thyroid gland is essential. The thyroid is palpated for fullness and nodules. The thyroid becomes transiently fuller during puberty, and it can resemble a truly enlarged gland. Other physical findings related to thyroid disorders are sought, including hair and skin changes, changes in heart rate, and deep tendon reflexes.

The importance of Tanner staging of breasts was discussed earlier, and a complete examination, including palpation, is necessary to differentiate between the irregular, dense consistency of ductal breast tissue and the smoother consistency of subcutaneous fat. Dark pigmentation of the areolae and nipples can suggest ingestion of synthetic estrogens in various forms such as oral contraceptive pills (OCPs), creams for hair or face and anabolic steroids. Milky or other secretions from the nipple should be noted as well.

Inspection of external genitalia is equally important to staging of breast development. In females, the clinician assesses if there is an estrogen effect (enlargement of labia minora, thickening of mucosa, dull pink color to vaginal mucosa, and a clear or whitish discharge) and the degree of that effect. In males, measurements of phallic and testicular sizes can be compared to norms. Initially, testicular volume is disproportionately larger than phallic size in normal puberty and CPP; however, in PPP or premature pubarche, phallic size may be greater and testes may be prepubertal in size. If the testes are asymmetrically enlarged, a neoplasm, such as a Leydig cell tumor, is considered.

A vaginal bimanual or speculum examination is often unnecessary and traumatic. An ultrasound examination is more sensitive for assessment of pubertal ovarian pathology, although a small, prepubertal ovary may reveal limited detail. An abdominal examination often identifies a mass, since a pelvic or abdominal mass is palpable in a majority of ovarian tumors.

In cases of premature pubarche it is important to seek out signs of virilization, such as voice change, hirsutism, clitoromegaly or increased phallic size, and an increase in muscle mass. These findings may suggest CAH or an adrenal tumor. In the case of solated premature pubarche, confirm the absence of breast development and other signs of estrogen effect. Looking at photos or videos from the past may be an excellent way to compare present and past appearances and body type. Finally, orthopedic history and examination provide information about fractures seen in McCune-Albright syndrome.

### Laboratory Studies

The decision to pursue imaging and laboratory studies is determined by the physical findings and history. A diagnostic flowchart for females is given in Figure 30-9.

The most useful initial test is a radiograph for bone age, which is advised in all categories of precocious puberty, as a minimal diagnostic workup. Bone age can help determine how extensive and urgent further workup should be. There is no consensus on whether to obtain bone age in equivocal cases; however, it is a noninvasive tool with modest cost and minimal risk. It involves taking a left hand and wrist radiograph, which is compared with standard atlases. It is best that the radiologist interpreting a bone age film is trained in pediatric radiology. In the United States the most commonly used reference standard for bone age is the Greulich and Pyle atlas. In the majority of patients who have CPP, the bone age is more than 2 years ahead of the chronologic age, whereas in cases of isolated precocious puberty, the bone age is only slightly advanced. The degree of advanced bone age in the case of PPP depends on the etiology.

Vaginal smears can confirm estrogen stimulation. If a greater percentage of cells are superficial, then there is a greater estrogen effect. Findings of greater than 40% superficial epithelial cells should lead to suspicion of an estrogen-secreting tumor or other source of estrogen.

Other common initial tests may include LH, FSH, estradiol, progesterone, DHEA, DHEAS, thyroid-stimulating hormone (TSH), AND, and free testosterone. More specific tests, depending on the differential diagnostic considerations, include 17-hydroxyprogesterone, a 24-hour free cortisol (if Cushing's syndrome is suspected), an adrenocorticotropic hormone (ACTH) stimulation test (if CAH is suspected), and a β-hCG (if an hCG-secreting tumor is suspected).

When CAH is strongly suspected, a 17-hydroxyprogesterone level should be obtained, which is best drawn between 7 and 9 AM because of diurnal variations. An ACTH stimulation test is then recommended for those patients with elevated 17-hydroxyprogesterone and adrenal androgens, as well as premature pubarche, with accelerated growth and advanced bone age. Patients with CAH caused by 21-hydroxylase deficiency have elevated 17-hydroxyprogesterone levels that decline with dexamethasone administration. The ACTH stimulation test involves measuring basal concentration and post-ACTH secretory response of the adrenal androgens, progesterone and cortisol. A bolus of 0.25 mg of ACTH is infused intravenously, and serum is sampled at baseline and at 30 or 60 minutes afterward.

Quantification of serum FSH and LH is important in the workup of precocious puberty, but it is not straightforward, as elucidated in Table 30-16. A single random sample is not always helpful.

Interpretation of estradiol, progesterone, and androgen levels also is problematic because of differences in quality control and different laboratory interpretations of normal levels. These

| Table 30-16 |
| --- |
| **Difficulties in Obtaining Random Serum LH and FSH Levels** |
| · FSH and LH are released in pulses |
| · Secretion is associated with sleep in early puberty |
| · Levels vary throughout normal menstrual cycles |
| · Levels are often prepubertal in the early stages of CPP |
| · FSH levels are less specific; they can be similar for CPP and isolated premature thelarche |
| · Assays and laboratories used vary in quality and normal values |
| CPP, Central precocious puberty; FSH, follicle-stimulating hormone; LH, luteinizing hormone. |

levels also change throughout the day, menstrual cycle, and stage of puberty. Therefore, it is important to review normal levels for age and stage of puberty and to know the reference values at the laboratory being utilized. Table 30-17 reviews the normal hormonal levels for males and females through the different stages of puberty.[29]

If there is pubertal development with accelerated growth and advanced bone age, without pubertal FSH and LH levels, and without virilization, then there may be an ovarian source causing these symptoms. A patient with an estradiol level above 100 pg/mL, low gonadotropin levels, and a suppressed GnRH response requires evaluation for an estrogen-secreting tumor. An hCG-producing tumor should also be considered in the diagnosis. An hCG-producing tumor can be confirmed by a quantitative serum immunoassay specific for the β subunit of hCG. In CPP the basal serum concentrations of estradiol may be low (<10 pg/mL) or appropriate for Tanner stage of breast development.

Serum testosterone in males with CPP is appropriate for Tanner stage but is markedly elevated in those with testicular tumors. Testosterone can also be increased in adrenal tumors secondary to direct secretion by the tumor or peripheral conversion that manifests as signs of virilization. Patients with adrenal tumors have significantly elevated DHEA, DHEAS, and AND, which cannot be suppressed by dexamethasone. Feminizing adrenal tumors usually secrete adrenal androgens, with mildly increased estradiol and suppressed FSH and LH. In testotoxicosis, there is a positive family history and mildly enlarged testes on examination (5 to 6 mL), pubertal testosterone levels, and an increase in testosterone after hCG stimulation. GnRH agonist does not typically suppress LH, FSH, or testosterone secretion in testotoxicosis.

The patient's fertility does not need to be evaluated in the workup of precocious puberty since sexual development does not depend on nor does it imply ovulatory capability. Complete sexual precocity, however, can lead to earlier ovulation with potential fertility.

Other studies may include MRI of the brain to exclude CNS structural abnormalities in CPP when the source of hormonal stimulation is not found with other tests. Chalumea et al have proposed a diagnostic tree to determine which girls with CPP require neuroimaging. They found that independent predictors of CNS pathology were age of onset of puberty less than 6 years and estradiol levels greater than 100 pmol/L.[30]

Pelvic and abdominal ultrasound examination provides a look at ovarian, uterine, and adrenal size, symmetry, and pathology.

# Pediatric and Adolescent Gynecology

**Table 30-17**
**Normal Female and Male Hormonal Levels Through the Stages of Puberty**

| Tanner Breast Stage | Female LH (IU/L) Basal | LH (IU/L) Post-GnRH | FSH (IU/L) Basal | FSH (IU/L) Post GnRH | Testosterone (ng/dL) | DHEAS (µg/dL) |
|---|---|---|---|---|---|---|
| I | 0.03 ± 0.03 | 2.0 ± 1.5 | 2.16 ± 1.14 | 21 ± 5.5 | 0.8 (0.5–2.0) | 40 (19–114) |
| II | 0.71 ± 1.04 | 21 ± 17 | 3.44 ± 1.58 | 10 ± 5.0 | 1.6 (1.0–2.4) | 72 (34–129) |
| III | 2.10 ± 2.33 | | 4.88 ± 2.11 | | 2.5 (0.7–6.0) | 88 (32–226) |
| IV | 3.67 ± 2.22 | 33 ± 20 | 6.19 ± 2.55 | 11 ± 3.3 | 4.7 (2.1–8.5) | 120 (58–260) |
| V | 2.88 ± 2.68 | | 4.92 ± 2.31 | | 11 (3:4–17) | 148 (44–248) |
| Adult | 5.76 ± 3.46 | | 6.63 ± 2.19 | | Foll 5.2 (3–10) Lut 13.0 (7–30) | 153 (60–255) |

| Tanner Genital Stage | Male LH (IU/L) Basal | LH (IU/L) Post-GnRH | FSH (IU/L) Basal | FSH (IU/L) Post GnRH | Testosterone (ng/dL) | DHEAS (µg/dL) |
|---|---|---|---|---|---|---|
| I | 0.70 ± 0.97 | 3.2 ± 3.0 | 2.52 ± 1.83 | 4.7 ± 2.2 | 4.9 (<3–10) | 36 (13–83) |
| II | 1.80 ± 1.30 | 15 ± 6.3 | 2.75 ± 1.84 | 3.4 ± 2.2 | 42 (18–50) | 93 (42–109) |
| III | 1.86 ± 1.41 | | 2.94 ± 1.55 | | 190 (100–320) | 122 (48–208) |
| IV | 2.65 ± 1.81 | 42 ± 23 | 4.47 ± 1.88 | 11 ± 5.6 | 372 (200–620) | 206 (102–385) |
| V | 2.76 ± 1.12 | | 7.64 ± 2.50 | | 546 (350–970) | 230 (120–370) |
| Adult | 4.51 ± 1.99 | | 4.91 ± 2.02 | | 627 (350–1030) | 270 (100–450) |

DHEAS, dehydroepiandrosterone sulfate; FSH, follicle-stimulating hormone; GnRH, gonadotropin-releasing hormone; LH, luteinizing hormone.
Data from Neely EK, Hintz RL, Wilson DM, et al: Normal ranges for immunochemiluminometric gonadotropin assays. J Pediatr 1995;127:40–46. The gonadotropin assays employed in this manuscript are ultrasensitive; the standards were human pituitary luteinizing hormone 80/522 and follicle-stimulating hormone 83/575.

Pelvic ultrasound or other sensitive imaging is needed when a peripheral sex hormonal source is suspected and in girls with vaginal bleeding that cannot be explained by physical examination, such as vaginal or uterine neoplasms. Ultrasound also provides evidence for estrogen effects on the size and maturity of pelvic organs. It is helpful in looking at or differentiating ovarian cysts or tumors. Pelvic ultrasound shows the size of the endometrial stripe or uterine lining and helps assess the risk of uterine bleeding. The uterus is enlarged for age in CPP but should be normal for the stage of puberty. Pelvic ultrasound in prepubertal and pubertal girls may be difficult to read depending on the resolution of the equipment and the skill and familiarity of the technician and radiologist. A bone scan or radiogram may be indicated when McCune-Albright syndrome is suspected.

The definitive diagnostic test for CPP, if suspected, is GnRH stimulation of gonadotropin response. Though the test is performed and interpreted by a pediatric endocrinologist, it is helpful to understand how it is done and when it is indicated (Table 30-18).

One way the test is performed is by administering 100 µg of GnRH subcutaneously and then measuring serum LH and FSH levels 40 minutes after injection. Figure 30-10 shows the serum LH and FSH levels after GnRH infusion. In cases of CPP, the LH rise will be 2 to 3 times higher than the prepubertal response and will greatly surpass the FSH response. Table 30-19 shows the LH/FSH ratio in response to GnRH. Prepubertal LH levels are consistent with PPP or isolated precocious puberty, but in some cases of early CPP post-GnRH LH values are still in the prepubertal range, and so these lab values need to be interpreted cautiously relative to other clinical and laboratory findings.

## Management and Treatment of Precocious Puberty
The management of precocious puberty depends on the etiology and diagnosis. Accurate identification of the cause and determination of its significance are crucial in managing precocious puberty of any etiology. In the cases of CPP, PPP, and often premature pubarche, the decisions will usually be made by the pediatric endocrinologist performing the diagnostic evaluation; however, it is helpful to anticipate the treatment options.

### Treatment of Idiopathic Central Precocious Puberty
True precocious puberty is characterized by the activation of the HPG axis, and standard treatment involves suppression of this axis with GnRH analog (GnRHa). Treatment goals include a decrease in the progression of pubertal changes, alleviation of associated behavioral problems, and an increase in linear growth

**Table 30-18**
**Determination of When to Administer a GnRH Stimulation Test**

- Early pubertal symptoms consistent with central precocious puberty
- Increased height velocity for age
- Advanced bone age
- Elevated luteinizing hormone and follicle-stimulating hormone levels

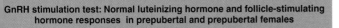

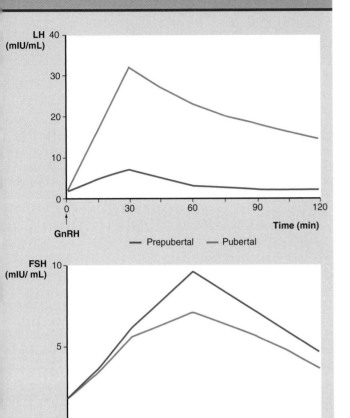

**Figure 30-10   Serum LH and FSH levels after GnRH stimulation.**
(From Mansfield JF: Precocious puberty. In Emans SJ, Laufer MR,
Goldstein DP [eds]: Pediatric and Adolescent Gynecology, 4th ed.
Philadelphia, Lippincott-Raven, 1998, p 116.)

potential. The main long-term complication of idiopathic CPP
is compromised final adult height. In deciding who to treat it
is important to establish an estimate of a child's projected
adult height based on the child's current height and comparing
this to mean parental height (MPH). Determination of what a
child's final height is likely to be based on MPH is shown in
Table 30-20. It is also important to determine the degree of
advancement in bone age.

| Table 30-19 |
| --- |
| **LH/FSH Response to GnRH Stimulation** |

- Prepubertal: LH/FSH ratio less than 1
- Pubertal: LH/FSH ratio greater than 1

FSH, follicle-stimulating hormone; LH, luteinizing hormone.

| Table 30-20 |
| --- |
| **Calculation of a Child's Final Adult Height Based on Mean Parental Height at 50%** |

**Girls**
[(Mother's + Father's height)/2] – 2.5 in. *or* 6.5 cm

**Boys**
[(Mother's + Father's height)/2] + 2.5 in. *or* 6.5 cm

### Determining Who to Treat

The approach to treatment differs among pediatric endocrinologists. However, girls less than 7 years old, with secondary
sexual development, markedly accelerated growth, and a bone
age that is advanced by more than 2 standard deviations are
usually treated. Most males with CPP are also treated, since
they typically have a markedly advanced bone age and rapidly
progressing pubertal development. Girls with less dramatic
findings are not consistently treated but may be followed closely
by a consulting pediatric endocrinologist. These are typically
girls with more slowly advancing sexual maturation, only mildly
advanced bone age, and a normal growth rate with good final
height potential.

Klein et al found that GnRHa therapy improved the final
height in children with rapidly progressing precocious puberty
treated before 8 years of age in girls and 9 years in boys.[31] They
found that GnRHa-treated girls between 6 and 8 years had a
greater average adult height than their pretreatment-predicted
height. Certain factors determine the degree of treatment
success (Table 30-21).

A more recent study demonstrates that height velocity
during GnRHa treatment is inversely related to the degree of
prior estrogen exposure. The authors propose that this impaired
growth is partly due to premature growth plate senescence
caused by earlier estrogen exposure.[32] Other studies have
demonstrated that intervening to improve final adult height is
not always indicated because often the final effect on adult
height is minimal and sometimes there is no difference.[33] However, in those girls who are not treated with GnRHa, close
follow-up is critical because occasionally a child with seemingly
slowly progressive precocious puberty may experience rapid
acceleration of skeletal maturation and be a candidate for treatment. If such girls are not followed closely, the opportunity to
treat may be minimized or lost. In 8- to 10-year-old girls with
"advanced puberty" characterized by development of secondary
sex characteristics, accelerated growth, and advanced bone age
(not more than 1.5 years), GnRHa has not proved beneficial in
altering final adult height.[34]

| Table 30-21 |
| --- |
| **Factors Determining GnRH-Agonist Treatment Success in Rapidly Progressing Precocious Puberty in Girls Less Than Age 8–9 years** |

- Less delay in onset of treatment
- Longer duration of treatment
- Lower chronological age
- Less advanced bone age

Other reasons to treat central precocious puberty include psychosocial or behavioral problems in a younger child with the early development of secondary sexual characteristics. These children and their families may experience undue stress because of the earlier and more rapid rate of pubertal development, and treatment can be beneficial by slowing the pace of pubertal development.

### Treatment of CPP with GnRHa

GnRHa works by initially stimulating gonadotropin release in the short term, which is then followed by desensitization and down-regulation of gonadotropin membrane GnRH receptors, ultimately leading to a marked decrease in gonadotropin and steroid production. Importantly, it is GnRH's pulsatile secretion that causes secretion of LH and FSH; however, when this pulsatile secretion is changed to a continuous infusion, LH and FSH secretion are suppressed. The same inhibition occurs when long-acting GnRHa is administered by intramuscular injection. As a result of a decline in gonadotropin and estrogen levels, most clinical characteristics of puberty, including accelerated growth and breast development, either regress or cease to progress. However, adrenarche progresses normally, since it is not under GnRH influence.

The treatment of choice, then, for central precocious puberty is GnRHa, and the most common form is depot leuprolide, which typically is administered as a subcutaneous sustained-release injection on a monthly basis. Other GnRH analogs approved for the treatment of CPP in the United States are histrelin and nafarelin. Shorter acting forms of GnRHa have been developed to be administered daily by subcutaneous injection or intranasal inhalation but are not as effective. Suppression of the HPG axis typically occurs 4 to 8 weeks after therapy is started in patients with central precocious puberty. In a few females vaginal bleeding may be seen in the first few weeks after initial treatment, but usually it does not persist.

The dose of GnRHa can be monitored by measuring estradiol levels in females (or testosterone levels in males), with the goal of keeping the sex hormone levels in the prepubertal range. Maintaining estradiol levels in the prepubertal range ensures efficacy of dose and treatment. A GnRH stimulation test and estradiol level is usually performed within the first 3 months after treatment has been started to confirm suppression. They can then be repeated every 6 months, along with bone age. Measurement of height, weight, and Tanner stage occurs regularly during treatment. Growth hormone treatment is sometimes added as supplemental treatment in patients with more substantial loss of growth potential and it has been found to significantly improve adult height in such cases. To date, there have been no reported adverse effects from simultaneous use of GH and GnRHa.[35]

Treatment is usually continued until girls are between 11 and 12 years of age and boys are between 12 and 13. Patients can then continue through puberty with their peers, and their growth potential is close to but does not exceed predicted height.

### Post-GnRH Treatment Outcomes and Possible Side Effects

Height potential may be lost if therapy is stopped too early or too late, or if a patient only has incomplete suppression of estrogen. For the latter reason, these patients must be monitored regularly or the main purpose of treatment is defeated. After treatment is stopped, the pubertal process quickly resumes and menstruation usually occurs within 6 to 18 months. Depot preparations of GnRHa therapy are convenient and safe with minor side effects. Hormonal suppression is reversible, with normal future reproductive function and often an improved final adult height. Rarely some patients develop sterile abscesses with IM depot leuprolide. The substitute treatment then becomes daily subcutaneous leuprolide injection.

Treatment with GnRHa has been associated with a decrease in bone mineral density (BMD), with patients treated with GnRHa having a lower BMD for bone age after 2 years of treatment although the BMD was normal for chronologic age.[36] Another study found that the bone age at discontinuation of GnRHa has an effect on final peak bone mass, in that the girls who stop therapy at a bone age of 11.5 have a markedly higher BMD than those who discontinue therapy at a bone age of 12.0 years ($1.22 \, g/cm^2 \pm 0.10$ and $1.04 \, g/cm^2 \pm 0.12$).[37]

An association has been observed between GnRHa treatment and an increase in BMI, whereas such an increase in BMI is not seen in controls. But this increase is reversible, with BMI equalizing between GnRH-treated and -untreated groups once final adult height is reached.

### Treatment of Other Causes of Central Precocious Puberty

Determining the treatment of choice for nonidiopathic CPP or other causes of precocious puberty depends on the underlying cause (Table 30-22). Regardless of the cause of CPP, GnRHa may be a short-term treatment recommendation, even if it is given until a CNS lesion is removed. In the case of hypothalamic hamartoma, GnRHa is the therapy of choice.

When precocious puberty is due to testotoxicosis or McCune-Albright syndrome, the patient is referred to a pediatric endocrinologist. The therapeutic goal is to decrease androgen or estrogen production or to inhibit its peripheral effects. Estimation of final adult height is important in deciding treatment options. Various treatments have been tried in testotoxicosis, including cyproterone acetate, ketoconazole, medroxyprogesterone acetate, spironolactone, and aromatase inhibitors (testolactone). Medications used to treat McCune-Albright syndrome have included aromatase inhibitors, ketoconazole, and medroxyprogesterone, with varying rates of success. Most of these medications have helped alleviate vaginal bleeding but have had no affect on improving growth potential. Recently, the selective estrogen receptor modulator used in breast cancer treatment, tamoxifen, has been studied in the treatment of McCune-Albright syndrome with significant success. In one study tamoxifen proved to be clinically effective in arresting vaginal bleeding, growth acceleration, and pubertal development.[38]

## Prognosis for Precocious Puberty

The prognosis for precocious puberty depends on the underlying cause. The prognosis for idiopathic CPP is excellent overall. The main adverse outcome is compromised final adult height. The prognosis for the other etiologies of precocious puberty vary (Table 30-23).

## Psychosocial Impact of Precocious Puberty

There has been no published demonstration to date that precocious puberty is associated with significant psychosocial roblems. Most children with precocious puberty have psycho-sexual, intellectual, and behavioral maturation in line with their chronological age. Unfortunately, parents, teachers, and peers can have unrealistic expectations of these mature-appearing children. It is therefore important to educate and provide counseling,

**Table 30-22**
**Treatment of Precocious Puberty**

I. Central precocious puberty (GnRH-dependent)
  A. Idiopathic
    1. Rapidly progressing (bone age ≥2 SD above the mean)
      a. Refer to pediatric endocrinology
      b. Likely GnRHa analog (GnRHa) and counseling
    2. Slowly progressing (less advanced bone age)
      a. Refer to pediatric endocrinology
      b. Likely observation* and counseling
  B. Hypothalamic hamartoma
    1. Refer to neurosurgeon or pediatric neurologist for seizure management
    2. Also refer to pediatric endocrinologist if CPP present
      a. Pedunculated (suspended from floor of third ventricle)—resect when possible
      b. Not pedunculated
        i. Treat symptoms
        ii. GnRHa usually helpful
  C. CNS pathology
    1. Tumor, congenital malformation, genetic, etc.
    2. Refer to specialist depending on MRI and laboratory test findings (neurosurgeon, oncologist, genetic specialist, etc.)
  D. CPP secondary to prolonged elevation of peripheral steroid
    1. Refer to specialist depending on source
    2. Treat underlying cause
    3. Someteimes GnRHa is indicated
II. Peripheral precocious puberty (GnRH-independent)
  A. Gonadal tumor—refer to surgery, pediatric endocrinology, gynecology, or oncology
  B. Adrenal tumor—Same as above
  C. hCG-secreting tumor—Same as above
  D. CAH
    1. Refer to pediatric endocrinology
    2. Possible glucocorticoid therapy and family evaluation
  E. Ovarian cyst—observe*
  F. Testotoxicosis
    1. Refer to pediatric endocrinology
    2. Inhibit testosterone synthesis
  G. McCune-Albright syndrome
    1. Refer to pediatric endocrinology
    2. Inhibit sex steroid synthesis
  H. Hypothyroidism
    1. Refer to or consult with pediatric endocrinology
    2. Hormone replacement
  I. Exogeneous steroid source—discontinue exposure
III. Isolated precocious puberty
  A. Premature thelarche—observe*
  B. Premature adrenarche
    1. Observe* and refer to pediatric endocrinology
    2. Long-term follow-up including evaluation of risk factors for future endocrine disease and other health risks
IV. Premature menarche
  A. Negative ultrasound (US)—observe*
  B. Positive US (cyst)—observe*,†
  C. Positive US (tumor)—refer to surgery
  D. Other cause of vaginal bleeding—treat or refer depending on suspected cause

* Frequency depends on age and rapidity of onset and progression. Initial follow-up recommended in 3 months. If there is evidence of growth velocity acceleration, pediatric endocrine referral is required.
† Recurrence or complication is an indication for consultation.

**Table 30-23**
**Prognosis for Precocious Puberty Based on Etiology**

I. Central precocious puberty (GnRH-dependent)
  A. Idiopathic—excellent prognosis
  B. CNS lesion—good prognosis if resection is possible, but typically depends on tumor type and histologic features
    1. Craniopharyngioma—partial resection and radiation therapy leads to remission for many years in most cases
    2. Glioma—worst prognosis
    3. Hypothalamic hamartomas—good prognosis
      a. Slowly growing; treat symptoms
      b. Often need GnRHa or seizure prophylaxis
  C. Genetic disorder (neurofibromatosis, etc.)
    1. Depends on other CNS or endocrine manifestations
    2. Growth potential and reproductive function generally normal
  D. CPP secondary to a peripheral source—depends on the source
II. Peripheral precocious puberty
  A. Adrenal tumor—depends on tumor type
  B. Ovarian (gonadal) tumor—depends on tumor type
  C. β-hCG-secreting tumor—depends on type and location
  D. CAH—good prognosis with glucocorticoid treatment but often adult short stature
  E. Hypothyroidism
    1. Symptoms resolve once hormonal replacement started
    2. Good prognosis
  F. Ovarian cyst—typically resolves on its own
  G. McCune-Albright syndrome
    1. Dependent on other manifestations of the disorder
    2. Growth potential may be compromised
    3. Reproductive function generally normal
  H. Testotoxicosis—good prognosis. Boys may be fertile earlier. Growth potential is variable.
  I. Exogenous sex steroid exposure—symptoms resolve once source is removed
III. Isolated precocious puberty
  A. Premature thelarche—excellent prognosis but can evolve into CPP
  B. Premature adrenarche—possibility of future endocrine disease
IV. Premature menarche—typically excellent prognosis for normal development

when necessary, for these children and their parents. They need to be informed that they are early, yet normal, developers. Also, there has been little evidence to support an earlier onset of heterosexual activity in children with precocious puberty.

## SUMMARY AND CONTROVERSIES

Puberty is a complex hormonal process, occurring in a specific pattern and manifested by certain clinical, emotional, and developmental characteristics that ultimately result in a sexually mature individual with the ability to procreate. Though trends in the earlier onset of puberty have been informally acknowledged, the widely accepted age of onset of puberty in females has been 8 years old, and an earlier onset has been considered precocious puberty. In response to the large, cross-sectional, practice-based PROS study supported by the AAP, a controversy among endocrinologists and other clinicians has arisen regarding the age-limited definition of precocious puberty. The data from the PROS and NHANES III studies suggest that puberty is beginning earlier than previously thought with a notable difference between ethnic groups. The impact of this data on the diagnosis of precocious puberty is still unfolding. However, it is clear that girls with early signs of puberty may be at increased risk for later endocrine disease. As a result, clinicians who are evaluating early signs of pubertal development in females should be wary of adhering to strict age limits in defining precocious puberty and approach each case individually.

It would be helpful for a large, prospective, population-based study to support the new guidelines for the evaluation of early pubertal onset. Until that time, the best approach to early or precocious puberty is a thorough history, complete physical examination, and a high level of concern, taking into account the many differential diagnostic possibilities. Utilizing subspecialty consultation is central to proper diagnosis and treatment in most cases. Pediatric endocrinologists are the most usual source of the required expertise. In some communities, specialists in adolescent medicine, pediatric gynecology, and neurosurgery may be available to assist with an initial diagnosis or some aspects of treatment.

## KEY TERMS

**Central precocious puberty (CPP) or true or complete precocious puberty:** early pubertal development that results from premature activation of the hypothalamic-pituitary-gonadal (HPG) axis and is GnRH-dependent.

**Constitutional early puberty:** early pubertal development that occurs in otherwise normal children who have a family history of early pubertal onset.

**Contrasexual precocious puberty:** peripheral precocious puberty characterized by female virilization or male feminization.

**Early puberty:** pubertal development that occurs early in relation to traditional norms but is not considered precocious. May or may not occur in families.

**Isolated menstruation or premature menarche:** one or two episodes of isolated vaginal bleeding without other signs of puberty, usually occurring at the beginning of what will be normal pubertal development.

**Isolated precocious puberty or incomplete precocious puberty:** includes premature thelarche and premature pubarche. These are usually self-limited signs, without marked growth acceleration. Isolated precocious puberty can overlap in classification schemes with PPP or be an early sign of CPP.

**Isosexual precocious puberty:** peripheral precocious puberty, which is characterized by sex-concordant secondary sexual development.

**Peripheral precocious puberty (PPP) or pseudoprecocious or incomplete precocious puberty:** early pubertal development that occurs secondary to gonadotropin and/or sex steroid secretion occurring independently of GnRH. PPP can be isosexual or contrasexual.

**Precocious puberty:** a more general term describing early pubertal development that may be an aberration from normal. The term frequently is used before the etiology is determined. It can be GnRH-independent or -dependent.

**Slowly progressive or nonprogressive precocious puberty:** term used by some authors that describes the course of most cases of isolated precocious puberty. The term also overlaps with early puberty and constitutional early puberty. It is usually used to describe a normal variant.

## REFERENCES

1. Palmert MR, Boepple PA: Variation in the timing of puberty: clinic spectrum and genetic investigation. J Clin Endocrinol Metab 200 86:2364–2368. **(IIa, B)**
2. Marshall WA, Tanner JM: Variations in pattern of pubertal changes i girls. Arch Dis Child 1969;44:291–303. **(IIb, B)**
3. Parente AS, Teilmann G, Juul A: The timing of normal puberty an the age limits of sexual precocity: variations around the world, secula trends, and changes after migration. Endocr Rev 2003;24:668–69 **(IIa, B)**
4. Anderson SE, Dallal GE, Must A: Relative Weight and race influenc average age at menarche: results from two nationally representativ surveys of US girls studied 25 years apart. Pediatrics 2003 111:844–850. **(IIa, B)**
5. Chamlea WC, Schubert CM, Roche AF: Age at menarche and racia comparisons in US girls. Pediatrics 2003;111:110–113. **(IIa, B)**
6. Herman-Giddens ME, Slora EJ, Wasserman RC: Secondary sexua characteristics and menses in young girls seen in office practice: a stud from the Pediatric Research in Office Settings Network. Pediatric 1997;99:505–512. **(IIab, B)**
7. Marti-Henneberg CM, Vizmanos B: The duration of puberty in girl is related to the timing of its onset. J Pediatr 1997;131:618–62 **(IIab, B)**
8. Apter D, Vihko R: Early menarche, a risk factor for breast cance indicates early onset of ovulatory cycles. J Clin Endocrinol Meta 1983;57:82–86. **(Ib–IIa, B)**
9. Troiano RP, Flegal KM, Kcuzmarski RJ: Overweight prevalence an trends for children and adolescents: The National Health and Nutritio Examination Surveys, 1963 to 1991. Arch Pediatr Adolesc Med 199 149:1085–1091. **(IIa, B)**
10. Kaplowitz PB, Oberfield SE: Reexamination of the age limit fc defining when puberty is precocious in girls in the United State implications for evaluation and treatment. Pediatrics 1999;104:936–94 **(IIa, B)**
11. Rosenfield RL, Bachrach LK, Chernausek SD: Current age of onset c puberty. Pediatrics 2000;106:622–623. **(IIa, B)**
12. Viner R: Splitting hairs. Arch Dis Child 2002;86:8–10. **(IIa, B)**
13. Midyett LK, Moore WV, Jacobson JD: Are pubertal changes in girl before age 8 benign? Pediatrics 2003;111:47–51. **(IIb, B)**
14. Halvarson LM, DeCherney AH: Inhibin, activin and follistatin i reproductive medicine. Fertil Steril 1996;65:459–469. **(IIb, B)**
15. Lloyd T, Andon MB, Rollings N: Calcium supplementation and bon mineral density in adolescent girls. JAMA 1993;270:841–844. **(Ib, A)**
16. Gilsanz V, Roe TF, Mora S: Changes in vertebral bone density in blac girls and white girls during childhood and puberty. N Engl J Me 1991;325:1597–1600. **(IIa, B)**
17. Berkey CS, Gardner JD, Frazner LA: Relation of childhood diet an body size to menarche and adolescent growth in girls. Am J Epidemic 2000;152:446–452. **(IIa, B)**
18. Mazur W, Adlercreutz H: Overview of naturally occurring endocrine active substances in the human diet in relation to human healtr Nutrition 2000;16:654–658. **(IIa, B)**
19. Palmert MR, Radovick S, Boepple PA: Leptin levels in children wit central precocious puberty. J Clin Endocrinol Metab 199 83:2260–2265. **(IIab, B)**
20. Kaplowitz PB, Slora EJ, Wasserman RC: Earlier onset of puberty i girls: relation to increased body mass index and race. Pediatrics 200 108:347–353. **(IIa, B)**
21. Davison DD, Susman EF, Birch LL: Percent body fat at age 5 predict earlier pubertal development among girls age 9. Pediatrics 2003 111:815–821. **(IIab, B)**
22. Rogan WJ, Ragan NB: Evidence of effects of environmental chemical on the endocrine system in children. Pediatrics 2003;112:247–252 **(IIb, B)**

23. Li ST, Lozano P, Grossman DC: Hormone-containing hair product use in prepubertal children. Arch Pediatr Adolesc Med 2002;156:85–86. **(III, C)**

24. Putnam F: Ten year research update review: child sexual abuse. J Am Acad Child Adolesc Psychiatry 2003;42:269–278. **(IIb, B)**

25. Ibanez L, Di Martino-Nardi J, Potau N: Premature adrenarche—normal variant or forerunner of adult disease? Endocr Rev 2000;21:671–696. **(IIab, B)**

26. Ibanez L, de Zegher F, Potau N: Anovulation after precocious pubarche: early markers and time course in adolescence. J Clin Endocrinol Metab 1999;84:2691–2695. **(IIa, B)**

27. Vuguin P, Linder B, Rosenfeld RG: The roles of insulin sensitivity, insulin-like growth facter-1 (IGF-1) and IGF-binding protein-1 and –3 in the hyperandrogenism of African American and Caribbean Hispanic girls with premature adrenarche. J Clin Endocrinol Metab 1999; 84:2037. **(IIb, B)**

28. Francois I, de Zegher F: Adrenarche and fetal growth. Pediatr Res 1997;41:440–442. **(IIa, B)**

29. Root A: Precocious puberty. Pediatr Rev 2000;21:10–19. **(IIb, B)**

30. Chalumea M: Central precocious puberty in girls: an evidence-based diagnostic tree to predict CNS abnormalities. Pediatrics 2002; 109:61–70. **(IIb, B)**

31. Klein KO, Barnes KM, Jones JV: Increased final height in precocious puberty after long-term treatment with LHRH agonists: the National Institutes of Health Experience. J Clin Endocrinol Metab 2001;86: 4711–4716. **(IIb, B)**

32. Weise M, Flor A, Barnes KM: Determinants of growth during gonadotropin-releasing hormone analog therapy for precocious puberty. J Clin Endocrinol Metab 2004;89:103–107. **(IIb, B)**

33. Lazar L, Kauli R, Pertzelan A: Gonadotropin-suppressive therapy in girls with early and fast puberty affects the pace of puberty but not total pubertal growth or final height. J Clin Endocrinol Metab 2002; 87:2090–2094. **(IIa, B)**

34. Bouvattier C, Coste J, Rodrigue D: Lack of effect of GnRH agonists on final height in girls with advanced puberty: a randomized long-term pilot study. J Clin Endocrinol Metab 1999;84:3575–3578. **(Ib, A)**

35. Pasquino AM, Pucarelli I, Segni M: Adult height in girls with central precocious puberty treated with gonadotropin-releasing hormone analogs and growth hormone. J Clin Endocrinol Metab 1999; 84:449–452. **(IIa, B)**

36. Boot AM, Keizer-Schrama SM, Pols HA: Bone mineral density and body composition before and during treatment with gonadotropin-releasing hormone agonist in children with central precocious puberty. J Clin Endocrinol Metab 1998;83:370–373. **(IIb, B)**

37. Bertelloni S, Baroncelli GI, Sorrentino MC: Effect of central precocious puberty and gonadotropin-releasing hormone and treatment on peak bone mass and final height in females. Eur J Pediatr 1998; 157:363–367. **(IIa, B)**

38. Eugster EA, Rubin SD, Reiter EO: Tamoxifen treatment for precocious puberty in McCune-Albright syndrome: a multicenter trial. J Pediatr 2003;143:61–67. **(IIb, B)**

# Chapter 31

# Delayed Puberty and Primary Amenorrhea

## Colleen Buggs, MD, PhD, and Robert L. Rosenfield, MD

### KEY POINTS

- Delayed puberty is defined as the lack of breast development by the chronologic age of 13 years in girls. Primary amenorrhea is defined as the absence of menses by 15 years of age.
- Girls who enter puberty later than the usual chronologic age most often have constitutional delay of growth and development, and the prognosis is excellent for normal stature and secondary sexual development.
- Constitutional delay of puberty is a benign variation of normal but can be mimicked by chronic disease and difficult to distinguish from causes of primary amenorrhea.
- After a thorough history and physical examination, the next step in the endocrine workup of a teenager with delayed puberty or amenorrhea is determination of gonadotropin, estradiol, and prolactin levels and bone age. Highly sensitive (third-generation) assays must be used for gonadotropin and estradiol determinations.
- Determining the stage of breast development (delayed or immature versus mature) is important in the algorithmic approach to the differential diagnosis and management of delayed puberty and primary amenorrhea.

Breast development (thelarche) is the first sign of true puberty in the vast majority of girls. In approximately 10% of girls, pubic hair development may occur first. The presence of pubic hair without breast development is *not* a sign of true puberty. This situation arises because adrenarche, which contributes to the onset of pubic hair development (pubarche), is an incomplete pseudo-puberty of the adrenal gland, which is gonadotropin-independent. The stages of breast and pubic hair development are shown in Figure 31-1.[1] Tanner stage I is prepubertal. Breast development stage II (B2) is the presence of a palpable sub-areolar bud. Enlargement and elevation of the whole breast is stage III (B3). Areolar mounding, which is very transient and may not necessarily appear, is stage IV (B4). The final stage, V (B5), is the attainment of mature breast contour. Presexual pubic hairs (stage II, PH2) are short, light, and straight and may not be obvious on cursory examination. Sexual pubic hairs (stage III, PH3) are long, dark, and curly, appearing on the labia majora before spreading to the pubis. Stage IV (PH4) is progression of pubic hair that does not spread to the medial surface of the thighs. The final stage is progression to the mature female escutcheon (inverted triangle pattern, stage V, PH5). Axillary hair usually appears about a year later than pubic hair and passes through similar stages.

For many years, the estimated onset of pubertal milestones was based on data from standards derived from North American children over 20 years ago.[2,3] Lately there has been considerable debate about whether the age of puberty has become earlier. The Third National Health and Examination Survey (NHANES III) has recently reported data obtained between 1988 and 1994. This study represented the total U.S. population, with intentional oversampling of non-Hispanic blacks (Blacks) and Mexican Americans to increase the reliability of these estimates relative to non-Hispanic whites (Whites). Trained physicians assessed pubic hair and breast stages by inspection in 2145 girls who were 8.0 to 19.0 years of age. Menarche was documented by questionnaire in 2510 girls who were 8.0 to 20.0 years of age. The median age of menarche was 12.43 years for the general population, not significantly different from that in the earlier National Health and Examination Survey (12.8 years). Current estimates are shown in Table 31-1.[4,5] Black girls were significantly earlier than white girls for all pubertal milestones, and Mexican-Americans were intermediate. A separate analysis showed that early sexual maturation was significantly positively associated with overweight and obesity in girls.[6]

## NORMAL PUBERTAL PHYSIOLOGY

The aspects of normal pubertal physiology that are key to understanding disorders of puberty are as follows:[1] (1) Childhood is a state of physiologic gonadotropin-releasing hormone (GnRH) deficiency due to the central nervous system (CNS) restraint that develops during infancy. (2) Pubertal gonadotropin secretion has a diurnal variation, with sleep-associated onset, and is cyclic in girls from the beginning. Luteinizing hormone (LH) levels are more indicative of the degree of pubertal maturation of the neuroendocrine system than are follicle-stimulating hormone (FSH) levels. (3) A certain level of general somatic maturity must normally be reached before the CNS permits pubertal GnRH and gonadotropin production. The bone age (the average age at which a given skeletal maturation begins) correlates with this maturity better than chronologic age, leading to the practical rule of thumb that puberty typically begins at a pubertal bone age (Table 31-2). Bone age is related to pubertal stage with 25% less variance than chronologic age. Height potential can be predicted from the bone age, too. Accurate bone age interpretation requires an experienced reader.

## DEFINITION AND EPIDEMIOLOGY

Puberty is delayed when breast bud development (B2) has not begun by 13.0 years of age.[1] On statistical grounds, this is approximately 2.0 standard deviations (SD) later than average

# Pediatric and Adolescent Gynecology

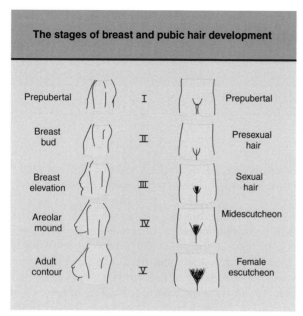

**The stages of breast and pubic hair development**

| | | |
|---|---|---|
| Prepubertal | I | Prepubertal |
| Breast bud | II | Presexual hair |
| Breast elevation | III | Sexual hair |
| Areolar mound | IV | Midescutcheon |
| Adult contour | V | Female escutcheon |

**Figure 31-1    Stages of breast and pubic hair development.** (From Rosenfield RL: Puberty in the female and its disorders. In Sperling M [ed]: Pediatric Endocrinology, 3rd ed. Philadelphia, W.B. Saunders, 2002, pp 455–518.)

(see Table 31-1).[4,5] Puberty is also considered delayed if it does not progress at a normal tempo, as indicated, for example, by arrested breast development or failure of menses to occur within 4.5 years of the onset of puberty. Typically, the chief complaint is lack of menstruation when girls enter high school at 14 years of age and realize that most of their friends are menstruating. Menarche will be delayed if pubertal onset is delayed; the average time from the onset of breast development to menarche is 2.3 ± 1.0 years, though there is a tendency for the tempo of puberty to be more rapid in those in whom it begins relatively late.[8,9] Primary amenorrhea is defined as the absence of menses by 15 years of age.

## ETIOLOGY

Normal function and interaction of the hypothalamus, pituitary, and ovary, as well as normal development of the genital tract and uterus, are required for appropriate pubertal development and

**Table 31-1**
**Current Estimates for Year of Onset of Pubertal Milestones in Girls in the United States***

| | Whites | | Blacks | |
|---|---|---|---|---|
| Pubertal Stage | Median | (5% to 95%) | Median | (5% to 95%) |
| Breast buds (B2) | 10.4 | (8.3–12.5) | 9.5 | (7.0–12.0) |
| Pubic hair, presexual (PH2) | 10.6 | (8.4–12.8) | 9.4 | (6.8–12.2) |
| Menarche | 12.55 | (11.0–14.1) | 12.06 | (10.1–14.0) |

*Italicized figures are estimated from fitted data.

**Table 31-2**
**Puberty Typically Begins at a Pubertal Bone Age**

- Certain level of general maturity must normally be reached before the CNS activates puberty
- Bone age corresponds to this maturity better than chronologic age

| | Girls | |
|---|---|---|
| **Examples** | | |
| Bone age | 11 yr | 13 yr |
| Pubertal stage | B2 | Menarche |
| Percent final height | 91 | 96 |

From Rosenfield RL: Delayed puberty. In Adashi EY, Rock JA, Rosenwaks Z (eds): Reproductive Endocrinology, Surgery, and Technology. Philadelphia, Lippincott-Raven, 1996, pp 1008–1015.

**Table 31-3**
**Causes of Delayed Puberty or Primary Amenorrhea**

| Hypothalamic-Pituitary-Gonadal (HPG) Disorders | Non-HPG Disorders |
|---|---|
| **Hypothalamic disorders** | **Uterus/outflow disorders** |
| Acquired | Aplasia |
|     Functional | Müllerian |
|         Constitutional delay of puberty | Vaginal |
|         Hypothalamic anovulation | Hymenal |
|     Organic | Ambiguous genitalia |
|         Tumors | Intersex syndromes |
|         Infiltrative | Pseudointersex |
| Congenital | |
| **Pituitary disorders** | **Adrenal disorders** |
| Gonadotropin deficiency | Androgen-secreting tumors* |
|     Congenital | Congenital adrenal hyperplasia* |
|         LH beta or FSH beta gene mutation | Cushing's syndrome |
|         GnRH receptor gene mutation | |
|     Organic | |
|         Prolactinoma | |
|         Non-prolactin-secreting tumor | |
|     Functional | |
|         Hypopituitarism | |
|         Hyper- or hypothyroidism | |
|         Hyperprolactinemia | |
| **Gonadal disorders** | **Chronic diseases** |
| Premature ovarian failure | Anemia |
|     Congenital | Gastrointestinal |
|         Chromosomal disorders | Liver |
|         Genetic disorders | Renal |
|         Resistant ovaries | |
|         Steroidogenic block | **Metabolic disorders** |
|     Acquired | |
|         Oophorectomy | |
|         Radiotherapy or chemotherapy | |
|         Oophoritis | |
|         Idiopathic | |
| Polycystic ovary syndrome (PCOS) | |
| Androgen-secreting tumors* | |
| Intersex syndromes | |

*Indicates disorders that can cause primary amenorrhea with incomplete sexual precocity.
From Rosenfield RL, Barnes RB: Menstrual disorders in adolescence. Endocrinol Metab Clin North Am 1993;22:491–505.

**Table 31-4**
**Characteristics of Constitutional Delay in Girls**

- No chronic illness or undernutrition
- Familial precedent (in about half)

**Before puberty begins**

- Puberty delayed, but begins before 16 years of age
- Puberty begins at a pubertal BA, before BA13
- Height velocity slows
- Routine endocrine tests resemble gonadotropin deficiency

**After puberty begins**

- Pubertal hormones and stages advance at normal tempo
- Pubertal growth advances at normal tempo
- Genetic height potential is achieved in late teenage years

From Rosenfield RL: Delayed puberty. In Adashi EY, Rock JA, Rosenwaks Z (eds): Reproductive Endocrinology, Surgery, and Technology. Philadelphia, Lippincott-Raven, 1996, pp 1008–1015.

menses to occur. Delayed puberty results from lack of pubertal maturation of the neuroendocrine-gonadal axis. It may result not only from neuroendocrine or ovarian disorders themselves but from chronic disorders of virtually any organ system because they affect the function of this axis (Table 31-3).[15]

## Constitutional Delay of Pubertal Development

Most commonly, delayed puberty occurs as an extreme variation of normal, which is termed *constitutional delay in growth and pubertal development*. For this discussion, the term constitutional delay of puberty (CDP) is used. CDP occurs in an otherwise healthy child but is eventually normal (Table 31-4).[7] It has familial precedents about half the time.[11–13] Therefore, a family history of delayed puberty is compatible with, but not diagnostic of, constitutional delay. Puberty onset is retarded to about the same extent as bone age and begins at a skeletal age appropriate for puberty, typically approximating 11 years. Although starting late, puberty begins by 16 years of age. When puberty does ensue, it is perfectly normal in tempo, and endocrinologic status is normal for the stage of puberty.

## DIFFERENTIAL DIAGNOSIS

It is important to distinguish CDP from the many disorders that can mimic it. It is most difficult to distinguish it from gonadotropin deficiency. Investigation should be begun for delayed puberty when breast development has not begun by the chronologic age of 13 years or if menses fails to occur within 4.5 years of the onset of puberty.

The evaluation should always begin with a history of current and previous medical problems and their treatment. An algorithmic approach to the differential diagnosis for delayed puberty and primary amenorrhea is dependent on the stage of breast development, as outlined in Figures 31-2 and 31-3, respectively. A girl may present with absent or immature breast development secondary to constitutional delay or primary amenorrhea (see Fig. 31-2), while a girl who has mature breast development may present with absence of menarche secondary to primary amenorrhea (see Fig. 31-3). Once breast development

has matured (B5), the breast contour does not substantially regress even in the absence of ovarian function. Particular focus should be directed at a history of growth retardation (all disorders that retard bone maturation retard the onset and progression of puberty), anosmia (suggestive of congenital gonadotropin deficiency), intracranial or visual symptoms (pituitary mass), radio- or chemotherapy (damage to neuroendocrine-gonadal axis), emotional or eating disorders (anorexia nervosa), and athletic activity (athletic amenorrhea). Use of corticosteroids, opiates, cocaine, or phenothiazine neuroleptics (hyperprolactinemia) can delay puberty.

## CLINICAL FEATURES

Key features of the physical examination are height and weight, with derivation of weight for height age or body mass index (BMI), and growth rate as well as vital signs (hypothermia, bradycardia, hypertension). Short stature is the rule, since the pubertal growth spurt has not occurred, but extreme short stature suggests extraovarian endocrinopathy (such as hypopituitarism, hypothyroidism, and Turner's syndrome).

Weight-for-height is an important clue to eating disorders and chronic disease. In prepubertal girls, undernutrition is defined by weight below the 10th percentile for height age. In pubertal girls, undernutrition should be considered if weight is below the 10th percentile of body fatness for height or BMI less than the 10th percentile. Body fat less than 10% to 15% of body mass is the critical parameter, and this may not be reflected accurately by weight-for-height parameters in athletes who have a disproportionately great muscle mass. Anorexia nervosa is a symptom complex consisting of amenorrhea, voluntary starvation, and a self-delusional disturbance in the perception of body fatness. Body fat determination by dual photon x-ray absorptiometry or bioimpedence monitoring may assist in the documentation of low body fat in girls with eating disorders (anorexia nervosa and bulimia nervosa).

Not only should the physician focus on clues from the history and review of systems, but the examination also should include evaluation of eye movements, visual fields, and optic fundi (for tumor or congenital abnormalities), as well as a search for midline facial defects (for acquired or congenital hypopituitarism). Patients should be evaluated for anosmia, which can be associated with hypogonadism (Kallmann syndrome). Pectoral hypoplasia may be a clue to breast aplasia (Poland's syndrome). Categorization of the stage of sexual development is essential. Careful examination of the introitus, hymen, and clitoris are important to identify the possibility of intersex or pseudointersex disorders.

### Laboratory Evaluation

A chronic disease panel, serum gonadotropins and estradiol, prolactin level, and bone age should be determined initially. It is essential that high-sensitivity ("third generation") assays be used for the FSH, LH, and estradiol determinations, as discussed following, rather than the rapid assays in routine gynecologic use. The latter are often too insensitive and thus too imprecise for this purpose. A chronic disease panel screens for the chronic endocrine, metabolic, and systemic disorders that attenuate or retard growth (Table 31-5).[7]

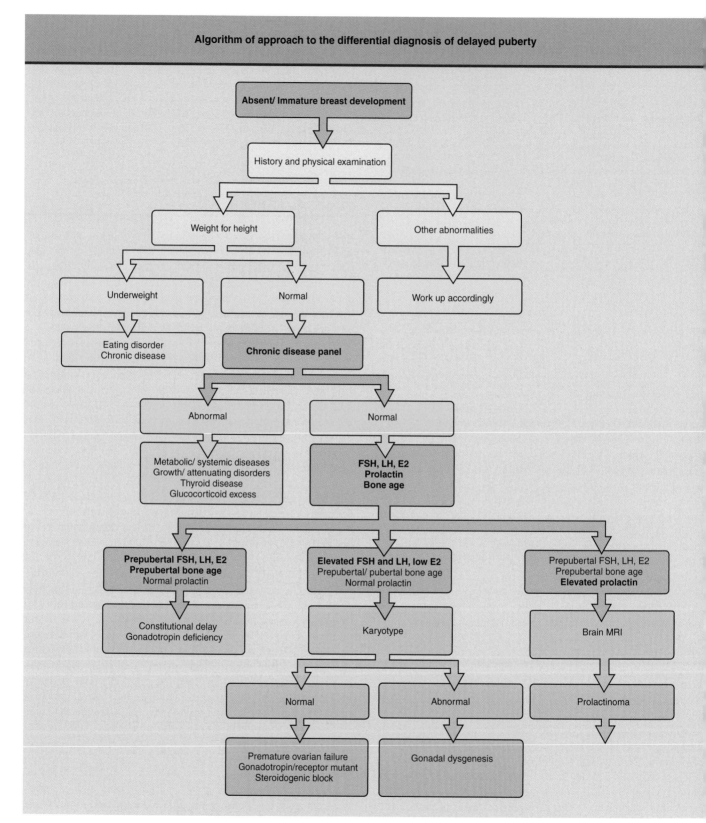

**Figure 31-2    Algorithm of approach to the differential diagnosis of delayed puberty.** E₂, estradiol. (From Rosenfield RL: Menstrual disorders and hyperandrogenism in adolescence. In Radovick S, MacGillivray MH [eds]: Pediatric Endocrinology: A Practical Clinical Guide. Totowa, NJ, Humana Press, 2003, pp 451–478.)

**Algorithm of approach to the differential diagnosis of primary amenorrhea in girls in whom puberty has been normal**

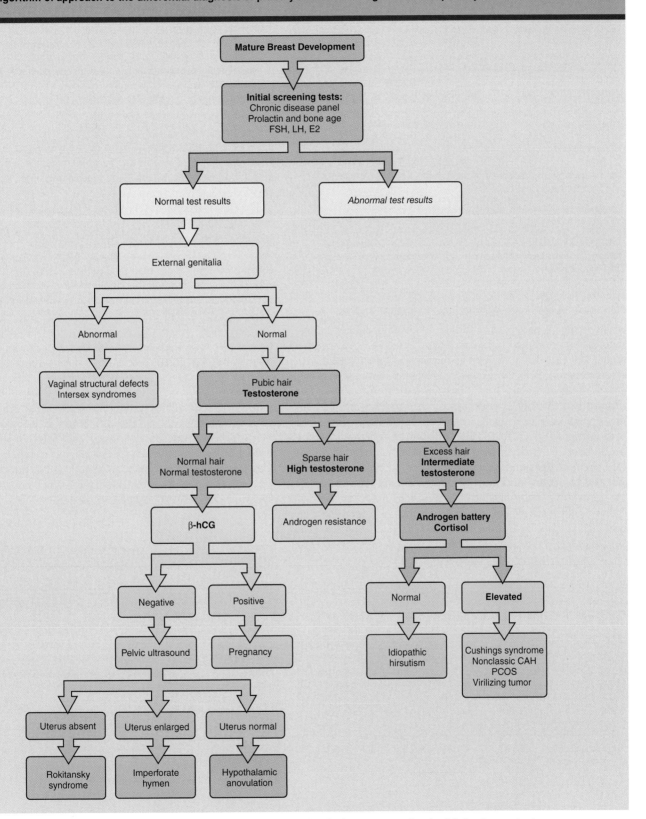

**Figure 31-3    Algorithm of approach to the differential diagnosis of primary amenorrhea in girls in whom puberty has been normal.** CAH, congenital adrenal hyperplasia, E$_2$, estradiol; PCOS, polycystic ovary syndrome. *See Figure 31-2. (Modified from Rosenfield RL: Menstrual disorders and hyperandrogenism in adolescence. In Radovick S, MacGillivray MH [eds]: Pediatric Endocrinology: A Practical Clinical Guide. Totowa, NJ, Humana Press, 2003, pp 451–478.)

# Pediatric and Adolescent Gynecology

## Table 31-5
## Chronic Disease Panel of Tests for Disorders That Delay Puberty

| Disorder | Tests |
|---|---|
| **Endocrinopathy** | |
| GH deficiency | Somatomedin C (IGF-1) |
| Hypothyroidism | Thyroid panel |
| Cushing's syndrome | Cortisol |
| **Metabolic disorders** | Comprehensive metabolic panel (CMP) |
| **Chronic disease** | |
| Anemia | Complete blood count (CBC) |
| Gastrointestinal, liver, renal disease | Erythrocyte sedimentation rate (ESR), celiac panel, CMP possibly |
| **Undernutrition** | Triiodothyronine ($T_3$), reverse $T_3$, prealbumin |

From Rosenfield RL: Delayed puberty. In Adashi EY, Rock JA, Rosenwaks Z (eds): Reproductive Endocrinology, Surgery, and Technology. Philadelphia, Lippincott-Raven, 1996, pp 1008–1015.

If the tests for undernutrition and chronic diseases are all negative, then gonadotropins, estradiol, prolactin, and a bone age should be determined. If marked prolactin excess is detected, a brain MRI study for a pituitary adenoma may be consistent with a prolactinoma. Prolactin excess is a potential, but rare, cause of gonadotropin deficiency; hypoestrogenic patients do not manifest galactorrhea. If FSH is not elevated in a prepubertal patient, determination of bone age is important in the interpretation of gonadotropin levels (Table 31-6).[15] If bone age is below 11 years, neuroendocrine puberty may not yet have occurred, in which case premature ovarian failure is not yet hypergonadotropic[15] and the physician must consider both primary and secondary hypogonadism (hypogonadotropic hypogonadism), as well as delayed puberty. Partial ovarian failure is the only other situation in which premature ovarian failure occurs in the presence of normal baseline gonadotropin levels; in these patients, GnRH or GnRH agonist testing will show exaggerated FSH responses.

If FSH is not elevated and the bone age is more than 11 years, proceed to determine the degree of estrogenization. Absence of

breast development ordinarily means lack of estrogen. On the other hand, immature breast development indicates that there has been estrogen exposure, but it does not mean that there is active feminization; estradiol levels are particularly important when there is concern that puberty has begun but has arrested. Diurnal variations must be taken into account in interpreting estradiol and gonadotropin levels in premenarcheal girls. Determination of vaginal hormonal cytology is most indicative of overall estrogen exposure but is not well tolerated by children and adolescents. If a girl with delayed puberty is well estrogenized and has no breast development, she has the rare disorder of breast aplasia; this may be associated with Poland's syndrome (hypoplasia of the pectoral muscles with rib deformities, webbed fingers, and radial nerve aplasia). Otherwise, the breast development is immature.

Daytime estradiol levels below 10 pg/mL, LH levels below 0.15 U/L, and FSH levels below 2.5 U/L are typical of the prepubertal state. However, these values do not rule out the onset of puberty, since they are found in some early pubertal normal children. A plasma estradiol level of 10 pg/mL or greater strongly suggests that puberty has begun, as does an LH level over 0.15 to 0.6 mIU/mL in a "third generation" monoclonal assay.[1] Daytime LH levels between 0.15 and 0.6 mIU/mL are "gray zone" values that suggest the onset of puberty but are not definitive. Estradiol levels of 20 pg/mL and LH levels of 1.0 mIU/mL or greater are clearly indicative of the onset of puberty.

Constitutional delay is the most likely diagnosis until the bone age reaches 13 years (see Table 31-6). If studies to this point show no pathology, the differential diagnosis is between idiopathic gonadotropin deficiency and delayed puberty. This distinction may be difficult. The parameters that help distinguish between gonadotropin deficiency and constitutional delay of puberty are summarized in Table 31-7.[15] Once puberty begins in constitutional delay, it goes to completion.

## Table 31-6
## Bone Age in Workup of Sexually Immature Girls with Prepubertal Gonadotropin Levels

| | Bone Age <11 yr | Bone Age 11–13 yr | Bone Age >13 yr |
|---|:---:|:---:|:---:|
| Hypergonadotropic hypogonadism | ✓ | | |
| Delayed puberty | ✓ | ✓ | |
| Hypogonadotropic hypogonadism | ✓ | ✓ | ✓ |

From Rosenfield RL, Barnes RB: Menstrual disorders in adolescence. Endocrinol Metab Clin North Am 1993;22:491–505

## Table 31-7
## Features Distinguishing Gonadotropin Deficiency from Constitutional Delay

In a healthy, delayed prepubertal girl with BA >11 yr and prepubertal FSH, gonadotropin deficiency is

**Possible if**

- Weight loss >5% to 8% (BMI <10th to 15th percentile for height age)
- Midline facial defect
- CNS dysfunction
- CT or MRI brain scan abnormal

**Probable if**

- BA >13 yr and LH <0.15 U/L in early daytime
- Anosmia or panhypopituitarism

**Diagnostic if**

- Sleep-associated increase in LH lacking
- GnRH (agonist) test → flat response
- Chronologic age >16 yr

From Rosenfield RL, Barnes RB: Menstrual disorders in adolescence. Endocrinol Metab Clin North Am 1993;22:491–505

GnRH testing may permit the differentiation between hypogonadotropic hypogonadism and constitutionally delayed puberty. The GnRH test, measuring the gonadotropin response to a 50- to 100-µg bolus, strongly suggests that the delayed puberty is a variation of normal if it elicits a brisk response of LH (7.0 IU/L or more by monoclonal assay). However, the GnRH test has limitations because some normal teenagers have minimal responses and because about one third of hypogonadotropic subjects have clear-cut responses. GnRH agonist testing, using 10 µg/kg of leuprolide, may discriminate between these disorders better and adds the dimension of assessing the gonadal secretory response to the secreted gonadotropins.[16] Normal sleep-associated increase of LH secretion into the pubertal range is the most definitive early hormonal evidence of puberty, but has not been proved to necessarily distinguish hypothalamic dysfunction from constitutional delay of puberty.[17] Thus, it may not be possible to definitively establish the diagnosis of gonadotropin deficiency until puberty fails to begin by 16 years of age. MRI of the hypothalamic-pituitary area is an important ancillary measure in the distinction of gonadotropin deficiency from constitutional delay.

Recent evidence suggests that constitutional delay of puberty can be better distinguished biochemically from hypogonadotropic hypogonadism by measuring GnRH-stimulated peak/basal ratio of the free α-subunit of the glycoprotein hormones.[18] Although this study included only boys and adult men, it is possible that free α-subunit measurements may improve the distinction between CDP and hypogonadotropic hypogonadism.

Congenital causes of hypogonadotropic hypogonadism are associated with cerebral, hypothalamic, or pituitary dysfunction or as an isolated defect.[1] Gonadotropin deficiency may be congenital or acquired, organic or functional. Congenital defects in hypothalamic-hypophyseal formation may be associated with midline facial defects. Congenital hypothalamic dysfunction may be associated with other neurologic or endocrine dysfunction, such as Prader-Willi syndrome (congenital hypotonia, neonatal failure to thrive followed by hypothalamic obesity, sometimes with hypopituitarism) or Laurence-Moon-Biedl syndrome (short stature, retinitis pigmentosa, obesity, polydactyly, renal anomalies, mental deficiency). Kallmann syndrome is the association of anosmia with gonadotropin deficiency and is less frequent in females than in males (1:5 sex ratio), reflecting the predominance of the X-linked disorder.[19] Mutations in the KAL1 gene on the pseudoautosomal region of the X chromosome account for half of the X-linked pedigrees, 1% to 5% of sporadic cases.[20,21] The cause in females is unknown. The KAL1 gene encodes a protein product with cellular adhesion function that is important for normal migration of olfactory nerves and GnRH neurons during development.[22] Eunuchoid body proportions (upper/lower body ratio <0.9 and arm span greater than height by more than 5 cm) is associated with Kallmann syndrome. In addition, there also are associated renal anomalies, cleft palate, dental agenesis, and mirror movements. Special MRI views often demonstrate absence of the olfactory tracts. In 10% of patients with Kallmann syndrome, mutations in the fibroblast growth factor receptor 1 (FGFR1, also known as KAL2) have been identified.[23] Patients with FGFR1/KAL2 mutations have typical Kallmann phenotype (hypogonadotropic hypogonadism and anosmia) with or without cleft palate and dental agenesis.[23]

Another genetic cause of gonadotropin deficiency has been associated with autosomal recessive mutations in PROP1, a gene important for pituitary development.[24,25] Patients with PROP1 mutations also have combined pituitary hormone deficiency.

Other causes of gonadotropin deficiency result from defects in the GnRH receptor, LH, FSH, or receptors for LH and FSH. To date, no mutations in the GnRH gene in humans have been identified as a cause for hypogonadotropic hypogonadism. Isolated gonadotropin deficiency arises from GnRH receptor mutations in about half of autosomal recessively inherited cases.[26] The degree of hypogonadism is variable, even within a family, with delayed puberty and delayed menarche as one presentation.[27-29] Isolated hypogonadotropic hypogonadism also has been reported in a woman homozygous for a nonsense mutation of the X-linked DAX1 gene, which was associated with adrenal insufficiency in her brother.[30] Isolated FSH deficiency caused by mutation in the β-subunit has been reported to cause primary amenorrhea in association with a unique test panel (low FSH, elevated LH, and low testosterone levels by immunoassay.) In contrast, the LHβ gene inactivating point mutation reported in a male was characterized by an elevated serum level of immunoreactive LH but low LH receptor binding activity. To date no mutations in the LHβ gene have been identified in females.

Mutations in a gene encoding a G protein–coupled receptor, GPR54, have been found in patients with idiopathic hypogonadotropic hypogonadism.[31] A GPR54 homozygous mutation was found in six members of a Saudi Arabian family who had hypogonadotropic hypogonadism. A compound heterozygous mutation was identified in a patient with normosomic idiopathic hypogonadotropic hypogonadism. To determine whether these mutations could alter the function of the receptor, wild type and mutant GPR54 constructs were transfected into kidney (COS-7) cells and phosphatidylinositol turnover was measured. Both mutations decreased phosphatidylinositol turnover by 65% to 67% after stimulation with a natural ligand for GPR54. Additional studies showed that the patient with the compound heterozygous mutation had reduced secretion of GnRH as indicated by low-amplitude pulses of LH and a leftward-shifted dose-response curve after intravenous administration of exogenous GnRH. Furthermore, studies in a GPR54-deficient mouse model showed normal responses to exogenous gonadotropins and GnRH, indicating that GPR54 is important for normal secretion of GnRH.[31]

Acquired gonadotropin deficiency may be secondary to a variety of organic CNS disorders, varying from hypothalamic-pituitary tumors (craniopharyngiomas, germinomas, or pituitary adenomas) to irradiation damage to empty sella syndrome. Hyperprolactinemia may be caused by prolactinomas, which secrete excess prolactin, or secondary to interruption of the pituitary stalk by large hypothalamic-pituitary tumors or other types of injury. The latter cause variable pituitary dysfunction, which may include secondary hypothyroidism. Medications, such as neuroleptic agents, can also cause hyperprolactinemia, which can also disrupt secretion of gonadotropins. In addition, infiltrative processes (granulomatous diseases and Langerhans cell histiocytosis) can cause acquired gonadotropin deficiency. Autoimmune hypophysitis is a rare disorder, sometimes accompanying a polyendocrine deficiency syndrome. The

# Pediatric and Adolescent Gynecology

prototypic form of functional gonadotropin deficiency is anorexia nervosa. Idiopathic hypogonadotropic deficiency may sometimes occur in families with anosmia, suggesting a relationship to Kallmann syndrome.

FSH elevation indicates premature ovarian failure (POF). The workup for POF should begin with determination of chromosomes to rule out Turner's syndrome and other forms of gonadal dysgenesis. Patients missing only a small portion of an X chromosome may not have the Turner syndrome phenotype. Indeed, among 45,X patients the classic Turner syndrome phenotype is found in less than one third (with the exception of short stature in 99%).[14] Ovarian function is sufficient for 10% to undergo some spontaneous pubertal development and for 5% to experience menarche.[14] Other chromosomal abnormalities associated with POF include mosaicism (45,X/46,XX) and deletions of the X chromosome.[32,33] Pubertal development and menstruation occur in 12% of 45,X/46,XX individuals. In addition, isolated premature ovarian failure with a genetic basis localized to the X chromosome has been associated with fragile X permutations. Other autosomal genetic disorders causing ovarian failure include trisomy 21, galactosemia, blepharophimosis, and myotonia dystrophica.

If there is no obvious explanation for the hypogonadism, autoimmune oophoritis should be considered. The patient should be assessed for autoimmune endocrinopathy, such as chronic autoimmune thyroiditis, diabetes mellitus, adrenal insufficiency, and hypoparathyroidism. Assays for antiovarian antibodies are not generally available. Rare congenital gene defects should also be considered in such cases. These include 17α-hydroxylase deficiency, which causes mineralocorticoid excess, classically associated with hypokalemic alkalosis and low renin hypertension, and mutations of the gonadotropins or their receptors. Pelvic ultrasound may demonstrate an absent uterus in intersex but cannot be relied upon to demonstrate hypoplastic ovaries in a girl with delayed puberty. Ovarian biopsy is seldom diagnostically useful, since histology is variable in premature ovarian failure.

Functional ovarian failure can also result from disorders in the ovary. Resistance to gonadotropin action (Savage syndrome) is a rare cause of functional hypogonadism. The ovary is resistant to both endogenous and exogenous gonadotropins. FSH levels are typically elevated and hyperrespond to GnRH testing. Ovarian histology shows a normal number of primordial follicles but a paucity of growing follicles. Certain hereditary defects in the biosynthesis of androgens and estrogens can also cause functional ovarian failure. Enzyme blocks can cause gonadal insufficiency in genetic males who are phenotypic females. This occurs in lipoid congenital adrenal hyperplasia (CAH), 17α-hydroxylase deficiency, 17,20-lyase deficiency, and 17β-HSD3 deficiency; all but the last two are associated with CAH. Lipoid CAH is unique in that the StAR mutation that underlies most cases has little direct impact on ovarian function, so that genetic females with this disorder can go through puberty, but the enzyme deficiency leads to gradual buildup of intraovarian lipid deposits that cause ovarian damage with late ovarian failure.

## Primary Amenorrhea

As stated earlier, if menarche does not occur by age 15 years or if no menses occur 4 to 5 years after the appearance of breast development, further workup for causes of primary amenorrhea should be pursued. Girls with extended delay in puberty will have primary amenorrhea. If breast development is immature, the algorithm shown in Figure 31-2 should be used to determine the cause of the delayed puberty.

On the other hand, if breast development is mature the differential diagnosis of primary amenorrhea proceeds according to the algorithm shown in Figure 31-3. As with delayed puberty, patients with primary amenorrhea should also have an initial screening evaluation for undernutrition, chronic diseases, and common endocrinologic disorders that can affect puberty (growth hormone deficiency, thyroid disease, glucocorticoid excess) and for prolactin excess. If initial screening test results are normal, then characterization of the stage of sexual development (pubic hair and external genitalia) is critical for diagnosing some causes of primary amenorrhea (see Fig. 31-3).

If the external genitalia are abnormal, intersex syndromes and structural abnormalities of the reproductive tract should be considered. Patients with intersex syndromes—those whose genitalia are ambiguous or inappropriate for their gonadal sex as a result of endocrinopathy—may come to a physician's attention for the first time at puberty. These syndromes are termed *true hermaphroditism* (if both ovarian and testicular tissue are present), *female pseudohermaphroditism* (if the genotype is female and there are only ovaries), and *male pseudohermaphroditism* (if the genotype is male and there are only testes). Patients with any of these disorders may undergo inappropriate puberty. They may present with clitoromegaly and be found upon examination to have a mild degree of genital ambiguity that was previously overlooked. Virilization beginning at puberty is sometimes the presenting complaint. True hermaphroditism or female pseudohermaphroditism due to CAH is compatible with fertility if treated appropriately. Testicular feminization syndrome may present as primary amenorrhea in an otherwise normal adolescent girl. In about 5% of females operated on for inguinal hernia, a testicular gonad will be found.

If the external genitalia are normal and a screening test for pregnancy is negative, then failure of the onset of menses can result from structural abnormalities of the genital tract that do not have an endocrinologic basis. The vagina may be aplastic or have an imperforate hymen; if the uterus is intact, hydrometrocolpos will occur. This type of structural defect that causes outflow obstruction should be considered if a girl complains of cyclic abdominal pain. The uterus may be congenitally aplastic in the presence of testicular tissue, which secretes antimüllerian hormone as seen in intersex syndromes (congenital deficiency of enzymes necessary for testosterone biosynthesis or metabolism, or androgen-insensitive syndrome/testicular feminization due to a defect in the androgen receptor). Uterine synechiae develop as the consequence of endometritis, which may result from infection or irradiation (Asherman's syndrome). Congenital absence of the vagina may be associated with varying degrees of uterine aplasia; this is the Rokitansky-Küster-Hauser syndrome. This syndrome seems to occur as a single-gene defect or as an acquired teratogenic event involving mesodermal development and the mesonephric kidney, the latter resulting in abnormalities of the genital tract and sometimes the urinary tract. The distal vagina may be normal, with aplasia of the upper vault, or there may be complete vaginal aplasia. When the vagina is blind and the uterus aplastic, this disorder must be distinguished from androgen resistance and, if the external genitalia are ambiguous, other causes of intersex.

In a girl with normal breast development and normal external genitalia, testosterone levels should be checked to exclude disorders of hyperandrogenism that may cause primary amenorrhea. Plasma total testosterone of a normal sexually mature female is 20 to 70 ng/dL (0.7 to 2.4 nM), and that of a normal adult male is greater than 320 ng/dL (>11 nM). Plasma free testosterone is a more accurate measure of the bioavailable testosterone. If testosterone levels are in the normal female range, then a screening test for pregnancy should be performed. If the patient is not pregnant, then a pelvic ultrasound should be performed to identify structural abnormalities of the genital tract. If testosterone levels are in the male range, androgen resistance should be suspected. Androgen resistance is characterized by a male plasma testosterone level (when sexual maturation has concluded), male karyotype (46,XY), and an absent uterus. External genitalia may be ambiguous (partial form) or normal female phenotype (complete form). If testosterone levels are intermediate or slightly elevated (70 to 320 ng/dL), then causes of hyperandrogenism should be sought, to exclude Cushing's syndrome, nonclassic CAH, virilizing tumors, and polycystic ovary syndrome (PCOS).

## MANAGEMENT

Underlying chronic and systemic disorders must be treated appropriately. When pubertal delay or primary amenorrhea is caused by the stress of eating disorders, behavioral modification and psychological counseling are indicated rather than estrogen replacement therapy. Surgical consideration is particularly important in the treatment of genital tract disorders, such as vaginal synechiae that do not lyse spontaneously with estrogenization, vaginal aplasia, or imperforate hymen. Most hypothalamic-pituitary tumors, with the exception of prolactinomas, require surgery with or without radiotherapy.

In the case of managing delayed puberty, two aspects of therapy are uniformly involved: psychological support and hormone administration.[1] Patients with delayed development that is a variation of normal should be reassured that there is nothing wrong, only a delay in timing of the onset of puberty. The wide normal variation in the pattern and time of the pubertal growth spurt should be explained in detail, and the girl should be informed of her predicted eventual height. The majority of children with delayed puberty do not have overt psychological symptoms. Complex compensations and sublimations obviously occur. However, peer group pressures may make adjustment to sexual infantilism especially difficult when the age of 13 is approached, and a poor self-image may lead to social withdrawal and feelings of hopelessness. Physical immaturity may prolong psychological immaturity. The physician should discuss the fact, when the evidence permits, that the odds are overwhelmingly in favor of the "timer in the subconscious area of the brain" eventually turning on. The length of time before this will happen can be approximated from the bone age, since maturation in constitutional delay proceeds at a normal pace. The physician should not hesitate to advise more intensive

psychological counseling if it becomes apparent that the concern about puberty is but one aspect of a more general maladjustment. Ultimately the decision as to whether to undertake treatment for delayed puberty is up to the patient and her family.

It is important to assure the teenager with an organic basis for hypoestrogenism that feminization will occur, although it will require appropriate hormone treatment. There are two caveats. Attainment of normal breast development in the girl with panhypopituitarism requires replacement of growth hormone and cortisol deficits. Also, it is difficult to induce secondary sex characteristics in some patients with systemic chronic inflammatory disease, such as lupus erythematosus.

In patients for whom short stature is a major concern, as in Turner's syndrome, other treatment modalities must be considered before undertaking estrogen replacement. Growth hormone is approved for the treatment of the short stature of Turner's syndrome and improves the adult height potential when started prepubertally.[34] Oxandrolone 0.0625 mg/kg/day does not seem to interfere with the realization of the genetic height potential and is synergistic with growth hormone. It is safest once the bone age reaches approximately 10 years. Clitoromegaly is ordinarily negligible on this dosage.

Some children with delayed puberty benefit from a short (6-month) course of physiologic estrogen treatment to help alleviate their anxieties; however, there are several challenges in using estrogen to induce puberty. First, estrogen should be given to mimic the normal changes in estrogen during puberty, with the intent to allow the patient to experience a normal progression through puberty. Second, since linear growth can be affected by estrogen therapy, careful examination of growth before and during treatment with estrogen is important to achieve the predicted adult height. Third, the bioavailability of oral synthetic estrogens can be variable owing to gastrointestinal absorption and hepatic metabolism. Fourth, delaying estrogen replacement can prevent achievement of normal peak bone mass. Finally, as discussed earlier, estrogen therapy can have a significant impact on socialization, personal development, and other psychological issues in girls with delayed puberty. Overall, estrogen therapy can be beneficial in the treatment of delayed puberty.

To induce puberty, estrogen can be administered orally, intramuscularly, or transdermally. Traditionally, oral synthetic estrogens have been the mainstay of therapy; however, they have potential disadvantages. For example, ethinyl estradiol is an analog of estradiol, the natural estrogen, that is, it has an ethinyl group covalently attached at the 17α position. This modification prevents metabolism of ethinyl estradiol to estradiol and allows it to bind to the estrogen receptor and be retained in tissues longer. Although oral estrogens are effective at inducing puberty, the commonly used dose of oral estrogens may not be optional for linear growth. This is because estrogen has been shown to have a biphasic effect on growth, and high doses inhibit growth and the generation of somatomedin C.[35,36]

The authors previously reported the use of intramuscular doses of depot estradiol compared with routine orally administered equine estrogens on linear growth in girls aged 12 to 15 years with Turner's syndrome who had been treated with growth hormone for 6 months or more.[37] After 2 years of treatment, girls given depot estradiol gained 2.6 cm more in height compared with those treated with routine estrogen. The most effective dose for growth was 0.2 mg to 0.6 mg of depot estradiol given monthly. In a previous study, growth was still achieved with a dose up to 1 mg of depot estradiol given monthly.

Therefore, estrogen replacement therapy can be started at a chronologic age of 12 years with a very low dose of synthetic estradiol to maximize both growth potential and age-appropriate feminization.[37] The authors recommend that a physiologic form of treatment is to begin with intramuscular depot estradiol 0.2 mg/month, which will usually induce breast budding; the dose can safely be increased by 0.2 mg every 6 months. (Midpubertal sex hormone production is approximated by delivering 1.0 to 1.5 mg of estradiol per month, which typically induces menarche within 1 year.[38]) Pubertal development and growth should be monitored every 6 months with bone age determinations at 6-month intervals to determine whether there is appropriate response to therapy.

A reasonable alternative regimen begins with 5 µg ethinyl estradiol (one fourth of the smallest available tablet) by mouth daily for 3 weeks out of 4.[39] Adult replacement doses of estrogen (20 mcg ethinyl estradiol or 0.625 mg conjugated estrogen daily) will stop growth.

One study has shown that estrogen can be administered transdermally to induce puberty. Transdermal estradiol patches have been recently shown to be an effective treatment for delayed puberty in girls aged 12 to 18 years by allowing the achievement of estradiol levels that mimic those seen during the normal onset of puberty.[40] In this study, a matrix patch of 17β-estradiol (25 µg per 24 hours) was cut into quarters (6.2 µg per 24 hours) and attached to the buttock overnight (10 PM to 8 AM). This low dose was used for 4 to 14 months and then increased subsequently to mimic estradiol levels in midpuberty. Breast development was observed 3 to 6 months after starting therapy in the majority of the girls treated. There was good correlation between serum 17β-estradiol levels with the 17β-estradiol patch dose, and the serum levels attained on one eighth (3.1 µg per 24 hours), one sixth (6.2 µg per 24 hours), or one quarter (6.2 µg per 24 hours) of a patch were similar to estradiol concentrations in normal girls undergoing spontaneous early puberty. Approximately 50% of girls on one half of a patch (12.5 µg per 24 hours) to three quarters of a patch (18.8 µg per 24 hours) achieved 17β-estradiol levels within the range for midpuberty. Therefore, low-dose estrogen administered transdermally in fractionated doses by patch seems to be an effective means of inducing puberty in girls with delayed puberty, although linear growth was not examined in this study.

Progestin should be added to estrogenic regimens 1 to 2 years after menarche or when bleeding begins to occur at unpredictable times, indicating endometrial proliferation. A simple regimen is to use 100 mg of natural progesterone (Prometrium) at bedtime for 7 to 14 days during the second to third week of estrogen therapy[1] or equivalent doses of medroxyprogesterone acetate (5 to 10 mg/day) or norethindrone acetate (5 mg/day). This will bring about normal menstruation during the week preceding resumption of estrogen therapy. The addition of progestin will decrease the risk of endometrial hyperplasia and endometrial carcinoma, but increase premenstrual symptoms.

Once optimal height is achieved, most patients can be managed effectively on birth control pills because these doses will halt growth. The pills containing the lowest dose of estrogen that will result in normal menstrual cycles are advisable. The lowest estrogen dosages currently available in the contraceptive pills with third-generation progestins in the United States contain 20 to 30 µg ethinyl estradiol.

After one 6-month course of therapy, it is advisable to wait 6 months for spontaneous puberty to occur if CDP is suspected. In the unlikely event that it does not occur, or if the patient has primary amenorrhea, then treatment depends on the underlying cause of the primary amenorrhea. Patients with gonadotropin deficiency, premature ovarian failure, androgen insensitivity, or XY gonadal dysgenesis will need lifelong estrogen therapy, and progestin should be added as previously discussed. In women with androgen insensitivity, XY gonadal dysgenesis, or uterine aplasia, estrogen replacement is needed but progesterone is not required. Once optimal height is achieved, patients may prefer to take oral contraceptives.

Adolescents with mature breast development and normal external genitalia who have primary amenorrhea first should be given a course of progesterone 100 mg or an equivalent progestin daily for 7 to 10 days. A positive response, withdrawal bleeding beginning a few days after completion of the course of therapy, will occur only if there is adequate estrogenization. This may occur especially if testosterone levels are elevated, as in the case of PCOS. In the perimenarcheal girls who respond well to this, progestin therapy may be repeated in 2- to 3-month cycles in order to detect the emergence of spontaneous menses that signals the resolution of physiologic anovulation of adolescence.

GnRH pulsatile treatment in patients with hypogonadotropic hypogonadism can induce puberty, but this type of therapy is not practical in adolescents and is used more frequently as therapy for infertility in adults.

## SUMMARY

The most common cause of delayed puberty is an extreme variation of normal, termed *constitutional*, delay of pubertal growth and development. Constitutional delay is a benign variation of normal, which is a prolongation of the functional gonadotropin deficiency of childhood. It can be mimicked by chronic disease, however, and can be difficult to distinguish from organic gonadotropin deficiency. In the early teenage years, before the bone age reaches a pubertal level, serum gonadotropin concentrations may not indicate POF. In the later teenage years, MRI imaging of the hypothalamic-pituitary area is a useful ancillary procedure to help distinguish constitutional delay from gonadotropin deficiency. Documentation of sleep augmentation of LH release is the most definitive finding, though imperfect, and gonadotropin responses to GnRH (or GnRH agonist) testing may be useful. Management requires anticipatory guidance and, occasionally, the use of low doses of estrogen that do not interfere with growth.

When there is an extended delay in puberty, or menarche does not occur by age 15, adolescents should be evaluated for causes of primary amenorrhea. Most of these adolescents may have mature breast development, unlike the majority of girls with delayed puberty. The diagnostic workup for CDP and primary amenorrhea is similar. The treatment options for both CDP and primary amenorrhea are also similar. Overall, exogenous hormone therapy is necessary for normal menstrual cycles, but the impact on future fertility is controversial.

## REFERENCES

1. Rosenfield RL: Puberty in the female and its disorders. In Sperling M (ed): Pediatric Endocrinology, 3rd ed. Philadelphia, W.B. Saunders, 2002, pp 455–518. **(IV, C)**

2. Tanner JM, Davies PS: Clinical longitudinal standards for height and height velocity for North American children [see comments]. J Pediatr 1985;107:317–329. **(III, B)**

3. Harlan W, Harlan E, Grillo G: Secondary sex characteristics of girls 12 to 17 years of age: The U.S. Health Examination Survey. J Pediatr 1980;96:1074–1078. **(III, B)**

4. Sun SS, Schubert CM, Chumlea WC, et al: National estimates of the timing of sexual maturation and racial differences among US children. Pediatrics 2002;110:911–919. **(III, B)**

5. Chumlea WC, Schubert CM, Roche AF, et al: Age at menarche and racial comparisons in US girls. Pediatrics 2003;111:110–113. **(III, B)**

6. Wang Y: Is obesity associated with early sexual maturation? A comparison of the association in American boys versus girls. Pediatrics 2002;110:903–910. **(III, B)**

7. Rosenfield RL: Delayed puberty. In Adashi EY, Rock JA, Rosenwaks Z (eds): Reproductive Endocrinology, Surgery, and Technology. Philadelphia, Lippincott-Raven, 1996, pp 1008–1015. **(IV, C)**

8. Marshall W, Tanner J: Variations in pattern of pubertal changes in girls. Arch Dis Child 1969;44:291. **(III, B)**

9. Marti-Henneberg C, Vizmanos B: The duration of puberty in girls is related to the timing of its onset. J Pediatr 1997;131:618–621. **(III, B)**

10. Barnes RB, Rosenfield RL: The polycystic ovary syndrome: pathogenesis and treatment. Ann Intern Med 1989;110:386–399. **(IV, C)**

11. Palmert MR: Variation in the timing of puberty: clinical spectrum and genetic investigation. J Clin Endocrinol Metab 2001;86:2364–2368. **(III, B)**

12. Sedlmeyer IL, Palmert MR: Delayed puberty: analysis of a large case series from an academic center. J Clin Endocrinol Metab 2002; 87:1613–1620. **(III, B)**

13. Sedlmeyer IL, Hirschhorn JN, Palmert MR: Pedigree analysis of constitutional delay of growth and maturation: determination of familial aggregation and inheritance patterns. J Clin Endocrinol Metab 2002; 87:5581–5586. **(III, B)**

14. Rosenfield RL: Menstrual disorders and hyperandrogenism in adolescence. In Radovick S, MacGillivray MH (eds): Pediatric Endocrinology: A Practical Clinical Guide. Totowa, NJ, Humana Press, 2003, pp 451–478. **(IV, C)**

15. Rosenfield RL, Barnes RB: Menstrual disorders in adolescence. Endocrinol Metab Clin North Am 1993;22:491–505. **(IV, C)**

16. Goodpasture J, Ghai K, Cara J, Rosenfield R: Potential of gonadotropin-releasing hormone agonists in the diagnosis of pubertal disorders in girls. Clin Obstet Gynecol 1993;36:773–785. **(III, B)**

17. Stanhope R, Pringle P, Brook C, et al: Induction of puberty by pulsatile gonadotropin releasing hormone. Lancet 1987;2:552.

18. Mainieri AS, Elnecave RH: Usefulness of the free alpha-subunit to diagnose hypogonadotropic hypogonadism. Clin Endocrinol 2003; 59:307–313. **(III, B)**

19. Jones J, Kemmann E: Olfacto-genital dysplasia in the female. Obstet Gynecol Ann 1976;5:443–466. **(III, B)**

20. Legouis R, Hardelin JP, Levilliers J, et al: The candidate gene for the X-linked Kallmann syndrome encodes a protein related to adhesion molecules. Cell 1991;67:423–435.

21. Franco B, Guioli S, Pragliola A, et al: A gene detected in Kallmann's syndrome shares homology with neural cell adhesion and axonal path-finding molecules. Nature 1991;353:529–536.

22. Layman LC: The molecular basis of human hypogonadotropic hypogonadism. Mol Genet Metab 1999;68:191–199. **(IV, C)**

23. Sato N, Katsumata N, Kagami M, et al: Clinical assessment and mutation analysis of Kallmann syndrome 1 (KAL1) and fibroblast growth factor receptor 1 (FGFR1 and Kal2) in five families and 18 sporadic patients. J Clin Endocrinol 2004;89:1079–1088. **(III, B)**

24. Wu W, Cogan JD, Pfaffle RW, et al: Mutations in PROP1 cause familial combined pituitary hormone deficiency. Nat Genet 1998;18:147–149. **(III, B)**

25. Cogan JD, Wu W, Phillips JAI, et al: The PROPR1 2-base pair deletion is a common cause of combined pituitary hormone deficiency. J Clin Endocrinol Metab 1998;83:3346–3349. **(III, B)**

26. Beranova M, Oliveira LM, Bedecarrats GY, et al: Prevalence, phenotypic spectrum, and modes of inheritance of gonadotropin-releasing hormone receptor mutations in idiopathic hypogonadotropic hypogonadism. J Clin Endocrinol Metab 2001;86:1580–1588. **(III, B)**

27. de Roux N, Young J, Misrahi M, et al: A family with hypogonadotropic hypogonadism and mutations in the gonadotropin-releasing hormone receptor. N Engl J Med 1997;337:1597–1602. **(III, B)**

28. Seminara SB, Beranova M, Oliveira LMB, et al: Successful use of pulsatile gonadotropin-releasing hormone (GnRH) for ovulation induction and pregnancy in a patient with GnRH receptor mutations. J Clin Endocrinol Metab 2000;85:556–562. **(III, B)**

29. de Roux N, Young J, Brailley-Tabard S, et al: The same molecular defects of the gonadotropin-releasing hormone receptor determine a variable degree of hypogonadism in affected kindred. J Clin Endocrinol Metab 1999;84:567–572. **(III, B)**

30. Merke DP, Tajima T, Baron J, Cutler GB Jr: Hypogonadotropic hypogonadism in a female caused by an X-linked recessive mutation in the DAX1 gene. N Engl J Med 1999;340:1248–1252. **(III, B)**

31. Seminara SB, Messager S, Chatzidaki EE, et al: The GPR54 gene as a regulator of puberty. N Engl J Med 2003;349(17):1589–1592. **(III, B)**

32. Reindollar RH, Byrd JR, McDonough PG: Delayed sexual development: a study of 252 patients. Am J Obstet Gynecol 1981;140:371–380. **(III, B)**

33. Rebar R, Connolly H: Clinical features of young women with hypergonadotropic amenorrhea. Fertil Steril 1990;53:804–810.

34. Rosenfeld RG, Frane J, Attie KM, et al: Six-year results of a randomized prospective trial of human growth hormone and oxandrolone in Turner syndrome. J Pediatr 1992;121:49–55. **(Ib, A)**

35. Blizzard R, Thompson R, Baghdassarian A, et al: The interrelationship of steroids, growth hormone, and other hormones on pubertal growth. In Grumbach M, Grave G, Mayer F (eds): Control of the Onset of Puberty. Airlie, Va, John Wiley & Sons; 1972, pp 342–359. **(IV, C)**

36. Cutler GB, Ross JL: Estrogen therapy in Turner's syndrome. Acta Paediatr Jpn 1992;34:195–202.

37. Rosenfield RL, Perovic N, Devine N, et al: Optimizing estrogen replacement treatment in Turner syndrome. Pediatrics 1998;102:486–488. **(IIa, B)**

38. Rosenfield RL, Fang VS: The effects of prolonged physiologic estradiol therapy on the maturation of hypogonadal teenagers. J Pediatr 1974; 85:830–837. **(III, B)**

39. Ross JL, Long LM, Skerda M, et al: The effect of low dose ethinyl estradiol on six monthly growth rates and predicted height in patients with Turner syndrome. J Pediatr 1986;109:950. **(III, B)**

40. Ankarberg-Lindgren C, Elfving M, Wikland KA, Norjavaara E: Nocturnal application of transdermal estradiol patches produces levels of estradiol that mimic those seen at the onset of spontaneous puberty in girls. J Clin Endocrinol 2001;86:3039–3044. **(III, B)**

# Medical Management of Gynecologic Problems in the Pediatric and Adolescent Patient

## Eduardo Lara-Torre, MD, and S. Paige Hertweck, MD

---

## KEY POINTS

### Gynecologic Examination of the Pediatric and Adolescent Patient
- Perform an overall physical assessment prior to completing a prepubertal genital examination.
- Prepubertal genital anatomy is not estrogenized and therefore is easily traumatized.
- Appropriate examination techniques and positioning assist the examiner in performing a prepubertal genital examination.
- Preventive health care visits for the adolescent should begin between ages 13 and 15.

### Vulvovaginal Dermatologic Conditions in the Pediatric Patient
- Vulvovaginal complaints or concerns are the most common reasons prepubertal girls see the gynecologist.
- The hypoestrogenic state of the prepubertal vulva and vagina predispose young girls to skin conditions of the external genitalia.
- Vulvovaginal conditions range from inflammatory to infectious to manifestations of systemic diseases.
- Many conditions, such as chronic nonspecific vaginitis and labial agglutination, resolve at puberty.

### Hirsutism
- In adolescents, hirsutism may be idiopathic or an early sign of a tumor or a pathologic condition of the ovary or adrenal gland.
- Hirsutism can be the first sign of impending virilization (clitoromegaly, temporal hair recession, deepening of the voice, changes in muscle pattern, breast atrophy).

### Adolescent Contraception
- Refusal to have a pelvic examination at an initial contraceptive visit should not be a barrier to prescribing hormonal contraception to an adolescent.
- An adolescent's selection of birth control should ideally include both a hormonal and a barrier method.
- Use of emergency contraception (EC) decreases risk of pregnancy from 8% to 1–2% after a single episode of unprotected coitus.
- An advance prescription of EC ensures increased use of method over EC counseling alone.

### Dysmenorrhea and Endometriosis
- Adolescents with worsening dysmenorrhea should have a pelvic assessment prior to treatment to rule out an outflow tract obstruction.
- Dysmenorrhea that is unresponsive to use of NSAIDs and OCPs may involve endometriosis.
- Atypical "clear" or "red" endometriotic lesions are common in the adolescent, as opposed to the typical "powderburn" or "chocolate" lesions seen in adults.

---

## GYNECOLOGIC EXAMINATION OF THE PEDIATRIC AND ADOLESCENT PATIENT

Examination of the external genitalia is a normal part of the routine physical examination. Assessment of the internal genitalia in pediatric patients is indicated in cases of genitourinary complaints or suspected cases of genitourinary pathology (Table 32-1). The proper, nontraumatizing office examination of the child or adolescent provides the gynecologist with the opportunity to establish an adequate relationship with the patient, allowing for the early diagnosis of common conditions found in this age group. Key components of any examination should be covered to the extent allowed by the patient and in no way should be forced either by the physician or by the parents, since it may prevent successful future gynecologic examinations in these patients.

### Prepubertal Female
The prepubertal examination should focus initially on obtaining the cooperation of the child. Explain what the examination will entail, and allow the child to have a sense of control to enlist their cooperation (e.g., give the child a choice of examination gown to wear). Perform an overall assessment of the child before initiating the genitalia examination.

Inspection of the genital region should follow a focused general examination. Initiating the examination with auscultation of heart and lung sounds will provide an opportunity for

| Table 32-1 |
| :-- |
| **Indications for Genital Examination in the Pediatric Patient** |
| Vaginal bleeding<br>Vaginal discharge<br>Vulvar trauma<br>Vulvovaginal cystic or solid masses<br>Vulvovaginal ulcerative/inflammatory lesions<br>Congenital anomalies<br>Sexual abuse |
| Modified with permission from Laufer MR, Emans SJ: Gynecologic examination of newborn and child. Up To Date. Available at: www.uptodate.com. |

the clinician to assess body habitus, hygiene, and presence of skin disorders while allowing the young patient to feel more comfortable in the examination room setting. It is also important to evaluate height and weight percentiles, assess breast development, and perform an abdominal and inguinal examination as part of the comprehensive examination. Once the patient is comfortable with the examiner, the genitalia may be examined.

### Positioning the Patient for Examination

Appropriate positioning is a key component to a successful pediatric gynecologic examination. Multiple positions have been described to allow adequate visualization of the area. In some situations more than one position may be required to adequately visualize the genitalia. The patient's age may determine the best position. The frog leg position is the most commonly used position in the younger patient and allows for the patient to have a direct view of the examiner and herself (Fig. 32-1). As the child grows older, the use of stirrups and the lithotomy position may provide the best visualization of the area. Having the mother hold her daughter on her lap may also be of assistance (Fig. 32-2). The knee-chest position is adjunctively helpful in

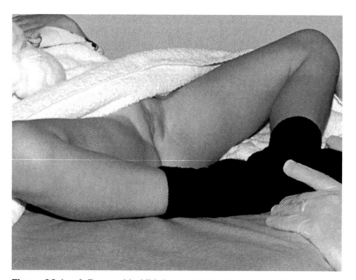

**Figure 32-1    A 5-year-old child demonstrating the supine "frog-leg" position.** (Used with permission from McCann JJ, Kerns DL: The Anatomy of Child and Adolescent Sexual Abuse: A CD-ROM Atlas/Reference. St. Louis, Mo, Intercort, Inc, 1999.)

**Child in lithotomy position on mother's lap**

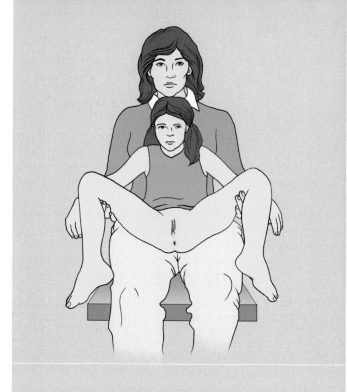

**Figure 32-2    Child in supine frog-leg position while in mother's lap.** (Used with permission from Finkel MA, Giardino AP [eds]: Medical Examination of Child Sexual Abuse: A Practical Guide, 2nd ed. Thousand Oaks, Calif, Sage Publications, 2002, pp 46–64.)

some cases in visualizing the lower and upper vagina with the use of an otoscope or other low power magnification.[1] This position may be especially helpful in those patients for whom a vaginal discharge or a foreign body may be a complaint (Figs. 32-3 and 32-4). In certain instances, even the most experienced examiner will be unable to complete the examination or get the patient to comply; in these patients, the emergent nature of the complaint and the clinical consequence of the pathology must be considered. A multivisit examination or an examination under anesthesia may be warranted.

### Using Appropriate Examination Techniques

The examiner must be careful not to cause any trauma or pain in the area, as it will promptly make the patient uncomfortable and possibly end the examination. In the prepubertal female, the unestrogenized nature of the hymeneal tissue makes it sensitive to touch and easily torn. The use of gentle traction with lateral and downward pulling may improve visualization while maintaining the integrity of the normal prepubertal genitalia (Figs. 32-5 through 32-7).

Although the evaluation of the internal pelvic organs may not be easy, the use of a recto-abdominal examination may assist in the palpation of the internal organs as well as possible pelvic

# Medical Management of Gynecologic Problems in the Pediatric and Adolescent Patient

**Child in knee-chest position for genital examination**

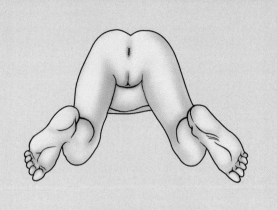

**Figure 32-3    Child in prone knee-chest position for genital examination.** (Used with permission from Finkel MA, Giardino AP [eds]: Medical Examination of Child Sexual Abuse: A Practical Guide, 2nd ed. Thousand Oaks, Calif, Sage Publications, 2002, pp 46–64.)

masses. This part of the examination is particularly important in cases of suspected vaginal foreign body, pubertal aberrancy, or pelvic pain for which the differential diagnosis includes a pelvic mass.

Proper nomenclature of the female genitalia should be used when reporting a pediatric examination to prevent confusion between examiners (Fig. 32-8). Components of such an examination include assessment of pubertal development (Tanner stage), visualization and measurement of the clitoris, and description of the labia majora and minora including any discoloration, pigmentation, or lesion. The urethra and the urethral

**Labial separation technique for examination of female genitalia**

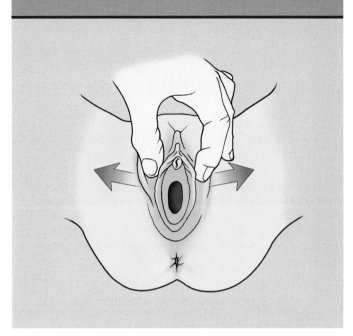

**Figure 32-5    Labial separation technique for examination of female genitalia in the supine frog-leg position.** (Used with permission from Finkel MA, Giardino AP [eds]: Medical Examination of Child Sexual Abuse: A Practical Guide, 2nd ed. Thousand Oaks, Calif, Sage Publications, 2002, pp 46–64.)

**Technique for examination of female genitalia in knee-chest position**

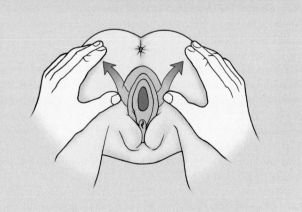

**Figure 32-4    Technique for examination of female genitalia in prone knee-chest position.** (Used with permission from Finkel MA, Giardino AP [eds]: Medical Examination of Child Sexual Abuse: A Practical Guide, 2nd ed. Thousand Oaks, Calif, Sage Publications, 2002, pp 46–64.)

**Labial traction technique for examination of female genitalia**

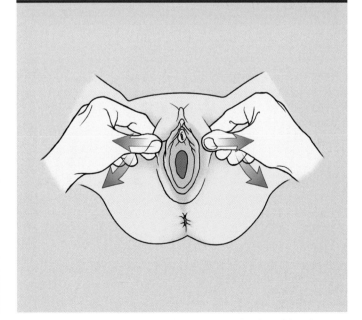

**Figure 32-6    Labial traction technique for examination of female genitalia in the supine frog-leg position.** (Used with permission from Finkel MA, Giardino AP [eds]: Medical Examination of Child Sexual Abuse: A Practical Guide, 2nd ed. Thousand Oaks, Calif, Sage Publications, 2002, pp 46–64.)

# Pediatric and Adolescent Gynecology

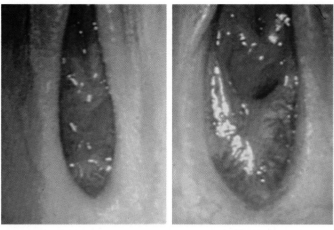

**Figure 32-7    Examples of the techniques of labial separation and lateral traction for viewing the hymen of a prepubertal girl.** (Used with permission from Yordan EE [ed]: The PediGYN Teaching Slide Set. Farmington, Conn, North American Society for Pediatric and Adolescent Gynecology, 1996.)

meatus should also be described. A proper description of the hymen, including type or shape, estrogen status, and abnormalities should be detailed. The prepubertal hymen is thin, red, and unestrogenized. Estrogenization at puberty thickens the hymen and it becomes pale pink and is often more redundant in its configuration. Normal and abnormal variants as well as common hymenal anomalies are shown in Figures 32-9 through 32-16. Other findings including presence of hemangiomas or

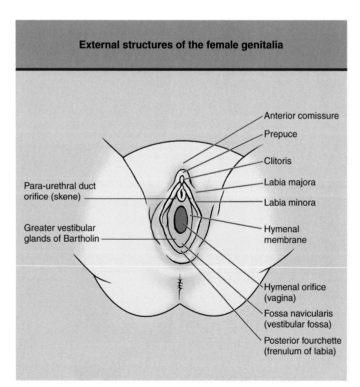

**External structures of the female genitalia**

- Anterior comissure
- Prepuce
- Clitoris
- Labia majora
- Labia minora
- Hymenal membrane
- Para-urethral duct orifice (skene)
- Greater vestibular glands of Bartholin
- Hymenal orifice (vagina)
- Fossa navicularis (vestibular fossa)
- Posterior fourchette (frenulum of labia)

**Figure 32-8    Proper nomenclature of the prepubertal external genitalia.** (Used with permission from Finkel MA, Giardino AP [eds]: Medical Examination of Child Sexual Abuse: A Practical Guide, 2nd ed. Thousand Oaks, Calif, Sage Publications, 2002, pp 46–64.)

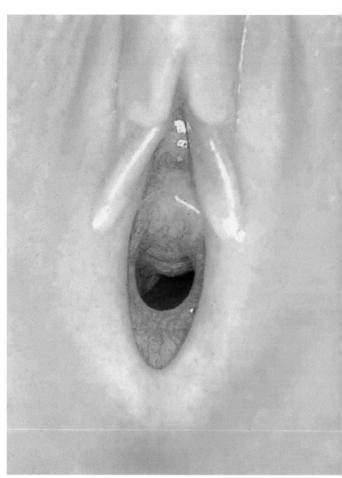

**Figure 32-9    Crescentic hymen.** (Used with permission from Perlman SE, Nakajima ST, Hertweck SP: Clinical Protocols in Pediatric and Adolescent Gynecology. London, Parthenon Publishing Group, 2004, p 132.)

other vulvar-vaginal lesions should also be described. If the cervix is visualized in the knee-chest position, it is important to document its appearance.

### Using Special Techniques to Obtain Specimens

When vaginal specimens for culture must be collected, moistened small Dacron swabs (male urethral size) may be used (Fig. 32-17). The hymenal aperture is small in this age group, and traditional large-sized cotton swabs create discomfort. Another helpful method is a catheter-within-a-catheter technique in which a four-inch intravenous catheter is inserted into the proximal end of a No. 12 red rubber bladder catheter. This is then connected to a fluid-filled syringe passed carefully into the vagina. The fluid is then injected and aspirated multiple times to allow a good mixture of secretions. These specimens may be sent for culture as needed (Fig 32-18).[2]

When suspected foreign bodies need to be flushed from the prepubertal vagina, a pediatric feeding tube connected to a 20-mL syringe may be used to irrigate the contents of the vagina and determine the nature of the foreign object. This can make the need for specula unnecessary in these prepubertal patients who have a small hymenal aperture that would be injured with insertion of a speculum.

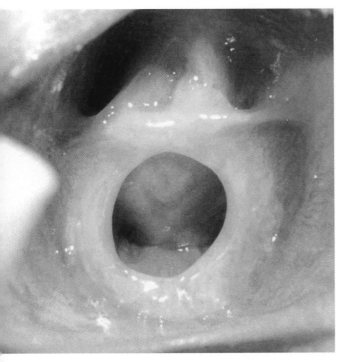

**Figure 32-10    Annular hymen.** (Used with permission from Perlman SE, Nakajima ST, Hertweck SP: Clinical Protocols in Pediatric and Adolescent Gynecology. London, Parthenon Publishing Group, 2004, p 132.)

### Documenting the Examination

Genital examinations in prepubertal girls should be documented and each genital structure that was examined listed to aid future examiners who may need previous examination results for the basis of their findings. This is particularly helpful in suspected cases of abuse in which a structure (e.g., the hymen) may have been altered by trauma. Therefore, the physician should document visualization of labia majora, labia minora, hymenal shape or variations (e.g., bumps, clefts) as well as urethral, vaginal, and rectal findings, even if normal. A clock face is helpful in delineating the location of any abnormal findings (Fig. 32-19). Findings and variations should be merely described and, importantly, no diagnostic descriptions should be made in the documentation of the examination. Conclusions (e.g., "an interrupted hymen suggestive of sexual abuse is seen") should be placed in the impression and plan portion of the documentation.

### Adolescent Gynecologic Examination

The peripubertal and adolescent patient may present a challenge for the examining practitioner. Although estrogenization may already have occurred, the patient's self-consciousness about her own body may make the examination even more difficult to perform. Extreme variation in psychosocial and sexual development at this age also contributes to the challenge of an examination. Teens develop at varying rates, for example, some are menarcheal at 10 while others may just be starting their pubertal development at 13; therefore, careful interviewing and counseling should precede an examination. The use of educational videos that explain the examination process and the common reasons why they are done may benefit your interaction with the patient. Delay of the genital examination, even if the patient is sexually active,

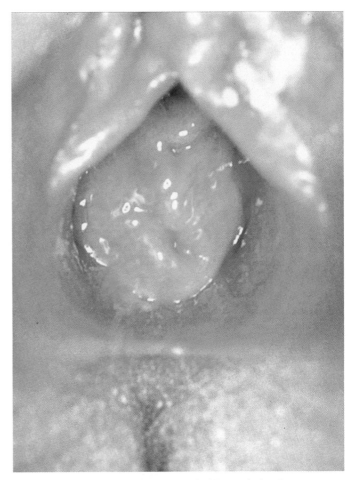

**Figure 32-11    Redundant hymen.** (Used with permission from Perlman SE, Nakajima ST, Hertweck SP: Clinical Protocols in Pediatric and Adolescent Gynecology. London, Parthenon Publishing Group, 2004, p 133.)

may prevent her from having reservations about her examiner. While some teens may like to know and see everything that will happen, some prefer not to look. These preferences should be taken into account to make the experience as nontraumatic as possible.

As for other patients, preventive health care should be part of the medical management in this age group. The initial visit to the obstetrician gynecologist should occur between 13 and 15 years of age.[3] During this visit, important components of general health such as immunizations, risk prevention, screening for tobacco and substance abuse, as well as depression and eating disorders should be completed. This visit does not necessarily include a pelvic examination. Table 32-2 lists indications

| Table 32-2 |
| :-- |
| **Indications for Pelvic Examination in the Adolescent** |
| Pubertal aberrancy |
| Abnormal bleeding |
| Abdominal/pelvic pain |
| History of vaginal coitus |

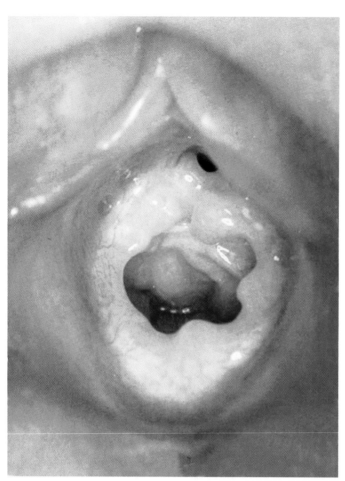

**Figure 32-12    Fimbriated hymen.** (Used with permission from Perlman SE, Nakajima ST, Hertweck SP: Clinical Protocols in Pediatric and Adolescent Gynecology. London, Parthenon Publishing Group, 2004, p 133.)

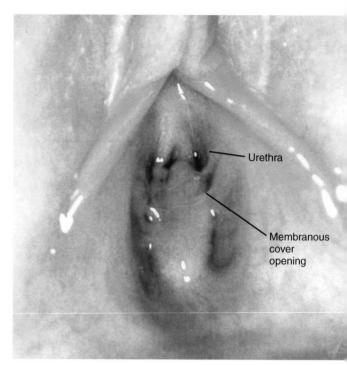

**Figure 32-13    Microperforate hymen.** (Used with permission from Perlman SE, Nakajima ST, Hertweck SP: Clinical Protocols in Pediatric and Adolescent Gynecology. London, Parthenon Publishing Group, 2004, p 137.)

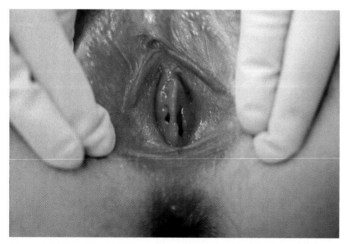

**Figure 32-14    Septate hymen.** (Used with permission from Perlman SE, Nakajima ST, Hertweck SP: Clinical Protocols in Pediatric and Adolescent Gynecology. London, Parthenon Publishing Group, 2004, p 139.)

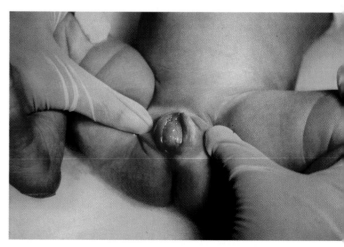

**Figure 32-15    Imperforate hymen.** (Used with permission from Perlman SE, Nakajima ST, Hertweck SP: Clinical Protocols in Pediatric and Adolescent Gynecology. London, Parthenon Publishing Group, 2004, p 136.)

Medical Management of Gynecologic Problems in the Pediatric and Adolescent Patient

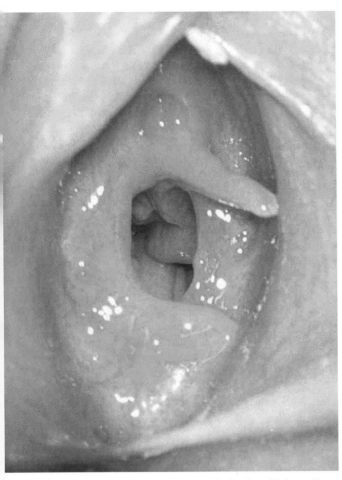

**Figure 32-16   Hymenal tag.** (Used with permission from McCann JJ, Kerns DL: The Anatomy of Child and Adolescent Sexual Abuse: A CD-ROM Atlas/Reference. St. Louis, Mo, InterCorp, Inc, 1999.)

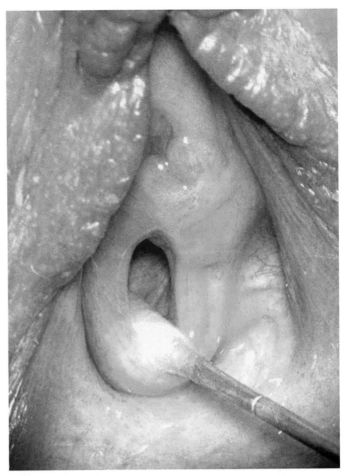

**Figure 32-17   Use of small Dacron swabs to obtain vaginal specimens.** (Used with permission from McCann JJ, Kerns DL: The Anatomy of Child and Adolescent Sexual Abuse: A CD-ROM Atlas/Reference. St. Louis, Mo, InterCorp, Inc, 1999.)

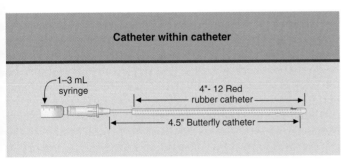

**Figure 32-18   Assembled catheter-within-a-catheter aspirator, as used to obtain samples of vaginal secretions from prepubertal patients.** (Used with permission from Pokorny SF, Stormer J: Atraumatic removal of secretions from the prepubertal vagina. Am J Obstet Gynecol 1987;156:581–582, ©1987 Mosby.)

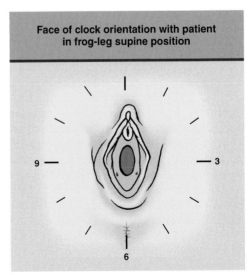

**Figure 32-19   Face-of-clock orientation with patient in frog-leg supine position.** (Used with permission from Finkel MA, Giardino AP [eds]: Medical Examination of Child Sexual Abuse: A Practical Guide, 2nd ed. Thousand Oaks, Calif, Sage Publications, 2002, pp 46–64.)

for a pelvic examination in the adolescent. After the initial gynecologic evaluation, annual/semiannual visits should be scheduled thereafter. Sexually active teens should be screened for sexually transmitted diseases (STDs) with each new sexual partner.

Adolescents are primarily interested in confidentiality from a consistent provider who will ask the questions that they won't (e.g., about STDs, contraception, acne, weight, menses, how their bodies work, and sexual behaviors such as kissing, petting, intercourse). To facilitate obtaining adequate screening for such issues as well as other risk-taking behaviors, the American College of Obstetricians and Gynecologists (ACOG) Tool Kit for Teen Care has a confidential screening questionnaire to be used at each visit and an adolescent-specific history and physical examination record (Fig 32-20).

With adolescents, if possible, it is important to meet initially with the adolescent/teen and her parents/guardian together to explain the concept of confidentiality and privacy. After both parent and teen have completed an initial history form together, the sensitive/confidential part of the history may be taken alone with the teen (e.g., alcohol, drug, and substance use; dating and sexual history). With sensitive questions, it may be helpful to give a wide range of acceptable answers. For example, "Some teens can talk about sex with their parents; others can't. How do you feel?" Creating a context for questions may be helpful, as in, "A lot of girls your age . . . how do you feel about that?" When screening, begin with less sensitive issues such as safety (e.g., seat belt use) prior to exploring more sensitive ones (e.g., sexuality).

Before completing the initial gynecologic examination, take time to explain the process. In all patients, assess height, weight, blood pressure, and body mass index (BMI). Examination of the neck including a thyroid and lymph node assessment followed by evaluation of skin and breast development should precede the pelvic examination. The external genitalia should be examined, if allowed, in all patients who come in for preventive care, as this will determine the presence of any genital anomalies as well as be the first step toward a pelvic examination. The initial pelvic examination may be delayed, although care should be taken to counsel the sexually active patient about the consequences of nondetection of sexually transmitted infections (STIs) such as asymptomatic chlamydia. Urine screening for STIs should be completed in sexually active teens who choose not to undergo a pelvic examination. Asymptomatic patients who are not sexually active may delay their initial pelvic examination up to the age of 21.[3] Papanicolaou (Pap) testing is required within 3 years of the onset of sexual activity. Annual Pap testing should be considered beginning with the initial visit in patients with multiple partners, who are immunocompromised, and for whom follow-up is unlikely.

The external genitalia should be thoroughly described as for the pediatric patient. Those who require a pelvic examination because of suspected pathology or for annual screening should be properly instructed in the methods used. Proper equipment for this age group should be available. The use of a speculum may be more acceptable in tampon-using adolescents. The use of a pediatric or a Huffman speculum ($\frac{1}{2}$ in. wide × 4 in. long) may be of help in those patients not sexually active. A Huffman

or Pederson speculum ($\frac{7}{8}$ in. wide × 4 in. long) may be used in patients who are sexually active or use tampons (Fig. 32-21).

Use of the "extinction of stimuli" may be of benefit in those undergoing their first pelvic examination. Using a finger to apply pressure to the perineal area, away from the introitus or thigh, will lessen or diffuse the sensation from the examiner's finger at the introitus. Once a finger has been placed in this area, the insertion of a speculum may be easier and the cervix and vagina can be visualized adequately. Once access to the cervix is gained, screening cervical cytology and cultures may be collected if indicated. A rectovaginal or single-digit bimanual examination should be used to palpate the internal organs. The approach will depend on the patient's preference, tolerance, and sexual history as well as the pathology suspected. All adolescents should be reassured that the examination, while uncomfortable, is not usually painful and will not alter their anatomy. This may reassure those who may believe that the examination will alter their "virginity."

After the examination, it is helpful to meet again with the family and the patient together to explain the examination findings and to plan further management. If confidentiality is a concern in the sexually active teen, first discuss findings with the patient alone while in the examination room. Make a plan together about how to discuss with the parent/guardian before meeting with the family together. Encourage the patient to allow the clinician to be the liaison between her and the family, stressing the benefits of informing everyone of her use of contraception and her situation. Ensure that the adolescent assumes the role of decision maker and help empower her to take charge of her own health care with the guidance and assistance of her parents and health care providers.

## VULVOVAGINAL DERMATOLOGIC CONDITIONS IN THE PEDIATRIC PATIENT

### Vulvovaginitis

#### Presentation, Etiology, and Risk Factors

Nonspecific vulvovaginitis accounts for 25% to 75% of the vaginitis seen in this age group.[4] Patients generally complain of vaginal discharge with or without a color or odor, vulvar pain, redness, itching, bleeding, or dysuria. Signs of irritation such as erythema and labial adhesions are seen commonly and may be the sole cause for the consultation. The etiology is unknown, but multiple contributing factors play a role in pathogenesis of the condition (Table 32-3). The use of tight nylon underpants and clothing, close fitting jeans, and leotards may contribute to the irritation and subsequent colonization of the unestrogenized skin. Although some bacteria such as Bacteroides and Peptostreptococcus have been seen more commonly in these patients, a true relationship has not been proved.[5]

As in adults, vulvitis in children may be caused by the presence of certain bacteria. Respiratory flora (group A Streptococcus [Fig. 32-22A and B], Haemophilus influenzae), enteric bacteria (Escherichia coli, Shigella, Yersinia), Candida (Fig 32-23), STDs, pinworms, and foreign bodies may also present with similar symptoms.[6] In many instances, the appearance of the vulva and the result of the diagnostic workup may be the only source of confirmation.

Text continued on p. 496

**CONFIDENTIAL FORM**    **DO NOT COPY**    **NOT FOR RELEASE**

## ADOLESCENT VISIT QUESTIONNAIRE

We strongly encourage you to discuss all issues of your life with your parent(s) or guardian(s). However, unless it is a life threatening issue, the information you give us on this form is confidential between our doctors and nurses and you. It will not be released without your written consent. If you would like help filling out this form, please let the nurse know. IF YOU DON'T FEEL COMFORTABLE ANSWERING A QUESTION, LEAVE IT BLANK AND YOUR DOCTOR OR NURSE WILL TALK WITH YOU ABOUT IT.

Name _____ Age _____ Today's Date _____

Why did you come into our office today? _____

**Please answer these general health questions. Ignore the last column. Your doctor or nurse will fill that out.**

| **Friends and Family** | | For doctor/nurse use |
|---|---|---|
| Can you talk with your parent(s) or guardian(s) about personal things happening in your life? | ❑ Yes ❑ No | |
| If no, is there another adult you trust and can talk to if you have a problem? | ❑ Yes ❑ No   Who? | |
| Who do you live with? (Please circle all that apply.) | Mother  Father  Guardian  Sibling(s) Other: | |
| Do you think your family has lots of fun together? | ❑ Yes ❑ No | |
| Do you think your parents care about you? | ❑ Yes ❑ No | |
| Do you have a best friend? | ❑ Yes ❑ No | |
| **School and Work** | | |
| Do you like school and do well in school? | ❑ Yes ❑ No       ❑ Not in school | |
| What grade are you in? | Grade:       ❑ Not in school | |
| What school do you go to? | School:       ❑ Not in school | |
| How often have you skipped school? | ❑ Never ❑ Once or twice ❑ A lot | |
| Do you have any learning problems? | ❑ Yes ❑ No | |
| Do you have a job? | ❑ Yes ❑ No   Doing what? | |
| Do you know what you want to be when you are older? | ❑ Yes ❑ No   What? | |
| **Appearance and Fitness** | | |
| Do you have any concerns or questions about the shape or size of your body or the way you look? | ❑ Yes ❑ No ❑ Not sure | |
| Do you want to gain or lose weight? | ❑ Gain ❑ Lose ❑ Neither | |
| Have you ever tried to lose weight or control your weight by throwing up, using diet pills or laxatives, or not eating for a day? | ❑ Yes ❑ No | |
| Have you ever had your body pierced (other than ears) or gotten a tattoo? | ❑ Yes ❑ No ❑ Considering | |
| Do you exercise or do a sport at least 5 times a week that makes you sweat or breathe hard for 30 minutes? | ❑ Yes ❑ No | |
| How many fruits and vegetables do you eat each day? | ❑ None ❑ 1–2 ❑ 3–4 ❑ 5–6 ❑ 7 or more | |
| How much milk, yogurt, ice cream do you eat each day? | ❑ None ❑ 1–2 ❑ 3–4 ❑ 5–6 ❑ 7 or more | |
| **Safety/Weapons/Violence** | | |
| Do you wear a seat belt when you ride in a car, truck, or van? | ❑ Yes ❑ No | |
| Do you wear a helmet when you use a bike, motorcycle, all-terrain vehicle, mini-bike, skateboard, rollerblades, or scooter? | ❑ Yes ❑ No | |
| Do you or does anyone you live with have a gun, rifle, or other firearm? | ❑ Yes ❑ No ❑ Not sure | |
| Have you ever carried a gun or weapon? | ❑ Yes ❑ No | |
| Have you ever been in trouble with the law? | ❑ Yes ❑ No | |
| Has anyone touched you in a way that made you uncomfortable? | ❑ Yes ❑ No ❑ Not sure | |
| Has anyone ever forced you to have sex? | ❑ Yes ❑ No ❑ Not sure | |
| Has anyone ever hurt you physically or emotionally? | ❑ Yes ❑ No ❑ Not sure | |

**Figure 32-20    ACOG Adolescent Visit Questionnaire and ACOG Adolescent Visit Record.**    *Continued*

Pediatric and Adolescent Gynecology

**ADOLESCENT VISIT QUESTIONNAIRE** *(continued)*

| Relationships | | For doctor/nurse use |
|---|---|---|
| Are you going out with anyone? | ❏ Yes ❏ No | |
| Who do you find yourself attracted to sexually? | ❏ Guys ❏ Girls ❏ Both | |
| Have you ever had sex with anyone? If yes, answer the questions in this section below.<br>    If no, do you plan to in the next year? When done answering this question, go to the section on tobacco, alcohol, and drugs below. | ❏ Yes ❏ No<br><br>❏ Yes ❏ No ❏ Not sure | |
| How many sexual partners do you have now? How many in the past? | Now:        Past: | |
| How old were you the first time you had sex (intercourse)? | Age: | |
| Have you ever had sex with a person of your same sex? | ❏ Yes ❏ No | |
| Do you use anything to prevent pregnancy? | ❏ Yes ❏ No<br>If yes, what do you use? | |
| Do you and your partner(s) always use a condom when you have sex? | ❏ Yes ❏ No | |
| Do you ever have sex for money or drugs? | ❏ Yes ❏ No | |
| Are you worried about your parents knowing that you are having sex? | ❏ Yes ❏ No | |
| Do you ever participate in other sexual activities, such as touching or oral or anal sex?<br>    If yes, do you use anything to prevent disease? | ❏ Yes ❏ No<br>❏ Yes ❏ No   If yes, what do you use? | |
| **Tobacco, Alcohol, and Drugs** | | |
| Have you or your close friends ever smoked cigarettes or cigars, used snuff, or chewed tobacco? | ❏ Yes, I have ❏ No, I haven't<br>❏ Yes, friends have ❏ No, friends haven't | |
| Have you or your close friends ever gotten drunk on wine, beer, or alcohol? | ❏ Yes, I have ❏ No, I haven't<br>❏ Yes, friends have ❏ No, friends haven't | |
| How much alcohol do you drink at one time? | ❏ Don't drink ❏ 1–2 glasses ❏ 3 or more | |
| Do you ever drink more than 5 drinks in a row? | ❏ Don't drink ❏ Yes ❏ No | |
| In the last year, have you been in a car or other motor vehicle when the driver is drunk or has been drinking alcohol or using drugs? (This includes when you were the driver as well as other people.) | ❏ Yes ❏ No | |
| Would you call your parent(s) or guardian(s) for a ride if you were stranded because the person who was supposed to drive you home had been drinking? (This includes when you were the driver as well as other people.) | ❏ Yes ❏ No ❏ Not sure | |
| Have you or your close friends ever used marijuana or other drugs (like cocaine, heroin, or ecstasy) or sniffed inhalants? | ❏ Yes, I have ❏ No, I haven't<br>❏ Yes, friends have ❏ No, friends haven't<br>❏ Not sure | |
| Have you ever used alcohol or drugs so much that you could not remember what happened? | ❏ Don't use drugs or alcohol ❏ Yes ❏ No | |
| Have you ever missed work or school because of use of alcohol or drugs? | ❏ Don't use drugs or alcohol ❏ Yes ❏ No | |
| **Emotions** | | |
| In the past few weeks, have you often felt sad and down or as though you have nothing to look forward to? | ❏ Yes ❏ No | |
| Have you ever seriously thought about killing yourself, made a plan or actually tried to kill yourself? | ❏ Yes ❏ No | |
| During the past year, have you had any major good or bad changes in your life (death of someone close, birth, graduation, significant change in close relationship)? | ❏ Good ❏ Bad ❏ No changes | |

What would you like to discuss with our nurses and doctors today?_____

Select questions have been taken directly or adapted from the following sources with permission. GAPS. Younger Adolescent Questionnaire. American Medical Association. 1998. Available at http://www.ama-assn.org/ama/pub/category/2280.html. Retrieved May 8, 2002. Middle-Older Adolescent Questionnaire. American Medical Association 1997. Available at http://www.ama-assn.org/ama/pub/category/2280.html. Retrieved May 8, 2002.

**Figure 32-20, cont'd    ACOG Adolescent Visit Questionnaire and ACOG Adolescent Visit Record.**

## Medical Management of Gynecologic Problems in the Pediatric and Adolescent Patient

Date: _____ Name: _____     Patient Addressograph
                              LAST              FIRST                    MIDDLE

Date of Birth: _____ Record Number: _____

Primary Physician: _____ Referral Source: _____

Insurance Carrier/Medicaid No.: _____

# ACOG ADOLESCENT VISIT RECORD

**I. General Information**

| Current age:                                | Complaint(s), if any: |
|---------------------------------------------|-----------------------|
| Current medications:                        |                       |

**Contact information**
(It should be determined who is aware of the teens sexual activity as this may affect where and/or how the teen wishes to be contacted with abnormal findings.)

**II. History**

| FOR PROBLEM VISIT ONLY—History of Present Illness (HPI) (please describe, if any): | FOR PROBLEM VISIT ONLY—HPI elements: |
|---|---|
| | ☐ Location ☐ Severity ☐ Timing ☐ Modifying factors |
| | ☐ Quality ☐ Duration ☐ Context ☐ Associated signs and symptoms |

Menstrual History

|  | Response | Details/Notes |  | Response | Details/Notes |
|---|---|---|---|---|---|
| Age at menarche | | | Last menstrual period | | |
| Length of periods | | | Normal/Abnormal | | |
| Cycle length | | | Cramping | | |

Past Medical and Family History

| Past Medical History | (+) Pos (0) Neg | Details/Remarks |
|---|---|---|
| Past illnesses (measles, mumps, rheumatic fever, chicken pox, hepatitis, cancer, sickle cell anemia) | | |
| Pulmonary (pneumonia, TB/lived with someone who has/had TB, asthma) | | |
| Surgical procedures | | |
| Trauma/violence | | |
| Injuries/accidents | | |
| Hospitalization | | |
| Allergies | | |
| Blood transfusions | | |
| Previous cervical cytology   Date: | Normal/Abnormal/ _____ | |
| Past family history | | |
| Blood clots | | |
| Parent with cholesterol >240 | | |
| Parent/grandparent death from heart attack/stroke at <55 years, coronary artery disease, peripheral vascular disease, cerebrovascular disease | | |
| Ethnic background related diseases (Tay–Sachs, sickle cell anemia, Thalessemia) | | |
| Cancer | | |
| Diabetes | | |

A nurse or nursing assistant, depending on staff capabilities and facilities, can complete all shaded areas of the record.

**Figure 32-20, cont'd    ACOG Adolescent Visit Questionnaire and ACOG Adolescent Visit Record.**     *Continued*

## Pediatric and Adolescent Gynecology

| Past Social History | Details/Notes |
|---|---|
| If sexually active, contraception/STD prevention method:<br><br>Frequency of method use: _____<br>Number of current partners: _____<br>Age of initial coitus: _____<br>Number of past partners:_____<br>Pregnancies: G _____ P _____ AB _____<br>STDs, including herpes simplex virus: _____ | |

CPT Levels of History

| Levels of History | Chief Complaint (CC) | History of Present Illness (HPI) | Review of Systems (ROS) | Past, Family, Social History (PFSH) |
|---|---|---|---|---|
| Problem focused | Required | Brief | Not required | Not required |
| Expanded problem focused | Required | Brief | Problem pertinent | Not required |
| Detailed | Required | Extended | Extended | Pertinent |
| Comprehensive | Required | Extended | Complete | Complete |

### III. Immunization

| Routine (a check mark indicates a positive response) | Notations |
|---|---|
| ❏ Tetanus Diphtheria (ideal booster at age 11–12, if not previously vaccinated within 5 years) | |
| ❏ Measles–mumps–rubella (ideal second dose at age 11–12, unless 2 vaccinations in early childhood) | |
| ❏ Hepatitis B vaccination (to be given at age 11–12, if previous recommended doses were missed) | |
| As indicated | |
| ❏ Hepatitis A (traveling/living in endemic community, chronic liver disease, or injecting drug users) | |
| ❏ Varicella vaccination (administered at age 11–12 to all unvaccinated patients or those lacking reliable history of chicken pox (susceptible patients age ≥ 13 receive 2 doses, at least 1 month apart) | |

### IV. Health Guidance/Counseling

| Positive from Adolescent Visit Questionnaire: | Details/Notes | Positive from Adolescent Visit Questionnaire: | Details/Notes |
|---|---|---|---|
| | | | |
| Routine as appropriate | | Routine as appropriate | |
| Tobacco | | Emergency contraception | |
| Alcohol and other drugs | | STDs, including HIV/AIDS | |
| Drinking and driving | | Sexual victimization risk reduction[2] | |
| Diet (calcium, weight management, folic acid) | | Pregnancy counseling (options, prenatal care, school) | |
| Exercise | | Violence | |
| Responsible sexual behavior (abstinence/contraception) | | Conflict resolution | |
| Condoms (how to acquire, use, and talk with partner) | | Seat belts/helmets | |
| Other | | Other | |

[1] Encourage adolescents and their parents to develop agreements for picking up adolescents who have consumed alcohol or other substances.
[2] Discuss role of alcohol and other drugs.

### V. Vital Signs

| Weight | Height | Blood Pressure |
|---|---|---|
| BMI[3] | Temperature | Pulse |

[3] Body mass index is computed as weight (in kilograms) divided by height in meters squared. Using pounds and inches, multiply the division results by 700. To determine prepregnancy weight-for-height status, go to the BMI chart.

A nurse or nursing assistant, depending on staff capabilities and facilities, can complete all shaded areas of the record.

**Figure 32-20, cont'd  ACOG Adolescent Visit Questionnaire and ACOG Adolescent Visit Record.**

## Medical Management of Gynecologic Problems in the Pediatric and Adolescent Patient

### VI. Review of Systems

| Systems | (+) Pos (0) Neg | Details/Notes |
|---|---|---|
| Constitutional (weight loss/gain, eating disorder) | | |
| Eyes | | |
| Ears, nose, mouth or throat problems | | |
| Cardiovascular | | |
| Respiratory | | |
| Gastrointestinal (eating behaviors indicating an eating disorder) | | |
| Genitourinary (urination problems, vaginal discharge) | | |
| Musculoskeletal (muscle/joint pain, scoliosis, broken bones) | | |
| Integumentary (severe acne) | | |
| Breast tenderness, mass | | |
| Neurologic (seizures/epilepsy, headaches/migraines) | | |
| Psychiatric disorders (depression) | | |
| Endocrine | | |
| Hematologic/lymphatic (blood disorder, anemia) | | |
| Allergic/immunologic | | |

### VII. Physical Examination. Leave blank if not examined (required if history indicates and at least once at ages 12–14, 15–17, and 18–21)

| Body Area/Organ System | Normal | Abnormal | Details/Notes | Body Area/Organ System | Normal | Abnormal | Details/Notes |
|---|---|---|---|---|---|---|---|
| Abdomen (masses, tenderness, hernia, HSM) | | | | Genitourinary | | | |
| Extremities | | | | Breasts Tanner stage: | | | |
| Neck (thyroid, masses) | | | | Pubic Hair Tanner stage: | | | |
| Cardiovascular (peripheral system/auscultation) | | | | Vulva/external genitalia | | | |
| Ears/Nose/Mouth/Throat (teeth) | | | | Kidney/bladder | | | |
| Eyes | | | | Vagina | | | |
| Gastrointestinal (digital rectal exam) | | | | Uterus | | | |
| Hematologic/Lymphatic/ Immunologic (lymph nodes) | | | | Adnexa | | | |
| Musculoskeletal | | | | Anus/perineum | | | |
| Neurologic | | | | Cervix | | | |
| Psychiatric | | | | Urethral Meatus | | | |
| Respiratory (effort, auscultation) | | | | Urethra | | | |
| Skin | | | | | | | |

#### CPT Levels of Physical Examination

| Level of Physical Examination | CPT Definitions |
|---|---|
| Problem focused | Limited examination of affected body area or organ system |
| Expanded problem focused | Limited examination of affected body area or organ system AND other symptomatic or related organ systems |
| Detailed | Extended examination of affected body area(s) AND other symptomatic or related organ systems |
| Comprehensive | General multi-system examination OR complete examination of single organ system |

A nurse or nursing assistant, depending on staff capabilities and facilities, can complete all shaded areas of the record.

**Figure 32-20, cont'd    ACOG Adolescent Visit Questionnaire and ACOG Adolescent Visit Record.**    *Continued*

## Pediatric and Adolescent Gynecology

### VIII. Testing Ordered/Performed

| | Tests | Date | Results |
|---|---|---|---|
| General | Cholesterol[1] <br> Lipoprotein profile[2] <br> Tuberculin[3] | | |
| Gynecologic | Cervical cytology[4] <br> Gonorrhea[5] <br> Chlamydia[5] <br> Syphilis[6] <br> HIV[7] | | |
| Other | | | |

[1]Adolescents with parental cholesterol >240 mg/dL should be screened for total blood cholesterol (nonfasting) at least once. Adolescents with either unknown family history, or multiple risk factors may be screened for total serum cholesterol level (nonfasting) at least once.

[2]Adolescents with parent/grandparent with coronary artery disease, peripheral vascular disease, cerebrovascular disease, or sudden cardiac death age <55 should be screened with a fasting lipoprotein profile.

[3]If have been exposed to active tuberculosis; have lived in a homeless shelter, been incarcerated, or lived in another long-term care facility; have lived in endemic area; currently working in health care setting; HIV positive; medically underserved or low-income; have history of alcoholism; have medical risk factors known to increase risk of disease if infected.

[4]Cervical cytology should be obtained no later than 3 years after first intercourse.

[5]Routine screening for chlamydial and gonorrheal infection should be performed for all sexually active adolescents.

[6]Serologic testing for syphilis should be conducted on sexually active adolescents who have a history of prior STDs, multiple sexual partners, exchanged sex for drugs or money, used illicit drugs, been admitted to jail or other detention facility, lived in an endemic area.

[7]Adolescents with the following risk factors should be offered HIV testing: multiple sexual partners, high-risk partner, prior STDs, exhanges sex for drugs or money, long-term residence or birth in an area with high prevalence of HIV infection, history of blood transfusion prior to 1985, use of intravenous drugs.

### IX. Assessment/Plan

| Assessment | Plan |
|---|---|
| | |

FOR PROBLEM VISIT ONLY—CPT Level of Medical Decision Making (Two of the three required elements must be met or exceeded.)

| Elements Included in Medical Decision Making Component | | | |
|---|---|---|---|
| Number of diagnoses or management options | Amount and/or complexity of data to be reviewed | Risk of complications and/or morbidity or mortality | Type of medical decision making |
| Minimal | Minimal or none | Minimal | Straightforward |
| Limited | Limited | Low | Low complexity |
| Multiple | Moderate | Moderate | Moderate complexity |
| Extensive | Extensive | High | High complexity |

**FOR PROBLEM VISIT ONLY—If E/M Code selected based on time:**

| Time spent counseling: | Physician signature: |
|---|---|
| Total time with patient: | |

**Figure 32-20, cont'd    ACOG Adolescent Visit Questionnaire and ACOG Adolescent Visit Record.**

Confidentiality in Adolescent Health Care

**Box 1. Confidential Agreement**

**Parent**

I, _____ (parent or guardian), allow

_____ (patient), to enter a confidential patient–physician relationship. I understand that she can make independent health care decisions, but that my input and involvement will be encouraged.

_____ (patient)has permission to schedule appointments and receive confidential reports from this office. I further understand that various laboratory tests may be necessary in medical protocols and accept responsibility for physician charges and laboratory fees.

_____
Parent or Guardian

_____
Physician

**Patient**

I, _____ (patient), am entering a confidential physician–patient relationship with

_____ (physician). I will make an effort to communicate with my parent(s) or guardian(s) about issues concerning my health. I accept the personal responsibility of being honest and will follow the health care recommendations my physician and I establish.

_____
Patient

_____
Physician

**Figure 32-20, cont'd ACOG Adolescent Visit Questionnaire and ACOG Adolescent Visit Record.** (Used with permission from American College of Obstetricians and Gynecologists [ACOG]: Tool Kit for Teen Care. Washington, DC, 2003,©ACOG.)

# Pediatric and Adolescent Gynecology

### Table 32-3
### Prepubertal Predisposing Risk Factors for Vaginitis

**Anatomic**

Lack of labial fat pads and pubic hair
Thin, sensitive vulvar skin
Thin, atrophic vaginal epithelium
Prepubertal hypoestrogenic state of vagina
Neutral pH of vagina
Closed proximity of vagina to anus

**Hygienic**

Poor hand washing
Inadequate cleansing of vulva after voiding or bowel movements
Exposure to vulvar irritants (e.g., dirt, sand, soaps)

**Infectious**

Upper respiratory infection in past month
Vulvovaginitis in past year

### Diagnosis and Treatment

The diagnostic approach in these patients should include a complete skin examination to look for other systemic manifestations of disease (e.g., varicella), a complete vulvar examination, and the appropriate use of culture media for the determination of the most common causes. The general treatment of these patients should include hygiene and local measures that prevent the continuing irritation of the area such as sitz baths, discontinuation of the use of chemicals and soaps in the area, cotton underpants, a protective barrier cream (e.g., zinc-oxide-containing diaper-rash creams), and use of laundry detergent free of deodorants or allergenic substances. If a particular infectious agent is identified, the proper antibiotic treatment should be instituted along with the measures listed in Table 32-4.

Further investigation may be necessary in patients when conservative management or the appropriate antibiotic does not resolve the symptoms, especially in the presence of purulent discharge or bleeding. Vaginal irrigation or vaginoscopy may be used in determining whether a foreign body or an anatomic lesion is causing the problem (Fig. 32-24). A treatment trial with mebendazole for pinworms or a bedtime dose of antibiotics may be of help if no other causes have been found, although no proof of efficacy is shown in the literature.

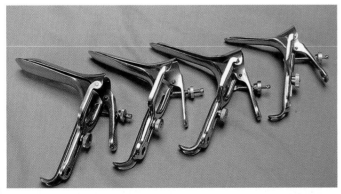

**Figure 32-21**   Types of specula (from left to right): Graves, Pederson, Huffman, infant.

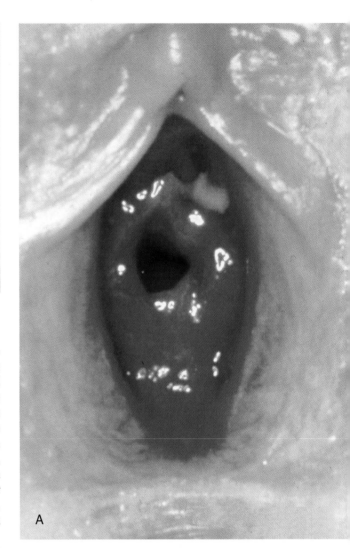

A

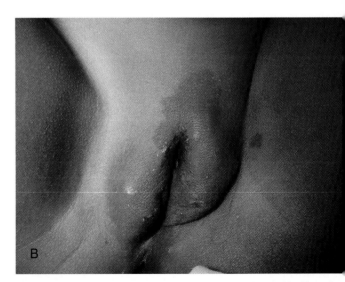

B

**Figure 32-22**   *A,* Prepubertal girl with streptococcal vaginitis. Note the purulent material near the urethra and gross erythema of the hymen obscuring normal vascular pattern. *B,* Group A *Streptococcus* vulvitis. (*A,* Used with permission from Yordan EE [ed]: The PediGYN Teaching Slide Set. Farmington, Conn, North American Society for Pediatric and Adolescent Gynecology, 1996.)

# Medical Management of Gynecologic Problems in the Pediatric and Adolescent Patient

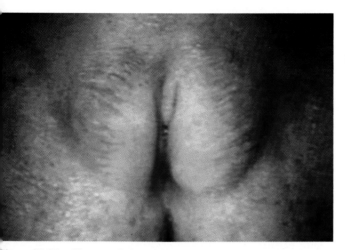

**Figure 32-23** **Diaper rash dermatitis and secondary *Candida* infection in a young girl receiving antibiotics.** (Used with permission from Yordan EE [ed]: The PediGYN Teaching Slide Set. Farmington, Conn, North American Society for Pediatric and Adolescent Gynecology, 1996.)

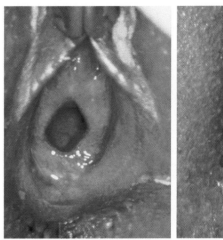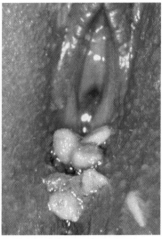

**Figure 32-24** **Girl with a vaginal discharge and bleeding.** The cause, initially unseen, was revealed to be small pieces of toilet paper. (Used with permission from Yordan EE [ed]: The PediGYN Teaching Slide Set. Farmington, Conn, North American Society for Pediatric and Adolescent Gynecology, 1996.)

**Table 32-4**
**Specific Causes and Treatment of Vulvovaginitis**

| Etiology | Drug | Dose | Route | Duration |
|---|---|---|---|---|
| *Streptococcus pyogenes* | Penicillin V | 250 mg tid | PO | 10 days |
| *Haemophilus influenzae* | Amoxicillin | 20–40 mg/kg/day divided every 8 hours | PO | 10 days |
| For resistant strains | Amoxicillin/clavulanate | 20–40 mg/kg/day divided every 8 hours | PO | 7–10 days |
| | Trimethoprim/sulfamethoxazole | 8 mg/40 mg/kg/day divided every 12 hours | PO | 10 days |
| *Staphylococcus aureus* | Cephalexin | 25–50 mg/kg/day divided every 12 hours | PO | 7–10 days |
| | Dicloxacillin | 25 mg/kg/day | PO | 7–10 days |
| | Amoxicillin/clavulanate | 20–40 mg/kg/day divided every 8 hours | PO | 7–10 days |
| | Cefuroxime axetil susp | 30 mg/kg/day bid (max 1 g) | PO | 10 days |
| | Cefuroxime axetil tabs | 250 mg bid | PO | 10 days |
| *Streptococcus pneumoniae* | Penicillin | | | |
| | Erythromycin | 50 mg/kg/day divided every 6 hours | PO | 10 days |
| | Trimethoprim/sulfamethoxazole | 8 mg/40 mg/kg/day divided every 12 hours | PO | 10 days |
| | Clarithromycin | 15 mg/kg/day divided every 12 hours | PO | 10 days |
| *Shigella* | Trimethoprim/sulfamethoxazole | 8 mg/40 mg/kg/day divided every 12 hours | PO | 10 days |
| For resistant strains | Cefixime | 8 mg/kg/day single dose | PO | 10 days |
| | Cetriaxone | 50 mg/kg/single dose (max 1 g) | IM | |
| If >45 kg | Ciprofloxacin | 250–500 mg every 12 hours | PO | 7–14 days |
| | Azithromycin | 1000 mg 1st day, then 500 mg every day | PO | 4 days |
| *Chlamydia trachomatis* | Erythromycin | 50 mg/kg/day | PO | 10–14 days |
| | Azithromycin | 20 mg/kg (max 1 g) | PO | One dose |
| If >age 8 years | Doxycycline | 100 mg bid | PO | 7 days |
| *Neisseria gonorrhoeae* | Ceftriaxone | 125 mg | IM | One dose |
| *Candida* | Nystatin | | Topical | 7 days |
| | Miconazole | | Topical | 7 days |
| | Clotrimazole | | Topical | 7 days |
| | Terconazole | | Topical | 7 days |
| *Trichomonas* | Metronidazole | 15 mg/kg/day tid (max 250 mg tid) | PO | 7–10 days |
| Pinworms | Mebendazole | One 100-mg tablet chewable repeat in 2 weeks | PO | |

Reprinted with permission from Perlman SE, Nakajima ST, Hertweck SP: Clinical Protocols in Pediatric and Adolescent Gynecology. London, Parthenon Publishing Group, 1994, Table 69-1, p 385.

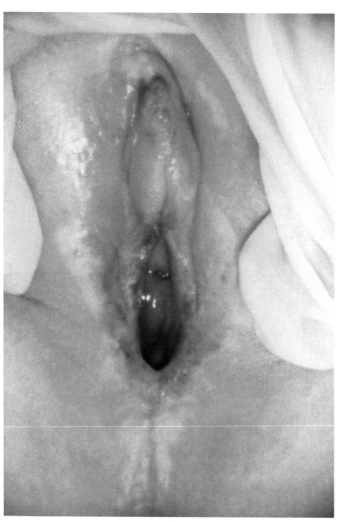

**Figure 32-25   Lichen sclerosus in a 5-year-old girl.** (Used with permission from Yordan EE [ed]: The PediGYN Teaching Slide Set. Farmington, Conn, North American Society for Pediatric and Adolescent Gynecology, 1996.)

## Lichen Sclerosus

Other common disorders of the vulva and vagina in this age group are related to primary disorders of the skin. One common condition, lichen sclerosus, may present in this age group with vaginal discharge, itching, and rarely bleeding. The characteristic appearance of the skin disorder (figure-of-eight distribution of parchment-like epithelium often with subepithelial hemorrhages) provides a clue about the etiology, and therefore in most cases a biopsy is not necessary (Fig. 32-25). The etiology of this condition is unknown. The use of hygiene measures is important to prevent scarring and continuing irritation of the area. Prevention of itching with systemic antihistamines may be a choice to decrease the patient's urge to scratch and further decrease scarring. The use of ultrapotent topical steroids (e.g., betamethasone dipropionate 0.05% or clobetasol 0.025% to 0.05% for up to 12 weeks) is the most efficacious treatment. It has even been shown to halt the progression of the disease in children and adolescents.[7] Close surveillance of these children is important to prevent long-term effects of local steroids including epithelial atrophy and telangiectasia. In mild cases, less potent steroids or tapered doses of high-dose topical steroids may also affect the disease positively. Long-term complications of this disease are those associated with scarring prior to treatment and multiple recurrences. In as many as 50% of patients the problem resolves after puberty.[8]

## Vulvar Ulcers

Ulcerative diseases (such as herpes), mononucleosis, and other viral diseases like Coxsackie A16 (hand-foot-and-mouth disease) or varicella may have vulvar presentations in this age group as well. *Behçet's syndrome*, an autoimmune disorder characterized by recurrent genital ulcers, eye lesions, and orocutaneous lesions, may be diagnosed in this age group (Fig. 32-26A and B). Although a viral etiology is suspected, the true origin of the disease is unknown. Therapeutic interventions such as corticosteroids, topical antibiotics, and anesthetics are the mainstay of treatment.

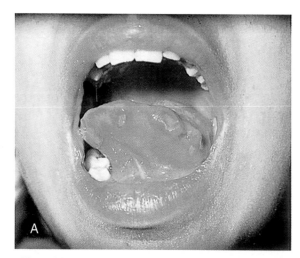
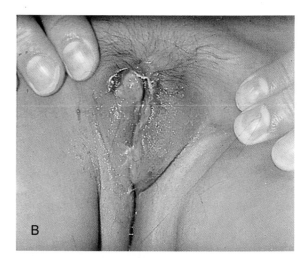

**Figure 32-26   Behçet's syndrome.** A, Oral lesions. B, Genital lesions. (From Weinberg S, Prose NS: Color Atlas of Pediatric Dermatology, 2nd ed. New York, McGraw-Hill, 1990, p 138. Reproduced with the permission of the McGraw-Hill Companies.)

## Labial Adhesions

Labial adhesions also present commonly in the prepubertal age group, primarily between the ages of 2 months and 6 years of age. These patients are generally seen because their parents have observed the "closed vagina" or they have been referred by their pediatricians because of frequent urinary infections or obstruction of urinary egress. The etiology of this condition is unknown, but chronic irritation along with the hypoestrogenic state of the vulva may predispose to the condition (Fig. 32-27). Most patients do not require treatment given the spontaneous resolution. Also, treatment may not be warranted given the high recurrence rate.[9] On the other hand, those patients with frequent urinary tract infections or urinary obstruction may require intervention. The use of estrogen cream may be efficacious and manual separation under local or general anesthesia may be necessary in the symptomatic patient refractory to medical or conservative management.[10] Recurrences are common, occurring in 25% of cases that have had manual separation.[11]

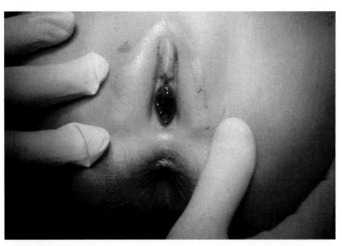

**Figure 32-28** Urethral prolapse in a prepubertal girl. (Used with permission from Yordan EE [ed]: The PediGYN Teaching Slide Set. Farmington, Conn, North American Society for Pediatric and Adolescent Gynecology, 1996.)

## Urethral Prolapse

Urethral prolapse is a common cause of vaginal bleeding in this age group. The classic friable, doughnut-shaped introital mass seen in these children confirms the diagnosis (Fig. 32-28). Pediatric and adolescent gynecologists advocate initial treatment with topical application of estrogen cream, reserving surgical removal for those cases that remain symptomatic and are associated with necrotic tissue.[12,13]

## Genital Neoplasms

Genital neoplasms may present in this age group and should be able to be recognized by the gynecologist. Hemangiomas of the vulva in general are of no clinical significance and typically resolve spontaneously between 2 and 5 years of age, requiring no further intervention. Large hemangiomas or trauma resulting in active bleeding may warrant careful removal or occlusion of the vessels of these lesions.[14] Sarcoma botryoides, although rare, is a classic pediatric diagnosis in prepubertal patients having a protruding vaginal mass and vaginal bleeding (Fig. 32-29). Primary chemotherapy after initial biopsy allows for excellent tumor control and limits the need for extensive extirpative surgical procedures while providing 5-year survival rates approaching 85%.[15]

## Inflammatory Vulvar Conditions

Other less common inflammatory processes of the vulva are also present in this age group such as eczema, seborrheic dermatitis, psoriasis, pemphigus, Stevens-Johnson syndrome, and Crohn's disease. Pigmentation defects such as vitiligo, acanthosis nigricans, and hyperpigmentation are vulvar manifestations of systemic diseases; the management of these conditions is outside the scope of this chapter.

# HIRSUTISM

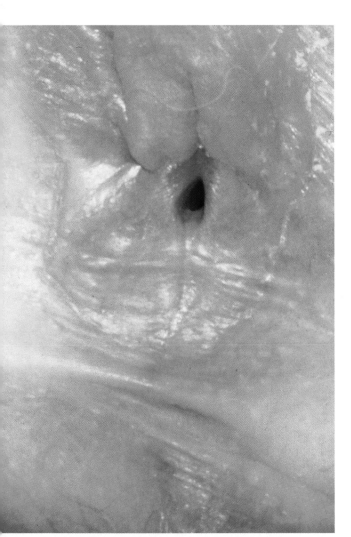

**Figure 32-27** Labial/vulvar agglutination in a 3-year-old girl. (Used with permission from Yordan EE [ed]: The PediGYN Teaching Slide Set. Farmington, Conn, North American Society for Pediatric and Adolescent Gynecology, 1996.)

Adolescents with complaints of androgen excess commonly come in with acne and occasionally excessive facial hair growth. Usually what concerns the adolescent the most is the distorted

# Pediatric and Adolescent Gynecology

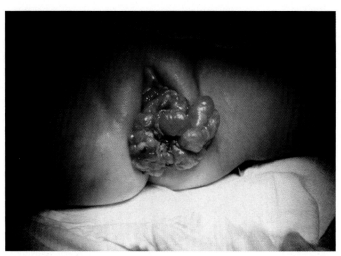

**Figure 32-29    Sarcoma botryoides (vulvovaginal rhabdomyosarcoma) protruding from the vagina of a 3-year-old girl.** (Used with permission from Yordan EE [ed]: The PediGYN Teaching Slide Set. Farmington, Conn, North American Society for Pediatric and Adolescent Gynecology, 1996.)

self-image associated with these conditions, which necessitates attention, evaluation, and possible treatment.

## Definition

Hirsutism is difficult to define given the interaction of the patient's interpretation of "normal." Hirsutism can be defined as the abnormal excess of terminal hair growth. Multiple causes are associated with this presenting symptom (Table 32-5). To determine the cause of hirsutism, a thorough history should be taken that identifies the speed and timing of hair growth (sudden vs.

long term), as well as the location and other associated androgenic symptoms including clitoromegaly, acne, and male baldness or voice deepening. The characteristics of menses as well as the use of medications (phenytoin) should be investigated to determine other conditions likely to cause hair growth and androgenization. Girls with low birth weight and a history of precocious pubarche in childhood are at high risk of polycystic ovary syndrome (PCOS) in adolescence.[16]

## Diagnosis

The physical examination should focus on anatomic as well as hormonal causes for androgen excess. Assessment of the thyroid, abdomen, and pelvis should be a part of the examination. Stigmata of Cushing's or hyperinsulinemia (e.g., acanthosis nigricans—darkly pigmented, velvety skin at the nape of the neck, axilla, waist) can sometimes be helpful in determining the source of the androgenic state, and the presence of a pelvic-abdominal mass could point toward an androgen-secreting tumor. Adequately documenting the amount and distribution of the hair can be used to standardize the classification of these patients and aids in determining progress after treatment initiation (Fig. 32-30A and B). The presence of clitoromegaly (clitoral glans >5 mm in diameter) should be documented.

The laboratory examination will assist in determining the cause of the hirsutism. While the presence of oligomenorrhea and long-standing hirsutism (>1 year) suggests PCOS, the menstrual history in the adolescent is limited to only a few years. The presentation of virilization or rapid-onset or exacerbation hirsutism may be a sign of significant pathology and requires initial laboratory evaluation.

Assessment of serum levels of testosterone, free testosterone, and dehydroepiandrosterone sulfate (DHEAS) is the best initial approach. Some patients may have an increased sensitivity to free testosterone, and even though the total amount is normal, the free component is elevated and is the cause of the hirsutism.[17] The presence of oligomenorrhea or amenorrhea may warrant evaluation of other conditions, and thyroid-stimulating hormone (TSH), follicle-stimulating hormone (FSH), human chorionic gonadotropin (hCG), and prolactin levels should be assessed. Levels of total testosterone higher than 200 ng/dL and of DHEAS above 700 µg/dL suggest the presence of an ovarian or adrenal tumor, respectively. Screen for late-onset congenital adrenal hyperplasia (CAH) with a 7 to 8 AM 17-hydroxyprogesterone (17-OHP) level. 17-OHP levels above 200 ng/dL have an 80% positive predictive value and 100% negative predictive value for 21-hydroxylase deficiency. If the level is greater than 1000 ng/dL, the diagnosis of late-onset CAH can be made without further testing.[18] In those patients with a mild elevation of 17-OHP, a modified ACTH stimulation test, using 0.25 mg of ACTH and measuring base-line and 60-minute levels of 17-OHP, is indicated to make the diagnosis. Levels higher than 1000 ng/dL and usually above 1500 ng/dL are seen.[19]

Some patients with PCOS may have a metabolic syndrome of hyperinsulinemia, abnormal glucose utilization, and abnormal lipid profiles. Consider screening these patients with a fasting lipid profile and glucose tolerance testing.

In the hirsute patient, the presence of a pelvic mass must be considered. In cases where an abdominopelvic examination is not definitive or laboratory tests indicate androgen-secreting

---

**Table 32-5**
**Causes of Hirsutism in Adolescents**

Ovarian disorders
  Polycystic ovary syndrome (PCOS)
  Hyperthecosis
  Tumors
  Enzyme deficiency (e.g., 17-ketosteroid reductase deficiency)
Adrenal disorders
  Congenital adrenal hyperplasia (21-hydroxylase, 11β-hydroxylase,
    3β-hydroxysteroid dehydrogenase deficiencies)
  Cushing's disease
  Tumors
Idiopathic hirsutism
Drugs (phenytoin, danazol, diazoxide, minoxidil, glucocorticoid excess,
  androgens, valproate)
Pregnancy
Hypothyroidism
Central nervous system injury
Hyperprolactinemia
Stress
Anorexia nervosa, malnutrition
Peripheral tissue
  Possible excessive activity of 5α-reductase and/or 17-ketosteroid reductase
Male pseudohermaphroditism, mixed gonadal dysgenesis

From Emans SJ: Endocrine abnormalities associated with hirsutism. In Emans SJ, Laufler MR, Goldstein DP (eds): Pediatric and Adolescent Gynecology, 4th ed. Philadelphia, Lippincott Williams & Wilkins, 1998, p. 265.

| Site* | Grade | Definition |
|---|---|---|
| 1. Upper Lip | 1 | A few hairs at outer margin |
| | 2 | A small moustache at outer margin |
| | 3 | A moustache extending halfway from outer margin |
| | 4 | A moustache extending to midline |
| 2. Chin | 1 | A few scattered hairs |
| | 2 | Scattered hairs with small concentrations |
| | 3 & 4 | Complete cover, light and heavy |
| 3. Chest | 1 | Circumareolar hairs |
| | 2 | With midline hair in addition |
| | 3 | Fusion of these areas, with three-quarters covered |
| | 4 | Complete cover |
| 4. Upper back | 1 | A few scattered hairs |
| | 2 | Rather more hair, still scattered |
| | 3 & 4 | Complete cover, light and heavy |
| 5. Lower back | 1 | A sacral tuft of hair |
| | 2 | With some lateral extension |
| | 3 | Three-quarters covered |
| | 4 | Complete cover |
| 6. Upper abdomen | 1 | A few midline hairs |
| | 2 | Rather more, still midline |
| | 3 & 4 | Half and full cover |
| 7. Lower abdomen | 1 | A few midline hairs |
| | 2 | A midline streak of hair |
| | 3 | A midline band of hair |
| | 4 | An inverted V-shaped growth |
| 8. Arm | 1 | Sparse growth affecting not more than a quarter of the limb surface |
| | 2 | More than a quarter of the limb surface affected |
| | 3 & 4 | Complete cover, light and heavy |
| 9. Forearm | 1, 2, 3, 4 | Complete cover of dorsal surface; 2 grades of light and 2 of heavy growth |
| 10. Thigh | 1, 2, 3, 4 | As for arm |
| 11. Leg | 1, 2, 3, 4 | As for arm |

*Grade 0 at all sites indicates absence of terminal hair.

**Figure 32-30   Hirsutism scoring sheet.** *A* and *B,* The Ferriman and Gallwey system for scoring hirsutism. A score of 8 or more indicates hirsutism. (Used with permission from Hatch R, Rosenfield RL, Kim MH, et al: Hirsutism: implications, etiology and management. Am J Obstet Gynecol 1981;149:815. Adapted from Ferriman D, Gallwey JD: Clinical assessment of body hair growth in women. J Clin Endocrinol Metab 1961;21:1440. *B,* Copyright 1961, The Endocrine Society.)

tumors, ultrasound imaging can detect ovarian masses and magnetic resonance imaging (MRI) can identify an adrenal tumor. Patients may also have idiopathic hirsutism (15%) characterized by regular ovulatory cycles and excess hair growth. This is a common diagnosis but one of exclusion.

## Treatment

The treatment of hirsutism is approached on two fronts. One is suppression of the androgen-producing entity and aims to decrease the amount of circulating androgens (surgery, medication). The other looks at the cosmetic component of the treatment, aiming to improve the appearance and confidence of the patient.

The surgical removal of androgen-producing tumors will diminish the amount of circulating androgens, but cosmetic help may still be needed. Medical management of hirsutism is more commonly used for non-neoplastic conditions and includes androgen suppression agents and peripherally acting agents.

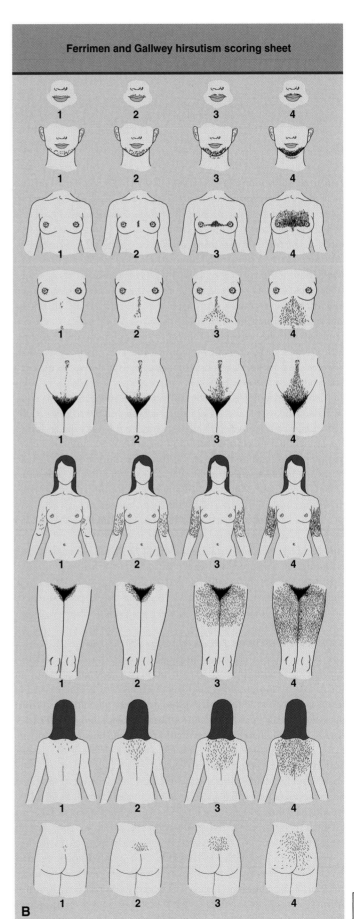

Ferrimen and Gallwey hirsutism scoring sheet

B

# Pediatric and Adolescent Gynecology

## Management of Excess Ovarian Androgen Production

Combination estrogen/progestin oral contraceptive pills (OCPs) are commonly used to treat hirsutism. Their mechanism of action is the associated increased levels of circulating sex hormone–binding globulin (SHBG) and suppressed ovarian androgen production that effectively decreases circulating unbound androgens. Generally 50% to 70% of patients improve with this treatment alone. Patients should be aware that this treatment primarily prevents future hair development and the existing hair may need to be cosmetically treated or removed. Gonadotropin-releasing hormone (GnRH) agonists may be used in cases of severe hirsutism refractory to conventional treatment. They function by suppressing luteinizing hormone (LH) levels and thereby ovarian androgen production.[20] Hormonal replacement in the form of norethindrone acetate is helpful in diminishing unwanted side effects such as hot flashes and decreased bone mineral density associated with GnRH agonist use.

Insulin-sensitizing agents, such as metformin, have been shown in adult women to decrease the amount of circulating androgens while improving other metabolic aspects of PCOS.[21]

Initial studies suggest that metformin may be useful in treating PCOS in the obese adolescent with insulin resistance; however, additional studies are needed to determine efficacy and long-term outcome.[22]

Recently, the use of metformin soon after menarche in a group of girls at high risk for PCOS (e.g., history of low birth weight and precocious pubarche) was shown to prevent progression to PCOS.[23] Although metformin monotherapy failed to fully normalize central fat masses, serum androgens, and SHBG, these might be further normalized by addition of an androgen-receptor blocker. Another pilot study has reported that low-dose flutamide (125 mg/day) with metformin improved body shape and body composition by decreasing central fat deposition without implementing any changes in diet, exercise, or lifestyle and without changing total body weight in nonobese adolescents with ovarian hyperandrogenism.[24]

These results indicate that the excess central fat in women with hyperinsulinemic hyperandrogenism is a consequence, rather than a cause, of their endocrine-metabolic state.

## Management of Excess Adrenal Androgen Production

The use of dexamethasone, although reported in the literature, has not been consistently shown to improve hirsutism. While steroids may be used in cases associated with CAH[25] its use is associated with osteoporosis. Since adolescents are accruing their peak bone mass in the teen years, more conservative methods of treatment (i.e., OCP use) are more commonly utilized.

## Management Directed at Hair Follicle

Peripheral suppression agents are commonly used to manage unwanted hair growth. Spironolactone, an aldosterone antagonist, is widely used in adults and adolescents and reported to be efficacious by binding to and blocking the androgen receptor in target tissues and by reducing androgen biosynthesis. Common dosage for this purpose is between 100 and 200 mg per day divided into two doses, and it generally can be added to the OCP regimen to improve the efficacy of both.[26] Cyproterone acetate, another antiandrogen similar in function to spironolactone but not available in the United States, has proved as efficacious as the combination of OCP and spironolactone.[27] The use of less commonly prescribed agents like finasteride, flutamide, and ketoconazole is limited by their side effects. A recent prospective randomized trial of the use of spironolactone, finasteride, and cyproterone acetate along with a combination OCP to treat idiopathic hirsutism in adults showed improvement rates to be similar at 12 months. At 1-year follow-up, the spironolactone group showed the most improvement.[28]

The cosmetic aspects of these patients may also be addressed in the form of laser therapy, electrolysis, bleaching, shaving, plucking, waxing, and depilatories for temporary hair removal. Topical treatment with eflornithine cream may also diminish unwanted hair.[29] Weight reduction to decrease the peripheral conversion of androstenedione and to increase the effective amount of SHBG may improve the hirsutism as would smoking cessation.[30]

# ADOLESCENT CONTRACEPTION

Teen pregnancy remains a major problem in the United States. Despite the fact that the rate of sexual activity among American teens is not different from that of other industrialized nations, the United States has the highest rate of teen pregnancy of any developed nation, a rate that is 50% higher than pregnancy rates in Europe and Canada.[31] For this reason, the use of appropriate contraception is especially important in this age group. As adolescents mature and become capable of reproduction, visits to their practitioner should include counseling on adequate methods of birth control targeting their needs and abilities to improve their compliance. Providing this information does not result in increased rates of sexual activity, earlier age of first intercourse, or greater number of sexual partners. On the contrary, when adolescents perceive that there is an obstacle to obtaining contraception, they are more likely to experience negative outcomes related to sexual activity.[32] Many factors play a role in adolescent contraception either motivating or inhibiting the teen from contraception (Table 32-6). One significant reason that adolescents hesitate or delay in obtaining family planning services or contraception is concern about confidentiality. While many states allow teens to consent to contraception without parental consent, health care providers need to be familiar with current state and local statutes on the rights of minors to

---

**Table 32-6**
**Motivating and Nonmotivating Factors for Adolescent Contraception**

**Motivating factors**

Perceiving pregnancy as a negative outcome
Having long-term educational goals
Being of older age
Experiencing a pregnancy scare or actual pregnancy
Having family, friends, or a clinician who approves of the use of contraception

**Nonmotivating factors**

Lack of parental monitoring
Fear that parents will find out
Ambivalence
Perception that birth control is dangerous

## Medical Management of Gynecologic Problems in the Pediatric and Adolescent Patient

consent to health care services, as well as the federal and state laws that affect confidentiality. This information must also be discussed with both the adolescent and, where appropriate, her parent or guardian. Likewise, it is important to inform office staff about policies and procedures to assist and ensure adolescent confidentiality.[33] Many teens also perceive the pelvic examination to be a barrier to accessing contraceptive services; therefore, the physical examination may be deferred until after initiation of contraceptives if requested by the patient and judged appropriate by the clinician. Postponement, not waiver, of a pelvic examination may be considered for an adolescent seeking contraception when she does not have genital complaints such as an abnormal vaginal discharge, pruritus, or odor. An explanation of the need for STD testing should be completed and the offer of urinary testing extended to those coitally active patients whose examination is not completed at the time of contraceptive initiation. The need for prevention of STDs as well as available contraceptive choices should be addressed. This section focuses on the appropriateness of various contraceptive methods available for adolescents as well as new approaches to contraception prescription.

### Abstinence

Abstinence is the most effective means of birth control. While many teenagers who request contraception are already sexually active, a review of abstinence as a choice should be part of any discussion of options available to the adolescent. The choice to remain or return to abstinence may be difficult for some adolescents. Those who choose abstinence should be encouraged and reminded of the advantages of decreased pregnancy and STD rates.

### Hormonal Contraceptive Methods

Hormonal methods of contraception primarily function via inhibition of ovulation through medication taken remote from the act of intercourse. As adolescent sexual activity tends to be sporadic, this contraceptive method provides a distinct and desired advantage. Of all other contraceptive methods, it is the hormonal methods that have undergone the most advance in the last few years. From pills to patches and injections, the variety available fits the profiles of most adolescents. These methods may be classified as combined methods with estrogen and progestin (i.e., OCP, patch, ring, injection) and progestin only (i.e., pill, injection, insert).

#### Combined Oral Contraceptive Pills

The combined OCP is the most commonly used method of contraception in the adolescent group, with rates of use approaching 50%.[34] The many available dosages ranging from 20 µg to 50 µg of estrogen (ethinyl estradiol), and multiple progestin components, make the choice of the best pill difficult. Despite the combination used, the contraceptive and non-contraceptive benefits of the pill are about the same, and the brand should be chosen based on side effect profile as well as practitioner's preference (Table 32-7). Other indications of use such as acne may also modify the choice. Combinations that contain norgestimate and levonorgestrel have been found to be efficacious for this indication.[35,36] Patient preference may also play a role in the selection of the OCP. The newly available

| Table 32-7 |
| --- |
| **Noncontraceptive Health Benefits of Oral Contraceptives** |
| Increased menstrual cycle regularity |
| Decreased incidence of dysmenorrhea, menorrhagia, iron-deficiency anemia, dysfunctional uterine bleeding, premenstrual syndrome |
| Decreased risk of benign breast disease |
| Decreased risk of pelvic inflammatory disease (and sequelae, including ectopic pregnancy) |
| Decreased risk of functional ovarian cysts |
| Decreased risk of acne and hirsutism |
| Decreased risk of ovarian cancer |
| Decreased risk of endometrial cancer |
| Decreased risk of colon cancer |
| Improved bone density |
| Decreased risk of rheumatoid arthritis |
| Used with permission from Sanfilippo JS, Muram D, Dewhurst J, Lee PA (eds): Pediatrc and Adolescent Gynecology, 2nd ed. Philadelphia, WB Saunders, 2001, Table 19-2, p 306. |

84/7 day package (30 µg ethinyl estradiol and 150 µg levonorgestrel) has shown similar efficacy and compliance with only mild increase in the incidence of breakthrough bleeding in the adult population and may be a new option for patients who desire less frequent menses such as athletes and military personal, although studies in adolescents are lacking.[37]

The initiation day of the pill has been controversial. Utilizing a "quick start" (same day as the visit) method versus the traditional Sunday start initiation seems to improve compliance and still maintain an acceptable side effect profile. This innovative method may be yet another way to encourage adolescent patients to take their method of birth control even before they leave the office with the hope of improving their compliance.[38]

#### New Hormonal Methods

The contraceptive transdermal patch uses the technology of a medicated adhesive that allows the skin to absorb and maintain a constant hormonal level, without the fluctuations seen with orally absorbed forms. In the adult population, failure rates and side effect profile are similar to those of combination OCPs. While studies are lacking in adolescents, this form may improve compliance by decreasing the dosing needed to once a week.[39]

The vaginal contraceptive ring (15 µg ethinyl estradiol/120 µg etonorgestrel) is another recently approved method of birth control. This method requires motivation from the patient to insert and remove the contraceptive device from the vagina once a month, and it has not been well studied in adolescents. The adult population studies have been reassuring, confirming the reliability of the method, low side effect profile, and acceptability by users.[40]

The monthly injectable combination contraceptive that combines 25 mg of medroxyprogesterone acetate and 5 mg of estradiol cypionate was recalled by the manufacturer and is not available for use in the United States. Previous studies of this product showed good efficacy, and the future release of a revised version of this method is anticipated.

#### Progestin-Only Methods

Progestin-only OCPs are available in the form of norgestrel or norethindrone. They are a choice for adolescents who are breastfeeding and for those with contraindications to the use of estrogen such as thrombophilias and certain other medical conditions. The efficacy of this product is similar to that of the combination OCP, and the failure rate may be due to patient noncompliance and short half-life, which requires taking the pill around the same time of the day (within 3 hours).[41] To enhance adolescent compliance, extensive education should be provided regarding irregular bleeding that may occur in the first 3 months and the need to take the pill at a similar time each day.

Depot medroxyprogesterone acetate (DMPA) is used by the adolescent population because of the minimal intervention on their part required to achieve compliance. The application of one intramuscular dose of 150 mg every 3 months increases convenience but still requires compliance to continue the method. Although its efficacy has been shown to be better than that of the OCP, most of its effect is probably related to compliance and ease of use. Weight gain and irregular bleeding are common and unpleasant side effects for adolescents. One concern has been the effect of the hypoestrogenic state on bone density in adolescents created by long-term use of DMPA. The use of DMPA has been shown to decrease bone mineral density in adolescent users when compared with normal menstrual controls and OCP users; however, the potential effect on future bone health is unknown.[42] The lack of long-term prospective trials, as well as the potential bone loss associated with pregnancy in the absence of contraception, make DMPA a valid and reliable method to prevent adolescent pregnancy until further data is obtained. Appropriate calcium intake (1200 to 1500 mg/day) and monitoring of bone density should be encouraged in adolescent long-term users, especially those who become and continue to be amenorrheic with use.

Progestin subdermal implants in the form of levonorgestrel were previously commonly used in the adolescent population because of the long-term contraception provided (5 years). The difficulty in removing the six rods as well as the voluntary recall of certain lots by the manufacturer during 1999 limited the use of this method. The introduction of a single etonogestrel implant with a 3-year contraceptive duration plus easy insertion and removal will make this an alternative for adolescents looking for long-term contraception. This product is completing its phase III trials in the United States and is awaiting Food and Drug Administration (FDA) approval.[43]

### Emergency Contraception

Emergency contraception (EC), the use of nonabortifacient, hormonal medications within 72 to 120 hours after unprotected/underprotected coitus for the prevention of unintended pregnancy, is an important part of the contraception counseling in adolescents. Use of EC decreases the risk of pregnancy from 8% to 1–2% after a single episode of unprotected coitus.[44,45] Two common regimens have been described. The Yuzpe regimen originally described in 1977 includes the use of 200 µg of ethinyl estradiol and 2 mg of dl-norgestrel taken within 72 hours after the episode of intercourse. This regimen is divided in two doses taken 12 hours apart.[44] The second method consists of levonorgestrel 1.5 mg divided into two doses taken 12 hours apart, and recent studies show that this regimen may be more effective in preventing pregnancy than the Yuzpe regimen.[45] Another

distinct advantage of this progestin-only regimen is the decrease in associated nausea and emesis as compared with the combination regimen. Timing is of importance, but recent studies have shown that even if more than 72 hours have passed, either regimen is efficacious and should be offered with the understanding that there may be an increase in the pregnancy rate the more remote from the unprotected coitus it is taken.[46] Dedicated products for emergency contraception may not be available in some pharmacies; therefore, commonly available combination oral contraceptives may be used to achieve the needed amount of hormone for efficacy. Each two doses must contain a minimum of 100 µg ethinyl estradiol and the equivalent of 0.50 mg levonorgestrel per dose (Table 32-8). Advance prescription of EC has been shown to increase the likelihood of use in young women and teens when needed and yet not increase sexual or contraceptive risk-taking behavior when compared with those receiving education only about EC.[47–52]

### Barrier Contraceptive Methods

Barrier methods include devices such as male condoms, female condoms, cervical caps, diaphragms, spermicidal and contraceptive foam, and ovules. Although effective, the use of these devices by adolescents is not consistent, even when chosen by them as their method to protect against STDs.[53] The need for application prior to each sexual encounter decreases the use of the method by "decreasing the spontaneity" of the act, as some teens explain. Latex condoms significantly reduce the transmission of STDs and should be used by all sexually active adolescents regardless of whether an additional method of contraception is used. Therefore, practitioners should encourage the use of barrier methods, such as the male and female condom. In addition to providing condom samples, education should be provided regarding the efficacy of barrier methods in decreasing the transmission of human immunodeficiency virus (HIV). Those adolescents who are most likely to use condoms understand that they can prevent HIV/acquired immunodeficiency syndrome (AIDS), carry them, are not embarrassed to use them, and are concerned about getting AIDS[54] (Table 32-9).

### Intrauterine Devices

The experience with intrauterine devices (IUDs) in adolescents is limited. Traditionally, use of IUDs has been avoided in adolescents as this population has the highest rates for STDs. Most practitioners feel that these patients may not be the best suited for this kind of contraception because of their risk of STDs and the possibility of ascending infection when the IUD is in place. However, no increase in infertility or STD incidence is seen with the use of these devices.[55] Most of the ascending infections are probably related to lack of condom use rather than the presence of the IUD facilitating it.[56] While not typically the first choice for adolescent contraception, with proper counseling and condom use, an IUD may be a viable option for some teens, regardless of their gravidity and parity status, and should be considered one of the available tools for contraception. STD prophylaxis at the time of insertion, if cultures are not available, may be of value for those patients in whom the STD incidence is higher than 5%.[57] Scheduling the first follow-up visit about 7 days later may allow detection of early infection.[58]

# Medical Management of Gynecologic Problems in the Pediatric and Adolescent Patient

| | | No. and Color of Tablets to Take Within | No. and Color of Tablets to Take |
|---|---|---|---|
| Brand Name | Generic Name and Dose | 120 Hours after Unprotected Coitus | 12 Hours after the First Dose |
| **Plan B** | Levonorgestrel 0.75 mg | 1 white | 1 white |
| **Yuzpe regimens** | | | |
| Preven | Levonorgestrel 0.25 mg/ethinyl estradiol 50 µg | 2 blue | 2 blue |
| Ovral | Norgestrel 0.5 mg/ethinyl estradiol 50 µg | 2 white | 2 white |
| Lo-Ovral | Norgestrel 0.3 mg/ethinyl estradiol 30 µg | 4 white | 4 white |
| Nordette or Levlen | Levonorgestrel 0.15 mg/ethinyl estradiol 30 µg | 4 light orange | 4 light orange |
| Levora | Levonorgestrel 0.15 mg/ethinyl estradiol 30 µg | 4 white | 4 white |
| Triphasil or Tri-Levlen | Levonorgestrel 0.125 mg/ethinyl estradiol 30 µg | 4 yellow | 4 yellow |
| Trivora | Levonorgestrel 0.125 mg/ethinyl estradiol 30 µg | 4 pink | 4 pink |
| Alesse or Levlite | Levonorgestrel 0.1 mg/ethinyl estradiol 20 µg | 5 pink | 5 pink |
| Ovrette | Norgestrel 0.075 mg | 20 yellow | 20 yellow |

**Table 32-8**
**Pharmacologic Methods of Emergency Contraception**

The earlier, the more effective.
Used with permission from Perlman SE, Nakajima ST, Hertweck PH: Emergency contraception. In Clinical Protocols in Pediatric and Adolescent Gynecology. London, Parthenon Publishing Group, 2004, pp 78–79.

---

**Table 32-9**
**Characteristics of Adolescents Likely to Use Condoms**

· Understand that condoms can prevent HIV/AIDS
· Carry condoms with them
· Not embarrassed to use condoms
· Worried about getting AIDS

## Assisting Adolescents in Choosing a Contraceptive

Health care practitioners should counsel and offer all these methods of contraception to their patients as part of their sexual counseling. From a developmental standpoint, younger adolescents tend to live for the moment, and methods of contraception that require planning and daily compliance may not be the first choice. Older adolescents have more decision-making skills and are more capable of higher level planning; therefore, daily contraception may be more appropriate. Certain medical conditions require specific types of contraceptives (Table 32-10). Despite high motivation and confidence in their ability to comply with medications, some patients, particularly postpartum adolescents, may not fully understand or possess the knowledge required for OCP use and may be better suited to longer acting contraceptives such as DMPA.[58,59]

## Enhancing Compliance and Continuation Rates in Adolescents

Adolescents may have difficulty in complying with contraception. Adolescent continuation rates for OCPs vary based on the population served. In free urban community and hospital-based clinics, rates of OCP use after 1 year range from 9% to 40%[60-62]; whereas in a suburban practice, OCP use after 1 year was 75%.[63] In addition to varying rates of continuation, various patterns of use that have also been described among adolescents include intermittent use of contraception, method switching, and periodic abstinence.[64]

To improve compliance and continuation rates, practitioners need to be aware of factors that are associated with incorrect or inconsistent use of contraception as well as factors that may inhibit or delay use of needed contraception (Table 32-11). It is equally important to remember that level of knowledge about how to use contraception effectively does not always correlate with consistent use.[58,65-70]

Adolescents have common difficulties in adhering with oral contraceptive compliance including not refilling OCP prescriptions, starting the next pill pack late, not using a back-up method when needed, and using pills sporadically. One study noted that up to one third of teens missed a pill in the previous 3 months of use.[71] All of this reinforces the need for simplified OCP instructions on when to start the pill, to take the pill at the same time every day, and to call with any questions. Contraceptive instruction and information should be reiterated and reinforced at frequent follow-up visits during the first year of contraceptive use until the patient matures enough to be compliant.

## DYSMENORRHEA AND ENDOMETRIOSIS

Pelvic pain and dysmenorrhea are common complaints in adolescents. The differential diagnosis can be quite challenging because of the multiple causes of acute and chronic pelvic pain in this age group (Tables 32-12 and 32-13). This section provides a

# Pediatric and Adolescent Gynecology

**Table 32-10**
**Contraceptive Options for Adolescent Women with Medical Conditions***

| Patient Disability | Contraceptive Options | Comment |
|---|---|---|
| Physical disability | Combination OC, progestin-only OC, DMPA, progestin implant, IUD | Small pill packages require dexterity<br>Partner or caregiver can assist<br>Combination OC is contraindicated in patients with immobility or impaired circulation |
| Mental disabilities and psychiatric illness | Combination OC, progestin-only OC, DMPA, implant, IUD | Long-acting progestins may be recommended to improve successful use<br>May be at increased risk for STDs |
| Epilepsy/seizure disorders | Combination OC, DMPA, IUD | Anticonvulsant therapy may increase catabolism in liver, prompting use of a higher dose combination OC |
| Systemic lupus erythematosus (SLE) | Progestin-only OC, DMPA, implant, IUD | Progestin-only OCs are not associated with increase in SLE flares |
| Chronic anticoagulation | Combination OC, progestin-only OC, DMPA, progestin implant, IUD | Use combination OCs only if underlying condition is not an absolute contraindication for estrogen use<br>Use caution with DMPA, progestin implant, and IUD owing to risk of bleeding |
| Hypercoagulable states associated with: Cardiovascular disease: history of venous or arterial thrombus; coagulopathies (activated protein C resistance, antithrombin III deficiency) | | |
| Anticoagulation | Combination OC, progestin-only OC, DMPA, implant, IUD | Use estrogen-containing OCs only if therapeutically anticoagulated<br>Give iron supplementation with IUD |
| Not anticoagulated | Progestin-only OC, DMPA, implant, IUD | Use of estrogen-containing method is contraindicated |
| Cardiovascular disorders: thrombophlebitis, thromboembolic disorders, coronary artery disease, myocardial infarction | Progestin-only OC, DMPA, implant, IUD | Estrogen promotes clotting and should not be used when patient is at increased risk for a thrombotic event |
| Dyslipidemia | Combination OC, progestin-only OC, DMPA, implant, IUD | In women with hypertriglyceridemia (TG ≤250 mg/dL), use less estrogen-dominant (lower estrogen dose or more androgenic progestin) combination OCs or other methods |
| Diabetes | Combination OC, progestin-only OC, DMPA, implant, IUD | Use low-dose combination OCs in normotensive, well-controlled diabetic women<br>Diabetic women using hormonal contraception should have periodic $HbA_{1c}$ glucose levels, annual fasting lipid profile |
| History of gestational diabetes | Combination OC, IUD<br>Progestin-only OC if not breastfeeding | Select low-estrogen dose OC with low dose of progestin<br>In breastfeeding women, do not use progestin-only OCs (associated with 3-fold increased risks of diabetes mellitus)<br>DMPA and implants are second-choice methods; if combination OCs are contraindicated and long-acting progestin is required for compliance, implant preferred over DMPA (owing to lack of carbohydrate metabolic effect)<br>Postpartum and annual diabetes testing<br>Achieve ideal body weight; encourage daily exercise |
| Human immunodeficiency virus (HIV) | Combination OC, progestin-only OC, DMPA, implant | Consistent and correct male condom use needed to prevent transmission of HIV<br>Combination OCs should not be used if migraine is with focal neurologic symptoms and there are other risk factors for stroke |

DMPA, depot medroxyprogesterone acetate; IUD, intrauterine device; OC, oral contraceptive.

*Barrier methods can be used by all women, but due to high failure rates, barrier methods are often not optimal for women with medical conditions. IUD use should only be by monogamous women with no risk of pelvic inflammatory disease.

Used with permission from Kjos SL: Contraceptive selection in women with medical conditions. Dialog Contracept 1999;5:1.

brief overview of the diagnosis and treatment of dysmenorrhea and endometriosis in adolescents; other causes of pain are covered in other chapters.

Dysmenorrhea is defined as painful menstruation. Primary dysmenorrhea is diagnosed in the absence of gross disease in the pelvic organs, while secondary dysmenorrhea is associated with a particular cause (e.g., endometriosis). An adolescent with dysmenorrhea, particularly lower abdominal pain that predates or begins at menarche, must be evaluated to rule out an outflow tract obstruction. In patients in whom a pelvic examination is not possible, a pelvic ultrasound is strongly advised. Although a

diagnosis of exclusion, primary dysmenorrhea is a treatable entity, with the treatment focus on preventing the release of prostaglandins prior to and during menses.

Nonsteroidal anti-inflammatory drugs (NSAIDs) and OCPs are the mainstay of treatment. NSAIDs such as ibuprofen, diclofenac, naproxen, mefenamic acid, and others have been well studied in the literature and provide adequate relief.[74] Cyclooxygenase (COX II) inhibitors such as rofecoxib, valdecoxib, and celecoxib have been shown to work as well as first-generation NSAIDs, but have not shown superiority; thus, they may be used as alternatives when first-generation

## Table 32-11
### Adolescent Factors Associated with Incorrect or Inconsistent, or Nonuse or Delay in Use of Contraception

**Incorrect or inconsistent**

Younger adolescents not involved in stable, long-term relationships
Youth involved in casual relationships
Adolescent subjected to involuntary sexual intercourse
Developmental factors
    Reluctance to acknowledge one's sexual activity
    Sense of invincibility
    Denial of possibility of pregnancy
Lack of education or misconception about appropriate contraceptive use
Those taking a virginity pledge
Those with older partners
Those who had a greater number of friends, who knew their first partner
Kissing and telling their partners they liked or loved them

**Nonuse or delay in use**

Lack of parental monitoring
Fear that parents will find out
Ambivalence
Perception that birth control is dangerous

## Table 32-12
### Causes of Acute Pelvic Pain in Adolescent Females

**Gynecologic causes**

Pregnancy complications (e.g., incomplete or threatened abortion, tubal pregnancy)
Infections (e.g., postabortal endometritis or acute pelvic inflammatory disease)
Ovarian cyst—rupture, torsion, or hemorrhage
Obstructive anomalies of the müllerian duct system (e.g., hematocolpos, complete transverse vaginal septum)

**Nongynecologic causes**

Gastrointestinal causes
    Acute appendicitis
    Volvulus
    Meckel's diverticulitis
    Intestinal obstruction
    Mesenteric adenitis
    Regional enteritis
    Ulcerative colitis
    Pancreatitis
Urinary tract causes
    Acute cystitis
    Acute pyelonephritis
    Ureteral calculus
Other causes
    Bone and joint infections of the sacrum, ileum, or hip
    Slipped femoral epiphysis
    Intra-abdominal abscess

Used with permission from Sanfilippo JS, Muram D, Dewhurst J, Lee PA (eds): Pediatric and Adolescent Gynecology, 2nd ed. Philadelphia, WB Saunders, 2001, Table 16-1, p 248.

## Table 32-13
### Causes of Recurrent Abdominal Pain in Adolescent Females

**Gynecologic causes**

Dysmenorrhea
Mittelschmerz
Pelvic inflammatory disease
Endometriosis
Müllerian obstructive anomalies
Ovarian cysts

**Nongynecologic causes**

Lactose malabsorption
Chronic constipation
Giardiasis
Crohn's disease
Irritable bowel syndrome
Unusual causes
    Meckel's diverticulum
    Midgut malrotation
    Schönlein-Henoch purpura
    Acute intermittent porphyria
    Uteropelvic junction obstruction
Abdominal wall trigger points
Psychogenic causes

Used with permission from Sanfilippo JS, Muram D, Dewhurst J, Lee PA (eds): Pediatric and Adolescent Gynecology, 2nd ed. Philadelphia, WB Saunders, 2001, Table 16-8, p 255.

# Pediatric and Adolescent Gynecology

NSAIDs fail.[73,74] The choice of formulation depends on the patient's characteristics as well as the side effect profile of each preparation. Once-a-day dosing with a COX II inhibitor may be preferable in certain patients not compliant with multiple dosing. The use of a scheduled dose prior to the initiation of menses (24 to 48 hours) may provide better relief by blocking prostaglandin substances already produced before the menstrual flow starts. Other options for treatment in patients who require contraception or for whom three cycles of NSAIDs have not provided relief may be the use of OCPs. The efficacy of this medication has been well documented and is an excellent choice for the sexually active adolescent.[75]

In cases where the combination of NSAIDs and OCPs for dysmenorrhea fails to relieve the pain, organic causes such as endometriosis should be strongly considered, and other diagnostic (i.e., laparoscopy) or therapeutic options (GnRH agonists) may be needed. Endometriosis is defined as the presence of endometrial glands and stroma outside the uterus. The prevalence in the adolescent population whom treatment with NSAIDs and OCPs fail has been reported as high as 70%.[76] Endometriosis was previously believed to affect only adult women but is increasingly being recognized in the adolescent population. In recent years, the increase in the use of laparoscopy as a diagnostic tool in adolescents has increased the awareness of this condition, and practitioners are more likely to include it in the differential diagnosis of pelvic pain.

Endometriosis in the adolescent differs from that of the adult in two ways: presentation and gross appearance. Whereas adults are diagnosed with endometriosis during a diagnostic evaluation for infertility, adolescents primarily present with pelvic pain in the form of acquired or progressive dysmenorrhea, acyclic pain, or dyspareunia. Interestingly, adolescents with endometriosis unresponsive to NSAIDs and OCPs most commonly have cyclic and acyclic pain (62.5%) as opposed to acyclic pain alone (28.1%) or cyclic pain alone (9.4%).[76] The gross appearance of adolescent endometriosis is more commonly clear or vesicular lesions (Fig. 32-31), sometimes referred to as "atypical" as opposed to the "classic" powderburn lesions seen in the adult.[77] Redwine has demonstrated that these atypical lesions occur at a mean age of 10 years earlier than the "black" lesions seen more commonly in adults.[78]

The treatment of endometriosis has always been controversial (Fig. 32-32). The use of laparoscopy for diagnosis and concomitant treatment by ablation or resection of implants if present has been suggested by many as the treatment of choice, followed by the use of continuous OCPs, progestins, NSAIDs, and/or GnRH agonists. Alternatively, the empiric use of a 3-month GnRH agonist as a diagnostic and therapeutic option in patients suspected of having endometriosis has proved beneficial in the adult population. In those patients who respond to the trial, endometriosis is present in up to 78%.[79] When these patients respond to this treatment, the long-term care is still difficult and not fully studied. The use of GnRH agonists for up to 1 year in the adult population, using "add-back" therapy with progestins, has been described without significantly affecting bone health.[80] Data regarding use of GnRH agonists in adolescents are not available. Owing to the lack of information and possible negative impact on bone mineral density in the adolescent, many reserve this option only for empiric use after age 18 and for cases of biopsy-proved endometriosis after age 16.[81] Other less adverse treatments may need to be considered for maintenance. Continuous OCPs combined with NSAIDs after treatment with GnRH agonists may be the treatment of choice, but in those patients with recurrence of pain despite these measures, laparoscopy may still be indicated. Other medications such as progestin-only pills and DMPA are alternatives when combination OCPs are contraindicated or unsuccessful in abating symptoms. Progestational agents commonly used include norethindrone acetate (15 µg daily by mouth), medroxyprogesterone acetate (30 to 50 mg daily by mouth), and DMPA (150 mg intramuscularly every 1 to 3 months). The use of progestins improves symptoms in 80% to 100% of patients with endometriosis.[81–83] Androgenic medications such as danazol, a 17α-ethinyltestosterone derivative, also have proven efficacy comparable to that of a variety of GnRH agonists, but dose-related side effects may limit their use in the adolescent patient population.[83]

Regardless of treatment used, supportive care is of the essence. Risk factors associated with worsening pelvic pain during their menses such as obesity, smoking, and alcohol consumption should be addressed and proper counseling given.[84] Behavioral therapy and support groups, transcutaneous electric nerve stimulation (TENS), and alternative medicine treatments, in the form of fish oils, may also be of benefit and may be offered to patients as supplements.[84,85]

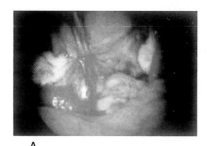
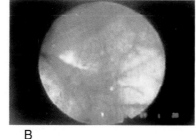
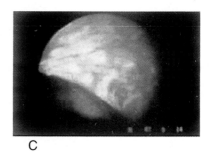

A          B          C

**Figure 32-31**    **ASRM Classification of endometriotic lesions.** *A*, Red. *B*, Clear. *C*, White. (Modified with permission from American Society for Reproductive Medicine: Revised American Society of Reproductive Medicine classification of endometriosis. 1996. Fertil Steril 1997;67:817.)

# Medical Management of Gynecologic Problems in the Pediatric and Adolescent Patient

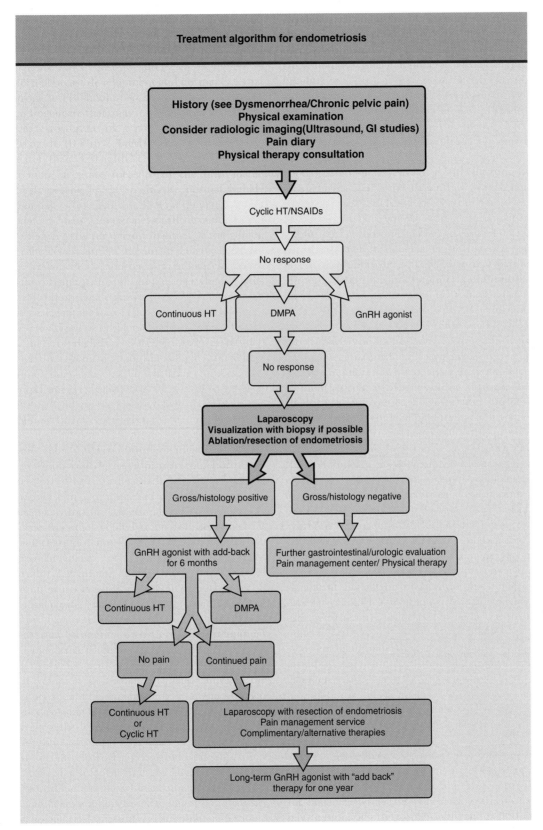

**Figure 32-32    Algorithm for endometriosis treatment.** Long-term GnRH agonist with add-back therapy for 1 year. Add-back, estrogen plus progestin or norethindrone acetate alone; DMPA, depot medroxyprogesterone acetate; GnRH, gonadotropin-releasing hormone; HT, hormonal therapy (oral contraceptive pills, estrogen/progestin contraceptive patch, estrogen/progestin contraceptive ring, norethindrone acetate); NSAIDs, nonsteroidal anti-inflammatory drugs. (From Laufer MR, Sanfilippo JS, Rose G: Adolescent endometriosis: diagnosis and treatment approaches. J Pediatr Adolesc Gynecol 2003;16[3 Suppl]:S3–S11. Copyright 2003. Reproduced by permission from the North American Society for Pediatric and Adolescent Gynecology.)

# REFERENCES

1. Emans SJ, Goldstein DP: The gynecologic examination of the prepubertal child with vulvovaginitis: use of the knee-chest position. Pediatrics 1980;65:758–760. **(IV, C)**
2. Pokorny SF, Stormer J: Atraumatic removal of secretions from the prepubertal vagina. Am J Obstet Gynecol 1987;156:581–582. **(IV, C)**
3. American College of Obstetricians and Gynecologists: ACOG Committee Opinion No. 292—Primary and preventive care: periodic assessments. Obstet Gynecol 2003;102:1117–1124. **(IV, C)**
4. Pierce AM, Hart CA: Vulvovaginitis: causes and management. Arch Dis Child 1992;67:509–512. **(IIb, B)**
5. Gerstner GJ, Grunberger W, Boschitsch E, Rotter M: Vaginal organisms in prepubertal children with and without vulvovaginitis: a vaginoscopy study. Arch Gynecol 1982;231:247–252. **(II, B)**
6. Cuadros J, Mazan A, Martinez R, et al: The aetiology of paediatric inflammatory vulvovaginitis. Eur J Pediatr 2004;163:105–107. **(IIb, B)**
7. Fischer G, Rogers M: Treatment of childhood vulvar lichen sclerosus with a potent topical corticosteroid. Pediatr Dermatol 1997;14:235–238. **(III, B)**
8. Berth-Jones J, Graham-Brown RA, Burns DA: Lichen sclerosus et atrophicus—a review of 15 cases in young girls. Clin Exp Dermatol 1991;16:14–17. **(III, B)**
9. Omar HA: Management of labial adhesions in prepubertal girls. J Pediatr Adolesc Gynecol 2000;13:183–185. **(IV, C)**
10. Nurzia MJ, Eickhorst KM, Ankem MK, Barone JG: The surgical treatment of labial adhesions in pre-pubertal girls. J Pediatr Adolesc Gynecol 2003;16:21–23. **(III, B)**
11. Bacon JL: Prepubertal labial adhesions: evaluation of a referral population. Am J Obstet Gynecol 2002;187:327–332. **(III, B)**
12. Emans SJ: Vulvovaginal problems in the prepubertal child. In Emans SJ, Laufer MR, Goldstein DP (eds): Pediatric and Adolescent Gynecology. Philadelphia, Lippincott-Raven, 1998, p 98. **(IV, C)**
13. Casale AJ, Austin PF: Urologic problems. In Sanfilippo JS, Muram D, Dewhurst J, Lee PA (eds): Pediatric and Adolescent Gynecology, 2nd ed. Philadelphia, WB Saunders, 2001, p 598. **(IV, C)**
14. Powell JL, Zwirek SJ, Sankey HZ: Hemangioma of the cervix managed with the Nd:YAG laser. Obstet Gynecol 1991;78:962–964. **(III, B)**
15. Andrassy RJ, Wiener ES, Raney RB, et al: Progress in the surgical management of vaginal rhabdomyosarcoma: a 25-year review from the Intergroup Rhabdomyosarcoma Study Group. J Pediatr Surg 1999; 34:731–734. **(I, A)**
16. Ibanez L, Potau N, Virdis R, et al: Post pubertal outcome in girls diagnosed of premature pubarche during childhood: increased frequency of functional ovarian hyperandrogenism. J Clin Endocrinol Metab 1993; 76:1599–1603. **(III, B)**
17. Emans SJ: Endocrine abnormalities associated with hirsutism. In Emans SJ, Laufler MR, Goldstein DP (eds): Pediatric and Adolescent Gynecology, 4th ed. Philadelphia, Lippincott Williams & Wilkins, 1998, p 281. **(IV, C)**
18. Azziz R, Zacur HA: 21-Hydroxylase deficiency in female hyperandrogenism: screening and diagnosis. J Clin Endocrinol Metab 1989; 69:577–584. **(IIa, B)**
19. Pang SY, Lerner AJ, Stoner E, et al: Late-onset adrenal steroid 3β-hydroxysteroid dehydrogenase deficiency. 1. A cause of hirsutism in pubertal and postpubertal women. J Clin Endocrinol Metab 1985; 60:428–439. **(IIb, B)**
20. Steingold KA, Judd HL, Nieberg RK, et al: Treatment of severe androgen excess due to ovarian hyperthecosis with a long-acting gonadotropin-releasing hormone antagonist. Am J Obstet Gynecol 1986; 154:1241–1248. **(III, B)**
21. Velazquez EM, Mendoza SG, Wang P, Glueck CJ: Metformin therapy in polycystic ovary syndrome reduced hyperinsulinemia, insulin resistance, hyperandrogenemia, and systolic blood pressure, while facilitating normal menses and pregnancy. Metabolism 1994;46:647–654. **(IIa, B)**
22. Glueck CJ, Wang P, Fontaine R, et al: Metformin to restore normal menses in oligo-amenorrhic teenage girls with polycystic ovary syndrome. J Adolesc Health 2001;29:160–169. **(III, B)**
23. Ibanez L, Ferrer A, Ong K, et al: Insulin sensitization early after menarche prevents progression from precocious pubarche to polycystic ovary syndrome. J Pediatr 2004;144:23–29. **(Ib, A)**
24. Ibanez L, Ong K, Ferrer A, et al: Low-dose flutamide-metformin therapy reverses insulin resistance and reduces fat mass in nonobese adolescents with ovarian hyperandrogenism. J Clin Endocrinol Metab 2003;88:2600–2606. **(IIb, B)**
25. Emans SJ, Grace E, Woods ER, et al: Treatment with dexamethasone of androgen excess in adolescent patients. J Pediatr 1988;112:821–826. **(III, B)**
26. Chapman MG, Dowsett M, Dewhurst CJ, Jeffcoate SL: Spironolactone in combination with an oral contraceptive: an alternative treatment for hirsutism. Br J Obstet Gynecol 1984;92:983–985. **(III, B)**
27. O'Brien RC, Cooper ME, Murray RM, et al: Comparison of sequential cyproterone acetate/estrogen versus spironolactone/oral contraceptive in the treatment of hirsutism. J Clin Endocrinol Metab 1991; 72:1008–1013. **(Ib, A)**
28. Lumachi F, Rondinone R: Use of cyproterone acetate, finasteride, and spironolactone to treat idiopathic hirsutism. Fertil Steril 2003; 79:942–946. **(Ib, A)**
29. Balfour JA, McClellan K: Topical eflornithine. Am J Clin Dermatol 2001;2:197–201. **(Ib, A)**
30. Guzick DS, Wing R, Smith D, et al: Endocrine consequences of weight loss in obese, hyperandrogenic, anovulatory women. Fertil Steril 1994; 61:598–604. **(Ia, A)**
31. Darroch JE, Singh S, Frost JJ: Differences in teenage pregnancy rates among five developed countries: the roles of sexual activity and contraceptive use. Fam Plann Perspect 2001;33:244–250. **(III, B)**
32. Smith CA: Factors associated with early sexual activity among urban adolescents. Soc Work 1997;42:334–346. **(III, B)**
33. Confidentiality in adolescent health care. In Health Care for Adolescents. American College of Obstetricians and Gynecologists, 2003. **(IV, C)**
34. Hewitt G, Cromer B: Update on Adolescent Contraception. Obstet Gynecol Clin North Am 2000;27:143–162. **(IV, C)**
35. Redmond GP, Olson WH, Lippman JS, et al: Norgestimate and ethinyl estradiol in the treatment of acne vulgaris: a randomized, placebo-controlled trial. Obstet Gynecol 1997;89:615–622. **(Ib, A)**
36. Leyden J, Shalita A, Hordinsky M, et al: Efficacy of a low-dose oral contraceptive containing 20 μg of ethinyl estradiol and 100 μg of levonorgestrel for the treatment of moderate acne: a randomized, placebo-controlled trial. J Am Acad Dermatol 2002;47:399–409. **(Ib, A)**
37. Anderson FD, Hait H: A multicenter, randomized study of an extended cycle oral contraceptive. Contraception 2003;68:89–96. **(Ib, A)**
38. Lara-Torre E, Schroeder B: Adolescent compliance and side effects with Quick Start initiation of oral contraceptive pills. Contraception 2002; 66:81–85. **(IIa, B)**
39. Archer DF, Bigrigg A, Smallwood GH, et al: Assessment of compliance with a weekly contraceptive patch (Ortho Evra/Evra) among North American women. Fertil Steril 2002;77:S27–S31. **(IIb, B)**
40. Novak A, de la Loge C, Abetz L, van der Meulen EA: The combined contraceptive vaginal ring, NuvaRing: an international study of user acceptability. Contraception 2003;67:187–194. **(IIb, B)**
41. Graham S, Fraser IS: The progestogen-only mini-pill. Contraception 1982;26:373–388. **(IV, C)**
42. Lara-Torre E, Edwards CP, Perlman SE, Hertweck SP: Bone mineral density in adolescent females using depot medroxyprogesterone acetate. J Pediatr Adolesc Gynecol 2004;17:17–21. **(Ib, A)**
43. Le J, Tsourounis C: Implanon: a critical review. Ann Pharmacother 2001;35:329–336. **(Ia, A)**
44. Yuzpe AA, Lancee WJ: Ethinylestradiol and dl-norgestrel as a postcoital contraceptive. Fertil Steril 1977;28:932–936. **(IIb, B)**
45. Task Force on Postovulatory Methods of Fertility Regulation: Randomized controlled trial of levenorgestrel versus the Yuzpe regimen

of combined oral contraceptives for emergency contraception. Lancet 1998;353:428–432. **(Ib, A)**

46. Piaggio G, von Hertzen H, Grimes DA, Van Look PF: Timing of emergency contraception with levonorgestrel or the Yuzpe regimen. Lancet 1999;353:721. **(Ib, A)**

47. Raine T, Harper C, Leon K, et al: Emergency contraception: advance provision in a young, high risk clinic population. Obstet Gynecol 2000; 96:1–7. **(IIa, B)**

48. Glaiser A, Baird D: The effects of self-administering emergency contraception. N Engl J Med 1998;339:1–4. **(Ib, A)**

49. Ellertson C, Ambardekar S, Hedley A, et al: Emergency contraception: randomised comparison of advance prescription and information only. Obstet Gynecol 2001;98:570–575. **(Ib, A)**

50. Jackson RA, Schwartz EB, Freedman L, et al: Advance supply of emergency contraception: effect on use and usual contraception—a randomized trial. Obstet Gynecol 2003;102:8–16. **(IIb, B)**

51. Belzer M, Uoshida E, Tejirian R, et al: Advanced supply of emergency contraception for adolescent mothers increased utilization without reducing condom or primary contraception use. J Adolesc Health 2003; 32:122–123. **(Ib, A)**

52. Blanchard K, Bungay J, Furedi A, et al: Evaluation of an emergency contraception advance provision service. Contraception 2003;67:343–348. **(III, B)**

53. Minnis AM, Shiboski SC, Padian NS: Barrier contraceptive method acceptability and choice are not reliable indicators of use. Sex Transm Dis 2003;30:556–561. **(IIb, B)**

54. Hingson RW, Strunin L, Berlin BM, Heeren T: Beliefs about AIDS, use of alcohol and drugs and unprotected sex among Massachusetts adolescents. Am J Public Health 1990;80:295–299. **(III, B)**

55. Stuart GS, Castano PM: Sexually transmitted infections and contraceptives: selective issues. Obstet Gynecol Clin North Am 2003; 30:795–808. **(IV, C)**

56. Grimes DA: Intrauterine device and upper-genital-tract infection. Lancet 2000;356:1013–1019. **(IV, C)**

57. Grimes DA, Schulz KF: Prophylactic antibiotics for intrauterine device insertion: a meta-analysis of the randomized controlled trials. Contraception 1999;60:57–63. **(Ia, A)**

58. Gilliam ML, Knight S, McCarthy M: Importance and knowledge of oral contraceptives in antepartum, low-income, African-American adolescents. J Pediatr Adolesc Gynecol 2003;16:355–360. **(III, B)**

59. Templeman CL, Cook V, Goldsmith LJ, Powell J, Hertweck SP: Postpartum contraceptive use among adolescent mothers. Obstet Gynecol 2000;95:770–776. **(IIb, B)**

60. Chacko MR, Kozinetz CA, Smith PB: Assessment of oral contraceptive pill continuation in young women. J Pediatr Adolesc Gynecol 1999; 12:143–148. **(III, B)**

61. Polaneczky M, Slap G, Forke C, et al: The use of levonorgestrel implants (Norplant) for contraception in adolescent mothers. N Engl J Med 1994;331:1201–1206. **(III, B)**

62. Berenson AB, Wiemann CM: Use of levonorgestrel implants versus oral contraceptives in adolescents: a case-control study. Am J Obstet Gynecol 1995;172:1128–1135. **(III, B)**

63. Woods ER, Grace E, Havens KK, et al: Contraceptive compliance with a levonorgestrel triphasic and a norethindrone monophasic oral contraceptive pill in adolescent patients. Am J Obstet Gynecol 1992; 166:901–907. **(IIa, B)**

64. Bearss N, Santelli JS, Papa P: A pilot program of contraceptive continuation in six school-based clinics. J Adolesc Health 1995;17:178. **(III, B)**

65. Diclemente R, Wingood G, Crosby R, et al: Parental monitoring: association with adolescents' risk behavior. Pediatrics 2001; 107:1363–1368. **(III, B)**

66. Brooks-Gunn J, Furstenburg FF: Adolescent sexual behavior. Am Psychol 1989;10:249–257. **(IV, C)**

67. Zabin LS, Stark HA, Emerson MR: Reasons for delay in contraceptive clinic utilization: adolescent clinic and nonclinic populations compared. J Adolesc Health 1991;12:225–232. **(IIb, B)**

68. Reddy DM, Fleming R, Swain C: Effect of mandatory parental notification on adolescent girls' use of sexual health services. JAMA 2002; 288:710–714. **(III, B)**

69. Manlove J, Ryan S, Franzetta K: Patterns of contraceptive use within teenagers' first sexual relationships. Perspect Sex Reprod Health 2003;35:246–255. **(III, B)**

70. Rock EM, Ireland M, Resnick MD: To know that we know what we know: perceived knowledge and adolescent sexual risk behavior. J Pediatr Adolesc Gynecol 2003;16:369–376. **(III, B)**

71. Emans SJ, Grace E, Woods ER, et al: Adolescents' compliance with the use of oral contraceptives. JAMA 1987;257:3377–3381. **(III, B)**

72. Zhang WY, Li Wan Po A: Efficacy of minor analgesics in primary dysmenorrhea: a systematic review. Br J Obstet Gynecol 1998; 105:780–789. **(Ia, A)**

73. Morrison BW, Daniels SE, Kotey P, et al: Rofecoxib, a specific cyclooxygenase-2 inhibitor, in primary dysmenorrhea: a randomized controlled trial. Obstet Gynecol 1999;94:504–508. **(Ib, A)**

74. Daniels SE, Talwalker S, Torri S: Valdecoxib, a cyclooxygenase-2-specific inhibitor, is effective in treating primary dysmenorrhea. Obstet Gynecol 2002;100:350–358. **(Ib, A)**

75. Robinson JC, Plichta S, Weisman CS, et al: Dysmenorrhea and use of oral contraceptives in adolescent women attending a family planning clinic. Am J Obstet Gynecol 1992;166:578–583. **(Ib, A)**

76. Laufer MR, Goitein L, Bush M, et al: Prevalence of endometriosis in adolescent women with chronic pelvic pain not responding to conventional therapy. J Pediatr Adolesc Gynecol 1997;10:199–202. **(IIb, B)**

77. Davis GD, Thillet E, Lindemann J: Clinical characteristics of adolescent endometriosis. J Adolesc Health 1993;14:362–368. **(III, B)**

78. Redwine DB: Age related evolution in color appearance of endometriosis. Fertil Steril 1987;48:1062–1063. **(III, B)**

79. Ling FW: Randomized controlled trial of depot leuprolide in patients with chronic pelvic pain and clinically suspected endometriosis. Pelvic Pain Study Group. Obstet Gynecol 1999;93:51–58. **(Ib, A)**

80. Surrey ES, Hornstein MD: Prolonged GnRH agonist and add-back therapy for symptomatic endometriosis: long-term follow-up. Obstet Gynecol 2002;99:709–719. **(IIb, B)**

81. Laufer MR, Sanfilippo J, Rose G: Adolescent endometriosis: diagnosis and treatment approaches. J Pediatr Adolesc Gynecol 2003;16(3 Suppl):S3–S11. **(IV, C)**

82. Vercellini P, De Giorgi O, Oldani S, et al: Depot medroxyprogesterone acetate versus an oral contraceptive combined with very low dose danazol for long-term treatment of pelvic pain associated with endometriosis. Am J Obstet Gynecol 1996;175:396–401. **(Ib, A)**

83. Harlow SD, Park M: A longitudinal study of risk factors for the occurrence, duration and severity of menstrual cramps in a cohort of college women. Br J Obstet Gynecol 1996;103:1134–1142. **(IIb, B)**

84. Dawood MY, Ramos J: Transcutaneous electrical nerve stimulation (TENS) for the treatment of primary dysmenorrhea: a randomized crossover comparison with placebo TENS and ibuprofen. Obstet Gynecol 1990;75:656–660. **(Ib, A)**

85. Harel Z, Biro FM, Kottenhahn RK, Rosenthal SL: Supplementation with omega-3 polyunsaturated fatty acids in the management of dysmenorrhea in adolescents. Am J Obstet Gynecol 1996;174:1335–1338. **(Ib, A)**

## KEY POINTS

- Proper evaluation and treatment of genital injuries is paramount to avoid significant long-term morbidity.
- Sexual assault should be considered in virtually all cases of genital injuries.
- Patients with severe genital injuries should be treated like trauma patients.
- A thorough evaluation must be performed to determine the extent of injury (i.e., involvement of bladder, bowel, abdominal cavity) in all patients.
- Surgical treatment should aim to restore both anatomy and function.
- Chronic pelvic pain should be evaluated via a multisystem approach, that is, gastrointestinal, genitourinary, gynecologic, musculoskeletal, and psychological/psychiatric.

## GENITAL INJURIES

Managing genital injuries in young girls can be a trying experience and one that causes much anxiety, but gynecologists should have the ability to evaluate and treat such injuries. These injuries induce so much anxiety for all involved because they present so many questions: "How will this impact her future fertility or her psychosexual development?" "How can we evaluate the injury without causing more trauma to the patient?" "Is this injury the result of an accident or sexual abuse?" Though most genital injuries do not result in an immediate threat to life, proper evaluation and treatment of genital injuries is paramount to avoid significant long-term morbidity.

It is difficult to assess the true incidence of genital injuries in the pediatric and adolescent population. This is secondary to a relative lack of data concerning the subject. The majority of publications written on the topic are anecdotal case reports or series drawn from skewed populations (e.g., suspected child abuse cases). Genital injuries in this population can be secondary to falls, straddle injuries, chemical or thermal burns, pelvic fractures, high-pressure liquid injection (e.g., ski douche injury), or penetration (sexual and nonsexual).[1] Though a significant portion of these injuries is secondary to sexual abuse, a more thorough discussion of this issue is beyond the scope of this chapter.

### Clinical Features

The clinical features associated with genital injuries are varied and depend on their cause and severity. Furthermore, the patient's age plays a role in the clinical presentation. Neonates and young toddlers have relatively high estrogen levels secondary to transplacental passage. The estrogen stimulates the vaginal and vulvar mucosa to thicken and become more elastic. This thickened, elastic mucosa is more resistant to bleeding when traumatized. As the child gets older, the estrogen level drops and the mucosa becomes more atrophic.[2] Owing to the rich blood supply of the external genitalia and the increased exposure of the underlying capillary beds, relatively minor injuries in this age group can lead to profuse bleeding.

The site of the injury can help classify genital injuries. A common type of genital injury is vulvar hematoma. Vulvar hematomas are usually the result of straddle injuries or blows to the area, such as falling on the crossbar of a bike or being kicked in the groin (Fig. 33-1). The force of the impact ruptures or tears blood vessels beneath the mucosa or skin, and the blood then dissects into the loose areolar tissue along the vaginal wall and along the fascial planes overlying the symphysis pubis and lower abdominal wall. In such accidents, the urethra, hymen, and inner vagina are usually spared injury because they are protected by the labia[1] (Fig. 33-2).

Vulvar hematomas can be of any size, with larger ones being greater than 15 cm in diameter and extending from the clitoris to the perineum. The size of the hematoma depends on the amount of subcutaneous bleeding. Patients usually come in with a round, tense, purple-red swelling in the vulvar region. These masses are quite painful, since they separate tissue planes as they expand. Very large hematomas exert pressure on the overlying skin and, if not treated promptly, can cause necrosis in this area leading to severe infections.[3]

Hematomas are usually the result of blunt trauma, whereas perineal and vulvar lacerations are secondary to sharp trauma or a penetrating injury. Most of these injuries involve only a limited portion of the perineum and vulva, but a thorough examination must be done to rule out injury to the bladder, urethra, upper vagina, or rectum. The location of simple lacerations is dependent on the child's position at the time of injury, the injuring object, and the force of the injury. The outer aspect of the labium majus is most often involved, and these injuries do not usually cause excessive blood loss.[3]

Vaginal injuries are usually due to penetrating trauma, and most are associated with some degree of vulvar injury. They often are the result of a fall onto sharp or pointed objects (Fig. 33-3). The penetration usually causes some degree of hymeneal tearing. The injury to the hymen, in general, does not cause much bleeding and does not require much treatment. The injury inside the vagina may be quite extensive owing to its thin, inelastic nature. An examination, usually under anesthesia, must be performed to rule out injury to other intrapelvic viscera. Many vaginal lacerations are superficial and involve only the mucosa

# Pediatric and Adolescent Gynecology

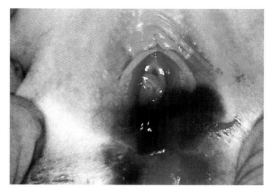

**Figure 33-1   Vulvar ecchymosis after a fall onto a bicycle crossbar.** (From Merritt DF, Rimza ME, Muram D: Genital injuries in the pediatric and adolescent female. In Sanfilippo JS, Muram D, Lee P, et al (eds): Adolescent Gynecology, 2nd ed. Philadelphia, WB Saunders, 2001. Used with permission from Diane F. Merritt, MD.)

and submucosa. These patients usually complain of very little pain, and bleeding may be minimal unless a major vessel was injured.[3,4]

When evaluating penetrating vaginal injuries, the physician must include sexual assault in the differential diagnosis. Injuries due to insertion of the penis often cause hymeneal tears between the 4 and 8 o'clock position and can also involve the posterior vaginal wall and perineum (Fig. 33-4). This is due to the posterior pressure exerted by the penis during penetration. If excessive, deep force is used, the tear can extend past the rectovaginal septum and into the rectum. Predisposing factors for vaginal injury during intercourse include first occurrence of penetration, congenital anomalies of the vagina, inebriation of either party, violence, and insertion of foreign objects.

Another type of vaginal injury is called a high-pressure insufflation injury. It is seen when the vagina is rapidly expanded, usually with water, and the distention results in tears to the vagina. These types of injuries are associated with falls from water skis or jet skis, sliding down water slides, and direct contact with spa jets.[1]

The most severe types of genital injury are those that involve other intrapelvic viscera (rectum or bladder) or entry into the

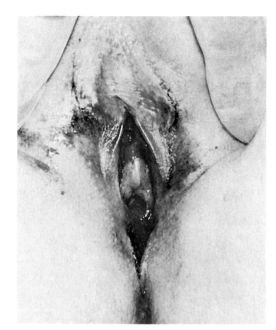

**Figure 33-3    This perineal laceration extended from the vagina into the rectum. It occurred when an 8-year-old girl slid down an incline onto a protruding nail.** (From Huffman JW, Dewhurst CJ, Capraro VJ: The Gynecology of Childhood and Adolescence. Philadelphia, WB Saunders, 1981.)

peritoneal cavity. This is often seen if the traumatizing force is excessive or if the penetrating object is longer than the length of the vagina. Once the peritoneal cavity is entered, there is the risk of evisceration through the site of trauma (Fig. 33-5). These patients are at high risk for peritonitis and hemorrhage. Depending on the amount of bleeding, these patients can quickly go into shock. This is usually seen when the injury extends above the pelvic floor and major blood vessels (i.e., the ovarian, uterine, iliacs) are lacerated. Once lacerated, these vessels retract into the abdominal cavity and cause massive hemorrhage into the retroperitoneal space.[5]

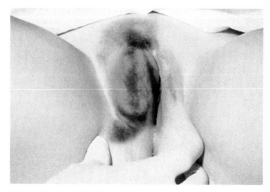

**Figure 33-2    Stable vulvar hematoma.** Hematomas of this size can be managed expectantly. (From Merritt DF, Rimza ME, Muram D: Genital injuries in the pediatric and adolescent female. In Sanfilippo JS, Muram D, Lee P, et al (eds): Adolescent Gynecology, 2nd ed. Philadelphia, WB Saunders, 2001. Used with permission from Diane F. Merritt, MD.)

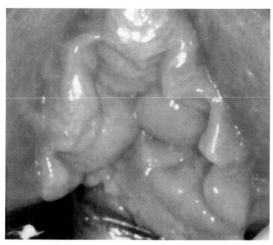

**Figure 33-4    Vaginal-hymenal tear at 8-o'clock secondary to sexual abuse.**

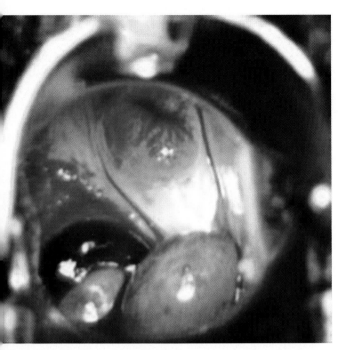

**Figure 33-5** **Evisceration of small bowel into the vagina after a penetrating injury of the posterior fornix.** (From Merritt DF, Rimza ME, Muram D: Genital injuries in the pediatric and adolescent female. In Sanfilippo JS, Muram D, Lee P, et al (eds): Adolescent Gynecology, 2nd ed. Philadelphia, WB Saunders, 2001. Used with permission from Diane F. Merritt, MD.)

Bowel injuries are usually of two types. The first is similar to fourth-degree obstetric tears. They extend from the vagina, through the rectal sphincter and rectovaginal septum, and into the rectum. These injuries can not only result from sharp trauma (e.g., falling onto an object), but also from blunt trauma. Blunt trauma, if forceful enough and directed posteriorly, can penetrate the relatively thin, weak rectovaginal septum into the rectum. The second type of bowel injury involves penetration of the abdominal cavity. After entering the abdomen, the penetrating object secondarily injures the bowel. In these types of injuries, the bowel can be directly injured or its mesentery injured. Direct injury to the bowel can result in spillage of contents into the abdominal cavity. This is a surgical emergency, and patients can present with peritoneal signs (rebound and guarding). If the mesentery is injured, clinical signs and symptoms can be delayed until the bowel becomes devitalized.

Urethral injuries are rarer in females than in males. This is secondary to the shorter length of the female urethra in comparison to the male urethra and its anatomic position. The female urethra is hidden behind the osseous pubic arch, and it is more mobile without significant attachment to the pubic bone. Injuries can occur as a result of pelvic fractures, with bone fragments from the ruptured pelvis causing urethral lacerations. They can also occur from blunt trauma or straddle injuries. With urethral stretching and bladder displacement, complete avulsion can occur. In the setting of a pelvic fracture, the clinician should have a high index of suspicion for a urethral injury. Clinical signs include blood at the introitus or meatus, hematuria, urethrorrhagia, inability to void in a conscious patient, or urine leakage through the vagina.[1,6]

Bladder injuries are relatively rare because of the position in the pelvis. The bladder is afforded protection by the bony pelvis. When the bladder is full though, it is more susceptible to injury because it now extends into the abdominal cavity. Bladder injuries can be classified as intra- and extraperitoneal injuries.

Intraperitoneal injuries involve rupture of the bladder into the abdominal cavity, with extravasation of urine into this space. This type of injury is seen most often with high-velocity trauma (e.g., motor vehicle accidents) with a full bladder, which results in rupture of the dome at its weakest point. Extraperitoneal injuries result in urine leakage limited to the perivesical and retroperitoneal space. This is almost always associated with pelvic fractures causing shearing forces or bony spicules to injure the bladder. Patients with these types of injuries complain of suprapubic or pelvic pain, dysuria, inability to void, or hematuria. On physical examination, blood can be seen at the urethral meatus, and patients may have a high, palpable intra-abdominal bladder.[1,5]

### Evaluation

When evaluating a child with genital injuries, the physician must take the clinical context into account. In a well-appearing child who just suffered a straddle injury on her bike, it is appropriate to obtain a history and build rapport with the patient prior to proceeding with the physical examination. On the other hand, a child who was involved in a motor vehicle accident and suffered a pelvic fracture requires prompt evaluation and/or intervention. Of paramount importance in all situations is ensuring the medical stability of the child.

Children with severe genital injuries are treated as trauma victims and are assessed as such. Their airway (A), breathing (B), and circulation (C) are assessed and addressed. Any child with bleeding must be evaluated immediately for hemodynamic stability. Once the patient has been deemed stable, a complete physical examination should be performed to ascertain the extent of injuries. The physician should be on the lookout for other, nongenital, injuries that may require attention.

In nonacute cases, the physician has a bit more time to evaluate the patient. As stated before, genital injuries are anxiety provoking for both the patient and her family. The physician should try to establish rapport with both prior to proceeding with the examination. The role of the history is to determine the cause of the injury and associated symptoms. These clues can often be used by the physician to guide the examination. The physician should be suspicious when the history and physical condition do not match, since this may be a sign of sexual abuse or assault.

Prior to the genital examination, the parents and patient should be informed of the nature and purpose of the examination. A decision then needs to be made as to the need for intravenous sedation or general anesthesia. Generally agreed upon indications for general anesthesia include extension of the injury through or above the hymen in a prepubertal child, vaginal lacerations that extend into the rectum or peritoneal cavity, unexplained vaginal bleeding, other injuries that require surgical management, and any obstacle to determining the full extent of the injury.[7] Physicians should have a low threshold of suspicion for examination under anesthesia because the morbidity associated with missed injuries is quite high, and serious injuries can often present without significant external findings.

# Pediatric and Adolescent Gynecology

When examining the pediatric patient with a genital injury, the physician must be aware of anatomic differences between children and adult patients. In the newborn, the labia minora, labia majora, and clitoris are all relatively large and prominent. As the child develops, their relative size decreases. Until puberty is reached, the vaginal wall is quite thin. At puberty, under the influence of estrogen and acid-forming bacteria (*Lactobacillus acidophilus*), the microenvironment of the vagina changes and the epithelium thickens. The internal reproductive organs also change as the patient develops. The uterus weighs only 14 to 17 g at puberty and grows to a final weight of 30 to 40 g in adulthood. The ovaries increase from 0.6 g (combined) in the infant to 5.0 g in the adult. The length of the vagina increases from 3 cm to over 8 cm. The central orifice of the hymen is about 0.4 cm in diameter at birth and enlarges to only about 0.5 cm in diameter at 5 years of age. The physician must keep these anatomic differences in mind and tailor the examination appropriately (e.g., using a nasal speculum to evaluate the vagina in a child with an intact hymen).[8]

Once the child has been made comfortable so that she may tolerate the examination, the physician should approach the examination in a systematic fashion. First, the physician should evaluate the external genitalia and vulva. All injured external structures should be thoroughly assessed and their extent determined. The physician should always have a high suspicion for involvement of other structures (bladder, rectum, etc.), and this possibility should always be investigated. Palpation can be used to determine the extent of hematomas, and an internal examination can help determine extension into spaces within the pelvis. If the physician cannot determine the extent of spread, imaging studies may be helpful. If the injury was caused by a penetrating object, the physician should request that the object be brought to the hospital. This allows the physician to determine if the traumatizing object has the potential length to penetrate above the pelvic floor. If the object has the potential to penetrate above the pelvic floor, a complete examination under anesthesia is likely warranted. If the object does not have projections, an external assessment is likely adequate.

Once the external genitalia have been investigated, the physician should evaluate the urinary and gastrointestinal (GI) systems before proceeding with the internal examination. Injuries to the external anal sphincter are rare without coincident injuries to the vulva and vagina. Tears of the sphincter usually are extensions from the vagina unless they are posterior in location. Digital palpation of the sphincter throughout its circumference and visual inspection of the capsule give a good assessment of the sphincter's integrity. Injuries that penetrate the rectovaginal septum can damage the rectum without violating the sphincter. These injuries can often be felt digitally, but in instances where the injury is more distal, proctoscopy may be necessary (Fig. 33-6).

An evaluation of the urethra and bladder is considered next if an injury to one of these organs is suspected. A urinalysis will often show hematuria with these injuries, but the sensitivity and specificity of hematuria for these injuries are poor. Therefore, if an injury is suspected, more accurate diagnostic tests are warranted. If an injury to the urethra is suspected, placement of a catheter prior to evaluation is inadvisable. This is because if a partial transection is present, traumatic catheterization may lead

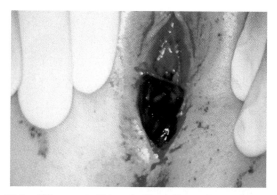

**Figure 33-6   This young girl impaled herself on a broom handle.** The point of entry was the perineum, with the exit wound being in the rectum. (From Merritt DF, Rimza ME, Muram D: Genital injuries in the pediatric and adolescent female. In Sanfilippo JS, Muram D, Lee P, et al (eds): Adolescent Gynecology, 2nd ed. Philadelphia, WB Saunders, 2001. Used with permission from Diane F. Merritt, MD.)

to a complete transection.[2] The evaluation for a urethral injury in female patients is more difficult than in male patients owing to the inability to perform accurate urethrography. A vaginal examination or vaginoscopy may be helpful in diagnosing a urethral injury if there is extension into the vagina or if there is a palpable hematoma, but urethroscopy remains the gold standard for the diagnosis of urethral injuries. After urethroscopy confirms an intact urethra, then a catheter can be placed.

Bladder injuries can be diagnosed with either computed tomography (CT) or conventional cystography, depending on the availability of the imaging modalities. With both, intraperitoneal bladder injuries show extravasation of contrast into the abdominal cavity with pooling of material around loops of bowel. Extraperitoneal bladder injuries, on the other hand, are associated with material contained within the pelvis, and the material can be best appreciated on postdrainage radiographs[5] (Fig. 33-7). If bladder and urethral injuries have been ruled out, the physician must assess whether the patient can void spontaneously prior to moving on to other parts of the examination. Often injuries to the vulva can cause spasms of the urethra or lead to obstructive swelling that can cause urinary retention. If this is the case, a Foley catheter should be placed until the condition resolves.

Examining the vagina is the next step in the evaluation and often the most difficult. Even with a patient under general anesthesia, the physician is often limited by the size of the introitus. In adolescents whose hymens are no longer intact, a speculum examination can be performed unhindered. It is in the pediatric population and in those whose hymen is intact that examination can be difficult. Nasal speculums are useful tools in younger girls but may not be long enough to expose the cervix and fornices in older girls. In these patients, special pediatric vaginal speculums can be used, or vaginoscopy may be required (Fig. 33-8). Whichever instrument is used, the physician must be sure that the entire vagina is inspected, especially the fornices. Often injuries to the vagina occur in the fornices and are hidden by redundant mucosa. A digital vaginal examination is performed only in those patients whose introitus allows such an examination. In some situations, a rectoabdominal examination may be substituted for a digital vaginal examination.

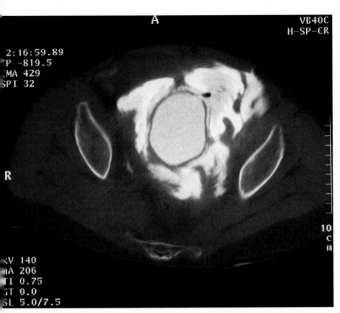

**Figure 33-7**   CT scan showing significant extraperitoneal bladder rupture after trauma. The dye is no longer contained by the bladder. (Brohi K: Classic cases: Lateral compression pelvic injury and extraperitoneal rupture of the bladder. Trauma.org, 2002(7:1). Available at http://www.trauma.org/cases/classic001.html. Accessed 5/19/05.)

Other portions of the evaluation must be tailored to the particular situation. Imaging modalities, such as ultrasonography or CT, may be utilized if the clinical picture dictates. An example would be the use of CT scanning to diagnose a retroperitoneal hematoma. If the peritoneal cavity is entered, laparotomy is indicated as part of the evaluation for intra-abdominal injuries. Some physicians have used laparoscopy instead of laparotomy in a limited number of cases. Though they have been successful, the procedure has not been evaluated thoroughly enough to be the standard of care.

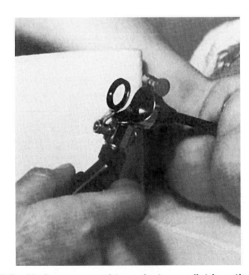

**Figure 33-8**   Vaginoscope used to evaluate a pediatric patient.

## Treatment

Many vulvar hematomas can be treated with expectant management, but some do require surgical intervention. Treatment is often determined by the size of the hematoma. Small hematomas (i.e., smaller than the size of an egg) can often be initially treated with pressure and an ice pack. The injured area should be observed in order to assess whether the hematoma is stable or expanding. In most small hematomas, the pressure created by the stretched vaginal mucosa will compress the bleeding vessel and limit its expansion.[4] Large or expanding hematomas must be opened to limit their expansion and prevent necrosis of the overlying skin (Fig. 33-9). An incision is made lateral to the vaginal orifice in the mucosa. Clot and devitalized tissue are removed, and an attempt to identify the bleeder is made. Absorbable mattress sutures can be placed to help control bleeding. If a specific bleeder is not identified, the hematoma cavity is packed with gauze and pressure is applied. The gauze is removed after 24 hours, at which point most bleeding has ceased. To close the defect created by the hematoma, placement of a suction drain may facilitate evacuation of transudates, exudates, and blood. While the drain is in place and the tissue healing, prophylactic antibiotics are given to prevent infection at the injury site. In all patients with hematomas, their ability to void should be assessed. Large hematomas may physically obstruct the urethra, and smaller hematomas may induce swelling in the region of the urethra leading to retention. If a patient experiences urinary retention, a Foley or suprapubic catheter should be placed until she is able to void spontaneously[1,3,7] (Fig. 33-10).

Treatment of vulvar and perineal lacerations begins with a thorough physical examination to rule out injury to adjacent

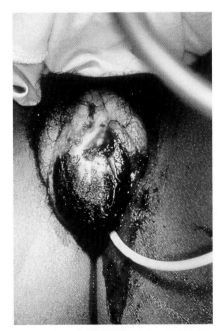

**Figure 33-9**   This large hematoma was not surgically drained, which led to necrosis of the overlying skin. (From Merritt DF, Rimza ME, Muram D: Genital injuries in the pediatric and adolescent female. In Sanfilippo JS, Muram D, Lee P, et al (eds): Adolescent Gynecology, 2nd ed. Philadelphia, WB Saunders, 2001. Used with permission from Diane F. Merritt, MD.)

# Pediatric and Adolescent Gynecology

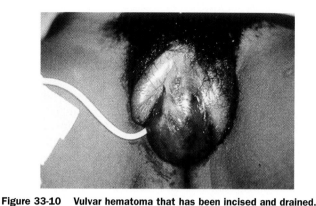

**Figure 33-10**  **Vulvar hematoma that has been incised and drained.**
Note incision, which has been closed with absorbable sutures, on medial
aspect of left labium. A urethral catherer is in place for bladder
decompression and closed suction drain exits the most dependent
aspect of the vulva. (From Merritt DF, Rimza ME, Muram D: Genital injuries
in the pediatric and adolescent female. In Sanfilippo JS, Muram D, Lee P,
et al (eds): Adolescent Gynecology, 2nd ed. Philadelphia, WB Saunders,
2001. Used with permission from Diane F. Merritt, MD.)

structures. If there is no evidence of any other injuries, the
wound site can be cleansed thoroughly and bleeding vessels
controlled. Deep injuries may require surgical repair, but the
surgeon should try to avoid sutures in the skin, especially those
not in the midline. Lateral sutures have a tendency to pull out
when placed under tension, which occurs when a young girl sits
and applies pressure to her perineum. Injuries to the lateral
walls of the vestibule heal quite well by secondary intention and
usually do not require surgical repair.[8]

As with other types of genital injuries, treatment of vaginal
injuries begins with evaluation of the patient for involvement
of the bladder, bowel, or other abdominopelvic viscera. Injuries
confined to the mucosa and submucosa can be treated with
absorbable sutures. The tissue is reapproximated and hemostasis
is obtained in a similar fashion to an obstetric repair. Care must
be taken to ensure that all bleeding points are controlled because
hematomas of the vaginal wall can occur if bleeding vessels are
not ligated prior to closing the mucosa.[4] Small fluid collections
can sometimes form in dead space within a repair. These collections can usually be drained in the office by releasing one or two
stitches. Once drained, the space should be left open to prevent
fluid reaccumulation. Prophylactic antibiotics are recommended
in repaired vaginal injuries.

Vaginal injuries that are superficial or inaccessible to surgical
repair can be treated with packing. The packing will apply
pressure to the site and stop bleeding. It is best if the gauze
is lubricated, especially with estrogen cream. Lubrication of the
gauze will make removal of the packing easier and inhibit
adherence of the gauze to the wound. Estrogen cream facilitates
healing of the mucosa and prevents the formation of granulation
tissue, which develops quite commonly on unestrogenized,
traumatized tissue. Estrogen cream can also be applied topically
to the vulva to aid in the healing of vaginal injuries.[2]

Treatment of injuries that involve abdominopelvic organs
usually requires surgical intervention. A vaginal or abdominal
approach is used depending on the severity and extent of the
injuries. After a thorough evaluation rules out extension of an

injury into the peritoneal cavity, a vaginal approach can be
attempted. This would include rectal injuries similar to fourth
degree obstetric tears and bladder injuries extending into the
vagina. The repair should reapproximate tissue in layers and have
as its objective the restoration of normal anatomy. A urologist or
colorectal surgeon should be consulted if necessary. Since strictures and scar tissue can have devastating long-term morbidity,
the physician should be vigilant for their formation. Vaginal
strictures can be released with the use of successively larger
dilators over a period of time. Severe cases may require surgical
intervention. If an injury results in a tear through the rectal
sphincter, stool softeners may be prescribed during the healing
period to reduce the effort required for bowel movements and
to decrease strain on the newly repaired tissue.

If there is any question about whether abdominal viscera are
involved from the injury, an abdominal approach is warranted.
A thorough assessment of the abdominal cavity should be performed in order to detect any concealed injuries. The bowel should
be run along its entire length to rule out any enterotomies, and
the mesentery of the small and large bowel should be evaluated
for any injury that may lead to devitalized tissue. Injured loops
of bowel can either be primarily repaired or resected, depending
on the extent of injury. The retroperitoneum should also be
explored, as an injury in this area can easily be hidden. An injury
to the vasculature can lead to a large hematoma, and the retroperitoneum is able to conceal a large quantity of blood. Common
vessels that are injured include the uterines, ovarians, and iliacs
(Figs. 33-11 and 33-12). If a hematoma is expanding or the patient
is becoming hemodynamically unstable, the retroperitoneum
should be entered and the bleeding vessel identified. Depending
on the vessel that is bleeding, it either can be ligated or require
repair by a vascular surgeon. Stable hematomas can be managed
expectantly, as the pressure from the hematoma will compress
and occlude the offending vessel.

Partial lacerations and contusions of the female urethra can
be effectively treated with prolonged catheterization. Larger
lacerations can be repaired by a layered closure over an indwelling
catheter. Because of the low incidence of complete urethral
avulsion or laceration, there has not been standardization of
treatment for these types of injury. Some surgeons favor a
staged approach, with initial urinary diversion through a suprapubic tube and subsequent reconstruction. Others favor immediate repair at the time of the injury. Ideally, to prevent the
long-term complications of strictures, incontinence, or fistulas,
these repairs should be undertaken with the help of a
urologist.[5,6]

Treatment of bladder injuries depends on the location (intra-
or extraperitoneal) and type of injury. All intraperitoneal bladder
ruptures require surgical exploration and direct repair through a
layered closure. Some surgeons recommend opening the bladder
in the midline to determine the size and location of all injuries.
Stent placement may be warranted to assess the position of
the ureteric orifices and the trigone prior to commencing with
the repair. Injuries are repaired in two layers and the bladder
decompressed for 2 weeks with either a Foley catheter or a
suprapubic tube. Drains (i.e., Jackson-Pratt) should also be left
in place near the area of repair. Prophylactic antibiotics are
recommended. Most extraperitoneal bladder ruptures can be
treated with Foley catheter drainage alone. Drainage should be

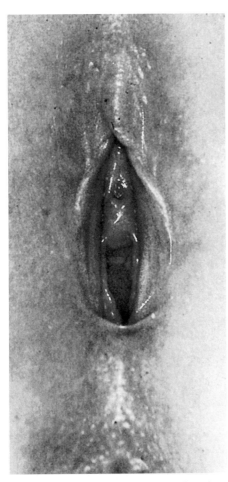

**Figure 33-11   A small tear in the hymen and vagina of a young girl.** This is the vulva of the patient depicted in Figure 33-12. This case illustrates the need for a high index of suspicion for intra-abdominal injuries in all patients with genital trauma, no matter how minor the trauma appears. (From Huffman JW, Dewhurst CJ, Capraro VJ: The Gynecology of Childhood and Adolescence. Philadelphia, WB Saunders, 1981.)

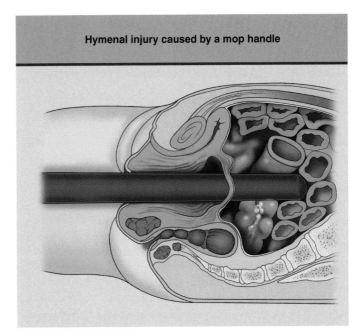

**Hymenal injury caused by a mop handle**

**Figure 33-12   Depiction of the injury sustained by the same patient as in Figure 33-11.** The mop handle impaled the girl through the pouch of Douglas and then ripped the peritoneum off the left common iliac vessels and tore 8 cm of mesentery away from a portion of the ileum.

for approximately 2 weeks, and the physician should be vigilant for blood clots that may obstruct the tube and worsen the rupture. If the patient's other wounds warrant laparotomy, then these injuries can be repaired at that time. Bladder injuries that are limited to the posterior wall and extend into the vagina can be closed transvaginally in two layers.

An important issue in the treatment of genital injuries is the prevention of such injuries. There is little literature concerning this topic, and prevention strategies are difficult to enforce as they may limit the normal active lifestyle of a child. Parents should be vigilant when buying toys with sharp points and avoid toys that may present a fall risk, such as sprinklers that encourage children to jump over them. Safety equipment should also be stressed. This includes wearing durable pants during jumping or climbing activities. Wet suits are recommended during water skiing to prevent the high-pressure insufflation injuries. Unfortunately, no matter what precautions are taken, genital injuries will occur; thus, it is important that clinicians be educated in the proper evaluation and treatment to reduce long-term morbidity.

## CHRONIC PELVIC PAIN IN ADOLESCENTS

The problem of chronic pelvic pain (CPP) often remains an enigma for clinicians dealing with this patient population. Defined as cyclic lower abdominal pain of at least 6 months' duration or noncyclic pain of 3 months' duration, either of which affects normal activities.[9] The International Association for the Study of Pain defines CPP as a "chronic or recurrent pelvic pain that has a gynecologic origin but for which no definitive lesion or etiology is identified." Four criteria are established that focus on the behavioral components related to CPP[10]:

1. Pain that is refractory to medical management
2. Significant impairment of physical function, including sexual function
3. Vegetative signs of depression
4. Patient's role within the family has changed secondary to the pain, or the family perceives the pain to be the "highest priority" problem

CPP is a common and serious problem with a prevalence of 14% to 16% of all women. In the adult it is a major indication for the hysterectomies performed annually in the United States. In the adolescent, the problem often proves to be burdensome to both patient and parent. It may be used as a way to gain attention.

The initial evaluation requires a detailed history and physical examination. At that time a multisystem approach encompassing evidence for a urinary tract, GI, musculoskeletal, gynecologic, or psychological etiology must be determined.

A general physical examination that includes a pelvic examination is recommended. Tenderness may be elicited in the cul

# Pediatric and Adolescent Gynecology

de sac, although this finding is far less common in the adolescent than in the adult. Determination of trigger points, straight-leg raising, and evaluation of gait are integral segments of the physical examination.

## Pathophysiology

### Cartesian and Gate Control Theories

One early theory of pain perception is that of the Cartesian model. In this model, stimulation of peripheral nerve pain fibers activates the pathway directly to the cerebral cortex with the end product being the perception of pain. Gate theory complements the Cartesian model and identifies transmission of nociceptive or discomfort signals reflecting innervation of several types of peripheral fibers, including C fibers, which are sensitive to heat, mechanical pressure, and chemical mediators of inflammation (Table 33-1). This association is predicated on bidirectional transmission of information from the periphery to the brain and from the brain to the spinal cord. Both motivational and affective states modulate the peripheral nociceptive signals. The modulation occurs via descending impulses, which release neuromodulators at the control transmission cells of the spinal cord.[11] The spinal cord acts as a "gate," regulating transmission of peripheral nociceptive signals to the brain by way of the spinothalamic pathways. According to the Gate theory, the longer the pain remains present, the less pertinent is the tissue damage that initially caused the release of neuromodulators.

### Operant Conditioning Model

Proposed by Fordyce, the operant conditioning model focuses on pain being based on communication between the patient and other individuals, either verbal or nonverbal. The communications are subject to reinforcement; that is, pain behaviors may be maintained by the responses elicited from others, such as attention, avoidance of undesirable activities, or financial compensation.[12]

### Cognitive Theories

Conscious thought processes or cognitions appear to be significant in influencing behavior and relationships as well as in modulating levels of pain. This theory expands the Gate theory. It provides a basis to understand the patient's thoughts as she experiences pain. Attributions regarding pain etiology as she perceives it, the meaning of it to her, all can heighten her perception of pain. Therapeutic interventions, from the psychological treatment perspective, may then be applied.

| Table 33-1 |
| --- |
| **Pain Neurotransmitters** |
| • Substance P |
| • Vasoactive intestinal peptide |
| • Somatostatin |
| • Cholecystokinin |
| • Prostaglandins |
| • Serotonin |

From Sanfilippo JS, Smith RP: Primary Care in Obstetrics & Gynecology: A Handbook for Clinicians. New York, Springer-Verlag, 1997, pp 107–111.

| Table 33-2 |
| --- |
| **Urologic Causes of Pelvic Pain** |
| **Acute causes** |
| Acute cystitis |
| Acute urethritis |
| Urethral diverticulum |
| Urolithiasis |
| Radiation cystitis |
| **Chronic causes** |
| Interstitial cystitis |
| Urethral syndrome |
| Urethral diverticulum |
| Urolithiasis |
| Radiation cystitis |
| Urethral caruncle |
| Neoplasm |
| Detrusor sphincter dyssynergia |

From Summitt RL Jr: Urogynecologic causes of pelvic pain. Obstet Gynecol Clin North Am 1993;20:688.

### Psychological Perspectives

There are "pain-prone personality" characteristics of individuals. Sexual abuse, including in one's childhood, may be one such factor. This as well as domestic violence must always be inquired about. Family or personal history of depression is important to determine. The latter may be the prime source, a predisposing factor, or a result of CPP. Alteration of endogenous opioid and serotonergic pathways is associated with the perception of pain. The pathways facilitate transmission of pain signals to the sensorium. Use of the Minnesota Multiphasic Personality Inventory (MMPI) allows determination of depression scales and personality assessment. Psychomimetric changes in these studies correlate with the severity and duration of the pain rather than severity per se.[13] Other problems include hypochondriasis, somatization, and somatic delusion.

### Urologic

Urethral syndrome, recurrent bacterial cystitis, and interstitial cystitis should be considered. See Table 33-2.

### Gastrointestinal

Constipation is a frequent problem in the adolescent with CPP. In part this may reflect dietary habits in this age group. In addition, the patient with changes in bowel habits, including constipation alternating with diarrhea, should be considered for irritable bowel disease. Clinical conditions such as Crohn's disease present in this age group. If there is a predominance of GI-related signs and symptoms the patient is best served by a GI consultation (Table 33-3). Extensive discussion of these entities is beyond the scope of this textbook.

### Musculoskeletal

Table 33-4 lists the musculoskeletal causes of pubic pain. The most common muscular problem responsible for pelvic pain is "pelvic floor tension myalgia."[14] It is associated with intermittent or constant contractions of the levator plate that are associated with intense pain.

## Surgical Problems in the Pediatric Patient

<table>
<tr><td colspan="1" align="center">

**Table 33-3**
**Gastrointestinal Causes of Pelvic Pain**

</td></tr>
</table>

**Irritable bowel syndrome**

Symptoms
  Crampy, colicky pain in lower abdomen
  Pain for hours or days
  Exacerbations: diet-related (high-fat diets), stress, anxiety, depression,
    menses
Treatment
  Reassurance, education, stress reduction
  Bulk-forming agents
  Anxiolytics
  Low-dose tricylic antidepressants
  Avoid anticholinergic agents

**Inflammatory bowel disease**

Crohn's disease
  Diagnosis
  Upper GI with small bowel follow-through
  Colonoscopy

**Ulcerative colitis**

Symptoms
  Acute pain
  Diarrhea
  Hematochezia
Diagnosis
  Sigmoidoscopy
  Rectal biopsy

**Diverticular disease**

Diverticulosis
Diverticulitis
Diagnosis
  Barium enema
  Colonoscopy

**Infectious enterocolitis**

**Intestinal neoplasms**

Carcinoma
  Colon and rectum
  Family history adenomatous polyps (frist-degree relatives)

**Appendicitis**

Hernia
Ischemic bowel disease
Intestinal endometriosis

From Sanfilippo JS, Smith RP: Primary Care in Obstetrics & Gynecology: A Handbook for Clinicians. New York, Springer-Verlag, 1997, pp 107–111.

---

Levator spasms are a "falling out" pressure sensation over the involved musculature. It is associated with dyspareunia and is primarily focused in the mid-vaginal area. The pain frequently radiates to the low back. Lying supine often relieves the pain and discomfort. On physical examination, tenderness to palpation and reoccurrence of the pain is associated with trigger point assessment.

Piriformis spasms are characterized by pain in the morning on arising. In addition, there is exacerbation when climbing stairs or driving a car. The physical findings include pain elicited with external rotation of the thigh. On palpation, tenderness is often noted over the involved musculature. This may manifest on pelvic examination.

Myofascial pain is focally located in the lower quadrants of the abdominal wall and reflects entrapment of the genito-femoral or ilioinguinal nerves. This problem is more commonly noted following a Pfannenstiel incision. Myofascial trigger points are elicited on abdominal palpation.[15] Fibromyalgia is associated with chronic fatigue, depression, and sleep disturbances.

### Gynecologic

Table 33-5 summarizes the gynecologic causes of pelvic pain.

#### Endometriosis

While theories of retrograde menstruation, totipotential müllerian rest cells, and hematogenous and lymphatic spread abound, the exact cause remains unknown. In the adolescent as well as in the adult, the exact incidence also remains unknown. Diagnosis is surgical and histopathologic. In adolescents with a history of CPP, studies have noted an incidence of 25% to 38% of endometriosis.[16-18]

In adolescents with persistent pelvic pain or dysmenorrhea despite medical therapy with oral contraceptives and non-steroidal anti-inflammatory drugs (NSAIDs), the prevalence of endometriosis may be as high as 70% to 73%.[19,20] The adolescent who is refractory to medical therapy, persists with CPP, and has had other possible etiologies ruled out is a candidate for operative laparoscopy. In one study evaluating adolescents with CPP, endometriosis was diagnosed in 25% of the 180 patients evaluated. Furthermore, ovarian cysts were noted in 7%, paraovarian cysts in 3%, pelvic inflammatory disease (PID) in 3%, and pelvic adhesions in 25%; notably, chronic PID–related findings were noted in 6%.[21] Of the adult patients presenting

---

<table>
<tr><td colspan="2" align="center">

**Table 33-4**
**Musculoskeletal Causes of Pelvic Pain**

</td></tr>
<tr><td>

**Musculoskeletal pain**

Identify trigger points
Referred pain
Poor posture

</td><td>

**Diagnostic assessment**

Physical therapy evaluation
History
Postural examination
Active and passive range of motion
Palpation examination
Muscle strength testing
Neurologic screening
Gait

</td></tr>
</table>

From Baker PK: Musculoskeletal origins of chronic pelvic pain. Obstet Gynecol Clin North Am 1993;20:719–742.

---

<table>
<tr><td align="center">

**Table 33-5**
**Gynecologic Causes of Pelvic Pain**

</td></tr>
<tr><td>

· Dyspareunia
· Atrophy
· Vulvar dystrophy
· Vulvovaginitis
· Vulvar vestibulitis
· Vulvodynia
· Urethritis
· Urethral syndrome
· Interstitial cystitis

</td></tr>
</table>

From Sanfilippo JS, Smith RP: Primary Care in Obstetrics & Gynecology: A Handbook for Clinicians. New York, Springer-Verlag, 1997, pp 107–111.

# Pediatric and Adolescent Gynecology

with pelvic pain in one other study, 70% were found to have endometriosis.[22] A study by Balasch and colleagues noted that 45% of patients with laparoscopy-proven endometriosis are asymptomatic.[23] Most clinicians agree that in the adolescent population biopsy of lesions believed to be endometriosis is recommended.

### Pelvic Adhesions

Pelvic adhesions can occur postoperatively or as a result of acute inflammatory processes, for example, acute PID or as a sequela to endometriosis. There is conflicting evidence about the relationship between pelvic adhesions and CPP as well as the benefits of adhesiolysis for symptom relief. A study of postappendectomy patients did not find a correlation between CPP and the presence of adhesions, whereas another study noted a higher rate of colon-to-colon as well as to side-wall adhesions in women with CPP compared with controls.[24,25] Of note, adhesions may be found in totally asymptomatic patients.[26] It is possible that a prerequisite for pelvic pain is that the adhesions restrict movement or distensibility of a pelvic or gastrointestinal organ. Little correlation exists between severity of pain and extent of adhesions.

The risks and benefits of adhesiolysis remain a point of discussion. A randomized clinical trial of adhesiolysis by laparotomy revealed no benefit in adhesiolysis when "light or moderate" pelvic adhesions were noted but benefit when there was lysis of severe adhesions.[27] Goldstein et al reported that 89% of adolescents with pelvic pain and documented adhesions had improvement in their symptoms following adhesiolysis.[28] One potential problem is that of re-formation of adhesions following lysis. Current surgical therapy continues to explore adhesion prevention agents for surgical intervention.

## Differential Diagnosis

The differential diagnosis is provided in Tables 33-1 to 33-5.

## History and Physical Examination

A pelvic pain assessment form (Fig. 33-13) is useful in evaluating patients with CPP.

## Treatment

Multidisciplinary pain centers are most helpful in management. These centers as a general rule do not set "cure" as a goal but rather establishment of a level of tolerance, at least at the beginning of therapy.

Management in large part is dependent on the underlying etiology. In the patient who is refractory to NSAIDs and suppressive therapy with oral contraceptives, operative laparoscopy is in order. At the time the diagnosis is established, ideally biopsy-proved, and appropriate ablative and/or excisional therapy applied. Controversy continues regarding the role of presacral neurectomy, which for the most part is reserved for patients with midline pelvic pain.

Other medical suppressive therapy may include use of gonadotropin-releasing hormone agonists. In essence a medical menopause is created with resultant ovarian suppression.

Adhesiolysis as treatment for established adhesions continues to be an area of controversy. The primary problem is recurrence of adhesions. One randomized study noted failure of significant improvement in pain symptoms following lysis of adhesions in comparison with a control group that did not undergo adhesiolysis. Only a subgroup of 15 patients with stage IV adhesions (criteria of Kapur) had symptomatic improvement.[29,30]

Irritable bowel syndrome (IBS) is best treated by elimination of dietary lactose, sorbitol, and fructose. Lactose intolerance can mimic IBS. On the other hand, 40% of patients with IBS also have lactose intolerance. Sorbitol is a common sweetener in "sugar-free" foods. Fructose is present in many processed foods. Caffeinated products and carbonated drinks also contribute to IBS-related discomfort.

Interstitial cystitis is a chronic inflammatory condition of the bladder and responsible for a segment of patients with CPP. It is best diagnosed with cystoscopy. The altered bladder permeability secondary to defective glycosaminoglycan mucous layer deficiency is responsible for the discomfort. The presence of Hunner's ulcers on cystoscopy and increased sensitivity on potassium intravesical instillation provide the basis for the diagnosis. Treatment remains controversial and includes bladder instillation of dimethylsulfoxide (DMSO), intravesical capsaicin, and placement of Calmette-Guérin bacillus into the bladder. Other treatment includes use of sodium pentosan polysulfate as well as cyclosporine and antihistamines such as hydroxyzine. Treatment focuses on the primary underlying etiology of CPP; for example, progestins including depot preparations can be administered when the cause is believed to be gynecologic.

## A — Pelvic Pain Assessment Form (Page 1)

**THE INTERNATIONAL PELVIC PAIN SOCIETY**
*Professionals engaged in pain management for women*

### Pelvic Pain Assessment Form

Physician: _____

*Initial History and Physical Exam*                     Date: _____

**Contact Information**
Name: _____   Birth Date: _____   Chart Number: _____
Phone: Work: _____   Home: _____
Is there an alternate contact if we cannot reach you? _____
Alternate contact phone number: _____

**Information About Your Pain**
Please describe your pain problem: _____
What do you think is causing your pain? _____
What does your family think is causing your pain? _____
Do you think anyone is to blame for your pain? ❑ Yes  ❑ No  If so, who? _____
Do you think surgery will be necessary? ❑ Yes  ❑ No
Is there an event that you associate with the onset of pain? ❑ Yes  ❑ No  If so, what? _____
How long have you had this pain? ❑ < 6 months  ❑ 6 months - 1 year  ❑ 1 - 2 years  ❑ > 2 years

*For each of the symptoms listed below, please "bubble in" your level of pain over the last month using a 10-point scale:*
0 – no pain        10 – the worst pain imaginable

| | 0 | 1 | 2 | 3 | 4 | 5 | 6 | 7 | 8 | 9 | 10 |
|---|---|---|---|---|---|---|---|---|---|---|---|
| How would you rate your present pain? | O | O | O | O | O | O | O | O | O | O | O |
| Pain at ovulation (mid-cycle) | O | O | O | O | O | O | O | O | O | O | O |
| Pain level just before period | O | O | O | O | O | O | O | O | O | O | O |
| Pain (not cramps) with period | O | O | O | O | O | O | O | O | O | O | O |
| Deep pain with intercourse | O | O | O | O | O | O | O | O | O | O | O |
| Pain in groin when lifting | O | O | O | O | O | O | O | O | O | O | O |
| Pelvic pain lasting hours or days after intercourse | O | O | O | O | O | O | O | O | O | O | O |
| Pain when bladder is full | O | O | O | O | O | O | O | O | O | O | O |
| Muscle/joint pain | O | O | O | O | O | O | O | O | O | O | O |
| Ovarian pain | O | O | O | O | O | O | O | O | O | O | O |
| Level of cramps with period | O | O | O | O | O | O | O | O | O | O | O |
| Pain after period is over | O | O | O | O | O | O | O | O | O | O | O |
| Burning vaginal pain with sex | O | O | O | O | O | O | O | O | O | O | O |
| Pain with urination | O | O | O | O | O | O | O | O | O | O | O |
| Backache | O | O | O | O | O | O | O | O | O | O | O |
| Migraine headache | O | O | O | O | O | O | O | O | O | O | O |
| What would be an acceptable level of pain? | O | O | O | O | O | O | O | O | O | O | O |

What is the worst type of pain that you have ever experienced?
❑ Kidney stone  ❑ Bowel obstruction  ❑ Migraine headache
❑ Labor & delivery  ❑ Current pelvic pain  ❑ Backache
❑ Broken bone  ❑ Surgery
❑ Other _____

(205) 877-2950        www.pelvicpain.org        (800) 624-9676 (if in the U.S.)

**A**

## B — Pelvic Pain Assessment Form (Page 2)

**Demographic Information**
Are you (check all that apply):
❑ Married  ❑ Widowed  ❑ Separated  ❑ Committed Relationship
❑ Single  ❑ Remarried  ❑ Divorced
Who do you live with? _____

Education:  ❑ Less than 12 years  ❑ High School graduate
❑ Bachelor's degree  ❑ Postgraduate degree

What kind of work are you trained for? _____
What type of work are you doing? _____

**Health Habits**
Do you get regular exercise? ❑ Yes  ❑ No        Type: _____
What is your diet like? _____
What is your caffeine intake (number per day, include coffee, tea, soft drinks, etc.)? ❑ 0  ❑ 1-3  ❑ 4-6  ❑ >6

How many cigarettes do you smoke per day? _____   How many years? _____
Have you ever felt the need to cut down on your drinking? ❑ Yes  ❑ No
Have you ever felt annoyed by criticism of your drinking? ❑ Yes  ❑ No
Have you ever felt guilty about your drinking, or about something you said or did while you were drinking? ❑ Yes  ❑ No
Have you ever taken a morning "eye-opener" drink? ❑ Yes  ❑ No

What is your use of recreational drugs? ❑ Never used  ❑ Used in past, but not now  ❑ Presently using  ❑ Choose not to answer
❑ Heroin  ❑ Amphetamines  ❑ Marijuana
❑ Barbiturates  ❑ Cocaine  ❑ Other
Have you ever received treatment for substance abuse? ❑ Yes  ❑ No

**Coping Mechanisms**
Who are the people you talk to concerning your pain, or during stressful times?
❑ Spouse/Partner  ❑ Relative  ❑ Support Group  ❑ Clergy
❑ Friend  ❑ Doctor/Nurse  ❑ Mental Health Professional  ❑ I take care of myself

How does your partner deal with your pain?
❑ Doesn't notice when I'm in pain  ❑ Takes care of me  ❑ Not applicable
❑ Withdraws  ❑ Feels helpless
❑ Distracts me with activities  ❑ Gets angry

What helps your pain?
❑ Meditation  ❑ Relaxation  ❑ Lying down  ❑ Music
❑ Massage  ❑ Ice  ❑ Heating pad  ❑ Hot bath
❑ Pain medication  ❑ Laxatives/enema  ❑ Injection  ❑ TENS unit
❑ Bowel movement  ❑ Emptying bladder  ❑ Nothing
❑ Other

What makes your pain worse?
❑ Intercourse  ❑ Orgasm  ❑ Stress  ❑ Full meal
❑ Bowel movement  ❑ Full bladder  ❑ Urination  ❑ Standing
❑ Walking  ❑ Exercise  ❑ Time of day  ❑ Weather
❑ Contact with clothing  ❑ Coughing/sneezing  ❑ Not related to anything
❑ Other

Of all of the problems or stresses in your life, how does your pain compare in importance?
❑ The most important problem  ❑ Just one of several/many problems

**B**

## C — Pelvic Pain Assessment Form (Page 3)

**Menses**
How old were you when your menses started? _____
Are you still having menstrual periods? ❑ Yes  ❑ No

**Answer the following only if you are still having menstrual periods:**
Periods are: ❑ Light  ❑ Moderate  ❑ Heavy  ❑ Bleed through protection
How many days between your periods? _____
How many days of menstrual flow? _____
Date of last menses: _____
Do you have any pain with your periods? ❑ Yes  ❑ No
Does pain start the day flow starts? ❑ Yes  ❑ No
Starts _____ days before flow starts: ❑ Yes  ❑ No
Are periods regular? ❑ Yes  ❑ No
Do you pass any clots in menstrual flow? ❑ Yes  ❑ No

**Bladder**
Do you experience any of the following:
Loss of urine when coughing, sneezing, or laughing? ❑ Yes  ❑ No
Frequent urination? ❑ Yes  ❑ No
Need to urinate with little warning? ❑ Yes  ❑ No
Difficulty passing urine? ❑ Yes  ❑ No
Frequent bladder infections? ❑ Yes  ❑ No
Frequency of nighttime urination: ❑ 0-1  ❑ 2 or more  Volume: ❑ Small  ❑ Medium  ❑ Large
Frequency of daytime urination: ❑ 8 or less  ❑ 9-15  ❑ >16  Volume: ❑ Small  ❑ Medium  ❑ Large
Do you still feel full after urination? ❑ Yes  ❑ No

**Bowel**
Is there discomfort or pain associated with a change in the consistency of the stool (i.e., softer or harder)? ❑ Yes  ❑ No
Would you say that at least one-fourth (_) of the occasions or days in the last 3 months you have had any of the following (Check all that apply)
❑ Fewer than three bowel movements a week (0–2 bowel movements)
❑ More than three bowel movements a day (4 or more bowel movements)
❑ Hard or lumpy stools
❑ Loose or watery stools
❑ Straining during a bowel movement
❑ Urgency – having to rush to the bathroom for a bowel movement
❑ Feeling of incomplete emptying after a bowel movement
❑ Passing mucus (white material) during a bowel movement
❑ Abdominal fullness, bloating, or swelling
The Functional Gastrointestinal Disorders, Drossman, et al. Chapter 4, "Functional Bowel Disorders and Functional Abdominal Pain". 1994.

**Gastrointestinal/Eating**
Do you have nausea? ❑ No  ❑ With pain  ❑ Taking medications
❑ With eating  ❑ Other
Do you have vomiting? ❑ No  ❑ With pain  ❑ Taking medications
❑ With eating  ❑ Other

Have you ever had an eating disorder such as anorexia or bulimia? ❑ Yes  ❑ No

**C**

## D — Pelvic Pain Assessment Form (Page 4)

**Short-Form McGill**
The words below describe average pain. Place a check mark (✓) in the column which represents the degree to which you feel that type of pain. Please limit yourself to a description of the pain in your pelvic area only.

What does your pain feel like?

| Type | None (0) | Mild (1) | Moderate (2) | Severe (3) |
|---|---|---|---|---|
| Throbbing | | | | |
| Shooting | | | | |
| Stabbing | | | | |
| Sharp | | | | |
| Cramping | | | | |
| Gnawing | | | | |
| Hot-Burning | | | | |
| Aching | | | | |
| Heavy | | | | |
| Tender | | | | |
| Splitting | | | | |
| Tiring-Exhausting | | | | |
| Sickening | | | | |
| Fearful | | | | |
| Punishing-Cruel | | | | |

*Melzack, R: The Short-Form McGill Pain Questionnaire, Pain 30:191–197, 1987.*

Which statement(s) below best describes how you cope with the pain? Check all that apply
❑ I count numbers in my head or run a song through my mind  ❑ I tell myself to be brave and carry on despite the pain
❑ I just think of it as some other sensation, such as numbness  ❑ I tell myself that it really doesn't hurt
❑ I pray to God it won't last long  ❑ I worry all the time about whether it will end
❑ I do something active, like household chores or projects  ❑ I take pain medication
❑ I ignore it as best I can  ❑ Other

**SF-36**
In general, would you say your health is:  ○ Excellent  ○ Very Good  ○ Good  ○ Fair  ○ Poor

Compared to one year ago, how would you rate your health in general now?
○ Much better now than one year ago  ○ Somewhat worse now than one year ago
○ Somewhat better now than one year ago  ○ Much worse now than one year ago
○ About the same as one year ago

The following items are about activities you might do during a typical day. Does your health now limit you in these activities? If so, how much?

| | Yes, limited a lot | Yes, limited a little | No, Not limited at all |
|---|---|---|---|
| Vigorous activities, such as running, lifting heavy object, participating in strenuous sports | | | |
| Moderate activities, such as moving a table, pushing a vacuum cleaner, bowling, or playing golf | | | |
| Lifting or carrying groceries | | | |
| Climbing several flights of stairs | | | |
| Climbing one flight of stairs | | | |
| Bending, kneeling, or stooping | | | |
| Walking more than a mile | | | |
| Walking several blocks | | | |
| Walking one block | | | |
| Bathing or dressing yourself | | | |

**D**

**Figure 33-13** *A–D,* Pelvic pain assessment form.        *Continued*

During the *past 4 weeks*, have you had any of the following problems with your work or other regular daily activities *because of your physical health*?

Cut down the amount of time you spent on your work or other activities ○ Yes ○ No
Accomplish less than you would like ○ Yes ○ No
Were limited in the kind of work or other activities ○ Yes ○ No
Had difficulty performing the work or other activities (for example, it took extra effort) ○ Yes ○ No

During the *past 4 weeks*, have you had any of the following problems with your work or other regular daily activities *because of any emotional problems* (such as feeling depressed or anxious)?

Cut down the amount of time you spent on your work or other activities ○ Yes ○ No
Accomplished less than you would like ○ Yes ○ No
Didn't do work or other activities as carefully as usual ○ Yes ○ No

During the *past 4 weeks*, to what extent has your physical health or emotional problems interfered with your normal social activities with family, friend, neighbors, or groups?
○ Not at all ○ Slightly ○ Moderately ○ Quite a bit ○ Extremely

How much bodily pain have you had during the past 4 weeks?
○ None ○ Very mild ○ Mild ○ Moderate ○ Severe ○ Very severe

During the 4 weeks, how much did pain interfere with your normal work (including both work outside the home and housework)?
○ Not at all ○ A little bit ○ Moderately ○ Quite a bit ○ Extremely

These questions are about how you feel and how things have been with you *during the past 4 weeks*. For each question, please give the one answer that comes closest to the way you have been feeling. How much of the time during *the past 4 weeks*:

| | All of the time | Most of the time | A good bit of the time | Some of the time | A little of the time | None of the time |
|---|---|---|---|---|---|---|
| Did you feel full of pep? | | | | | | |
| Have you been a very nervous person? | | | | | | |
| Have you felt so down in the dumps that nothing could cheer you up? | | | | | | |
| Have you felt calm and peaceful? | | | | | | |
| Did you have a lot of energy? | | | | | | |
| Have you felt downhearted and blue? | | | | | | |
| Did you feel worn out? | | | | | | |
| Have you been a happy person? | | | | | | |
| Did you feel tired? | | | | | | |

During the *past 4 weeks*, how much of the time has your *physical health or emotional problems* interfered with your social activities (like visiting with friends, relatives, etc.?
○ All of the time ○ Most of the time ○ Some of the time ○ A little of the time ○ None of the time

How TRUE or FALSE is each of the following statements for you?

| | Definitely True | Mostly True | Don't Know | Mostly False | Definitely False |
|---|---|---|---|---|---|
| I seem to get sick a little easier than other people | | | | | |
| I am as healthy as anybody I know | | | | | |
| I expect my health to get worse | | | | | |
| My health is excellent | | | | | |

E

---

*Personal History*

What would you like to tell us about your pain that we have not asked? Comments: _____
_____

What types of treatments have you tried in the past for this pain?    ❑ Acupuncture ❑ Homeopathic medicine ❑ Physical therapy
❑ Anesthesiologist          ❑ Lupron, Zoladex, Synarel    ❑ Psychotherapy
❑ Anti-seizure medications  ❑ Massage                     ❑ Rheumatologist
❑ Antidepressants           ❑ Meditation                  ❑ Skin magnets
❑ Biofeedback               ❑ Narcotics                   ❑ Surgery
❑ Birth control pills       ❑ Naturopathic medications    ❑ TENS unit
❑ Danazol (Danocrine)       ❑ Nerve blocks                ❑ Trigger point injections
❑ Depo-Provera              ❑ Neurosurgeon                ❑ Other _____
❑ Family Practitioner       ❑ Nonprescription medicine
❑ Herbal medication         ❑ Nutrition/diet

What physicians or health care providers have evaluated or treated you for chronic pelvic pain? Include all healthcare professionals, whether they were physicians or not. Do you have any objections to me contacting these healthcare providers? ❑ Yes ❑ No

| Physician/Provider | City, State |
|---|---|
| | |
| | |
| | |
| | |

Who is your primary care physician? _____

Please list all surgical procedures you've had (*related to this pain*):

| Year | Procedure | Surgeon |
|---|---|---|
| | | |
| | | |
| | | |

Please list all other surgical procedures:

| Year | Procedure | Year | Procedure |
|---|---|---|---|
| | | | |
| | | | |

Please list pain medications you've taken for your pain condition in the past 6 months, and the physicians who prescribed them (use separate page if necessary):

| Medication | Physician | Did it help? |
|---|---|---|
| | | ❑ Yes ❑ No |
| | | ❑ Yes ❑ No |
| | | ❑ Yes ❑ No |
| | | ❑ Yes ❑ No |
| | | ❑ Yes ❑ No |
| | | ❑ Yes ❑ No |
| | | ❑ Yes ❑ No |
| | ❑ I have written more medications on a separate page | |

F

---

Have you ever been hospitalized for anything besides surgery or childbirth? ❑ Yes ❑ No    If yes, explain: _____

Have you had major accidents such as falls or back injury? ❑ Yes ❑ No

Have you ever been treated for depression? ❑ Yes ❑ No  Treatments: ❑ Medication ❑ Hospitalization ❑ Psychotherapy

Birth control method:  ❑ Nothing    ❑ Pill      ❑ Vasectomy   ❑ Hysterectomy
                       ❑ IUD        ❑ Rhythm    ❑ Diaphragm   ❑ Tubal Ligation
                       ❑ Condom     ❑ Other: _____
Is future fertility desired? ❑ Yes ❑ No

How many pregnancies have you had? _____
Resulting in (#): _____ Full 9 month _____ Premature _____ Abortions (miscarriage) _____ # living children
Any complications during pregnancy, labor, delivery, or post partum period?
❑ 4° Episiotomy        ❑ C-section     ❑ Post-partum hemorrhaging
❑ Vaginal lacerations  ❑ Forceps       ❑ Medication for bleeding
❑ Other: _____

Has anyone in your family ever had:  ❑ Fibromyalgia           ❑ Chronic pelvic pain    ❑ Scleroderma
                                     ❑ Endometriosis          ❑ Lupus                  ❑ Interstitial cystitis
                                     ❑ Cancer                 ❑ Depression             ❑ Irritable Bowel Syndrome
                                     ❑ Recurrent Urinary Tract Infections

Place an "X" at the point of your most intense pain.
Shade in all other painful areas.

G

---

*Sexual and Physical Abuse History*
Have you ever been the victim of emotional abuse? This can include being humiliated or insulted.  ❑ Yes  ❑ No  ❑ No answer

| | | As a child (13 and younger) | | As an adult (14 and over) | |
|---|---|---|---|---|---|
| | Circle an answer for *both* as a child and as an adult. | | | | |
| 1a. | Has anyone ever exposed the sex organs of their body to you when you did not want it? | Yes | No | Yes | No |
| 1b. | Has anyone ever threatened to have sex with you when you did not want it? | Yes | No | Yes | No |
| 1c. | Has anyone ever touched the sex organs of your body when you did not want this? | Yes | No | Yes | No |
| 1d. | Has anyone ever made you touch the sex organs of their body when you did not want this? | Yes | No | Yes | No |
| 1e. | Has anyone ever forced you to have sex when you did not want this? | Yes | No | Yes | No |
| 1f. | Have you had any other unwanted sexual experiences not mentioned above? If yes, please specify: | Yes | No | Yes | No |
| 2 | When you were a child (13 or younger), did an older person do the following: | | | | |
| a. | Hit, kick, or beat you? | Never | Seldom | Occasionally | Often |
| b. | Seriously threaten your life? | Never | Seldom | Occasionally | Often |
| 3 | Now that you are an adult (14 or older), has any other adult done the following: | | | | |
| a. | Hit, kick, or beat you? | Never | Seldom | Occasionally | Often |
| b. | Seriously threaten your life? | Never | Seldom | Occasionally | Often |

Leserman, J., Drossman, D., Li, Z: The Reliability and Validity of a Sexual and Physical Abuse History Questionnaire in Female Patients with Gastrointestinal Disorders. Behavioral Medicine 21:141–148, 1995

H

**Figure 33-13, cont'd    *E–H,* Pelvic pain assessment form.**

*Physical Examination – For Physician Use Only*

Name: _____  Chart Number: _____

Height: _____ Weight: _____ BP: _____ LMP: _____ Temp: _____ Resp: _____

ROS, PFSH Reviewed: ☐ Yes ☐ No  Physician Signature _____

General: ☐ WNL ☐ Walk ☐ Facial expression
☐ Color ☐ Alterations in posture ☐ Other _____

**NOTE: Mark "Not Examined" as N/E**

HEENT ☐ WNL _____ Chest ☐ WNL _____ Heart ☐ WNL _____ Breasts ☐ WNL _____

Abdomen
☐ Non-tender ☐ Incisions ☐ Trigger Points ☐ Ovarian point tenderness
☐ Inguinal tenderness ☐ Inguinal bulge ☐ Suprapubic tenderness ☐ Other ____

Back
☐ Non-tender ☐ Tenderness ☐ Altered ROM ☐ Alterations in posture

Extremities
☐ WNL ☐ Edema ☐ Varicosities ☐ Neuropathy ☐ Range of motion

Neuropathy
☐ Iliohypogastric ☐ Ilioinguinal ☐ Genitofemoral ☐ Pudendal ☐ Altered sensation

EGBUS/Vagina
☐ WNL ☐ Lesions
☐ Wet prep:
☐ Local tenderness:
☐ Vaginal mucosa:
☐ Posterior fourchette:
☐ Discharge:
Cultures:
☐ GC ☐ Chlamydia ☐ Fungal ☐ Herpes

Unimanual pelvic exam
☐ WNL ☐ Cervix
☐ Introitus ☐ Cervical motion
☐ Uterine-cervical junction ☐ Parametrium
☐ Urethra ☐ Vaginal cuff
☐ Bladder ☐ Cul de sac
☐ R ureter ☐ L ureter
☐ R inguinal ☐ L inguinal
☐ Muscle awareness ☐ Clitoral tenderness

Rank muscle tenderness on 0-4 scale
☐ R obturator _____
☐ L obturator _____
☐ R piriformis _____
☐ L piriformis _____
☐ R pubococcygeus _____
☐ L pubococcygeus _____
☐ Total pelvic floor score _____

*Patient rates allodynia produced by Q-tip for each circle (0-4).*
Total Score: _____

© 1999, The International Pelvic Pain Society  Page 9

Bimanual pelvic exam ☐ Absent
Uterus: ☐ Tender ☐ Non-tender
Position ☐ Anterior ☐ Posterior ☐ Midplane
Size ☐ Normal ☐ Other _____
Contour ☐ Regular ☐ Irregular ☐ Other
Consistency ☐ Firm ☐ Soft ☐ Hard
Mobility ☐ Mobile ☐ Hypermobile ☐ Fixed
Support ☐ Well supported ☐ Prolapse

Adnexae
Right  Left
☐ Absent ☐ Absent
☐ WNL ☐ WNL
☐ Tender ☐ Tender
☐ Fixed ☐ Fixed
☐ Enlarged _____ cm ☐ Enlarged _____ cm

Rectovaginal
☐ WNL ☐ Nodules ☐ Guaiac positive
☐ Tenderness ☐ Mucosal pathology (negative with
☐ Not examined quality control)

Trigger Points  Fibromyalgia

Assessment: _____

Diagnostic Plan: _____

Therapeutic Plan: _____

Page 10  © 1999, The International Pelvic Pain Society

**Figure 33-13, cont'd** *I–J, Pelvic pain assessment form.* (From Scialli A, Barbiere R, Glasser M, et al: Chronic Pelvic Pain: An Integrated Approach. APGO Educational Series on Women's Health Issues. Washington, DC, Association of Professors of Gynecology and Obstetrics, 2000. © 1999, International Pelvic Pain Society.)

**Acknowledgment**

The authors wish to acknowledge Dr. Diane Merritt and Dr. David Muram for providing figures as noted in the legends.

**REFERENCES**

1. Merritt DF, Rimza ME, Muram D: Genital injuries in the pediatric and female adolescent. In Sanfilippo JS, Muram D, Lee P, et al (eds): Pediatric and Adolescent Gynecology, 2nd ed. Philadelphia, WB Saunders, 2001. **(IV, C)**
2. Pokorny SF: Genital trauma. Clin Obstet Gynecol 1997;40:219–225. **(IV, C)**
3. Huffman JW, Dewhurst CJ, Capraro VJ: The Gynecology of Childhood and Adolescence. Philadelphia, WB Saunders, 1981. **(IV, C)**
4. Mendez DR: Straddle injury. UpToDate, 2003. **(IV, C)**
5. Dreitlein D, Suner S, Basler J: Genitourinary trauma. Emerg Med Clin North Am 2001;19:569–590. **(III, B)**
6. Hartanto V, Nitti V: Recent advances in management of female lower urinary tract trauma. Curr Opin Urol 2003;13:279–284. **(III, B)**
7. Muram D, Levitt CJ, Frasier CD, et al: Genital injuries. J Pediatr Adolesc Gynecol 2003;16:149–155. **(IV, C)**
8. Merritt D: Evaluating and managing acute genital trauma in premenarchal girls. J Pediatr Adolesc Gynecol 1999;12:237–238. **(IV, C)**
9. Scialli A, Barbiere R, Glasser M, et al: Chronic Pelvic Pain: An Integrated Approach. APGO Educational Series on Women's Health Issues. Washington, DC, Association of Professors of Gynecology and Obstetrics, 2000. **(IV, C)**
10. Steege J, Metzger D, Levy B: Chronic Pelvic Pain: Integrated Approach. New York, WB Saunders, 1997. **(IV, C)**
11. Melzack R: Neurophysiological foundations of pain. In Sternbach RA (ed): The Psychology of Pain, 2nd ed. New York, Raven Press, 1986, pp 1–24. **(IV, C)**
12. Fordyce W: Behavioral Methods of Control of Chronic Pain and Illness. St Louis, Mo, Mosby, 1976. **(IV, C)**
13. Bernstine R, Stome C, Waldron J: Post PID sequelae and pain: assessment, management and new findings. Med Aspects Hum Sex 1987; 21(11):46–54. **(III, B)**
14. Sinaki M, Merritt J, Stillwell G: Tension myalgia of the pelvic floor. Mayo Clin Proc 1977;52:717–722. **(IV, C)**
15. Slocumb J: Neurological factors in chronic pelvic pain: trigger points and the abdominal pelvic pain syndrome. Am J Obstet Gynecol 1984; 149:536–543. **(IV, C)**
16. Ballweg ML, Laufer MR: Adolescent Endometriosis: State of the art Forum. J Pediatr Adolesc Gynecol June 2003 (Suppl). **(IV, C)**
17. Kontoravdis A, Hassan E, Hassiakos D, et al: Laparoscopic evaluation and management of chronic pelvic pain during adolescence. Clin Exp Obstet Gynecol 1999;26:76–77. **(IV, C)**
18. Vercellini P, Fedele L, Arcaini L, et al: Laparoscopy in the diagnosis of chronic pelvic pain in adolescent women J Reprod Med 1989; 34:827–830. **(III, B)**
19. Laufer M, Goiten B, Bush M, et al: Prevalence of endometriosis in adolescent women with chronic pelvic pain not responding to conventional therapy. J Pediatr Adolesc Gynecol 1997;10:199–202. **(IV, C)**
20. Reese K, Reddy S, Rock J: Endometriosis in an adolescent population: the Emory experience. J Pediatr Adolesc Gynecol 1996;9:125–128. **(III, B)**

# Pediatric and Adolescent Gynecology

21. Howard FM: The role of laparoscopy in chronic pelvic pain: promises and pitfalls. Obstet Gynecol Surv 1993;48:357–387. **(IV, C)**

22. Koninckx P, Meuleman C, Demeyere S, et al: Suggestive evidence that pelvic endometriosis is a progressive disease, whereas deeply infiltrated endometriosis is associated with pelvic pain. Fertil Steril 1991; 55:759–765. **(III,B)**

23. Balasch J, Creus M, Fabregues F, et al: Visible and non-visible endometriosis at laparoscopy for infertility and in patients with chronic pelvic pain: a prospective study. Hum Reprod 1996;11:387–391. **(I, A)**

24. Lehmann-Willenbrock E, Mecke H, Riedel HH: Sequelae of appendectomy with special reference to intra-abdominal adhesions, chronic abdominal pain and infertility. Gynecol Obstet Invest 1990;29:241–245. **(III, B)**

25. Sohn N, Weinstein M, Robins R: The levator syndrome and its treatment with high voltage electrogalvanic stimulation Am J Surg 1982; 144:580–582. **(IIa, B)**

26. Trimbos J, Trimbos-Kemper G, Peters A, et al: Findings in 200 asymptomatic women having a laparoscopic sterilization. Arch Gynecol Obstet 1990;247:121–124. **(IIb, B)**

27. Steege J, Stout A: Resolution of chronic pelvic pain after lysis of adhesions. Am J Obstet Gynecol 1991;165:278–283. **(III, B)**

28. Goldstein D, deCholnoky C, Emans SJ, Levanthal JM: Laparoscopy in the diagnosis and management of pelvic pain in adolescents. J Reprod Med 1980;24:251–256. **(III, B)**

29. Kapur B, Rai P, Gulati S: Prevention of experimental peritoneal adhesions by low molecular weight dextran. Int Surg 1967;48:264 **(IIa, B)**

30. Peters A, Trimbos-Demper G, Admiral C, Trimbos J: A randomized clinical trial on the benefit of adhesiolysis in patients with intraperitoneal adhesions and chronic pelvic pain. Br J Obstet Gynaecol 1992;99:59–62. **(Ib, A)**

# Chapter 34

# Laparoscopic Instrumentation

Raedah Al-Fadhli, MD, Togas Tulandi, MD, MHCM, and
Eric J. Bieber, MD, MHCM

## KEY POINTS

- The laparoscopic surgeon should be familiar with a number of instruments for performing laparoscopic surgery.
- High-flow insufflators facilitate operative laparoscopy.
- The laparoscopic surgeon should be comfortable placing several different types of trocars.
- Multiple surgical devices are available for tissue incision and dissection, including unipolar, bipolar, ultrasonic, and laser. Device choice largely depends on surgeon preference.
- Electric tissue morcellators facilitate removal of large masses.
- Robotic surgery is presently being investigated for use in gynecology.
- Virtual reality trainers allow improvement in hand-eye coordination that may enhance performance of surgery.

Proper instrumentation is required for the ease and safe conduct of any procedure. This is especially essential for advanced laparoscopic surgery. Equally important is the surgeon's familiarity with the equipment and instruments. There are a plethora of laparoscopic instruments, but basic principles apply to the use of all of them. Depending on the volume of patients, a minimum of two complete sets of laparoscopic instruments per operating room is needed. Basic instruments for a single laparoscopic set are depicted in Table 34-1 and Figure 34-1. This chapter focuses on basic instruments required for operative laparoscopy.

## INSTRUMENTS REQUIRED FOR OPERATIVE LAPAROSCOPY

### Camera and Monitor

High-quality visualization of the operating field is crucial during laparoscopic surgery. Image quality may be enhanced with the use of a three-chip endovision video camera, high-intensity light, and a high-resolution video monitor. A three-dimensional camera is also available, but it remains unclear if this facilitates surgery.

The modern camera should be lightweight; have a zoom lens, automatic color setting, and high-speed shutter to decrease or eliminate overexposure; and should be easily sterilized. The number of pixels on a chip determines the resolution capacity of the camera. A single-chip camera with 450 lines per inch provides fair quality resolution; a three-chip camera with 700 lines per inch provides better resolution and color accuracy.

Although laparoscopic surgery can be performed with a single monitor between the patient's legs, having at least two monitors in the operating room may decrease surgeon fatigue. This allows viewing of each monitor by both the surgeon and the assistant in a comfortable position (Fig. 34-2). A properly designed imaging trolley should accommodate the monitor at a convenient height (Fig. 34-3). It should have space for the camera control unit, light source, video recorder, printer, and the insufflators. The use of antifogging solution or laparoscopic warming devices helps prevent condensation of fog that might obscure the field.

Some surgeons use three or more flat-screen monitors attached to the ceiling with an adjusting unit for better placement. A video recorder to record the conduct of the procedure can be utilized for documentation and for teaching purposes. More recently it has become possible to digitally record surgeries on hard drives. Printers should be available in the operating room (Fig. 34-4) and may be most helpful in later discussing the surgical findings with the patient and in maintaining the patient's chart. Alternatively, the image could be recorded on a floppy disk in digital mode, which can be then enhanced with the computer for printing. This may ultimately be stored in a digital format in an electronic medical record.

### Light Source

The best illumination for laparoscopic surgery is by xenon light (Fig. 34-5). It is associated with minimal heat conduction via a light cable to the laparoscope. However, direct contact of the cable with a patient's skin or operating drapes can result in a thermal burn. The light should only be turned on after the light cable is attached to the laparoscope. Most of the light sources available are capable of manual and automatic adjustment for optimal illumination. The light cables may be fiberoptic or liquid gel with a diameter between 3.5 mm and 6 mm, with the length ranging from 180 to 350 cm. These cables have a limited life span and should be treated carefully because the individual fibers may break, ultimately diminishing the amount of transferred light to the endoscope.

### High-flow Insufflators

The availability of a high-flow electronic insufflator that can administer several liters of $CO_2$ gas per minute is mandatory for advanced laparoscopic surgery (Fig. 34-6). Frequent instrument changes, as well as irrigation and aspiration during a procedure, lead to a rapid loss of pneumoperitoneum. Gas will only flow into the peritoneal cavity under pressure. The higher the pressure, the greater the risk of gas being forced into the circulation, with

# Minimally Invasive Surgery

**Table 34-1**
**Basic Laparoscopic Instruments for a Single Laparoscopic Set**

| Instrument | Number |
|---|---|
| Laparoscopes | |
| 10-mm straight forward 0-degree laparoscope | 2 |
| 5-mm 0- or 30-degree laparoscope | 1 |
| Trocars | |
| 10-mm primary trocar | 1 |
| 10-mm secondary trocar | 1 |
| 5-mm secondary trocars | 2 |
| 20-mm trocar for the morcellator | 1 |
| 10 to 5 mm, 20 to 10 mm, and 20 to 5 mm reduction sleeves | 3 |
| Suction irrigation system | 1 |
| Bipolar forceps with cable | |
| Bipolar grasping forceps | 2 |
| Bipolar microforceps for tubal surgery | 1 |
| Unipolar instrument with cable | |
| 1-mm needle electrode for ectopic pregnancy | 1 |
| Unipolar scissors for myomectomy | 1 |
| Forceps | |
| Atraumatic grasping forceps | 1 |
| 5-mm grasping forceps with 2 × 2 teeth | 2 |
| 10-mm claw forceps | 1 |
| Scissors | |
| Metzenbaum scissors | 1 |
| Hook scissors | 1 |
| Microdissecting scissors | 1 |
| Suture and ligature | |
| Needle holder | 1 |
| Assistant needle holder | 1 |
| Suture manipulator (knot pusher) | 1 |
| 5-mm laparoscopic aspiration needle | 1 |
| Optional | |
| Morcellator, possibly in a separate set for myomectomy or hysterectomy | 1 |
| Disposable scissors, laparoscopic pouch, pretied ligature, lens defogger | Separate |

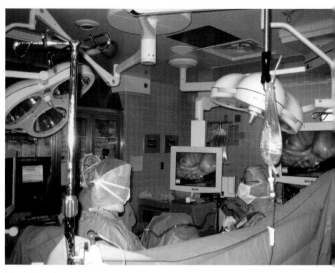

**Figure 34-2    Operating room setup for advanced laparoscopic surgery.** The surgeon views one monitor and the assistant views another. The third monitor can be used for teaching or viewing by other operating room personnel.

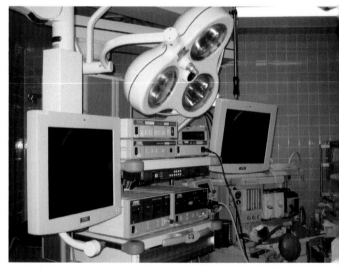

**Figure 34-3    Laparoscopic trolley with a camera unit, light source, and insufflator.** (Courtesy of Karl Storz Endoscopy, Tuttlingen, Germany.)

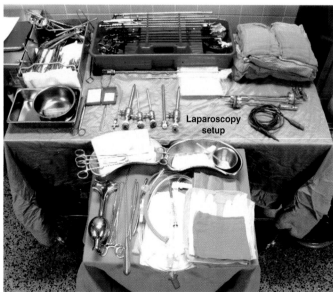

Laparoscopy setup

**Figure 34-1    Basic laparoscopic set.**

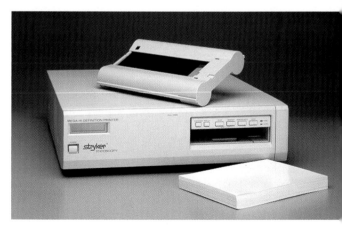

**Figure 34-4    An electronic controlled unit available for circulating nurses to document all the procedures in the operating room.** (Courtesy of Stryker Corporation, San Jose, CA)

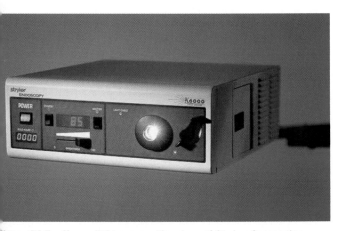

**Figure 34-5  Xenon light source.** (Courtesy of Stryker Corporation, San Jose, CA)

possible risk of gas embolism. A pressure of 10 to 15 mm Hg is usually adequate.

During initial insufflation a small amount of gas should be instilled to ascertain appropriate placement. Once this has occurred and trocars are in place, insufflation may be set to as much as 40 L/min.

More recently, insufflators that allow heating of gas before entry into the peritoneal cavity have been developed. These bring the gas to core temperature, which may decrease hypothermia and improve patient recovery.[1]

### Laparoscope

Different diameter laparoscopes are available, ranging from 1.8 to 12 mm. The straight forward telescopes with 0-degree angle are generally preferred by gynecologists as they look into the pelvic cavity because there is a large viewing angle.

However, the choice of telescope depends on the surgical procedure. For laparoscopy under conscious sedation a small laparoscope is preferable, whereas a larger one is usually used for procedures under general anesthesia or where tissue removal will be required.

Laparoscopes do not magnify the image as does a microscope, but the closer the scope is to the tissue the greater the magnification. Depending on the camera, zoom capability, and the distance between the lens and the tissue, magnification of up to 40× can be achieved. This is especially important for procedures such as tubal reanastomosis.

Having both a 5- and 10-mm laparoscope available on the tray may be beneficial to the surgeon, because many surgeons use a larger 10-mm or greater port infraumbilically and 5-mm ancillary ports. This allows the surgeon the ability to readily move from one port to another with either size laparoscope.

Foreoblique laparoscopes may also be of value in performing advanced laparoscopy. For example, a 30-degree laparoscope may be helpful in performing work deep in the pelvis or in patients with substantial adhesive disease.

Another option is an operative laparoscope, which contains an operating channel through which various grasping and other laparoscopic instruments may be placed. Some surgeons prefer this type of instrument because it may decrease the need for an additional ancillary trocar. Other surgeons feel that the necessary diminution in the size of the endoscope to allow the operating channel, as well as the inability to move the operating instrument used through this channel outside of the axis of the instrument, limit its usefulness.

### Veress Needle

Although some surgeons choose to use either direct or open trocar insertion, many gynecologists prefer using a Veress needle for insufflation prior to trocar insertion. There are disposable and nondisposable types of Veress needle. The Veress is a long needle with a blunt hollow spring-loaded trocar in its center. The blunt trocar springs back at and through the resistance of the abdominal wall, and springs out again to protect the viscera from the needle once the resistance disappears within the abdominal cavity. Gas flows through the hollow to create the initial pneumoperitoneum. The bore of the needle limits the initial flow during insufflation. The surgeon will have tactile sensation to feel the entrance of the needle through the abdominal wall, especially the fascia and the peritoneum. This may be limited if the patient has had prior surgery and significant scarring exists.

More recently, radially dilating devices have been developed that allow dilation to be performed outward after placement of the device (Fig. 34-7). In essence these are a hybrid of a Veress needle and a trocar.

### Trocars, Reducers, and Access Devices

A variety of disposable and reusable trocars are available. The cannula or port is a tubular device through which operative access is obtained. Many cannulae have a sharp trocar to facilitate passage through the abdominal wall and a valve or membrane to prevent the leakage of gas when no instrument is in place.

Most of the cannulae have a rubber seal at the top through which telescope and instruments may be passed without the loss of pneumoperitoneum. There are three general types of trocars: a conical trocar, which is less traumatic to the tissue but requires greater force for entry; a pyramidal trocar that makes it easier to enter the abdominal wall with less force; and a Hasson cannula, a blunt trocar that is used for the open laparoscopy technique.[2]

Many surgeons use three or more trocars when performing advanced laparoscopy, a 10-mm primary trocar at the infraumbilical area for the laparoscope and two secondary 5-mm

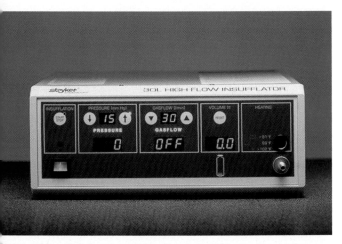

**Figure 34-6  High-flow insufflator.** (Courtesy of Stryker Corporation, San Jose, CA)

# Minimally Invasive Surgery

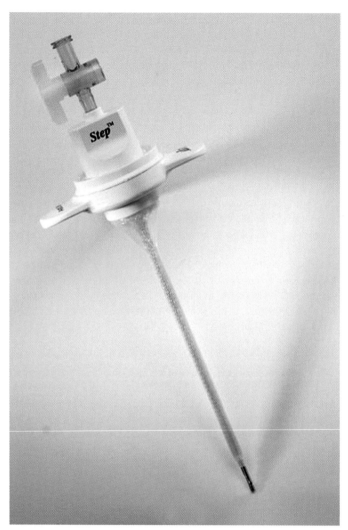

**Figure 34-7  Radially dilating trocar with needle.** (Courtesy of U.S. Surgical, Norwalk, CT.)

trocars. One of the two secondary trocars may be 10 mm or larger if removal of a specimen is anticipated. For removal of a large or solid mass such as a uterus or myoma, a 15- or 20-mm trocar is used to accommodate a morcellator.

More recently, blunt-tip nonbladed trocars have been developed that are able to penetrate through the various layers of the abdominal wall (Fig. 34-8). In some cases this penetration may be performed with a laparoscope in place to observe the trocar moving through the tissues. Unfortunately, no large com-

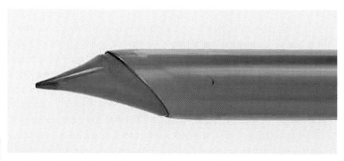

**Figure 34-8    Blunt-tip trocar.** (Courtesy of Taut, Inc., Geneva, IL)

parative trials exist to better define if a specific trocar type is inherently safer than another.

### Suction-Irrigation

The addition of simple suction and irrigation devices was important historically for the evolution to advanced endoscopic techniques. With modern irrigators we are able to quickly evacuate blood, fluid, and ovarian cysts, markedly facilitating surgery. A powerful suction-irrigator that can deliver pressure of up to 800 mm Hg is thus invaluable for operative laparoscopy. The suction-irrigation probe should have a single channel for both functions, with the flow controlled by a hand-valve system (Fig. 34-9).

### Laparoscopic Aspiration Needle

A 5-mm aspiration needle is used to aspirate peritoneal fluid for cytology (alternatively the suction-irrigator may be used). It can also be used to inject vasopressin into the uterus or myoma, or saline solution for hydrodissection.

### Bipolar and Unipolar Instruments

The main principles of a good electrosurgical system are to cut, coagulate, and vaporize tissue (Fig. 34-10). The electrosurgical tool uses electrons in a closed electrical circuit. In the bipolar system, the active electrode and the neutral electrode (grounding pad) are built into the tip of the instrument. Thus interaction is limited to a small area of tissue, which may result in safer and lower energy input. A bipolar grasping forceps should always be available for hemostasis at any laparoscopic surgery. These cannot be substituted by unipolar forceps or laser. Most bipolar forceps are available in a 5-mm diameter. A microbipolar forceps allows precise and limited coagulation during delicate surgery such as laparoscopic tubal anastomosis. One such device, the Ligasure, has been developed. It uses the principles of the bipolar system and can be used as a grasping or clamping instrument (Fig. 34-11). Another variation is the "tripolar device," in which a sharp blade is passed through bipolar forceps once tissue has been coagulated (Fig. 34-12).

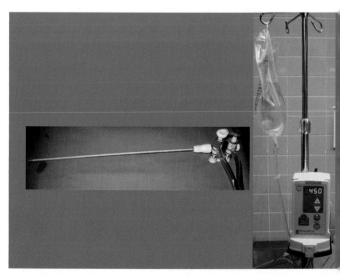

**Figure 34-9    Disposable unit of suction-irrigation system.**

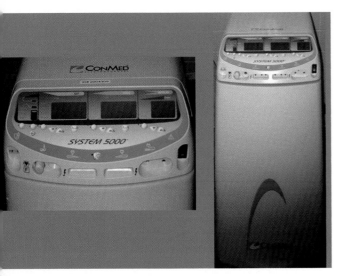

**Figure 34-10    Bipolar/unipolar generator.** (Courtesy of ConMed Corporation, Utica, NY.)

Unipolar forceps are rarely used today. However, many other types of unipolar instruments may be safely and effectively used during laparoscopic surgery. In this system, electrons flow from the electrosurgical unit to the active electrode. From the tip of the electrode, the current will flow through the air to the tissue. The current then will be conducted through the body to the ground plate attached to the patient and returns to the electrosurgical unit. Some examples of unipolar instruments include unipolar needle electrodes to perform salpingostomy for ectopic pregnancy and occasionally for laparoscopic ovarian drilling and unipolar scissors to make a uterine incision during myomectomy or lysis of adhesions.

### Laser

There are several types of surgical lasers, including $CO_2$, argon, potassium titanium phosphate (KTP), and neodymium:yttrium aluminium garnet (Nd:YAG). Their properties depend on the characteristics of the laser beam, the nature and the color of the

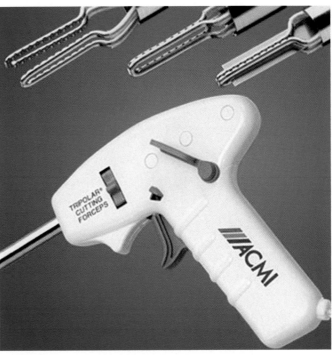

**Figure 34-12    "Tripolar" device.** (Courtesy of Circon-ACMI, Stamford, CT.)

structure in its path, the irradiation spot size, and the exposure time. Lasers with long wavelength are more effective for tissue vaporization but poor for coagulation. Lasers with short wavelength, on the other hand, have good coagulation but poor vaporization properties.

Studies have shown that the results of laser surgery are similar to those with conventional laparoscopic instruments. Therefore, use will depend on surgeon preference and experience.

### Ultrasonic Vibrating Scalpel (Harmonic Scalpel)

The ultrasonic scalpel consists of a generator and a handpiece that houses the ultrasonic transducer (Fig. 34-13). When activated, the scalpel blade moves longitudinally at 55,000 vibrations per

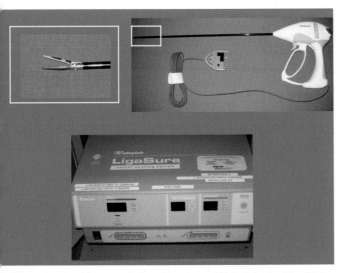

**Figure 34-11    Ligasure device.** (Courtesy of Valleylab, Boulder, CO.)

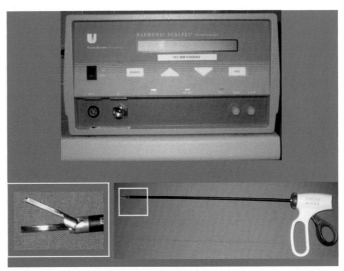

**Figure 34-13    Harmonic scalpel.** (Courtesy of Gynecare, a division of Ethicon, Inc., a Johnson & Johnson company, Somerville, NJ.)

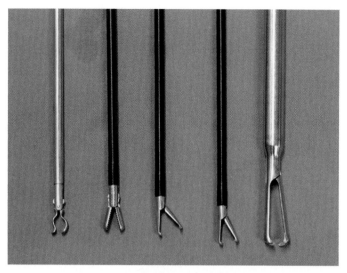

**Figure 34-14    Different types of laparoscopic forceps.**

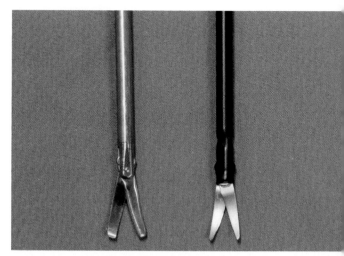

**Figure 34-16    Reusable scissors.**

second. This allows several different tissue effects, including the ability to cut through tissue as well as seal vessels. Because little heat is produced (usually under 80°C), necrosis and charring are minimal. Initially the ultrasonic scalpel was available only in larger handpieces, but newer technology has allowed development of 5-mm handpieces, which no longer require control with a footswitch.

### Dissecting and Grasping Forceps
Grasping instruments are available in different sizes, shapes, and forms (Fig. 34-14). There are two types of grasping forceps: traumatic or atraumatic. Traumatic forceps, such as the 5-mm grasping forceps with 2 × 2 teeth, allows secure grasping of tissue. Babcock atraumatic forceps are invaluable for gentle handling of fallopian tubes. A 10-mm claw forceps used with a morcellator permits efficient removal of a solid specimen. There are also many different types of handles: scissors type, angled, or non-angled. Their use depends on surgeon preference.

### Scissors
It is important to have scissors that cut and do not tear the tissue. A wide variety of scissors is available (Figs. 34-15 and 34-16). The curved-jaw scissors are multipurpose but are usually used for dissection. Fine-pointed curved or straight micro-scissors are used for microdissection. Hooked scissors are used for cutting ligated vessels. In practice, all these instruments are used interchangeably.

A combination of cutting and coagulating can be obtained by incorporating unipolar current to the scissors. Nondisposable scissors used many times tend to become dull; therefore, many surgeons prefer to use disposable scissors.

### Instruments for Laparoscopic Suturing
Laparoscopic suturing is needed in several procedures, including myomectomy, tubal anastomosis, or closure of the vaginal cuff during laparoscopic total hysterectomy (Fig. 34-17). Suturing might also be needed to repair intestinal laceration and ureteral or bladder injury.

#### Needle Holder
Besides a longer shaft, the design for the needle holder used in laparoscopic suturing is similar to that used for conventional surgery. The handles could be offset aligned or aligned in the axis as the shaft. The offset alignment is beneficial if the surgeon's arm is extended, whereas the in-line variety is useful for suturing near the anterior abdominal wall.

The jaw could be aligned with the shaft or curved. Side-loading needle holders are available for curved needles; however

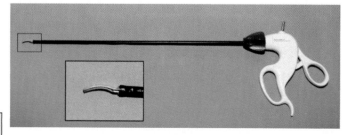

**Figure 34-15    Disposable scissors.**

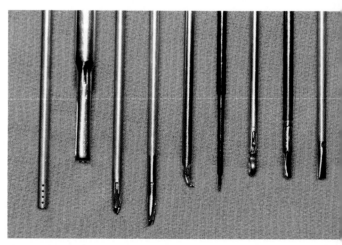

**Figure 34-17    Basic instruments for a single laparoscopic set.**
Instruments for suturing are not shown.

he handle is often very stiff. Most needle holders are 3 to 5 mm in diameter.

### Needles and Sutures

The type and size of needles and sutures depend on the procedure. For example, a curved needle with 1-0 suture is used to repair a uterine defect after a myomectomy, and 6-0 to 8-0 sutures are needed for laparoscopic tubal anastomosis. Conventional laparoscopic suturing can be done using ski or straight needles with 3-0 or 4-0 sutures.

### Knot Pusher

Sutures can be tied intracorporeally or extracorporeally. The use of a knot pusher or suture/knot manipulator allows extracorporeal knot tying. Compared to an open-end knot pusher, the closed end ensures that the suture stays connected to the end of the device. After suturing, the needle is extracted from the abdominal cavity and inserted into the fenestration of a closed-end knot pusher. The surgeon makes a knot and the knot is pushed into the abdominal cavity.

### Ligature

Endoloop (Ethicon, Somerville, NJ) is a loop with a preformed slipknot that can be positioned around the tissue to be removed. These are best used when a tissue pedicle exists. In the absence of this commercial product, a piece of suture material with or without the needle attached may be used to ligate. Alternatively, the surgeon can ligate a structure using a self-made slipknot prepared extracorporeally and inserted into the abdominal cavity using a knot pusher.

### Clips and Staples

A single- or multiple-clip applier should be available for emergency situations, such as rapid occlusion of an isolated bleeding vessel. They are made of metal or absorbable plastic. In addition, endoscopic GIA staplers have now been readily available for well over a decade. These come in multiple different forms with several sizes of staples.

### Morcellator

Use of electronic morcellators has supplanted handheld morcellation devices. Electronic morcellators are able to quickly and efficiently remove large amounts of solid tissue from the abdominal cavity. This is especially helpful during laparoscopic myomectomy or supracervical hysterectomy. In a time and cost analysis, Carter and McCarus found power morcellators to be cost effective.[3]

Tissues are held by the grasping forceps, morcellated in pieces, and subsequently removed. Morcellators are available in multiple different versions and a range of sizes (Fig. 34-18). Generally the morcellator is placed at the site of one of the secondary trocars. It is important when using these devices that tissue is brought toward the morcellator and that the morcellator is not moved toward the tissue where vascular or other injury may occur.[4]

### Laparoscopic Pouch

Removal of an intact cyst using a disposable extraction pouch prevents spillage of the contents of the cyst into the abdominal

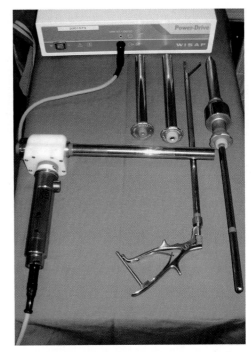

**Figure 34-18**  **Instruments for morcellation.** (Courtesy of WISAP, Munich, Germany)

cavity and contamination of the abdominal wall during extraction of the specimen (Fig. 34-19). They are also useful in removing ovaries, adnexa, or other larger pieces of tissue from the abdomen. Multiple different pouches are available in a range of sizes and materials from a number of manufacturers. Care should be used when extracting these bags through small-diameter incisions to avoid rupture of the bag and loss of the contents back into the abdominal cavity.

### Standard Dilation and Curettage Set

This set should contain a weighted speculum, tenaculum, uterine sound, dilators, and a uterine manipulator. Disposable and non-disposable uterine manipulators (Fig. 34-20) allow chromopertubation, anteversion, retroversion, and rotation to maximize surgical access. Another manipulator, the Rumi manipulator (Fig. 34-21), articulates around the cervix and is equipped with two balloons. The intrauterine balloon anchors the instrument within the uterus and seals the cervix, and an intravaginal balloon prevents escape of $CO_2$ gas at the completion of total laparoscopic hysterectomy.

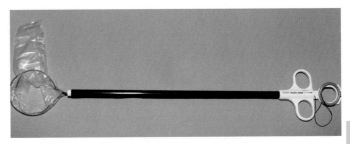

**Figure 34-19**  **Endoscopic pouch.**

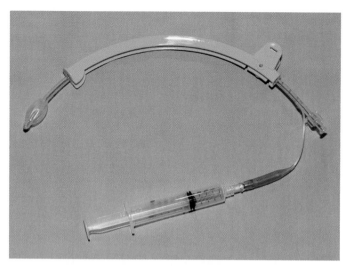

**Figure 34-20    A disposable uterine manipulator.** (Courtesy of Cooper Surgical Inc., Trumbull, CT)

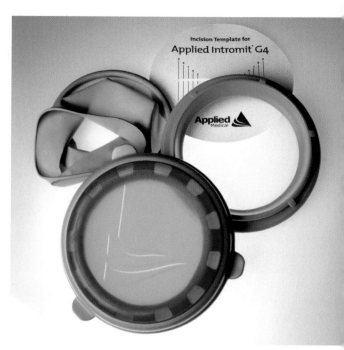

**Figure 34-22    Novel access device to allow intra-abdominal hand placement.** (Courtesy of Applied Medical, Rancho Santa Margarita, CA.)

## Hand Assistance

A novel variation on standard laparoscopy has been the development of devices to allow the endoscopic surgeon the advantage of placing a hand intra-abdominally without the loss of the pneumoperitoneum (Fig. 34-22). This offers the advantage of performing procedures where actually touching tissue with the surgeon's fingers aids the surgery while still keeping the incisions very small. A further modification has been the development of specialized retractors that allow mini-laparotomy to be used either instead of, or sometimes after a portion of the procedure is performed laparoscopically (Fig. 34-23). These devices may also be combined to give further surgical options (Fig. 34-24).

## Other Disposable Instruments

Today, many laparoscopic instruments are available in both reusable and disposable forms. Disposables tend to be lighter than reusable instruments, but questions remain regarding cost efficacy. Compared to reusable scissors and trocars, which could become dull with frequent usage, disposable trocars and scissors are always sharp.

Due to the high expense of disposable instruments, some hospitals use reusable instruments. In any event, disposable instruments should be available in the operating theatre as a backup. The final position of the patient and the surgeons is seen in Figure 34-25 and is discussed further in Chapter 36.

## Robotics

The most recent enhancement of laparoscopic surgery is the introduction of robotics into the operating room.[5] Many surgeons today use voice recognition technology to raise and lower light levels, increase insufflation, and capture digital images. An addition has been the use of systems such as the daVinci Robotic Surgical System (Fig. 34-26). These systems allow the operator to work at a distance from the patient (generally within the same operating room but not necessarily; transcontinental surgeries have now been performed). The robotic instruments have multiple articulating points, which allow approximation of normal surgical movements.

It has been suggested that robotics may allow a surgeon to perform more difficult surgery such as fine suturing (Fig. 34-27). The true cost efficacy, as well as clinical enhancements transferring to improved patient outcomes, are still being evaluated in gynecologic surgery.[6,7] It may be that only some surgeries are enhanced whereas others may be slowed or otherwise encumbered by this technology. A different issue is how to train and credential surgeons in the postgraduate environment on this instrumentation. One group evaluated performance of a standard tubal ligation (once laboratory and didactic training had been given) as a means to train surgeons in a graded manner.

## Simulation and Virtual Reality

Efforts have been directed to enhancing surgeon experience either before or in addition to hands-on training. With the

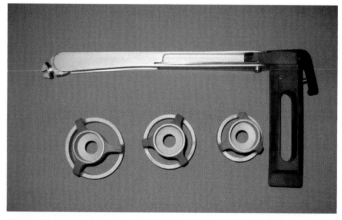

**Figure 34-21    Rumi uterine manipulator.** (Courtesy of Superior Medical, Toronto, Canada)

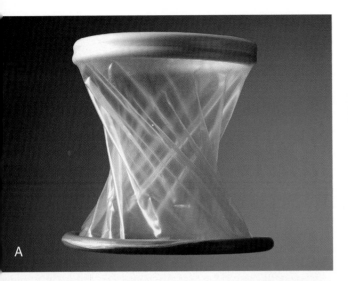

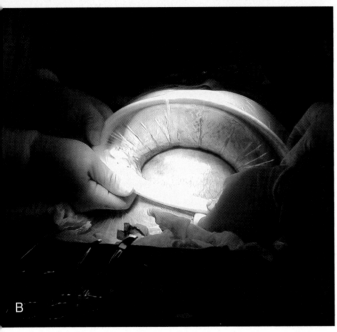

Figure 34-23    A and B, Retractors for mini-laparotomy. (Courtesy of Applied Medical, Rancho Santa Margarita, CA.)

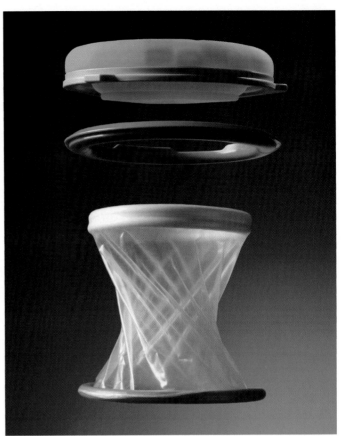

Figure 34-24    Device for hand placement and mini-laparotomy combined. (Courtesy of Applied Medical, Rancho Santa Margarita, CA.)

associated with training in an animal laboratory. At present, several manufacturers are developing specific programs to model laparoscopic, hysteroscopic, and other procedures. Although development is still in its infancy, programs have become increasingly lifelike. There may come a day when residents will

advent of superfast microprocessors, the technology now exists to attempt to recapitulate the actual surgical experience outside of the operating room (Fig. 34-28). Early trials suggest devices that allow surgeons to improve hand-eye coordination in simulators might improve surgical function in the operating room.[8] In a randomized trial that used blinded and independent reviewers, surgical trainees were scored during a laparoscopic cholecystectomy. Trainees then underwent virtual reality training versus a control group, which received no additional training. Following this, the participants were again scored on an additional case. The experimental group was noted to be significantly faster, with greater improvement in error and economy of movement.[9]

An additional consideration is that often animals have been used to train surgeons. Use of virtual reality trainers may limit the use of animals while also decreasing the substantial costs

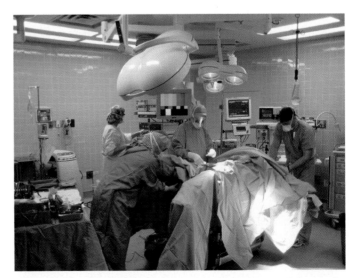

Figure 34-25    The position of the patient, the surgeon, and the scrub technician during the preparation for surgery. (Courtesy of Applied Medical, Rancho Santa Margarita, CA.)

## Minimally Invasive Surgery

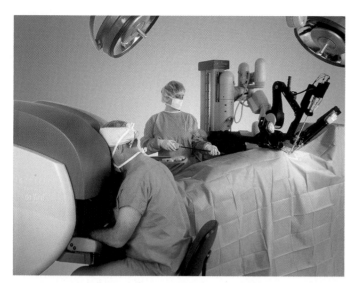

**Figure 34-26    DaVinci surgical robot.** (Courtesy of Intuitive Surgical, Sunnyvale, CA.)

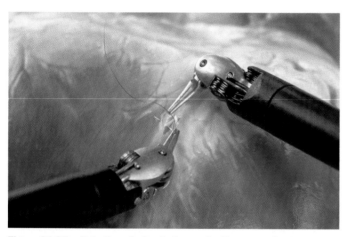

**Figure 34-27    Robotic suturing instruments.** (Courtesy of Intuitive Surgical, Sunnyvale, CA.)

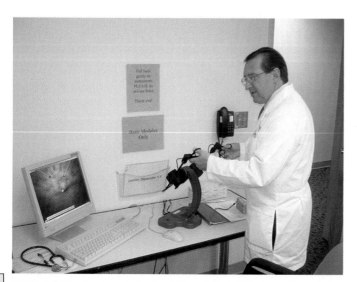

**Figure 34-28    Laparoscopic simulation station.** (Courtesy of Immersion Medical, Gaithersburg, MD.)

begin their surgical training using only simulators until specific thresholds are met. This may also offer an opportunity for post graduate training when new procedures are developed and aid in establishing credentialing guidelines in the future.

## REFERENCES

1. Lenhardt R, Marker E, Goll V, et al: Mild intraoperative hypothermia prolongs post anesthetic recovery. Anesthesiology1997;87:1318–1323. **(Ib, A)**
2. Hasson HM, Rotman C, Rana N, Kumari N: Open laparoscopy: 29-year experience. Obstet Gynecol 2000;96:763–766. **(IV, C)**
3. Carter JE, McCarus SD: Laparoscopic myomectomy. Time and cost analysis of power vs. manual morcellation. J Reprod Med 1997; 42:383–388. **(IIa, B)**
4. Milad MP, Sokol E: Laparoscopic morcellator-related injuries. J Amer Assoc Gynecol Lap 2003;10:383–385. **(IV, C)**
5. Ferguson JL, Beste TM, Nelson KH, Daucher JA: Making the transition from standard laparoscopy to robotic laparoscopy. J Soc Lap Surg 2004;8:326–328. **(IIb, B)**
6. Goldberg JM, Falcone T: Laparoscopic microsurgical tubal anastomosis with and without robotic assistance. Hum Reprod 2003;18:145–147. **(IIa, B)**
7. Elliott DS, Frank I, Dimarco DS, Chow GK: Gynecologic use of robotically assisted laparoscopy: sacrocolpopexy for the treatment of high-grade vaginal vault prolapse. Am J Surg 2004;188:52S–56S. **(IV, C)**
8. Lehmann KS, Ritz JP, Maass H, et al: A prospective randomized study to test the transfer of basic psychomotor skills from virtual reality to physical reality in a comparable training setting. Ann Surg 2005; 241:442–449. **(Ib, A)**
9. Grantcharov TP, Kristiansen VB, Bendix J, et al: Randomized clinical trial of virtual reality simulation for laparoscopic skills training. Br J Surg 2004;91:146–150. **(Ib, A)**

# Chapter 35

# Hysteroscopic Instrumentation

## Frank M. Wittmaack, MD, and Eric J. Bieber, MD, MHCM

## KEY POINTS

- Hysteroscopy is a diagnostic or operative procedure in which the distended uterine cavity is examined with an endoscope passed through the cervix.
- A wide selection of equipment and distention media are commercially available.
- Use of hysteroscopes with separate inflow and outflow channels allows improved visualization.
- Systems to monitor inflow and outflow volumes should be in place prior to operative hysteroscopic procedures.
- A common source of inadequate visualization during hysteroscopic surgery is inadequate fluid distention and inadequate outflow.

The invention of endoscopes dates back some 200 years to 1807 when Bozzini used a mechanical light conductor for inspection of body cavities.[1] Pantaleoni, however, performed the first hysteroscopic procedure in 1850. The early endoscopes were rigid and used oil lamps as the light source. Later, small electric filament bulbs produced light. Unfortunately, neither light source was satisfactory because of dim images and significant heat generation. For this reason, hysteroscopy fell into disfavor, and dilation and curettage became the standard of care for evaluation of the uterine cavity up until recent times. Modern hysteroscopic equipment has benefited by advances in high-intensity light sources, fiber optic cables, camera and video equipment, and distention media. No longer should a surgeon look into a "sea of red"; images should be clear with excellent diagnostic and operative capabilities.

## FLEXIBLE HYSTEROSCOPES

Flexible endoscopes have been used extensively in gastrointestinal medicine to view the stomach and colon. The flexible tip can bend 120 to 160 degrees and allow visualization around irregularly shaped structures.

A deflection control is found on the body of the hysteroscope (Fig. 35-1). Light and image bundles inside the scope carry light into the uterus and back to the eyepiece or video chip (Fig. 35-2). Diagnostic flexible hysteroscopes have one channel for the distention medium, while operative flexible hysteroscopes have an additional channel for instrumentation. The outer diameter ranges in size from 3.1 mm to 5 mm. Because of their narrow diameter and flexible tip, introduction into the uterine cavity can often be accomplished without anesthesia, which makes it an attractive office procedure.

## RIGID HYSTEROSCOPES

Rigid hysteroscopes are not flexible and contain a complex optical telescope element (Fig. 35-3). Glass lenses and spacers are precisely aligned between the ocular lens (eyepiece) and objective lens at the distal tip. The diameter of the telescope ranges from 1.9 mm (micro-hysteroscope) to 4 mm. Viewing angles typically range from 0 to 30 degrees. Oblique angle telescopes such as 12- and 30-degree hysteroscopes help visualize uterine cornua and lateral walls and may be useful when a resectoscope is employed or operative procedures such as tubal cannulation are performed. The outer diameter of the hysteroscope sheath ranges from 3 to 8 mm. Initially diagnostic hysteroscopes included only one inflow channel for passage of a distention media. Now, most hysteroscopic systems include at least one discrete inflow and outflow channel. This is particularly important when using fluid media and allows the surgeon to quickly clear even a relatively bloody field to achieve excellent visualization. Rigid, semirigid, or flexible instruments can be passed through the sheath such as scissors, forceps, biopsy instruments, or catheters (Fig. 35-4). They come in various sizes, allowing the combination of different telescope sizes and operative tools.

## RESECTOSCOPES

The hysteroscopic resectoscope is a modification of the urologic resectoscope. Original reports describe the use of the urologic resectoscope for gynecologic procedures.[2-5] The gynecologic resectoscope consists of a rigid hysteroscope, a working element with spring handle, and an inner and outer sheath (Fig. 35-5). The working element can be loaded with various attachments such as resection loops, rollerballs, roller bars, and point electrodes (Fig. 35-6). These tools can be advanced past the sheath of the resectoscope by pushing the working element handle forward. The passive spring mechanism allows for retraction of the tool while it exerts the desired tissue effect. The loop electrodes are used primarily to remove myomas and polyps. The needle electrode can be used for septum resection or lysis of intrauterine adhesions. The barrel or ball electrode is suitable for endometrial ablation. Electrode surface area is inversely proportional to energy density, with thin electrodes producing cutting or vaporizing effects while wide electrodes produce coagulation. Monopolar cautery is typically used, which requires nonconducting distention media and the patient to be grounded. With low viscosity distention media and continuous flow resectoscopes, adequate flushing of the uterine cavity can be achieved, allowing for good visualization and safe surgical technique.

# Minimally Invasive Surgery

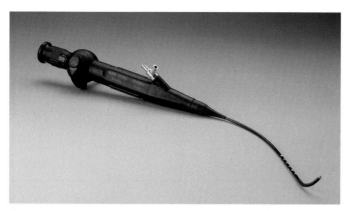

**Figure 35-1 Control body of flexible endoscope.** (From Richard Wolf Medical Instrument Company Clinical Resource Manual: Care and Handling of Flexible Endoscopes, p 2.)

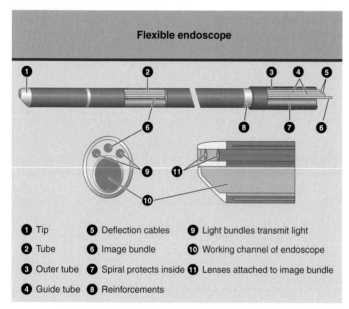

**Flexible endoscope**

- ❶ Tip
- ❷ Tube
- ❸ Outer tube
- ❹ Guide tube
- ❺ Deflection cables
- ❻ Image bundle
- ❼ Spiral protects inside
- ❽ Reinforcements
- ❾ Light bundles transmit light
- ❿ Working channel of endoscope
- ⓫ Lenses attached to image bundle

**Figure 35-2 Schematic view of flexible endoscope.** (From Richard Wolf Medical Instrument Company Clinical Resource Manual: Care and Handling of Flexible Endoscopes, p 1.)

A bipolar electrosurgery system has been developed to avoid the risks associated with the use of hypotonic solutions. The VersaPoint system comes with a variety of electrodes. Energy is delivered from the generator to the tissue through an active electrode. The energy then seeks the path of least resistance through the saline distention media to the return electrode and back to the bipolar generator.

## DISTENTION MEDIA

Adequate distention is essential for visualization of the uterine cavity. The minimum amount of pressure necessary to achieve this is 40 to 50 mm Hg. Pressures between 70 and 80 mm Hg routinely produce good visualization for a hysteroscopic survey. The higher the intrauterine pressure, the higher the risk of medium absorption. This can be minimized by not exceeding the patient's mean arterial pressure. A variety of distention media are available. Their advantages and risks are summarized in Table 35-1.

### Carbon Dioxide

Carbon dioxide ($CO_2$) is a safe[6] gas medium with excellent optical properties. Its low viscosity allows easy flow through the inflow portals of small hysteroscopes and makes it a good choice for diagnostic studies. However, it does not mix with blood, which makes operative hysteroscopic procedures difficult as view-obscuring bubbles form. $CO_2$ is delivered through dedicated hysteroscopic insufflators with flow rates of 60 to 80 mL/min and preset pressure between 80 and 100 mm Hg. Laparoscopic insufflators should never be used for hysteroscopy, since high flow rates can cause a $CO_2$ pulmonary embolism. Historically $CO_2$ was widely used during office hysteroscopy. Now with refined, small-diameter, dual-channel hysteroscopes, many surgeons prefer a liquid medium.

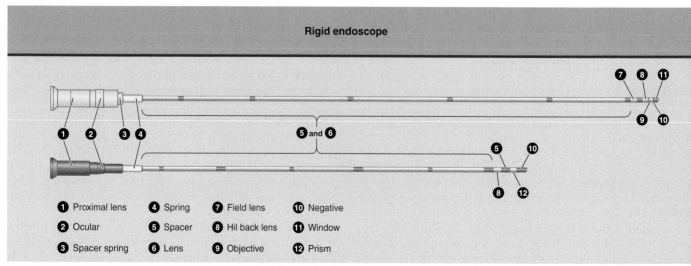

**Rigid endoscope**

- ❶ Proximal lens
- ❷ Ocular
- ❸ Spacer spring
- ❹ Spring
- ❺ Spacer
- ❻ Lens
- ❼ Field lens
- ❽ Hil back lens
- ❾ Objective
- ❿ Negative
- ⓫ Window
- ⓬ Prism

**Figure 35-3 Anatomy of rigid endoscope.** (From Richard Wolf Medical Instrument Company Clinical Resource Manual: Care and Handling of Flexible Endoscopes, p 2.)

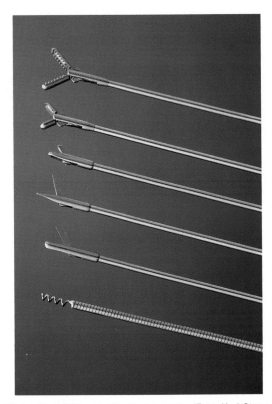

**Figure 35-4 Semirigid operative instruments.** (From Karl Storz endoscopy catalog.)

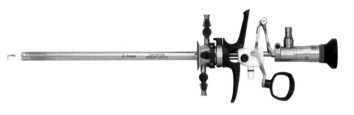

**Figure 35-5 Resectoscope.** (From Olympus catalog.)

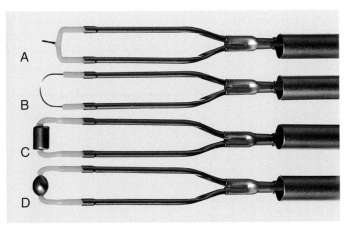

**Figure 35-6 Basic electrode designs for resectoscopy.** *A,* Needle point. *B,* Loop. *C,* Barrel. *D,* Ball. (From Olympus catalog.)

**Table 35-1**
**Comparison of Hysteroscopic Distention Media**

| Medium | Advantage | Disadvantage | Risks |
|---|---|---|---|
| $CO_2$ | Safe[6] Easy to use Rapidly absorbed | Poor visibility in the presence of bleeding | $CO_2$ pulmonary embolism if flow rate exceeds 100 mL/min |
| Normal saline Lactated Ringer's | Isotonic | Not suitable for monopolar electrosurgery | Fluid overload |
| Glycine 1.5% Sorbitol Mannitol 5% | Electrolyte free Nonconductive | Hypotonic[7] | Hypotonic fluid overload Hyponatremia |
| Dextran 32% (Hyskon) | Electrolyte free Nonconductive Immiscible with blood[9] | Highly viscous Difficult to deliver | Hypertonic fluid overload Anaphylactic reaction |

## Normal Saline and Lactated Ringer's Solutions

Normal saline and lactated Ringer's solutions are isotonic, which greatly reduces the risk of hyponatremia in the event of intravasation. However, fluid overload can still occur, making it important to keep track of inflow and outflow during the hysteroscopic procedure. Normal saline and lactated Ringer's also are low-viscosity solutions with good optical characteristics. They readily mix with blood and keep the operative field clear when used with a continuous flow instrument. Unfortunately they do not allow electrosurgical operations with monopolar current, since the electrolyte solution will disperse electrosurgical current in the uterine cavity. Because of this shortcoming, a bipolar electrosurgery system was developed. These solutions should be the media of preference for operative hysteroscopic procedures such as adhesiolysis for which electrosurgery is not required.

## Glycine

Glycine is an amino acid mixed as a 1.5% solution in water. This low-viscosity fluid is supplied in 3-L bags, making it economical and convenient for longer operative procedures. It has been used for decades by urologists for transurethral resections of the prostate because of its excellent optical properties and lack of electrolytes. However, it is a hypotonic solution and carries the risk of volume overload with concurrent hyponatremia.[7] Glycine metabolism generates ammonia, with the potential for encephalopathic changes in patients with underlying liver abnormalities, although the risk appears small. There have been instances of transient visual disturbances following surgery but no documented cases of persistent findings.[8] It is believed that glycine acts as a neuroinhibitory substance at the retina, causing these reversible changes.

## Sorbitol and Mannitol

Sorbitol and mannitol are 6-carbon carbohydrates with similar chemical structures. Their solutions in water are electrolyte free and therefore nonconductive. Similarly to glycine, significant hypoglycemia can occur in the event of fluid overload. While

# Minimally Invasive Surgery

sorbitol is metabolized to glucose and fructose, mannitol is rapidly excreted by the kidney and acts as an osmotic diuretic. This gives it a theoretical advantage for prevention of fluid overload. A concentration of 5% mannitol has been suggested as a close-to-ideal distention medium.[7] It has an osmolarity of 274 mosm/L, similar to that of serum (280 mosm/L).

## Dextran 32% (Hyskon)

Hyskon is a high-viscosity solution composed of dextran 70 (32% w/v) in 10% dextrose (w/v). It is electrolyte free, non-conductive, and immiscible with blood.[9] Its viscous nature helps prevent loss of fluid through fallopian tubes and cervix. Typically 100 mL is sufficient to distend the uterine cavity. The drawback to its high viscosity is difficult delivery of the solution through the small inflow channels of the hysteroscope. Furthermore, the hysteroscopic instruments must be washed immediately in warm water following procedures to prevent crystallization of the fluid and blockage of stopcocks. There have been reports of allergic reactions, pulmonary edema, and deaths.

## AVAILABILITY OF INSTRUMENTS

When preparing for hysteroscopic surgery, it may behoove the surgeon to have different types of instruments available. A continuous-flow, small-caliber diagnostic instrument will allow passage in all but the most stenotic of cervixes (Fig. 35-7). Availability of an operative hysteroscope with a larger sheath improves the ability to clear the cavity because of the greater inflow/outflow capacity of the larger bore sheath. It is important that all these instruments have discrete inflow and outflow channels. Multiple instruments should be readily available

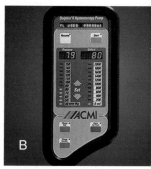
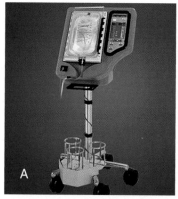

**Figure 35-8   ACMI fluid monitoring system.** *A* and *B*, Dolphin hysteroscopic fluid management system (ACMI), demonstrating fluid input/output digitally.

including scissors, graspers, and biopsy forceps. When a larger operative hysteroscope is used, these other instruments may be slightly larger and more robust. Finally, a smaller pediatric resectoscope as well as a standard resectoscope (26–28F) should be available in case the surgeon encounters a large polyp, fibroid, and so on. Multiple electrodes are available for these various sized resectoscopes. In this way the surgeon is able to treat any pathology appropriate for hysteroscopic management and to readily switch between instruments.

## FLUID PUMPS AND FLUID MONITORING

It is critical during operative hysteroscopic or resectoscopic procedures to monitor fluid inflow and outflow. While little risk exists for substantial fluid overload during a diagnostic procedure, such small procedures often change to operative procedures. Simple systems such as a flow sheet to document input and output may be made part of the operative record. A nurse or one of the operating team may be assigned this critical responsibility. At regular timed intervals the values should be reported, and extra vigilance should be paid if there is a discrepancy of more than 500 mL in a healthy patient. More recently, pump systems have been developed that monitor and visually report inflow/outflow and any deficit (Fig. 35-8). This may be helpful to the operating surgeon who will have a continuous sense of fluid status and be able to terminate the operative procedure should the threshold be passed.

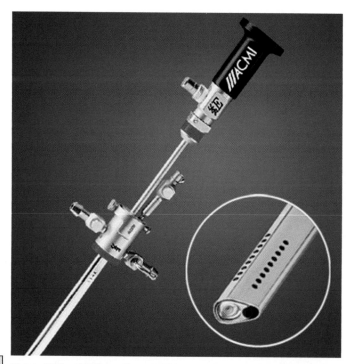

**Figure 35-7   ACMI small operative hysteroscope with continuous inflow/outflow.**

## REFERENCES

1. Bozzini P: Der Lichtleiter oder Beschreibung einer einfachen Vorrichtung und ihrer Anwendung zur Erleuchtung innerer Hoehlen und Zwischenraeume des lebenden animalischen Koerpers. Weimar, Landes-Industrie-Comptoir, 1807. **(IV, C)**
2. Neuwirth RS: A new technique for and additional experience with hysteroscopic resection of submucous fibroids. Am J Obstet Gynecol 1978;131:91–94. **(IV, C)**
3. Haning RV, Harkins, PG, Uehling DT: Preservation of fertility by transcervical resection of a benign mesodermal uterine tumor with a resectoscope and glycine distending medium. Fertil Steril 1980; 33:209–210. **(IV, C)**

4. DeCherney AH, Polan ML: Hysteroscopic management of uterine lesion and intractable uterine bleeding. Obstet Gynecol 1983;61:392–397. **(IIb, B)**

5. DeCherney AH, Russell JB, Graebe RA, et al: Resectoscopic management of müllerian fusion defects. Fertil Steril 1986;45:726–728. **(IIb, B)**

6. Rubin IC: Uterotubal insufflation. St. Louis, CV Mosby, 1947. **(IIb, B)**

7. Baggish MS, Brill AI, Rosensweig B, et al: Fatal acute glycine and sorbitol toxicity during operative hysteroscopy. J Gynecol Surg 1993;9:137–143. **(III, B)**

8. Mizutam AR, Parker J, Katz J, Schmidt J: Visual disturbances, serum glycine levels, and transurethral resection of the prostate. J Urol 1990; 144:697–699. **(IIb, B)**

9. Amin HK, Neuwirth RS: Operative hysteroscopy utilizing dextran as a distending medium. Clin Obstet Gynecol 1983;26:277–284. **(IV, C)**

# Chapter 36

# Surgical Setup for Minimally Invasive Surgery

## Ronald L. Levine, MD, and Resad Pasic, MD, PhD

## KEY POINTS

- Minimally invasive surgery (MIS) requires a different operating room (OR) configuration than that of open surgery.
- Instruments for MIS should be positioned in a standard setup within each hospital OR.
- The OR personnel, including a biotechnician, make up the team that can expedite surgery in the most efficient and cost-effective manner.

MIS has literally become the modus operandi of the practicing gynecologist. However, multiple ORs still have not adapted to routine instrument setups as they have for open abdominal cases, neither for the general surgeons nor for the gynecologists. Similarly many ORs are also not configured for MIS. ORs that are structured for a particular use or specialty can decrease turnover times and increase the efficiency of the personnel, significantly saving costs.[1,2]

Although many articles have been published, mainly by nursing personnel, there are no randomized controlled trials comparing various standardized setups.[3-7] Unfortunately, the setup of instruments and ancillary equipment in the OR varies widely from hospital to hospital, from scrub nurse to scrub nurse and from surgeon to surgeon, depending on their personal routines. In this setting randomized clinical trials are made more difficult.[8]

Previous chapters address the necessary instrumentation utilized in both hysteroscopic and laparoscopic surgery. The question then becomes how to prepare and set up the instruments and the operating suite for the employment of these instruments in the most expeditious manner for the surgeon, the OR nurses, and the patient. Although most scrub personal will adroitly place more than 100 instruments around the back tables of an open case, laparoscopic instruments may often all be in a large pan placed in no discernible order. Another problem that is engendered by endoscopic surgery is the necessity for a large array of electronic equipment and other "gadgets" that are frequently used in this modality. The choice of the instruments also varies greatly from surgeon to surgeon. An additional complicating factor is the plethora of new instruments that become available almost daily as this highly technology driven surgery continues to gain acceptance.

The authors can only give recommendations based on a long anecdotal experience of teaching and performing laparoscopic surgery over more than 30 years. As equipment changes so must the set-up of the room, to meet the exigencies of the time.

## ROOM SETUP

### Personnel

The overall goal of the OR setup should be to perform safe surgery in the most expeditious manner possible; this can only be achieved by utilizing a team approach. The traditional surgical team present during open surgery remains the same during endoscopic surgery (a circulating nurse and a scrub nurse or technician) with one exception, the addition of a biotechnician. The biotechnician is a relatively new constituent of the operating suite and is becoming a standard fixture in many hospitals. This individual should be trained to address any instrument, video, or electrosurgical problems that may occur. The biotechnician need not be a nurse but should be extremely familiar with all of the multiple complex instruments that are utilized in modern endoscopic surgery. The biotechnician frequently acts as a troubleshooter in the care and assembly of the instruments employed in endoscopic surgery and may act as an assistant to the circulator by obtaining materials that may not be in the OR. This individual can shorten OR time by decreasing downtime that occurs owing to failed instrument function. It is imperative that the biotechnician be trained regarding OR procedures such as antisepsis and the standard rules of OR etiquette and behavior.[9]

The instruments that are used in open surgery are for the most part of simple construction with few if any movable components, whereas in endoscopy, many of the instruments have complex interchangeable parts, connections, and moving pieces, making them more subject to failure of one or more parts. Many surgeons have faced the frustration of a bipolar forceps that does not work at a crucial moment. This can be for multiple reasons: a malfunctioning electrosurgical generator, a poor connection from instrument to generator, a broken component within the forceps, or the forceps not being reassembled correctly after cleaning and sterilization. Although it should be mandatory for the surgeon to know all the instruments and be able to troubleshoot, this is not always the case. Another major problem in gynecologic endoscopy is the plethora of new instruments and energy modalities that are marketed almost daily that make it almost impossible for the surgeon to be knowledgeable of all the changes. The role of the biotechnician is to troubleshoot technical problems in order to reduce OR time. This person therefore is a cost-effective part of the OR team.

# Minimally Invasive Surgery

Many surgical nurses and scrub technicians were trained prior to the current ubiquitous use of endoscopy. It is therefore necessary for these members of the team to receive some type of postgraduate instruction in the complexities of gynecologic endoscopy. An ongoing program of in-service education should be required in a modern endoscopic surgery operating suite.

## Position of Operating Table, Equipment, and Lights for Laparoscopy

Often, little thought is given to the placement of the operating table in relation to the room. Several conditions must be met:

1. The table should be oriented so that the doors of the room are located at the head of the table or at the side of the table so that when the patient is in the lithotomy position she is not exposed to the door opening (Fig. 36-1).
2. The monitors and video equipment are best suspended from ceiling mounts. This avoids clutter and keeps the myriad of wires and connections off the floor (Fig. 36-2). The table has to be placed so that monitors can be positioned for the best view by the surgeon and the assistant. If two monitors are employed, then one may be on each side of the patient's feet, but if only one monitor is used, then it is best located between the abducted legs.

Although the OR lights are usually turned down or off during laparoscopy, they need to be positioned so that one light is over the abdomen for placement of ports and for suturing and another can be directed at the vaginal area (Fig. 36-3).

## Position of Table and Lights for Hysteroscopy

There are only minor differences in positioning from laparoscopy to hysteroscopic surgery. Since all hysteroscopic surgery is performed vaginally, the monitors are placed near the patient's side, or in the case of suspended monitors, a single monitor may be placed just over the abdomen in the midline. In either case, the monitor must be positioned for easy visual access by the hysteroscopist. The OR lights are positioned to illuminate the

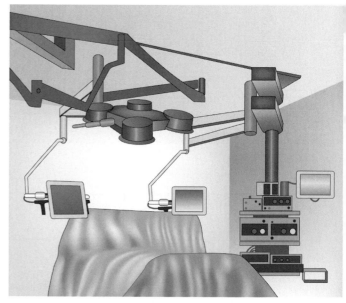

**Figure 36-2  The ideal MIS operating suite utilizes modular units that are suspended from the ceiling and capable of moving to various positions.** This keeps the myriad of wires and cables off the floor and reduces both clutter and entanglement while increasing visual acquisition.

vagina, so they should be shining from behind and above the surgeon (Fig. 36-4).

## Position of Surgeons and Staff for Laparoscopy

Traditionally, in laparoscopy prior to the use of cameras and video, the operating surgeon stood at the left side of the patient so that his or her right hand would be free to use the instruments. However, in the modern OR, the surgeon may stand on either side, often depending on which hand is the dominant one. In laparoscopy the surgeon should be able to use either hand

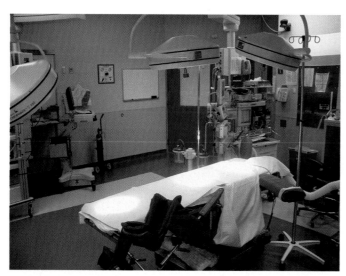

**Figure 36-1  The operating table should always be placed so that the entrance to the OR is either at the head of the table or at the side to limit exposure of the patient when the door is opened.**

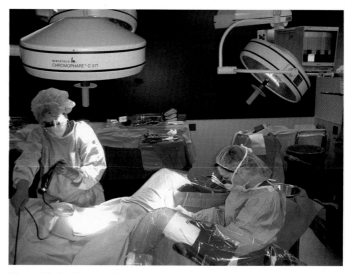

**Figure 36-3  The position of OR lights is important for the expeditious performance of surgery. If the lights are positioned prior to the onset of the operation, it saves time.** Note that one light is used for the vaginal portion of the case, while the other is directly over the abdomen for port placement and site closure.

## Surgical Setup for Minimally Invasive Surgery

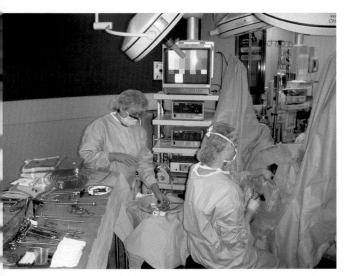

**Figure 36-4   During hysteroscopy the only necessary light is shining into the vaginal area.** In this picture, the monitor is part of a modular unit, so it is to the side of the patient, but when only the monitor is suspended, it is best placed over the patient's abdomen directly in front of the surgeon.

effectively, and often the surgeon may switch sides in order to manipulate the instruments in an expeditious manner unless there is an assistant who has similar skills. If the assistant and the surgeon operate as a team, the surgery often is a beautiful ballet of the hands, and it is frequently difficult for an observer watching the screen to discern whose hands are controlling which instruments. This team approach produces the best surgical result.

As noted previously, the assistant usually stands on the opposite side of the surgeon, and the scrub person may be either between the patient's legs or behind the surgeon in the more traditional placement (Fig. 36-5).

### Position of Surgeons and Staff for Hysteroscopy

During hysteroscopy, it is often unnecessary to have a formal assistant, since the scrub person can assist in the holding of instruments. In this case, the scrub person stands alongside the surgeon, who usually is sitting. The necessary instruments may be on a Mayo stand next to the scrub person.

### Position of Patient for Laparoscopy

The laparoscopic surgical patient should be positioned well down on the operating table with her buttocks just over the edge to allow for the placement of a uterine manipulator that can be moved in the most advantageous manner. The feet should be placed in a well-padded boot stirrup that can be adjusted from a position in which there is no flexion of the thigh relative to the abdomen to a position in which the thigh is almost at a 90-degree angle to the abdomen to permit vaginal surgery (Fig. 36-6).

The patient's arms can be tucked in at her sides by utilizing the sides of the lift sheet. Some ORs use a plastic or metal curved shield to hold the arm close to the body. The OR personnel must be careful to protect the patient's fingers from injury when the table end is either dropped or brought back to the full position. This can be accomplished by placing and taping the hand into the bottom portion of a plastic IV bottle that has the top cut off (Fig. 36-7). The goal is to have the arms out of the way of the operating surgeon without injuring the patient. However, especially if the patient is obese, this may be difficult to accomplish and may require the arm with the IV in place to be out on an arm board. It is often possible to bring the arm up over the chest and to secure it in this position so that it is safely out of the way and there is no danger of causing injury to the brachial plexus.

### Position of Patient for Hysteroscopy

The positioning of the patient for hysteroscopy requires placing the patient in the traditional lithotomy position, either using

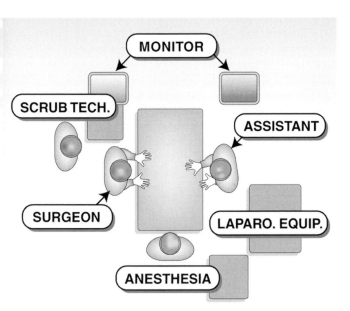

**Figure 36-5   If two monitors are available, one should be on each side of the patient's legs.** The surgeon and assistant are positioned as described in the text.

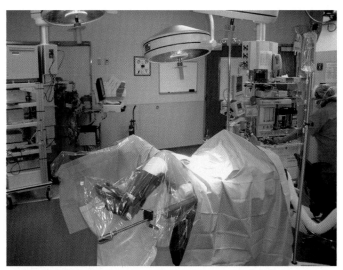

**Figure 36-6   The legs should be placed in a boot type stirrup that puts the weight of the leg primarily on the sole of the foot.** The boot stirrup can be adjusted to either raise up for the vaginal portion of the surgery or drop so that the thigh is virtually even with the abdomen.

# Minimally Invasive Surgery

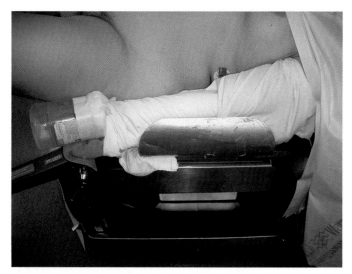

**Figure 36-7 The patient's arm may be held close to the body with the use of a metal or plastic shield.** The fingers are protected by use of half of a plastic bottle taped in place.

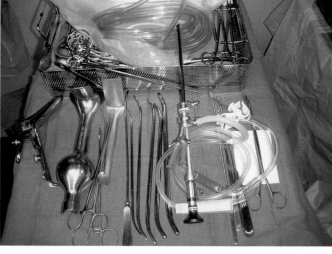

**Figure 36-9 Instruments are placed on the back table or a Mayo stand in the approximate order of use.** These instruments are used during the vaginal portion of a case.

candy cane stirrups or boot stirrups. If candy canes are used, then one must be careful in positioning the lower extremities so as not to place too much stretch on the femoral nerve. Boot stirrups may be preferable for longer operative hysteroscopic cases.

## Instrument Layout for Laparoscopy

Instruments on the back table for laparoscopy should be set up in relative order of use. They should generally be in a standardized placement for the institution (Fig. 36-8). It is important that the scrub nurse be able to be relieved during an operation by other personnel without causing confusion regarding the location of instruments, particularly in the dimmed light of the OR. Individual surgeons should have a preference card on file, with a plastic-coated copy available in the OR for reference if needed by the scrub personnel (Fig. 36-9).

A general guide for the order of use of instruments prior to the performance of the pneumoperitoneum is as follows:

1. Vaginal specula: bivalve and weighted
2. Vaginal retractors (side wall)
3. Single-tooth tenaculum
4. Uterine sound
5. Pratt dilators
6. Sponge stick
7. Uterine manipulator

The preceding instruments may be placed in order on a back table. A Mayo stand may hold the following (Fig. 36-10):

1. Light cable
2. Camera head
3. Insufflation tubing

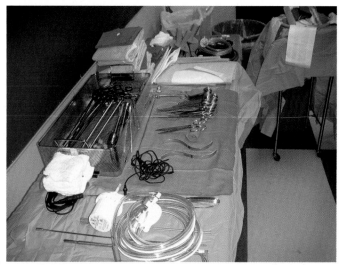

**Figure 36-8 The instruments on the back table are placed in an orderly fashion that may change from institution to institution.**

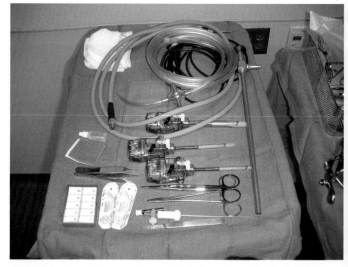

**Figure 36-10 A Mayo stand holds the instruments that are used during the entry phase of the laparoscopy.**

4. Scopes (5 mm and 10 mm)
5. Electro-cable (for electrosurgical generator)
6. Veress needle
7. Trocars
8. Suction tubing
9. Scalpel

As stated earlier, there are a great number of laparoscopic surgical instruments and variations among them. They may be placed on the back table in a standard order for the individual OR, but they may be grouped according to use and size.

Five-millimeter instruments:

1. Graspers: traumatic and atraumatic
2. Dissectors
3. Scissors: curved and straight

A similar method can then be used for instruments of other sizes (3 mm or 10–12 mm).

The next group of instruments is those needed for closure of the incisional sites. They may be grouped on the back table. These should include the following:

1. Small S-shaped retractors
2. Needle holders
3. Suture
4. Hemostats
5. Suture scissors

Many surgeons use some newer technology pieces such as harmonic energy instruments or electrosurgery systems that require their own specialized unit to supply the energy. This type of equipment also uses an array of disposable instruments and cables that may require a single Mayo stand to hold all of the supply in one place.

## Instrument Layout for Hysteroscopy

Hysteroscopy requires many fewer instruments than laparoscopy. Instruments may be divided into three distinct sets: diagnostic, operative, and global ablative. However, the hysteroscopes may be interchangeable in all three sets unless they are matched or if the OR is lucky enough to have several scopes in each category of viewing angle. Each set minimally needs a 12-degree and a 25- or 30-degree scope.[10]

### Diagnostic Hysteroscopy

Diagnostic hysteroscopy requires very few instruments. The tray containing these instruments is Spartan compared with a laparoscopic setup. Often, diagnostic hysteroscopy is accomplished in the office or clinic with a small-caliber flexible hysteroscope using a syringe of saline as the uterine distending mechanism. The same technique may be used in the OR, but a rigid hysteroscope can be substituted for the flexible if needed. Rigid hysteroscopy may require some cervical dilatation, so the setup should include a dilation and curettage set that contains several types of specula (weighted and bivalves of various sizes), a uterine sound, a tenaculum, and cervical dilators.

Diagnostic hysteroscopy can be performed with either $CO_2$ gas, which requires a specialized insufflator, or with just saline or other physiologic media for fluid distention. The saline may be instilled with 60-mL syringes connected to the scope sheath

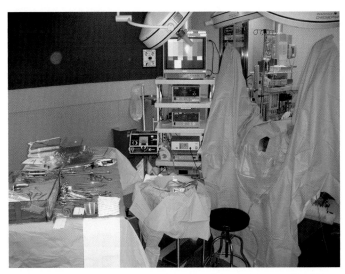

**Figure 36-11 The fluid management system should be positioned in easy view of the surgeon.** A bag is in place to collect the distention fluid that is returned.

with IV tubing or alternatively as a 500- or 1000-mL bag. The entire setup may be placed on a Mayo stand.

### Operative Hysteroscopy

The setup for operative hysteroscopy may entail the use of a resectoscope and also requires fluid monitoring. Many surgeons use a diagnostic setup to begin their operative cases and then proceed to an operative setup. The use of a resectoscope usually requires a fluid collection system placed under the patient's buttocks with tubing that returns all fluid for an accurate accounting of input and outputs (I&Os). Newer fluid management systems may aid the surgeon and operating team in tracking fluid I&Os (Fig. 36-11). The management system should be in close proximity to the patient's side and well within the view of the operator. It is often helpful to have the electrosurgical generator on the opposite side to decrease the amount of tubing, cables, and so on, coming from this area (camera cable, fluid management tubes, electrosurgical cable, suction tubing). The position of the video monitor was described earlier.

### Global Ablative Surgery

Currently many global ablative techniques are available, and each has an individualized setup. Some, such as the balloon technology, require very little equipment as they do not require the use of a hysteroscope and a camera. Others, such as the hydrothermal ablator, need essentially the same setup as required for diagnostic hysteroscopy.

## SUMMARY

It is worthwhile to make an effort to standardize both laparoscopic and hysteroscopic setups across obstetrics and gynecology departments. Evaluation of actual use of individual instruments may identify little used instruments or opportunities for surgeons to agree on one instrument or another for their setup. Elimination of redundancy may decrease costs for instrument cleaning, decrease time spent reassembling trays, and decrease cost of eventual instrument replacement after multiple use cycles.

# REFERENCES

1. Kenyon TA, Urbach DR, Speer JB, et al: Dedicated minimally invasive surgery suites increase operating room efficiency. Surg Endosc 2001; 15:1140–1143. **(III, C)**
2. Mangum S, Cutler K: Increased efficiency through OR redesign and process simplification. AORN J 2002;76:1041–1046. **(IV, C)**
3. Standards, Recommended Practices, and Guidelines with Official AORN Statements. Denver, CO, AORN, 2005.
4. Winer WK, Operating room personnel: In Sanfilippo JS, Levine RL (eds): Operative Gynecologic Endoscopy, 2nd ed. New York, Springer-Verlag, 1996, pp 412–422. **(IV, C)**
5. Winer WK: The role of the operating room staff in operative laparoscopy. J Am Assoc Gynecol Laparosc 1993;1:86–88. **(IV, C)**
6. Winer WK, Lyons TL: Suggested set-up and layout of instruments and equipment for advanced operative laparoscopy. J Am Assoc Gynecol Laparosc 1995;2:231–234. **(IV, C)**
7. Winer WK: The set-up for operative endoscopy. Laser Nurs 1991; 5:139–145. **(IV, C)**
8. Kadar N: Randomized trials involving laparoscopic surgery: valid research strategy or academic gimmick? J Gynecol Endosc 1994; 3:69–73. **(IV, C)**
9. Warren JM: Preparation of nonmedical personnel in the operating room environment. Med Instrum 1981;15(3):156–158. **(IV, C)**
10. Levine RL: Hysteroscopic instruments. In Pasic R, Levine RL (eds): A Practical Manual of Hysteroscopy and Endometrial Ablation Techniques: A Clinical Cookbook. London, Parthenon Publishing, 2004, pp 13–24. **(IV, C)**

# Chapter 37

# Laparoscopic Procedures

Farr Nezhat, MD, FACOG, FACS, Ali Mahdavi, MD, FACOG, and Tanja Pejovic, MD, PhD

## KEY POINTS

- Diagnostic laparoscopy is the most commonly performed laparoscopic gynecologic procedure. The main indications are infertility, pelvic pain, pelvic inflammatory disease, and suspected pelvic mass or ectopic pregnancy.
- Bipolar coagulation is the most commonly used laparoscopic tubal occlusion method in the United States. Mechanical methods make microsurgical reversal more likely to succeed.
- Laparoscopic linear salpingostomy is the method of choice for surgical management of most tubal pregnancies.
- Although clinical examination and the results of preoperative workup often indicate the benign or malignant nature of an ovarian cyst, only histologic study can provide the absolute diagnosis. Therefore, as clinically indicated for laparoscopic management of adnexal masses, the availability of immediate histologic diagnosis with frozen section is crucial.
- For women who require abdominal hysterectomy, the laparoscopic approach offers the benefit of less postoperative discomfort, shorter hospital stay, and quicker recovery.
- Laparoscopic hysterectomy is not cost effective compared with vaginal hysterectomy.
- Laparoscopic myomectomy is associated with accelerated postoperative recovery compared with laparotomy. The incidence of uterine rupture and recurrence can be slightly higher compared with an open procedure.
- If standard surgical techniques are followed, laparoscopic procedures for stress urinary incontinence and pelvic organ prolapse should have similar outcomes and cure rates compared with an open approach.
- In experienced hands, laparoscopic pelvic and para-aortic lymphadenectomy appears to be a safe, adequate, and feasible procedure, with a low complication rate.
- Surgical therapy is warranted as the first line of treatment for women with endometriosis who have pain symptoms and desire to become pregnant as soon as possible.

Gynecologic applications of laparoscopy have contributed greatly to the popularization of laparoscopic surgery. Laparoscopic gynecologic surgery has many accepted applications, from diagnostic use to facilitation of hysteroscopy and reconstructive pelvic surgery. Gynecologic oncologists also have embraced laparoscopic techniques that are now being evaluated in prospective randomized trials. According to the American Association of Gynecologic Laparoscopists (AAGL) survey of members regarding patterns in the use of laparoscopic procedures, diagnostic laparoscopy was the most commonly performed laparoscopic procedure.[1]

## INDICATIONS FOR LAPAROSCOPY

The main indications for diagnostic gynecologic laparoscopy include infertility, pelvic pain, pelvic inflammatory disease, suspected pelvic masses, and ectopic pregnancy. The evaluation of pelvic pain and infertility focuses on identification of endometriosis, adhesions, or tubal blockage. Less common indications for diagnostic laparoscopy include evaluation of possible uterine perforation during dilation and curettage, evaluation of early postoperative complications, removal of foreign bodies, and evaluation of pelvic tumors before laparotomy. The workup prior to performing diagnostic laparoscopy for acute pelvic pain should include documentation of the location, severity and duration of symptoms, last menstrual period, pregnancy test, urinanalysis, and complete blood count.[2]

## ADHESIOLYSIS

Peritoneal adhesions may cause pelvic pain, infertility, and bowel obstruction. Formation of intra-abdominal adhesions between the operative scar and the underlying viscera is a common consequence of laparotomy. Patients with midline incisions have more adhesions than those with Pfannenstiel incisions.[3] Patients with midline incisions performed for gynecologic indications also have more adhesions than patients with any abdominal incisions for obstetric indications.[4] Adhesions to the bowel are more common after supraumbilical midline incisions.[5]

Impairment of fertility has been a major indication for adhesiolysis, and severity of adhesions is considered an inverse prognostic factor in the success of infertility surgery.[6] After adhesiolysis, pregnancy rates vary according to the extent of adnexal damage and, to a lesser degree, the severity of the adhesions.[7]

### Formation of Adhesions

Normal fibrinolytic activity usually prevents formation of fibrinous attachments during the first 72 to 96 hours after injury. Mesothelial repair starts within 5 days after trauma when a

# Minimally Invasive Surgery

single layer of mesothelium covers the raw area, replacing the fibrinous exudates. However, if the fibrinolytic activity of the peritoneum is suppressed, fibroblasts will proliferate and form adhesions with collagen deposition and vascular proliferation. Factors that suppress fibrinolytic activity and promote postoperative adhesion formation are ischemia, drying of serosal surfaces, excessive suturing, traction of the peritoneum, blood clots in the peritoneal cavity, infection, prolonged surgery, and adnexal trauma.[3]

The current opinion is that operative laparoscopy may be more efficient than laparotomy in treating postoperative adhesions and should be the initial step in their management when clinically appropriate. Several animal and clinical studies compared the formation of postoperative adhesions after fertility-promoting operations by laparotomy and laparoscopy. With few exceptions, laparoscopy resulted in the development of fewer re-formed adhesions and new (de novo) adhesions.[8,9]

Decreased adhesion formation after laparoscopic surgery has been attributed to the reduced presence of foreign bodies within the peritoneal cavity that usually stimulate dense and more numerous adhesions. The type of injury to the peritoneum also influences the formation of adhesions. The potential to form adhesions is much higher in visceral than in parietal peritoneum.[10] Transperitoneal laparoscopy induced fewer adhesions than transperitoneal laparotomy. Also, there is a presumed advantage of the extraperitoneal approach in avoidance of adhesion formation because peritoneum remains intact and direct contact with intra-abdominal structures is thereby avoided. However, when the peritoneum is dissected off the abdominal wall, it is partially devascularized, leading to potential scars and adhesions. Interestingly, in a murine model, the totally extraperitoneal approach did not completely prevent the formation of adhesions.[11]

Three or four abdominal puncture sites are necessary to perform adequate adhesiolysis: an infraumbilical site for the videolaparoscope and two lower quadrant and one suprapubic trocar for the instruments. Through the lateral trocar at the assistant's side, an atraumatic grasping forceps is inserted to hold the adhesion, stretch it, and identify its boundaries and avascular planes. The opposite trocar is used for scissors or the suction-irrigation probe. Adhesions are cut close to the involved organ at both ends and may be removed from the abdominal cavity if possible. Vascular adhesions are coagulated with laser or microelectrodes before being cut. Intestinal adhesions may be cut first, followed by parovarian and peritubal adhesions. This approach allows for progressive exposure of the pelvic structures. Grasping forceps are essential for applying traction to the ovary, tubes, bowel, and the abdominal wall to identify a free plane of dissection. Whenever possible, either the adhesions or the ovarian ligaments are grasped rather than the ovarian cortex to reduce trauma to the ovary. Once the ovaries are mobilized, the peritubal adhesions are freed. Adhesions can be safely coagulated and incised with a $CO_2$ laser, superpulse (40 W) laser, ultrapulse (20–80 W and 25–200 mJ) fiber laser (15–25 W), or microelectrode (15–20 W in cutting mode).[3] In the case of dense adhesions, hydrodissection with a suction-irrigator may be useful to create tissue planes before dissection. Once the pelvic structures are freed, the cul-de-sac is filled with lactated Ringer's solution and the adnexa are allowed to float. Filmy adhesions become visible and can be removed from their attachments by microdissection. Fimbrial folds also float and disperse in the fluid, and their adhesions become visible and amenable to dissection with fine scissors or the ultrapulse laser. Laser beams other than ultrapulse are greater than 1 mm and therefore too wide for these adhesions. Thermal damage may occur with electrosurgery or the fiber laser and thus may not be optimal in these delicate procedures.

## STERILIZATION

The use of laparoscopy as a safe outpatient sterilization technique has contributed greatly to the popularity of laparoscopy in gynecology. Single, double, and triple puncture techniques have been described. Techniques for tubal occlusion have included electrocoagulation, mechanical methods, and ligation methods. Bipolar coagulation is now the most commonly used laparoscopic occlusion method in the United States.[12] To maximize the effectiveness of bipolar coagulation, at least 3 cm of the isthmic portion of the fallopian tube must be completely coagulated by use of sufficient energy (25 W) delivered in a cutting waveform. Use of a current meter, rather than a visual endpoint or a defined period, has been suggested to indicate complete coagulation. Mechanical occlusion devices commonly used in the United States include the silicone rubber band (Falope ring), the spring-loaded clip (Hulka-Clemens clip), and the titanium clip lined with silicone rubber (Filshie clip). Mechanical methods have no associated risk of electrical burn and destroy less of the fallopian tube (5 mm for clips and 2 cm for rings), making microsurgical reversal more likely to succeed. The silicone band can only be applied to a fallopian tube that is sufficiently mobile to allow it to be drawn into the applicator; tubal adhesions or a thickened or dilated fallopian tube increase the risk of misplacement and subsequent failure. Techniques for laparoscopic ligation and resection of portions of both tubes have also been described.

The 5-year and 10-year pregnancy rates, respectively, for different methods are as follows[13]: bipolar coagulation: 16.5 and 24.8 per 1000 procedures, silicone band methods: 10 and 17.7 per 1000 procedures, and spring clip: 31.7 and 36.5 per 1000 procedures.

The risk of ectopic pregnancy varies substantially with the method and timing of sterilization. Based on CREST (U.S. Collaborative Review of Sterilization) study data,[13] bipolar coagulation had the highest cumulative probability of ectopic pregnancy (17.1/1000), and postpartum partial salpingectomy had the lowest cumulative probability (1.5/1000).

## ECTOPIC PREGNANCY

The treatment of ectopic pregnancy has been dramatically changed over the last 15 years by the use of operative laparoscopy and chemotherapy (see Chapter 15). Initially the management included salpingo-oophorectomy; thereafter, salpingectomy by laparotomy. With the development of laparoscopic techniques, linear salpingostomy became the method of choice for surgical management of an unruptured tubal pregnancy. Tubal salvage has been further improved by the use of methotrexate in selected hemodynamically stable patients.[14] Today, ruptured tubal pregnancies are treated successfully by endoscopy if the bleeding has

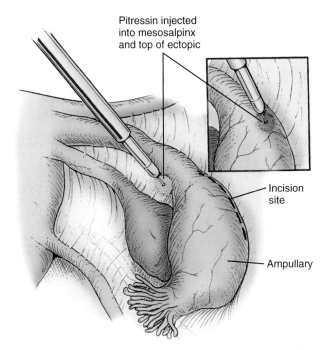

**Figure 37-1** Injection of vasopressin into the mesosalpinx and the incision site.

the antimesenteric surface of the tubal segment containing the gestational products (Fig. 37-1). With a laser, microelectrode, or scissors, a linear incision is made on the antimesenteric surface extending 1 to 2 cm over the thinnest portion of the tube containing the pregnancy (Fig. 37-2). The gestational products usually protrude through the incision and slowly slip out of the tube; it is then removed by use of hydrodissection or laparoscopic forceps (Figs. 37-3 and 37-4). Oozing from the tube is common but usually ceases spontaneously. Occasionally, coagulation is necessary with a defocused laser beam or an electrocoagulator. Salpingectomy is preferable to salpingostomy in the presence of uncontrolled bleeding, tubal destruction, or a recurrent pregnancy in the same tube.[15]

Salpingectomy is done by progressively desiccating and cutting the mesosalpinx, beginning with the proximal isthmic portion and progressing to the fimbriated end of the tube (Figs. 37-5 to 37-7). The isolated segment containing the gestational tissue is removed intact or in sectioned parts through the 10-mm trocar sleeve. Products of conception can be placed in an endoscopic bag (endo-bag) and removed. Adhesions or other pathologic processes such as endometriosis are treated after removal of the tubal pregnancy. The pelvic cavity should be irrigated and washed to entirely remove the gestational tissue, since reimplantation of this tissue can occur. Usually, the patient is discharged home subsequently on the day of surgery.

## FALLOPIAN TUBE SURGERY

Tubal abnormalities cause infertility in 20% of infertile couples. Pelvic inflammatory disease (PID), previous pelvic operations, ruptured appendix, and endometriosis are the principal causes.

Diagnostic laparoscopy is routinely used to diagnose acute PID in Europe.[16] Laparoscopic procedures to treat pelvic abscesses have been described by several authors.[17,18] The abscesses are

ceased or is stopped adequately. A 10-mm suction instrument quickly cleanses the abdominal cavity. Forced irrigation with lactated Ringer's solution dislodges clots and trophoblastic tissue from the serosa with minimal trauma.

For unruptured tubal pregnancies, the tube is identified and mobilized. To reduce bleeding, 5 to 7 mL of diluted vasopressin (20 units in 100 mL normal saline) is injected with a 20-gauge spinal or laparoscopic needle into the mesosalpinx and over

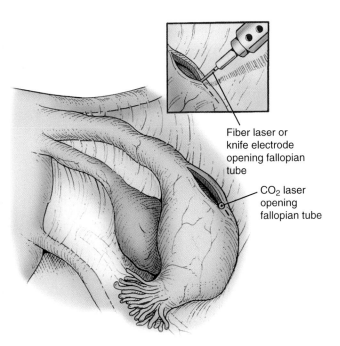

**Figure 37-2** Salpingostomy is made with a $CO_2$ laser, knife electrode, or fiber laser.

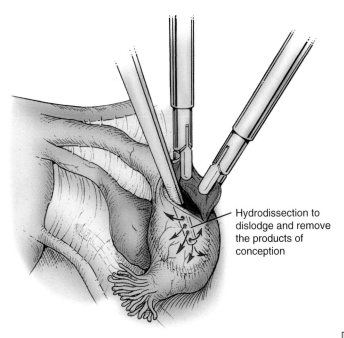

**Figure 37-3** Hydrodissection is performed to dislodge the ectopic pregnancy.

551

# Minimally Invasive Surgery

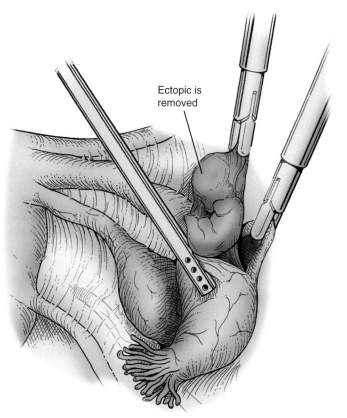

**Figure 37-4    The ectopic pregnancy is removed from the tube.**

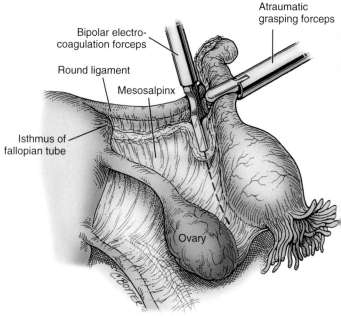

**Figure 37-6    The tube is separated from the uterus.**

dense walls. The bowel often adheres to pelvic organs and is dissected with difficulty. The adnexa may appear as a dense mass, making it difficult to distinguish between the pyosalpinx and the ovary. In these cases, adhesiolysis is technically difficult and associated with a high risk of complications.[20]

Distal tubal obstruction has been treated with microsurgical techniques with pregnancy rates of 20% to 30%, 2 years post-operatively.[21] Fimbrioplasty and lysis of peritubal and parovarian adhesions result in the best outcome (Figs. 37-8 and 37-9).

A hydrosalpinx results from distal tubal occlusion and is characterized by a dilated tube filled with clear fluid. The presence of numerous fixed adhesions and thick tubal wall are associated with poor pregnancy rates and therefore are

separated by means of a combination of sharp and blunt dissection and hydrodissection. After the abscess is mobilized, it is drained.[19] Its walls are removed in sections by the use of 5-mm graspers. The upper abdomen is also irrigated, and the remainder of the fluid is aspirated with the patient in a reverse Trendelenburg position. In contrast to the adhesions associated with an acute abscess, chronic tubo-ovarian abscesses have

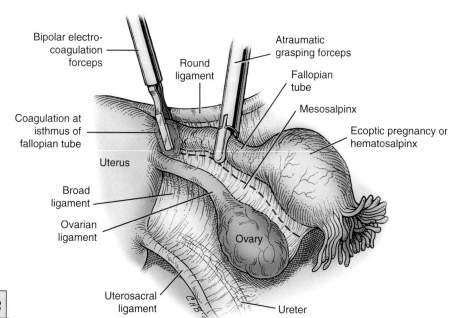

**Figure 37-5    Coagulation of the mesosalpinx is performed for complete salpingectomy.** Inset shows transection of mesosalpinx with scissors or $CO_2$ laser.

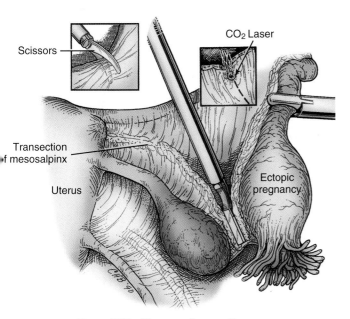

Figure 37-7    The procedure continues.

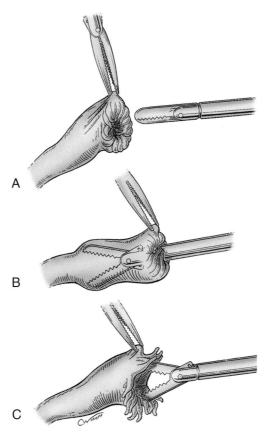

Figure 37-9    **Steps in performing fimbrioplasty.** *A*, Introduction of grasping forceps. *B*, Opening the forceps. *C*, Withdrawing the forceps.

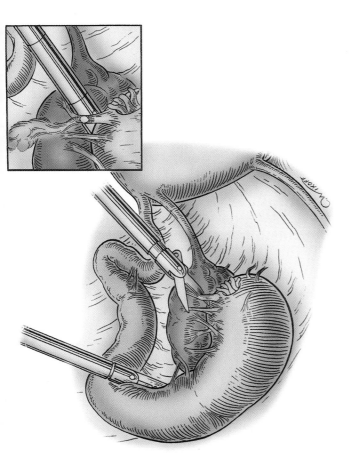

Figure 37-8    **Sharp microscissors or an ultrapulse $CO_2$ laser is used for fimbrioplasty.** The tube is under traction.

contraindications to tuboplasty. For neosalpingostomy, after the adhesions surrounding the tubes and ovaries are released, the distal portion of the tube is manipulated into position with the grasper and the uterine fundus is used as a shelf.[19] Fluid distention of the tube with chromopertubation allows identification of the avascular central point that is the thinnest portion of the tube. A cruciate incision using the $CO_2$ laser or scissors creates several flaps (Fig. 37-10). The edges are flared back by use of the defocused laser (10 W) (Fig. 37-11). If the tube is thick and does not flare back with the laser, the edges are sutured to the tubal serosa by use of 4-0 to 6-0 polydioxanone. Tubal patency is confirmed by injection of diluted indigo carmine through the uterine cannula.

The goal of fimbrioplasty is to expose the fimbria to restore normal function. Tubal phimosis results from fimbrial agglutination and adhesions that bind the fimbriated end to the ovary or cover the distal end. Chromopertubation distends the tube. If adhesions cover the ostia, they are incised with scissors and separated with a $CO_2$ laser, microscissors, a fiber laser, or a fine electrode tip (see Fig. 37-8). The tube is immobilized by using the uterus as a shelf or by steadying its position with a blunt probe. To lyse adhesions around the fimbria, a closed 3-mm forceps is inserted into the fallopian tube through the phimotic opening. The jaws of the forceps are opened within the tube; the opened forceps are withdrawn (see Fig. 37-9). This procedure is repeated until satisfactory deglutination of the fimbria is obtained. Gentle manipulation decreases the chance of bleeding.

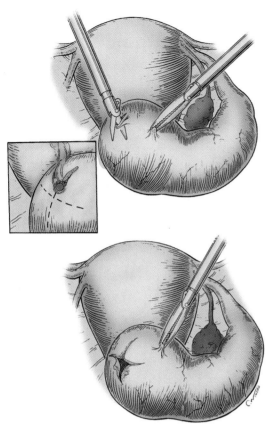

**Figure 37-10    Cruciate incisions in distal end of the tube.** Sharp microscissors or an ultrapulse $CO_2$ laser is used.

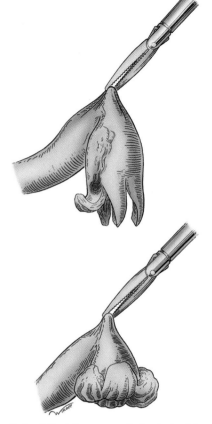

**Figure 37-11    Ends of the tube are everted using a defocused laser beam.**

The selection of patients who can benefit from tubal reconstructive operations is mostly based on the results of a preoperative hysterosalpingogram (HSG) and the laparoscopic appearance of the tubes. Although mucosal folds can be seen on HSG, the correlation between radiologic studies and endoscopy in assessing the tubal mucosa has been poor in many instances. Henry-Suchet et al,[22] in a study of 231 tubes during tubal microsurgery, demonstrated that salpingoscopy was more accurate in detecting tubal mucosal abnormalities than was HSG. Laparoscopic salpingoscopy permits detailed examination of the ampullary endosalpinx. The surgeon should examine and decide on treatment of the contralateral tube in a woman with tubal pregnancy.

With advances in laparoscopic microinstruments, refinement of three-dimensional video cameras, and further improvement of surgical skills, microsurgical tubal anastomosis has become possible entirely by laparoscopy. Robotic assistance may facilitate laparoscopic tubal anastomosis by filtering tremors, reducing the surgeon's fatigue, and scaling the maneuvers.[23]

# ADNEXAL MASS

## Etiology
Suspected ovarian neoplasm is a common clinical problem affecting women of all ages. Although the majority of adnexal masses in reproductive-age women are due to benign processes,

the primary goal of the diagnostic evaluation is the exclusion of malignancy. Extrapolating from the data of ovarian cancer, it can be estimated that approximately 5% to 10% of women in the United States will undergo a surgical procedure for a suspected ovarian neoplasm during their lifetime.

The most common adnexal masses in reproductive-age women are benign functional cysts of the ovaries, and these tend to regress spontaneously. These include follicular cysts, corpus luteum cysts, theca-lutein cysts, and polycystic ovaries. The other benign conditions include endometriosis (with ovarian endometriotic cysts), inflammatory enlargements of the fallopian tubes and ovaries (hydrosalpinges, tubo-ovarian abscess) due to pelvic infection, ectopic pregnancy, and trophoblastic disease.

True benign ovarian neoplasms can also cause adnexal enlargement. These include serous or mucinous cystadenoma and benign cystic teratomas. It is unclear whether these are precursors of malignant neoplasms, although some changes may represent true ovarian intra-epithelial neoplasia. Other neoplastic processes include parovarian cysts, pedunculated fibroids, and ovarian and fallopian tube cancers. In certain instances, the mass is clinically indeterminate and may be due to nongynecologic causes such as full bladder, stool in colon, distended cecum, peritoneal cyst, appendiceal abscess, diverticular abscess, Crohn's disease, ectopic kidney, urachal cyst, abdominal wall tumor, lymphoma, retroperitoneal sarcoma, metastatic tumor to the ovaries, and malignant diseases of the gastrointestinal system.

## Clinical Presentation and Evaluation

The majority of patients have symptoms related to compression of the pelvic organs. Less commonly, an ovarian mass is discovered during a routine pelvic examination. In patients with a malignant process, the most common clinical symptom is abdominal discomfort due to ascites. In several surgical series, the reported incidence of ovarian malignancy in patients with a preoperative diagnosis of ovarian mass ranges from 13% to 21%. The most important predictor of malignancy is the age of the patient. In fact, the risk that an ovarian neoplasm is malignant increases 12-fold from ages 12 to 29 and 60 to 69.

The evaluation of a woman with a suspected adnexal mass consists of a clinical history, including a gynecologic history and family history of ovarian or breast cancer. The physical examination should include an abdominal, pelvic, and rectovaginal examination. However, physical examination alone is often inaccurate in determining whether an adnexal mass is benign or malignant, unless there are associated findings of disseminated disease. Imaging studies are usually required for further evaluation.

There are no universally accepted criteria for the sonographic description of ovarian disease. No single gray-scale or Doppler sonographic feature allows distinction between benign and malignant adnexal masses. Although most comparison studies have found that gray-scale is superior to Doppler sonography or that Doppler offers no significant improvement over gray-scale sonography, a minority of studies report Doppler features to be superior. Sassone et al[24] evaluated an ultrasound scoring system to predict ovarian malignancy. Transvaginal sonographic pelvic images of 143 patients were correlated with surgicopathologic findings. The variables in the scoring system included the inner wall structure of the adnexal cyst, wall thickness, presence and thickness of septa, and echogenicity. The scoring system was useful in distinguishing benign from malignant masses, with specificity of 83%, sensitivity of 100%, and positive and negative predictive values of 37% and 100%, respectively. Subsequently, Alcazar and Jurado[25] developed a logistic model to predict malignancy based on menopausal status, ultrasound morphology, and color Doppler findings in 79 adnexal masses. The authors derived a mathematical formula to estimate preoperatively the risk of malignancy of a given adnexal mass in a simple and reproducible way. When this formula was applied prospectively, 56 of 58 (96.5%) adnexal masses were correctly classified.

In general, a CT scan is not indicated routinely for the evaluation of the adnexal mass. However, it is probably indicated in the evaluation of a patient with a hard, fixed, lateralized mass; ascites; abnormal liver function tests; or a palpable abdomino-pelvic mass.

### Tumor Markers

Serum tumor markers for malignant germ cell tumors, lactic dehydrogenase (LDH), beta human chorionic gonadotropin (β-hCG), and α-fetoprotein should be obtained in the young patient with a cystic-solid or solid adnexal mass. Serum CA 125 and carcinoembryonic antigen (CEA) should also be obtained in patients suspected of gynecologic or GI cancer, respectively. However, in premenopausal women, CA 125 is elevated in a variety of benign conditions and may cloud, rather than clarify, the differential diagnosis of ovarian mass.

## Management

The crucial decisions regarding management of a premenopausal woman with an adnexal mass are 2-fold: to observe the patient or proceed with surgical removal of the mass, and if surgical removal is indicated, when is a laparoscopic approach justified?

During the reproductive years, cystic adnexal masses that are less than 8 cm in diameter may be followed expectantly in the asymptomatic patient, since 70% of these masses will resolve spontaneously. The patient should undergo repeat physical examination and pelvic ultrasound at a specified time interval. A common practice is to suppress ovulation with the oral contraceptive pill, but the value of this strategy remains unproved. Indications for surgery include persistence of the mass, change in ultrasonic characteristics to a more complex appearance, solid enlargement, or evidence of ascites. However, if the mass remains less than 8 cm, is simple in ultrasound appearance, and causes no symptoms, continued follow-up is a reasonable option. In the reproductive-age woman with an adnexal mass greater than 8 cm in diameter, solid appearance on ultrasound, bilaterality, and presence of ascites, surgical evaluation is indicated.

Once surgery is decided upon, keep in mind the goal of the operation: for most patients, it is the exclusion of ovarian malignancy. If a malignant ovarian neoplasm is discovered, the current standard of care is the performance of a comprehensive surgical staging procedure, followed in most cases by adjuvant chemotherapy.

Many surgeons now use the laparoscopic approach for the management of the adnexal mass in reproductive-age women. In a 1990 survey by the American Association of Gynecologic Laparoscopists,[26] operative laparoscopy was accomplished in most patients and there were only 53 cases of unsuspected ovarian cancer in 13,739 cases (0.04%). The benefits of laparoscopic surgery include shorter length of hospital stay, decreased postoperative pain and recovery time, and probably reduced cost. However, there are understandable persisting concerns about the laparoscopic management of adnexal masses. These include the failure to diagnose ovarian malignancies, tumor spillage, inability to proceed immediately with a staging procedure, and delay in therapy. On balance, laparoscopic surgery can be attempted for selected reproductive-age women requiring operative treatment of an adnexal mass provided there is no evidence of metastatic disease, frozen section diagnosis is available, and the patient has signed consent for comprehensive surgical staging for ovarian cancer, including laparotomy. Postoperatively, the patient should follow up with the physician to determine the need for further therapy based on the results of full pathologic evaluation of the surgical specimen. Future studies in reproductive-age women should focus on decreasing the number of patients undergoing a surgical procedure, and in patients who require surgery, further evaluation of laparoscopy as a safe, cost-effective means of treatment.

## ENDOMETRIOSIS

Endometriosis is a progressive disease that affects 10% to 15% of women of childbearing age. It is the second most frequent gynecologic disorder, with leiomyomas, affecting one third of women in their reproductive years, being more frequent. Endometriosis is the presence of the glands and stroma of the lining of the uterus in an aberrant location. The etiology of endometriosis is uncertain and may involve retrograde menstruation, metaplasia, vascular dissemination, genetic predisposition, and immunologic factors. The etiology, diagnosis, and treatment are discussed in Chapter 13.

## LAPAROSCOPIC MYOMECTOMY

Uterine leiomyomas are the most common tumor of the female reproductive tract. Although traditionally noted in 20% of women over the age of 35, leiomyomas have been noted in 50% of women at time of autopsy examination. Myomas develop from benign transformation and proliferation of smooth muscle cells and can develop in any area with smooth muscle cells of müllerian origin.

### Clinical Features
Uterine myomas can cause abnormal uterine bleeding, abdominal and pelvic pain and pressure, urinary symptoms, and constipation. The severity of these symptoms is dependent on the number of tumors, their size, and their location. Although not primarily the cause of infertility, myomas have been linked to fetal wastage and premature delivery.

### Diagnosis and Preoperative Evaluation
It is imperative to know the size, location, and number of uterine myomas. This is especially important in a laparoscopic approach to myomectomy, since tactile feedback is diminished. Ultrasonography is the most commonly used imaging technique in the preoperative assessment. In cases in which ultrasound results are suspect, magnetic resonance imaging also can be used to map the myomas. Before the procedure or at the time of myomectomy, the endometrial cavity must be evaluated by hysterosonogram, hysteroscopy, or hysterosalpingogram.[27] Before surgery, hematologic status must be evaluated. The use of gonadotropin-releasing hormone (GnRH) analogs is an option for anemic patients because it may restore a normal hematocrit, decrease the size of the myoma, and reduce the need for transfusion. Patients should be counseled about the potential for intraoperative and postoperative bleeding and the possible need for blood transfusion, conversion to laparotomy, and chance of hysterectomy.

### Treatment and Surgical Technique
If myomas are thought to be unrelated to reproductive dysfunction or if they are asymptomatic, no treatment is indicated. The indications for myomectomy are summarized in Table 37-1.

Laparoscopic myomectomy (LM) has recently gained wide acceptance. This procedure remains technically demanding and concerns have been raised regarding the prolonged time of anesthesia, increased blood loss, and possible higher risk of postoperative uterine rupture of the pregnant uterus. However, in carefully selected cases, LM is a safe and efficient alternative to myomectomy by laparotomy.

The required instruments for LM include $CO_2$ or fiber laser, unipolar electrode or harmonic scalpel for cutting, bipolar Kleppinger forceps for achieving hemostasis, and clawed grasping forceps.

In cases of pedunculated subserosal myoma, dilute vasopressin (20 units in 50 mL normal saline) is injected at the base of the stalk. The myoma is removed by coagulating and cutting the stalk. For subserosal and intramural myomas, dilute vasopressin is injected in multiple sites between the myometrium and the fibroid capsule (Fig. 37-12). An incision is made on the serosa overlying the leiomyoma, using a $CO_2$ laser, monopolar electrode, fiber laser, or harmonic scalpel (Fig. 37-13). The incision is extended until it reaches the capsule. The myometrium retracts as the incision is made, exposing the tumor. The suction-irrigator is used as a blunt probe to shell the myoma from its capsule. Traction is applied using a myoma screw that is inserted into the tumor (Fig. 37-14). Bleeding points are controlled with electrocoagulation, and the uterine defect is irrigated. The edges of the uterine defect are approximated by suturing. If the defect is deep or large, the myometrium and serosa are approximated (Fig. 37-15). After repair, the uterine surface is irrigated. Myomas can be removed from the abdominal cavity by means of an electromechanical morcellator, through a posterior colpotomy, or via minilaparotomy.[28]

Laparoscopically assisted myomectomy (LAM) is a safe alternative to LM and is less difficult and less time consuming.[29] LAM can be used for large (>8 cm), multiple, or deep intramural myomas. By means of a combination of laparoscopy and a

| Table 37-1 |
| Indications for Myomectomy |
| --- |
| 1. Iron deficiency anemia |
| 2. Abnormal uterine bleeding (most frequently menorrhagia) |
| 3. Rapid growth of myoma or growth after menopause |
| 4. Infertility or recurrent pregnancy loss |
| 5. Abdominal or pelvic pain or pressure symptoms |
| 6. Urinary tract symptoms or obstruction |

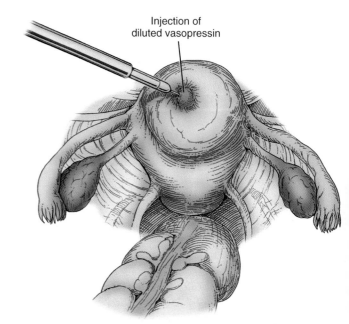

Injection of diluted vasopressin

**Figure 37-12** The serosa overlying the myoma is injected with dilute vasopressin.

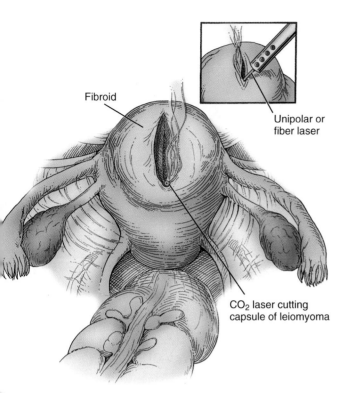

**Figure 37-13    Incision of the myometrium to remove an intramural myoma.**

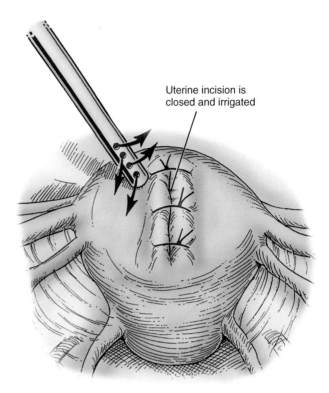

**Figure 37-15    Uterine incision is closed and irrigated.**

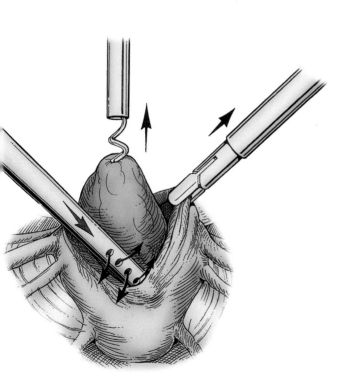

**Figure 37-14    Myoma removal using the suction-irrigator as a blunt probe and also for hydrodissection.**

2- to 4-cm abdominal incision, the uterine defect can be closed in two or three layers to reduce the risk of uterine dehiscence and fistula and adhesion formation.

Following LM or LAM, most patients are observed in an outpatient unit and discharged the morning after the operation. Women who desire future fertility and require myomectomy for an intramural tumor may benefit from LAM to ensure proper closure of the myometrial incision. Cesarean delivery is recommended in patients who have deep intramural or multiple intramural myomas even if the endometrial, cavity is not entered.

**Pitfalls and Controversies**

Four aspects of LM make it technically more difficult compared with an approach by laparotomy[27]:

1. Finding a deep intramural myoma may be difficult with laparoscopy due to lack of tactile sensation.
2. Enucleation of a myoma is sometimes difficult in the laparoscopic setting.
3. Laparoscopic suturing is technically more difficult and time consuming than laparotomy suturing.
4. Myoma extraction adds to the complexity of LM.

Laparoscopy is associated with a reduction in adhesion formation. Since fertility preservation is a primary goal of myomectomy, the potential reduction of adhesion formation by LM may provide a advantage over laparotomy.[30]

The incidence of uterine rupture after LM is unknown, since the procedure is relatively new. However, the incidence was estimated to be approximately 1% (95% CI 0.0–5.5) in a follow-up study of 100 cases by Dubuisson et al. In another study,[31] spontaneous uterine rupture was not noted during pregnancy in any of the 40 women with a history of LM.

The recurrence of myomas has been reported to be higher after laparoscopic surgery in some studies, but not all. Nezhat et al[33] reported a recurrence rate of 33% after a mean interval of 27 months after LM. They concluded that although LM was associated with less morbidity than removal by laparotomy, the recurrence of myomas might be higher with a laparoscopic approach. The reported recurrence after a randomized clinical trial[34] between laparoscopy and laparotomy was the same at approximately 21%. In this study, the operative time was not significantly different between the two groups; postoperative morbidity was less and recovery was faster in the laparoscopy group. Pregnancy rates, abortion rates, preterm delivery, and the use of cesarean section were similar between the two groups. No uterine rupture was reported. Several recent studies further address these issues. In one randomized clinical trial,[35] operative time was significantly longer for LM; however, the laparoscopic approach was associated with faster postoperative recovery compared with laparotomy.

In a recent case-control study, Silva et al[36] compared laparoscopic with abdominal approaches to myomectomy. Median length of hospital stay (30.5 vs 65.0 hours) and duration of postoperative intravenous narcotic use (14.8 vs 24.0 hours) were significantly shorter for laparoscopic group. The laparoscopic cases required a longer median operative time; however, no difference was detected in estimated blood loss from surgery.

## Summary

Two randomized clinical trials and many observational studies have shown that LM is associated with an accelerated postoperative recovery compared with laparotomy. In the hands of skilled surgeons, the incidence of uterine rupture and recurrence may be the same as with an open procedure. There are no specific limitations regarding the size or number of myomas, but clinical judgment and experience should determine the surgeon's personal limits.

# LAPAROSCOPIC HYSTERECTOMY

Hysterectomy is a common operation, with up to 550,000 and 100,000 procedures undertaken annually in the United States and United Kingdom, respectively. The advent of laparoscopic approaches to hysterectomy offers the prospect of improved outcomes and gains in cost effectiveness through reduced severity of convalescence and shorter length of hospital stay. The main indications for hysterectomy for nonmalignant disease in the United States include fibroids (35%), abnormal uterine bleeding (22%), and chronic pelvic pain (18%). For women who require hysterectomy, the appropriate route of surgery is determined by anatomic considerations, the type of pathologic condition expected, patient preference, and physician experience and training.

## Laparoscopically Assisted Vaginal Hysterectomy
### Definition and Indications
The term *laparoscopically assisted vaginal hysterectomy* (LAVH) has been applied to various operations that include portions of the procedure performed vaginally. In this procedure, the uterine vessels are ligated either vaginally or laparoscopically. According to an American College of Obstetricians and Gynecologist (ACOG) criteria set,[37] LAVH is indicated to assist in the performance of a vaginal hysterectomy in situations in which an abdominal approach might otherwise be indicated. These conditions include previous pelvic surgery, endometriosis or pelvic inflammatory disease requiring lysis of adhesions, ligation of the infundibulopelvic ligaments for ovarian removal allowing completion by vaginal hysterectomy, and presence of a pelvic mass and malignancies that require evaluation.

### Risks, Benefits, and Possible Complications
In the first randomized clinical trial, Nezhat et al[38] compared the perioperative and postoperative courses for 10 women who underwent total abdominal hysterectomy and 10 who underwent LAVH. Although LAVH took longer (160 vs 102 min), the women undergoing it had a shorter duration of hospitalization (2.4 vs 4.4 days), more rapid recuperation (3 vs 5 weeks), and fewer complications. They concluded that in the hands of experienced surgeons, LAVH is preferable to abdominal hysterectomy for selected candidates.

A multicenter randomized clinical trial[39] compared intraoperative and postoperative outcomes between LAVH and abdominal hysterectomy among patients who were not eligible for vaginal hysterectomy. Sixty-five women at three institutions underwent LAVH (n = 34) or abdominal hysterectomy (n = 31). Three patients in the laparoscopic group required conversion to abdominal hysterectomy. Mean operating time was significantly longer for LAVH (179.8 vs 146 min). There were no differences in blood loss or incidence of intraoperative complications. There was a higher incidence of wound complications in the abdominal hysterectomy group, but no significant difference in the frequency of other postoperative complications. LAVH required a significantly shorter mean hospital stay (2.1 days) and convalescence (28 days) than abdominal hysterectomy (4.1 days and 38 days, respectively). There were no significant differences in mean hospital charges between the study groups (laparoscopic $8161, abdominal $6974).

A prospective randomized clinical trial[40] of LAVH (n = 24) versus abdominal hysterectomy (n = 24) was carried out in a tertiary care setting. The LAVH group had longer operative times (180 vs 130 min), lower requirement for postoperative intravenous analgesia, shorter length of hospital stay (1.5 vs 2.5 days), and quicker return to work. Both procedures had similar hospital costs.

A randomized clinical trial[41] showed that LAVH took longer (120 vs 64 min) and had higher cost ($7905 vs $4891) compared with vaginal hysterectomy. There was no difference in complications, length of stay, and postoperative recovery between the two groups. The authors concluded that the vaginal approach should be preferred for hysterectomy whenever feasible.

Kovac[42] conducted a prospective cohort study in 142 women who underwent abdominal hysterectomy, LAVH, or vaginal hysterectomy. Length of stay was longer after abdominal hysterectomy than for LAVH or vaginal hysterectomy (P <0.001), hospital charges were lower for vaginal hysterectomy than for either LAVH or abdominal hysterectomy (P <0.001), and postoperative complications were higher for abdominal hysterectomy ($P < 0.001$). He concluded that the vaginal route of hysterectomy should be considered when disease is confined to the uterus and estimated uterine weight is less than 280 g.

The frequency and cause of aborted LAVH were studied in a retrospective cohort study[43] of 78 patients. Of the aborted LAVH procedures, 11.1% were converted to abdominal hysterectomy, the most frequent reason for conversion being large uterine size followed by significant intraperitoneal adhesions and intraoperative bleeding.

## Total Laparoscopic Hysterectomy

### Definition and Indications

In total laparoscopic hysterectomy (TLH), all vascular pedicles and uterine attachments are ligated and excised laparoscopically. The vaginal cuff may be repaired laparoscopically or vaginally.

TLH is indicated when vaginal hysterectomy is not possible because of little or no vaginal access to uterine vessels or presence of intraperitoneal pathology. Contraindications to TLH include a uterine mass suspicious for cancer that cannot be removed intact, medical conditions that prohibit surgery such as severe cardiac and pulmonary diseases, and inadequate training and experience in advanced laparoscopic surgery on the part of the staff.

### Risks, Benefits, and Possible Complications

In two parallel randomized clinical trials, one comparing laparoscopic with abdominal hysterectomy and the other comparing laparoscopic with vaginal hysterectomy in 1346 patients, Garry et al[44] showed that TLH was associated with higher rate of major complications than abdominal hysterectomy (11.1% vs 6.2%) and also took longer to perform (84 vs 50 min) but was less painful and resulted in shorter hospital stay after the operation (3 vs 4 days). In the vaginal trial, they found no evidence of a difference in major complication rates between TLH and vaginal hysterectomy (9.8% vs 9.5%). LH took longer to perform (72 vs 39 min) and was associated with a higher rate of detection of unexpected pathology.

A Finnish prospective cohort study[45] compared the operation-related morbidity and postoperative complications of abdominal, vaginal, and total laparoscopic hysterectomies. In a total of 10,110 hysterectomies, infection and hemorrhagic events were similar in the three groups. However, ureteral injuries were more frequent in the laparoscopic group (RR = 7.2) compared with the abdominal group, whereas bowel injuries were most common in the vaginal group (RR = 2.5). Surgeons who had performed more than 30 laparoscopic hysterectomies had a significantly lower incidence of ureter and bladder injuries (0.5% and 0.8%, respectively) than those who had performed fewer than 30 operations (2.2% and 2.0%, respectively). A decreasing trend of bowel complications was also seen with increasing experience in vaginal hysterectomy.

When a retrospective comparative study[46] evaluated the frequency of complications of TLH performed in the first and then more recent years of surgeons' experience, they found substantial decreases in major complication rates in the more recent group (1.3% vs 5.6%). It was concluded that LH was safe, effective, and reproducible after training and with current technique had a low rate of complications.

Recently, Sculpher and colleagues[47] assessed the cost-effectiveness (U.S. dollars) of LH compared with conventional abdominal and vaginal hysterectomies in the United Kingdom. LH cost an average of $708 more than vaginal hysterectomy and $328 more than abdominal hysterectomy. They concluded that LH was not cost effective relative to vaginal hysterectomy and was comparable to abdominal hysterectomy.

### Preoperative Evaluation

Routine preoperative tests may include complete blood count, serum electrolytes, and blood type and antibody screen. More comprehensive blood studies, electrocardiogram, chest x-ray and endometrial biopsy are performed as indicated. A mechanical or sometimes antibiotic bowel preparation is advised depending on the clinical situation. A GnRH analog may be considered if anemia is present. Informed consent is obtained after a thorough explanation of the procedure, its potential risks and benefits, the possibility of laparotomy, and therapeutic alternatives.

### Surgical Technique

The patient is placed in a dorsolithotomy position with the buttocks extended over the end of the table. We prefer Allen universal stirrups with thighs in a flexed (120-degree) position to allow instrument manipulation. An oral gastric tube is inserted for decompression of the stomach prior to instrumentation of the abdomen. After insertion of a Foley catheter, a uterine manipulator is placed into the cervix and uterine cavity to properly manipulate the uterus during the procedure. A 5- or a 10-mm trocar is inserted infraumblically and two to four accessory trocars are positioned suprapubically or as needed depending on the anatomy. After exploration of the abdominal and pelvic cavities and treatment of any associated pathology such as endometriosis or adhesions, the direction and location of both ureters are identified from pelvic brim to the cardinal ligaments and their locations are marked lateral to the uterosacral ligaments (Fig. 37-16). If needed, the peritoneum is opened above the ureter and hydrodissection is carried out (Fig. 37-17). With the ureters retracted laterally, the uterosacral ligaments can be dissected at their connections to the back of the cervix at this time or later. If adnexectomy is indicated, after electrocoagulation and cutting of the round ligament 2 to 3 cm from the uterus (Figs. 37-18 and 37-19), the infundibulopelvic ligament is isolated and electrodesiccated. Using hydrodissection, the anterior leaf of the broad ligament is opened toward the vesicouterine fold and the bladder flap is developed (Fig. 37-20). The anterior leaf of the broad ligament is grasped, elevated, and dissected from the anterior lower uterine segment. After the bladder is dissected from the anterior cervix, the uterine vessels are identified, desiccated, and cut to free the lateral borders of the uterus (Fig. 37-21). At the of the cardinal ligaments, the ureter and descending branches of the uterine artery are close to one another and the cervix. Once the ureter is displaced laterally, the cardinal ligament tissue closest to the cervix is desiccated (Fig. 37-22). A folded wet gauze in a sponge forceps or the tip of a right-angle retractor marks the anterior and posterior vaginal fornix. The vaginal wall is tented and transected horizontally (Fig. 37-23). The uterus is removed through the vagina or abdominally using an electromechanical morcellator. The vaginal cuff is closed vaginally or laparoscopically. To ensure

# Minimally Invasive Surgery

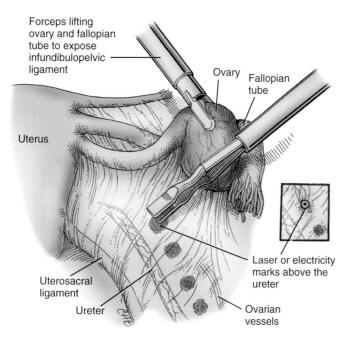

Forceps lifting ovary and fallopian tube to expose infundibulopelvic ligament

Ovary

Fallopian tube

Uterus

Uterosacral ligament

Ureter

Laser or electricity marks above the ureter

Ovarian vessels

**Figure 37-16** Marking the direction and location of the ureter by making a superficial peritoneal coagulation above it.

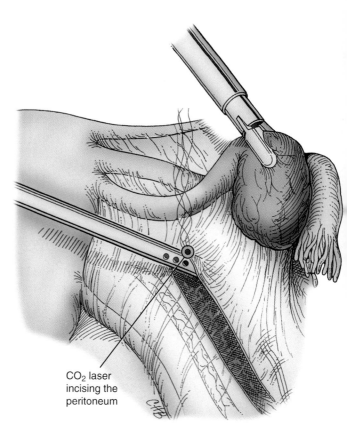

$CO_2$ laser incising the peritoneum

**Figure 37-17** **Ureter dissection.** With the suction irrigator probe used as a backstop, an opening is made above the ureter with a $CO_2$ laser. Using blunt dissection and hydrodissection, the ureter is dissected from the pelvic brim to the back of the bladder.

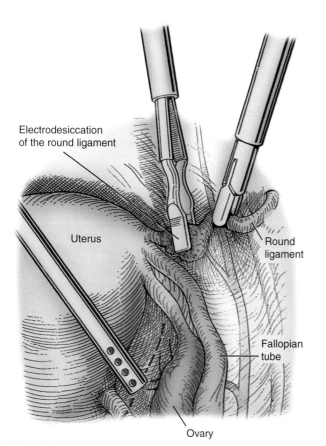

Electrodesiccation of the round ligament

Uterus

Round ligament

Fallopian tube

Ovary

**Figure 37-18** The round ligament is electrodesiccated and cut 2 to 3 cm lateral to the uterus.

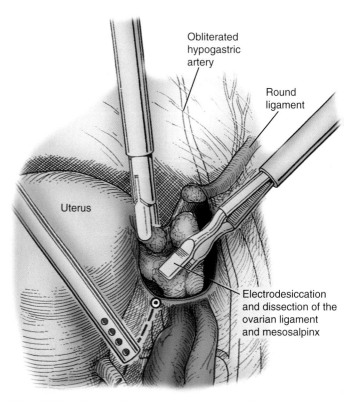

Obliterated hypogastric artery

Round ligament

Uterus

Electrodesiccation and dissection of the ovarian ligament and mesosalpinx

**Figure 37-19** The proximal tube, mesosalpinx, and utero-ovarian ligament are electrodesiccated and cut.

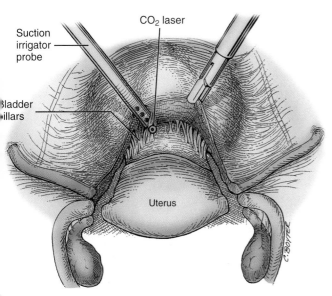

Figure 37-20    The bladder pillars are identified and cut close to the cervix with a $CO_2$ laser.

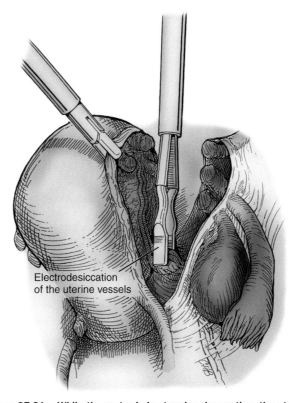

Figure 37-21    While the ureter is kept under observation, the uterine vessels are skeletonized, electrodesiccated, and cut.

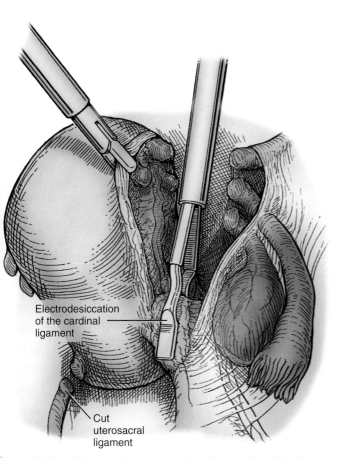

Figure 37-22    While the uterus is pulled to the opposite side, the cardinal ligament is electrodesiccated and cut. The ureter must be observed to ensure its integrity.

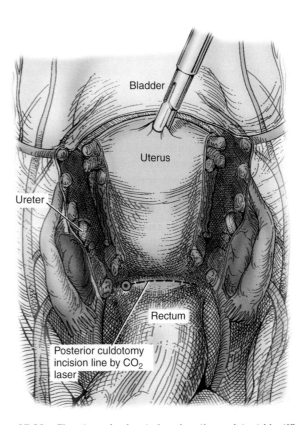

Figure 37-23    The uterus is elevated, and as the assistant identifies the posterior fornix, laparoscopic posterior culdotomy is performed. The surgeon must ensure that the correct location is selected and that the rectum is not involved.

# Minimally Invasive Surgery

hemostasis, the pelvis is partially filled with lactated Ringer's solution and the vaginal cuff is viewed by submerging the laparoscope under water. If indicated, cystoscopy may be performed to ensure ureteral patency and bladder integrity.[48]

## Laparoscopic Supracervical Hysterectomy

Laparoscopic supracervical hysterectomy (LSH) may be offered to patients in whom hysterectomy is indicated and the following conditions are ruled out: endometrial or cervical cancer or recent cervical dysplasia, pelvic floor relaxation, and severe endometriosis of the uterosacral ligaments as well as in any patient who cannot be expected to continue cytologic surveillance. The real risk of cervical disease is no greater than in patients with an intact uterus, but the patient should be counseled concerning the importance of continued Papanicolaou (Pap) smear screening.

Milad et al[49] performed a prospective cohort analysis comparing 27 patients who underwent LSH with 105 who underwent LAVH. Patients undergoing LSH had significantly shorter operating times (181 vs 220 min), briefer hospital stays (1 vs 2 days) and less blood loss (125 vs 400 mL). None of the patients submitted to LSH experienced morbidity as compared with a 13% morbidity rate for those who underwent LAVH. They concluded that the practice of routine cervicectomy at laparoscopic hysterectomy should be reconsidered.

A retrospective study[50] of 70 patients assessed the long term outcome of LSH. Seventeen women (24.3%) reported symptoms related to the cervical stump, and all required further surgery. The cervical stump was removed in 16 (22.8%). Histologic analysis showed normal cervical tissue in six (35.3%), endometriosis in four (23.5%), residual endometrium in another four, and chronic cervicitis, CIN I, and a mucocele in three patients. They concluded that symptoms related to the cervical stump requiring further surgery frequently occurred following LSH. Discussion of possible complications should be included in the preoperative counseling.

Overall, data on LSH are equivocal. It may be considered in cases where there is difficult dissection, distorted anatomy, compromised medical conditions, and patient desire to preserve the cervix. Careful evaluation to rule out any cervical dysplasia is required prior to LSH.

## Laparoscope-Assisted Radical Vaginal Hysterectomy

Advanced operative laparoscopy in gynecologic oncology developed after advances in laparoscopic retroperitoneal surgery, particularly pelvic and para-aortic lymphadenectomy. The radical vaginal hysterectomy (Schauta) was historically associated with a reduction in postoperative mortality compared with abdominal radical hysterectomy. However, with the popularization of complete pelvic lymphadenectomy in the surgical management of cervical cancer, the Schauta operation became less popular. Dargent is credited with reviving this operation through a combined laparoscopic retroperitoneal lymphadenectomy and radical vaginal hysterectomy. Abu-Rustum[51] summarized 11 reports on 382 laparoscope-assisted radical vaginal hysterectomies (LARVHs) and pelvic and para-aortic lymphadenectomies. The operative time was 225 to 380 minutes with 4 to 5 days of hospital stay. Intra- and postoperative complications included 4% to 5% cystotomy, 1% to 2% ureteral and 1% to 2% vascular injuries, 1% to 2% absces and 1% to 2% hematoma formation, and 6% to 7% transfusion These results appear to be comparable to those of standard ope technique.

## Total Laparoscopic Radical Hysterectomy

Total laparoscopic radical hysterectomy (TLRH) with pelvic and para-aortic lymph node dissection was first reported by Nezhat et al in 1992.[52,53] No randomized trials are available ye comparing TLRH with abdominal radical hysterectomy; how ever, more than 150 patients have so far been reported, with encouraging results. Abu-Rustum[51] has recently reviewed eight reports on 146 patients who underwent TLRH with pelvic and para-aortic lymphadenectomy. The mean operative time wa 300 minutes with hospital stay of 4 days. Complications included 3% to 4% conversion to laparotomy, 2% to 3% cystotomy, 2% to 3% ureteral injury, and 1% to 2% transfusion. It appears that the overall complication rate is acceptable with no compromise in outcome. However, randomized clinical trials are needed before the role of laparoscopy in gynecologic oncology is well established.

# RETROPERITONEAL LYMPHADENECTOMY

Since the initial report by Dargent and colleagues[54] in the late 1980s, laparoscopic lymphadenectomy has been utilized in the management of gynecologic and urologic malignancies as well as of some lymphomas. Nezhat et al[52] described the first para-aortic lymphadenectomy performed laparoscopically for cancer of the uterine cervix. Over recent years, the literature has been expanding regarding outcomes and complications of laparoscopic lymphadenectomy.

Lymph node status is the most important prognostic factor in gynecologic cancer, and surgical removal of pelvic or para-aortic lymph nodes for histologic assessment is an integral part of staging for gynecologic malignancies. Additionally, removal of the bulky lymph nodes may have therapeutic benefit.

## Surgical Technique

Pelvic lymphadenectomy performed either laparoscopically or by laparotomy begins with identification of the ureter coagulation and cutting of the round ligament, and opening of the posterior peritoneum and the pelvic side wall. The common iliac and external iliac nodes are dissected with care taken to avoid the genitofemoral nerve, which lies medial on the psoas muscle. The nodes are dissected from the common iliac artery bifurcation to the circumflex iliac vein caudally (Fig. 37-24) After development of the paravesical space between the obliterated hypogastric artery and external iliac artery and vein the obturator space is opened and the obturator nerve and vessels are identified (Fig. 37-25). Although the majority of patients have both the obturator artery and vein dorsal to the obturator nerve, 10% will have an aberrant obturator vein arising from the external iliac vein. The obturator lymph nodes are

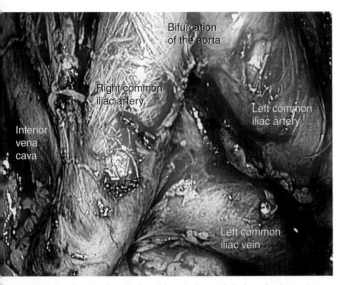

**Figure 37-24**  Anatomic relationships during pelvic lymphadenectomy on the left side.

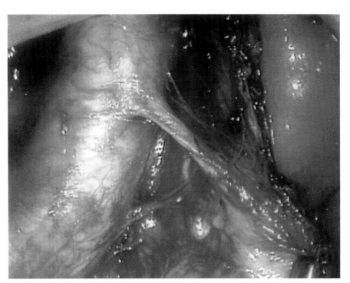

**Figure 37-26**  Anatomic relationships of the lower para-aortic region.

grasped just under the external iliac vein and traction is applied medially. The node chain is thereby separated from the obturator nerve and vessels and the nodes are dissected cephalad to the hypogastric artery. Finally, the hypogastric lymph nodes are removed up to the common iliac artery with care to avoid injury to hypogastric vein. For the para-aortic dissection, the peritoneum is incised over the sacral promontory or right common iliac artery with the right ureter in view. This incision is extended up to the inferior mesenteric artery or up to the left renal vein in cases of ovarian or fallopian tube carcinoma. The lymph node packages are retrieved along the common iliac vessels, along the aorta and vena cava with careful attention to the ovarian vessels, ureters, renal vessels, and inferior mesenteric artery (Fig. 37-26).

## Risks, Benefits, and Possible Complications

Technically there are multiple benefits of the laparoscopic approach to pelvic and para-aortic lymphadenectomy. The

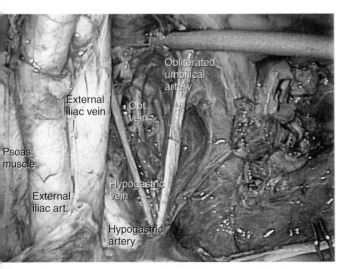

**Figure 37-25**  Anatomic relationships of the aorta and inferior vena cava.

laparoscope provides 7- to 10-fold magnification of the operative field, allowing identification of small tributary vessels. Additionally, the pneumoperitoneum facilitates the development of pelvic spaces and decreases venous oozing, thereby maintaining a clean operative dissection with good visualization of nodal bundles.

Complications of laparoscopic lymphadenectomy belong in two general categories. The first includes the complications that are intrinsic to laparoscopy, regardless of the specific procedure being performed. These include complications such as subcutaneous emphysema or laceration of the abdominal wall and trocar injuries to inferior epigastric vessels, the bowel, or major retroperitoneal vessels. The second group of complications includes those that are intrinsic to the procedure regardless of the method by which it is performed. These include the following:

### Vascular Injury

Vascular injuries related to lymphadenectomy are potentially life-threatening. In a series of laparoscopic lymphadenectomies,[55] seven of nine vascular complications occurred as the result of trocar injury to the anterior abdominal wall vasculature. Potential vascular compromise specific to pelvic lymphadenectomy includes injury to the obturator, internal iliac, external iliac, or common iliac vessels. Vessels at risk for injury during para-aortic lymphadenectomy include the aorta and vena cava, as well as the common iliac, inferior mesenteric, lumbar, ovarian, and renal vessels. In one of the largest studies[56] of more than 300 pelvic lymphadenectomies, injury to major pelvic vessels was a rare event. The vessel most likely to be injured was the aberrant obturator vein emerging from the obturator canal, across the nodal bundle, to empty into the external iliac vein. Laparoscopic management of vascular injuries varies according to the type (artery or vein) and the size of the vessel injured. The modalities utilized in managing these vascular injuries include pressure, monopolar and bipolar electricity, clips, and sutures. Depending on the caliber of the injured vessel, any of these modalities may achieve hemostasis satisfactorily.

### Genitourinary Injury

Cystotomy during trocar insertion, adhesiolysis, or dissection with endoscopic scissors with or without electrocautery has been described as a complication of laparoscopic lymphadenectomy, although it is not specific to this procedure. Cystotomy can occur when the paravesical and pararectal spaces are opened if the obliterated umbilical artery is not retracted medially. Ureterovaginal and vesicovaginal fistulae, as well as injury to the patent urachus, are other potential complications. Pelvic lymphadenectomy places the ureter at risk for sharp, crush, and thermal injury. The lumbar portion of the ureter is at risk during para-aortic lymphadenectomy. If such an injury is recognized intraoperatively, it can be managed laparoscopically. A transurethral stent is placed, the ureteral defect is oversewn, and a retroperitoneal drain is placed laparoscopically. Though it is an area of current investigation, there is no proven role for prophylactic ureteral stent placement prior to laparoscopic lymphadenectomy.

### Neurologic Injury

Genitofemoral nerve injury can occur during removal of the lateral pelvic lymph nodes. Such an injury results in medial thigh numbness but is otherwise of little clinical consequence. It is arguably the most common injury encountered by the gynecologic oncologist. Injury of the obturator nerve is a rare complication of laparoscopic pelvic lymphadenectomy. It manifests as adductor weakness and decreased sensation of the anteromedial thigh.

### Abdominal Wall Metastases and Peritoneal Tumor Dissemination

Abdominal wall metastases, also called port or wound site metastases, have been reported after both laparoscopy and laparotomy. The incidence has been 1% after laparotomy and 1% to 3% after laparoscopy.[57] Port sites are contaminated during tumor extraction or withdrawal of contaminated ports. The risk of contamination is higher if abdominal insufflation is lost during tumor extraction or port withdrawal. Although port site recurrences may be disfiguring and difficult to treat, there is no prospective evidence that port site metastases worsen prognosis. To prevent this complication, removal of all specimens using an endo-bag, removal of all ports while the abdomen is still insufflated, immediate local treatment of the contaminated ports with a cytotoxic agent, and closure of the peritoneum and fascia of all trocar sites is highly recommended.

### Complications Requiring Laparotomy

Complications resulting in laparotomy have been related to damage to the ureter, bladder, bowel, and vascular structures. The incidence of conversion to laparotomy in 150 cases reported by Passover et al[58] was 2.7% (see also Chapter 38).

### Adequacy of Node Retrieval

Lymphadenectomy is primarily performed to evaluate for micrometastasis in the setting of a malignancy. It is therefore essential that the lymph node dissection achieve adequate node retrieval by laparotomy or laparoscopy. The gynecologic oncology group (GOG) protocol 9207 examined laparoscopic para-aortic lymph node sampling and therapeutic pelvic lymphadenectomy in women with stages IA, IB, and IIA cervical cancer. In 69 patients, across seven institutions, the average lymph node retrieval was up to 70 (mean of 32) for pelvic nodes, and up to 37 (mean of 12) for para-aortic nodes. The complication rate was 10% for vascular injury and 1.4% for ureteral injury. The study concluded that laparoscopic approach is a feasible alternative for retroperitoneal lymphadenectomy by laparotomy.

### Summary

Laparoscopic lymphadenectomy is an evolving technique that may play an increasingly important role in the management of gynecologic malignancies. Laparoscopic pelvic and para-aortic lymphadenectomy appears to be a safe, adequate, and feasible procedure, with a low complication rate. The risks include those traditionally attributed to laparoscopy as well as those inherent in open lymphadenectomy. The use of simple preventive measures allows the patient to benefit from this technique while diminishing the likelihood of complications.

## PELVIC RECONSTRUCTIVE PROCEDURES

Laparoscopic approach to pelvic reconstructive procedures has been made possible by recent advances in minimally invasive surgery. Laparoscopy allows better visualization of the retropubic space because of magnification, insufflation effects, and better hemostasis. The laparoscopic technique for Burch urethropexy is identical to the open approach. After induction of general anesthesia, the patient is placed in the lithotomy position using Allen stirrups, and a Foley catheter is inserted. A 5- or a 10-mm videolaparoscope is introduced intraumbilically, and three 5-mm accessory cannulas are inserted. The middle cannula is 5 to 6 cm above the pubic symphysis, and the other two cannulas are 3 cm medial to and above the anterior superior iliac spines. After the intraperitoneal cavity is thoroughly inspected for any pelvic disease, the anterior abdominal wall peritoneum, 5 to 6 cm above the pubic symphysis, is pulled down by means of grasping forceps and a transverse incision is made with a laser, scissors, or harmonic scalpel. The midline cannula entry and anatomic landmarks, including the round ligament and the internal ring, are used to avoid injury to the bladder. The retropubic space is dissected mostly bluntly. The incision should remain close to the back of the pubic bone to drop the anterior bladder wall, vaginal wall, and the urethra downward (Fig. 37-27). Dissection is limited over the urethra in the midline to approximately 2 cm lateral to the urethra to protect its delicate neuromusculature. An assistant does a vaginal examination with one finger on each side of the catheterized urethra, elevating the lateral vaginal fornix. The overlying fibrofatty tissue is cleared from the anterior vaginal wall under laparoscopic magnification. The thin-walled venous plexus is identified and protected from trauma. The pubic symphysis, urethrovesical junction, obturator neuromuscular bundle, Cooper's ligament, and arcus tendineus fasciae pelvis are visualized bilaterally. If paravaginal wall defects are present, the lateral margins of the pubocervical fascia will be detached from the pelvic side wall at the arcus tendineus fasciae pelvis (white line). Unilateral or bilateral defects may be present. It is recommended to complete the paravaginal repair prior to the Burch colposuspension. To repair the paravaginal defect,

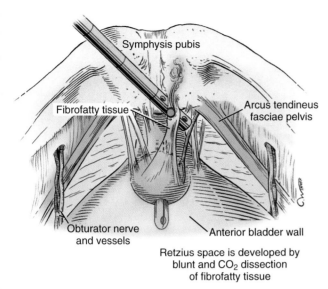

Retzius space is developed by
blunt and $CO_2$ dissection
of fibrofatty tissue

**Figure 37-27** **The space of Retzius is developed by means of blunt and sharp dissection of fibrofatty tissue.** Care is taken to avoid obturator nerve and vessel injury.

2-0 nonabsorbable sutures are placed sequentially along the paravaginal defects from the ischial spine toward the urethrovesical junction. By performing the paravaginal defect repair first, normal anatomical support of the anterior vaginal segment is recreated, reducing the chance of overelevation of the paraurethral Burch sutures and subsequent voiding dysfunction. With elevation of the vaginal fingers, the Burch sutures are placed in the vaginal wall excluding the vaginal epithelium, 2 cm lateral to the urethrovesical junction. No. 0 nonabsorbable suture is placed in a figure-of-eight stitch incorporating the entire thickness of anterior vaginal wall. The suture is then passed through the ipsilateral Cooper ligament and tied with either intracorporeal or extracorporeal knots (Fig. 37-28). A second suture is placed at the level of the mid-urethra. The procedure is repeated on the opposite side. In tying the sutures, the surgeon should not reapproximate the vaginal wall to Cooper's ligament or place too much tension on the vaginal wall. A suture bridge of 1.5 to 2 cm is common. Cystoscopy is performed to assess ureteral patency and integrity of the bladder wall. A suprapubic or an indwelling

bladder catheter is placed, and the peritoneum of the retropubic space may be closed with a running absorbable suture. Voiding trials begin on the first postoperative day. The suprapubic tube is clamped when the patient is awake. The patient voids with urge or every 3 hours. The patient is allowed to unclamp the suprapubic tube at night. Once the patient has voided 80% of total bladder volume during two serial attempts (voids must be greater than 150 mL), the catheter is removed. Patients are instructed to refrain from having sexual intercourse and from lifting objects greater than 10 pounds for at least 6 weeks.

If the laparoscopic technique parallels the open retropubic urethropexy, the laparoscopic procedure should have similar cure rates. Buller and Cundiff[59] reviewed 50 papers that collectively included 1867 patients who underwent laparoscopic surgery for the treatment of genuine stress incontinence. At a mean follow-up of 17 months, a cure rate of 89% was observed. Only 30.8% of studies reported objective outcome data, and a wide variety of laparoscopic techniques were used. Three prospective, randomized clinical trials have compared open and laparoscopic retropubic urethropexies. Burton[60] showed lower objective and subjective cure rates for laparoscopic colposuspension, which decreased from 1 year (73% vs 97%) to 3 years (60% vs 93%). The use of absorbable suture in this study must be questioned. Su and colleagues[61] showed a lower 1-year objective cure rate for laparoscopic Burch colposuspension (80.4%), compared with the open group (95.6%); however, only one suture was placed bilaterally in the laparoscopic group, compared with two or three sutures placed bilaterally in the open group. Summitt et al[62] subsequently found similar objective cure rates for laparoscopic and transabdominal Burch procedures at 3 months (100% vs 97%) and 1 year (92.8% vs 88.2%). Two stitches were placed bilaterally in all patients using permanent sutures.

The indications and surgical techniques for laparoscopic enterocele, vaginal apex prolapse, and rectocele repair are not new; it is the route by which they are performed that differs. The choice of laparoscopic route is determined by surgeon and patient preference and the laparoscopic skill of the surgeon. There are a small number of reports of laparoscopic repair of vaginal apex prolapse. Nezhat et al[63] reported a series of 15 patients who underwent laparoscopic sacral colpopexy in whom the mean operative time was 170 minutes and mean blood loss was 226 mL. The mean hospital stay was 2.3 days, excluding a case converted to laparotomy for presacral hemorrhage. The cure rate for apical prolapse was 100% at 3 and 40 months. Ross[64] evaluated 19 patients with posthysterectomy vaginal apex prolapse who underwent laparoscopic sacral colpopexy, Burch colposuspension, and modified culdeplasty. The cure rate at 1 year was 100% for vaginal apex prolapse and 93% for genuine stress incontinence, although two patients were lost to follow-up.

## UTEROSACRAL TRANSECTION AND ABLATION AND PRESACRAL NEURECTOMY

Laparoscopic uterosacral nerve ablation (LUNA) can be performed in patients with chronic pelvic pain in whom laparoscopy reveals either no pathology or mild endometriosis; however, reported long-term relief with this procedure is variable. The

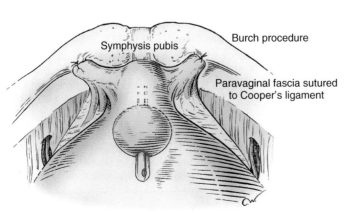

**Figure 37-28** **Sutures are tied, extracorporeally or intracorporeally, elevating the urethrovesical angle.**

# Minimally Invasive Surgery

Lee-Frankenhauser sensory nerve plexuses and parasympathetic ganglia in the uterosacral ligaments carry pain from the uterus, cervix, and other pelvic structures. Interruption of these nerve trunks by LUNA may alleviate the pain. However, the balance between benefits and risks has not been reliably assessed, and many surgeons no longer perform this surgery because of the controversy regarding its indications.

Presacral neurectomy is indicated for patients who have disabling midline dysmenorrhea and pelvic pain who have not responded to appropriate and adequate management. The success rate is difficult to predict, although the operation is likely to relieve pain in 50 to 75% of patients.[65,66] Primary dysmenorrhea or dysmenorrhea caused by endometriosis may be an indication for endoscopic corrective procedures followed by presacral neurectomy. In most patients, dyspareunia is decreased and chronic pain is alleviated.[65,66]

## CONCLUSION

Recent advances in endoscopic surgery have revolutionized our approach to gynecologic surgery. Most reproductive operations can be done by laparoscopy. It appears that laparoscopic gynecologic surgery, when performed by an experienced endoscopist, is feasible and effective and provides the patient with benefits of less postoperative pain, faster recovery, and better cosmesis.

## REFERENCES

1. Hulka JF, Levy BS, Luciano AA, et al: 1997 AAGL membership survey: practice profiles. J Am Assoc Gynecol Laparosc 1998;5:93–96. **(IV, C)**
2. American College of Obstetricians and Gynecologists: Diagnostic laparoscopy. ACOG Criteria Set 25. Washington, DC, July 1997. **(IV, C)**
3. Nezhat C: Laparoscopic adhesiolysis. In Nezhat C, Siegler A, Nezhat F, et al (eds): Operative Gynecologic Laparoscopy: Principles and Techniques, 2nd ed. New York, McGraw-Hill, 2000, pp 123 –131. **(IV, C)**
4. DiZerega GSD, Holtz G: Cause and prevention of postsurgical pelvic adhesions. In Osofsky H (ed): Advances in Clinical Obstetrics and Gynecology. Baltimore, Williams & Wilkins, 1982. **(IV, C)**
5. Brill AI, Nezhat F, Nezhat CH, et al: The incidence of adhesions after prior laparotomy: a laparoscopic appraisal. Obstet Gynecol 1995; 85:269–272. **(III, B)**
6. Caspi E, Halperin Y, Bukovski I: The importance of periadnexal adhesions in tubal reconstruction surgery for infertility. Fertil Steril 1979;31:296–300. **(III, B)**
7. Nezhat CR, Nezhat FR, Metzger DA, et al: Adhesion formation following reproductive surgery by videolaparoscopy. Fertil Steril 1990;53:1008–1011. **(III, B)**
8. Lundorff P, Hahlin M, Kallfelt B, et al: Adhesion formation after laparoscopic surgery in tubal pregnancy: a randomized trial versus laparotomy. Fertil Steril 1991;55:911–915. **(Ib, A)**
9. Schippers E. Tittel A, Ottonger A, et al: Laparoscopy versus laparotomy: Comparison of adhesion formation after bowel resection in a canine model. Fertil Steril 1998;15:145–147. **(Ib, A)**
10. Wallwiener D, Meyer A, Bastert G: Adhesion formation of the visceral and parietal peritoneum: an explanation for the controversy on the use of autologous and alloplastic barriers. Fertil Steril 1998; 69:132–137. **(IV, C)**
11. Halverson AL, Barrett WL, Bhanot P, et al: Intraabdominal adhesion formation after preperitoneal dissection in the murine model. Surg Endosc 1999;13:14–16. **(III, B)**
12. American College of Obstetricians and Gynecologists: Benefits and risks of sterilization. ACOG Practice Bulletin No. 46. Washington, DC Sep 2003. **(IV, C)**
13. Peterson HB, Xia Z, Hughes JM, et al: The risk of pregnancy after tubal sterilization. Am J Obstet Gynecol 1996;174:1161–1168. **(III, B)**
14. Morlock RJ, Lafata JE, Eisenstein D: Cost-effectiveness of single-dose methotrexate compared with laparoscopic treatment of ectopic pregnancy. Obstet Gynecol 2000; 95:407–412. **(III, B)**
15. Nezhat C: Management of ectopic pregnancy. In Nezhat C, Siegler A Nezhat F, et al. (eds): Operative Gynecologic Laparoscopy: Principles and Techniques, 2nd ed. New York, McGraw-Hill, 2000, pp 211–231. **(IV, C)**
16. Henry-Suchet L, Soler A, Loffredo V: Laparoscopic treatment of tubo ovarian abscesses. J Reprod Med 1984;8:579. **(IV, C)**
17. Walker CK, Landers DV: Pelvic abscesses: new trends in management Obstet Gynecol Surg 1991;46:615–624. **(IV, C)**
18. Anducci JE: Laparoscopy in the diagnosis and treatment of pelvic inflammatory disease with abscess formation. Int Surg 1981;66:359 **(IV, C)**
19. Nezhat C: Operations on the fallopian tube. In Nezhat C, Siegler A Nezhat F, et al (eds): Operative Gynecologic Laparoscopy: Principles and Techniques, 2nd ed. New York, McGraw-Hill, 2000, pp 233–259 **(IV, C)**
20. Mecke H, Semm K, Freys I, et al: Pelvic abscesses: pelvicoscopy or laparotomy. Gynecol Obstet Invest 1991;31:231. **(IV, C)**
21. Bateman BG, Nunley WC, Kitchin JD: Surgical management of distal tube obstruction: are we making progress? Fertil Steril 1987;48:523 **(IV, C)**
22. Henry-Suchet J, Loffredo V, Tesquier L, et al: Endoscopy of the tube: its prognostic value for tuboplasties. Acta Eur Fertil 1985;16:139. **(IV, C)**
23. Falcone T, Goldberg J, Garcia-Ruiz A, et al: Full robotic assistance for laparoscopic tubal anastomosis. J Laparoendosc Adv Surg Tech 1999 9:107. **(III, B)**
24. Sassone A., Timor-Tritsch I, Artner A, et al: Transvaginal sonographic characterization of ovarian disease: evaluation of a new scoring system to predict ovarian malignancy. Obstet Gynecol 1991;78:70. **(III, B)**
25. Alcazar JL, Jurado M: Prospective evaluation of a logistic model based on sonographic morphologic and color Doppler findings developed to predict adnexal malignancy. J Ultrasound Med 1999;18:837. **(IIb, B)**
26. Hulka J, Parker W, Surrey M, et al: American Association of Gynecologic Laparoscopists survey of management of ovarian masses in 1990 J Reprod Med 1992;7:599. **(IV, C)**
27. Miller CE: Myomectomy: comparison of open and laparoscopic techniques. Obstet Gynecol Clin North Am 2000;27:407–420. **(IV, C)**
28. Nezhat C: Laparoscopic operations on the uterus. In Nezhat C, Siegler A Nezhat F, et al (eds) Operative Gynecologic Laparoscopy: Principles and Techniques, 2nd ed. New York, McGraw-Hill, 2000, pp 261–272 **(IV, C)**
29. Seidman DS, Nezhat CH, Nezhat F, et al: The role of laparoscopic-assisted myomectomy (LAM). J Soc Laparoendosc Surg 2001 5:299–303. **(IV, C)**
30. Koh C, Janik G: Laparoscopic myomectomy: the current status. Curr Opin Obstet Gynecol 2003;15:295–301. **(IV, C)**
31. Dubuisson JB, Chavet X, Chapron C, et al: Uterine rupture during pregnancy after laparoscopic myomectomy. Hum Reprod 1995 10:1475–1477. **(III, B)**
32. Nezhat CH, Nezhat F, Roemisch M, et al: Pregnancy following laparoscopic myomectomy: preliminary results. Hum Reprod 1999 14:1219–1221. **(III, B)**
33. Nezhat FR, Roemisch M, Nezhat CH, et al: Recurrence rate after laparoscopic myomectomy. J Am Assoc Gynecol Laparosc 1998 5:237–240. **(III, B)**
34. Seracchioli R, Rossi S, Govoni F, et al: Fertility and obstetric outcome after laparoscopic myomectomy of large myomata: a randomized comparison with abdominal myomectomy. Hum Reprod 2000;15:2663–2668 **(Ib, A)**
35. Mais V, Ajossa S, Guerriero S, et al: Laparoscopic versus abdominal myomectomy: a prospective randomized trial to evaluate benefits in early outcome. Am J Obstet Gynecol 1996;174:654–658. **(Ib, A)**

6. Silva BA, Falcone T, Bradley L, et al: Case-control study of laparoscopic versus abdominal myomectomy. J Laparoendosc Adv Surg Tech 2000; 10:191–197. **(III, B)**

7. American College of Obstetricians and Gynecologists: ACOG criteria set: laparoscopically assisted vaginal hysterectomy. Int J Gynecol Obstet 1996;53:91–92. **(IV, C)**

8. Nezhat F, Nezhat C, Gordon S, et al: Laparoscopic versus abdominal hysterectomy. J Reprod Med 1992;37:247–250. **(IV, C)**

9. Summitt RL, Jr, Stovall TG, Steege JF, Lipscomb GH: A multicenter randomized comparison of laparoscopically assisted vaginal hysterectomy versus abdominal hysterectomy in abdominal hysterectomy candidates. Obstet Gynecol 1998;92:321–326. **(Ib,A)**

10. Falcone T, Paraiso MF, Mascha E: Prospective randomized clinical trial of laparoscopically assisted vaginal hysterectomy versus total abdominal hysterectomy. Am J Obstet Gynecol 1999;180:955–962. **(Ib, A)**

11. Summitt RL, Stovall TG, Lipscomb GH, et al: Randomized comparison of laparoscopically assisted vaginal hysterectomy with standard vaginal hysterectomy in an outpatient setting. Obstet Gynecol 1992;80:895–901. **(Ib, A)**

12. Kovac SR: Hysterectomy outcomes in patients with similar indications. Obstet Gynecol 2000;95:787–793. **(III, B)**

13. Cristoforoni PM, Palmieri A, Gerbaldo D, et al: Frequency and cause of aborted laparoscopic-assisted vaginal hysterectomy. J Am Assoc Gynecol Laparosc 1995;3:33–37. **(III, B)**

14. Garry R, Fountain J, Mason S, et al: The eVALuate study: two parallel trials, one comparing laparoscopic with abdominal hysterectomy, and the other comparing laparoscopic with vaginal hysterectomy. BMJ 2004;328:129. **(IIa, B)**

15. Makinen J, Johansson J, Tomas C, et al: Morbidity of 10110 hysterectomies by type of approach. Hum Reprod 2001;16:1473–1478. **(III, B)**

16. Wattiez A, Soriano D, Cohen SB, et al: The learning curve of total laparoscopic hysterectomy. J Am Assoc Gynecol Laparosc 2002; 9:339–345. **(III, B)**

17. Sculpher M, Manca A, Abbott J, et al: Cost effectiveness analysis of laparoscopic hysterectomy compared with standard hysterectomy: results from a randomized trial. BMJ 2004;328:134. **(Ib,A)**

18. Nezhat C: Hysterectomy. In Nezhat C, Siegler A, Nezhat F, et al (eds): Operative Gynecologic Laparoscopy: Principles and Techniques, 2nd ed. New York, McGraw-Hill, 2000, pp 272–299. **(IV, C)**

19. Milad MP, Morrison K, Sokol A, et al: A comparison of laparoscopic supracervical hysterectomy versus laparoscopically assisted vaginal hysterectomy. Surg Endosc 2001;15:286–288. **(III, B)**

50. Okaro EO, Jones KD, Sutton C: Long term outcome following laparoscopic supracervical hysterectomy. BJOG 2001;108:1017–1020. **(III,B)**

51. Abu-Rustum NR: Laparoscopy 2003: oncologic perspective. Clin Obstet Gynecol 2003;46 61–69. **(III, B)**

52. Nezhat CR, Burrell MO, Nezhat FR, et al: Laparoscopic radical hysterectomy with para-aortic and pelvic node dissection. Am J Obstet Gynecol 1992;166:864–865. **(III, B)**

53. Nezhat CR, Nezhat FR, Ramirez CE, et al: Laparoscopic radical hysterectomy and laparoscopic assisted vaginal radical hysterectomy with pelvic and paraaortic node dissection. J Gynecol Surg 1993;9:105. **(III, B)**

54. Dargent D, Salvat J: L'envahissement ganglionnaire pelvien: place de la pelviscopie retroperitoneale. Medsi, Paris, McGraw-Hill, 1989. **(III, B)**

55. Kavoussi LR, Sosa E, Chandhoke P, et al: Complications of laparoscopic pelvic lymph node dissection. J Urol 1993;149:322–325. **(III, B)**

56. Childers JM, Hatch KD, Surwit EA: Laparoscopic para-aortic lymphadenectomy in gynecologic malignancies. Obstet Gynecol 1993; 82:741–747. **(III, B)**

57. Kruitwagen RF, Swinkels BM, Keyser KG, et al: Incidence and effect on survival of abdominal wall metastases at trocar puncture sites following laparoscopy or paracentesis in women with ovarian cancer. Gynecol Oncol 1996;60:233–237. **(III, B)**

58. Passover M, Krause N, Paul K, et al: Laparoscopic para-aortic and pelvic lymphadenectomy: experience with 150 patients and review of the literature. Gynecol Oncol 1998;71:19–28. **(III, B)**

59. Buller JL, Cundiff GW: Laparoscopic surgeries for urinary incontinence. Clin Obstet Gynecol 2000;43:604–618. **(III, B)**

60. Burton G: A three-year prospective randomized urodynamic study comparing open and laparoscopic colposuspension. Neurourol Urodyn 1997;16:353–354. **(Ib,A)**

61. Su T, Want K, Hsu C, et al: Prospective comparison of laparoscopic and traditional colposuspensions in the treatment of genuine stress incontinence. Acta Obstet Gynecol Scand 1997;76:576–582. **(IIa,B)**

62. Summitt RL, Lucente V, Karram MM, et al: Randomized comparison of laparoscopic and transabdominal Burch urethropexy for treatment of genuine stress incontinence. Obstet Gynecol 2000;95(4 Suppl):2S. Abstract. **(Ib, A)**

63. Nezhat CH, Nezhat F, Nezhat C: Laparoscopic sacral colpopexy for vaginal vault prolapse. Obstet Gynecol 1994;84:885. **(III, B)**

64. Ross JW: Apical vault repair, the cornerstone of pelvic floor reconstruction. J Am Assoc Gynecol Laparosc 1997;4:173. **(IV, C)**

65. Polan ML, DeCherney A: Presacral neurectomy for pelvic pain in infertility. Fertil Steril 1980;34:557–560. **(III, B)**

66. Perez JJ: Laparoscopic presacral neurectomy: results of the first 25 cases. J Reprod Med 1990;35:625–630. **(III, B)**

# Hysteroscopic Procedures

Eric J. Bieber, MD, MHCM

Hysteroscopy has evolved over the past several decades to become the gold standard for diagnosing and treating abnormalities of the endometrial cavity. Many procedures previously requiring laparotomy, such as removal of uterine septa or submucous myomata, are now able to be performed hysteroscopically, saving the patient from undergoing major surgery as well as the morbidity and expense associated with such surgery. This chapter focuses on the various procedures that are now possible with the hysteroscope.

## DIAGNOSTIC HYSTEROSCOPY

Diagnostic hysteroscopy has supplanted D&C as the standard for evaluating the endometrial cavity and ultimately obtaining tissue for biopsy. Few D&Cs are performed in modern gynecology other than for obstetric purposes. Ultrasound and sonohysterography (SHG) are extremely useful tests for evaluating the uterus and pelvic organs (see Chapter 8), but only hysteroscopy allows concomitant treatment if an underlying abnormality is identified.

Multiple types of hysteroscopes are available in the marketplace today (see Chapter 35). An ideal operating room setup includes a small-diameter hysteroscope (approximately 3 mm) with sheaths that allow continuous inflow and outflow. A larger 4-mm hysteroscope should also be available with operative channels; finally, a resectoscope should be available. Use of small diagnostic hysteroscopes allows the surgeon to pass through small-diameter endocervical canals. They are also useful in the office setting to decrease patient discomfort.

For many years we have chosen to use fluid media, even for office and diagnostic evaluation. A small bag of 250 to 500 mL normal saline solution is attached to large-bore tubing, which is then connected to the hysteroscope. A small pressure bag may be used if necessary to allow adequate distention of the cavity because with diagnostic and basic operative cases there is less concern regarding fluid overload. The patient should be examined before starting the procedure to ascertain the position of the uterus. Generally the cervix is stabilized with a tenaculum, which also allows the endometrial canal to be straightened, although some authors have reported successful hysteroscopic examinations without the use of a tenaculum.[1] The media should be run through the tubing and the hysteroscope to decrease air in the line as well as subsequent bubbles in the endometrial cavity. The hysteroscope is then placed into the external os under direct visualization and is used to first examine the endocervical canal, identifying the internal os and carefully entering the endometrial canal. We attempt not to sound the uterus or dilate the cervix unless cervical stenosis precludes this, preferring direct visualization instead. Use of a fore-oblique hysteroscope with 12- or 30-degree offset easily allows the entire cavity to be visualized. This also allows the surgeon to rotate around the axis of the endometrial canal and avoids overmanipulation and torque of the instrument, which may cause patient discomfort as well as overdilation of the cervix. The ostia should be readily visible; with rotation the anterior, posterior, and sidewalls are easily inspected.

Various options exist for anesthesia when performing diagnostic hysteroscopy. Often, use of nonsteroidal anti-inflammatory agents alone is adequate for analgesia for simple office cases in a parous patient; more difficult cases or those that may become operative are best performed in an operative setting with general anesthesia readily available.

## THERAPEUTIC HYSTEROSCOPY

### Polypectomy

Endometrial polyps are commonly identified in patients with abnormal bleeding as well as infertility. SHG or hysterosalpingogram (HSG) readily identifies a discrete intrauterine mass, although on occasion small myomata may be mistaken for a polyp (Fig. 38-1). The patient's symptoms may range from nonexistent to menorrhagia. Polyps may also range in size from very tiny and of limited clinical significance to very large. Tamoxifen has been implicated as causing endometrial polyps, some of which may be quite large (Fig. 38-2).

Once diagnostic hysteroscopy has identified the polyp(s), if necessary the surgeon needs to change to an operative instrument with at least one operating channel. An alternative is to use polyp forceps after identification, although reevaluation of the cavity with hysteroscopy should occur to ensure that the lesion has been removed in its entirety. Hysteroscopic scissors may be used to incise the base of the polyp or stalk until only a small portion remains to anchor the lesion. At this point, the scissors may be exchanged for a grasping instrument, which can grasp the lower portion of the lesion. The distention media should be turned off and the lesion slowly removed at the same time as the hysteroscope. This method allows even large polyps to be removed through an undilated cervix. Unless the operating channel is large or the polyp is small, attempting to bring the polyp into the operative channel will cause it to be lost from the jaws of the grasper. If the entire lesion is incised and released into the cavity, it can become difficult to grasp while floating in the fluid media. An alternative to use of the operative hysteroscope is use of a resectoscope to excise the polyp. In one of the largest series published to date, Preutthipan and Herabtya retrospectively evaluated 240 premenopausal and postmenopausal women who underwent polypectomy.[2] They noted a higher recurrence rate with use of forceps versus the resectoscope to perform the polypectomy. They also noted no differences in reproductive outcome when small (<2.5 cm) versus large (>2.5 cm) polyps were removed. Complete extraction of the polyp or lesion is likely more important than the particular methodology employed for removal. However, even when lesions are removed in their entirety, patients may still return with a recurrence and new lesion.

Gebauer and colleagues prospectively evaluated postmenopausal patients who presented with an abnormal ultrasound or bleeding.[3] Patients initially underwent hysteroscopy,

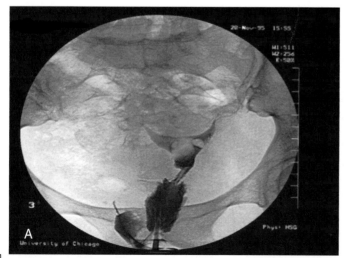
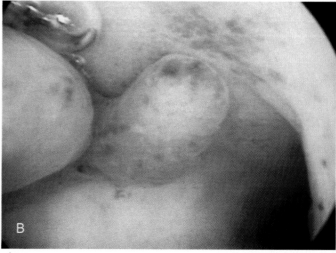

**Figure 38-1**  *A,* Hysterosalpingogram demonstrates intracavitary abnormality. Note: only a small amount of dye, which readily outlines the lesion, has been injected at this point. *B,* On hysteroscopy, the lesion is easily seen as a polyp.

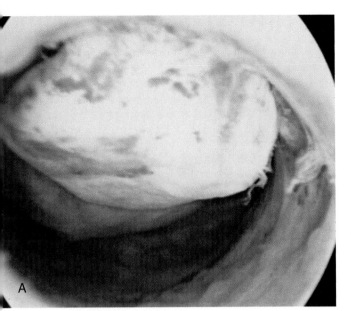
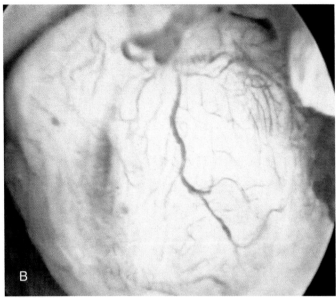

**Figure 38-2** *A,* Patient on tamoxifen who presented with postmenopausal bleeding. Hysteroscopy demonstrates a small lesion near the endocervix. *B,* Once the two smaller polyps were removed, a large polyp remains. These were all benign.

then a second blinded team performed curettage and passage of Randall polyp forceps; a repeat hysteroscopy was then performed with removal of any remaining polyps. They noted that curettage revealed the polyp in only 43% of cases, and the addition of the polyp forceps significantly improved the yield. However, use of hysteroscopy was found to be superior, especially in patients with thickened endometrium. Tjarks and Van Voorhis evaluated patients who had presented with abnormal bleeding and an abnormal SHG suggestive of endometrial polyp and found polypectomy with or without concomitant endometrial ablation or myomectomy significantly decreased bleeding and led to patient satisfaction[4] (Table 38-1). Chalas and colleagues evaluated the benign gynecologic conditions in patients from the large Breast Cancer Prevention Trial that compared the use of tamoxifen versus placebo for breast cancer prevention.[5] They noted that tamoxifen increased the risk not only of endometrial

polyps in premenopausal and postmenopausal patients, but also of leiomyomata and procedures such as curettage and hysterectomy (Table 38-2).

## Myomectomy

Uterine fibroids may be very amenable to hysteroscopic treatment, depending on depth of penetration into the endometrial cavity. Figure 38-3 demonstrates the natural evolution of a myoma from intramural to partly intracavitary to completely intracavitary to prolapsing.

Often, as endometrial distortion increases, menorrhagia will ensue and the patient may be significantly anemic. SHG is an excellent preoperative method for ascertaining what amount of the myoma is intracavitary versus intramural. It also allows an assessment of overall size as well as allowing the physician to determine if other myomata exist within the uterus. Leone and

---

**Table 38-1**
**Patient Satisfaction with Treatment**

| Procedure | *n* | Mean age (year) | Mean Length of Follow-up (mo) | Satisfaction Score* | Satisfied (%) | Percentage Having Another Procedure |
|---|---|---|---|---|---|---|
| Polypectomy | 26 | 52 ± 12 | 12 ± 5 | 3 (0–4) | 65 | 15 |
| Polypectomy with ablation | 8 | 47 ± 4 | 12 ± 4 | 4 (0–4) | 63 | 0 |
| Polypectomy with myomectomy | 8 | 46 ± 6 | 15 ± 2 | 3.5 (0.4) | 63 | 13 |
| Hysterectomy | 7 | 45 ± 12 | 14 ± 5 | 4 (3–4) | 100 | 0 |
| Medical treatment | 7 | 48 ± 10 | 14 ± 5 | 2 (1–3) | 43 | 14 |

*Satisfaction rating: 0 = very dissatisfied, 1 = dissatisfied, 2 = neither satisfied nor dissatisfied, 3 = satisfied, 4 = very satisfied. Satisfaction scores are reported as the median value with the range in parentheses.
From Tjarks M, Van Voorhis BJ: Treatment of endometrial polyps. Obstet Gynecol 2000;96:886–889.

# Minimally Invasive Surgery

**Table 38-2**
**Relative Risk\* for Patients Treated with Tamoxifen for Gynecologic Conditions and Procedures**

| | Premenopausal | Postmenopausal | Total |
|---|---|---|---|
| Endometrial polyps | 1.9 (1.55–2.41) | 2.4 (1.76–3.24) | 2.1 (1.74–2.45) |
| Leiomyomata | 1.3 (1.14–1.55) | 1.4 (1.04 –1.80) | 1.3 (1.17–1.54) |
| Curettage | 1.5 (1.23–1.77) | 3.8 (2.86–5.09) | 2.0 (1.74–2.35) |
| Hysterectomy | 1.6 (1.29–1.88) | 2.2 (1.60–3.13) | 1.7 (1.46–2.02) |

\*95% confidence interval
Adapted from Chalas E, Costantino JP, Wickerham DL, et al: Benign gynecologic conditions among participants in the Breast Cancer Prevention Trial. Am J Obstet Gynecol 2005;192:1230–1237.

colleagues found that using a strict SHG methodology, they were able to as effectively evaluate the extent of intramural versus submucous involvement of the myoma with SHG as with hysteroscopy.[6] Figures 38-4 and 38-5 demonstrate the SHG appearance of various types of myomata and how the authors evaluated the amount of endometrial extension. Figure 38-6 demonstrates the hysteroscopic appearance of a G2 type myoma, with only a portion of the myoma seen protruding into the cavity.

The surgical technique for removal generally involves the use of the resectoscope, although historically lasers and other devices were used. Loffer described the process of resection, whereby the active electrode is placed behind the myoma and strips of myoma are removed as the electrode is brought toward the resectoscope (Fig. 38-7).[7] If a portion of the myoma is

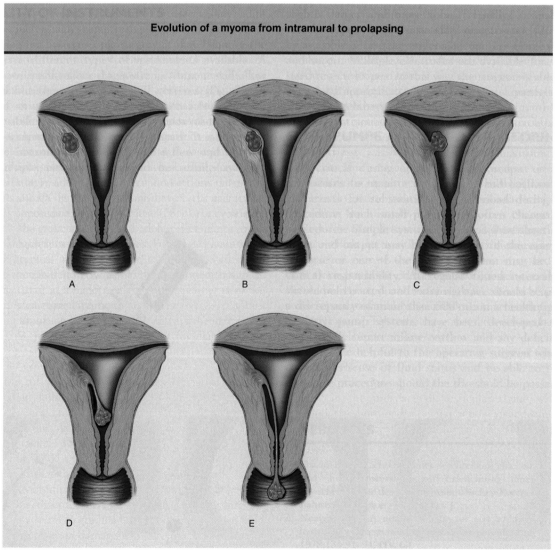

**Evolution of a myoma from intramural to prolapsing**

A    B    C

D    E

**Figure 38-3**    Demonstration of the evolution of a myoma from intramural (A), to partly intracavitary (B), to completely intracavitary with a sessile base (C), to pedunculated intracavitary myoma (D), to prolapsing myoma on a thin pedicle (E). (From Bieber EJ, Maclin VM [eds]: Myomectomy. Boston, Blackwell Science, 1998, chap. 7, fig. 1.)

**Schematic drawing of the sonographic criteria**

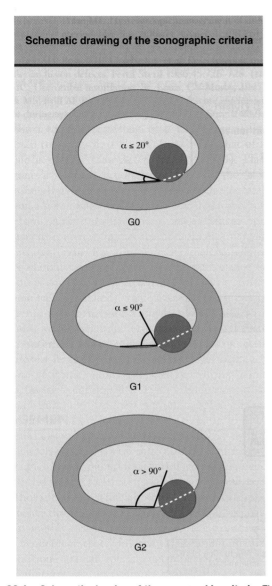

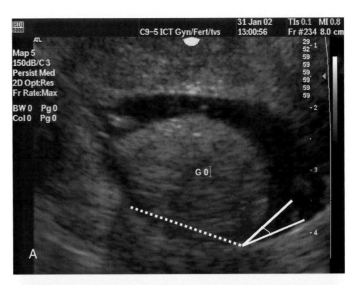

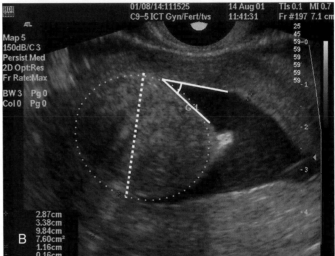

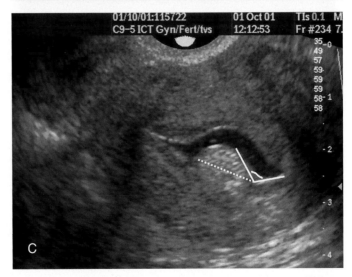

**Figure 38-4    Schematic drawing of the sonographic criteria.** The white dotted line depicts the line joining the two myoma–endomyometrial edges of the myoma, which allows the percentage of intracavitary and intramural portions of the myoma to be determined. The black lines show the angle between the endometrium and the circumference of the fibroid on the same plane. (From Leone FP, Lanzani C, Ferrazzi E: Use of strict sonohysterographic methods for preoperative assessment of submucous myomas. Fertil Steril 2003;79:998–1002.) Copyright 2003. Reprinted with permission from the American Society for Reproductive Medicine.

intramural, as the resection proceeds myometrial contractility will "push" the intramural portion of the myoma toward the cavity, allowing more of the myoma to be removed (Fig. 38-8). Generally, we do not resect below the level of the endometrium. This same technique may be applied to polyps or other intra-uterine abnormalities such as adenomyomata (Fig. 38-9), which would otherwise be impossible to remove. As myoma chips accumulate and obscure vision, they are removed and retained to send for pathology. Fluid input and output is always important to observe during any operative hysteroscopy. The process of resecting myomata may quickly open large vessels, which then

**Figure 38-5    Submucous myomas.** *A,* Submucous myoma classified as G0 on sonohysterogram (SHG). *B,* Submucous myoma classified as G1 on SHG. *C,* Submucous myoma classified as G2 on SHG. (From Leone FP, Lanzani C, Ferrazzi E: Use of strict sonohysterographic methods for preoperative assessment of submucous myomas. Fertil Steril 2003;79:998–1002.) Copyright 2003. Reprinted with permission from the American Society for Reproductive Medicine.

# Minimally Invasive Surgery

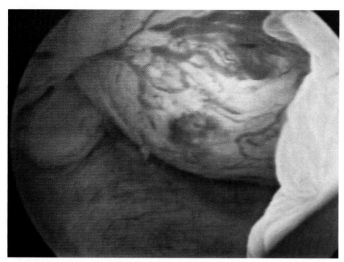

**Figure 38-6    A partly intracavitary myoma is seen on hysteroscopy in a patient who presented with anemia and menorrhagia.** The majority of the myoma is intramural.

will allow fluid intravasation and quick loss of media, so vigilance during these procedures is especially important. Figure 38-10 demonstrates a patient who had presented with significant bleeding and had been placed on high-dose oral contraceptives for an extended period. An entirely intracavitary myoma is seen with underlying striations of musculature and a very thin endometrium from use of the oral contraceptives. Figure 38-11 demonstrates a patient who presented with profound anemia and an intracavitary myoma. With removal of the intrauterine mass her menorrhagia resolved completely.

A newer alternative to this technique is the use of bipolar instrumentation, which allows vaporization of a portion of the

myoma.[8] In this situation, normal saline may be used as a distending media. A portion of the myoma should still be retained for pathology.

Resectoscopic myomectomy appears to have an excellent success rate in patients presenting with menorrhagia. More than 90% of patients will experience immediate relief after these procedures. Vercellini and colleagues evaluated results in 108 women who underwent hysteroscopic myomectomy, finding a 3-year recurrence rate of 34% and a return of menorrhagia at 3 years of 30%.[9] They found that extent of intramural extension was correlated with need for additional procedures for complete removal but did not influence long-term success. In a larger case series, Emanuel and colleagues reported on 285 patients who underwent hysteroscopic myomectomy.[10] Median follow-up was 46 months, with 14.5% of patients having a repeat surgery. Both uterine size and number of submucous myomata were independent prognosticators for recurrence, with 90.3% of patients with an initial normal size uterus and two or fewer myomata recurrence-free.

Results after hysteroscopic myomectomy in infertility patients are less well investigated but appear to have similar results to open myomectomy. Vercellini and colleagues reported a 3-year cumulative pregnancy rate of 49%, 36%, and 33% in patients with pedunculated, sessile, and partly intramural myomata, respectively.[9]

Limitations of hysteroscopic myomectomy may include the size of the submucous myoma, with myomata greater than 4 cm being somewhat difficult to remove in a single operative session. In addition, risk of fluid overload may increase with increasing myoma size. Another difficult situation is when the myoma has begun to prolapse through the cervix making distention impossible (Fig. 38-12). In these settings, if the myoma is on a stalk, rotating the myoma repetitively may allow it to be freed from its underlying attachment. Care must also be exercised

**Increasing the length of chips removed by movement of electrode and resectoscope**

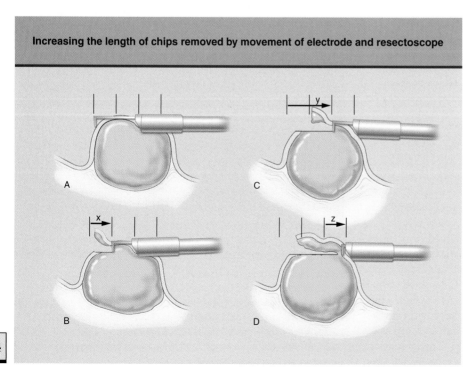

**Figure 38-7    Increasing the length of chips removed by movement of both the electrode and the resectoscope.** *A,* The loop is placed fully extended. *B,* The loop is partially closed resecting a portion *(x)* of the chip. *C,* The resectoscope is then withdrawn without further closing of the loop thus enlarging the length of the chip to *y. D,* Finally, the loop is closed into the resectoscope completing the formation of a long chip by resecting to *z.* (From Bieber EJ, Loffer FD [eds]: Hysteroscopy, Resectoscopy and Endometrial Ablation. New York: Parthenon, 2003, p 102, fig. 4.)

**Figure 38-8    Incomplete fibroid resection.** *A,* A sessile myoma before partial removal is prevented from becoming pedunculated by counterpressure from the opposite uterine wall. *B,* The myoma is shaved flush with the uterine wall during the resectoscope procedure. *C,* After the uterine cavity is emptied of distending medium to retrieve the chips, the uterine muscle fibers beneath the myoma contract and push the myoma out of its base so that a lip of the myoma visibly protrudes beyond the level of the uterine cavity *(arrow).* (From Loffer FD: Removal of large symptomatic intrauterine growths by the hysteroscopic resectoscope. Obstet Gynecol 1990;76:836–840 fig. 1.)

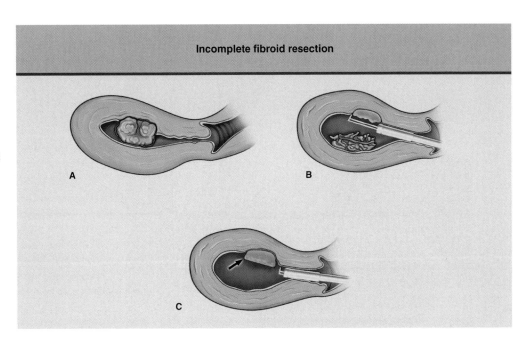

Incomplete fibroid resection

when resecting myomata that are either fundal or near the cornua. When resecting near the fundus, it may be difficult to move the electrode toward the instrument effectively; it may require a back-and-forth motion. When resecting near the cornua, care must be taken because this area may be thin and thus predisposed to perforation. Consideration may be given to concomitant laparoscopy in selected cases, although in many cases it will not be required.

### Resection/Incision of Uterine Septum

Historically, the septate uterus had been managed with a laparotomy and Tompkins or Jones metroplasty. These procedures required inpatient hospitalization and the morbidity of a laparotomy, with concern regarding formation of adhesions, as well as the need for subsequent mandatory cesarean section should pregnancy ensue. Fortunately, the advent of hysteroscopy has allowed effective transcervical treatment of this müllerian abnormality. Patients may present with habitual pregnancy loss or infertility and are generally identified on SHG or HSG. The clinician must determine that the abnormality is not a bicornuate uterus, a condition not amenable to hysteroscopic management.

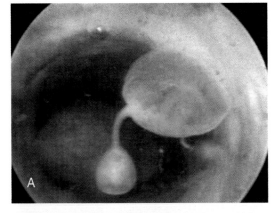

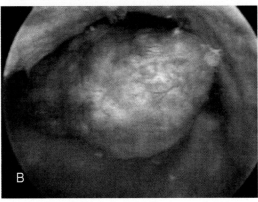

**Figure 38-9**    *A,* A small bizarre-looking polyp is seen in the lower uterine segment. *B,* Beyond this polyp a large adenomyoma is present in a patient who presented with menorrhagia.

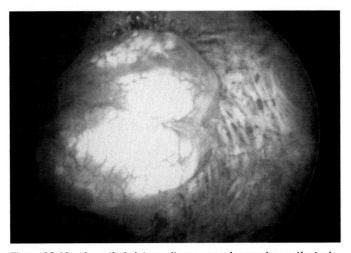

**Figure 38-10    An entirely intracavitary myoma is seen in a patient who had been treated with extended high-dose oral contraceptives.** Little endometrium is identified and underlying myometrial striations are seen.

# Minimally Invasive Surgery

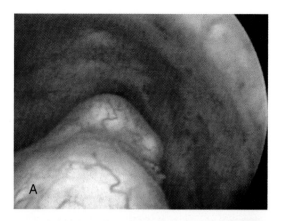

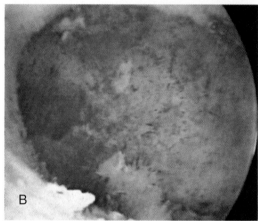

**Figure 38-11** **Patient who had prior laparotomy myomectomy who presented with profound anemia.** *A,* A discrete intracavitary myoma is identified. *B,* A normal cavity after resection of the myoma. The patient resumed normal menses following the surgery.

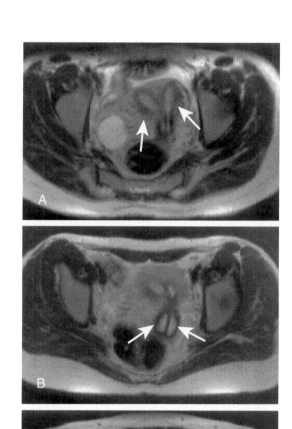

**Figure 38-13** *A,* High-resolution, T$_2$-weighted axial MRI, demonstrating a normal uterine contour, a uterine septum, two separate endometrial cavities *(arrows),* and two cervices. Incidental note is made of a right ovarian cyst. *B,* T$_2$-weighted axial MRI of same patient, which further demonstrates two distinct cervices *(arrows). C,* High-resolution T$_2$-weighted MRI of another patient, demonstrating a mixed müllerian anomaly with partial uterine septum, fused uterine horns, small indentation at the fundus, and two distinct cervices. (From Chang AS, Siegel CL, Moley KH, et al: Septate uterus with cervical duplication and longitudinal vaginal septum:a report of five new cases. Fertil Steril 2004;81:1133–1136.) Copyright 2004. Reprinted with permission from the American Society for Reproductive Medicine.

Magnetic resonance imaging studies may be useful in this regard (Fig. 38-13).[11] If the patient has presented with habitual pregnancy loss, a complete workup should be performed before surgery even if an abnormality is seen early on in the evaluation on HSG. Many variations of uterine septa exist, ranging from small septa to complete septation to the cervix or even an associated vaginal septum (Fig. 38-14).

Interestingly, most uterine septa do not require excision but instead require incision. Multiple different devices and energy modalities have been used to accomplish incision, including

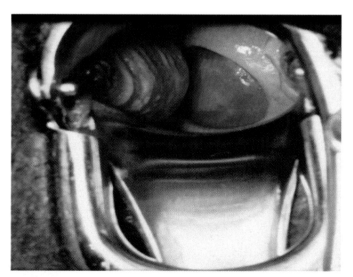

**Figure 38-12** **Patient with dilated cervix and myoma beginning to prolapse through the cervix.** (From Bieber EJ, Maclin VM [eds]: Myomectomy. Boston, Blackwell Science, 1998.)

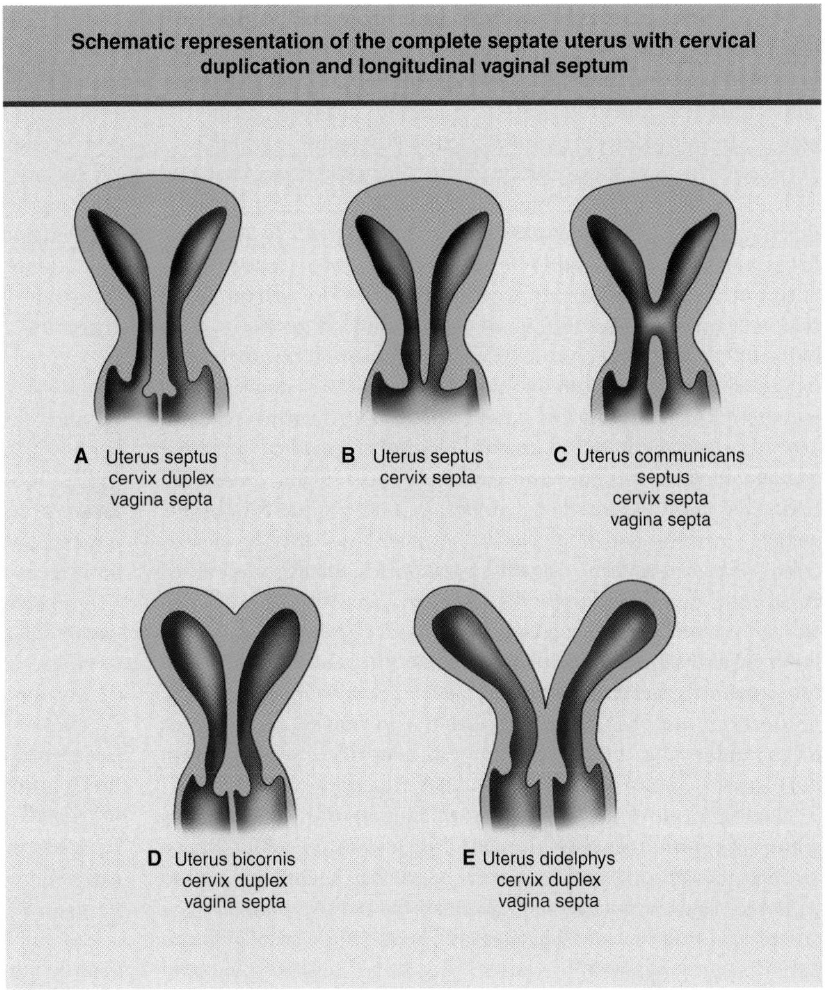

**Schematic representation of the complete septate uterus with cervical duplication and longitudinal vaginal septum**

**Figure 38-14  Complete septate uterus with cervical duplication and longitudinal vaginal septum and other uterine anomalies for which it may be mistaken.** *A,* Schematic representation. *B,* Complete septate uterus with single cervix. *C,* Complete septate uterus and single cervix with midseptal perforation (atrium communicans) and vaginal septum; *D,* Bicornuate uterus with double cervix and longitudinal vaginal septum. *E,* Didelphic uterus. (From Patton PE: The diagnosis and reproductive outcome after surgical treatment of the complete septate uterus, duplicated cervix, and vaginal septum. Am J Obstet Gynecol 2004;190:1669–1678.)

**A  Uterus septus cervix duplex vagina septa**

**B  Uterus septus cervix septa**

**C  Uterus communicans septus cervix septa vagina septa**

**D  Uterus bicornis cervix duplex vagina septa**

**E  Uterus didelphys cervix duplex vagina septa**

laser, scissors, knife or point electrodes, or the resectoscope with a 180-degree loop. Each has different pros and cons, and no one modality has been found to be more effective than another.

The surgical technique involves identification of the extent of the septum and evaluation of the two subcavities that it separates. If a vaginal septum is present, this may need to be incised prior to the hysteroscopic portion of the procedure. The ostia should be identified in each of the cavities. Concomitant laparoscopy is often employed both to ascertain that the anomaly is amenable to hysteroscopic treatment and to evaluate the extent of incision. The chosen modality is then used to begin to incise the septum. As this occurs the cavity begins to open. It is important to stay in the center of the septum and not cut toward the anterior or posterior wall because bleeding may ensue. Incising small amounts of the septum at a time will optimize this. Care should be taken not to overextend the incision into the uterine fundus because this may weaken the area and allow subsequent perforation during pregnancy (see Chapter 39). If a laparoscope is in place, the surgeon may be able to access the remaining fundal thickness by turning the laparoscope illumination to a low level and viewing the transmission of light from the hysteroscope through the uterine fundus.

Postoperatively various regimens have been used to decrease the formation of intrauterine adhesions in the denuded area of the septal incision. Few good studies exist to determine if any of these, including use of an antibiotic, intrauterine device (IUD), or estrogens, have value.[12] Nawroth and colleagues evaluated a small number of patients who underwent septal resection and were placed on no therapy, cyclical hormone replacement therapy (HRT) and IUD, or HRT alone and noted no improvement with either of the active treatments.[13] Given the limited data, in a patient with no contraindications, we generally place the patient on unopposed estrogen for a month followed by progestin withdrawal. Fortunately, few patients will form adhesions and the area appears to heal quickly. After several cycles the cavity should be reassessed by HSG or hysteroscopy. On occasion, a small fundal indentation may still exist where the larger septum was lysed. These appear to have little clinical consequence when smaller than 1 cm.

Reproductive outcome after lysis of uterine septa is very good and comparable to that achieved through the successful but more invasive open procedures. It is generally believed that while a uterine septum may interfere with the ability to sustain a pregnancy, it may have a limited impact on fertility. Unfortunately, to date no well-performed randomized, controlled trial exists regarding treatment of a uterine septum. Valle reported on a case series of 124 patients with partial or complete uterine septa who had 299 pregnancies, of which 87% were miscarried and 10% were delivered prematurely.[14] After hysteroscopic

# Minimally Invasive Surgery

removal of the septum, 81% of patients achieved pregnancy, with 83% delivered at term, 7% preterm, and 12% first-trimester losses. Homer and colleagues evaluated a number of case series and found that collectively the 658 patients with recurrent loss had an 88% miscarriage rate prior to metroplasty, which was decreased to 14% after surgery.[15] Smaller case series by Valli and colleagues and by Verturoli and colleagues found similar improvements.[16,17]

Lavergne and colleagues retrospectively evaluated patients with uterine anomalies and noted a lower rate of implantation that improved when patients with a uterine septum were treated.[18] Many surgeons who initially would not treat patients until they had one or more miscarriage have reevaluated this paradigm and will now treat patients desiring fertility prior to any losses. Indeed, it is recommended that patients pursuing in vitro fertilization have uterine septa lysed before beginning treatment with assisted reproductive technology. Hopefully, in the future randomized, controlled trials will provide similar compelling information regarding the efficacy of septolysis as the multitude of case series have suggested.

## Lysis of Intrauterine Adhesions (Asherman's Syndrome)

Hysteroscopy has also revolutionized the treatment of intra-uterine adhesions. Historically the clinician simply performed a D&C with the hope of breaking apart the adhesive bands and preventing them from re-forming. Modern hysteroscopy allows a more rationale approach to this difficult surgery.

Patients typically present with amenorrhea having undergone an antecedent procedure such as D&C for a missed abortion or postpartum. However, the range of presentations also includes patients with hypomenorrhea or eumenorrhea who may only present with infertility. Valle and Sciarra reported that in 183 of 187 patients with intrauterine adhesions, these adhesions were associated with a prior obstetric curettage.[19] Westendorp and colleagues prospectively evaluated 50 patients who had undergone curettage for placental remnants more than 24 hours after delivery or a repeat curettage after D&C for incomplete abortion.[20] Hysteroscopy performed 3 months later demonstrated that 20 of 50 (40%) patients had adhesions ranging from mild to severe.

Typically, HSG will document an abnormal cavity that may be small, misshapen, or filled with discrete intracavitary abnormalities consistent with adhesions. The fallopian tubes may or may not be patent on HSG; adhesive disease can range from a single adhesion to an entirely obliterated cavity.

Surgery for Asherman's syndrome may be the most difficult hysteroscopic procedure, with the highest level of concomitant risk of complications (see Chapter 39). Unless the case is deemed to be simple with a small number of adhesions, laparoscopy may be considered and performed during the hysteroscopic portion of the procedure on a separate video monitor. During the initial phase of the hysteroscopy we prefer a small-size hysteroscope. The endocervical canal is evaluated first and then exploration of the uterine cavity is begun (if possible). Visualization of the ostia may or may not be possible but when seen they provide excellent landmarks. Adhesions are identified and transected in the middle. Again, various modalities have been used, including laser, resectoscope, and various electrodes. It is believed that avoiding

energy sources that may cause lateral thermal damage offers an advantage, although no trials exist to demonstrate the superiority of one modality over another. Zikopoulos and colleagues reported on a 10-year experience using either the resectocope or the Versapoint system and found similar rates of success.[21] We prefer scissors placed through the operative hysteroscope with a large enough sheath to allow adequate pressures for distention and outflow should any bleeding be encountered. If distention is inadequate, it may be more difficult to appreciate the origin and insertion of the adhesive bands. This process is continued until the adhesive bands are freed and the uterus attains a reasonably normal configuration. At this point, if tubal patency was not initially visible, it should be reevaluated.

Postoperatively most surgeons treat with unopposed estrogen for a period followed by progestin withdrawal unless contraindicated. Others have used IUD (nonmedicated) as an alternative or in addition to estrogen. Unfortunately, little information exists on what postoperative treatments (if any) optimize success and limit the re-formation of adhesions. Ultimately HSG, hysteroscopy, or both should be performed to reevaluate the cavity for the possibility of adhesion reformation.

Valle and Sciarra reported one of the first large series of hysteroscopic intervention in patients with Asherman's syndrome.[19] Only 9.6% of patients initially had normal menses, but after intervention 89% reported normal menstrual function. Successful term pregnancy correlated with extent of adhesions, with 81% of patients successful with mild adhesions but only 32% success with severe adhesions. Katz and colleagues specifically evaluated patients who had a minimum of two prior pregnancies with a prior early loss or a preterm delivery with subsequent loss who underwent hysteroscopic adhesiolysis.[22] Prior to intervention, only 18% of pregnancies were delivered at term, with 62% first-trimester losses. After adhesiolysis, success was seen in 64% of pregnancies. Capella-Allouc and colleagues reported on hysteroscopic adhesiolysis in patients with severe Asherman's syndrome.[23] In 15 of 31 cases, two, three, or even four procedures were required to free the cavity and at least one ostia area. A live birth rate of 32% was ultimately achieved, although success was higher (62.5%) in patients younger than age 35.

Patients undergoing these surgeries should understand the potential need for further surgery to attain a cavity with a normal configuration and that in some cases, this may not be possible. In addition, subsequent pregnancies may have placental abnormalities such as placenta accreta, which may cause significant bleeding at the time of delivery and even necessitate hysterectomy.[19,21,23]

## Hysteroscopic Sterilization

For a number of years, multiple clinical trials have evaluated hysteroscopic methodologies for sterilization. In November 2002 one of these methods became available in the United States. Multiple technical issues made the development of such a device quite difficult, including the need to easily place the device in uteri of different shapes as well as the need for occlusion in all patients.

The Essure device that is presently available is made of polyethelyne (PET) fibers in a coil (Fig. 38-15). The device is delivered through the operative channel of the hysteroscope and

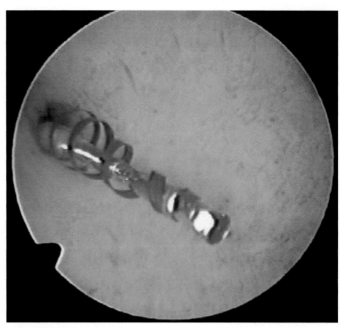

Figure 38-15 **An Essure insert.** (Courtesy of Conceptus, Inc., Mountain View, CA.)

is placed within the ostia. Release of the device allows the coils to unwind, anchoring them at the level of the uterotubal junction (Fig. 38-16). When ideally placed a small number of coils are visible within the uterine cavity while the majority of the coils are located within the tubal lumen (Fig. 38-17). The PET fibers cause a local inflammatory response with subsequent occlusion of the tubal lumen. Patients are recommended to use a reliable form of contraception for the next 3 months and then undergo subsequent HSG to document tubal occlusion (Fig. 38-18). Some authors have suggested that a follow-up ultrasound may be adequate for assessing the location of the inserts.[24]

Data from the pivotal trial of the Essure device as well as ongoing evaluation document an effectiveness of more than 99% in patients who have the devices placed appropriately and have evidence of tubal occlusion at follow-up evaluation. Patients do need to be aware that the implants may be extruded, perforation may occur, and uterine or tubal abnormalities may preclude placement. If placement of the device is unsuccessful, some patients will opt for laparoscopic tubal sterilization.

Figure 38-17 **Essure coils visible in the ostia after hysteroscopic placement.** (Courtesy of Conceptus, Inc., Mountain View, CA.)

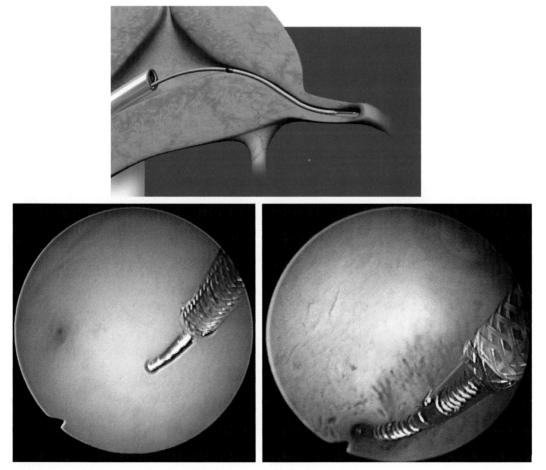

Figure 38-16 **An Essure device being placed into the fallopian tube.** (Courtesy of Conceptus, Inc., Mountain View, CA.)

# Minimally Invasive Surgery

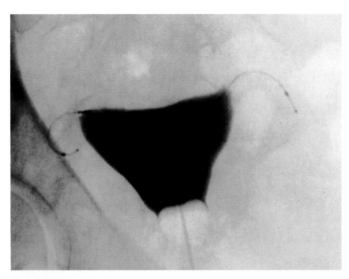

**Figure 38-18    Hysterosalpingogram (HSG) demonstrates tubal occlusion with both Essure devices visible at the uterotubal junctions.**

In the Phase III clinical trial, the microinserts were able to be bilaterally placed in 92% of patients and at 3 months tubal occlusion was confirmed in 92%.[25] In this study, 449 of 518 (87%) patients were able to rely on this device for permanent contraception. In another report 98% of patients at 2 years after surgery reported their tolerance of the microinsert as very good or excellent.[26] Follow-up studies have documented significant satisfaction with the procedure and quick recovery with little morbidity. No significant change in menstrual function has been seen to date.

The significant advantage of a hysteroscopic approach for sterilization is the avoidance of entry into the abdominal cavity, which may be very relevant for patients with prior surgery as well as obese patients or those at higher surgical risk for laparoscopy. The Essure device should not be placed in persons who are allergic to nickel. Clinical investigations are ongoing into other methods of hysteroscopic sterilization, which may become available in the future.

## Treatment of Proximal Tubal Occlusion

Proximal tubal occlusion may be seen in patients seeking fertility treatment with up to 15% of HSGs demonstrating tubal occlusion. Historically these patients were treated with laparotomy and resection and reanastomosis or reimplantation of the affected tube. Hysteroscopic treatment allows a much less invasive technique with similar rates of patency and pregnancy. At HSG, a false-positive finding of tubal occlusion may occur with tubal spasm. When Sulak and colleagues evaluated sections of tube excised for a diagnosis of proximal tubal occlusion, they noted that in 11 of 18 cases no occlusion could be demonstrated and in 6 cases amorphous material was contained within the tubal lumen that they called "plugs."[27]

Novi and colleagues reported on use of a transcervical catheter and inner flexible guidewire placed either via hysteroscopy or fluoroscopy to treat proximal tubal occlusion.[28] Hysteroscopy and concomitant laparoscopy allow documentation that proximal occlusion is present and that concomitant distal disease is not present. An operative hysteroscope is then used to introduce

the initial catheter, which has an angulation that allows it to preferentially come in proximity with the ostia. At this point methylene blue may be reintroduced in direct proximity to the ostia to again document that proximal tubal occlusion exists. Once reconfirmed, the inner wire is inserted through the initially placed catheter in an attempt to break through the area of blockage. The use of concomitant laparoscopy facilitates viewing the lateral passage of the inner catheter through the tube as well as helping the surgeon avoid perforation of the tube if the blockage is severe. If the catheter passes through the blockage, methylene blue is again used to document that tubal patency has been restored.

Another alternative to this technique has been the performance of the procedure using similar catheter systems with radiographic assistance. Similar rates of success have been reported in the literature. A potential limitation of the fluorographic technique is that, without documentation of the normality of the distal tube, an abnormal tube that would not have been operated on endoscopically and that would instead have prompted the gynecologist to recommend in vitro fertilization could be opened. In reality, both techniques appear effective.

Al-Jaroudi and colleagues evaluated 7 years of data on patients presenting for bilateral tubal occlusion at a single institution.[29] On reevaluation, they noted that over 14% of patients had bilateral patent tubes and 12% had at least one patent tube. Using fluoroscopic techniques, they were able to recannulize at least one tube in 61% of patients, with an overall pregnancy rate of 31.9%. This data is consistent with a review of 1079 patients by Thurmond and colleagues demonstrating a crude pregnancy rate of 30%.[30]

## Endometrial Ablation/Resection

DeCherney and Polan first reported on use of the resectoscope to treat critically ill patients with abnormal uterine bleeding.[31] Since this first report, thousand of patients have undergone endometrial ablation with a multitude of technologies. Initial reports used either the laser, or ball, barrel, or loop electrodes to cause endometrial destruction. More recently, global methodologies have supplanted hysteroscopic endometrial ablation. These technologies include cryoablation, microwave ablation, bipolar ablation, thermal balloon ablation, hysteroscopic thermal ablation, and other rapidly developing devices.

Hysteroscopic endometrial ablation remains a viable alternative for some patients. In a patient with an enlarged or abnormally shaped uterus, this option may be preferable to a global technology. Patients may be pretreated with medical agents before endometrial ablation. The most recent Cochrane review suggests that use of gonadotropin-releasing hormone analogs may improve operating conditions and short-term outcomes.[32] Unfortunately, little information is available regarding long-term outcomes or use of agents with global techniques.

Most surgeons use a small ball electrode with a standard resectoscope. This requires use of a nonelectrolyte-containing media such as glycine unless bipolar technology is used. Initially the cornua are ablated, followed by the fundus, anterior, and sidewalls and finally the posterior uterus. If the uterus has been well prepared before surgery, there should be little tissue present. Variation exists among surgeons regarding the use of a pure cutting current versus coagulation or blended current. Visual feedback during the ablation suggests whether an adequate effect is being achieved. An alternative to use of a ball electrode is endometrial resection, in which a loop electrode is used to remove a large portion of the endometrium. Interestingly, this technique seems to be favored in Europe whereas coagulation ablation is the favored technique in the United States.

Rauramo and colleagues performed a 3-year open randomized trial of endometrial resection versus the levonorgestrel intrauterine system (IUS) for long-term treatment of menorrhagia.[33] They found both markedly reduced menstrual bleeding and noted a 63% continuation rate in the IUS group. Zupi and colleagues randomized 180 patients to endometrial resection or laparoscopic supracervical hysterectomy and found decreased operative time in the hysteroscopic group but greater patient satisfaction in the hysterectomy group.[34] Pellicano and colleagues evaluated endometrial resection versus thermal ablation and noted thermal ablation to have a higher satisfaction rate, with a decreased operative time, blood loss, and need for reintervention.[35] Interestingly, Boujida and colleagues evaluated 120 women with menorrhagia who had undergone endometrial ablation via coagulation or resection and found no difference in frequency of complications between the groups.[36] However, only 15% of patients subsequently failed their ablation and underwent hysterectomy, while another 15% underwent a second endometrial ablation. Similar reductions in blood loss and patient satisfaction were also noted in both groups. In a case series of 240 women undergoing roller ball endometrial ablation, Dutton and colleagues reported that the probability of no hysterectomy at 5 years was 71% and that repeat ablation and ablation at a younger age were risk factors for failure.[37] Confirming the significant and sustained reduction in blood loss, Teirney and colleagues evaluated menstrual blood loss after roller ball ablation.[38] Using alkaline hematin technique, they reported a decrease in menstrual bleeding from 90 mL before surgery to 3.8 mL at 3 months, 1.8 mL at 6 months, and 3.3 mL at 5 to 6 years after endometrial ablation.

Endometrial ablation has been compared to hysterectomy in several trials, including one conducted by the Aberdeen Endometrial Ablation Trials Group.[39] They randomized 204 women to hysterectomy or endometrial ablation; patients were followed for a minimum of 4 years. Of women randomized to the endometrial ablation group, 38% required further surgery, with 24% undergoing hysterectomy. Both groups had overall high patient satisfaction—80% for endometrial ablation and 89% for hysterectomy. When all factors were considered, ablation was still less expensive, but over time this difference had narrowed from initially after surgery. A 2000 Cochrane review of endometrial resection versus hysterectomy for menorrhagia suggested that improvement in heavy menstrual bleeding and overall satisfaction up to 4 years after surgery was weighted toward hysterectomy.[40] They did state that major and minor adverse events were more likely after hysterectomy, although these differences were markedly diminished on discharge to home.

These data suggest that endometrial ablation remains an appropriate therapy in selected patients with menorrhagia. Up to one third of these patients may require further intervention, with one quarter or more likely to undergo subsequent hysterectomy when viewed over a number of years. It appears that global methods of performing endometrial ablation are as

successful as the more difficult hysteroscopic procedures but may not be applicable to all patients; in addition, overall there is less long-term data related to them. Endometrial resection is a more complicated procedure to perform, although in experienced hands it appears to produce good results. Consideration may be given to alternatives such as the levonorgestrel-containing IUS if appropriate or even hysterectomy if definitive treatment is preferable.

### Endometrial Cancer

Hysteroscopy has been used for several decades as an adjuvant to D&C in the evaluation of patients with abnormal or postmenopausal bleeding. An advantage of hysteroscopy is that the surgeon may identify a lesion, which may then be directly sampled. Figure 38-19 demonstrates complex hyperplasia with atypia with numerous abnormal vessels, which contained a discrete lesion that was a well-differentiated adenocarcinoma. Clark and colleagues, in a review of the literature, found

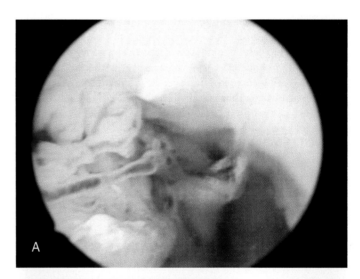

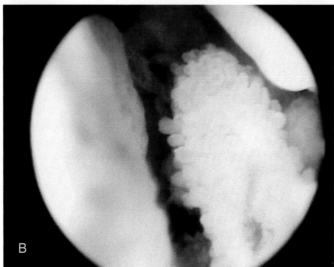

**Figure 38-19** *A,* Patient with postmenopausal bleeding who is seen to have markedly abnormal vessels and tissue, which was atypical hyperplasia with atypia. *B,* Same patient; focus of well-differentiated adenocarcinoma within the endometrial hyperplasia.

hysteroscopy to have 86% sensitivity and 99% specificity for endometrial cancer.[41] They noted that hysteroscopy had high diagnostic accuracy for endometrial cancer and moderate accuracy for endometrial disease (endometrial cancer and hyperplasia). Litta and colleagues also found hysteroscopy to be of value in evaluating postmenopausal bleeding and differentiating benign lesions such as polyps and myomata.[42] They suggest the synergistic value of transvaginal ultrasound along with hysteroscopy and endometrial biopsy in clearly obtaining a diagnosis.

A persistent question has been the issue of dissemination of endometrial cancer cells during the performance of hysteroscopy, especially with the use of fluid media. Bradley and colleagues retrospectively evaluated 256 charts from patients who had endometrial cancer and found positive peritoneal cytology in 6.9% of patients who initially underwent endometrial biopsy or D&C versus 13.5% in those who underwent hysteroscopy.[43] Sainz de la Cuesta and colleagues randomly assigned patients to hysteroscopy immediately before laparotomy for endometrial cancer or to no hysteroscopy and found a small increase in risk of positive peritoneal cytology in the fluid hysteroscopy group but no change in prognosis.[44] In contrast, multiple authors have reported no increase in incidence of positive peritoneal washings or change in prognosis.[45,46] Further prospective studies may help to address the question of whether hysteroscopy actually increases the dissemination of cells more than standard D&C and if this is clinically relevant for disease prognosis.

## CONCLUSION

Hysteroscopy remains the most efficient technology for both evaluating and treating intrauterine disease. In modern gynecologic surgery, hysteroscopy has supplanted many of the gold standard procedures. Rarely today are there indications for Jones or Tompkins metroplasty or laparotomy for proximal tubal disease. Even standard laparoscopic tubal ligation may give way to less invasive hysteroscopic sterilization.

## REFERENCES

1. Bettocchi S, Nappi L, Ceci O, Selvaggi L: Office hysteroscopy. Obstet Gynecol Clin North Am 2004;31:641–654. **(IV, C)**
2. Preutthipan S, Herabtya Y: Hysteroscopic polypectomy in 240 premenopausal and postmenopausal women. Fertil Steril 2005; 83:705–709. **(III, C)**
3. Gebauer G, Hafner A, Siebzehnrubl E, Lang N: Role of hysteroscopy in detection and extraction of endometrial polyps: results of a prospective study. Am J Obstet Gynecol 2001;184:59–63. **(IIa, B)**
4. Tjarks M, Van Voorhis BJ: Treatment of endometrial polyps. Obstet Gynecol 2000;96:886–889. **(IIb, B)**
5. Chalas E, Costantino JP, Wickerham DL, et al: Benign gynecologic conditions among participants in the Breast Cancer Prevention Trial. Am J Obstet Gynecol 2005;192:1230–1237. **(Ib, A)**
6. Leone FP, Lanzani C, Ferrazzi E: Use of strict sonohysterographic methods for preoperative assessment of submucous myomas. Fertil Steril 2003;79:998–1002. **(IIb, B)**
7. Loffer FD: Removal of large symptomatic intrauterine growths by the hysteroscopic resectoscope. Obstet Gynecol 1990;76:836–840. **(III, B)**
8. Clark TJ, Mahajan D, Sunder P, Gupta JK: Hysteroscopic treatment of symptomatic submucous fibroids using a bipolar intrauterine system: a feasibility study. Eur J Obstet Gynecol Reprod Biol 2002;100:237–242. **(IIb, B)**
9. Vercellini P, Zaina B, Yaylayan L, et al: Hysteroscopic myomectomy: long term effects on menstrual pattern and fertility. Obstet Gynecol 1999;94:341–347. **(III, B)**
10. Emanuel MH, Wamsteker K, Hart AA, et al: Long–term results of hysteroscopic myomectomy for abnormal uterine bleeding. Obstet Gynecol 1999;93:743–748. **(III, B)**
11. Chang AS, Siegel CL, Moley KH, et al: Septate uterus with cervical duplication and longitudinal vaginal septum: a report of five new cases. Fertil Steril 2004;81:1133–1136. **(III, B)**
12. Dabirashrafi H, Mohammad K, Moghadami-Tabrizi N, et al: Is estrogen necessary after hysteroscopic incision of the uterine septum? J Am Assoc Gynecol Lap 1996;3:623–625. **(III, B)**
13. Nawroth F, Schmidt T, Freise C, et al: Is it possible to recommend an "optimal" postoperative management after hysteroscopic metroplasty? A retrospective study of 52 infertile patients showing a septate uterus. Acta Obstet Gynecol Scand 2002;81:55–57. **(III, B)**
14. Valle RF: Hysteroscopic treatment of partial and complete uterine septum. Int J Fertil Menop Stud 1996;41:310–315. **(III, B)**
15. Homer HA, Li TC, Cooke ID: The septate uterus: a review of management and reproductive outcome. Fertil Steril 2000;73:1–14. **(III, B)**
16. Valli E, Vaquero E, Lazzarin N, et al: Hysteroscopic metroplasty improves gestational outcome in women with recurrent spontaneous abortion. J Am Assoc Gynecol Lap 2004;11:240–244. **(III, B)**
17. Verturoli S, Colombo FM, Vianello F, et al: A study of hysteroscopic metroplasty in 141 women with a septate uterus. Arch Gynecol Obstet 2002;266:157–159. **(III, B)**
18. Lavergne N, Aristizabal J, Zarka V, et al: Uterine anomalies and in vitro fertilization: what are the results? Eur J Obstet Gynecol Reprod Biol 1996;68:29–34. **(III, B)**
19. Valle RF, Sciarra JJ: Intrauterine adhesions: hysteroscopic diagnosis, classification, treatment and reproductive outcome. Am J Obstet Gynecol 1988;158:1459–1470. **(III, B)**
20. Westendorp IC, Ankum WM, Mol BW, Vonk J: Prevalence of Asherman's syndrome after secondary removal of placental remnants or a repeat curettage for incomplete abortion. Hum Reprod 1998; 13:3347–3350. **(IIb, B)**
21. Zikopoulos KA, Kolibianakis EM, Platteau P, et al: Live delivery rates in subfertile women with Asherman's syndrome after hysteroscopic adhesiolysis using the resectoscope or the Versapoint system. Reprod Biomed Online 2004;8:720–725. **(III, B)**
22. Katz Z, Ben-Arie A, Lurie S, et al: Reproductive outcome following hysteroscopic adhesiolysis in Asherman's syndrome. Int J Fertil Menop Stud 1996;41:462–465. **(III, B)**
23. Capella-Allouc S, Morsad F, Rongieres-Bertrand C, et al: Hysteroscopic treatment of severe Asherman's syndrome and subsequent fertility. Hum Reprod 1999;14:1230–1233. **(III, B)**
24. Kerin JF, Levy BS: Ultrasound: an effective method for localization of the echogenic Essure sterilization micro-insert: correlation with radiologic findings. J Min Inv Gynecol 2005;12:50–54. **(IIb, B)**
25. Cooper JM, Carignan CS, Cher D, Kerin JF: Microinsert nonincisional hysteroscopic sterilization. Obstet Gynecol 2003;102:59–67. **(IIa, B)**
26. Kerin JF, Cooper JM, Price T, et al: Hysteroscopic sterilization using microinsert device: results of a multicentre phase II study. Hum Reprod 2003;18:1223–1230. **(IIa, B)**
27. Sulak PJ, Letterie GS, Coddington CC, et al: Histology of proximal tubal occlusion. Fertil Steril 1987;48:437–440. **(III, B)**
28. Novi MJ, Thurmond AS, Patton P, et al: Diagnosis of cornual obstruction by transcervical fallopian tube cannulation. Fertil Steril 1988;50:434–440. **(III, B)**
29. Al-Jaroudi D, Herba MJ, Tulandi T: Reproductive performance after selective tubal catheterization. J Min Inv Gynecol 2005;12:150–152. **(III, B)**
30. Thurmond AS, Machan L, Maubon AJ, et al: A review of selective salpingography and fallopian tube catheterization. Radiograph 2000; 20:1759–1768. **(III, B)**

31. DeCherney A, Polan ML: Hysteroscopic management of intrauterine lesions and intractable uterine bleeding. Obstet Gynecol 1983; 61:392–397. **(III, B)**

32. Sowter MC, Lethaby A, Singla AA: Pre-operative endometrial thinning agents before endometrial destruction for heavy menstrual bleeding. Cochrane Database Systemic Rev 2002:CD001124. **(Ia, A)**

33. Rauramo I, Elo I, Istre O: Long-term treatment of menorrhagia with levonorgestrel intrauterine system versus endometrial resection. Obstet Gynecol 2004;104:1314–1321. **(Ib, A)**

34. Zupi E, Zullo F, Marconi D, et al: Hysteroscopic endometrial resection versus laparoscopic supracervical hysterectomy for menorrhagia: a prospective randomized trial. Am J Obstet Gynecol 2003;188:7–12. **(Ib, A)**

35. Pellicano M, Guida M, Acunzo G, et al: Hysteroscopic transcervical endometrial resection versus thermal destruction for menorrhagia: a prospective trial on satisfaction rate. Am J Obstet Gynecol 2002; 187:545–550. **(IIa, B)**

36. Boujida VH, Philipsen T, Pelle J, Joergensen JC: Five-year follow-up of endometrial ablation: endometrial coagulation versus endometrial resection. Obstet Gynecol 2002;99:988–992. **(III, B)**

37. Dutton C, Ackerson L, Phelps-Sandall B: Outcomes after rollerball endometrial ablation for menorrhagia. Obstet Gynecol 2001;98:35–39. **(III, B)**

38. Teirney R, Arachchi GJ, Fraser IS: Menstrual blood loss measured 5 to 6 years after endometrial ablation. Obstet Gynecol 2000;95:251–254. **(IIa, B)**

39. Aberdeen Endometrial Ablation Trials Group: A randomized trial of endometrial ablation versus hysterectomy for the treatment of dysfunctional uterine bleeding: outcome at four years. Br J Obstet Gynaecol 1999;106:360–366. **(Ib, A)**

40. Lethaby A, Shepperd S, Cooke I, Farquhar C: Endometrial resection and ablation versus hysterectomy for heavy menstrual bleeding. Cochrane Database System Rev 2000:CD000329. **(Ia, A)**

41. Clark TJ, Voit D, Gupta JK, et al: Accuracy of hysteroscopy in the diagnosis of endometrial cancer and hyperplasia: a systematic quantitative review. JAMA 2002;288:1610–1621. **(III, B)**

42. Litta P, Merlin F, Saccardi C, et al: Role of hysteroscopy with endometrial biopsy to rule out endometrial cancer in postmenopausal women with abnormal uterine bleeding. Maturitas 2005;50:117–123. **(III, B)**

43. Bradley WH, Boente MP, Brooker D, et al: Hysteroscopy and cytology in endometrial cancer. Obstet Gynecol 2004;104:1030–1033. **(III, B)**

44. Sainz de la Cuesta R, Espinosa JA, Crespo E, et al: Does fluid hysteroscopy increase the stage or worsen the prognosis in patients with endometrial cancer? A randomized controlled trial. Eur J Obstet Gynecol Reprod Biol 2004;115:211–215. **(Ib, A)**

45. Biewenga P, de Blok S, Birnie E: Does diagnostic hysteroscopy in patients with stage I endometrial carcinoma cause positive peritoneal washings? Gynecol Oncol 2004;93:194–198. **(III, B)**

46. Kudela M, Pilka R: Is there a real risk in patients with endometrial carcinoma undergoing diagnostic hysteroscopy? Eur J Gynecol Oncol 2001;22:342–344. **(IIa, B)**

# Chapter 39

# Laparoscopic and Hysteroscopic Complications

## Eric J. Bieber, MD, MHCM

## KEY POINTS

- Operative laparoscopy has an overall 1% to 2% complication rate.
- The majority of complications in laparoscopy occur during attempted entry with Veress needle or trocar.
- Even under direct visualization, placement of ancillary trocars may still cause injuries.
- Patients with prior midline surgery have a 60% chance of midline adhesions.
- Alternative sites, such as the left upper quadrant, may be used to gain abdominal entry in selected cases.
- No one method of entry (closed, direct, open) has been demonstrated to be better or safer.
- The inferior epigastric vessels have a dual blood supply.
- A Foley catheter may be placed through a trocar sleeve to tamponade bleeding from epigastric vessels.
- Instill dilute methylene blue to document integrity of bladder if there is a question of perforation.
- The ureter is in close proximity to the infundibulopelvic ligaments.
- The right and left pelvis are not mirror images.
- Increasing abdominal/pelvic pain more than 48 hours after surgery should raise suspicion regarding injury.
- If significant vascular injury occurs during laparoscopy, consider midline laparotomy.
- Approximately 50% of hysteroscopic complications are entry related.
- Track input and output throughout all operative hysteroscopies.
- Stop the hysteroscopic procedure once the threshold for fluid deficit has been reached.
- Be aware of risks of air embolism during hysteroscopy.
- Endometrial ablation is not a sterilization procedure.
- Diagnostic hysteroscopy has a much lower rate of complications than operative hysteroscopy.
- Lysis of intrauterine adhesions, hysteroscopic myomectomy, and septal lysis have the highest risk of hysteroscopic complications.

Laparoscopic and hysteroscopic complications may occur in even the simplest of cases. This chapter reviews the various risks associated with these gynecologic endoscopic procedures and offers suggestions for avoidance and treatment when complications occur (Tables 39-1 and 39-2). It has been stated that even the best surgeon on the best day may have a complication. Thus, preparation for managing complications when they inevitably occur is critical. This may begin as early as the initial visit to discuss surgery and the informed consent process and continues into the operating room and subsequent postoperative care.

Few good studies exist from which to glean information regarding likelihood of risk. However, multiple salient points begin to emerge from analysis of published data that may be useful in preparing for endoscopic surgery.

## LAPAROSCOPIC COMPLICATIONS

### General Background Information

Chapron and colleagues reported on almost 30,000 laparoscopic cases performed in seven busy French centers.[1] This case series included all laparoscopic cases and found a low overall complication rate of 0.464% and a low conversion rate to laparotomy of 0.32%. Importantly, 29% of complications were not diagnosed intraoperatively. They also noted a trend, over the 9 years of case collection, of decreasing bowel injuries but increasing bladder injuries.

In another large case series, Jansen and colleagues reported on 25,764 laparoscopies performed at 72 hospitals.[2] They noted a complication rate of 0.57%, which included two patient deaths, and a 0.33% conversion to laparotomy. They noted increasing complication rates commensurate with difficulty of surgery, with diagnostic laparoscopy at 0.27%, laparoscopic sterilization at 0.45%, and operative laparoscopy having a 1.79% complication rate. As with other case reports, they noted that 57% of complications occurred during attempts at intraperitoneal entry, including those using both trocars and insufflation needles.

A large Finnish study evaluated records from 32,205 gynecologic laparoscopies occurring over a period of 2 years. This included all Finnish hospitals where laparoscopic surgery was performed.[3] They found a total of 130 major complications, for an overall complication rate of 0.4%. However, diagnostic and sterilization procedures had very low major complication rates of 0.06% and 0.05%, respectively. Operative cases were noted to have a much higher complication rate of 1.26%.

Several smaller case studies have demonstrated similar results. Mirhashemi and colleagues reported on 843 consecutive nontubal ligation laparoscopies and found an overall complication rate of 1.9%.[4] They found a 4.7% conversion rate to laparotomy consistent with the report being comprised of more difficult operative surgeries. Complications were distributed as follows: 14 bowel, 2 bladder, 1 ureter, 2 vascular, and 5 abdominal wall

# Minimally Invasive Surgery

**Table 39-1**
**Laparoscopic Complications, by Organ**

| Type of Complication | Incidence (%) |
|---|---|
| Bowel | 0.08–0.33 |
| Bladder | 0.2–8.3 |
| Ureter | 0.38–2.0 |
| Vascular | 0.05–0.07 |
| Inferior epigastric vessels | 0.2–2.0 |

**Table 39-2**
**Laparoscopic Complications, by Procedure**

| Type of Complication | Incidence (%) |
|---|---|
| Diagnostic laparoscopy | 0.06–0.27 |
| Laparoscopic sterilization | 0.05–0.45 |
| Operative laparoscopy | 1.26–1.9 |
| Conversion to laparotomy | 0.32–4.7 |

injuries. They also noted a surprisingly high rate of laparoscopic-assisted vaginal hysterectomy (LAVH) complications, 12.5%, which may be consistent with this study occurring early in the history of the procedure. Leonard reported on 1033 cases from a tertiary care center, of which 80% of cases were operative.[5] They noted a 1.2% conversion to laparotomy and also found that 55% of complications occurred during attempted entry. Surprisingly, they found that only 23.5% of these entry-related complications were with the initial port/needle placement, while 76.5% were with the placement of ancillary trocars.

## Entry Techniques

The previously noted trials suggest that entry complications play a major part in laparoscopic complications in general. Unfortunately there is little agreement regarding the best methodology for obtaining the safest abdominal entry.

Many gynecologists prefer to establish a pneumoperitoneum prior to trocar placement. Jansen's report[2] demonstrates that even a small-bore Veress needle may cause injury. It is recommended that patients be placed supine before initial needle and/or trocar placement and that the bladder be empty. If patients have undergone prior surgery, consideration may be given to placement of the needle or trocar in an area other than the infraumbilical region (Fig. 39-1). Studies have shown that 59% of patients with a prior midline incision were noted to have adhesions.[6] In addition, patients with prior Pfannenstiel incisions might also have adhesions reaching to the level of the umbilicus. The left upper quadrant appears to be a suitable alternative for placement of Veress needle or trocars in patients who have not had surgery in this region or who have underlying splenic abnormalities. However, the surgeon is not limited to this alternative because other areas may also be suitable for placement in different situations.

During placement of a Veress needle, the needle should be directed toward the pelvis in all but the most obese patients. This allows a safe distance from underlying major vasculature. Once the needle has been placed, a syringe with saline aspiration and hanging drop technique should be used to ascertain that a vessel or viscus has not been entered. Abdominal pressures should be low (<10 mm Hg) once insufflation has begun. There are reports of insufflation of major vasculature that can cause a $CO_2$ embolus. Proceeding with insufflation in the face of elevated pressures may cause a large pneumo-omentum or insufflation of the preperitoneal space. Either of these may make subsequent attempts at establishing an actual pneumoperitoneum very difficult.

Alternatives to needle placement in the abdomen include use of the posterior cul-de-sac to gain entry or transuterine insufflation. Large case series exist for both techniques. Contraindications for posterior cul-de-sac placement include prior vaginal surgery, cul-de-sac obliteration, prior history of pelvic inflammatory disease (PID), and severe cervical or vaginal infection. Contraindications for a transuterine approach are uterine fibroids, patients at risk for uterine adhesion (i.e., prior myomectomy), history of PID, and need for chromopertubation.

Direct trocar placement is an alternative to use of the Veress needle. Several large series suggest that in appropriately selected patients, a pneumoperitoneum is not necessary before trocar placement. The primary advantages of this technique are that it eliminates the risk associated with Veress needle placement and also thereby improves time efficiency. At least one randomized

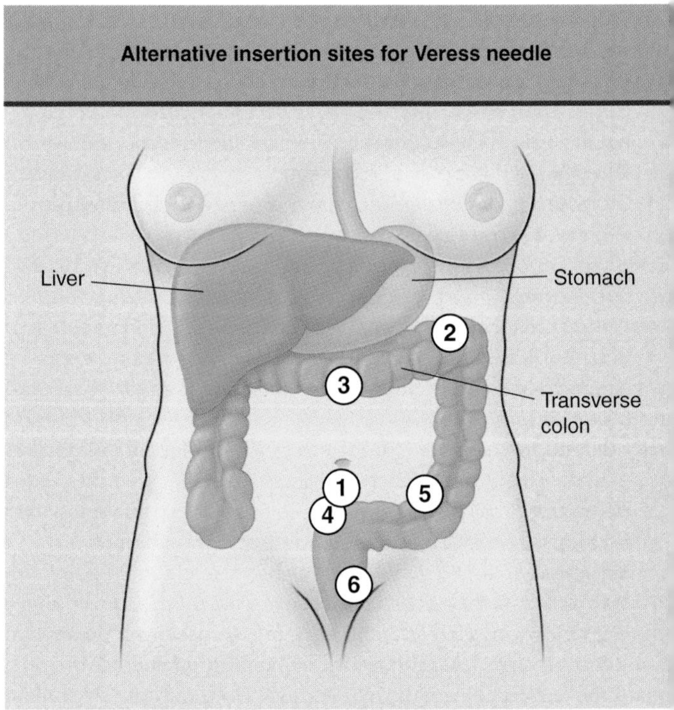

**Alternative insertion sites for Veress needle**

**Figure 39-1  Alternative sites for Veress needle insertion.**
1, infraumbilical or intraumbilical; 2, left upper quadrant, midclavicular line; 3, supraumbilical; 4, midline suprapubic; 5, left lower quadrant; 6, transcervical through the uterine fundus or transvaginal through the posterior fornix into the abdominal cavity. (From Nezhat CR, Nezhat FR, Luciano AA, et al: Operative Gynecologic Laparoscopy Principles and Techniques. New York, McGraw Hill, 1995, p 84, fig.8-8.)

comparison showed decreased minor complications such as preperitoneal insufflation with use of the technique.[7]

Open laparoscopy is another widely used technique for entry into the abdominal cavity. Hasson and colleagues reported on his large case series over almost three decades with this technique.[8] This included 5284 patients and only 27 complications. He noted no method failure and reported success in patients with multiple surgeries as well as increased weight (>98 kg). Other authors have not noted the same results with this technique, finding similar or even increased rates of complication.[9,10] The opportunity to evaluate these various techniques in a large randomized prospective trial still remains. Until that time, no one technique will meet all needs; thus the laparoscopic surgeon should be familiar and comfortable with several options for abdominal entry, realizing that this part of the procedure may be associated with the greatest risk.

## Inferior Epigastric Injury

The inferior epigastric artery and vein generally are identified in the lateral third of the rectus muscles. Superiorly they anastomose with the superior epigastric vessels and inferiorly with the external iliac most of the time. Saber and colleagues used computed tomography (CT) to map the epigastric vessels of 100 patients.[11] The results demonstrate the variation in distance from the midline to the epigastric vessels from superior to inferior, as well as the fact that the anatomy on the right is not a mirror image of the left (Table 39-3). Given where ancillary trocars are generally placed, epigastric vessels are at risk of injury that has been estimated at 0.2% to 2%. These vessels can rarely be transilluminated when viewing the abdominal wall from the outside. This is in contradistinction to the superficial epigastric vessels, which can usually be identified. Hurd and colleagues prospectively evaluated the ability to identify these vessels during laparoscopic surgery and found that transillumination was successful in 64% of cases for identifying superficial epigastric vessels and in 82% of cases, laparoscopic visualization identified the inferior epigastric vessels.[12] Increasing weight dimished the effectiveness for identifying both superficial

| Table 39-4 |
| --- |
| **Management of Inferior Epigastric Vessel Bleeding** |

- Identification of vessel
- Possible placement of Foley catheter through trocar sleeve to tamponade bleeding
- Consideration of bipolar/electrosurgery vs. suture to control bleeding
- Remember dual blood supply to epigastric vessels

and inferior epigastric vessels, and darker skin color decreased the ability to effectively transilluminate the superficial vessels. Notably, the superficial and inferior epigastric vessels do not run in parallel with one another; thus the surgeon must identify both vessels independently. Often the inferior epigastric vessels are not readily visible and may be identified only as a slight protuberance on the anterior peritoneum. One method for identifying the vessels is through identifying the insertion of the round ligament at the canal of Nuck and creating an imaginary line superior from this point. Often the vessels are in close proximity to this region.

If the inferior epigastric vessels are transected or injured, significant bleeding may ensue (Table 39-4). Placing a small Foley catheter through the trocar, inflating the balloon, and pulling back on the balloon to tamponade the bleeding may quickly control this. Small nicks in the vessel may then seal; however, significant injury will require suture placement. Various needle devices exist to facilitate passage of a suture on either side of the blood vessel. It is relevant to remember that there is a dual blood supply to these vessels and thus if transected two sutures may be required (i.e., superiorly and inferiorly) to completely control bleeding. A sizable hematoma and even hemorrhage may occur if this is not done.

When removing trocars at the conclusion of surgery, it is worthwhile to view the trocar site. Occasionally, the trocar itself will tamponade bleeding during the case only to have bleeding resume after removal of the trocar.

### Bladder Injury

Bladder injury may occur during classic open gynecologic surgery, but the techniques involved in diagnostic and operative laparoscopy may increase the rate of injury to this organ. Because the bladder is positioned in the midline in the same angle as that in which the Veress needle and trocars are being placed, it is at risk. Decompression of the bladder through catheterization may decrease this risk. A review of published studies demonstrated a 0.02% to 8.3% incidence of bladder injury in series reported in the literature.[13] Unfortunately, in this report, 47% of bladder injuries were not made intraoperatively. They also noted that the bladder dome was the most common area of injury. Although it is often easy to discern the margins of the bladder on the anterior surface of the uterus and peritoneum, this is not always true.[12] In addition, prior surgery may make it difficult to delineate the boundaries of the bladder.

Multiple reports have documented injury during laparoscopic surgery ranging from simple diagnostic cases, in which a Veress needle, primary trocar, or secondary trocar injured the bladder, to more complicated cases such a bladder neck suspension or

| Table 39-3 |
| --- |
| **CT Scan Mapping of Epigastric Vessels** |

| | | Distance from Midline | |
| --- | --- | --- | --- |
| **Vessel** | **Location** | **Right** | **Left** |
| Superior epigastric | Xiphoid | 4.41 ± 0.13 cm | 4.53 ± 0.14 cm |
| Superior epigastric | Midway xiphoid/umbilicus | 5.50 ± 0.16 cm | 5.36 ± 0.16 cm |
| Epigastric | Umbilicus | 5.88 ± 0.14 cm | 5.55 ± 0.13 cm |
| Inferior epigastric | Midway umbilicus/symphysis | 5.32 ± 0.12 cm | 5.25 ± 0.11 cm |
| Inferior epigastric | Symphysis pubis | 7.47 ± 0.10 cm | 7.49 ± 0.09 cm |

From Saber AA, Meslemani AM, Pimentael R: Safety zones for anterior abdominal wall entry during laparoscopy: a CT scan mapping of epigastric vessels. Ann Surg 2004;239:182–185.

---

**Table 39-5**
**Evaluation and Treatment of Bladder Injury**

- Instill dilute methylene blue through Foley catheter
- Identify size of defect
- Identify position of defect
- If question of trigone, cystoscopy
- Consult urology if necessary
- Suture defect if size requires
- Drainage with Foley or suprapubic catheter
- Possible antibiotics

LAVH. A recent prospective comparison of LAVH techniques demonstrated that whereas laparoscopic colpotomy was associated with decreased blood loss and operating time, vaginal colpotomy had a much lower rate of bladder injury (2.9% vs. 0.4%).[14] It is possible that blunt dissection versus classic sharp dissection of the bladder from the underlying uterus and cervix may predispose to this type of injury.

It is important to recognize a bladder injury during surgery so that repair may be performed at that time (Table 39-5). A common presentation for bladder injury is gross hematuria, but this may not always be present.[15] Oliguria is another finding in patients with bladder injury. Instillation of methylene blue or other agents into the bladder may facilitate recognition and identification of the area of disruption. Very small defects such as that created by a Veress needle may require no treatment or merely drainage for a limited period. Larger defects may require suture repair. It is also important to define where the defect has occurred and that the trigone is not involved. Cystoscopy should be employed as needed. Depending on the nature of the defect and the skill of the surgeon, repair may be performed laparoscopically or via laparotomy. Various closures ranging from single-layer to multilayer have been reported in the literature, although no comparisons using laparoscopic techniques have been published to date. Drainage with a Foley or suprapubic catheter is generally continued for some days after surgery, although the specific timing of removal varies throughout the literature. Prophylactic antibiotics are often used concomitantly; however, little information exists regarding the utility of this practice and the length of time for treatment.

## Ureter Injury

There are few good reports in the literature regarding ureter injury and methods to decrease its occurrence. Because of the location of the ureters as they descend through the pelvis, they are at particular risk during operative procedures such as oophorectomy, excision of pelvic endometriosis, and LAVH or laparoscopic hysterectomy.

The ureters are likely at greatest risk in the following three locations: as they pass near the infundibulopelvic ligament, under the uterine vessels, and as they pass lateral to the vaginal fornices. The location at the pelvic brim, near the common iliac vessels, may also be a high-risk area. It may be because of this anatomy that LAVH is a particularly difficult laparoscopic procedure, with a higher risk of ureter injury. Nezhat and colleagues evaluated anatomic relationships at the time of laparoscopy and also found that right and left pelvic anatomy are not mirror images.[16] They also noted (as many anatomists have) the proximity of the ureter to the infundibulopelvic and uterosacral ligaments (Table 39-6).

Interestingly, Tamussino and colleagues reviewed 790 operative laparoscopic procedures and found a ureteral injury rate of 0.38%, all occurring during LAVH.[17] Johnson and colleagues, in reviewing published trials on mode of hysterectomy, also found that laparoscopic hysterectomy was associated with a higher risk of urinary tract injury versus abdominal hysterectomy (odds ratio, 2.61).[18]

Ostrzenski and colleagues reviewed the published literature on laparoscopic ureteral complications and reported injury rates ranging from less than 1% to 2%.[19] They noted that in many of the reviewed series, critical information such as initial procedure, type of injury, and location were not reported. They did note that in series that provided information, LAVH was the most common antecedent procedure (Table 39-7). Also, diagnosis was made postoperatively in 70% of cases.

---

**Table 39-6**
**Mean Distances Between Selected Anatomic Structures**

| Body Mass Index | Medial Umbilical Ligament to Inferior Epigastric Vessels | | Midline to Inferior Epigastric Vessels | | Infundibulopelvic Ligament to Ureter | | Ipsilateral Uterosacral Ligament to Ureter | |
|---|---|---|---|---|---|---|---|---|
| | Right | Left | Right | Left | Right | Left | Right | Left |
| ≤20 kg/m² (n = 25) | 2.3 ± 1.8 | 1.6 ± 0.8 | 5.9 ± 1.9 | 5.1 ± 0.8 | 2.3 ± 0.7 | 2.6 ± 0.8 | 2.1 ± 0.8 | 2.5 ± 0.7 |
| 21–25 kg/m² (n = 55) | 1.9 ± 0.9 | 1.7 ± 1.0 | 5.1 ± 1.5 | 5.0 ± 1.4 | 2.2 ± 0.6 | 2.7 ± 0.6 | 1.7 ± 0.8 | 2.4 ± 0.8 |
| ≥26 kg/m² (n = 23) | 1.7 ± 0.8 | 1.6 ± 0.7 | 4.4 ± 1.5 | 4.2 ± 1.7 | 2.3 ± 0.7 | 2.60 ± 0.59 | 1.6 ± 1.1 | 2.5 ± 0.8 |
| Total (n = 103) | 2.9 ± 1.3* | 1.7 ± 1.0 | 5.5 ± 2.25* | 5.1 ± 2.0 | 2.2 ± 0.7 | 2.6 ± 0.8† | 1.8 ± 0.9† | 2.4 ± 0.9 |

All distances are rounded to nearest 0.1 cm and are given as mean ± standard deviation.
*Mean distances between the structures on the right side were significantly greater than the left.
†Mean distances between the structures on the right side were significantly less than the left.
From Nezhat CH, Nezhat F, Brill A, Nezhat C: Normal variations of abdominal and pelvic anatomy evaluated at laparoscopy. Obstet Gynecol 1999;94:238–242.

**Table 39-7**
**Most Common Associations with Ureteral Injury and a Comparison with the Number of Unspecified Associations in Total Reviewed Cases**

| Reviewed Category | Most Common Associated with Injury* | Specified Instances | Unspecified Instances |
|---|---|---|---|
| Procedure | LAVH | 14 (20%) | 18 (25.7%) |
| Time of diagnosis | Postoperative | 49 (70%) | 15 (21.4%) |
| Type | Transection | 14 (20%) | 36 (51.4%) |
| Location | At or above pelvic brim | 10 (14.3%) | 46 (65.7%) |
| Mode of repair | Laparotomy | 43 (61.4%) | 15 (21.4%) |
| Instrumentation | Electrocautery | 17 (24.3%) | 34 (48.6%) |

LAVH, laparoscopically assisted vaginal hysterectomy.
*When data has been available for review.
From Ostrzenski A, Radolinski B, Ostrzenska KM: A review of laparoscopic ureteral injury in pelvic surgery. Obstet Gynecol Surv 2003;58:794–799.

Ureteral injury may be difficult to diagnose intraoperatively. This may underscore the need for the gynecologic surgeon to be very familiar with the pelvic sidewall and retroperitoneal anatomy. However, even opening the retroperitoneal space and evaluating the path of the ureter does not guarantee freedom from inadvertent injury. Unlike the bladder, which may be readily evaluated for injury via cystoscopy or instillation of methylene blue, the ureter is less amenable to inspection. Parenteral injection of indigo carmine in association with cystoscopy can identify jets of the dye emanating from each ureteral orifice, signifying the ureters are intact.

## Bowel Injury

Bowel injury is a constant threat to the gynecologic laparoscopic surgeon. Given the size of the bowel and its location throughout the abdomen and pelvis as well as the propensity for bowel to form adhesions to the anterior abdominal wall, significant care must be taken during entry into the abdomen and throughout laparoscopic surgery. van der Voort and colleagues evaluated multiple studies comprising 329,935 laparoscopic procedures and noted a bowel injury rate of 0.13%.[20] Unfortunately, as with other complications, the diagnosis may not be straightforward. They noted that the diagnosis of injury was made at the time of surgery or within 24 hours 67% of the time, which may explain the 3.8% mortality rate with this complication. The small intestine was most frequently injured (55.8%), with the large bowel accounting for 38.6% of the injuries (Table 39-8). Trocars or the Veress needle were identified as the inciting instrument in 42% of bowel injuries (Table 39-9).

Shen and colleagues reviewed a large series of LAVH cases and found a rate of small bowel injury of 0.19%.[21] In evaluating the literature, Brosens and collegaues similarly found a low incidence of injury, with diagnostic and minimal laparoscopic procedures carrying a risk of 0.08% and operative laparoscopy a risk of 0.33%.[22] They noted that delay in diagnosis may occur in up to 15% of cases with a 20% chance of death with this delay. They also state that at times, "… even in experienced hands injury during access can not be avoided."

Vilos evaluated 40 litigated cases of bowel injury that occurred over almost a decade in Canada.[23] Consistent with other reports, injury was related to entry difficulties in 55% of cases—of which three cases of bowel injury occurred with the "open" technique. Injury was only recognized intraoperatively in 55% of cases, although surprisingly the ultimate outcome was not different for large versus small bowel injury or in cases where diagnosis was made intraoperatively versus postoperatively. There may be significant bias in these results, because intraoperative recognition could lead to a better outcome and thus less litigation.

**Table 39-8**
**Location of Laparoscopy-induced Gastrointestinal Bowel Injuries**

| Location | No. of Injuries (n = 407) |
|---|---|
| Stomach | 16 (3.9) |
| Small intestine | 227 (55.8) |
| Large intestine | 157 (38.6) |
| Unknown | 7 (1.7) |

Values in parentheses are percentages.
From van der Voort M, Heijnsdijk EA, Gouma DJ: Bowel injury as a complication of laparoscopy. Br J Surg 2004;91:1253–1258.

**Table 39-9**
**Instruments Causing Bowel Injury During Laparoscopy**

| Instrument | No. of Injuries (n = 273) |
|---|---|
| Trocar or Veress needle | 114 (41.8) |
| Coagulator or laser | 70 (25.6) |
| Grasping forceps | 3 (1.1) |
| Scissors | 2 (0.7) |
| Other | 84 (30.8) |

Values in parentheses are percentages.
From van der Voort M, Heijnsdijk EA, Gouma DJ: Bowel injury as a complication of laparoscopy. Br J Surg 2004;91:1253–1258.

# Minimally Invasive Surgery

It appears that one of the keys to avoidance of bowel injury during laparoscopy is the recognition that entry poses the greatest risk for bowel injury and that prior surgery may predispose the patient to a higher risk of injury secondary to adhesions to the anterior abdominal wall. Preoperative use of mechanical bowel preparation solutions such as GoLYTELY (polyethylene glycol) may occur in the day prior to surgery. It is best to begin these types of preparations early in the day and to maintain excellent hydration of the patient up until the time she must be NPO. Alternatives such as Fleets Phospho-Soda (sodium phosphate enema) may also be used. The addition of antibiotics to these regimens has fallen out of favor. It is best to have discussions with your general or colorectal surgeon, who might be involved if the need arises, to ascertain their biases regarding preoperative preparation.

The possibility of delayed diagnosis of bowel injury should be considered if patients complain of increasing pelvic or abdominal pain (with or without rebound), fever and elevated white blood cell (WBC) count, abdominal distention, and kidney-ureter bladder x-rays or CT scans suggestive of ileus or continued free air more than 24 to 48 hours after surgery. Unfortunately, depending on the site of injury, few, some, or all of these findings may be present. Indeed, in the septic patient, WBC counts will no longer be elevated and may at times be depressed.

## Vascular Injury

Injury to a major abdominal vessel is an uncommon complication of gynecologic laparoscopic surgery. When this complication occurs, identification and quickness of response become critical in reducing patient morbidity and mortality. Often this complication is a result of a misadventure during either needle or trocar placement and underlies the importance of use of correct technique during this pivotal portion of the surgery.

A large French study of over 100,000 laparoscopies reported 47 cases of major vascular injury.[24] Unfortunately eight patients died of this complication, yielding a mortality rate of 17%. Chapron and colleagues reported 21 vascular injuries in 29,966 cases, with 85% occurring during initial trocar placement.[1] Baggish similarly analyzed 31 cases of major vessel injury and noted that 90% were related to complications during entry; 78% of the cases involved injury to the iliac vessels, and blood loss in these cases ranged from 1000 to 7000 mL.[25]

Investigations into distances from point of entry to major vessels have been performed in several studies. Hurd and colleagues evaluated magnetic resonance imaging and CT studies of women and noted increasing distance from abdomen to aorta with increasing body mass index (BMI).[26] Narendran and Baggish prospectively evaluated distances from entry point to key vascular structures in patients who were undergoing laparoscopy.[27] They noted that as BMI increased, both abdominal wall thickness as well as distance to aortic bifurcation increased. Distance to the iliac vessels or bladder increased relative to the patient's height but did not change when patients were placed in Trendelenburg position.

An understanding of normal anatomy as well as normal variation, along with an understanding of distance from entry point to these areas, may be helpful in reducing injury. Entry may become especially challenging as BMI increases. Pre-

| Table 39-10 |
| :-- |
| **Vascular Injury Management** |

- Alert anesthesia
- Exploratory laparotomy – ideally with midline incision
- Obtain baseline and serial labs: CBC
- Type and cross-match for 4–6 units
- Cell saver if available
- Insert additional large-bore IV lines
- Summon surgeon–vascular surgeon STAT
- Compress aorta if necessary

peritoneal insufflation may be particularly problematic in these cases because it exacerbates the difficulty in traversing the distance from entry to peritoneum. There may also be a concomitant decrease in the distance from the peritoneum to the major vascular structures as well as bowel and bladder. In these settings, changing to an open laparoscopic approach, moving to another area such as the left upper quadrant, or converting to laparotomy may be required.

Should vascular injury occur during the course of surgery, the surgeon and the surgical team should be prepared to quickly mobilize to attend to the situation (Table 39-10). Immediately and concurrently a vascular surgeon or surgeon with experience repairing vascular structures should be called, a complete blood count and other baseline laboratory studies should be obtained along with a type and crossmatch for 4 to 6 units of blood. If available a cell saver device should be summoned. The anesthesia department should be made aware of the potential for significant blood loss, and additional large-bore lines should be placed. Laparotomy should be performed through a vertical incision to aid in quickly entering the abdomen as well as maximizing visualization to aid in isolation of the injured vessel(s). Aortic compression may also be required until a vascular or general surgeon is available. In this situation, often other injuries have occurred, including multiple vascular injuries as well as injuries to bowel and bladder, for example. Ultimately all structures should be systematically evaluated to ensure that no injuries are left unrepaired at the completion of the surgery.

In this situation, surgeons may delay some of these necessary steps because they believe they can manage the problem either expectantly or laparoscopically. Large hematomas should not be observed, because it is difficult to ascertain the amount of blood loss and access the stability. In addition, as a hematoma enlarges further anatomic distortion ensues, making subsequent identification of the injury all the more difficult.

## Conclusion

Laparoscopy is generally a safe and well-tolerated procedure. Like all invasive procedures, there are certain risks associated with the technique. The most significant risk for injury to any structure occurs during the entry phase of the procedure. An understanding of the available options for entry and knowledge of the inherent risks will hopefully help the surgeon minimize the chance of injury or facilitate recognition and treatment when injury occurs. Unfortunately, the significant anatomic variation that exists both within and between patients creates challenges for even the most skilled surgeon.[16]

## HYSTEROSCOPIC COMPLICATIONS

Hysteroscopic complications may be divided between problems associated with entry into the endometrial canal, difficulties with fluid distention, and procedural/postoperative complications. Although many of these complications may be more innocuous than laparoscopic complications, significant morbidity and even mortality may occur. As with most complications, recognition of the problem may decrease subsequent additional morbidity.

### Complications Associated with Entry

In one of the few large studies of hysteroscopic complications, Jansen and colleagues evaluated data from 82 hospitals and 13,600 hysteroscopies and noted that entry-related complications occur infrequently, yet are the most common hysteroscopic complication—representing 50% of all complications.[28] Specific risk factors are noted in Table 39-11. Most hysteroscopists have had experience with postmenopausal patients with a stenotic cervix or cervix that is flush with the vagina. Similar situations may also be seen in some patients after cone biopsy. In such cases, cervical lacerations may also occur as dilation is attempted. Use of very small hysteroscopes (i.e., 3.5 to 5 mm) and placement under direct visualization can decrease these risks but do not eliminate the problem. Campo and colleagues prospectively evaluated the use of a 3.5-mm versus a 5-mm hysteroscope for office diagnostic hysteroscopy and found less pain, better visualization, and higher success rates with the use of the smaller scope.[29] In some cases the surgeon is easily able to identify the external os and the canal up to the internal os but is unable to maneuver past this point. It is quite easy to create a false passage at the level of the obstruction and into the myometrium. This will appear as striations of musculature as the false passage is distended and has a markedly different appearance than the endometrial cavity itself. If the ostia cannot be visualized, it is unlikely that the uterine cavity has been entered. Once a false passage has been developed, it may be quite difficult for entry to be gained into the actual cavity, because the hysteroscope or dilators tend to follow the path of least resistance. Carefully removing the hysteroscope and continuously viewing the passage in a circumferential fashion can occasionally allow the actual passage to be visualized. Transabdominal ultrasound may be used, but in these difficult situations we have found this of limited assistance.

Cervical dilation and softening may be attempted before a procedure. *Laminaria* have been used as well as cervical ripening agents such as misoprostol. Several studies have evaluated the use of both vaginal (200 µg 12 hours prior to surgery) and oral (400 µg 12 hours prior to surgery) misoprostol and found

success.[30,31] Unfortunately if the cervix becomes over dilated, the surgeon may have difficulty with distention.

Uterine perforation may occur through either a false passage or through the endometrial cavity. Once this has occurred, further uterine distention becomes very difficult and distention media will be lost into the peritoneal cavity. This may be problematic if hypo-osmolar media are being used. The surgeon generally is able to identify the perforation because enteric structures are visualized. Significantly anteverted or retroverted uteri may be susceptible to perforation because even placement of a tenaculum and downward traction may not be able to straighten the canal. Care must be taken to note that a bladder or bowel perforation has not occurred. If necessary, cystoscopy or sigmoidoscopy may be performed. Generally bleeding from small fundal perforations is self-limited and may require no further action. If a larger instrument such as a resectoscope has caused the perforation, the patient may need to be observed over a period of time for hemodynamic stability. Consideration should be given to further evaluation with laparoscopy or laparotomy in the following situations: if there is any question regarding enteric injury, if the resectoscope was being activated electrosurgically at the time of perforation, if there is a question of lateral damage that may include the uterine vessels, and if uncontrollable bleeding has resulted from a hysteroscopic procedure.

### Complications Associated with Distention Media

The various types of distention media have been reviewed in Chapter 35. One key facet to the successful performance of hysteroscopy is the appropriate use of the correct distention media, which allows optimal visualization. Unfortunately, significant morbidity may occur secondary to intravasation of media into the vasculature.

In the past, carbon dioxide was a commonly used media for hysteroscopy. More recently, many hysteroscopists have switched to use of fluid media even for simple diagnostic cases. However, $CO_2$ may still be successfully employed for diagnostic hysteroscopy and has a long track record of safety. If a change to an operative case is required, this is not an optimal media given the inability of gas to be miscible with blood. $CO_2$ is also relatively unforgiving if the surgeon is not careful during entry and examination of the endometrial cavity. Discrete hysteroscopic delivery systems exist for $CO_2$, which are markedly different and not interchangeable with laparoscopic insufflators. These allow low flow but higher pressures, the opposite of most laparoscopic insufflators. Pellicano and colleagues evaluated $CO_2$ versus normal saline use during diagnostic hysteroscopy in infertility patients in a prospective, randomized trial.[32] They noted decreased abdominal pain and vasovagal reactions, as well as decreased operative time when saline was used as the distention media.

Fluid media have also been associated with various complications. Use of any media, whether hypotonic or not, may lead to fluid overload, pulmonary edema, and congestive heart failure (CHF). Once adequate distention has been achieved, further increases in intracavitary pressure will not lead to better visualization, only to an increased risk of fluid absorption. A patient's inherent ability to withstand this type of fluid challenge will determine if CHF will result. Patients with underlying medical

---

**Table 39-11**
**Risk Factors for Uterine Perforation**

- Nulliparity
- Severely anteverted or retroverted uterus
- Menopause
- Prior cervical surgery
- Use of GnRH agonist
- Cervical stenosis

| Table 39-12 |
| --- |
| Treatment of Fluid Overload with Hyponatremia |

- Terminate procedure
- Alert anesthesia
- Send stat electrolytes
- Administer diuretic
- Central monitoring as needed
- Track input/output carefully
- Follow serial electrolytes until sodium normalized
- Comanagement with anesthesia and/or critical care team

conditions may be at higher risk and unable to withstand fluid absorption versus a young healthy patient who will easily tolerate a transient fluid challenge.

A more risky situation is the compounding of fluid overload with hyponatremia, as seen when using hypotonic solutions such as 1.5% glycine or 3% sorbitol, which are commonly used in operative hysteroscopic/resectoscopic procedures. In this situation the fluid itself has a tonicity of less than 200 mOsm, which is well below physiologic range. Because these fluids contain no electrolytes, absorption of the media will dilutionally decrease sodium and other electrolytes. Table 39-12 details the steps necessary when this occurs. Key to avoidance of this complication is to continuously track fluid input and output during surgery. It is important to be aware that the patient may quickly go from absorbing very little fluid to a situation in which more than 1 liter of fluid has been absorbed. If input exceeds output above a predetermined limit (usually 1000 mL in a healthy patient), the procedure should be stopped. Blood should be drawn to evaluate electrolytes immediately and diuretics administered as necessary. The process of diuresis will quickly begin to correct the underlying problem, which is excess free water. In some situations, central monitoring is necessary and should be managed jointly with anesthesia and a critical care team. Unlike

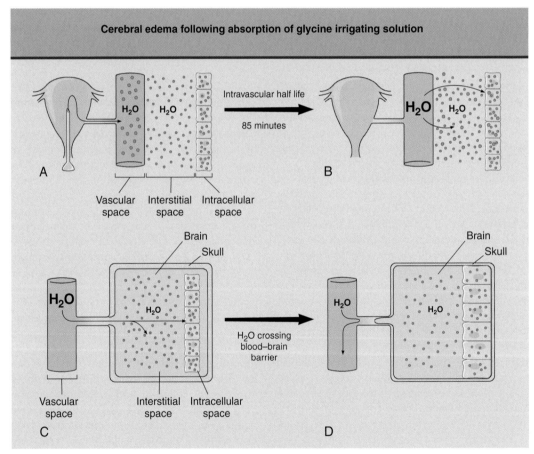

**Figure 39-2** **Cerebral edema following absorption of glycine irrigating solution.** *A,* Intravascular osmolarity is initially maintained by glycine molecules (G) contained in the intravascular space. *B,* When glycine moves from the intravascular space into the cell, intravascular osmolarity falls. The concentration of water ($H_2O$) is greater in the intravascular space than in the interstitial space. As a result, water moves from the vascular space into the interstitial and intracellular space *(arrows). C,* Because of the intravascular hypo-osmolar state, water moves across the blood-brain barrier into the interstitial and intracellular space. *D,* Cerebral edema develops with compression of the brain against the skull. Water will continue to move into the brain until the hydrostatic pressure of the brain offsets the osmotic force. (From Witz CA, Silverberg KM, Burns WN, et al: Complications associated with the absorption of hysteroscopic fluid media. Fertil Steril 1993;60:745–756, fig. 1. Copyright 1993. Reprinted with permission from the American Society for Reproductive Medicine.)

he situation of chronic hyponatremia, sodium levels may quickly be reversed and care should be taken not to overshoot during sodium replenishment and cause hypernatremia. The significant fluid shifts that occur with profound hyponatremia may cause cerebral edema and the most significant morbidity Fig. 39-2).[33] Quickly recognizing the problem and instituting treatment should help to minimize this risk (see Table 39-12).

Previously, Dextran 70 or Hyskon was used widely for hysteroscopic surgery. The consistency of the solution allowed excellent visualization even in the presence of blood. Unfortunately, the unique characteristics of Hyskon may have also been the cause of complications during hysteroscopic surgery. Reports of anaphylactic shock have been intermittently published. In addition, "dextran syndrome" has been reported, with anemia, coagulopathy, hypotension, shock, and noncardiogenic pulmonary edema.[34] Because of the large molecular size of dextran 70, intravasation of the media during hysteroscopy may cause an intravascular fluid shift, creating fluid overload. Limiting the amount of media used and, if necessary, aggressively managing patients with overload should decrease these risks.

## Procedural and Postoperative Complications

Intraoperative bleeding may occasionally occur during operative hysteroscopic surgeries. This may be more common with hysteroscopic myomectomy or endometrial resection than with other types of surgery. Agostini and colleagues reviewed 2116 operative hysteroscopies and found a 0.61% incidence of hemorrhage, with lysis of adhesions and myoma resection having the great risk (RR=5.2 and 6.5, respectively).[35] If abnormal bleeding occurs during hysteroscopy, care should be taken to note that a false passage has not been created and that a major vessel has not been lacerated. If necessary, a Foley catheter may be placed within the cavity for several hours. The balloon may then be deflated while leaving the catheter in place to access any further bleeding. If none occurs, the catheter may be removed. If bleeding continues, the catheter may be re-inflated and left in place for approximately 24 hours of in-house observation. The surgeon should be cognizant of not missing an expanding broad ligament hematoma in the case of major vessel injury.

Infection is an unusual complication of any hysteroscopic procedure. Several large series report rates of infection of less than 1%.[36] It is reasonable to obtain cervical cultures in patients who may be at risk for *Chlamydia* or other infections. Although little data is available regarding antibiotic prophylaxis, most authors recommend use of antibiotics during longer procedures and in patients with underlying fertility issues.

Care should be taking during the use of any media to purge the line of all air. Recent case reports have focused attention on the significant morbidity and mortality associated with air embolism occurring during hysteroscopic procedures.[37] $CO_2$ is readily absorbed and buffered in the bloodstream, whereas air is not, thus creating the potential for embolism. Besides removing the air that may exist in tubing, several other techniques have been suggested to reduce the risk of air embolism, including minimizing use of steep Trendelenburg position, covering the vaginal or cervical opening when changing instruments, and limiting the movement of instruments in and out of the cervix. Key to avoiding morbidity in this situation is awareness by the anesthetist. Common signs and symptoms exhibited by patients with air embolism include tachypnea, hypotension, hypoxia, hypercapnea, arrhythmias, pulmonary hypertension, and decreasing end-tidal $CO_2$. It is critical in this situation that the procedure be terminated, appropriate anesthetic measures begun, the patient be turned to the left lateral decubitis position, and a central venous catheter be used to aspirate the gas if necessary (Table 39-13).

Intrauterine and intracervical adhesions may form after any procedure but are less likely following simple diagnostic or operative procedures. Endometrial ablation has been associated with the formation of intrauterine adhesions as well as cervical stenosis. Some authors had even recommended sounding or curette passage in the office after the procedure to attempt to reduce these risks.[38] A variation of intrauterine adhesions is the "postablation tubal sterilization" syndrome that was first reported by Townsend and colleagues.[39] Patients were noted to have hematometra, with no point of egress given their prior tubal ligation, and may present with cyclic pain or abnormal uterine bleeding some months after endometrial ablation. Ultrasound will demonstrate a hematometra generally located near one of the cornua. It is unclear if the different modalities for performing endometrial ablation (e.g., cryoablation, thermal balloon ablation) impact on the risk of subsequent adhesions or hematometra. It has been suggested that limiting ablation to the active endometrium and not ablating near the internal os and cervix may decrease the risk of subsequent stenosis. Intrauterine adhesions may also form after submucous myomectomy. A special case may occur when multiple myomata are juxtaposed within the cavity. In this circumstance, it may be preferable to resect only one myoma at a time so as to not have two denuded areas in contact with one another.

Pregnancy complications have also resulted after hysteroscopy or endometrial ablation. During lysis of intrauterine adhesions, submucous myomectomy, or hysteroscopic metroplasty, the myometrium may be entered with or without eventual perforation. Although rare, uterine rupture during labor has been reported in patients who have undergone operative hysteroscopic procedures.[40] Generally, it has been felt that most patients undergoing these procedures will not require an elective cesarean section; however, individualization should occur depending on the nature of the prior procedure.

Pregnancies have also resulted after endometrial ablation. The exact incidence is unclear but may be as high as 1% to 2%.[41] For this reason, patients should understand that endometrial ablation is not a sterilization procedure. In addition, various

| Table 39-13 Air Embolism | |
|---|---|
| **Diagnosis** | **Treatment** |
| · Hypoxia | · Stop procedure |
| · Hypercapnea | · Administer 100% oxygen, stop any |
| · Tachypnea | nitrous oxide |
| · Pulmonary hypertension | · Turn patient to left lateral decubitis |
| · Arrhythmias | position |
| · Hypotension | · If necessary, aspirate gas with |
| · Drop in end-tidal $CO_2$ | central venous catheter |

# Minimally Invasive Surgery

complications have been reported in pregnancies after endometrial ablation, including intrauterine growth restriction, preterm labor, placental abruption, and placentation abnormalities, such as placenta accreta, placenta increta, and placenta percreta (Table 39-14).[42]

Overall hysteroscopy appears to have a low complication rate. The Jansen report demonstrated only 38 complications in 13,600 procedures, for a complication rate of only 0.28%. This rate was lowered further for diagnostic procedures (0.13%) and slightly increased for operative procedures (0.95%). Intrauterine adhesiolysis was associated with the greatest rate of complications in this trial (4.48%), whereas endometrial resection, myomectomy, and polypectomy all had complication rates less than 1% (Table 39-15). Propst and colleagues evaluated 925 hysteroscopies and noted a slightly higher overall complication rate of 2.7%.[43] They found that hysteroscopic myomectomy and resection of uterine septum had increased odd ratios for complications (OR=7.4 and 4.0, respectively), although the latter did not reach statistical significance (Table 39-16). Surprisingly, they noted that use of gonadotropin-releasing hormone agonists as well as cases being performed by a reproductive endocrinologist were associated with increased risk of complication, possibly because in both situations, more difficult and complex procedures were being performed (Table 39-17).

Hysteroscopy appears to be a well-tolerated procedure with a relatively low rate of complications. An understanding and awareness of the various problems that the surgeon may encounter while performing surgery will alert the clinician when an unusual situation or complication does arise. Management of distention media with vigilant observation of fluid input and output are critical to decreasing patient morbidity. In addition, the previously noted trials suggest a need for care during the entry phase of the procedure.

**Table 39-14**
**Table of Pregnancy-associated Complications Following Endometrial Ablation**

- Spontaneous abortion
- Intrauterine growth restriction
- Abnormal fetal presentation
- Placental accreta, increta, percreta
- Placenta previa
- Premature rupture of membranes
- Placental abruption
- Preterm labor
- Ectopic pregnancy
- Preterm delivery
- Hysterectomy

**Table 39-15**
**Surgical Complications During Operative Hysteroscopic Procedures**

| Procedure | n | Complication | Rate (per 100) |
|---|---|---|---|
| Adhesiolysis | 134 | 6 | 4.5 |
| Endometrial ablation* | 494 | 4 | 0.8 |
| Myomectomy | 798 | 6 | 0.8 |
| Polypectomy | 784 | 3 | 0.4 |
| Rest[†] | 305 | 0 | 0 |
| Total | 2515 | 19 | 0.8 |

Comparison of rates showed statistical significance for adhesiolysis ($P < 0.001$) versus other procedures. No statistical significance was found for resection versus myomectomy versus polypectomy ($P = 0.39$).

*Ablation included procedures of endometrium resection ($n = 155$), rollerball ($n = 116$), and combination ($n = 223$).

[†] Removal corpus alienum ($n = 180$), sterilization ($n = 81$), septum resection ($n = 40$), rest ($n = 4$)

From Jansen FW, Vredevoogd CB, Ulzen KV, et al: Complications of hysteroscopy: a prospective multicenter study. Obstet Gynecol 2000;96:266–270.

**Table 39-16**
**Odds of Operative Complications, by Selected Patient Characteristics**

| Variable | Number | Age-Adjusted OR (95% CI) |
|---|---|---|
| Age 35–50 yr* | 510 | 0.5 (0.2, 1.4) |
| Age > 50 yr* | 308 | 0.2 (0.1, 0.8) |
| Premenopausal[†] | 606 | 2.8 (0.6, 12.9) |
| Preoperative GnRH-α therapy | 42 | 6.6 (2.5, 17.6) |
| Reproductive endocrinologist[†] | 253 | 2.9 (1.2, 6.8) |
| General gynecologist[†] | 632 | 0.4 (0.2, 1.0) |
| 1 or 2 live births[§] | 254 | 1.3 (0.5, 3.2) |
| >2 live births[§] | 173 | 1.2 (0.4, 4.0) |
| Weight > 200 lbs[‖] | 81 | 0.4 (0.1, 3.2) |
| History of cesarean delivery | 101 | 0.3 (0.0, 2.4) |
| Previous myomectomy | 43 | 0.8 (0.1, 5.9) |
| Cervical stenosis | 55 | 1.5 (0.4, 6.8) |

CI, confidence interval; GnRH-α, gonadotropin-releasing hormone agonist; OR, odds ratio.

*Relative to those ≤ 34 years. Not age-adjusted.

[†]Relative to postmenopausal women.

[‡]Relative to all surgeons.

[§]Relative to nulliparity (207 of 925 patients did not have parity information).

[‖]Relative to women ≤ 200 pounds.

From Propst AM, Liberman RF, Harlow BL, Ginsburg ES: Complications of hysteroscopic surgery: predicting patients at risk. Obstet Gynecol 2000;96:517–520.

**Table 39-17**
**Operative Time, Glycine Use, and Complications**

| Procedure | Number* | Mean Length of Surgery (minute) | Mean Total Glycine (mL) | Mean Deficit (mL) | Complications† n (%) | Complications† OR (95% CI) |
|---|---|---|---|---|---|---|
| Myomectomy | 128 | 64.6 | 6155 | 311 | 13 (10.2%) | 7.4 (3.3, 16.6) |
| Septum resection | 21 | 35.3 | 2200 | 233 | 2 (9.5%) | 4.0 (0.9, 19.6) |
| Lysis of adhesions | 20 | 34.7 | 1695 | 150 | 1 (5.0%) | 1.9 (0.2, 15.0) |
| Hysteroscopy and/or curettage | 410 | 21.4 | 522 | 38 | 7 (1.7%) | 0.5 (0.2, 1.1) |
| Endometrial ablation | 78 | 36.7 | 2660 | 92 | 1 (1.3%) | 0.4 (0.1, 3.3) |
| Polypectomy | 270 | 27.9 | 1214 | 55 | 1 (0.4%) | 0.1 (0.0, 0.7) |

CI, confidence interval; OR, odds ratio.

*Total number of procedures up to 927 because two of 925 patients had more than one primary procedure.

†Complications odds ratio relative to all 925 patients.

From Propst AM, Liberman RF, Harlow BL, Ginsburg ES: Complications of hysteroscopic surgery: predicting patients at risk. Obstet Gynecol 2000;96:517–520.

# REFERENCES

1. Chapron C, Querleu D, Bruhat MA, et al: Surgical complications of diagnostic and operative gynaecological laparoscopy: a series of 29,966 cases. Hum Reprod 1998;13:867–872. **(III, B)**
2. Jansen FW, Kapiteyn K, Trimbos-Kemper T, et al: Complications of laparoscopy: a prospective multicentre observational study. Br J Obstet Gynecol 1997;104:595–600. **(IIb, B)**
3. Harkki-Siren P, Sjoberg J, Kurki T: Major complications of laparoscopy: a follow-up Finnish study. Obstet Gynecol 1999;94:94–98. **(III, B)**
4. Mirhashemi R, Harlow BL, Ginsburg ES, et al: Predicting risk of complications with gynecologic laparoscopic surgery. Obstet Gynecol 1998;92:327–331. **(III, B)**
5. Leonard F, Lecuru F, Chasset S, et al: Perioperative morbidity of gynecological laparoscopy. A prospective monocenter observational study. Acta Obstet Gynecol Scand 2000;79:129–134. **(IIb, B)**
6. Levrant SG, Bieber EJ, Barnes RB: Anterior abdominal wall adhesions after laparotomy or laparoscopy. J Am Assoc Gynecol Lap 1997;4:353–356. **(III, B)**
7. Byron JW, Markenson G, Miyazawa K: A randomized comparison of Veress needle and direct trocar insertion for laparoscopic surgery. Surg Gynecol Obstet 1993;177:259–262. **(Ib, A)**
8. Hasson H, Rotman C, Rana N, Kumari NA: Open laparoscopy: 29-year experience. Obstet Gynecol 2000;96:763–766. **(IV, C)**
9. Jansen FW, Kolkman W, Bakkum EA, et al: Complications of lparoscopy: an inquiry about closed- versus open-entry technique. Am J Obstet Gynecol 2004;190:634–638. **(IIb, B)**
10. Chapron C, Cravello L, Chopin N, et al: Complications during set-up procedures for laparoscopy in gynecology: open laparoscopy does not reduce the risk of major complications. Acta Obstet Gynecol Scand 2003;82:1125–1129. **(III, B)**
11. Saber AA, Meslemani AM, Pimentael R: Safety zones for anterior abdominal wall entry during laparoscopy: a CT scan mapping of epigastric vessels. Ann Surg 2004;239:182–185. **(IIb, B)**
12. Hurd WW, Amesse LS, Gruber JS, et al: Visualization of the epigastric vessels and bladder before laparoscopic trocar placement. Fertil Steril 2003;80:209–212. **(III, B)**
13. Ostrzenski A, Ostrzenska KM: Bladder injury during laparoscopic surgery. Obstet Gynecol Surv 1998;53:175–180. **(III, B)**
14. Horng SG, Huang KS, Lo TS, Soong YK: Bladder injury after LAVH: a prospective randomized comparison of vaginal and laparoscopic approaches to colpotomy during LAVH. J Am Assc Gynecol Lap 2004;11:42–46. **(Ib, A)**
15. Godfrey C, Wahle GR, Schilder JM, et al: Occult bladder injury during laparoscopy: report of 2 cases. J Lapro Adv Surg Tech 1999;9:341–345. **(IV, C)**
16. Nezhat CH, Nezhat F, Brill AI, Nezhat C: Normal variations of abdominal and pelvic anatomy evaluated at laparoscopy. Obstet Gynecol 1999;94:238–242. **(III, B)**
17. Tamussino KF, Lang PFJ, Breinl E: Ureteral complications with operative gynecologic laparoscopy. J Urol 1998;160:2313–2314. **(III, B)**
18. Johnson N, Barlow D, Lethaby A, et al: Methods of hysterectomy: systematic review and meta-analysis of randomized controlled trials. Br Med J 2005;330:1478. **(Ia, A)**
19. Ostrzenski A, Radolinski B, Ostrzenska KM: A review of laparoscopic ureteral injury in pelvic surgery. Obstet Gynecol Surv 2003;58:794–799. **(III, B)**
20. van der Voort M, Heijnsdijk EA, Gouma DJ: Bowel injury as a complication of laparoscopy. Br J Surg 2004;91:1253–1258. **(III, B)**
21. Shen CC, Wu MP, Lu CH, et al: Small intestinal injury in laparoscopic-assisted vaginal hysterectomy. J Am Assoc Gynecol Lap 2003;10:350–355. **(III, B)**
22. Brosens I, Gordon A, Campo R, Gordts S: Bowel injury in gynecologic laparoscopy. J Am Assoc Gynecol Lap 2003;10:9–13. **(III, B)**
23. Vilos G: Laparoscopic bowel injuries: 40 litigated gynaecologic cases in Canada. J Obstet Gynecol Can 2002;24:224–230. **(IV, C)**
24. Champault G, Cazacu F, Taffinader N: Serious trocar accidents in laparoscopic surgery: a French survey of 103,852 operations. Surg Lap Endoscop 1996;6:367–370. **(IIb, B)**
25. Baggish MS: Analysis of 31 cases of major vessel injury associated with gynecologic laparoscopy operations. J Gynecol Surg 2003;19:63–73.
26. Hurd WW, Bude RO, Delancey JOL, et al: Abdominal wall characterization by MRI and CT imaging: the effect of obesity on laparoscopic approach. J Reprod Med 1991;36:473. **(IIb, B)**
27. Narendran M, Baggish MS: Mean distance between primary trocar insertion site and major retroperitoneal vessels during routine laparoscopy. J Gynecol Surg 2002;18:121–127. **(IIb, B)**
28. Jansen FW, Vredevoogd CB, Ulzen KV, et al: Complications of hysteroscopy: a prospective multicenter study. Obstet Gynecol 2000;96:266–270. **(III, B)**
29. Campo R, Molinas CR, Rombauts L, et al: Prospective multicentre randomized controlled trial to evaluate factors influencing the success rate of office diagnostic hysteroscopy. Hum Reprod 2005;20:258–263. **(Ib, A)**
30. Preutthipan S, Herabuty Y: Vaginal misoprostol for cervical priming before operative hysteroscopy: a randomized controlled trial. Obstet Gynecol 2000;96:890–894. **(Ib, A)**

31. Thomas JA, Leyland N, Durand N, Windrim RD: The use of oral misoprostol as a cervical riping agent in operative hysteroscopy: a double-blind, placebo-controlled trial. Am J Obstet Gynecol 2002; 186:876–879. **(Ib, A)**

32. Pellicano M, Guida M, Zullo F, et al: Carbon dioxide versus normal saline as a uterine disternsion medium for diagnostic vaginoscopic hysteroscopy in infertile patients: a prospective, randomized, multi-center study. Fertil Steril 2003;79:418–421. **(Ib, A)**

33. Witz CA, Silverberg KM, Burns WN, et al: Complications associated with the absorption of hysteroscopic fluid media. Fertil Steril 1993;60:745–756. **(IV, C)**

34. Ellingson TL, Aboulafia DM: Dextran syndrome. Acute hypotension, noncardiogenic pulmonary edema, anemia, and coagulopathy following hysteroscopic surgery using 32% dextran 70. Chest 1997;111:513–518. **(III, B)**

35. Agostini A, Cravello L, Desbriere R, et al: Hemorrhage risk during operative hysteroscopy. Acta Obstet Gynecol Scand 2002;81:878–881. **(III, B)**

36. Agostini A, Cravello L, Shojai R, et al: Postoperative infection and surgical hysteroscopy. Fertil Steril 2002;77;766–768. **(III, B)**

37. Behnia R, Holley HS, Milad M: Successful early intervention in air emoblism during hysteroscopy. J Clin Anesth 1997;9:248–250. **(IV, C**

38. Goldrath MH: Use of danazol in hysteroscopy surgery for menorrhagia J Reprod Med 1990;35:91–92. **(III, B)**

39. Townsend DE, McCausland V, McCausland A, et al: Postablation tubal sterilization syndrome. Obstet Gynecol 1993;82:422–423. **(III, B)**

40. Angell NF, Tan DJ, Siddiqi N: Uterine rupture at term after uncomplicated hysteroscopic metroplasty. Obstet Gynecol 2002;100 1098–1099. **(III, B)**

41. Pinette M, Katz W, Drouin M, et al: Successful planned pregnancy following endometrial ablation with the YAG laser. Am J Obstet Gynecol 2001;185:242–3 **(III, B)**

42. Rogerson L, Gannon B, O'Donovan P: Outcome of pregnancy following endometrial ablation. J Gynecol Surg 1997;13:155–160. **(III, B)**

43. Propst AM, Liberman RF, Harlow BL, Ginsburg ES: Complications of hysteroscopic surgery: predicting patients at risk. Obstet Gynecol 2000;96:517–520. **(III, B)**

# Chapter 40

# Breast Carcinoma

Padma C. Nadella, MD, Karen Godette, MD, Monica Rizzo, MD, Toncred M. Styblo, MD, and Ruth M. O'Regan, MD

## KEY POINTS

- Breast cancer is the second most common cause of cancer-related mortality in women in the United States.
- Screening with mammography is recommended for all women over age 40 years.
- Mortality from breast cancer has been decreasing over the last decade.
- Newer surgical and radiation techniques have decreased treatment-related morbidity.
- Chemotherapy and hormonal therapies reduce recurrence rates and improve survival from early stage-breast cancer.
- Systemic therapies improve quality of life in metastatic breast cancer.

Breast cancer is the most common cancer and the second most common cause of cancer-related mortality in women in the United States. It is estimated that 1 in 8 women in the United States will develop breast cancer during their lifetime. However, mortality from breast cancer has been decreasing over the last decade because of earlier diagnosis and better treatments. Screening with mammography is recommended for all women over the age of 40, and newer screening methods, including MRI,[1] are being actively researched. Although several risk factors for breast cancer have been identified, in most cases there is no identifiable cause. However, the discovery of two breast cancer genes[2] has allowed identification of women at very high risk of breast cancer and ovarian cancer.

New surgical techniques, in particular, the widespread use of sentinel lymph node biopsies, have decreased surgery-related morbidity. Additionally, new radiation techniques, for example, brachytherapy, are under investigation and offer the possibility of improved tolerability and convenience. Over the past decade, the use of adjuvant therapies, including both chemotherapy and hormonal therapies, have reduced recurrence rates and improved survival from early-stage breast cancer.[3,4] Although tamoxifen has been the mainstay of treating all stages of hormone-responsive breast cancer, selective aromatase inhibitors offer the possibility of increased efficacy,[5-7] with an improved side effect profile.

Metastatic breast cancer remains incurable; however, the use of chemotherapy and hormonal therapies has been shown to improve quality of life. Additionally, the identification of the HER2/neu receptor and the subsequent development of trastuzumab, a monoclonal antibody that targets the extracellular domain of this receptor, have resulted in survival advantages in patients with poor prognostic metastatic breast cancer.[8] Lastly, bisphosphonates have been demonstrated to reduce complications relating to bone metastases in patients with breast cancer.[9,10]

## EPIDEMIOLOGY

Breast cancer is the most common neoplasm affecting women in the United States.[11] It is the second leading cause of cancer-related mortality in women. An estimated 215,990 women will be given a diagnosis of breast cancer in 2004 in the United States, resulting in approximately 40,110 deaths. The incidence rate of breast cancer increased by approximately 4% during the 1980s but leveled off to 100.6 cases per 100,000 women in the 1990s. The death rates from breast cancer also declined significantly between 1992 and 1996, with the largest decreases among younger women. It is estimated that the lifetime risk of breast cancer is 12%.

## RISK FACTORS

Several factors that increase an individual's risk of breast cancer have been identified. The most important risk factors for breast cancer are increasing age and family history. The risk of breast cancer increases with the number of relatives who have the disease. The likelihood of carrying one of the two breast cancer genes, BRCA1 and BRCA2, increases based on the factors shown in Table 40-1. Carriers of BRCA1 have a significantly high risk of developing breast cancer, both primary and secondary, and of ovarian cancer, while carriers of BRCA2 have a similar risk of breast cancer but a lower—but still increased—risk of ovarian cancer.[2,12-14] Individuals of Ashkenazi Jewish descent have an increased likelihood of carrying both BRCA genes. Preventive maneuvers for individuals who carry BRCA genes range from observation to prophylactic surgeries, both mastectomies and oophorectomies.[15,16] Recently, a specific gene expression has been noted in breast cancers in patients who carry BRCA1.[17]

The association between hormonal factors and breast cancer was identified over a century ago.[18] Early menarche and late menopause have been demonstrated to increase the risk of breast cancer.[19,20] The earlier a woman has her first child, the

**Table 40-1**

**Factors Associated with Increased Likelihood of Having a *BRCA* Mutation**

- Relative with breast cancer at a young age
- Multiple relatives with breast cancer
- Relative or personal history of bilateral breast cancer
- Relative or personal history of ovarian cancer
- Relative with male breast cancer
- Ashkenazi Jewish descent

lower her risk of breast cancer, and a woman who has her first child after the age of 35 has the same risk of developing breast cancer as a nulliparous woman.[20] Recent evidence suggests that the longer a woman breastfeeds, the lower her risk of breast cancer.[21] Exogenous estrogens have been clearly associated with an increased risk of breast cancer.[22,23] The use of combined estrogen and progestin hormone replacement therapy increases the risk of breast cancer, with longer durations resulting in greater risks of breast cancer.[22,23] Interestingly, birth control pills only marginally increase breast cancer risk and appear protective against ovarian cancer.[24,25]

Although dietary fat intake has not been conclusively shown to increase the risk of breast cancer, obesity in postmenopausal women is associated with increased breast cancer risk, likely due to increased conversion of androgens to estrogens in adipose tissue.[26] Alcohol use in excess of 2 units per day is associated with an increased risk of breast cancer, and there is evidence to suggest that folic acid may abrogate this risk.[27]

Certain breast diseases clearly are associated with an increased risk of breast cancer. Lobular carcinoma in situ is a nonmalignant condition that increases the risk of breast cancer, both ductal and lobular, in both breasts.[28] Likewise, atypical hyperplasia is associated with an increased risk of breast cancer. In both these conditions, the selective estrogen receptor modulator (SERM) tamoxifen reduces the risk of breast cancer.[29]

## PREVENTION

Using the risk factors for breast cancer mentioned above, it is possible to determine whether a woman is at increased risk of breast cancer. The Gail model[30] (Table 40-2) utilizes age, family history, hormonal factors including age of menarche and age at birth of first child, number of prior breast biopsies, and presence of hyperplasia to estimate a woman's 5-year and lifetime risk of breast cancer. Any woman with an estimated 5-year risk of developing breast cancer of greater than 1.66% is considered

**Table 40-2**

**Gail Model for Increased Risk of Breast Cancer**

- Race
- Age
- Age of menarche
- Age at birth of first child
- Number of first-degree relatives with breast cancer
- Number of previous breast biopsies
- Atypical hyperplasia (Yes/No)

at high enough risk to receive chemoprevention. However, the Gail model probably underestimates the influence of family history, as it accounts for only first-degree relatives and puts too much emphasis on hormonal factors.

The National Surgical Adjuvant Breast and Bowel Project (NSABP) Prevention (P-1) trial[29] randomized women with a 5-year risk of breast cancer of greater than 1.66% to tamoxifen or placebo for 5 years. Following the accrual of 13,000 women, a significantly reduced number of breast cancers were noted in women receiving tamoxifen. The rates of ductal carcinoma in situ and of invasive breast cancers were reduced by 50% and 49%, respectively. As would be expected, tamoxifen only significantly reduced the rate of estrogen receptor (ER)–positive breast cancers and had no impact on ER-negative breast cancers. Based on the results of this large trial, and despite two other negative trials[31,32] in Europe, tamoxifen was approved for the prevention of breast cancer in women at high risk in 1998. A follow-up trial from the NSABP is comparing tamoxifen with another SERM, raloxifene, in women at high risk. It is hoped that raloxifene will be as effective as tamoxifen in reducing the incidence of breast cancer, without the associated increase in uterine cancer seen with tamoxifen.

How effective tamoxifen is in reducing the incidence of breast cancer in women with hereditary breast cancer is unclear. The majority of breast cancers in women who carry *BRCA1* are ER-negative[33]; therefore, the rate of breast cancer would be unlikely to be affected by the use of tamoxifen. This is corroborated by the finding of a specific gene expression pattern in breast cancers occurring in *BRCA1* carriers.[34] This gene expression pattern is designated as basilar type, is ER-negative, and carries a poor prognosis.[34] However, bilateral oophorectomies have been demonstrated to not only reduce the risk of ovarian cancer but also to reduce the risk of breast cancer by 50% in women who carry *BRCA1*.[15] Additionally, bilateral prophylactic mastectomies are effective in preventing breast cancer in *BRCA1* carriers.[16] In contrast to *BRCA1*, the majority of breast cancers in *BRCA2* carriers are ER-positive,[33] so tamoxifen may be effective in reducing breast cancer incidence in these patients.[35]

## STAGING

Staging of breast cancer is based on tumor size, extent of breast involvement, axillary lymph node involvement, and distant metastases (the TNM system). The most important changes in the 2003 American Joint Committee on Cancer (AJCC) classification compared with the 1998 classification include a reclassification of nodal status by the number of involved axillary lymph nodes, size-based discrimination between micrometastases and isolated tumor cells, and classification of metastasis to internal mammary nodes and supraclavicular nodes as N3 rather than M1 disease.[36] These changes in the staging system dramatically affect stage-specific survival.[37] AJCC staging system is summarized in Table 40-3.

## PROGNOSTIC FACTORS

Stage IV breast cancer remains incurable, and treatment of this disease remains palliative. Several prognostic factors have been identified in early-stage breast cancer. The most important is

**Table 40-3**
**American Joint Committee on Cancer (AJCC) Staging System**
**for Breast Cancer**

**Primary Tumor (T)**

TX—Primary tumor cannot be assessed
T0—No evidence of primary tumor
Tis—Carcinoma in situ: intraductal carcinoma, lobular carcinoma in situ, or
　　Paget's disease of the nipple with no tumor
T1—Tumor 2 cm or less in greatest dimension
T2—Tumor more than 2 cm but not more than 5 cm in greatest dimension
T3—Tumor more than 5 cm in greatest dimension
T4—Tumor of any size with direct extension to the chest wall (a), skin (b),
　　both (c), inflammatory carcinoma (d)

**Regional Lymph Nodes (N) (Pathologic)**

NX—Regional lymph nodes cannot be assessed
N0—No regional lymph node metastasis
N1—Metastasis in 1 to 3 axillary lymph nodes, and/or in internal mammary
　　nodes with microscopic disease detected by sentinel lymph node dissection
　　but not clinically apparent
N1mi—Micrometastasis (>0.2 mm but ≤2.0 mm)
N2—Metastasis in 4 to 9 axillary lymph nodes, or in clinically apparent internal
　　mammary lymph nodes in the absence of axillary lymph node metastasis
N3—Metastasis in 10 or more axillary lymph nodes, or in infraclavicular lymph
　　nodes, or in clinically apparent ipsilateral internal mammary lymph nodes in
　　the presence of one or more axillary lymph nodes; or in more than 3 axillary
　　lymph nodes with clinically negative microscopic metastasis in internal
　　mammary lymph nodes; or in ipsilateral supraclavicular lymph nodes

**Metastasis (M)**

M1—Distant metastasis

**Stage Groupings**

| 0 | TisN0M0 |
|---|---|
| I | T1N0M0 |
| IIA | T0N1M0, T1N1M0, T2N0M0 |
| IIB | T2N1M0, T3N0M0 |
| IIIA | T0N2M0, T1N2M0, T2N2M0, T3N1M0, T3N2M0 |
| IIIB | T4 N0M0, T4N1M0, T4N2M0 |
| IIIC | Any T N3 |
| IV | Any T any N M1 |

From Singletary SE, Allred C, Ashley P, et al: Revision of the American Joint Committee on cancer staging system for breast cancer. J Clin Oncol 2002;20:3628–3636.

status of the axillary lymph nodes, and the greater the number of lymph nodes involved, the worse the prognosis. Another important prognostic factor is tumor size, with larger tumors having a worse prognosis. Less important prognostic factors include tumor grade, hormone receptor status,[4] HER2/neu status,[38] and S phase. Using known prognostic factors, it is possible to estimate likelihood of recurrence and to make decisions regarding the appropriateness of adjuvant therapies. An on-line model, ADJUVANT!, is available to estimate the prognosis of a patient's disease and its likelihood of recurrence with and without adjuvant therapies.[39] Newer molecular techniques are becoming available that may add to existing prognostic factors utilized in breast cancer.

Despite advances in determining prognoses, the majority of patients in the United States receive adjuvant therapy. Therefore, the identification of factors that *predict* outcome from adjuvant therapies is becoming more important than *prognostic* factors. The most important predictive factors in current use include hormone receptors, which predict the likelihood of recurrence following hormonal therapies.[4] Other predictive factors include HER2/neu, which not only predicts response to trastuzumab,[8] a monoclonal antibody that targets this receptor, but also may predict lack of response to tamoxifen.[40] Newer molecular tools are being researched that may be able to determine more accurately the likelihood of responding to both chemotherapy and hormonal agents.

## TREATMENT OF EARLY-STAGE BREAST CANCER

### Local Therapy
#### Surgical Management of Breast Cancer

Surgery has been the primary treatment for breast cancer for thousands of years. In 1889, William Halstead originated an operation named "the radical mastectomy" for the treatment of breast cancer, based on his theory of tumor biology and tumor metastases.[41] For the next 100 years, it was the gold standard and a life-saving operation for women, many of whom had advanced breast cancer by today's standards. With increasing knowledge of tumor biology, newer and less extensive surgical approaches for breast cancer were evaluated in a scientific manner. These trials demonstrated that limited surgical procedures could result in good local control and the same overall survival as more extensive surgical procedures. Modified radical mastectomy refers to several different operative procedures, all of which include complete removal of the breast tissue, the underlying fascia of the pectoralis major muscle, and some but not all of the axillary lymph nodes. Breast conservation is surgical removal of the tumor followed by radiation therapy. In addition, the importance of micrometastatic disease and the role of adjuvant therapies in increasing survival were noted.[3] In 1990, the National Institutes of Health Consensus Development Conference on Treatment of Early-Stage Breast Cancer brought together surgical, radiation, and medical oncologists, biostatisticians, psychologists, nurses, and other health care professionals as well as the public to address the role of mastectomy versus breast conservation, the role of adjuvant therapy, and the use of prognostic indicators in the treatment and management of early-stage breast cancer. Following 2 days of presentations by experts and discussion by the audience, a consensus panel weighed the evidence and prepared their consensus statement. Among their findings, the panel recommended that breast conservation treatment is an appropriate method of primary therapy for the majority of women with Stages I and II breast cancer and is preferable because it provides survival equivalent to total mastectomy and axillary dissection while preserving the breast.[42]

There are some patients for whom primary surgical therapy is not appropriate. These patients include those with locally advanced breast cancer (T4 lesions including skin edema peau d'orange, skin ulceration, satellite nodules, and/or infiltration, or N2 fixed or matted axillary lymph nodes). If these patients are treated with mastectomy alone, local recurrence rates are greater than 50% and few survive more than 5 years.[43] An alternative approach for these patients is primary or preoperative chemotherapy. It is clear from multiple studies[44] that the use of primary chemotherapy results in a down-staging of the primary tumor with a subsequent increase in surgical tumor resection rates. Many patients can then proceed to surgical resection of the tumor, which would not have been possible prior to the administration of primary chemotherapy. (The use of preoperative chemotherapy in resectable breast cancer is discussed in the section on neoadjuvant chemotherapy.)

Axillary lymph node dissection (ALND) has remained an integral part of breast cancer management for more than a century. Among patients with T1/T2 tumors, up to 70% have a negative axillary dissection, and more than 50% of these node-negative patients develop morbidity related to ALND.[45] Shoulder stiffness and numbness and paresthesias in the upper arm are common complaints following ALND, impacting on quality of life. The likelihood of arm edema is higher in women who undergo more extensive axillary lymphadenectomy and combined axillary surgery and RT. More recently, sentinel lymph node biopsy has replaced axillary dissection for staging. The sentinel lymph node is identified using lymphazurin, a blue dye, radiolabeled colloid, or both. The sentinel lymph nodes are excised and pathologically evaluated. If there are no tumor metastases in the nodes, then no additional nodes are removed. This reduces the morbidity of complete axillary dissection (arm edema and neuropathy).[46]

### Radiation Therapy

Radiation therapy is an integral part of the management of patients with breast cancer. It can be utilized definitively, in breast conservation therapy, or following mastectomy. It can also be used to for palliation in advanced stage of disease. With new technologies impacting the treatment planning and the delivery of radiation, there have been advances in the historical way that breast cancer patients were traditionally treated with irradiation. The integration of radiation therapy with surgery and systemic therapies has also changed.

#### Breast Conservation for Invasive Cancer

Several randomized trials in the United States and Europe have confirmed that breast conservation consisting of lumpectomy followed by adjuvant radiation therapy yields survival rates that are equal to mastectomy in women who have tumors up to 5 cm in diameter.[47] NSABP-06 trial randomized patients to total mastectomy, lumpectomy, and lumpectomy followed by irradiation. There was no significant difference in disease-free survival, distant disease-free survival, and overall survival in these three groups. Irradiation reduced the risk of recurrence in the ipsilateral breast from 39.2% to 14.3% in patients who had a lumpectomy.[48]

Absolute contraindications to irradiation are first or second trimester of pregnancy, prior irradiation, diffuse-appearing microcalcifications, presence of persistent positive margins especially with extensive intraductal component, and two or more lesions in separate quadrants. Relative contraindications to breast irradiation are a history of collagen vascular disease, multiple tumors in the same quadrant, a large tumor in a small breast, and very large or pendulous breasts.

Efforts have been made to identify a subgroup of patients with invasive breast cancer who do not require breast irradiation. In a recent article the authors concluded that lumpectomy plus adjuvant therapy with tamoxifen alone is a reasonable choice for the treatment of women 70 years of age or older who have early estrogen receptor–positive breast cancer. There was a 3% difference in local or regional recurrence but no difference in

distant metastases or overall survival at 5 years.[49] In contrast, another study reconfirmed that women under age 70 still do require irradiation and tamoxifen to reduce the risk of recurrence in the breast or axilla in women with T1 node-negative hormone receptor–positive tumors.[50]

#### Technique and Regional Irradiation

A treatment-planning CT scan of the chest enables the physician to define the underlying structures and to limit the volume of these structures encompassed in the radiation portal. The breast is treated in its entirety through medial and lateral tangents, usually with 6 MV photons. This field is treated to 4500–5000 cGy in daily fractions of 180–200 cGy per day for 25 to 28 treatments for over a course of 5 to 6 weeks. A boost of 10–16 cGy is then delivered over 5 to 8 days just to the tumor bed. Lymph nodes in the axilla and supraclavicular fossa are treated if there is a suboptimal axillary dissection, gross disease in the axilla, or gross extracapsular extension.

#### Breast Conservation for Noninvasive Cancer

The management of ductal carcinoma in situ (DCIS) is controversial. NSABP-17 trial demonstrated that irradiation after lumpectomy is more beneficial than lumpectomy alone in women with DCIS. This was due to a reduction in risk of developing invasive (13.4% to 3.9%) and noninvasive cancers (13.4% to 8.2%) at 8-year follow-up.[51] Further subgrouping of the various histologies would help define a subgroup of these patients who might be treated effectively with excision alone.

#### Postmastectomy Irradiation

Multivariate analysis showed that four or more positive nodes and tumor size up to 5 cm were associated with an increased risk of locoregional recurrence.[52] Two well-publicized trials examined the role of adjuvant irradiation in premenopausal, node-positive women. Both studies found a survival advantage from post-mastectomy radiation therapy (PMRT). In both trials all regional nodes were treated.[53,54] The radiotherapy techniques, types of surgery, and systemic treatments varied, and because of this there is disagreement about the optimal radiation therapy field. American Society of Clinical Oncology guidelines recommend PMRT for patients with four or more positive axillary lymph nodes and suggest it for patients with T3 tumors with positive axillary lymph nodes and operable Stage III tumors. With PMRT the chest wall should always be treated and the supraclavicular field added in patients with four or more nodes positive after adequate dissection. Irradiation of the internal mammary nodes should be individualized, with the morbidity of treatment weighed against the possible benefit.[55]

#### Side Effects of Irradiation

The risk of moderate arm edema is 5% to 25%.[47,56] The quoted incidence varies depending on the definition of the term and the extent of surgery. Brachial plexopathy, symptomatic pneumonitis, and pericarditis are seen in less than 1% of patients.[55,56] Rib fracture has been noted in 2% to 7% of patients who received chemotherapy along with irradiation.[55] Although the data conflict, a recent meta-analysis of 40 randomized trials demonstrated a decrease in breast cancer mortality but an increase in cardiac-related deaths after irradiation in early-stage breast cancer.[57] Another meta-analysis published that same year showed a decrease in overall mortality.[58] However, the different techniques used to deliver the radiation treatment (many now outdated), the type of surgical procedures performed, and the type and duration of chemotherapeutic agents must be taken into account.

### Newer Techniques

The traditional gold standard for breast conservation is external beam irradiation to the entire breast for 5 to 6 weeks following lumpectomy and axillary dissection. Three-dimensional conformal treatment planning is now routinely used. Intensity-modulated radiation therapy (IMRT), in which the intensity of irradiation varies within the beam, improves dose homogeneity[59] and may decrease toxicity to underlying structures in selected cases. Active breathing control devices can reduce the amount of heart treated within the radiation portal.[60] For many patients, treatment time, geographic inaccessibility, and cost of therapy and side effects of treatment may act as deterrents to breast conservation therapy. Studies examining recurrence after breast conservation therapy show that the majority of failures occur within or close to the tumor cavity.[61] An exciting and viable option is accelerated partial breast irradiation with external irradiation or brachytherapy. Brachytherapy catheters may be placed at the time of surgery and then after-loaded with iridium sources. The local failure rates at 5 years are comparable to results from external beam irradiation.[62] The MammoSite is a brachytherapy applicator consisting of a balloon catheter, which is inserted in the tumor cavity. Early studies are promising.[63]

## Systemic Therapy

### Neoadjuvant Therapy

The use of neoadjuvant or preoperative chemotherapy for treating breast cancer is increasing in the United States. The NSABP B-18 trial[64] demonstrated that both disease-free and overall survival are similar in patients with resectable breast cancer treated with preoperative chemotherapy, as compared with postoperative chemotherapy. This trial also demonstrated that preoperative chemotherapy can be used to down-stage breast tumors, allowing less extensive surgery.[64] Additionally, patients who had a complete pathologic response had significantly better disease-free and overall survival, compared with patients with any invasive cancer in the breast after chemotherapy.[65] Subsequent trials have demonstrated that complete pathologic response rates can be increased by the sequencing of non-resistant chemotherapy regimens.[66] The investigational use of preoperative chemotherapy may allow the identification of specific tumor profiles that may be used to predict response to specific agents. The uses of preoperative hormonal agents and of trastuzumab are currently being researched.

### Hormonal Therapy

Five years of adjuvant tamoxifen therapy reduces the recurrence rate and decreases mortality from ER-positive early-stage breast cancer[4] (Fig. 40-1). Five years of tamoxifen appear superior to shorter durations in reducing breast cancer recurrence.[4] Additionally, tamoxifen reduces the rate of breast cancer events, both preinvasive and invasive, in patients with ductal carcinoma in situ.[67] Unfortunately, tamoxifen is associated with potentially

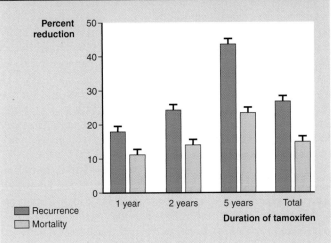

**Figure 40-1** Proportional reduction of recurrence and mortality from tamoxifen in estrogen receptor (ER)–positive early-stage breast cancer.

serious side effects, including a 4-fold increase in uterine cancer in postmenopausal patients[29] and a significant increase in thromboembolic events and cerebrovascular events.[7,29] Additionally, many patients treated with tamoxifen experience disease recurrence because of the development of resistance.

The aromatase inhibitors (Fig. 40-2) are a newer type of hormonal agent that are now being used as adjuvant therapies in

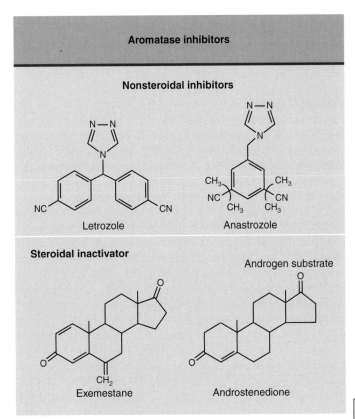

**Figure 40-2** Aromatase inhibitors.

early-stage breast cancer. These agents inhibit the conversion of androgens to estrogens in postmenopausal women and are ineffective in women with intact ovarian function. Anastrozole, a selective, nonsteroidal, competitive aromatase inhibitor, has been demonstrated to significantly improve disease-free survival, compared with tamoxifen, in postmenopausal patients with early-stage breast cancer[5,6] and has been approved as an alternative to tamoxifen for this indication. A recent trial[7] compared 5 years of adjuvant tamoxifen with 2 to 3 years of tamoxifen followed by the selective aromatase inactivator exemestane for the remainder of the 5 years in postmenopausal patients with early-stage breast cancer. Changing to the aromatase inhibitor resulted in superior disease-free survival at 30 months, compared with continuing tamoxifen for a total of 5 years.[7]

An extension to the NSABP B-14 trial[68] demonstrated no advantage to continuing tamoxifen through 10 years, compared with stopping the drug at 5 years, in patients with early-stage node-negative breast cancer. Based on the results of this trial, the National Cancer Institute recommended administering tamoxifen for no longer than 5 years. Two trials were initiated to examine the use of aromatase inhibitors following 5 years of adjuvant tamoxifen. The MA-17 trial randomized patients to the selective, competitive aromatase inhibitor letrozole, or to placebo, following 5 years of adjuvant tamoxifen. This trial was discontinued prematurely after a significantly improved disease-free survival was noted at a follow-up of 24 months in the patients randomized to receive the aromatase inhibitor.[69,70] Final analysis of this trial, at a follow-up of 30 months, demonstrates an improved disease-free and overall survival in patients with involved axillary lymph nodes treated with letrozole.[70]

Five years of tamoxifen remains the adjuvant therapy of choice for premenopausal patients with early-stage breast cancer. However, several trials are evaluating the use of aromatase inhibitors, along with ovarian ablation, by oophorectomy or luteinizing hormone–releasing hormone agonists, compared with tamoxifen, in premenopausal patients.

### Adjuvant Chemotherapy

Polychemotherapy produced significant proportional reductions in recurrence in women under 50 years of age by 35% and in women aged 50 to 69 years by 20%.[3] Few women aged 70 or over had been studied. For mortality, the reductions were also significant both among women aged under 50 (27%) and among those aged 50 to 69 (11%). Applying the proportional mortality reduction in women less than 50 years old would translate into an absolute 10-year survival benefit of 7% for those with node-negative disease and of 11% for those with node-positive disease. The smaller proportional mortality reduction observed in women aged 50 to 69 at randomization would translate into smaller absolute benefits—2% for those with node-negative disease and 3% for those with node-positive disease. The greater impact of chemotherapy in younger women might be partly attributable to premature menopause. This hypothesis is supported by some studies that demonstrated better outcome for women with drug-induced amenorrhea than for women whose menses persist following adjuvant chemotherapy.[71-74]

The reduction in the relative risk of recurrence and death with adjuvant systemic therapy is similar in node-negative and node-positive disease. However, patients with the lowest risk of

recurrence are least likely to benefit from systemic therapy when the lower absolute benefit and associated toxicities are considered. Women with node-negative tumors that are over 1 cm should be considered for chemotherapy if the tumors are associated with poor histologic features. There are no prospective clinical trials in women with tumors smaller than 1 cm. However, a retrospective analysis of tumors less than 1 cm suggested a benefit from adjuvant chemotherapy in tumors with poor-risk features.[75] The degree of risk reduction and risks of chemotherapy should be discussed with patients so they can make informed choices.

Several chemotherapy regimens are used for breast cancer (Table 40-4). The benefit of anthracycline over nonanthracycline regimens is controversial. Doxorubicin and cyclophosphamide (AC) for four cycles is equivalent in efficacy to the oral cyclophosphamide, methotrexate, and fluorouracil (CMF) regimen for six cycles.[76] However, in the overview analysis, compared with CMF, anthracycline-based regimens were associated with a modest but significant reduction in disease recurrence and death.[3] Seven hundred and ten premenopausal women with node-positive disease were randomized to six courses of oral CMF or cyclophosphamide, epirubicin, and fluorouracil (CEF).[77] With 59-month median follow-up, women receiving

| Table 40-4 Commonly Used Adjuvant Chemotherapy Regimens and Toxic Effects | |
|---|---|
| **Regimen** | |
| Oral CMF | Cyclophosphamide 100 mg/m² PO on days 1–14<br>Methotrexate 40 mg/m² IV on days 1 and 8<br>Fluorouracil 600 mg/m² IV on days 1 and 8<br>Repeat every 28 days |
| AC | Doxorubicin 60 mg/m² IV on day 1<br>Cyclophosphamide 600 mg/m² IV on day 1<br>Repeat every 21 days |
| CAF | Cyclophosphamide 500 mg/m² IV on day 1<br>Doxorubicin 50 mg/m² IV on day 1<br>Fluorouracil 600 mg/m² IV on day 1<br>Repeat every 21–28 days |
| Oral CEF | Fluorouracil 50 mg/m² IV on days 1 and 8<br>Epirubicin 60 mg/m² IV on days 1 and 8<br>Cyclophosphamide 75 mg/m² PO on days 1–14<br>Repeat every 28 days |
| AC → T | Paclitaxel 175 mg/m² IV on day 1 after 4 cycles of AC<br>Repeat every 21 days |
| TAC | Docetaxel 75 mg/m² IV on day 1<br>Doxorubicin 50 mg/m² IV on day 1<br>Cyclophosphamide 500 mg/m² IV on day 1 |

| **Common toxicities** | **Uncommon toxicities** |
|---|---|
| Nausea and vomiting | Febrile neutropenia (common with TAC) |
| Alopecia | Thrombosis |
| Fatigue | Hemorrhagic complications |
| Mucositis | Cardiomyopathy from anthracyclines |
| Weight gain | Secondary leukemia |
| Premature menopause | |
| Neuropathy from taxanes | |
| Myalgias from taxanes | |

IV, intravenously; PO, orally.

CEF had significantly better relapse-free survival (RFS) and overall survival (OS); however, CEF was associated with a higher likelihood of chemotherapy-induced amenorrhea and more cases of acute leukemia. When oral cyclophosphamide, doxorubicin, and fluorouracil (CAF) and oral CMF were compared in high-risk women, CAF was marginally superior to CMF for both RFS and OS; however, CAF was also associated with more toxicity.[78]

Since taxanes have shown benefit in the metastatic setting, several studies have been designed to look at their benefit in the adjuvant setting. The addition of paclitaxel for four cycles following the AC regimen was associated with a statistically significant 17% reduction in the risk of disease recurrence at 5 years and an 18% reduction in risk of death compared with AC alone.[79] In another study, the addition of paclitaxel to AC resulted in a significant improvement in disease-free survival but not in overall survival.[80] The addition of docetaxel was studied in BCIRG study. Patients treated with a combination of docetaxel, doxorubicin, and cytoxan (TAC) had a statistically significant 30% reduction in the risk of both recurrence and death.[81] Febrile neutropenia was more common with TAC.

Dose-dense therapy is a method of administering chemotherapy with shorter intertreatment intervals to minimize the potential of tumor regrowth. CALGB trial 9741 compared sequential therapy with doxorubicin, paclitaxel, and cyclophosphamide versus concurrent AC followed by paclitaxel administered at either 14-day (with filgrastim on days 3 to 10) or 21-day intervals in 2005 women with node-positive disease.[82] The dose-dense arm was associated with significant improvements in 4-year disease-free survival and 3-year overall survival compared with the standard arm.

## TREATMENT OF METASTATIC BREAST CANCER

Despite earlier diagnosis and better adjuvant therapies, many patients develop metastatic disease. Metastatic or Stage IV breast cancer remains, in almost all cases, an incurable disease. However, it is a heterogeneous disease, and some patients can live for 10 years with a good quality of life. The goals of therapy, therefore, are to improve quality of life and attempt to improve survival. Common sites of distant metastases include bone, lung, liver, and brain. Patients with bone-only disease do better than if visceral metastases are present. Therapy options include local therapy with surgery and irradiation and systemic therapy with endocrine therapy, chemotherapy, and novel approaches. These options can be used in combined or sequential fashion. Hormonal therapy and antibody treatment offer the advantage of excellent toxicity profiles and should be used when possible.

Broadly, metastatic breast cancer can be classified according to expression of hormone receptors and HER2/neu. HER2/neu is a member of the epidermal growth factor receptor (EGFR) family, which contains four transmembrane receptors. All the receptors have extracellular domains, which can be targeted with antibodies, such as trastuzumab, which targets HER2/neu. Additionally, each of the EGF receptors except HER3 has an intracellular tyrosine kinase domain, which can be targeted with small molecules, such as gefitinib.

### Treatment of Hormone Receptor–Positive Metastatic Breast Cancer

Metastatic breast cancer expressing ER and/or PR should be treated with hormonal agents. The only indication for chemotherapy as first-line treatment in this setting is a life-threatening visceral disease such as diffuse liver metastasis. Tamoxifen continues to be widely used in the treatment of hormone-responsive metastatic breast cancer, and the likelihood of responding can be predicted by the hormone receptor status of a patient's tumor. Patients are most likely to respond if their tumor expresses both ER and PR, but patients with tumor expressing one or other of the receptors benefit from hormonal therapy in 30% to 40% of cases.[83] A patient who benefits from one hormonal therapy can benefit from second-, third-, and even fourth-line hormonal therapy.

Recent trials have demonstrated that aromatase inhibitors are at least as effective as tamoxifen as first-line therapies for hormone-responsive metastatic breast cancer.[84–88] Newer agents, such as fulvestrant, which down-regulates ER and PR, are effective in patients whose cancer has progressed on tamoxifen.[89] Progestins, such as megestrol acetate, estrogens, and androgens can be used as third- and fourth-line agents in patients who continue to benefit from hormonal therapy.

### Treatment of HER2/neu-positive Metastatic Breast Cancer

HER2/neu is overexpressed in approximately 30% of breast cancers and may be associated with an aggressive course.[38] Trastuzumab is a monoclonal antibody that targets HER2/neu and has demonstrated survival advantages in metastatic breast cancer. When it is used as a single agent as first-line therapy,[90] approximately 50% of patients with HER2/neu-positive metastatic breast cancer benefit. Trastuzumab has marked synergy in preclinical studies with several chemotherapy agents on HER2/neu-positive breast cancer cell lines.[91,92] A pivotal trial randomized patients with HER2/neu-positive metastatic breast cancer to chemotherapy alone or chemotherapy plus trastuzumab.[8] Patients who received trastuzumab had longer disease-free and overall survival compared with those treated with chemotherapy alone. An unexpected side effect of trastuzumab was an increased incidence of cardiomyopathy, particularly in patients who received the drug concomitantly with anthracyclines. Therefore, trastuzumab is currently approved as a single agent, and with paclitaxel, for patients with HER2/neu-positive metastatic breast cancer. Several other agents, including docetaxel and vinorelbine, appear synergistic with trastuzumab. Adjuvant trials examining trastuzumab in early-stage breast cancer are ongoing.

### Treatment of Metastatic Breast Cancer with Chemotherapy

Several different antineoplastic agents have shown benefit in breast cancer (Table 40-5). Even though with first-line chemotherapy response rates are 50% to 60%, only 10% will have complete remission. Average duration of response is 6 to 12 months. Significant palliation can be achieved with chemotherapy. Subsequent chemotherapy agents used in sequential fashion produce fewer responses, which are short-lived. Even though several trials have shown significant response benefit of combination

**Table 40-5**
**Chemotherapy Agents Commonly Used in Metastatic Breast Cancer**

| | |
|---|---|
| Doxorubicin | Response rates of 35% to 50% in previously untreated metastatic disease |
| Epirubicin | Less cardiotoxicity compared with doxorubicin |
| Liposomal doxorubicin | Reduced cardiotoxicity and comparable efficacy to doxorubicin in first-line treatment[96] Not FDA-approved for breast cancer |
| Paclitaxel | Weekly administration has better efficacy with less myelosuppression but more neurotoxicity than higher doses given every 3 weeks[97,98] |
| Docetaxel | Compared with paclitaxel, has significantly better response rate, median time to progression, and median overall survival Greater toxicity than paclitaxel[98] |
| Capecitabine | Response rates are 20% to 27% in taxane-pretreated patents Better efficacy than CMF[99] |
| Vinorelbine | Response rates of 25% to 50% even in heavily pretreated patients |
| Gemcitabine | Response rates of 14% to 37% |
| Cyclophosphamide | Response rate of 25% |
| Trastuzumab in HER2-over expressing tumors | 50% response rate in combination with chemotherapy[8] |

chemotherapy over single-agent chemotherapy,[93,94] no clinical trial has shown a benefit of combination chemotherapy over sequential use of different chemotherapy agents. However, combination therapy is appropriate when immediate response is needed, for example, in women with rapidly progressive tumor growth. Bisphosphonates have utility in advanced breast cancer patients with bone metastasis. Intravenous pamidronate delays the appearance of clinical skeletal complications and reduces the proportion of women with skeletal complications.[95]

## REFERENCES

1. Kriege M, Brekelmans CT, Boetes C, et al: Efficacy of MRI and mammography for breast-cancer screening in women with a familial or genetic predisposition. N Engl J Med 2004;351:427–437. **(IIa, B)**
2. King MC: Breast cancer genes: how many, where and who are they? Nat Genet 1992;2:89–90. **(IV, C)**
3. Polychemotherapy for early breast cancer: an overview of the randomised trials. Early Breast Cancer Trialists' Collaborative Group. Lancet 1998; 352:930–942. **(Ia, A)**
4. Tamoxifen for early breast cancer: an overview of the randomised trials. Early Breast Cancer Trialists' Collaborative Group. Lancet 1998; 351: 1451–1467. **(Ia, A)**
5. Baum M, Budzar AU, Cuzick J, et al: Anastrozole alone or in combination with tamoxifen versus tamoxifen alone for adjuvant treatment of postmenopausal women with early breast cancer: first results of the ATAC randomised trial. Lancet 2002;359:2131–2139. **(Ib, A)**
6. Baum M, Buzdar A, Cuzick J, et al: Anastrozole alone or in combination with tamoxifen versus tamoxifen alone for adjuvant treatment of postmenopausal women with early-stage breast cancer: results of the ATAC (Arimidex, Tamoxifen Alone or in Combination) trial efficacy and safety update analyses. Cancer 2003;98:1802–1810. **(Ib, A)**
7. Coombes RC, Hall E, Gibson LJ, et al: A randomized trial of exemestane after two to three years of tamoxifen therapy in postmenopausal women with primary breast cancer. N Engl J Med 2004;350: 1081–1092. **(Ib, A)**
8. Slamon DJ, Leyland-Jones B, Shak S, et al: Use of chemotherapy plus a monoclonal antibody against HER2 for metastatic breast cancer that overexpresses HER2. N Engl J Med 2001;344:783–792. **(Ib, A)**
9. Rosen LS, Gordon DH, Dugan W, Jr., et al: Zoledronic acid is superior to pamidronate for the treatment of bone metastases in breast carcinoma patients with at least one osteolytic lesion. Cancer 2004;100:36–43. **(Ib, A)**
10. Lipton A: Bisphosphonates and breast carcinoma: present and future. Cancer 2000;88(12 Suppl):3033–3037. **(IV, C)**
11. Jemal A, Tiwari RC, Murray T, et al: Cancer statistics, 2004. CA Cancer J Clin 2004;54:8–29. **(IV, C)**
12. Easton DF, Ford D, Bishop DT, et al: Breast and ovarian cancer incidence in BRCA1 mutation carriers. Am J Hum Genet 1995; 56:265–271. **(III, B)**
13. Metcalfe K, Lynch HT, Ghadirian P, et al: Contralateral breast cancer in BRCA1 and BRCA2 mutation carriers. J Clin Oncol 2004;22: 2328–2335. **(III, B)**
14. Ford D, Easton DF, Stratton M, et al: Genetic heterogeneity and penetrance analysis of the BRCAI and BRCA2 genes in breast cancer families. Am J Hum Genet 1998;62:676–689. **(III, B)**
15. Rebbeck TR, Levin AM, Eisen A, et al: Breast cancer risk after bilateral prophylactic oophorectomy in BRCA1 mutation carriers. J Natl Cancer Inst 1999;91:1475–1479. **(IIa, B)**
16. Rebbeck TR, Friebel T, Lynch HT, et al: Bilateral prophylactic mastectomy reduces breast cancer risk in BRCA1 and BRCA2 mutation carriers: the PROSE Study Group. J Clin Oncol 2004;22:1055–1062. **(IIa, B)**
17. Perou CM, Sorlie T, Eisen MB, et al: Molecular portraits of human breast tumours. Nature 2000;406:747–752. **(IIb, B)**
18. Beatson G: On the treatment of inoperable cases of carcinoma of the mamma: suggestions for a new method of treatment, with illustrative cases. Lancet 1896;2:104–107. **(III, B)**
19. Paffenbarger RS Jr, Kampert J, Chang HG: Characteristics that predict risk of breast cancer before and after menopause. Am J Epidemiol 1980;112:258–268. **(IIa, B)**
20. Rosner B CG: Nurses' Health Study: log-incidence mathematical model of breast cancer incidence. J Natl Cancer Inst 1996;88:359–364. **(IIb, B)**
21. Breast cancer and breastfeeding: collaborative reanalysis of individual data from 47 epidemiological studies in 30 countries, including 50302 women with breast cancer and 96973 women without the disease. Lancet 2002;360:187–195. **(IIa, B)**
22. Grady D, Herrington D, Bittner V, et al: Cardiovascular disease outcomes during 6.8 years of hormone therapy: Heart and Estrogen/progestin Replacement Study follow-up (HERS II). JAMA 2002;288: 49–57. **(Ib, A)**
23. Anderson GL, Limacher M, Assaf AR, et al: Effects of conjugated equine estrogen in postmenopausal women with hysterectomy: the Women's Health Initiative randomized controlled trial. JAMA 2004; 291:1701–1712. **(Ib, A)**
24. Potential risks, benefits of progestins in birth control pills outlined. Contracept Technol Update 1984;5:71. **(IV, C)**
25. Ursin G, Ross RK, Sullivan-Halley J, et al: Use of oral contraceptives and risk of breast cancer in young women. Breast Cancer Res Treat 1998;50:175–184. **(IIa, B)**
26. Huang Z, Willett WC, Colditz GA, et al: Waist circumference, waist:hip ratio, and risk of breast cancer in the Nurses' Health Study. Am J Epidemiol 1999;150:1316–1324. **(IIb, B)**
27. Hankinson SE, Willett WC, Manson JE, et al: Alcohol, height, and adiposity in relation to estrogen and prolactin levels in postmenopausal women. J Natl Cancer Inst 1995;87:1297–1302. **(IIb, B)**
28. Goldschmidt RA, Victor TA: Lobular carcinoma in situ of the breast. Semin Surg Oncol 1996;12:314–320. **(III, B)**
29. Fisher B, Costantino JP, Wickerham DL, et al: Tamoxifen for prevention of breast cancer: report of the National Surgical Adjuvant Breast and Bowel Project P-1 Study. Journal of the National Cancer Institute 1998;90:1371-88. **(Ib, A)**

30. Gail MH, Brinton LA, Byar DP, et al: Projecting individualized probabilities of developing breast cancer for white females who are being examined annually. J Natl Cancer Inst 1989;81:1879–1886. **(IIb, B)**

31. Powels T, Eeles R, Ashley S, et al: Interim analysis of the incidence of breast cancer in Royal Marsden Hospital tamoxifen randomised chemoprevention trial. Lancet 1998;352:98–101. **(Ib, A)**

32. Veronesi U, Maisonneuve P, Costa A, et al: Prevention of breast cancer with tamoxifen: preliminary findings from the Italian randomised trial among hysterectomised women. Lancet 1998;352:93–97. **(Ib, A)**

33. Robson M, Gilewski T, Haas B, et al: BRCA-associated breast cancer in young women. J Clin Oncol 1998;16:1642–1649. **(IIb, B)**

34. Sorlie T, Tibshirani R, Parker J, et al: Repeated observation of breast tumor subtypes in independent gene expression data sets. Proc Natl Acad Sci USA 2003;100:8418–8423. **(IIb, B)**

35. King MC, Wieand S, Hale K, et al: Tamoxifen and breast cancer incidence among women with inherited mutations in BRCA1 and BRCA2: National Surgical Adjuvant Breast and Bowel Project (NSABP-P1) Breast Cancer Prevention Trial. JAMA 2001;286:2251–2256. **(Ib, A)**

36. Singletary SE, Allred C, Ashley P, et al: Revision of the American Joint Committee on Cancer staging system for breast cancer. J Clin Oncol 2002;20:3628–3636. **(IV, C)**

37. Woodward WA, Strom EA, Tucker SL, et al: Changes in the 2003 American Joint Committee on Cancer staging for breast cancer dramatically affect stage-specific survival. J Clin Oncol 2003;21: 3244–3248. **(IIb, B)**

38. Slamon DJ, Clark GM, Wong SG, et al: Human breast cancer: correlation of relapse and survival with amplification of the HER-2/neu oncogene. Science 1987;235:177–182. **(IIb, B)**

39. Ravdin PM, Siminoff LA, Davis GJ, et al: Computer program to assist in making decisions about adjuvant therapy for women with early breast cancer. J Clin Oncol 2001;19:980–991. **(IIb, B)**

40. Ellis MJ, Coop A, Singh B, et al: Letrozole is more effective neoadjuvant endocrine therapy than tamoxifen for ErbB-1- and/or ErbB-2-positive, estrogen receptor-positive primary breast cancer: evidence from a phase III randomized trial. J Clin Oncol 2001;19:3808–3816. **(Ib, A)**

41. Halstead W: The results of radical operations for the cure of carcinoma of the breast. Ann Surg 1907;46:1–19. **(III, B)**

42. Early stage breast cancer. Consens Statement 1990;8:1–19. **(III, B)**

43. Haagensen CD, Stout AP: Carcinoma of the breast. 2. Criteria of operability. Ann Surg 1943;118:1032–1051. **(IV, C)**

44. Jacquillat C, Weil M, Baillet F, et al: Results of neoadjuvant chemotherapy and radiation therapy in the breast-conserving treatment of 250 patients with all stages of infiltrative breast cancer. Cancer 1990; 66:119–129. **(IIb, B)**

45. Giuliano AE: Mapping a pathway for axillary staging: a personal perspective on the current status of sentinel lymph node dissection for breast cancer. Arch Surg 1999;134:195–199. **(IV, C)**

46. Golshan M, Martin WJ, Dowlatshahi K: Sentinel lymph node biopsy lowers the rate of lymphedema when compared with standard axillary lymph node dissection. Am Surg 2003;69:209–211, 212. **(IIa, B)**

47. Morrow M, Harris J: Local management of invasive cancer: breast. In Harris J, Lippman ME, Morrow M, et al (eds): Diseases of the Breast, 3rd ed. Philadelphia, Lippincott Williams & Wilkins, 2004. **(IV, C)**

48. Fisher B, Anderson S, Bryant J, et al: Twenty-year follow-up of a randomized trial comparing total mastectomy, lumpectomy, and lumpectomy plus irradiation for the treatment of invasive breast cancer. N Engl J Med 2002;347:1233–1241. **(Ib, A)**

49. Hughes KS, Schnaper LA, Berry D, et al: Lumpectomy plus tamoxifen with or without irradiation in women 70 years of age or older with early breast cancer. N Engl J Med 2004;351:971–977. **(Ib, A)**

50. Fyles AW, McCready DR, Manchul LA, et al: Tamoxifen with or without breast irradiation in women 50 years of age or older with early breast cancer. N Engl J Med 2004;351:963–970. **(Ib, A)**

51. Fisher B, Dignam J, Wolmark N, et al: Lumpectomy and radiation therapy for the treatment of intraductal breast cancer: findings from National Surgical Adjuvant Breast and Bowel Project B-17. J Clin Oncol 1998;16:441–452. **(Ib, A)**

52. Fowble B, Gray R, Gilchrist K, et al: Identification of a subgroup of patients with breast cancer and histologically positive axillary nodes receiving adjuvant chemotherapy who may benefit from postoperative radiotherapy. J Clin Oncol 1988;6:1107–1117. **(Ib, A)**

53. Ragaz J, Jackson SM, Le N, et al: Adjuvant radiotherapy and chemotherapy in node-positive premenopausal women with breast cancer. N Engl J Med 1997;337:956–962. **(Ib, A)**

54. Overgaard M, Hansen PS, Overgaard J, et al: Postoperative radiotherapy in high-risk premenopausal women with breast cancer who receive adjuvant chemotherapy. Danish Breast Cancer Cooperative Group 82b Trial. N Engl J Med 1997;337:949–955. **(Ib, A)**

55. Recht A, Edge SB, Solin LJ, et al: Postmastectomy radiotherapy: clinical practice guidelines of the American Society of Clinical Oncology. J Clin Oncol 2001;19:1539–1569. **(IV, C)**

56. Fowble BL, Solin LJ, Schultz DJ, et al: Ten year results of conservative surgery and irradiation for stage I and II breast cancer. Int J Radiat Oncol Biol Phys 1991;21:269–277. **(IIb, B)**

57. Favourable and unfavourable effects on long-term survival of radiotherapy for early breast cancer: an overview of the randomised trials. Early Breast Cancer Trialists' Collaborative Group. Lancet 2000; 355:1757–1770. **(Ia, A)**

58. Whelan TJ, Julian J, Wright J, et al: Does locoregional radiation therapy improve survival in breast cancer? A meta-analysis. J Clin Oncol 2000; 18:1220–1229. **(Ia, A)**

59. Vicini FA, Sharpe M, Kestin L, et al: Optimizing breast cancer treatment efficacy with intensity-modulated radiotherapy. Int J Radiat Oncol Biol Phys 2002;54:1336–1344. **(III, B)**

60. Remouchamps VM, Letts N, Vicini FA, et al: Initial clinical experience with moderate deep-inspiration breath hold using an active breathing control device in the treatment of patients with left-sided breast cancer using external beam radiation therapy. Int J Radiat Oncol Biol Phys 2003;56:704–715. **(III, B)**

61. Freedman G, Hanlon A, Anderson P: Pattern of local recurrence after conserving surgery and whole-breast irradiation: implications for partial breast irradiation. Proc Am Soc Ther Radiat Oncol 2003;57. Abstract 79. **(IIb, B)**

62. Vicini FA, Kestin L, Chen P, et al: Limited-field radiation therapy in the management of early-stage breast cancer. J Natl Cancer Inst 2003; 95:1205–1210. **(IIa, B)**

63. Keisch M, Vicini F, Kuske RR, et al: Initial clinical experience with the MammoSite breast brachytherapy applicator in women with early-stage breast cancer treated with breast-conserving therapy. Int J Radiat Oncol Biol Phys 2003;55:289–293. **(IIb, B)**

64. Fisher B, Bryant J, Wolmark N, et al: Effect of preoperative chemotherapy on the outcome of women with operable breast cancer. J Clin Oncol 1998;16:2672–2685. **(Ib, A)**

65. Wolmark N, Wang J, Mamounas E, et al: Preoperative chemotherapy in patients with operable breast cancer: nine-year results from National Surgical Adjuvant Breast and Bowel Project B-18. J Natl Cancer Inst Monogr 2001;96–102. **(Ib, A)**

66. Smith IC, Heys SD, Hutcheon AW, et al: Neoadjuvant chemotherapy in breast cancer: significantly enhanced response with docetaxel. J Clin Oncol 2002;20:1456–1466. **(Ib, A)**

67. Fisher B, Dignam J, Wolmark N, et al: Tamoxifen in treatment of intraductal breast cancer: National Surgical Adjuvant Breast and Bowel Project B-24 randomised controlled trial. Lancet 1999;353(9169): 1993–2000. **(Ib, A)**

68. Fisher B, Dignam J, Bryant J, et al: Five versus more than five years of tamoxifen for lymph node-negative breast cancer: updated findings from the National Surgical Adjuvant Breast and Bowel Project B-14 randomized trial. J Natl Cancer Inst 2001;93:684–690. **(Ib, A)**

69. Goss PE, Ingle JN, Martino S, et al: A randomized trial of letrozole in postmenopausal women after five years of tamoxifen therapy for early-stage breast cancer. N Engl J Med 2003;349:1793–1802. **(Ib, A)**

70. Goss PE: Updated results of MA-17 trial. Special presentation, American Society of Clinical Oncology (ASCO), New Orleans, June 8, 2004. **(Ib, A)**

71. Jonat W, Kaufmann M, Sauerbrei W, et al: Goserelin versus cyclophosphamide, methotrexate, and fluorouracil as adjuvant therapy in premenopausal patients with node-positive breast cancer: The Zoladex Early Breast Cancer Research Association Study. J Clin Oncol 2002;20:4628–4635. **(Ib, A)**

72. Bianco AR, Del Mastro L, Gallo C, et al: Prognostic role of amenorrhea induced by adjuvant chemotherapy in premenopausal patients with early breast cancer. Br J Cancer 1991;63:799–803. **(III, B)**

73. Goldhirsch A, Gelber RD, Castiglione M: The magnitude of endocrine effects of adjuvant chemotherapy for premenopausal breast cancer patients. The International Breast Cancer Study Group. Ann Oncol 1990;1:183–188. **(Ib, A)**

74. Richards MA, O'Reilly SM, Howell A, et al: Adjuvant cyclophosphamide, methotrexate, and fluorouracil in patients with axillary node-positive breast cancer: an update of the Guy's/Manchester trial. J Clin Oncol 1990;8:2032–2039. **(Ib, A)**

75. Fisher B, Dignam J, Tan-Chiu E, et al: Prognosis and treatment of patients with breast tumors of one centimeter or less and negative axillary lymph nodes. J Natl Cancer Inst 2001;93:112–120. **(Ib, A)**

76. Fisher B, Brown AM, Dimitrov NV, et al: Two months of doxorubicin-cyclophosphamide with and without interval reinduction therapy compared with 6 months of cyclophosphamide, methotrexate, and fluorouracil in positive-node breast cancer patients with tamoxifen-nonresponsive tumors: results from the National Surgical Adjuvant Breast and Bowel Project B-15. J Clin Oncol 1990;8:1483–1496. **(Ib, A)**

77. Levine MN, Bramwell VH, Pritchard KI, et al: Randomized trial of intensive cyclophosphamide, epirubicin, and fluorouracil chemotherapy compared with cyclophosphamide, methotrexate, and fluorouracil in premenopausal women with node-positive breast cancer. National Cancer Institute of Canada Clinical Trials Group. J Clin Oncol 1998; 16:2651–2658. **(Ib, A)**

78. Hutchins L, Green S, Ravdin P, et al: CMF versus CAF with and without tamoxifen in high-risk node-negative breast cancer patients and a natural history follow-up study in low-risk node-negative patients: first results of Intergroup Trial INT 0102. Proc Am Soc Clin Oncol 1998. Abstract 2. **(Ib, A)**

79. Henderson IC, Berry DA, Demetri GD, et al: Improved outcomes from adding sequential Paclitaxel but not from escalating Doxorubicin dose in an adjuvant chemotherapy regimen for patients with node-positive primary breast cancer. J Clin Oncol 2003;21:976–983. **(Ib, A)**

80. Mamounas EP, Bryant J, Lembersky BC, et al: Paclitaxel (T) following doxorubicin/cyclophosphamide (AC) as adjuvant chemotherapy for node-positive breast cancer: results from NSABP B-28. Proc Am Soc Clin Oncol 2003;22:4. Abstract 12. **(Ib, A)**

81. Martin M, Pienkowski T, Mackey J, et al: TAC improves disease free survival and overall survival over FAC in node positive early breast cancer patients, BCIRG 001: 55 months follow-up. Breast Cancer Res Treat 2003;85.2. Abstract 43. **(Ib, A)**

82. Citron ML, Berry DA, Cirrincione C, et al: Randomized trial of dose-dense versus conventionally scheduled and sequential versus concurrent combination chemotherapy as postoperative adjuvant treatment of node-positive primary breast cancer: first report of Intergroup Trial C9741/Cancer and Leukemia Group B Trial 9741. J Clin Oncol 2003; 21:1431–1439. **(Ib, A)**

83. Horwitz KB, McGuire WL, Pearson OH, et al: Predicting response to endocrine therapy in human breast cancer. Science 1975;189:726–727. **(IIb,B)**

84. Mouridsen H, Gershanovich M, Sun Y, et al: Phase III study of letrozole versus tamoxifen as first-line therapy of advanced breast cancer in post-menopausal women: analysis of survival and update of efficacy from the International Letrozole Breast Cancer Group. J Clin Oncol 2003; 21:2101–2109. **(Ib, A)**

85. Mouridsen H, Gershanovich M, Sun Y, et al: Superior efficacy of letrozole versus tamoxifen as first-line therapy for postmenopausal women with advanced breast cancer: results of a phase III study of the International Letrozole Breast Cancer Group. J Clin Oncol 2001; 19:2596–2606. **(Ib, A)**

86. Nabholtz JM, Buzdar A, Pollak M, et al: Anastrozole is superior to tamoxifen as first-line therapy for advanced breast cancer in post-menopausal women: results of a North American multicenter randomized trial. J Clin Oncol 2000;18:3758–3767. **(Ib, A)**

87. Paridaens R, Therasse P, Dirix L, et al: First line hormonal treatment for metastatic breast cancer with exemestane or tamoxifen in post-menopausal patients—a randomized phase III trial of the EORTC Breast Group. Proc Am Soc Clin Oncol 2004;22(14S). Abstract 515. **(Ib, A)**

88. Bonneterre J, Thurlimann B, Robertson JF, et al: Anastrozole versus tamoxifen as first-line therapy for advanced breast cancer in 668 post-menopausal women: results of the Tamoxifen or Arimidex Randomized Group Efficacy and Tolerability study. J Clin Oncol 2000;18: 3748–3757. **(Ib, A)**

89. Howell A, Robertson JF, Quaresma Albano J, et al:, formerly ICI 182,780, is as effective as anastrozole in postmenopausal women with advanced breast cancer progressing after prior endocrine treatment. J Clin Oncol 2002;20:3396–3403. **(Ib, A)**

90. Vogel CL, Cobleigh MA, Tripathy D, et al: Efficacy and safety of trastuzumab as a single agent in first-line treatment of HER2-overexpressing metastatic breast cancer. J Clin Oncol 2002;20: 719–726. **(Ib, A)**

91. Pegram M, Hsu S, Lewis G, et al: Inhibitory effects of combinations of HER-2/neu antibody and chemotherapeutic agents used for treatment of human breast cancers. Oncogene 1999;18:2241–2251. **(IIb, B)**

92. Pegram MD, Finn RS, Arzoo K, et al: The effect of HER-2/neu over-expression on chemotherapeutic drug sensitivity in human breast and ovarian cancer cells. Oncogene 1997;15:537–547. **(IIb, B)**

93. O'Shaughnessy J, Miles D, Vukelja S, et al: Superior survival with capecitabine plus docetaxel combination therapy in anthracycline-pretreated patients with advanced breast cancer: phase III trial results. J Clin Oncol 2002;20:2812–2823. **(Ib, A)**

94. Albain KS, Nag S, Calderillo-Ruiz G, et al: Global phase III study of gemcitabine plus paclitaxel (GT) vs. paclitaxel (T) as frontline therapy for metastatic breast cancer (MBC): first report of overall survival. Proc Am Soc Clin Oncol 2004;22(14S). Abstract 510. **(Ib, A)**

95. Theriault RL, Lipton A, Hortobagyi GN, et al: Pamidronate reduces skeletal morbidity in women with advanced breast cancer and lytic bone lesions: a randomized, placebo-controlled trial. Protocol 18 Aredia Breast Cancer Study Group. J Clin Oncol 1999;17:846–854. **(Ib, A)**

96. O'Brien ME, Wigler N, Inbar M, et al: Reduced cardiotoxicity and comparable efficacy in a phase III trial of pegylated liposomal doxorubicin HCl (CAELYX/Doxil) versus conventional doxorubicin for first-line treatment of metastatic breast cancer. Ann Oncol 2004;15: 440–449. **(Ib, A)**

97. Seidman AD, Berry D, Cirrincione C, et al: CALGB 9840: Phase III study of weekly (W) paclitaxel (P) via 1-hour (h) infusion versus standard (S) 3h infusion every third week in the treatment of meta-static breast cancer (MBC), with trastuzumab (T) for HER2 positive MBC and randomized for T in HER2 normal MBC. Proc Am Soc Clin Oncol 2004;22(14S). Abstract 512. **(Ib, A)**

98. Jones S, Erban J, Overmoyer B, et al: Randomized trial comparing docetaxel and paclitaxel in patients with metastatic breast cancer. Breast Cancer Research and Treatment; 2003;85.2. Abstract 10. **(Ib, A)**

99. Oshaughnessy JA, Blum J, Moiseyenko V, et al: Randomized, open-label, phase II trial of oral capecitabine (Xeloda) vs. a reference arm of intravenous CMF (cyclophosphamide, methotrexate and 5-fluorouracil) as first-line therapy for advanced/metastatic breast cancer. Ann Oncol 2001;12:1247–1254. **(Ib, A)**

# Breast Cancer Screening

Victoria L. Green, MD, MBA, JD

## KEY POINTS

- Mammary (or breast) gland development is noted in both male and female fetuses at the fifth or sixth week of development.
- The sentinel lymph node is the first node draining from the tumor site. Pathology within this node determines the necessity for further axillary evaluation.
- Witch's milk may occur in both newborn females and males as a result of transplacental transfer of maternal hormones (primarily estrogen).
- Breast cancer is the most common cancer in women and is second only to lung cancer in cancer deaths for women.
- A history of multiple affected first-degree relatives, bilateral disease, early or premenopausal age of onset, a family history of both ovarian and breast cancer, or male breast cancer increases the probability of having an inherited predisposition to breast cancer.
- Breast self-examination has not been shown in randomized, controlled trials to decrease mortality associated with breast cancer.
- Ultrasound, magnetic resonance imaging, digital mammography, and computer-assisted diagnosis have insufficient data to justify support in breast cancer screening.
- The sensitivity of ductal lavage in detecting breast cancer is low; however, it may be helpful in detection of preneoplastic cells in women at high risk for the development of breast cancer.

Issues surrounding breast diseases are one of the most pervasive concerns of women today. From abnormal development to mastitis, discussions about breast maladies are widespread. Moreover, breast health and treatment are among the most controversial subject matters of the day. From estrogen therapy and breast cancer risk to mammographic screening, women are bombarded with decisions related to breast health, which may have important outcomes and significant impact on their future quality of life. Thus, disorders of the breast are of particular importance to those who function as primary caregivers for women from reproductive age through the perimenopause, the specialty of obstetrics and gynecology.

Because gynecologists continue to assume a position of extensive importance with respect to diagnosing and treating breast diseases in women, the diagnosis of breast cancer in its most curable forms lies within this specialty for large numbers of women. To effectively respond to the challenge of this profound medical responsibility, physicians must have an understanding of the natural history as well as the contemporary diagnostic and screening modalities for both benign and malignant disorders of the breast.

This chapter reviews the anatomy and physiology of the breast and examines recent advances in breast cancer knowledge, with emphasis on mammographic screening recommendations, alternative imaging modalities, assessment of risk factors, breast cancer susceptibility testing, and chemoprevention in high-risk women. Women who develop breast cancer require a multidisciplinary team approach, which includes the gynecologist, general surgeons, radiation oncologists, and medical oncologists. Thus, the gynecologist must be a knowledgeable participant in treatment planning.

## EMBRYOLOGY

Embryologic differentiation of the paired mammary glands begins at the fifth or sixth week of fetal development in both genders. Thickened ectoderm (known as *mammary ridges* or *milk lines*) develops from the area of the future axilla to the future inguinal region. During normal development, regression of the ridges results in persistence of only one gland bilaterally at the level of the thorax. Failure of regression may give rise to accessory mammary glands (polymastia) or accessory nipples (polythelia) along the original mammary ridge. This minor congenital anomaly may occur in both sexes, with an estimated frequency of about 1%.[1,2]

Extension of the remaining ectoderm into the underlying mesenchyme initiates development of the primary bud. From 15 to 20 secondary buds develop as outgrowths of each primary bud and extend into the surrounding connective tissue of the chest wall. Canalization of these epithelial cords (under the influence of placental sex steroids) during the third trimester heralds the development of the lactiferous ductal system. Proliferation of basal mesenchymal cells initiates transformation into the fully formed nipple. Continued elevation is supported by both expansion of underlying connective tissue and smooth muscle development in the areolar gland. Failure of elevation of the nipple above the skin level occurs in 2% to 4% of the population, resulting in inverted nipples.

### Anatomy

The breast, or mammary gland, is a highly modified sudoriferous (sweat) gland situated between two layers of superficial fascia on the pectoralis major, serratus anterior, and external oblique muscles. The second rib and the sixth intercostal space in the vertical plane, and the sternum and the midaxillary line in the horizontal plane, border it. It is composed of 15 to 20 lobes, with the greatest volume of glandular tissue located in the upper outer quadrant. The breast lobes branch into lobules and then into terminal duct lobular units, which are thought to be the originating site for breast cancer. Each lobe terminates in a lactiferous duct, which opens onto the nipple.

Cooper's (or suspensory) ligaments are fibrous septa that interdigitate between the tissue to connect the two fascial layers. Cancerous invasion of Cooper's ligament may result in skin retraction or dimpling.

The nipple contains smooth muscle fibers, which is the only muscle "within" the breast tissue. Stimulation of these muscle fibers in response to various sensory stimuli accounts for erection of the nipple. The vast array of sensory nerve cell endings provide the neurohumoral pathway necessary for milk letdown during suckling. The areola consists of many sweat, sebaceous, and accessory glands. During pregnancy, accessory glands called *Montgomery tubercles* become very prominent.

The breast tissue is well supplied by an extensive system of arteries and veins. The medial and central aspect of the breast is supplied by the anterior perforating branches of the internal thoracic (internal mammary) artery. A branch of the axillary artery, the lateral thoracic artery, supplies the upper outer quadrant. The two vessels combined also provide the major blood supply to the nipple. Other vessels of the extensive arterial and venous system include the anterior and lateral branches of the intercostals, the pectoral branch of the thoracoacromial artery and other branches of the axillary artery, and the subscapular and thoracodorsal arteries.

Venous and lymphatic drainage follows the course of the arteries. The principal venous drainage of the breast is the internal thoracic vein medially, the axillary vein superolaterally, and the intercostal veins, which drain to the vertebral and azygos veins posteriorly. This drainage pathway explains the frequent sites of metastasis, because breast cancer will enter the venous system and metastasize to the lungs through the axillary or intercostal veins or to thoracic, abdominal, and pelvic organs by way of the vertebral vein. Similarly, the primary lymph node drainage is initially into the axillary region, but additional drainage can proceed to the infraclavicular and supraclavicular and mediastinal (parasternal) areas, thus suggesting the need to extend the routine breast examination to the bony margins (rather than simply the breast tissue) to assure adequate coverage of these potential cancer-bearing areas. The lymphatic plexus is divided into levels based on the relation to the pectoralis minor muscle. Level one nodes are located lateral to the muscle and level three nodes are located medically. Level two nodes are located deep or posterior to the pectoralis minor muscle. The sentinel lymph node, which has gained important significance in breast cancer treatment over the past decade, is the first node draining from the tumor site. Pathology within this node determines the necessity of further axillary evaluation.

## PHYSIOLOGY

The anterior lobe of the pituitary gland and the ovaries orchestrate the development and physiologic functioning of the breast. This development is a lifelong process that begins in utero. A transient enlargement of the breast bud and/or associated milk-like nipple secretion (witch's milk) may occur in both newborn females and males as a result of transplacental transfer of maternal hormones (primarily estrogen). The fluid secretion may appear for a week postpartum, but subsequent involution of the tissue results by the third or fourth week postpartum.

Before the transformation that occurs at puberty, the function and histology of the human breast is identical in males and females. During puberty in the female, the rudimentary gland buds proliferate and increase in size while the nipple and areola become pigmented. The ductal system develops as a consequence of estrogen stimulation, and the lobular–alveolar system develops due to progesterone secretion.

Menstruation, pregnancy, and menopause are sentinel events in breast development. Before the onset of menstruation, breast development begins with ductal branching and proliferation of interductal stroma. With each menstrual cycle ductal proliferation occurs under the influence of estrogen. Under the influence of progesterone, proliferation of the terminal duct structure and increased mitotic activity in the basal epithelial cells occur in the secretory phase. Stromal proliferation and edema, in response to the hormonal milieu, account for the sense of fullness or tenderness experienced premenstrually. The fall in hormones that occurs with menstruation is associated with the disappearance of stromal edema, desquamation of epithelial cells, atrophy of intralobular connective tissue, and overall shrinkage in the size of the ducts.

Further maturation of the breast occurs with pregnancy. Significant growth of glandular tissues and decrease in the surrounding stroma portends reversal of the previous stromal predominance within the stromal/glandular relation seen before this stage. After pregnancy these changes regress but do not return completely to their prepregnancy state. Menopause heralds a further reduction and shrinkage of the ducts, gland buds, and surrounding stroma.

### Lactation

Hormonal and structural changes that occur during pregnancy prime the breast for future milk production. Increased estrogen and progesterone secretion in early pregnancy results in ductal development and maturation as well as enlargement of lobular size. During the latter half of pregnancy, glandular epithelium is transformed into secretory epithelium as a result of hormonal stimulation, including insulin, thyroxine, growth hormone, and corticosteroids. Human placental lactogen and prolactin also play critical roles in breast development during pregnancy. Paradoxically, despite considerable increases in prolactin, this hormone's functioning is inhibited at the alveolar level by progesterone. Thus lactation does not occur until the rapid decline of estrogen and progesterone at the time of delivery.

At delivery, simulation of the afferent neural arc suppresses prolactin-inhibiting hormone, allowing release of prolactin-releasing hormone and further elevation of the prolactin concentration. Not only breast suckling, but also auditory and visual stimuli, stimulate the neural arc. Prolactin-inhibiting hormone is thought to be dopamine and prolactin-releasing hormone is thought to be thyrotropin or thyrotropin-releasing hormone. Additionally, stimulation of the neural arc triggers release of oxytocin by involving the paraventricular and supraoptic nuclei of the hypothalamus. Oxytocin release from the posterior pituitary induces contraction of the myoepithelial cells surrounding the nipple ducts, resulting in milk letdown. Continued suckling induces additional prolactin secretion as well as replenishment of the milk supply. Discontinuation of suckling results in increased levels of prolactin-inhibiting hormone, which inhibits prolactin production. Ultimately, lactation will cease, with resultant decrease in size of the alveoli.

## BREAST CANCER

Although the etiology of most breast symptoms is a benign disorder, the fear of cancer is often the motivating factor for women seeking evaluation of breast symptomatology. Breast cancer remains the most common cancer in women, with the American Cancer Society (ACS) estimating nearly 215,990 new cases of invasive breast cancer in the United States during 2004. Startlingly, approximately 1450 men will be afflicted with breast cancer as well.[3] Moreover, an estimated 40,580 deaths from breast cancer (40,110 women, 470 men) are anticipated during the same period. Cancer of the breast is second only to lung cancer in the number of cancer deaths in women, making it an especially dreadful adversary. Although breast cancer incidence rates have continued to increase since 1980 (albeit the rate of increase slowed in the 1990s), mortality rates have declined by 2.3% per year since 1990.[3] This decline is surmised to be directly attributable to increased utilization of screening mammography, resulting in earlier detection, improved treatment, and a heightened awareness of breast cancer symptoms among women.[4] Further advances in hormonal treatment, deciphering of genetic etiologies, and risk reduction therapies has thrust breast health issues into the forefront of the media and medical technology. The zeal to achieve the ideal cure or prevention strategy persists unabated in the medical profession and remains an ongoing challenge. A thorough understanding of the evaluation of breast disease is essential for the practicing gynecologist.

### Risk Factors

Breast cancer prevention is now an achievable medical objective; thus, an understanding of the epidemiology of breast cancer is critical in assessing the individual's risk for development of the disease. Breast cancer risk factors are covered in detail in Chapter 40, but a brief review is appropriate at this juncture.

The etiology of breast cancer is multifactorial; although numerous risk factors have been identified, fewer than 15% of patients with breast cancer have an identifiable risk factor, which means nearly 85% of women with breast cancer have no identifiable risk factors other than gender and age. Thus, all women should be considered at risk for breast cancer.[5]

Age is the most significant risk factor, because the risk of breast cancer increases with advancing age. Additional risk factors include nulliparity, delayed childbearing (childbirth before age 18 portends one third the risk of breast cancer of a woman delivering at age 35), a personal or family history of breast cancer, benign proliferative breast disease (ductal or lobular hyperplasia, particularly with atypia), obesity in postmenopausal women, alcohol intake, early menarche (before age 12), late menopause (after age 53), and higher socioeconomic status. Breast cancer susceptibility genes account for approximately 5%

to 10% of breast cancer cases. Genetic etiologies associated with breast cancer are discussed later in this chapter.

Breast cancer rates vary among racial and ethnic groups. For all ages combined, white women have a higher incidence of breast cancer (are more likely to develop breast cancer), yet African American women have a higher mortality (are more likely to die) from breast cancer. Native Americans have the lowest incidence of breast cancer, nearly one third the rate of white women. In addition, Native American and Asian women have approximately one third the breast cancer mortality of African American women.[6]

Family history is the most widely recognized epidemiologic risk factor.[7] First-degree female relatives of women with breast carcinoma have 2 to 3 times the general population risk of developing the disease. The risk increases even more if the affected relative was premenopausal with bilateral breast disease on diagnosis (eightfold increased risk) compared to a postmenopausal affected relative with only unilateral disease (up to twofold increased risk). First-degree relatives include the patient's mother, sister, or daughter. Second-degree relatives include grandmothers, nieces, and aunts. Due to information we now have regarding breast cancer susceptibility genes and their possible inheritance from the paternal side of the family, a careful paternal family history must be obtained, including relatives with prostate and brain cancers as well.

### Screening
#### History
A thorough clinical history is a vital aspect of the initial evaluation, because it identifies the patient's personal and family health history, which is useful in assessing risk. The practitioner should obtain detailed information regarding the patient's complaint, if any (duration, onset), and pertinent positive and negative symptoms related to the complaint. The clinical history also provides an important opportunity to explain the benefits and limitations of the breast examination. The valuable information useful in assessing breast health includes age; menstrual, gynecologic, sexual, reproductive, and lactation history; and any family history of breast disorders. In addition, a total body review of systems (e.g., headache, blurred vision for macroadenomas) focused to the patient's complaint should be included. The patient's menopausal status; timing and specific nature of her symptoms and their relation to the menstrual cycle; onset, duration, and growth pattern of any masses; presence of pain; relief measures that have been attempted or have succeeded; alleviating or aggravating factors; use of hormone replacement therapy or oral contraceptives; and presence or absence of risk factors for breast cancer are vitally important. All previous breast imaging, diagnostic procedures, and surgical procedures should be documented. One should not forget to review the patient's past medical and surgical history, as well as her current medications and social history (including smoking, alcohol use, and educational level). Because most breast complaints in reproductive-age women are associated with a benign etiology, reassurance may be an important aspect in reducing anxiety. However, the practitioner should be careful to notify the patient of any concerns regarding the history and examination to ensure that the patient understands the significance of follow-up and does not misconstrue the practitioner's reassurance to mean the diagnostic workup is completed.

## ROLE OF RISK ASSESSMENT IN BREAST CANCER SCREENING

Truly individualized breast cancer risk assessment would require the identification of a histopathologic or serologic marker indicating that this particular woman's breast tissue has initiated the preneoplastic process, thus providing clinicians an opportunity to intervene in the natural history of malignant development. Hence, studies have documented the most consistent pathologic feature, the presence of atypical hyperplasia. Cellular atypia has been found to be predictive of an increased risk of developing breast cancer, especially in women with a family history of breast cancer.[8-10] Recent studies indicate that breast cancer incidence may be substantially reduced in high-risk cohorts by treatment with tamoxifen, prophylactic oophorectomy, and prophylactic mastectomy.[11-13] (This is discussed in more detail in Chapter 40.) In the NSABP-P1 (National Surgical Adjuvant Breast and Bowel Project) study, patients with atypical ductal hyperplasia had the greatest benefit from tamoxifen chemoprophylaxis, with an 86% lower incidence of breast cancer among this group of patients. This highlights the need for accurate risk stratification as women contemplate the utilization of these invasive procedures. Further studies are needed to elucidate the optimal management of these patients. In the absence of consensus about which risk level is best suited to which option, decisions about risk reduction depend as much on an individual's priorities and risk aversion as on numerical risk estimates. In the field of research, high priority is being placed on the development of accurate short-term risk models so that women most likely to benefit from preventive strategies can be readily identified. Risk assessment is likely to offer the greatest potential benefit for women younger than age 40, based on greatest gain in life expectancy offered by existing risk reduction options.

Several algorithms have been developed to estimate a woman's risk of developing breast cancer, with the best known of these being the Gail and Claus models.[14,15] The Gail Model Risk Assessment Tool (Fig. 41-1) incorporates the patient's race, current age, age at menarche, age at first live birth, number of first-degree relatives with breast cancer, number of previous breast biopsies, and pathology results in generating an estimate of breast cancer risk. Conversely, the Claus model utilizes fewer categories, including only the number of relatives with breast cancer, their relationship to the patient, and the relative's age at cancer diagnosis. Although helpful in diagnosis, models are often inapplicable to the proband. In particular, the Gail model cannot be used for women younger than age 35 (because these age groups were not included in the initial validation studies) and is less accurate in those with second-degree affected relatives, those with *BRCA* mutations, those with a personal history of

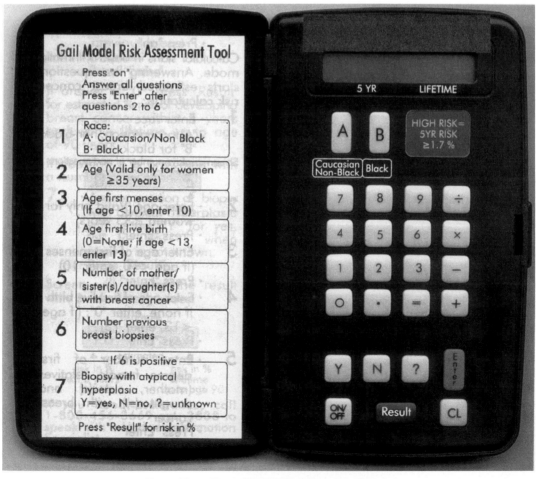

**Figure 41-1   The Gail Model Risk Assessment Tool.**

breast cancer, and those who do not obtain annual mammograms. Several studies have shown a lack of correlation in minority patients. BRCAPro is another helpful model, which estimates an individual's likelihood of harboring a *BRCA* mutation. This model incorporates additional factors, including bilaterallity of breast disease and history of ovarian cancer. Although initial policy statements suggested testing for those with a probability greater than 10%, current recommendations are less stringent.[16] Unlike the Gail model, neither the BRCAPro nor the Claus model have been validated in clinical studies. Counseling must stress that these figures are estimates and not absolute risks and thus balance the magnitude of risk for the individual patient.

Moreover, those patients carrying germ line mutations have a dramatically higher risk for ipsilateral recurrence or contra-lateral primary cancer after a diagnosis of breast or ovarian cancer (Table 41-1). Thus, genetic testing is integral in tailoring surveillance, chemoprevention, and surgical management plans for patients (and their families) at risk of hereditary cancer syndromes. Obstetrician/gynecologists will play a pivotal role in eliciting detailed personal and family histories from patients, determining which of those histories is suggestive of an individual at significantly high risk, facilitating referrals for genetic counseling and testing or risk assessment procedures (such as ductal lavage or periareolar fine-needle aspiration), and incorporating the results of testing into the patient's short- and long-term management plans.

## Testing for *BRCA1* and *BRCA2*

The past decade has witnessed an explosion of knowledge in the arena of cancer genetics and inherited susceptibility to cancer syndromes. Approximately 5% to 10% of breast cancers are thought to be inherited in an autosomal dominant pattern (Fig. 41-2). Two breast and ovarian cancer susceptibility genes have been identified and mapped to chromosomes 17q and 13q, namely *BRCA1* and *BRCA2*.[17,18] They are thought to be tumor suppressor genes, which become ineffective in suppression of cancerous proliferation if mutation in both copies evolves.

BRCA1 is a very large protein, encoding for 1863 amino acid pairs. Several hundred different mutations have been found in both the *BRCA1* and *BRCA2* genes.[19] A *BRCA1* mutation is believed to account for nearly half of all inherited breast cancer cases and nearly 90% of hereditary ovarian cancer cases. Similarly, *BRCA2* mutations are responsible for approximately 40% of familial breast cancer and 5% to 10% of familial ovarian cancer. Li-Fraumeni syndrome,[20] *TP53* mutations, *HRAS* mutations, ataxia-telangiectasia,[21] and other genetic changes as yet

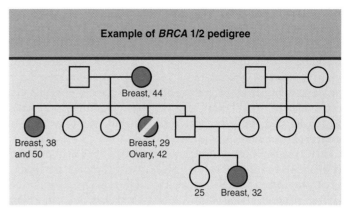

**Example of *BRCA* 1/2 pedigree**

**Figure 41-2** Affected individuals are often seen in each generation with a *BRCA1/BRCA2* mutation.

undetected appear to account for the other cases of inherited breast cancer.

Initial studies suggested the lifetime risk of developing breast cancer in families with *BRCA1* and *BRCA2* mutations was approximately 80% to 90%, and the risk of ovarian cancer was approximately 10% to 60%. The overall lifetime risk of developing breast or ovarian cancer was nearly 100%.[22] However, population-based studies (versus studies based on specific families) now suggest that the actual overall lifetime cancer risk for mutation carriers is closer to 56% for breast cancer and 16% for ovarian cancer, based on knowledge regarding penetrance and modification of penetrance and risk factors by other genes. Further longitudinal studies may resolve this question.

Interestingly, *BRCA* mutation carriers not only have an increased overall risk of developing cancer, but also commonly have a younger age of onset and a greater probability of second tumors. Accordingly, although the inherited *BRCA* mutations account for only 5% to 10% of all breast cancers, they account for nearly 25% of breast cancer cases diagnosed before age 30. Thus, knowledge of *BRCA* status may impact the type of surgery suggested for mutation carriers (lumpectomy versus mastectomy, including associated contralateral prophylactic mastectomy).

Eligibility criteria for testing for *BRCA* status vary among institutions. Most agree the likelihood of harboring a *BRCA* gene is elevated (and thus these women are eligible for testing) in women with histories suggestive of an autosomal dominant pattern of inheritance and/or with a known *BRCA*-positive individual in the immediate family. They often differ as to the number of relatives with breast cancer that prompt concern or the age of onset (some suggest testing in families with ovarian cancer at any age). The ACS would offer testing to those with two or more relatives with breast or ovarian cancer in addition to the previously cited criteria.[23]

Not only are the *BRCA* genes associated with increased risk of female malignancies, but they have also been shown to be a marker for hereditary cancer syndromes in males. Interestingly, male breast cancer is much more common in *BRCA2* mutation carriers compared to the general population.[24] In addition, mutation carriers may be at increased risk for other malignancies, such as laryngeal, prostate, gallbladder, stomach, and pancreatic cancer; malignant melanoma; and primary peritoneal

---

| Table 41-1 |
|---|
| **Characteristics Suggestive of a Germ Line Mutation** |
| Two or more relatives with breast or ovarian cancer |
| Personal or family history of breast cancer occurring before age 50 |
| Relatives with both breast and ovarian cancer |
| Breast and ovarian cancer in the same individual |
| Relatives with bilateral disease or two independent breast cancers |
| Male relatives with breast cancer |
| A family history of breast or ovarian cancer and Ashkenazi Jewish heritage |

# Gynecologic Oncology

carcinoma.[17,25-29] Hence, the BRCA mutation may be transferred through a male or female relative. It is therefore important to elicit a history of all related malignancies from both sides of the family, including age of onset, bilaterality, and history of multiple primary cancers in an individual family member, not just a family history of breast and ovarian cancer. Patients are often unaware that the risk of transmission of a BRCA mutation is equally high from the paternal side and do not volunteer information about cancers from that side.

The frequency of a BRCA1 mutation in the general population is estimated to be 1/500 to 1/1000 (with BRCA2 mutations occurring somewhat less frequently), although it appears to be higher in certain ethnic groups , such as Ashkenazi Jews, in whom it is estimated to be 1%.[30] In the Ashkenazi Jewish population (of Eastern or Central European origin), three different founder mutations have been identified: 185delAG and 5382insC in BRCA1, and 6174delT in BRCA2. Estimates indicate that 1 in 40 Ashkenazi individuals carry one of these founder mutations, and they are responsible for 25% of cases of early-onset breast cancer in this population.[31,32] Current investigations indicate the estimated gene frequency in the general population may be artificially high due to ascertainment bias in the initial studies of high-risk families.

The benefit of genetic testing remains hypothetical because there is no proof that testing and increased surveillance or other risk reduction initiatives would translate into a decrease in breast and ovarian cancer mortality. The accuracy of screening tests (the sensitivity and specificity of the test) is affected by the prior probability of having the condition.[33,34] Given the current cost of testing ($2900; $350 for specific mutations) and the fact that its benefits remain unproven, physicians should discourage individuals from undergoing testing in the absence of a strong family history or early disease. Moreover, the ability to reassure those with negative tests is limited by the possible existence of other as-yet undiscovered genes.

It is preferable to test an affected family member to document the particular familial BRCA1 or BRCA2 mutation. A negative result is most meaningful in a situation in which the family member has previously tested positive. In this scenario—the absence of the detectable mutation in the proband—the patient may be reassured that she does not share the high risk for cancer seen in her family. She should be counseled, however, that she still has the baseline risk of cancer seen in the general population (1 in 8 for women who live to age 85) and that she should continue usual care, such as mammography, and consider breast self-examination (BSE). Present techniques do not identify all disease-causing mutations, and patients need to be informed of the limitations of present technology.

## CLINICAL SCREENING FOR BREAST CANCER

Breast cancer remains one of the most dreaded diseases of the millennium. As statistics state that 1 in 8 women will be affected, mass attention has been focused on determining the cause and prevention. Because 80% of patients with breast cancer have no risk factors other than gender and age, early identification of those at highest risk for developing the disease is difficult. Thus, one of the most important aspects in combating this disease is diagnosis at an early stage when the prognosis for

cure is greatest. The three-pronged approach of breast imaging, clinical breast examination (CBE), and BSE has become the hallmark of early breast cancer detection. But breast cancer screening is not without risks. The potential benefit must be carefully weighed against the potential harm, including radiation exposure, false-positive testing, and overdiagnosis resulting in anxiety and unnecessary breast biopsies (Tables 41-2 through 41-4).

Not only is increasing breast cancer surveillance suggested for BRCA mutation carriers, ovarian surveillance is also recommended. Patients may receive annual CA 125 and vaginal probe ultrasounds beginning between age 25 and 35 (based on the age of the affected relative). Patients and practitioners should, however, realize that current recommendations have not been shown to decrease mortality from breast or ovarian cancer; thus, clinical evidence for support is minimal.[35] Guidelines suggest that women with positive BRCA status and those at increased risk for the development of breast cancer may benefit from these alternative screening strategies, such as earlier initiation of screening, shorter screening intervals, or the use of adjunctive screening modalities in conjunction with mammography and

**Table 41-2**
**American Cancer Society Guidelines for Early Breast Cancer Detection, 2003**

Average risk (asymptomatic)
Age 20–40
   BSE monthly (optional)
   CBE every 1–3 years
Age over 40
   BSE monthly (optional)
   CBE annually or biannually
   Mammography annually

BSE, breast self-exam; CBE, clinical breast exam.
Modified from Smith RA, Saslow D, Sawyer KA, et al: American Cancer Society guidelines for breast cancer screening: Update 2003. CA Cancer J Clin 2003;53:141–169.

**Table 41-3**
**American College of Obstetricians and Gynecologists: Breast Cancer Screening Guidelines, 2000**

Average risk (asymptomatic)
Age 20–39
   BSE monthly
   CBE annually
Age 40–49
   BSE monthly
   CBE annually
   Mammography every 1–2 years*
Age 50 and over
   BSE monthly
   CBE annually
   Mammography annually

BSE, breast self-exam; CBE, clinical breast exam.
*Unless mammographic or physical findings suggest more frequent evaluation.
Modified from the American College of Obstetricians and Gynecologists. Primary and preventive care: periodic assessments. ACOG Committee Opinion 246. Washington, DC:ACOG, 2000.

**Table 41-4**
**Breast Cancer Surveillance for Women with *BRCA1* and *BRCA2***

Age 18–20
  BSE monthly
Beginning between age 20 and 35 years
  CBE semiannually
Beginning between age 25 and 35 years
  Mammography annually

BSE, breast self-exam; CBE, clinical breast exam.
Modified from the NCCN 2003 genetic/familial high-risk assessment clinical practice guidelines in oncology, version 1, 2003.
Available at: http://www.nccn.org. Accessed October 2004.

physical examination, such as ultrasound or magnetic resonance imaging (MRI). However, there are no randomized, controlled trials supporting their benefit.[23]

All women in their twenties should have an opportunity to become informed about the benefits, limitations, and potential harms associated with regular breast cancer screening. Clinicians must emphasize the importance of prompt reporting of any breast symptomatology. Those who choose to do BSE should receive instruction and have their technique reviewed regularly. It is acceptable for women to choose not to do BSE or to do it irregularly. Whether to continue screening in older women should be individualized based on the potential benefits and risks of mammography considering their current health status and estimated life expectancy. However, the ACS suggests continuation of annual mammographic screening after 40 years of age as long as a woman is in reasonably good health and would be a candidate for cancer treatment.

Mammography is the only widely accepted imaging modality used to screen for early, otherwise occult breast cancer. Although mammography is especially valuable as an early detection tool, significant controversy surrounds the efficacy of mammographic screening in decreasing breast cancer mortality. Early detection of malignant disease has usually resulted in a more favorable outcome. However, a systematic review of the literature regarding screening with mammography did not show a survival benefit of mass screening for breast cancer; the evidence was inconclusive for breast cancer mortality. This may be secondary to earlier detection of ductal carcinoma in situ lesions, detection of early breast cancers that may not have been aggressive and thus may not have caused death, or detection of lesions in older patients who may die from causes unrelated to the breast cancer. It has therefore been questioned whether screening with mammography does more good than harm.

The appropriate age for commencing annual mammography has generated substantial debate. The American Medical Association,[36] ACS,[23] the American College of Radiology,[37] the American College of Surgeons, and the American Society of Clinical Oncology advocate annual mammographic screening in women beginning at age 40. In contrast, the Canadian Task Force on Preventive Health Care[38,39] and the American College of Preventive Medicine espouse annual surveillance beginning at age 50 (although the Canadian Task Force does not suggest the inclusion or exclusion of mammography in the periodic health examination of women age 40 to 49 at average risk for breast

cancer). The American Academy of Family Physicians[40] and the American College of Obstetricians and Gynecologists (ACOG)[41] promote 1- to 2-year screening intervals beginning at age 40 corroborated by evidence-based analysis of published screening trials. A 1997 Consensus Development Panel convened by the National Institutes of Health concluded that the evidence was insufficient to determine the benefits of mammography among women aged 40 to 49. This panel recommended that women in this age group should be counseled about potential benefits and harms before making a decision about mammography screening.[42] General screening guidelines are not intended to apply to women at increased risk of breast cancer, symptomatic women undergoing diagnostic mammography, or women with a history of breast cancer receiving follow-up mammograms.

**Breast Self-Examination**

Women have been trained in the technique of BSE for years, with the goal of earlier detection of breast abnormalities. An additional goal of BSE is to increase awareness of normal breast composition (i.e., topography, structure, design), which may heighten awareness of changes that may be detected during BSE. The value of heightened awareness, however it may be achieved, is commonly acknowledged based on the value of earlier treatment of both nonpalpable and palpable breast cancers. Studies show that breast cancers detected while practicing BSE are diagnosed at an earlier stage and tend to be smaller than those diagnosed in the absence of any screening. In addition, women are more likely to find their tumor themselves when practicing BSE regularly.[23] However, data documenting the efficacy of BSE in reducing breast cancer mortality is lacking. Moreover, many clinicians criticize this technique because of concerns that it creates excessive fear of cancer in some women and may result in unnecessary surgery for benign conditions.[43–45] It may represent the only viable alternative for women who do not meet screening eligibility requirements, however, or for whom mammography services are simply unavailable. Furthermore, Shen and Zelen analyzed data from selected mamography screening trials and found the sensitivity of BSE to be appreciable (39%–59%).[46]

To review the evidence, one recent study randomized over 250,000 women in Shanghai to intensive BSE instruction compared with no intervention. This was followed by reinforcement sessions at 1 and 3 years and medically supervised BSE practice at least 12 times in a 5-year period. The study found no reduction in mortality.[45] In the routine health care group (no intervention), nearly 65% of the women received one or more annual examinations. No mammographic screening was available to women in the study population, and the level of clinical breast examination activity was low. The results, however, suggested that teaching BSE did enhance a woman's level of awareness and ability to find lumps in her own breasts. In addition, a slightly higher percentage of breast cancers in the instruction group than in the control group were diagnosed at either the Tis (carcinoma in situ) stage or the T1 (≤ 2 cm in diameter) stage. Diagnosis of tumors at these early stages was weakly associated with level of attendance at study activity sessions. Furthermore, a high proportion of women in the instruction group reported that they had found their breast cancer as a result of practicing BSE, and they sought medical

# Gynecologic Oncology

attention after detecting their tumor in somewhat less time than did women in the control group. However, in spite of these apparent successes of the BSE teaching program, as many cancers in the instruction group as in the control group were diagnosed with axillary lymph nodal metastases.

In a randomized trial in Russia, more cancers were found in the instruction group than in the control group (RR, 1.24; 95% CI, 1.09 to 1.41); this was not the case in Shanghai (RR, 0.97; 95% CI, 0.88 to 1.06).[47] Yet, these trials review BSE instruction, not the practice of BSE, because this information could not be reliably obtained from self-report. The implication of these results for women who have periodic mammograms is unclear. Further randomized trials reviewing SBE in conjunction with mammography are warranted. Accordingly, promotion of BSE as a single screening method is often not recommended. Conversely, to negate SBE as an important component of overall personal health care seems inappropriate if there is any possibility to affect the survival rate in women. In breast disease, where early detection is so clearly related to improved survival, the value of this relatively simple, economical, and minimally inconvenient technique should not be underemphasized. With this in mind, ACOG and the ACS continue to recommend performance of BSE monthly beginning at age 20.

Therefore, literature on the effectiveness of BSE as a detection modality has shown mixed results, but recent evidence reviews have focused on the absence of direct evidence of benefit in two randomized controlled trials and on data indicating that the rate of benign biopsy is higher in women who regularly perform BSE compared with women who do not do so. The U.S. Preventive Services Task Force concluded that the evidence is insufficient to recommend for or against teaching or performing routine BSE. The Canadian Task Force on Preventive Health Care went further and recommended against routine instruction in BSE in periodic health examinations on the basis of evidence showing lack of benefit and evidence of harm, primarily increased false-positive results. The Canadian Task Force agreed with the ACS in recommending that women should be taught to report any breast changes or concerns and should be provided with careful instruction and information about risks, benefits, and limitations of BSE. Conversely, in an accompanying editorial, Nekhlyudov and Fletcher argued that the existing data did not provide a sound basis for dismissing the value of BSE based on both the limitations in the randomized, controlled trial data and on the basis of the principle that when evidence is lacking, it is best to err on the side of prudence.[43,45,48–50]

Effective instruction of patients in the technique of BSE incorporates description of the procedure while the patient views the providers' performance of the examination or demonstrates the technique using models. Additionally, having the patient reiterate her understanding of what has been taught and then demonstrating her mastery of the technique using manufactured breast models further solidifies compliance. Ensure that the patient understands the significance of breast inspection in various positions as well as the utility of breast palpation in the standing and supine positions. The circular method of breast palpation is routinely the easiest to master, although for patients with pendulous breasts, positional changes to ensure positioning of the breast tissue on the chest wall must be emphasized. The

best time to perform the examination is usually the week after the menses, although menopausal women should pick a convenient time of the month, such as their birth date or the first of each month. After hysterectomy, patients with continued estrogenic support of the ovaries should observe for breast fullness or tenderness. Breast examination should then be performed 7 to 10 days after maximal breast symptoms.

## Clinical Breast Examination

As with BSE, clinical breast examination (CBE) seeks to detect breast abnormalities at an earlier stage of disease, when treatment options are more numerous, include less invasive alternatives, and are generally more effective than treatment options for cancers detected at later stages. However, of the commonly employed methods of breast cancer screening, CBE has received the least attention in the medical literature. In actual fact, CBE is a common component of current comprehensive preventive health maintenance with widespread performance across the United States. Moreover, tools to assist practitioners in improving performance of the examination may be of particular importance in the arena of breast cancers because failure to diagnose breast cancer is a primary cause of action for malpractice claims. It is also the second-leading reason for payments to claimants.[51] Obstetrician/gynecologists should not abdicate their responsibilities by relying on previous examinations performed by other specialists. The practitioner must be concerned with protecting him/herself from future lawsuits due to errors of omission.

A recent committee of national and international experts well versed in CBE, comprised of representatives from the ACS advisory group, the Breast Cancer Early Detection Guideline Review Physical Examination Working Group, the Centers for Disease Control and Prevention, and the National Cancer Institute, published recommendations to enhance CBE performance and reporting.

Each portion of the breast examination may be performed in both the sitting and supine positions because positional changes will often expose a lesion that was otherwise masked by the patient's normal anatomic variations. CBE should begin with visual inspection of the breasts. The practitioner should assess the breast for erythema, skin retraction, rashes, nipple retraction/deviation, and breast asymmetry. Use of the acronym BREAST may assist providers in remembering critical physical signs associated with advanced breast cancer, including Breast mass, Retraction, Edema, Axillary mass, Scaly nipple, and Tender breast.[52] While seated, the patient should press hands firmly on her hips to tighten the pectoral muscles and enhance identification of asymmetries. Not only does this allow visualization of the lateral aspects of the breast (which are often obscured by excess arm girth), but it also provides a superior view of the skin on the undersurface of the breast (inframammary ridge). In patients with rheumatoid arthritis or other conditions that prevent pressure on the hip joint, more comfortable options are available. The patient may grasp her fingertips at a level near the waistline while pulling laterally or may press her palms together while extending her arms above her head. Because the breast lies on the pectoral muscle and Cooper's ligaments are attached to the muscle and the skin, tension on the muscle will accentuate carcinoma invading these structures. Additional positions, such as hands overhead and at her side, may further assist identification of symmetries, but the committee did not feel they added substantively to the single position described previously. Nipple inversion is generally significant only when developed secondarily and unilaterally. If gentle manual eversion may be accomplished, the inversion is likely a normal variation.

An alternative position for breast inspection that is especially helpful in women with pendulous breasts is to have the woman lean forward while placing her hands on the practitioner's shoulders. Palpation of the breast in this position (while the breast tissue is away from the chest wall) is helpful to differentiate chest wall pain from true breast pain.

Several postures are helpful for evaluation of the axilla in both the seated and supine positions. The physician may hold the patient's elbow or wrist in his/her hand, with the patient's arm at a 90-degree angle and slightly abducted from her side (or gently across the front of the patient's torso). The opposite hand is then used to evaluate the axilla. Another position rests the patient's hand on the shoulder of the practitioner while asking the patient to relax her elbow. This allows the examiner to utilize both hands in evaluation of the axillary area. Adequate evaluation of the axilla in the supine position requires the patient's arm to be at a right angle rather than posterior to the head. For all positions, one must ensure that the patient's shoulder girdle is relaxed to allow proper assessment of the axilla. Following evaluation of the axilla, one should palpate the infraclavicular and supraclavicular lymph nodes, which are important sites for breast cancer metastasis.

Next, the patient should be placed in a comfortable supine position with her arm on the same side as the breast being examined and raised above her head to evenly distribute the breast over the chest wall, thereby making its deeper regions more easily assessed. Care must be taken to ensure that the patient is properly gowned with only the area being examined exposed. The patient must be positioned (by tilting her hips and torso) to allow the portion of the breast tissue being examined to lie directly on the chest wall. For patients with pendulous breasts, this may require three to four positional changes for each breast. The pads of the fingers (and not the fingertips) are the most sensitive and should be used in examination. Three overlapping dime-sized circular motions are made with the pads of the middle three fingers using three levels of pressure (superficial, medium, and firm) on each $1 cm^2$ area of the breast. Not only will this improve mass detection, but it also prevents masking a lesion through excessive pressure. The perimeter of the examination should incorporate the midaxillary line, one to two ribs below the inframammary ridge, the sternum, across the clavicle, and through the axillary area to ensure nodal involvement in these areas is discernible.

Although the circular pattern is the most frequently used in practice to evaluate the asymptomatic patient, the vertical strip pattern has been shown to have greater thoroughness of coverage when studied during BSE.[53] During the vertical strip search pattern the provider will begin the overlapping circular motions in the axilla, extending inferiorly (1 cm at a time) to one to two ribs below the breast tissue. The fingers are then moved inward 1 cm and the pattern of search is extended superiorly, in a straight line, to the clavicle. This pattern is continued until the sternum is reached (Fig. 41-3). The patient's position may have

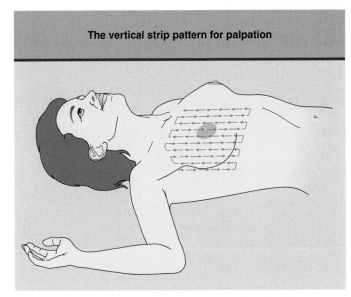

**The vertical strip pattern for palpation**

Figure 41-3  The vertical strip pattern for palpation.

to be changed several times during this portion of the examination to ensure that the tissue being examined lies directly on the chest wall. With the circular method of palpation, the breast tissue is examined with the pads of the fingers. The examination proceeds clockwise around the full circumference of the breast at its perimeter and gradually moves inward toward the nipple (Fig. 41-4). The wheel-and-spoke method requires radially palpating from the clavicle, sternum, and other bony margins and palpating toward the nipple (Fig. 41-5). Each method should be mastered, because they may be helpful in certain clinical and diagnostic situations, such as in patients with large breasts. Most practitioners use two hands to perform the breast examination, although a thorough and systematic use of a single hand is satisfactory (especially for an asymptomatic screening examination) and is recommended by The Mammocare method

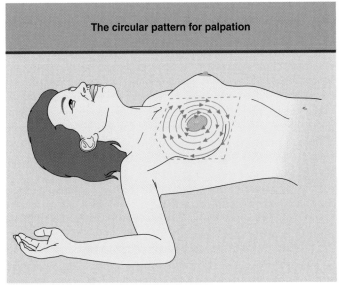

**The circular pattern for palpation**

Figure 41-4  The circular pattern for palpation.

# Gynecologic Oncology

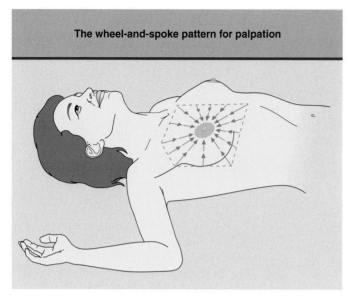

**The wheel-and-spoke pattern for palpation**

**Figure 41-5    The wheel-and-spoke pattern for palpation.**

of breast examination and the consensus committee.[54] When using two hands, the second hand follows behind in the same pattern as the first hand, thus providing dual evaluations of each area.

If the patient presents with breast complaints, it is advisable to palpate the unaffected breast first, because it provides the physician a "tactile baseline" with which to compare the involved breast and prevents omitting lesions in the unaffected breast. Regardless of the pattern of breast examination used, the importance of using a consistent and methodical pattern of evaluation and allowing sufficient time for a thorough assessment should not be underemphasized as factors that will increase detection capabilities.

Routine evaluation of the nipple for discharge is controversial. Some authors do not recommend this as a routine portion of the breast examination in women without nipple discharge or complaints. It is well known that excessive breast manipulation may lead to a nipple discharge. If one excludes this as a routine part of the examination, one must ensure that a detailed history is obtained to rule out any nipple complaints. Patients will often have such complaints but forget to relate this information to the practitioner, particularly if she has experienced the symptoms for an extended period. In general, only spontaneous nipple discharge will render abnormal pathology.[55] Squeezing the nipple may actually obstruct the ductal orifice and impede any discharge from coming to the surface. Utilizing a milking technique will improve your ability to elicit a nipple discharge; slide the fingers from the outer quadrant in a clockwise fashion toward the nipple and document the location of any fluid accumulation.

Not surprisingly, the committee's final recommendation is a call for research into particular questions that will provide a firmer foundation for decisions about the practice of CBE as a component of women's health care.

Generally, CBE has been shown to increase the sensitivity of mammography, has fewer false-positives than mammography, and is more effective in detecting cancers in younger women than mammography. However, the impact of these advantages

on breast cancer survival and mortality is not known. Moreover, the sensitivity of CBE was estimated in a recent meta-analysis to be only 54%.[56] As stated, the evidence supporting the value of CBE as a method of reducing breast cancer mortality is limited and mostly inferential, because there is no definitive prospective randomized, controlled trial evidence from which to draw conclusions. Thus, current recommendations rely on existing evidence[57] and expert opinion.

Screening CBE targets asymptomatic women, as opposed to a diagnostic CBE, which is performed on a woman with breast complaints. In the primary care setting, screening CBE is more commonly performed than diagnostic CBE. Authors have argued, therefore, that screening CBE demands greater care and attention than diagnostic CBE because the patient's symptoms do not guide the examination.[58] Strategies to improve a practitioner's ability to detect a mass include increasing the time devoted to the examination, using a technique with variable degrees of pressure, and developing a systematic, consistent search mode. The size of the lesion, of course, also correlated with the practitioner's ability to detect the mass.[59] The appropriate duration for a through examination is based on a variety of factors including proficiency, breast size, tenderness, lumpiness, body weight, and risk factors.

The ACS and the ACOG recommend CBE and mammography for women age 40 and older, because randomized, controlled trials and demonstration projects have established that CBE is able to detect some cancers that were not detected on mammography and, when used in combination with mammography, results in decreased mortality from breast cancer.[60–63] Conversely, the U.S. Preventive Services Task Force declined to recommend either for or against breast cancer screening with CBE alone and also recommend mammography with or without CBE, concluding that there is insufficient evidence to quantify the incremental benefits of adding CBE to mammography. This decision is based on the fact that the randomized, controlled trial data incorporating CBE into the screening program derives from a period predating modern breast imaging. With advancements in technology, the proportion of breast cancers not visible with modern mammography may be considerably lower than in the past.

In this increasingly litigious society, breast assessment demands careful documentation of the history, examination, and disposition of the case. A clear and legible note should record all findings from the breast examination, noting texture, size, consistency, and a detailed description (including diagrams) of abnormal and suspicious findings as well as the plan for follow-up. Although abnormal findings are very important, it is equally important to list negative findings in the medical record as well. Appropriate clinical follow-up is of utmost importance as based on patient's age, clinical suspicion, proficiency of the provider, and other patient characteristics, including risk factors. One third of all breast malpractice cases involve inadequate chart documentation. Because 75% of successful malpractice lawsuits involve the specialties of family medicine, internal medicine and obstetrics and gynecology, the importance of documentation becomes evident.[5]

## Mammography

A German surgeon, Albert Solomon, used conventional radiography equipment to image mastectomy specimens in

1913, thus beginning the history of modern breast imaging. Dedicated film mammography was introduced by Robert Egan, a radiologist from Texas, nearly a half century later. As mammography became associated with excellent breast cancer detection rates in the 1970s, use of dedicated equipment for screen-film mammography became widely adopted by most breast imaging facilities in the United States in the 1980s.

Despite recent controversy surrounding the efficacy of mammographic screening, it remains the only imaging study that has been extensively evaluated in randomized controlled trials and has been shown, in many cases, to reduce breast cancer mortality (Fig. 41-6).[64,65] Eight randomized prospective trials have examined the impact of screening mammography on breast cancer mortality: the Health Insurance Plan (HIP) of New York trial, the Swedish Two-County trial, the Gothenburg trial, the Stockholm trial, the Malmö trial, the Edinburgh trial,[66] and the Canadian National Breast Screening Study (CNBSS) I and II trials. These trials were conducted in North America and Europe beginning in the 1960s and involving a combined total of nearly 500,000 women, with mortality as the endpoint for each study. The studies vary greatly in terms of design. Lower age limit for enrollment varied from 40 to 50 years. Some screenings consisted of the standard two-view mammograms; others, of a single view. The screening interval varied from 12 to 33 months, and the number of rounds of screening ranged from two to six. Moreover, four of the eight trials (HIP, Edinburgh, and CNBSS I and II) also included CBE as a screening modality. Meta-analysis of the results from these studies has shown a statistically significant reduction in mortality from breast cancer on the order of 25% to 30% among screened populations compared with controls after 5 to 7 years.[67] Based on the results of these trials, routine mammography has become established as a valuable screening tool for breast cancer detection.

The HIP of New York trial, initiated in 1963, sparked the controversy that continues today. Over 60,000 enrollees were randomized to either screening with mammography and CBE or routine health examinations; however, none received mammography alone. After 10 years of follow-up a 29% reduction in breast cancer mortality was noted in the screened group.[68]

An overview of randomized studies in Sweden demonstrated at least a 25% reduction in mortality in a screened population (an even greater reduction—35%—was seen in the cohort aged 45 to 46 at entry into the study).[69–71] Three other trials (Malmö, Stockholm, and Gothenburg) found nonsignificant reductions in breast cancer deaths of 19%, 20%, and 14%, respectively.[72]

Subsequently, findings of the Breast Cancer Detection Demonstration Project (BCDDP), a nonrandomized trial, demonstrated that mammography conducted in optimal surroundings had a true-positive rate greater than 90% and was significantly more accurate than clinical examination in detecting small cancers.[73] In both the HIP and BCDDP studies, 80% of those patients who had carcinomas detectable only by mammogram had no axillary nodal disease. In contrast, patients who had clinically detected breast cancer were more likely to have axillary node involvement (50%). When breast cancer is detected before the axillary nodes are involved, the 5-year survival rate is 97%. If there are regional nodal metastases at the time of breast cancer detection, the survival rates drops to 78.7% and more drastically to 23.3% with even more distant metastases.[3] In recently updated information of the Swedish two-county screening trial, Tabar and colleagues reported that 50% of screen-detected cancers were in the good prognostic category (generally stage 0 or 1, depending on histologic type), as opposed to 19% in the clinically detected group.[74] Earlier stage disease requires less aggressive therapy options, thus highlighting the importance of early detection.

The controversy intensified when the results of the Canadian National Breast Screening Study (NBSS), a randomized clinical trial that enrolled nearly 90,000 women ages 40 to 59, were published in late 1992.[75] The data did not demonstrate a reduction in mortality from breast cancer among women undergoing yearly mammography without an established baseline as compared with women who had a baseline breast examination. Updated results were reported in 2000 and 2002 for NBSS-1 and NBSS-2. Miller and colleagues reported 13-year follow-up results that compared annual two-view mammography and CBE with annual CBE only in women age 50 to 59 at randomization. The authors reported no difference in the breast cancer mortality rate between the groups and concluded that mammography provided no additional advantage compared with carefully conducted CBE. NBSS updated additional results comparing annual mammography and CBE with usual care in women age 40 to 49; after 11 to 16 years of follow-up there was no difference in breast cancer mortality in the group invited to mammography screening compared with usual care. Even before the initial paper on NBSS-1 was published, serious questions were raised by mammographers about the validity of the study results. Criticisms were leveled regarding poor imaging technique, technically unacceptable films, bias in the randomization process, short follow-up times, and inadequate interpretation of the final results. The Kaiser Permanente Study Group has also reported no mortality differences in a screened population.[76]

A meta-analysis of the most recent results of the eight studies showed a 16% to 24% mortality reduction associated with "an invitation to screening."[77,78]

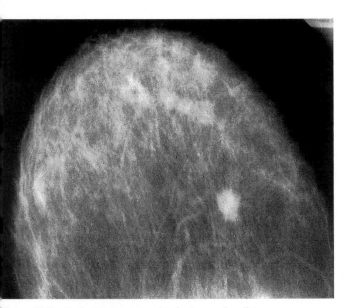

**Figure 41-6** Typical mammographic features of malignancy are seen in this lesion, with stellate "fingers" extending into the surrounding stroma and irregular borders.

| Table 41-5 |
| :-- |
| **Reasons for False-Negative Mammograms** |
| Failure to image the region of interest |
| Poor image quality |
| Errors of perception |
| Breast cancer indistinguishable from normal breast tissue |
| Poor image quality due to overlying breast tissue |

The controversy regarding screening in younger women is multifold. Reduction of mortality rates in this younger cohort as a result of screening is a subject of debate; the cost-effectiveness when compared with older women is unknown; finally, the frequency of screening intervals has become a point of disagreement among the committees that issue imaging guidelines. Authors have argued that mammograms performed in women younger than age 50 are not useful because younger women have more radiographically dense breast tissue that obscures abnormalities. By contrast, some investigators have strongly advocated yearly mammograms for all women age 40 to 49 because breast cancer is often more aggressive and faster growing in younger women.[79] Though the initial overview of Swedish randomized trials failed to show an advantage of screening women younger than age 50,[70] a follow-up study showed a 23% reduction in breast cancer mortality in women age 40 to 49.[80] The most recent meta-analysis, published by Hendrick and colleagues, found a statistically significant mortality reduction of 18% for women invited to screening in their forties. With increasing length of follow-up, successive meta-analyses have shown progressively greater, statistically significant mortality reductions for women age 40 to 49, regardless of whether the NBSS results are included or excluded.[81]

Based on an observed 45% reduction in breast cancer mortality among women age 39 to 49 offered screening every 18 months in the Gothenburg trial, Feig suggested that mortality from breast cancer could be reduced by as much as 65% if all women age 40 and older were screened annually with mammography and physical examination. The authors based their assumptions on the observed 80% compliance rate and estimated even higher mortality reductions of 75% if a 100% compliance rate could be attained.[82] Moreover, Michaelson and colleagues suggested a 51% reduction in breast cancer deaths with annual mammography in this age group using a computer simulation of biologic data from cancer growth rates and metastatic spread.[83] It is suspected that improved screening with detection of smaller tumors will expand the population of women for whom breast-preserving surgery is an option and reduce the need for systemic therapy.

The meta-analysis of Gotzsche and Olsen, published in 2001, rekindled the acrimonious debate over the efficacy of mammography. This meta-analysis reviewed the methodologic rigor of the then seven existing randomized, controlled trials of screening mammography, deeming five trials seriously flawed and only two trials as having adequate methods. Thus, the meta-analysis based their negative findings (no reduction of breast cancer mortality with screening mammography) on only these two "adequate" trials.[84,85] In their assessment, the authors cited differences in the ages of women in the screened and control groups (range, 1 to 5 months) as indicative of serious flaws in randomization. However, the age distributions of the women in the two studies judged to be "adequately randomized" (Canadian and Malmö) were not known. Practitioners must realize that no study has ever been performed entirely without flaws or questions regarding methodologic validity. However, to discount and nullify the results of studies based solely on small differences in age between study groups seems unjustified. Despite the scathing articles by Olsen and Gotzsche, the National Cancer Institute in early 2002 reiterated their recommendation that women of average risk for breast cancer begin mammographic screening at age 40, and the U.S. Preventive Services Task Force lowered their recommendation for commencing screening from age 50 to age 40.[86,87]

Accuracy of mammography depends on a number of factors including expertise of the technician, size and density of the breast, and the location of the lesion. False-negative results occur even in the best installations (Table 41-5). Routinely, a false-negative rate of 10% to 15% is quoted; therefore, a normal mammographic examination does not rule out the presence of breast cancer. A palpable mass requires further evaluation despite a "negative" mammographic examination.

The American College of Radiology established the Breast Imaging Reporting and Data System (BI-RADS) to assist in standardization of mammography reporting (Table 41-6).[88] The likelihood of finding a malignancy at the time of core biopsy with findings suspicious or highly suggestive of malignancy is listed. BI-RADS category zero should not be construed as a normal report because additional testing, such as ultrasound, spot compression, or magnification views, is necessary before

| Category | Assessment Category | Follow-up | Likelihood of Malignancy or Atypia |
| :--: | :-- | :-- | --: |
| 0 | Incomplete | Additional imaging needed | |
| 1 | Negative | Routine (annual) | |
| 2 | Benign | | |
| 3 | Probably benign | Short interval follow-up at 6 months for ipsilateral breast, followed by both breasts at 1, 2, and 3 years after initial mammogram | <3% |
| 4 | Suspicious for malignancy | Consider biopsy | 9% |
| 5 | Highly suggestive of malignancy | | 54% |

Table 41-6
Breast Imaging Reporting and Data System

inal disposition. BI-RADS has revolutionized reporting of mammography films in providing common diagnostic terminology to better compare different treatment outcomes and to assist in follow-up and treatment planning. Unfortunately, this standardization does not improve variability of mammographic interpretation or its accuracy.[89]

Although mammography remains the gold standard for breast cancer screening and diagnosis, it often cannot differentiate benign from malignant disease and is less accurate in patients with dense glandular breasts, with diffuse involvement of the breast with tumor, and in those taking hormone replacement therapy. From 10% to 20% of breast cancers detectable by physical examination are not visible radiographically. Furthermore, of the women who are referred for biopsy based on mammographic findings, only 20% to 40% of lesions actually prove to be malignant.[90] Clearly, there is room for improvement in both breast cancer detection and lesion characterization.

## Ultrasound

Ultrasonography is used routinely as an adjunct to mammography and has an established role in the evaluation of the breast; namely, to help differentiate benign from malignant lesions and cystic from solid lesions and to provide guidance for interventions. Ultrasound is also helpful where mammographic sensitivity is decreased, such as in radiographically dense breast tissue and noncalcified masses, and for locations in the breast that may not be included in mamography because of the limitations of mammographic positioning. Ultrasound has evolved into a highly specialized imaging technique that is useful as a primary imaging modality for younger women and for pregnant or lactating patients (Fig. 41-7). More recent uses include assisting in staging of breast cancer and intraoperative evaluation of surgical margins. Although touted as an appropriate screening modality in asymptomatic women, it is currently not widely accepted for this use.

Breast ultrasound is usually performed using a linear array high-frequency transducer of 7.5 MHz or higher. In North America, breast ultrasound is most often a targeted examination (limited to the area of concern based on palpation or mammography); conversely, whole breast (or survey) real-time scanning has been more prevalent in Europe. Improper technique can affect interpretation of breast lesions. Although the Mammography Quality Standards Act of 1992 set standards for screening mammography that decreased faulty radiographic technique,[91] there are no such laws for breast ultrasound. However, the American College of Radiology has guidelines for imaging with sonography.[92] Noncompliance with the standards has been shown to result in misinterpretation of findings.[93]

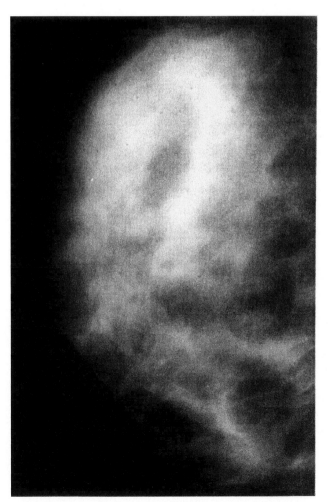
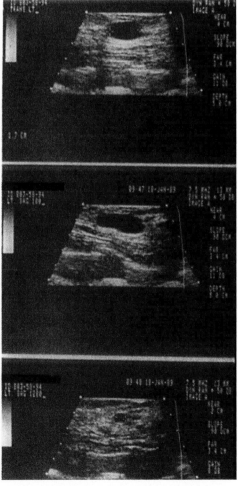

**Figure 41-7**  Ultrasound was useful in detecting a simple cyst in this patient with dense breasts and a negative mammogram in the face of a palpable mass.

Several recent studies have evaluated the relatively new sonographic techniques of spatial compound imaging,[94] tissue harmonics imaging,[95] and three-dimensional imaging[96–98] in breast disorders. Compound imaging of the breast has been shown to increase the conspicuousness of the lesion by enhancing soft tissue contrast, improving the definition of tumor margins, and improving evaluation of the internal architecture and surrounding distortion. Use of tissue harmonics imaging also improves lesion conspicuousness and overall image quality. Lastly, three-dimensional imaging has been shown to have a higher specificity for diagnosing malignancy over two-dimensional imaging (86.9% vs. 64.1%). However, three-dimensional imaging is cumbersome and time consuming. Moreover, if a lesion has suspicious features on two-dimensional imaging, regardless of the three-dimensional results, intervention is warranted. To date these newer sonographic techniques do not appear to offer improved accuracy or diagnostic value over current modalities.[99]

Advocates of ultrasonography have touted its use as a screening tool for the general population. Unfortunately, ultrasound is limited as an imaging modality by its inability to detect microcalcifications, its fairly labor-intensive methodology, and its dependence on operator skill. Nonetheless, promising data is emerging indicating aptitude in certain subpopulations. Ultrasound screening in the asymptomatic population has been evaluated primarily in younger women who have mammographically dense breast tissue or are considered to be at elevated risk of breast cancer.[100–104] Kolb and colleagues reported a 97% sensitivity rate for the combination of whole-breast ultrasound and mammography in screening 4897 BI-RADS category II and IV cases compared with 74% for the combination of mammography and physical examination.[105] Kaplan reported a 0.3% cancer detection rate when sonography was used in women previously found to have a normal mammogram and CBE.[106] The results suggest that ultrasound may be more sensitive but less specific that mammography in this specific subset of women. Thus, ultrasound used as an adjunct to mammography detects additional cancers, but also increases the false-positive rate. The theoretical benefit of detecting and treating these mammographically occult cancers may be decreased mortality or decreased rate of recurrence. The controversies lie in weighing the benefits against the cost and assessing whether detection of these otherwise occult cancers will result in increased patient survival.

In addition to the incidentally found cancers, in three studies ultrasound detected an additional 2088 benign lesions, resulting in more biopsies. But the radiologist was not blinded to the results of the mammogram, which may impact the sensitivity and specificity of the method. The added cost, both financial and psychological (of performing the test, potentially increasing patient anxiety and discomfort, and potentially increasing morbidity from increased number of benign biopsies), must be weighed against the benefits of finding these solely sonographically detected cancers in addition to evaluating this modality's ability to reduce breast cancer mortality.

## Magnetic Resonance Imaging

Breast MRI is an emerging technology that has certain advantages over conventional screen-film mammography, including omission of ionizing radiation, improved image quality, and lack of known radiobiological hazards. However, its low capacity to detect microcalcifications, which may provide evidence of early carcinoma, severely limits its usefulness as a screening method. Although the images produced have similar criteria for the diagnosis of benign and malignant disease as does mammography, they lack sufficient resolution to identify small lesions. Moreover, there is considerable overlap between benign and malignant tissue, which significantly reduces the potential of MRI to detect early breast cancer. The cost of MRI and the time required to perform it will likely be prohibitive to its use for screening evaluation of the breast.

Breast MRI technology relies almost exclusively on the fact that tumors generate neovascularity to support their growth. Thus in theory, administration of an intravenous contrast agent such as gadolinium-diethylenetriamine penta-acetic acid (Gd-DTPA) results in rapid uptake in malignant tissue compared to benign entities. Detection of invasive breast carcinoma is extremely reliable on MRI, with sensitivity approaching 100%. False-negative results have been reported with well-differentiated invasive ductal and lobular lesions.[107] Despite its sensitivity in detection of invasive cancers (especially in dense breast tissue), sensitivity in noninvasive lesions such as ductal carcinoma in situ has been reported to be as low as 40%, possibly secondary to more variable angiogenesis in these lesions.[108] False-positive results (seen with fibroadenoma, lobular carcinoma in situ, ductal atypia, fibrocystic changes, proliferative changes, papilloma, sclerosing adenosis, and duct hyperplasia) account for the lack of reliability of MRI, with specificities ranging from 37% to 97%.[109]

Currently, MRI of the breast has proven most useful in patients with proven breast cancer to assess for multifocal/multicentric disease, chest wall involvement, and chemotherapy response or tumor recurrence or to identify the primary site in patients with occult breast cancer. It has also been helpful in evaluation of silicone breast prostheses for rupture. Enhanced detection is also noted in women with dense breasts.[110]

### MRI Screening in High-Risk Populations

Despite its limitations, the robustness of this technique has generated considerable enthusiasm for screening women at high risk for breast cancer (usually on the basis of genetic mutations or a strong family history of breast cancer; Fig. 41-8). Although

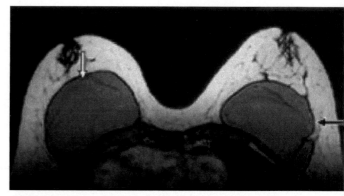

**Figure 41-8** Magnetic resonance imaging may be helpful in evaluation of patients with dense breasts and in those with implants (*arrows*), as seen here.

ot proven, early diagnosis as a result of intensive surveillance may decrease the rate of death from breast cancer in this select group. In a recent study of over 200 women with *BRCA1* and *BRCA2* mutations who underwent one to three annual screening examinations, consisting of MRI, mammography, and ultrasound in addition to biannual CBE, authors detected 77% (17 of 22) of cancers using MRI. This compares to 36%, 33%, and 9.1% detection using mammography, ultrasound, and CBE, respectively. All four screening modalities combined had a sensitivity of 95% versus 45% for mammography and CBE combined.[111] Although two of the cancers were detected by ultrasound alone, including ultrasound in the protocol resulted in more additional biopsies than MRI after the first year of screening. Whether the benefit of including ultrasound is justified in light of the high false-positive rate remains to be observed. The authors did not observe any benefit from the addition of CBE over and above the combination of the three imaging modalities.

In another similar study, the sensitivity of MRI for detecting invasive breast cancer was 79.5%, compared to 33.3% and 17.9% using mammography and CBE, respectively. The specificity was 68.1%, 95.0%, and 89.8%, respectively.[112] The results suggest that MRI is more sensitive than mammography in selected populations but may also have a lower specificity. Thus, these studies demonstrate that the addition of annual MRI and possibly ultrasound to mammography and CBE may significantly improve the sensitivity of screening for early detection of breast cancer.[103,113] Clinicians must realize, however, that there were less than 40 cancers in all studies combined.

No randomized, controlled trials are available that demonstrate a mortality benefit from employing MRI in current screening regimens for high-risk individuals. However, the preceding authors[103,112,113] state the finding of increased sensitivity for cancer detection in this high-risk subgroup suggests that women with *BRCA* mutations should be offered such screening. Nonetheless, clinicians must be cognizant that both sensitivity and specificity of screening MRI may be substantially less than described based on the technical capabilities at each institution using MRI technologies. For instance, if different imaging protocols are followed or if experienced radiologists and suitable technology, including the capability to perform magnetic resonance–guided biopsies, are not available, similar sensitivities may not be seen.

Although these results are encouraging, application of this technology to the high-risk population at large or to the general low-risk population is not advocated at this time until larger studies are performed to validate these data. Ultimately, the false-negative and false-positive rates as well as cost effectiveness need to be addressed before generalized use of MRI for screening in the average population is instituted. Currently several trials are being conducted in the United Kingdom, Europe, and the United States to assess the role of MRI in breast screening.[114]

### Digital Mammography

Digital mammography is a rapidly evolving technology that has the potential to improve on and/or function as a complement to conventional screen-film mammography for the early detection of breast cancer.[115–118] Digital mammography is an advanced form of screening that offers detection of breast disease secondary to improved efficiency of absorption of x-ray photons, greater contrast resolution over a larger dynamic range, especially in dense breast tissue (Fig. 41-9), and electronic archiving of breast studies. In screen-film mammography, x-ray photons cause light emission from a phosphor screen, which then imprints an image on the film emulsion. The image is then processed photographically and produces a permanent film image that is the final mammogram. In digital mammography, x-ray photons strike the digital detector and are absorbed by a phosphor material, which is then converted in an electronic (rather than a light) charge. The charge signal is then digitized and results in a computer-generated image.[119] Rather than an unalterable, permanent image as provided with screen-film mammography, digital mammography allows for postacquisition image processing and manipulation. Radiologists have the ability to manipulate the image by changing the brightness and contrast and to enlarge specific areas, either the entire breast or focal areas within the breast. These unique aspects of digital mammography create a significant advantage over screen-film mammography because it provides diagnostic information without exposing the patient to additional radiation (recalls) or the discomfort of further compression and has the potential to eliminate the huge film storage issue, thereby lowering ultimate screening costs associated with breast cancer screening.

In addition, these electronic images may be transmitted to radiologists for remote interpretation, thus facilitating second-opinion consultations by telemammography under near real-time circumstances. In addition, they also offer the potential value of computer-aided interpretations. *Telemammography* refers to the rapid transmission of high-quality mammographic images in digital format from one site to another. Telemammography can be used to enhance the performance of mobile mammography units by eliminating the need to transport films and may allow the off-site radiologist to monitor image quality and direct the technologist in obtaining additional views.

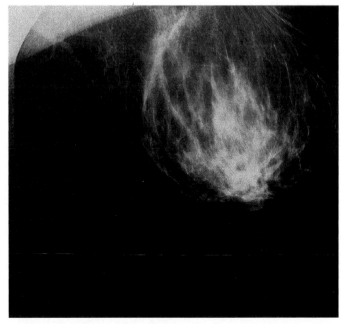

**Figure 41-9   Digital mammography.** This allows manipulation of the image to increase mass detection. Here the image is normal.

# Gynecologic Oncology

One study screened 4489 average-risk women age 40 and older and found digital mammography to have a lower overall sensitivity (64.3%) than conventional mammography (78.6%) in detection of invasive cancer. However, despite the lower sensitivity, digital mammography does identify additional cancers not identified on conventional mammography and thus results in an incremental gain in sensitivity of 21.4%. Digital mammography was also reported to have a recall rate of 11.8%, which was significantly lower ($P < 0.001$) than the recall rate of conventional mammography (14.9%).[120] However, incremental improvement in sensitivity will not necessarily translate into an absolute benefit, because the new technology may be selectively detecting cancers that are biologically inconsequential. In addition, characterization of morphologic details is inferior with the digital system, presumably due to reduced spatial resolution; also some lesions were not detected by digital detectors but were visualized on conventional film-screen mammography. Moreover, no statistically significant difference was found in the differentiation of benign from malignant lesions with this technique.[121,122]

The major limitation preventing widespread conversion to digital mammography programs is the considerable expense of purchasing the advanced equipment. Systems may cost $500,000, compared to $50,000 to $70,000 for screen-film mammography units. Ancillary costs include training staff in its use and maintenance, costs of laser printers and display monitors, retraining radiologists, and redesign of imaging facilities; these must be considered in any benefit analysis.

Digital mammography imaging allows multiple images to be shifted electronically, combined into three-dimensional views (tomosynthesis), and subtracted from one another. Areas of active research include tomosynthesis, stereomammography, dual-energy subtraction mammography, and contrast-medium mammography.[123] Ultimately such systems may substantially improve diagnostic accuracy by reducing obscuration by overlying structures, eliminating false-positive findings, and offering assistance with interventional procedures. Dual-energy mammography may improve accuracy by rendering calcifications more obvious in dense breast tissue.

Finally, expanding on the advantages of breast MRI, which compares the differential blood flow of malignancies and normal tissue, digital mammography should be able to depict subtle differences in contrast uptake by tumors, compared with background tissue. Therefore, it may be possible to detect cancers at a smaller size than those currently detected with conventional film-screen mammography as well as improve the accuracy of detection of the extent of cancer invasion.

Major technical challenges remain, and further clinical studies are necessary to determine the actual clinical value of this modality as a probable adjunct to conventional mammography primarily in the dense breast tissue. The diagnostic mammography trial, funded by the Office of Women's Health, will be of considerable assistance in determining the true efficacy of this evolving technology. Early analysis of data revealed approximately equal sensitivity of screen-film and digital mammography. However, digital mammography was shown to significantly lower the recall rate and offer a higher true-positive biopsy rate over conventional mammography in the population studied. As with all research studies caution should be applied because preliminary results are based on only a limited amount of data.

## Computer-Aided Diagnosis

The digital computer revolution at the end of the 20th century played a significant role in advances in medical technology and automation. The field of radiology was a major beneficiary of this knowledge. The sophisticated cross-sectional imaging modalities on which radiology, and much of medicine, now relies would not be possible without high-speed computing capabilities.

The early manifestations of breast cancer can be very subtle and difficult to detect. Moreover, they are portrayed on a complex and variable pattern of normal anatomy. In addition, the limitations of conventional screening mammography are well documented with an average false-negative rate of 10% to 15%. With the enhanced tools provided by computer assistance radiologists now need sophisticated assistance in image review.

Sophisticated computer techniques have been applied to the interpretation of radiologic images with ever-increasing success (Fig. 41-10). Computer-aided detection is the detection of potential abnormality by means of computer analysis of the mammogram. Computer-aided detection is aimed at reducing the false-negative rate of screening mammography by marking the perceived abnormal areas and directing the interpreting radiologist to re-review these areas, as well as reducing the false-positive rate thereby reducing the number of biopsies performed on benign lesions. Computer-aided detection is essentially a tool to prompt the radiologist to look again at potential abnormalities and is complementary to mammography. In the context of the mass screening program, it is potentially equal to another reader; that is, a second reading by a computer to increase the yield of screening mammography for the detection of early breast cancer. Several investigators have demonstrated improved radiologist performance in lesion detection and characterization when a computer-aided detection system is used with digitized screen film mammograms. The computer-aided detection enhancement of digital mammography appears highly promising; however further clinical studies are needed to evaluate the relative efficacy of different computer-aided detection methods. Moreover, the medicolegal status of computer-aided detection is uncertain at present and needs to be clarified.

Computer-aided detection has been assessed in several studies with over 650 cancers. However, only one of these studies was prospectively conducted.[124] All of the studies examined the incremental value of computer-aided detection and showed improved sensitivity, but the evidence on specificity is conflicting. It is not clear to what extent the improvement compares to other maneuvers, such as having an actual second film reader.

Many image analysis algorithms have been shown to outperform general radiologists in characterizing lesions as malignant or benign, with sensitivities for malignancy as high as 100% described.[125] Computer diagnoses have also been observed to be more specific than radiologists when operating at the high levels of sensitivity required in clinical practice,[126] with one report of an 83% positive predictive value for biopsy at 100% sensitivity, better than both experienced mammographers and general radiologists taking part in the study.[127] Such greater specificity has the potential to aid radiologists in decreasing the number of biopsies done for benign lesions.

Overall, with these imaging techniques (ultrasound, MRI, digital mammography, and computer-aided detection) being used as screening modalities, the evidence is promising but currently

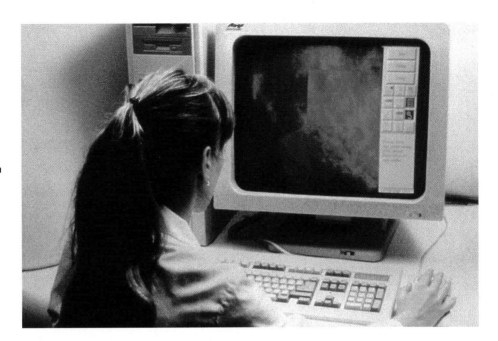

Figure 41-10    Computers may function as a second reader to prompt radiologists.

## Positron Emission Tomography

Positron emission tomography (PET) scanning is a noninvasive nuclear medicine imaging modality in existence for more than 30 years (Fig. 41-11). It is rapidly gaining acceptance in oncologic imaging especially in identifying recurrent or metastatic breast, lung, colorectal, and esophageal cancers. The technique involves injection of a short-lived positron-emitting radiopharmaceutical, fluorodeoxyglucose (FDG), which is the most commonly used agent for PET imaging, as well as the only such agent approved by the Food and Drug Administration (FDA). Decay of this glucose analog releases positively charged energy (positron). PET imaging captures the energy emitted from the body when a positron encounters an electron. Rapidly dividing neoplastic cells display higher metabolism of glucose than the surrounding nonneoplastic cells and, hence, preferential uptake of FDG. Malignant lesions appear visually as areas of increased activity, termed *hot spots* on a PET scan.[129,130] Inflammation or infection may also result in increased FDG uptake, resulting in a false-positive interpretation.[131,132]

Other radiologic studies, such as mammography, sonography, computed tomography, and MRI, provide detailed anatomic information about the size and location of masses, but not the unique metabolic information available with PET imaging. This distinctive characteristic affords PET imaging several advantages over anatomic modalities, including possible earlier detection of malignancy, differentiation of scar or benign disease from active malignancy; detection of metastatic disease in normal size lymph nodes, detection of locoregional recurrence or distant metastases, and assessment of early tumor treatment response (Fig. 41-12). Theoretically, earlier recognition of ineffective therapy could allow a change to an alternative, hopefully more effective chemotherapeutic regimen. Thus, the information obtained from PET imaging can be used to minimize drug toxicity, the costs of ineffective treatment, and delay in initiation of more effective treatment. Studies have shown PET to be better than mammography or ultrasound in initial tumor detection and more sensitive early in the course of effective therapy, but less sensitive for detection of residual tumor measuring less than 1 cm.[133]

Meta-analysis of nonrandomized studies found a sensitivity of 89% and specificity of 80% for PET scans in diagnosing breast cancer. Reported sensitivities range from 80% to 96% and specificities from 83% to 100%.[134-136] Because of limitations of spatial resolution, the sensitivity of PET depends largely on lesion size; thus PET is not accurate in detecting lesions less than 1 cm in diameter. It is also limited in identifying ductal carcinoma in situ. Hence, the authors noted flaws in most of these studies,

insufficient to support their use in population screening, but would support further evaluation.[128]

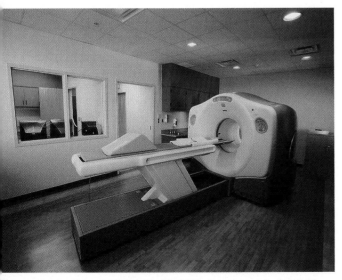

Figure 41-11    This multimodality CT/PET scanner may be helpful in assessing both anatomic and metabolic information about the size and location of masses.

623

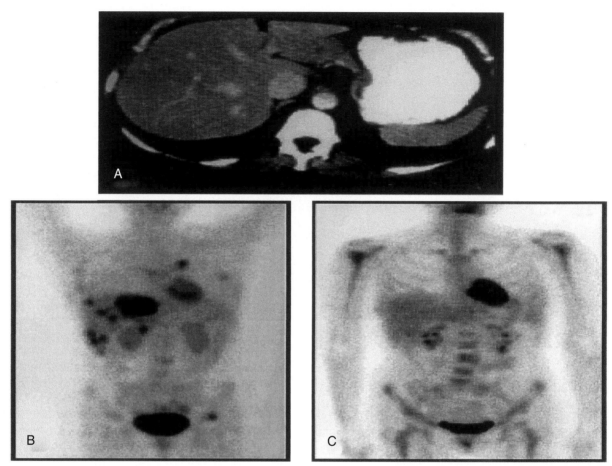

**Figure 41-12** Here the PET scan shows evidence of subdiagphragmatic metastasis in a patient with a normal MRI scan.

the most significant of which were small study sizes, large mean tumor sizes (2 to 4 cm), and the high prior probability of malignancy in subjects studied with PET.

Positron emission tomography imaging shows promise in identifying regional nodal and distant metastases in a patient with known primary breast cancer and in monitoring treatment response. However, it is currently recommended as an adjunct to mammography rather than as an alternative technique due to high false-negative results.[137] PET imaging is not suitable for breast cancer screening because both the scanners and radiopharmaceuticals are expensive. Current PET scanners can cost from $1 million to $1.75 million. However, PET imaging may be cost effective in offering an alternative to surgery/biopsy.

Because the technology has not undergone sufficient clinical testing, its use in screening for breast cancer would not be justified. However, of particular interest is the observation that early PET findings appear to predict long-term outcome. Smith and colleagues, in a study of 30 patients with cancers larger than 3 cm in diameter, found that PET imaging after a single pulse of chemotherapy was predictive of complete pathologic response, with sensitivity of 90% and specificity of 74%.[138] Schelling and colleagues found similar results in a study of 22 patients. After the first course of chemotherapy, patients responding to treatment were identified with sensitivity of 100% and specificity of 85%.[139]

## Sestamibi Scintimammography

This technique, like PET scanning, requires cellular activity and reflects metabolic activity. Technetium-99m-sestamibi is currently the only FDA-approved scintigraphic agent for breast imaging. It is a cationic lipophilic compound that is transferred across the cell membrane into the cytoplasm and mitochondria and retained because of electrical potentials across membranes. Selective uptake by cancer cells depends on cellular perfusion, mitochondrial uptake, and transmembrane electronegativity. Similar to PET scanning, false-negative and false-positive results can occur secondary to radiobiologic potentials. Slow-growing tumors and those of low cellularity often do not demonstrate significant tracer uptake; conversely, infection, inflammation, and benign tumors such as papillomas, hyperproliferative fibrocystic disease, and fibroadenomas may show increased uptake.[140] In clinical study, sensitivities range from 85% to 89%, specificities from 52% to 89%, positive predictive values from 61% to 89%, and negative predictive values from 67% to 92%. Detection of lesions less than 1 cm was limited in nearly all studies.[141–145]

Sestamibi scintimammography is also not used as a screening tool due to its high cost and limited ability to detect lesions smaller than 1 cm. It has been studied as an adjunct to standard imaging modalities in obviating "unnecessary" biopsies, detecting axillary nodal metastases, and monitoring treatment. Several studies have shown that sestamibi scintimammography is more specific than mammography, ultrasound, or MRI of palpable masses[146-149]; however, the negative predictive value remains insufficiently high to replace biopsy.

The cost effectiveness of these newer modalities remains to be evaluated, but all have the potential to significantly advance the diagnosis, and management of women with breast cancer. Research continues on other technologies. A National Institutes of Health–sponsored project is reviewing a laser-imaging system, which may provide more accurate views of breast tissue. Initial reports showed the system was able to detect some growths that were not seen on traditional film-screen mammography. In addition, this system was successful in predicting whether tumors were benign or malignant, which could lead to a reduction in the huge number of unnecessary biopsies performed.

## Ductal Lavage

The initial fervor over ductal lavage, which obtains tissue to check for initiation of the preneoplastic process, appears to be declining swiftly among the clinical community. Dooley and colleagues were successful in performing ductal lavage in 92% of women yielding nipple aspirate fluid[150] (Fig. 41-13). This and other risk assessment procedures have been mistaken as screening for cancer rather than screening for preneoplastic processes is labeled. Sensitivity in detecting breast cancer is low[151]; however, 20% of women in one study were shown to have precancerous or cancerous changes.[150]

Breast carcinoma is thought to have its earliest expression in the epithelial cells lining the terminal ductal lobular units that comprise the ductal system of the breast,[152,153] yet until recently, we have not had direct access to this area for pathologic correlation other than by blindly removing tissue by core biopsy or fine-needle aspiration. Ductal lavage is a safe, minimally invasive office procedure performed on women considered to be at high risk for breast carcinoma. Ductal lavage is used to collect breast ductal epithelial cells in the terminal ductal lobular units for cytologic analysis to provide further risk stratification. In a clinical trial of 507 high-risk women, cells collected through

ductal lavage allowed clinicans to detect the presence of precancerous and cancerous changes in 20% of the women. Each participant in the study had a normal mammogram or physical examination within 1 year of enrollment.[150,154] Moreover, this procedure yielded fewer acellular samples compared with nipple aspirates (22% vs. 73%). The presence of these changes correlated with a fivefold to 18-fold increased risk of developing breast cancer, depending on family history and the patient's risk of breast cancer development as determined by the Gail model.[8,155-157] The procedure involves the insertion of a microcatheter approximately 1.5 cm into the nipple orifice after topical anesthesia, lavaging the cannulated ductal system with normal saline, and analyzing the collected lavage effluent for the presence of normal, atypical, or malignant breast ductal cells.

Ductal lavage may not only be a helpful adjunct to determine which high-risk women require closer, more active management, but also may be used to track cell status in particular ducts over time. Because breast cancer may have insidious progression over time and can be present nearly 6 years before earliest detection on mammography, availability of this technique is surmised to provide practitioners with a tool to detect precancerous and cancerous breast cells before they become imageable, palpable cancers, thus allowing closer surveillance, surgical intervention, or chemoprevention. Studies in patients undergoing mastectomy has shown ductal lavage to have low sensitivity for carcinoma in situ in breasts containing invasive carcinoma.[158] Thus patients should have continued close follow-up. This procedure may be considered for women with a prior history of breast cancer and women at high risk for development of breast cancer, as defined by Gail Index score, family history, BRCA mutation, or previous benign breast biopsies.[16] Many institutions utilize other combinations of epidemiologic risk factors to determine eligibility.

Although reports of benefit in reducing the incidence of breast cancer from pharmaceuticals and surgery are encouraging, chemopreventive therapy and prophylactic surgery are expensive and have inherent side effects. Moreover, the only validated risk assessment model (the Gail model)[159,160] was used clinically primarily in white women who underwent annual mammography screening. Although the Gail model is used to determine eligibility for these risk management options, it has been shown to be woefully inadequate in detecting a particular woman's risk for the development of disease, although it is helpful in population risk assessment.[161-168] Conversely, ductal lavage and similar procedures may be a reasonable option for further evaluation of patients who already have clinical evidence of increased breast cancer risk, but for whom additional evidence is sought to facilitate decisions regarding these therapies. The finding of cytologic atypia on ductal lavage may provide a woman with additional information regarding her individualized risk of developing breast cancer. This information may assist the woman and her physician in weighing the risks and benefits of hormone replacement therapy, antiestrogen therapy (tamoxifen and possibly other selective estrogen receptor modulators or estrogen receptor down-regulators in the near future) and, in very-high-risk women, prophylactic surgery. In a study from the Memorial Sloan-Kettering Cancer Center, Port and colleagues found that fewer than 5% of high-risk women counseled about tamoxifen therapy accepted the chemoprevention option, whereas 61%

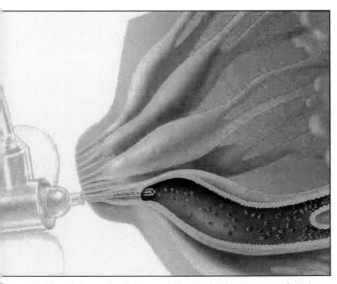

**Figure 41-13  Schematic diagram of the ductal lavage procedure to access intraductal cells.** (Courtesy of Cytec Corporation and affiliates.)

remained undecided and 35% declined definitely.[169] Detection of atypia seems to be a more convincing element in motivating high-risk women to pursue chemoprevention, as documented by Vogel and colleagues.[170] Recent assessment of women screened for participation in the Study of Tamoxifen and Raloxifene (STAR) trial revealed that overall, 21% of risk-eligible women agreed to randomization. For the subset of risk-eligible women who also had atypia, however, 36% agreed to randomization.[170]

Ductal lavage has also been studied in conjunction with intensive screening utilizing biannual CBE, annual mammography, and breast MRI in a high-risk cohort. Breast MRI identified high-grade ductal carcinoma in situ and high-risk lesions that were missed by mammography. Ductal lavage detected cytologic atypia in an individual with a normal MRI and mammogram. Additional research is necessary not only to determine the sensitivity and specificity of this method but also to determine whether the identification of malignant and high-risk lesions at an early stage will affect breast carcinoma incidence and mortality.[171]

### Random Periareolar Fine-Needle Aspiration

Fine-needle aspiration is a simple, fast, sensitive, and cost-effective method for evaluating breast lesions whereby tumor markers such as DNA ploidy, G-actin, p53, *HER2/Neu*, and c-*myc* can be analyzed and quantitated.[172] Multiple biomarker analysis may be helpful in individual risk assessment of breast cancer development.[173] Random periareolar fine-needle aspiration is a modification of fine-needle aspiration and has been touted as a technique to obtain breast tissue repeatedly over time for risk assessment in a high-risk cohort or for measurement of response to preventive interventions. Fabian and colleagues found this procedure to be inexpensive, and noted that it could be performed repeatedly with minimum morbidity.[174,175] In addition the majority of samples are cellular in these high-risk premenopausal and postmenopausal women in contrast where even in experienced hands approximately 40% of nipple aspirates are acellular.[8,176]

During this procedure, women at increased epidemiologic risk on the basis of family history of breast cancer, a prior breast cancer, or precancerous biopsy undergo a variation of the routine fine-needle aspiration procedure. Under local anesthesia, a 21-gauge needle attached to a 10- to 12-mL syringe is used to aspirate in eight different positions per breast at the 3:00 and 9:00 locations. Tissue is probed deeply to sample the terminal lobular–ductal units. Authors were able to predict those women who later developed cancer based on evidence of hyperplasia with atypia in the initial periareolar fine-needle aspiration and a 10-year Gail projected probability of developing breast cancer.

Ductal lavage has obvious advantages over periareolar fine-needle aspiration in that it is less invasive and enables localization of atypical or malignant cells to an individual ductal structure, whereas random periareolar fine-needle aspiration evaluates a pooled sample of multiple aspirates. An NIH-sponsored trial is under way to compare nipple aspirate versus ductal lavage versus periareolar fine-needle aspiration and determine the sensitivity, specificity and positive predictive value of each method. There are currently insufficient data to recommend either procedure as an independent screening modality or in combination with screening mammography.

## THE FUTURE

Future advances in technology that are presently being studied could revolutionize screening for breast carcinoma. An experimental breast cancer vaccine may eventually help treat or prevent nearly 80% of breast cancers.[177] The vaccine is based on a novel breast cancer-associated antigen, mammaglobin-A, which is expressed in 80% of breast tumors and amazingly absent (or found at only low levels) in normal breast cells. Administration of the vaccine to mice bred to have breast cancer resulted in more than a 30% reduction in tumor volume. The vaccine is thought to work by stimulating the immune system to attack breast cancer tumor cells.[178] Clearly, further research is needed to avoid potentially dangerous side effects in normal breast tissue.

Proteomic and genomic technology is rapidly advancing with definition and refinement of biomarkers that vary with level of risk and response to preventive interventions. Gene profiles and microarray technology have detected several genes and proteins that define specific cancer biology. These markers, which include mammographic breast density, serum insulin-like growth factor and its binding protein, insulin-like growth factor-binding protein-3, serum levels of estradiol and testosterone in postmenopausal women, and breast tissue markers[174,175] have been biologically and statistically significantly associated with cancer development. Thus techniques have been developed to quantify and standardize endpoint markers to be used to refine risk estimates based on epidemiologic models and to measure response to prevention interventions.

## REFERENCES

1. Romrell LJ, Bland KI: Anatomy of the breast, axilla, chest wall, and related metastatic sites. In Bland KI, Copeland EM III (eds): The Breast: Comprehensive Management of Benign and Malignant Diseases, 2nd ed. Philadelphia: Saunders, 1998, pp 19–37. **(IV, C)**
2. Schwartz SI, Shires GT, Spencer FC (eds): Principles of Surgery, 6th ed. New York: McGraw-Hill, 1994. **(IV, C)**
3. American Cancer Society: Cancer Facts and Figures 2004. Atlanta: ACS, 2004. **(IV, C)**
4. American Cancer Society: Cancer Prevention and Early Detection Facts and Figures 2004. Atlanta: ACS, 2004. **(IV, C)**
5. Fiorica J: Prevention and treatment of breast cancer. Obstet Gynecol Clin 2001;28:711–726. **(III, B)**
6. Ries IAG, Fisner MP, Kosary CI, et al: SEER Cancer Statistics Review 1973–1997. Bethesda, Md.: National Cancer Institute, 2000. **(III, B)**
7. Hansen N, Morrow M: Breast disease. Med Clin North Am 1998; 82:203–222. **(III, B)**
8. Wrensch MR, Petrakis NL, King EB, et al: Breast cancer incidence in women with abnormal cytology in nipple aspirates of breast fluid. Am J Epidemiol 1992;135:130–141. **(III, B)**
9. Dupont WD, Page DL: Risk factors for breast cancer in women with proliferative breast disease. N Engl J Med 1985;312:146–151. **(III, B)**
10. Dupont WD, Parl FF, Hartmann WH, et al: Breast cancer risk associated with proliferative breast disease and atypical hyperplasia. Cancer 1993;71:1258–1265. **(III, B)**
11. Fisher B, Costantino JP, Wickerham DL, et al: Tamoxifen for prevention of breast cancer: report of the National Surgical Adjuvant Breast and Bowel Project P-1 Study. J Natl Cancer Inst 1998; 90:1371–1388. **(Ib, A)**
12. Hartmann LC, Schaid DJ, Woods JE, et al: Efficacy of bilateral prophylactic mastectomy in women with a family history of breast cancer. N Engl J Med 1999;14:71–84. **(IIa, B)**

13. Rebbeck TR, Levin AM, Eisen A, et al: Breast cancer risk after bilateral prophylactic oophorectomy in *BRCA1* mutation carriers. J Natl Cancer Inst 1999;91:1475–1479. **(IIa, B)**

14. Gail MH, Brinton LA, Byar DP, et al: Projection individualized probabilities of developing breast cancer for white females who are being examined annually. J Natl Cancer Inst 1989;81:1879–1996. **(III, B)**

15. Claus EB, Risch N, Thompson WD: Autosomal dominant inheritance of early-onset breast cancer: implications for risk prediction. Cancer 1994;73:643–651. **(III, B)**

16. NCCN guidelines. www.nccn.org/professionals/physician_gls/f_guidelines.asp?button=I+Agree. Accessed October 2004. **(IV, C)**

17. Wooster R, Bignell G, Lancaster J, et al: Identification of the breast cancer susceptibility gene *BRCA2*. Nature 1995;378:789–792. **(III, B)**

18. Berchuck A, Carney M, Lancaster JM, et al: Familial breast–ovarian cancer syndromes: *BRCA1* and *BRCA2*. Clin Obstet Gynecol 1998;41:157–166. **(IV, C)**

19. Collins FS: *BRCA1*—lots of mutations, lots of dilemmas. New Engl J Med 1996;334:186–188. **(IV, C)**

20. Malkin D, Li FP, Strong LC, et al: Germ line *p53* mutations in a familial syndrome of breast cancer, sarcomas, and other neoplasia. Science 1990;250:1233–1238. **(III, B)**

21. Swift M, Reitnauer PJ, Morrell D, et al: Breast and other cancers in families with ataxia–telangiectasia. N Engl J Med 1987;316:1289–1294. **(III, B)**

22. Warmuth MA, Sutton LM, Winer EP: A review of hereditary breast cancer: from screening to risk factor modification. Am J Med 1997;102:407–415. **(IV, C)**

23. Smith RA, Saslow D, Sawyer KA, et al: Amern Cancer Society guidelines for breast cancer screening: update 2003. CA Cancer J Clin 2003;53:141–169. **(Ia, A)**

24. Karp SE: Clinical management of *BRCA1* and *BRCA2*-associated breast cancer. Semin Surg Oncol 2000;18:296–304. **(IV, C)**

25. Ford D, Easton DF: The genetics of breast and ovarian cancer. Br J Cancer 1995;72:805–812. **(IV, C)**

26. Easton DF, Ford D, Bishop DT: Breast and ovarian cancer incidence in *BRCA1*-mutation carriers. Breast Cancer Linkage Consortium. Am J Hum Genet 1995;56:265–271. **(IV, C)**

27. Berchuck A, Carney M, Lancaster JM, et al: Familial breast ovarian cancer syndromes: *BRCA1* and *BRCA2*. Clin Obstet Gynecol 1998;41:l57–161. **(IV, C)**

28. Arason A, Barkardottir RB, Egilsson V: Linkage analysis of chromosome 17q markers and breast–ovarian cancer in Icelandic families, and possible relationship to prostate cancer. Am J Hum Genet 1993;52:711–717. **(III, B)**

29. Ford D, Easton DF, Bishop DT, et al: Risk of cancer in *BRCA1*-mutation carriers. Lancet 1994;343:692–695. **(III, B)**

30. Strewing JP, Abeliovich D, Peretz T, et al: The carrier frequency of the *BRCA1* 185delAG mutation is approximately 1 percent in Ashkenazi Jewish individuals. Nat Genet 1995;11:198–200. **(III, B)**

31. Easton DF: Cancer risks in A-T heterozygotes. Int J Radat Biol 1994;66:S177–S182. **(III, B)**

32. Wooster R, Ford D, Mangion J, et al: Absence of linkage to the ataxia–telegiectasia locus in familial breast cancer. Hum Genet 1993;92:91–94. **(III, B)**

33. Mulvihill JJ, Stadler MP: Breast cancer risk analysis and counseling. Clin Obstet Gynecol 1996;39:851–859. **(IV, C)**

34. Sattuck-Eidens D, McClure M, Simard J, et al: A collaborative survey of 80 mutations in the *BRCA1* breast and ovarian cancer susceptibility gene. JAMA 1995;273:535–541. **(III, B)**

35. Burke W, Daly M, Garber J, et al: Recommendations for follow-up care of individuals with an inherited predisposition to cancer. II. *BRCA1* and *BRCA2*: Cancer Genetics Studies Consortium. JAMA 1997;277:997–1003. **(IV, C)**

36. American Medical Association: Report 16 of the Council on Scientific Affairs (A-99). Mammographic screening for asymptomatic women. June 1999. Available at: http://www.ama-assn.org/ama/pub/article/2036-2346.html. Accessed October 2004. **(Ia, A)**

37. Feig SA, D'Orsi CJ, Hendrick RE, et al: American College of Radiology guidelines for breast cancer screening. Am J Roentgenol 1998;171:29–33. **(IV, C)**

38. Canadian Task Force on Periodic Health Examination: Ottawa (Canada): Health Canada; 1994:788–795 (reaffirmed by the Canadian Task Force on the Periodic Health Examination 1999). Available at: http://www.ctfphc.org/index.html. Accessed October 2004. **(Ia, A)**

39. Ringash J: Preventive health care, 2001 update: screening mammography among women aged 40–49 years at average risk of breast cancer. Can Med Assoc J 2001;164:469–476. **(IIb, B)**

40. Periodic Health Examinations: Summary of AAFP Policy Recommendations and Age Charts. August 2003 Available at: http://www.aafp.org/enform.xml. Accessed October 2004. **(Ia, A)**

41. American College of Obstetricians and Gynecologists: Primary and preventive care: periodic assessments. ACOG Committee Opinion 246. Washington, DC: ACOG, 2000. **(Ib, A)**

42. Breast Cancer Screening for women ages 40–49. NIH Consensus Statement Online. 1997 Jan 21-23;15:1–35. Available at: http://odp.od.nih.gov/consensus/cons/103/103_statement.htm. Accessed October 2004. **(Ia, A)**

43. Baxter N: Preventive health care, 2001 update: should women be routinely taught breast self-examination to screen for breast cancer? Can Med Assoc J 2001;164:1837–1846. **(IIa, B)**

44. Hackshaw AK, Paul EA: Breast self-examination and death from breast cancer: a meta-analysis. Br J Cancer 2003;88:1047–53. **(IIa, B)**

45. Thomas DB, Dao LG, Ray RM, et al: Randomized trial of breast self examination in Shanghai: final results. J Natl Cancer Inst 2002;94:1445–1457. **(Ib, A)**

46. Shen Y, Zelen M: Screening sensitivity and sojourn time from breast cancer early detection clinical trials: mammograms and physical examinations. J Clin Oncol 2001;19:3490–3499. **(III, B)**

47. Semiglazov VF, Moiscenko VM, Manikhas AG, et al: Interim results of a prospective randomized study of self-examination for early detection of breast cancer (Russia/St. Petersburg/WHO). Vopr Onkol 1999;45:265–271. **(Ib, A)**

48. Kosters JP, Gotzsche PC: Regular self-examination or clinical examination for early detection of breast cancer. The Cochrane database of systematic reviews. The Cochrane Library, Volume 2, 2004. **(Ia, A)**

49. Nekhlyudov L. Fletcher SW: Is it time to stop teaching breast self-examination? Can Med Assoc J 2001;164:1851–1852. **(IV, C)**

50. U.S. Preventive Services Task Force: Screening for breast cancer: recommendations and rationale. Ann Intern Med 2002;137:347–360. **(IV, C)**

51. Physician Insurers Association of America: Breast cancer study—2002. Rockville, Md., Physician Insurers Association of America, 2002. **(IV, C)**

52. Coleman EA, Heard JK: Clinical breast examination: an illustrated educational review and update. Clin Excell Nurse Pract 2001;5:197–204. **(IV, C)**

53. Saunders KJ, Pilgrim CA, Pennypacker HS: Increased proficiency of search in breast self examination. Cancer 1986;58:2531–2537. **(III, B)**

54. Saslow D, Hannan J: Osuch J, et al: Clinical breast examination: practical recommendations for optimizing performance and reporting. CA Cancer J Clin 2004;54:327–344. **(IV, C)**

55. Dixon J, Ma B, Nigel J: Management of disorders of the ductal system and infections. In Harris JR (ed): Diseases of the Breast. Philadelphia: Lippincott Williams & Wilkins, 2000, 47–55. **(IV, C)**

56. Barton MB, Harris R, Fletcher SW: The rational clinical examination. Does this patient have breast cancer? The screening clinical breast examination: Should it be done? How? JAMA 1999;282:1270–1280. **(Ia, A)**

57. McDonald S, Saslow D, Alciati MH: Performance and reporting of clinical breast examination: a review of the literature. CA Cancer J Clin 2004;54:345–361. **(III, B)**

58. Mittra I: Breast cancer screening by physical examination. In Jatoi I (eds): Breast Cancer Screening. Austin, Tex.: Landes Bioscience, 1997, pp 97–110. **(IIb, B)**

**627**

59. Fletcher SW, O'Malley MS, Bunce LA: Physicians' abilities to detect lumps in silicone breast models. JAMA 1985;253:2224–2228. **(III, B)**

60. Alexander FE, Anderson TJ, Brown HK, et al: 14 years of follow-up from the Edinburgh randomized trial of breast-cancer screening. Lancet 1999;353:1909–1914. **(Ib, A)**

61. Shapiro S, Venet W, Strax P, et al: Periodic screening for breast cancer: the Health Insurance Plan project and its sequelae. Baltimore: Johns Hopkins Press, 1988. **(Ib, A)**

62. Seidman H, Gelb SK, Silverberg E, et al: Survival expediency in the breast cancer detection demonstration project. CA Cancer J Clin 1987;37:258–290. **(IIb, B)**

63. Shapiro S, Strax P, Venet L: Periodic breast cancer screening in reducing mortality from breast cancer. JAMA 1971;215:1777–1785. **(IIb, B)**

64. International Agency for Research on Cancer: IARC Handbooks on Cancer Prevention: Breast Cancer Screening. Lyon: IARC, 2002, pp 34–39. **(IV, C)**

65. Nystrom L, Andersson I, Bjurstam N, et al: Long-term effects of mammography screening: updated overview of the Swedish randomized trials. Lancet 2002;359:909–919. **(Ib, A)**

66. Alexander FE, Anderson RJ, Brown HK, et al: 14 years of follow up from the Edinburgh randomized trial of breast cancer screening. Lancet 1999;353:1903–1908. **(Ib, A)**

67. Kerlikowske K, Grady D, Rubin SM, et al: Efficacy of screening mammography: a meta-analysis. JAMA 1995;273:149–54. **(Ia, A)**

68. Chur KC, Smart CR, Tarone RE: Analysis of breast cancer mortality and state distribution by age of the Health Insurance Clinical Trial. J Natl Cancer Inst 1988;80:1125–1132. **(Ib, A)**

69. Tabar L, Fagerber CJ, Gad A, et al: Reduction in mortality from breast cancer after mass screening with mammography: randomized trial from the breast cancer screening work group of the Swedish National Board of Health and Welfare. Lancet 1985;1:829–832. **(Ib, A)**

70. Nystrom L, Rutqvist LE, Wall S, et al: Breast cancer screening with mammography: overview of Swedish randomized trials. Lancet 1993; 341:973–978. **(Ib, A)**

71. Tabar L, Fagerberg G, Chen HH, et al: Efficacy of breast cancer screening by age: new results from the Swedish Two County Trial, Cancer 1995;75:2507–2517. **(Ia, A)**

72. Fletcher SW, Black W, Harris R, et al: Report of the International Workshop on Screening for breast cancer. J Natl Cancer Inst 1993; 85:1644–1656. **(Ia, A)**

73. Baker LH: Breast Cancer Detection Demonstration Project: Five year summary report. CA Cancer J Clin 1982;32:194. **(IIa, B)**

74. Tabar L, Vitak B, Chen H–H, et al: The Swedish Two-County Trial twenty years later. Radiol Clin North Am 2000;38:625–652. **(Ib, A)**

75. Miller AB, Baines CJ, To T, et al: Canadian National Breast Screening Study. Breast cancer detection and death rates among women aged 40–49 years. Can Med Assoc J 1992;147:1459–1476. **(Ib, A)**

76. Dales LG, Friedman GD, Collen MF: Evaluating periodic multi-phasic health check ups: a controlled trial. J Chronic Dis 1979;2:385–404. **(IIa, B)**

77. Humphrey LL, Helfand M, Chan BK, et al: Breast cancer screening: a summary of the evidence for the U.S. Preventive Services Task Force. Ann Intern Med 2002;137:347–360. **(Ia, A)**

78. Tabar L, Smith RA, Duffy SW: Update on effects of screening mammography. Lancet 2002;360:337–340. **(Ia, A)**

79. Moskowitz M: Breast cancer: age specific growth rates and screening strategies. Radiology 1986;161:37–41. **(III, B)**

80. Larsson L, Anderson I, Bjurstam N, et al: Update overview of the Swedish randomized trails in breast cancer screening with mammography: age group 40–49 at randomization. J Natl Cancer Inst Monogr 1997;22:57–61. **(Ia, A)**

81. Hendrick RE, Smith RA, Rutledge JH 3rd, Smart CR: Benefit of screening mammography in women aged 40–99: a new meta-analysis of randomized controlled trials. J Natl Cancer Inst 1997;22:87–92.

82. Feig SA: Increased benefit from shorter screening mammography intervals for women ages 40–49 years. Cancer 1997;80:2035–2039. **(III, B)**

83. Michaelson JS, Halpern E, Kopans DB: Breast cancer compute simulation methods for estimation of optimal intervals for screening Radiology 1999;212:551–560. **(III, B)**

84. Gotzsche PC, Olsen O: Is screening for breast cancer wit mammography justifiable? Lancet 2000;355:129–134. **(Ib, A)**

85. Olsen O, Gotzsche PC: Cochrane review on screening for breas cancer with mammography. Lancet 2001;358:1340–1342. **(Ia, A)**

86. National Cancer Institute: NCI Statement on Mammograph Screening. Office of Communications/Mass Media Branch. Bethesda Md.: National Institutes of Health, 21 February, 2002. **(Ib, A)**

87. Screening for Breast Cancer. Recommendations and Rationale Rockville, Md.: Agency for Health Care Research and Quality, 2002 **(Ib, A)**

88. Kopans DB (ed): Breast Imaging Report: Data Management, False Negative Mammography, and the Breast Imaging Audit in Breast Imaging, 2nd ed. Philadelphia: Lippincott-Raven, 1998, pp 761–796 **(IV, C)**

89. Kerlikowske D, Grady D, Barclay J, et al: Variability and accuracy ir mammographic interpretation using the American College o Radiology Breast Imaging Reporting And Data System. J Natl Cancer Inst 1998;90:1801–1809. **(III, B)**

90. Schilling RB, Cox JD, Sharma SR: Advanced digital mammography J Digit Imaging 1998;11(3 Suppl 1):163–165. **(IV, C)**

91. Mammography Quality Standards Act of 1992. Pub L No. 102–539 1992.

92. American College of Radiology: American College of Radiology Standards. Reston, Va., American College of Radiology, 2002.

93. Baker JA, Soo MS: Breast US: assessment of technical quality and image interpretation. Radiology 2002;223:229–238. **(III, B)**

94. Entrekin RR, Porter BA, Sillesen HH, et al: Real-time spatial compound imaging: application to breast, vascular, and musculoskeletal ultrasound. Semin Ultrasound CT MR 2001;22:50–64. **(III, B)**

95. Rosen EI, Soo MS: Tissue harmonic imaging sonography of breast lesions: improved margin analysis, conspicuity, and image quality compared to conventional ultrasound. Clin Imaging 2001;25:379–384 **(IIb, B)**

96. Downey DD, Fenster A, Williams JC: Clinical utility of three-dimensional US. Radiographics 2000;220:559–571. **(III, B)**

97. Huber S, Wagner M, Medl M, et al: Real-time spatial compound imaging in breast ultrasound. Ultrasound Med Biol 2002;28:155–163 **(II, B)**

98. Rotten D, Levaillant JM, Zerat L: Analysis of normal breast tissue and of solid breast masses using three-dimensional ultrasound mammography. Ultrasound Obstet Gynecol 1999;14:114–24. **(III, B)**

99. Mehta TS: Current uses of ultrasound in the evaluation of the breast. Radiol Clin North Am 2003;41:841–856. **(IV, C)**

100. Hou MF, Chuang HI, Yang FO, et al: Comparison of breast mammography, sonography and physical examination for screening women at high risk of breast cancer in Taiwan. Ultrasound Med Biol 2002;28:415–520. **(III, B)**

101. Kolb TM, Lichy J, Newhouse JH: Occult cancer in women with dense breasts: detection with screening US-diagnostic yield and tumor characteristics. Radiol 1998;207:191–199. **(III, B)**

102. O'Driscol D, Warren R, Mackay J, et al: Screening with breast ultrasound in a population at moderate risk due to family history. J Med Screen 2001;8:106–109. **(III, B)**

103. Warner E, Plewes DB, Shumak RS, et al: Comparison of breast magnetic resonance imaging, mammography and ultrasound for surveillance of women at high risk for hereditary breast cancer. J Clin Oncol 2001;19:3524–3521. **(III, B)**

104. Buchberger W, DeKoekkoek-Doll P, Springer P, et al: Incidental findings on sonography of the breast: clinical significance and diagnostic workup. Am J Roentgenol 1999;173:921–927. **(III, B)**

105. Kolb TM, Lichy J, Newhouse JH: Comparison of the performance of screening mammography, physical examination, and breast US and evaluation of factors that influence them: an analysis of 27,825 patient evaluations. Radiology 2002;225:165–175. **(III, B)**

106. Kaplan SS: Clinical utility of bilateral whole-breast US in the evaluation of women with dense breast tissue. Radiology 2001;221:641–649. **(III, B)**

107. Morris EA: Breast cancer imaging with MRI. Radiol Clin North Am 2002;40:443–466. **(IIb, B)**

108. Orel SG, Medonca MH, Reynolds C, et al: MR imaging of ductal in situ. Radiology 1997;202:413–420. **(III, B)**

109. Klimberg VS, Harms SE, Henry-Tillman RS: Not all MRI techniques are created equal. Ann Surg Oncol 2000;7:404–405. **(III, B)**

110. Weinstein SP, Orel SG, Heller R, et al: MR imaging of the breast in patients with invasive lobular breast cancer. Am J Radiol 2001;176:399–406. **(III, B)**

111. Warner E, Plewes DB, Hill KA, et al: Surveillance of *BRCA1* and *BRCA2* mutation carriers with magnetic resonance imaging, ultrasound, mammography and clinical breast examination. JAMA 2004;292:1317–1325. **(III, B)**

112. Kriege M, Brekelmans CTM, Boetes C, et al: Efficacy of MRI and mammography for breast cancer screening in women with a familial or genetic predisposition. New Engl J Med 2004;351:427–437. **(III, B)**

113. Stoutjesdijk MJ, Boetes C, Jager GJ, et al: Magnetic resonance imaging and mammography in women with a hereditary risk for breast cancer. J Natl Cancer Inst 2001;93:1095–1102. **(III, B)**

114. U.S. MRI Breast Screening Study Advisory Group, 2000. http://www.acrin.org/current_protocols.html. Accessed 3 October 2004. **(IIa, B)**

115. Edell SL, Eisen MD: Current imaging modalities for the diagnosis of breast cancer. Delaware Med J 1999;71:377–382. **(IV, C)**

116. Reynolds HE: Advances in breast imaging. Hematol Oncol Clin North Am 1999;13:333–348. **(IV, C)**

117. Hogge JP, Artz DS, Freedman MT: Update in digital mammography. Crit Rev Diagn Imaging 1997;38:89–113. **(IV, C)**

118. Pisano ED, Yaffe MJ, Hemminger BM, et al: Current status of full-field digital mammography. Acad Radiol 2000;7:266–280. **(IV, C)**

119. Feig SA, Yaffe MJ: Digital mammography. Radiographics 1998;18:893–901. **(IV, C)**

120. Lewin JM, D'Orsi CJ, Hendrick RE, et al: Clinical comparison of full-field digital mammography and screen-film mammography for detection of breast cancer. Am J Roentgenol 2002;179:671–677. **(IIb, B)**

121. Perlet C, Becker C, Sittel H, et al: A comparison of digital luminescence mammography and conventional film-screen system: preliminary results of clinical evaluation. Eur J Med Res 1998;3:165–171. **(III, B)**

122. Preliminary data presented at the San Antonio Breast Conference. December 2000. **(III, B)**

123. Niklason LT, Christian BT, Niklason LE, et al: Digital tomosynthesis in breast imaging. Radiology 1997;205:399–406. **(III, B)**

124. Freer TW, Ulissey MR: Screening mammography with computer-aided detection: prospective study of 12,860 patients in a community breast center. Radiology 2001;220:781–786. **(IIb, B)**

125. Wu Y, Giger ML, Doi K, et al: Application of neural networks in mammography: applications in decision making in the diagnosis of breast cancer. Radiology 1993;187:81. **(III, B)**

126. Jiang Y, Metz CE, Nishikawa RM: A receiver operating characteristic partial area index for highly sensitive diagnostic tests. Radiology 1996;201:745. **(III, B)**

127. Huo Z, Giger ML, Vyborny CJ, et al: Automated computerized classification of benign and malignant masses on digital mammograms. Acad Radiol 1998;5:155. **(IV, C)**

128. Irwig L, Houssami N, van Vliet C: New technologies in screening for breast cancer: a systematic review of their accuracy. Br J Cancer 2004;90:2118–2122. **(IIa, B)**

129. Brown RS, Leung JY, Fisher SJ, et al: Intratumoral distribution of tritiated-FDG in breast carcinoma: correlation between GLUT-1 expression and FDG uptake. J Nucl Med 1996;37:1042–1047. **(III, B)**

130. Higashi K, Clavo AC, Wahl RL: Does FDG uptake measure proliferative activity of human cancer cells? In vitro comparison with DNA flow cytometry and tritiated thymidine uptake. J Nucl Med 1993;34:414–419. **(III, B)**

131. Bakheet SMG, Powe J, Kandil A, et al: $F^{18}$ FDG uptake in breast infection and inflammation. Clin Nucl Med 2000;25:100–103. **(III, B)**

132. Hoh CK, Hawkins RA, Glaspy JA, et al: Cancer detection with whole-body PET using [$^{18}$F]fluoro-2-deoxy-D-glucose. J Comput Assist Tomogr 1993;17:582–589. **(III, B)**

133. Bassa P, Kim EE, Inoue T, et al: Evaluation of preoperative chemotherapy using PET with fluorine-18-flurodeoxy-D-glucose to predict the pathologic response of breast cancer to primary chemotherapy. J Clin Oncol 2000;18:1676–1688. **(III, B)**

134. Kim TS, Moon WK, Lee DS, et al: Fluorodeoxyglucose positron emission tomography for detection of recurrent or metastatic breast cancer. World J Surg 2001;25:829–834. **(III, B)**

135. Samson DJ, Flamm CR, Pisano E, et al: Should FDG PET be used to decide whether a patient with an abnormal mammogram or breast finding at physical examinations should undergo biopsy? Acad Radiol 2002;9:773–783. **(III, B)**

136. Greco M, Crippa F, Agresti R, et al: Axillary lymph node staging in breast cancer by 2-fluoro-2-deoxy-D-glucose-positron emission tomography: clinical evaluation and alternative management. J Natl Cancer Inst 2001;93:630–635. **(III, B)**

137. Kelemen PR, Lowe V, Phillips N: Positron emission tomography and sentinel lymph node dissection in breast cancer. Clin Breast Cancer 2002;3:73–77. **(III, B)**

138. Smith IC, Welch AE, Hutcheon AW, et al: Positron emission tomography using [$^{18}$F]fluoro-2-deoxy-D-glucose to predict the pathologic response of breast cancer to primary chemotherapy. J Clin Oncol 2000;18:1676–1688. **(III, B)**

139. Schelling M, Avril N, Nahrig J, et al: Positron emission tomography using [$^{18}$F]fluoro-2-deoxy-D-glucose for monitoring primary chemotherapy in breast cancer. J Clin Oncol 2000;18:1689–1695. **(III, B)**

140. Leung JW: New modalities in breast imaging: digital mammography, positron emission tomography, and sestamibi scintimammography. Radiol Clin North Am 2002;40:467–482. **(III, B)**

141. Taillefer R: The role of $^{99m}$Tc-sestamibi and other conventional radiopharmaceuticals in breast cancer diagnosis. Semin Nucl Med 1999;29:16–40. **(III, B)**

142. Flanagan DA, Gladding SB, Lovell FR: Can scintimammography reduce "unnecessary" biopsies? Am Surg 1998;64:670–673. **(III, B)**

143. Cwikala JB, Buscombe JR, Kelleher SM, et al: Comparison of accuracy of scintimammography and x-ray mammography in the diagnosis of primary breast cancer in patients selected for surgical biopsy. Clin Radiol 1998;53:274–280. **(IIb, B)**

144. Prats E, Aisa F, Abos MD, et al: Mammography and $^{99m}$Tc-MIBI scintimammography in suspected breast cancer. J Nucl Med 1999;40:296–301. **(IIb, B)**

145. Buscombe JR, Cwikla JB, Holloway B, et al: Prediction of the usefulness of combined mammography and scintimammography in suspected primary breast cancer using ROC curves. J Nucl Med 2001;42:3–8. **(IIb, B)**

146. Imbriaco M, Del Vecchio S, Riccardi A, et al: Scintimammography with $^{99m}$Tc-MIBI versus dynamic MRI for non-invasive characterization of breast masses. Eur J Nucl Med 2001;28:56–63. **(IIb, B)**

147. Klaus AJ, Klingensmith WC III, Parker SH, et al: Comparative value of $^{99m}$Tc-sestamibi scintimammography and sonography in the diagnostic workup of breast masses. Am J Radiol 2000;174:1779–1783. **(IIb, B)**

148. Palmedo H, Grunwald F, Bender H, et al: Scintimammography with technetium-99m methoxyisobutylisonitrile: comparison with mammography and magnetic resonance imaging. Eur J Nucl Med 1996;23:940–946. **(IIb, B)**

149. Tiling R, Sommer H, Pechmann M, et al: Comparison of technetium-99m-sestamibi scintimammography with contrast-enhanced MRI for diagnosis of breast lesions. J Nucl Med 1997;38:58–62. **(IIb, B)**

150. Dooley W, Veronesi U, Phillips R, et al: Detection of pre-malignant and malignant breast cells by ductal lavage: results from a multicenter trial. Submitted for publication. **(III, B)**

151. Kilgore C: Ductal lavage not a sensitive screening tool for breast cancer, study suggests. OB GYN News. November 15, 2004. **(IV, C)**

152. Wellings SR, Jensen HM, Marcum RG: An atlas of subgross pathology of the human breast with special reference to possible precancerous lesions. J Natl Cancer Inst 1975;55:231–273. **(IV, C)**

153. Wellings SR: A hypothesis of the origin of human breast cancer from the terminal ductal lobular unit. Pathol Res Pract 1980; 166:515–535.**(IV, C)**

154. Preliminary data presented to the American Society of Clinical Oncology Annual meeting, May 2000 and the Second Annual Lynn Sage Breast Cancer symposium, Chicago, September 2000. **(III, B)**

155. Page DL, Dupont WD, Rogers LW, Rados MS, et al: Atypical hyperplastic lesions of the female breast. Cancer 1985;55:2698–2708. **(III, B)**

156. Dupont W, Page D: Risk factors for breast cancer in women with proliferative breast disease. N Engl J Med 1985;312:146–151. **(III, B)**

157. Dupont WD, Parl FF, Hartmann WH, et al: Breast cancer risk associated with proliferative breast disease and atypical hyperplasia. Cancer 1993;71:1258–1265. **(III, B)**

158. Brogi E, Robson M, Panageas KS, et al: Ductal lavage in patients undergoing mastectomy for mammary carcinoma: a correlative study. Cancer 2003;98:2170–2176. **(III, B)**

159. Gail MH, Brinton LA, Byar DP, et al: Projecting individualized probabilities of developing breast cancer for white females who are being examined annually. J Natl Cancer Inst 1989;81:1879–1886.**(III, B)**

160. Bondy MO, Lustbader ED, Halabi S, et al: Validation of a breast cancer risk assessment model in women with a positive family history. J Natl Cancer Inst 1994;86:620–625. **(III, B)**

161. Costantino JP, Gail MH, Pee D, et al: Validation studies for models projecting the risk of invasive and total breast cancer incidence. J Natl Cancer Inst 1999;91:1541–1548. **(III, B)**

162. Gail MH, Benichou J: Validation studies on a model for breast cancer risk [editorial][published erratum appears in J Natl Cancer Inst 1994;86:803]. J Natl Cancer Inst 1994;86:573–575. **(III, B)**

163. Spiegelman D, Colditz GA, Hunter D, et al: Validation of the Gail et al. model for predicting individual breast cancer risk. J Natl Cancer Inst 1994;86:600–607. **(IIb, B)**

164. Boyle P, Mezzetti M, La Vecchia C, et al: Contribution of three components to individual cancer risk predicting breast cancer risk in Italy. Eur J Cancer Prev 2004;13:183–191. **(III, B)**

165. Tartter PI, Gajdos C, Smith SR, et al: The prognostic significance of Gail model risk factors for women with breast cancer. Am J Surg 2002;184:11–15. **(III, B)**

166. Mackarem G, Roche C, Hughes K: The effectiveness of the Gail model in estimating risk for development of breast cancer in women under 40 years of age. Breast J 2001;7:34–39. **(III, B)**

167. Bondy ML, Newman LA: Breast cancer risk assessment models applicability to African-American women. Cancer Suppl 2003 97:230–235. **(III, B)**

168. Kaur JS, Roubidoux MA, Sloan J, et al: Can the Gail model be useful in American Indian and Alaska native populations? Cancer 2004 100:906–912. **(III, B)**

169. Port ER, Montgomery LL, Heerdt AS, et al: Patient reluctance toward tamoxifen use for breast cancer primary prevention. Ann Surg Oncol 2001;8:580–585. **(III, B)**

170. Vogel VG, Costantino JP, Wickerham DL, et al: Re:Tamoxifen for prevention of breast cancer: report of the National Surgical Adjuvant Breast and Bowel Project P-1 Study. J Natl Cancer Inst 2002;94:1504. **(III, B)**

171. Hartman AR, Daniel BL, Kurian AW, et al: Breast magnetic resonance image screening and ductal lavage in women at high genetic risk for breast carcinoma. Cancer 2004;100:479–489. **(III, B)**

172. Rao JY, Apple SK, Hemstreet GP, et al: Single cell multiple biomarker analysis in archival breast fine-needle aspiration specimens: quantitative fluorescence image analysis of DNA content, p53, and G-actin as breast cancer biomarkers. Cancer Epidemiol Biomarkers Prev 1998;7:1027–1033. **(III, B)**

173. Rao JY, Apple SK, Jin Y, et al: Comparative polymerase chain reaction analysis of c-*myc* amplification on archival breast fine-needle aspiration materials. Cancer Epidemiol Biomark Prev 2000;9:175–179. **(III, B)**

174. Fabian CJ, Zalles C, Kamel S, et al: Prevalence of aneuploidy, overexpressed ER, and overexpressed EGFR in random breast aspirates of women at high and low risk for breast cancer. Breast Cancer Res Treat 1994;30:263–274. **(III, B)**

175. Fabian CJ, Kamel S, Kimler DR, et al: Potential use of biomarkers in breast cancer risk assessment and chemoprevention trials. Breast J 1995;1:236–242. **(III, B)**

176. Sauter ER, Ross E, Daly M, et al: Nipple aspirate fluid: a promising non-invasive method to identify cellular markers of breast cancer risk. Br J Cancer 1997;76:494–501. **(III, B)**

177. Warner J: New breast cancer vaccine passes first hurdle: experimental breast cancer vaccine halts tumors in Mice. Available at http://my.webmd.com/content/article/94/102645.htm. Accessed 28 September 2004. **(IIc, B)**

178. Narayanan K, Jaramillo A, Benshoff ND, et al: Response of established human breast tumors to vaccination with mammaglobin-A cDNA. J Natl Cancer Inst 2004;96:1388–1396. **(IIb, B)**

# Chapter 42

# Vulvar Carcinoma

## Alan N. Gordon, MD

## KEY POINTS

- Carcinoma in situ is usually asymptomatic.
- Careful inspection and biopsy of suspicious lesions is central to managing carcinoma in situ.
- Treatment of carcinoma in situ should be guided with an aim to preserve anatomy and function.
- Lesion size and depth of invasion predict for nodal involvement in invasive vulvar cancer.
- Nodal spread is predictive of survival.
- An adequate surgical margin is essential to prevent local recurrence.
- Draining inguinal-femoral nodes must be treated unless there is less than 1 mm of invasion.

Vulvar cancer is a relatively rare neoplasm that accounts for less than 5% of all gynecologic cancers. Because of the relatively small number of cases, it has taken considerable time to accrue significant series of patients and analyze the outcomes of prior therapies to see what effect they may have had on survival and complications. Therefore, changes in therapy have been slow to be instituted relative to other gynecologic cancers.

From 90% to 95% of vulvar cancers are squamous cell carcinoma arising from the native epithelial covering of the vulva (Table 42-1). Other malignant lesions that can arise along the vulva include melanoma, Paget's disease of the vulva, and adenocarcinomas arising from the glandular components of the epithelium and sarcomas arising from the mesenchymal component of the vulva. These cumulatively account for less than 10% of invasive vulvar neoplasms. This chapter therefore focuses on the natural history, diagnosis, and treatment of squamous cell carcinoma of the vulva.

## PREINVASIVE DISEASE

### Epidemiology, Risk Factors, and Pathogenesis

Previously, it was felt that lichen sclerosus et atrophicus was the precursor lesion to invasive vulvar cancer. Retrospective analyses of patients treated for vulvar cancer in the mid-1900s found that lichen sclerosus was adjacent to most of the vulvar cancers resected, leading to accaptance of the conclusion that lichen sclerosus was indeed a precursor lesion to invasive squamous cell cancers. Several clinicians advocated total vulvectomy for lichen sclerosis to prevent the development of invasive cancer.[1] However, it has been found that this conclusion was far from true, in that only a small percentage of patients who had lichen sclerosus actually went on to develop invasive vulvar cancer. Today, treatment of lichen sclerosus aims to control symptoms while carefully observing for the development of new lesions, which might indicate invasive cancer in a small minority of patients.

Although not very commonly seen in the United States, several infectious lesions can cause epithelial abnormalities to arise within the overlying dermis and eventually develop into squamous cell cancers of the vulva. Most notably, this has been seen with lymphogranuloma venereum and granuloma inguinale. These disease processes need to be considered, especially when evaluating and treating patients from tropical environments.

Squamous cell carcinoma in situ is by far the most common precursor lesion for squamous cell carcinoma of the vulva in the United States and other developed countries at this time. The incidence of carcinoma in situ did appear to increase significantly during the latter half of the twentieth century, but this increase was not accompanied by any significant change in the incidence of invasive squamous cancers of the vulva. One possible explanation may be that not all cases of carcinoma in situ are capable of progressing into invasive squamous cell cancer. This phenomenon may also be partly due to the increased recognition of the disease as clinicians became aware of it and actively evaluated patients for its presence. Because patients with squamous cell carcinoma in situ are largely asymptomatic, the lesions may go unnoticed in the absence of a careful systematic search of the vulva.

Although the vulvar epithelium is directly contiguous with the vaginal epithelium and squamous epithelium of the cervix, these tissues are not necessarily identical in their response to external stimuli. It has been seen that, as with cervical lesions, an increase in cigarette smoking has accounted for an increase in the incidence of squamous cell lesions involving the vulva.[2] However, although almost all cervical cancers appear to be related to infection with himan papillomavirus (HPV), studies in squamous lesions involving the vulva have shown various degrees of association with HPV. One possible explanation may be that two distinct forms of this disease occur. In younger patients, multifocal lesions are more common, even multiple confluent lesions that may cover the vulva; these are more commonly associated with HPV (Table 42-2). However, in older

| Table 42-1 Cancer of the Vulva | |
|---|---|
| Squamous cell carcinoma | 95% |
| Melanoma | 3% |
| Adenocarcinoma | 1% |
| Sarcoma | 1% |

631

| Table 42-2 Carcinoma in Situ—Two Different Diseases | | | | | |
|---|---|---|---|---|---|
| | | **Type of Lesion** | | | |
| **Age** | **No. of Patients** | *Multifocal* | *Unifocal* | *Diffuse* | *Unknown* |
| <30 | 12 | 66% | 33% | | |
| 30–50 | 33 | 26% | 70% | 2% | 2% |
| >50 | 36 | 25% | 44% | 11% | 20% |

From Benedet JL, Murphy KJ: Squamous carcinoma in situ of the vulva. Gynecol Oncol 1982;14:213.

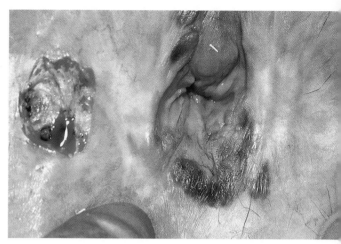

**Figure 42-1    Carcinoma in situ.** Note the pigmented lesion involving the perineal body.

patients, carcinoma in situ tends to be more unifocal, the lesions are less condylomatous in appearance, and lesions are far less likely to be associated with HPV infection.[2,3]

### Clinical Features

As previously discussed, most patients with carcinoma in situ of the vulva will be asymptomatic. These patients are largely discovered as part of a routine examination or for follow-up of prior squamous disease that involved the upper portion of the genital canal. The most common symptom seen in association with squamous carcinoma in situ is pruritus (Table 42-3). The lesions are usually quite pruritic; patients occasionally develop ulcerations and bleeding secondary to scratching at the lesions. Bleeding, however, is relatively unusual with squamous carcinoma in situ unless scratching has led to disruptions of the epithelium. If patients do present with bleeding as their main complaint in the absence of pruritus, the practitioner should be concerned with the possibility of an invasive lesion rather than carcinoma in situ. Some patients will occasionally notice a lump or growth due to the condylomatous nature of their lesions or the development of plaque-type areas in lesions that are hyperkeratotic.

The clinical appearance of lesions on the vulva is highly variable. Lesions may be multiple; this is more commonly the case in the younger patient population. In the older patient population, a single lesion is more frequently seen. The different appearance of these lesions has led in the past to the use of different terms to describe the various clinical appearances of carcinoma in situ, such as Bowen's disease or erythroplasia of Queyrat. The difference in appearance of the lesions is due to

differing histologic architecture and not to any difference in biological behavior. Multiple lesions are more often condylomatous in nature; this type is often associated with HPV infection. Lesions can be hyperpigmented due to excess deposition of melanin within the basement membrane of the epithelium (Fig. 42-1). Other lesions may appear thickened and white or hyperkeratotic due to an excess of keratin deposition in the superficial epithelial layers (Figs. 42-2 and 42-3). The absence of keratinization accompanied by a lack of melanin within the basement membrane and the presence of parakeratosis accounts for the red appearance of other lesions (see Fig. 42-2). All of these different lesion types are characterized by a lack of

| Table 42-3 In Situ Disease: Symptoms and Clinical Appearance |
|---|
| **Symptoms** |
| Pruritus |
| Bleeding |
| None; discovered on follow-up for prior cervical disease |
| **Lesion characteristics** |
| Macular or papular |
| White, red, or hyperpigmented |

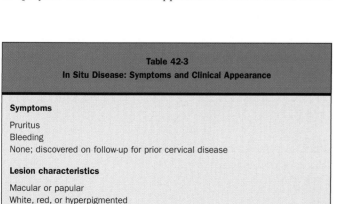

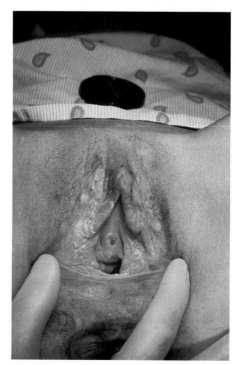

**Figure 42-2    Carcinoma in situ.** Multiple white hyperkeratotic and multiple red lesions are present.

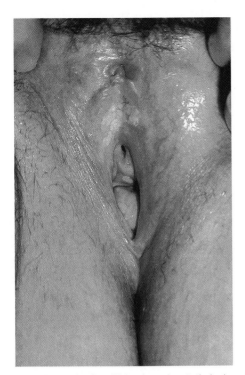

**Figure 42-3    Carcinoma in situ.** White, hyperkeratotic lesions in the interlabial fold.

maturation of the epithelial cells going toward the surface layer; with full thickness involvement by immature cells, the classic picture of carcinoma in situ is seen.

## Diagnosis

The key to diagnosis is careful inspection of the entire vulvar epithelium. The interlabial folds and other skin creases must be fully opened and exposed to evaluate all skin surfaces. Additionally, the perineal body itself should also be carefully examined, because this disease affects squamous epithelium and can extend into the anal canal up to the dentate line. Some have advocated the use of stains as an aid in detecting in situ lesions. However, nuclear stains such as toluidine blue can be associated with false-positive results. If excoriations or breaks in the skin are present, these areas will also produce positive results. Additionally, in hyperkeratotic areas, because the stain is unable to penetrate to the cells, false-negative results are obtained. The use of a dilute acetic acid and magnification, i.e., vulvoscopy, can also yield false positives and false negatives for many of the same reasons. Therefore, careful close inspection is the most important element in diagnosis. Confirmation must be obtained by biopsy of any suspicious skin areas, which is usually easily accomplished through the use of intradermal lidocaine for local anesthesia and the use of a 4.0 or 6.0-mm Keyes biopsy punch. The punch biopsy should be taken down into the immediate subcutaneous tissues, but because the practitioner is looking to determine intraepithelial disease or the presence of early invasion, it is not necessary to go deeper into the subcutaneous tissues, which can lead to significant hemorrhaging. With a small core biopsy limited to the immediate subcutaneous tissues, hemostasis can usually be obtained through the use of silver nitrate stick or, at most, some ferric subsulfate solution and local

pressure. It would be unusual to need to resort to a suture at the biopsy site.

## Treatment

Therapy for in situ carcinoma of the vulva can generally be thought of as falling into one of two techniques[3] (Table 42-4). These consist of either excisional therapy or use of topical agents, such as 5-fluorouracil or trichloroacetic acid, or other techniques such as laser vaporization or the ultrasonic surgical aspirator.

Excisional therapy consists of wide local excision of single lesions or several lesions in the case of extensive multifocal disease. This therapy may even necessitate the use of a skinning vulvectomy, the removal of all of the involved vulvar skin down to the level of the dartos fascia but sparing the subcutaneous tissues and thereby preserving the architecture, and through the use of a split-thickness skin graft to give an aesthetic result.

Topical agents or other destructive techniques are alterations that may be used when the risk of invasion is low. With any of these methods, an attempt should be made to obtain an approximately 1.0-cm margin around the lesions to prevent local recurrence.

Choice of therapy will often depend on the patient's age, the desire to maintain as normal an anatomic appearance as possible, and the location of the disease. Disease in the nonhair-bearing areas, where the skin is quite thin, is readily amenable to laser vaporization and other destructive techniques. With minimal destruction of the underlying dermis, healing is rapid and usually cosmetic. However, in hair-bearing areas, where the epithelial abnormality can extend into the hair follicles and therefore into the deeper subcutaneous tissues, use of these destructive therapies necessitates penetration into the deeper levels of the dermis, which may result in scarring that actually produces a worse cosmetic outcome than excisional therapy. Where concern about the possibility of underlying invasive cancer exists, it would be best to defer to excisional therapy to allow complete histologic evaluation of the entire specimen and margins. Chafe and colleagues reported on the risk of invasion in patients treated with wide local excision.[4] In a group of 69 patients thought to have intraepithelial disease only who underwent wide local excision, invasive disease was found in 13 patients, or 18.8%. In eight of the 13 patients, this was found to be microinvasion of less than 1.0 mm. However, four patients had invasion greater than 1.0 mm; an additional patient was found to have a verrucous carcinoma of the vulva.

| Table 42-4 |
| :-- |
| **Therapeutic Modalities for Carcinoma in Situ** |

**Destructive**

Topical 5 fluorouracil.
Laser vaporization.
CUSA.

**Excisional**

Wide local excision.
Skinning vulvectomy with or without split-thickness skin graft.

Gynecologic Oncology

With therapy, approximately 90% of patients will be rendered disease-free after a single therapeutic session. Regardless of the mode of therapy employed, approximately 10% of patients will "recur" and therefore must be subject to long-term follow-up. These recurrences most likely are actually the occurrence of new disease in an adjacent area of skin, especially in those patients who had adequate margins of resection at therapy. Under close follow-up, it is unlikely that patients will develop invasive disease. A previous report by Buscema and colleagues, which studied 102 patients followed for up to 15 years, revealed that only 4 patients subsequently developed invasive disease under observation after therapy.[5] Of these patients, 2 were postmenopausal, and two were receiving immunosuppression therapy for autoimmune diseases. It would appear that in those patients with lowered immunity, increased surveillance for the possible development of invasive disease is warranted.

## INVASIVE VULVAR CANCER

### Natural History and Pattern of Spread

Stanley Way addressed the American Gynecologic Society in the early 1960s, stating that failure to adequately treat vulvar cancer was due to incomplete removal of the primary lesion and/or a totally inadequate attack on the draining lymph nodes. As a result of his work along with that of others, standard care for vulvar cancer became an en bloc radical vulvectomy with bilateral inguinal-femoral lymphadenectomy and bilateral pelvic lymphadenectomy to completely excise the primary lesion, the skin at risk for recurrence, and all of the draining lymph node groups. The large skin excisions were also necessary due to the large size of the primary lesions and in many cases the associated clinically positive inguinal nodes that were commonly seen at the time. However, as experience accumulated and large series of cases were carefully examined, the natural history of the disease along with its mechanisms of spread became clearer, eventually allowing for improvements in the care and management of patients with vulvar cancer.

The primary mechanism of disease spread is via direct extension. The lesions tend to expand concentrically along mucosal surfaces and by invasion into the dermis and then deeper underlying structures. As lesions expand, they may also encroach on adjacent structures, notably the urethra, vagina, or anus; this is reflected in the staging system, with increasing stage being assigned, based first on the overall size and then on involvement of adjacent structures.

Secondary spread of vulvar cancer occurs via the draining lymphatics (Fig. 42-4). The vulvar skin actually migrates during fetal development from the lower abdomen into its final position. The primary lymphatic drainage follows along the external pudendal vessels to the inguinal lymph nodes. This group of nodes, also commonly referred to as the inguinal-femoral nodes, consist of the first level of lymph nodes, which are those above the cribriform fascia, commonly referred to as the superficial inguinal nodes (Fig. 42-5), and the femoral lymph nodes, which are located below the cribriform fascia and medial to the femoral artery and overlying the femoral vein. Lymphatic drainage then proceeds cranially through the inguinal ligament to the ipsilateral pelvic lymph nodes. An extensive anastomotic network surrounds the midline structures, theoretically allowing

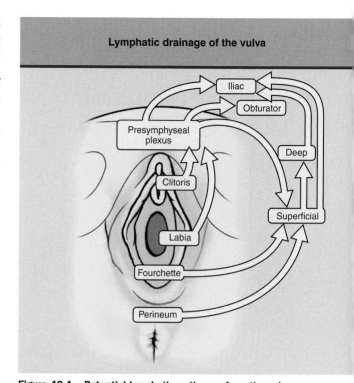

**Figure 42-4 Potential lymphatic pathways from the vulva.**
(From Plentl AA, Friedman EA: Lymphatic System of the Female Genitalia. Philadelphia: WB Saunders, 1971, p. 25 with permission.)

for drainage from either side to the contralateral inguinal-femoral lymph node group. However, extensive clinical experience has demonstrated that involvement of the contralateral nodes is extremely rare, unless there is primary involvement of the draining ipsilateral inguinal-femoral lymph nodes. Lesions that involve or approach the midline can, however, spread to either side with equal ease. Additionally, although it is theoretically possible for direct spread to occur to the pelvic lymph nodes along the dorsal artery and vein and internal pudendal vessels, which are direct branches of the anterior division of the internal iliac vessels, clinical experience has also found that direct involvement of the pelvic lymph nodes rarely occurs, even with midline lesions, unless there has been initial involvement of the inguinal-femoral lymph nodes on either side.

The current staging system for vulvar cancer utilizes surgical findings that reflect the spread pattern of the disease as it is now understood (Table 42-5). Stage increases based on the increasing size of the lesion and the involvement of adjacent structures. Stage also increases with any inguinal-femoral lymph node involvement, with further increases for either bilateral inguinal-femoral node involvement, or secondary pelvic lymph node involvement. In addition, stage increases with distant disease spread, which is rarely seen.

Various clinical parameters have been held out as prognostic factors for patients with carcinoma of the vulva. These have included size of the lesion, depth of invasion of the lesion, location, and status of the inguinal-femoral or pelvic lymph nodes.[6–9] When a factor is designated as prognostic, it is important to consider what it is prognostic for (Table 42-6). Although there is at least indirect correlation with all of the above factors and risk of recurrence or death, the most important factor in

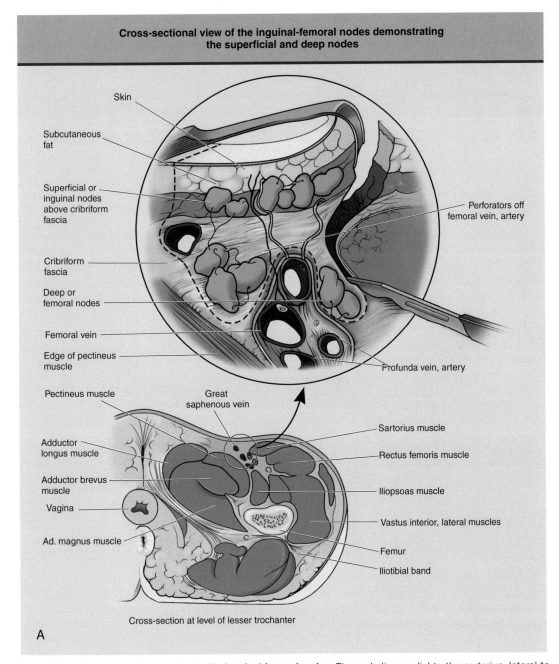

**Cross-sectional view of the inguinal-femoral nodes demonstrating the superficial and deep nodes**

Skin

Subcutaneous fat

Superficial or inguinal nodes above cribriform fascia

Cribriform fascia

Deep or femoral nodes

Femoral vein

Edge of pectineus muscle

Perforators off femoral vein, artery

Profunda vein, artery

Pectineus muscle

Great saphenous vein

Adductor longus muscle

Adductor brevus muscle

Vagina

Ad. magnus muscle

Sartorius muscle

Rectus femoris muscle

Iliopsoas muscle

Vastus interior, lateral muscles

Femur

Iliotibial band

Cross-section at level of lesser trochanter

A

**Figure 42-5  *A,* Anatomic landmarks for the inguinal-femoral nodes.** The node lies medial to the sartorius, lateral to the adductor longus, and above the pectineus muscles.                    *Continued*

predicting survival is the status of the inguinal-femoral lymph nodes. Additionally, the number of involved nodes is also highly predictive for survival. Patients who have more than two positive inguinal-femoral nodes show a marked decrease in survival relative to those patients with two or fewer positive nodes. The other clinical prognostic factors are indirectly associated with risk of recurrence; increasing size, increasing depth, and lesion location (bordering or involving the clitoris, urethra, or anus) may be associated with an increased risk of spread to the inguinal-femoral nodes.

The primary draining node group, the ipsilateral inguinal-femoral nodes, predicts for the possibility of spread to the pelvic node group or to the contralateral groin. Patients with two or more positive nodes are more likely to have microscopic spread to the other node groups.[10] As a result of this further spread along the lymphatic chains, they are also more likely to develop pelvic recurrences or distant disease that is unlikely to be amenable to further salvage therapies currently available (Table 42-7).

With the knowledge that the status of the inguinal nodes predicts not only the possibility of metastasis to the pelvic lymph nodes, but also an increased risk of pelvic recurrence and distant disease, the value of pelvic lymphadenectomy as a therapeutic procedure was questioned. This is especially important in light of the fact that additional node dissection can result in severe

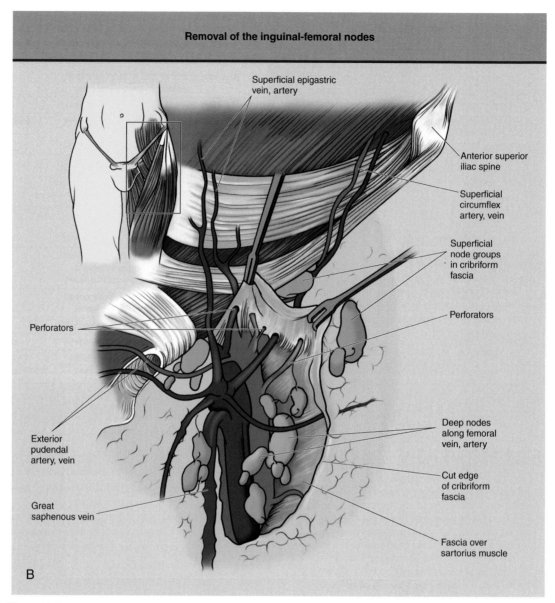

**Removal of the inguinal-femoral nodes**

Superficial epigastric
vein, artery

Anterior superior
iliac spine

Superficial
circumflex
artery, vein

Superficial
node groups
in cribriform
fascia

Perforators

Perforators

Deep nodes
along femoral
vein, artery

Exterior
pudendal
artery, vein

Cut edge
of cribriform
fascia

Great
saphenous vein

Fascia over
sartorius muscle

B

**Figure 42-5, cont'd** *B,* **View of the cribriform fascia separating the deep from the superficial nodes.** The deep
nodes can be seen around the femoral vessels.

increased morbidity, such as lymphedema and lymphangitis, added operative time, and carries the immediate risk of the surgical procedure itself. The Gynecologic Oncology Group (GOG) conducted a prospective randomized trial to evaluate the role of pelvic lymphadenectomy versus postoperative radiation therapy to potentially involved nodes in patients at risk.[11] Patients who were found to have positive inguinal-femoral nodes were randomized intraoperatively to either pelvic lymph node dissection or to postoperative radiation therapy to the pelvic lymph nodes after wound healing. Results showed that survival was significantly improved in the group that received radiation therapy (Fig. 42-6). The radiation therapy patients had fewer complications and significantly less lymphedema and other postoperative complications. This demonstration of both a survival benefit and significantly lower morbidity with postoperative radiation therapy led to the discontinuation of standard

pelvic lymphadenectomy. All patients with positive inguinal nodes are currently treated with adjuvant postoperative radiation therapy to the pelvic nodes.

### Treatment of the Inguinal-femoral Lymph Nodes
In treatment of invasive vulvar cancer, it is imperative that the inguinal-femoral nodes, as the primary draining nodes, be evaluated. Bilateral node dissection is indicated for lesions that approach the midline. For well-lateralized lesions, dissection of the contralateral inguinal-femoral nodes is indicated only if there is evidence of involvement of the nodes in the ipsilateral groin. Most clinicians currently would perform an ipsilateral node dissection only at the time of initial treatment and then a contralateral node dissection at a later date if indicated.

As part of the previous standard en bloc therapy, dissection of the inguinal-femoral nodes had traditionally been carried out

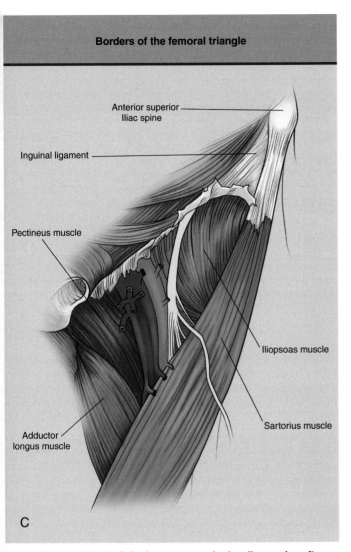

**Borders of the femoral triangle**

Anterior superior Iliac spine

Inguinal ligament

Pectineus muscle

Iliopsoas muscle

Sartorius muscle

Adductor longus muscle

C

**Figure 42-5, cont'd    C, Only the neurovascular bundle remains after complete dissection.** (From Copeland LJ, Jarrell JF: Textbook of Gynecology, 2nd ed. Philadelphia, WB Saunders, 1999, Fig. 53-4, 53-5.)

**Table 42-5**
**FIGO Staging of Carcinoma of the Vulva**

| | |
|---|---|
| T1 | Tumor confined to the vulva and/or perineum 2 cm or less in greatest dimension |
| T2 | Tumor confined to the vulva and/or perineum greater than 2 cm in greatest dimension |
| T3 | Tumor of any size with adjacent spread to the lower urethra and/or the vagina, and/or the anus |
| T4 | Tumor of any size invading the upper urethra, bladder mucosa, rectal mucosa, or pelvic bone |
| N0 | No lymph node metastasis |
| N1 | Unilateral regional lymph node metastasis |
| N2 | Bilateral regional lymph node metastasis |
| M0 | No clinical metastasis |
| M1 | Distant metastasis (including pelvic lymph node metastasis) |
| Stage I | T1 N0 M0 |
| IA | T1 ≤ 1 mm |
| IB | T1 > 1 mm |
| Stage II | T2 N0 M0 |
| Stage III | |
| IIIA | T3 N0 M0 |
| IIIB | T3 N1 M0 |
| | T2 N1 M0 |
| | T1 N1 M0 |
| Stage IV | |
| IVA | T4 N0 M0 |
| IVB | TX N2 M0 |
| | TX NX M1 |

**Table 42-6**
**Prognostic Factors in Invasive Vulvar Cancer**

**For nodal involvement**

Size
Depth of invasion
Lesion thickness
Grade
Vascular space involvement

**For survival**

Positive inguinal nodes
Positive pelvic nodes

**Table 42-7**
**Importance of Inguinal Node Status: Recurrence Site and Survival**

| Nodes Positive | Vulva | Groin | Pelvis | Systemic | Deaths |
|---|---|---|---|---|---|
| <3+ | 5.8% | 2.9% | 0% | 3.8% | 6.7% |
| ≥3+ | 33% | 33% | 44% | 66% | 88% |

with the excision of the skin bridge and the en bloc resection of the nodes. This was done because of the belief that the tumor could permeate into the lymphatics and that therefore an attempt to excise all the intervening skin was important to remove any tumor in transit in these lymphatic channels. Excision of the skin bridge often resulted in wound breakdown, infection, and prolonged hospitalizations. As it became clear that tumor embolizes to the primary lymph nodes rather than permeating the lymphatics, a thinner and thinner bridge was excised. Eventually, this resulted in the use of separate incisions for the node dissections, without resection of any intervening skin bridge.[12,13] There has not been a randomized prospective trial evaluating the use of separate incisions versus an en bloc resection, but comparison of patients treated via the triple, or separate, incision approach has clearly shown significant decreases in operative time and blood loss and, most importantly, a significant decrease in the incidence of breakdown of the wounds overlying the groin, which has resulted in significantly shorter postoperative stay (Table 42-8).

Attempts to eliminate inguinal-femoral node dissection have been fraught with hazard. Early detection of inguinal-femoral node metastasis would still allow for a possible cure; unfortunately, later detection of a recurrence in the groin in the inguinal-femoral node group is almost uniformly fatal. Hacker and colleagues[15] have shown, in a series of patients who had

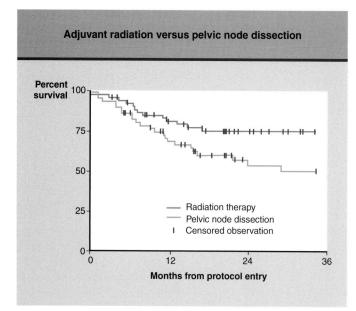

**Figure 42-6** Survival curve from GOG showing improved survival for those patients treated with radiation therapy rather than pelvic node dissection. (From Homesley HD, Bundy BN, Sedlis A, Adcock L: Radiation therapy versus pelvic node resection for carcinoma of the vulva with positive groin nodes. Obstet Gynecol 1986;68:733–740.)

undergone node dissection for clinically nonsuspicious nodes, that approximately 10% were found to have nodal metastasis; all of these patients were able to be salvaged. However, in a group of patients in whom node dissection was omitted, there was a 10% incidence of recurrence in the groin; none of these patients could be salvaged due to development of widespread disease. Therefore, early detection of involved inguinal-femoral nodes is important to allow for treatment before dissemination of disease to the secondary node groups and subsequent systemic spread can occur. An alternative to surgical therapy is radiation therapy to the groins at risk (bilaterally for midline lesions, unilateral for lateral lesions). When the GOG compared these techniques in a randomized trial, the trial was closed early due to the improvement in outcome (lower recurrences rates in the groins) in the patients undergoing surgical excision.[16] However, the greater failure rate in the radiation group may have been due to a failure to deliver an adequate dose to the appropriate depth in the groin tissues.[17]

| Table 42-8 Triple Incisions Versus En bloc Resection | | | |
|---|---|---|---|
| | Separate | Single | *p* |
| Operative time | 134 | 191 | 0.009 |
| Blood loss (mL) | 424 | 733 | 0.004 |
| Postop stay (days) | 9.7 | 17.2 | 0.012 |
| Breakdown | 3% | 19% | 0.045 |

From Helm CW, Hatch K, Austin JM, et al: A matched comparison of single- and triple-incision techniques for the surgical treatment of carcinoma of the vulva. Gynecol Oncol 1992;46:150–156.

A group of patients for whom the incidence of node metastasis is so low that inguinal-femoral node dissection can be omitted has now been established. Although the risk of nodal metastasis increases with increasing depth of invasion, as is seen in cervical cancers, there is an 8% to 10% incidence of nodal metastasis with lesions of 3.0 mm or less invasion in vulvar cancer, which is quite different from the less than 1% incidence of metastasis with less than 3.0 mm invasion in cervical cancer. The International Society for the Study of Vulvovaginal Diseases has defined *microinvasion* as those lesions that exhibit less than 1.0 mm of stromal invasion. This depth of invasion is measured from the top of the nearest uninvolved dermal papillae, because as other points of reference can alter the measurement (Fig. 42-7).

Lymph node dissection has typically been carried out through the use of a border technique, which involves defining all of the borders of dissection and then removing all of the nodes confined within those borders. The superior border of dissection is along the edge of the inguinal ligament. The medial border is defined as the lateral aspect of the adductor longus muscle, and the lateral border is along the medial aspect of the sartorius muscle. The apex of the dissection is where the adductor longus and sartorius intersect, forming the top of Hunter's canal. The superficial group of nodes lies deep to Camper's fascia and above the cribriform fascia that lies over the femoral vessels. The saphenous vein enters into the femoral vein as it passes through the fossa ovale in the cribriform fascia. The deep group of nodes lies along the medial aspect of the femoral artery and overlies the femoral vein, and drainage then extends cranially through the inguinal ligament into the pelvic node group. By carefully staying medial of the femoral artery, the clinician can avoid the femoral nerve, which lies outside the sheath. Preservation rather than transection of the saphenous vein during the dissection will allow for better collateral flow and will help prevent subsequent lymphedema.

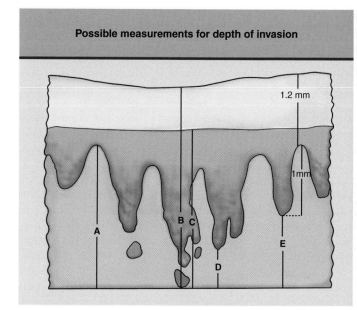

**Figure 42-7** Possible sites from which depth of invasion could be measured. (From Wilkinson, EJ: Superficial invasive carcinoma of the vulva. Clin Obstet Gynecol 1985;28:188.)

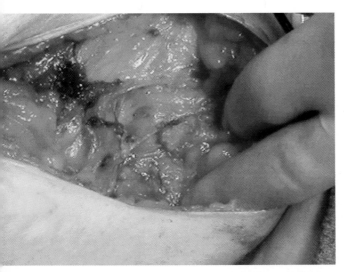

**Figure 42-8** Blue dye localized in a sentinel node in the superficial inguinal nodes.

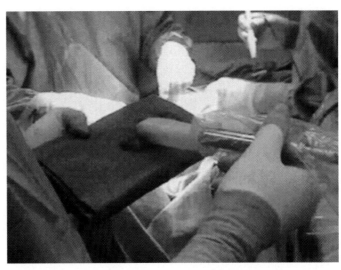

**Figure 42-10** A gamma counter is used to confirm that the labeled node has been excised.

Recent efforts have focused on an effort to identify the sentinel node, that node which would be the first to be subject to metastasis and which could then predict for the positivity or negativity of the entire inguinal-femoral node group.[18,19] In theory, if this node is negative, there would be no need for a further, complete node dissection. Before surgery, the leading edge of the tumor is injected subcutaneously with either a radioactive tracer of technetium or a blue-colored lymphophilic dye, which will then follow the draining lymphatics, allowing identification of the sentinel node by either direct visual inspection, in the case of the blue dye (Fig. 42-8) or through localization of the radioactivity in the case of the technetium colloid (Figs. 42-9 and 42-10). For lesions that approach the midline, both leading edges and both groins will obviously need to be examined. In almost 90% of cases that have been evaluated, the sentinel node is able to be identified, isolated, and examined. To date, most reports have also indicated good correlation between the status of the sentinel node and the status of the remaining inguinal-femoral nodes after a complete dissection. At this time, however, there is not enough data to allow for treatment decisions based on the status of the sentinel node alone. Further confirmation of its ability to predict the status of the residual nodes and absence of recurrence in the inguinal-femoral group is still required.

### Treatment of the Primary Lesion

Universal treatment of the primary lesion by radical vulvectomy resulted in resection of large amounts of normal tissue, especially in patients with smaller localized lesions. The larger defects would therefore be associated with increasing incidence of breakdown, wound infection, and long hospitalizations to allow for secondary healing of the surgical bed. Additionally, very few subclinical lesions were noted in the radical vulvectomy specimens, questioning the need for the prophylactic resection of normal vulvar tissue. In lesions that were lateralized or well situated either anteriorly or posteriorly along the vulva, initial efforts focused on a radical hemivulvectomy to remove the lesion with wide margins. Investigators also began to look at a radical local excision for smaller lesions (Fig. 42-11). In such an excision, an attempt was made to obtain margins at a minimum of 1 cm around the primary lesion, with a depth of excision extending down to the inferior fascia of the urogenital diaphragm, as with the standard en bloc radical vulvectomy.[13,15,20,21] Lesions that were far enough removed from either the anal mucosa, vaginal mucosa, or urethral orifice should be able to be widely resected with either the en bloc or radical local excision techniques. However, when lesions were closely approximating any of these structures, the difficulty in obtaining an adequate margin would be equivalent for either technique, and additional excision of the lateral tissues would not improve the ability to obtain an adequate margin. Retrospective evaluation of groups of patients treated by radical excision rather than the en bloc technique has

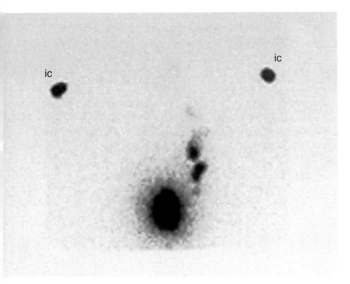

**Figure 42-9** Technetium-99 scan after injection of the vulvar lesion. The center spot at the bottom represents excreted label. Two sentinel nodes can be seen just above and to the left of the bladder. IC, illiac crest.

639

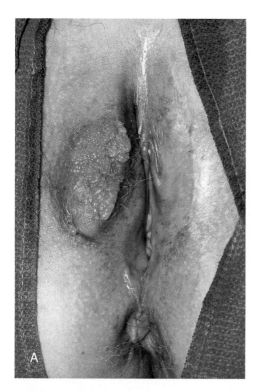

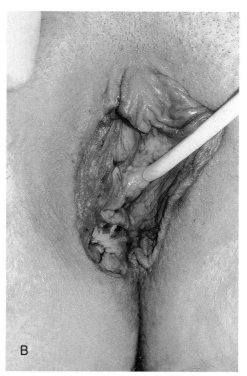

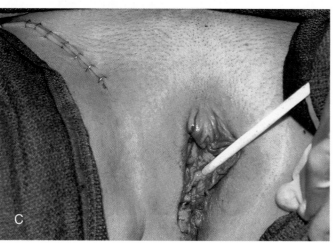

**Figure 42-11    Cancer of the vulva.** *A*, A T1 lesion on the right side of the vulva. *B*, Defect after excision of the primary lesion. *C*, Postoperative results after closure and node dissection via separate incisions.

shown equivalent rates of local control with similar rates of local recurrence.[15] In fact, the best predictor of local control is the adequacy of the margin on the surgical specimen (Table 42-9),[22] and as previously noted this will depend on the lesion's proximity to the anal, vaginal, or urethral orifices. Extending the margins beyond a minimum of 1 cm doesn't improve local control rates and only results in larger defects.

Problems arise whenever a lesion extends to involve the vagina, urethra, or anus. This could result from a lesion arising in proximity to one of these structures or may be due to neglect of a lesion that spreads along the epithelial surface and eventually involves one of these structures. If an attempt is made to obtain an adequate margin, it would necessitate an exenteration, with subsequent loss of bowel, bladder, or sexual function. Reconstruction might return some, but certainly not all, function. To try to preserve function and anatomy, radiation therapy was given prior to surgical excision; approximately 75% of patients

had regression sufficient to allow preservation of sphincter or vaginal function.[23] Most patients can therefore be saved from an exenteration. However, if local recurrence occurs in the radiated area, an exenteration would offer the only possibility for a cure. In an effort to improve the local control achieved with radiation

| Table 42-9 Value of the Margin | | |
| --- | --- | --- |
| **Margin** | **Patients** | **Local Recurrences** |
| <1 cm | 44 | 21 |
| >1 cm | 91 | 0 |

From Heaps JM, Fu YS, Montz FJ, et al: Surgical pathologic variables predictive of local recurrence in squamous cell carcinoma of the vulva. Gynecol Oncol 1990;38:309–314.

| Table 42-10 Efficacy of Synchronous Chemoradiation | | |
| --- | --- | --- |
| | **Number** | **Percent** |
| Patients | 71 | 100% |
| Clinical chemoradiation | 33 | 46% |
| Pathologic chemoradiation | 22 | 31% |
| No exenteration | 68 | 96% |

From Moore DH, Thomas GM, Montana 65, et al: Preoperative chemoradiation for advanced vulvar cancer: a phase II study of the GOG. Int J Radiat Oncol Biol Phys 1998;42:79–85.

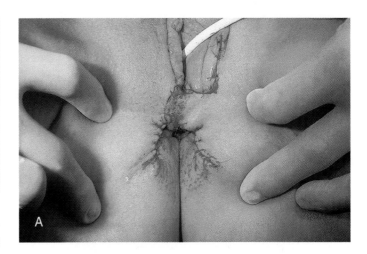

therapy, recent studies have focused on the addition of synchronous chemotherapy,[24,25] usually with platinum-containing regimens, as a radiation sensitizer, especially given the improvement that was seen in advanced squamous cancers of the cervix. In the GOG study reported by Moore,[24] 48% of patients had a complete clinical response to combined chemoradiation, and almost all were managed without an exenterative procedure (Table 42-10).

Even with a conservative approach, with an attempt to obtain adequate margins, a radical local excision can result in a large defect that is difficult to close primarily. Historically, large defects were allowed to close by secondary intention, resulting in prolonged hospitalizations. If the defect is not very large, local flaps or Z-plasties could be used to advance skin and provide a blood supply in the area to aid in closure[26] (Fig. 42-12). In the case of a large defect or when there has been prior radiation to reduce the size of a large lesion, a myocutaneous flap is necessary to not only fill the defect, but also bring in a new blood supply to aid in healing. Using the gracilis myocutaneous flap from the medial aspect of the thigh can allow for coverage of the vulva and also for filling in a portion of the vagina, if necessary, by rotating the flap superiorly and medially into the defect.[27]

## RECURRENT DISEASE

Disease recurrence can be manifest either locally, in the groins, or distally (including pelvic lymph node recurrence). Local recurrence is either due to an inadequate margin at initial therapy or new disease in another area of the vulva. The treatment of a local recurrence is guided by the same principles as the treatment of a primary lesion. Groin recurrence is almost inevitably fatal,[10] as previously discussed (see Table 42-7). If the groin has not been previously radiated, it might be possible to excise grossly positive nodes or use radiation to the groin for palliation. If, however, radiation has been used already or in the case of distant disease, palliative chemotherapy is the only treatment option. Chemotherapy is usually based around platinum, either alone or in combination, as with squamous cancers of the cervix.

## OTHER VULVAR NEOPLASMS

Malignant melanoma is the second most common malignancy arising on the vulva, yet it accounts for only 5% of vulvar malignancies, and these are relatively uncommon to begin with. Therefore, most experience with these lesions has come from

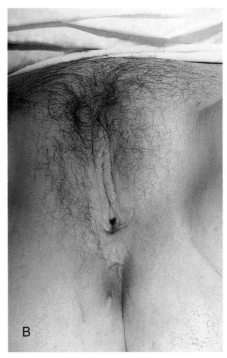

**Figure 42-12  Cancer of the vulva.** *A*, A rhomboid flap has been used to close the perineal defect. *B*, Result at 3 months' postsurgery.

small series of patients accumulated over a fairly long period. Most patients will initially present with some form of growth or abnormal bleeding. An analysis of patients treated with at least a radical hemivulvectomy revealed that the 1992 American Joint Committee on Cancer (AJCC) staging correlated best with progression-free survival, followed by Breslow's staging based on thickness of the tumor.[28] As most patients had initially presented with advanced tumors, radical surgeries were often proposed to try to treat the lesions and the draining inguinal-femoral nodes, only to have patients fail with distant disease. This, along with the findings from the GOG study, which indicated that vulvar melanoma tends to behave similarly to other cutaneous melanomas,[28] has prompted a more conservative management, as with other cutaneous melanomas. The primary lesion is treated by radical local excision with reconstruction of the defect; groin node dissection may be performed depending on the clinical status of the nodes and on Breslow's staging.

Cancer arising in Bartholin's gland can have several different appearances. Almost all patients will present with a lump appearing in the area of the gland and occasionally with bleeding. Squamous cancers can arise from the duct opening, whereas transitional cell lesions can arise from the remainder of the duct. Adenocarcinoma, including the adenoid cystic variant, can arise from the gland itself. Therapy for these lesions is also guided by the current treatment principles for squamous cancers of the vulva. The goal is for a radical resection of the primary lesion along with lymphadenectomy in the ipsilateral groin. Due to the location of the gland, deep within the vuvlar tissue, overlying the urogenital diaphragm, there is a greater probability of a compromised deep margin and the need for postoperative radiation as a result.

Extramammary Paget's disease can also arise on the vulva and usually presents as a brick-red fiery lesion that is usually intensely pruritic. Most cases of Paget's disease are intraepithelial, and invasion and metastases are uncommon. However, as with Paget's disease of the breast, a significant association with the development of a second neoplasm exists. This could be an associated underlying adenocarcinoma in the vulvar tissue or, more commonly, a second neoplasm in the breast or colon (about 25% of patients).[29]

# REFERENCES

1. Taussig FJ: Cancer of the vulva: An analysis of 155 cases (1911–1940). Amer J Obstet Gynecol 1940;40:764. **(III, B)**
2. Brinton LA, Nasca PC, Mallin K, et al: Case-control study of cancer of the vulva. Obstet Gynecol 1990;75:859–866. **(IIa, B)**
3. Kaufman RH: Intraepithelial neoplasia of the vulva. Gynecol Oncol 1995;56:8–21. **(IV, C)**
4. Chafe W, Richards A, Morgan L, et al: Unrecognized invasive carcinoma in vulvar intraepithelial neoplasia (VIN). Gynecol Oncol 1988;31:154–165. **(IIa, B)**
5. Buscema J, Woodruff JD, Parmley T, et al: Carcinoma in situ of the vulva. Obstet Gynecol 1980;55:225–230. **(IV, C)**
6. Homesley HD, Bundy BN, Sedlis A, et al: Prognostic factors for groin node metastasis in squamous cell carcinoma of the vulva (a GOG study). Gynecol Oncol 1993;49:279–283. **(IIa, B)**
7. Sedlis A, Homesley H, Bundy BN, et al: Positive groin lymph nodes in superficial squamous cell vulvar cancer. Am J Obstet Gynecol 1987;156:1159. **(IIa, B)**
8. Rutledge FN, Mitchell MF, Munsell MF, et al: Prognostic indicators for invasive carcinoma of the vulva. Gynecol Oncol 1991;42:239–244. **(II, B)**
9. Binder SW, Huang I, Fu YS, Hacker NF, Berek JS: Risk factors for the development of lymph node metastasis in vulvar squamous cell carcinoma. Gynecol Oncol 1990;37:9–16. **(III, B)**
10. Hacker NF, Berek JS, Lagasse LD, Leuchter RS, Moore JG: Management of regional lymph nodes and their prognostic influence in vulvar cancer. Obstet Gynecol 1983;61:408–412. **(III, B)**
11. Homesley HD, Bundy BN, Sedlis A, Adcock L: Radiation therapy versus pelvic node resection for carcinoma of the vulva with positive groin nodes. Obstet Gynecol 1986;68:733–740. **(Ib, A)**
12. Stehman FB, Bundy BN, Dvoretsky PM, Creasman T: Early Stage I carcinoma of the vulva treated with ipsilateral superficial inguinal lymphadenectomy and modified radical hemivulvectomy: a prospective study of the GOG. Obstet Gynecol 1992;79:490–497. **(IIa, B)**
13. Burke TW, Levenback C, Coleman RC, et al: Surgical therapy of T1 and T2 vulvar carcinoma: further experience with radical wide excision and selective inguinal lymphadenectomy. Gynecol Oncol 1995;57:215–220. **(IV, C)**
14. Helm CW, Hatch K, Austin JM, et al: A matched comparison of single and triple incision techniques for the surgical treatment of carcinoma of the vulva. Gynecol Oncol 1992;46:150–156. **(IIb, B)**
15. Hacker NF, Berek JS, Lagasse LD, et al: Individualization of treatment for Stage I squamous cell vulvar carcinoma. Obstet Gynecol 1984;63:155–162. **(III, B)**
16. Stehman F, Bundy B, Thomas G, et al: Groin dissection versus groin radiation in carcinoma of the vulva: a GOG study. Int J Radiat Oncol Biol Phys 1992;24:389–396. **(Ib, A)**
17. Koh WJ, Chiu M, Stelzer KJ, et al: Femoral vessel depth and the implications for groin node radiation. Int J Radiat Oncol Biol Phys 1993;27:969–974. **(III, B)**
18. DeHullu JA, Hollema H, Piers DA, et al: Sentinel lymph node procedure is highly accurate in squamous cell carcinoma of the vulva. J Clin Oncol 2000;18:2811–2816. **(IIa, B)**
19. Levenback C, Coleman RL, Burke TW, Bodurka-Bevers D, Wolf JK, Gershenson DM: Intraoperative lymphatic mapping and sentinel node identification with blue dye in patients with vulvar cancer. Gynecol Oncol 2001;83:276–281. **(IIa, B)**
20. DiSaia PJ, Creasman WT, Rich WM. An alternative approach to early cancer of the vulva. Am J Obstet Gynecol 1979;133:825–832. **(IV, C)**
21. Berman ML, Soper JT, Creasman WT, et al: Conservative surgical management of superficially invasive Stage I vulvar carcinoma. Gynecol Oncol 1989;35:352–357. **(III, B)**
22. Heaps JM, Fu YS, Montz FJ, et al: Surgical pathologic variables predictive of local recurrence in squamous cell carcinoma of the vulva. Gynecol Oncol 1990;38:309–314. **(III, B)**
23. Boronow RC, Hickman BT, Reagan MT, Smith A, Steadham RE: Combined therapy as an alternative to exenteration for locally advanced vulvovaginal cancer: II. Results, complications and dosimetric and surgical considerations. Am J Clin Oncol 1987;10:171–181. **(III, B)**
24. Moore DH, Thomas GM, Montana GS, et al: Preoperative chemoradiation for advanced vulvar cancer: a phase II study of the GOG. Int J Radiat Oncol Biol Phys 1998;42:79–85. **(IIa, B)**
25. Koh WJ, Wallace HJ, Greer BE, et al: Combined radiotherapy and chemotherapy in the management of local-regionally advanced vulvar cancer. Int J Radiat Oncol Biol Phys 1993;26:809–816. **(III, B)**
26. Hoffman MS, LaPolla JP, Roberts WS, Fiorca JV, Cavanagh D. Use of local flaps for primary anal reconstruction following perianal resection for neoplasia. Gynecol Oncol 1990;36:348–352. **(III, B)**
27. Burke TW, Morris M, Roh MS, Levenback C, Gershenson DM: Perineal reconstruction using single gracilis myocutaneous flaps. Gynecol Oncol 1995;57:221–225. **(III, B)**
28. Phillips GL, Bundy BN, Okagaki T, Kucera PR, Stehman FB: Malignant melanoma of the vulva treated by radical hemivulvectomy. A prospective study of the Gynecologic Oncology Group. Cancer 1994;73:2626–2632. **(IIa, B)**
29. Feuer GA, Shevchuk M, Calanog A: Vulvar Paget's disease: the need to exclude an invasive lesion. Gynecol Oncol 1990;38:81–89. **(III, B)**

## KEY POINTS

- The majority of malignancies involving the vagina are metastatic lesions.
- Primary vaginal carcinoma represents approximately 1% to 2% of all gynecologic malignancies.
- Most primary vaginal carcinomas present with some type of vaginal bleeding or discharge.
- Radiation therapy is the mainstay of treatment for primary vaginal carcinomas, but because of their rarity, treatment of these tumors must be individualized.

## ANATOMY

The vagina is a tubelike muscular structure averaging 6 to 8 cm in length that is located between the uterus/cervix and the vulva, anterior to the rectum, and posterior to the bladder. The vagina is composed of three layers: an inner mucosal layer, a muscularis layer, and an outer adventitial layer. The mucosal layer is a nonkeratinizing squamous epithelium with no glands. An inner circular layer and an outer longitudinal layer of smooth muscle make up the muscularis layer. The adventitial layer is made of connective tissue that is contiguous with the other organs of the pelvis.

The vagina is composed of a rich network of lymphatic channels, and drainage to regional lymph node chains depends on location within the vagina itself. The middle to upper vaginal lymphatics anastomose with the lymphatics of the cervix and primarily drain to the pelvic lymph nodes (obturator, external iliac, and internal iliac nodes). The lower vagina drains similar to the vulva, going initially to the inguinal nodes. Lymphatics from the posterior vagina communicate to the rectal, gluteal, and sacral node chains.

## EPIDEMIOLOGY

Primary vaginal carcinoma represents only about 1% to 2% of all gynecologic malignancies. The majority of malignancies involving the vagina are metastatic lesions. These metastatic lesions most commonly arise from the cervix and vulva or occur as a result of hematogenous or lymphatic spread. There are expected to be approximately 2140 new cases of primary vaginal cancer diagnosed in 2005 in the United States.[1] A decreased incidence of primary vaginal carcinomas has been noted in the recent past, most likely secondary to earlier detection of premalignant conditions with cervicovaginal cytology. To be considered a primary vaginal cancer the lesion must arise in the vagina and not involve the external cervical os or the vulva. Most of these primary vaginal carcinomas, approximately 85% to 90%, are squamous subtype. The mean age at diagnosis of the squamous subtype is approximately 60 years. Adenocarcinomas, melanomas, sarcomas, and lymphomas have also been shown to arise primarily from the vagina (Table 43-1).[2-9] This chapter discusses premalignant lesions of the vagina and primary vaginal carcinoma.

### Vaginal Intraepithelial Neoplasia

Vaginal intraepithelial neoplasia is much less common than intraepithelial neoplasia of the cervix or vulva. The classification of vaginal intraepithelial neoplasia is similar to that of cervical lesions: vaginal intraepithelial neoplasia 1 (mild dysplasia), vaginal intraepithelial neoplasia 2 (moderate dysplasia), vaginal intraepithelial neoplasia 3 (severe dysplasia). Some patients with vaginal intraepithelial neoplasia may present with vaginal bleeding or discharge, but the majority of patients are asymptomatic. It is most commonly found during the evaluation of an abnormal Papanicolau (Pap) smear. An abnormal Pap smear in a patient with no abnormal cervical pathology or in a patient without a cervix should prompt investigation of the vaginal mucosa. It is more common for the proximal vagina to be involved. Most patients with vaginal intraepithelial neoplasia have a prior history of lower genital tract neoplasia, previously involving the cervix or vulva. Like cervical and vulvar intraepithelial neoplasia, vaginal intraepithelial neoplasia is also associated with human papillomavirus (HPV).

Colposcopy of the vagina is performed in a manner similar to colposcopy of the cervix, and colposcopic abnormalities of the vagina are similar to those described in the cervix. It can be quite difficult to adequately visualize the entire vagina when evaluating an abnormal Pap smear. It is usually necessary to manipulate the speculum during examination to view the entire vaginal mucosa secondary to the vaginal folds. Lugol's solution (aqueous iodine) can often aid in demarcating abnormal vaginal mucosa and can be utilized for both diagnosis and treatment (Fig. 43-1). Biopsy of an abnormal-appearing area can usually be accomplished as an office procedure without anesthesia.

The management of vaginal intraepithelial neoplasia depends on the degree of abnormality and the location of the disease. Vaginal intraepithelial neoplasia 1 is usually managed by observation. It is not uncommon for vaginal intraepithelial neoplasia 2 and 3 to involve the vagina in a multifocal nature, secondary to the HPV effect. Vaginal intraepithelial neoplasia 2 and 3 are premalignant conditions and can be treated in various ways. Traditionally, treatment modalities for vaginal intraepithelial neoplasia 2 and 3 consisted of surgical excision (vaginectomy) or vaginal irradiation. These modalities have been associated with significant morbidity, including vaginal shortening, vaginal

# Gynecologic Oncology

| Table 43-1 |  |
| --- | --- |
| **Primary Vaginal Carcinoma Histologic Distribution** | |
| **Histologic Subtype** | **Percentage** |
| Squamous | 85–90 |
| Adenocarcinoma | 8–10 |
| Sarcoma | 2–4 |
| Melanoma | 1 |
| Other | 1 |

Data from Benedet JL, Murphy KJ, Fairey RN, et al: Primary invasive carcinoma of the vagina. Obstet Gynecol 1983;62:715–719; Peters WA, Kumar NB, Morley GW: Carcinoma of the vagina: factors influencing treatment. Cancer 1985;55:892–897; Rubin C, Young J, Mikuta JJ: Squamous carcinoma of the vagina: treatment, complications, and long-term follow-up. Gynecol Oncol 1985;20:346–353; Kucera H, Langer M, Smekol G, et al: Radiotherapy of primary carcinoma of the vagina: management and results of different therapy schemes. Gynecol Oncol 1985;21:87–93; Eddy GL, Marks RD II, Miller MC, et al: Primary invasive vaginal carcinoma. Am J Obstet Gynecol 1991;165:292–296; Stock RG, Chen AS, Seski J: A 30-year experience in the management of primary carcinoma of the vagina: analysis of prognostic factors and treatment modalities. Gynecol Oncol 1995;56:45–52; Kirkbride P, Fyles A, Rawlings GA, et al: Carcinoma of the vagina: experience at the Princess Margaret Hospital (1974–1989). Gynecol Oncol 1995;56:435–443; and Chyle N, Zagars GK, Wheeler JA, et al: Definitive radiotherapy for carcinoma of the vagina: outcome and prognostic factors. Int Radiat Oncol Biol Phys 1996;35:891–905.

scarring, and problems with postoperative sexual function. More contemporary therapy has been to use $CO_2$ laser in the treatment of vaginal intraepithelial neoplasia. Chemical treatment with 5-fluorouracil can also be utilized. Cavitron ultrasonic surgical aspirator has also been used to treat vaginal intraepithelial neoplasia.[10]

The $CO_2$ laser treatment is favored by most. This method provides an excellent cosmetic result and enables the physician to more easily treat multifocal disease with limited morbidity. The vaginal mucosa should be treated to a depth of up to 1 mm. Larger spot sizes and the superpulse mode are used to avoid deep penetration and the conduction of excessive heat. Power settings used range between 10 and 40 watts. The potential disadvantage of using the $CO_2$ laser for the treatment of vaginal intraepithelial neoplasia is that this ablative therapy provides no tissue specimen; therefore, liberal biopsy is recommended before employing the $CO_2$ laser to rule out an invasive process.

## SQUAMOUS CELL CARCINOMAS

The majority of primary vaginal carcinomas are exophytic squamous lesions and present with vaginal bleeding and/or discharge (Fig. 43-2). Presenting symptoms such as pelvic pain or changes in bowel/bladder habits usually suggest a more advanced process. Most vaginal carcinomas occur in older women and arise in the upper one third of the vagina, especially the posterior wall. It is mandatory to inspect and palpate the entire vagina during a pelvic examination, especially when unexplained vaginal bleeding is present. This often involves rotating the speculum as smaller more proximal tumors at the vaginal apices may go unnoticed. Verrucous carcinoma is a rare variant of squamous cell carcinoma that can arise in the vagina. Grossly these tumors present as a cauliflower-like mass.

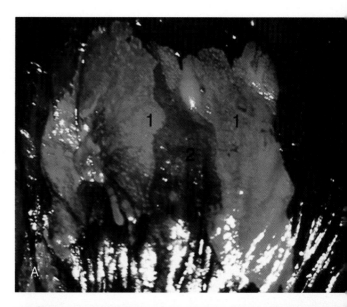

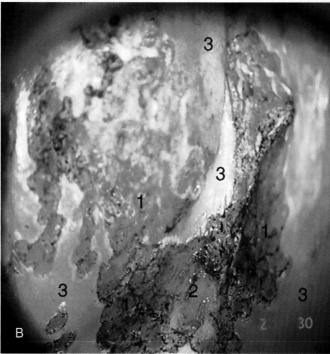

**Figure 43-1** *A*, The upper vagina after application of Lugol's solution. Areas labeled 1 do not stain and represent dysplastic precancerous changes. Areas labeled 2 are normal squamous mucosa of the vagina. *B*, Areas of vaginal mucosa after treatment with $CO_2$ laser (labeled 1 and 2). Untreated normal squamous mucosa of the vagina is labeled 3. (From Singer A, Monaghan J [eds]: Lower Genital Tract Precancer, Colposcopy, Pathology and Treatment, 2nd ed. London, Blackwell Science, 2000, pp 224 and 228.)

### Diagnosis

Direct biopsy of the vaginal tumor can almost always be accomplished with office punch biopsy. Abnormal cytologic findings on Pap smear (Fig. 43-3) or routine pelvic examination should prompt further evaluation. The range of patients who develop primary vaginal cancer after a previous hysterectomy

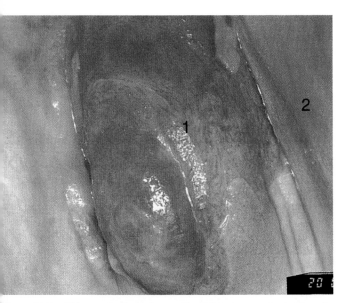

**Figure 43-2    This exophytic lesion on the right upper vaginal sidewall is a squamous cell vaginal cancer.** (From Singer A, Monaghan J [eds]: Lower Genital Tract Precancer, Colposcopy, Pathology and Treatment, 2nd ed. London, Blackwell Science, 2000, pp 224 and 228.)

varies between 36% and 59%.[11,12] A significant number of these patients have a prior history of lower genital tract neoplasia.

Vaginal carcinoma is a clinically staged disease. International Federation of Gynecology and Obstetrics (FIGO) staging can be seen in Table 43-2. Most primary vaginal carcinomas have spread beyond the vaginal mucosa at the time of diagnosis (Fig. 43-4). Stage II vaginal carcinoma can further be subdivided into IIa (submucosal involvement without parametrial involvement) and IIb (submucosal involvement with parametrial involvement).

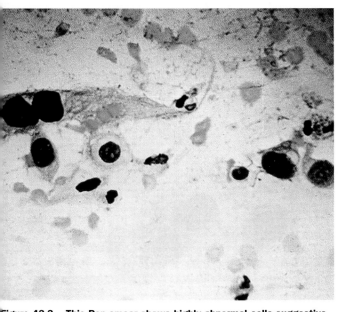

**Figure 43-3    This Pap smear shows highly abnormal cells suggestive of malignancy.** (From Baggish M [ed]: Colposcopy of Cervix, Vagina, and Vulva: A Comprehensive Textbook. St. Louis: Mosby, 2003, p 20.)

| Table 43-2 FIGO Staging for Vaginal Carcinoma | |
|---|---|
| Stage 0 | Carcinoma in situ |
| Stage I | Limited to the vaginal wall |
| Stage II | Subvaginal tissue not involving pelvic sidewall |
| Stage III | Carcinoma extending to pelvic sidewall |
| Stage IVa | Carcinoma involves mucosa of bladder or rectum and/or extends beyond the true pelvis |
| Stage IVb | Distant metastasis |

Once vaginal carcinoma is diagnosed, workup usually includes examination under anesthesia, cystoscopy, proctoscopy, and chest x-ray. Abdominopelvic computed tomography scan or magnetic resonance imaging are often done to evaluate for metastatic disease and to assist in treatment planning. Additional evaluation with endocervical curettage, endometrial curettage, intravenous pyelogram, barium enema, positron-emission tomography or a pretreatment laparotomy may also be beneficial in treatment planning.

The incidence of clinically positive lymph nodes at the time of diagnosis varies between 3% and 20% (Table 43-3).[9,13,14] Involved lymph node chains can vary and include pelvic, inguinal, or sacral/rectal, depending mostly on the location of the primary lesion.

### Risk Factors

The cause of squamous cell carcinoma of the vagina is unknown. It is believed that most squamous vaginal carcinomas share the same etiology as squamous cervical carcinomas. Because of their relative rarity, primary vaginal carcinomas are much less studied than their cervical counterparts. A recent report by Daling and colleagues identified several risk factors for vaginal carcinoma similar to previously identified cervical carcinomas risk factors.[15] These authors reported prior HPV infection, more than five lifetime sexual partners, onset of intercourse before age 17, and smoking to be associated with primary vaginal carcinoma.

Also shown to be at risk were those patients who have undergone hysterectomy. Other potential risk factors for primary

| Table 43-3 Clinically Positive Pelvic Nodes in Carcinoma of the Vagina | | |
|---|---|---|
| Reference | Patients with Clinically Positive Nodes (N) | Patients with Clinically Positive Node (%) |
| Plentl et al. | 141/679 | 20.8 |
| Perez et al. | 6/113 | 5.3 |
| Chyle et al. | 14/301 | 5.0 |

Plentl AA, Friedman EA: Lymphatic System of the Female Genitalia: The Morphologic Basis of Oncologic Diagnosis and Therapy. Philadelphia, WB Saunders, 1971, p 51; Perez CA, Camel HM, Galakatos AE, et al: Definitive irradiation in carcinoma of the vagina: long-term evaluation of results. Int J Radiat Oncol Biol Phys 1988;15:1283–1290; and Chyle V, Zagars GK, Wheeler JA, et al: Definitive radiotherapy for carcinoma of the vagina: outcome and prognostic factors. Int J Radiat Oncol Biol Phys 1996;35:891–905.

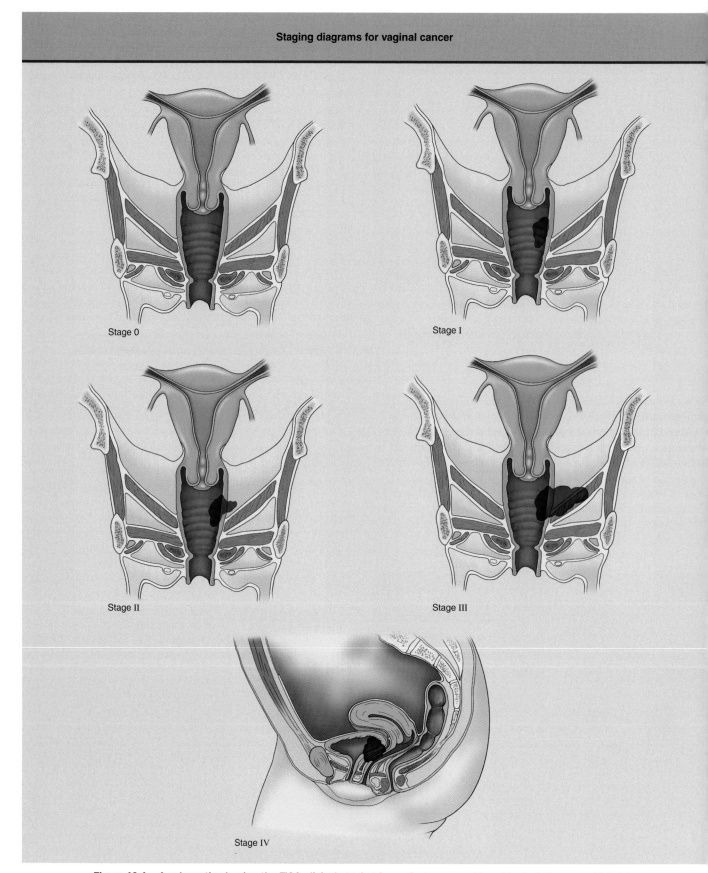

**Staging diagrams for vaginal cancer**

Stage 0

Stage I

Stage II

Stage III

Stage IV

**Figure 43-4  A schematic showing the FIGO clinical staging for vaginal cancers.** (From Disaia P, Creasman W [eds]: Clinical Gynecologic Oncology. St. Louis: Mosby, 1997, p 236.)

vaginal carcinoma include low socioeconomic status, vaginal trauma, and vaginal discharge/irritation. Prior irradiation has been considered a risk factor, but this remains controversial.

## Prognostic Factors

As with all other gynecologic malignancies, stage of disease is the most important prognostic factor in primary vaginal carcinoma. Overall survival based on stage of disease is shown in Table 43-4.[2,4-6,8] Primary tumors arising in the upper vagina have been shown by Chyle and colleagues to portend a better prognosis.[9] Others, however, have not shown this same trend.[13] Grade, patient age, and gross tumor appearance have not been shown to be of independent prognostic significance.

## Treatment

Radiation therapy is the cornerstone of treatment for primary squamous cell vaginal carcinoma; however, because of the low overall incidence of this disease, therapy must be individualized based on stage of disease and location of the tumor. Surgery is usually reserved for small stage I lesions or in patients with stage IVa disease or patients with a centralized recurrence, in whom a pelvic exenteration may be necessary. Some clinicians favor the use of chemoradiation with radiosensitizing agents such as cisplatin or 5-fluorouracil, extrapolating data from the treatment of locally advanced cervical cancer.

The majority of patients with primary vaginal carcinoma are treated with radiotherapy. Achieving a total tumor dose of 7000 cGy has been shown to improve local tumor control.[9] This most commonly involves a combination of teletherapy and intracavitary/interstitial therapy. Some small stage I and II lesions may be adequately treated with intracavitary/interstitial therapy alone. Larger (>2 cm) stage I and II lesions are customarily treated initially with teletherapy to a dose of 4000 to 5000 cGy. Pelvic lymph nodes are included in this external radiation field; this technique usually decreases tumor size, such that subsequent treatment can be performed with intracavitary/interstitial implants. If the tumor is distally located in the lower vagina the

inguinal lymph nodes are more frequently involved and should be treated either with surgical excision or radiotherapy.

When surgery is utilized to treat selected stage I lesions (usually involving the upper vagina), a radical hysterectomy, partial vaginectomy, and pelvic lymphadenectomy are performed. In those patients who have undergone a previous hysterectomy a radical upper vaginectomy with pelvic lymphadenectomy is done.

Regardless of the therapy that is instituted, serious complications are seen in up to 10% to 15% of cases. These can include the following: vesicovaginal or rectovaginal fistula, rectal stricture, rectal ulceration, and radiation-induced necrosis of the vagina. Less severe and more common side effects of treatment include cystitis, proctitis, and radiation fibrosis of the vagina.

### Survival and Recurrent Disease

The overall 5-year survival rate is approximately 40% to 45% (see Table 43-4).[2,4-6,8] The overall survival is lower than that for cervical and vulvar cancers. This is thought to be secondary to more advanced disease at the time of diagnosis and the technical difficulty in treating these tumors.

Most recurrences from primary vaginal cancer occur within 2 years of treatment and occur in the pelvis. Pelvic exenteration can be performed in appropriate candidates with central pelvic recurrences. Chemotherapy has usually been reserved for recurrence at distant sites. The treatment results with chemotherapy for recurrent disease are generally quite poor.

## ADENOCARCINOMAS

Adenocarcinomas of the vagina are much less common than squamous carcinomas. Adenocarcinomas can affect women of all ages; however, a clear cell variant affecting younger females has been extensively described. When an adenocarcinoma of the vagina is found in a postmenopausal female consideration should be given to a metastatic process originating in the uterus, ovary, fallopian tube, colon, or rectum.

In 1971, Herbst and colleagues were the first to report an association between in utero diethylstilbestrol (DES) exposure and clear cell carcinoma of the vagina in young women.[16] More commonly these women were found to develop vaginal adenosis, or benign structural abnormalities such as a cervical collar, a cockscomb cervix, or a transverse vaginal septum. Herbst and Scully found that the majority of women with clear cell cancer of the vagina had a documented in utero exposure to DES. With the discontinuation of DES usage in the early 1970s this clear cell variant has become much less common.

The incidence of clear cell vagina carcinoma in those who were exposed to DES prenatally is approximately 1 in 1000. The median age at diagnosis is approximately 19 years, and more than 90% of these tumors are diagnosed early in stages I and II. The risk has been shown to be greatest in those women who were exposed in the first 20 weeks of gestation. Clear cell vaginal carcinomas are most frequently observed in the upper anterior vaginal wall, in contrast to squamous lesions, which are mostly in the upper posterior vagina.

Adenocarcinoma of the vagina is generally treated in a manner similar to squamous carcinoma of the vagina; however, because of the rarity of these tumors treatment is often

**Table 43-4**
**Overall Survival in Primary Vaginal Carcinoma**

| Stage | Number of Patients | 5-yr Survival (%) |
|---|---|---|
| I | 194 | 71 |
| II | 310 | 47 |
| III | 196 | 33 |
| IV | 78 | 19 |
| Total | 778 | 42 |

From Benedet JL, Murphy KJ, Fairey RN, et al: Primary invasive carcinoma of the vagina. Obstet Gynecol 1983;62:715–719; Rubin SC, Young J, Mikuta JJ: Squamous carcinoma of the vagina: treatment, complications, and long-term follow-up. Gynecol Oncol 1985; 20:346–353; Kucera H, Langer M, Smekal G, et al: Radiotherapy of primary carcinoma of the vagina: management and results of different therapy schemes. Gynecol Oncol 1985;21:87–93; Eddy GL, Marks RD II, Miller MC, et al: Primary invasive vaginal carcinoma. Am J Obstet Gynecol 1991;165:292–296; and Kirkbride P, Fyles A, Rawlings GA, et al: Carcinoma of the vagina—experience at the Princess Margaret Hospital (1974–1989). Gynecol Oncol 1995;56:435–443.

individualized. In younger patients who are diagnosed, high regard should be given to both vaginal and ovarian preservation. Early-stage tumors involving the upper vagina may be treated with radical hysterectomy, pelvic lymphadenectomy, and upper vaginectomy. Radiation therapy may be employed if surgical excision is local and/or less radical. In those cases in which less radical surgery is the only treatment modality employed, the risk of local recurrence is greater. The use of radiation therapy as the sole means of treatment is usually reserved for more extensive tumors and tumors involving the lower vagina.

The overall prognosis for adenocarcinoma of the vagina is directly dependent on the stage of disease. Those patients with the clear cell variant, who are generally younger and more likely to present with early-stage disease, generally have very good outcomes. The 5-year overall survival for this group of patients ranges between 75% and 80%. The outcomes for non–clear cell adenocarcinomas of the vagina not related to in utero DES exposure are generally less favorable compared to the squamous carcinomas.[9] As with the squamous subtypes recurrent disease is most likely to occur locally. Treatment for recurrent adenocarcinoma is also individualized and depends on location of the recurrence and the type of treatment used primarily.

## SARCOMAS

Most vaginal sarcomas arise submucosally. Many different subtypes of sarcoma have been described, including fibrosarcomas, rhabdomyosarcomas, leiomyosarcomas, endometrial stromal sarcomas, angiosarcomas, and malignant histiosarcomas. Poor prognostic factors include size greater than 3 cm, greater than 5 mitoses per 10 HPF, and cytologic atypia.[17] These tumors are best treated by surgical excision with adjuvant irradiation recommended for those with poor prognostic features or positive surgical margins.

Sarcoma botryoides is an embryonal rhabdomyosarcoma that affects young children. This variant of sarcoma is the most common malignancy of the vagina in children. The majority of these occur in children younger than age 5, and they often present with a grapelike vascular-appearing mass in the vagina. Historically these tumors were treated with radical surgery. More contemporary therapy now includes preoperative or postoperative chemotherapy and irradiation. The implementation of combination chemotherapy with vincristine, dactinomycin, and cyclophosphamide has improved overall survival for this tumor type.[18]

## MELANOMAS

Primary melanomas arising in the vagina are rare, representing approximately 0.5% to 1% of all vaginal malignancies. They are most common in the lower anterior vagina and can vary in color, size, shape, and pattern of growth. They usually present in postmenopausal females with vaginal bleeding, vaginal discharge, or a vaginal mass. As with cutaneous melanomas, several classification schemata can be used (Breslow, Chung, Clark), and tumor depth is the best predictor of overall survival.

The treatment for vaginal melanoma usually entails a radical surgical approach. For proximal lesions a radical hysterectomy,

partial vaginectomy, and pelvic lymphadenectomy can be utilized, whereas distal vaginal melanomas may require partial vaginectomy, partial or total vulvectomy, and inguinofemoral lymphadenectomy. Irradiation (both external and intracavitary) is primarily reserved for the adjuvant setting or more advanced vaginal tumors. Chemotherapy has not been shown to be effective, and the use of immunotherapy has not been proven.

Overall survival depends on the depth of invasion and is generally poor. Buchanan and colleagues found only 18 of 197 patients to survive more than 5 years from the time of diagnosis.[19] Recurrence is most common locally or in the lungs, and prognosis is universally poor; mean survival is approximately 8 months in these cases.

## LYMPHOMAS

Most primary vaginal lymphomas present as a submucosal mass. They are most commonly of diffuse large-cell type. Lymphomas of the vagina can be primary in origin or they may represent a metastatic process. Combination chemotherapy depending on the cell type should be utilized to treat these tumors.

## REFERENCES

1. Jemal A, Ward E, Murray T, et al: Cancer statistics, 2005. CA Cancer J Clin 2005;55:10–30. **(IV, C)**
2. Benedet JL, Murphy KJ, Fairey RN, et al: Primary invasive carcinoma of the vagina. Obstet Gynecol 1983;62:715–719. **(IV, C)**
3. Peters WA, Kumar NB, Morley GW: Carcinoma of the vagina. Factors influencing treatment. Cancer 1985;55:892–897. **(IV, C)**
4. Rubin SC, Young J, Mikuta JJ: Squamous carcinoma of the vagina: treatment, complications, and long-term follow-up. Gynecol Oncol 1985;20:346–353. **(IV, C)**
5. Kucera H, Langer M, Smekal G, et al: Radiotherapy of primary carcinoma of the vagina: management and results of different therapy schemes. Gynecol Oncol 1985;21:87–93. **(IV, C)**
6. Eddy GL, Marks RD II, Miller MC, et al: Primary invasive vaginal carcinoma. Am J Obstet Gynecol 1991;165:292–296. **(IV, C)**
7. Stock RG, Chen AS, Seski J: A 30-year experience in the management of primary carcinoma of the vagina: analysis of prognostic factors and treatment modalities. Gynecol Oncol 1995;56:45–52. **(IV, C)**
8. Kirkbride P, Fyles A, Rawlings GA, et al: Carcinoma of the vagina—experience at the Princess Margaret Hospital (1974–1989). Gynecol Oncol 1995;56:435–443. **(IV, C)**
9. Chyle V, Zagars GK, Wheeler JA, et al: Definitive radiotherapy for carcinoma of the vagina: outcome and prognostic factors. Int J Radiat Oncol Biol Phys 1996;35:891–905. **(IV, C)**
10. Robinson JB, Sun CC, Bodurka-Bevers D, et al: Cavitational ultrasonic surgical aspiration for the treatment of vaginal intraepithelial neoplasia. Gynecol Oncol 2000;78:235–241. **(IV, C)**
11. Bell J, Sevin BU, Averette H, et al: Vaginal cancer after hysterectomy for benign disease: value of cytologic screening. Obstet Gynecol 1984;64:699–702. **(IV, C)**
12. Ball HG, Berman ML: Management of primary vaginal carcinoma. Gynecol Oncol 1982;14:154–163. **(IV, C)**
13. Perez CA, Camel HM, Galakatos AE, et al: Definitive irradiation in carcinoma of the vagina: long-term evaluation of results. Int J Radiat Oncol Biol Phys 1988;15:1283–1290. **(IV, C)**
14. Plentl AA, Friedman EA: Lymphatic system of the female genitalia: the morphologic basis of oncologic diagnosis and therapy. Philadelphia: WB Saunders, 1971, p 51. **(IV, C)**

15. Daling JR, Madeleine MM, Schwartz SM, et al: A population-based study of squamous cell vaginal cancer: HPV and cofactors. Gynecol Oncol 2002;84:263–270. **(IIa, B)**

16. Herbst AL, Ulfelder H, Poskanzer DC, et al: Adenocarcinoma of the vagina. Association of maternal stilbestrol therapy with tumor appearance in young women. N Engl J Med 1971;284:878–882. **(IV, C)**

17. Tavassoli FA, Norris HJ: Smooth muscle tumors of the vagina. Obstet Gynecol 1979;53:689–693. **(IV, C)**

18. Friedman M, Peretz BA, Nissenbaum M, et al: Modern treatment of vaginal embryonal rhabdomyosarcoma. Obstet Gynecol Surv 1986; 41:614–618. **(IV, C)**

19. Buchanan DJ, Schlaerth J, Kurosaki T: Primary vaginal melanoma: thirteen-year disease-free survival after wide local excision and review of recent literature. Am J Obstet Gynecol 1998;178:1177–1184. **(IV, C)**

# Cervical Carcinoma

Zoyla Almeida-Parra, MD, Manuel Peñalver, MD, and
Luis E. Mendez, MD

## KEY POINTS

- Human papillomavirus is a carcinogen directly linked to dysplasias and cervical cancer, and has been detected in greater than 90% of cancer tissues.
- The Bethesda System was revised in 2001 based on multiple studies to provide uniform nomenclature and therapeutic guidelines. The new Bethesda System subdivides atypical squamous cells (ASC) into atypical cells of undetermined significance (ASC-US) and atypical cells cannot exclude high-grade intraepithelial lesion (ASC-H).
- Management of abnormal Pap smears depends on their classification. Most abnormal Pap smears should be evaluated with colposcopic-directed biopsies. HPV testing has an important role to play in ASC-US workups but does not help with other types of abnormal Pap smears.
- Cervical cancer staging is based on size and extension of tumor. It is staged clinically rather than surgically.
- Treatment of cervical cancer depends on size of lesion. Microinvasive disease may be treated with less extensive surgery. Stage IA1 may be treated with a cone biopsy versus simple hysterectomy (after cone biopsy). The treatment for IA2 is a type II hysterectomy. Stage IB1, IB2, and IIA can be treated with either a type III hysterectomy or chemoradiation.
- Adjuvant chemoradiation is given to patients with poor prognostic factors, as determined by surgical pathology. Poor prognostic factors include lymph node involvement, lymphovascular involvement, parametrial involvement, depth of invasion, vaginal margins, and size of tumor.
- Concomitant chemotherapy, specifically cisplatin, results in a superior progression-free survival compared to radiation alone (approximately 50%).
- Surveillance for recurrence is extremely important. Irradiation is the treatment for local recurrence after surgery. Patients with local central recurrence after radiation therapy may be explored for possible exenteration. Pelvic exenterations are morbid and patient selection is important. Distal recurrence can be treated with palliative chemotherapy.

## EPIDEMIOLOGY

In the early 1970s, approximately 75% to 80% of cases of cervical cancer in the United States were invasive at the time of diagnosis. Today, most cases of cervical cancer are diagnosed at the in situ stage (78%). The incidence and mortality for invasive cervical cancer has declined approximately 40% since the 1970s. This decline is due to effective cytologic screening with the advent of the Pap smear, introduced in the 1940s by Dr. George Papanicolaou. This screening test has not undergone much modification in the past 50 years (Fig. 44-1). Screening guidelines for cervical cancer are given in Table 44-1.

There were an estimated 10,520 new cases of cervical cancer for 2004, with a higher prevalence among minorities. The incidence is 12.7/100,000 among African Americans versus 8.0/100,000 among whites (Fig. 44-2). Although Pap smears for cervical cancer prevention are highly effective, use among minorities is significantly lower than among white women (85.6%). Hispanics are least likely to undergo Pap smears (82.6%), whereas 88.9% of black women reported undergoing a Pap smear.[3]

## ETIOLOGY

Risk factors for cervical cancer and clinical features are listed in Table 44-2. Cervical cancer is strongly linked to the human papillomavirus (HPV). HPV are small DNA viruses from the Papovaviridae family that contain 7900 base pairs (Fig. 44-3). There are more than 100 different types affecting different body areas. HPV is associated with condylomas, dysplasias, and cervical and anal cancers. The exact incidence of HPV is unknown for several reasons. Infections are many times subclinical and there is a lack of reporting of overt infections. In addition, detection techniques are difficult and complicated. HPV cannot grow ex vivo. Detection methods include in situ hybridization, southern transfer hybridization, hybrid capture, dot blot, filter hybridization, and polymerase chain reaction.

Human papillomavirus types are subdivided into low, intermediate, and high risk. The high-risk HPV types most associated with cervical cancer are 16 and 18.

### Molecular Biology

In 1995, The World Health Organization (WHO) declared HPV as carcinogenic in humans from the biologic and epidemiologic points of view. There is strong evidence to support the role of HPV pathogenesis in cervical dysplasias and cervical cancer.[4] HPV DNA has been detected in greater than 90% cervical cancer tissues.

The HPV genome encodes for the following proteins[5]:

- 6 E (early) proteins—gene regulation and cell transformation
- 2 L (late) proteins—shell of the virus
- 1 region—regulation of DNA sequences

The HPV proteins E6 and E7 are important viral oncogenes involved in the pathogenesis of cervical cancer. These oncogenes

# Gynecologic Oncology

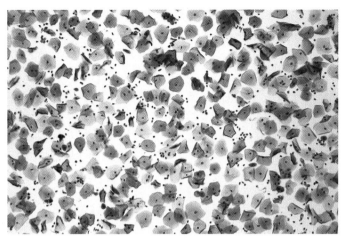

**Figure 44-1    Normal Pap smear used for cervical cancer screening.**

| Table 44-1 | |
|---|---|
| **ACOG Screening Guidelines for Cervical Cancer** | |
| Initial screening | Should begin approximately 3 years after first sexual intercourse or by age 21, whichever comes first |
| Until age 30 | Annual screening |
| At age 30 or older | · Annual screening<br>· Every 2 to 3 years, if patient has had 3 consecutive negative results<br>· Combination of cytology with high-risk HPV testing; if both tests are negative, combined tests no more frequently than every 3 years, if one test is negative, more frequent testing. |

Exceptions:
· Women at high risk, such as those having a history of cervical cancer, immunosuppression, HIV, or cervical dysplasias, should be screened more often according to their diagnosis.
· Women with their cervix removed for benign reasons do not need annual screening. If the patient had a history of dysplasia, testing may be discontinued after three consecutive negative screening tests.
Data from American College of Obstetricians and Gynecologists.[1,2]

have transforming properties that interact with growth-regulating proteins. Their continued expression is necessary for malignant transformation. It is important to point out that there are different levels of oncogenicity of E6 and E7, depending on their base pairs. E7 has more oncogenic properties on HPV16 than on HPV6.

The molecular processes by which these proteins cause malignant transformation involve the p53 and retinoblastoma systems (Rb). Normally p53 is a negative regulator of cell growth. When there is chromosomal damage, p53 allows DNA repair enzymes to function. The E6 protein binds and degrades p53, thus allowing the accumulation of mutations without DNA repair and thereby causing "unchecked" cellular cycling.[6] Apoptosis is therefore inhibited (Fig. 44-4).

The Rb protein is involved in inducing cell apoptosis in response to DNA damage.[7,8] Rb binds to E2F transcription factor and inactivates E2F, which is involved with promoting the S phase of cell division. E7 bind to the Rb protein, which causes E2F to be released and allows cell division and bypasses the "check" system with p53. E6 and E7 are also involved in apoptotic inhibition and cell transformation through other mechanisms.

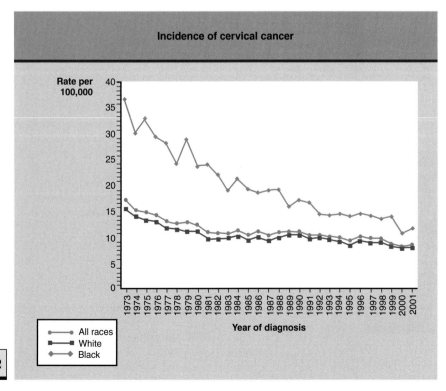

**Figure 44-2    Incidence of cervical cancer.** (Based on National Cancer Institute's Surveillance, Epidemiology and End Results [SEER], Facts and Figures, 2004.)

### Table 44-2
### Risk Factors and Clinical Features of Cervical Cancer

| Risk Factors | Clinical Features and Symptoms | |
| --- | --- | --- |
| | Early Stage | Late Stage |
| Early age at first intercourse | No symptoms | Abdominal pain |
| Multiple partners | Screening with Pap smears | Unilateral leg edema/pain |
| Sexually transmitted diseases, HPV, HIV, HSV | Vaginal bleeding | Heavy vaginal bleeding |
| Oral contraception use | Postcoital bleeding | |
| Cigarette smoking | Abnormal discharge | |
| Low socioeconomic status | | |
| Increased number of sexual partners of the current male partner | | |

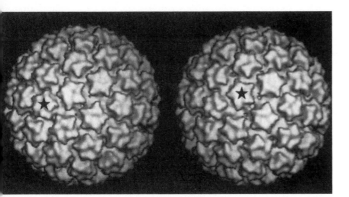

**Figure 44-3    Depiction of the human papillomavirus.** (From Baker TS, Newcom WW, Olson NH, et al: Structures of bovine and human papillomaviruses. Analysis by cryoelectron microscopy and three-dimensional image reconstruction. Biophys J 1991;60:1445–1456.)

## CLASSIFICATION AND SURGICAL CONSIDERATIONS

The incidence of abnormal Pap smears is approximately 1.5% to 6%.[9] With this, there has also been an increase in HPV-associated disease. Currently, HPV is the most common sexually transitted disease in the United States. The most widely used system to describe cervical lesions is the Bethesda System for Reporting Cervical Cytology, which emphasizes histologic description rathe than predictors for neoplastic potential.

In 1991, the National Cancer Institute revised the criteria for cytologic interpretation and the reporting of results. The Bethesda System (Table 44-3) was created to improve communication and to provide uniform therapeutic guidelines. Several revisions have been made based on new studies and on the most recent consensus conference in 2001.

A Pap smear specimen is considered adequate if the following criteria are met:

- Estimated 8000 to 12,000 well-visualized squamous cells in conventional smears
- Estimated 5000 squamous cells for liquid-based preparations
- Transformation zone should be at least 10 well-preserved endocervical or squamous metaplastic cells

If more than 75% of epithelial cells are obscured, the specimen is considered unsatisfactory (Figs. 44-5 and 44-6).

**Figure 44-4    Hypothetical mechanism for cervical cancer tumorigenesis by the human papillomavirus.**

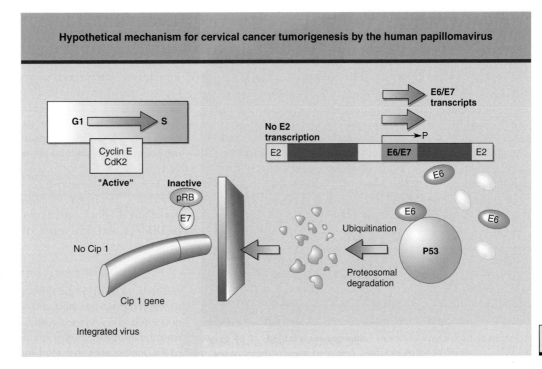

Hypothetical mechanism for cervical cancer tumorigenesis by the human papillomavirus

## Thin Prep Pap test

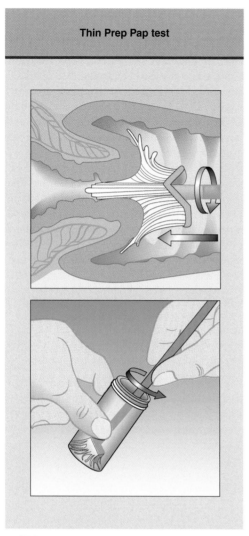

Figure 44-5    Liquid-based cytology, the Thin Prep Pap Test.

### Table 44-3
### Bethesda System 2001

**Squamous epithelial cell abnormalities**

ASC: atypical squamous cells
ASC-US: atypical cells of undetermined significance
ASC-H: atypical cells, cannot exclude high-grade squamous intraepithelial
    lesions
LSIL: low grade squamous intraepithelial lesions
Includes HPV, mild dysplasia, CIN I
HSIL: high grade squamous intraepithelial lesion
Includes moderate and severe dysplasia, CIN II, CIN III

**Glandular epithelial cell abnormalities**

AGC: atypical glandular cells; specify endocervical, endometrial, or glandular
    cells
AGC-N: atypical glandular cells, favoring neoplasia; specify endocervical or not
    otherwise specified
AIS: endocervical adenocarcinoma in situ

Data from Solomon D, Davey D, Kurman R, et al: The 2001 Bethesda System: terminology
for reporting results of cervical oncology. JAMA 2002;287:2114–2119.

Endometrial cells were only reported in postmenopausal women. However, the 2001 revision notes endometrial cells present in women younger than age 40. Pertinent history is not always known when the Pap smears are read. Endometrial cells other than menses should not be present; this could indicate an endometrial abnormality.

The importance of proper classification is to manage these lesions appropriately. Multiple reports are available indicating the natural history of cervical cancer precursors. Several studies have looked at the average age of a lesion and have extrapolated that it takes more than 10 years for a dysplastic lesion to become carcinoma in situ or an invasive cancer.[10,11] Although many studies have determined progression of different grades of dysplasia, the more severe lesions have a higher likelihood of progression.

The category ASC (atypical squamous cells) has been divided into two categories with the purpose of detecting higher grade lesions. It has been estimated that 10% to 20% of women have underlying CIN II or CIN III and that 1/1000 may have invasive cancer. Specificity of ASC should aid in detecting CIN II and CIN III more rapidly (Fig. 44-7).[12]

There are different approaches to managing ASC. One alternative is to repeat the Pap smear in 4 to 6 months. Once two are negative, follow with routine Pap smear screening. If positive colposcopy should be done. Antoher approach calls for HPV testing. If results are negative, the Pap smear is repeated in 12 months. If HPV results are positive, colposcopy should be done. If the colposcopy is negative, repeat Pap smears should be performed every 6 to 12 months or repeat HPV testing in 12 months. Refer for colposcopy if Pap smear or HPV testing is positive. A final option is initial colposcopy. If it is negative repeat Pap smear in 12 months. If results of the colposcopy are positive, manage appropriately. Excisional procedures should be

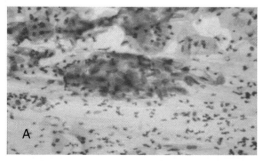
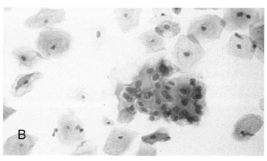

A          B

Figure 44-6    Comparison between the conventional Pap smear (A) and the Thin Prep Pap Test (B).

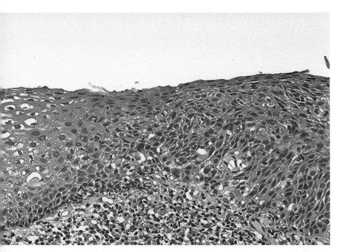

Figure 44-7   Cervical biopsy depicting moderate to severe dysplasia.

voided, and all immunosupressed patients should undergo colposcopy regardless of viral load or CD4 count.

The category ASC-H (atypical squamous cells, cannot exclude high grade squamous intraepithelial lesion) should be referred for colposcopic evaluation:

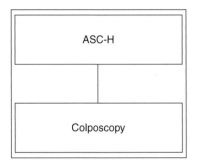

The SIL categories are divided into LSIL and HSIL to differentiate the two entities. LSIL refers to a transient infection with HPV. HSIL refers to a higher risk group associated with persistent viral infection and a higher risk of progression.

The majority of LSIL lesions will regress (47%) or persist (37%). Only 16% of patients will develop more severe lesions.[13] HSIL has a higher incidence of progression to CIS. From 32% to 43% of HSIL lesions will regress, 22% to 56% will progress, and lesions that are CIN III have the highest progression rate to invasive cancer (16% to 36%).[14] (See the flowchart at the bottom of page.)

Low-grade SIL has been managed with repeat Pap smears. Although acceptable, this approach is associated with poor compliance and the possibility for delaying diagnosis of a more severe lesion; therefore, colposcopy is recommended. HPV testing does not seem to be useful because up to 83% of women will test positive for HPV.[15]

High-grade SIL has been managed with colposcopy with directed biopsies. If results of the colposcopy are unsatisfactory, an excisional procedure is recommended. HPV testing for triage purposes has no role in the management of HSIL (Fig. 44-8).

Colposcopy is recommended for the management of atypical glandular cells (AGC) or endocervical carcinoma in situ (AIS). Endometrial biopsy should be performed if the woman is older than age 35 or abnormal bleeding is present. If colposcopy is negative for AGC NOS (not of significance), a repeat Pap smear should be performed every 4 to 6 months until the patient has had four consecutive negative Pap smears. If colposcopy is negative for AGC favoring neoplasia, an excisional procedure is recommended. There is not enough data to warrant HPV testing.

The 2001 revision changed the term *AGUS* (atypical glandular cells of undetermined significance) to differentiate this from ASCUS. There are a much higher number of high-grade diseases in this group. High-grade lesions may be seen in 10% to 39% of this group. For cases that are not sufficient to be called

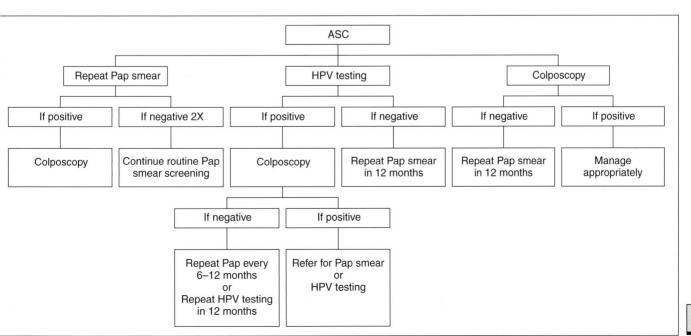

# Gynecologic Oncology

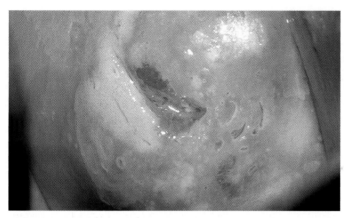

**Figure 44-8   Colposcopic image of the cervix.** The transformation zone is seen completely. There are punctate lesions equivalent to CIN II seen at 8 o'clock.

| Stage | Qualification |
|---|---|
| | **Table 44-4** |
| | **FIGO Staging System for Cervical Cancer** |
| 0 | Carcinoma in situ, intraepithelial carcinoma. Cases of Stage 0 should not be included in any therapeutic statistics for invasive carcinoma. |
| I | The carcinoma is strictly confined to the cervix (extension to the corpus should be disregarded). |
| IA | Invasive cancer identified only microscopically. All gross lesions, even with superficial invasion, are Stage IB cancers. Invasion is limited to measured stromal invasion with a maximum depth of 5 mm and no wider than 7 mm. (The depth of invasion should not be more than 5 mm taken from the base of the epithelium, either surface or glandular, from which it originates.) Vascular space involvement, either venous or lymphatic, should not alter the staging. |
| IA1 | Measured invasion of stroma no greater than 3 mm in depth and no wider than 7 mm |
| IA2 | Measured invasion of stroma 3 to 5 mm in depth and no wider than 7 mm |
| IB | Clinical lesions confined to the cervix or preclinical lesions greater than IA |
| IB1 | Clinical lesions no greater than 4 mm in size |
| IB2 | Clinical lesions greater than 4 mm in size |
| II | The carcinoma extends beyond the cervix but has not extended onto the pelvic wall; the carcinoma involves the vagina but not as far as the lower third. |
| IIA | No obvious parametrial involvement |
| IIB | Obvious parametrial involvement |
| III | The carcinoma has extended onto the pelvic wall; on rectal examination there is no cancer-free space between the tumor and the pelvic wall. The tumor involves the lower third of the vagina. All cases with a hydronephrosis or nonfunctioning kidney should be included, unless they are known to be due to other cause. |
| IIIA | No extension onto the pelvic wall, but involvement of the lower third of the vagina |
| IIIB | Extension onto the pelvic wall or hydronephrosis or nonfunctioning kidney |
| IV | The carcinoma has extended beyond the true pelvis or has clinically involved the mucosa of the bladder or rectum. |
| IVA | Spread of the growth to adjacent organs |
| IVB | Spread to distant organs |

AIS, a separate category has been created, atypical endocervical cells, favor neoplastic.

High-grade lesions, including CIN II, CIN III, AIS, or invasive cancer, have been found in 9% to 41% of women with AGC NOS, compared with 27% to 96% of women with AGC favoring neoplasia. Endocervical adenocarcinoma in situ is associated with AIS in 48% to 69% of cases and underlying invasive cervical carcinoma in 38% of cases.

## Microinvasive Cancer

Historically there has been much debate over the proper definition of microinvasive disease. In 1974, the Society of Gynecologic Oncologists defined *microinvasive carcinoma* as invasion with a depth of 3 mm or less. This definition was not adopted worldwide until the International Federation of Gynecology and Obstetrics (FIGO) did so in 1994 (Table 44-4).[16] Stage IA1 was defined as a tumor that invaded at a depth of 3 mm or less. Stage IA2 was defined as having a depth of 3 mm to 5 mm. Both stages had a horizontal spread of up to 7 mm. The purpose of this definition was to standardize treatment worldwide.

### Stage IAI

Treatment of Stage IA1 cervical cancer is conservative; it may be treated by a cone biopsy if the patient desires fertility or by an extrafascial hysterectomy if childbearing has been completed. Management is conservative secondary to the low incidence of lymph node involvement (0.5%) and low rate of recurrence (2%).[17]

Treatment for microinvasion on a cone biopsy depends on the margins. The surgical margins at both the endocervix and ectocervix must be negative. If there is dysplasia at the margins, a reconization is necessary. Both Greer and colleagues and Roman and colleagues demonstrated residual disease in patients with positive margins.[18,19] The incidence of residual disease was 33% versus 4% if both margins were positive. If the endocervical margin was positive, 22% of women with positive margins had residual disease.

Involvement of the lymphovascular space may be present in approximately 10% of cases. Presently there is no standard treatment for these patients, although most gynecologic oncologists will agree that a more aggressive management is warranted secondary to an increased risk of lymph node positivity.

### Stage IA2

Stage IA2 cervical cancer requires more extensive surgery and i treated by a modified radical hysterectomy with pelvic lymph adenectomy. The incidence of lymph node metastasis is 7.3% with a 3% recurrence. Pelvic lymph node dissection is sufficient unless the lymph nodes are suspicious, which then should includ dissection of the periaortic region.

If the patient desires fertility, a radical trachelectomy may b considered with nodal dissection. These are highly selected case and patients must be counseled appropriately.

### Stage IB and IIA

Stage IB is subdivided into IB1 (tumor size <4 cm) and IB (tumor size >4 cm; Fig. 44-9). This subdivision was created b

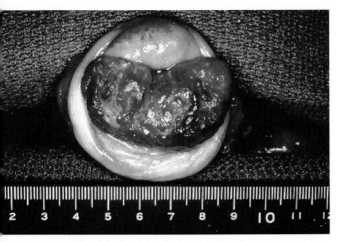

**Figure 44-9    Cervical cancer Stage IB.**

based on the experience and comfort level of the gynecologic oncologist. The advantages of surgery are to determine prognostic factors more accurately and to preserve ovarian function and vaginal elasticity. Cure rates are equal between both groups.

Although surgery may preserve ovarian function and vaginal elasticity, there are patients who will require adjuvant radiation therapy. Surgicopathologic prognostic factors include lymph node involvement, lymphovascular involvement, parametrial involvement, depth of invasion, vaginal margins, and the size of the tumor. These prognostic factors affect survival and thus may indicate the need for adjuvant therapy with chemotherapy and radiation.

Surgical management allows for these pathologic factors to be identified, allowing for more accurate prognosis and therapeutic recommendations. In addition, surgery affords lymph node debulking. If the patient has enlarged nodes, removing these allows the patient a better chance to respond to radiation therapy.

Complications that may occur from a radical hysterectomy are mostly related to urinary tract morbidity and bleeding. The average blood loss with a radical hysterectomy is 800 to 1500 mL.[20] The most common immediate postoperative complication is a urinary tract infection secondary to prolonged catheterization. In addition, many patients may have hypotonic bladder dysfunction with urine retention.

Complications occurring with radiation are related to injury to the surrounding tissues. These patients are at risk for vesicovaginal and rectovaginal fistulas. The incidence of these fistulas ranges from 0.9% to 1.6%.[21] In addition, many experience sexual dysfunction due to decreased caliber and vaginal elasticity. These

IGO in 1994 because of an increase in evidence indicating that size correlated directly with prognosis.

Generally, Stage IB1 cervical cancer is treated by a radical hysterectomy (type III). A type III hysterectomy entails removing the parametrium from where the uterine artery originates from the hypogastric artery. In addition, the upper third of the vagina is excised. There are several modifications of this technique. Removal of 2 cm of the vagina below the cervix is considered adequate margin (Fig. 44-10). For patients who are poor surgical candidates, chemoradiation therapy is another alternative.

Cervical cancer may be treated by either surgery or chemoradiation therapy. The decision is mostly institution-based or

**Figure 44-10    Diagram indicating the extent of surgical resection for different types of hysterectomy.**

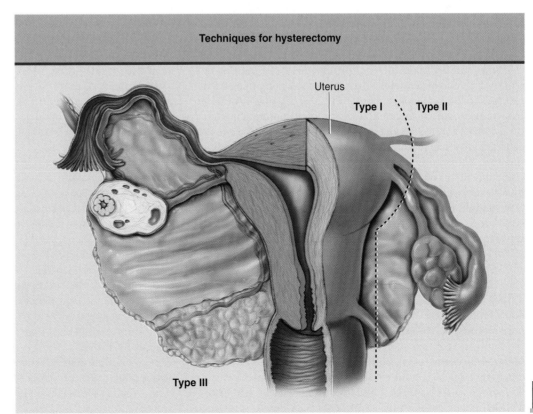

Techniques for hysterectomy

Uterus

Type I      Type II

Type III

# Gynecologic Oncology

fistulas are difficult to manage and often require additional surgical intervention such as colostomy and bladder diversions and reconstructions.

Treatment for stage IB2 and IIA cervical cancers needs to be tailored to the patient's medical comorbidities and desire for sexual function preservation.

Candidates for fertility preservation are those patients with Stage IB1 cervical cancer with lesions smaller than 2 cm. If lymph nodes and lymphovascular space involvement are negative, these patients may undergo a radical trachelectomy with laparoscopic lymph node dissection. Cerclage placement should be done at the time of surgery.

In patients with bulky stage IB2 and IIA cervical cancer, many institutions prefer irradiation over surgery. One main reason to perform surgery in these patients is to "debulk" the disease. The tumor may extend beyond the radiation fields and thus not be treated optimally. These patients have a more aggressive tumor and recurrence rates of up to 30%.

### Stage IIB to IV

Treatment for advanced-stage cervical cancer consists of irradiation, both external beam therapy and brachytherapy, usually with radiation-sensitizing doses of chemotherapy. The extent of disease must always be evaluated, first by computed tomography and possibly by surgery for staging and resection of bulky lymph nodes that may not respond to radiotherapy. The surgical approach consists of extraperitoneal lymph node dissection to decrease morbidity and simultaneously evaluate and resect extensive nodal disease. If periaortic lymph nodes are positive, extended-field radiation is warranted.[22] The incidence of periaortic lymph node involvement ranges from 21% to 31%, based on stage.

Besides defining the extended field of radiation, radiation sensitizers have been proven to have an impact on treatment and survival. Several Gynecologic Oncology Group (GOG) studies have looked into different radiosensitizers such as hydroxyurea, cisplatin, and fluorouracil. Hydroxyurea was one of the first agents studied as a chemosensitizer and was found to increase the progression-free interval and survival.[23] A comparison between hydroxyurea and concomitant cisplatin and fluorouracil found the combination to produce superior improvement.[24] Rose and colleagues compared three different groups receiving radiation therapy.[25] Group 1 used only cisplatin; Group 2 combined cisplatin, fluorouracil, and hydroxyurea; and Group 3 used hydroxyurea only. Groups 1 and 2 showed similar progression-free survival at 24 months (64% to 77%) versus a 24% survival in Group 3. Therefore, this study proved that the cisplatin-based regimen had a superior progression-free survival. Currently, the standard is to give weekly cisplatin during radiation therapy for advanced cervical cancer.

# TREATMENT PLAN FOR LOCALLY ADVANCED (STAGES IIB TO IVA) CERVICAL CANCER

Treatment consists of both external beam radiation and brachytherapy. The total external beam dose is approximately 45 Gy over 4 to 6 weeks. This is then followed by one or two low-density radiation implants or serial high-density radiation.

The total amount given with brachytherapy is 85 to 90 Gy, and treatment usually lasts 6 to 8 weeks. Delays should not extend treatment past 10 weeks.

The method most commonly used is the Manchester system. This system defines two important points that will delineate the treatment area. Point A is a point 2 cm lateral and superior to the external cervical os within the plan of the implant, and Point B is 3 cm lateral with respect to point A. Point A theoretically reflects the parametria, and Point B reflects the pelvic sidewall. Other factors to take into account are the type of implant, the distance from the bladder and rectum, tumor volume, and the patient's habitus.

## Radiation Therapy

In general, radiation therapy is delivered in three different ways: teletherapy, brachytherapy, and interstitial therapy.

### Teletherapy or External Beam Therapy

*Teletherapy* is defined as radiation delivered from a distance through a linear accelerator. The linear accelerator produces photon beams with accelerated electrons. Several factors influence dose distribution, including voltage of the energy beam, size of the radiation field, distance between the patient and the beam, angle of the field being treated, patient habitus, and use of other devices. To deliver appropriate treatment, computer calculations are made that account for all these factors.

The radiation plan usually will consist of two or more beams for dose distribution. The goal is to produce a homogeneous dose that will maximize treatment and minimize exposure to uninvolved tissues.

### Brachytherapy or Intracavitary Treatment

Brachytherapy is radiation therapy given at a short distance, and may be given as low dose rate (LDR) or as high dose rate (HDR) treatment. Most centers will give LDR. HDR treatment consists of treatment given over minutes rather than hours and is done in an outpatient setting. Most HDR regimens consists of 5.5 to 6 Gy to point A given in five fractions. Although this kind of treatment seems more practical, there is resistance to treating patients with HDR because the optimal dosing is not quite known and there are insufficient randomized studies comparing both modalities.

Brachytherapy is an important tool for treating cervical tumors because external beam radiation is not sufficient to sterilize large tumor volumes. Most of the applications are directed toward a smaller and more specific area. Different applicators may be used, consisting of a hollow tube usually called the *tandem* and side applicators usually called *ovoids*. The applicator used most commonly is the Fletcher-Suit-Delclos, which has a pear-shaped isodose curve (Fig. 44-11).

It is essential that these applicators are properly positioned under anesthesia with radiographic confirmation. Care must be taken to avoid excessive dose to the rectum and bladder. The applicators are loaded after confirmation of placement and are usually loaded with $^{137}$cesium. The delivery dose is 40 to 60 cGy/hr. Treatment plan is 72 to 96 hours. Due to specific or unique patient characteristics, brachytherapy may be administered in two applications. This divided application does not affect the overall cumulative radiation dose.

## Tandem and ovoids for intracavitary radiation

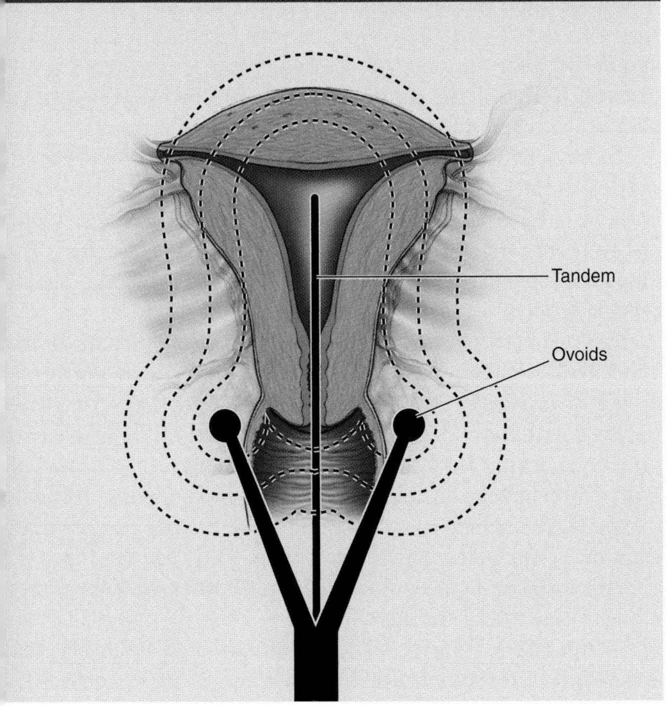

**Figure 44-11    Tandem and ovoids for intracavitary radiation.** (From Galjanovic MS, Hunter TB: Special report: Gallery of medical devices. Part 2: Devices of the head, neck, spine, chest, and abdomen. Radiographics 2005;25:1119–1132.)

### Interstitial Radiation Therapy

With interstitial radiation therapy, the radioactive sources are placed directly into the tissue rather than in an applicator. Sources of radiation for interstitial implants are usually [192]iridium and [125]iodine. These sources can be placed as permanent seeds, temporary implants, or transperineal implants. This technique allows a high dose of radiation to be delivered within a small area. Placement needs to be accurate to avoid normal tissue damage. Transperineal implants have not been shown to be superior to intracavitary implants. Studies are equivocal for both modalities. Intracavitary implants are more practical and less painful than interstitial implants.

### Radiation Therapy Fields for Cervical Cancer

The borders of the anteroposterior (A/P) and posteroanterior (P/A) pelvic fields are the following:

- *Superior border*—a transverse line between L4 and L5. This will include the common iliac nodes. If the patient is low risk for metastatic nodal disease, the superior border may be L5–S1.
- *Inferior border*—a transverse line below the obturator foramen or ischial tuberosity (midpubis) or 2 cm below inferiormost extent of disease (if vaginal involvement is noted).
- *Lateral border*—2 cm lateral to the widest aspect of true pelvic diameter.

Note: If the lower one third of the vagina is involved, the groin nodes should be included in the treatment fields and irradiated to approximately 45 Gy at 1.8 Gy per fraction.

Custom blocking shields the small bowel and femoral heads without shielding the common or external iliac nodes (allow at least 1 cm margin). These borders help to minimize the high-dose treatment but adequately treat the tumor.

The four-field box technique is more effective and specific than the parallel technique (A/P, P/A). Lateral fields may also be important for patients who are receiving chemotherapy and should be able to preserve as much bone marrow as possible.

Specific areas may need a boost dose. In general, parametrial and/or nodal boosts will be given by A/P or P/A (>10 MV) technique. All fields will be treated on a daily basis with 1.8 Gy prescribed to Point B (a point 3 cm lateral to Point A) to bring the cumulative dose to these prescription point to 55 Gy to 70 Gy (+/–5%):

- *Parametrial/Nodal Boost*—Central blocking should measure at least 4 cm and should be tailored to the Point A isodose line from the LDR brachytherapy.
- *Nodal boosts*—These should measure at least 4 × 4 cm and maintain a margin of 1 cm from involved nodes.

### Toxicity

Side effects from cumulative radiation therapy for cervical cancer include fatigue, diarrhea, rectal irritation, urinary frequency and burning, loss of pubic hair, darkening of skin in the region within the irradiated fields, and low blood counts. Common long-term side effects include vaginal narrowing and shortening and pain during sexual intercourse. Uncommon long-term side effects may include rectal bleeding, diarrhea, rectal ulcer, urinary burning, urinary frequency, urinary bleeding, and tissue breakdown of the vagina. Rare long-term side effects include bowel obstruction, ureteral obstruction, and fistula formation between the bladder and the vagina or between the rectum and the vagina.

### Surveillance and Follow-up Care

Postradiation monthly visits are prescribed for the initial 3 months to ensure tumor regression. Should the tumor progress then surgery can be entertained. Otherwise, follow-up visits should consist of the following:

The patient should be assessed for presence of pain, bleeding, and leg edema. Bladder and rectal function should be assessed. Pap and pelvic examination should be performed every 3 months for 2 years, then every 4 to 6 months for the next year, and then every 6 months until 5 years. Routine Pap smears are important because most recurrences are asymptomatic, but will have abnormal cytology. Detection and treatment of recurrence before symptoms seem to have an improvement in survival.

The supraclavicular and inguinal nodes should be assessed for metastasis. Abdominal examination; complete visual inspection of the vagina, cervix, and urethra; and a rectovaginal examination for masses and parametrial nodularity should be performed.

Imaging is physician dependent. Computed tomography scans and chest x-rays may be useful for assessing recurrences and for treatment plans.

Tumors markers that may be used are carcinogenic embryonic antigen, CA 125, and SCA, but these are not used routinely in cervical cancer.

# RECURRENT CERVICAL CANCER

The majority of recurrences occur within the first 2 years after treatment (including surgery and primary radiation therapy). Perez and colleagues[26] reported pelvic failures as follows:

- Stage IB—10%
- Stage IIA—17%
- Stage IIB—23%
- Stage III—42%
- Stage IVA—74%

The 10-year incidence of distant metastatic disease was reported by Fagundes and colleagues[27] as follows:

- Stage IA—3%
- Stage IB—16%
- Stage IIA—31%
- Stage IIB—26%
- Stage III—39%
- Stage IVA—75%

The sites of recurrence were as follows:

- Lung—21%
- Bone—16%
- Periaortic nodes—11%
- Abdominal cavity—8%
- Supraclavicular nodes—7%

There are different types of recurrences. Treatment depends on location and on forms of initial treatment.

If the recurrence occurs after a radical hysterectomy, without adjuvant treatment (chemoradiation), the treatment consists of chemoradiation. If the recurrence is only at the vaginal cuff, a vaginal cylinder may be used.

Recurrences after radiation therapy are best treated by surgery only if is the recurrence is in the central pelvis. This entails an exenteration, either complete or partial. The extent of the surgery depends on the location and extent of the recurrence. It may involve the bladder and/or rectum and may be above or below the levator plate.

A small group of patients may undergo a radical hysterectomy, but the morbidity is high, up to 50%. Morbidity consists of different types of fistulas, such as vesicovaginal, rectovaginal, and ureterovaginal fistula. These individuals must have a very small recurrence that is confined to the cervix to be candidates for a more conservative approach. These patients must have a lesion smaller than 2 cm with an original early-stage tumor to qualify for a radical hysterectomy. Few if any patients can be salvaged by chemotherapy.

## Exenterations

A pelvic exenteration is a challenging procedure for both the patient and surgeon. The patient must be prepared psychologically and should receive ostomy nursing care. Only 50% of patients who are candidates will actually undergo the procedure.

Preoperative workup includes confirmation of central recurrence, as well as complete imaging of the lungs, abdomen, and pelvis. An evaluation of renal function must be performed, as well as a sexual evaluation to include the possibility of vaginal reconstruction. Ostomy teaching must be provided. The patient must also receive psychological support.

There are essentially three parts to a pelvic exenteration: careful exploration and evaluation to make the decision to resect, the actual procedure, and reconstruction.

Exploration entails complete inspection of the avascular spaces to secure complete resection with negative margins. Aortic and pelvic node sampling are necessary to exclude disseminated disease. If any of the nodes or spaces are involved, very little benefit is achieved from such a morbid procedure.

The procedure itself depends on the extent of the disease. If the lesion only involves the cervix, a supralevator exenteration may be performed. However, if there is extensive vaginal involvement, the dissection must go below the levator plate. Depending on the size and location, the rectum or the bladder may be spared.

The reconstructive aspect depends on the patient's desires. Whenever possible, a low colorectal anastomosis is performed to avoid a colostomy. Urinary diversion must be considered for each patient individually. Either continent or incontinent urinary diversions may be done. The continent urinary diversion offer better quality of life if the patient is a suitable candidate. In addition, vaginal reconstruction may be performed if the exenteration is below the levator plate. This may be done with a rectus abdominis myocutaneous flap or other neovaginal techniques (Figs. 44-12 through 44-14).

Recuperation from a pelvic exenteration is extensive, with a postoperative complication rate of up to 50%, including mortality rate of 1%. Immediate complications include postoperative bleeding, infection, pulmonary embolism, deep venous thrombosis, and renal problems. Complications that may occur later include ureteral strictures, ostomy problems, and chronic wound healing difficulties.

### Radiation Therapy

Radiation may be used for palliation in the setting of vaginal bleeding or pelvic pain. Caution must be exercised when re irradiating an area because of increased morbidity. Radiation may be administered in large fractions to other areas of metastasis such as the brain and bony lesions that are not in the previous area of radiation.

### Palliative Chemotherapy

Chemotherapy in the setting of recurrence poses several problems. Most of these patients have received radiation therapy and many of these will have received adjuvant chemotherapy. These patients have a decreased bone marrow reserve and decreased vascular supply in the pelvis due to these previous therapies. In addition, many will have ureteral stricture, which will impair their renal function or the ability to renally excrete certain chemotherapy agents.

Several different agents have been shown to have some activity against cervical cancer. The most active is cisplatin, with an overall response rate of 23%. Other agents that have some activity against cervical cancer are ifosfamide (22%), topotecan (19%), paclitaxel (17%), and vinorelbine (15%). Response rates depend on the site of recurrence. If the recurrence is outside the field of radiation, such as the lungs or liver, response rates may be up to 25%. However, if the recurrence is in the site of radiated tissue such as the pelvis, the response rate is only 5%.

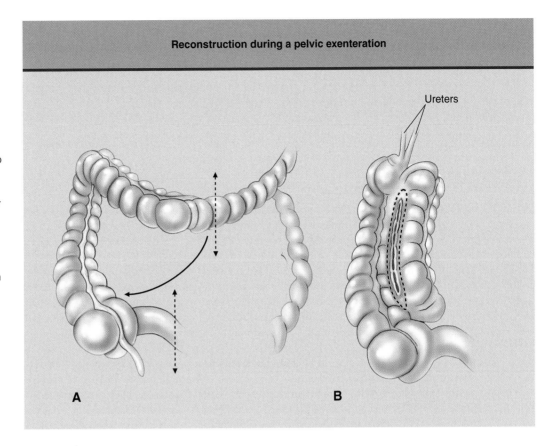

**Reconstruction during a pelvic exenteration**

Ureters

A  B

**Figure 44-12   Diagram for reconstruction during a pelvic exenteration.** Appoximately 12 to 15 cm of distal ileum, cecum, ascending colon, and half of the transverse colon are resected for the construction of the Miami pouch. *A,* Segment used for ileocolonic continent reconstruction: distal ileum, ascending and half of the transverse colon. *B,* Pouch seen after detubularization and reconstruction with ureters visualized.

Several GOG trials have demonstrated that the use of multi-agent chemotherapy has a better response rate and slightly improved survival rate than single agents.

Omura and colleagues[28] randomized 418 patients to cisplatin alone or combined with ifosfamide or mitolactol. Response rates were higher in the cisplatin and ifosfamide group (33%) versus the cisplatin alone group (19%). Time to progression was also better in the combination group than the single-agent group (4.6 months versus 3.2 months). There was not a significant difference in overall survival.

In another GOG trial,[29] 280 women were randomized to receive cisplatin alone or in combination with paclitaxel. The combination group had a higher response rate (36% vs. 19%) and higher progression-free survival (4.8 months vs. 2.8 months), with no difference in overall survival.

Another GOG trial has preliminary results showing an increased overall survival in the combination group. This trial randomized 356 women to receive cisplatin alone versus in combination with topotecan versus MVAC (methotrexate, vinblastine, doxorubicin, and cisplatin). The cisplatin/topotecan

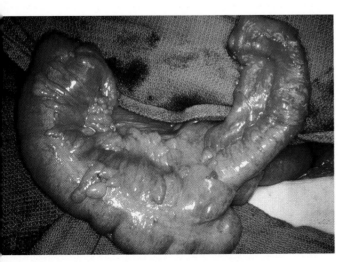

**Figure 44-13    Ileocolonic continent conduit, Miami pouch reconstruction.**

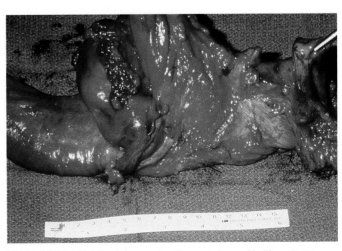

**Figure 44-14    Total pelvic exenteration specimen: bladder, uterus, cervix, and rectum.**

group had a higher response rate (26% vs. 13%), with a progression-free survival of 4.6 months compared to 2.9 months. The median survival difference for the cisplatin/topotecan group was 9.2 months versus 7 months.

Although several GOG trials have demonstrated a significant advantage of using combination agents versus single agents, treatment should be tailored to the patient's overall situation. Combination treatments have a higher incidence of neutropenia, renal toxicity, and peripheral neuropathy.

## BEST SUPPORTIVE CARE

In the past, palliative care was defined as care to be given during the final stages of life when treatment had failed. Currently, newer models incorporate palliative care during the initial stages of cancer treatment. In this manner, the patient has a more active role in fighting her illness. If the patient does not respond to her treatment, early introduction of palliative care may give her more autonomy and a better quality of life. It is essential for the patient to be involved from the beginning with her diagnosis, treatment plan, and decision making. Proper communication between the physician, nurses, and other caregivers is very important. In addition, psychological support should be available as well as other forms of supportive treatment.

Patients with end-stage cervical cancer may present with several different clinical presentations and symptoms, such as pain from bony metastasis, respiratory distress from lungs metastasis, and renal failure secondary to tumor growth.

Depending on a patient's wishes, tests should be done to alleviate symptoms as soon as possible. Bone metastasis can be treated with analgesics, bisphosphonates, and physical therapy. Respiratory disease may be alleviated by pleuracentesis, oxygen support, and withholding toxic treatment to give only supportive care. With regards to renal failure, involvement of the patient is essential. Some patients would rather not undergo percutaneous nephrostomies and die of uremia; others may want to continue all efforts because of fear or the need for more time. For this to be fair to the patient, complete information should be given and informed consent should be obtained. It is difficult for decisions to be made during a time of crisis. Many times, less intervention renders the patient with better quality of life.

During the final stages of illness, there should be proper support with regards to the transition toward death. Hospice care may be an option for some patients, but others may refuse. It is important to explore the patient's wishes before the final stages. In this manner, the patient has had an active role in planning her wishes as opposed to family members taking this decision from her. In addition, there must always be sensitivity to religious and culture beliefs added to any decision making.

### Pain Management

Pain has been defined by the International Association for the Study of Pain as "an unpleasant sensory or emotional experience associated with actual or potential tissue damage or described in terms of such damage." There are different forms of assessing and treating pain. One common method is the visual acuity scale, which is a simple, effective way to manage pain and assess treatment efficacy.

Pain management is adjusted to each patient's needs; full assessment is always indicated. Other symptoms must be assessed, such as anxiety, depression, and physical tissue involvement. Once must not hesitate to use other modalities such as psychological support, integrative therapy, music therapy, and pet therapy.[30]

The WHO[31] uses a systematic ladder approach[32] when treating cancer pain. The first line of medications should be nonsteroidal anti-inflammatory drugs (NSAIDs) or the newer cyclo-oxygenase-2 (COX-2) inhibitors. These work by inhibiting the enzyme cyclo-oxygenase, thus reducing prostaglandins, which affect the nociceptive primary afferent neurons. NSAIDs have to be used with caution in patients with a history of gastric ulcer and renal disease. In addition, they have a ceiling effect.

The second line of drugs used to treat cancer pain is opioids, preferably agonists such as morphine. These medications do not have a ceiling. An understanding of individual pharmacodynamics of these agents, such as half-life, peak effect, and duration, is important to provide efficacious pain relief. In addition, depending on the severity of pain, different combinations may be used with NSAIDs. Presently there are alternatives to oral administration for patients who have difficulty swallowing or persistent nausea and vomiting; these routes consist of transdermal, intravenous, intraspinal, buccal, and rectal. When having difficulty managing pain, a consult from anesthesia pain experts should be obtained. In addition, patients input, perception, and wishes should always be taken into consideration.

Although many times hospice facilities manage the last moments or days of life, the physician should know how to manage this time as well and ease the pain not only for the patient, but also for the family. Agitation, anxiety, and pain may all be displayed in the final stages. Many times, patients are not able to communicate, and alleviation of symptoms may be challenging. Morphine pumps, anxiolytics, and proper hygiene care are important strategies for care in the final stages. Once again, involvement of the patient and family as much as possible provides peace and dignity to the dying patient.

## REFERENCES

1. ACOG Practice Bulletin #45: Cervical cytology screening, August 2003. Int J Gynaecol Obstet 2003;83:237–247. (IIa, B)
2. ACOG Practice Bulletin #45: Clinical management guidelines for obstetrician-gynecologists, August 2003. Cervical cytology screening (replaces committee opinion # 152, March 1995). Obstet Gyneco 2003;102:417–427. (IIa, B)
3. American Cancer Society. Facts and Figures, 2004. Atlanta, American Cancer Society, 2004. (IV, C)
4. Zur Hausen H: Papillomaviruses causing cancer: evasion from host-cell control in early event in carcinogenesis. J Natl Cancer Inst 2000, 92:690–698. (Ib, A)
5. Palefsky JM, Holly EA: Molecular virology and epidemiology of human papillomavirus and cervical cancer. Cancer Epid Biomarkers Prev 1995, 4:415–428. (Ib, A)
6. Havre PA, Yuan J, Hedrick L, et al: P53 inactivaton by HPV E16 results in increased mutagenesis in human cells. Cancer Res 1995, 55:4420–4424. (IIb, B)
7. Tommasino M, Adamczewski JP, Carlotti F: HPV 16 E7 associates with the protein kinase p33CDK2 and cyclin A. Oncogene 1993;8:195–202. (IIb, B)

8. Demers GW, Foster SA, Halbert CL, et al: Growth arrest by induction of p53 in DNA damaged keratinocytes is bypassed by human papillomavirus 16 E7. Proc Natl Acad Sc USA 1995;91:4382–4386. **(IIb, B)**

9. Jones HW: The Bethesda System. Cancer 1995;76(Suppl):1994. **(III, B)**

0. Barron BA, Richart RM: A statistical model of the natural history of cervical carcinoma based on a prospective study of 557 cases. J Natl Cancer Inst 1968;41:1343. **(III, B)**

1. Barron BA, Richart RM: A statistical model of the natural history of cervical carcinoma II. Estimates of the transition from dysplasia to carcinoma in situ. J Natl Cancer Inst 1970;45:1025. **(III, B)**

2. Solomon D, Davey D, Kurman R, et al: The 2001 Bethesda System: terminology for reporting results of cervical oncology. JAMA 2002;287:2114–2119. **(IV, C)**

3. Ostor AG: Natural history of cervical intraepithelial neoplasia: a critical review. Int J Gynecol Path 1993;12:186–192. **(IV, C)**

4. Mitchell MF, Tortolero-Luna G, Wright T, et al: Cervical human papillovirus infection and intraepithelial neoplasia. J Natl Cancer Inst 1996,21:17. **(III, B)**

5. Atypical squamous cells of undetermined significance/Low-grade squamous intraepithelial lesions Triage Study (ALTS) Group: Human papillomavirus testing for triage of women with cytologic evidence of low-grade squamous intraepithelial lesions. J Natl Cancer Inst 2000;92:397–402. **(Ib, A)**

6. Creasman WT: New gynecologic cancer staging. Gynecol Oncol 1995;58:157–158. **(IV, C)**

7. Ostor AG: Pandora's box or Ariadne's thread? Definition and prognostic significance of microinvasion in the uterine cervix: squamous lesions. Pathol Annual 1995;30(pt 2):103–136. **(III, B)**

8. Greer BE, Figge DC, Tamimi HK, et al: Stage IA2, squamous carcinoma of the cervix: difficult diagnosis and therapeutic dilemma. Am J Obstet Gynecol 1990;162:1406–1409. **(III, B)**

9. Roman LD, Felix JD, Muderspach LI, et al: Risk of residual invasive disease in women with microinvasive squamous cancer in conization specimen. Obstet Gynecol 1997;90:759–764. **(III, B)**

0. Samlal RAK, van der Velden J, Ketting BW, et al: Disease-free interval and recurrence pattern after the Okabayashi variant of Wertheim's radical hysterectomy for stage IB and IIA cervical carcinoma. Int J Gynecol Cancer 1996;6:120–127. **(III, B)**

21. Perez CA, Grisby PW, Camel HM, et al: Irradiation alone or combined with surgery in stage IB, IIA, and IIB carcinoma of uterine cervix: update of a nonrandomized comparison. Int J Radiat Oncol Biol Phys 1995;31:703–716. **(IIa, B)**

22. Downey GO, Potish RA, Adcock LL, et al: Pretreatment surgical staging in cervical carcinoma: therapeutic efficacy of pelvic lymph node resection. Am J Obstet Gynecol 1989;160:1055–1061. **(III, B)**

23. Stehman FB, Bundy BN, Thomas G, et al: Hydroxyurea vs misonidazole with radiation in cervical carcinoma: long term follow up of a Gynecologic Oncology Group trial. J Clin Oncol 1993;11:1523–1528. **(Ib, A)**

24. Whitney CW, Sause W, Bundy BN, et al: Randomized comparison of fluorouracil plus cisplatin versus hydroxyurea as an adjunct to radiation therapy in stage IIB-IVA carcinoma of the cervix with negative para-aortic lymph nodes: a Gynecologic Oncology Group and Southwest Oncology Group study. J Clin Oncol 1999;17:1339–1348. **(Ib, A)**

25. Rose PG, Bundy BN, Watkins EB, et al: Concurrent cisplatin-based radiotherapy and chemotherapy for locally advanced cervical cancer. N Engl J Med 1999;340:1144–1153. **(Ib, A)**

26. Perez CA, Grigsby PW, Camel HM, et al: Irradiations alone or combined with surgery in stage IB, IIA, and IIB carcinoma of uterine cervix: update of a nonrandomized comparison. Int J Radiat Oncol Biol Phys 1995;31:703–716. **(III, B)**

27. Fagundes H, Perez CA, Grigsby PW, Lockett MA: Distant metastasis after irradiation alone in carcinoma of the uterine cervix. Int J Radiat Oncol Biol Phys 1992;24:197–204. **(III, B)**

28. Omura GA, Blessing JA, Vacarello L, et al: Randomized trial of cisplatin versus cisplatin plus mitolactol versus cisplatin plus ifosfamide in advanced or recurrent squamous cell carcinoma of the cervix: a Gynecologic Oncology Group study. J Clin Oncol 1997;15:165–171. **(Ib, A)**

29. Moore DH, Blessing JA, McQuellon RP, et al: Phase III study of cisplatin with or without paclitaxel in Stage IVB, recurrent, or persistent squamous cell carcinoma of the cervix: a Gynecologic Oncology Group study. J Clin Oncol 2004;22:3113–3119. **(Ib, A)**

30. Cleary JF: Cancer pain management. Cancer Control 2000;7:120–131. **(IV, C)**

31. World Health Organization: Cancer Pain Relief, 2nd ed. Geneva: World Health Organization, 1996. **(IV, C)**

32. Ventafridda V, Saita L, Ripamonti C, et al: WHO guidelines for the use of analgesics in cancer pain. Int J Tissue React 1985;7:93–96. **(IV, C)**

# Endometrial Carcinoma

## Enrique Hernandez, MD, and Karen L. Houck, MD

## KEY POINTS

- Endometrial carcinoma is the most common gynecologic malignancy.
- The most common presenting symptom is vaginal bleeding in postmenopausal women.
- Diagnosis is made by endometrial biopsy.
- Total abdominal hysterectomy, bilateral salpingo-oophorectomy, pelvic and periaortic lymph node sampling, peritoneal washing, and omental biopsy in selected cases is the cornerstone of therapy.
- The stage of cancer is determined by the surgicopathologic findings.
- The need for adjuvant therapy (radiation and/or chemotherapy) is determined by the histologic type, tumor grade, and stage.

## EPIDEMIOLOGY, PATHOGENESIS, AND RISK FACTORS

Cancer of the uterine corpus is the most common gynecologic cancer in the United States, with approximately 40,000 cases diagnosed annually. Endometrial carcinoma is by far the most common of the uterine cancers. Other malignancies of the uterus include leiomyosarcomas, carcinosarcomas, and endometrial stromal sarcomas.

The mean and median age at diagnosis of women with endometrial carcinoma is 61 years.[1] Less than 5% of cases occur in women younger than age 40, and 90% occur in women older than age 50.[2]

### Histology

Endometrial carcinoma is divided into several histologic types; endometrioid adenocarcinoma is the most common (Table 45-1). The endometrioid adenocarcinomas can have areas of squamous metaplasia (adenoacanthoma) or areas of squamous carcinoma (adenosquamous carcinoma). In these cases the preferred histopathologic diagnosis is endometrial adenocarcinoma with benign or malignant squamous differentiation. The prognosis in cases of endometrioid endometrial adenocarcinoma with squamous differentiation is associated with the grade of the glandular component rather than the presence of a malignant squamous component. However, a malignant squamous component is usually associated with a grade 3 endometrioid adenocarcinoma; this is associated with a higher stage of cancer and a worse prognosis. Pure squamous cell carcinomas of the endometrium are extremely rare. Other histologic types, such as papillary serous and clear cell carcinomas, which are associated with a more aggressive behavior than endometrioid carcinomas, account for 5% to 10% of endometrial cancers. These rare types of endometrial carcinoma include mucinous adenocarcinoma, secretory adenocarcinoma, and transitional cell carcinoma. The uterine papillary serous carcinomas must be distinguished from the endometrioid carcinomas with papillary architecture. The latter, also known as a villoglandular adenocarcinoma, is a well-differentiated endometrioid adenocarcinoma. In general, villoglandular endometrial adenocarcinoma is associated with a good prognosis, and uterine papillary serous carcinomas are not.

Estrogen induces mitotic activity of the endometrial epithelial and stromal cells. Under estrogenic influence the endometrium proliferates and the glandular epithelium becomes pseudostratified. Persistent estrogen stimulation unopposed by progesterone leads to endometrial hyperplasia. Depending on the architectural complexity of the glands, the hyperplasia is described as simple or complex (Fig. 45-1). The hyperplasia is further stratified by the presence or absence of cytologic atypia. Therefore, endometrial hyperplasia is classified as simple hyperplasia with or without atypia or complex hyperplasia with or without atypia (Fig. 45-2). In untreated patients endometrial hyperplasia can progress to adenocarcinoma. This has been reported to occur in 1% of cases of simple hyperplasia without atypia, 3% of complex hyperplasia without atypia, 8% of cases of simple hyperplasia with atypia, and 29% of complex hyperplasia with atypia.[3,4] Endometrial adenocarcinoma frequently coexists with endometrial hyperplasia. Furthermore, 20% to 50% of patients who undergo a hysterectomy a few weeks after endometrial sampling shows atypical simple or complex endometrial hyperplasia are found to have endometrial adenocarcinoma in the hysterectomy specimen.[5]

It has been suggested that there are two types of endometrial carcinoma, type I and II (Table 45-2). Type I are estrogen-induced, well-differentiated, superficially invasive tumors. They frequently coexist with endometrial hyperplasia, respond to treatment with progestins, and are associated with a good prognosis. Type II endometrial carcinoma may not be associated with unopposed estrogen stimulation of the endometrium. It occurs in women older than those who develop type I. It is characterized by poorly differentiated tumors (i.e., grade 3) or aggressive histologic types (e.g., papillary serous, clear cell) that deeply invade the myometrium. Type II endometrial carcinoma is associated with a poorer prognosis than type I.

### Risk Factors

More than 75% of endometrial carcinomas are type I. Many of the identified risk factors for endometrial adenocarcinoma are associated with an excess of unopposed estrogen. Obesity of 13 to 22 kg over ideal body weight is associated with a threefold

| Table 45-1 |
| --- |
| Histologic Types of Endometrial Carcinoma |
| Clear cell |
| Endometrioid |
| Mucinous |
| Papillary serous |
| Secretory |
| Squamous |
| Transitional cell |

| Table 45-2 |
| --- |
| Types I and II Endometrial Carcinoma |
| **Type I** |
| • Grade 1–2 |
| • Superficial or no myometrial invasion |
| • Coexisting endometrial hyperplasia |
| • Perimenopausal |
| • Induced by estrogen |
| • Responds to progestins |
| • Good prognosis |
| **Type II** |
| • High grade (grade 3, papillary serous, clear cell) |
| • Deep myometrial invasion |
| • Postmenopausal women |
| • Not induced by estrogen |
| • Does not respond to progestins |
| • Poor prognosis |

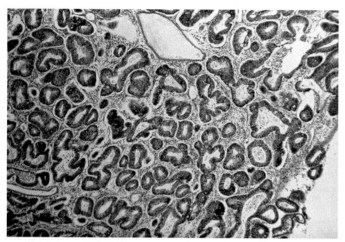

**Figure 45-1   Simple endometrial hyperplasia.** Glandular proliferation is present; there are more glands and they are closer together than seen in normal proliferative endometrium. Plenty of endometrial stroma is still present between the glands. Some of the glands are mildly convoluted; most are round, but a few are dilated.

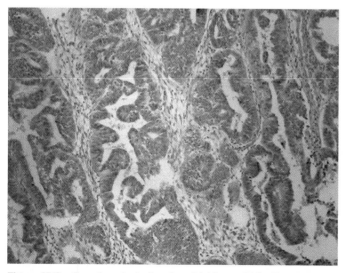

**Figure 45-2   Complex atypical endometrial hyperplasia.** The glands are hyperplastic, with complex infolding of the glandular epithelium into the gland's lumen. Back-to-back glands with little intervening endometrial stroma are seen on the right. The nuclear atypia is not well appreciated at this magnification.

increase in the relative risk of developing endometrial adeno carcinoma[6]; the increase in relative risk is 10-fold in women who are 23 kg overweight. Peripheral conversion of androstenedione to estrone by the fibroblasts in the fat accounts for the increased risk. Nulliparity is associated with a twofold increase in the relative risk of developing endometrial adenocarcinoma. This is probably related to the absence of progesterone in women who are infertile secondary to anovulation resulting in unopposed estrogen stimulation of the endometrium.

Other situations associated with the development of endo metrial adenocarcinoma include hypertension (1.5-fold increase in relative risk), diabetes mellitus (1.8-fold increase in relative risk), use of unopposed estrogen replacement therapy (fourfold increase in relative risk), and the presence of complex atypical endometrial hyperplasia (29-fold increase in relative risk). Endometrial adenocarcinoma is found in 5% to 15% of women with ovarian tumors that produce estrogen (e.g., granulosa-theca cell tumor). Ten percent of women with ovarian adenocarcinoma are found to have a synchronous endometrial adenocarcinoma. In more than 50% of these cases the histologic type of both tumors is endometrioid, making it difficult for the pathologist to distinguished between metastasis or the presence of two primary cancers.[8–10]

The use of tamoxifen also increases the risk of developing endometrial adenocarcinoma and carcinosarcoma. In the North American breast cancer clinical trials, the use of 20 mg/d of tamoxifen resulted in a 7.5-fold increase in the relative risk of developing endometrial adenocarcinoma.[6] In women taking placebo the annual incidence of endometrial adenocarcinoma was 0.2/1000; in women who took tamoxifen it was 1.6/1000. Since the expected mortality from endometrial adenocarcinoma is 15% (i.e., 0.24/1000 women taking tamoxifen), annual screening of the thousands of women who take tamoxifen could potentially prevent death from endometrial adenocarcinoma in only a small fraction of them. Routine screening for endometrial carcinoma in women taking tamoxifen is not recommended. However, endometrial sampling should be done in women who experience vaginal bleeding while on tamoxifen.[4]

Endometrial adenocarcinoma is more common among members of families with hereditary nonpolyposis colorectal cancer (HNPCC).[4,11] HNPCC is also known as Lynch syndrome and is subdivided into Lynch I and Lynch II. The Lynch I syndrome is characterized by early-onset (median age, 46 years) colorectal cancer that shows a predilection (60% to 70%) for the proximal colon and has a high rate of multiple primary colorectal carcinomas. The Lynch II syndrome has all of the preceding features, but in addition includes a number of extracolonic cancers (endometrial, ovarian, small intestine, gastric, pancreas, transitional cell carcinoma of the ureter and renal pelvis), the most common of which is endometrial adenocarcinoma.

Mutations of DNA mismatch repair genes in chromosome 2p (hMSH2) and chromosome 3p (hMLH1) account for 90% of HNPCC cases. This disturbance in DNA mismatch repair leads to genetic instability in somatic cells.

The lifetime risk for developing endometrial carcinoma for HNPCC gene carriers may be as high as 30%. It is recommended that, starting at age 30, women from HNPCC families undergo annual endometrial sampling.[12] These women should also undergo a colonoscopy every 2 years from age 20 to 35 and annually thereafter. At present, it is also recommended that starting at age 30 they undergo annual transvaginal sonographic examination of the ovaries and serum CA 125 determination. Prophylactic oophorectomy should be considered if preserving fertility is not an issue.

A number of studies have shown that full-term pregnancies and the use of oral contraceptives provide a degree of protection from endometrial carcinoma. A linear inverse relationship exists between the number of full-term pregnancies and the relative risk of developing endometrial carcinoma.[13,14] The use of oral contraceptives has been consistently associated with an approximately 50% reduction in the relative risk of developing endometrial carcinoma.[15]

The risk factors for type II endometrial carcinoma have not been as thoroughly studied as those for type I. Studies of patients with uterine papillary serous carcinoma and clear cell carcinoma do not show an association with estrogen use, obesity, diabetes mellitus, or hypertension.[16,17]

## DIAGNOSIS

Abnormal uterine bleeding (e.g., menometrorrhagia, postmenopausal bleeding) is the typical presenting symptom in women with endometrial hyperplasia or carcinoma. Some patients may complain of bloody-tinged, sometimes purulent (in cases of carcinoma) vaginal discharge. Rarely, the diagnosis is made while investigating a Papanicolaou smear showing abnormal glandular cells. On occasion the endometrial hyperplasia or carcinoma is found in a uterus removed for some other condition.

In a woman with postmenopausal bleeding, sampling of the endometrial cavity is mandatory; it should be strongly considered in women older than age 40 who have abnormal menses or intermenstrual bleeding. This could be done by traditional dilatation and curettage (D&C). However, a number of endometrial sampling devices that do not require cervical dilatation and that are appropriate for the clinical office setting (Fig. 45-3) offer the same sensitivity for detecting endometrial hyperplasia or adenocarcinoma as D&C.[18] Office endometrial sampling has now become routine for the evaluation of women with abnormal uterine bleeding. Dilatation and curettage samples about 50%

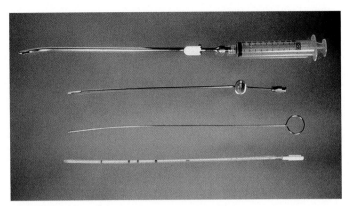

**Figure 45-3  Several endometrial sampling devices.** A, Novak curette attached to a syringe. B and C, Hofmeister curet, a thinner, metal curette with stylet. D, the plastic Pipelle (Unimar, Wilton, CT) or similar device is the most popular endometrial sampling device in use today. It is 3 mm in diameter and 25 cm long. After the operator inserts the Pipelle into the endometrial cavity to the fundus, the inner plastic stylet is withdrawn. This creates suction. As the Pipelle is slowly withdrawn and rotated, endometrium is suctioned into the hollow of the device.

of the endometrial cavity, but the most commonly used suction endometrial sampling devices sample less than 15%. Therefore, a D&C should be performed if the endometrial biopsy detects hyperplasia. A neighboring adenocarcinoma may have been missed by the limited sample obtained by the endometrial aspiration device.

Hysteroscopy does not offer better sensitivity for detecting endometrial hyperplasia or adenocarcinoma than an endometrial biopsy. However, if the endometrial biopsy is negative or inconclusive and the patient continues to experience vaginal bleeding, hysteroscopy should be considered. Hysteroscopy is better than D&C at detecting endometrial polyps and submucosal fibroids.[19] Sonohysterography can also detect these lesions, but hysteroscopy/D&C might still be necessary since endometrial hyperplasia or cancer can be found, although infrequently, in endometrial polyps.[20]

The probability of finding endometrial cancer in the endometrial curettings from a woman with postmenopausal bleeding is age dependent. The frequency of endometrial cancer in women age 50 to 59 with postmenopausal bleeding is 9%; in women age 60 to 69, 16%; in women age 70 to 79, 28%; and in women older than age 80, 60%.[21] Although some have tried to predict the presence of endometrial adenocarcinoma in women with postmenopausal bleeding based on the risk factors discussed previously, the models proposed are not sufficiently sensitive.[22] In the rare situation in which endometrial sampling cannot be accomplished, transvaginal ultrasonography is of value. At a threshold of 5 mm for endometrial thickness, the negative predictive value of transvaginal sonography is 99%. However, the positive predictive value for detecting any abnormality is only 9%.[23]

## TREATMENT

### Endometrial Hyperplasia

After excluding an estrogen-producing tumor as the cause of endometrial hyperplasia, treatment with progestins can prevent

# Gynecologic Oncology

the development of endometrial adenocarcinoma. For treatment purposes patients with endometrial hyperplasia can be divided into those with atypical hyperplasia (who are at higher risk for developing carcinoma) and those without atypia. Women with simple or complex endometrial hyperplasia without atypia are treated with either cyclic (e.g., medroxyprogesterone 10 mg/d the first 14 days of every month) or continuous (e.g., megestrol 20 mg bid) progestins. However, laboratory data suggests that the cyclic administration may be more effective.[24] The successful treatment of endometrial hyperplasia using a progestin-releasing intrauterine device (IUD) has also been reported.[25] An endometrial biopsy obtained after 3 to 6 months of therapy should reveal a normal endometrium with progestational changes. After resolution of the hyperplasia, women at risk for pregnancy who do not desire one are placed on oral contraceptives, if not contraindicated. Those who are anovulatory and desire to become pregnant can undergo ovulation induction. Those who are not at risk for pregnancy can continue on cyclic progestin therapy. The disappearance of withdrawal bleeding after 14 days of progestin would indicate that there is no longer enough circulating estrogen to stimulate the endometrium and progestin therapy can be discontinued.

As stated previously, women with atypical endometrial hyperplasia (simple or complex) are at risk for harboring a coexistent adenocarcinoma. If they have completed their family, a hysterectomy should be considered. If they want to preserve their uterus or have comorbid conditions that significantly increase the risk of surgical complications, treatment with continuous progestins is instituted. Megestrol acetate (20 to 40 mg bid) is one option. Alternatives include the use of depot medroxyprogesterone or a progestin-containing IUD.[25] The endometrium is sampled 3 to 6 months after the initiation of therapy. If the hyperplasia persists and the patient is at high risk for surgical complications, a pelvic magnetic resonance imaging (MRI) study will help exclude a coexistent endometrial adenocarcinoma with myometrial invasion. If the MRI shows a normal junctional zone, intracavitary radiation (i.e., brachytherapy) could be considered.

Surgery is the cornerstone of therapy for endometrial carcinoma. Most patients with endometrial cancer undergo surgical staging. The pretreatment evaluation, when surgery is to be performed by a gynecologic oncologist, can be limited to a chest radiograph and routine blood studies. Pretreatment studies such as cystoscopy, sigmoidoscopy, intravenous pyelogram, and barium enema have been found to be unnecessary.[26] Preoperative computed tomography (CT) has a poor positive predictive value (50%) and poor sensitivity (57%) for detecting lymph node metastasis.[26] The CT findings seldom alter the treatment plan.

## Presurgical Evaluation of Carcinoma

Patients with stage IA or IB, grade 1 endometrial adenocarcinoma are at low risk of having lymph node metastasis. In these patients there is little to gain by doing a lymphadenectomy and there are some risks associated with it. These patients can have their surgery performed by a gynecologic generalist. A preoperative pelvic MRI can determine the absence of myometrial invasion.[27-29] In addition, the probability of finding extrauterine disease with a serum CA 125 of less than 20 U/mL is close to 0%.[30] Therefore, a preoperative MRI and a CA 125 in a woman with clinical stage I, grade 1 endometrial adenocarcinoma can

identify patients that can be treated with a hysterectomy only (i.e., normal junctional zone on gadolinium-enhanced MRI, CA 125 < 20 U/mL). In this select group of patients a transvaginal hysterectomy can be considered.[30]

## Staging Endometrial Carcinoma

The International Federation of Gynecology and Obstetrics (FIGO) staging of endometrial carcinoma in use today was adopted in 1988 (Table 45-3). It requires surgery and careful pathologic evaluation of the removed tissues. The clinical staging classification used before 1988 is an alternative if the patient cannot be surgically staged (Table 45-4).

**Table 45-3**
**FIGO Staging of Endometrial Carcinoma**

| Stage | Description |
|---|---|
| I | Confined to the body of the uterus |
| IA | No myometrial invasion |
| IB | Invades myometrium to <50% |
| IC | Invades the myometrium to 50% depth or more |
| II | Involves the uterus and the cervix |
| IIA | Cancer in the cervix is no deeper than the endocervical glands |
| IIB | Cancer in the cervix invades the stroma below the endocervical glands |
| III | Cancer invades the uterine serosa, adnexa, retroperitoneal nodes, or vagina and/or positive peritoneal cytology |
| IIIA | Positive peritoneal cytology, uterine serosal and/or adnexal involvement with cancer |
| IIIB | Cancer present in the vagina |
| IIIC | Cancer present in the pelvic and/or periaortic lymph nodes |
| IV | Intra-abdominal metastasis, metastasis outside of the abdomen and pelvis to include to the inguinal nodes and/or rectal or bladder mucosa invasion by the cancer |
| IVA | Rectal and/or bladder mucosa invasion by the cancer |
| IVB | Intra-abdominal metastasis (e.g., metastasis to omentum) metastasis to inguinal nodes, distant metastasis (e.g., metastasis to lungs) |

The stage also includes the tumor grade
| Grade 1 | 5% or less of the tumor is solid |
| Grade 2 | 6% to 50% of the tumor is solid |
| Grade 3 | >50% of the tumor is solid |

In cases of significant nuclear atypia, the cancer is upgraded one grade. In patients who cannot undergo surgery, the clinical staging system in place before 1988 is used.

**Table 45-4**
**Clinical Staging of Endometrial Cancer in Use Before 1988***

| Stage | Description |
|---|---|
| I | Confined to the uterus |
| IA | Uterus sounds to ≤8 cm |
| IB | Uterus sounds to >8 cm |
| II | Cancer extends to the cervix |
| III | Cancer involves other pelvic organs, other than the bladder or rectum |
| IVA | Invasion into bladder and/or rectal mucosa |
| IVB | Distant metastasis |

*This classification is used for patients who cannot undergo surgicopathologic staging.

The surgicopathologic staging classification correlates better than clinical staging with the risk for nodal metastasis and prognosis. For each stage, the grade of the tumor is included. The FIGO grading system for endometrial adenocarcinoma is based on the architectural features of the tumor. In grade 1 endometrial adenocarcinomas, 5% or less of the tumor is solid. Grade 2 tumors are 6% to 50% solid, and grade 3 tumors are more than 50% solid. In tumors with a squamous cell carcinoma component (i.e., adenosquamous), the grading is based on the glandular component. Tumors with significant cytologic atypia are upgraded one grade higher than their architectural grading would suggest. In papillary serous and clear cell carcinomas nuclear grading takes precedence, but these histologic types are usually considered grade 3.

In patients with surgicopathologic stage I disease, the endometrial carcinoma is confined to the corpus. If there is no myometrial invasion it is stage IA. If invasion is limited to the inner half of the myometrium (<50%), it is stage IB. If the carcinoma invades the outer half of the myometrium (≥ 50%), it is stage IC. There is a direct correlation between the depth of myometrial invasion and the proportion of patients found to have pelvic or periaortic nodal metastasis (Table 45-5).[31] Eleven percent of patients with deep myometrial invasion and grade 1 endometrial adenocarcinoma have pelvic node metastasis. Pelvic node metastases are found in 19% of patients with grade 2 deeply invasive tumors and in 34% with grade 3 deeply invasive tumors. Periaortic node metastases are found in 6% of patients with deep myometrial invasion and grade 1 adenocarcinoma. They are found in 14% of patients with deeply invasive grade 2 adenocarcinomas and in 23% of patients with deeply invasive grade 3 tumors. However, metastases to the pelvic or periaortic lymph nodes are negligible in patients with grade 3 tumors with no myometrial invasion.

Stage II tumors involve the uterine corpus and the cervix. If the tumor does not invade any deeper than the normal location of the endocervical glands it is classified as stage IIA. If there is cervical stromal invasion below the endocervical glands it is classified as stage IIB. Patients with stage IIA endometrial adenocarcinoma have a better prognosis than patients with stage IIB.

Stage IIIA endometrial carcinoma includes a heterogeneous group of patients. These patients may have invasion of the carcinoma to the uterine serosa, involvement of the adnexa, or positive peritoneal washings. Patients with one of these findings and those with two or three of them are still classified as having stage IIIA endometrial carcinoma. However, the prognosis worsens as the number of factors that would classify a patient as having stage IIIA disease increases. Among women with stage IIIA endometrial adenocarcinoma, those with positive peritoneal cytology have a better prognosis than those with adnexal metastasis or uterine serosal involvement.[32]

In 1981, Creasman and collaborators reported on 167 patients with clinical stage I endometrial cancer.[33] Malignant cells were identified in the peritoneal washings of 15% of these patients. Patients with positive peritoneal cytology had a poorer probability of survival than those with negative washings. This was true in the presence or absence of identified extrauterine cancer. However, not all patients underwent systematic surgical staging. At the Roswell Park Cancer Institute women with stage I endometrial adenocarcinoma received a prehysterectomy intrauterine radioactive implant. Of 93 patients reported by Yazigi and colleagues[34] in 1983, 10 had positive peritoneal cytology. There was no statistically significant difference in survival probability between patients with negative or positive peritoneal washings. In 1992, Kadar and collaborators reported on 269 women with clinical stage I or II endometrial adenocarcinoma who underwent systematic surgical staging. Thirty-four (13%) were found to have positive peritoneal cytology.[35] No difference in the probability of survival was found between patients with positive or negative peritoneal cytology who had no extrauterine metastasis. However, the cumulative 5-year survival of patients with extrauterine metastasis (e.g., metastasis to periaortic lymph nodes) and positive peritoneal cytology was 13%, whereas it was 73% if the cytology was negative. This correlates with Gynecologic Oncology Group (GOG) data that showed that in women with clinical stage I and II endometrial adenocarcinoma who underwent surgical staging, recurrences occurred in 64 (11%) of 611 with negative washings and in 25 of 86 (29%) of those with positive washings.[36] However, recurrences occurred in only 6 (19%) of 32 women with positive peritoneal cytology without other risk factors. The preceding data suggest that the presence of positive peritoneal cytology is of most clinical significance in patients with endometrial adenocarcinoma who have extrauterine spread.

Endometrial carcinoma that invades the bladder or rectal mucosa is classified as stage IVA. If intra-abdominal, extra-abdominal, or inguinal lymph nodes metastases are present, the disease is classified as stage IVB. Extrapelvic peritoneal metastases are found in approximately 10% of patients with clinical stage I, grade 2 or 3 endometrioid adenocarcinoma or high-risk histologic types (i.e., papillary serous, clear cell).[37] In most, the metastases are macroscopic. This highlights the importance of careful exploration of the entire peritoneal cavity.

## Treatment of Endometrial Carcinoma

Although surgery is the cornerstone of therapy for endometrial cancer, patients who are not surgical candidates can be effectively treated with radiation. To obtain results similar to those obtained in patients who undergo primary surgical therapy, both

**Table 45-5**
**Percentage of Patients with Pelvic and Periaortic Node Metastasis in Endometrial Carcinoma***

| Depth of Invasion | Grade 1 (N=180) | | Grade 2 (N=288) | | Grade 3 (N=153) | |
|---|---|---|---|---|---|---|
| | Pelvic (%) | PA (%) | Pelvic (%) | PA (%) | Pelvic (%) | PA (%) |
| None (N=86) | 0 | 0 | 3 | 3 | 0 | 0 |
| Inner 1/3 (N=281) | 3 | 1 | 5 | 4 | 9 | 4 |
| Mid 1/3 (N=115) | 0 | 5 | 9 | 0 | 4 | 0 |
| Out 1/3 (N=139) | 11 | 6 | 19 | 14 | 34 | 23 |

PA, periaortic nodes.
*Based on histologic grade and depth of myometrial invasion.
From Creasman WT, Morrow CP, Bundy BN, et al: Surgical pathologic spread of endometrial cancer. Cancer 1987;60:2035–2041.

external beam (teletherapy) and intracavitary irradiation (brachytherapy) should be used.[38] Pretreatment evaluation with CT and/or MRI is performed. Patients with grade 1 adenocarcinoma, no myometrial invasion on MRI, and a CA 125 of less than 20 U/mL can be treated with brachytherapy only. Women with well-differentiated endometrial adenocarcinoma who are not fit to undergo brachytherapy or women who are young and desire to preserve their fertility can be treated with progestins.[39] An MRI of the pelvis and a serum CA 125 determination are obtained before taking this approach. Approximately 70% of women with a grade 1 endometrial adenocarcinoma who are treated with progestins will have a complete response.[39] Megestrol acetate (80 mg bid) is one treatment option. Sampling of the endometrium is done after 3 to 6 months of therapy.

Most women with endometrial cancer are treated primarily by total abdominal hysterectomy and bilateral salpingo-oophorectomy. The abdomen is opened through a low vertical midline incision that can be extended above the umbilicus if periaortic lymph node dissection is to be performed. On entering the abdomen, pelvic washings are obtained utilizing at least 200 mL of saline. Laparoscopic-assisted vaginal hysterectomy (LAVH) and bilateral salpingo-oophorectomy is an alternative to laparotomy. If LAVH is done, peritoneal washings are obtained early in the procedure. If necessary a laparoscopic pelvic and/or periaortic node dissection can be done.

Although the status of the pelvic and periaortic lymph nodes is considered in FIGO staging, most patients with endometrial adenocarcinoma do not undergo lymphadenectomy. The National Cancer Institute's Survival, Epidemiology, and End Results (SEER) database has 23,258 women with "stage I" endometrial adenocarcinoma treated between 1998 and 2000. Only 6371 (27%) underwent lymph node dissection.[40] Lymphadenectomy is routinely performed by only 54% of gynecologic oncologists in North America who took part of a survey in 1994.[41] This is so because the need for adjuvant therapy directed at the pelvic lymph nodes can be determined by the grade of the tumor and the depth of myometrial invasion. One study showed that no patient with stage IA or IB, grade 1 or 2 endometrial adenocarcinoma with greatest surface dimension of 2 cm or less had positive lymph nodes or died of cancer.[42] It has been shown that when adjuvant whole pelvis irradiation is limited to patients at risk for pelvic node metastasis, the recurrence rate is 10%.[43] The cumulative 5-year survival of patients with endometrial adenocarcinoma at low risk of pelvic node metastasis treated with surgery only is not statistically different from that of patients who are at higher risk of pelvic node metastasis and who receive adjuvant whole pelvis irradiation after surgery.[44] In addition, 38% of patients who do not receive postsurgical adjuvant irradiation and who develop a recurrence are salvaged by radiation therapy.[45] This means that even if 10% of patients with low-risk endometrial adenocarcinoma were to recur, the cure rate for this group of patients would be at least 93%.

The GOG showed that 9% of women with clinical stage I endometrial adenocarcinoma have pelvic node metastasis.[31] Ninety-five percent of the pelvic node metastasis occurs in patients with deeply invasive tumors or grade 2 or 3 adenocarcinomas. Pelvic node metastasis is found in 5% or less of patients with grade 1 or 2 adenocarcinoma that does not invade the myometrium or in which the invasion is limited to the inner third (see Table 45-5). In contrast, 11% of patients with grade 1 endometrial adenocarcinomas that invaded to the outer third of the myometrium have pelvic node metastasis. Therefore, adjuvant whole pelvis irradiation should be considered for patients with stage IC endometrial adenocarcinoma of any grade.

Some advocate the performance of pelvic and periaortic lymphadenectomy in all patients with endometrial adenocarcinoma grossly confined to the uterus[46]; others suggest that it is not necessary to perform the lymphadenectomy in patients with stage IA or IB, grade 1 adenocarcinoma.[47] Orr and colleagues[46] reported on 69 patients with stage IC endometrial adenocarcinoma who underwent pelvic and periaortic lymphadenectomy and did not receive radiation. Their cumulative 5-year survival was 93%. Larson and colleagues[47] performed pelvic and periaortic lymphadenectomy in 123 patients with clinical stage I, grade 2 or 3 endometrial adenocarcinoma, or stage I, grade 1 with invasion to the outer half of the myometrium. Of these patients, 105 (85%) had negative nodes and a median follow-up of 39 months. Their cumulative 5-year survival was 91%. Of the 18 patients with metastasis to the lymph nodes, 5 had estrogen receptor-positive tumors and received 320 mg of megestrol acetate daily. Thirteen had estrogen receptor-negative tumors and were treated with chemotherapy (cyclophosphamide, doxorubicin, and cisplatin). With a median follow-up of 51 months, the cumulative 5-year survival of these 18 patients is 85%.

Orr and colleagues[46] did not show a clinically significant increase in the morbidity associated with performing a pelvic and periaortic lymphadenectomy. In contrast, investigators from Duke University did show that women with endometrial adenocarcinoma who underwent pelvic lymph node sampling sustained increased blood loss and transfusions, longer operative time, and increased morbidity.[48] In addition, Lewandowski and colleagues[49] showed an increase in intestinal complications in patients who received whole pelvis radiation after pelvic and periaortic lymphadenectomy. Eleven percent of patients who received whole pelvis radiation after total abdominal hysterectomy, bilateral salpingo-oophorectomy, and pelvic and periaortic lymphadenectomy developed intestinal complications. Intestinal complications were not reported among women who received postoperative whole pelvis radiation and who did not undergo lymphadenectomy.

Periaortic node metastases are present in 5% of women with clinical stage I endometrial adenocarcinoma.[31] Ninety-four percent of patients with periaortic node metastasis have grade 2 or 3 tumors or grade 1 adenocarcinomas that invade deeply into the myometrium. Less than 5% of patients whose tumors do not penetrate any deeper than the inner one third of the myometrium have periaortic node metastasis (see Table 45-5).

The Postoperative Radiation Therapy for Endometrial Carcinoma (PORTEC) study group randomized patients with endometrial carcinoma after total abdominal hysterectomy and bilateral salpingo-oophorectomy without lymph node dissection to receive 4600 cGy to the pelvis or to observation.[50] This is the only published randomized trial with long-term follow-up that studies the value of adjuvant pelvic radiation therapy in patients with endometrial carcinoma with intermediate risk factors. The PORTEC trial was limited to women with stage IC, grade 1 or 2 endometrial adenocarcinoma or stage IB, grade 2 or 3 disease.

Patients with stage IC, grade 3 tumors were not included. Patients with stage IA, any grade, or stage IB, grade 1 carcinoma were also excluded.

In this group of patients with endometrial adenocarcinoma with intermediate risk of recurrence who did not undergo a lymphadenectomy the actuarial 8-year survival rate is no different for the adjuvant radiation therapy group and the observation group, 71% and 77%, respectively. The 8-year actuarial locoregional failure rate was higher in the observation group (15%) than in the adjuvant radiation group (4%). Most recurrences in the observation group occurred in the vagina (32 of 41). Of the patients in the observation group with vaginal recurrences, 30 received treatment for the recurrence with curative intent. Twenty-six of the 30 achieved a complete response and 20 were without disease at last follow-up. The actuarial 5-year survival rate after vaginal recurrence in the observation group and in the radiation therapy group is 65% and 43%, respectively.

A similar study by the GOG, with a median follow-up of 69 months, randomized surgically staged women with stage IB, IC, and II (occult disease) endometrial adenocarcinoma to adjuvant whole pelvis irradiation or observation.[51] This study also shows no difference in survival. The estimated 4-year survival was 86% in the observation group and 92% in the radiation arm ($P = 0.557$).

The PORTEC study found that the rate of locoregional failure was significant (>10%) only among women older than age 60 and among those with grade 2 deeply invasive tumors and stage IB, grade 3 tumors. In a retrospective study, investigators from the Mayo Clinic identified lymphovascular invasion (LVI) as another significant risk factor for local failures.[52] Others have shown that tumor size (>2 cm) is also a significant risk factor.[53] Therefore, patients with stage IB, grade 3 tumors who are age 60 or older, have tumors with LVI, and/or tumors larger than 2 cm may benefit from adjuvant whole pelvis irradiation, especially if the periaortic nodes are histologically negative.

Based on the preceding data, the therapeutic approach to endometrial adenocarcinoma that offers the best therapeutic index (minimizes morbidity and maximizes cure rate) is the following (Tables 45-6 and 45-7). On entering the abdomen peritoneal cytology is obtained. A total hysterectomy and bilateral salpingo-oophorectomy is performed. An omental biopsy is obtained in cases of papillary serous or clear cell carcinoma. Lymphadenectomy is not performed in patients with grade 1 tumors that on gross examination and/or frozen section of the uterine specimen show less than 33% myometrial invasion.

In selected patients (not obese, low surgical risk) with grade 2 or 3 tumors or deeply invasive grade 1 carcinomas, a bilateral pelvic lymphadenectomy and periaortic node sampling is performed. If metastases in lymph nodes are found (i.e., stage IIIC), chemotherapy with cisplatin and doxorubicin has been recently found to offer a survival advantage over whole abdominal radiation.[54] An ongoing GOG study could show that the addition of chemotherapy to a smaller radiation field (whole pelvis with or without periaortics) improves the probability of survival.[38]

In patients with deeply invasive grade 1 adenocarcinomas and patients with grade 2 or 3 adenocarcinoma, periaortic node dissection might discover extrapelvic disease. Adjuvant whole pelvis radiation is given to patients who have stage IC adeno-

carcinoma of any grade or stage IB, grade 3 adenocarcinoma and who were considered poor candidates for a pelvic lymphadenectomy (see Table 45-6). The addition of intravaginal radioactive implant (i.e., brachytherapy) to adjuvant whole pelvis irradiation has been shown to increase the rate of therapy-induced toxicity and has no impact on local control or the probability of survival.[55] If periaortic node metastasis is discovered, chemotherapy with cisplatin and doxorubicin or carboplatin and paclitaxel can be given. Alternatively, these patients can be entered in a clinical trial. One such trial randomizes patients to receive cisplatin and doxorubicin versus cisplatin, doxorubicin, and paclitaxel after whole pelvis irradiation with or without radiation to the periaortic area, as indicated.[38]

**Table 45-6**
**Guidelines for Adjuvant Therapy of Endometrial Cancer after Total Abdominal Hysterectomy, Bilateral Salpingo-oophorectomy, and Periaortic Node Dissection Without Pelvic Node Dissection**

| Stage | Adjuvant Therapy | Rationale |
|---|---|---|
| IA grade 1–3 | None | Positive nodes, recurrence rate <5% |
| IB grade 1 & 2 | None | Locoregional failure <5% |
| IB grade 3 <60 yo no LVI <2 cm* | None or WP XRT | Low locoregional failure (but based on limited data) |
| IB grade 3 >60 yo LVI >2 cm | WP XRT | Locoregional failure, pos. pelvic nodes >10% |
| IC grade 1* | Individualize, consider WP XRT | Locoregional failure—7% 11% positive pelvic nodes with outer third myometrial invasion |
| IC grade 2–3 | WP XRT | Locoregional failure—15% >10% positive pelvic nodes |
| As above, with positive periaortic (stage IIIC) | Chemotherapy | Better survival probability with chemotherapy than with WAR |
| | Consider whole pelvis and periaortic irradiation followed by chemotherapy | Under investigation |

LVI, lymphovascular invasion; WAR, whole abdominal radiation; WP XRT, whole pelvis radiation.
*In these patients, pelvic lymphadenectomy could offer the best therapeutic index.

**Table 45-7**
**Guidelines for Adjuvant Therapy of Endometrial Carcinoma after Total Abdominal Hysterectomy, Bilateral Salpingo-oophorectomy, and Pelvic and Periaortic Lymphadenectomy**

| Stage | Adjuvant Therapy |
|---|---|
| IA–C, grade 1–3 | None (consider vaginal brachytherapy in grade 3 or with LVI) |
| IIA-B, grade 1–3 | Vaginal radiation implant |
| IIIC and IVB | Chemotherapy |
| IIIA, IIIB, IVA | See text |

LVI, lymphovascular invasion.

# Gynecologic Oncology

Patients with stage I papillary serous carcinoma have a poorer survival probability than patients with endometrioid adenocarcinoma.[4] Their survival probability seems to improve if they are treated aggressively following surgery with radiation and platinum-based chemotherapy.[56] Patients with advanced or recurrent uterine papillary serous carcinoma respond to carboplatin and paclitaxel better than to any other chemotherapy combination.[57] The combination of carboplatin and paclitaxel is increasingly being used in these cases.

Patients with clinically obvious cervical involvement by the endometrial adenocarcinoma (i.e., stage IIB) can be treated with a radical hysterectomy, bilateral salpingo-oophorectomy, bilateral pelvic lymphadenectomy, and periaortic node dissection.[58] In most cases a preferable alternative is to deliver preoperative external-beam whole pelvis radiation and one intrauterine radioactive implant followed 6 weeks later by an extrafascial total abdominal hysterectomy, bilateral salpingo-oophorectomy, and periaortic node dissection.[38] If extrapelvic metastases are found, chemotherapy (e.g., cisplatin and doxorubicin, carboplatin and paclitaxel) is given. Patients with occult stage IIA or IIB endometrial carcinoma found in the hysterectomy specimen receive postoperative adjuvant radiation therapy if a pelvic lymphadenectomy was not done. An intravaginal radioactive implant can be done in patients with occult stage IIA or IIB endometrial adenocarcinoma who were treated by simple hysterectomy and bilateral pelvic lymphadenectomy.[59] This approach can decrease the rate of local recurrences.

Patients with stage IIIA endometrial adenocarcinoma based only on positive peritoneal cytology could be treated with megestrol acetate 160 mg to 320 mg daily.[60] Patients with stage IIIA endometrial adenocarcinoma based on adnexal and/or serosal involvement are treated with chemotherapy (e.g., doxorubicin and cisplatin, carboplatin and paclitaxel). In these patients the entire abdominal cavity is at risk for recurrence. The use of chemotherapy has been found to offer a survival advantage over whole abdominal irradiation.[54] Patients with vaginal metastasis (stage IIIB) receive pelvic irradiation (external beam and intravaginal implant) followed by a hysterectomy and periaortic node dissection. Radiation to the inguinal nodes is given in cases of metastasis to the distal third of the vagina. Chemotherapy is given if more advanced disease is found at the time of the hysterectomy. Another approach, depending on the size and location of the vaginal metastasis, is to perform the surgical staging first and, if more advanced disease (i.e., stage IIIC or IVB) is found, to treat the patient with chemotherapy with or without radiation for control of the vaginal lesions.

Patients with intra-abdominal metastasis (i.e., stage IVB) who are surgically rendered free of macroscopic disease can be treated with whole abdominal radiation, chemotherapy, or hormonal therapy (megestrol and/or tamoxifen). Recent data shows that treatment with cisplatin and doxorubicin results in improved disease-free survival and overall survival than treatment with radiation.[54] Patients with extra-abdominal metastasis or with residual intra-abdominal disease can be treated with chemotherapy (e.g., doxorubicin and cisplatin, carboplatin and paclitaxel) or hormones (megestrol and/or tamoxifen). A recently published GOG study showed a 33% (CI, 21% to 46%) response rate with tamoxifen 40 mg/d given without break and medroxyprogesterone 200 mg/d or 100 mg twice a day, orally, for one week.[61] Another study of patients with recurrent or advanced endometrial adenocarcinoma showed a 27% (CI, 17% to 38%) response rate with megestrol (160 mg/d for 3 weeks) followed by tamoxifen (40 mg/d for 3 weeks).[62] Patients with positive inguinal nodes (stage IVB) and no extrapelvic disease could receive whole pelvis and inguinal irradiation. Alternatively, they could be treated with chemotherapy. Most patients with known stage IVB endometrial adenocarcinoma will still benefit from undergoing a hysterectomy.[63] Selected patients with stage IVA (i.e., bladder or rectal invasion) endometrial adenocarcinoma may benefit from a pelvic exenteration. However, because these patients tend to be older, obese, and with multiple comorbidities, most are treated with pelvic irradiation with or without surgery. The surgery may be a diverting colostomy or urostomy if a fistula develops. In patients with stage IVA endometrial adenocarcinoma that have periaortic node metastasis, chemotherapy, periaortic irradiation, and/or hormonal therapy are also used.

## Treatment of Recurrences

If a recurrence occurs, treatment will depend on the site or sites of recurrence and on the previous therapy. In patients with clinical stage I carcinoma, the vagina is the most frequent site of recurrence.[50,51] A confirmed isolated vaginal recurrence can be treated by surgical excision followed by whole pelvic and intravaginal radiation. If pelvic radiation was used at the time of primary therapy, an intravaginal radiation implant can be used after surgical excision of the recurrence. The actuarial 5-year survival rate after treatment of a vaginal recurrence is approximately 50%.[50] Pelvic sidewall recurrences and extrapelvic recurrences are associated with a low probability of 5-year survival. If no prior radiation therapy has been given, a pelvic recurrence or a periaortic recurrence can be treated with radiation, chemotherapy, or a combination of the two. A patient receiving radiation therapy can receive cisplatin at a dose of $50 \text{ mg/m}^2$ every 21 days concomitant with radiation. Once radiation therapy is completed, several courses of carboplatin and paclitaxel are given. Doxorubicin, an active agent against endometrial carcinoma, can result in increased radiation-induced skin toxicity. Patients who have previously received radiation to the area of the recurrence are treated with chemotherapy. The combination of carboplatin and paclitaxel has shown a high response rate when used to treat women with advanced-stage or recurrent endometrial carcinoma.[57] Topotecan at a dose of $1.5 \text{ mg/m}^2/\text{d}$ for 5 days on a 21-day cycle has shown activity in the treatment of recurrent endometrial carcinoma.[64] However, this dose and schedule are associated with unacceptable bone marrow toxicity. A lower dose of $1 \text{ mg/m}^2$ in patients who had not received prior radiation and $0.8 \text{ mg/m}^2$ for those with a history of prior radiation is being investigated. Hormonal therapy may also be effective. Megestrol at a dose of 160 to 320 mg/d has been used, with complete responses observed, especially in patients with lung metastases.[65] Estrogen increases the expression of progesterone receptors. A combination of progesterone and tamoxifen may result in a higher response rate, as previously discussed.[61,62]

## FOLLOW-UP

Most endometrial carcinoma recurrences occur within the first 2 years after therapy. For this reason, patients undergo a pelvic examination with or without vaginal cytology every 3 months during the first 2 years. An annual chest radiograph should be considered. The yield is higher if the chest radiograph is obtained 2 years after therapy. Most recurrences are detected when the clinical evaluation is directed by the patient's symptoms.[66] In years three, four, and five a pelvic examination is performed every 6 months and vaginal cytology is obtained at least annually. Thereafter, the patient is examined annually. In patients considered at risk for intraperitoneal recurrences (e.g., stage IIIA adenocarcinoma, uterine papillary serous carcinoma), serum for CA 125 levels is periodically sent.[67] This follow-up scheme has not been shown to have a statistically significant impact on the salvage rate of patients with endometrial cancer recurrence. However, it offers the patient psychological support during a period of great anxiety. It also allows the clinician to screen for other cancers (e.g., breast, colon) and to offer other health maintenance services (e.g., smoking cessation, serum lipid determinations, calcium supplementation).

## Management of Menopausal Symptoms

After treatment of endometrial adenocarcinoma, some women may need estrogen replacement therapy for the treatment of vaginal atrophy. Estrogen replacement therapy most likely has no impact on the probability of survival in women who had early-stage endometrial adenocarcinoma. However, a GOG prospective randomized clinical trial that attempted to answer this question was closed before achieving its accrual goal of 2108 patients. An analysis of 1234 evaluable patients (618 randomized to receive estrogen, 616 randomized to receive placebo) was presented at the 35th annual meeting of the Society of Gynecologic Oncologists.[68] The median follow-up for all patients was 30.8 months. Of the 618 patients randomized to receive estrogen, only 12 (1.9%) experienced a recurrence. Of the 616 patients randomized to receive placebo, 9 (1.5%) developed a recurrence. Therapies other than estrogen are available for the management of menopausal changes other than genital atrophy. Hot flashes can be managed with progestins, clonidine, or venlafaxine. Osteoporosis can be prevented with raloxifene or bisphosphonates, in addition to calcium supplementation and weight-bearing exercise.

## Endometrial Carcinoma Survival

Most women with endometrial adenocarcinoma in the United States have stage I disease at diagnosis. Data for 1994 and 1995 reported from 1578 hospitals to the American College of Surgeons' Commission on Cancer show that 63% of patients

had stage I disease, 7.4% stage II, 10.5% stage III, and 6% stage IV (http://web.facs.org/ncdbbmr). The reported 5-year survival is stage I, 81%; stage II, 61%; stage III, 39%; and stage IV, 11%. The probability of 5-year survival by substage according to international statistics is shown in Table 45-8.

## REFERENCES

1. Creasman W, Odicino F, Maisonnenve P, et al: Carcinoma of the corpus uteri. J Epidemiol Biostat 1998;3:35–61. **(III, B)**
2. Farhi DC, Nosanchuk J, Silverberg SG: Endometrial adenocarcinoma in women under 25 years of age. Obstet Gyencol 1986;68:741–745. **(III, B)**
3. Kaminski PF, Podczaski ES: Premalignant and malignant conditions of the uterus. In Hernandez E, Atkinson BF (eds): Clinical Gynecologic Pathology. Philadelphia, WB Saunders, 1995, pp 287–359. **(IV, C)**
4. Irvin WP, Rice LW: Advances in the management of endometrial adenocarcinoma. A review. J Reprod Med 2002;47:173–190. **(IV, C)**
5. Xie X, Wei-Guo L, Da-Feng Y, et al: The value of curettage in diagnosis of endometrial hyperplasia. Gynecol Oncol 202;84:135–139. **(IIb, B)**
6. Barakat RR: Contemporary issues in the management of endometrial cancer. Ca—A Cancer J Clin 1998;48:299–314. **(IV, C)**
7. Kaminski PF, Podczaski ES: Benign conditions of the uterus. In Hernandez E, Atkinson BF (eds): Clinical Gynecologic Pathology. Philadelphia, WB Saunders, 1995, pp 223–286. **(IV, C)**
8. Choo Y, Naylor B: Multiple primary neoplasms of the ovary and uterus. Int J Gynaecol Obstet 1982;20:327–334. **(III, B)**
9. Eifel P, Hendrickson M, Ross J, et al: Simultaneous presentation of carcinoma involving the ovary and the uterine corpus. Cancer 1982;50:163–170. **(III, B)**
10. Zaino R, Whitney C, Brady MF, et al: Simultaneously detected endometrial and ovarian carcinomas—a propective clinicopathologic study of 74 cases: a Gynecologic Oncology Group study. Gynecol Oncol 2001;83:355–362. **(III, B)**
11. Menko FH, Wijnen JT, Vasen HFA, Oosterwijk MH: Genetic counselling in hereditary nonpolyposis colorectal cancer. Oncology 1996;10:71–76. **(IV, C)**
12. Lynch HT, Lynch J: Genetic counselling for hereditary cancer. Oncology 1996;10:27–34. **(IV, C)**
13. Brinton LA, Berman ML, Mortel R, et al: Reproductive, menstrual, and medical risk factors for endometrial cancer: results from a case-control study. Am J Obstet Gynecol 1992;167:1317–1325. **(IIa, B)**
14. Kalandini A, Tzonou A, Lipwirth L, et al: Case-control study of endometrial cancer in relation to reproductive, somatometric, and life-style variables. Oncology 1996;53:354–359. **(IIa, B)**
15. Jick SS, Walker AM, Jick H: Oral contraceptives and endometrial cancers. Obstet Gynecol 1993;82:931–936. **(IIa, B)**
16. Cirisano FD II, Robboy SJ, Dodge RK, et al: Epidemiologic and surgicopathologic findings of papillary serous and clear cell endometrial cancers when compared to endometrioid carcinoma. Gynecol Oncol 1999;74:385–394. **(IIb, B)**
17. Dunton C, Balsara G, McFarland M, et al: Uterine papillary serous carcinoma: a review. Obstet Gynecol Surv 1991;46:97–102. **(IV, C)**
18. Reddington L, Hernandez E, Balsara G, et al: The effectiveness of the Masterson curette in sampling the endometrial cavity. J Natl Med Assoc 1995;87:877–880. **(III, B)**
19. Gimpelson RJ, Rappold HO: A comparative study between panoramic hysteroscopy with directed biopsies and dilatation and curettage: a review of 276 cases. Am J Obstet Gynecol 1988;158:489–492. **(IIa, B)**
20. Savelli L, DeIaco P, Santini D, et al: Histopatholoic features and risk factors for benignity, hyperplasia, and cancer in endometrial polyps. Am J Obstet Gynecol 2003;188:927–931. **(III, B)**
21. Rose PG: Endometrial carcinoma. N Engl J Med 1996;335:640–649. **(IV, C)**

| Table 45-8 Five-Year Probability of Survival for Women with Endometrial Carcinoma According to International Statistics ||||
|---|---|---|---|
| **Stage I** | **Stage II** | **Stage III** | **Stage IV** |
| A 89% | A 80% | A 63% | A 20% |
| B 90% | B 72% | B 39% | B 17% |
| C 81% | | C 51% | |

Creasman WT, Odicino F, Maisonneuve P, et al: Carcinoma of the corpus uteri. J Epidemiol Biostat 2001;6:45–86.

22. Weber AM, Belinson JL, Piedmonte MR: Risk factors for endometrial hyperplasia and cancer among women with abnormal bleeding. Obstet Gynecol 1999;93:594–598. **(IIa, B)**

23. Langer RD, Pierce JJ, O'Hanlan KA, et al: Transvaginal ultrasonography compared with endometrial biopsy for the detection of endometrial disease. N Engl J Med 1997;337:1792–1798. **(IIa, B)**

24. Wang S, Pudney J, Song J, et al: Mechanisms involved in the evolution of progestin resistance in human endometrial hyperplasia—precursor of endometrial cancer. Gynecol Oncol 2003;88:108–117. **(IIb, B)**

25. Wildemeersch D, Dhont M: Treatment of nonatypical endometrial hyperplasia with levonorgestrel-releasing intrauterine system. Am J Obstet Gynecol 2003;188:1297–1299. **(III, B)**

26. Lindell LK, Anderson B: Routine pretreatment evaluation of patients with gynecologic cancer. Obstet Gynecol 1987;69:242–246. **(III, B)**

27. Connor JP, Andrews JI, Anderson B, et al: Computed tomography in endometrial carcinoma. Obstet Gynecol 2000;95:692–696. **(IIb, B)**

28. Chen SS, Rumanick WM: Magnetic resonance imaging in stage I endometrial carcinoma. Obstet Gynecol 1990;75:274–277. **(IIb, B)**

29. Todo Y, Sakuragi N, Nishida R, et al: Combined use of magnetic resonance imaging, CA 125 assay, histologic type, and histologic grade in the prediction of lymph node metastasis in endometrial carcinoma. Am J Obstet Gynecol 2003;188:1265–1272. **(IIb, B)**

30. Sood AK, Buller RE, Burger RA, et al: Value of preoperative CA 125 level in the management of uterine cancer and prediction of clinical outcome. Obstet Gynecol 1997;90:441–447. **(IIb, B)**

31. Creasman WT, Morrow CP, Bundy BN, et al: Surgical pathologic spread patterns of endometrial cancer. Cancer 1987;60:2035–2041. **(IIb, B)**

32. Preyer O, Obermair A, Forman E, et al: The impact of positive peritoneal washings and serosal and adnexal involvement on survival in patients with stage IIIA uterine cancer. Gynecol Oncol 2002;86:269–273. **(IIb, B)**

33. Creasman WT, DiSaia PJ, Blessing J, et al: Prognostic significance of peritoneal cytology in patients with endometrial cancer and preliminary data concerning therapy with intraperitoneal radiopharmaceuticals. Am J Obstet Gynecol 1981;141:921–929. **(IIb, B)**

34. Yazigi R, Piver MS, Blumenson L: Malignant peritoneal cytology as a prognostic indicator in stage I endometrial cancer. Obstet Gynecol 1983;62:359–362. **(IIb, B)**

35. Kadar N, Homesley HD, Malfetano JH: Positive peritoneal cytology is an adverse factor in endometrial carcinoma only if there is other evidence of extrauterine disease. Gynecol Oncol 1992;46:145–149. **(IIb, B)**

36. Morrow CP, Bundy BN, Kurman RJ, et al: Relationship between surgical-pathological risk factors and outcome in clinical stage I and II carcinoma of the endometrium: a Gynecologic Oncology Group study. Gynecol Oncol 1991;40:55–65. **(IIb, B)**

37. Marino BD, Burke TW, Tornos C, et al: Staging laparotomy for endometrial carcinoma: assessment of peritoneal spread. Gynecol Oncol 1995;56:34–38. **(III, B)**

38. Grigsby PW: Update on radiation therapy for endometrial cancer. Oncology 2002;16:777–786. **(IV, C)**

39. Gotlieb WH, Beiner ME, Salmon B, et al: Outcome of fertility-sparing treatment with progestins in young patients with endometrial cancer. Obstet Gynecol 2003;102:718–725. **(III, B)**

40. Plaxe SC: The prognostic value of staging lymphadenectomy for patients with stage I endometrial cancer is independent of number of nodes removed. Gynecol Oncol 2004;95:408 (abstr). **(IIb, B)**

41. Maggino T, Romagnolo C, Candoni F, et al: An analysis of approaches to the management of endometrial cancer in North America. Gynecol Oncol 1998;68:274–279. **(III, B)**

42. Mariani A, Webb MJ, Keeney GL, et al: Low-risk corpus cancer: Is lymphadenectomy or radiotherapy necessary? Am J Obstet Gynecol 2000;182:1506–1519. **(IIb, B)**

43. Belinson JL, Lee KR, Badger GJ, et al: Clinical stage I adenocarcinoma of the endometrium: analysis of recurrence and the potential benefit of staging lymphadenectomy. Gynecol Oncol 1992;44:17–23. **(III, B)**

44. Kucera H, Vavra N, Weghaupt K: Benefits of external irradiation in pathologic stage I endometrial carcinoma: a prospective clinical trial of 605 patients who received postoperative vaginal irradiation and additional pelvic irradiation in the presence of unfavorable prognostic factors. Gynecol Oncol 1990;38:99–104. **(Ib, A)**

45. Ackerman I, Malone S, Thomas G, et al: Endometrial carcinoma: relative effectiveness of adjuvant irradiation vs. therapy reserved for relapse. Gynecol Oncol 1996;60:177–183. **(IIb, B)**

46. Orr JW Jr, Holimon JL, Orr PF: Stage I corpus cancer: is teletherapy necessary? Am J Obstet Gynecol 1997;176:777–789. **(III, B)**

47. Larson DM, Broste SK, Krawisz BR: Surgery without radiotherapy for primary treatment of endometrial cancer. Obstet Gynecol 1998;91:305–359. **(III, B)**

48. Cilby WA, Clarke-Pearson DL, Dodge R, et al: Acute morbidity and mortality associated with selective pelvic and para-aortic lymphadenectomy in the surgical staging of endometrial carcinoma J Gynecol Tech 1995;1:19–26 **(IIb, B)**

49. Lewandowski G, Torrisi J, Poktul RK, et al: Hysterectomy with extended surgical staging and radiotherapy versus hysterectomy alone and radiotherapy in stage I endometrial cancer: a comparison of complication rates. Gynecol Oncol 1990;36:401–404. **(IIb, B)**

50. Creutzberg CL, vanPutten WLJ, Keper PC, et al: Survival after relapse in patients with endometrial cancer: results from a randomized trial. Gynecol Oncol 2003;89:201–209. **(Ib, A)**

51. Keys HM, Roberts JA, Brunetto VL, et al: A phase III trial of surgery with or without adjunctive external pelvic radiation therapy in intermediate risk endometrial adenocarcinoma: a Gynecologic Oncology Group study. Gynecol Oncol 2004;92:744–751. **(Ib, A)**

52. Mariani A, Keeny G, Webb MJ, Podratz KC: Stage I endometrial cancer: assessment of vaginal failure. Gynecol Oncol 2003;88:184 (abstr). **(IIb, B)**

53. Schink JC, Rademaker AW, Miller DS, Lurain JR: Tumor size in endometrial cancer. Cancer 1991;67:2791–2794. **(IIb, B)**

54. Randall ME, Brunetto G, Muss H, et al: Whole abdominal radiotherapy versus combination doxorubicin-cisplatin chemotherapy in advanced endometrial carcinoma: a randomized phase III trial of the Gynecologic Oncology Group. Proc Am Soc Clin Oncol 2003;22:2 (abstr 3). **(Ib, A)**

55. Irwin C, Levin W, Fyles A, et al: The role of adjuvant radiotherapy in carcinoma of the endometrium: results of 550 patients with pathologic stage I disease. Gynecol Oncol 1998;70:247–254. **(IIb, B)**

56. Bancher-Todesca D, Neunteufel W, Williams KE, et al: Influence of postoperative treatment on survival in patients with uterine papillary serous carcinoma. Gynecol Oncol 1998;71:344–347. **(III, B)**

57. Hoskins PJ, Swenerton KD, Pike JA, et al: Paclitaxel and carboplatin, alone or with irradiation, in advanced or recurrent endometrial cancer: a phase II study. J Clin Oncol 2001;19:4048–4053. **(III, B)**

58. Mariani A, Webb MJ, Keeney GL, et al: Role of wide/radical hysterectomy and pelvic lymph node dissection in endometrial cancer with cervical involvement. Gynecol Oncol 2001;83:72–80. **(IIb, B)**

59. Ng TY, Nicklin JL, Perrin LC, et al: Postoperative vaginal vault brachytherapy for node-negative stage II (occult) endometrial carcinoma. Gynecol Oncol 2001;81:193–195. **(III, B)**

60. Piver MS, Recio FO, Baker TR, et al: A prospective trial of progesterone therapy for malignant peritoneal cytology in patients with endometrial carcinoma. Gynecol Oncol 1992;47:373–376. **(III, B)**

61. Whitney CN, Brunetto VL, Zaino RJ, et al: Phase II study of medroxyprogesterone acetate plus tamoxifen in advanced endometrial carcinoma: a Gynecologic Oncology Group study. Gynecol Oncol 2004;92:4–9. **(III, B)**

62. Fiorica JV, Brunetto VL, Hanjani P, et al: A phase II trial of alternating courses of megestrol acetate and tamoxifen in advanced endometrial carcinoma: a Gynecologic Oncology Group study. Gynecol Oncol 2004;92:10–14. **(III, B)**

63. Bristow R, Zerbe MJ, Rosenshein NB, et al: Stage IVB endometrial carcinoma: the role of cytoreductive surgery and determinants of survival. Gynecol Oncol 2000;78:85–91. **(IIb, B)**

64. Wadler S, Levy DE, Lincoln ST, et al: Topotecan is an active agent in the first-line treatment of metastatic or recurrent endometrial carcinoma: Eastern Cooperative Oncology Group study E#E93. J Clin Oncol 2003;21:2110–2114. **(III, B)**

65. Herzog TJ: What is the clinical value of adding tamoxifen to progestins in the treatment of advanced or recurrent endometrial cancer? Gynecol Oncol 2004;95:1–3 (edit). **(IV, C)**

66. Reddoch JM, Burke TW, Morris M, et al: Surveillance for recurrent endometrial carcinoma: development of a follow-up scheme. Gynecol Oncol 1995;59:221–225. **(III, B)**

67. Rose PG, Sommers RM, Reale FR, et al: Serial serum CA 125 measurements for evaluation of recurrence in patients with endometrial carcinoma. Obstet Gynecol 1994;84:12–16. **(III, B)**

68. Barakat RR, Bundy BN, Spirtos NM, et al: A prospective randomized double-blind trial of estrogen replacement therapy versus placebo in women with stage I or II endometrial cancers: a Gynecologic Oncology Group study. Gynecol Oncol 2004;92:393 (abstr). **(Ib, A)**

## Chapter 46

# Uterine Sarcomas

## Valena Soto-Wright, MD, and Robert McLellan, MD

**KEY POINTS**

- Uterine sarcomas are a rare group of hetereogeneous uterine tumors that comprise less than 4% of all uterine cancers.
- Most uterine sarcomas present with common gynecologic symptoms of abnormal bleeding and pelvic pain that result in the recommendation for surgical intervention.
- Despite the use of Pap tests, endometrial biopsies, and ultrasound, the majority of cases are diagnosed by final surgical pathology.
- Unlike other Stage I gynecologic cancers (endometrial, cervical, vulvar, ovarian), where 5-year survival is about 90%, patients with Stage I uterine sarcoma have less than 50% 5-year survival.

Uterine sarcomas are a heterogeneous group of malignancies that arise from the mesenchymal tissue within the uterus. These tumors may consist of mesenchymal tissue alone or in combination with benign or malignant epithelial tissue (adenosarcoma, carcinosarcoma). Uterine sarcomas are rare, comprising 3% to 5% of all malignancies arising from the uterus. These malignancies behave in a variety of fashions, and their management is often poorly understood, because many studies in the peer review literature combine the various subtypes of uterine carcinoma in the reporting data. Uterine sarcomas are aggressive malignancies with a 5-year survival rate of less than 50% in patients with clinical Stage I disease.

## EPIDEMIOLOGY, RISK FACTORS, AND PATHOGENESIS

Uterine sarcomas are rare, with an annual worldwide incidence of 0.5 to 3.3 cases per 100,000 women per year.[1,2] The Surveillance, Epidemiology, and End Results program (SEER) provides the most accurate data in the United States with a range of 1.2 to 2.3 cases per 100,000 women. Harlow's analysis of the SEER data demonstrates that carcinosarcoma occurs in 0.8 cases/100,000 women, followed by leiomyosarcoma (0.64 cases/100,000 women), endometrial stromal sarcoma (0.19 cases/100,000 women), and unclassified sarcomas (0.05 cases/100,000 women), respectively.[3]

Uterine sarcomas are about twice as common in black women relative to white women. The more common endometrial adenocarcinoma occurs more often in white women. Although few reports suggest a history of pelvic radiation in leiomyosarcoma or endometrial stromal sarcoma, exposure to pelvic irradiation appears to be a risk factor for the development of carcinosarcoma and adenosarcoma. In multiple series of carcinosarcoma, antecedent radiation was identified in up to 29% of cases.[4-10] Although some of these reports have described sarcomas that arise in an irradiated field behaving in a particularly aggressive fashion, the small number of reported cases do not allow reliable conclusions to be drawn regarding their behavior. Data regarding age of menarche, menopause, and parity as risk factors are inconsistent in the literature.

In 1978 tamoxifen (Nolvadex) was introduced for the treatment of breast cancer. As of April 2001, 43 cases of uterine sarcoma were reported among breast cancer patients treated with tamoxifen in the United States, and a further 116 women in other countries developed sarcomas.[11,12] The median duration of tamoxifen use in these patients was 5 years, with the primary histology being carcinosarcoma. Although data regarding risk factors and staging was not complete, 27 of 86 patients on whom such data were available had FIGO Stage III or IV disease according to International Federation of Gynecology and Obstetrics (FIGO) staging criteria. Long-term follow-up of women enrolled in tamoxifen trials suggests an increased incidence of uterine sarcoma of 0.17 cases per 1000 women per year. The advanced stage of uterine sarcomas associated with tamoxifen use is in marked contrast to the early stage of uterine adenocarcinomas that have been reported in tamoxifen users.

Uterine sarcomas are derived from mesoderm and may arise in uterine smooth muscle, endometrial stroma, or blood and lymphatic vessel walls. The International Society of Gynecological Pathologists (ISGYP) has adopted the classification system outlined in Table 46-1 that divides sarcomas into two groups.[13] The first represents pure nonepithelial uterine sarcomas; the second represents mixed epithelial and nonepithelial sarcomas. The descriptive terms *homologous* and *heterologous* refer to sarcomas containing tissue elements indigenous to the uterus and sarcomas with tissue elements such as bone or cartilage that are not normally found in the uterus (i.e., chondrosarcoma), respectively. There appear to be no difference in the clinical behavior of homologous and heterologous müllerian sarcomas. The term *malignant mixed müllerian sarcoma* is equivalent to carcinosarcoma. For practical purposes, the four most common uterine sarcomas in order of decreasing frequency are carcinosarcoma, leiomyosarcoma, endometrial stromal sarcoma, and adenosarcoma. The natural history of sarcomas varies based on the histologic subtypes outlined by the ISGYP classifications system.[13]

# Gynecologic Oncology

**Table 46-1**
**Classification of Uterine Sarcomas**

**Pure nonepithelial sarcomas**

Endometrial stromal tumors
   Stromal nodule
   Low-grade stromal sarcoma
   High-grade stromal sarcoma
Leiomyosarcoma

**Mixed epithelial and nonepithelial sarcomas**

Adenosarcoma
   Homologous
   Heterologous
Carcinosarcoma
   Homologous
   Heterologous

Modified from Clement P, Scully RE: Pathology of uterine sarcomas. In Coppleson M (ed): Gynecologic Oncology. New York, Churchill Livingstone, 1981, p 591.

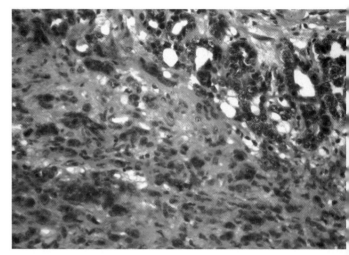

**Figure 46-1**   **Carcinosarcoma.** Endometrial adenocarcinoma associated with malignant stroma.

## CLINICAL FEATURES

### Carcinosarcoma

Carcinosarcomas (mixed müllerian sarcomas) are the most common type of uterine sarcomas, representing 43% of all sarcomas in one study.[14] These tumors consist of endometrial adenocarcinoma in association with malignant mesenchymal tissue (Fig. 46-1). The debate regarding the histogenesis of these tumors has focused on whether the origin is from a common multipotential stem cell versus distinct malignant mesenchymal and epithelial cells. Immunohistochemical staining of carcinosarcoma and poorly differentiated uterine carcinoma show extensive overlap, suggesting a common cell of origin. It has also been observed that metastases of carcinosarcoma are frequently composed of only the carcinomatous component. Compared to adenocarcinomas these tumors grossly appear more fleshy and bulky. The classic presentation of painful postmenopausal bleeding associated with the clinical finding of friable tumor prolapsing through a dilated cervix should raise concern for a presumptive diagnosis of carcinosarcoma.

Doss and colleagues[5] reported that gross tumor at the cervical os was present in 36 of 49 patients presenting with carcinosarcoma. Abnormal vaginal bleeding occurs in 95% of patients presenting with carcinosarcoma, and about 30% of patients describe pain.[14-16] Up to 50% of patients will have the clinical finding of uterine enlargement or a palpable pelvic mass.[4,16,17] A study by Doss and coauthors showed that a mean interval of 3.7 months passed from the onset of symptoms to the subsequent diagnosis of early-stage carcinosarcoma.[5] Hematogenous and lymphatic metastases are common in carcinosarcoma. Doss and colleagues reported on 18 patients with carcinosarcoma and lymphatic metastasis: 6 periaortic, 6 pelvic, 3 supraclavicular, and 1 each of inguinal, colonic, or mesenteric.[5] Fleming, in a summary of 10 previously reported autopsy studies, showed that widespread intra-abdominal and pelvic disease was commonplace for women who died of uterine sarcoma.[18] Tubo-ovarian metastases are also frequent when intra-abdominal metastases are present. In 14 patients with extra-uterine disease, 10 were found to have adnexal metastases in a study by Norris and colleagues.[19] Of the 14 patients with intra-abdominal and adnexal metastases, only 2 had vaginal wall metastasis. A relatively high rate of pulmonary metastatic disease has also been noted in autopsy studies.[18,20]

### Leiomyosarcoma

Leiomyosarcoma is the second most common form of uterine sarcoma, accounting for about 1% of all uterine carcinomas. In premenopausal women, leiomyosarcoma is more common than carcinosarcoma. Leiomyosarcoma is a malignancy thought to arise de novo from uterine smooth muscle. Grossly, leiomyosarcoma has been described as a whitish gray or pale pink cancer similar in appearance to a benign leiomyoma. Like benign leiomyomas, areas of the leiomyosarcoma may show cystic or hemorrhagic degeneration or areas of coagulative necrosis.

Dinh and Woodruff reported a series of 43 cases of leiomyosarcoma; the carcinoma was a solitary lesion in 45% of the women studied but also was associated with multiple myomas in 42% of cases.[21] They emphasize that in the remaining 13% of cases the leiomyosarcoma was not recognized grossly but only identified as an infiltrative process in the final hysterectomy specimen. The location of the sarcoma was thought to be prognostic based on 5-year survival rates for submucosal, intramural, and subserosal sarcomas, which ranged from 80% to 100%, in contrast to a 5-year survival rate of 25% for sarcomas occurring de novo in the myometrium without a definite mass. Patients in their series with extrauterine disease had a 33% overall 5-year survival. Favorable prognostic features included premenopausal status of the patient, confinement of the tumors within a myoma, low mitotic count, absence of necrosis, and presumed hyalinization in adjacent tissue. Forty-one of the 43 patients were followed up 2 or more years. The overall 5-year survival was 73%.[21]

The histopathology of leiomyosarcoma, according to the classic paper by O'Connor and Norris,[22] is based on the mitotic count and the degree of atypia of tumor cells, with no attention paid to the cellularity of the neoplasm. Figure 46-2 demonstrates

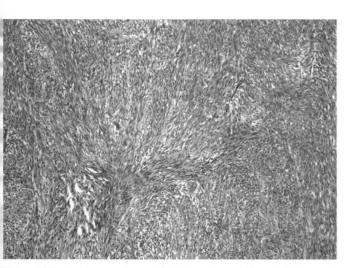

**Figure 46-2    Leiomyosarcoma.** Interlacing pleomorphic spindle-shaped smooth muscle cells containing hyperchromic nuclei.

the cellular pleomorphic spindle-shaped smooth muscle cells with hyperchromatic nuclei and numerous mitotic figures characteristic of leiomyosarcoma. Tumors with 1 to 4 mitoses/10 high-power field (HPF), independent of the degree of atypia, are grouped as leiomyoma. Tumors with 5 to 9 mitoses/10 HPF with grade 1 atypia are of uncertain malignant potential. A similar mitotic count but with grade 2 or 3 atypia or any tumor with 20 mitoses/10 HPF is considered a malignant leiomyosarcoma. An alternative approach that takes into consideration the mitotic count, degree of atypia, and the presence or absence of coagulative necrosis has been advocated by Hendrickson and Kempson at Stanford.[23] Figure 46-3 demonstrates a leiomyosarcoma with coagulative necrosis, which the Stanford group feels is both of diagnostic and prognostic significance. In this more complex diagnostic schema, which includes coagulative necrosis, five categories exist; it remains unclear if this approach will be validated by better prognostic or therapeutic outcomes of clinical significance in the future.

Leiomyosarcoma most commonly presents with abnormal bleeding, with symptoms often attributed to the presumed

diagnosis of leiomyoma. The clinical pearl that a presumed uterine leiomyoma rapidly increasing in size (defined as a doubling in size over 3 to 6 months of observation) should raise concern regarding possible leiomyosarcoma has not been substantiated by recent review. In a study of 1332 women admitted for myomectomy or hysterectomy for presumed uterine leiomyoma, the incidence of sarcoma was 0.23%. Furthermore, among the 341 women with rapidly enlarging leiomyoma, only 0.27% had uterine sarcoma.[24] More commonly, the rapid increase in size is due to cystic or hemorrhagic degeneration of a benign leiomyoma rather than malignant growth. Because leiomyosarcoma arises from the myometrium, the ability to diagnose this tumor preoperatively may be elusive.

The clinical characteristics of 208 patients with uterine leiomyosarcoma outlined in Table 46-2 are reported in a retrospective series at the Mayo Clinic from 1976 to 1999 conducted by Giuntoli and colleagues.[25] The age at diagnosis for women with leiomyosarcoma ranged from 23 to 89.3 years, with a median of 50.9 years. Abnormal bleeding, a pelvic mass, or pain occurred in 56%, 54%, and 22% of the patients, respectively. The median uterine sarcoma measured 9 cm. Most patients (130 of 208, 62%) had Stage I disease. Notably, Stage IV disease on the basis of lung metastasis was the second most common stage, occurring in 41 patients (20%). This reflects the propensity for hematogenous and lymphatic spread other than the direct peritoneal extension more commonly seen in epithelial gynecologic cancer.

### Endometrial Stromal Sarcoma

Endometrial stromal sarcoma is composed of cells resembling the endometrial stroma in the proliferative phase of the menstrual cycle (Figs. 46-4 and 46-5). The tumor typically grows into the endometrium and is usually diagnosed by endometrial sampling. Traditionally, endometrial stromal sarcoma has been divided into low-grade and high-grade stromal sarcomas on the basis of less

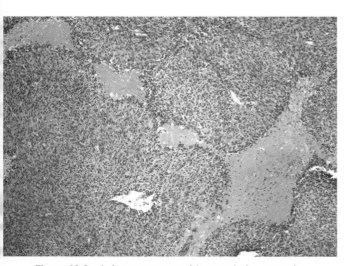

**Figure 46-3    Leiomyosarcoma with coagulative necrosis.**

| Table 46-2 Characteristics of 208 Patients with Leiomyosarcoma of the Uterus | |
|---|---|
| **Characteristic** | **Value** |
| Age at diagnosis (range), years | 50.9 (23.0–89.3) |
| Follow-up, years | 4.02 |
| Follow-up for survivors, years | 7.7 |
| Maximal dimension (±SD), cm | 9 ± 5.1 |
| | **No. (%)** |
| Prior history of pelvic radiation therapy | 1 (0.5) |
| Preoperative symptoms | |
|    Abnormal bleeding | 117 (56) |
|    Pelvic mass | 112 (54) |
|    Pain | 46 (22) |
| Stage | |
|    I | 130 (62) |
|    II | 13 (6) |
|    III | 18 (9) |
|    IV | 41 (20) |

Modified from Giuntoli RL 2nd, Metzinger DS, DiMarco CS, et al: Retrospective review of 208 patients with leiomyosarcoma of the uterus: prognostic indicators, surgical management and adjuvant therapy. Gynecol Oncol 2003;89:460–469.

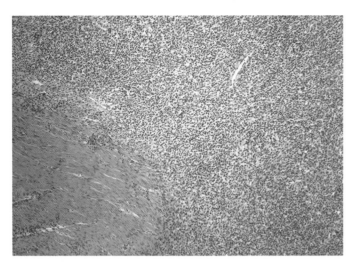

**Figure 46-4    Endometrial stromal sarcoma.** Tumor infiltrating through myoma.

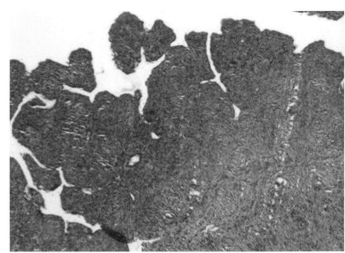

**Figure 46-6    Adenosarcoma.** Papillary structures with cystic spaces covered by endometrial-type epithelial cells.

than 10 mitoses/10 HPF or greater than 10 mitoses/10 HPF, respectively. Within the high-grade endometrial stromal sarcoma group, many of the tumors had anaplastic cells that did not show endometrial stromal differentiation. Debate exists whether this subgroup of tumors with anaplastic cells would be better classified as poorly differentiated sarcoma.[26,27]

Endometrial stromal sarcoma is observed mainly in premenopausal women. Amant and coworkers reported on a series from 1990 to 2002; it involved 16 women with a median age of 34 (range, 18 to 53 years). In 6 of 15 (40%) of the women the original diagnosis was missed and was established only after consultation with a pathologist with a special interest in gynecologic pathology.[28] Lesions to be considered in the differential diagnosis of endometrial stromal sarcomas include cellular leiomyoma, cellular intravenous leiomyomatosis, and adenomyosis with sparse glands, metastatic carcinoma, and lymphoma.

Endometrial stromal sarcomas may be associated with an indolent growth pattern, with lung metastases often occurring late. Low-grade endometrial stromal sarcomas may be rich in

estrogen and progesterone receptors and generally respond to progestins. Complete response to the aromatase inhibitor aminoglutethimide (500 mg q.i.d.) has been reported.[29] Removal of the ovaries is recommended for endometrial stromal sarcoma, because the recurrence rate in patients with retained ovaries was 100% (6 of 6) compared to 6 of 13 in those who underwent initial oophorectomy.[30]

## Adenosarcoma

Adenosarcoma is a mixed form of uterine sarcoma characterized by the presence of benign glandular epithelium mixed with a sarcomatous stroma. Histologically broad papillary structures, clefts, glands, and cystic structures are lined by endometrial-type epithelium with minor areas of focal cytologic atypia (Fig. 46-6). The stromal component is condensed beneath the surface epithelium, forming a "cambium layer" that most often resembles endometrial stromal sarcoma or less commonly leiomyosarcoma.

Adenosarcomas are considered a low-grade malignancy but do recur about 20% of the time after surgical therapy. Figure 46-7 demonstrates recurrent metastatic adenosarcoma to the lung after progestational therapy 6 years after the patient's primary tumor was excised. This patient remains alive with disease 8 years from her original diagnosis and 2 years from the first documented lung recurrence.

## DIAGNOSIS

Most women with uterine sarcomas present with abnormal bleeding and pelvic pain. Initial evaluation may include Papanicolaou (Pap) smear, pelvic ultrasound, and/or endometrial biopsy, depending on the age of the patient. The sensitivity of these tests in diagnosing uterine sarcoma is poor and varies with the histologic subtype of uterine sarcoma. Carcinosarcoma, due to its malignant glandular component arising in the endometrial cavity, is much more likely to be diagnosed by endometrial biopsy than leiomyosarcoma, which arises from the myometrium.[31] The majority of women with leiomyosarcoma have not had a preoperative endometrial biopsy.[14] Of those women with

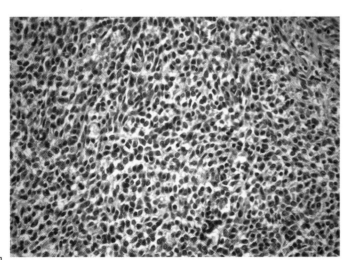

**Figure 46-5    Endometrial stromal sarcoma.** The higher magnification shows small uniform cells with bland nuclei.

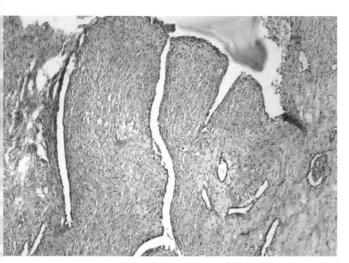

**Figure 46-7**    Metastatic pulmonary adenosarcoma after medroxyprogesterone acetate therapy.

leiomyosarcoma biopsied, only 25% to 50% of cases were diagnosed correctly before hysterectomy. Most women with leiomyosarcomas are diagnosed after hysterectomy performed for the management of presumed leiomyoma. Many women have had additional testing, such as computed tomography (CT) scan or magnetic resonance imaging (MRI), but in disease confined to the uterus the findings are not specific and may not raise concern regarding a possible malignancy. MRI findings suggestive of uterine sarcoma include a heterogeneous medium and high-signal intensity within a uterine mass or hematometra with high-signal intensity on $T_1$ and $T_2$.[32]

In women with a diagnosis of uterine sarcoma made pre-operatively, evaluation should focus on determining the extent of disease. A careful history may identify patients with pulmonary or abdominal symptoms suggestive of metastatic disease. A complete physical examination is indicated, with special attention given to a careful lymph node survey, including the supra-clavicular lymph nodes, auscultation of the chest, and palpation of the abdomen and inguinal-femoral nodes. Gynecologic examination should include inspection of the entire vaginal vault and cervix, bimanual examination, and rectovaginal examination. Rectovaginal examination and occult blood testing may identify otherwise occult involvement of the rectovaginal septum by direct tumor extension. Preoperative radiographic studies include a posteroanterior (PA) and lateral chest x-ray. A CT scan of the abdomen and pelvis may identify extrauterine disease, such as lymphatic or peritoneal metastases. Chest CT scan may be useful postoperatively when pathological diagnosis is confirmed because both carcinosarcoma and leiomyosarcoma metastasize to the lung. Punnonen reported 14 isolated pulmonary recurrences in 21 patients diagnosed with recurrent leiomyosarcoma.[33] Women with isolated pulmonary metastasis from leiomyosarcoma A are candidates for thoracotomy, with 5- and 10-year survival of 43% and 35%, respectively.[34,35]

Figure 46-8 demonstrates the importance of preoperative chest radiography, PA and lateral. An 11-mm right upper lobe nodule is seen on the PA view, but only on the lateral film is a second, retrocardiac lesion identified. The patient underwent a total hysterectomy and bilateral salpingo-oophorectomy for presumed leiomyoma. Her intraoperative findings, however, were worrisome for uterine sarcoma; final surgical pathology demonstrated a high-grade endometrial stromal sarcoma involving the uterus, with metastatic disease present to the adnexa bilaterally. Postoperative metastatic workup included a chest and abdominal pelvic CT scan. The chest CT scan identified the right upper lobe 11-mm nodule but also clearly defined a 2-cm mass abutting the right side of the heart that was only a subtle finding on the lateral chest x-ray (Fig. 46-9). The abdominal pelvic CT scan shown in Figure 46-10 demonstrates a 5.5-cm soft tissue mass at the level of the left common iliac bifurcation that was felt to represent necrotic lymphadenopathy versus metastatic implant of soft tissue sarcoma to the peritoneal surface. Figure 46-11 demonstrates the fluoro-2-deoxy-D-glucose ($^{18}$FDG) positron emission tomography (PET) scan of the patient with endometrial stromal sarcoma whose chest x-ray and CT scans have been shown in Figures 46-9 and 46-10, respectively. $^{18}$FDG is an analog of glucose that engages in cellular metabolism, allowing a distinction to be made between benign and malignant tissues. The whole-body scan demonstrates increased uptake at two sites in the lung in addition to the left periaortic nodes, left external iliac nodes, and right external iliac nodes, correlating well with the CT scan findings. The rarity of uterine sarcomas limits assessing the sensitivity or specificity of PET scan, but in soft tissue sarcoma of other sites, Schwarzbach and colleagues reported a sensitivity and specificity of 91% and 88%, respectively.[36] PET scans have also been shown to be of value in staging, restaging, and prognosis in soft tissue sarcomas.[37]

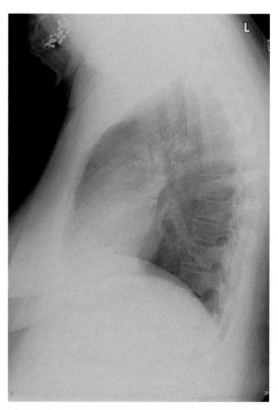

**Figure 46-8**    Lateral chest radiograph with a retrocardiac lesion not seen on PA view, representing metastatic high-grade endometrial stromal sarcoma.

# Gynecologic Oncology

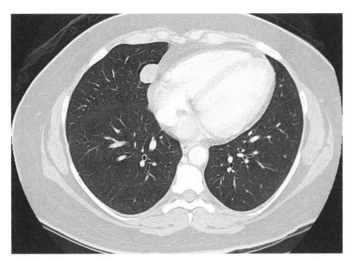

**Figure 46-9   Chest CT scan documenting 2-cm metastatic pulmonary nodule of high-grade endometrial stromal sarcoma.**

This diagnostic workup reflects the aggressive nature of the majority of uterine sarcomas and the importance of meticulous preoperative evaluation.

## TREATMENT

Surgery is the only treatment for curative intent in patients with carcinosarcoma. The traditional procedure consists of an exploratory laparotomy through a midline abdominal incision. Peritoneal washings for cytology are obtained followed by careful inspection and palpation of the diaphragm, liver, spleen, stomach, small and large bowel, omentum, peritoneal surfaces, and retroperitoneal structures. When a thorough laparotomy is performed, extrauterine disease may be found in 12% to 40% of patients with carcinosarcoma who otherwise had clinical findings to suggest disease confined to the uterus.[4,5,8,10,38] The pattern of spread may mimic poorly differentiated endometrial cancer with direct serosal extension, metastasis to the fallopian tube or ovary, and intraperitoneal dissemination.[39] The

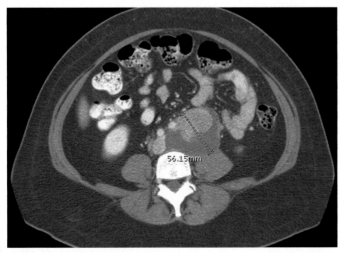

**Figure 46-10   Abdominopelvic CT scan with 5.5-cm soft tissue mass at the left common iliac bifurcation.**

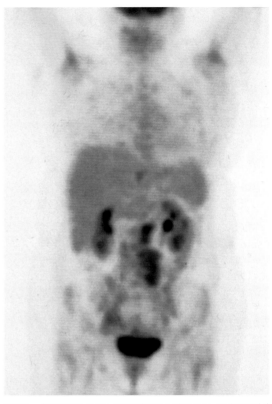

**Figure 46-11   FDG-PET scan.** Metastatic high-grade endometrial stromal sarcoma with increased uptake in the left periaortic nodes and left iliac nodes.

Gynecologic Oncology Group, in a prospective surgical staging study, reported that 17% of all patients with carcinosarcoma had pelvic and/or periaortic nodal disease.[40] Accordingly, in patients with no evidence of extrauterine disease nodal sampling should be considered because additional prognostic information may be gained. Although cytoreductive surgery has not been shown to improve survival in patients with carcinosarcoma, if intestinal obstruction is present from metastatic disease, palliative bypass is appropriate.

As in carcinosarcoma, patients with leiomyosarcoma are treated with curative intent with extrafascial abdominal hysterectomy with a bilateral salpingo-oophorectomy. When leiomyosarcoma is diagnosed on final pathology after myomectomy for presumed benign fibroids, total hysterectomy should be considered. Berchuck and colleagues reported three patients who had myomectomy followed by hysterectomy, with two of the three having residual leiomyosarcoma in the final hysterectomy specimen.[41] Fertility-sparing surgery for young, nulliparous women has been reported by Lissoni and colleagues.[42] After myomectomy, all patients had normal hysteroscopy, pelvic ultrasound, abdominal pelvic CT scan or MRI, and normal chest radiography. Of the eight women studied, with a median follow-up of 42 months, three live births were recorded, but one patient died of recurrent disease. Patients must be informed of the risks of fertility-sparing surgery and the limited data available to support a conservative approach. In young patients who have had hysterectomy for leiomyosarcoma, the role of bilateral salpingo-oophorectomy has been analyzed in a case-control series by Giuntoli.[25] Of 25 women with functioning ovaries in whom one or both ovaries had been preserved compared to similarly staged women whose ovaries had been resected, no significant difference in disease-specific survival was noted.

In patients with a diagnosis of leiomyosarcoma established at the time of surgery, generally bilateral salpingo-oophorectomy has been performed. Prospectively acquired surgical staging data from Memorial Sloan-Kettering Cancer Center documented 3.9% (4 of 1080) and 8.1% (3 of 37) incidence of ovarian and nodal metastasis, respectively.[43] No patients with Stage I or II disease had positive lymph nodes. (The presence of gross extra-uterine disease was the only factor predictive of nodal involvement.) In the retrospective series by Giuntoli and colleagues, lymph node involvement was reported in 11% (4 of 39) with leiomyosarcoma. Three of the four patients had extrauterine disease, but the remaining patient had no clinically suspicious nodes or extrauterine disease.[25] Therefore, although lymph node dissection provides prognostic information, it is not felt to be therapeutic and may be omitted unless required by treatment protocol.

Palliative radiation therapy has been employed when patients present with symptomatic locally advanced disease with or without known metastatic disease that cannot be resected with adequate surgical margins. The Radiation Therapy Oncology Group (Protocol #8502) demonstrated in a Phase II trial that a split-course radiation schedule effectively relieved symptoms with minimal short- or long-term complications. The schedule consisted of 3.7 Gy of external beam radiation delivered twice daily for 2 days, followed by a 2- to 4-week rest before a similar repeat course. This regimen may be repeated twice for a total pelvic dose of 44.4 Gy.

## Adjuvant Treatment

Radiation, chemotherapy, and combined chemoradiation have all been reported as adjuvant or postoperative treatment for women with uterine sarcoma. The European Organization for the Research and Treatment of Cancer (EORTC) reports the only randomized trial in the peer-reviewed literature for adjuvant therapy of uterine sarcoma.[44] The trial evaluated observation versus postoperative adjuvant pelvic radiotherapy. Enrolled patients had undergone a minimum of total abdominal hysterectomy with bilateral salpingo-oophorectomy and cytology. The trial took 13 years to accrue 124 patients reflecting the rarity of uterine sarcomas and the need for collaborative multicentered trials. All histologic types were permitted with 103 LM, 91 CS, and 28 endometrial stromal sarcomas. Patients were randomized to pelvic radiation or observation. There was no effect on overall survival or progression-free survival. A decrease in local recurrence was noted in patients with CS who received radiotherapy without any benefit noted for treated patients with LMS. Similar to the EORTC data, most authors describe decreased local recurrence but have not demonstrated improved overall survival. This may reflect the extent of unrecognized microscopic disease or metastatic disease outside the pelvic treatment fields that remains after laparotomy. Extended field or whole abdominal radiation may prevent abdominal/pelvic recurrence but it is unknown if this influences survival.[45,46] Future study designs of adjuvant therapy will need to consider the histologic subtypes of sarcomas based on the EORTC trial data.

## Chemotherapy

To improve survival in women with uterine sarcoma, active chemotherapeutic agents are needed to prevent both local and systemic recurrence. No studies to date have shown efficacy for adjuvant chemotherapy despite the known recurrence rate of 50% for clinical Stage I disease. Because 90% of uterine sarcomas are either carcinosarcoma or leiomyosarcoma, meaningful trial data are available for only these histologic subtypes. Chemotherapy is employed for patients with metastatic or recurrent disease with drug choice guided by histology, based on data from GOG trials (Table 46-3).

The most active single agent against carcinosarcoma identified, with a response rate of about 32%, is ifosfamide. Sutton and colleagues reported a response rate of 5 complete and 4 partial responders among 28 patients who had not received prior chemotherapy, receiving a 5-day schedule of ifosfamide at a dose of 1.5 mg/day every 4 weeks.[47] The GOG reported a response rate of 34.8% in a Phase II trial of ifosfamide in 23 patients with carcinosarcoma.[47] The GOG also identified cisplatin as an active agent, but with a response rate of only 19% in 63 previously untreated patients with carcinosarcoma.[48] The GOG compared combination therapy with ifosfamide and cisplatin to single-agent ifosfamide in a Phase III trial in 194 evaluable patients with carcinosarcoma.[49] Despite an overall response rate of 54% and 36%, respectively, and median progression-free survival of 6 months and 4 months, respectively, which favored combination therapy, the cost of increased morbidity, particularly myelosuppression, has limited the use of this combination.

The GOG conducted a Phase II trial evaluating the clinical activity of paclitaxel in patients with persistent or recurrent carcinosarcoma of the uterus.[50] All patients had failed previous treatments, 15 patients had received previous radiation therapy, and 33 patients had failed prior chemotherapy. All patients had histologically confirmed carcinosarcoma with measurable disease. Eight of 44 patients responded to paclitaxel administered at a dose of 170 mg/m$^2$ (135 mg/m$^2$ in those patients with prior radiation therapy). Four patients (9.1%) had a complete response and four had a partial response. Neutropenia was the most common toxic effect. The authors concluded that Paclitaxel had moderate activity in patients with carcinosarcoma of the uterus. Currently the GOG is accruing patients for a Phase III trial comparing ifosfamide with or without paclitaxel in the treatment of recurrent carcinosarcoma (GOG #161).

The use of chemoradiation for patients with optimally debulked advanced carcinosarcoma is the subject of GOG

---

**Table 46-3**
**Recommendations for Chemotherapy in Advanced or Recurrent Uterine Sarcomas**

| Histology | Recommendation |
|---|---|
| Carcinosarcoma | Ifosfamide or ifosfamide/cisplatin |
| Leiomyosarcoma | Doxorubicin |
| Other histologies | Data inconclusive |

Modified from Rubin SC (ed): Chemotherapy of Gynecologic Cancers, 2nd ed. Philadelphia, Lippincott Williams & Wilkins, 2004, Table 4.9, p 18.

# Gynecologic Oncology

#150, a Phase III randomized trial, which uses whole abdominal radiation with combination ifosfamide and cisplatin.

In contrast to carcinosarcoma, leiomyosarcoma has only modest response to ifosfamide and negligible response to cisplatin. The highest response rates in leiomyosarcoma, about 25%, are achieved with doxorubicin.[51,52] Phase II trials continue to focus on identification of active drugs for leiomyosarcoma. More recent data has documented that combination chemotherapy with gemcitabine and docetaxel in leiomyosarcoma patients showed an overall response rate of 53%, including three complete responders.[53] In this study 50% of patients previously treated with doxorubicin with or without ifosfamide responded. Grade 3 or 4 neutropenia developed in 27% of patients despite the use of granulocyte colony-stimulating factor.

In summary, the use of chemotherapy in uterine sarcoma in recurrent or metastatic disease is palliative, not curative. Experimental protocols may be considered versus palliative care programs based on the patient's performance status. Although a number of active agents have been identified, a large study of 1042 uterine sarcoma patients reported to the Cancer Registry of Norway from 1956 to 1992 showed no improvement in 5-year survival after the introduction of chemotherapy into treatment protocols.[54] The rarity of uterine sarcomas and the difference in clinical response between the two major histologic types has limited randomized trial data to guide therapy. In view of these obstacles and the lack of highly active regimens in advanced disease no trials for chemotherapy in the adjuvant setting are currently under way.

## PROGNOSIS

Malignant uterine sarcomas are aggressive tumors with a poor prognosis. Surgical stage is the most important prognostic variable. Even if the tumor is Stage I at presentation, the overall 5-year survival is only 50%. If extrauterine disease is present, 5-year survival is about 20% with little change despite postoperative treatment. Among the three main histologic subtypes of uterine sarcoma, sites of disease recurrence and survival rates are similar after correcting for stage of disease.[21,48]

## REFERENCES

1. Hajnal-Papp R, Szilagyi I: Malignant müllerian tumors of the uterus. Arch Gynecol Obstet 1988;241:209–219. (III, B)
2. Kvale G, Heuch I, Ursin G: Reproductive factors and the risk of cancers of the uterine corpus: a prospective study. Cancer Res 1988; 48:6217–6221. (IIb, B)
3. Harlow BL, Weiss NS, Lofton S: The epidemiology of sarcomas of the uterus. J Natl Cancer Inst 1986;76:399–402. (III, B)
4. Dinh TV, Slavin RE, Bhagavan BS, et al: Mixed müllerian tumors of the uterus: a clinicopathologic study. Obstet Gynecol 1989;74:388–392. (III, B)
5. Doss LL, Llorens AS, Hernandez EM: Carcinosarcoma of the uterus: a 40-year experience from the state of Missouri. Gynecol Oncol 1984; 18:43–53. (III, B)
6. George M, Pejovic MH, Kramer A: Gynecologic Cooperating Group of French Oncology Centers. Uterine sarcomas: prognostic factors and treatment modalities study on 209 patients. Gynecol Oncol 1986; 24:58–67. (IIb, B)
7. Marchese MJ, Liskow AS, Crum CP, et al: Uterine sarcomas: a clinicopathologic study, 1965–1981. Gynecol Oncol 1984;18:299–312. (III, B)
8. Nielsen SC, Podratz KC, Scheithauer BW, O'Brien PC: Clinicopathologic analysis of uterine malignant mixed müllerian tumors. Gynecol Oncol 1989;34:372–378. (III, B)
9. Norris HJ, Taylor HB: Mesenchymal tumors of the uterus. III. A clinical and pathologic study of 31 carcinosarcomas. Cancer 1966; 19:1459–1465. (III, B)
10. Peters WA, Kumar NB, Fleming WP, Morley GW: Prognostic features of sarcomas and mixed tumors of the endometrium. Obstet Gynecol 1984;63:550–556. (III, B)
11. Wickerman DL, Fisher B, Wolmark, N, et al: Association of tamoxifen and uterine sarcoma. J Clin Oncol 2002;20:2758–2760. (Ib, A)
12. Wysowski DK, Honig SF, Beitz J: Uterine sarcoma associated with tamoxifen use. N Eng J Med 2002;346:1832–1833. (Ib, A)
13. Clement P, Scully RE: Pathology of uterine sarcomas. In Coppleson M (ed): Gynecologic Oncology. New York, Churchill Livingstone, 1981, p 591. (IV, C)
14. Kahanpaa KV, Wahlstrom T, Grohn P, et al: Sarcomas of the uterus: a clinicopathologic study of 119 patients. Obstet Gynecol 1986; 67:417–424. (III, B)
15. Dreisler A, Lykkesfeldt G: Sarcoma of the uterus: a retrospective clinical study of 56 cases. UgeskrLaeger 1985;147:3698–3701. (III, B)
16. Geraci P, Maggio S, Adragna F, et al: Uterine sarcomas: a retrospective study of 17 cases. Eur J Gynaecol Oncol 1988;9:497–501. (III, B)
17. Larson B, Silverware C, Nilsson B, Pettersson F: Mixed müllerian tumors of the uterus—prognostic factors: a clinical and histopathologic study of 147 cases. Radiother Oncol 1990;17:123–132. (III, B)
18. Fleming WP, Peters WA, Kumar NB, et al: Autopsy findings in patients with uterine sarcoma. Gynecol Oncol 1984;19:168–172. (III, B)
19. Norris HJ, Roth E, Taylor HB: Mesenchymal tumors of the uterus. II. A clinical and pathologic study of 31 mixed mesodermal tumors. Obstet Gynecol 1966;28:57–63. (III, B)
20. Rose PG, Piver MS, Tsukada Y, Lau T: Patterns of metastasis in uterine sarcoma. Cancer 1989;63:935–938. (III, B)
21. Dinh TV, Woodruff JD: Leiomyosarcoma of the uterus. Am J Obstet Gynecol 1982;144:817–823. (III, B)
22. O'Connor DM, Norris HJ: Mitotically active leiomyomas of the uterus. Hum Pathol 1990;21:223–227. (III, B)
23. Hendrickson MR, Kempson RL: Pure mesenchymal tumours of the uterine corpus. In Fox H (ed): Haines and Taylor: Textbook of Obstetrical and Gynecological Pathology, 4th ed. Edinburgh, Churchill Livingstone, 1995, p 519. (IV, C)
24. Parker WH, Fu YS, Berek JS: Uterine sarcoma in patients operated on for presumed leiomyoma and rapidly growing leiomyoma. Obstet Gynecol 1994;83:414–418. (III, B)
25. Giuntoli RL 2nd, Metzinger DS, DiMarco CS, et al: Retrospective review of 208 patients with leiomyosarcoma of the uterus: prognostic indicators, surgical management and adjuvant therapy. Gynecol Oncol 2003;89:460–469. (III, B)
26. Evans HL: Endometrial stromal sarcoma and poorly differentiated endometrial sarcoma. Cancer 1982;50:2170–2182. (III, B)
27. Oliva E, Clement PB, Young RH: Endometrial stromal tumors: an update on a group of tumors with a protean phenotype. Adv Anat Pathol 2000;7:257–281. (III, B)
28. Amant F, Moerman P, Cadron I, et al: The diagnostic problem of endometrial stromal sarcoma: report on 6 cases. Gynecol Oncol 2003; 90:37–43. (III, B)
29. Spano JP, Sovia JC, Kambouchner M, et al: Long-term survival of patients given hormonal therapy for metastatic endometrial stromal sarcoma. Med Oncol 2003;20:87–93. (III, B)
30. Schwartz SM, Thomas DB: The World Health Organization: Collaborative study of neoplasia and steroid contraceptives. Cancer 1989;64:2487–2492. (III, B)
31. Leibsohn S, d'Ablaing G, Mishell DR, Schlaerth JB: Leiomyosarcoma in a series of hysterectomies performed for presumed uterine leiomyomas. Am J Obstet Gynecol 1990;162:968–976. (III, B)

32. Shapiro LG, Hricak H: Mixed müllerian sarcoma of the uterus: MR imaging findings. Am J Roentgenol 1989;153:317–319. **(III, B)**

33. Punnonen R, Lauslahti K, Pystynen P, Kauppila O: Uterine sarcomas. Ann Chir Gynaecol Suppl 1985;197:11–14. **(III, B)**

34. Mountain CF, McMurtrey MJ, Hermes RE: Surgery for pulmonary metastasis: 20-year experience. Ann Thorac Surg 1984;38:323–330. **(III, B)**

35. Levenback C, Rubin SC, McCormack PM, et al: Resection of pulmonary metastases from uterine sarcomas. Gynecol Oncol 1992;45:202–205. **(III, B)**

36. Schwarzbach MH, Dimitrakopoulou-Strauss A, Willeke F, et al: Clinical value of (18-F) fluorodeoxyglucose positron emission tomography imaging in soft tissue sarcoma. Ann Surg 2000; 231:380–386. **(III, B)**

37. Israel-Mardirosian N, Adler LP: Positron emission tomography of soft tissue sarcomas. Curr Opin Oncol 2003;15:327–330. **(III, B)**

38. Silverberg SG, Major FJ, Blessing JUA, et al: Carcinosarcoma (malignant mixed mesodermal tumor) of the uterus: a Gynecologic Oncology Group pathologic study of 203 cases. Int J Gynecol Pathol 1990; 9:1–19. **(III, B)**

39. Podczaski ES, Woomert CA, Steven CH III, et al: Management of malignant, mixed mesodermal tumors of the uterus. Gynecol Oncol 1989;32:240–244. **(III, B)**

40. Major FJ, Blessing JA, Silverberg SG, et al: Prognostic factors in early-stage uterine sarcoma: a Gynecologic Oncology Group study. Cancer 1993;71:1702–1709. **(III, B)**

41. Berchuck A, Rubin SC, Hoskins WJ, et al: Treatment of uterine leiomyosarcoma. Obstet Gynecol 1988;71:845–850. **(III, B)**

42. Lissoni A, Cormio G, Bonazzi C, et al: Fertility sparing surgery in uterine leiomyosarcoma. Gynecol Oncol 1998;70:348–350. **(III, B)**

43. Leitao MM, Sonoda Y, Brennan MF, et al: Incidence of lymph node and ovarian metastases in leiomyosarcoma of the uterus. Gynecol Oncol 2003;91:209–212. **(III, B)**

44. Echt G, Jepson J, Steel J, et al: Treatment of uterine sarcomas. Cancer 1990;66:35. **(III, B)**

45. Reed NS, Magioni C, Malmstrom H, et al: First results of a randomized trial comparing radiotherapy versus observation postoperatively in patients with uterine sarcomas. An EORTC-GCG Study [Abstract]. Intl J Gynecol Cancer 2003;13(Suppl 1):A-PL 4,12.

46. Hoffman W, Schmandt S, Kortmann RD, et al: Radiotherapy in the treatment of uterine sarcomas: a retrospective analysis of 54 cases. Gynecol Obstet Invest 1996;42:49–57. **(III, B)**

47. Sutton GP, Blessing JA, Rosenheim N, et al: Phase II trial of ifosfamide and mesna in mixed mesodermal tumors of the uterus (a Gynecologic Oncology Group study). Am J Obstet Gynecol 1989;161:309–312. **(IIa, B)**

48. Thigpen JT, Blessing JA, Beecham J, et al: Phase II trail for cisplatin as first-line chemotherapy in patients with advanced or recurrent uterine sarcomas (a Gynecologic Oncology Group study). J Clin Oncol 1991; 9:962–966. **(IIa, B)**

49. Sutton GP, Brunetto, Berchuck A, et al: Treatment of uterine leiomyosarcoma. Obstet Gynecol 1988;71:845–850. **(III, B)**

50. Curtin JP, Blessing JA, Soper JT, et al: Paclitaxel in the treatment of carcinosarcoma of the uterus: a Gynecologic Oncology Group study. Gynecol Oncol 2001;83:268–270. **(IIa, B)**

51. Hannigan EV, Freedman RS, Elder KW, et al: Treatment of advanced uterine sarcoma with Adriamycin. Gynecol Oncol 1983;16:101–104. **(IIa, B)**

52. Omura GA, Major FJ, Blessing JA, et al: A randomized study of Adriamycin with and without dimethyl triazinoimidazole carboxamide in advanced uterine sarcomas. Cancer 1983;52:626–632. **(Ib, A)**

53. Hensley ML, Maki R, Venkatraman E, et al: Gemcitabine and docetaxel in patients with unresectable leiomyosarcoma: results of a phase three trial. J Clin Oncol 2002;20:2824–2831. **(Ib, A)**

54. Nordal RR, Thoprensen SO: Uterine sarcomas in Norway 1956–1991: incidence, survival and mortality. Eur J Cancer 1997;33:907–911. **(III, B)**

# Chapter 47

# Fallopian Tube Carcinoma

Harriet O. Smith, MD, Steven C. Eberhardt, MD, Claire F. Verschraegen, MD, and Thèrése E. Bocklage, MD

## KEY POINTS

- Primary fallopian tube carcinoma is relatively rare (0.1% to 1% of all female genital tract malignancies).
- Treatment for fallopian tube carcinoma is similar to that for ovarian carcinoma. Initial treatment is surgical staging (peritoneal washings and biopsies, omentectomy, pelvic/periaortic lymphadenectomy). For advanced disease, tumor debulking to less than 1 cm residual disease followed by chemotherapy is advocated.
- Chemotherapy includes six cycles of a platinum-based compound combined with paclitaxel. Newer agents active in epithelial ovarian cancer may have comparable efficacy in fallopian tube carcinoma.
- Survival appears to be higher than for ovarian cancer, probably because fallopian tube carcinoma is usually detected at an earlier stage.
- Women with genetic susceptibility to ovarian and breast cancer (especially *BRCA1* carriers) are at increased risk for fallopian tube carcinoma. In women undergoing prophylactic surgery to prevent ovarian cancer, careful gross and microscopic assessment of the fallopian tubes may be indicated.

Primary carcinoma of the fallopian tube is relatively rare, accounting for approximately 1% of all female genital tract malignancies. Etiologic factors are largely unknown, but are probably similar to those for epithelial ovarian cancer. Histologically, most fallopian tube carcinomas are pure adenocarcinomas. The most commonly identified histology is serous, although other epithelial subtypes (e.g., endometrioid, clear cell, transitional cell, carcinosarcoma) have been reported. In this chapter, we outline the clinical presentation and current management of fallopian tube carcinoma. Recently, case reports and a few epidemiologic studies have demonstrated a link to fallopian tube carcinoma in women at increased risk for hereditary breast and ovarian carcinoma. In light of this, an algorithm that addresses risk, current guidelines for surveillance, and the role and type of prophylactic surgery under investigation is provided.

## EPIDEMIOLOGY

Primary fallopian tube carcinoma accounts for 0.1% to 1.1% of all genital malignancies,[1] with a prevalence of about 3.6 per million women per year.[2] According to data derived from the Surveillance, Epidemiology, and End Results (SEER) program, from 1973 to 1984, incidence rates in the United States have remained stable, and age-specific incidence follows a pattern similar to that for ovarian and endometrial tumors. In the United States, whites were found to have a slightly higher, although not a statistically different, incidence rate per million women (3.5 vs. 3.1; RR, 1.14; 95% CI, 0.7 to 1.8).[3] In contrast, a study from the Finnish Cancer Registry (1953–1997) reported a 4.5-fold increase in incidence, from 1.2 per million women in 1953 to 1957 to 5.4 per million women in 1993 to 1997.[4] As has been shown for ovarian cancer, higher living standards may be a contributing factor; women of higher socioeconomic classes have a 1.8-fold higher incidence rate (95% CI, 1.2 to 2.6) than women within the lowest classes. Also like ovarian cancer, comparing women from rural versus urban areas and unemployed women versus women in academic or clerical occupations, rates are approximately 50% higher in the latter groups.[4]

In the United States, based on SEER data, considerable differences in population-based incidence rates occur by geographic region, from as low as 2.7 per million women up to 6.5 per million women. This may be a reflection of true regional differences; more likely, it is due to differences in the frequency of misclassification of fallopian tumors as ovarian neoplasms.[4] In the Finnish study, incidence rates per million white women compared to other ethnicities were slightly higher (5.4 vs. 3.3) and were otherwise similar, other than that the peak in age-specific rates in Finland was in women between ages 60 and 64, compared to between ages 70 and 74 in the United States.[3,4] Many factors may account for the trend in higher rates overall and in more socioeconomically advantaged women; these include better detection, improved awareness, better access to gynecologic oncology specialty care, and earlier diagnosis. In advanced and inoperable cases, it is often difficult and sometimes impossible to discriminate between an ovarian and a fallopian tube primary carcinoma. Because the ovaries, uterus, and fallopian tubes are all of müllerian origin, neoplasms arising in any of these sites are histologically identical. Thus, especially in advanced cases, because fallopian tumors mimic these more common neoplasms both histologically and in patterns of spread, the likelihood of misdiagnosis is increased.[4,5]

According to a number of epidemiologic studies, the prognosis for fallopian tube carcinoma may be better than that for ovarian cancer. In the United States (SEER data, 1990–1997) primary fallopian tube carcinoma patients stage for stage were found to have a better 5-year relative survival than ovarian cancer patients diagnosed in the same time period (Table 47-1).[3] Similar results have been reported by the Austrian Cooperative

# Gynecologic Oncology

**Table 47-1**

**Relative Survival (5-Year) for Fallopian Tube Carcinoma Compared with Epithelial Ovarian Cancer [SEER, 1990–1997]**

| FIGO Stage | FC (N) | FC 5-year Survival (%) | OC (N) | OC 5-Year Survival (%) |
|---|---|---|---|---|
| I | 102 | 95 | 2044 | 88 |
| II | 29 | 75 | 675 | 65 |
| III | 52 | 69 | 2728 | 31 |
| IV | 151 | 45 | 3233 | 19 |
| Unstaged | 82 | 66 | — | |

*FC, Fallopian tube cancer; OC, ovarian cancer.
Fallopian tube cancer, total of 334 cases; epithelial ovarian cancer, total of 9032 cases.
Adapted from Kosary C, Trimble EL: Treatment and survival for women with fallopian tube carcinoma: a population-based study. Gynecol Oncol 2002;86:190–191.

Study Group for Fallopian Tube Carcinoma (Stage I/II, 50%; Stage III/IV 19%),[5] the Norwegian Radium Hospital (Stage I, 73%; Stage II, 37%; Stage III, 29%; Stage IV, 12%),[6] and by the International Federation for Gynecology and Obstetrics (FIGO: Stage I, 69%; Stage II, 58%; Stage III, 20%; Stage IV, 22%).[7] On the other hand, Rosen and colleagues, in a nationwide retrospective analysis of Stage I and II fallopian tube carcinoma versus ovarian cancer, reported that survival was worse for the fallopian tube carcinoma patients (5-year survival, 50.8% vs. 77.5%).[8]

## CLINICAL FEATURES

### Clinical Signs and Symptoms

The most common symptoms associated with fallopian tube cancer are abdominal pain, abnormal vaginal bleeding, and an abdominal or pelvic mass. The classic presentation is colicky abdominal pain, often relieved with passage of a profuse watery vaginal discharge, and a mass on examination, a triad of symptoms termed *hydrops tubae profluens*, considered pathognomonic for fallopian tube carcinoma. According to most series, however, this presentation is found in only 5% to 10% of patients. The most common symptoms include abnormal vaginal bleeding (42% to 62%), abdominal pain (28% to 48%), and watery vaginal discharge (20%).[1,5,9-11] An abdominal mass discovered on ultrasound or computed tomography (CT) scan (33%) is a more common presentation than incidental finding of a pelvic mass on examination (5%)[9]; in 14% of cases, ascites is suspected based on radiographic studies or examination.[6] Rarely (about 1% of cases), patients present with acute abdomen with torsion and/or intra-abdominal bleeding.[1,11] About 15% to 20% of patients experience no symptoms.[1,6]

### Biological Markers, Cervical Cytology, and Radiographic Studies

Few reports address the utility of CA 125 either for screening or predicting outcome in patients with fallopian tube cancer.[12-14] In one series, CA 125 levels were elevated in 70% of all cases, but in only 20% of those with Stage I disease[12]; other studies indicate that CA 125 levels in Stage I fallopian tube cancer, as in ovarian cancer, are not elevated in at least half of the cases studied.[13,14] The largest available review demonstrated that pretreatment serum CA 125 was a prognostic predictor of disease-free and overall survival, regardless of tumor stage. Pretreatment levels correlated with stage, but not lymph node survival or tumor grade. In 90% of patients, an elevated CA 125 preceded clinical or radiographic evidence of recurrence. During posttreatment surveillance, serial CA 125 determinations had a 92% sensitivity in detecting recurrent disease,[14] consistent with other studies, which found that initial elevated levels corrrelate with stage of disease and prognosis.[12,15] Cervical cytology has not been shown to be predictive (8% to 25%) in diagnosing fallopian tube carcinoma.[9,12] However, positive cervical cytology has identified tubal cancer in patients following hysterectomy.[16] Endometrial aspiration cytology has been found to be positive in 50% of fallopian tube cancer cases, and 85% of cases were found to have either an elevated CA 125 or positive endometrial sampling.[12] In a recent larger series, in 13% of cases, the presumptive preoperative diagnosis was endometrial cancer based on abnormal uterine curettage.[15]

Retrospective studies of fallopian tube cancer indicate that diagnosis is most often made intraoperatively, often at laparotomy for benign conditions, including torsion, uterine leiomyomata, and/or hematoperitoneum, or as previously mentioned, for presumed ovarian or endometrial cancer.[1] Newer imaging studies (color Doppler ultrasound, positron emission tomography [PET]/CT scanning, and magnetic resonance imaging [MRI]) have also accurately predicted tubal malignancy preoperatively.[17-23] Conventional transvaginal ultrasonography can detect a tubal mass and distinguish tubal from ovarian masses, as illustrated in Figure 47-1, but there is a high degree of overlap in the appearance of benign and malignant tubal pathology. Although not specific, reported features include a sausage-shaped mass, cystic spaces with mural nodules, and a multilocular mass with a "cog and wheel" appearance.[17] Transvaginal color and pulsed Doppler ultrasound with low impedance to blood flow (RI = 0.34 to 0.40) correctly identified eight cases of fallopian tube carcinoma preoperatively, including two patients with no gross evidence of malignancy detected intraoperatively.[18] Three-dimensional static and power Doppler sonography has been shown to depict irregularities of the tubal wall and vascular architecture, consistent with malignant growth.[19] Fallopian tube adenocarcinoma often has a nonspecific appearance on CT scan (Fig. 47-2) and is easily confused with advanced ovarian carcinoma (Figs. 47-3 and 47-4).[20] However, the presence of a hydrosalpinx associated with a soft tissue mass can suggest the diagnosis preoperatively.[21] MRI technology correctly identified a prominent tubal mass (T$_2$-weighted) separate from the ovary preoperatively, in a patient with fallopian tube carcinoma with normal serum markers (CA 125, CA 19-9).[22] MRI technology requires further investigation, but shows promise as a potential tool for preoperative detection of fallopian tube carcinoma. PET scanning fused with CT imaging also warrants further study in this clinical setting. Available data is limited and retrospective; however, PET/CT correctly detected and localized metastatic recurrent disease in 62% of cases, including those with normal CA 125 levels, laparoscopy, and CT scan.[23]

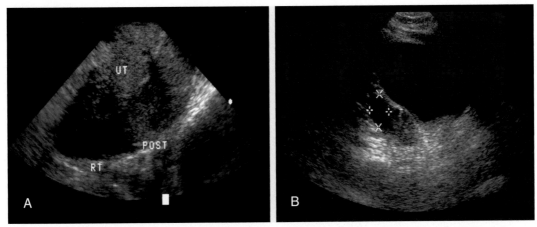

**Figure 47-1    A 62-year-old woman who presented with copious watery vaginal discharge (Latzke sign).**
Transvaginal ultrasonography identified a mass in the pouch of Douglas with cystic and solid components (3 cm transverse × 8 cm AP × 3 cm superior to inferior) posterior (POST) to the uterus (UT) and compressing the right ovary (RT). Differential diagnosis included a complex adnexal mass or, less likely, an exophytic uterine leiomyomata.

# PATHOLOGY

## Patterns of Spread

Fallopian tube carcinoma spreads in the abdominal cavity in a manner similar to ovarian carcinoma, by invasion of adjacent organs, by lymphatic pathways and, less commonly, by hematogeneous spread.[1,8] In most series, at least half of fallopian tube carcinomas were diagnosed in early-stage disease (47% to 51% of fallopian tube cases, Stage I–II).[3,5,24–26] This is quite different from the usual stage distribution of ovarian cancer, in which at best a third have localized disease and two thirds are diagnosed with advanced disease, either within the peritoneal cavity or the retroperitoneal lymphatics. A higher rate of lymph node metastasis for fallopian tube carcinoma relative to that found for ovarian carcinoma has been reported in some series.[27,28] Lymph node metastases, however, rarely occur in patients with tumor confined to the tube or highly differentiated (grade 1) tumors, even in patients with peritoneal disease.[28–30] Radical lymphadenectomy has been reported to increase the likelihood of accurately detecting nodal involvement (42%), and in a retrospective analysis was shown to significantly increase overall survival (43 months; 95% CI, 20 to 66 vs. 21 months; 95% CI, 10 to 32) as well as disease-free survival.[30] Rarely, tumors involving the proximal tube can metastasize in the lymphatics of the round ligament to the inguinal nodes.[31] Tumors in the ampullary/fimbriated portion of the tube are more likely to spread to pelvic and periaortic lymph nodes.[28]

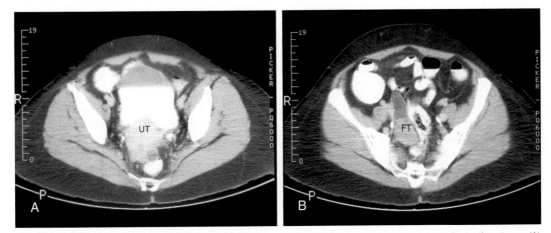

**Figure 47-2    Pelvic CT scan of patient described in Figure 47-1.** Irregular complex mass posterior to the uterus (A) and anterior to the sigmoid colon and a separate fluid attenuation structure extending right superolateral to the uterine bladder of uncertain etiology (B). Laparotomy confirmed this structure to be a dilated, occluded right fallopian tube (FT) with a 2-cm mass at the fimbriated end. A separate solid mass was identified in the cul-de-sac that invaded the sigmoid colon muscularis. Total abdominal hysterectomy, bilateral salpingo-oophorectomy, sigmoid resection with primary anastomosis, infracolic omentectomy, and pelvic and periaortic lymphadenectomy were performed.

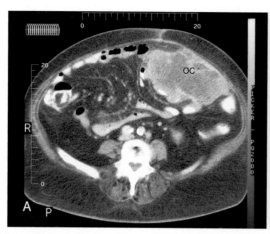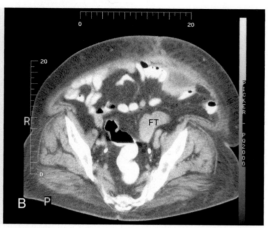

**Figure 47-3    A 68-year-old woman who underwent exploratory laparotomy, total abdominal hysterectomy, bilateral salpingo-oophorectomy, omentectomy, small bowel resection, and pelvic/periaortic lymphadenectomy for presumed ovarian cancer.** Final pathology revealed high-grade papillary tumor occupying 95% of the tube with transmural penetration. Both ovaries were grossly and microscopically atrophic and without tumor. *A,* The 14 × 9 × 15 cm anterior abdominal mass found on preoperative CT scan was a large omental cake (OC). *B,* At laparotomy, there was a 7 × 3 cm dilated fallopian tube (FT) with a tumor at the fimbriated end; preoperatively this lesion was described as an ill-defined adnexal mass.

## Gross Appearance and Histopathology

Benign and malignant tumors of the fallopian tube are both rare. The typical appearance of localized tubal carcinoma is that of a dilated tube that can resemble a hydrosalpinx or tubo-ovarian abscess. On cut section, the tube may be filled with papillary or solid tumor. In up to 50% of cases, the fimbriated end is occluded, potentially reducing peritoneal spread. In 26% of cases, tubal involvement is bilateral.[32] Criteria for the histologic diagnosis of fallopian tube carcinoma, first proposed by Hu and colleagues[33] and modified by Sedlis,[32] are depicted in Table 47-2. Although initially papillary features were a required histologic feature,[33] almost any histologic variant consistent with müllerian/epithelial/stromal tumors has been described; tubal neoplasms are classified by the World Health Organization into epithelial, mixed epithelial, and mesenchymal tumors, although the vast majority are serous.[34–36] Histologic features of fallopian tube carcinomas are illustrated in Figures 47-5 through 47-8.

Unlike ovarian carcinoma, fallopian tube carcinoma includes an in situ variant. Carcinoma in situ of the fallopian tube is characterized by atypical epithelial cells with loss of polarity and mitotic activity, that form papillae, but the basement membrane is intact (see Fig. 47-5).[37] Fallopian tube cancer is rarely found in the in situ stage, but in carefully studied sections, in situ disease is often found adjacent to invasive tumor.

**Figure 47-4    A 68-year-old woman with Stage IIC ovarian carcinoma; this case illustrates the difficulty sometimes encountered in distinguishing ovarian from fallopian tube cancer preoperatively.** This patient presented with elevated CA 125 and a history of serosanguinous vaginal discharge. A preoperative endometrial biopsy was negative for malignancy. At laparotomy, a 4 × 4 cm left ovarian mass was found, but it was unclear grossly if the tumor originated in the dilated fallopian tube (FT) or the ovary. Solid arrows indicate dilated end of fallopian tube; stippled arrows, the ovarian mass.

---

**Table 47-2**
**Histologic Criteria for the Diagnosis of**
**Primary Fallopian Tube Carcinoma**

1. Grossly, the main tumor is within the fallopian tube. .
2. Microscopically, the mucosa should be involved, and should show a papillary pattern.
3. If the tubal wall is extensively involved, the transition between benign and malignant tubal epithelium should be demonstrable.
4. The endometrium or ovaries are normal, or at least the volume of tumor in these organs is less extensive than that within the tube.

Adapted from Hu CY, Taymor ML, Hertig AT: Primary carcinoma of the fallopian tube. Am J Obstet Gynecol 1950;59:58–67; Sedlis A: Carcinoma of the fallopian tube. Surg Clin North Am 1978;58:121–129.

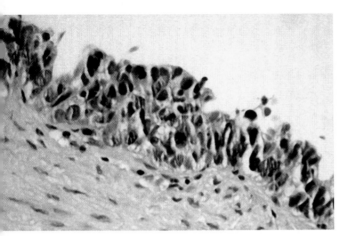

**Figure 47-5** **Carcinoma in situ.** Dysplastic cells are disorganized and heaped up, with marked nuclear pleomorphism. Atypical mitotic figures (not shown) may be present.

## STAGING AND RISK FACTORS FOR RECURRENCE

As with ovarian and endometrial cancer, surgical staging of fallopian tube carcinoma is considered essential to deliver optimal care and to compare treatment strategies. The current staging schema for fallopian tube carcinoma (FIGO and TNM) is outlined in Table 47-3.[38] Carcinoma in situ is included in the FIGO staging system as Stage 0. Invasion into the submucosa, muscularis, and extension into and beyond the serosa can be identified histologically and affects survival; this is now incorporated into the staging system. Like ovarian cancer, cases with malignant ascites in the absence of pelvic or extrapelvic extension identified histologically are denoted as Stage IC.

Pathologic factors that influence survival include tumor grade. In one series, patients with grade 1 tumors had a 5-year survival of 58% compared with 47% for grade 2 or 3 lesions.[5] Extent of lymphadenectomy performed may also influence survival.[30] In this clinical setting, initial and serial CA 125 determinations appear to have the same significance as a surrogate marker for response and recurrence as they do in ovarian carcinoma.[14]

Univariate and multivariate analysis of survival in Stage I and II fallopian tube cancer has identified tumor grade, use of radiation therapy, and chemotherapy as significant factors influencing survival.[8] Cormio and colleagues reported that in addition to stage and grade, the presence of positive peritoneal cytology, node positivity, and residual disease after surgery all significantly reduced survival, whereas age at diagnosis and depth of tubal infiltration were not significant variables.[10] In the series by Alvarado-Cabrero and colleagues, significant prognostic factors included stage and, to a lesser extent, absence of fimbriated-end closure. In Stage I cases, depth of tumor within the tube and location (fimbrial or nonfimbrial) appeared to be prognostically important.[15] Very few studies address the relevance of histologic

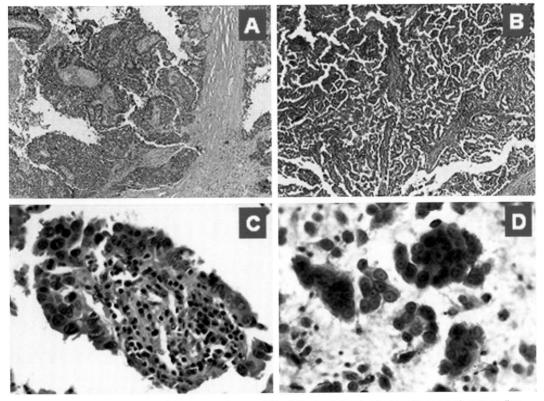

**Figure 47-6** **Histologic features of serous carcinoma of the fallopian tube.** *A,* Micropapillary growth pattern (low magnification view of hierarchical layers of papillae). *B,* Complex arborizing papillary growth. *C,* Still higher magnification of tumor papilla with chronic (lymphoplasmacellular) inflammation of the stalk and moderate nuclear atypia. *D,* Fine-needle aspiration specimen showing loose, 3-D clusters of malignant tumor cells with moderate nuclear atypia.

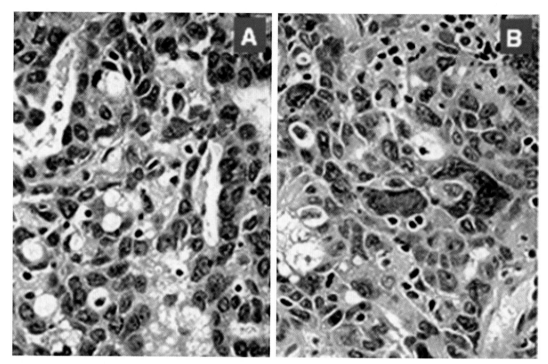

**Figure 47-7    Poorly differentiated (grade 3) serous carcinoma of the fallopian tube.** Histologic sections demonstrate signet ring cells *(A)* and markedly pleomorphic tumor giant cells *(B)*.

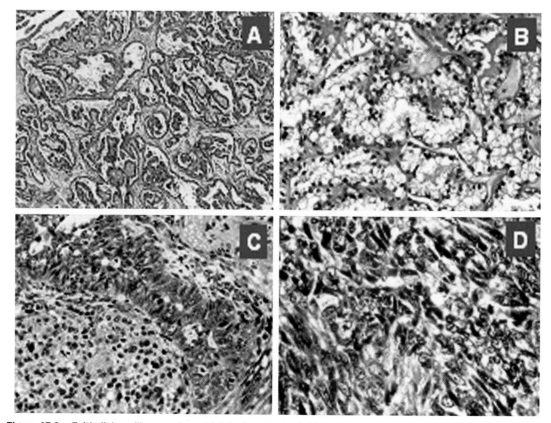

**Figure 47-8    Epithelial papilloma and rare histologic variants.** Epithelial papillomas or polyps are rare, and their malignant potential is uncertain. *A,* Papillae are formed by a single layer of cells, with no invasion into the submucosa or muscularis of the fallopian tube. *B,* Clear cell carcinoma. This is an unusual low-grade type of primary fallopian tube carcinoma (the clearing is most likely due to glycogen). *C,* Malignant mixed mesodermal tumors (MMMT, carcinosarcomas) containing both malignant epithelial and mesenchymal elements. *D,* Pure sarcomatoid area comprising malignant spindle cells.

**Table 47-3**
**Surgical Staging of Carcinoma of the Fallopian Tube**

| | FIGO Staging Classification* | TNM Classification |
|---|---|---|
| Primary tumor cannot be assessed | — | TX |
| No evidence of primary tumor | — | T0 |
| Carcinoma in situ (preinvasive carcinoma) | 0 | Tis |
| Tumor confined to fallopian tube(s) | I | T1 |
|   Tumor limited to one tube, without penetrating the serosal surface, no ascites | IA | T1a |
|   Tumor confined to both tubes, without penetrating the serosal surface, no ascites | IB | T1b |
|   Tumor limited to one or both tubes with extension onto or through the tubal serosa, or with malignant cells in ascites or peritoneal washings | IC | T1c |
| Tumor involves one or both fallopian tubes with pelvic extension | II | T2 |
|   Extension and/or metastasis to uterus and/or ovaries | IIA | T2a |
|   Extension to other pelvic structures | IIB | T2b |
|   Pelvic extension (IIA or IIB) and malignant cells in ascites or washings | IIC | T2c |
| Tumor involves one or both fallopian tubes with peritoneal implants outside the pelvis and/or positive regional lymph nodes | III | T3 and/or N1 |
|   Microscopic peritoneal metastasis outside the pelvis | IIIA | T3a |
|   Macroscopic peritoneal metastasis outside the pelvis ≤ 2 cm in maximal size | IIIB | T3b |
|   Peritoneal metastasis over 2 cm in greatest dimension and/or positive regional lymph nodes | IIIC | T3 and/or N1 |
| Distant metastasis (excluding peritoneal metastasis) | IV | M1 |

*Stage III classification is based on initial findings, not residual disease at the end of debulking; liver serosal involvement is designated Stage III; inguinal nodal metastases are designated Stage III; pleural effusions must have malignant cells to be designated Stage IV.

*Regional lymph nodes (N):* Nx—regional lymph nodes cannot be assessed; N0—No regional lymph node metastasis; N1—regional lymph node metastasis

*Distant metastasis (M):* MX—Distant metastasis cannot be assessed; M0—no distant metastasis; M1—distant metastasis

*Histopathologic grades (G):* Gx—Grade cannot be assessed; G1—well differentiated; G2—moderately differentiated; G3—poorly or undifferentiated

Adapted from Benedet JL, Bender H, Jones H III et al: FIGO staging classifications and clinical practice guidelines in the management of gynecologic cancers. FIGO Committee on Gynecologic Oncology. Int J Gynaecol Obstet 2000;70:209–262.

subtype, but endometrial histology cases tend to be noninvasive or superficially invasive only and have a generally favorable prognosis.[39,40]

As previously mentioned, even in patients with peritoneal metastases, grade 1 tumors rarely disseminate into the lymphatics.[29,30] Fallopian tube carcinomas biologically are similar to ovarian in the proportion of cases expressing c-*erb*-b2 and *TP53* gene mutations as detected by immunohistochemistry.[41] In some series, the authors could not demonstrate a prognostic relevance for these markers,[41–43] but in other series, altered *TP53* expression identified a subset with poorer survival as an independent marker.[44,45] Mutations in the 12th codon of K-*ras* were found in six of eight patients analyzed, suggesting that mutations in this proto-oncogene may be important in fallopian tube mutagenesis.[46]

Angiogenic tumor vascularity, as measured using the endothelial cell marker CD34, indicates that tumor angiogenesis is a molecular marker for adverse outcome.[47] The similarities in genomic alterations for fallopian tube serous ovarian tumors provides strong support for common molecular etiopathogenesis.[48] One series evaluated hormonal receptor status in fallopian tube carcinoma. Approximately 42% were found to be estrogen-receptor positive and 26% progesterone-receptor positive, but receptor status did not correlate with survival. However, a positive inflammatory reaction correlated with significantly better outcome.[49]

An Italian Cooperative Task Force study reported that the overall 5-year survival was 57%, results similar to most of the other series comparing ovarian and fallopian tube survival.

However, they observed a unique difference in patterns of recurrence; fallopian tube carcinoma was more likely to recur in retroperitoneal nodes and at distant sites.[50]

## TREATMENT

### Surgery

The current management of fallopian tube carcinoma mimics that for ovarian cancer. For cases with disease visibly confined to the fallopian tube, the standard procedure includes exploratory laparotomy, visual inspection of all peritoneal surfaces, total abdominal hysterectomy, bilateral salpingo-oophorectomy, pelvic and periaortic lymphadenectomy, omentectomy, and multiple peritoneal biopsies, including both subdiaphragmatic surfaces, paracolic gutters, and pelvic peritoneum.[38] There is sufficient data to demonstrate that volume of residual disease influences survival.[1,3,5,10,38] There are no comparative trials of optimal cytoreduction in fallopian tube carcinoma. However, when this data was included, most retrospective series indicated that patients with small volume disease had significantly better outcomes.

Because survival is improved in patients with minimum residual tumor,[50] it seems prudent whenever feasible to follow ovarian carcinoma surgical guidelines, that is, tumor debulking if possible to at most 1 cm residual disease. The role of conservative therapy (conservation of the uterus and contralateral fallopian tube) in patients desiring preservation of reproductive function is not well studied, but recurrence following conservative management has been reported.[51] Given recent data that women with familial breast and ovarian cancer do carry an increased risk for fallopian tube carcinoma and that ovarian carcinogenesis in these women occurs typically a decade younger than for nonfamilial disease, these women should be cautioned even further regarding the potential risk of conservative therapy and should receive genetic counseling.[52]

The role, if any, of second-look surgery in women with fallopian tube cancer is unclear. Most of the series that include cases undergoing second-look surgery do not include a subset analysis of recurrence or survival differences in patients undergoing second-look surgery versus observation.[53] In the series by Cormio and colleagues, four patients (31%) experienced a recurrence after a negative second-look procedure (median follow-up, 49 months).[53] In the series by Gadducci and colleagues, seven (46.7%) undergoing second-look surgery experienced a recurrence (median, 18 months; range, 9 to 41 months).[50] These data are similar to data in ovarian cancer; for ovarian cancer, second-look surgery is considered the best predictor of response to therapy and disease recurrence.

## Chemotherapy

Twenty years ago, 5-year survival rates for advanced disease were considered poor (<20%).[54] Again mirroring results from ovarian cancer trials for primary treatment, combination therapy with a platinum compound, Adriamycin (doxorubicin), and cyclophosphamide (PAC regimen) resulted in significantly better responses (complete response rate in various trials of 67%,[54] 64.4%,[50] 80%,[55] and 67%[56]) and 5-year survival rates of 19%,[56] 38%,[55] and 48%.[57] In the series by Gadducci and colleagues, the 5-year survival rate was 57%, and the chemotherapy regimens utilized were all platinum-based (PAC, cisplatin + epirubicin + cyclophosphamide [PEC]).[50] As with ovarian carcinoma, Phase II data indicate that combination therapy that includes paclitaxel improves survival over combination platinum-based therapies developed before the discovery of paclitaxel. Gemignani and colleagues reported a series of 24 patients with all stages of disease that included 8 patients who underwent suboptimum cytoreduction. Patients were treated with paclitaxel in combination with either cisplatin or carboplatin (or paclitaxel alone, one patient). These patients had a median progression-free survival at 3 years of 67%, and overall survival of 90% at 3 years (median follow-up, 24 months; range, 1 to 73 months). There were fewer recurrences in patients undergoing optimal cytoreduction (88% vs. 31%).[58] In another Phase I study, although response was not a primary endpoint, 79% of previously untreated patients were in complete remission after a regimen consisting of paclitaxel (175 mg/m$^2$ given over 3 hours), carboplatin (AUC = 5), and prolonged oral etoposide, and the progression-free survival was 17 months.[59] In inoperable patients, the combination regimen of carboplatin followed by dose-intense paclitaxel, followed by maintenance paclitaxel resulted in an overall 2-year survival of 48% (95% CI, 34% to 62%).[60] In recent years, cooperative group trials and institutional series have tended to lump advanced ovarian, primary peritoneal, and fallopian tube carcinomas as a single entity, at least for advanced diseased trials and in recurrent disease, because response to chemotherapy and tumor biology are similar.[59–65]

As salvage therapy, single-agent liposomal doxorubicin has been shown to have modest activity (4/44 patients, 9%) in patients with platinum- and paclitaxel-refractory tumors.[6] In a Phase III study of recurrent ovarian, fallopian tube, and primary peritoneal carcinoma, the response rate at 40 mg/m$^2$ and 50 mg/m$^2$ as single-agent therapy was 13.5% and 7.7% respectively.[62] In patients who had previously received at least one platinum- and one paclitaxel-based regimen, liposomal doxorubicin (20 mg/m$^2$) in combination with prolonged oral etoposide (50 mg/m$^2$/day for 12 days) was associated with a 29% response rate (95% CI, 13% to 53%).[63] Docetaxel has been investigated as second-line therapy in patients with platinum- and paclitaxel-refractory disease, and has a response rate of 10%.[64] Because of this, docetaxel is beginning to be investigated as front-line therapy for ovarian, fallopian tube, and primary peritoneal carcinoma. In one Phase II study, the combination of carboplatin (AUC = 6) and docetaxel (60 mg/m$^2$) as front-line therapy had an objective response rate of 81%; the median progression-free interval at the time of publication was unknown.[65] Topotecan has activity for fallopian tube carcinoma; a complete response in a patient with recurrent fallopian tube carcinoma has been reported.[66] Almost no data are available regarding topotecan in the front-line setting for this disease. A Phase II trial (again, combining fallopian tube with other müllerian types) of sequential doublets (carboplatin and paclitaxel, doublet 1; cisplatin and gemcitabine, doublet 2; doxorubicin and topotecan, doublet 3) indicated that sequential doublet therapy is feasible, with a pathologic complete response rate of 38%.[67]

## Radiation Therapy and Radiation Compared with Chemotherapy

Chemotherapy and radiation therapy were equally effective in achieving response in early-stage disease and were more effective than observation. In the largest study of its type, survival was higher in patients receiving combination chemotherapy (57 months—95% CI, 33 to 81 months vs. 73 months—95% CI, 68 to 78 months). However, this difference did not reach statistical significance.[68] Wolfson and colleagues, in a multi-institutional retrospective study, argued that relapses outside of typical whole abdominal fields were uncommon (6/40 patients, 15%).[24] Whole abdominal radiation therapy for microscopic and small-volume disease is associated with excellent disease-free survival, but in patients with residual disease, treatment failures are high (5-year survival for Stage I, 76.9%; Stage II, 55.6%; Stage III, 20%; gross residual disease >2 cm in size, 0%).[69] Brown and colleagues advocated whole abdominal radiation therapy in patients with residual disease less than 2 cm, although they found chemotherapy an acceptable alternative in patients with early-stage disease.[70] Together, these data indicate that although whole abdominal radiation therapy may be an effective option,[24,70,71] the best responses and disease-free survival are achieved with platinum-based combination regimens containing paclitaxel.[58,72]

## GENETIC SUSCEPTIBILITY

In women with autosomal dominant patterns of genetic susceptibility, the lifetime risk of ovarian cancer approaches 40%, and *BRCA1* and *BRCA2* mutations may account for as much as 90% of hereditary ovarian cancer. Women with *BRCA1* and *BRCA2* mutations have also been found to be at increased risk for fallopian tube cancer.[52,73-79] Current epidemiologic evidence indicates that fallopian tube cancer should be considered a clinical component of familial (BRCA1, BRCA2) cancer. In one study, 11% of fallopian tube carcinoma patients were positive for BRCA1 and 5% for BRCA2 mutations. First-degree relatives of these women were found to be at increased risk for ovarian cancer (RR, 2.2; 95% CI, 0.4 to 6.3) and early-onset breast cancer (RR, 2.4; 95% CI, 0.6 to 9.1).[80] In addition to breast and ovarian cancer, carriers of BRCA2 mutations are also at increased risk for nonmüllerian cancers, including prostate, pancreatic, gallbladder and biliary tract, stomach, and malignant melanoma.[81] Genetic counseling should therefore be offered to women who present with fallopian tube carcinoma.[80-82] The lifetime risk of fallopian tube carcinoma in these families has not yet been fully delineated. However, it has been estimated to be from 1.1% to 3.0%, compared to an estimated 0.025% lifetime risk of fallopian tube carcinoma in the general population.[82] Fallopian tube carcinoma in situ[83] and dysplastic changes in prophylactically removed fallopian tubes of women predisposed to developing ovarian carcinoma, have been described.[84] Salpingo-oophorectomy in women with BRCA1 mutations reduces the risk of subsequent breast cancer development by 50% and also significantly reduces the risk of ovarian cancer.[85] The role of chemoprevention to reduce the risk of ovarian carcinoma in familial cancer is uncertain; at this juncture, the role of chemoprevention in this disease setting is unknown.[86-88]

## SUMMARY

Survival rates for fallopian tube carcinoma appear to be improving. Compared with early ovarian carcinoma, early-stage fallopian tube carcinoma appears to have a better survival but a higher propensity for retroperitoneal spread and distant metastasis. Treatment requires appropriate surgical staging, debulking where possible, and systemic combination chemotherapy using a platinum-based regimen with paclitaxel. Fallopian tube carcinoma is part of the spectrum of genetically linked müllerian (BRCA1/BRCA2) and other tumors (BRCA2). Therefore, patients with fallopian tube carcinoma should undergo genetic counseling for familial cancer prevention. When prophylactic surgery is performed, the fallopian tubes must be removed and carefully sectioned.

## REFERENCES

1. Nordin AJ: Primary carcinoma of fallopian tube: a 20-year literature review. Obstet Gynecol Surv 1994;49:349–361. (IV, C)
2. Rosenblatt KA, Weiss NS, Schwartz SM: Incidence of malignant fallopian tube tumors. Gynecol Oncol 1989;35:236–239. (IIa, B)
3. Kosary C, Trimble EL: Treatment and survival for women with fallopian tube carcinoma: a population-based study. Gynecol Oncol 2002; 86:190–191. (IIa, B)
4. Riska A, Leminen A, Pukkala E: Sociodemographic determinants of incidence of primary fallopian tube carcinoma, Finland 1953–1997. Int J Cancer 2003;104:643–645. (IIa, B)
5. Rosen AC, Klein M, Hafner E, et al: Management and prognosis of primary fallopian tube carcinoma. Gynecol Obstet Invest 1999; 47:45–51. (III, B)
6. Baekelandt M, Jorunn Nesbakken AJ, Kristensen GB, et al: Carcinoma of the fallopian tube. Clinicopathologic study of 151 patients treated at the Norwegian Radium Hospital. Cancer 2000;89:2076–2084. (IIa, B)
7. Heinz AP, Odicino F, Maisonneuve P, et al: Carcinoma of the fallopian tube. Int J Gynaecol Obstet 2003;83:119–133. (IIa, B)
8. Rosen AC, Sevelda P, Klein M, et al: A comparative analysis of management and prognosis in stage I and II fallopian tube carcinoma and epithelial ovarian cancer. Br J Cancer 1994;69:577–579. (IIa, B)
9. Obermair A, Taylor KH, Janda M, et al: Primary fallopian tube carcinoma: the Queensland experience. Int J Gynecol Cancer 2001; 11:69–72. (IIa, B)
10. Cormio G, Maneo A, Gabriele A, et al: Primary carcinoma of the fallopian tube. A retrospective analysis of 47 patients. Ann Oncol 1996;7:271–275. (III, B)
11. Azodi M, Langer A, Jenison EL: Primary fallopian tube carcinoma with isolated torsion of involved tube. Eur J Gynaecol Oncol 2000; 21:364–367. (IV, C)
12. Takeshima N, Hirai Y, Yamauchi K, et al: Clinical usefulness of endometrial aspiration cytology and CA-125 in the detection of fallopian tube carcinoma. Acta Cytol 1997;41:1445–1450. (III, B)
13. Rosen AC, Klein M, Rosen HR, et al: Preoperative and postoperative CA-125 serum levels in primary fallopian tube carcinoma. Arch Gynecol Obstet 1994;255:65–68. (IIb, B)
14. Hefler LA, Rosen AC, Graf AH, et al: The clinical value of serum concentrations of cancer antigen 125 in patients with primary fallopian tube carcinoma: a multicenter study. Cancer 2000;89:1555–1560. (IIa, B)
15. Alvarado-Cabrero I, Young RH, Vamvakas EC, et al: Carcinoma of the fallopian tube: a clinicopathological study of 105 cases with observations on staging and prognostic factors. Gynecol Oncol 1999; 72:367–379. (IIa, B)
16. Warshal DP, Burgelson ER, Aikins JK, et al: Post-hysterectomy fallopian tube carcinoma presenting with a positive Papanicolaou smear. Obstet Gynecol 1999;94(Pt 2):834–836. (IV, C)
17. Yuen JH, Wong GC, Lam CH: Preoperative sonographic diagnosis of primary fallopian tube carcinoma. J Ultrasound Med 2002; 21:1171–1173. (IV, C)
18. Kurjak A, Kupesic S, Ilijas M, et al: Preoperative diagnosis of fallopian tube carcinoma. Gynecol Oncol 1998;68:29–34. (IIb, B)
19. Kurjak A, Kupesic S, Sparac V, et al: Preoperative evaluation of pelvic tumors by Doppler and three-dimensional sonography. J Ultrasound Med 2001;20:829–840. (IIb, B)
20. Santana P, Desser TS, Teng N: Preoperative CT diagnosis of primary fallopian tube carcinoma in a patient with a history of total abdominal hysterectomy. J Comput Assist Tomogr 2003;27:361–363. (III, B)
21. Slanetz PJ, Whitman GJ, Halpern EF: Imaging of fallopian tube tumors. AJR Am J Roentgenol 1997;169:1321–1324. (IIb, B)
22. Takagi H, Matsunami K, Noda K, et al: Primary fallopian tube carcinoma: a case of successful preoperative evaluation with magnetic resonance imaging. J Obstet Gynaecol 2003;23:455–456. (III, B)
23. Makhija S, Howden N, Edwards R, et al: Positron emission tomography/computed tomography imaging for the detection of recurrent ovarian and fallopian tube carcinoma: a retrospective review. Gynecol Oncol 2002;85:53–58. (IIb, B)
24. Wolfson AH, Tralins KS, Greven KM: Adenocarcinoma of the fallopian tube: results of a multi-institutional retrospective analysis of 72 patients. Int J Radiation Oncology Biol Phys 1998;40:71–76. (IIb, B)
25. Heintz AP, Odicino F, Maisonneuve P, et al: Carcinoma of the fallopian tube. J Epidemiol Biostat 2001;6:89–103. (IIb, B)
26. Schneider C, Wight E, Perucchini D, et al: Primary carcinoma of the fallopian tube. A report of 19 cases with literature review. Eur J Gynaecol Oncol 2000;21:578–582. (IIb, B)
27. Wang P-H, Chaao H-T, Yen M-S, Ng H-T: Outcome of advanced primary fallopian tube adenocarcinoma. Chin Med J (Taipei) 1999;62:782–786. (III, B)
28. Klein M, Rosen A, Lahousen M: Lymphogenous metastasis in the primary carcinoma of the fallopian tube. Gynecol Oncol 1994; 55:336–338. (IIb, B)

29. Klein M, Graf AH, Rosen A, et al: Tumor progression, histologic grading and DNA-ploidy as predictive factors of lymphogenous metastasis in primary carcinoma of the fallopian tube. Cancer Lett 2002;177:209–214. (IIb, B)

30. Klein M, Rosen AC, Lahousen M, et al: Lymphadenectomy in primary carcinoma of the fallopian tube. Cancer Lett 1999;147:63–66. (IIb, B)

31. Winter-Roach BA, Tjalma WA, Nordin AJ, et al: Inguinal lymph node metastasis: an unusual presentation of fallopian tube carcinoma. Gynecol Oncol 2001;81:324–325. (III, B)

32. Sedlis A: Carcinoma of the fallopian tube. Surg Clin North Am 1978;58:121–129. (IV, C)

33. Hu CY, Taymor ML, Hertig AT: Primary carcinoma of the fallopian tube. Am J Obstet Gynecol 1950;59:58–67. (IIb, B)

34. Rabczynski J, Ziolkowski P, Kochman A, et al: Primary fallopian tube carcinoma. Histopathology of 46 cases. Pol J Pathol 1998;49:285–292. (IIb, B)

35. Scully RE, Henson DE, Nielsen ML, et al: Protocol for the examination of specimens from patients with carcinoma of the fallopian tube. A basis for checklists. Cancer Committee, College of American Pathologists. Arch Pathol Lab Med 1999;123:33–38. (IV, C)

36. Scully RE: Protocol for the examination of specimens from patients with carcinoma of the vagina: a basis for checklists. Cancer Committee, College of American Pathologists. Arch Pathol Lab Med 1999;123:62–67. (IV, C)

37. Minato H, Shimizu M, Hirokawa M, et al: Adenocarcinoma *in situ* of the fallopian tube. A case report. Acta Cytol 1998;42:1455–1457. (III, B)

38. Benedet JL, Bender H, Jones H III, et al: FIGO staging classifications and clinical practice guidelines in the management of gynecologic cancers. FIGO Committee on Gynecologic Oncology. Int J Gynaecol Obstet 2000;70:209–262. (IV, C)

39. Navani SS, Alvarado-Cabrero I, Young RH, et al: Endometrioid carcinoma of the fallopian tube: a clinicopathologic analysis of 26 cases. Gynecol Oncol 1996;63:371–378. (IIb, B)

40. Alvarado-Cabrero I, Navani SS, Young RH, et al: Tumors of the fimbriated end of the fallopian tube: a clinicopathologic analysis of 20 cases, including nine carcinomas. Int J Gynecol Pathol 1997;16:189–196. (IIb, B)

41. Lacy MQ, Hartmann LC, Keeney GL, et al: c-erbB-2 and p53 expression in fallopian tube carcinoma. Cancer 1995;75:2891–2896. (IIb, B)

42. Chung TK, Cheung TH, To KF, et al: Overexpression of p53 and HER-2/neu and c-myc in primary fallopian tube carcinoma. Gynecol Obstet Invest 2000;49:47–51. (IIb, B)

43. Hellström AC, Blegen H, Malec M, et al: Recurrent fallopian tube carcinoma: TP53 mutation and clinical course. Int J Gynecol Pathol 2000;19:145–151. (IIb, B)

44. Zheng W, Sung CJ, Cao P, et al: Early occurrence and prognostic significance of p53 alteration in primary carcinoma of the fallopian tube. Gynecol Oncol 1997;64:38–48. (IIb, B)

45. Rosen AC, Ausch C, Klein M, et al: P53 expression in fallopian tube carcinomas. Cancer Lett 2000;156:1–7. (IIb, B)

46. Mizuuchi H, Mori Y, Sato K: High incidence of point mutation in K-ras codon 12 in carcinoma of the fallopian tube. Cancer 1995;76:86–90. (IIb, B)

47. Bancher-Todesca D, Rosen A, Graf A, et al: Prognostic significance of tumor angiogenesis in primary fallopian tube cancer. Cancer Lett 1999;141:179–186. (IIb, B)

48. Pere H, Tapper J, Seppälä M, et al: Genetic alterations in fallopian tube carcinoma: comparison to serous uterine and ovarian carcinomas reveals similarity suggesting likeness in molecular pathogenesis. Cancer Res 1998;58:4274–4276. (IIb, B)

49. Rosen AC, Reiner A, Klein M: Prognostic factors in primary fallopian tube carcinoma. Austrian Cooperative Study Group for Fallopian Tube Carcinoma. Gynecol Oncol 1994;53:307–313. (IIb, B)

50. Gadducci A, Landoni F, Sartori E, et al: Analysis of treatment failures and survival of patients with fallopian tube carcinoma: a Cooperation Task Force (CTF) study. Gynecol Oncol 2001;81:150–159. (IIb, B)

51. Adolph A, Le T, Khan K, et al: Recurrent metastatic fallopian tube carcinoma in pregnancy. Gynecol Oncol 2001;81:110–112. (III, B)

52. Colgan TJ: Challenges in the early diagnosis and staging of fallopian tube carcinomas associated with BRCA mutations. Int J Gynecol Pathol 2003;22:109–120. (IV, C)

53. Cormio G, Gabriele A, Maneo A, et al: Second-look laparotomy in the management of fallopian tube carcinoma. Acta Obset Gynecol Scan 1997;76:369–372. (IIb, B)

54. Muntz HG, Tarraza HM, Goff BA, et al: Combination chemotherapy in advanced adenocarcinoma of the fallopian tube. Gynecol Oncol 1991;40:268–273. (IIb, B)

55. Cormio G, Maneo A, Gabriele A, et al: Treatment of fallopian tube carcinoma with cyclophosphamide, adriamycin, and cisplatin. Am J Clin Oncol 1997;20:143–145. (IIb, B)

56. Wagenaar HC, Pecorelli S, Vergote I, et al: Phase II study of a combination of cyclophosphamide, adriamycin and cisplatin in advanced fallopian tube carcinoma. An EORTC gynecological cancer group study. European Organization for Research and Treatment of Cancer. Eur J Gynaecol Oncol 2001;22:187–193. (IIa, B)

57. Pectasides D, Barbounis V, Sintila A, et al: Treatment of primary fallopian tube carcinoma with cisplatin-containing chemotherapy. Am J Clin Oncol 1994;17:68–71. (IIa, B)

58. Gemignani ML, Hensley ML, Cohen R, et al: Paclitaxel-based chemotherapy in carcinoma of the fallopian tube. Gynecol Oncol 2001;80:16–20. (IIa, B)

59. Rose PG, Rodriguez M, Waggoner S, et al: Phase I study of paclitaxel, carboplatin, and increasing days of prolonged oral etoposide in ovarian, peritoneal, and tubal carcinoma: a Gynecologic Oncology Group study. J Clin Oncol 2000;18:2957–2962. (IIa, B)

60. Markman M, Glass T, Smith HO, et al: Phase II trial of single-agent carboplatin followed by dose intense paclitaxel, followed by maintenance paclitaxel therapy in stage IV ovarian, fallopian tube, and peritoneal cancers: a Southwest Oncology Group Trial. Gynecol Oncol 2003;88:282–288. (IIa, B)

61. Markman M, Kennedy A, Webster K, et al: Phase 2 trial liposomal doxorubicin (40 mg/m$^2$) in platinum-/paclitaxel-refractory ovarian and fallopian tube cancers and primary carcinoma of the peritoneum. Gynecol Oncol 2000;78:369–372. (IIa, B)

62. Rose PG, Maxson JH, Fusco N, et al: Liposomal doxorubicin in ovarian, peritoneal, and tubal carcinoma: a retrospective comparative study of single-agent dosages. Gynecol Oncol 2001;82:323–328. (IIa, B)

63. Rose PG, Rodriguez M, Walker J, et al: A phase I trial of prolonged oral etoposide and liposomal doxorubicin in ovarian, peritoneal, and tubal carcinoma: a Gynecologic Oncology Group study. Gynecol Oncol 2002;85:136–139. (IIa, B)

64. Markman M, Kennedy A, Webster K, et al: Combination chemotherapy with carboplatin and docetaxel in the treatment of cancers of the ovary and fallopian tube and primary carcinoma of the peritoneum. J Clin Oncol 2001;19:1901–1905. (IIa, B)

65. Markman M, Zanotti K, Webster K, et al: Phase 2 trial of single agent docetaxel in platinum and paclitaxel-refractory ovarian cancer, fallopian tube cancer, and primary carcinoma of the peritoneum. Gynecol Oncol 2003;91:573–576. (IIa, B)

66. Dunton CJ, Neufeld J: Complete response to topotecan of recurrent fallopian tube carcinoma. Gynecol Oncol 2000;76:128–129. (III, B)

67. Matulonis U, Campos S, Duska L, et al: A phase II trial of three sequential doublets for the treatment of advanced mullerian malignancies. Gynecol Oncol 2003;91:293–298. (IIa, B)

68. Klein M, Rosen A, Lahousen M, et al: The relevance of adjuvant therapy in primary carcinoma of the fallopian tube, stages I and II: irradiation vs. chemotherapy. Int J Radiat Oncol Biol Phys 2000;48:1427–1431. (IIa, B)

69. Kojs Z, Urbanski K, Reinfuss M, et al: Whole abdominal external beam radiation in the treatment of primary carcinoma of the fallopian tube. Gynecol Oncol 1997;65:473–477. (III, B)

70. Brown MD, Kohorn EI, Kapp DS, et al: Fallopian tube carcinoma. Int J Radiat Oncol Biol Phys 1985;11:583–590. (III, B)

71. Klein M, Graf AH, Rosen A, et al: Analysis of treatment failures and survival of patients with fallopian tube carcinoma: a cooperative task force study. Gynecol Oncol 2002;84:351–352. (IV, C)

72. Cormio G: Experience at the Memorial Sloan-Kettering Cancer Center with paclitaxel-based combination chemotherapy following primary cytoreductive surgery in carcinoma of the fallopian tube. Gynecol Oncol 2002;84:185–186. **(IIa, B)**

73. Stratton JF, Thompson D, Bobrow L, et al: The genetic epidemiology of early-onset epithelial ovarian cancer: a population-based study. Am J Hum Genet 1999;65:1725–1732. **(IIa, B)**

74. Paley PJ, Swisher EM, Garcia RL, et al: Occult cancer of the fallopian tube in BRCA-1 germline mutation carriers at prophylactic oophorectomy: a case for recommending hysterectomy at surgical prophylaxis. Gynecol Oncol 2001;80:176–180. **(III, B)**

75. Rose PG, Shrigley R, Wiesner GL: Germline BRCA2 mutation in a patient with fallopian tube carcinoma: a case report. Gynecol Oncol 2000;77:319–320. **(III, B)**

76. Zweemer RP, van Diest PJ, Verheijen RHM, et al: Molecular evidence linking primary cancer of the fallopian tube to BRCA1 germline mutations. Gynecol Oncol 2000;76:45–50. **(IIa, B)**

77. Levine DA, Argenta PA, Yee CJ, et al: Fallopian tube and primary peritoneal carcinomas associated with BRCA mutations. J Clin Oncol 2003;21:4222–4227. **(IIa, B)**

78. Leeper K, Garcia R, Swisher E, et al: Pathologic findings in prophylactic oophorectomy specimens in high-risk women. Gynecol Oncol 2002;87:52–56. **(IIa, B)**

79. Peyton-Jones B, Olaitan A, Murdoch JB: Incidental diagnosis of primary fallopian tube carcinoma during prophylactic salpingo-oophorectomy in BRCA2 mutation carrier. BJOG 2002;109:1413–1414. **(III, B)**

80. Aziz S, Kuperstein G, Rosen B, et al: A genetic epidemiological study of carcinoma of the fallopian tube. Gynecol Oncol 2001;80:341–345. **(IIa, B)**

81. The Breast Cancer Linkage Consortium: Cancer risks in BRCA2 mutation carriers. JNCI 1999;91:1310–1316. **(IIa, B)**

82. Quillin JM, Boardman CH, Bodurtha J, et al: Preventive gynecologic surgery for BRCA1/2 carriers—information for decision-making. Gynecol Oncol 2001;83:168–170. **(III, B)**

83. Sonnendecker HEM, Cooper K, Kalian KN, et al: Primary fallopian tube adenocarcinoma in situ associated with adjuvant tamoxifen therapy for breast cancer. Gynecol Oncol 1994;52:402–407. **(III, B)**

84. Piek JM, van Diest PJ, Zweemer RP, et al: Dysplastic changes in prophylactically removed fallopian tubes of women predisposed to developing ovarian cancer. J Pathol 2001;195:451–456. **(IIa, B)**

85. Rebbeck TR: Prophylactic oophorectomy in BRCA1 and BRCA2 mutation carriers. Eur J Cancer 2002;38:S15–S17. **(IIa, B)**

86. Modan B, Hartge P, Hirsh-Yechezkel G, et al: National Israel Ovarian Cancer Study Group. Parity, oral contraceptives, and the risk of ovarian cancer among carriers and noncarriers of a BRCA1 or BRCA2 mutation. N Engl J Med 2001;345:235–240. **(IIa, B)**

87. Narod SA, Risch H, Moslehi R, et al, for the Hereditary Ovarian Cancer Clinical Study Group: Oral contraceptives and the risk of hereditary ovarian cancer. N Engl J Med 1998;339:424–428. **(IIa, B)**

88. Partridge EE, Barnes MN: Epithelial ovarian cancer: prevention, diagnosis, and treatment. CA Cancer J Clin 1999;49:297–320. **(IV, C)**

# Chapter 48

# Ovarian Carcinoma

## Denise Uyar, MD, and Peter G. Rose, MD

## KEY POINTS

- Because ovarian cancer is often associated with nonspecific symptoms, a high clinical suspicion and thorough examination, including a pelvic examination, are necessary.
- Ovarian cancer stage is one of the most important prognostic factors for survival; it is especially important that complete staging be performed in early-stage disease.
- The majority of patients present with epithelial ovarian malignancies and advanced-stage disease.
- Advanced-stage ovarian cancer is managed with a combination of surgical cytoreduction and chemotherapy.
- One of the most important advances in ovarian cancer therapy has been the addition of platinum-based chemotherapy.
- Currently there is no cancer screening strategy for ovarian cancer that has demonstrated an impact on mortality in the general population.
- Several controversies remain in the management of patients with ovarian cancer, including the role of neoadjuvant chemotherapy, consolidation chemotherapy, and intraperitoneal chemotherapy.

## EPIDEMIOLOGY AND RISK FACTORS

### Incidence and Mortality

Ovarian cancer has the highest fatality-to-case ratio (63%) and is the most challenging of the gynecologic cancers. The American Cancer Society estimates that approximately 22,220 women will be diagnosed with ovarian cancer in 2005, and nearly 16,210 women will die of this disease.[1] In terms of incidence, it has been estimated that in the United States 1 in 70 women will be diagnosed with ovarian cancer and that 1 in 100 women will die of this disease.[2]

This chapter focuses on epithelial tumors, which comprise the vast majority (85% to 90%) of malignant primary ovarian tumors. Malignant germ cell tumors, stromal tumors, and metastatic tumors almost equally make up the remaining 10% to 15%. These different histologies have dramatically different presentations and prognoses. For epithelial ovarian cancers, approximately 70% of patients are found to have advanced-stage disease at the time of diagnosis, likely due to its direct access to the peritoneal cavity, absence of symptoms, and lack of effective screening.

Over the past 2 decades, however, there have been advances in the management of ovarian cancer. The current median survival after diagnosis has increased from 6 to 12 months to 36 months.[3] The 5-year overall survival increased from 36% (1970s) to 50% in 1996.[4] However, marked differences in survival still exist based on age and stage of disease.

### Patient-Related Risk Factors

Advanced age is the foremost patient-related risk factor for ovarian cancer. The mean age at diagnosis is age 63, women age 70 to 74 represent the peak ages of incidence; up to 57 per 100,000 women in that age group are diagnosed with ovarian cancer.[2]

The second greatest risk factor for the development of ovarian cancer is family history. A female with a single first-degree relative or two or three relatives with ovarian cancer has a lifetime relative risk of 3.6 and 5.5, respectively, for the development of ovarian cancer compared to the general population.[5]

Although 90% to 95% of cases of ovarian cancer are sporadic (unknown etiology), 5% to 10% of cases are linked to identifiable inherited mutations in specific genes. Three familial ovarian cancer syndromes have been identified: site-specific ovarian cancer syndrome, hereditary breast/ovarian cancer syndrome (HBOC), and hereditary nonpolyposis colorectal cancer syndrome (HNPCC), which account for 10% to 15%, 65% to 75%, and 10% to 15% of hereditary ovarian cancers, respectively.[6] Genetic linkage analyses performed in the early 1990s led to the identification of two specific genes, BRCA1 and BRCA2, which are primarily linked to HBOC. Women with mutations of BRCA1, BRCA2 and MSH2 and MLH1 (associated with HNPCC) may carry a lifetime risk for developing ovarian cancer of up to 44%, 27%, and 12% by age 70, respectively.[7–9]

Ovarian cancer is most often diagnosed in white women living in industrialized countries. The highest lifetime risk of developing ovarian cancer is noted in Sweden (1.73%), followed by the white population of the United States (1.53%), the United Kingdom (1.25%), Southern Europe (1.11%), South America (0.87%), India (0.75%), and Japan (0.47%).[2] For unexplained reasons, the incidence of ovarian cancer is generally lower for African American women. African American women have a lifetime risk of developing ovarian cancer of 1.08%, compared to 1.86% for white women living in the United States.

It has been noted that the risk of ovarian cancer increases for women who migrate from a country with a low-risk incidence to a country with a higher-risk incidence of ovarian cancer. This leads to the assumption that diet, environmental factors, and behavioral factors play a significant role in the pathogenesis of ovarian cancer.

The western diet has a considerably greater contribution from animal fat than diets of other regions; this has been suggested as one of the factors supporting the development of ovarian cancer in some industrialized countries. As the diets of countries with lower incidences of ovarian cancer (such as Japan) increase in their consumption of dietary fat, an increase in the incidence of ovarian cancer has been noted. Lending support to this theory are several studies[10,11] that have demonstrated an association between the consumption of whole milk and ovarian cancer risk. The theory hypothesizes that galactose, a metabolite of the milk sugar lactose, may be responsible for affecting the normal development of oocytes. However, follow-up studies have failed to provide substantial evidence definitively establishing the link between lactose consumption and increased cancer risk.[12] No associations have been found between ovarian cancer and coffee, tobacco, or alcohol use.

### Exposure-Related Mechanisms of Carcinogenesis

The incessant ovulation hypothesis forms the basis of a theory by Fathalla,[13] whereby cellular injury and inflammation precipitated by ovulation result in disordered repair and potential neoplastic change. Local inflammation at the level of the epithelium may be associated with oxidant production, which may promote subsequent DNA damage. This theory generated much concern over the intended induction of hyperovulation resulting from the use of infertility drugs. Although conflicting results have been published, results of several case-control studies[5,14] have suggested that women with infertility who had or were taking fertility medications have an increased risk for ovarian cancer. A meta-analysis of eight case-control studies did not find an association between use of fertility drugs and invasive cancer, although some evidence of an increased incidence of borderline ovarian malignancies was noted.[15]

The premise that environmental toxins incite ovarian epithelial injury via retrograde transmission from the vagina has also been posited. Retrograde ovarian exposure to perineal talc has been implicated as a possible ovarian carcinogen, owing to the previous contamination of talc with asbestos, a known carcinogen. Although the carcinogenic potential of talc is unclear, the current literature consensus does not show a significant association between its use and the development of ovarian cancer.

Theoretically, cessation of the retrograde pathway should decrease the risk of ovarian cancer. This premise was demonstrated by prospective cohort data from the Nurses' Health Study (NHS),[16] in which women who had undergone tubal ligation experienced a nearly 70% decrease in the risk of ovarian cancer. This decrease may be attributed to decreased ovarian exposure to toxins, but other possibilities include decreased ovarian blood supply as a result of the ligation and ovulation suppression owing to decreased estradiol and progesterone levels.

The NHS also demonstrated the protective effects of parity. Evidence from this study established that a woman's first full-term pregnancy reduced her ovarian cancer risk by 20% to 40%, and each subsequent pregnancy reduced ovarian cancer risk by an additional 14%. According to cohort studies, this protective effect of pregnancy is also conferred on women with a family history significant for ovarian cancer.[17]

To a lesser degree, lactation has also demonstrated a protective effect against ovarian cancer. Lactation inhibits pituitary

luteinizing hormone, which in turn suppresses ovulation. Longer duration of lactation does not correlate with greater benefit.

The effect of oral contraceptive pills (OCPs) on ovarian cancer risk has also been extensively studied. The Cancer and Steroid Hormone (CASH)[18] study conducted by the Centers for Disease Control and Prevention and the National Institutes of Health, a case-control study, revealed a 40% decrease in the development of ovarian cancer after 3 to 6 months of OCP use. This protective effect increased with increasing duration of use and persisted after discontinuation of OCPs. Narod and colleagues[19] performed a follow-up study combining the CASH and SEER (Surveillance, Epidemiology, and End Results) data and noted that the protective effect of OCP use was also significant for women who had a family history of ovarian cancer. In this case-control study of women with hereditary *BRCA1* or *BRCA2* mutation, a 50% decrease in ovarian cancer risk was associated with any past use of OCPs. Expert consensus agrees that 5 years of OCP use will significantly reduce ovarian cancer risk without an appreciable increase in the risk of breast cancer.[20] However, the exact mechanism by which OCPs decrease ovarian cancer risk is unknown.

## SCREENING AND PREVENTION

### General Population

The World Health Organization has outlined general principles regarding the development of screening programs. Factors considered favorable for the development of a screening program include pathology that poses a significant health problem with a well-defined precursor lesion and known natural history; pathology with a high prevalence in the screened population; demonstrable survival benefit of early diagnosis; accessible, simple testing with high specificity that is able to be performed at designated intervals; and a balanced cost-to-benefit ratio.

Proposed strategies for ovarian cancer screening thus far have had difficulty meeting these criteria. Currently available testing has primarily incorporated the serum CA 125 test and transvaginal ultrasound.

The CA 125 tumor marker is an antigenic determinant derived from coelomic epithelium. It is located on a high molecular weight glycoprotein recognized by the mouse monoclonal antibody (OC 125) developed by using an ovarian cancer cell line as an immunogen.[21] Overexpression of this antigen is noted in 25% of Stage I ovarian cancer patients.[22] Unfortunately, levels are also elevated in several benign and malignant gynecologic and nongynecologic conditions, which limit its utility as a screening test. However, sensitivity is markedly improved with serial determinations.[23] Several large prospective studies have evaluated the utility of the CA 125 as a screening test. One of the largest studies was orchestrated by Jacobs,[24] who performed the first randomized controlled study to assess screening with sequential CA 125 testing. The positive predictive value of screening was 20.7%. Median survival time of women with index cancer in the screened group was 72.9 months compared to 41.8 months for women with index cancers in the control group. However, no difference in overall mortality was demonstrated.

Ultrasonography has been studied as a potential screening modality for several decades. Initially transabdominal ultrasound was utilized, but specificity has been improved with the use of transvaginal ultrasonography and incorporation of morphologic criteria to categorize pelvic mass characteristics. Characteristics disclosed by ultrasound, such as thick septa, solid components, multicystic patterns, nodularity, or the presence of excrescences are associated with a greater malignant potential. Ultrasonography alone lacks sufficient sensitivity and specificity to be an adequate screening method, however. Doppler flow analysis was incorporated to help differentiate malignant and benign masses; it is valuable because malignant masses tend have increased blood flow during diastole compared to benign masses, but the interpretation of such studies is subjective.[25]

Sequential multimodality screening can improve specificity and positive predictive value, but the optimal screening strategy and interval are unknown. Current proposed screening measures have not demonstrated an impact on decreased mortality in any clinical trials. High false-positive rates are costly, because they may require an invasive procedure to rule out carcinoma. As a result, cancer screening for the general population is not currently recommended.

### High-Risk Population

Due to the higher lifetime risk of ovarian cancer in women with *BRCA1* and *BRCA2* mutations, screening with serum CA 125 measurements and transvaginal ultrasounds has been recommended in this population,[26] despite the diversity among the data published to date. These recommendations are based on the consensus of expert opinions and have not demonstrated an impact on mortality. Women in this population need extensive counseling on the limitations of current screening recommendations.

Prophylactic oophorectomy has been suggested for over 2 decades as a preventive surgical intervention for women with a family history of ovarian cancer. Primary peritoneal carcinoma, which has an identical embryologic origin, disease presentation, and prognosis as ovarian carcinoma, has been reported in 2% to 11% of patients undergoing prophylactic oophorectomy.[27] Recent prospective studies in women who are carriers of the *BRCA1* or *BRCA2* mutations have demonstrated that prophylactic oophorectomy reduces the risk for both BRCA-associated gynecologic cancer as well as breast cancer.[28]

A recent prospective case cohort study by Rebbeck and colleagues demonstrated a 96% reduction in the risk of ovarian cancer and a 53% reduction in the risk of breast cancer with prophylactic oophorectomy. Mean age at the time of oophorectomy was 42 years. Peritoneal cancer subsequently occurred in only 2 of 259 (0.8%) patients at 3.8 and 8.6 years after oophorectomy.[29]

Several questions remain regarding prophylactic oophorectomy, such as the optimal timing of oophorectomy and whether it should universally include a hysterectomy. Hysterectomy has been advocated by some investigators to ensure the removal of the fallopian tube in its entirety and to reduce the risk of uterine malignancy incurred with prophylactic tamoxifen therapy. Recent evidence also suggests that women with *BRCA* mutations may be at an increased risk of developing fallopian tube carcinoma as well.[30]

The issue of hormone replacement in both high and low risk populations is still the subject of much debate. Epidemiologic studies have yielded conflicting results regarding the association between hormone use and ovarian cancer. The Cancer Prevention Study II found a positive association only after more than 10 years of use.[31]

## CLINICAL FEATURES

A thorough history and physical examination, including a pelvic and rectovaginal examination, is necessary during evaluation of all women. The suspicion of malignancy must be especially high in a postmenopausal female with a symptomatic and palpable pelvic mass.

Most women with early ovarian cancer are asymptomatic. If a pelvic mass is large enough to produce compression of the bowel or bladder, the patient may complain of urinary frequency or changes in bowel habits. In very advanced disease, patients may have symptoms related to the presence of ascites or metastatic disease, which may include abdominal distension, abdominal pain, bloating, constipation, nausea, emesis, weight loss, anorexia, reflux, or early satiety. If a pleural effusion is present, symptoms may also include cough or shortness of breath. Less commonly, patients may experience abnormal vaginal bleeding, which is more often seen in premenopausal patients with ovarian cancer.

## DIAGNOSIS

Although findings on physical examination may lead one to suspect malignancy, and radiologic studies may confirm these findings, the definitive diagnosis of ovarian cancer is a pathologic one and requires tissue diagnosis. A serum CA 125 may be useful depending on the clinical setting. As opposed to a premenopausal patient, in a postmenopausal patient with a pelvic mass, an elevated serum CA 125 (>65 U/mL) had a sensitivity of 97% and a specificity of 78% for ovarian cancer.[32]

Before a planned exploration, routine blood work is obtained, including a complete blood count and electrolytes, along with additional tests as indicated. Chest x-ray and electrocardiogram may be obtained if indicated. Additional imaging may be useful, such as a computed tomography scan, ultrasound, or magnetic resonance imaging, but these are not strict requisites.

Disease with metastasis to the ovaries should also be on the differential diagnosis in a patient with pelvic masses, an elevated carcinogenic embryonic antigen, and normal CA 125. These patients should undergo endoscopic or radiologic studies to exclude a gastrointestinal or biliary primary neoplasia. If extensive rectosigmoid involvement is suspected on examination, a barium enema may be useful for surgical planning. Abnormal vaginal bleeding should be evaluated with speculum examination, endometrial biopsy, and colposcopy if indicated.

## PATTERNS OF DISEASE SPREAD

Ovarian cancer tends to spread primarily by direct extension to adjacent organs, via transcoelomic routes, as the ovarian cancer cells are shed into the peritoneal cavity, and via lymphatics that provide drainage for the adnexae. A significant number of ovarian cancers have lymphatic involvement which accompanies either the ovarian vessels to the periaortic lymph nodes, the

# Gynecologic Oncology

---

**Table 48-1**
**Carcinoma of the Ovary: FIGO Nomenclature**

| | | |
|---|---|---|
| Stage I | | Growth limited to the ovaries |
| | IA | Growth limited to one ovary |
| | IB | Growth limited to both ovaries |
| | IC | Stage IA or IB with tumor on surface of ovaries, with capsule ruptured, or with ascites present containing malignant cells |
| Stage II | | With pelvic extension |
| | IIA | Extension to reproductive organs |
| | IIB | Extension to other pelvic tissues |
| | IIC | Stage IIA or IIB with tumor on surface of ovaries, with capsule(s) ruptured, or with ascites present containing malignant cells |
| Stage III | | Tumor outside the pelvis or positive retroperitoneal or inguinal nodes |
| | IIIA | Microscopic seeding of abdominal peritoneal surfaces |
| | IIIB | Macroscopic disease measuring < 2 cm in diameter |
| | IIIC | Macroscopic disease measuring > 2 cm in diameter or positive retroperitoneal or inguinal nodes |
| Stage IV | | Extra-abdominal extension |
| | | If a pleural effusion is present, there must be positive cytology; parenchymal liver metastasis |

---

**Table 48-3**
**Surgical Staging for Advanced Ovarian Cancer**

- Laparotomy via vertical midline incision
- Exploration
- Peritoneal washings or ascites for cytology
- Total abdominal hysterectomy, bilateral salpingo-oophorectomy
- Omentectomy
- Pelvic and periaortic lymphadenectomy, except for Stage IIIC and IV, in which case clinically involved lymph nodes are excised
- Excision of any suspicious lesions, including radical tumor resection if indicated

---

broad ligament to the external and internal iliac lymph nodes, or the round ligament to the inguinal lymph nodes. Hematogeneous spread of ovarian cancer is a less common route of metastasis.

## STAGING AND PROGNOSTIC FACTORS

### Surgical Staging

Ovarian cancer is a surgically staged disease. An international staging system determined by the International Federation of Gynecology and Obstetrics (FIGO) represents the current surgical and pathologic criteria[33] (Table 48-1).

The surgical approach to ovarian cancer involves defining the extent of disease and removing the primary tumor. Defining the extent of disease involves careful exploration and assessment of the entire abdominal and pelvic cavities. If preservation of fertility is not a consideration, the removal of the primary tumor usually involves a total hysterectomy and bilateral salpingo-oophorectomy via an adequate vertical midline incision. In the absence of advanced disease, if the preservation of fertility is a primary concern, a fertility-sparing procedure that incorporates adequate staging may be performed with appropriate patient counseling (Tables 48-2 and 48-3).

Disease stage is one of the most important prognostic factors for survival (Table 48-4) in epithelial ovarian cancer, yet staging is often inaccurate. Emphasis should be placed on the performance of adequate staging in women with seemingly early disease because approximately one third will be staged higher as the result of histopathologic evaluation[34] (see Table 48-1).

### Optimal and Suboptimal Debulking

The current management of patients with presumed advanced ovarian cancer is surgical exploration and cytoreductive, or debulking, surgery. Although prospective trials are lacking, retrospective data consistently associates low volume of residual disease with prolonged survival.[36]

The definition of maximal cytoreduction has varied, but currently optimal cytoreductive surgery is the removal of all resectable tumors to a residual volume of less than 1 cm.[37] Unlike the approach seen with other solid tumors, aggressive cytoreduction, especially in the cases of advanced disease, has resulted in prolonged disease-free and overall survival in patients with ovarian cancer. Hoskins and colleagues found that patients with residual volume less than 1 cm had a 5-year survival of 30% to 50% compared with patients with bulky residual disease, who had a 5-year survival of 10% to 20%.[38]

Cytoreductive surgery has additional benefits, including alleviation of symptoms from tumor mass effect. In addition, removal of large necrotic tumor masses may improve perfusion to remaining lesions and possibly maximize the cell kill (fractional cell kill hypothesis) of chemotherapy treatments. Small-volume tumors may also be less likely to develop chemotherapy resistance (Goldie-Coldman hypothesis).

---

**Table 48-2**
**Complete Surgical Staging for Early Ovarian Cancer**

- Peritoneal washings or ascites for cytology
- Total abdominal hysterectomy with bilateral oophorectomy and intact tumor removal; however, unilateral oophorectomy may be performed in selected patients with Stage I disease who desire fertility and wish to defer definitive surgery
- Omentectomy
- Pelvic and periaortic lymph node sampling
- Peritoneal biopsies: cul de sac, rectal and bladder serosa, right and left pelvic sidewalls, right and left paracolic gutters, right and left diaphragms, and any adhesions
- Excision of any suspicious lesions
- Appendectomy, if indicated

---

**Table 48-4**
**Ovarian Cancer Survival by Stage at Diagnosis**

| Stage | 5-Year Survival Rate (%) |
|---|---|
| I | 85–90 |
| II | 80 |
| III | 20 |
| IV | 5 |

From Hensley ML, Alektiar KM, Chi D: Ovarian and fallopian tube cancer. In Barakat RR, Bevers MW, Gershenson DM, Hoskins WJ (eds): Handbook of Gynecologic Oncology. London: Martin Dunitz Pub, 2000, pp 243–263.

## Prognostic Factors

Tumor grade and histology play a significant prognostic role in early ovarian cancer. Patients with Stage I disease and poorly differentiated or clear cell histology have a significantly worse prognosis than those with Stage I disease and grade 1 or grade 2 serous histology, with 5-year overall survival rates of 60% and 90%, respectively.[39]

The level of CA 125 at the time of diagnosis may correlate with the volume of disease in some patients; however, it is not thought to be an independent prognostic factor. Conversely, in the setting of postoperative chemotherapy, the rate of decline of the CA 125 marker and normalization of this marker with therapy has been shown to be an independent prognostic factor.[40]

Younger patients have been found to have a slightly more favorable stage distribution and may, therefore, have an improved prognosis. Even when corrected for stage, survival rates are improved for younger women (ages 40 to 50) diagnosed with ovarian cancer versus older women.[41,42] It has also been observed, however, that up to 40% of older patients may not have received definitive treatment. Among 2085 patients who participated in prospective clinical trials evaluating combination therapy with a platinum compound and paclitaxel, age and performance status remained significant prognostic factors for progression-free and overall survival.[42]

DNA ploidy has been studied as a prognostic indicator. Vergote and colleagues conducted a study in Stage I tumors, which concluded that ploidy was more predictive of outcome than other factors, such as adhesions, ascites, rupture, and extracystic growth.[43]

## PATHOLOGY

### Histologic Types of Ovarian Cancer

Approximately 90% of ovarian cancers are epithelial ovarian carcinomas. Epithelial malignancies are adenocarcinomas. In this type of cancer, a malignant tumor originates in the surface epithelium tissue, which is the lining on the outside of the ovary. Epithelial ovarian cancer can be further subdivided into several histologic cell types, including serous, mucinous, endometrioid, clear cell, transitional, and undifferentiated carcinomas. Serous carcinomas are the most common comprising approximately 60%, followed by endometrioid (20%), clear cell (8% to 10%), and mucinous tumors (approximately 3%).[44] Clear cell and mucinous histologies have significantly worse prognoses than other forms of ovarian cancer.

### Tumor Grade

Classically, epithelial ovarian cancers were graded according to their degree of differentiation. Well-differentiated tumors have maintained their glandular appearance and are categorized as grade 1. Poorly differentiated tumors, or grade 3 tumors, no longer have the appearance of glandular features and have instead solid sheets of cells. Intermediate grade tumors (grade 2) have a combination of grade 1 and grade 3 features. All clear cell carcinomas are considered grade 3 tumors.

Although some studies have shown grade to be an independent prognostic factor in early-stage disease, reproducibility has been problematic. A universal grading system has been developed to alleviate the inconsistency by incorporating mitotic score, nuclear atypia, and cellular architecture.[45] Further revisions of this system are aimed at simplifying the criteria and improving its prognostic ability.

### Tumors of Low Malignant Potential

Noninvasive epithelial ovarian neoplasms account for approximately 15% to 25% of epithelial tumors and are classified as borderline malignancies, tumors of low malignant potential, or more recently as atypical proliferative tumors.[44] These tumors may be serous, mucinous, endometrioid, or, rarely, clear cell type. This heterogeneous subclass of tumors is identified by careful histologic evaluation for the absence of overtly malignant characteristics. Clinically, these tumors are characterized by diagnosis at a lower average age than frankly malignant tumors, early stage at diagnosis, infrequent or late recurrences, and long survival even with residual or recurrent disease. Prognosis of atypical proliferative tumors relies heavily on whether the implants that are often found on or outside of the primary tumor are invasive or noninvasive. Women diagnosed with atypical proliferative tumors have an excellent prognosis, with a 7-year overall survival of 100% in the absence of invasive implants.[44]

## TREATMENT

### Chemotherapy

#### Early-Stage Ovarian Cancer

Early-stage ovarian cancer has an overall excellent prognosis. Women with Stage IA or IB well-differentiated or moderately differentiated tumors are considered to have a very favorable prognosis and have 5-year survival rates nearing 90%.[46] Adjuvant chemotherapy is often given to patients with early-stage disease meeting highrisk criteria (Table 48-5); however, the definition of *high risk* varies and the benefit of such an approach is the subject of controversy.

A systematic review of the literature reveals a total of eight randomized trials of early-stage ovarian cancer that include a comparison of adjuvant chemotherapy with no further treatment. Four of these trials include melphalan or other nonplatinum-based therapy, which is considered of limited relevance to current clinical practice. The four remaining studies incorporating platinum-based therapy versus no further treatment are summarized in Table 48-6. The largest and most recent parallel randomized trials—the International Collaborative Ovarian Neoplasms (ICON)-1 trial[47] and the Adjuvant ChemoTherapy in Ovarian Neoplasm (ACTION)[48] trial in patients with early ovarian cancer—compared platinum-based adjuvant chemotherapy with observation following surgery. Although parallel in

---

**Table 48-5**
**High-Risk Criteria for Early-Stage Ovarian Cancer**

- Stage IA or IB with poorly differentiated tumors
- Tumor on external capsule
- Ruptured capsule
- Ascites or positive washings
- All Stage II

**Table 48-6**
**Adjuvant Platinum-Based Treatment versus No Further Therapy for Early Ovarian Cancer**

| Study, Year | (n) | Intervention | 5-Year OS (%) |
|---|---|---|---|
| Bolis et al., 1995[70] | 85 | Adjuvant cisplatin (50 mg/m$^2$) × 6 cycles | 88 |
| | | vs | |
| | | no further treatment | 82 |
| Trope et al., 2000[71] | 162 | Adjuvant carboplatin (AUC = 7) × 6 cycles | 86 |
| | | vs | |
| | | treatment at progression | 85 |
| ICON 3, 2003[53] | 447 | Immediate adjuvant platinum-based chemotherapy | 79 |
| | | vs | |
| | | treatment on progression | 70 |
| ACTION, 2003[49] | 448 | Immediate adjuvant platinum-based chemotherapy | 85 |
| | | vs | |
| | | treatment on progression | 78 |

OS, overall survival.

many respects, these trials did differ significantly in their inclusion criteria. Specifically, the ACTION trial required surgical staging, whereas the ICON 1 trial did not. The results of these trials are subject to several interpretations. In summary, adjuvant chemotherapy improved overall and disease-free survival in nonoptimally staged patients but did not show a significant benefit in optimally staged patients. The results of these studies support the importance of complete surgical staging in apparent early-stage ovarian cancer. In the event that complete staging has not been performed and restaging cannot be completed, adjuvant chemotherapy is indicated to treat potential residual tumor, which exists in approximately 25% to 30% of cases.

### Advanced-Stage Ovarian Cancer

Because most patients are diagnosed with advanced-stage disease, the need for effective chemotherapy after cytoreductive surgery is apparent. In the United States, the standard of therapy for advanced epithelial ovarian cancer has largely been the result of a series of randomized trials orchestrated by the Gynecologic Oncology Group (GOG). One of the most important advancements in ovarian cancer has been the addition of platinum-based chemotherapy for women with ovarian cancer. Adjuvant therapy regimens based on platinum offer overall response rates up to 80%, with complete response rates as high as 50%.[49] Several randomized prospective trials have been conducted, which have culminated in the current standard first-line therapy consisting of carboplatin and paclitaxel. These trials are summarized in Table 48-7.

During the platinum era (since the 1970s), the gold standard of treatment for advanced ovarian cancer had been cyclophosphamide and cisplatin. When paclitaxel was noted to have activity in the second-line setting in patients with platinum-resistant disease, it was deemed appropriate for testing in the first-line setting. The GOG performed a randomized study (GOG 111)[50] in suboptimally debulked Stage III or IV ovarian cancer assigned to either cyclophosphamide (750 mg/m$^2$) and cisplatin (75 mg/m$^2$) or paclitaxel (135 mg/m$^2$ in 24-hour infusion) and cisplatin (75 mg/m$^2$). Both regimens were given every 3 weeks for six cycles. The objective response rates,

progression-free survival, and overall survival were superior in the paclitaxel/platinum arm (see Table 48-7). A larger confirmatory trial (OV 10)[51] was performed in Europe and Canada. This study used the same doses for the cyclophosphamide/cisplatin arm, but the comparison arm contained paclitaxel (175 mg/m$^2$ in 3-hour infusion) and cisplatin (75 mg/m$^2$). Although protocol differences between the two trials existed, response rates, progression-free survival, and overall survival were superior in the paclitaxel/cisplatin arm. These findings were similar to GOG 111; however, a greater degree of neuropathy was noted, which was attributed to the 3-hour paclitaxel infusion time. The GOG also evaluated the efficacy of single-agent paclitaxel (200 mg/m$^2$) therapy versus single-agent cisplatin (100 mg/m$^2$) versus a combination paclitaxel (135 mg/m$^2$) and cisplatin (75 mg/m$^2$) in patients with suboptimal Stage III and IV ovarian cancer in GOG 132. Objective responses were inferior in the single-agent paclitaxel arm compared to the other two arms of the study. Patient tolerance of the combination arm was superior; the authors subsequently concluded that the combination of cisplatin and paclitaxel was the preferred initial treatment for advanced ovarian cancer.

While these studies were being completed, evaluation of cisplatin versus the newer platinum analog carboplatin was also being performed in the ICON 2,[52] ICON 3,[53] and GOG 158[54] studies. The cisplatin and carboplatin compounds were compared in combination therapy; the regimens containing the carboplatin compound were found to be equivalent in efficacy and associated with less nephrotoxicity, less nausea and vomiting, less neurotoxicity, but greater myelosuppression. These studies led to the favoring of carboplatin over cisplatin for first-line therapy.

The current standard of chemotherapy for previously untreated patients with Stage III/IV ovarian cancer who have undergone optimal or suboptimal cytoreductive surgery leaves room for improvement in terms of response rate and both progression-free and overall survival. GOG 182–ICON 5[55] is a five-arm international collaborative study designed to improve on the efficacy of standard platinum/taxane therapy by incorporating newer cytotoxic agents (gemcitabine, topotecan, and pegylated liposomal doxorubicin) in sequential doublet and

**Table 48-7**
**Randomized Trials of First-Line Treatment of Ovarian Cancer**

| Study | Regimen | (n) | OS (mo) |
|---|---|---|---|
| GOG 111[50] | Cisplatin (75 mg/m$^2$) + cyclophosphamide (750 mg/m$^2$) | | 24 |
| | vs | 410 | |
| | cisplatin (75 mg/m$^2$) + paclitaxel (135 mg/m$^2$) | | 38 |
| OV 10[51] | Cisplatin (75 mg/m$^2$) + cyclophosphamide (750 mg/m$^2$) | | 25.8 |
| | vs | 680 | |
| | cisplatin (75 mg/m$^2$) + paclitaxel (175 mg/m$^2$) | | 35.6 |
| GOG 132[72] | Cisplatin (75 mg/m$^2$) + paclitaxel (135 mg/m$^2$) | | 26.6 |
| | vs | | |
| | cisplatin (100 mg/m$^2$) | 614 | 30.2 |
| | vs | | |
| | paclitaxel (200 mg/m$^2$ over 24 hours) | | 26.0 |
| ICON 3[53] | Carboplatin (AUC > 5) + paclitaxel (175 mg/m$^2$) | | 36.1 |
| | vs | | |
| | carboplatin (AUC > 5) | 2705 | 35.4 |
| | OR | | |
| | cyclophosphamide (500 mg/m$^2$) + doxorubicin (50 mg/m$^2$) + platinum (50 mg/m$^2$) | | |
| SCOTROC[73] | Carboplatin (AUC = 5) + paclitaxel (175 mg/m$^2$) | | |
| | vs | 1077 | NR* |
| | carboplatin (AUC = 5) + docetaxel (75 mg/m$^2$) | | |

OS, overall survival.
*5-year OS NR (not reported); 2-year OS 69.8% with paclitaxel; 65.4% with docetaxel.

triplet combinations. This trial is currently completing accrual, and the benefits of additional cytotoxic agents will need to be evaluated.

## Second-Look Surgery

Second-look laparotomy originally described for colon cancer is a careful laparotomy with extensive cytologic and pathologic sampling to determine if residual disease is present. Second-look laparotomy for ovarian cancer was first introduced in the mid-1960s as a way to determine if the chemotherapy effect had been complete and chemotherapy could be stopped. Until 1999 all trials sponsored by the National Cancer Institute required a second-look procedure to determine the true response rate. However, due to the perception that second-look laparotomy, although identifying good or poor responders, had little effect on the overall prognosis, the NCI stopped mandating this procedure. In the first study without a mandated second-look laparotomy (GOG 158), approximately 400 patients chose to have and 400 not to have a second-look laparotomy. Despite the earlier identification of disease and institution of immediate therapy, there was no significant effect on progression-free or overall survival. As a result second-look laparotomy is not indicated outside of an investigational setting.

## Radiation Therapy

Several studies have been performed evaluating the potential of radiation therapy as consolidation treatment (treatment following initial chemotherapy). Whole abdominal radiation (WAR) therapy in patients with ovarian carcinoma has been evaluated in several prospective, randomized trials. No large studies have demonstrated a statistically significant difference in overall survival between WAR, further chemotherapy, or observation in patients with complete response to initial chemotherapy. Radiation toxicity (specifically bowel) may be significant in this population owing to prior surgeries and chemotherapy.

## PROGNOSIS

After the completion of initial therapy, patients are placed under careful surveillance. Examinations are performed every 3 months for at least the first 3 years. This includes physical and pelvic examinations and serial CA 125 measurements, if initially elevated. Radiologic evaluation may be performed according to symptoms, examination findings, or at designated intervals.

## Recurrent Ovarian Cancer

The overall response rate to primary platinum-based chemotherapy nears 75%. Ultimately, 25% of patients do not respond to primary therapy and in many other patients the response is short-lived, with relapse occurring within 3 years. Unfortunately, for patients with persistent disease after primary therapy or recurrent disease cure is no longer possible; however, induction of a second remission is still a realistic goal. Management of patients with recurrent disease is a challenge owing to the delicate balance between the maintenance of the patient's quality of life and minimization of treatment-related toxicity.

The role of surgery in patients with recurrent ovarian cancer needs to be individualized. In the event of late recurrent disease that may be chemotherapy-sensitive and focal disease, surgical cytoreduction may be of benefit. This observation, however, has not been conclusively established by large randomized prospective trials. Recurrent disease is often multifocal and associated with bowel obstruction. The decision to surgically manage a bowel obstruction attributed to recurrent disease should be considered on an individual basis, taking into account response to prior chemotherapy.

The role of chemotherapy for patients with recurrent ovarian cancer is more complex. Patients who have experienced a durable response for longer than 6 months from completion of initial platinum-based therapy are considered potentially "platinum sensitive."[56] Platinum-sensitive patients may be re-treated with platinum agents (cisplatin or carboplatin). Response rates of 20% to 60% have been demonstrated in this population. Which agent or agents to use is controversial. In a platinum-sensitive population, defined in one study as a platinum-free interval of 12 months, Cantu and colleagues[57] demonstrated an improved progression-free interval with initiating therapy with a platinum-based regimen over nonplatinum-based therapy, in this case paclitaxel. Even with a crossover design, patients who initiated second-line therapy with a platinum regimen had improved survival.

In potentially platinum-sensitive patients, two large randomized trials have evaluated single-agent therapy with carboplatin versus carboplatin in combination. The first trial[58] compared single-agent carboplatin to carboplatin and paclitaxel. An improvement in both progression-free and overall survival was noted. Subgroup analysis suggested the greatest improvement was in patients whose treatment-free interval was 12 months or greater. This study was criticized because not all the patients were treated with paclitaxel primarily and in subgroup analysis only patients not pretreated with paclitaxel had a statistical benefit.

In a second study[59] comparing single-agent carboplatin with carboplatin and gemcitabine, combination therapy was again associated with an improved progression-free survival but the study could not evaluate overall survival differences.

Patients who do not respond to initial therapy or recur in less than 6 months from completion of initial platinum-based therapy are considered "platinum refractory."[56] Chemotherapy options for patients with platinum-refractory disease have primarily focused on potential agents that are noncross-resistant with platinum therapy. Several options are available for alternative agents (Table 48-8), but there is no clear data to support the choice of one agent over another. Preexisting comorbidities from prior chemotherapy will often dictate the choice of future therapy. The response rates for patients with platinum refractory disease are generally between 10% to 30%.[60] Combination therapy in this setting has not demonstrated improved

progression-free survival; thus, single-agent therapy is employed in an attempt to minimize toxicity. Patient preferences, quality of life, and performance status must be taken into consideration in the setting of recurrent disease.

Radiation therapy may be beneficial as symptom palliation for patients with recurrent ovarian cancer. The duration of palliation varies, but many have reported successful complete palliation of symptoms.

## Controversies

### Cytoreductive Surgery

As noted, multivariate analysis has revealed that residual tumor is a significant prognostic factor for ovarian cancer. Despite its prominent place in the treatment of ovarian cancer, the benefits of cytoreductive surgery remain controversial. The primary criticisms of cytoreductive surgery include the lack of randomized prospective data to confirm its theoretical benefits. The ability to perform maximal cytoreduction may be a function of the biology of the tumor. Remaining tumor volume or distribution may be more important than an absolute measurement of maximum diameter, meaning that the presence of miliary disease may be an indicator of a worse prognosis than a single focus of disease measuring greater than 1 cm. In addition, the morbidity from radical debulking surgery increases the risk of complications, decreases the patient's quality of life, and possibly delays the initiation of chemotherapy.

### Neoadjuvant Chemotherapy and Interval Debulking Surgery

Many patients are unable to receive maximum cytoreductive surgery owing to several reasons, including coexisting medical morbidities that preclude surgery, the extent of disease, the experience of the surgeon, and possibly the tumor biology itself. A possible advantage of postponing surgical intervention until after chemical cytoreduction is decreased operative morbidity. However, even though neoadjuvant chemotherapy is offered to patients whose disease is considered potentially inoperable, there are no prospective randomized data to demonstrate equivalent results between neoadjuvant chemotherapy and the standard management of surgery followed by chemotherapy.

Two randomized trials have evaluated the role of a secondary interval debulking surgery for patients with suboptimal residual ovarian cancer with a volume greater than 1 cm. A trial performed by the European Organization for Research and Treatment of Cancer (EORTC) Gynecologic Cancer Cooperative Group evaluated interval debulking surgery.[61] In this study, patients who underwent initial suboptimal cytoreduction following three cycles of cisplatin and cyclophosphamide were randomized to either three additional cycles of chemotherapy versus a repeat exploratory laparotomy with a second attempt at cytoreduction followed by three additional cycles of chemotherapy. Among 319 patients those who received interval debulking surgery had a 33% (CI, 95%) reduction in risk of death at 2 years and a significant improvement in progression-free survival ($p = 0.01$).

The GOG performed a similar study,[62] GOG 152, in which 550 patients who had undergone suboptimal cytoreduction were treated with three cycles of paclitaxel/cisplatin after initial surgery. In the absence of progressive disease, patients were then randomly assigned to three additional cycles of chemotherapy

---

**Table 48-8**
**Single-Agent Therapy for Patients with Recurrent Ovarian Cancer**

Platinum (if ≥6 months from initial therapy)
Topotecan
Pegylated liposomal doxorubicin
Gemcitabine
Oral etoposide
Docetaxel
Vinorelbine
Irinotecan
Hexamethylmelamine
Tamoxifen

versus a second cytoreduction and three cycles of chemotherapy. Results did not demonstrate a difference in median progression-free survival (10.5 vs. 10.8 months) or median overall survival (32 vs. 33 months) for the chemotherapy versus the interval debulking surgery arms, respectively. The European study was primarily criticized for the less aggressive primary surgery, correlating with a greater volume of residual disease bulk before study entry. It appears that interval debulking surgery can only improve outcomes for patients who did not receive maximal cytoreduction at the initial surgical procedure.

### Intraperitoneal Chemotherapy

Ovarian cancer usually remains confined to the peritoneal cavity, growing along its surface. The portal circulation, which bypasses the liver, is largely responsible for drug uptake from the peritoneal cavity. For these reasons intraperitoneal (IP) chemotherapy, the administration of cytotoxic agents directly into the peritoneal cavity, provides a potential pharmacokinetic advantage over systemic therapy by enhancing locoregional drug delivery. In theory, IP therapy may allow for greater concentrations administered locally, without a concomitant increase in dose-limiting systemic toxicities. However, it has also been shown in preclinical models that the depth of penetration of IP therapy into tumor nodules is limited, which clinically translates into a limited population (small-volume residual disease) in whom IP therapy may be of therapeutic benefit.

Several drugs have been examined for their potential efficacy when used via the IP route. Cisplatin has been one of the more extensively studied agents due to its pivotal role in the treatment of ovarian cancer. Three large randomized prospective trials have examined the benefits of IP therapy in the treatment of ovarian cancer (Table 48-9).

In the first trial conducted by the Southwest Oncology Group and subsequently joined by the GOG,[63] patients received cyclophosphamide (600 mg/m$^2$ IV) and cisplatin (100 mg/m$^2$ IV or IP). A statistical improvement in complete response as determined by second-look laparotomy and survival, was noted in the intraperitoneal arm. The study has been criticized on three bases. First, when analysis after completing the intended accrual demonstrated a lack of statistical benefit, the study was reopened

for further accrual. Second, despite this the intended risk reduction of 33% was never achieved. Last, patients with residual disease measuring between 0.5 and 2 cm had the greatest improvement in outcome when the expected improvement was for those with disease measuring less than 0.5 cm.

The second large randomized trial conducted by the GOG[64] compared intravenous cisplatin and paclitaxel for six cycles to moderately high-dose carboplatin (AUC = 9) for two cycles followed by intraperitoneal cisplatin and intravenous paclitaxel for six cycles. One-tailed statistical analysis demonstrated an improvement in progression-free survival ($p = 0.01$) and a marginal improvement in survival ($p = 0.05$). However, this study had three variables—the use of intraperitoneal therapy, the administration of moderately high-dose carboplatin, and the administration of eight cycles of therapy in the experimental arm—which confounds its interpretation.

The third most recently completed study[65] compared intravenous cisplatin and paclitaxel with a regimen of intraperitoneal cisplatin and intravenous paclitaxel on day 1 and intraperitoneal paclitaxel on day 8. This experimental arm had an improvement in complete response as determined by second-look laparotomy and progression-free survival, but survival data is immature. This regimen was significantly more toxic, which has limited its general acceptance.

Collectively, these studies have failed to convince the medical community to routinely use intraperitoneal therapy as the standard of care. The confusing design of the studies, with multiple variables used simultaneously, left the impact of the IP route uncertain. Yet IP therapy remains an active area of investigation. To further address this issue, the GOG has elected to study IP carboplatin due to its greater tolerability and to develop a study evaluating the IP route as the only variable modified. Current practices await the maturation of the data from this trial.

Observed survival benefits likely cannot be attributed to surgical debulking alone; unrecognized tumor factors play a considerable role as well. It is also interesting to note that, although believed to be a significant prognostic variable, volume of residual disease is not incorporated into the current staging system, largely owing to the fact that a reproducible and accurate measurement for this volume is not available.

**Table 48-9**
**Randomized Trials of Intraperitoneal versus Intravenous Chemotherapy**

| Study | (n) | Residual Disease | Regimen | PFS (mo) | OS (mo) |
|---|---|---|---|---|---|
| GOG 104[63] | 546 | ≤2 cm | IV cisplatin (100 mg/m$^2$) + IV Cytoxan (600 mg/m$^2$) vs IP cisplatin (100 mg/m$^2$) + IV Cytoxan (600 mg/m$^2$) | N/A | 41 vs 49 ($p < 0.02$) |
| GOG 114[64] | 462 | ≤1 cm | IV cisplatin (75 mg/m$^2$) + IV paclitaxel (135 mg/m$^2$) vs IV carboplatin (AUC-9) + IP cisplatin (75 mg/m$^2$) + IV paclitaxel (135 mg/m$^2$) | 22 vs 28 ($p = 0.01$) | 63 vs 52 ($p = 0.05$) |
| GOG 172[65] | 416 | <1 cm | IV cisplatin (75 mg/m$^2$) + IV paclitaxel (135 mg/m$^2$) vs IV paclitaxel (135 mg/m$^2$) on day 1 + IP cisplatin (100 mg/m$^2$) on day 1 + IP paclitaxel (80 mg/m$^2$) on day 8 | 19 vs 24 ($p < 0.29$) | N/A |

OS, overall survival; PFS, progression-free survival.

### Consolidation Therapy

*Consolidation therapy* is defined as chemotherapy given after induction of initial chemotherapy to reduce the number of cancer cells. The role of consolidation therapy for patients with ovarian cancer who have achieved a complete clinical response after initial surgery and platinum-based chemotherapy is controversial. Because so many patients relapse after a seemingly complete response, it is clear that microscopic disease is likely present but cannot be detected by current imaging methods. In an effort to improve the durable responses to therapy and decrease the relapse rate after initial treatment, a study (GOG 178/SWOG 9701) was performed by the GOG and the Southwest Oncology Group (SWOG). This study compared 12 months versus 3 months of paclitaxel consolidation therapy in patients with advanced ovarian cancer who were considered to be in complete clinical response after platinum/paclitaxel chemotherapy.[66] With half of the planned 450 patients accrued, the primary endpoint of progression-free survival advantage was achieved. The study was closed in October 2001 by the Data and Safety Monitoring Committee after an interim analysis. A statistically significant difference in progression-free survival was observed at 28 months in the 12-cycle arm versus 21 months in the 3-cycle arm. However, overall survival benefit cannot be determined because the study was discontinued and patients in the 3-cycle arm were allowed to cross over to the 12-cycle arm.

This has led many to question whether the initiation of therapy immediately after primary treatment (maintenance therapy) is superior to withholding treatment until there is evidence of progression (second-line therapy). The lack of benefit in the two other randomized trials, which utilized topotecan for four cycles versus observation, is also of concern because these agents are equivalent in randomized trials as second-line therapy. Further studies of consolidation therapy evaluating the risks, benefits, optimal agents, and dosing strategies are needed.

### Nonepithelial Ovarian Tumors

#### Germ Cell Tumors

Germ cell tumors account for less than 5% of all ovarian cancers and originate in the egg-producing cells found within the ovary.[67] A variety of pure germ cell histologies have been described. With the exception of dysgerminoma and low grade immature teratoma, the prognosis of the germ cell histologies is similar, with an approximate 50% recurrence rate for Stage I tumors treated with surgery alone. When treated with adjuvant chemotherapy the recurrence rate for these tumors is 22% following chemotherapy with vincristine, actinomycin-D, and cyclophosphamide (VAC), and 3% following chemotherapy with bleomycin, etoposide, and Platinol (cisplatin; BEP). Mixed germ cell tumors should be treated based on the histologic component with the poorest prognosis. This type of ovarian cancer can occur in women of any age, but approximately 80% are diagnosed in women under age 30.

#### Stromal Cell Tumors

Sex cord stromal tumors, which account for approximately 5% of all ovarian cancers, develop in the connective tissue that holds the ovary together and produces the female hormones—estrogen and progesterone. A variety of pure stromal cell histologies have been described. Sex cord stromal tumors are usually low-grade malignancies, and observation following initial surgery is the standard practice, with the exception of those with extraovarian metastasis or poorly differentiated Sertoli-Leydig cell tumors. Granulosa cell tumors comprise 70% of the neoplasms in this category.[68] The time to recurrence varies widely, with a median of 8 years, but may be up to 20 years after removal of the original tumor. As with other nonepithelial ovarian tumors, the BEP chemotherapy regimen has been the most commonly used. The GOG studied 38 patients with advanced or recurrent granulosa cell tumor treated with this regimen followed by second-look surgery and noted a 37% response rate.[69] Paclitaxel has been reported to demonstrate activity as well and is currently being evaluated by the GOG.

#### Sarcomas

Ovarian sarcomas are difficult to diagnose intraoperatively and as a result are only recognized on permanent pathology. For patients with disease spread beyond the ovary the prognosis is poorer than for epithelial tumors. In view of the high grade of most of these tumors, systemic chemotherapy based on other soft tissue sarcomas could be considered.

## FUTURE DIRECTIONS

The 20% to 30% 5-year survival rate for advanced disease clearly leaves room for improvement. Most patients present in an advanced stage, and cure rates remain low despite improvements in progression-free and overall survival. The clinical challenges that remain regarding the care of women with ovarian cancer demand further refinement of current screening measures, imaging modalities, serum markers, and control of metastatic disease.

## REFERENCES

1. Jemal A, Murray T, Samuels A, et al: American Cancer Society cancer statistics, 2005. CA Cancer J Clin 2005;55:10–30. **(III, B)**
2. World Health Organization: World Health Statistics Annuals 1987–1992. Geneva, Switzerland, WHO, 1987–1992. **(III, B)**
3. McGuire WP, Brady MF, Ozols RF: The Gynecologic Oncology Group experience in ovarian cancer. Ann Oncol 1999;10(Suppl 1):29–34. **(Ia, A)**
4. Landis SH, Murray T, Bolden S, et al: Cancer statistics, 1999. CA Cancer J Clin 1999;49:8–31. **(III, B)**
5. Whittemore AS, Harris R, Itnyre J: Characteristics relating to ovarian cancer risk: collaborative analysis of 12 US case-control studies. II. Invasive epithelial ovarian cancers in white women. Collaborative Ovarian Cancer Group. Am J Epidemiol 1992;136:1184–1203. **(III, B)**
6. Werness BA, Eltabbakh GH: Familial ovarian cancer and early ovarian cancer: biologic, pathologic, and clinical features. Int J Gynecol Pathol 2001;20:48–63. **(IIb, B)**
7. Easton DF, Ford D, Bishop DT: Breast and ovarian cancer incidence in BRCA1-mutation carriers. Breast Cancer Linkage Consortium. Am Hum Genet 1995;56:265–271. **(III, B)**
8. Greenlee RT, Murray T, Bolden S, et al: Cancer statistics, 2000. CA Cancer J Clin 2000;50:7–33. **(III, B)**
9. Aarnio M, Sankila R, Pukkala E, et al: Cancer risk in mutation carriers of DNA-mismatch-repair genes. Int J Cancer 1999;81:214–218. **(III, B)**
10. Mettlin CJ, Piver MS: A case-control study of milk-drinking and ovarian cancer risk. Am J Epidemiol 1990;132:871–876. **(III, B)**

11. Cramer DW, Harlow BL, Willett WC, et al: Galactose consumption and metabolism in relation to the risk of ovarian cancer. Lancet 1989; 2:66–71. **(III, B)**

12. Cramer DW, Greenberg ER, Titus-Ernstoff L, et al: A case-control study of galactose consumption and metabolism in relation to ovarian cancer. Cancer Epidemiol Biomarkers Prev 2000;9:95–101. **(III, B)**

13. Fathalla MF: Factors in the causation and incidence of ovarian cancer. Obstet Gynecol Surv 1972;27:751–768. **(IIa, B)**

14. Venn A, Watson L, Bruinsma F, et al: Risk of cancer after use of fertility drugs with in-vitro fertilisation. Lancet 1999;354:1586–1590. **(IIa, B)**

15. Ness RB, Cramer DW, Goodman MT, et al: Infertility, fertility drugs, and ovarian cancer: a pooled analysis of case-control studies. Am J Epidemiol 2002;155:217–224. **(III, B)**

16. Hankinson SE, Colditz GA, Hunter DJ, et al: A prospective study of reproductive factors and risk of epithelial ovarian cancer. Cancer 1995;76:284–290. **(IIa, B)**

17. Vachon CM, Mink PJ, Janney CA, et al: Association of parity and ovarian cancer risk by family history of breast or ovarian cancer in a population-based study of postmenopausal women. Epidemiol 2002; 13:66–71. **(III, B)**

18. The reduction in risk of ovarian cancer associated with oral-contraceptive use. The Cancer and Steroid Hormone Study of the Centers for Disease Control and the National Institute of Child Health and Human Development. N Engl J Med 1987;316:650–655. **(Ia, A)**

19. Narod SA, Risch H, Moslehi R, et al: Oral contraceptives and the risk of hereditary ovarian cancer. Hereditary Ovarian Cancer Clinical Study Group. N Engl J Med 1998 Aug 13;339(7):424–428. **(III, B)**

20. Narod SA, Boyd J: Current understanding of the epidemiology and clinical implications of *BRCA1* and *BRCA2* mutations for ovarian cancer. Curr Opin Obstet Gynecol 2002;14:19–26. **(Ia, B)**

21. Bast RC II, Feeney M, Lazarus H, et al: Reactivity of a monoclonal antibody with human ovarian carcinoma. J Clin Invest 1981;68:1331–1337. **(IIb, B)**

22. Mann WJ, Patsner B, Cohen H, et al: Preoperative serum CA-125 levels in patients with surgical stage I invasive ovarian adenocarcinoma. J Natl Cancer Inst 1988;80:208–209. **(III, B)**

23. Skates SJ, Xu FJ, Yu YH, et al: Toward an optimal algorithm for ovarian cancer screening with longitudinal tumor markers. Cancer 1995; 76(Suppl 10):2004–2010. **(Ib, A)**

24. Jacobs IJ, Skates SJ, MacDonald N, et al: Screening for ovarian cancer: a pilot randomised controlled trial. Lancet 1999;353:1207–1210. **(Ib, A)**

25. Carter JR, Lau M, Fowler JM, et al: Blood flow characteristics of ovarian tumors: implications for ovarian cancer screening. Am J Obstet Gynecol 1995;172:901–907. **(IIb, B)**

26. National Institutes of Health Consensus Development Panel on Ovarian Cancer: Ovarian cancer: screening, treatment, and follow-up. JAMA 1997;277:491–497. **(Ia, A)**

27. Lynch HT, Casey MJ: Current status of prophylactic surgery for hereditary breast and gynecologic cancers. Curr Opin Obstet Gynecol 2001;13:25–30. **(Ib, A)**

28. Risch HA, McLaughlin JR, Cole DE, et al: Prevalence and penetrance of germline *BRCA1* and *BRCA2* mutations in a population series of 649 women with ovarian cancer. Am J Hum Genet 2001;68:700–710. Epub 2001 Feb 15. **(III, B)**

29. Rebbeck TR, Lynch HT, Neuhausen SL, et al, for the Prevention and Observation of Surgical End Points Study Group: Prophylactic oophorectomy in carriers of *BRCA1* or *BRCA2* mutations. N Engl J Med 2002; 346:1616–1622. Epub 2002 May 20. **(IIa, B)**

30. Zweemer RP, van Diest PJ, Verheijen RH, et al: Molecular evidence linking primary cancer of the fallopian tube to *BRCA1* germline mutations. Gynecol Oncol 2000;76:45–50. **(III, B)**

31. Rodriguez C, Patel AV, Calle EE, et al: Estrogen replacement therapy and ovarian cancer mortality in a large prospective study of US women. JAMA 2001 Mar 21;285:1460–1465. **(IIa, B)**

32. Malkasian GD II, Knapp RC, Lavin PT, et al: Preoperative evaluation of serum CA 125 levels in premenopausal and postmenopausal patients with pelvic masses: discrimination of benign from malignant disease. Am J Obstet Gynecol 1988;159:341–346. **(IIa, B)**

33. Staging Announcement FIGO Cancer Committee. Gynecol Oncol 1986;25:383. **(Ia, A)**

34. Piver M, Barlow J, Lele S: Incidence of subclinical metastasis in stage I and II ovarian carcinoma. Obstet Gynecol 1978;52:100–108. **(IV, C)**

35. Hensley ML, Alektiar KM, Chi D: Ovarian and fallopian tube cancer. In Barakat RR, Bevers MW, Gershenson DM, Hoskins WJ (eds): Handbook of Gynecologic Oncology. London, Martin Dunitz, 2000, pp 243–263. **(Ia, A)**

36. Bristow RE, Tomacruz RS, Armstrong DK, et al: Survival effect of maximal cytoreductive surgery for advanced ovarian carcinoma during the platinum era: a meta-analysis. J Clin Oncol 2002;20:1248–1259. **(III, B)**

37. Omura G, Brady M, Homesley H, et al: Long term follow-up and prognostic factor analysis in advanced ovarian carcinoma: the Gynecologic Oncology Group experience. J Clin Oncol 1991;9:1138–1150. **(Ib, A)**

38. Hoskins WJ, McGuire WP, Brady MF, et al: The effect of diameter of largest residual disease on survival after primary cytoreductive surgery in patients with suboptimal residual epithelial ovarian carcinoma. Am J Obstet Gynecol 1994;170:974–980. **(IIb, B)**

39. Winter-Roach B, Hooper L, Kitchener H: Systematic review of adjuvant therapy for early stage (epithelial) ovarian cancer. Int J Gynecol Cancer 2003;13:395–404. **(Ia, A)**

40. Markman M: The role of CA-125 in the management of ovarian cancer. Oncologist 1997;2:6–9. **(IIa, B)**

41. Pecorelli S: 1998 FIGO annual report of the treatment in gynecological cancer. J Epidemiol Biostat 3:1–168. **(Ia, A)**

42. Winter WE, Maxwell L, Tian C, et al: Prognostic factors for advanced epithelial ovarian cancer: a Gynecologic Oncology Group study. Gynecol Oncol 2004;92:412, abstract 41. **(IIb, B)**

43. Vergote IB, Kaern J, Abeler VM, et al: Analysis of prognostic factors in stage I epithelial ovarian carcinoma: importance of degree of differentiation and deoxyribonucleic acid ploidy in predicting relapse. Am J Obstet Gynecol 1993;169:40–52. **(III, B)**

44. Seidman JD, Kurman RJ: Pathology of ovarian carcinoma. Hematol Oncol Clin North Am 2003;17:909–925, vii. **(III, B)**

45. Silverberg SG: Histopathologic grading of ovarian carcinoma: a review and proposal. Int J Gynecol Pathol 2000;19:7–15. **(III, B)**

46. Richardson GS, Scully RE, Nikrui N, et al: Common epithelial cancer of the ovary (2). N Engl J Med 1985;312:415–424. **(Ib, A)**

47. Colombo N, Guthrie D, Chiari S, et al, for the International Collaborative Ovarian Neoplasm (ICON) collaborators: International Collaborative Ovarian Neoplasm trial 1: a randomized trial of adjuvant chemotherapy in women with early-stage ovarian cancer. J Natl Cancer Inst 2003;95:125–132. **(Ib, A)**

48. Trimbos JB, Vergote I, Bolis G, et al, for the EORTC-ACTION collaborators: Impact of adjuvant chemotherapy and surgical staging in early-stage ovarian carcinoma: European Organisation for Research and Treatment of Cancer-Adjuvant ChemoTherapy in Ovarian Neoplasm trial. Natl Cancer Inst 2003;95:113–125. **(Ib, A)**

49. Cannistra SA: Cancer of the ovary. N Engl J Med 1993;329:1550–1559. **(Ib, A)**

50. McGuire WP, Hoskins WJ, Brady MF, et al: Cyclophosphamide and cisplatin compared with paclitaxel and cisplatin in patients with stage III and stage IV ovarian cancer. N Engl J Med 1996;334:1–6. **(Ia, A)**

51. Piccart MJ, Bertelsen K, James K, et al: Randomized intergroup trial of cisplatin/paclitaxel versus cisplatin/cyclophosphamide in women with advanced epithelial ovarian cancer: 3-year results. J Natl Cancer Inst 2000;92:699–708. **(Ib, A)**

52. ICON Collaborators: ICON2: randomised trial of single-agent carboplatin against three-drug combination of CAP (cyclophosphamide, doxorubicin, and cisplatin) in women with ovarian cancer. International Collaborative Ovarian Neoplasm Study. Lancet 1998;352:1571–1576. **(Ib, A)**

53. International Collaborative Ovarian Neoplasm Group: Paclitaxel plus carboplatin versus standard chemotherapy with either single-agent carboplatin or cyclophosphamide, doxorubicin, and cisplatin in women

with ovarian cancer: the ICON3 randomised trial. Lancet 2002; 360:505–515. (Ib, A)

54. Ozols RF, Bundy BN, Greer BE, et al: Phase III trial of carboplatin and paclitaxel compared with cisplatin and paclitaxel in patients with optimally resected Stage III ovarian cancer: a Gynecologic Oncology Group study. J Clin Oncol 2003;21:3194–3200. Epub 2003 Jul 14. (Ib, A)

55. Copeland LJ, Bookman M, Trimble E: Gynecologic Oncology Group Protocol GOG 182-ICON5. Clinical trials of newer regimens for treating ovarian cancer: the rationale for Gynecologic Oncology Group Protocol GOG 182-ICON5. Gynecol Oncol 2003;90(Pt 2):S1–S7. (Ia, A)

56. Thigpen JT, Blessing JA, Ball H, et al: Phase II trial of paclitaxel in patients with progressive ovarian carcinoma after platinum-based chemotherapy: a Gynecologic Oncology Group study. J Clin Oncol 1994;12:1748–1753. (Ib, A)

57. Cantu MG, Buda A, Parma G, et al: Randomized controlled trial of single-agent paclitaxel versus cyclophosphamide, doxorubicin, and cisplatin in patients with recurrent ovarian cancer who responded to first-line platinum-based regimens. J Clin Oncol 2002;20:1232–1237. (Ib, A)

58. Parmar MK, Ledermann JA, Colombo N, et al, for the ICON and AGO Collaborators: Paclitaxel plus platinum-based chemotherapy versus conventional platinum-based chemotherapy in women with relapsed ovarian cancer: the ICON4/AGO-OVAR-2.2 trial. Lancet 2003; 361:2099–2106. (Ib, A)

59. du Bois A, Luck HJ, Pfisterer J, et al: Second-line carboplatin and gemcitabine in platinum sensitive ovarian cancer—a dose-finding study by the Arbeitsgemeinschaft Gynakologische Onkologie (AGO) Ovarian Cancer Study Group. Ann Oncol 2001;12:1115–1120. (IIa, B)

60. DuPont J: Management of ovarian cancer: balancing medical and quality of life. Oncology Spec Ed 2004;7:191–198. (Ia, A)

61. van der Burg ME, van Lent M, Buyse M, et al: The effect of debulking surgery after induction chemotherapy on the prognosis in advanced epithelial ovarian cancer. Gynecological Cancer Cooperative Group of the European Organization for Research and Treatment of Cancer. N Engl J Med 1995;332:629–634. (Ib, A)

62. Rose PG, Nerenstone S, Brady M, et al: A Phase III randomized study of interval secondary cytoreduction in patients with advanced stage ovarian carcinoma with suboptimal residual disease: a Gynecologic Oncology Group study. Proc Am Soc Clin Oncol 2002;21:201a. (Ib, A)

63. Alberts DS, Liu PY, Hannigan EV, et al: Intraperitoneal cisplatin plus intravenous cyclophosphamide versus intravenous cisplatin plus intravenous cyclophosphamide for stage III ovarian cancer. N Engl J Med 1996;335:1950–1955. (Ib, B)

64. Markman M, Bundy BN, Alberts DS, et al: Phase III trial of standard-dose intravenous cisplatin plus paclitaxel versus moderately high-dose carboplatin followed by intravenous paclitaxel and intraperitoneal cisplatin in small-volume stage III ovarian carcinoma: an intergroup study of the Gynecologic Oncology Group, Southwestern Oncology Group, and Eastern Cooperative Oncology Group. J Clin Oncol 2001; 19:1001–1007. (Ib, A)

65. Armstrong DK, Bundy BN, Baergen R, et al: Randomized Phase III study of intravenous paclitaxel and cisplatin versus IV paclitaxel, intraperitoneal cisplatin and IP paclitaxel in optimal stage III epithelial ovarian cancer: a Gynecologic Oncology Group Trial (GOG 172). Proc Am Soc Clin Oncol 2002;21:201a. (Ib, A)

66. Markman M, Liu PY, Wilczynski S, et al, for the Southwest Oncology Group and the Gynecologic Oncology Group: Phase III randomized trial of 12 versus 3 months of maintenance paclitaxel in patients with advanced ovarian cancer after complete response to platinum and paclitaxel-based chemotherapy: a Southwest Oncology Group and Gynecologic Oncology Group trial. J Clin Oncol 2003;21:2460–2465. (Ib, A)

67. Abu-Rustum NR, Aghajanian C: Management of malignant germ cell tumors of the ovary. Semin Oncol 1998;25:235–242. (Ia, A)

68. Schumer ST, Cannistra SA: Granulosa cell tumor of the ovary. J Clin Oncol 2003;21:1180–1189. (Ia, A)

69. Homesley HD, Bundy BN, Hurteau JA, et al: Bleomycin, etoposide, and cisplatin combination therapy of ovarian granulosa cell tumors and other stromal malignancies: a Gynecologic Oncology Group study. Gynecol Oncol 1999;72:131–137. (Ib, A)

70. Bolis G, Colombo N, Pecorelli S, et al: Adjuvant treatment for early epithelial ovarian cancer: results of two randomised clinical trials comparing cisplatin to no further treatment or chromic phosphate (32P). GICOG: Gruppo Interregionale Collaborativo in Ginecologia Oncologica. Ann Oncol 1995;6:887–893. (Ib, A)

71. Trope C, Kaern J, Hogberg T, et al: Randomized study on adjuvant chemotherapy in stage I high-risk ovarian cancer with evaluation of DNA-ploidy as prognostic instrument. Ann Oncol 2000;11:281–288. (Ib, A)

72. Muggia FM, Braly PS, Brady MF, et al: Phase III randomized study of cisplatin versus paclitaxel versus cisplatin and paclitaxel in patients with suboptimal stage III or IV ovarian cancer: a Gynecologic Oncology Group study. J Clin Oncol 2000;18:106–115. (Ib, A)

73. Kaye SB, Vasey PA: Docetaxel in ovarian cancer: phase III perspectives and future development. Semin Oncol 2002;29(Suppl 12):22–27. (Ib, A)

# Chapter 49

# Gestational Trophoblastic Disease

## Inbar Ben-Shachar, MD, and Larry J. Copeland, MD

---

### KEY POINTS

- Gestational trophoblastic disease (GTD) comprises a spectrum of interrelated conditions originating from the placenta.
- Histologically four distinct clinicopathologic forms are recognized: complete and partial hydatidiform moles, invasive mole, choriocarcinoma, and placental site trophoblastic tumor.
- Diagnosis and management can be based solely on history, elevated levels of human chorionic gonadotropins, and metastatic workup.
- Three main systems have been used to categorize patients with gestational trophoblastic disease: the WHO prognostic index score, the anatomic FIGO classification, and the clinical classification system.
- Recently FIGO revised its classification to include both the anatomic stages and a modified WHO prognostic score. The new FIGO risk index also standardized the radiologic studies to be used for determining the number and size of metastases.
- At present with quantitative assays for β-hCG and the use of different protocols of chemotherapy, most women with gestational trophoblastic disease can be cured and their reproductive function preserved even when the disease is widely disseminated.

---

GTD, or gestational trophoblastic neoplasia (GTN), includes a spectrum of diseases with a wide range of neoplastic potential and is among the rare solid human malignancies that can be cured even when widely disseminated. Reasons for this success include a sensitive marker, beta-human chorionic gonadotropin (β-hCG), and sensitivity to various chemotherapy agents and other modalities such as surgery and radiation. Although four distinct clinicopathologic forms are recognized—complete or partial hydatidiform mole, invasive mole (chorioadenoma destruens), placental site trophoblastic tumor (PSTT), and choriocarcinoma—diagnosis and management can be based solely on history, elevated levels of β-hCG, and metastatic workup. This approach, in which a disease is treated by cytotoxic drugs based on clinical classification without cytologic or pathologic documentation of malignancy, is unique.

## HYDATIDIFORM MOLE

### Epidemiology

The precise incidence of molar pregnancy is difficult to derive, because in most reports neither the total number of pregnancies nor the total number of hydatidiform moles (HM) in a defined population are known. The most reliable studies suggest that the incidence of HM is slightly less than 1 out of 1000 pregnancies in most of the world and possibly as high as 1 out of 500 pregnacies in the Far East. It is possible that the higher risk in the Far East is the result of bias caused by reporting data from hospital-based studies rather than population based studies. Because many normal deliveries occur at home in these countries, hospital-based studies result in a bias overestimation of the true incidence of hydatidiform mole. The reported incidence of hydatidiform mole varies among ethnic groups; in the United States white women are twice as likely to develop hydatidiform mole as black women. In a study from Hawaii,[1] the incidence was lower in white and native Hawaiian populations (7.7 to 8 of every 1000 pregnancies) and highest in Filipino and Japanese populations (16.5 to 17.5 of every 1000 pregnancies); whether this difference is of genetic or cultural origin is unknown. Familial molar pregnancies were reported as well. The incidence of hydatidiform mole is clearly related to maternal age and is reported to be higher in women younger than age 15 or older than age 40. Women older than age 50 have a 300- to 400-fold increased risk of hydatidiform mole compared to women ages 25 to 29. Patients with a prior history of a molar pregnancy have an increased risk of trophoblastic disease. The risk of hydatidiform mole after one previous molar pregnancy is 1 out of 76; after two previous molar pregnancies, the risk increases to 1 out of 6.5; and after three molar pregnancies the likelihood for a live birth is almost 0.

Unconfirmed risk factors include Rh-positive blood type, artificial insemination, nulliparity, consanguinity, diet (low in protein, folate, vitamin A), history of prior spontaneous abortions, and professional occupation[2] (Table 49-1).

### Classification

Hydatidiform mole (from the Latin *hydatis*—watery vesicle, *moles*—shapeless mass) can be classified as either complete or partial on the basis of gross morphology, histopathology, and karyotype (Table 49-2).

#### Complete Hydatidiform Mole

The complete hydatidiform mole (Figs. 49-1 and 49-2) is characterized by lack of identifiable embryonic or fetal tissues, gross vesicular swelling involving all the placental villi, and diffuse cytotrophoblastic and syncytiotrophoblastic hyperplasia. Cellular anaplasia may also be present.

Complete hydatidiform moles usually have a 46,XX karyotype entirely of paternal origin. Complete mole appears to arise from an empty or inactivated ovum that has been fertilized by a single sperm carrying 23 chromosomes. The haploid set of

| Table 49-1 |
|---|
| **Factors Associated with GTD Occurrence and Corresponding Relative Risks** |

| Risk Factor | OR Complete Mole (%) |
|---|---|
| Prior molar gestation | 20–40 |
| Maternal Age <br>   <20 years <br>   >40 years | <br> 1.5 <br> 5.2 |
| Prior spontaneous abortion | 1.9–3.3 |
| Current smoking | 2.2 |
| Vitamin A in diet above control median | 0.6 |
| Parity >1, abortions 0 | 0.2–0.6 |

From Smith HO: Gestational trophoblastic disease epidemiology and trends. Clin Obstet Gynecol 2003;46:541–546.

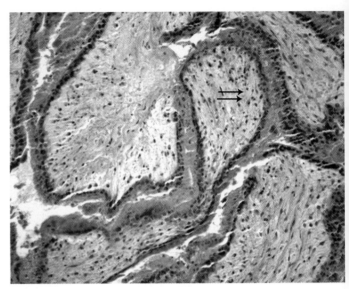

**Figure 49-1** **Early complete hydatidiform mole.** Note characteristic stromal karyorrhexis *(arrows)*. (Courtesy Dr. Ilana Ariel, Hadassah Medical Center, Jerusalem.)

chromosomes reduplicate to give a 46 karyotype. This process, called *androgenesis*, results in a homozygous conceptus. Although most complete moles have a 46,XX chromosomal pattern, approximately 10% have a 46,XY karyotype. Chromosomes in a 46,XY complete mole also appear to be entirely of paternal origin, but in these circumstances an apparently empty egg is fertilized by two sperm, one carrying the X and the other the Y chromosome. The risk of malignancy is similar in the XX and XY subset. Kovacs and colleagues,[3] using molecular genetic fingerprinting methods in 20 consecutive complete moles, found 12 (60%) to be of homozygous androgenetic origin, 4 (20%) to be of heterozygous androgenetic origin, and 4 (20%) to be of heterozygous biparental origin. The latter heterozygous biparental complete mole appears to be associated with an autosomal recessive condition predisposing to molar pregnancies. Because they are pathologically indistinguishable from androgenetic complete hydatidiform mole, biparental complete hydatidiform moles are likely to result from defects in genomic imprinting.

There is evidence that the gene mutation in this condition, provisionally mapped to 19q13.3–13.4, may be important in setting the maternal imprint in the ovum. Women with biparental complete hydatidiform mole have a much higher risk of recurrent hydatidiform mole than women with androgenetic complete hydatidiform mole; they also have an appreciable risk of persistent trophoblastic disease.[4] Other studies have shown that complete moles were 50% diploid, 43% tetraploid, and 3.6% polyploid.

### Partial Hydatidiform Mole
Partial hydatidiform mole (Figs. 49-3 and 49-4) is invariably associated with an embryo or fetus, cord, or membranes.

| Table 49-2 |
|---|
| **Features of Complete and Partial Hydatiform Moles** |

| Feature | Complete Mole | Partial Mole |
|---|---|---|
| Synonyms | Classic, true | Incomplete |
| Fetal or embryonic tissue or membranes | Absent | Usually present |
| Villous capillaries | Usually absent; when present, no fetal blood cells | Usually present; may contain fetal blood cells |
| Hydatidiform swelling of chorionic villi | Diffuse | Focal |
| Trophoblastic hyperplasia | Usually present | Mild and focal |
| Malignant potential | 15%–25% | 5%–10% |
| Karyotype | 46,XX;46,XY | 69,XXX;69,XXY |

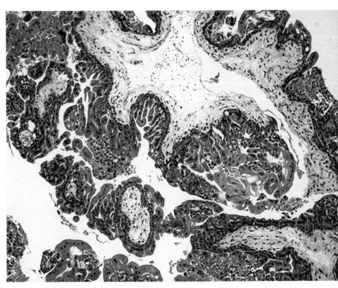

**Figure 49-2** **Complete hydatidiform mole.** Note hydropic degeneration with formation of central cisterns and prominent circumferential trophoblastic hyperplasia. (Courtesy Dr. Ilana Ariel, Hadassah Medical Center, Jerusalem.)

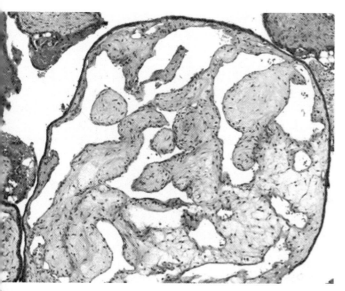

**Figure 49-3    Partial hydatidiform mole.** Labyrinthine vascular pattern. (Courtesy Dr. Ilana Ariel, Hadassah Medical Center, Jerusalem.)

Although the embryo usually dies by 9 weeks' gestation, it may survive to the second and rarely even to the third trimester. The characteristic pathologic features are chorionic villi of varying size with focal hydatidiform swelling and cavitations; marked villous scalloping; focal trophoblastic hyperplasia, usually limited to the syncytial trophoblastic cells; development of functioning capillaries manifested by the presence of erythrocytes; and prominent stromal trophoblastic inclusions.

Partial hydatidiform moles usually have a triploid karyotype (69 chromosomes), containing two sets of paternal and one set of maternal chromosomes. Partial moles may be confused with triploid embryos with a diploid set of maternal DNA and haploid set of paternal DNA.[5] Until these cytologic differences

became recognized, incidence rates were probably falsely elevated, because inclusion of triploid abortus cases resembling partial hydatidiform moles was likely.

### Clinical Features

The presenting symptoms and signs of complete and partial molar pregnancy are provided in Table 49-3.

Essentially all patients with complete hydatidiform mole have delayed menses, and most patients are considered pregnant. Although in the past it was stated that only 50% of hydatidiform moles are diagnosed before expulsion of the typical grape-like vesicles, with the widespread use of sonography to assess early pregnancy and first-trimester bleeding, most molar pregnancies are currently diagnosed before the appearance of symptoms.

According to the Trophoblastic Disease Registration Centre database at Charing Cross Hospital in London, the risk of molar pregnancy is increased in both upper and lower extremes of maternal age ($\geq 45$ years and $\leq 15$ years). This association is strongest for complete moles, and the degree of risk is much greater with older rather than younger maternal age.

Because most of cases of complete hydatidiform mole are currently diagnosed in the first or early second trimester, the classic signs and symptoms of excessive uterine size, hyperemesis, anemia, pre-eclampsia, clinical hyperthyroidism, and acute respiratory distress described in Table 49-3 are no longer commonly seen. Soto-Wright and colleagues[6] have described the changing clinical presentation of complete hydatidiform mole. In their series between 1988 and 1993 none of the patients with complete hydatidiform mole had respiratory distress or clinical hyperthyroidism; however, patients continue to present with vaginal bleeding and markedly elevated hCG levels.

As a rule patients with partial hydatidiform mole do not have the clinical features characteristic of patients with complete mole. Most patients with partial molar pregnancy present with vaginal bleeding in the late first trimester, with signs and symptoms suggestive of threatened or spontaneous abortion. The diagnosis of partial mole is generally considered only after histologic review of the curetting specimens. Clinical findings usually include a uterus small or equal to gestational age;

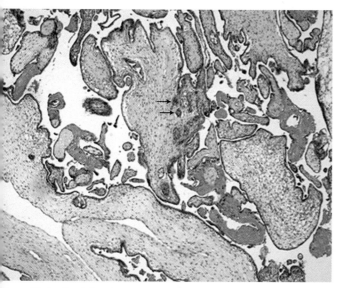

**Figure 49-4    Partial hydatidiform mole.** Note two populations of villi: small fibrotic and large hydropic villi. The large villi are characterized by scalloped borders and round trophoblastic inclusions (*arrows*). (Courtesy Dr. Ilana Ariel, Hadassah Medical Center, Jerusalem.)

| Table 49-3 | | |
| :-- | :-- | :-- |
| **Presenting Symptoms and Signs in Patients with Complete and Partial Molar Pregnancy** | | |
| **Sign** | **Complete Mole (%)** | **Partial Mole (%)** |
| Vaginal bleeding | 97 | 73 |
| Enlarged uterine size | 51 | 4 |
| Hyperthyroidism | 7 | 0 |
| Pre-eclampsia | 27 | 3 |
| Hyperemesis gravidarum | 26 | 0 |
| Theca-lutein cysts | 50 | 0 |
| Acute respiratory distress | 2 | 0 |

Reproduced from Berkowitz RS, Goldstein DP: Gestational trophoblastic neoplasia. In Berek JS, Hacker NF (eds): Practical Gynecologic Oncology. Philadelphia: Lippincott Williams & Wilkins, 2000; p 617

excessive uterine size or toxemia are the presenting signs in only 6% of patients.

## Clinical Diagnosis

The diagnosis of hydatidiform mole should be suspected in any woman with first- or second-trimester bleeding with any of the clinical features described. Ultrasonography is a simple, sensitive, and reliable approach for the diagnosis of molar pregnancy. The characteristic "snowstorm" pattern, caused by the diffuse hydatidiform swelling of complete moles, is usually easy to identify in a uterus greater than 14 weeks in size. Most complete hydatidiform moles are now diagnosed in the first trimester; the typical sonographic appearance is a complex, echogenic, intrauterine mass containing many small cystic spaces with prominent flow (Fig. 49-5).

The mean serum hCG value for molar pregnancy is about 200,000 mIU/mL compared to a peak value of 50,000 to 100,000 mIU/mL for normal pregnancy. A single hCG determination, however, is not diagnostic because both high hCG titer with normal singleton pregnancy and a normal hCG level in molar pregnancy can be seen. In clinical situations in which sonographic findings are not convincing, serial hCG determinations should be performed. Before ultrasound was available, amniocentesis combined with amniography was the diagnostic test most widely used to confirm the diagnosis of hydatidiform mole. This approach is seldom needed today.

The usual clinical diagnosis of partial mole is similar to missed or incomplete abortion. The ultrasonographic findings may show focal cystic spaces in the placental tissues, but more commonly findings are suggestive of abortion. The pre-evacuation hCG levels in partial mole patients are usually lower than in those with complete mole. Values rarely exceed 100,000 mIU/mL and tend to return to normal promptly.

A partial mole is a pathologic diagnosis, and clinical diagnosis should not be performed without pathologic conformation.

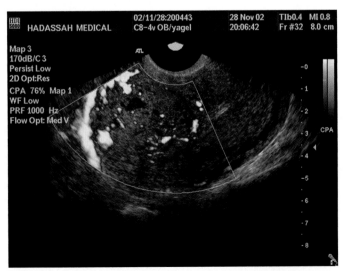

**Figure 49-5** Typical sonographic appearance of complete mole, showing complex, echogenic, intrauterine mass containing many small cystic spaces with prominent flow. (Courtesy Dr. Simcha Yagel, Hadassah Medical Center, Jerusalem.)

## Natural History

The risk of postmolar trophoblastic disease is reported to range from 5.7% to 36% in complete hydatidiform mole. Both local invasion and distant spread may occur. Risk factors for malignant sequelae include a uterus large for dates, ovarian cysts larger than 6 cm, serum hCG level greater than 100,000 mIU/mL, previous history of molar pregnancy, and age above 40. Goldstein and colleagues[7] noted that patients with symptoms of marked trophoblastic growth (hCG >100,000 mIU/mL, excessive uterine size for dates, and prominent theca-lutein cysts) are at high risk for persistent GTD.

The natural history of twin conceptions consisting of complete hydatidiform mole and a coexisting fetus was studied by the New England Trophoblastic Disease Center (NETDC).[8] Eight cases of twin pregnancy with complete hydatidiform mole and coexisting fetus were compared to 71 patients with singleton complete hydatidiform mole. Five of the eight patients in this series developed persistent gestational trophoblastic neoplasia requiring chemotherapy. Three of these five patients developed metastases and required multiagent chemotherapy to achieve remission. The authors' conclusions were that patients with complete hydatidiform mole and coexisting fetus are at high risk for developing persistent gestational trophoblastic neoplasia.

Partial hydatidiform mole carries a better prognosis than complete mole; invasive disease or metastasis rarely develops. The risk for persistent postmolar trophoblastic disease after partial molar pregnancy is approximately 2% to 4%. Since making a distinction between partial hydatidiform mole and complete hydatidiform mole using histologic criteria alone may be difficult, the reliability of this finding is in question. Cheung and colleagues[9] used fluorescent microsatellite genotyping following laser-capture microdissection and chromosome in situ hybridization to perform genetic analysis of six patients with histologically diagnosed partial hydatidiform mole who subsequently developed metastatic gestational trophoblastic neoplasia. It was found that four of the six patients had a diploid karyotype and no maternal alleles; thus, their neoplasms actually were complete hydatidiform mole. Although this study supports the belief that most aggressive trophoblastic diseases are derived from complete hydatidiform mole, a small number of partial hydatidiform moles do progress to metastatic disease; however, no distinctive clinical or pathologic risk factors have been identified.

## Treatment

As soon as diagnosis is made, evaluation of the associated medical problem should be performed and preparations for termination of the pregnancy should be carried out.

### Suction Curettage

The evacuation method of choice for patients who desire to preserve their fertility is suction curettage, regardless of uterine size. If there is heavy bleeding, plans for immediate evacuation should be made and an oxytocin drip should be started. When bleeding is absent or mild, intravenous oxytocin can be held until surgical intervention has been started.

The suction curettage technique includes dilatation of the cervix to permit insertion of a 10- to 12-mm suction curette just past the internal os. The suction is initiated and uterine content are evacuated by gently rotating the curette without inserting it further. The surgeon may also perform a fundal massage to stimulate uterine contractions. This technique reduces the risk of uterine perforation, especially if there is a focus of invasive mole and in cases of a large uterus. After completion of the suction evacuation, sharp curettage should be performed to remove any residual molar tissue. This procedure may be done under sonographic imaging using an abdominal probe to reduce the risk of uterine perforation and remaining trophoblastic tissue in the uterine cavity.

### Hysterectomy

Termination of molar pregnancy by primary hysterectomy (with the mole in situ) may be performed in patients who are good surgical candidates and who desire sterilization. Although hysterectomy eliminates the risk of local invasion and the risk of distant metastases is remote, these patients should also be followed with repeated hCG titers.

### Treatment of Non-neoplastic Medical Complications

Hyperthyroidism is present in 2% to 7% of patients with complete mole. Elevated levels of total $T_4$ or free $T_4$ compared to normal pregnancy levels can be found in as many as 25% to 50% of patients. If hyperthyroidism is suspected, it is important to administer a beta-adrenergic antagonist before the induction of anesthesia for molar evacuation because of the risk of precipitated thyroid storm.

Acute pulmonary insufficiency is a dramatic, life-threatening complication that develops in approximately 2% of patients. This condition may be related to high output cardiac failure or pulmonary edema. The latter may be caused by excessive fluid administration or, less likely, to trophoblastic tissue embolization to the pulmonary vasculature. The signs and symptoms of respiratory distress usually occurs within 4 hours postevacuation and resolve within 72 hours with cardiopulmonary support. Most cases are reported in patients with a uterus 16 weeks' gestational size or larger.

Because both invasive and noninvasive molar trophoblasts demonstrate the presence of $Rh_0D$ antigen, Rh-negative patients should receive RhoGam if no anti-$Rh_0D$ antibodies are detected.

### Prophylactic Chemotherapy

Prophylactic chemotherapy, the administration of single-agent chemotherapy immediately before or after evacuation, is controversial. Several studies suggest that this approach reduces the risk of postmolar trophoblastic disease from 15% to 20% to 0% to 2%. The agents that are mostly used are actinomycin D (dactinomycin) and methotrexate. Goldstein and Berkowitz[10] performed a large case-control study comparing 247 patients with complete molar pregnancy who received a single course of actinomycin at the time of evacuation and 858 control patients with complete molar pregnancy who did not receive prophylactic chemotherapy. Focal uterine invasion subsequently developed in 4% and 14.6% of the patients, respectively, and distant metastases in 0% and 4%, respectively. No serious toxicity was observed. Kim and colleagues[11] prospectively randomized 71 patients with complete hydatidiform mole into two groups; one group was treated with a single course of methotrexate and

citrovorum factor rescue as chemoprophylaxis and the other group was not treated. After molar evacuation, persistent trophoblastic disease developed in 10% and 31% of the patients in the treated and untreated groups, respectively. All 14 patients with persistent trophoblastic disease achieved complete remission with therapeutic chemotherapy. More courses of chemotherapy were required until complete remission in the treated group than in the untreated group. These findings suggest that even though chemoprophylaxis reduces the incidence of persistent trophoblastic disease in high risk patients, it increases tumor resistance and morbidity. In view of these experiences it seems reasonable to limit prophylactic chemotherapy treatment to patients who have high risk complete molar pregnancies and who may be noncompliant for hCG follow-up surveillance.

### Follow-up

After evacuation of the molar tissue or hysterectomy with the mole in situ, patients require weekly determinations of β-hCG levels until these are within normal limits for 3 consecutive weeks. The titers are then observed at monthly intervals for 6 to 12 months. The normal regression curve for β-hCG after molar evacuation is shown in Figure 49-6.

Within the first 8 weeks 65% to 70% of patients should enter into spontaneous regression. From 10% to 15% will continue to show decline in titers, whereas 15% to 20% will show a plateau or rise. The latter group is considered to have postmolar GTD or malignant gestational trophoblastic disease.

Although serial hCG value determinations are the most important part of postmolar pregnancy surveillance, it is important to perform a gynecologic examination postevacuation to evaluate uterine size, adnexal masses, and evidence of metastases to the genital tract (vulva, vagina, cervix, urethra).

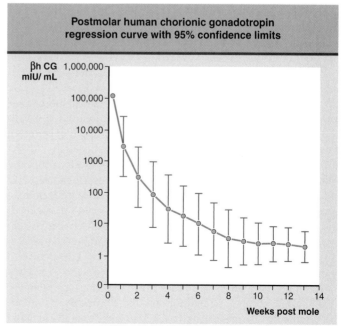

**Figure 49-6    Postmolar hCG regression curve, with 95% confidence limit.** (From Morrow CP, et al: Clinical and laboratory correlates of molar pregnancy and trophoblastic disease. Am J Obstet Gynecol 1977;128:424.)

## Human Chorionic Gonadotropin Assay

Human chorionic gonadotropin, an obligate secretory product of the syncytiotrophoblast, is a glycoprotein composed of two dissimilar subunits, $\alpha$ and $\beta$, held together by charge interaction. The smaller $\alpha$ subunit is nearly identical to the subunits of luteinizing hormone (LH), follicle-stimulating hormone, and thyrotropin. The $\beta$ subunit gives these hormones their biologic and immunologic specificities. hCG is an unusual glycoprotein in that as little as 65% of its molecular weight is due to amino acids or protein. The balance is due to large sugar side chains. hCG is not a single molecule but a mixture of regular hCG, large carbohydrate variants of hCG, nicked hCG, hCG missing the $\beta$ subunit C-terminal peptide, free subunits, and fragments of each of these forms of hCG. This is particularly important in gestational trophoblastic disease, in which one of these hCG variants or its free subunits is commonly the principal molecule in the blood samples. Most tests use the multi-antibody immunometric assay method. These tests use multiple antibodies against different sites on hCG and related molecules. A small number of laboratories continue to use the competitive radioimmunoassay (RIA) method. All tests, whether RIA or modern immunometric assays, use at least one antibody against the $\beta$ subunit to differentiate hCG and LH, which share indistinguishable $\alpha$ chains. Considering the heterogenicity of hCG, especially with regard to trophoblastic disease, it is essential to use an hCG test that measures all forms of hCG and its free subunits.

## Phantom hCG

Rarely patients present with persistently elevated hCG levels but are subsequently found to have a false-positive hCG assay result, sometimes after receiving unnecessary chemotherapy or surgery for presumed malignant GTD. Most of these patients have a mild elevation of their hCG serum levels, but occasionally values higher than 200 to 300 mIU/mL are seen. The false-positive hCG values result from interference with the hCG immunometric sandwich assay caused by nonspecific heterophil antibodies in the patient's sera. Most of these patients have undefined previous pregnancy events and do not have radiographic evidence of metastatic disease. Serial hCG levels usually do not vary and are unresponsive to surgery or chemotherapy. Phantom hCG may also present after evacuation of a hydatidiform mole or clearly defined pregnancy. The diagnosis of phantom hCG relies on the absence of hCG immunoreactivity in the urine and the lack of parallel dilution of hCG levels with serial dilution of the patient's serum.[12] Persistent low levels of hCG following a pregnancy or hydatidiform mole are related to a noninvasive condition, quiescent GTD, or remain unexplained. Two recommended strategies to differentiate between malignant GTD and the benign conditions are: (1) Follow the pattern of hCG rise; if hCG levels rise consistently or sharply, this will indicate a higher risk for persistent or invasive disease. A shallow rise and plateau pattern are more likely to represent quiescent trophoblastic disease, a condition that most probably should not be treated by chemotherapy.[13] (2) Use the hyperglycosylated hCG test. Hyperglcosylated hCG is produced only by invasive cytotrophoblast cells and therefore can be an invaluable second marker to differentiate malignant GTD from benign conditions.

## Contraception

Because hCG produced by the neoplastic trophoblast is indistinguishable from the hCG produced during normal pregnancy, it is important to avoid pregnancy in the entire interval of hCG follow-up. Pregnancy may also limit treatment options should malignant sequelae develop. In the absence of contraindications, oral contraceptives are the method of choice. Because ovulation may occur soon after evacuation (4 weeks or less), the patient should be encouraged to start oral contraception as soon as possible. Other methods of contraception are possible but intrauterine devices should be avoided before normal hCG levels are obtained because of the risk for perforation. Data from both the NETDC[14] and the Gynecologic Oncology Group (GOG)[15] revealed no association between the use of oral contraceptives and risk of requiring chemotherapy. In addition, the contraceptive method did not influence the mean hCG regression time.

## Reproductive Sequelae

Patients who have been diagnosed with molar pregnancy can anticipate normal reproductive function in subsequent pregnancies. Sebire and colleagues[16] recently published a retrospective review of a large supraregional database of registrations for gestational trophoblastic disease. Of 2578 complete moles, further pregnancy was observed in 1417 patients and the subsequent pregnancy was affected by hydatidiform mole in 27 (1.9%) cases, including 22 (81%) complete moles and 5 (19%) partial moles. Of 2627 partial moles, further pregnancy was observed in 1512 patients and the subsequent pregnancy was also molar in 25 (1.7%) cases, including 17 (68%) partial moles and 8 (32%) complete moles. Overall recurrence risk for molar pregnancy was 1.8% (1 in 55), or a 20-fold increase over the background risk. Of 27 cases with repeat complete moles, 3 had further complete moles, suggesting the recurrence risk following two previous complete moles is approximately 10%. No other significant differences in pregnancy outcome were observed between patients with previous complete or partial hydatidiform mole and an unselected obstetric population. The authors concluded that women having a pregnancy affected by a histologically confirmed complete or partial hydatidiform mole may be counseled that the risk of repeat mole in a subsequent pregnancy is about 1 in 60; in addition, if this were to occur, the majority of cases would be of the same type of mole as the preceding pregnancy. However, more than 98% of women who become pregnant following a molar conception will not have a further hydatidiform mole, and these pregnancies are at no increased risk of other obstetric complications. Current recommendations for patients with a history of molar pregnancy who plan another pregnancy include the following: (1) an early ultrasound to confirm normal gestational development and dates, (2) a chest x-ray to screen for occult metastasis masked by the hCG rise of pregnancy, (3) histologic examination of the placenta or products of conception at the time of delivery or evacuation for evidence of occult GTD, and (4) hCG levels 6 weeks after evacuation or delivery to confirm normalization.

## Diagnostic Criteria for Postmolar Gestational Trophoblastic Disease

The risk of post molar GTD ranges from 3% to 25%, including both partial and complete hydatidiform moles, and as noted

**Table 49-4**
**FIGO Criteria for the Diagnosis of Postmolar Gestational Trophoblastic Disease**

- Four values or more of hCG documenting a plateau (± 10% of hCG values) over at least 3 weeks: days 1, 7, 14, 21
- A rise of hCG of 10% or greater for three values or longer over at least 2 weeks: days 1, 7, 14
- The presence of histologic choriocarcinoma
- Persistence of hCG 6 months after mole evacuation

previously the risk for postmolar GTD is higher among patients with complete compared to partial hydatidiform moles (20% vs. 5%, respectively). The risk of metastatic disease at the time of postmolar GTD diagnosis is 6% to 25%. Because criteria for the diagnosis of postmolar GTD varied between North America and Europe, an attempt was recently made by the Society of Gynecologic Oncologists, the International Society for the Study of Trophoblastic Diseases, the International Gynecologic Cancer Society, and the International Federation for Gynecology and Obstetrics (FIGO) to standardize these criteria.[17] The current FIGO criteria for the diagnosis of postmolar GTD are summarized in Table 49-4.

Although the revised FIGO criteria did not address the issue of metastatic disease, in most centers the diagnosis of metastasis is sufficient for the diagnosis of postmolar GTD and a cause for initiating chemotherapy.

### Repeated Uterine Curettage

Patients with postmolar GTD may present with vaginal bleeding, signifying persistent or recurrent trophoblastic disease in the uterine cavity. The bleeding is very often attended by an enlarged uterus and abnormal hCG regression. The issue of secondary curettage is controversial; it is not recommended on a routine basis. Although some investigators report that secondary curettage obviates the need for chemotherapy in 10% to 20% of cases,[18] this approach is not without risks; uterine perforation (8% of repeated curettage), intra-abdominal hemorrhage, and the occasional need for transfusion and hysterectomy have been reported. In view of this information, secondary D&Cs are recommended only in patients with life-threatening hemorrhage, and most other patients with bleeding can be managed with chemotherapy. An algorithm for molar pregnancy management after evacuation or hysterectomy is illustrated in Figure 49-7.

## OTHER FORMS OF GESTATIONAL TROPHOBLASTIC DISEASE

### Invasive Mole (Chorioadenoma Destruens)

Complete and partial moles can invade the myometrium or blood vessels and produce a condition designated *invasive mole.* Based on hysterectomy specimens it is estimated that between 5% and 10% of all molar pregnancies contain myometrial invasion, but because this process is clinically occult, and usually does not necessitate hysterectomy it is difficult to accurately assess the frequency of this clinical entity. Invasive mole is the most common form of persistent GTD following a molar pregnancy and is probably 6 to 10 times more common than choriocarcinoma.

### Pathology

Grossly, invasive mole appears as hemorrhagic, erosive masses, and perforation is possible when the full thickness of the uterine wall is penetrated. Histologically, invasive mole is characterized by hydrophilic villi and proliferating trophoblastic epithelium invading the uterine muscle and blood vessels, with associated hemorrhage and necrosis. In extrauterine sites, the distinction from choriocarcinoma is based on the presence of villi, which can be sparse in number, and the presence of masses within blood vessels without significant invasion into the surrounding tissue.

### Clinical Features

Clinically the hallmark of the disease is hemorrhage; both severe vaginal and intraperitoneal bleeding may occur. The most common sites for metastases are the vagina and lung, although rare instances of secondary lesions in the brain and spinal cord have been documented. Invasive mole is a self-limited disease; if no bleeding or serious complications occur, the tumor may regress spontaneously, including in patients with metastatic disease.

### Treatment

In the absence of metastatic disease, patients require post-surgical surveillance and treatment similar to patients with complete or partial moles. Additional therapy in the form of chemotherapy is indicated when metastases are present or abnormal regression of serum hCG levels is observed.

### Choriocarcinoma

Gestational choriocarcinoma is a highly malignant tumor, developing in relation to a gestational event, and must be distinguished from a nongestational choriocarcinoma, which typically arises in extrauterine sites. Choriocarcinoma is preceded by molar pregnancy in 50% of cases, by spontaneous abortion in 25%, by normal pregnancy in 22.5%, and by ectopic pregnancy in 2.5% of patients.

Metastases are common with a predisposition to hematogeneous spread, and the organs that are most frequently involved (in decreasing order of frequency) are the lung, lower genital tract (cervix, vagina, vulva), brain, liver, kidney, and gastrointestinal tract.

### Pathology

Grossly choriocarcinoma are extremely hemorrhagic neoplasms, often resembling a friable segment of placenta. Microscopically, the tumor is characterized by hemorrhage and necrosis, clusters and sheets of poorly differentiated cytotrophoblastic cells, surrounded and encased by multinucleated syncytiotrophoblast cells, and by the absence of villi.

### Clinical Features

The clinical presentation of patients with choriocarcinoma is related to disease spread. The strong propensity of trophoblastic cells to disrupt normal vascular integrity, leading to focal hemorrhage, usually leads to the symptoms of the disease. Local disease may resemble threatened abortion or ectopic pregnancy, with amenorrhea followed by vaginal bleeding. Some cases are manifested by intraperitoneal bleeding secondary to uterine perforation, liver or spleen rupture, bleeding from ovarian tissue,

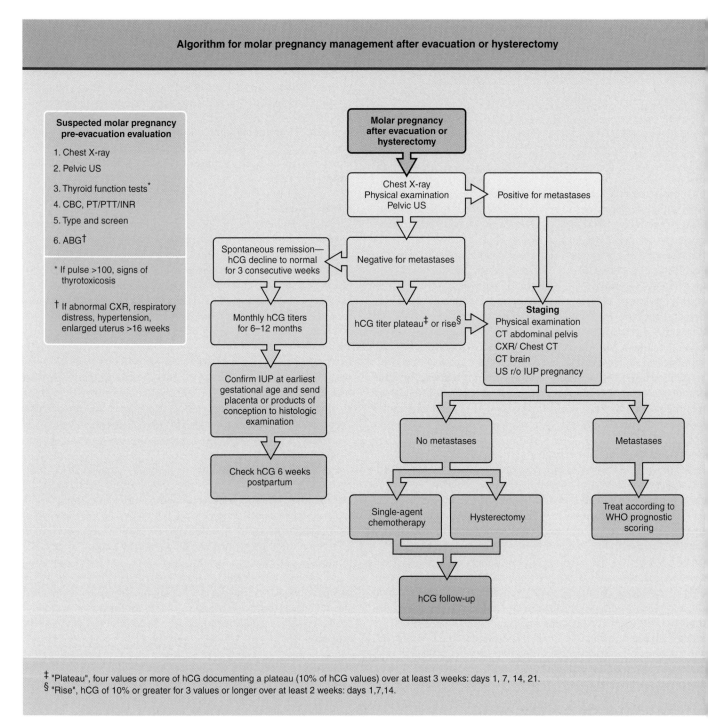

**Figure 49-7  Algorithm for molar pregnancy management after evacuation or hysterectomy.** CXR, Chest X-ray; UP; intrauterine pregnancy; US, ultrasound.

or ruptured theca-lutein cyst. Other manifestations may be cough, hemoptysis, pleuritic pain, and dyspnea in cases of pulmonary involvement; anemia, melena, or massive gastrointestinal bleeding in patients with gastrointestinal involvement; and focal neurologic signs caused by spinal or intracranial metastases.

*Diagnosis*

The diagnosis of metastatic choriocarcinoma may be considered in any woman of reproductive age who presents with metastatic

disease from an unknown primary tumor. Diagnosis is often based on history, imaging, and serum hCG determinations. Histologic confirmation is not mandatory for diagnosis and treatment. The two main risks associated with an attempt to obtain histologic confirmation are bleeding from the biopsy site and failure to achieve satisfactory tissue for diagnosis because of tissue necrosis and hemorrhage obscuring the disease, possibly contributing to a delay in treatment. A diagnosis based predominantly on hCG alone should raise the question of phantom hCG.

Choriocarcinoma in situ is a rare finding and is diagnosed when a focus of choriocarcinoma is discovered on a routine microscopic examination of placenta. In these cases both the mother and the fetus need hCG monitoring.

## Placental Site Trophoblastic Tumor

Placental site trophoblastic tumor (PSTT) is a malignant tumor derived from intermediate trophoblast. Intermediate trophoblast is mostly extravillous and is a biologically unique cell type that performs an important function in placentation. Initially the disease was thought to be a nonneoplastic syncytial endometritis, but subsequent reports identified the malignant potential of this tumor. Over the past two decades, approximately 100 cases of PSTT have been reported, in numerous case reports and small case series.[19]

### Pathology

Grossly, PSTT are generally well-circumscribed, solid masses within the myometrium, although polypoid components projecting into the uterine cavity are frequently observed. In contrast to choriocarcinoma, hemorrhage and necrosis are focal or absent. Microscopically the cells of PSTT are mononuclear with abundant cytoplasm and strongly resemble intermediate trophoblast of the implantation site. A characteristic feature of the tumor is a nondestructive pattern of infiltration into the myometrium. Immunohistochemical staining demonstrates strong expression of human placental lactogen (hPL) and little or no expression of hCG. Distinction of PSTT from normal implantation site is based on the presence of a grossly or radiographically detectable tumor and the presence of mitotic activity, both of which are more common in PSTT. PSTT should also be distinguished from placental site nodule, usually an incidental finding in a hysterectomy specimen performed for uterine fibroids.

### Clinical Features

Women of reproductive age are at risk, although diagnosis is occasionally made in the sixth decade of life. Patients usually present with vaginal bleeding after amenorrhea of variable duration. Most patients present following normal pregnancy, but antecedent hydatidiform molar pregnancy or spontaneous abortion have been reported. hCG values are usually less than 1000 mIU/mL; serum hPL has not proven to be a reliable serum marker, despite the reliability of hPL tissue staining.[20] Nephrotic syndrome, with its distinctive renal lesion, and virilization have also been reported to be associated with the disease. Most patients are diagnosed in Stage I when disease is confined to the uterus and metastases usually occur late. More common sites of metastases are the lung, vagina, and lymph nodes.

### Diagnosis

Diagnosis is usually based on uterine curettage or hysterectomy specimen showing diffuse immunohistochemical positive staining for hPL and focally positive for hCG.

### Treatment

Because this disease tends to metastasize late and is fairly resistant to chemotherapy, surgical excision (hysterectomy) is the primary treatment for patients with PSTT. Management of patients who wish to preserve fertility is more difficult and includes systemic chemotherapy, regional infusion chemotherapy, hysteroscopic tumor resection, and uterine curettage. In patients with metastatic disease, hysterectomy may offer little or nothing in terms of improved survival.

Only 5% of early-stage PSTT patients will have recurrence of disease, whereas 70% to 90% of Stage IV disease will be diagnosed with recurrence. Because recurrence has been reported after an interval of 5 years, longer follow-up is indicated in these patients. However, the diagnosis of PSTT more than 2 years after the suspected gestational source carries a poor prognosis.

## Malignant Gestational Trophoblastic Disease

### Diagnosis

It is crucial to diagnose malignant GTD with no delay because such a delay may increase the patient's risk and adversely affect response to treatment. Patients with GTD should undergo a metastatic workup, and clinically prognostic factors should be identified.

One half to two thirds of cases of malignant GTD occur following evacuation of complete or partial hydatidiform moles.[21] Because most patients are treated based on hCG levels with no tissue diagnosis, the exact histologic distribution of the lesions is not precisely known. Approximately 50% to 70% of patients with malignant GTD have persistent or invasive mole; 30% to 50% have postmolar gestational choriocarcinoma.[21] Women diagnosed with GTD after evacuation of molar pregnancy are usually identified earlier in the course of the disease because they are followed with serial hCG blood tests. In contrast, patients with malignant GTD diagnosed after nonmolar pregnancies are usually diagnosed secondary to a variety of gynecologic or nongynecologic symptoms. Therefore, the possibility of malignant GTD should be suspected in any women of reproductive age who presents with metastatic disease of unknown primary site or unexplained cerebral hemorrhage.[22]

Diagnosis of malignant GTD is based on the following[17]:

- Abnormal pattern of hCG regression after evacuation of hydatidiform mole
- Histologic result showing choriocarcinoma on curettage or hysterectomy specimens
- Presence of metastasis with unknown primary site in the presence of positive serum hCG after excluding pregnancy.

Identification of metastases on examination or imaging is an indication for chemotherapy treatment in most centers, although some centers in the United Kingdom would follow pulmonary metastases conservatively as long as serum hCG levels regress properly.

### Clinical Features

Pretherapy evaluation (Table 49-5) of patients with malignant GTD includes history assessment for clinical risk factors, thorough physical examination, laboratory evaluation, and imaging survey for possible sites of metastases. Clinical risk factors include the duration of disease as determined by the interval from the antecedent pregnancy, the type of antecedent pregnancy, and previous treatment.

Physical examination may identify vaginal lesions. The lesions are most often dark blue, soft nodules. Ulceration and active

# Gynecologic Oncology

| Table 49-5 |
| --- |
| **Staging Workup for Malignant Gestational Trophoblastic Disease** |
| · History, physical and neurologic examination<br>· Pelvic ultrasound to exclude pregnancy<br>· Chest CT/Chest x-ray<br>· CT/MRI of brain, abdomen, and pelvis<br>· Liver, renal, and thyroid function tests<br>· Complete blood count<br>· Serum hCG levels |

| Table 49-6 | |
| --- | --- |
| **Anatomic FIGO Staging of Malignant Gestational Trophoblastic Disease, 1992** | |
| Stage I | Disease confined to uterus |
| Stage II | Metastases to pelvis and vagina |
| Stage III | Metastases to the lung |
| Stage IV | Distant metastases |
| A, No risk factors; B, One risk factor; C, Two risk factors | |
| Risk factors | hCG levels >100,000 mIU/mL |
| For any stage | Antecedent pregnancy >6 months |

bleeding may necessitate vaginal packing or selective embolization; because of the vascular nature of the lesions, it is suggested not to biopsy these lesions, especially not in the outpatient clinic.

Labaratory evaluation should include serum hCG level, blood counts, and renal and liver function tests to determine baseline functions before chemotherapy initiation.

Imaging should include computed tomography (CT) scan of the brain, chest, abdomen, and pelvis. Although some studies recommend performing chest x-ray and more advanced evaluation in the case of an abnormal x-ray finding, other studies showed a 29% to 41% false-negative rate with chest x-ray. In patients in whom the use of contrast material is contraindicated, magnetic resonance imaging (MRI) may be used. Ultrasound of the pelvis should be used to exclude pregnancy and to identify intrauterine tumors and foci of myometrial invasion (Fig. 49-8).

Although operative procedures may be used in the course of treatment of patients with malignant GTD, surgery is rarely required for diagnosis or staging. Routine endometrial curettage is therefore not indicated before chemotherapy.

## Staging and Classification

The staging and classification of malignant GTD have changed significantly over the past 40 years. The three main systems used are the anatomic staging system, the clinical classification system, and the prognostic scoring system; the latter system includes variables that predict the likelihood of drug resistance. The more recent staging systems combine these systems. An anatomic staging system for malignant GTD was adopted by FIGO in the early 1980s. This staging system was revised in 1992 (Table 49-6) to include additional risk factors: hCG levels greater than 100,000 mIU/mL and time from antecedent pregnancy greater than 6 months.

The clinical classification system (Table 49-7) is frequently used in United States.[23] In this classification patients with nonmetastatic disease are not assigned into prognostic groups because of the good outcome that can be achieved with single-agent chemotherapy in nonmetastatic disease. The risk factors used in this system were originally identified by retrospective analysis to predict resistance to single-agent chemotherapy among women with metastatic GTD at the National Institutes of Health.

Another prognostic scoring system was developed by the World Health Organization (WHO) in the early 1980s. This system was based on the experience from Charing Cross Hospital in London published by Bagshawe[24] and included nine

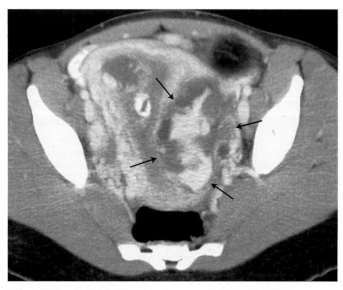

**Figure 49-8    Computed tomography scan of pelvis, showing heterogeneous mass in enlarged uterus with vascular enhancement.** The mass extends into the uterine wall (invasive GTD). The uterus, the mass, and the surrounding tissues are commonly very vascular. (Courtesy Dr. Tamar Sella, Hadassah Medical Center, Jerusalem.)

| Table 49-7 | |
| --- | --- |
| **Clinical Classification System for Patients with Malignant Gestational Trophoblastic Disease** | |
| **Category** | **Criteria** |
| Nonmetastatic GTD | Not assigned to prognostic category |
| Metastatic GTD | Any extrauterine metastases |
| Good prognosis metastatic GTD | No risk factors<br>    Short duration (<4 months)<br>    Pretherapy hCG <40,000 mIU/mL<br>    No brain or liver metastases<br>    No antecedent term pregnancy<br>    No prior chemotherapy |
| Poor prognosis metastatic GTD | Any risk factors<br>    Long duration (>4 months)<br>    Pretherapy hCG >40,000 mIU/mL<br>    Brain or liver metastases<br>    Antecedent term pregnancy<br>    Prior chemotherapy |
| GTD, Gestational trophoblastic disease. | |

prognostic factors identified among patients treated with simple chemotherapy regimens. The WHO prognostic index applies a weighted score to each of these factors, and the sum of component scores is then used to determine the individual patient's risk category.

In 2000, FIGO revised their staging[25] with the addition of a risk factor score that modified from the original WHO prognostic index score (Table 49-8). Patients are categorized as either low or high risk. Although some patients assigned to the low risk category will need additional and occasionally intensive therapy, the ultimate outcome is not compromised. Importantly, mortalities rarely occur in the low-risk group, thus validating this system of classification.

It is hoped that this updated scoring system will encourage objective comparison of data among various centers and will be the basis for standardization of treatment protocols for GTD patients in the future.

### Low-Risk Malignant Gestational Trophoblastic Disease

The following groups of patients are considered to have low-risk malignant GTD:

- Nonmetastatic GTD
- Metastatic malignant GTD with good prognosis (other than brain or liver metastases)
- FIGO stage I, II, or III
- FIGO 2000 scoring system = 6

**Role of Hysterectomy.** Patients categorized with malignant GTD and found to have a nonmetastatic form may be offered a hysterectomy if the patient no longer wishes to preserve fertility. It is acceptable to preserve the ovaries in these cases because ovarian metastases are extremely rare in the absence of other metastatic disease. Because the remote risk of hCG-producing germ cell tumor of the ovary presenting as GTD cannot be ruled out, it is important for the clinician to evaluate any suspicious mass on the ovary at the time of hysterectomy.

Adjuvant single-agent chemotherapy at the time of hysterectomy is recommended by the NETDC for three reasons: (1) to reduce the likelihood of disseminating viable tumor cells at the time of surgery, (2) to maintain a toxic level of chemotherapy during surgery in the event of hematogeneous spread of viable tumor cells, and (3) to treat any occult metastases that may already be present at the time of surgery. Because no survival benefit has been demonstrated with this approach, it is not widely used.

After hysterectomy, patients are followed over time for normalization of their hCG levels. If the hCG levels do not resolve, the patient should be assigned to low-risk chemotherapy treatment protocols.

Hysterectomy for low-risk metastatic disease has been advocated by some authors to reduce the amount of cytotoxic chemotherapy and the likelihood of recurrence; however, because these patients will always need some amount of chemotherapy this approach is not uniformly accepted. Hysterectomy is also performed in all patients with placental site trophoblastic tumor. Because these tumors are resistant to chemotherapy, hysterectomy for presumed nonmetastatic disease is the only curative method.

**Chemotherapy for Low-Risk Gestational Trophoblastic Disease.** Patients diagnosed with malignant GTD and categorized as low risk are almost always cured using modern chemotherapy regimens. Patients with nonmetastatic disease will have cure rates of virtually 100% with single-agent therapy. Patients with low-risk metastatic disease have a higher failure rate with initial single-agent chemotherapy, but their overall cure rate approaches 100%. Methotrexate, dactinomycin, and etoposide, used singly, have demonstrated clearcut superiority to all other cytotoxic drugs in the treatment of malignant GTD. The more common treatment protocols are summarized in Table 49-9.

Methotrexate is the most commonly used single agent. The decreased toxicity associated with alternate-day folinic acid treatments may be attributed to both the scheduling interval of methotrexate and to the rescue effect of the folinic acid.

Patients with nonmetastatic and low risk metastatic disease are treated with single-agent therapy at 10- to 14-day intervals, waiting for the major toxicities (usually granulocytopenia and stomatitis) to clear. Chemotherapy is continued until hCG serum levels are down to normal. Usually at least one additional treatment cycle is then given before discontinuing treatment; patients are followed with close observation of their hCG values. Table 49-10 summarizes the management and follow-up of patients with low risk malignant GTD.

From 10% to 30% of patients with low-risk malignant GTD will demonstrate resistance to single-agent therapy. If the disease is confined to the uterus, the resistant focus is usually located deep in the myometrium. These patients are more likely to have high hCG levels at initiation of treatment and a longer interval since the antecedent pregnancy compared to those who do not demonstrate drug resistance. When hCG levels fail to drop significantly during two consecutive treatment courses, or if

#### Table 49-8
#### FIGO 2000 Scoring System*,†

| FIGO Score | 0 | 1 | 2 | 4 |
|---|---|---|---|---|
| Age | <39 | >39 | | |
| Antecedent pregnancy | HM | Abortion | Term pregnancy | |
| Interval from index pregnancy (months) | <4 | 4–6 | 6–12 | >12 |
| Pretreatment hCG (mIU/mL) | <1000 | $10^3$–$10^4$ | >$10^4$–$10^5$ | >$10^6$ |
| Largest tumor size, including uterus (cm) | 3–5 | ≥5 | | |
| Sites of metastases | | Spleen, kidney | GI tract | Brain, liver |
| Number of metastases† | 0 | 1–4 | 4–8 | >8 |
| Previous failed chemotherapy | | | Single drug | ≥2 drugs |

Total score: 0–6, low risk; ≥7, high risk
HM, hydatiform mole, GI, gastrointestinal.
*Under the new FIGO system, reporting of patients will inlcude both anatomic stage (see Table 49–6) and FIGO risk score.
† Number of lung metastases should be assessed by chest x-ray and not CT; intra-abdominal metastases should be assessed by CT; brain MRI is superior to CT scanning.
‡ Histologically diagnosed PSTT patients should be reported separately.

# Gynecologic Oncology

**Table 49-9**
**Chemotherapy Options for Low-Risk Malignant Gestational Trophoblastic Disease**

| Agent(s) | Dosage and Route of Administration | Toxicities |
|---|---|---|
| Methotrexate (MTX) | • 20–25 mg (0.4 mg/kg) or 16 mg/m² IM/IV q day × 5 days (repeat in 7–14 days)<br>• 30–50 mg/m² IM (repeat weekly) | More common: myelosuppression, gastrointestinal effects (mucosities, nausea), alopecia, rashes<br>Less common: hepatotoxicity, nephrotoxicity, pleuritis, pulmonary fibrosis |
| MTX and folinic acid (FA) | • MTX 1 mg/kg IM/PO days 1, 3, 5, 7 alternating with FA 0.1 mg/kg days 2, 4, 6, 8 (repeat q 14 days)<br>• MTX 300–500 mg/m² IV followed by FA 15 mg q6h × 4 doses (repeat q 14 days) | As described for MTX, but usually milder and last for <5 days |
| Dactinomycin | • 9–13 µg/kg IV qod × 5 days (repeat q 14 days)<br>• 1.25 mg/m² IV bolus (repeat q 14 days) | Myelosuppression, gastrointestinal effects (nausea, vomiting, stomatitis), alopecia<br>Less systemic toxicity compared to MTX |
| MTX and dactinomycin | • MTX 20–25 mg (0.4 mg/kg) IM qod × 5 days in week 1 alternating with dactinomycin 9–13 µg/kg IV qod × 5 days in week 2 (repeat q 14 days) | Cumulative toxicity is reduced compared to MTX or dactinomycin alone |
| 5-fluorouracil | • 28–30 mg/kg/day (continuous 10-day infusion) | More common: gastrointestinal effects (nausea, vomiting, stomatitis, diahrrea, pseudomembranous colitis), hepatotoxicity<br>Less common: cerebellar ataxia |
| Etoposide | • 100–200 mg/m² PO for 5 days (repeat q 2 weeks) | More common: myelosuppression, gastrointestinal effects (nausea, vomiting), alopecia<br>Less common: acute myelogenous leukemia (0.6%; chromosomal damage: 11q23) |

Modified from Carney ME: Treatment of low risk gestational trophoblastic disease. Clin Obstet Gynecol 2003;46:579–592.

more than 8 weeks are required to induce titer remission, a change to dactinomycin or methotrexate, depending on which drug was initially used, is usually successful in eradicating the disease. If the tumor fails to respond to this change, use of oral etoposide or one of the combination chemotherapy regimens for high-risk malignant GTD is recommended.[26]

**Table 49-10**
**Management and Follow-up of Single-Agent Chemotherapy**

1. Chemotherapy regimen as described in Table 49–8.
   Check CBC, liver and renal functions before chemotherapy administration.
   Repeat chemotherapy according to protocol and toxicity.
   Start oral contraception (if not contraindicated).
2. Chemotherapy continued until hCG titer is normal, usually, 1–3 courses are additionally given.
3. Chemotherapy should be switched if:
   hCG titers rise
   hCG titers plateau
   New metastases
4. Chemotherapy is held if:
   WBC <3000/µL
   ANC <1500/µL
   Platelets <100,000/µL
   Abnormal liver or kidney functions
   Toxicity develops (e.g., oral or gastrointestinal ulceration, neutropenic fever)
5. Remission defined as three consecutive normal weekly hCG
6. Follow-up includes:
   hCG titers every 2 weeks for 3 months, then monthly for 3 months, then every 2 months for 6 months, then every 6 months
   Frequent pelvic examination
7. Contraception should be continued for at least 6 months.

### High-Risk Malignant Gestational Trophoblastic Disease

The following groups of patients are considered to have high risk malignant GTD:

- Metastatic malignant GTD with poor prognosis (i.e., long duration [>4 months], pretherapy hCG > 40000 mIU/mL brain or liver metastases, antecedent term pregnancy, o prior chemotherapy)
- FIGO stage IV
- FIGO 2000 scoring system = 7

Patients with high-risk malignant GTD preferably should b treated by physicians who are experienced in the managemen of this disease. Although chemotherapy with multidrug regimen is the cornerstone of treatment, both surgery and irradiation have been used to achieve a curative outcome.

**Chemotherapy for High-Risk Gestational Trophoblasti Disease.** Women with high-risk gestational trophoblastic diseas should be treated initially with multidrug combination chemo therapy. The superiority of combination chemotherapy protocol over single-drug regimens was demonstrated in the early 1970s.[2]

The first multidrug regimen for high-risk GTD to b extensively evaluated was MAC: methotrexate (15 mg IV/IM) actinomycin D (dactinomycin; 8 to 10 µg/kg IV) and chlorambuci (8 to 10 mg PO), all given daily for 5 days with an interval o 10 to 14 days between courses. Cyclophosphamide (3 mg/kg/da IV) is often substituted for chlorambucil in the MAC regime because the latter cannot be given parenterally. The reporte remission rates for primary treatment with these triple regimen range from 50% to 73%. The variation in the reported result most probably reflects patient tumor factors rather tha differences in the treatment protocols. Because of the relatively high failure rates, Bagshawe and coworkers from the Charing Cross Hospital proposed the seven-drug CHAMOCA regimen, consisting of cyclophosphamide, hydroxyurea, actinomycin D (dactinomycin), methotrexate, Oncovin (vincristine), citrovorum factor, and Adriamycin (doxorubicin).[28] When the CHAMOCA and MAC regimens were compared by the GOG in a prospective, randomized trial, the cure rates were 70% and 96%, respectively. The MAC regimen was also found to be significantly less toxic; the authors concluded that this regimen has a more favorable therapeutic index.[29] Newlands and colleagues[30] were the first to introduce the EMA-CO protocol and reported a complete response rate of 80% and overall survival of 82% to 89% in high-risk GTD patients. The new protocol consisted of etoposide, metotrexate, actinomycin D (dactinomycin), cyclophosphamide, and Oncovin (vincristine). Since its introduction it has generally replaced MAC as the treatment of choice for high-risk disease because of greater efficacy and lower risk of serious toxicity (Table 49-11).

Whatever combination regimen is used to treat high-risk malignant GTD patients, chemotherapy should be continued three courses past the first normal hCG titer to minimize the risk of relapse. The risk of recurrence after 12 months of normal hCG levels is less than 1% but pregnancy should be postponed for 2 years after remission.

**Salvage Chemotherapy.** Salvage therapy for recurrent disease has improved significantly since the late 1970s. The reported salvage rate after 1978 is reported to be 83%.

Regimens containing cisplatin and etoposide are commonly employed for the treatment of persistent or relapsed trophoblastic tumor. Newlands and colleagues[31] reported their experience with the EMA-EP regimen, consisting of etoposide, methotrexate, actinomycin D (dactinomycin), and cisplatin. The overall survival rate for their series was 88%; myelosuppression was significant, causing treatment delay and dosage adjustment in 88% and 38% of the patients, respectively. Other regimens used include the PVB (Platinol [cisplatin], vinblastine, and bleomycin) regimen, BEP (bleomycin, etoposide, and Platinol

[cisplatin]) regimen, and the combination of high dose chemotherapy with autologous bone marrow transplantation.

**Management of Metastatic Sites.** Brain metastases occur in about 10% of women with metastatic GTD. The most common presenting clinical symptoms are headaches, paresis, vomiting, and seizures. Unfortunately many women with brain metastases from choriocarcinoma die without receiving therapy because of late diagnosis. The presence of brain or spinal metastases can be evaluated by either CT or MRI; measurements of hCG levels in the cerebrospinal fluid are rarely needed. The most common management strategy for CNS lesions in the United States is the addition of whole brain irradiation (total dose, 3000 cGy) to the EMA-CO chemotherapy protocol. This approach doubles the survival rate (50% vs. 24% without irradiation). Protocols for the management of CNS lesions in the United Kingdom include administration of intrathecal metothrexate (12.5 mg every 2 weeks). Craniotomy is performed in a select group of patients with drug-resistant lesions, when intracranial hemorrhage occurs, or when edema decompression is needed.

Liver metastases are reported to occur in 5% to 20% of poor prognosis patients; poor prognosis is related to hemorrhagic sequelae. The survival rate for these patients is 26% to 33%. Several authors advocate whole liver irradiation (2000 cGY over 10 days) to reduce the risk of bleeding. Liver metastases can also be managed with hepatic artery embolization and partial hepatectomy.

Lung metastases are relatively common ($\approx$50%) in malignant high-risk GTD patients. Most of these patients can be cured by chemotherapy. Thoracotomy with wedge resection or partial lobectomy may be considered in patients with focal resistant disease. Patients who present with extensive pulmonary disease are at risk for an early respiratory death after the initiation of chemotherapy. Progressive hypoxia may be related to interstitial bleeding or edema. In patients who develop early respiratory failure from diffuse metastatic GTD, mechanical ventilation with low tidal volumes and a pressure-targeted approach should be considered in combination with chemotherapy.[32] Correction of anemia and extracorporeal perfusion are important aspects of management; unfortunately, extracorporeal perfusion requires complete therapeutic anticoagulation and therefore is dangerous in this setting (Fig. 49-9).

Although the placenta is the site of origin of gestational choriocarcinoma, even when complicating term pregnancy, the primary intraplacental choriocarcinoma is rarely detected and metastases to the fetus are seldom seen. When transplacental metastasis occurs, the prognosis is poor. Consideration should be given to hCG testing of the infant when maternal diagnosis is made.

**Follow-up and Outcome.** Follow-up recommendation is similar to that for low-risk malignant GTD patients; long-term follow-up indicates a 5-year survival rate of 86% for this group of women. The most common causes of death are hemorrhage and pulmonary insufficiency.

### Pregnancy after Chemotherapy for Malignant Gestational Trophoblastic Disease

Because malignant GTD can be cured with chemotherapy, preserving an intact reproductive system, the issue of the effects

**Table 49-11**
**EMA-CO Regimen for High-Risk Malignant Gestational Trophoblastic Disease**

| Day | Agent | Dose and Route |
|-----|-------|----------------|
| 1 | Etoposide | 100 mg/m², IV infusion over 30 minutes |
| | Methotrexate | 100 mg/m², IV bolus |
| | | 200 mg/m², IV infusion over 12h |
| | D actinomycin | 350 μg/m², IV bolus |
| 2 | Etoposide | 100 mg/m², IV infusion over 30 minutes |
| | D actinomycin | 350 μg/m², IV bolus |
| | Folinic acid | 15 mg, PO/IM q12h × 4 doses, 24h after MTX bolus |
| 8 | Cyclophosphamide | 600 mg/m², IV infusion over 30 minutes |
| | Vincristine | 1 mg/m², IV bolus |
| 15 | Begin next cycle | |

Toxicities: Neutropenia and thrombocytopenia are the most common toxicity (27%). Stem cell support may be required. Post-therapy AML: 0.4%–2.4%

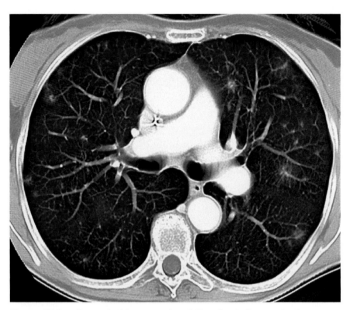

**Figure 49-9    Computed tomography of the chest, demonstrating hematogeneous spread of malignant trophoblastic neoplasia.** The most common site of spread is the lungs. These pulmonary metastases tend to be hemorrhagic; therefore, they may have a fuzzy border.    (Courtesy Dr. Tamar Sella, Hadassah Medical Center, Jerusalem.)

of cytotoxic drugs on fertility and the genetic well-being of the oocytes is important. Several researchers have examined fertility as well as fetal health following chemotherapy for malignant GTD. The majority of these series conclude that there is no detrimental effect in either outcome after chemotherapy. Rustin and colleagues[33] reported that only 3% of patients who tried to conceive after chemotherapy for GTD failed to do so and that 86% had at least one live birth. The ability to conceive was not worse for patients older than age 30, but was slightly lower in patients receiving multiagent chemotherapy. Both the use of gonadotropin-releasing hormone analogs and oral contraception during chemotherapy to protect the ovaries from premature ovarian failure and the rule of 1-year pregnancy delay from treatment to permit clearance of damaged oocytes are speculative. Pregnancies should not be attempted until 12 months after conclusion of treatment, because although pregnancies occurring before completion of hCG follow-up tend to do well, the patient is at risk for delayed diagnosis of a relapse.[34]

## REFERENCES

1. Matsuura J, Chiu D, Jacobs PA, Szulman AE: Complete hydatidiform mole in Hawaii: an epidemiological study. Genet Epidemiol 1984; 1:271–284. **(III, B)**
2. Smith HO: Gestational trophoblastic disease epidemiology and trends. Clin Obstet Gynecol 2003;46:541–556. **(III, B)**
3. Kovacs BW, Shahbahrami B, Tast DE, Curtin JP: Molecular genetic analysis of complete hydatidiform moles. Cancer Genet Cytogenet 1991;54:143–152. **(IIb, B)**
4. Fisher RA, Hodges MD: Genomic imprinting in gestational trophoblastic disease—a review. Placenta 2003;24(Suppl A):S111–S118. **(IIb, B)**
5. Lage JM, Wolf NG: Gestational trophoblastic disease. New approaches to diagnosis. Clin Lab Med. 1995;15:631–664. **(III, B)**
6. Soto-Wright V, Bernstein M, Goldstein DP, Berkowitz RS: The changing clinical presentation of complete molar pregnancy. Obstet Gynecol 1995;86:775–779. **(III, B)**
7. Goldstein DP, Berkowitz RS, Bernstein MR: Management of molar pregnancy. J Reprod Med 1981;26:208–212. **(III, B)**
8. Steller MA, Genest DR, Bernstein MR, et al: Natural history of twin pregnancy with complete hydatidiform mole and coexisting fetus. Obstet Gynecol 1994;83:35–42. **(IIb, B)**
9. Cheung AN, Khoo US, Lai CY, et al: Metastatic trophoblastic disease after an initial diagnosis of partial hydatidiform mole: genotyping and chromosome in situ hybridization analysis. Cancer 2004;100:1411–1417 **(IIb, B)**
10. Goldstein DP, Berkowitz RS: Prophylactic chemotherapy of complete molar pregnancy. Semin Oncol 1995;22:157–160. **(IIa, B)**
11. Kim DS, Moon H, Kim KT, et al: Effects of prophylactic chemotherapy for persistent trophoblastic disease in patients with complete hydatidiform mole. Obstet Gynecol 1986;67:690–694. **(Ib, A)**
12. Cole LA: Phantom hCG and phantom choriocarcinoma. Gynecol Oncol 1998;71:325–329 **(III, B)**.
13. Khanlian SA, Smith HO, Cole LA: Persistent low levels of human chorionic gonadotropin: a premalignant gestational trophoblastic disease. Am J Obstet Gynecol 2003;188:1254–1259. **(III, B)**
14. Berkowitz RS, Goldstein DP, Marean AR, Bernstein M: Oral contraceptives and postmolar trophoblastic disease. Obstet Gynecol 1981; 58:474–477. **(Ib, A)**
15. Curry SL, Schlaerth JB, Kohorn EI, et al: Hormonal contraception and trophoblastic sequelae after hydatidiform mole (a Gynecologic Oncology Group Study). Am J Obstet Gynecol 1989;160:805–809. **(Ib, A)**
16. Sebire NJ, Fisher RA, Foskett M, et al: Risk of recurrent hydatidiform mole and subsequent pregnancy outcome following complete or partial hydatidiform molar pregnancy. Br J Obstet Gynecol 2003;110:22–26 **(III, B)**
17. Kohorn EI, Goldstein DP, Hancock BW, et al: Workshop Report: Combining the staging system of the International Federation of Gynecology and Obstetrics with the scoring system of the World Health Organization for Trophoblastic Neoplasia. Report of the Working Committee of the International Society for the Study of Trophoblastic Disease and the International Gynecologic Cancer Society. Int J Gynecol Cancer 2000;10:84–88. **(III, B)**
18. Schlaerth JB, Morrow CP, Rodriguez M: Diagnostic and therapeutic curettage in gestational trophoblastic disease. Am J Obstet Gynecol 1990;162:1465–1470. **(III, B)**
19. Feltmate CM, Genest DR, Wise L, et al: Placental site trophoblastic tumor: a 17-year experience at the New England Trophoblastic Disease Center. Gynecol Oncol 2001;82:415–419. **(III, B)**
20. Rhoton-Vlasak A, Wagner JM, Rutgers JL, et al: Placental site trophoblastic tumor: human placental lactogen and pregnancy-associated major basic protein as immunohistologic markers. Hum Pathol 1998; 29:280–288. **(IIb, B)**
21. Soper JT: Staging and evaluation of gestational trophoblastic disease. Clin Obstet Gynecol 2003;46:570–578. **(III, B)**
22. Tidy JA, Rustin GJ, Newlands ES, et al: Presentation and management of choriocarcinoma after nonmolar pregnancy. Br J Obstet Gynaecol 1995;102:715–719. **(IIb, B)**
23. Soper JT, Lewis JL II, Hammond CB: Gestational trophoblastic disease. In Hoskins WJ, Perez CA, Young R (eds): Principles and Practice of Gynecologic Oncology, 2nd ed. Philadelphia: Lippincott-Raven, 1996, pp1039–1077. **(III, B)**
24. Bagshawe KD: Risk and prognostic factors in trophoblastic neoplasia. Cancer 1976;38:1373–1385. **(III, B)**
25. Kohorn EI: The new FIGO 2000 staging and risk factor scoring system for gestational trophoblastic disease: description and critical assessment. Int J Gynecol Cancer 2001;11:73–77. **(III, B)**
26. Carney ME: Treatment of low risk gestational trophoblastic disease. Clin Obstet Gynecol 2003;46:579–592. **(III, B)**
27. Hammond CB, Borchert LG, Tyrey L, et al: Treatment of metastatic trophoblastic disease: good and poor prognosis. Am J Obstet Gynecol 1973;115:451–457. **(III, B)**

28. Bagshawe KD: Treatment of high–risk choriocarcinoma. J Reprod Med 1984;29:813–820. **(IIa, B)**

29. Curry SL, Blessing JA, DiSaia PJ, et al: A prospective randomized comparison of methotrexate, dactinomycin, and chlorambucil versus methotrexate, dactinomycin, cyclophosphamide, doxorubicin, melphalan, hydroxyurea, and vincristine in "poor prognosis" metastatic gestational trophoblastic disease: a Gynecologic Oncology Group study. Obstet Gynecol 1989;73(3 Pt 1):357–362. **(Ib, A)**

30. Newlands ES, Bagshawe KD, Begent RH, et al: Developments in chemotherapy for medium- and high-risk patients with gestational trophoblastic tumours (1979–1984). Br J Obstet Gynaecol 1986; 93:63–69. **(III, B)**

31. Newlands ES, Mulholland PJ, Holden L, et al: Etoposide and cisplatin/ etoposide, methotrexate, and actinomycin D (EP/EMA) chemotherapy for patients with high-risk gestational trophoblastic tumors refractory to EMA/cyclophosphamide and vincristine chemotherapy and patients presenting with metastatic placental site trophoblastic tumors. J Clin Oncol 2000;18:854–859. **(III, B)**

32. Vaccarello L, Apte SM, Diaz PT, et al: Respiratory failure from metastatic choriocarcinoma: a survivor of mechanical ventilation. Gynecol Oncol 1997;67:111–114. **(IV, C)**

33. Rustin GJ, Booth M, Dent J, et al: Pregnancy after cytotoxic chemotherapy for gestational trophoblastic tumours. Br Med J 1984; 288:103–106. **(III, B)**

34. Tuncer ZS, Bernstein MR, Goldstein DP, Berkowitz RS: Outcome of pregnancies occurring before completion of human chorionic gonadotropin follow-up in patients with persistent gestational trophoblastic tumor. Gynecol Oncol 1999;73:345–347. **(III, B)**

## KEY POINTS

- Effective analgesic therapies are available for cancer patients.
- Large numbers of patients are dissatisfied with pain control.
- Morphine plus multidimensional therapy is encouraged for relief of cancer pain.
- Interventional therapy should be considered sooner rather than later.
- Accurate pain assessment is essential for effective management of cancer pain.
- Identification of barriers to implementation of effective therapies is the key to success.

Perhaps more is known today about the mechanisms of pain and its exacerbation than during any other period in medical history. This is combined with the availability of more evidence-based analgesic medications and procedures than ever before. However, the most palpable improvement in cancer pain management has been the willingness of physicians to routinely prescribe potent opioid medications for extended periods of time and their recognition that inducing opioid addiction in this population is the exception rather than the rule. Titration of potent opioid medications has become the standard of care for managing moderate to severe cancer pain in North America and many other developed regions of the world. Despite widespread use of morphine and other opioids and the development of new methods to administer these drugs, it has become apparent that many patients still do not achieve satisfactory pain relief.[1] This is occurring even in environments where opioids are prescribed readily to control pain. Now that the barrier of limited access to opioid medications is falling, other obstructions that block the path toward consistent relief of symptoms must be identified and dismantled.

One clinical variable that makes achieving adequate analgesia for patients difficult is the presence of comorbid symptoms. Multiple symptom incidents are typical in cancer patients, particularly in late stages of the disease. Distressing nonpainful symptoms tend to cluster and potentially exacerbate the intensity and impact of painful symptoms (e.g., depression, anxiety, insomnia, fatigue) on life quality.[2,3] Rather than an isolated experience, pain must be viewed globally in the context of multiple undesirable symptoms in a single patient; as such, multiple therapies should be prescribed simultaneously when appropriate. The mechanism for the "pain" itself typically is multifactorial as well. Hence, a multidimensional approach to controlling symptoms is warranted for most patients. This is particularly important and relevant when pain intensity is perceived to be moderate or greater.

Another affront to effective symptom management is limited assessment of symptom complaints. For a variety of reasons, many cancer patients will not complain or reveal the gravity of their symptom intensity until after they are incapacitated.[4,5] Cancer patients in particular need to be queried systematically about symptoms so that appropriate treatment actions can be triggered early. Symptom complaints should be evaluated and managed aggressively, preferably long before the intensity of the symptom becomes severe. This chapter discusses specific therapies for cancer pain management. Options that clinicians should consider in their clinical decision making to improve cancer pain management are discussed.

## A MODEL FOR QUALITY OF LIFE ENHANCEMENT

Many components go into developing and maintaining a high quality of living for cancer patients. The ingredients necessary to experience high-quality living include intimacy, creativity, productivity, and independence. Health care providers can be key participants in achieving these goals by eliminating or controlling undesirable symptoms. During the patient's illness, there are at least four legs of support that the patient stands on in order to maintain a high-quality life experience. The first is the health care system. Ideally, cancer patients have access to health care providers who bring a broad knowledge base and experience to symptom management and are able to respond to specific needs rapidly and compassionately. Second, patients have access to effective symptom control measures (analgesics and techniques in the case of pain). Third, patients are greatly advantaged if they are given a sense of empowerment through understanding of the mechanisms of their disease and the therapies used to treat symptoms. Fourth, a symptom management regimen works best when it can be tailored to the patient's particular circumstances and needs. In the Quality of Life model presented in Figure 50-1, the tabletop represents quality of life. Quality of life is supported on the strength of the four legs described here. Quality of life falls along a continuum. As the supporting legs fail, quality of life diminishes. Strengthening of these key supports will improve the impact of services rendered for all patients in need of care.

## EPIDEMIOLOGY

In 2002 the nation's leading cancer organizations reported that Americans' risk of getting and dying from cancer continued to decline and that survival rates for many cancers continue to

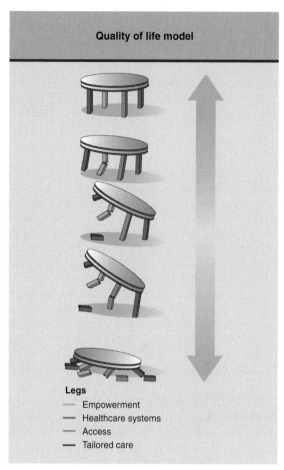

**Quality of life model**

Legs
— Empowerment
— Healthcare systems
— Access
— Tailored care

**Figure 50-1    Quality of life model.**

improve. The Annual Report to the Nation on the Status of Cancer, 1975–2001, found that overall observed cancer incidence rates dropped 0.5% per year from 1991 to 2001, whereas death rates from all cancers combined dropped 1.1% per year from 1993 to 2001.[6] According to the report's authors, the new data reflect progress in prevention, early detection, and treatment; however, not all segments of the U.S. population have benefited equally from the advances.[7-10] Disparities in this arena are a blight on our medical system and must be addressed and eliminated. Disparities notwithstanding, there is good news to report overall. For the first time, lung cancer incidence rates among women are on the decline. Incidence rates decreased for 5 additional cancers out of the top 15 in women (colon, cervix, pancreas, ovary, and oral cavity). Only breast, thyroid, bladder, and kidney cancer and melanoma rates are rising among women.[6]

Increased survival from cancer can be a double-edged sword for many patients. Residual effects from the disease or toxicities from the treatment can sometimes lead to chronic pain. The prevalence of pain in cancer patients is extremely high, occurring in more than three fourths of patients with advanced disease. Despite optimism generated from clinical trial data, uncontrolled pain in cancer patients remains unacceptably high.[4,6] This leads to the conclusion that available effective therapies are not being utilized to the fullest extent. The solution to this problem is not necessarily to increase the units of morphine administered per cancer patient in pain, but first to make an assessment of

systemic and individual barriers to good analgesia that attenuate the efficacy of treatment.

## ANATOMY OF PELVIC CANCER PAIN

A variety of anatomic sites, including viscera, nerves, muscles, ligaments, and skeletal structures, give rise to painful sensations in the pelvis during progression of cancer. Seldom is the disease confined to only one type, and commonly the most troublesome tissue can be identified based on imaging studies and clinical presentation. This is important to consider because some analgesic approaches have specific indications. Pelvic and perineal cancer pain broadly are classified as visceral, neuropathic, and somatic. *Visceral pain* is the result of but not limited to spasms of the smooth muscle of a hollow viscus, distortions of the capsule of a solid organ, inflammation, ischemic conditions, and visceral encroachment by tumor growth.[11,12]

Neuropathic pain may occur from tumor invasion of the nearby lumbosacral plexus and peripheral nerves. Irritation and destruction of nerves result from extension of tumor or from secondary complications of radiation and chemotherapy. Neuropathic pain is particularly difficult to treat and too often slow to reverse, even if the disease is eradicated. Somatic pain occurs with stimulation of pain fibers *(nociceptors)* in the peripheral structures, such as striated muscles, bones, and joints.

Sympathetic and parasympathetic nerves supply the viscera of the pelvis. Both contain afferent and efferent fibers. The aortic plexus contributes fibers for the formation of the superior and inferior hypogastric plexus, which in turn supply all of the pelvic viscera. Neurolysis of these structures can be an effective means to analgesia and opioid reduction. The somatic structures of the perineum are predominately innervated by branches of the pudendal nerve, which originates from sacral nerve roots. Figure 50-2 illustrates the anatomy of this neural network, as well as anatomic sites for injection of neurolytic agents to locally disrupt painful transmissions related to advancing tumor involving the pelvis and lower abdominal structures.

## CONDITIONS RELEVANT TO CANCER PAIN MANAGEMENT

### Breakthrough Pain and Incident Pain
*Breakthrough pain* is a transitory flare of pain that occurs on a background of well-controlled baseline pain. Breakthrough pain is highly prevalent among patients with cancer and predicts more severe pain, pain-related distress and functional impairment, and relatively poor quality of life.

*Incident pain* also is a transitory flare of pain but is associated or initiated by a specific activity, such as activation of visceral functions and movement of the offended body part. Lack of control of incident pain can be particular debilitating, especially when avoidance of the activity further reduces quality of life.

Rescue medications are rapid-onset, short-acting medications (typically opioids) used concurrently with controlled-release or long-acting opioids to control breakthrough and incident pain.

### Physical Dependence and Addiction
*Physical dependence* is the physiological adaptation of the body to the presence of an opioid. It is defined by the development of

**Nerve fibers to the female pelvis**

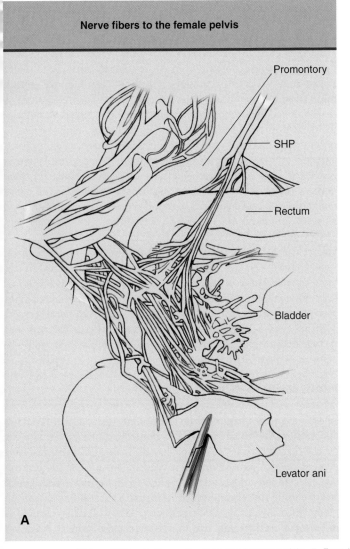

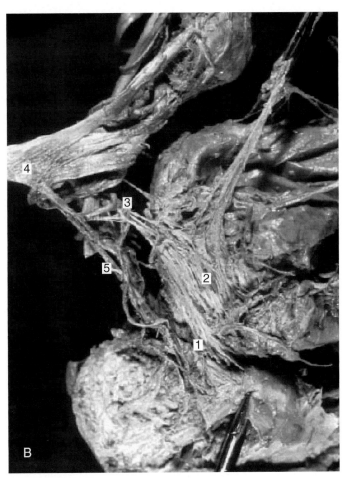

**Figure 50-2** *A,* Nerve fibers to the female pelvis. *B,* Female adult, right side; shows the sacral plexus reflected posteriorly (4), giving rise to the pudendal nerve (5) and pelvic splanchnic nerves (3). Both connect to the inferior hypogastric plexus (2). Furthermore, the most inferior parts of the inferior hypogastric plexus contribute to a neurovascular bundle (1). The hemostat shown in the right upper corner holds the superior hypogastric plexus. (From Baader M, Herrmann B: Clinical Anatomy 2003;16:119–130.)

withdrawal symptoms when opioids are discontinued, when the dose is reduced abruptly, or when an antagonist (e.g., naloxone) or an agonist–antagonist (e.g., pentazocine) is administered. It is not synonymous with addiction.

*Addiction* is compulsive use of drugs for nonmedical reasons despite potential harm; it is characterized by a craving for the mood-altering drug effects. Tolerance and physical dependence are physical changes in the body, but addiction is defined by aberrant changes in behavior. Addiction means dysfunctional behavior, in sharp contrast to the improved function and quality of life that result from pain relief. Aberrant behaviors that indicate addiction may include denial of drug use, lying, forgery of prescriptions, theft of drugs from other patients or family members, selling and buying drugs on the street, and using prescribed drugs to get "high."

It should not be assumed that cancer patients are exempt from the reinforcing properties of opioid medications, and drug diversion does occur in this population. However, a true drug addiction rarely develops after prescription of opioids to treat cancer-related pain unless prior risk factors for addiction exist.[13]

*Pseudoaddiction* describes what happens when health care workers inappropriately perceive as addictive behavior a pain patient's requests for more or stronger pain medications. In fact, the patient's behavior may be a response to inadequate pain management.

### Incomplete Cross-tolerance

Although all morphine receptor agonists are associated with tolerance following repeated usage and exhibit cross-tolerance to other opioids acting at the receptor, the degree of cross-tolerance varies widely. Indeed, clinicians use incomplete cross-tolerance to restore analgesic sensitivity in highly tolerant patients.[14]

Opioid rotation takes advantage of the concept of incomplete cross-tolerance. It is the process of switching a patient who is highly tolerant to one opioid-selective drug to another to restore analgesia. It has been reported that analgesia may be restored by the second drug at doses 50% below the predicted equivalent dose determined by relative potency studies in naive subjects.[14]

## MAJOR RISK FACTORS FOR CHRONIC SEVERE CANCER PAIN

### Bone Metastasis

Metastatic bone disease is a major risk factor for severe pain and is a common cause of deterioration in quality of life in cancer patients. Breast cancers more commonly metastasize to bone, but malignancies involving the pelvis may also cause bone pain via vascular spread to distant sites and via direct tumor spread into surrounding bony structures. Bone metastases to the vertebral column can be particularly troubling because of the possibility of structural collapse, bone fracture, and nerve compression.

The painful bone lesions are the result of a complex pathophysiological process between host and tumor cells leading to cellular invasion, migration, and adhesion and stimulation of osteoclastic and osteoblastic activity. External beam radiation therapy remains the mainstay of pain palliation of solitary lesions, and bone-seeking radiopharmaceuticals have entered the therapeutic armamentarium for the treatment of multiple painful osseous lesions. Bisphosphonates act by inhibiting osteoclast-mediated resorption and have been increasingly used in treatment of painful bone metastases. Deformation of the periosteum is thought to generate an intense, sharp, stabbing pain. Bisphosphonates reduce the destruction, and should significantly reduce movement-evolved pain.[15]

Several sequelae occur as a result of osseous metastases, and resulting bone pain can lead to significant debilitation. Pain associated with osseous metastasis is thought to be distinct from neuropathic or inflammatory pain. Several mechanisms—such as invasion of tumor cells, spinal cord gliosis, and sensitization of the nervous system—have been postulated to cause pain. A significant reorganization of the spinal cord that received sensory input from the cancerous bone occurs, and this reorganization generates a neurochemical signature of bone cancer pain, which is both dramatic and significantly different from that observed in mouse and rat models of chronic neuropathic or inflammatory pain.

Bone scan is the most effective screening procedure to determine vertebral involvement, and magnetic resonance imaging (MRI) effectively shows epidural involvement. Front-line therapy for this problem is control of tumor activity when possible. Treatments include hormonal therapy, chemotherapy, bisphosphonates, and radiation therapy. Analgesic approaches are applied simultaneously, but too often are ineffective when given alone.

### Neuropathic Pain

Neuropathic pain is a chronic pain syndrome with characteristic clinical symptoms including the feeling of pins and needles; burning, shooting, and/or stabbing pain with or without throbbing; and numbness. Neuropathic pain is caused directly by cancer-related pathology (compression/infiltration of nerve tissue, combination of compression/infiltration) or by diagnostic and therapeutic procedures (surgical procedures, chemotherapy, radiotherapy). Neuropathy is infrequently associated with major pelvic surgery. The usual etiology is direct surgical trauma, stretch injury, suture entrapment, or retractor injury.

Neuronal hyperexcitability represents the hallmark cellular mechanism involved in the underlying pathophysiology of neuropathic pain. Pathophysiological mechanisms are very complex and are still not completely understood. Neuropathic pain is generated by electrical hyperactivity of neurons along the pain pathways. Peripheral mechanisms (primary sensitization of nerve endings, ectopically generated action potentials within damaged nerves, abnormal electrogenesis within sensory ganglia) and central mechanisms (loss of input from peripheral nociceptors into dorsal horn, aberrant sprouting within dorsal horn, central sensitization, loss of inhibitory interneurons, mechanisms at higher centers) are involved. The most frequent sites of neurologic injury for pelvic cancer are nerve roots, the spinal cord and cauda equina, lumbosacral plexus, and peripheral nerves. Typically, painful neuropathic lesions are difficult to treat and resistant to opioid therapy. Breakthrough and incident pain are commonly present.

## PAIN ASSESSMENT

In addition to determining the location of pain, intensity of pain, and its response to current analgesic medications, an assessment of the patient's medical experiences, social background, and current mental state should be undertaken. An evaluation of the patient's mood and cognitive ability, daily activity, nutritional status, family/social support system, and spiritual beliefs can be useful in designing a treatment plan. Mood disorders, such as depression and anxiety, can greatly affect the intensity of pain and other troublesome symptoms.[3] In the author's opinion, patients who have significant depression or major anxiety occurring in conjunction with severely painful symptoms, rarely find satisfactory relief of the pain for extended periods. Patients who are paranoid and disoriented are very difficult to manage and assess going forward. Subtle disorientation may not be appreciated at first. Family can help decipher normal and abnormal behavior and cognitive ability for the patient. The nutritional status and daily activity assessment reveals a great deal about the general physical condition of the patient. Patients who are unable to tolerate food by mouth, have very poor appetites and spend most of their time in bed are generally in poor mental and physical health. This leads ultimately to overwhelming fatigue and malaise and difficulty in controlling painful symptoms. It is always desirable to have good family support systems in place. Patients who are concerned with spiritual matters should be encouraged to practice their beliefs. A psychosocial assessment upfront will help shape and tailor the treatment regimen for a given patient.

The patient's pain history is an important determinant in the assessment (Table 50-1). It is important to note if the patient has visceral versus peripheral/somatic pain symptoms. Visceral symptoms may be treatable with sympathetic ganglion modulation. Neuropathic pain involving peripheral regions of the body

| Table 50-1 |
| --- |
| Pain History Considerations |

Visceral pain vs. peripheral/somatic pain
Somatic pain vs. neuropathic pain
Acute pain vs. chronic pain
Intermittent pain vs. unrelenting pain
Incident pain vs. nonincident pain

can often be controlled with adjuvant therapies such as anti-convulsants and neurotransmitter-modulating medications. Acute exacerbations, because they may be short-lived, are amenable to short-term aggressive analgesic approaches, such as epidural analgesia or high-dose, high-potency opioid therapy for several days. During this rest period, radiation therapy and other palliative approaches can be implemented to provide a longer-term solution. Chronic pain should set in motion formulation of a long-term analgesic regimen. Intermittent pain might be best treated with potent medications administered in varying dosages on an as-needed basis. Incident pain can be particularly problematic if the source of the insult cannot be stabilized. When incident pain does not improve spontaneously, interventional approaches should be considered.

Current medications, duration of therapy, and effect on pain are critical components of pain assessment. Patients with an acute pain syndrome on top of a chronic pain disorder usually necessitate variation in the treatment approach.

## TREATMENT CONSIDERATIONS

Because opioid analgesics are generally effective in controlling cancer pain, it is important to evaluate opioid effectiveness, dosage, duration of use, and side effect profile in every patient before launching a new regimen. A history that evaluates use of adjuvant drugs and interventional therapies also help develop the analgesic plan. Table 50-2 outlines a potential course of action as these data are analyzed.

### Psychiatric Therapy

The psychological dimensions of pain control should not be underestimated in cancer patients. The diagnosis of cancer places a great burden on one's psyche, and the strain of it will exacerbate the impact of unrelenting symptoms, particularly pain. Symptom clustering (e.g., pain, depression, and fatigue) is a common occurrence in cancer patients, and each should be rigorously treated simultaneously to maximize improvement in quality of life.[16]

### Sympathetic Ganglionic Neurolytic Blockade

Sympathetic ganglionic blockade has been shown to significantly reduce the intensity of cancer pain, decrease opioid consumption, improve quality of life, and significantly reduce the incidence of drug-induced undesirable side effects when compared to a control group of patients treated with opioids only.[17] The majority of reports related to sympatholysis for cancer pain relate to the effectiveness of this technique against pain due to pancreatic adenocarcinoma. Positive results have also been

demonstrated for pelvic malignant diseases.[18,19] A more recently published controlled study showed difficulty in reducing the intensity of pain in the control group in spite of the weekly increase in opioid dosage.[20] Sympathetic procedures for pain conditions due to pancreatic and pelvic cancers should be intended as adjuvant techniques to reduce analgesic consumption and not as a panacea, given that multiple pain mechanisms are often involved because progression of disease can change underlying pain mechanisms. Pancreatic pain seems to maintain visceral characteristics amenable to sympathetic block more than pain due to pelvic cancer.

### Technique (Superior Hypogastric Plexus Neurolysis)

A number of different specialists are capable of performing this procedure, including trained anesthesiologists, surgeons, and physiatrists. The hypogastric plexus is the target of sympathetic neurolysis for painful lesions involving the pelvic viscera. The preganglionic fibers of the hypogastic plexus originate primarily in the lower thoracic and upper lumbar region of the spinal cord. These fibers interface with the lumbar sympathetic chain via the white communicantes. Postganglionic fibers exit the lumbar sympathetic chain and, together with fibers from the para-sympathetic sacral ganglion, make up the superior hypogastric plexus. The plexus lies in front of L4 as a coalescence of fibers and passes downward in front of the L5–S1 interspace. This location marks the site of needle placement for neurolytic injection. The needle is guided to position via computed tomography (CT), fluoroscopy, or under direct vision at surgery. Incremental

| Table 50-2 | | |
| --- | --- | --- |
| Development of an Analgesic Treatment Plan | | |
| Analgesic Therapeutic History | | Potential Consideration When Analgesia Inadequate |
| Opioid-responsive pain? | Yes | Alter timing, route of administration, or dosing of medication. |
| | No | Opioid-resistant symptom (e.g., neuropathic pain), inadequate dosing (too little or too much opioid medication) |
| High-dose opioid required? | Yes | Opioid-resistant symptom (e.g., neuropathic pain), inadequate dosing (too little or too much opioid medication): Switch opioid medication. Add adjuvant or intervention approach if not done. |
| | No | Increase dose or potency of medication. |
| Long-term opioid history? | Yes | Analgesic tolerance; depression; anxiety |
| | No | Adjust dosing schedule. |
| Adjuvant therapy responsive | Yes | Assess patient compliance; is dosing adequate? |
| | No | Add adjuvant therapy. |
| Severe side effects to therapy? | Yes | Add adjuvant therapy; reduce dosage; counter side effect. |
| | No | Make notation in patient record. |
| Interventional approach considered? | Yes | Evaluate if performed optimally. |
| | No | Add intervention. |
| Concomitant symptom control therapy on board? | Yes | Evaluate and treat. |
| | No | Make notation in patient record. |

# Gynecologic Oncology

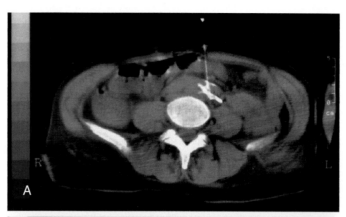

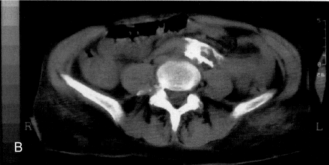

**Figure 50-3  Computed tomography scans show anterior approach to superior hypogastric block in a woman with extensive uterine carcinoma.** *A,* Injection of 1 mL contrast medium to confirm the exact position of needle. *B,* Spread of alcohol solution around iliac vessels.

doses of absolute alcohol or 6.5% aqueous phenol are injected to achieve neurolysis (Fig. 50-3).

Hypogastric neurolysis performed either with radiologic guidance or under direct visualization has the potential of producing undesirable nerve damage leading to loss of lower extremity mobility as well as bladder and bowel control. Also, given the proximity of vital viscera, including the ureters, unwanted destruction of vital organs is possible. The incidence of major complications is very low, however. Case reports for a variety of complications are assessable. Interestingly, no such complications have been reported in the few controlled clinical trials that have been performed. The potential benefit from this procedure greatly overshadows the potential side effects. Unfortunately, these procedures are considered very late in the course of the patient's disease. It is the authors' opinion that these procedures should be performed earlier. There is no apparent downside to early neurolysis,[17] and complications from advancement of tumor frequently complicate or prevent the use of these techniques late in the disease.

## Intraspinal Analgesic Therapy

Soon after it was shown that opioid analgesia could be activated in the spinal cord independent of cerebral site activation, techniques were developed to administer intraspinal opioids (monotherapy) for acute pain and chronic pain therapy. Intraspinal implantable drug delivery systems deliver small doses of drug directly to the spinal fluid, achieving pain relief with much smaller doses than are possible with oral or parenteral routes. The

technology used to deliver the medication has received most of the attention, as compared to drug discovery and development. Clonidine has been developed for intraspinal use in humans and is Food and Drug Administration (FDA) approved for epidural administration.[21] Ziconotide (Prialt), a snail conotoxin peptide derivative, has been shown to effectively control cancer pain and is currently under review by the FDA.[22] Many different drugs and drug combinations are used for intrathecal analgesia. Morphine continues to be the standard by which other drugs are compared. To date morphine is the only FDA-approved agent for long-term intrathecal administration to control pain.

The analgesic drug solution is placed in the reservoir of a battery-powered programmable or a bladder-driven nonprogrammable pump, both of which can be refilled percutaneously as needed (Fig. 50-4). The pump is implanted under the skin of the abdomen and connected to a small catheter tunneled to the site of spinal entry. The cost-effectiveness of this intervention has not yet been formally studied in cancer patients but it could work to reduce cost by cutting significantly the total number of hospital visits and the need for other medications, while providing better pain relief than conventional therapies.

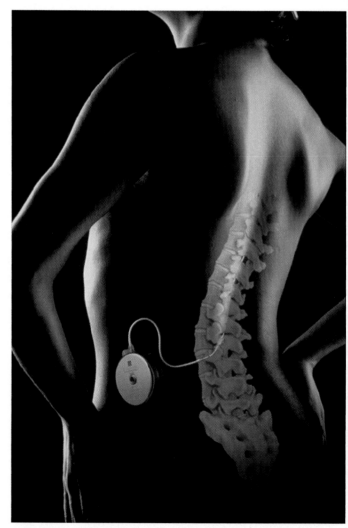

**Figure 50-4  An implanted pump and catheter system for intraspinal analgesic administration.** (From Medtronic Inc., Minneapolis, MN.)

Emerging data provided by randomized controlled studies offer evidence that this approach can be highly efficacious,[23,24] although more study is necessary as direction in patient selection is lacking and methods to assure sustained relief after implantation continue to be elusive. Before implantation of the system, a trial is performed, and patients are asked if they experienced 50% or greater relief of their symptoms. No standard approach has been used to conduct this trial; the ideal method is intrathecal infusion of the analgesic drug through a temporary intrathecal catheter and pump system for at least several days. Long-term therapy should be considered if the pain relief is sustained. Single-shot trials are commonly used, but these may be prone to more false-positive and false-negative test results. Another challenge to the use of intrathecal analgesic therapy is the high likelihood that tolerance to the analgesic drug will occur and that disease progression in the cancer patient will limit the effectiveness of the analgesic over time. When the correct patient has been matched with the appropriate drug and dosage, excellent analgesia can be achieved.[21] The reversibility of the technique and its efficacy at multiple body sites and for different types of pain are important advantages.

## Systemic Opioid Therapy

Opioid medications such as morphine are age-old therapies for treating severe pain. These molecules work via activation of opioid receptors located throughout the body. The locations associated with analgesia are found deep in the brain and in the dorsal horn of the spinal cord. The varieties of opioid products differ in pharmacokinetics and affinity/potency at the opioid receptor-binding site. The side effect profiles for the different agents are similar, but the incidence and severity of a particular effect may differ between agents (Table 50-3). It has been demonstrated that patients started on strong opioids required

significantly fewer changes in therapy, had greater reduction in pain when a change was initiated, and reported greater satisfaction with treatment than the comparison group. Strong opioids were safe and well-tolerated, with no development of tolerance or serious adverse events. These data suggest the utility of strong opioids for first-line treatment of pain in patients with terminal cancer.[4]

Opioids remain the cornerstone of pharmacotherapy for cancer pain. We are currently benefiting from a proverbial explosion of products that increase the range of opioid agents and formulations available for the treatment of cancer pain. Analgesic regimens involving opioids can be tailored to suit the individual circumstances for each patient. Short half-life drugs, such as morphine, hydromorphone, fentanyl, oxycodone, and oxymorphone, are common front-line agents because they are easier to titrate than long half-life agents and have a record for being effective. Long-acting opioid and controlled-release preparations can provide convenience and reduce around-the-clock administration of drugs with a short duration of action. In recent years several new formulations have been developed, including controlled-release morphine suppositories and suspensions; controlled-release tablets of oxycodone, hydromorphone, and codeine; and transdermal fentanyl, a patch that allows 3-day dosing and avoids the first-pass effect of the liver. The efficacy of opioid medications for the control of cancer pain is well established both from experience and clinical trials, particularly for treating mild to moderately intense pain. The difficulty occurs when the pain is very severe and extremely high doses are required. Appropriate strategies must be tailored to suit the patient's requirements and a series of trials are required. This can be complicated further when the mechanism of the pain is neuropathic in nature, when higher than typical dosing regimens are required. Of course, the risk of severe side effects is increased

**Table 50-3**
**Opioid Medications**

| Drug | Recommended Starting Dose (Adults) | | Comments |
|------|------|------|------|
| | Oral | Parenteral | |
| Morphine | | | |
|   Immediate release | 15–30 mg q 3–4 hr | 4–10 mg q 3–4 hr | Prototype opioid analgesic. Available in a variety of preparations. |
|   Extended release | 15–30 mg q 12 hr | | |
| Hydromorphone | 2–6 mg q 3–4 hr | 1–2 mg q 3–4 hr | Extended-release preparation under review by FDA. |
| Oxycodone | | | |
|   Immediate release | 5–10 mg q 3–4 hr | — | No parenteral formulation is available. Oral formulation available |
|   Extended release | 10–20 mg q 12 hr | — |   plain or in combination with aspirin or acetaminophen. |
| Levorphanol | 2–4 mg q 6–8 hr | 1–2 mg q 6–8 hr | Long half-life may lead to drug accumulation. |
| Meperidine | — | 50–100 mg q 3–4 hr | Oral preparation generally not effective. First-order metabolite, normeperidine, can accumulate if renal function compromised, leading to CNS toxicity, including seizures. |
| Oxymorphone | | | |
|   Immediate release | — | | |
|   Extended release | 10–20 mg q 12 hr | 0.5–1 mg q 3–4 hr | Under review by FDA. |
| Fentanyl | | | |
|   Patch | 25–50 µg/hr q 3 day | | Patch designed for transdermal administration. 25, 50, 75, 100 µg/hr dose units available. |
|   Oral dispenser | 200 µg q 3–4 hr | | Oral dispenser designed for severe breakthrough pain in opioid tolerant cancer patients. 200, 400, 600, 800, 1200, and 1600 µg dose units available |

as the dosage of medications is increased. Effects are not confined to analgesia. Other effects include euphoria, respiratory depression, sedation, slowing of bowel motility, sphincter contraction (glands), dysphoria, and hyperalgesia (exaggerated pain responses).

Potent agonist opioid analgesics are in focus here. Mixed agonist–antagonist opioids (e.g., butorphanol) are sometimes prescribed for chronic pain. These drugs are not typically prescribed for treatment of cancer pain because of their antagonistic effects at the mu receptor. Likewise, partial agonists (e.g., buprenorphine) have a ceiling effect of analgesia and should not be used to treat moderate to severe cancer pain or mild pain that could escalate in intensity.

### Commonly Prescribed Opioid Agents

#### Morphine

Morphine is a relatively selective mu receptor agonist with which other opioid and nonopioid analgesics are compared. Morphine is a moderately lipid-soluble molecule and is available in a variety of preparations, including immediate- and extended-release tablets, elixir, suppository, and intravenous and intrathecal (preservative-free) solutions. The extended-release preparation provides even plasma concentrations of drug to control ongoing background chronic pain and minimizes the need for frequent analgesic dosing. The bioavailability of orally administered morphine is 25% to 30%. There is significant first-pass metabolism in the liver. The minor metabolite is active, but accumulation is slow if normal renal function is preserved. Morphine is considered to have strong potency, but other commercially available agents have much greater potency. The side effect profile is very similar to other opioids. Morphine can cause greater histamine release, resulting in significant pruritus.

#### Hydromorphone

Hydromorphone is a synthetic opioid agonist that was originally synthesized and promoted as a safe, nonaddicting substitute for morphine. It is structurally related to morphine but is approximately 5 to 10 times as potent. It is currently available as an immediate-release tablet, oral elixir, rectal suppository, and injectable solution. When taken orally, the onset of analgesia occurs within 15 minutes and lasts 3 to 5 hours. An application has been submitted to the FDA for an extended-release tablet. Orally administered drug has a bioavailability of 50%. Hydromorphone is primarily used to control breakthrough pain and is commonly used in combination with long half-life or extended-release opioid preparations.

#### Oxycodone

Oxycodone is a synthetic opioid agonist with equianalgesic potency to morphine when given parenterally. Oxycodone has twice the potency of morphine because of a significantly greater bioavailability in comparison to morphine (less first-pass metabolism). Oxycodone is produced as an oral solution, and in immediate- and extended-release tablets. Parenteral preparations are not commercially available. OxyContin, an extended-release preparation, has been associated with a disturbing number of drug diversion cases across the United States, prompting investigations from the FDA and other agencies. Some suggest that oxycodone may have greater abuse potential relative to other legally prescribed opioids, but the evidence is lacking to this point.

#### Fentanyl

Fentanyl (and congeners) is a synthetic opioid mu receptor agonist and is about 100 times more potent than morphine as an analgesic. Fentanyl has been a popular drug in anesthesia as an intravenous agent, but is now commonly administered to manage cancer pain via a transdermal patch device (Duragesic). The available patches come in four dose formulations, 25, 50, 75, and 100 μg/hr. Used patches are replaced every 3 days. Interruptions in steady-state analgesia can be avoided by changing patches every other day in some patients. Fentanyl is also formulated for oral transmucosal administration (Actiq). Six different available dosages are available: 200, 400, 600, 800, 1200, and 1600 μg. Actiq is used only to control severe breakthrough pain and should not be used as the primary analgesic for persistent symptoms. Careful titration of this formulation is needed to avoid severe, potentially lethal, side effects. The time to peak analgesic effect after intravenous administration of fentanyl is minutes. Likewise, the duration of action (offset of analgesia) is fast (1 to 2 hours).

#### Methadone

Methadone is a long-lasting mu receptor agonist with pharmacologic properties similar to morphine. In addition to the mu opioid receptor agonist effects, methadone has an antagonist at the N-methyl-D-aspartate (NMDA) receptor. NMDA blockade effectively prevents and reverses opioid analgesic tolerance in animal preparations. This effect has not been clearly shown to occur in humans,[25] but clinical experience suggests benefit from adding methadone to opioid-tolerant patients.[26] This benefit could be explained by incomplete cross-tolerance. The main clinical consideration in using this drug is its long half-life. Miotic and respiratory depressant effects can be detected for more than 24 hours after a single dose. The long half-life of this drug can be an advantage, however, for cancer patients who require constant plasma concentrations of a potent opioid to control pain. The onset of analgesia occurs 10 to 20 minutes after parenteral administration and 30 to 60 minutes after oral medication. Accumulation of the drug can occur because of the prolonged half-life. Despite a long terminal plasma half-life, methadone, when used to control cancer pain, is frequently administered in divided doses, two to three times per day, although theoretically once-daily doses should be adequate. Care must be taken when escalating the dosage. A number of sudden death cases have been associated with the use of methadone. Hypoventilation is a possible cause of these deaths, but methadone has also been shown to lengthen the QT interval and therefore may be arrhythmogenic in high doses (>150 mg/day).

Opioid agents can induce severe side effects, including death. The primary means of death is respiratory depression. Fortunately, death from opioid medications is rare for cancer patients. The dosing regimen typically is titrated to levels that provide an acceptable balance between side effects and analgesia. Fairly soon after initiation of daily usage of opioid medications (1 week), patients develop tolerance to the respiratory effects of the drug at the prescribed level. If the regimen is increased, the body must adjust to the higher dosage; respiratory depression and oversedation is a possibility but the risk is reduced. Constipation, reduced libido, and reduced ability to concentrate are common side effects. Altered sleeping patterns and muscle jerking are also major concerns to patients.

Use of these drugs may be limited by inappropriate fears of addiction, drug abuse, and misuse. Unpublished data suggest that at least 10% of cancer survivors are concerned about developing addiction to morphine. This is in addition to physician bias concerning addiction potential and legal liabilities. All patients taking opioids will develop tolerance to the drug to some degree. The significance of analgesic tolerance without evidence of advancing disease is an area of controversy. More recent data suggest that we can reach a level of opioid administration at which the patient becomes hyperalgesic and that additional opioid administration would paradoxically exacerbate the painful symptom. No specific guidelines are available, but for many patients who are treated with extremely high doses of opioid may improve with respect to their pain complaints if the daily dosage is reduced.

### Dosing Strategies

There are no rigid dosing strategies that practitioners must adhere to in order to be within the standard of practice in the community, but there are a few principles that might enhance analgesic performance. Typically, a long-acting drug or a sustained-release preparation is administered with a fast-acting, shorter-duration drug to treat "breakthrough" pain. This is commonly necessary because pain intensity is rarely static but rather waxes and wanes over time. Activity is a common reason for increased pain, but pain may increase or decrease without apparent cause.

### Opioid Switching

Anecdotal observations suggest that opioid switching is a useful practice that will improve pain relief and drug tolerability. Some practitioners schedule switching of opioid medications after 2 to 3 months of therapy. It is also acceptable to switch after effectiveness begins to wane or when unacceptable side effects manifest. Constipation seems to be the only side effect that is equivalent across the board.

Morphine is typically the first-line strong opioid of choice for treating severe pain. Although most patients achieve adequate analgesia with morphine, a significant number suffer either intolerable side effects, inadequate pain relief, or both. Switching these patients to an alternative opioid is becoming established clinical practice. For patients with inadequate pain relief and intolerable opioid-related toxicity/adverse effects, a switch to an alternative opioid may be the only option for symptomatic relief. However, the evidence to support this practice is largely anecdotal or based on observational and uncontrolled studies. Randomized trials, including "N of 1" studies, where a patient acts as their own control, are needed: first, to establish the true effectiveness of this clinical practice; second, to determine which opioid should be used first-line or second-line; and third, to standardize conversion ratios when switching from one opioid to another.[27]

Opioid-containing medications are age-old remedies for controlling cancer-related pain. Among the important advances in the past decade in the treatment of cancer pain is the realization that the goals of care and the best means of achieving them differ not only among individuals, but also for a single patient throughout a long course of care. Physicians must not only be knowledgeable, but also flexible in their approach to managing cancer pain. An understanding of the range of opioid agents and the formulations available can allow physicians to maintain the best possible quality of life for their patients with chronic pain.

## Adjuvant Therapies

### Nonsteroidal Anti-inflammatory Drugs

On the basis of limited data, nonsteroidal anti-inflammatory drugs (NSAIDs) appear to be more effective than placebo for cancer pain. Clear evidence to support superior safety or efficacy of one NSAID compared with another is lacking. Trials of combinations of an NSAID with an opioid have disclosed either no significant difference or at most a slight but statistically significant advantage compared with either single entity.[28] The cyclooxygenase-2 (COX-2) selective inhibitors are not expected to be any more efficacious than the standard NSAIDs, but have less gastrointestinal irritation. Rofecoxib (Vioxx) was pulled from the market because evidence indicated that this agent increased the risk of cardiac ischemia and cerebrovascular incidents. It remains to be seen what impact, if any, this will have on the remaining COX-2 inhibitors under study.

### Steroids

Spinal cord and nerve root compression following epidural metastasis is a dreaded complication of metastatic cancer. Severe pain is the most common presentation. Steroids can provide significant relief of pain and improve the patient's quality of life. Glucocorticosteroids are believed to exert their influence on brain tumors mainly by reducing the tumor-associated vasogenic edema, probably by decreasing the increased capillary permeability of the blood-brain barrier. Although some prefer methylprednisolone, dexamethasone is the glucocorticosteroid given to most neuro-oncology patients, at an empirically chosen dosage of 4 mg four times a day; lower doses in a twice-daily regimen may be sufficient. Side effects may be divided into three groups: those originating from the mineralocorticoid activity, from withdrawal of the drug, and from chronic excess glucocorticosteroid administration. Steroid myopathy is the most frequent occurring serious side effect in neuro-oncology patients. Others include gastrointestinal perforation and hemorrhage, opportunistic infections, steroid diabetes, and skin and facial changes. The most important interaction is that with phenytoin. Phenytoin uniformly decreases the levels of dexametrasone, accelerating its metabolism through induction of hepatic microsomal enzymes.[29]

### Anticonvulsants

Anticonvulsant adjuvant medications are used primarily to treat pain secondary to neural damage or irritation. Nerve injury pain and sympathetically maintained pain are treated more frequently with adjuvant analgesics, especially antidepressants and anticonvulsants. For many years this anticonvulsant was used off label for control of neuropathic pain syndromes. Gabapentin has stood the test of time and continues to be the medication of choice when neuropathic pain is suspected because of its favorable side effect profile. Efficacy has been demonstrated in control trials for use in small-fiber neuropathy and other neuropathic pain related to cancer invasion and treatment.[30]

### Bisphosphonates

Bisphosphonates are potent inhibitors of osteoclast-mediated bone resorption. It is well accepted that tumor cells in bone can stimulate osteoclast formation and activity, leading to the release of growth factors or cytokines, which will further stimulate cancer cell growth and secretion of osteolytic factors. Bisphosphonates are now the standard treatment for cancer hypercalcemia. Clodronate is the most potent drug available in this class and has a longer lasting effect. It has been reported that pamidronate infusions exert clinically relevant analgesic effects in more than half of patients with metastatic bone pain, but randomized, controlled trials have yet to definitively show efficacy of these agents as analgesics for bone pain.[31,32] Perhaps nonresponding patients should be treated with higher doses.

### Psychostimulants

A variety of psychostimulants have been studied and are used clinically as adjuvant therapy for uncontrolled pain. Typically these drugs are used with opioid medications to counter sedative effects and fatigue complaints. Methylphenidate and dextroamphetamine have been the primary agents used in this regard. A number of studies have been conducted to estimate expected benefits and side effects of these adjuncts. In a recent publication, Bruera and colleagues showed that not only were fatigue complaints improved with methylphenidate (5 mg q 2 hours p.r.n.), but that anxiety, appetite, pain, nausea, depression, and drowsiness also all improved significantly.[33] This is in keeping with the concept that a multidimensional approach is essential to good analgesia in cancer patients.

## CONCLUSION

The cancer patient with chronic painful symptoms that resist initial efforts at symptom control presents a complex conundrum, requiring a multidimensional approach to seize control and relieve the pain. Patients with severe pain often have multiple mechanisms that produce the painful symptoms, each requiring a different approach for relief. Many patients expect complete relief of their pain or other symptoms, and many doctors believe that increasing the dose of the opioid can relieve all pain. The reality is that not all pain complaints can be completely purged in all circumstances, but if barriers to good analgesic techniques can be reduced and a multidimensional approach can be the rule, most patients can enjoy a reduction in their pain and an improvement in their quality of life. It is recommended that an aggressive approach on all fronts as early as possible in the course of a patient's management. The evidence suggests that attention to psychosocial issues, aggressive opioid and adjuvant regimens, and application of interventional therapy early in the course of the patient's complaints offer the best opportunity for relief and satisfaction for both the patient and the health care provider.

## REFERENCES

1. Patrick DL, Ferketich SL, Frame PS, et al: National Institutes of Health State-of-the-Science Conference Statement: Symptom management in cancer: pain, depression, and fatigue, July 15 to 17, 2002. J Natl Cancer Inst Monogr 2004;9–16. (IV, C)
2. Fleishman SB: Treatment of symptom clusters: pain, depression, and fatigue. J Natl Cancer Inst Monogr 2004;119–123. (IV, C)
3. Miaskowski C, Dodd M, Lee K: Symptom clusters: the new frontier in symptom management research. J Natl Cancer Inst Monogr 2004; 17–21. (IV, C)
4. Portenoy RK, Lesage P: Management of cancer pain. Lancet 1999; 353:1695–1700. (Ib, A)
5. Strasser F, Sweeney C, Willey J, et al: Impact of a half-day multidisciplinary symptom control and palliative care outpatient clinic in a comprehensive cancer center on recommendations, symptom intensity, and patient satisfaction: a retrospective descriptive study. J Pain Symptom Manage 2004;27:481–491. (III, B)
6. Edwards BK, Howe HL, Ries LA, et al: Annual report to the nation on the status of cancer, 1973–1999, featuring implications of age and aging on U.S. cancer burden. Cancer 2002;94:2766–2792. (IV, C)
7. Green CR, Anderson KO, Baker TA, et al: The unequal burden of pain: confronting racial and ethnic disparities in pain. Pain Med 2003; 4:277–294. (Ib, A)
8. Payne R, Medina E, Hampton JW: Quality of life concerns in patients with breast cancer: evidence for disparity of outcomes and experiences in pain management and palliative care among African-American women. Cancer 2003;97:311–317. (IV, C)
9. Tammemagi CM, Neslund-Dudas C, Simoff M, et al: Lung carcinoma symptoms—An independent predictor of survival and an important mediator of African-American disparity in survival. Cancer 2004; 101:1655–1663. (IV, C)
10. Vaishampayan UN, Do H, Hussain M, et al: Racial disparity in incidence patterns and outcome of kidney cancer. Urology 2003;62:1012–1017. (IIb, B)
11. Mercadante S, Fulfaro F, Casuccio A: Pain mechanisms involved and outcome in advanced cancer patients with possible indications for celiac plexus block and superior hypogastric plexus block. Tumori 2002; 88:243–245. (IIb, B)
12. Rigor BM: Pelvic cancer pain. J Surg Oncol 2000;75:280–300. (III, B)
13. Davis MP, Walsh D: Epidemiology of cancer pain and factors influencing poor pain control. Am J Hosp Palliat Care 2004;21:137–142. (III, B)
14. Mercadante S: Opioid rotation for cancer pain: rationale and clinical aspects. Cancer 1999;86:1856–1866. (Ia, A)
15. Sevcik MA, Luger NM, Mach DB, et al: Bone cancer pain: the effects of the biophosphonate alternative on pain, skeletal remodeling, tumor growth, and tumor necrosis. Pain 2004;111:169–180. (Ib, A)
16. Paice JA: Assessment of symptom clusters in people with cancer. J Natl Cancer Inst Monogr 2004;98–102. (IV, C)
17. de Oliveira R, dos Reis MP, Prado WA: The effects of early or late neurolytic sympathetic plexus block on the management of abdominal or pelvic cancer pain. Pain 2004;110:400–408. (Ib, A)
18. Cariati M, De Martini G, Pretolesi F, et al: CT-guided superior hypogastric plexus block. J Comput Assist Tomogr 2002;26:428–431. (III, B)
19. Leon-Casasola OA, Kent E, Lema MJ: Neurolytic superior hypogastric plexus block for chronic pelvic pain associated with cancer. Pain 1993; 54:145–151. (IIb, B)
20. de Oliveira R, dos Reis MP, Prado WA: The effects of early or late neurolytic sympathetic block on the management of abdominal or pelvic cancer pain. Pain 2004;110:400–408. (Ia, A)
21. Eisenach JC, DuPen S, Dubois M, et al: Epidural clonidine analgesia for intractable cancer pain. The Epidural Clonidine Study Group. Pain 1995;61:391–399. (Ib, A)

22. Staats PS, Yearwood T, Charapata SG, et al: Intrathecal ziconotide in the treatment of refractory pain in patients with cancer or AIDS: a randomized controlled trial. JAMA 2004;291:63–70. **(Ib, A)**

23. Smith TJ, Staats PS, Deer T, et al: Randomized clinical trial of an implantable drug delivery system compared with comprehensive medical management for refractory cancer pain: impact on pain, drug-related toxicity, and survival. J Clin Oncol 2002;20:4040–4099. **(Ib, A)**

24. Staats P, Smith T, Deer T, et al: Randomized comparison of Medtronic intrathecal drug delivery systems (IDDS) plus comprehensive medical management (CMM) vs. CMM for unrelieved cancer pain. Pain Med 2001;2:251–252. **(Ib, A)**

25. Gottschalk A, Schroeder F, Ufer M, et al: Amantadine, a N-methyl-D-aspartate receptor antagonist, does not enhance postoperative analgesia in women undergoing abdominal hysterectomy. Anesth Analg 2001; 93:192–196. **(Ib, A)**

26. Mercadante S, Casuccio A, Agnello A, et al: Morphine versus methadone in the pain treatment of advanced-cancer patients followed up at home. J Clin Oncol 1998;16:3656–3661. **(Ib, A)**

27. Quigley C: Opioid switching to improve pain relief and drug tolerability. Cochrane Database Syst Rev 2004;CD004847. **(Ia, A)**

28. McNicol E, Strassels S, Goudas L, et al: Nonsteroidal anti-inflammatory drugs, alone or combined with opioids, for cancer pain: a systematic review. J Clin Oncol 2004;22:1975–1992. **(Ia, A)**

29. Lackner TE: The interaction of dexamethasone with phenytoin. Pharmacotherapy 1991;11:344–347. **(IV, C)**

30. Caraceni A, Zecca E, Bonezzi C, et al: Gabapentin for neuropathic cancer pain: a randomized controlled trial from the Gabapentin Cancer Pain Study Group. J Clin Oncol 2004;22:2909–2917. **(Ia, A)**

31. Carr DB, Goudas LC, Balk EM, et al: Evidence report on the treatment of pain in cancer patients. J Natl Cancer Inst Monogr 2004; 23–31. **(Ia, A)**

32. Small EJ, Smith MR, Seaman JJ, et al: Combined analysis of two multicenter, randomized, placebo-controlled studies of pamidronate disodium for the palliation of bone pain in men with metastatic prostate cancer. J Clin Oncol 2003;21:4277–4284. **(Ia, A)**

33. Bruera E, Driver L, Barnes EA, et al: Patient-controlled methylphenidate for the management of fatigue in patients with advanced cancer: a preliminary report. J Clin Oncol 2003;21:4439–4443. **(Ib, A)**

# Chapter 51

# Cancer Genetics

## Oliver Dorigo, MD, PhD, and Jonathan S. Berek, MD, MMSc

### KEY POINTS

- Cancer is a genetic disease that results from a series of mutations in various cancer genes.
- Cancer gene mutations affect genes that are responsible for control of normal cell proliferation and cell death (gatekeeper genes), and genes that control genomic stability (caretaker genes).
- Cancer predisposing genes are categorized into oncogenes, tumor suppressor genes, and stability genes.
- The majority of gynecologic malignancies are a result of sporadic mutations.
- Hereditary syndromes in gynecologic cancers include genomic mutations in *BRCA1* and *BRCA2* genes (ovarian cancer), and mismatch repair gene alterations (endometrial cancer).

Cancer is caused by the accumulation of various genetic mutations that lead to the transformed phenotype. A tumor may arise through the accumulation of somatic mutations or the inheritance of one or more mutations through the germline followed by additional somatic mutations. Mutations in genes that are directly involved in normal cellular growth and proliferation can lead to the development of uncontrolled cell growth, invasion, and metastasis.

All cells in a tumor arise from a single cell in which the regulatory mechanisms of proliferation have been disrupted. Based on the Knudson hypothesis, first described in children with hereditary retinoblastoma, two hits or mutations are required within the genome of a cell to develop into the malignant phenotype.[1] In hereditary cancer, the first hit is present in the genome of every cell, therefore requiring only one additional hit to disrupt the correct function of the second cancer gene allele. In contrast, sporadic cancers develop in cells that don't harbor mutations in the cancer-predisposing alleles. In this case, both hits must occur in a single somatic cell that disrupts both cancer gene alleles[2] (Fig. 51-1).

Cancer-causing mutations include gain of function mutations that convert proto-oncogenes into oncogenes, loss of function mutations that inactivate tumor suppressor genes, and disruption of cellular mechanisms that preserve genomic integrity. Epigenetic changes such as DNA methylation of, for example, "promoter" sequences of tumor suppressor genes might also contribute to malignant transformation. Promoter methylation can impair the transcription of the following open reading frame of a gene and therefore cause reduced or absent expression of that particular gene. These genetic and epigenetic changes are collectively responsible for the development of cancer characterized by growth factor independence, diminished susceptibility to *apoptosis* (programmed cell death), the ability to invade and metastasize, induction of angiogenesis, and escape from immunity and senescence.

Mathematical models based on age-specific cancer incidence and spontaneous mutation rates have shown that most adult solid tumors require 5 to 10 rate-limiting mutations to acquire the malignant phenotype. The most compelling evidence for the mutagenic tumor development process is that the age-specific incidence rates for most human epithelial tumors increase at roughly the fourth to eighth power of elapsed time. Although the precise number of mutations in solid tumors is unknown, it is important to distinguish between mutations that cause the cancer phenotype and other mutations, which might be considered bystander mutations (e.g., the amplification of genes that are adjacent to an oncogene).

## CANCER GENES

About 300 human genes are implicated in tumorigenesis, accounting for more than 1% of genes from the human genome.[3] The molecular effects of cancer genes are mediated by proteins. Overall, approximately 90% of cancer genes show somatic mutations and up to 20% show germline mutations. In general, the spectrum of neoplasms associated with germline mutations in a particular gene is similar to that reported with somatic mutations. Exceptions include the neoplasms related to the tumor suppressor gene *TP53* and *BRCA1/BRCA2*. *TP53* mutations are found in about 50% of colorectal cancers, yet germline mutations, as observed in the Li-Fraumeni syndrome, do not cause a predisposition to colorectal cancer. In contrast, germline mutations of the *BRCA1* and *BRCA2* genes confer a high incidence of breast and ovarian cancer, but somatic mutations are found very infrequently in sporadic cancers of the same type.

Most somatic mutations involve chromosomal translocations that result in chimeric transcripts, with juxtaposition of one gene to the regulatory region of another gene. This mutation type is most commonly reported in leukemias, lymphomas, and mesenchymal tumors. The Philadelphia chromosome in chronic myeloid leukemia, for example, is the result of a reciprocal translocation between one chromosome 9 and one chromosome 22. This translocation results in one chromosome 9 that is longer than normal and one chromosome 22 that is shorter than normal. The DNA sequence removed from chromosome 9 contains the proto-oncogene *ABL* and inserts into the *BCR* gene sequence on chromosome 22 *(Philadelphia chromosome)*. The resulting chimeric *bcr-abl* gene product functions as a constitutively active tryrosine kinase and stimulates cellular proliferation, for example,

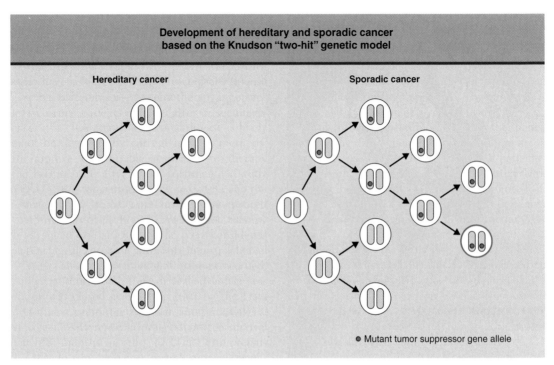

**Figure 51-1    Development of hereditary and sporadic cancer based on the Knudson "two-hit" genetic model.** In hereditary cancers, all cells harbor one mutant tumor suppressor gene allele. The loss of the second allele will result in the malignant phenotype. In contrast, sporadic cancers develop in cells with normal genomes, therefore requiring both alleles to be inactivated (two hits).

via an increase of growth factors. Epithelial neoplasms such as thyroid papillary carcinoma and breast secretory carcinomas have been reported to harbor chromosomal translocations that are likely responsible for the development of the malignant phenotype. Other cancer gene mutations involve base substitutions that can result in missense amino acid changes, non-sense changes, and alterations in splice sites. Insertions or deletions in coding sequences or splice sites can cause in-frame or frame-shifting mutations, resulting in loss of protein function. Increased gene copy numbers can lead to overexpression of proteins like proto-oncogenes. In contrast, decreased gene copy numbers result in loss of sufficient protein function (Table 51-1).

### Gatekeepers and Caretakers
Cancer susceptibility genes are divided into gatekeepers and caretakers. Gatekeeper genes act directly to control cellular proliferation. They are divided into oncogenes, which elicit a stimulatory effect on growth and proliferation, and tumor suppressor genes, which suppress cell growth.[4] Gatekeepers directly prevent the development of tumors by inhibiting growth

or promoting cell death. Mutations of a gatekeeper gene result in a risk of developing cancer at least 100 times greater than in the general population. Examples of gatekeeper genes include the tumor suppressor genes *TP53* and the *RB1* (retinoblastoma) gene (Table 51-2).

Caretaker genes (stability genes) preserve the integrity of the genome and are involved in DNA repair and maintenance of genomic integrity. The inactivation of caretakers facilitates the development of mutations in gatekeeper genes and other cancer-related genes. Caretakers, like gatekeepers, may be tissue specific, but mutation in the caretaker is neither necessary nor sufficient for the development of cancer. The DNA mismatch repair genes *MLH1*, *MSH2*, and *MSH6* are examples of caretaker genes.

### Oncogenes
Oncogenes comprise a family of genes that result from gain of function mutations of their normal counterparts, proto-oncogenes. The normal function of proto-oncogenes is to drive cell proliferation in the appropriate context. Activated oncogenes act in a dominant fashion to stimulate cell proliferation or

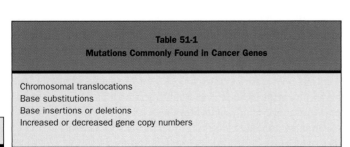

| Table 51-1 |
| --- |
| **Mutations Commonly Found in Cancer Genes** |
| Chromosomal translocations |
| Base substitutions |
| Base insertions or deletions |
| Increased or decreased gene copy numbers |

| Table 51-2 |
| --- |
| **Classification of Cancer Genes** |
| **Gatekeeper genes:** control of cell proliferation and cell death |
|    Oncogenes: stimulate cell growth |
|    Tumor suppressor genes: induce cell growth arrest |
| **Caretaker genes:** preserve genomic stability |
| **Stability genes** |

development of the malignant phenotype. It is important to note that this requires the mutation of only one allele.

Oncogenes were initially discovered via the mechanism of retroviral tumorigenesis. Viral transduction of mammalian cells can lead to integration of the viral sequences into the proto-oncogene sequence of the host cell. The integrated viral promoter activates transcription from the surrounding DNA sequences, including the proto-oncogene. Subsequent overexpression of the proto-oncogene sequences results in the expression of growth factors, growth factor receptors, signal transduction proteins, nuclear proto-oncogenes, and transcription factors. The resulting cellular effect is stimulation of cell proliferation. One of the most important group of viral oncogenes is the family of *RAS* genes, which include c-H(Harvey)-*ras*, c-K(Kirsten)-*ras*, and N(neuroblastoma)-*ras*. Human homologs of c-H-*ras* and c-K-*ras* murine sarcoma virus oncogenes were identified using in vitro assays to screen for active transformation of mouse fibroblasts. The third, N-*ras*, was found in human neuroblastoma and fibrosarcoma cell lines.

Proto-oncogene growth factors include platelet-derived growth factor (PDGF), epidermal growth factor (EGF), insulin-like growth factors I and II (IGF-I and IGF-II), and transforming growth factor α and β (TGF-α and TGF-β). Growth factor receptors mediate the stimulatory effect of growth factors and the intracellular signaling pathways. Examples include the two transmembrane receptor protein tyrosine kinases RET and MET, which are mutated in multiple endocrine neoplasia type II and familial papillary renal cancer. Proto-oncogene signaling includes membrane-associated guanine nucleotide proteins such as *RAS* and membrane-associated cytoplasmic protein tyrosine kinases (e.g., *ABL* and *SRC*). The *MYC* genes are examples of nuclear proto-oncogenes. Amplification of the *MYC* genes has been found in a variety of tumor types, including ovarian cancer.

## Tumor Suppressor Genes

Tumor suppressor genes are involved in the development of most cancers and are usually inactivated in a two-step process in which both copies of the tumor suppressor gene are mutated or inactivated by epigenetic mechanisms such as methylation.[5] The most commonly mutated tumor suppressor gene in human cancers is *TP53*. The p53 protein regulates transcription of other genes involved in cell-cycle arrest such as *P21*. Up-regulation of *TP53* expression is induced by DNA damage and contributes to cell-cycle arrest, allowing DNA repair to occur. *TP53* also plays an important role in the initiation of apoptosis. Interestingly, the most common mechanism of inactivation of *TP53* differs from the classic two-hit model. In most cases, missense mutations that change a single amino acid in the DNA-binding domain of *TP53* results in overexpression of nonfunctional p53 protein in the nucleus of the cell.

The identification of tumor suppressor genes has been facilitated by positional cloning strategies. The main approaches are cytogenetic studies to identify chromosomal alterations in tumor specimens, DNA linkage techniques to localize genes involved in inherited predisposition to cancer, and examination for loss of heterozygosity or allele among studies in sporadic tumors. Comparative genomic in situ hybridization allows fluorescence identification of chromosome gain and loss in human cancers within a similar experiment.

## Stability Genes

The third class of cancer genes, called stability genes, promote tumorigenesis in a way that differs from tumor suppressor genes or amplified oncogenes. Stability genes function mainly to preserve the correct DNA sequence during DNA replication (caretaker function). Mistakes made during normal DNA replication or induced by exposure to mutagens can be repaired by a variety of mechanisms that involve mismatch repair genes, nuclear-type excision repair, and base excision repair genes. Inactivation of stability genes leads to a higher mutation rate in potentially all genes. However, only mutations in oncogenes and tumor suppressor genes influence cell proliferation and confer a selective growth advantage to the mutant cell. As with tumor suppressor genes, both alleles of stability genes must be activated to cause loss of function.

## HEREDITARY CANCER

A small number of cancers arise on a heritable genomic background. Germline mutations require additional mutations at one or more loci for tumorigenesis. These mutations can be acquired via either environmental factors such as ionizing radiation or mutations of stability genes, further increasing the chance of spontaneous mutations. Hereditary cancers are characterized by a relatively early age of onset compared with similar sporadic tumors. The germline mutations in hereditary cancer might confirm a phenotype in multiple tissues. The production of multiple phenotypic effects by a single mutant gene is called *pleiotropy*. Different manifestations among members of a family with the same genetic defect is also called *variable expressivity*. Because the development of cancer is a multistep process involving more than the germline mutation, genetically cancer-prone individuals might not develop a phenotype because of insufficient somatic hits. The event of a gene carrier escaping all manifestations of disease is called a *nonpenetrant carrier*. This concept might explain why some women with *BRCA1* or *BRCA2* mutations do not develop breast or ovarian cancer during their lifetime yet are at high risk for development of these diseases.

Several multisystem genetic syndromes with a high risk of cancer have been described. The Li-Fraumeni syndrome with germline mutations in *TP53* and the *CHEK2* gene is associated with early-onset breast cancer, childhood soft tissue sarcoma, osteosarcoma, brain tumors, adrenocortical carcinoma, and acute leukemia. The hereditary nonpolyposis colorectal cancer syndrome (HNPCC) is an autosomal dominant disorder that confers a high lifetime risk of colon, endometrial, stomach, ureteral, and ovarian cancer. The genes responsible for the phenotype of the HNPCC syndrome involve mutations in mismatch repair genes such as *MLH1*, *MSH2*, and *MSH6*. Table 51-3 summarizes hereditary cancer syndromes that are associated with gynecologic tumors.

## CANCER GENETICS IN GYNECOLOGIC CANCERS

### Genetics of Breast and Ovarian Cancer

Ovarian carcinoma is generally a monoclonal disease that originates in the ovaries. Both familial and sporadic cases of ovarian cancer require the accumulation of genetic mutations.

**Table 51-3**
**Hereditary Tumor Syndromes Associated with Gynecologic Tumors**

| | Hereditary Syndrome | Associated Tumors |
|---|---|---|
| **Tumor suppressor genes** | | |
| TP53, CHEK2 | Li-Fraumeni syndrome | Breast cancer, soft tissue sarcoma, adrenocortical carcinoma, brain tumor |
| PTEN | Cowden syndrome<br>Bannayan-Zonana syndrome | Breast cancer, hamartoma, glioma, endometrial cancer |
| Menin | Multiple endocrine neoplasia type I | Cancer of thyroid, pancreas, and pituitary; ovarian carcinoid |
| PRKARIA | Carney complex | Cardiac and cutaneous myxoma, adrenal adenoma, thyroid, testes, ovary |
| STK11 | Peutz-Jeghers syndrome | Gastrointestinal hamartomatous polyps; tumors of the stomach, duodenum, and colon; ovarian sex cord tumor with annular tubules (SCTAT) |
| **Stability genes** | | |
| BRCA1, BRCA1 | Hereditary breast and ovarian cancer | Cancer of breast, ovary, and fallopian tube |
| MLH1, MSH2, MSH3, MSH6, PMS2 | Hereditary nonpolyposis colorectal cancer (HNPCC) | Cancer of colon, endometrium, ovary, stomach, small bowel, and urinary tract |
| **Oncogenes** | | |
| RET | Multiple endocrine neoplasia type II | Cancer of thyroid and parathyroid; pheochromocytoma, ovarian carcinoid |

The mechanism of these mutations is unclear. However, the frequency of ovulation has been correlated with the incidence of epithelial ovarian cancer. In general the inhibition of ovulation (e.g., during pregnancy or contraceptive use) protects against the development of ovarian cancer. It is unclear how ovulation leads to mutations in the ovarian surface epithelial cells. Mutations in the ovarian surface epithelium might result in errors in DNA synthesis during the repair of ovulatory defects because spontaneous mutations are more likely to occur in cells that are proliferating compared to cells at rest. Although DNA repair mechanisms usually maintain high-grade fidelity of DNA synthesis, the efficiency of DNA repair systems may vary among individuals and therefore result in persistent mutagenic changes.

### Family History of Breast and Ovarian Cancer

Approximately 5% to 10% of women in the general population have a first-degree relative with breast cancer, and about twice as many have either a first-degree or a second-degree relative with breast cancer. The relative risk of breast cancer conferred by a first-degree relative with breast cancer is about 2.1.[6] The relative risk is dependent on the age of diagnosis: the younger the affected relative, the greater the risk to the related individual. Other important factors that influence the relative risk are the number of affected relatives and the closeness of their biologic relationship. The larger the number of affected relatives and the closer the biologic relationship, the greater the risk.

The lifetime risk for developing ovarian cancer in the United States is approximately 1 in 70, or 1.4%. The single greatest ovarian cancer risk factor is a family history of the disease. Several studies have evaluated the risk of developing ovarian cancer in relatives of ovarian cancer cases compared with controls. In a meta-analysis that included the Cancer and Steroid Hormone (CASH) study, the relative risk for ovarian cancer was 3.1 for a woman with a single first-degree relative with ovarian cancer and 4.6 for a woman with two or three

relatives with ovarian cancer. This translates into lifetime probabilities for ovarian cancer of 5.0% and 7.2%, respectively.[7] About 12% of invasive ovarian cancer results from a hereditary predisposition. The family characteristics that suggest hereditary breast and ovarian cancer predisposition include the occurrence of cancer at an earlier age than in sporadic cases, two or more primary cancers in a single individual, and cases of male breast cancer (Table 51-4).

### BRCA1 and BRCA2

No single gene conferring increased susceptibility to ovarian cancer alone has been isolated. The majority of germline mutations that control the risk for ovarian and breast cancer occur in the BRCA1 and BRCA2 genes. Genetic linkage initially identified a susceptibility gene for breast cancer on the long arm of chromosome 17. Subsequent positional cloning identified the BRCA1 gene. The second breast cancer susceptibility gene, BRCA2, was localized to the long arm of chromosome 13 through linkage studies of 15 families with multiple cases of breast cancer that were not linked to BRCA1. Mutations in BRCA2 are not only associated with breast and ovarian cancer, but are also linked to male breast cancer, prostate cancer, and pancreatic cancer.

The risk estimates of developing breast and ovarian cancer in patients with mutations in BRCA1 and BRCA2 vary. The range of risk estimates is caused by a number of different factors,

**Table 51-4**
**Family Characteristics Suggestive of Hereditary Breast and Ovarian Cancer**

Early age of onset
Two or more primary breast and/or ovarian cancers in a single individual
Cases of male breast cancer

including the variable penetrance of different mutations. For example, *BRCA2* mutations that occur in families with a high risk of ovarian cancer are clustered in the central portion of the gene, which has been termed the ovarian cancer cluster region (OCCR), between nucleotides 3059 to 4075 and 6503 to 6629. Mutations in this region are associated with a significantly lower risk of breast cancer and a significantly higher risk of ovarian cancer. Based on recent studies, the lifetime risk of breast cancer among female *BRCA1/BRCA2* mutation carriers is up to 87%, which is similar to risks in families with many cases. For ovarian cancer, lifetime risk estimates range between 44% and 68% by age 70. In a recent study, the risk to develop ovarian cancer was found to be 54% for *BRCA1* and 23% for *BRCA2* mutation carriers, respectively.[8]

In the general population, *BRCA1/BRCA2* mutations occur at a frequency of about 1 in 250 women, with probably 250,000 carriers in the United States. Most *BRCA1/BRCA2* mutation carriers are identified in ovarian cancer patients with a family history significant for early age of diagnosis, dual primary cancers of the breast and ovaries, or relatives affected by breast and ovarian cancer. The occurrence of at least two cases of ovarian cancer and at least two cases of breast cancer relates to an estimated likelihood of 56% to 63% for *BRCA1* mutations. Among cases identified from the Cancer Surveillance System of Western Washington, the frequency of *BRCA1* mutations was highest in cases diagnosed before age 30 (23%) and in those with more than three relatives with breast cancer (20%). A family history of ovarian cancer in a first-degree relative was also associated with an increased prevalence of *BRCA1* mutations (25%). In another study of 263 women with familial breast cancer, *BRCA1* mutations were found in 7% of families with site-specific breast cancer, 18% of families with bilateral breast cancer, and 40% of families with both breast and ovarian cancer. In a population-based series of incident cases of ovarian cancer in Canada, the overall prevalence of *BRCA1/BRCA2* mutations was 11.7%.

The occurrence of specific *BRCA1/BRCA2* mutations in multiple apparently unrelated families is consistent with a "founder effect." These mutations can be traced back from a contemporary population to an early small group of founders. For example, two *BRCA1* mutations (185delAG and 5382insC) and one *BRCA2* mutation (6174delT) have been reported to be common in Ashkenazi Jews of Central and Eastern European descent. The overall frequency of these three mutations is about 2.5% among Ashkenazi Jews; they account for up to 90% of both breast and ovarian cancer in families with multiple cases. In contrast, in the general Jewish population, carrier frequencies for these mutations are lower: 0.9% for the 185delAG mutation, 0.3% for the 5382insC mutation, and 1.3% for the *BRCA2* 6174delT mutation. Additional founder mutations have been described in other ethnic groups, including from the Netherlands (*BRCA1* 2804delAA and several large deletion mutations), Iceland (*BRCA2*, 995del5), and Sweden (*BRCA1*, 3171ins5).[9]

### Biologic Functions of BRCA1 and BRCA2 Proteins

The *BRCA1* gene contains 24 exons that encode a protein of 1863 amino acids. The *BRCA2* protein is even larger, with 3418 amino acids. The *BRCA* genes were initially classified as tumor suppressor genes based on several observations. First, the hered-

itary breast and ovarian cancer syndrome is an autosomal dominant condition with one normal and one mutated *BRCA1* or *BRCA2* allele. In most breast and ovarian cancers that develop in mutation carriers, deletion of the normal allele with subsequent loss of *BRCA1/BRCA2* function is observed. The loss of the second allele in the process of carcinogenesis is a classic characteristic of tumor suppressor genes, suggesting a recessive function. Second, overexpression of the *BRCA1* protein leads to tumor growth suppression in vitro and in mouse models, another feature commonly associated with tumor suppressor genes.

However, based on recent biochemical evidence and data from knockout models, both *BRCA1* and *BRCA2* proteins play a much more complex role and are implicated in various cellular pathways that regulate DNA repair, cell-cycle progression, ubiquitination, and transcriptional regulation.[10] Cells deficient in BRCA1/BRCA2 sustain spontaneous aberrations of chromosome structures as seen, for example, in murine cells in culture. Similar structural aberrations occur in *BRCA1/BRCA2*-deficient human cancer cells. Gross chromosomal rearrangements might include triradial or quadriradial structures, markers of defective mitotic recombination. Collectively, these findings suggest that *BRCA* genes are essential for preserving chromosome structure and suppressing genome instability (caretaker function).

One of the common functions of both proteins is their role in homologous recombination as an important DNA repair mechanism. On DNA damage by ionizing radiation or chemotherapy, for example, the BRCA2 protein binds to the RAD51 protein, which is central for the repair of double-stranded breaks via homologous recombination. BRCA2 regulates the availability and activity of RAD51 in this key reaction. Phosphorylation of the BRCA2–RAD51 complex allows RAD51 to bind to the site of DNA damage and in conjunction with several other proteins to mediate repair of DNA by homologous recombination. In contrast, BRCA1 is involved more proximally in the cellular response to a double-stranded break. BRCA1 has a complex network of protein–protein interactions mediating DNA repair by homologous recombination and regulating transcription via the BRCA1-associated surveyant complex.

It is still unclear how cells deprived of BRCA1 and BRCA2 physiological functions develop into the malignant phenotype. Mice deprived of either protein by transgenic deletion of gene expression are embryonically lethal, suggesting that BRCA1 is critical for normal development. Most mutant strains exhibit an embryonic lethal phenotype due to cellular proliferation defects, genomic instability, and developmental retardation. Generally, mutations are found in every cell of the body, yet *BRCA1/BRCA2* mutations confer a malignant phenotype mainly for breast and ovarian cancer. The specificity of malignant transformation on a BRCA1-deficient background is still unclear. It is possible that the BRCA proteins play a much more important role in tumor suppression in breast and ovarian tissue compared to other tissues in the body that use alternative mechanisms for tumor suppression, even in the absence of BRCA protein function.

### Genetic Testing for Breast and Ovarian Cancer Syndrome

Genetic screening of high risk families provides useful prognostic information. Genetic testing to identify patients with germline

# Gynecologic Oncology

mutations should always be preceded by genetic counseling. The careful evaluation of an individual's medical and family history is crucial to estimate the likelihood for the presence of a cancer-predisposing mutation. Several algorithms are available to help calculating this likelihood. BRCAPRO, for example, is a statistical model that calculates the probability that an individual carries a germline mutation of the *BRCA1* and *BRCA2* genes. The model is based on family history of breast and ovarian cancer and uses a mendelian approach that assumes autosomal dominant inheritance.

The presence of specific mutations for certain populations allows testing for "ethnic-specific" alleles, facilitating genetic screening. In the Ashkenazi Jewish population, only 15% of *BRCA1* and *BRCA2* mutations are nonfounder mutations. However, in countries with ethnically mixed populations, such as the United States, the range of genetic variations is wide, making the search for cancer-causing genes more difficult. In general, the high frequency of mutations and the necessity to accurately communicate risks to patients before offering preventive options necessitates the estimation of penetrance of certain mutations. However, the penetrance of many mutations is still unclear. For example, the lifetime risk of developing breast or ovarian cancer is usually higher in *BRCA1* mutation carriers compared to carriers of the *BRCA2* mutation. In addition, the risk of ovarian cancer is not the same for all *BRCA2* mutations. Mutations in the central part of the gene, the OCCR, seem to confer a higher lifetime risk.

### Clinical Implications for BRCA1/BRCA2 Mutation Carriers

The identification of *BRCA1/BRCA2* mutation carriers has important clinical implications that pertain to risk reduction interventions and characteristic features of *BRCA*-associated cancers. Several studies have by now confirmed the effect of prophylactic salpingo-oophorectomy to reduce the incidence of ovarian and breast cancer in women with *BRCA1* and *BRCA2* mutations.[11] In one of the largest trials to date, 551 women carrying mutations in the *BRCA1* or *BRCA2* gene underwent either surveillance or bilateral prophylactic oophorectomy. The incidence of ovarian cancer in the surveillance group was 19.9% after 9 years' follow-up. In the group who underwent bilateral prophylactic oophorectomy, early-stage ovarian cancer was identified at the time of surgery in 2.3% of women and primary peritoneal cancer developed in two other patients (0.8%). This data shows a significant risk reduction with prophylactic surgery. Interestingly, the incidence of breast cancer in these predisposed individuals was also shown to be significantly reduced, from 42.3% in the surveillance group to 21.2% in the prophylactic oophorectomy group, likely due to a deprivation of ovarian hormone stimulation to the breast tissue.

Ovarian cancers that develop on a *BRCA1/BRCA2* mutation background are usually serous papillary carcinomas, although endometrioid and clear cell carcinomas have also been described. Borderline ovarian carcinomas rarely harbor mutations in either gene. Compared to sporadic ovarian cancers, *BRCA1/BRCA2*-associated ovarian cancers seem to be more sensitive to chemotherapeutic agents, particularly DNA damage-inducing agents. Carboplatin, for example, induces double-stranded DNA breaks. Cancer cells that lack the correct function of BRCA proteins cannot efficiently repair these DNA breaks and are therefore more sensitive to DNA damage. Several studies have shown an improved survival of patients with *BRCA1*-associated ovarian cancers compared to sporadic controls.[12] However, other studies have found no difference in survival.

## Genetics of Hereditary Endometrial Cancer

Approximately 5% to 10% of endometrial cancers are believed to be hereditary. The most important familial syndrome with a genetic predisposition for endometrial cancer is the hereditary nonpolyposis colorectal cancer (HNPCC) syndrome.[13] HNPCC, also known as Lynch II syndrome, is the most commonly occurring hereditary syndrome that predisposes to colorectal carcinoma. It accounts for approximately 2% to 7% of colorectal carcinoma diagnosed in the United States annually.[14]

Various extracolonic malignancies have been described in HNPCC families. Table 51-5 compares the incidence of HNPCC-associated cancers with the incidence of sporadic cancers. Individuals diagnosed with HNPCC have an up to 80% lifetime risk of colorectal cancer, a risk to develop endometrial cancer of about 60%, and a 12% lifetime risk of ovarian cancer. Another hallmark of HNPCC-affected individuals is the high incidence of second primary tumors. The most pronounced difference between endometrial cancer with genetic predisposition based on human mismatch repair gene mutations and sporadic cancer is the early age of onset in hereditary disease. The mean age of onset of endometrial cancer is about age 45 in women with HNPCC and age 68 for women with sporadic endometrial cancer.

HNPCC is caused by germline mutations of human mismatch repair genes like *MLH1*, *MSH2*, *MSH3*, *MSH6*, and *PMS2*.[15] The primary function of the mismatch repair genes is to eliminate base mismatches and insertion deletion loops that may arise during DNA replication. Repair of single base mismatches and insertion deletion loops requires at least six different mismatch repair proteins. For mismatched base recognition, the MSH2 protein forms a heterodimer with either MSH6 or MSH3. The proteins MLH1 and PMS2 form a heterodimer that coordinates the interplay between the mismatched recognition complex and other proteins necessary for mismatch repair.

| Table 51-5 Cancer Risk for *MLH1* and *MSH2* Mutation Carriers |||
|---|---|---|
| **Site** | **Population Risk** | **Hereditary Risk** |
| Colon | Risk of colon cancer 0.25% by age 50 2.0% by age 70 Risk of second cancer 3% within 10 yrs 5% within 15 yrs | Risk of colon cancer >25% by age 50 80% by age 70 Risk of second cancer 30% within 10 yrs 50% within 15 yrs |
| Endometrium | 0.2% by age 50 1.5% by age 70 | 20% by age 50 61% by age 70 |
| Stomach | 1% by age 70 | 13% by age 70 |
| Ovary | 1.2% by age 70 | 12% by age 70 |
| Urinary tract | <1% by age 70 | 4% by age 70 |
| Biliary tract | <1% by age 70 | 2% by age 70 |
| Small intestine | <1% by age 70 | 5% by age 70 |

Loss of DNA mismatch repair in cells leads to an accumulation of replication errors and genetic instability at short tandem repeat sequences known as *microsatellites*. This molecular phenotype, called *microsatellite instability*, is found in the majority of HNPCC-associated cancers and is a hallmark of DNA mismatch repair. Microsatellite instability has been demonstrated in 30% to 75% of endometrial and up to 100% of ovarian cancers from members of HNPCC families. In contrast, microsatellite instability is found in only 10% to 17% of sporadic ovarian cancers and 17% to 32% of sporadic endometrial cancers.[16] The decreased genomic stability in the absence of a correctly functioning mismatch repair system results in an elevated rate of mutations throughout the genome, including defects in tumor suppressor genes and inactivation of genes involved in DNA double-strand break repair. These mutations ultimately lead to the malignant phenotype. Germline mutations in one of the four major HNPCC-associated mismatch repair genes—*MLH1*, *MSH2*, *MSH6*, and *PMS2*—are detected in up to 80% of affected families. More than 400 different predisposing mismatch repair gene mutations are known, with 50% affecting *MLH1*, 40% *MSH2*, and 10% *MSH6*. Mutations in *PMS2* account for less than 5%.

### Genetic Screening for Hereditary Nonpolyposis Colerectal Cancer

HNPCC is one of the most common cancer syndromes in humans. Cancers are usually diagnosed at an early age and transmitted as an autosomal dominant trait. The international diagnostic criteria for HNPCC are known as Amsterdam I criteria (based on colorectal cancer) and Amsterdam II criteria (based on extracolonic cancers from the endometrium, small bowel, ureter, and renal pelvis). The majority of families that fulfill the clinical criteria also meet the molecular definition of the syndrome, which requires the demonstration of a heritable defect in mismatch repair genes. Molecular identification involves testing for microsatellite instability and sequencing of mismatch repair genes.

Current recommendations for women with HNPCC involve annual screening with endometrial biopsies, transvaginal ultrasound, and CA 125.[17] Prophylactic hysterectomy should be considered after completion of childbearing. In addition, initiation of annual full colonoscopy is recommended between ages 20 and 25. Ongoing trials are investigating the effects of oral contraceptives and progestins on the prevention of endometrial cancer in HNPCC women. Correction of the genetic defects in HNPCC families is a long-term goal that will require the development of efficient stem cell gene therapeutic approaches.

The following is the Amsterdam II Criteria for the identification of HNPCC families:

- Three or more relatives with HNPCC-associated cancers, including colorectal cancer or cancer of the endometrium, small bowel, ureter, or renal pelvis, plus all of the following
- One affected person is a first-degree relative of the other two
- Two or more successive generations are affected
- Cancer in one or more affected relatives diagnosed before age 50
- Exclusion of familial adenomatous polyposis in any cases of colorectal cancer
- Tumors verified by pathologic examination

## TUMOR ONCOGENES

Oncogenes encode proteins that are able to transform cells in cultures or induce cancer in animals. The word stems from the Greek work *onkos*, meaning a bulk or mass. Most oncogenes derive from genes whose products play a role in normal cell growth. Oncoproteins are either mutant forms or the same as the associated proto-oncogene product. A variety of oncogenes have been found to play a role in gynecologic malignancies (Table 51-6).

### K-RAS

The *RAS* genes acquire transforming activity either by enhanced expression or by a single point mutation. The predominant single base pair mutation site in ovarian tumors is found at codons 12 and 13. Mucinous ovarian neoplasms exhibit a higher incidence of K-*ras* mutations compared to the serous tumors.[18] K-*ras* codon 12 and 13 point mutations are found in up to 70% of mucinous ovarian neoplasms, including borderline tumors. In contrast, only about 10% of serous ovarian tumors harbor K-*ras* mutations. K-*ras* activation also plays a role in endometrial cancer, because expression of K-*ras* is found in endometrial hyperplasia and in invasive endometrial cancer. Mutations are found in 10% to 30% of endometrial cancer specimens and are associated with

**Table 51-6**
**Tumor Oncogenes in Gynecologic Malignancies**

| Gene | Protein | Function | Activation |
|------|---------|----------|------------|
| K-ras | G protein | Activation of signal transduction proteins | Mutation, overexpression |
| Akt | Protein kinase | Phosphorylation and activation of various proteins that promote cell survival and decrease apoptosis | Amplification |
| PIK3CA | Phosphoinositide 3 kinase | Phosphorylation of membrane-bound lipids | Amplification |
| c-myc (MYC) | Transcription factor | Transcriptional activation of genes that promote cell proliferation, regulation of apoptosis | Overexpression |
| HER-2/neu | Transmembrane tyrosine kinase | Activation of signal transduction pathways involved in regulation of cellular proliferation, differentiation, and survival | Amplification, overexpression |

the presence of lymph node metastasis. In cervical cancer, mucin-producing tumors have a greater incidence of K-*ras* mutations compared to nonmucin-secreting tumors.

## PIK3CA

Activation of the phosphatidylinositol 3-kinase (PI3-kinase) pathway either via down-regulation of *PTEN* expression or increased PI3-kinase activity plays an important role in certain subtypes of ovarian cancer. The *PIK3CA* gene encodes for the p110α subunit of PI3-kinase and is found at increased copy numbers in ovarian cancer specimens. *PIK3CA* functions as an oncogene, increasing the expression of PI3-kinase and subsequently the activation of Akt.[19] Activation of Akt is found in about one third of ovarian cancer specimens, with highest frequency in serous adenocarcinomas.

## HER2/Neu

The *HER2/Neu* proto-oncogene, also known as *ERBB2* and *HER2*, is located on the long arm of chromosome 17 and encodes a 185 kDa transmembrane glycoprotein with intrinsic tyrosine kinase activity. It belongs to a family of transmembrane receptor genes that includes the epidermal growth factor receptor *(ERBB1)*, *ERBB3*, and *ERBB4*. *HER2/Neu* has complex activation pathways and interacts with a variety of different cellular proteins that in general increase cell proliferation. Overexpression of *HER2/Neu* has been demonstrated in about 30% of breast cancers, 20% of advanced ovarian cancers, and up to 50% of endometrial cancers.[20] High tissue expression of *HER2/Neu* is correlated with a decreased overall survival, particularly in patients with endometrial cancer. Monoclonal antibodies against *HER2/Neu* can decrease growth of breast and ovarian cancer cells and have shown significant antitumor responses in breast cancer patients.

## c-myc

The c-*myc (MYC)* oncogene plays an important role in the malignant transformation of a variety of tumors, including breast, colon, and small cell lung cancers and lymphoma. The *MYC* gene encodes a transcription factor that in general activates genes that are involved in growth, protein synthesis, and mitochondrial function. Amplification and overexpression of the *MYC* gene is associated with poor prognosis and decreased survival. In ovarian cancer, amplification of the *MYC* gene is found in about 50%of cancers, particularly in advanced stages.[21] *MYC* is also implicated in the pathogenesis of cervical cancer.

## TUMOR SUPPRESSOR GENES

Tumor suppressor genes oppose the action of oncogenes via different pathways. In general, tumor suppressor activity is a result of inhibition of cell-cycle progression, stimulation of apoptosis, or promotion of senescence. Tumor suppressor genes are recessive and require biallelic inactivation for loss of function. They are frequently found to be inactivated in cancers and play a causal role in the initiation and progression of cancer. The reconstitution of tumor suppressor gene function in a cancer cell can reverse the malignant phenotype and induce growth arrest and cell death. Transgenic mouse models have provided insight

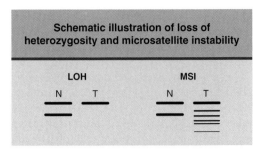

**Figure 51-2   Schematic illustration of loss of heterozygosity (LOH) and microsatellite instability (MSI).** DNA from tumor tissue (T) and normal tissue (N) can be analyzed using specific allelic markers. Separation of the DNA using gel electrophoresis will produce a specific band pattern for LOH and MSI. LOH is evident in DNA from tumor tissue compared to normal control tissue as lack of one of the allelic bands. In MSI, additional allelic bands are visible in the tumor tissue.

into critical pathways affected by tumor suppressor genes. For example, abrogation of *TP53* expression in *p53* knockout mice results in the development of various tumors by age 4 to 6 months. This model is similar to the human Li-Fraumeni syndrome.

A hallmark signature of tumor suppressor genes is an event known as *loss of heterozygosity* (LOH). LOH might be defined as a genetic event that can occur in the dividing cells of a diploid organism heterozygous for one or more markers, in which a daughter cell becomes homozygous or hemizygous for one or more alleles through mitotic recombination, deletion, or gene conversion. In the case of tumor suppressor genes, a cell heterozygous for one mutant and one normal allele loses heterozygosity if either the mutant or the normal allele is deleted. If the normal allele is lost, the correct function of the tumor suppressor activity for this gene is abrogated. Screening for LOH in tumor specimens using markers for specific DNA sequences is a common technique used to identify novel tumor suppressor gene (Fig. 51-2).

Tumor suppressor genes play a significant role in gynecologic malignancies. The most common genes, their proteins, and associated functions are summarized in Table 51-7. The

| Table 51-7 Tumor Suppressor Genes in Gynecologic Malignancies |||
| --- | --- | --- |
| **Gene** | **Protein** | **Function** |
| TP53 | Nuclear protein p53 | Transcription factor, involved in various cellular processes, including apoptosis, DNA damage response, angiogenesis |
| PTEN | Dual specificity phosphatase | Dephosphorylation of both lipids and proteins, down-regulation of the PI3-kinase/Akt pathway with negative effect on cell growth |
| P16INK4a (CDKN2A) | P16 | Binds to cyclin–CDK4 complex inhibiting cell-cycle progression |
| FHIT | Fragile histidine triad gene | Tumor suppressor function via unknown mechanisms |

mportance of individual tumor suppressor genes in gynecologic
cancers depends on the tissue of origin and its histology. For
example, the *TP53* tumor suppressor gene plays a significant
role in a large percentage of ovarian cancers, but only a few
endometrial cancers harbor *TP53* mutations. In contrast, *PTEN*
is found to be mutated in a high percentage of endometrioid
adenocarcinomas of the uterus, but does not play a significant
role in uterine papillary serous cancers or most other epithelial
ovarian cancers. The *FHIT* gene is a frequent integration site
for the human papillomavirus (HPV) and is of considerable
importance in cervical cancers but is not likely to be a major
factor in endometrial and ovarian cancer.

## TP53

The *TP53* tumor suppressor gene is located on chromosome
17p13.1 and encodes for a phosphoprotein that is generally
detectable in the nucleus of normal cells. On DNA damage, *p53*
can arrest cell-cycle progression to allow the DNA to be repaired
or undergo apoptosis. The lack of function of normal *p53* within
a cancer cell results in a loss of control of cell proliferation, with
inefficient DNA repair and genetic instability.

Mutations of the *TP53* gene occur in 40% to 80% of
epithelial ovarian cancers, but these mutations are not present in
borderline malignancy, benign tumors, or normal surface
epithelium.[22] Mutant *TP53* functions as a dominant negative
oncogene because introduction of mutant *TP53* into cancer cells
can lead to transformation into a more aggressive phenotype.
*TP53* overexpression is seen in approximately 4% to 17% of
borderline tumors, 10% to 15% of early cancers, and 40% to
50% of advanced cancers. Overexpression of mutant *TP53* is
significantly higher in advanced stages of ovarian cancer (40% to
50%) relative to expression of *TP53* in early stages (10% to
20%), suggesting that this is a late event in ovarian carcinogenesis.[23] Furthermore, mutant *TP53* overexpression has been
associated with worse survival, poor histologic grade and differentiation, and a high proliferative fraction. One explanation for
the poorer survival is possibly the chemoresistant phenotype in
*TP53* mutated tumors.

## PTEN

The *PTEN* (phosphatase and tensin homolog deleted on
chromosome 10) gene is a tumor suppressor gene that is located
on chromosome 10q23 and encodes a dual-specificity
phosphatase for both lipid and protein substrates. Germline
mutations have been identified in patients with Cowden
syndrome and Bannayan-Zonana syndrome, two rare, autosomal
dominant familial cancer syndromes with multiple abnormalities, including hamartomas and breast cancer.[24] Somatic
mutations of *PTEN* have been found in glioblastomas, melanomas,
and prostate, endometrium, and ovarian cancer.

The PTEN protein is an important factor in the PI3-kinase
pathway, an important pathway that promotes the proliferation
of cancer cells in vitro and in vivo[25] (Fig. 51-3). Activation of
PI3-kinase by various ligands such as PDGF and IGF results in
an increase of intracellular, membrane-bound phosphatidylinositol-
3,4-diphosphate (PIP$_2$) and phosphatidylinositol-3,4,5-
triphosphate (PIP$_3$). Akt is recruited to the membrane-bound
PIP$_3$ with its N-terminal Pleckstrin homology domain and is
phosphorylated by PIP$_3$-dependent kinase 1 (PDK-1) at

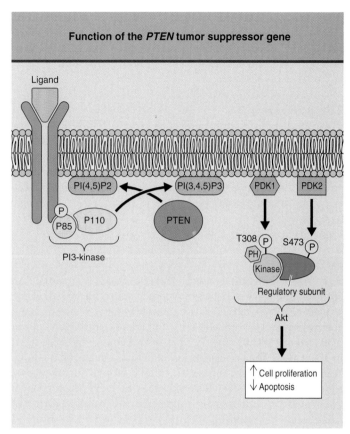

**Figure 51-3    Function of the *PTEN* tumor suppressor gene.** Activation
of PI3-kinase by various ligands, such as platelet-derived growth factor
or insulin growth factor, results in an increase of intracellular, membrane-
bound phosphatidylinositol-(3,4)-diphosphate (PIP2) and
phosphatidylinositol-(3,4,5)-triphosphate (PIP3). Akt is recruited to the
membrane bound PIP3 with its N-terminal Pleckstrin homology (PH)
domain and is phosphorylated by PIP3-dependent kinase 1 (PDK-1) at
threonine 308 (T308) and PKD-2 kinase at serine 473 (S473) for full
activation. Activated Akt is released from the membrane and elicits
downstream effects by phosphorylating signal-transduction proteins.
*PTEN* acts as a dual-specificity phosphatase that can dephosphorylate
proteins and phospholipids. In the PI3K/Akt pathway, *PTEN*
dephosphorylates PIP2 and PIP3 and, therefore, counteracts the function
of PI3K.

threonine 308 (T308) and PDK-2 kinase at serine 473 (S473)
for full activation. Activated Akt is released from the membrane
and elicits downstream effects by phosphorylating signal
transduction proteins. These effects lead to an increase in cell
proliferation, prevention of apoptosis, invasiveness, drug resistance, and neoangiogenesis.[26] *PTEN* acts as a dual-specificity
phosphatase that can dephosphorylate proteins and phospholipids.
In the PI3K/Akt pathway, *PTEN* dephosphorylates PIP$_2$ and
PIP$_3$ and therefore counteracts the function of PI3K.

Mutations of the *PTEN* gene have been identified as the most
frequently mutated tumor suppressor pathway in endometrial
cancer. Among the endometrioid histologic subtype of endometrial cancer, up to 50% contain mutations of *PTEN*. *PTEN*
mutations are also found in about 20% of endometrial cancer
precursors such as complex atypical hyperplasia, suggesting that
*PTEN* plays a role in early pathogenesis of these tumors. In

# Gynecologic Oncology

ovarian cancer, mutations of *PTEN* have been described in about 7% to 21%, with a higher frequency in the endometrioid subtype.[27] Other studies in human ovarian cancer specimens have shown frequent loss of PTEN protein expression.

## TGF-β Receptor 2

The transforming growth factor-β receptor 2 *(TGF-βR2)* tumor suppressor gene is part of the TGF-β growth inhibitory pathway. Mutations in the *TGF-βR2* genes cause loss of growth inhibition and enhance tumorigenicity in epithelial tumor cells. Mutations are found in about 25% of ovarian cancer cases and are more frequent in endometrioid carcinomas than other histologic subtypes.[28]

## FHIT

The fragile histidine triad *(FHIT)* gene is located on chromosome 3p14.2, the most common active fragile site of the human genome.[29] *FHIT* is a common target of chromosomal aberrations and a frequent HPV integration site involving the long arm of chromosome 3. It has been found to be inactivated in about 60% of all malignancies, including cancers of the lung, stomach, breast, and kidney. The FHIT protein functions as a tumor suppressor gene. Reconstitution of FHIT expression in FHIT-negative tumor cells suppresses the tumorigenicity of these cells and induces apoptosis. The exact mechanism of tumor suppression is still under investigation.

Alterations in the *FHIT* gene are found in various precursor lesions, including early cervical lesions. About 20% to 50% of high-grade squamous epithelial lesions show loss of *FHIT* function, suggesting an important role for *FHIT* in cervical carcinogenesis. An important mechanism that might explain the loss of *FHIT* function in cervical epithelium is related to the frequent infection with HPV. HPV can insert its genome into the chromosome 3 fragile site FRA3B and delete DNA sequences, including the *FHIT* gene.

## P16

The *p16INK4a (CDKN2A)* gene encodes for the p16 protein, which functions as a negative cell-cycle regulator. P16 binds to the cyclin-dependent kinase CDK4, inhibiting the catalytic activity of the CDK4–cyclin D complex. Mutations in the *p16INK4A* gene are rare in gynecologic cancers. The lack of p16 protein expression is, however, found in 20% to 70% of ovarian and endometrial cancers and is mostly a consequence of hypermethylation. In endometrial cancer, the loss of p16 protein expression has been associated with a higher proliferative index and poorer survival.[30]

## REFERENCES

1. Knudson AG II: Mutation and cancer: statistical study of retinoblastoma. Proc Natl Acad Sci USA 1971;68:820–823. **(IIa, B)**
2. Knudson AG: Two genetic hits (more or less) to cancer. Nat Rev Cancer 2001;1:157–162. **(IIa, B)**
3. Futreal PA, Coin L, Marshall M, et al: A census of human cancer genes. Nat Rev Cancer 2004;4:177–183. **(IIa, B)**
4. Vogelstein B, Kinzler KW: Cancer genes and the pathways they control. Nat Med 2004; 10:789–799. **(Ib, A)**
5. Sherr CJ: Principles of tumor suppression. Cell 2004;116:235–246.
6. Pharoah PD, Day NE, Duffy S, Easton DF, Ponder BA: Family history and the risk of breast cancer: a systematic review and meta-analysis. Int J Cancer 1997;71:800–809. **(Ia, A)**
7. Stratton JF, Pharoah P, Smith SK, et al: A systematic review and meta-analysis of family history and risk of ovarian cancer. Br J Obstet Gynaecol 1998;105:493–499. **(Ia, A)**
8. King MC, Marks JH, Mandell JB: Breast and ovarian cancer risks due to inherited mutations in *BRCA1* and *BRCA2*. Science 2003; 302:643–646. **(IIa, B)**
9. Arason A, Jonasdottir A, Barkardottir RB, et al: A population study of mutations and LOH at breast cancer gene loci in tumours from sister pairs: two recurrent mutations seem to account for all *BRCA1/BRCA2* linked breast cancer in Iceland. J Med Genet 1998;35:446–449. **(IIa, B)**
10. Narod SA: Modifiers of risk of hereditary breast and ovarian cancer. Nat Rev Cancer 2002;2:113–123.
11. Rebbeck TR: Prophylactic oophorectomy in BRCA1 and BRCA2 mutation carriers. Eur J Cancer 2002;38(Suppl 6):S15–S17. **(IIa, B)**
12. Boyd J, Sonoda Y, Federici MG, et al: Clinicopathologic features of BRCA-linked and sporadic ovarian cancer. JAMA 2000; 283:2260–2265. **(IIa, B)**
13. Berends MJ, Wu Y, Sijmons RH, et al: Toward new strategies to select young endometrial cancer patients for mismatch repair gene mutation analysis. J Clin Oncol 2003; 21:4364–4370. **(IIb, B)**
14. Lynch HT, de la Chapelle A: Hereditary colorectal cancer. N Engl J Med 2003;348:919–932. **(IIa, B)**
15. Peltomaki P: Role of DNA mismatch repair defects in the pathogenesis of human cancer. J Clin Oncol 2003;21:1174–1179. **(IIa, B)**
16. Drake AC, Campbell H, Porteous ME, Dunlop MG: The contribution of DNA mismatch repair gene defects to the burden of gynecological cancer. Int J Gynecol Cancer 2003;13:262–277. **(IIa, B)**
17. Lynch HT, Riley BD, Weissman SM, et al: Hereditary nonpolyposis colorectal carcinoma (HNPCC) and HNPCC-like families: problems in diagnosis, surveillance, and management. Cancer 2004;100:53–64. **(IIa, B)**
18. Gemignani ML, Schlaerth AC, Bogomolniy F, et al: Role of K-RAS and BRAF gene mutations in mucinous ovarian carcinoma. Gynecol Oncol 2003;90:378–381. **(IIa, B)**
19. Shayesteh L, Lu Y, Kuo WL, et al: PIK3CA is implicated as an oncogene in ovarian cancer. Nat Genet 1999;21:99–102. **(IIa, B)**
20. Hogdall EV, Christensen L, Kjaer SK, et al: Distribution of HER-2 overexpression in ovarian carcinoma tissue and its prognostic value in patients with ovarian carcinoma: from the Danish MALOVA Ovarian Cancer Study. Cancer 2003;98:66–73. **(IIa, B)**
21. Aunoble B, Sanches R, Didier E, Bignon YJ: Major oncogenes and tumor suppressor genes involved in epithelial ovarian cancer (review). Int J Oncol 2000;16:567–76.

22. Feki A, Irminger-Finger I: Mutational spectrum of p53 mutations in primary breast and ovarian tumors. Crit Rev Oncol Hematol 2004; 52:103–116. **(IIa, B)**

23. Kmet LM, Cook LS, Magliocco AM: A review of *p53* expression and mutation in human benign, low malignant potential, and invasive epithelial ovarian tumors. Cancer 2003;97:389–404. **(IIa, B)**

24. Marsh DJ, Coulon V, Lunetta KL, et al: Mutation spectrum and genotype–phenotype analyses in Cowden disease and Bannayan-Zonana syndrome, two hamartoma syndromes with germline *PTEN* mutation. Hum Mol Genet 1998;7:507–515. **(IIa, B)**

25. Franke TF, Hornik CP, Segev L, et al: *PI3K/Akt* and apoptosis: size matters. Oncogene 2003;22:8983–8998. **(IIa, B)**

26. Sansal I, Sellers WR: The biology and clinical relevance of the *PTEN* tumor suppressor pathway. J Clin Oncol 2004;22:2954–2963.

27. Kurose K, Zhou XP, Araki T, et al: Frequent loss of *PTEN* expression is linked to elevated phosphorylated Akt levels, but not associated with p27 and cyclin D1 expression, in primary epithelial ovarian carcinomas. Am J Pathol 2001;158:2097–2106. **(IIa, B)**

28. Lynch MA, Nakashima R, Song H, et al: Mutational analysis of the transforming growth factor beta receptor type II gene in human ovarian carcinoma. Cancer Res 1998;58:4227–4232. **(IIa, B)**

29. Pekarsky Y, Palamarchuk A, Huebner K, Croce CM: *FHIT* as tumor suppressor: mechanisms and therapeutic opportunities. Cancer Biol Ther 2002;1:232–236. **(IIa, B)**

30. Salvesen HB, Das S, Akslen LA: Loss of nuclear p16 protein expression is not associated with promoter methylation but defines a subgroup of aggressive endometrial carcinomas with poor prognosis. Clin Cancer Res 2000;6:153–159. **(IIa, B)**

# Chapter 52

# Female Infertility and the Evaluation of the Infertile Couple

Ertug Kovanci, MD, and Sandra A. Carson, MD

The desire to produce an offspring is a basic human instinct that facilitates the continuity of our species. However, people have suffered from infertility for as long as the human species has existed. Social, medical, and economic aspects of infertility have evolved throughout history as the condition has gone from being considered a source for disgrace, as in the case of Rachel in the Book of Genesis, to merely another medical condition. Advances in medicine and science have revolutionized the diagnosis and treatment of infertility and allowed couples who could not have reproduced two decades ago an opportunity to be parents. However, infertility treatments do have limitations and potential undesired effects that couples should understand before undertaking treatment.

## EPIDEMIOLOGY, RISK FACTORS, AND PATHOGENESIS

Although infertility does not pose a serious public health risk, it has significant psychological and economic consequences at both personal and societal levels. Therefore, U.S. public health organizations perform infertility data surveillance to improve prevention and treatment. Standard fertility terminology is utilized by these organizations and other investigators to classify infertility, follow its prevalence, and determine treatment efficacy (Table 52-1).

The number of women who require infertility services has been increasing over the past decade. In the United States, the proportion of women between ages 15 and 44 who received any kind of infertility service was approximately 15% of all women, about 9 million, in 1995 compared to 12% in 1988. Of those, 1% underwent advanced fertility treatments. About 7% of married couples, 2.1 million, reported that they were infertile in 1995.[1]

Fertility rates in the United States have also been declining since 1980 and reached the lowest rate, 64.8 births per 1000 women aged 15 to 44, in 2002.[2] The birth rate for women ages 35 to 39 has been increasing over the past three decades and peaked at 41.4 births per 1000 women in 2002, despite the overall U.S. birth rate reaching its lowest point ever—13.9 births per 1000 total population—during that year. At the same point, women aged 40 to 44 had the highest birth rate in three decades, 8.3 births per 1000 women. Postponement of marriage, delayed childbearing, increased use of birth control, availability of new infertility treatments, and increased media attention to treatments have contributed to the infertility epidemic. The

U.S. Department of Health and Human Services' objective is to reduce impaired fecundity to 10% by the year 2010.[3]

The *fecundability rate* (i.e., the probability of becoming pregnant in one menstrual cycle) is about 20% to 25% in normal couples. Mathematically, 25% of normal couples are expected to get pregnant in one cycle. Of women who did not get pregnant (75% of the initial group), 25% will get pregnant in the following cycle. Therefore, 43.75% of the initial couples will conceive after 2 months. In the third cycle, 25% of the remaining women (56.25% of the initial group) who did not get pregnant in the first two cycles will get pregnant. Cumulative pregnancy rate after 3 months will be approximately 58%, and 98% of the couples should be expected to conceive in 13 cycles. However, fecundability rate declines in normal populations after the first 2 to 3 months. This is likely due to the heterogeneity of the initial population. The couples with high fecundability rates conceive rapidly, leaving the couples with low fecundability rates, thus decreasing the fecundability rate for the remainder of the population.

Multiple systems work in harmony to achieve an optimal fecundability rate. Close interaction among the ovary, pituitary, and hypothalamus is necessary to develop a mature oocyte. This interaction encompasses ovarian negative and positive feedback actions on the pituitary, as well as the pituitary response to these feedbacks. Initially decreased estradiol levels after menses stimulate follicle-stimulating hormone (FSH) secretion, which induces follicular growth. When one of the follicles reaches maturation, the ovary signals the pituitary to secrete increased amounts of luteinizing hormone (LH), establishing the LH surge and triggering ovulation. Thus, the "ovarian clock" enables selection of the mature oocyte. Following ovulation, the fallopian tube picks up the released mature oocyte to introduce it to the waiting sperm, which have traveled through the cervical mucus, uterus, and fallopian tube after deposition in the vagina. The sperm should also be produced in sufficient quality and quantity by the male gonad. After fertilization of the oocyte, the resulting embryo is propelled to the uterus. The endometrium, prepared by the sequential cascade of ovarian hormones, allows implantation and embryo growth. Potential problems at any level of this complex process may impair fertility.

### Cervical Factor Infertility

The cervix plays a number of roles in human fertility. Cervical mucus enhances the transport of sperm from the vagina to the uterus during the ovulation window by forming parallel channels

# Reproductive Endocrinology and Infertility

| Table 52-1 Standard Fertility Terminology | |
|---|---|
| Fertility rate | The ratio of livebirths in an area to the number of women aged 15 to 44; expressed per 1000 population per year |
| Birth rate | The ratio of live births in an area to the population of that area; expressed per 1000 population per year |
| Fecundability | The probability of achieving a pregnancy in one menstrual cycle |
| Fecundity | The capacity for bringing forth young; fertility |
| Cumulative pregnancy rate | The probability of becoming pregnant within a given time, e.g., over 1 year |

of micelles. It facilitates sperm capacitation and serves as a reservoir for normal sperm. Developmental anomalies, trauma, and cervical procedures such as cone biopsy may impair mucus production or may cause cervical stenosis. The resultant hostile environment for sperm may block sperm transport to the upper genital tract altogether. However, diagnosis and treatment of cervical factor remains controversial.

## Uterine Factor Infertility

Sperm is transported toward the oocyte faster than can be accounted for by its motility alone. Uterine and tubal peristalsis/contractility is responsible for this rapid transport of the sperm to the upper genital tract. The uterus is also the site for the implantation of the embryo. Therefore, a normal uterine cavity is important for fertility. Uterine fibroids, depending on their location and size, may distort the uterine cavity and may impair implantation or cause pregnancy wastage. Submucosal fibroids and intramural fibroids measuring greater than 7 cm in diameter have been associated with infertility and pregnancy loss.

It is not surprising that fibroids distorting the uterine cavity decrease pregnancy rates in women undergoing in vitro fertilization (IVF).[4–7] Pregnancy rates in women with fibroids compared to women with no fibroids were 30% versus 41%, respectively, but the odds ratio (OR) was 0.73 (95% CI, 0.49 to 1.19, $p = 0.2$) after controlling for age and other risk factors.[7] However, even fibroids in the presence of a normal cavity reduced success rates in IVF.[8–10] Hart and colleagues, in a prospective study, found that intramural fibroids with no distortion of the uterine cavity reduced ongoing pregnancy rates from 28% to 15% compared to controls (OR, 0.46; 95% CI, 0.24 to 0.88, $p = 0.02$).[8] In contrast, Jun and colleagues, in their retrospective study, showed that fibroids smaller than 7 cm in diameter with a normal uterine cavity do not decrease pregnancy rates in women undergoing IVF. Therefore, the effect of subserosal and small intramural fibroids on fertility is controversial, although submucosal and large intramural fibroids distorting the cavity are clearly associated with decreased fertility.

Developmental anomalies of the reproductive tract, such as a septate uterus, bicornuate uterus, and didelphic uterus, also appear to be associated with delayed spontaneous conception

and are correlated with poor pregnancy outcome, including pregnancy loss and preterm delivery.[11] Müllerian duct aplasia syndromes result in infertility because oocyte and sperm proximity cannot be attained and a uterus is not present.

## Tubal Factor Infertility

The fallopian tubes are essential for transport of the oocyte, sperm, and embryo. Damaged tubes preclude the marriage of oocytes and sperm. Pelvic inflammatory disease (PID), adhesions from previous tubal or pelvic surgery, endometriosis, ruptured appendix, and septic abortion are risk factors for tubal disease. After three PID episodes, the rate of infertility has been estimated to exceed 50%.[12] Silent chlamydia infections are also strongly correlated with tubal damage. Up to 86% of women with tubal infertility have been reported to have serum IgG antibodies against Chlamydia trachomatis, which is significantly higher than the percentage of fertile women with the same type of antibodies.[13]

Previous abdominal surgery is a strong risk factor for pelvic adhesions. Approximately 23% of women who had undergone abdominal surgery were found to have significant pelvic adhesions during laparoscopic sterilization, compared to 2.7% of controls.[14] Adhesion formation can occur in up to 60% of women after tubal surgery for infertility.[15] Also, tubal polyps and intratubal debris or mucus plug may cause transient tubal occlusion. The incidence of tubal polyps is approximately 3% to 11%.[16,17] Salpingitis isthmica nodosa is characterized by bilateral diverticula of the tubal epithelium in the isthmic region. It is associated with pelvic infections and tuberculosis leading to mucosal damage and may involve the muscular layer, leading to occlusion of the tubal lumen.

## Endometriosis

Endometriosis is the presence of endometrial tissue outside the uterus. The most common sites for endometriosis are peritoneal surfaces covering the posterior cul-de-sac, uterosacral ligaments, pelvic side walls, bladder, and uterus. Tubes and ovaries are also frequently involved. The American Society for Reproductive Medicine (ASRM) has developed a staging system to determine the degree of endometriosis. This system divides the disease into four stages. Stages III and IV reflect the most severe cases, with extensive pelvic adhesions and anatomic distortion of the pelvic structures, including tubes and ovaries. A cause and effect relationship is clear in women with Stages III or IV endometriosis, when anatomical distortion interferes with oocyte release from the ovary, tubal pickup of the oocyte, and sperm transport to the proximity of the oocyte. However, the relationship with infertility is less clear in Stages I and II (minimal to mild) endometriosis, when such distortion is absent. Therefore, functional abnormalities have been suggested.

The proposed mechanisms of impaired infertility in the presence of mild to moderate endometriosis include changes in the contents of the peritoneal fluid that may interfere with sperm function, fertilization, and tubal function. Decreased oocyte quality and impaired implantation have also been implicated in the reduced fertility that may be associated with minimal to mild endometriosis.[18,19] Some investigators have suggested that impaired endometrial receptivity may be responsible for the decreased implantation rates.[20] However, when donor oocytes are used in patients with and without endometriosis, pregnancy rates have been found to be similar.[21] Women with endometriosis also have a similar response to gonadotropins compared to women without the disease.[22,23] Numerous studies reported that peritoneal fluid activated macrophage concentrations and that their secretory products, including interleukin-1, tumor necrosis factor, and proteases, are elevated in endometriosis.

Impaired sperm function due to the detrimental effects of peritoneal fluid from women with endometriosis has also been postulated. However, multiple studies in the literature reporting on sperm motility after culture with peritoneal fluid from endometriosis patients have conflicting results. In their well-designed study, Stone and Himsl showed that peritoneal recovery of motile sperm did not change in the presence of endometriosis compared to controls.[24] A detrimental effect of peritoneal fluid on embryo development, so-called *embryotoxicity*, has also been suggested. However, when donor oocytes are used, attainment of similar pregnancy rates in women with endometriosis compared to controls appears to oppose the embryotoxicity hypothesis.[25] Even though mild endometriosis is more commonly encountered in patients with infertility compared to controls[26] and the probability of pregnancy is lower in women with minimal to mild endometriosis compared to women with unexplained infertility,[27] improved pregnancy rates after medical or surgical treatment of minimal to mild endometriosis have been reported in only one multicenter study.[28] Therefore, the association between infertility and minimal or mild endometriosis remains controversial.

## Ovarian Factor Infertility

Anovulation is the most common etiologic factor in infertility. Various conditions may lead to anovulation which can be divided into three groups: hypogonadotropic, eugonadotropic, and hypergonadotropic anovulation. The most common type is eugonadotropic anovulation, which includes polycystic ovary syndrome (PCOS). PCOS, defined as oligomenorrhea and hyperandrogenism, accounts for approximately 75% of anovulatory infertility.[29] Although tonic levels of LH and inadequate FSH secretion lead to follicular maturation arrest, LH and FSH levels remain within the normal range. PCOS is discussed in detail in Chapter 61.

Other causes of anovulation include hypothalamic dysfunction, pituitary disease, premature ovarian failure, and endocrine disorders. Hypothalamic anovulation is caused by impaired pulsatile gonadotropin-releasing hormone (GnRH) secretion. This, in turn, results in decreased LH and FSH secretion. Without cyclic gonadotropin production, the ovarian follicles do not mature the oocyte and anovulation occurs. Extreme weight loss, vigorous exercise, and emotional stress may induce hypothalamic anovulation. Infiltrating diseases such as histiocytosis X and sarcoidosis or tumors localized in the hypothalamic-pituitary region may rarely lead to hypothalamic anovulation. *Functional hypothalamic anovulation* is defined as the cessation of ovulation with no identifiable organic causes. Insufficient caloric intake induced by diet or exercise, eating disorders, and emotional stress caused by performance pressure and dysfunctional attitudes may act synergistically to disrupt pulsatile GnRH secretion, causing functional hypothalamic amenorrhea.[30]

Kallmann syndrome, an inherited disorder with X-linked, autosomal dominant, and autosomal recessive variants, is characterized by isolated GnRH deficiency induced by impaired migration of GnRH neurons from the olfactory placode to the basal hypothalamus during embryonic development. Both genders can be involved. Patients with Kallmann syndrome present with absent or incomplete puberty and show irregular or low GnRH pulse amplitude and frequency. Kallmann syndrome is often associated with anosmia or hyposmia and midline defects such as cleft palate.

Elevated serum prolactin (PRL) levels inhibit pituitary LH and FSH secretion, thus causing anovulation. Pituitary PRL secretion is controlled by the tonic inhibitory effects of dopamine. Any central nervous system lesion or drug that impairs dopamine secretion may cause elevated PRL levels. However, hyperprolactinemia is most commonly induced by PRL-producing pituitary tumors, or prolactinomas. The majority of these tumors are microadenomas (i.e., <10 mm in diameter). Elevated PRL levels inhibit pulsatile secretion of GnRH and cause hypogonadotropic anovulation. Hypothalamic dopamine and opioid dysfunction may play a role in the inhibition of GnRH secretion. Other tumors of the pituitary, pituitary stalk transection, empty sella syndrome, and drugs such as antipsychotics (phenothiazines, butyrophenones) and centrally acting antihypertensives (reserpine, methyldopa) may induce hyperprolactinemia.

Sheehan's syndrome is characterized by hypopituitarism due to pituitary necrosis following severe postpartum hemorrhage. The degree of Sheehan's syndrome ranges from partial hypopituitarism involving only growth hormone and/or gonadotropin deficiency to panhypopituitarism with lack of all pituitary hormones. Hypogonadotropic anovulation is frequently present. This condition can be life-threatening and may require replacement of multiple hormones.

*Premature ovarian failure* is defined as the irreversible cessation of ovulation and menses before age 40. The prevalence of premature ovarian failure is approximately 1%. Genetic or autoimmune disorders may result in the loss of ovarian follicles and premature ovarian failure. Fragile X syndrome and 45,X (Turner's syndrome) are the most commonly identified genetic abnormalities that may cause premature ovarian failure. When autoimmunity is the underlying factor, premature ovarian failure is frequently associated with other autoimmune disorders including hypothyroidism, insulin-dependent diabetes mellitus (IDDM), adrenal insufficiency, pernicious anemia, and hypoparathyroidism. The most common autoimmune disorder occurring in women with premature ovarian failure is hypothyroidism. However, no underlying factor can be identified in many premature ovarian failure patients.

## Age

Today, many women delay parenthood until their fourth and fifth decades of life, and age-related fertility decline in women is well-documented by multiple studies on natural populations.[31] This decline accelerates markedly after age 35. Women undergoing donor sperm insemination demonstrate marked fertility decline starting at age 35.[32,33] However, Dunson and colleagues reported that pregnancy probability starts decreasing after age 26.[34] Unfortunately, this study utilized arbitrary age groups, such as age 19 to 26, age 27 to 34, and age 35 to 39. Therefore, it is difficult to interpret at exactly what age fertility begins to decline. Miscarriage rates also increase with maternal age. Baseline miscarriage rate is approximately 15% to 17%. This rate exceeds 30% by age 40 and 50% by age 45.[35,36]

Several mechanisms are involved in the detrimental effects of aging on fertility. The number of follicles significantly declines with age. This decline starts in utero and continues throughout reproductive life. The number of oogonia is approximately 6 to 7 million in the second trimester; during the third trimester this number declines, reaching approximately 2 million oogonia at birth. This attrition of germ cells continues after birth, resulting in only 300,000 oocytes at puberty. Oocyte exhaustion accelerates after age 35. The quality of oocytes is also impaired by age. Oocytes obtained from older women demonstrate higher rates of meiotic spindle and microtubular abnormalities compared to younger women, 47% versus 25%, respectively.[37] This may be one of the factors that cause the increased incidence of chromosomal aneuploidy in older women. Significantly lower pregnancy rates in older animals that received oocytes from younger animals suggest that impaired uterine receptivity might play a role in age-related infertility. Early IVF studies also demonstrated lower pregnancy rates in older women undergoing oocyte donation compared to younger women. However, a later study showed that older and younger patients had similar pregnancy rates when they received oocytes from the same donor,[38] which was confirmed by other studies. Intercourse frequency also declines with advancing age, which may contribute to the decreased fecundity in older couples.

### Endocrine Disorders and Infertility

Any endocrine disorder that affects the hypothalamic-pituitary-ovarian axis may cause anovulation and infertility.

The most common endocrine disorder that causes menstrual irregularity, anovulation, and infertility is thyroid disease. Both hypothyroidism and hyperthyroidism may lead to menstrual irregularity and infertility. Menstrual irregularity in thyroid disease ranges from amenorrhea to polymenorrhea.

The prevalence of hypothyroidism in reproductive age women is approximately 2% to 4%. Autoimmune thyroid disease is the most common etiologic factor. The frequency of menstrual irregularity in hypothyroidism ranges from 23% to 80%.[39] Overt hypothyroidism is usually associated with oligoamenorrhea, and subclinical hypothyroidism generally causes menorrhagia, which may precede hypothyroidism symptoms. Infertility due to anovulation is more common in severe hypothyroidism than milder forms. Increased thyrotropin-releasing hormone (TRH) levels in long-standing primary hypothyroidism and decreased dopamine secretion in the hypothalamus may also stimulate PRL secretion, which can further contribute to anovulatory infertility in hypothyroidism. The prevalence of galactorrhea in women with hypothyroidism is 1% to 3%, which can be reversed with thyroid hormone replacement.

Menstrual irregularity in hyperthyroidism was first noted by von Basedow in 1840. The frequency of menstrual disturbances in hyperthyroidism ranges from 21% to 64%.[39,40] The most common menstrual abnormality is oligomenorrhea, followed by amenorrhea and polymenorrhea. Increased sex hormone–binding globulin production in hyperthyroidism leads to elevated estrogen and total testosterone levels in serum. LH and FSH secretion is also increased, and midcycle LH peak is lost in hyperthyroidism, leading to anovulation. These changes in gonadotropin metabolism may be due to hypersensitivity of the pituitary to GnRH. The frequency of infertility in patients with hyperthyroidism is not well-established, although one study reported that approximately 6% of women with hyperthyroidism experienced infertility.[40]

The association between thyroid antibodies and infertility is controversial. Some investigators reported a higher incidence of thyroid antibodies in women with infertility compared to controls (17% vs. 8%, respectively),[41] but other investigators did not confirm this finding (19% vs. 15%, respectively).[42] Furthermore, the presence of thyroid antibodies does not affect pregnancy rates in infertile women undergoing assisted reproductive technology (ART) such as IVF.[43] Therefore, thyroid antibodies are unlikely to play a role in the pathogenesis of infertility.

Women with untreated IDDM may also suffer from hypogonadism, amenorrhea, and infertility. Insulin and gonadotropin metabolisms are closely intertwined. Numerous animal studies have shown that streptozotocin-induced diabetes leads to loss of LH surge and blunted LH response to GnRH. Insulin administration reverses this effect and lowers the frequency of reproductive problems. The effects of insulin appear to be central; intracerebroventricular insulin injection in rats with streptozotocin-induced diabetes is able to restore LH surge.[44] Similarly, hyperinsulinemic disorders such as PCOS result in increased LH pulse frequency and amplitude. When the insulin receptor was knocked out in the mouse central nervous system, elevated plasma insulin levels along with exaggerated LH response to exogenous GnRH was also observed.[45] Moreover, approximately 50% of women with noninsulin-dependent diabetes mellitus demonstrate PCOS features, including menstrual irregularity and hyperandrogenism.[46] Thus, either insufficient or increased amounts of insulin may interfere with the hypothalamic-pituitary-ovarian axis, leading to anovulatory infertility.

Both adrenal insufficiency and adrenal hyperplasia may also lead to hypothalamic-pituitary-ovarian axis dysfunction and infertility. Gonadotropin secretion and LH response to GnRH are suppressed in congenital adrenal hyperplasia (CAH) and Cushing's syndrome because of hyperandrogenemia and hyperadrenocorticism, respectively. Sexual dysfunction and anatomic defects may also contribute to infertility in CAH. Adrenal insufficiency may be associated with amenorrhea in 25% of women secondary to weight loss, chronic illness, or autoimmune premature ovarian failure. Libido is also decreased in adrenal insufficiency. Both adrenal hyperplasia and insufficiency may result in hyperprolactinemia, which may also suppress ovulation.

Acromegaly is caused by a growth hormone–secreting pituitary adenoma in most cases. Pituitary mass effect of these adenomas may result in suppressed gonadotropin secretion and anovulation. Hyperprolactinemia may also accompany acromegaly.

### Unexplained Infertility

Unexplained infertility is defined as the inability to conceive with no identifiable causes for infertility using standard investigations. Numerous factors may contribute to unexplained infertility. Couples who are at the lower limits of the normal fecundability distribution curve may fall into this category, although the duration of infertility is similar in these couples compared to those with other infertility diagnoses. Female partner age greater than 30 years may also be responsible for decreased fertility. However, the age distribution of couples with unexplained infertility does not differ significantly from that of couples with other infertility diagnoses.[47] The majority of couples with unexplained infertility probably suffer from a defect that is undetectable by current diagnostic approaches.

### Genetics of Infertility

Multiple mutations and chromosomal abnormalities affecting the hypothalamic-pituitary-ovarian axis have been described. Some of these mutations are very rare and reported as case series, whereas others affecting the gonads, such as 45,X, can be as common as 1:2500 live female births.

Mutations involving the hypothalamic function include mutations of *KAL1, KAL2*, leptin *(LEP)*, and leptin receptor *(LEPR)* genes.[48–51] Mutations in the *KAL1* and *KAL2* genes are the etiologic factor with hypogonadotropic hypogonadism and anosmia, (Kallmann syndrome) in some women. X-linked, autosomal dominant, and autosomal recessive inheritance modes have been suggested in Kallmann syndrome. *LEP* and *LEPR* mutations are associated with hypogonadotropic hypogonadism, obesity, and hyperinsulinemia. However, these mutations are extremely rare.

Gene mutations interfere with pituitary functions. GnRH receptor gene *(GNRHR)* mutations result in hypogonadotropic hypogonadism, ranging from partial function loss of the receptor to the complete loss of function.[52] The mutations of the genes coding the beta subunit of the gonadotropins have also been described. *FSHβ* gene mutations cause infertility, with primary amenorrhea in females and azoospermia in males[53] There has been one case report with the *LHβ* gene mutation,[54] a male who presented with delayed puberty, low testosterone, and small testes. Gonadotropin levels were elevated in this patient because of a missense mutation of the *LHβ* gene. Mutations of other genes such as *PROP1, HESX1*, and *LHX3* also result in lack of gonadotropins or combined pituitary hormone deficiency.

Multiple mutations and chromosomal abnormalities involve both the female and male gonad, causing gonadal failure and infertility. Pubertal development is normal in most men with gonadal infertility whereas it is usually impaired in women. The mutations involving the gonads can be gonosomal or autosomal. The most common gonosomal mutations in men involve the *SRY, DAZ, DDX3Y*, and *USP9Y* genes[55] The most common gonosomal chromosomal abnormalities or mutations in women include 45,X and mutations of the *FMR1, POF1*, and *DIAPH2* genes.[55] FSH receptor *(FSHR)* and LH receptor *(LHR)* gene mutations are autosomal and result in infertility in both women and men.[56–59] Other autosomal mutations that cause infertility in women and men involve multiple genes, including *CYP17, CYP19, AIRE, WT1, NR5A1*, and *DHH*.[55]

Women with müllerian duct agenesis have vaginal aplasia and a rudimentary uterus with normal functioning ovaries. Mutations involving genes such as hepatic nuclear factor 1β, or the transcription factor 2 *(TCF2)* gene and Kaufman-McKusick syndrome *(MKKS)* gene may cause müllerian agenesis.[60] However, molecular defect in other müllerian agenesis syndromes,

including Mayer-Rokitansky-Küster-Hauser syndrome, is unknown. Mutations involving cystic fibrosis transmembrane conductance regulator *(CFTR)* gene may result in congenital bilateral absence of vas deferens (CBAVD).[61] The majority of men with CBAVD are compound heterozygotes, which is defined as having a single copy of two different mutations. These men present with obstructive azoospermia and normal spermatogenesis although they do not have cystic fibrosis.

### Male Factor Infertility

Multiple genetic or acquired disorders may lead to male factor infertility. Endocrine disorders, genetic disorders, varicocele, cryptorchidism, disorders of ejaculation and erection, male aging, exposure to environmental toxins, and outflow obstruction are the etiologic factors that may cause male infertility. However, the cause of infertility can be identified in only 50% of infertile men. This topic is discussed in detail in Chapter 53.

## CLINICAL FEATURES AND DIAGNOSIS

Infertility is defined as the inability to conceive after 12 or more months of regular unprotected intercourse. An investigation should be started after 1 year of unsuccessful trying unless medical history or physical examination findings support an earlier evaluation or treatment (Table 52-2). Often, in women over age 35 an infertility evaluation is started after 6 months. A detailed history and physical examination should be performed in all couples because etiologic factors such as sexually transmitted diseases, uterine fibroids, and endometriosis may be revealed.

**Table 52-2**
**Diagnostic Evaluation of the Infertile Couple**

| | Diagnostic Test | Recommendation |
|---|---|---|
| Cervical factor | Postcoital test | Routine use unnecessary |
| Uterine factor | Hysterosalpingography, ultrasound, hysteroscopy | An integral part of the evaluation |
| Tubal factor | Hysterosalpingography, sonohysterography, laparoscopy with chromopertubation | An integral part of the evaluation |
| Endometriosis | Ultrasound, laparoscopy | Indicated if strong suspicion |
| Ovarian factor | Menstrual history, basal body temperature, serum progesterone, urinary luteinizing hormone, serial transvaginal ultrasound and/or endometrial biopsy | An integral part of the evaluation |
| Age | Day 3 follicle-stimulating hormone level | Indicated in women older than age 35 and poor responders |
| Endocrine | Thyrotropin level, prolactin level | Indicated if suspicion |
| Male factor | Semen analysis | An integral part of the evaluation |

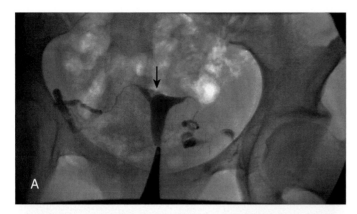

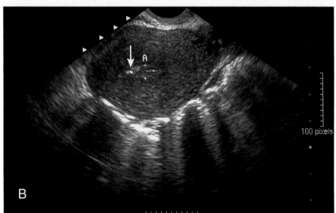

**Figure 52-1** *A,* A filling defect in the right fundal region of the uterus on hysterosalpingography. *B,* The appearance of the same filling defect on ultrasound; hyperechoic area in the fundus.

## Cervical Factor Infertility

Women with cervical factor infertility may present with a history of a cervical procedure, trauma, or exposure to drugs such as diethylstilbestrol. Physical examination may reveal anatomic distortion of the cervix. One of the most controversial diagnostic tests in female infertility is the postcoital test, which is also the oldest one, introduced by James Marion Sims in 1866. However, there is still no consensus on the correct timing of the postcoital test, cutoff for a normal result, and treatment

for an abnormal result. A multinational study reported a large variation in the timing of the postcoital test, both with reference to the menstrual cycle and time after intercourse.[62] Moreover, the microscopic magnification used and the definition of a normal result varied significantly; more than 10 different treatment strategies were utilized among different centers. Sensitivity and specificity of the postcoital test also show a large variation, ranging from 10% to 97%. A well-designed randomized controlled study revealed similar pregnancy rates between women who underwent postcoital test and the control group.[63] Furthermore, widespread use of intrauterine insemination (IUI) and IVF have rendered the postcoital test ineffective in the prediction of pregnancy. Although the postcoital test is no longer part of the standard infertility evaluation, it may be useful in some couples to ascertain the ability to have timed intercourse and to confirm that the sperm is entering the cervical mucus.

## Uterine Factor Infertility

A history of increased menstrual flow and frequency, pelvic pressure, or enlarged abdominal girth may be present in women with uterine fibroids. Endometrial polyps may also cause irregular vaginal bleeding. Physical examination may reveal an enlarged uterus with an irregular contour in women with fibroids. Pelvic ultrasound is the preferred imaging modality for evaluation of uterine fibroids. Size, location, and number of fibroids can be identified using ultrasound imaging. If a more thorough analysis of the fibroids is desired, magnetic resonance imaging (MRI) is the most accurate imaging modality.[64] Some investigators advocate routine use of hysterosalpingography (HSG) or hysteroscopy as part of an infertility evaluation to image the uterus because 10% to 45% of women with infertility may have an intrauterine lesion.[65,66] Submucosal fibroids, endometrial polyps, or intrauterine synechia may be visualized as filling defects on HSG (Fig. 52-1). Hysteroscopy is recommended to characterize the lesion when HSG shows an abnormal cavity. Furthermore, submucosal fibroids or endometrial polyps can be removed using operative hysteroscopy (Fig. 52-2).

## Tubal Factor Infertility

A careful history may reveal a past history of sexually transmitted diseases (STD) or past symptoms of STD. Although

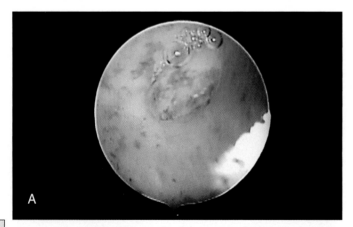

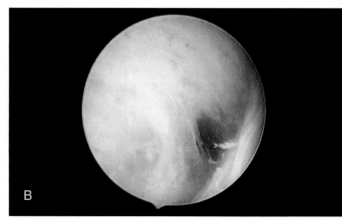

**Figure 52-2** *A,* A submucosal fibroid visualized via hysteroscopy. *B,* Intrauterine synechia developed after dilatation and curettage visualized via hysteroscopy.

clinical usefulness of history taking in tubal factor infertility has been questioned due to the low specificity (29%) and sensitivity (84%),[67] many investigators strongly recommend a detailed history taking as an integral part of infertility evaluation.[68,69] Chlamydia antibody testing has been proposed to evaluate tubal patency noninvasively. However, sensitivity values ranging from 50% to 75% and restricted information obtained from antibody testing limit its use.

Hysterosalpingography is the most commonly used imaging modality to evaluate tubal patency, although laparoscopy with chromopertubation is considered the gold standard. A meta-analysis found that the sensitivity and specificity of HSG are 65% and 83%, respectively for the prediction of tubal patency compared to diagnostic laparoscopy.[70] Thus, it is a good predictor of tubal obstruction but not tubal patency. HSG also was not reliable for the evaluation of peritubal adhesions. However, a later study reported that after a normal HSG, laparoscopy was not likely to reveal tubal disease.[71] Of the 794 patients who underwent HSG and laparoscopy in this prospective study, only 12 had patent tubes on HSG and bilaterally blocked tubes during laparoscopy, although the best predictor of future fertility was laparoscopy. The sensitivity and specificity of HSG were 72% and 82%, respectively, for the detection of bilateral obstruction. HSG can be performed using oil-soluble or water-soluble contrast media. Water-soluble contrast media is superior to oil-soluble media in the evaluation of tubal structure. Oil-soluble media also has a higher incidence of complications, such as granulomatous inflammation of the tubes and pulmonary embolism, especially in women with tubal pathology. However, a meta-analysis reported higher pregnancy rates after flushing the tubes with oil-soluble media.[72] Therefore, flushing the tubes with oil-soluble media is recommended after HSG is found to be normal using water-soluble media. The advantages of HSG over laparoscopy with chromopertubation include the annulment of surgical morbidity and complications, the lack of necessity for anesthesia and increased chances of spontaneous pregnancy after HSG.

Sonohysterography is an alternative imaging modality to HSG for the assessment of the uterine cavity and tubal patency. Ultrasound imaging of the uterus and tubes after insufflating with a contrast media such as normal saline, a galactose solution, or air-contrast after normal saline injection has comparable sensitivity and specificity to HSG,[73] but is usually reserved for women with iodine allergy. Sonohysterography offers the advantage of the ability to detect other uterine and adnexal abnormalities, including intramural or subserosal fibroids and ovarian masses. However, complete tubal anatomy usually cannot be evaluated during sonohysterography. Salpingoscopy, the visualization of the tubal mucosa using a rigid or flexible endoscope, has also been introduced. Although comparable results to HSG have been reported, this procedure has not gained widespread use because of the technical difficulties and high rates of incomplete procedures.

## Endometriosis

Chronic pelvic pain, dyspareunia, and dysmenorrhea are frequently encountered in endometriosis. The frequency of endometriosis in women with chronic pelvic pain ranges from 15% to 32%.[74,75] Dyspareunia in endometriosis is usually deep

and associated with rectovaginal involvement of the disease. Pain after intercourse may also be reported by women with endometriosis. Dysmenorrhea is considered the most common symptom in endometriosis.[76] The risk of endometriosis is associated with the total number of menstrual cycles. Endometriosis is less frequently diagnosed in women who have longer menstrual cycles (>27 days) or a higher number of pregnancies compared to women with shorter cycles or nulliparity. Women with a family history of endometriosis are more likely to have endometriosis compared to controls; a polygenic/ multifactorial inheritance has been suggested.[77] Rarely, symptoms related to the extrapelvic involvement of endometriosis, such as intestinal tract, urinary tract, lungs, and central nervous system involvement, may be encountered.

A wide range of physical examination findings have been reported in endometriosis, including uterosacral nodularity and pain, reduced uterine mobility, deviated or retroverted uterus, cervical motion tenderness, and adnexal mass. However, these findings have poor sensitivity and specificity.[78,79] Even if the endometriosis is deeply infiltrating, a palpable nodule is noted in only 43% of women.[80] Therefore, a normal physical examination does not rule out endometriosis. Moreover, the presence of the physical signs is not diagnostic.

Laboratory tests such as CA 125, CA 15-3, and CA 19-9 have been suggested as diagnostic tools. However, none of them has adequate sensitivity and specificity. A meta-analysis showed that CA 125 has a poor sensitivity for endometriosis and a high false-positive rate, 50% and 28%, respectively.[81]

A recent review of eight studies that evaluated the accuracy of ultrasound in the diagnosis of endometriosis reported moderate accuracy, with a high likelihood ratio (LR; 7.6–29.8) to rule in the diagnosis of endometrioma.[82] The sensitivity of ultrasound in the same review ranged from 64% to 89%; specificity ranged from 89% to 100% (Fig. 52-3). However, ultrasound has a limited role in the diagnosis of superficial peritoneal lesions and adhesions.

Magnetic resonance imaging has also been evaluated for the diagnosis of endometriosis. The sensitivity and specificity of MRI in the detection of all stages of endometriosis are 69% and 75%, respectively.[83] MRI has a better sensitivity and specificity in the detection of endometriomas, 90% and 98%, respectively.[84]

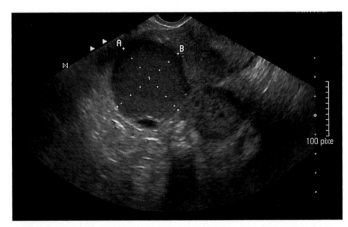

**Figure 52-3  The appearance of an endometrioma on ultrasound; cystic structure with internal echoes.**

# Reproductive Endocrinology and Infertility

However, a recent study showed that rectal endoscopic ultrasound has a better sensitivity and negative predictive value in the diagnosis of deeply infiltrating rectovaginal endometriosis compared to MRI, 97% versus 76% and 97% versus 85%, respectively.[85]

The gold standard for the diagnosis of endometriosis is laparoscopy with biopsy for histologic examination. The classic appearance of endometrial peritoneal implants is characterized by blue-black powder-burn lesions. However, endometrial implants have multiple appearances, including nonpigmented white lesions, red flamelike lesions, papular or vesicular lesions with serous or hemorrhagic content, peritoneal defects or pockets, and subovarian adhesions. The implants are commonly encountered over the uterosacral ligaments, posterior cul-de-sac, pelvic side walls, and ovarian fossa. Endometriomas, ovarian cysts filled with old blood of endometriosis, can be identified readily during laparoscopy.

## Ovarian Factor Infertility

A history of regular menstrual cycles suggests normal ovulation in greater than 90% of cycles.[86] Anovulation normally results in oligomenorrhea. In the absence of pregnancy, secondary amenorrhea, the cessation of menses after menarche, may be caused by PCOS, hyperprolactinemia, hypothalamic amenorrhea, or other endocrine disorders. Symptoms such as galactorrhea, hirsutism, and acne are helpful in the differential diagnosis. Physical examination is focused on the signs of these disorders, such as hair and skin changes, nipple discharge, and body composition.

Initial laboratory evaluation in secondary amenorrhea should include serum thyrotropin, PRL, and FSH levels to rule out thyroid disorders, hyperprolactinemia, and premature ovarian failure.

Multiple methods have been investigated for the detection or prediction of ovulation, such as basal body temperature (BBT) charts, midluteal progesterone levels, ultrasound, and LH levels. BBT charts may be useful in women who have regular cycles without ovulation. The rectal or oral temperature should be taken in the morning before getting out of bed. The BBT is usually lower than 98.6°F in the follicular phase. It reaches a nadir around the time of LH surge, although it is generally difficult to detect this nadir. A temperature rise is noted after ovulation because of the increased progesterone levels. However, monophasic or uninterpretable graphs can be noted in approximately 20% of ovulatory cycles.[87] Moreover, interpretation of the charts is often difficult; at any rate, BBT cannot identify ovulation prospectively.

Serial transvaginal ultrasound scanning has been used as an accurate predictor of ovulation since the early 1980s.[88] The mean follicular diameter 1 day prior to ovulation is approximately 21 mm, and decreases dramatically after ovulation.[89] Ultrasound predicts ovulation in 85% to 96% of regularly cycling women.[87,90] The disadvantages of ovulation prediction using ultrasound are its high cost and the requirement for serial visits to the ultrasound center.

Another method is the measurement of midluteal (7 days prior to the next period) progesterone. A concentration greater than 3 ng/mL is consistent with ovulation. The sensitivity of a single midluteal progesterone measurement for ovulation detection is approximately 80%, because progesterone is secreted in a pulsatile manner and the luteal phase length may vary.[87]

Histologic examination of endometrial biopsy material obtained using a plastic suction cannula is also a reliable method to detect ovulation. However, endometrial biopsy performed in the luteal phase identifies ovulation retrospectively, similar to serum progesterone.

The World Health Organization (WHO) task force in 1980 selected serum LH surge as the best marker for impending ovulation and serum estradiol rise as the sign of the potentially fertile period.[91] However, serial daily serum LH measurements are not practical; this has been replaced by daily urine LH testing, based on data from later studies funded by WHO.[92] The sensitivity of urine LH testing is approximately 100% in infertile women with regular cycles.[87] Urine LH testing predicts ovulation approximately 20 hours before it occurs. However, ovulation may take place 14 to 26 hours after a positive test.[93] The highest probability of clinical pregnancy is achieved with intercourse 1 day prior to ovulation. Randomized controlled trials comparing IUI cycles by urine LH testing, BBT charts, ultrasound, or timing of hCG administration showed these methods to be equally effective.[94-96] Numerous one-step urine LH kits are commercially available, all easy to use.

Other less commonly applied methods to detect ovulation include monitoring of salivary ferning, cervical mucus score and urinary estrone-3-glucuronide measurement. However, these methods have not gained popularity because of the low accuracy and difficulty of use.

## Age

Women older than age 35 experience a rapid decline in fertility. The length of menstrual cycles becomes shorter after age 35 indicating diminished luteal phase length and oocyte quality. The intercourse frequency and sexual function should be elicited during the medical history. Decline in frequency and sexual dysfunction may contribute to the diminished fertility in older couples.

Numerous methods have been proposed to determine the ovarian reserve in older women, including female age, cycle day 3 or basal serum FSH level, cycle day 3 serum estradiol level, cycle day 3 serum inhibin B level, GnRH agonist stimulation test, the clomiphene citrate challenge test, exogenous FSH ovarian reserve test, total antral follicle count, ovarian stromal blood flow, ovarian volume, and ovarian biopsy. All these tests have similar efficacy in the prediction of a clinical pregnancy. Female age alone is not a good predictor of ovarian response to treatment, although it is an important factor in the infertility prognosis. If age 40 is selected as the threshold, the LR of not becoming pregnant is very high (12.5).[97] The two most commonly used tests are the basal serum FSH level and the clomiphene citrate challenge test. Basal serum FSH level is a single measurement obtained on day 3 of the menstrual cycle. In the clomiphene citrate challenge test, clomiphene citrate at 100 mg is administered daily between cycle day 5 and 9; this is followed by a serum FSH measurement on day 10. Many investigators also obtain a day 3 FSH level with the clomiphene citrate challenge test. Various threshold values have been proposed for each test. These values range from 10 to 17 IU/L for basal serum FSH and 10 to 26 IU/L for the clomiphene citrate challenge test. A recent meta-analysis comparing these two methods revealed that both tests have poor sensitivities, 6.6% and 25.9%, respectively, and high specificities, 99.6% and 98.1%, respectively.[98] Therefore, a normal result from either test does not rule out poor ovarian response, however, an abnormal result indicates that ovaries will not respond to treatment.

## Endocrine Disorders and Infertility

Signs and symptoms of endocrine disorders may be helpful in establishing the diagnosis. Women with hypothyroidism may present with the following signs and symptoms: fatigue, weight gain in the presence of decreased appetite, cold intolerance, hair loss, dry skin, constipation, prolonged relaxation of the deep tendon reflexes, and intellectual slowness or depression. A serum thyrotropin level above the reference range with a serum free $T_4$ concentration below the reference range indicates hypothyroidism.

The signs and symptoms of hyperthyroidism include tremors, heat intolerance, tachycardia, palpitations, increased appetite with weight loss, and frequent stools. A serum thyrotropin level below the reference range with a serum free $T_4$ level above the reference range is consistent with hyperthyroidism.

The classic symptoms of diabetes mellitus are polyuria, polydipsia and weight loss. Fasting plasma glucose concentration greater than 125 mg/dL is consistent with diabetes; a concentration between 110 and 125 mg/dL indicates impaired glucose tolerance. Similarly, plasma glucose concentration between 140 and 200 mg/dL 2 hours after ingestion of 75 g of glucose is indicative of impaired glucose tolerance, and a concentration above 200 mg/dL is diagnostic for diabetes.

The classic features of Cushing's syndrome include amenorrhea, central obesity, moon facies, hirsutism, and purple striae. Diagnosis is usually established with an elevated 24-hour urinary free cortisol. Females with CAH may present with various signs and symptoms, ranging from in utero virilization in the classic salt-wasting form to adult hirsutism in the nonclassic form. Women with congenital lipoid adrenal hyperplasia usually present with abnormal pubertal development or premature ovarian failure. An elevated morning 17-hydroxyprogesterone level above 800 ng/dL is diagnostic. Clinical features of adrenal insufficiency include fatigue, anorexia, weight loss, hyperpigmentation, hypotension, and gastrointestinal symptoms such as nausea and vomiting. A corticotropin stimulation test is performed to confirm the diagnosis.

Typical presentation of patients with acromegaly is characterized by enlarged extremities and facial changes, such as frontal skull bossing, prognathism, enlarged nose, and tongue. An elevated morning level of growth hormone is diagnostic for acromegaly.

## Unexplained Infertility

Unexplained infertility is a diagnosis of exclusion that occurs in 15% of infertility evaluations. It should be considered in a couple with ovulatory cycles, patent tubes, and a normal semen analysis. Ovulation can be confirmed with measurement of serum progesterone in the luteal phase. Tubal patency is usually assessed by HSG or laparoscopy. A normal semen analysis, including sperm concentration, motility, and morphology, is sufficient to rule out male infertility.

The use of other infertility tests such as the postcoital test, antisperm antibodies, varicocele assessment, *Chlamydia* testing, and sperm function tests such as zona-free hamster egg penetration test to confirm unexplained infertility are controversial because these tests do not correlate consistently with pregnancy.[99] Moreover, many of these tests are interdependent, which increases false-positive results exponentially when multiple tests are performed. They are also rarely helpful to establish a treatment plan. Therefore, it is prudent to avoid expensive unnecessary tests and procedures that will not have an effect on the management plan.

## Male Factor Infertility

Semen analysis is an integral part of the evaluation of the infertile couple. The basic parameters of a semen analysis include sperm concentration, motility, and morphology. Sperm morphology may be assessed under low magnification without staining using standard WHO criteria. A more precise method is to evaluate sperm morphology under high magnification after staining of the sperm head using Kruger criteria. This method, known as *strict morphology*, has been shown to correlate with fertilization rates.[100]

Any abnormal semen analysis value should prompt additional clinical and laboratory evaluation of the patient. This may include physical examination, endocrine testing (FSH, testosterone), postejaculatory urinalysis, scrotal ultrasound, specialized semen and sperm tests ($\alpha$-glucosidase, fructose, antisperm antibodies, sperm viability and penetration tests, and the zona-free hamster egg penetration test), and genetic screening depending on the abnormality detected.

All semen and sperm tests have the same pitfalls. Men who fall outside the reference ranges may be fertile; conversely, men with normal values may be infertile. Moreover, application of these tests precludes the use of the same sperm for ART. Nondestructive sperm tests are needed to select good-quality sperm for use in ART.

Evaluation of male infertility is discussed at length in Chapter 53.

# TREATMENT

Recent advances in medicine and science often generate unrealistic expectations regarding pregnancy rates. These expectations increase the pressure on physicians and frequently result in application of empirical therapy, such as the treatment of minimal to mild endometriosis, varicocelectomy, and IVF. However, infertility specialists have much more to offer to their patients today compared to two decades ago (Table 52-3). Nonetheless, the basic principles of diagnosis-directed evidence-based treatment should guide the choice of therapy.

## Cervical Factor Infertility

If cervical stenosis is suspected, dilatation of the cervix is performed. Intrauterine insemination is recommended when a history of cervical surgery, cryotherapy, or other anatomic defects are present and no sperm is detected on the postcoital test. If other factors are involved in infertility such as tubal factors and male factors, IVF is the preferred treatment.

# Reproductive Endocrinology and Infertility

**Table 52-3**
**Most Commonly Used Assisted Reproductive Technologies**

| Type of ART | Procedure | Main Indication |
|---|---|---|
| Intrauterine insemination | Placement of washed sperm into uterus | Unexplained infertility |
| In vitro fertilization | Retrieval of superovulated eggs and placement of sperm with these eggs outside body, followed by transfer of resultant embryos into uterus | Tubal factor infertility |
| In vitro fertilization with intracytoplasmic sperm injection | Retrieval of superovulated eggs and injection of each egg with a single sperm followed by transfer of resultant embryos | Male factor infertility |

ART, assisted reproductive technology.

## Uterine Factor Infertility

Submucosal fibroids and endometrial polyps are best confirmed and removed via hysteroscopy. When intramural or subserosal fibroids are present, myomectomy may be considered, depending on the size and location of the fibroids. Treatment strategy for developmental anomalies is based on the type of anomaly. When a septate uterus is detected, hysteroscopic resection of the septum is recommended. Other anomalies, such as bicornuate and didelphic uterus, are managed expectantly. Surgery may be considered if the couple is unable to become pregnant or miscarry recurrently. The only option for women with vaginal aplasia and uterine hypoplasia is surrogacy.

## Tubal Factor Infertility

Surgical tubal reconstruction such as fimbrioplasty, lysis of adhesions, and salpingoneoplasty used to be the only option for women with tubal damage. However, low pregnancy rates after surgery and the advent of IVF rendered tubal reconstruction a choice only for selected couples who are known to have normal tubal mucosa and are adverse to IVF.

In vitro fertilization is now the preferred therapy for couples with tubal factor infertility. Of 99,989 women who started ART treatment in 2000, 39,437 underwent IVF for etiologies other than male factor infertility such as tubal factor and unexplained infertility. Pregnancy and delivery rates per oocyte retrieval were 35% and 29%, respectively.[101] Removal of tubes prior to IVF is recommended in women with hydrosalpinx; as a recent meta-analysis reported that laparoscopic salpingectomy increases pregnancy and live birth rates significantly in these women (OR, 1.75; 95% CI, 1.07 to 2.86; and OR, 2.13; 95% CI, 1.24 to 3.65, respectively).[102] Increased risks for multiple pregnancy, ovarian hyperstimulation syndrome, ectopic pregnancy and preterm delivery are encountered with IVF therapy.

## Endometriosis

Medical treatment of minimal to mild endometriosis with ovulation-suppressing agents, including medroxyprogesterone acetate, oral contraceptive pills (OCPs), GnRH agonists and danazol offers no benefit to infertile women because these therapies do not increase pregnancy rates but delay potential spontaneous pregnancies or successful treatment with IVF.[103]

Laparoscopic ablation or removal of minimal to mild endometriosis using electrocautery or laser to improve pregnancy rates has been debated. There are only two contradicting randomized clinical trials in the literature. Marcoux and colleagues in their larger multicenter trial showed an improvement in pregnancy rates after surgical intervention[28] whereas Gruppo Italiano reported no significant improvement.[104] A meta-analysis combining the two showed increased pregnancy rates.[105] However, 8 women need to undergo surgery to achieve 1 additional pregnancy. Therefore, laparoscopic therapy offers modest improvement in pregnancy rates compared to no therapy.

When endometriosis is advanced, with significant pelvic adhesive disease and tubal damage, IVF is the best therapy available. However, removal of endometriomas prior to IVF has been controversial. Some authors advocate the resection of endometriomas because surgery did not negatively affect the ovarian response during IVF,[106] whereas others reported no improvement in pregnancy rates or poor ovarian response after surgery.[107,108] Postoperative medical treatment does not improve pregnancy rates. Therefore, it is not recommended. Therapy for endometriomas should be individualized based on patient history and physical examination findings.

## Ovarian Factor Infertility
### Eugonadotropic Anovulation

The majority of anovulatory women with normal gonadotropin levels have PCOS. Diet and exercise resulting in 10% decline in the BMI may resume ovulation in up to 90% of patients.[109] However, difficulty in achieving weight loss drives women and physicians to use readily available ovulation-inducing medications. Clomiphene citrate, an estrogen antagonist, remains the first-line agent for anovulatory infertility in PCOS for some clinicians. Clomiphene citrate stimulates FSH secretion by the pituitary, resulting in the development of mature follicles. The starting dose of clomiphene citrate is usually 50 mg/day between cycle days 3 and 7. Ovulation usually occurs 7 days after the last pill. If there is no response, the dose may be increased by 50-mg increments up to 200 to 250 mg/day. Approximately 75% of pregnancies with clomiphene citrate occur in the first three treatment cycles; 50% of patients conceive at the 50-mg dose.[110]

Recently, the use of metformin, an insulin-sensitizing agent, for ovulation induction has dramatically changed the treatment of chronic anovulation in PCOS. Its mechanism of action on insulin metabolism is unknown. However, metformin improves insulin sensitivity, resulting in lower serum insulin and glucose levels. It does not induce hypoglycemia because insulin levels are not elevated. A meta-analysis including 13 randomized clinical trials comparing metformin to placebo or clomiphene citrate reported improved pregnancy rates, with metformin replacing clomiphene citrate as a first-line agent[111] Metformin is usually administered 500 mg three times daily by mouth. However, a starting dose of 500 mg daily gradually increased by 500-mg increments may be considered because of the gastrointestinal side effects such as nausea, vomiting, and bloating. Side effects of metformin are discussed in detail in chapter 61. Other insulin-sensitizing agents, including troglitazone, rosiglitazone, and pioglitazone, are peroxisome proliferator activator receptor γ inhibitors. Troglitazone was withdrawn from the market because of hepatic side effects, but the largest randomized trial involving an insulin-sensitizing agent reported that troglitazone was effective in ovulation induction.[112] There is only limited data on the other two agents.

Gonadotropins are administered in women who do not respond to metformin or clomiphene citrate. However, these women are at risk for ovarian hyperstimulation syndrome and multiple pregnancy when they respond to gonadotropins. Low-dose, step-up FSH therapy has been suggested to prevent ovarian hyperstimulation syndrome and multiple pregnancy.[113]

Another agent that has gained attention recently is the aromatase inhibitor, letrozole, which blocks the conversion of androgens to estrogens and therefore acts in a similar way with clomiphene citrate. However, only preliminary studies have been conducted to date. Dexamethasone treatment in combination with clomiphene citrate has been shown to be effective in women with elevated dehydroepiandrosterone sulfate levels. The addition of metformin may be preferable to dexamethasone because of its better side effect profile. The combination of metformin with gonadotropins has also been suggested to improve pregnancy rates and decrease ovarian hyperstimulation syndrome. However, current preliminary data is not sufficient to make definitive conclusions on the combination therapy.

Ovarian wedge resection, once used to treat clomiphene citrate-resistant PCOS patients, can result in significant postoperative peritubal and periovarian adhesion formation. Recently, a less invasive technique, laparoscopic ovarian drilling using electrocautery or laser, has been suggested. However, recombinant FSH alone was more effective than ovarian drilling in a randomized trial. Because the multiple pregnancy rate was significantly lower in women treated with ovarian drilling compared to the recombinant FSH group,[114] this technique may be useful for couples who desire to avoid multiple pregnancy.

### Hypergonadotropic Anovulation (Premature Ovarian Failure)

There is no treatment available to resume ovulation after ovarian failure, although spontaneous pregnancies may occur even in women taking OCPs or hormone replacement therapy. IVF with donor oocytes and adoption are the only options for these couples. However, women who underwent IVF with donor oocytes had the highest pregnancy and delivery rates, 51% and 43% per embryo transfer, respectively, among women who underwent ART nationwide in 2000.[101]

### Hypogonadotropic Anovulation

Hypothalamic anovulation and other central etiologies may cause hypogonadism with resultant anovulation. Treatment of underlying etiology, such as weight gain, cessation of strenuous exercise, or treatment of the infiltrating disease or tumor, should be considered initially. If medical therapy is necessary for ovulation induction, gonadotropins are the first-line agents. Most women become pregnant on gonadotropins. Pulsatile GnRH therapy has been investigated for hypothalamic anovulation. Although pulsatile GnRH administration is very cumbersome, it is successful in achieving pregnancy and has the advantage of a relatively low multiple pregnancy rate.

### Hyperprolactinemic Anovulation

The classic treatment for hyperprolactinemia is bromocriptine. Bromocriptine is a dopamine agonist that acts through the stimulation of dopamine ($D_2$) receptors. It decreases PRL synthesis and adenoma size. Normoprolactinemia and ovulatory cycles are achieved in 80% to 90% of the women[115] The starting dose of bromocriptine is 2.5 to 5.0 mg/day by mouth, which can be titrated after normoprolactinemia is achieved. The most common side effects are nausea and vomiting. Headache, dizziness, orthostatic hypotension, and depression are the other side effects of dopamine agonists. The dose may be gradually increased or administered intravaginally to minimize the side effects. Cabergoline is another ergot derivative with a longer half-life and better side effect profile. The usual dose is 0.5 to 1 mg twice weekly by mouth. It may be administered intra-vaginally to minimize side effects. A multicenter randomized trial showed that normoprolactinemia and the resumption of menses were achieved in 83% and 91% of women, respectively, on twice-weekly cabergoline compared to 59% and 83% for the bromocriptine group, respectively.[116] Moreover, cabergoline was better tolerated than bromocriptine. However, there is less data on the fetal safety of cabergoline compared to bromocriptine.

### Age

If initial attempts at ovulation induction and IVF fail because of poor ovarian response or the day 3 FSH value is elevated, as occurs more commonly in women older than age 35, the use of donor oocytes or adoption should be considered. Spontaneous abortion rates remain unchanged in women who use donor oocytes, whereas they increase exponentially in women who undergo IVF with their own eggs after age 36.[117]

### Endocrine Disorders and Infertility

Treatment of the underlying endocrine disorder is the goal of therapy. If ovulation is not restored, ovulation induction can be achieved using various agents ranging from clomiphene citrate to gonadotropins depending on the patient's presentation.

### Unexplained Infertility

Expectant management may be considered in couples who have been infertile for less than 3 years and the female age is younger than age 35. Approximately 32% of couples with unexplained infertility become pregnant within the first 3 years of infertility. However, the chances of pregnancy decline significantly after 3 years. Clomiphene citrate and IUI may be considered as the initial treatment in unexplained infertility. The pregnancy rate with this approach is 9.5% per cycle.[118] A multicenter randomized trial reported a pregnancy rate of 9% per cycle with FSH stimulation and IUI, which was significantly higher than pregnancy rates with FSH stimulation and intracervical insemination, intracervical insemination only, and IUI only (4%, 2%, and 5% per cycle, respectively).[119] Approximately 33% of the couples who received FSH stimulation and IUI became pregnant. However, increased risk of multiple pregnancy is a disadvantage of FSH stimulation. If pregnancy is not achieved with clomiphene citrate and IUI or FSH and IUI, IVF is recommended.

# Reproductive Endocrinology and Infertility

## Male Factor Infertility

Contrary to female infertility, the underlying problem, such as hypogonadotropic hypogonadism, disorders of ejaculation and erection, and obstructive azoospermia, can be treated in a small percentage of infertile men. The majority of men with abnormal semen parameters require IVF with intracytoplasmic sperm injection (ICSI). This topic is discussed in detail in Chapter 53.

## CLINICAL COURSE AND PROGRESSION

The duration of infertility, female age, and a history of a previous pregnancy are important prognostic determinants for an infertile couple. However, it is not possible to predict whether a couple will become pregnant with or without treatment. After 3 years of infertility, pregnancy rates decrease significantly every month (by 2%) in couples with unexplained infertility.[47] Treatment success also declines in repeated cycles. Couples have the highest chances of pregnancy in the first three or four cycles of treatment regardless of the type of treatment. It is prudent to avoid the exploitation of the couple with repeated cycles of unsuccessful therapies before exploring other options such as donor oocytes, donor sperm, and adoption. Some couples may become pregnant spontaneously even after adopting a child. However, pregnancy rates after adoption is not different from that for nonadopting couples.[120]

An association between infertility and cancer has been suggested. Treatment for infertility has also been investigated as a risk factor for female cancers. Two recent multicenter retrospective studies involving the same patient population (12,193 women) have investigated the ovarian cancer risk in women with infertility and women who received ovulation-stimulating agents.[121,122] Overall, infertile women had a significantly higher risk for developing ovarian cancer than the general population (standardized incidence ratio, 1.98; 95% CI, 1.4 to 2.6). This risk was even higher in women with primary infertility or endometriosis. However, infertility treatment—defined as the use of clomiphene citrate or gonadotropins—did not increase the risk of ovarian cancer (standardized incidence ratios, 0.82; 95% CI, 0.4 to 1.5; and 1.09; 95% CI, 0.4 to 2.8, respectively).

These investigators also examined the risk of breast cancer in the same population.[123] Infertile women had a higher risk for breast cancer compared to the general population (standardized incidence ratio, 1.29; 95% CI, 1.1 to 1.4), whereas treatment with clomiphene citrate or gonadotropins did not affect the risk of breast cancer (standardized incidence ratios, 1.02 and 1.07, respectively). A different group of investigators from Europe confirmed that the treatment for infertility did not increase the breast cancer risk (RR, 0.95; 95% CI, 0.82 to 1.11).[124]

## PITFALLS AND CONTROVERSIES

Advances in the treatment of infertility have enabled many couples to have children who otherwise would not be able to experience parenthood. The goal of infertility treatment is the birth of a singleton healthy baby by a healthy mother.

However, treatment of infertility is not risk free. Ovarian hyperstimulation syndrome, multiple pregnancy, low birth weight, preterm delivery, and plausible risk for chromosomal anomalies are potential complications that may lead to morbidity and mortality in both the baby and mother. Moreover, men with severe oligospermia or azoospermia have an increased risk of chromosomal anomalies or single gene mutations. IVF with ICSI enables these men to have children. Therefore, one can argue that genetically caused infertility may be perpetuated using infertility treatment. However, these children will have access to the same, if not better, treatment, and attempts at improving the genetic quality of the population may have eugenic implications. Infertility interest groups support the idea that having a child is a basic biologic value and every person's right.[125] The ASRM describes infertility as a disease.[126] Therefore, one can argue that it is the infertile couples' right to give informed consent for infertility treatments that may result in potential complications, just as any other therapy with side effects or complications.

Another debated issue is the accessibility of infertility treatments. Although infertility treatment with ART is no longer an experimental procedure, couples still do not have universal access to ART because of the lack of comprehensive insurance coverage for infertility. Lack of comprehensive insurance coverage may also have an impact on ART outcome. Limited patient resources preclude more than one attempt at treatment. But adequate coverage may relieve the pressure on physicians to achieve pregnancy in one attempt, leading to a decrease in the number of embryos transferred. This may improve multiple pregnancy rates as the number of embryos transferred is strongly correlated with the success rate and multiple pregnancy rate. However, insurance coverage alone cannot diminish the multiple pregnancy rate. Although the need for the regulation of infertility treatment is clear, a strict government control, as seen in Europe, can be counterproductive because it may lead to suboptimal practices, such as the transfer of two embryos in a 42-year-old woman with a history of failed IVF cycles.[127] Rigorous regulations by professional societies and health organizations such as The American Society for Reproductive Medicine and the Centers for Disease Control and Prevention may be the best approach to minimize the risks of infertility treatment and improve pregnancy rates.

## REFERENCES

1. Abma JC, Chandra A, Mosher WD, et al: Fertility, family planning, and women's health: new data from the 1995 National Survey of Family Growth. Vital Health Stat 23 1997;1–114. **(III, B)**
2. Martin JA, Hamilton BE, Sutton PD, et al: Births: final data for 2002. Natl Vital Stat Rep 2003;52:1–113. **(III, B)**
3. U.S. Department of Health and Human Services: Healthy People 2010: Understanding and Improving Health, 2nd ed. Washington DC, U.S. Government Printing Office, 2000, pp 9-28–9-29. **(IV, C)**
4. Farhi J, Ashkenazi J, Feldberg D, et al: Effect of uterine leiomyomata on the results of in vitro fertilization treatment. Hum Reprod 1995; 10:2576–2578. **(III, B)**
5. Ramzy AM, Sattar M, Amin Y, et al: Uterine myomata and outcome of assisted reproduction. Hum Reprod 1998;13:198–202. **(III, B)**
6. Surrey ES, Lietz AK, and Schoolcraft WB: Impact of intramural leiomyomata in patients with a normal endometrial cavity on in vitro fertilization–embryo transfer cycle outcome. Fertil Steril 2001;75: 405–410. **(III, B)**

7. Jun SH, Ginsburg ES, Racowsky C, et al: Uterine leiomyomas and their effect on in vitro fertilization outcome: a retrospective study. J Assist Reprod Genet 2001;18:139–143. **(III, B)**

8. Hart R, Khalaf Y, Yeong CT, et al: A prospective controlled study of the effect of intramural uterine fibroids on the outcome of assisted conception. Hum Reprod 2001;16:2411–2417. **(III, B)**

9. Eldar-Geva T, Meagher S, Healy DL, et al: Effect of intramural, sub-serosal, and submucosal uterine fibroids on the outcome of assisted reproductive technology treatment. Fertil Steril 1998;70:687–691. **(III, B)**

10. Stovall DW, Parrish SB, Van Voorhis BJ, et al: Uterine leiomyomas reduce the efficacy of assisted reproduction cycles: results of a matched follow-up study. Hum Reprod 1998;13:192–197. **(III, B)**

11. Grimbizis GF, Camus M, Tarlatzis BC, et al: Clinical implications of uterine malformations and hysteroscopic treatment results. Hum Reprod Update 2001;7:161–174. **(III, B)**

12. Westrom L: Incidence, prevalence, and trends of acute pelvic inflammatory disease and its consequences in industrialized countries. Am J Obstet Gynecol 1980;138:880–892. **(III, B)**

13. Osser S, Persson K, Liedholm P: Tubal infertility and silent chlamydial salpingitis. Hum Reprod 1989;4:280–284. **(III, B)**

14. Szigetvari I, Feinman M, Barad D, et al: Association of previous abdominal surgery and significant adhesions in laparoscopic sterilization patients. J Reprod Med 1989;34:465–466. **(III, B)**

15. DeCherney AH, Mezer HC: The nature of post-tuboplasty pelvic adhesions as determined by early and late laparoscopy. Fertil Steril 1984;41:643–646. **(III, B)**

16. Lisa JR, Gioia JD, Rubin IC: Observations on the interstitial portion of the fallopian tube. Surg Gynecol Obstet 1954;92:159–169. **(III, B)**

17. Wansaicheong GK, Ong CL: Intramural tubal polyps—a villain in the shadows? Singapore Med J 1998;39:97–100. **(III, B)**

18. Simon C, Gutierrez A, Vidal A, et al: Outcome of patients with endometriosis in assisted reproduction: results from in vitro fertilization and oocyte donation. Hum Reprod 1994;9:725–729. **(III, B)**

19. Arici A, Oral E, Bukulmez O, et al: The effect of endometriosis on implantation: results from the Yale University in vitro fertilization and embryo transfer program. Fertil Steril 1996;65:603–607. **(III, B)**

20. Lessey BA, Castelbaum AJ, Sawin SW, et al: Aberrant integrin expression in the endometrium of women with endometriosis. J Clin Endocrinol Metab 1994;79:643–649. **(III, B)**

21. Diaz I, Navarro J, Blasco L, et al: Impact of stage III–IV endometriosis on recipients of sibling oocytes: matched case-control study. Fertil Steril 2000;74:31–34. **(III, B)**

22. Geber S, Paraschos T, Atkinson G, et al: Results of IVF in patients with endometriosis: the severity of the disease does not affect outcome, or the incidence of miscarriage. Hum Reprod 1995;10:1507–1511. **(III, B)**

23. Olivennes F, Feldberg D, Liu HC, et al: Endometriosis: a stage by stage analysis—the role of in vitro fertilization. Fertil Steril 1995;64:392–398. **(III, B)**

24. Stone SC, Himsl K: Peritoneal recovery of motile and nonmotile sperm in the presence of endometriosis. Fertil Steril 1986;46:338–339. **(IIb, B)**

25. Sung L, Mukherjee T, Takeshige T, et al: Endometriosis is not detrimental to embryo implantation in oocyte recipients. J Assist Reprod Genet 1997;14:152–156. **(III, B)**

26. Strathy JH, Molgaard CA, Coulam CB, et al: Endometriosis and infertility: a laparoscopic study of endometriosis among fertile and infertile women. Fertil Steril 1982;38:667–672. **(III, B)**

27. Akande VA, Hunt LP, Cahill DJ, et al: Differences in time to natural conception between women with unexplained infertility and infertile women with minor endometriosis. Hum Reprod 2004;19:96–103. **(III, B)**

28. Marcoux S, Maheux R, Berube S: Laparoscopic surgery in infertile women with minimal or mild endometriosis. Canadian Collaborative Group on Endometriosis. N Engl J Med 1997;337:217–222. **(Ib, A)**

29. Balen AH, Braat DD, West C, et al: Cumulative conception and live birth rates after the treatment of anovulatory infertility: safety and efficacy of ovulation induction in 200 patients. Hum Reprod 1994;9:1563–1570. **(III, B)**

30. Marcus MD, Loucks TL, Berga SL: Psychological correlates of functional hypothalamic amenorrhea. Fertil Steril 2001;76:310–316. **(III, B)**

31. Menken J, Trussell J, Larsen U: Age and infertility. Science 1986;233:1389–1394. **(III, B)**

32. Schwartz D, Mayaux MJ: Female fecundity as a function of age: results of artificial insemination in 2193 nulliparous women with azoospermic husbands. Federation CECOS. N Engl J Med 1982;306:404–406. **(III, B)**

33. Stovall DW, Toma SK, Hammond MG, et al: The effect of age on female fecundity. Obstet Gynecol 1991;77:33–36. **(III, B)**

34. Dunson DB, Colombo B, Baird DD: Changes with age in the level and duration of fertility in the menstrual cycle. Hum Reprod 2002;17:1399–1403. **(III, B)**

35. Warburton D, Kline J, Stein Z: Cytogenetic abnormalities in spontaneous abortions of recognized conceptions. In Wiley HA (ed): Perinatal Genetics: Diagnosis and Treatment. New York, Academic Press, 1990, p 133. **(III, B)**

36. FIVNAT: Fécondation in vitro après 40 ans. Contracept Fertil Sex 1993;21:367–370. **(III, B)**

37. Plachot M, De Grouchy J, Junca AM, et al: Chromosomal analysis of human oocytes and embryos in an in vitro fertilization program. Ann NY Acad Sci 1988;541:384–397. **(III, B)**

38. Navot D, Bergh PA, Williams MA, et al: Poor oocyte quality rather than implantation failure as a cause of age-related decline in female fertility. Lancet 1991;337:1375–1377. **(III, B)**

39. Krassas GE: Thyroid disease and female reproduction. Fertil Steril 2000;74:1063–1070. **(III, B)**

40. Joshi JV, Bhandarkar SD, Chadha M, et al: Menstrual irregularities and lactation failure may precede thyroid dysfunction or goitre. J Postgrad Med 1993;39:137–141. **(III, B)**

41. Poppe K, Glinoer D, Van Steirteghem A, et al: Thyroid dysfunction and autoimmunity in infertile women. Thyroid 2002;12:997–1001. **(III, B)**

42. Kutteh WH, Yetman DL, Carr AC, et al: Increased prevalence of antithyroid antibodies identified in women with recurrent pregnancy loss but not in women undergoing assisted reproduction. Fertil Steril 1999;71:843–848. **(III, B)**

43. Poppe K, Glinoer D, Tournaye H, et al: Assisted reproduction and thyroid autoimmunity: an unfortunate combination? J Clin Endocrinol Metab 2003;88:4149–4152. **(III, B)**

44. Kovacs P, Parlow AF, Karkanias GB: Effect of centrally administered insulin on gonadotropin-releasing hormone neuron activity and luteinizing hormone surge in the diabetic female rat. Neuroendocrinol 2002;76:357–365. **(IIa, B)**

45. Bruning JC, Gautam D, Burks DJ, et al: Role of brain insulin receptor in control of body weight and reproduction. Science 2000;289:2122–2125. **(IIa, B)**

46. Conn JJ, Jacobs HS, Conway GS: The prevalence of polycystic ovaries in women with type 2 diabetes mellitus. Clin Endocrinol (Oxf) 2000;52:81–86. **(III, B)**

47. Collins JA, Rowe TC: Age of the female partner is a prognostic factor in prolonged unexplained infertility: a multicenter study. Fertil Steril 1989;52:15–20. **(III, B)**

48. Franco B, Guioli S, Pragliola A, et al: A gene deleted in Kallmann's syndrome shares homology with neural cell adhesion and axonal pathfinding molecules. Nature 1991;353:529–536. **(III, B)**

49. Dode C, Levilliers J, Dupont JM, et al: Loss-of-function mutations in *FGFR1* cause autosomal dominant Kallmann syndrome. Nat Genet 2003;33:463–465. **(III, B)**

50. Strobel A, Issad T, Camoin L, et al: A leptin missense mutation associated with hypogonadism and morbid obesity. Nat Genet 1998;18:213–215. **(III, B)**

51. Clement K, Vaisse C, Lahlou N, et al: A mutation in the human leptin receptor gene causes obesity and pituitary dysfunction. Nature 1998;392:398–401. **(III, B)**

52. de Roux N, Young J, Misrahi M, et al: A family with hypogonadotropic hypogonadism and mutations in the gonadotropin-releasing hormone receptor. N Engl J Med 1997;337:1597–1602. **(III, B)**

53. Layman LC, Porto AL, Xie J, et al: *FSH-β* gene mutations in a female with partial breast development and a male sibling with normal puberty and azoospermia. J Clin Endocrinol Metab 2002;87: 3702–3707. **(III, B)**

54. Weiss J, Axelrod L, Whitcomb RW, et al: Hypogonadism caused by a single amino acid substitution in the beta subunit of luteinizing hormone. N Engl J Med 1992;326:179–183. **(III, B)**

55. Layman LC: Genetic causes of human infertility. Endocrinol Metab Clin North Am 2003;32:549–572. **(III, B)**

56. Aittomaki K, Lucena JL, Pakarinen P, et al: Mutation in the follicle-stimulating hormone receptor gene causes hereditary hyper-gonadotropic ovarian failure. Cell 1995;82:959–968. **(III, B)**

57. Tapanainen JS, Aittomaki K, Min J, et al: Men homozygous for an inactivating mutation of the follicle-stimulating hormone *(FSH)* receptor gene present variable suppression of spermatogenesis and fertility. Nat Genet 1997;15:205–206. **(III, B)**

58. Kremer H, Kraaij R, Toledo SP, et al: Male pseudohermaphroditism due to a homozygous missense mutation of the luteinizing hormone receptor gene. Nat Genet 1995;9:160–164. **(III, B)**

59. Toledo SP, Brunner HG, Kraaij R, et al: An inactivating mutation of the luteinizing hormone receptor causes amenorrhea in a 46,XX female. J Clin Endocrinol Metab 1996;81:3850–3854. **(III, B)**

60. Kobayashi A, Behringer RR: Developmental genetics of the female reproductive tract in mammals. Nat Rev Genet 2003;4:969–980. **(III, B)**

61. Mercier B, Verlingue C, Lissens W, et al: Is congenital bilateral absence of vas deferens a primary form of cystic fibrosis? Analyses of the *CFTR* gene in 67 patients. Am J Hum Genet 1995;56:272–277. **(III, B)**

62. Oei SG, Keirse MJ, Bloemenkamp KW, et al: European postcoital tests: opinions and practice. Br J Obstet Gynaecol 1995;102:621–624. **(III, B)**

63. Oei SG, Helmerhorst FM, Bloemenkamp KW, et al: Effectiveness of the postcoital test: randomised controlled trial. BMJ 1998;317: 502–505. **(Ib, A)**

64. Ascher SM, Jha RC, Reinhold C: Benign myometrial conditions: leiomyomas and adenomyosis. Top Magn Reson Imaging 2003;14: 281–304. **(III, B)**

65. Nawroth F, Foth D, Schmidt T: Minihysteroscopy as routine diagnostic procedure in women with primary infertility. J Am Assoc Gynecol Laparosc 2003;10:396–398. **(III, B)**

66. Oliveira FG, Abdelmassih VG, Diamond MP, et al: Uterine cavity findings and hysteroscopic interventions in patients undergoing in vitro fertilization–embryo transfer who repeatedly cannot conceive. Fertil Steril 2003;80:1371–1375. **(III, B)**

67. Hubacher D, Grimes D, Lara-Ricalde R, et al: The limited clinical usefulness of taking a history in the evaluation of women with tubal factor infertility. Fertil Steril 2004;81:6–10. **(IIb, B)**

68. Tulandi T, Platt R: The art of taking a history. Fertil Steril 2004;81: 11–12. **(IV, C)**

69. Donnez J, Jadoul P: Taking a history in the evaluation of infertility: obsolete or venerable tradition? Fertil Steril 2004;81:16–17. **(IV, C)**

70. Swart P, Mol BW, van d V, et al: The accuracy of hysterosalpingography in the diagnosis of tubal pathology: a meta-analysis. Fertil Steril 1995; 64:486–491. **(Ia, A)**

71. Mol BW, Collins JA, Burrows EA, et al: Comparison of hysterosalpingography and laparoscopy in predicting fertility outcome. Hum Reprod 1999;14:1237–1242. **(IIb, B)**

72. Vandekerckhove P, Watson A, Lilford R, et al: Oil-soluble versus water-soluble media for assessing tubal patency with hysterosalpingography or laparoscopy in subfertile women. Cochrane Database Syst Rev 2000;CD000092. **(Ia, A)**

73. Holz K, Becker R, Schurmann R: Ultrasound in the investigation of tubal patency. A meta-analysis of three comparative studies of Echovist-200 including 1007 women. Zentralbl Gynakol 1997;119: 366–373. **(IIb, B)**

74. Kresch AJ, Seifer DB, Sachs LB, et al: Laparoscopy in 100 women with chronic pelvic pain. Obstet Gynecol 1984;64:672–674. **(III, B)**

75. Mahmood TA, Templeton A: Prevalence and genesis of endometriosis. Hum Reprod 1991;6:544–549. **(III, B)**

76. Mahmood TA, Templeton AA, Thomson L, et al: Menstrual symptoms in women with pelvic endometriosis. Br J Obstet Gynaecol 1991; 98:558–563. **(III, B)**

77. Simpson JL, Elias S, Malinak LR, et al: Heritable aspects of endometriosis. I. Genetic studies. Am J Obstet Gynecol 1980;137: 327–331. **(III, B)**

78. Matorras R, Rodriguez F, Pijoan JI, et al: Are there any clinical signs and symptoms that are related to endometriosis in infertile women? Am J Obstet Gynecol 1996;174:620–623. **(IIb, B)**

79. Eskenazi B, Warner M, Bonsignore L, et al: Validation study of non-surgical diagnosis of endometriosis. Fertil Steril 2001;76:929–935. **(IIb, B)**

80. Chapron C, Dubuisson JB, Pansini V, et al: Routine clinical examination is not sufficient for diagnosing and locating deeply infiltrating endometriosis. J Am Assoc Gynecol Laparosc 2002;9:115–119. **(III, B)**

81. Mol BW, Bayram N, Lijmer JG, et al: The performance of CA 125 measurement in the detection of endometriosis: a meta-analysis. Fertil Steril 1998;70:1101–1108. **(IIb, B)**

82. Moore J, Copley S, Morris J, et al: A systematic review of the accuracy of ultrasound in the diagnosis of endometriosis. Ultrasound Obstet Gynecol 2002;20:630–634. **(IIb, B)**

83. Stratton P, Winkel C, Premkumar A, et al: Diagnostic accuracy of laparoscopy, magnetic resonance imaging, and histopathologic examination for the detection of endometriosis. Fertil Steril 2003;79: 1078–1085. **(IIb, B)**

84. Togashi K, Nishimura K, Kimura I, et al: Endometrial cysts: diagnosis with MR imaging. Radiology 1991;180:73–78. **(III, B)**

85. Chapron C, Vieira M, Chopin N, et al: Accuracy of rectal endoscopic ultrasonography and magnetic resonance imaging in the diagnosis of rectal involvement for patients presenting with deeply infiltrating endometriosis. Ultrasound Obstet Gynecol 2004;24:175–179. **(III, B)**

86. Wilcox AJ, Weinberg CR, Baird DD: Timing of sexual intercourse in relation to ovulation. Effects on the probability of conception, survival of the pregnancy, and sex of the baby. N Engl J Med 1995;333: 1517–1521. **(III, B)**

87. Guermandi E, Vegetti W, Bianchi MM, et al: Reliability of ovulation tests in infertile women. Obstet Gynecol 2001;97:92–96. **(III, B)**

88. Queenan JT, O'Brien GD, Bains LM, et al: Ultrasound scanning of ovaries to detect ovulation in women. Fertil Steril 1980;34:99–105. **(III, B)**

89. Vermesh M, Kletzky OA, Davajan V, et al: Monitoring techniques to predict and detect ovulation. Fertil Steril 1987;47:259–264. **(III, B)**

90. Ecochard R, Marret H, Rabilloud M, et al: Sensitivity and specificity of ultrasound indices of ovulation in spontaneous cycles. Eur J Obstet Gynecol Reprod Biol 2000;91:59–64. **(III, B)**

91. WHO: Temporal relationships between ovulation and defined changes in the concentration of plasma estradiol-17 beta, luteinizing hormone, follicle-stimulating hormone, and progesterone. I. Probit analysis. World Health Organization, Task Force on Methods for the Determination of the Fertile Period, Special Programme of Research, Development and Research Training in Human Reproduction. Am J Obstet Gynecol 1980;138:383–390. **(III, B)**

92. Temporal relationships between indices of the fertile period. Fertil Steril 1983;39:647–655. **(III, B)**

93. Miller PB, Soules MR: The usefulness of a urinary LH kit for ovulation prediction during menstrual cycles of normal women. Obstet Gynecol 1996;87:13–17. **(III, B)**

94. Barratt CL, Cooke S, Chauhan M, et al: A prospective randomized controlled trial comparing urinary luteinizing hormone dipsticks and basal body temperature charts with timed donor insemination. Fertil Steril 1989;52:394–397. **(Ib, A)**

95. Robinson JN, Lockwood GM, Dalton JD, et al: A randomized prospective study to assess the effect of the use of home urinary luteinizing hormone detection on the efficiency of donor insemination. Hum Reprod 1992;7:63–65. **(Ib, A)**

96. Deaton JL, Clark RR, Pittaway DE, et al: Clomiphene citrate ovulation induction in combination with a timed intrauterine insemination: the value of urinary luteinizing hormone versus human chorionic gonadotropin timing. Fertil Steril 1997;68:43–47. **(III, B)**

97. Scott RT, Opsahl MS, Leonardi MR, et al: Life table analysis of pregnancy rates in a general infertility population relative to ovarian reserve and patient age. Hum Reprod 1995;10:1706–1710. **(III, B)**

98. Jain T, Soules MR, Collins JA: Comparison of basal follicle-stimulating hormone versus the clomiphene citrate challenge test for ovarian reserve screening. Fertil Steril 2004;82:180–185. **(III, B)**

99. Crosignani PG, Rubin BL: Optimal use of infertility diagnostic tests and treatments. The ESHRE Capri Workshop Group. Hum Reprod 2000;15:723–732. **(IV, C)**

100. Coetzee K, Kruge TF, Lombard CJ: Predictive value of normal sperm morphology: a structured literature review. Hum Reprod Update 1998;4:73–82. **(III, B)**

101. Assisted reproductive technology in the United States: 2000 results generated from the American Society for Reproductive Medicine/ Society for Assisted Reproductive Technology Registry. Fertil Steril 2004;81:1207–1220. **(III, B)**

102. Johnson N, Mak W, Sowter M: Surgical treatment for tubal disease in women due to undergo in vitro fertilisation. Cochrane Database Syst Rev 2004;3:CD002125. **(Ia, A)**

103. Hughes E, Fedorkow D, Collins J, et al: Ovulation suppression for endometriosis. Cochrane Database Syst Rev 2003;CD000155. **(Ia, A)**

104. Parazzini F: Ablation of lesions or no treatment in minimal to mild endometriosis in infertile women: a randomized trial. Gruppo Italiano per lo Studio dell'Endometriosi. Hum Reprod 1999;14:1332–1334. **(Ib, A)**

105. Jacobson TZ, Barlow DH, Koninckx PR, et al: Laparoscopic surgery for subfertility associated with endometriosis. Cochrane Database Syst Rev 2002;CD001398. **(Ia, A)**

106. Marconi G, Vilela M, Quintana R, et al: Laparoscopic ovarian cystectomy of endometriomas does not affect the ovarian response to gonadotropin stimulation. Fertil Steril 2002;78:876–878. **(IIa, B)**

107. Garcia-Velasco JA, Mahutte NG, Corona J, et al: Removal of endometriomas before in vitro fertilization does not improve fertility outcomes: a matched, case-control study. Fertil Steril 2004;81: 1194–1197. **(IIb, B)**

108. Ho HY, Lee RK, Hwu YM, et al: Poor response of ovaries with endometrioma previously treated with cystectomy to controlled ovarian hyperstimulation. J Assist Reprod Genet 2002;19:507–511. **(III, B)**

109. Clark AM, Thornley B, Tomlinson L, et al: Weight loss in obese infertile women results in improvement in reproductive outcome for all forms of fertility treatment. Hum Reprod 1998;13:1502–1505. **(IIb, B)**

110. Gysler M, March CM, Mishell DR II et al: A decade's experience with an individualized clomiphene treatment regimen including its effect on the postcoital test. Fertil Steril 1982;37:161–167. **(III, B)**

111. Lord JM, Flight IH, Norman RJ: Metformin in polycystic ovary syndrome: systematic review and meta-analysis. BMJ 2003;327: 951–953. **(Ia, A)**

112. Azziz R, Ehrmann D, Legro RS, et al: Troglitazone improves ovulation and hirsutism in the polycystic ovary syndrome: a multicenter, double blind, placebo-controlled trial. J Clin Endocrinol Metab 2001;86: 1626–1632. **(Ib, A)**

113. Christin-Maitre S, Hugues JN: A comparative randomized multi-centric study comparing the step-up versus step-down protocol in polycystic ovary syndrome. Hum Reprod 2003;18:1626–1631. **(Ib, A)**

114. Bayram N, Van Wely M, Kaaijk EM, et al: Using an electrocautery strategy or recombinant follicle stimulating hormone to induce ovulation in polycystic ovary syndrome: randomised controlled trial. BMJ 2004;328:192–196. **(Ib, A)**

115. Molitch ME: Medical management of prolactin-secreting pituitary adenomas. Pituitary 2002;5:55–65. **(III, B)**

116. Webster J, Piscitelli G, Polli A, et al: A comparison of cabergoline and bromocriptine in the treatment of hyperprolactinemic amenorrhea. Cabergoline Comparative Study Group. N Engl J Med 1994;331: 904–909. **(Ib, A)**

117. Schieve LA, Tatham L, Peterson HB, et al: Spontaneous abortion among pregnancies conceived using assisted reproductive technology in the United States. Obstet Gynecol 2003;101:959–967. **(III, B)**

118. Deaton JL, Gibson M, Blackmer KM, et al: A randomized, controlled trial of clomiphene citrate and intrauterine insemination in couples with unexplained infertility or surgically corrected endometriosis. Fertil Steril 1990;54:1083–1088. **(Ib, A)**

119. Guzick DS, Carson SA, Coutifaris C, et al: Efficacy of superovulation and intrauterine insemination in the treatment of infertility. National Cooperative Reproductive Medicine Network. N Engl J Med 1999; 340:177–183. **(Ib, A)**

120. Weir WC, Weir DR: Adoption and subsequent conceptions. Fertil Steril 1966;17:283–288. **(III, B)**

121. Brinton LA, Lamb EJ, Moghissi KS, et al: Ovarian cancer risk associated with varying causes of infertility. Fertil Steril 2004;82:405–414. **(III, B)**

122. Brinton LA, Lamb EJ, Moghissi KS, et al: Ovarian cancer risk after the use of ovulation-stimulating drugs. Obstet Gynecol 2004;103: 1194–1203. **(III, B)**

123. Brinton LA, Scoccia B, Moghissi KS, et al: Breast cancer risk associated with ovulation-stimulating drugs. Hum Reprod 2004;19:2005–2013. **(III, B)**

124. Gauthier E, Paoletti X, Clavel-Chapelon F: Breast cancer risk associated with being treated for infertility: results from the French E3N cohort study. Hum Reprod 2004;19:2216–2221. **(III, B)**

125. Hofmann B: Technological assessment of intracytoplasmic sperm injection: an analysis of the value context. Fertil Steril 2003;80: 930–935. **(IV, C)**

126. American Society for Reproductive Medicine Practice Committee Opinion: Definition of Infertility. Birmingham, AL, 1993. **(IV, C)**

127. Alper MM: In vitro fertilization outcomes: why doesn't anyone get it? Fertil Steril 2004;81:514–516. **(IV, C)**

# Chapter 53

# Assisted Reproductive Technologies/ In Vitro Fertilization

## Randall S. Hines, MD, and Bryan D. Cowan, MD

---

### KEY POINTS

- In vitro fertilization (IVF) has become a common infertility therapy.
- Age is the most powerful predictor of IVF success.
- Hydrosalpinx and uterine myoma may impair IVF success.
- Gonadotropins combined with GnRH agonists or antagonists provide the best pregnancy rates.
- Ovarian hyperstimulation and multiple pregnancy are the two most important complications of IVF.

IVF was a remarkable medical breakthrough in 1978 that resulted in the birth of Louise Brown. This revolutionary technique consists of medical stimulation of the ovaries, transvaginal oocyte retrieval, in vitro gamete processing, embryo culture, and embryo transfer, and it has become a common therapy around the world. Estimates of children born from this procedure are at 1.2 million worldwide, and there were over 115,000 treatment cycles and over 45,000 infants born from IVF in the year 2002 based on data collected by the Society for Assisted Reproductive Technology (SART, a subsociety of the American Society for Reproductive Medicine).[1] This approach to the treatment of infertility has made it possible to establish families in couples for whom reproduction appeared hopeless. Advances in techniques have led to new approaches for other conditions, such as preimplantation genetic diagnosis for inherited disorders. We address the IVF process, from patient preparation to advances in laboratory techniques.

The goal of any IVF program should be to provide patient friendly and successful therapy for assisted reproduction. Because IVF is often an expensive and complex therapy, efforts to reduce obstacles to patient care become paramount. In many parts of the United States, insurance coverage for infertility is limited and out-of-pocket expenses for IVF are high. In addition, the IVF process can be an emotionally trying experience for many couples. Innovations that simplify treatment protocols and lessen the strain on patients are important.

IVF success has increased dramatically over the years, with current pregnancy rates in many clinics at 40% to 50% per embryo transfer. Pregnancy rates per retrieval in patients under 35 years of age increased from 28.4% in 1996 to 33% in 2000.[2]

## PREPARATION FOR IN VITRO FERTILIZATION CYCLE

### Patient Selection

In vitro fertilization has become such a routine and successful part of the infertility practice, an argument could be made that any patient with infertility not caused by anovulation is a candidate for this therapy. While IVF is restricted to more entrenched infertility in most practices, IVF has become the final common pathway for patients who do not achieve pregnancy via other means. Standard indications include tubal disease and male factor (Fig. 53-1). With patent fallopian tubes ovulation disorders are treated first with ovulation induction agents, but when these fail IVF is offered.

### Age and Success

Age is the most powerful predictor of success in an IVF treatment cycle. Historical information from populations attempting spontaneous pregnancies without the availability of contraception demonstrates the impact of age on natural fecundity. In the Mormon population, pregnancy rates fall dramatically at age 35 (Fig. 53-2).

In IVF, the same effect of age is seen. Data from the SART registry reveals a significant decline in pregnancy rates for women over age 35 and an abrupt decline for women over age 40 (Fig. 53-3). Based on the SART 2000 data, women over age 40 had a 70% lower chance of delivery than women less than 35 years of age.[2] Pregnancies in women over age 45 are rare. Advancing age is also associated with increasing rates of miscarriage and a small but significant increase in the risk of chromosomal abnormalities in liveborns.

These dramatic changes with age lead some clinicians to offer donor oocyte cycles at age 40. Clinics vary with regard to specific recommendations, but as the expected endogenous pregnancy rate falls below 10%, the donor oocyte rate of 50% to 60% becomes an attractive option for many patients. Finally, there is an effect of paternal age on IVF success, although this effect is not so dramatic as that seen in women[3] (see Fig. 53-3).

### Uterine Evaluation

Candidates for IVF should have an imaging study to evaluate the uterine cavity. Endometrial polyps, uterine myoma, and congenital uterine abnormalities such as uterine septum should

# Reproductive Endocrinology and Infertility

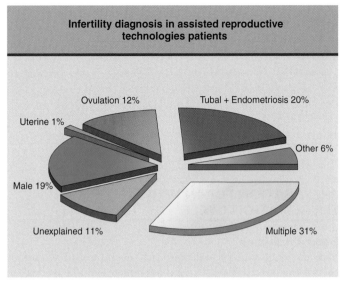

**Figure 53-1    Infertility diagnosis reported among couples who had assisted reproductive technologies (ART) procedures using fresh nondonor eggs or embryos in 2002.** Diagnosis procedures may vary from one clinic to another, so the categorization may be inexact. (Modified from Centers for Disease Control: 2002 Assisted Reproductive Technology Success Rates. Dec 2004. Available at http://www.cdc.gov/reproductivehealth/ART02/index.htm. Accessed 5/22/05.)

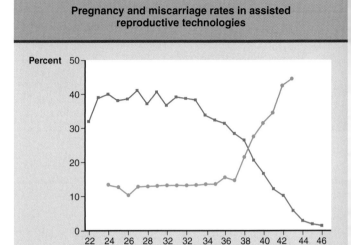

**Figure 53-3    Pregnancy and miscarriage rates adjusted for age during treatment cycles in women undergoing assisted reproductive technologies (ART) procedures using fresh nondonor eggs or embryos in 2002.** Pregnancy rate per IVF cycle is in blue, and miscarriage rate is in green. (Modified from Centers for Disease Control: 2002 Assisted Reproductive Technology Success Rates. Dec 2004. Available at http://www.cdc.gov/reproductivehealth/ART02/index.htm. Accessed 5/22/05.)

be diagnosed prior to beginning the IVF treatment cycle. Hysterosalpingography was commonly utilized in the early days of IVF, but sonohysterography (SHG) is now the most widely used technique for uterine screening. SHG requires vaginal ultrasound and a uterine catheter for saline instillation, is not expensive, and is well tolerated by the patient. Office hysteroscopy has also been used.

In a study of 72 women undergoing IVF, SHG appeared to be effective and was less expensive than other uterine screening methods, although not all patients were evaluated by multiple

techniques.[4] Uterine lesions were detected in 11% of cases. When hysteroscopy was performed on those cases of uterine abnormalities, six of eight cases were confirmed. IVF pregnancy rates were not different for patients undergoing SHG as compared with those patients in the same time period who had a uterine evaluation by a different method. The estimated cost savings per patient undergoing sonohysterography instead of in-office hysteroscopy was $275.

## Surgical Adjuncts to In Vitro Fertilization

If uterine myoma are detected on SHG, the location and size of the myoma often dictate the need for surgical therapy. Submucosal myomas are thought to impair implantation, and there is universal acceptance that hysteroscopic resection is indicated before the IVF cycle.[5] Subserosal myomas do not impair pregnancy and are generally not treated unless symptoms are significant. Management of intramural myomas is controversial. The proximity to the endometrial cavity, size, and number of myomas may influence the decision for myomectomy. In a retrospective study, women with subserosal myomas had the same pregnancy rate as controls, women with submucosal myomas had a low implantation and pregnancy rate, and women with intramural myomas had pregnancy rates between the subserosal and submucosal groups.[6]

For some time, it has been recognized that patients with hydrosalpinx had a lower than expected pregnancy rate when undergoing IVF therapy. Since IVF was created for patients with tubal disease, this finding was surprising. The reasons for the decrease in expected pregnancy rates in patients with hydrosalpinx are not completely known. Hypotheses include a mechanical

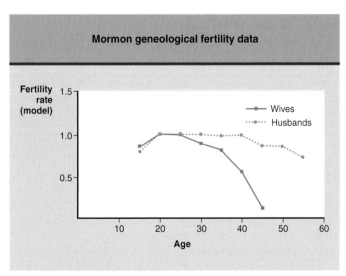

**Figure 53-2    Mormon genealogical fertility data.** (From Mineau GP, Trussell J: A specification of marital fertility by parents' age, age at marriage and marital duration. Demography 1982;19:335–350.)

effect of fluid regressing into the cavity and a toxic effect from fluid on embryo development. A multicenter, randomized controlled trial demonstrated improvement in the pregnancy rate for patients with hydrosalpinx who underwent surgery for salpingectomy, or at least proximal tubal occlusion, before the IVF treatment cycle.[7] Although the overall pregnancy rate was improved with surgery, it did not reach statistical significance. However, the subgroup analysis indicated a dramatic and statistically significant improvement in pregnancy rates for those patients with bilateral hydrosalpinges documented by ultrasound who underwent surgical intervention before IVF. A follow-up of this same study group confirmed the efficacy of this approach.[8] In the follow-up study, patients who had previously been randomized to IVF without surgery and then were unable to achieve pregnancy were taken to surgery for salpingectomy and had subsequent IVF cycles. The pregnancy rate in this group was statistically improved.

The current recommendation is to counsel patients known to have hydrosalpinx that their best chance of success is to proceed with surgical removal or occlusion and then undergo IVF. This poses a dilemma for the practicing obstetrician/gynecologist, who must now include in the consent for laparoscopy, the possibility of salpingectomy for significant tubal disease in the patient who desires future fertility. An important factor in making the decision for salpingectomy is the fact that pregnancy rates following neosalpingostomy may be as low as 5%. Another option for tubal occlusion currently being tested is a hysteroscopic approach.

## Laboratory Testing

General hormonal testing is unlikely to be of benefit prior to IVF. During an infertility evaluation for anovulation, prolactin and thyroid-stimulating hormone measurements are warranted. Without specific complaints or physical manifestations, hormonal testing should be limited.

Diminished ovarian reserve is the inability of the ovary to respond to stimulation and produce mature oocytes resulting in healthy embryos and pregnancies. In preparation for an IVF cycle, the evaluation of ovarian function is designed to identify patients who may have a poor response. This information could then be used to counsel patients on expected prognosis, alter treatment protocols, or offer patients alternative therapy such as donor oocyte cycles. Denying therapy to patients on the basis of such testing is not recommended.

Ovarian reserve testing is now common practice although the choice of testing is debated. The modalities currently employed include cycle day 3 follicle-stimulating hormone (FSH), clomiphene citrate challenge test (CCCT), antral follicle counts (AFCs), and inhibin B testing. CCCT consists of day 3 FSH followed by clomiphene citrate at 100 mg on days 5 to 9. Day 10 FSH completes the test. An abnormal test may be defined by different values depending on the assay used, but a value over 16 mIU/mL is usually abnormal. CCCT is typically reserved for patients over age 35 or over age 30 with unexplained infertility. In a study of some 500 patients attempting pregnancy through a variety of methods, the pregnancy rate for those with a normal CCCT was 40% and for those with an abnormal test, 5%.[9] Day 3 FSH values, independent of age, are advocated by some IVF clinics to identify patients with abnormal ovarian

reserve. Other screening modalities include AFC in the early follicular phase.

A study investigating the predictive accuracy and clinical value of various ovarian reserve tests compared a single or a repeated CCCT in predicting poor response in IVF versus day 3 FSH, inhibin B, and AFC in 63 patients undergoing their first IVF cycle.[10] A first CCCT was performed in which FSH and inhibin B levels were measured on cycle day 10. A second CCCT was performed after a washout period of one cycle. In all patients the tests were followed by an IVF treatment cycle. Parameters examined included poor response (<4 oocytes or cancellation due to impaired [<3 follicles] or absent follicular growth). Both the single day 3 FSH as well as the repeated CCCT markers had rather good discriminative potential for the prediction of poor response, with day 10 FSH and day 10 inhibin B demonstrating similar efficacy. This compared well with the performance of the basal markers (FSH, inhibin B, and AFC). In a multivariate analysis on only the basal variables, FSH day 3 and AFC were selected. Only stepwise forward analysis on the repeated CCCT variables revealed a better discriminating potential for the prediction of poor response. At a specificity level of approximately 0.97, sensitivity and the positive predictive value were marginally improved in the CCCT models. The authors concluded that performing CCCT (single or repeated) has a good ability to predict poor response in IVF. The use of basal FSH and AFC appeared to be as predictive. In a meta-analysis to evaluate pregnancy with treatment, a normal test was not helpful, but an abnormal test strongly predicted a failed outcome.[11]

Ovarian reserve testing is best used in counseling the patient prior to IVF treatment. An older patient who has a low probability of pregnancy might choose donor oocytes if she also has diminished ovarian reserve. A younger patient with abnormal testing may benefit from a different stimulation protocol. Unfortunately, there is no one best treatment protocol for the poor responder.

### Male Evaluation

The precycle IVF evaluation requires an assessment of male factor infertility. Standard semen analysis with attention to count, morphology, and motility will identify many patients requiring intracytoplasmic sperm injection (ICSI), although subtle male factor infertility can exist even with normal numbers. Additional testing in the form of a sperm chromatin structure assay is now being offered.[12] Abnormal testing in light of an otherwise normal semen analysis is felt to be another indication for ICSI. Males with azoospermia can undergo surgical sperm retrieval in the form of epididymal aspiration or testicular biopsy in an outpatient setting. Pregnancy rates for males with severe oligospermia are equivalent to the pregnancy rates seen in other diagnoses, particularly if there is not an additional female factor.

## STIMULATION PROTOCOLS

### Follicular Stimulation

At the beginning of a menstrual cycle, gonadotropin-releasing hormone (GnRH) stimulates the anterior pituitary to release a mixture of FSH and LH (luteinizing hormone). The effect of these rising hormones on the ovary is to recruit a group of

# Reproductive Endocrinology and Infertility

primordial follicles. As the follicles grow, FSH (and LH) receptor activity is increased in the follicles. As a result of the increase in FSH receptor activity in the follicular phase, estradiol is secreted in higher concentrations. The rising estradiol has a negative feedback effect on release of FSH, and FSH falls. The combined effect of (1) follicle acquisition of increased sensitivity to FSH and (2) the negative effect of estradiol on FSH secretion results in follicle dominance by which follicles recruited earlier in the cycle with high FSH levels are now unable to continue growth when estradiol-mediated FSH levels fall and only one (usual) follicle develops. In essence, the follicle that acquires the greatest (and crescendo) sensitivity to FSH will continue to increase estradiol production, and the less sensitive follicles will perish when FSH levels diminish (Fig. 53-4).

Pharmaceutical preparations that are generally available for follicular development include FSH, LH, and modified GnRH analogs. These preparations have been used nationally and internationally to produce multiple, mature fertilizable oocytes for assisted reproduction in IVF.

## Natural Cycle

Many factors influence the success of in vitro fertilization–embryo transfer (IVF-ET) including the age of the female partner, evidence of ovarian reserve, and the number of oocytes retrieved. An important determinant of IVF-ET success is the ovarian stimulation regimen employed. Successful fertilization of a human oocyte resulted in the birth of a baby girl, Louise Brown, in 1978.[13]

The first birth from IVF-ET used a single oocyte obtained from a natural cycle. Recent studies demonstrate that the pregnancy rate is low when natural cycles are compared with follicular stimulation cycles. IVF success was compared using a natural

cycle versus a clomiphene citrate–stimulated cycle. In the group of women with natural cycles, no pregnancies occurred, and 6% of the clomiphene group achieved a pregnancy. This low success rate makes natural cycle IVF-ET unsuitable for clinical use, except in unusual cases (Table 53-1).

Clomiphene citrate as a single agent has been evaluated for ovarian stimulation in IVF-ET in few clinical trials.[14] These pregnancy rates are lower than those achieved by stimulation protocols that use exogenous gonadotropins for ovarian stimulation. Clomiphene has also been used in conjunction with pulsatile administration of GnRH, resulted in several large follicles, and can be associated with pregnancy. Use of pulsatile GnRH requires a programmable infusion pump and chronic parenteral access, which has limited its use in IVF-ET.

## Gonadotropins

Most IVF programs now utilize exogenous gonadotropins for ovarian stimulation. Gonadotropin preparations that are commonly used include human menopausal gonadotropins (Bravelle, Repronex, Ferring), and recombinant FSH (Gonal-F, Serono; Follistim, Organon). There are few randomized clinical trials that evaluate the efficacy of exogenous gonadotropins against clomiphene or natural cycles alone in IVF-ET.[15] However, in IVF-ET, ovarian stimulation regimens that include human gonadotropins are routinely associated with pregnancy rates per cycle in the range of 20% to 60%. These pregnancy rates are far greater than those observed when clomiphene or natural cycles are used (Table 53-2).

Hormonal control of reproductive function is mediated by LH and FSH, glycosylated proteins with a molecular weight of

**Table 53-1**
**Type of Ovarian and Hormonal Responses During Follicular Stimulation for IVF-ET**

| Follicular Stimulation | Follicles | Pregnancy Rate | Inhibition of LH surge |
|---|---|---|---|
| Normal | 1–2 | 0–6 | No |
| Clomiphene | 2–4 | 6–10 | No |
| FSH | Multiple | 20–50 | No |
| FSH with GnRH agonist | Multiple | 30–60 | Yes |

FSH, follicle-stimulating hormone; IVF-ET, in vitro fertilization–embryo transfer; LH, luteinizing hormone.

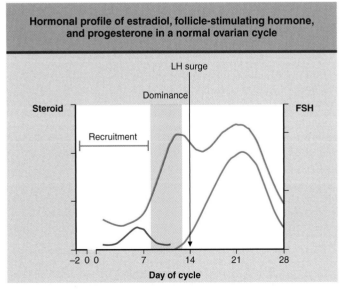

**Hormonal profile of estradiol, follicle-stimulating hormone, and progesterone in a normal ovarian cycle**

**Figure 53-4 Hormonal profile of estradiol ($E_2$), follicle-stimulating hormone (FSH), and progesterone in a normal ovarian cycle.** Follicular recruitment is determined by the rise of FSH in the early follicular phase, and follicular dominance is determined by the decline of FSH when $E_2$ begins to rise. Recruitment usually starts 1 to 2 days before the onset of a new cycle. $E_2$ is in red; progesterone is in green; and FSH is in blue.

**Table 53-2**
**Classification of Different Types of Human FSH Preparations**

| | Menopausal Urine | FSH/LH Ratio | Administration |
|---|---|---|---|
| u-FSH | Yes | 1:1 | Intramuscular |
| HP-FSH | Yes | 75:1 | Intramuscular or subcutaneous |
| r-FSH | No | No LH | Intramuscular or subcutaneous |

FSH, follicle-stimulating hormone; HP, highly purified (monoclonal antibody); LH, luteinizing hormone; r, recombinant; u, urine.

28,000 to 30,000 Da. Both have an alpha and beta subunit, and the alpha subunit (92 amino acids) is common to LH, hCG, and TSH. Neither subunit has any biological activity individually. Secreted FSH has a plasma half-life about 149 minutes, which is five times longer than the approximate 30-minute half-life of LH. Once secreted, FSH is bound by granulosa cell receptors and increases follicular aromatase activity, which transforms theca-derived androgens (under LH stimulation) into estradiol.

To prepare pharmacologic preparations of FSH,[16] human menopausal urine is centrifuged, filtered, chromatographed, and biologically tested. Approximately 4 to 5 L of urine is needed to make a 75-unit ampule of urinary FSH (u-FSH). To improve the purity of FSH preparations (by isolating FSH) a highly specific monoclonal antibody to FSH was developed. The product derived from this extraction (HP-FSH) could be injected subcutaneously.

Worldwide demand led to an increase in the collection of postmenopausal urine and nearly exhausted its supply. As a result, Ares-Serono collaborated with an American laboratory, Integrate Genetics, to synthesize human gonadotropins FSH, LH, and hCG using genetic engineering techniques. The first step was to construct the entire DNA sequences required to produce recombinant human FSH (r-FSH). The second step was to develop a clonal cell line that synthesizes FSH (see Table 53-2). In 1988, r-FSH was successfully expressed in a hamster ovary cell line, and in 1991 the first clinical pharmacology tests began with a twin pregnancy born one year later.

Daya and Gumby[17] published a meta-analysis of 12 trials (2875 cases, of which 1556 were treated with r-FSH and 1319 with u-FSH) that compared the use of r-FSH with u-FSH in women undergoing treatment for an IVF or ICSI cycle. The overall conclusion was that r-FSH significantly increased clinical pregnancies. In several studies r-FSH was more effective than HP-FSH or u-FSH to reduce FSH requirements, days of stimulation, and successful egg recovery.

## GnRH Analogs

Approximately 20% of stimulated cycles within an IVF program are canceled owing to premature LH surges when gonadotropins are used as the sole medication. Most reproductive infertility clinics attempt to minimize this premature LH surge by using pituitary down-regulation. To achieve this, GnRH agonists were introduced into IVF superovulation regimens in the late 1980s and have become established as a component of standard regimens in most centers worldwide. GnRH is a decapeptide (pGlu-His-Trp-Ser-Tyr-Gly-Leu-Arg-Pro-Gly.NH2) and is secreted in a pulsatile fashion to stimulate the secretion of LH and FSH (Table 53-3). The amino acids of GnRH with crucial functions have been substituted (analogs) at positions 1, 2, 3, 5, 6, and 10. Position 6 is involved in enzymatic cleavage, positions 2 and 3 affect gonadotropin release, and positions 1, 6, and 10 impose the three-dimensional structure. Agonists initially stimulate release followed by suppression, while antagonists immediately suppress gonadotropin release (Fig. 53-5).

Many randomized clinical trials demonstrate that in IVF-ET, the combination of exogenous gonadotropin and a GnRH agonist is associated with higher pregnancy rates than is the use of gonadotropins without a GnRH agonist.[18,19] Most GnRH agonist analogs differ from the native decapeptide GnRH in amino acid positions 6 and 10 and are resistant to degradation by endopeptidases. In addition, the GnRH agonist analogs have high affinity for the receptor and long receptor occupancy. The initial administration of GnRH agonist analogs is associated with an increase in LH and FSH secretion (agonist phase). The addition of GnRH agonist analogs to regimens of gonadotropin stimulation for IVF-ET appears to be associated with an increase in the number of oocytes retrieved, the number of embryos transferred, and the clinical pregnancy rate. Thus, available data support the routine use of pituitary suppression in assisted reproduction including IVF-ET.

**Table 53-3**
**Structure and Amino Acid Substitutions of GnRH Agonist and Antagonist Medications**

| Medication | 1 | 2 | 3 | 4 | 5 | 6 | 7 | 8 | 9 | 10 |
|---|---|---|---|---|---|---|---|---|---|---|
| **Agonist** | | | | | | | | | | |
| GnRH | pGlu | His | Trp | Ser | Tyr | Gly | Leu | Arg | Pro | Gly-NH2 |
| Buserelin | | | | | | D-Ser | | | | |
| Goserelin | | | | | | D-Ser | | | | AzGly |
| Leuprolide | | | | | | D-Ser | | | | |
| Triptorelin | | | | | | D-Ser | | | | |
| Nafarelin | | | | | | D-Nal | | | | |
| **Antagonist** | | | | | | | | | | |
| Cetrorelix | D-Nal | D-Phe | D-Pal | | | D-Cit | | | | D-Ala |
| Nal-Glu | D-Nal | D-Phe | D-Pal | | Arg | D-Glu | | | | D-Ala |
| Antide | D-Nal | D-Phe | D-Pal | | Lys | D-NicLys | | Lys | | D-Ala |
| Ganirelix | D-Nal | D-Phe | D-Pal | | | D-hArg | | Arg | | D-Ala |
| Azaline B | D-Nal | D-Phe | D-Pal | | Phe | D-Phe | | Lys | | D-Ala |
| Degarelix | D-Nal | D-Cpa | D-Pal | | Aph | D-Aph | | Lys | | D-Ala |

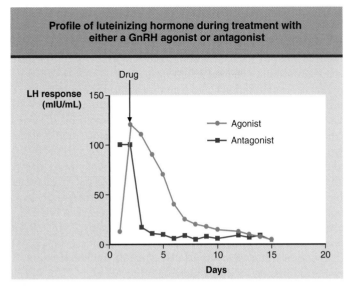

**Figure 53-5    Profile of luteinizing hormone (LH) during treatment with either a GnRH agonist or a GnRH antagonist.** The action of the antagonist is seen *(blue)* when women with elevated gonadotropins (menopausal) are treated. The LH levels fall immediately. Cycling women *(red)* are treated with an agonist, and the "agonist" phase of the preparation increases hormone release and is followed by down-regulation.

Figure 53-6 is a common protocol combining GnRH agonist suppression of pituitary gonadotropin secretion with exogenous gonadotropin administration to stimulate ovarian follicular growth. Surges of LH that occur before full follicle maturity may cause premature luteinization of the granulosa cells. In addition, a premature surge of LH may disrupt oocyte maturation. The inclusion of a GnRH agonist in ovarian stimulation protocols for assisted reproductive technologies (ART) has resulted in significant improvements in outcome (see Table 53-1). Use of the GnRH agonist to prevent LH surges in IVF-ET cycles decreased the cancellation rate to about 2% and concomitantly increased the IVF and pregnancy rate (PR) per cycle. The agonists, after an initial stimulatory effect (flare-up), led to desensitization of

the gonadotropin-secreting cells and a reduction in the number of GnRH-Rs on the cell membrane (down-regulation). Several treatment schedules currently are in use, and the long protocol begins with GnRH agonists in the luteal phase of the cycle preceding follicular stimulation.

GnRH antagonists inhibit the reproductive system through competition with endogenous GnRH for the receptor and are used in control of follicular stimulation in IVF.[20] Synthetic GnRH with a deletion or substitution of the histidine in position 2 is a GnRH antagonist. Additional substitutions at positions 1, 3, 6, 8, and 10 in the molecule have resulted in progressive increases in antagonistic potency. Thus, the structures of the antagonists, unlike the agonists, substantially differ from that of GnRH (see Table 53-3).

The clinical usefulness of the GnRH agonist drugs is based on their ability to reversibly block pituitary gonadotropin secretion, thereby preventing a premature surge of LH. The mechanisms of action of GnRH antagonists are completely different. The antagonists produce an immediate effect by competitive blockade of the GnRH-R. The adenohypophysis maintains its responsiveness to a GnRH stimulus (pituitary response). Owing to competitive blockage of GnRH-R by antagonist administration, LH (and to a lesser extent FSH) levels drop rapidly. Fortunately, pituitary function normalizes immediately following cessation of the antagonist. The direct and rapid action of GnRH antagonists, the dose-dependent suppression of LH and FSH, and the rapid restoration of hypophyseal function after cessation of the use of antagonists may simplify IVF follicular stimulation.

The first generation of GnRH antagonists had the disadvantage of producing adverse side effects including anaphylactic reactions due to histamine release. This side effect was greatly reduced by substituting amino acids at positions 5, 6, and 8 (see Table 53-3). Multidose treatment rapidly decreased serum levels of gonadotropins and estradiol ($E_2$). Ongoing pregnancies have been reported in older women who received oocyte donation from young donors using a GnRH antagonist with human menopausal gonadotropin (hMG) and hCG to complete oocyte maturation. IVF patients older than 40 years undergoing IVF-ET cycles were treated with mid-cycle GnRH antagonists. Cancellation rates were significantly lower with GnRH antagonists (about 20%)

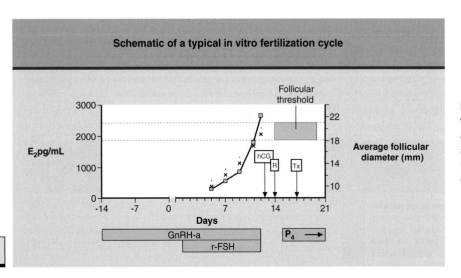

**Figure 53-6    Schematic of a typical in vitro fertilization (IVF) treatment cycle using a GnRH agonist and recombinant gonadotropins.** Depicted are the approximate time frames, representative ultrasound and estradiol ($E_2$) measurements, and duration of medication.

compared with gonadotropin only (about 70%). However, the number of embryos transferred, cumulative embryo scores, implantation rates, and ongoing pregnancy rate did not differ from those of controls. Although these results were preliminary, the addition of GnRH antagonists avoided ovarian suppression at the start of follicular stimulation and prevented the premature LH surge at mid-cycle.

## Oocyte Retrieval

In the early days of IVF, surgical retrieval of oocytes required laparoscopy. Transabdominal approaches using the bladder window were also used. Today, almost all retrievals follow a transvaginal approach made possible by the use of high-resolution transvaginal scanners and attached needle guides (Fig. 53-7). Aspiration of the follicular fluid is possible with a small-gauge needle attached to suction. Oocyte recovery ranges from 50% to 80% of follicles producing oocytes. The retrieval is quick, often accomplished in 20 to 30 minutes, and complications are infrequent.

The type of anesthesia used ranges from conscious sedation with midazolam and fentanyl, to deeper sedation with propofol, and in some clinics general anesthesia is used. The choice hinges on patient and physician preference, but light intravenous (IV) sedation provides adequate pain relief and is cost effective.

Retrieval is most often accomplished in a room adjacent to the embryo culture room, for rapid transport of the follicular fluid to the laboratory environment. Postoperative recovery time is short and depends on the type of anesthesia used.

## Embryo Transfer

Embryo transfer is the final step in the IVF process and has received considerable attention as a possible factor in pregnancy success. Obviously, embryos must be successfully transferred for pregnancy to occur. A gray area surrounds the significance of the type of transfer catheter, the use of ultrasound, the exact location in the cavity for embryo placement, and other factors that potentially contribute to this process. Clinical experience reveals that the most difficult transfers are sometimes successful, while other factors presumably prevent pregnancy in the majority of smooth, atraumatic transfers.

Debate continues about the value of trial or mock transfer. In many clinics, trial transfer is used to preset the length of the transfer catheter for a more efficient transfer. In addition, patients with a potentially difficult transfer can be identified ahead of time. For some cases, alternative transfer catheters can be selected. Mock transfers have been performed with and without sonogram guidance. While randomized trials are lacking, a number of studies have looked at the distance from the fundus

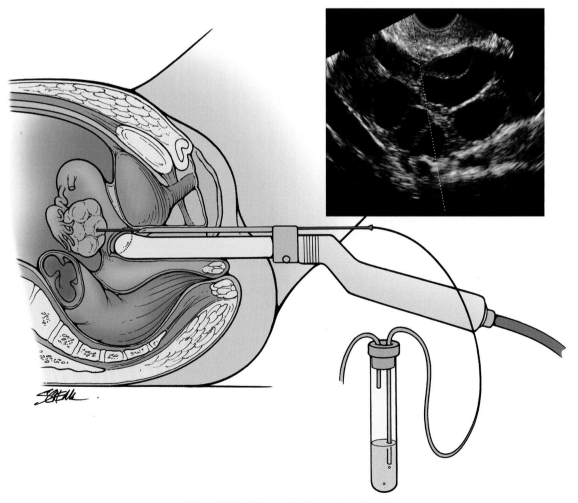

**Figure 53-7    Transvaginal oocyte retrieval.**

# Reproductive Endocrinology and Infertility

for embryo placement. In a retrospective study involving 699 embryo transfers, distance from the fundus as measured by ultrasound was better correlated with pregnancy than was the distance derived by clinical touch at mock transfer.[21] These authors concluded that ultrsound-guided trial or mock transfer was beneficial.

At the time of actual embryo transfer, randomized controlled trials indicate a benefit in the use of ultrasound to guide the transfer catheter.[22,23] In addition, this factor has been examined with the use of cryopreserved embryos. In a study of 184 randomized patients undergoing thawed embryo transfer cycles with hormone replacement under pituitary suppression, ultrasound-guided transfer was compared with clinical touch.[24] Both pregnancy and implantation rates in the ultrasound group (34.4% and 19.8%, respectively) were significantly higher than the corresponding values (19.7% and 11.9%, respectively) in the clinical touch group.

## Luteal Support

Luteal support is important for IVF success. Long GnRH agonist protocols appear to create a luteal phase defect. The most common modalities used have been oral, vaginal, and intramuscular (IM) progesterone. A meta-analysis suggests that of these routes of administration, oral progesterone is the least effective.[25] IM progesterone carries a slight benefit over the vaginal route, although there is a fair amount of disagreement on this point. In comparison with placebo, delivery rates were improved with the addition of IM progesterone, with an RR of 5.50 (95% CI 1.25–35.53). In the meta-analysis, delivery rates were compared between IM and vaginal progesterone, and the IM route conferred an RR of 2.06 (95% CI 1.48–2.88). The most common vaginal progesterones used have been micronized progesterone capsules and gel preparation (Crinone), the latter an FDA-approved product. Luteal support with hCG has been used and produced excellent ongoing pregnancy rates. However, the rate of hyperstimulation was unacceptable, and this practice has largely been abandoned. Other forms of progesterone, including a progesterone-containing vaginal ring and 17-hydroxycaproate, appear to be effective. The duration of therapy has not been adequately determined, and studies have examined use from as short as the first positive pregnancy test through the first 12 weeks of pregnancy.

## COMPLICATIONS OF IN VITRO FERTILIZATION

### Ovarian Hyperstimulation Syndrome

Ovarian hyperstimulation syndrome (OHSS) is an exaggerated response to ovulation induction therapy.[26] OHSS is associated with exogenous gonadotropin stimulation followed by hCG and is rarely observed with other agents (clomiphene citrate and GnRH). Clinicians who prescribe ovulation-inducing agents must recognize and manage OHSS.[27–29] Fortunately, OHSS usually is a self-limiting disorder that resolves spontaneously, but it may persist for longer periods in conception cycles.

### Pathophysiology

The hallmark of OHSS is an increase in capillary permeability resulting in a fluid shift from the intravascular space to third space compartments.[30,31] Vascular endothelial growth factor (VEGF) has emerged as one of the factors most likely involved in the pathophysiology of OHSS.[32] Other factors including angiotensin II, insulinlike growth factor 1 (IGF-1), epidermal growth factor (EGF), transforming growth factor (TGF) , basic fibroblast growth factor (BFGF), platelet-derived growth factor (PDGF), interleukin 1 (IL-1), and interleukin 6 (IL-6)[33] may also be involved.

### Risk Factors

The following factors increase the risk for developing OHSS[34]:

- Young age
- Low body weight
- Polycystic ovary syndrome (PCOS)
- High doses of gonadotropins
- Rapidly rising serum estradiol levels
- Previous episodes of OHSS

Risk also increases when repeated doses of exogenous hCG are administered in superovulation and ART cycles (for luteal-phase support) and decreases when exogenous progesterone, rather than hCG, is used to support the luteal phase. Pregnancy increases the likelihood, duration, and severity of OHSS symptoms.

### Clinical Features

OHSS has been classified as mild, moderate, or severe.[35] However, the clinical symptoms and signs of OHSS exhibit a continuum of scope and severity that defies attempts at specific classification or staging. Mild manifestations of OHSS are relatively common and include transient lower abdominal discomfort, mild nausea, vomiting, diarrhea, or abdominal distention. Moderate illness is recognized when symptoms persist, worsen, or include ascites that may be demonstrated by increasing abdominal girth or ultrasound evaluation. Serious illness exists when extreme pain occurs with rapid weight gain, tense ascites, hemodynamic instability, and respiratory difficulty, oliguria, or laboratory abnormalities. Risk of thromboembolism is increased as a result of hemoconcentration, diminished peripheral blood flow, and inactivity due to abdominal distention and pain. Life-threatening complications of OHSS include renal failure, adult respiratory distress syndrome (ARDS), hemorrhage from ovarian rupture, and thromboembolism.

### Outpatient Management

Patients with mild manifestations of OHSS can be managed with oral analgesics. Intercourse should be avoided. Daily weight measurements and serial laboratory assessment of hematocrit, electrolytes, and serum creatinine can monitor progression.

Recommendations for the outpatient management of persistent and worsening OHSS include the following:

- Oral fluid intake (commercially available electrolyte-supplemented drink) should be maintained at more than 1 L/day.
- Strenuous physical activity should be avoided.
- Weight should be recorded daily.
- Weight gain of more than 2 pounds per day or decreasing urinary frequency (output) should prompt an evaluation.

## Hospitalization

Hospitalization is required based on severity of symptoms, analgesic requirements, and other social considerations (availability of responsible adult supervision, support, and assistance with child care).[36,37] Given the scope of symptoms and the potential for complications, most women with severe OHSS merit hospitalization for more treatment.

### Fluid Management

Hospitalized patients require IV fluid management to address the acute need for volume expansion while also considering the marked increase in vascular permeability that accompanies severe OHSS. Renal and pulmonary function must be carefully monitored. Rapid initial hydration may be accomplished with a bolus of IV fluid (500 to 1000 mL). Fluids should be administered in the volumes necessary to maintain adequate urine output (>20 to 30 mL/h). Five percent dextrose in normal saline is preferable to lactated Ringer's solution. Correction of hypovolemia, hypotension, and oliguria has the highest priority, given that fluid administration may contribute to the accumulation of ascites.

### Paracentesis

Ultrasound-guided paracentesis or transvaginal culdocentesis may be indicated for patients with ascites that causes pain, compromised pulmonary function, or oliguria/anuria. Rapid removal of large volumes of ascitic fluid has been observed to trigger dangerous compensatory fluid shifts in elderly patients with malignant ascites, but the risk of this complication in women with OHSS is small. Serial paracentesis may be required to maintain adequate renal and pulmonary function.

### Complications

Thromboembolism is a life-threatening complication of severe OHSS. Full-length venous support stockings or an intermittent pneumatic compression device are recommended, and prophylactic heparin therapy (5000 U subcutaneously every 12 hours) should be seriously considered. Patients with severe OHSS who may require surgery for a ruptured ovarian cyst with hemorrhage, torsion, or an ectopic pregnancy present a unique challenge for the anesthesiologist who is unlikely to be familiar with the pathophysiology of the syndrome and must minimize the additional risks involved.

### Prevention

The keys to preventing OHSS are experience with ovulation induction therapy and recognition of risk factors for OHSS. Withholding further gonadotropin stimulation and delaying hCG administration until estradiol levels plateau or decrease significantly can reduce risks of OHSS.[38] Available evidence suggests that such "coasting" does not adversely affect outcome in IVF cycles unless it is prolonged (>3 days).[39] Given the evidence suggesting that hCG may play a pivotal role in the development of OHSS, a lower dose of hCG (e.g., 5000 IU vs. the standard 10,000 IU dose) may be prudent for patients judged to be at high risk for OHSS. Alternatively, a GnRH agonist (e.g., leuprolide 0.5 to 1.0 mg subcutaneously) rather than hCG might be used to stimulate an endogenous LH surge to promote final oocyte maturation and induce ovulation. This approach would be useful only in cycles not involving previous down-regulation or use of a GnRH antagonist (e.g., ganirelix, cetrorelix). Regardless of whether hCG or a GnRH agonist is administered at midcycle, the use of progesterone for luteal phase support rather than supplemental doses of hCG may further reduce the risk of OHSS. Prophylactic IV administration of albumin at oocyte retrieval has been suggested as a means to reduce the risk of OHSS.[40] Studies of its efficacy have mixed results, and albumin treatment risks exacerbation of ascites, allergic reactions, and virus/prion transmission. However, albumin infusion may be expected to prevent one case of severe OHSS for every 18 women at risk who are treated.

## Multifetal Pregnancy

The incidence of multiple pregnancy and delivery has increased dramatically over the past decades in many developed countries. In IVF, the usual practice of transferring two or more embryos to achieve higher pregnancy rates results in a high incidence of multiple births. In the World Collaborative Report on IVF figures for 1995 showed that 24.7% of the pregnancies were twin, 4.1% were triplet, and 0.2% were quadruplet. Multiple pregnancy carries additional risks for both mother and offspring and requires more elaborate monitoring of the pregnancy. Obstetric complications associated with multiple pregnancy include prenatal screening problems, an increased incidence of preeclampsia and eclampsia, antepartum hemorrhage, preterm labor, intrauterine growth retardation, and surgical and assisted delivery. Among neonatal complications the most common are low birth weight due to prematurity or placental dysfunction and congenital malformations. The perinatal mortality is five to six times higher among twins compared with singletons.

The pregnancy and neonatal complications observed in IVF pregnancies were almost entirely due to multiple pregnancies, the majority of which were twin pregnancies. The rate of prematurity (<37 weeks) among twin pregnancies was 47.3% compared with 11.2% among singletons.

## Malformations

Multiple pregnancies are also associated with infant and childhood morbidity such as cerebral palsy and mental retardation.[41] Two recent studies of the incidence of cerebral palsy reported dramatically increased risks in multiple births: twins had risks approximately 5 times higher and triplets 17 times higher than singletons, and the risk of producing at least one child with cerebral palsy was estimated to 1% to 5% for twin, 8% for triplet, and almost 50% for quadruplet pregnancies.[42,43]

Most studies of child development after IVF carried out to date include relatively small numbers of children and have a limited period of follow-up, and consequently the risks for long-term handicap are not well established.

Which methods are available today to reduce the number of multiple births after ART? An overall change in transfer policy to transfer only one embryo at a time would certainly result in mainly singletons.[44,45] This might be unacceptable to both patients and practitioners, who aim at the best possible rates of success. An alternative to an overall one-embryo transfer would be an individualized embryo transfer policy. It seems possible to identify a subgroup of patients having an increased risk of multiple birth and offer them one-embryo transfers. In a recent publication, elective one-embryo transfer showed a satisfactory pregnancy rate (29.7% per transfer) in a selected group of patients, the pregnancy rate being similar to that of the routine two-embryo transfer program.

Embryo/fetal reduction, as a third strategy to reduce the number of multiple births, has been used worldwide.[46] Despite the fact that collaborative data have reported satisfactory outcome for the children and limited risks for the mother, this kind of intervention raises serious ethical and psychological problems. It may be indicated in cases of particularly high-order multiple pregnancies but can never be justified for reduction of twins.

## LABORATORY TECHNIQUES

Despite all the effort and research devoted to follicular stimulation, retrieval, and embryo transfer, the most important part of any IVF program is the laboratory. The initial laboratory steps in an IVF treatment cycle are oocyte identification and preparation for fertilization. The technique of combining oocyte and sperm in the laboratory has evolved over the years. Standard insemination occurs in the Petri dish and may be facilitated by insemination under oil. The most remarkable change in assisted reproductive technology in the last decade has been the development and universal adoption of intracytoplasmic sperm injection (ICSI). Initial attempts at micromanipulation led to the development of subzonal insertion and breaching of the zona pellucida. In 1990 the first use of direct injection of sperm into the cytoplasm of the oocyte was reported. Fertilization rates with ICSI are 80% to 90% and produce excellent pregnancy rates in couples with male infertility. In cases where there is only a single factor, male infertility can be corrected in more successful fashion than almost any other diagnosis. The additional use of surgical retrieval of sperm in cases of azoospermia has created a remarkable change from the time when male factor infertility had no effective therapy. Surgical sperm retrieval includes percutaneous aspiration of the vas deferens and testicular biopsy. Males with cystic fibrosis provide the classic indication for testicular biopsy, since they have normal sperm production but an ejaculatory obstruction.

Laboratory changes in culture media have led to longer in vitro culture periods. Embryos are now routinely transferred after 3 days of culture when the embryos may be at the 6- to 12-cell stage. Alternatively, blastocyst stage transfer on days 5 to 6 has also been effective. A number of randomized trials have been performed, and overall the pregnancy rates with blastocyst transfer are not different, although multiple pregnancy rates do differ. Day 3 transfers are often performed with a higher number of embryos, yielding higher multiple pregnancy rates. When the number of embryos transferred is the same, pregnancy and multiple pregnancy rates do not differ[47] Cancellation rates for transfer are higher when embryo culture is extended to the blastocyst stage, and most clinics use specific criteria before moving to blastocyst transfer.

Excess embryos resulting from an IVF cycle are cryopreserved for future attempts at pregnancy. Embryos that are frozen have a lower probability of implanting, and typical pregnancy rates are half those of "fresh" embryo transfer pregnancy rates. Cryopreservation of oocytes has been problematic, but pregnancies have been reported from frozen eggs.[48]

Assisted hatching is a laboratory technique that holds promise for improving fertility in certain populations. The blastocyst develops within the zona pellucida, and this membrane must break down in order for the trophoblast to invade the decidua and establish pregnancy. Assisted hatching was conceived to help with this process and has been demonstrated to improve implantation rates.[49] In large studies, assisted hatching has not been shown to be beneficial when used in all IVF populations.[50] It does seem to be effective in selected cases of advanced maternal age, thick zonae, and repeated implantation failure.[51] The use of a laser for assisted hatching, in place of chemical or mechanical means, may offer some advantages.[52]

The efforts to enhance laboratory techniques and quality control have led to accreditation of laboratories and to certification of laboratory directors in IVF programs. Evidence of certification of the laboratory by the College of American Pathologists (CAP) and the Clinical Laboratory Improvement Act (CLIA), as well as a designation as a High Complexity Laboratory Director for the embryologist in charge by the American Board of Bioanalysts, is critical in today's environment. Mechanisms for quality control have created a great deal of standardization of pregnancy rates in laboratories around the United States among patients who are expected to have a good outcome.

### Complex Reproductive Solutions

The advent of improved laboratory techniques and the enhancement of clinical IVF has given clinicians and patients the ability to create pregnancies in ways that were previously not recognized. One of the earliest approaches in circumventing reproductive disorders with a complex solution was the use of donor sperm for azo- or oligospermia. This technique has been accepted worldwide for some time, and for many years the use of frozen sperm has improved the safety and convenience of this approach. Donor insemination has to some degree been replaced by advances in ICSI and surgical sperm retrieval but remains a valid option for couples with male factor infertility.

Donor oocyte cycles are a solution for poor egg quality or failed ovarian function. Oocytes obtained from a donor in an IVF treatment cycle are fertilized with sperm from the recipient's husband, and embryos resulting from this process are transferred to the recipient. All the clinical steps in this approach are part of the routine IVF protocol. The legal and ethical issues are the aspects of this treatment that can be complicated. Fortunately, there rarely are legal disputes over gametes, unlike the situation in pregnancies resulting from gestational carriers. Donor oocytes can be from either known or anonymous donors, depending on the wishes of the couple. While pregnancies have been reported in recipients over age 50, most programs favor restricting this practice to recipients who have yet to go through natural menopause.

If the fertility problem lies not with the ovary but with the uterus, then either a gestational carrier or a surrogate can be used. These cases have drawn the attention of the public, since disputes over parenthood do occur when the woman delivering the child is not the genetic parent. Gestational carriers are the recipients of an embryo transfer, usually in a case where the embryo is created by eggs and sperm from an infertile couple. Most commonly, this technique would be used in the case of an extreme uterine abnormality or absence of the uterus. The couple would go through standard IVF with oocyte retrieval and fertilization occurring with their eggs and sperm. The resulting embryos would then be transferred to the gestational carrier, and pregnancy and delivery would be routine. This process, while requiring attention to legal and social issues, does not present any unusual clinical approaches. Gestational surrogates are typically used when both the uterus and the ovary are defective in the infertile woman. In surrogacy, the woman carrying the pregnancy is impregnated via insemination and, once pregnant, carries and delivers a child that is genetically related.

Cryopreservation of embryos is an important technique for enhancing pregnancy rates, by allowing all the mature oocytes from a cycle to be inseminated, and then allowing biology to dictate which oocytes will produce healthy embryos. This eliminates the need to restrict the fertilization process at a biological point in time when judging quality may be difficult. Once fertilized, most programs then utilize all healthy embryos for either a "fresh" transfer or for freezing and subsequent frozen/thawed embryo transfer. Embryos resulting from this process may become available for embryo donation, if the couple creating the embryos is finished with childbearing or their relationship is dissolved. Embryo donation follows the same clinical steps as a routine frozen embryo transfer: preparation of the recipient with hormonal stimulation and then embryo transfer. Embryo donation can be a responsible and ethical solution for the difficult problem of "excess" embryos.

## IN VITRO FERTILIZATION CASE HISTORY

To understand the IVF treatment process, consider a 32-year-old gravida 0 who presents for an infertility evaluation. Her prior record includes a hysterosalpingogram revealing bilateral hydrosalpinges, and semen analysis reveals restrictive oligospermia. Ultrasound confirms fluid-filled adnexal structures consistent with tubal pathology. The patient reports regular cycles and has a midluteal progesterone of 20 ng/mL. Infectious disease screening is negative.

She elects to proceed with IVF and ICSI secondary to tubal disease and male factor. The pretreatment sonohysterogram and trial transfer are normal, and she had bilateral salpingectomy prior to therapy.

A long down-regulation protocol is chosen for follicular stimulation, and the patient receives GnRH agonist subcutaneously from day 21 of a cycle prior to gonadotropin stimulation. Two weeks later, she reports menses, and an ultrasound of the reproductive tract is unremarkable. Daily injections of r-FSH are started in addition to the concomitant GnRH agonist. On day 5 of stimulation, estradiol measurement confirms a brisk response to stimulation and the patient decreases her gonadotropin dose. On day 8 and again on day 10, ultrasound and estradiol measurements confirm a rise in estradiol and growth of the follicles at approximately 2 mm per day (see Fig. 53-6). When an estradiol measurement reflects 300 pg/mL per mature follicle, and follicular measurements demonstrate at least two follicles that are 18 mm or greater, the patient is scheduled for transvaginal oocyte retrieval. She self-administers hCG (10,000 IU) 37 hours prior to her planned procedure and stops the GnRH agonist on

the day of hCG administration. hCG will trigger final maturation of the oocyte so that metaphase II oocytes are obtained at the time of retrieval.

Immediately after oocyte retrieval, ICSI is performed on mature oocytes because of the history of a restrictive male factor. The following day (day 1), fertilization is confirmed when two extruded polar bodies and two pronuclei are identified within the zygote. In this case, a check for cleavage the next day confirmed that 80% of the zygotes have now become embryos at the 2- to 4-cell stage. On day 3, an embryo transfer of two, 8-cell embryos was performed, and four additional dividing embryos were cryopreserved for potential later attempts at pregnancy. Progesterone supplementation for luteal support, started on the day after retrieval (day 1), is continued past the positive pregnancy test and typically maintained until the ovarian-placental shift of hormone production occurs (around week 8 to 10 of gestation). An ultrasound confirms a single intrauterine pregnancy.

## REFERENCES

1. Centers for Disease Control and Prevention, National Center for Chronic Prevention and Health Promotion, Division of Reproductive Health: 2002 Assisted Reproductive Technology Success Rates, National Summary and Fertility Clinic Reports. U.S. Department of Health and Human Services, 2004. **(III, B)**
2. Society for Assisted Reproductive Technology; American Society for Reproductive Medicine: Assisted reproductive technology in the United States: 2000 results generated from the American Society for Reproductive Medicine/Society for Assisted Reproductive Technology Registry. Fertil Steril 2004;81:1207–1220. **(III, B)**
3. Klonoff-Cohen HS, Natarajan L: The effect of advancing paternal age on pregnancy and live birth rates in couples undergoing in vitro fertilization or gamete intrafallopian transfer. Am J Obstet Gynecol 2004;191:507–514. **(IIa, B)**
4. Kim AH, McKay H, Keltz MD, et al: Sonohysterographic screening before in vitro fertilization. Fertil Steril 1998;69: 841–844. **(IIa, B)**
5. Farhi J, Ashkenazi J, Feldberg D, et al: Effect of uterine leiomyomata on the results of in-vitro fertilization treatment. Hum Reprod 1995;10:2576–2578. **(IIa, B)**
6. Eldar-Geva T, Meagher S, Healy DL, et al: Effect of intramural, subserosal, and submucosal uterine fibroids on the outcome of assisted reproductive technology treatment. Fertil Steril 1998;70:687–691. **(IIa, B)**
7. Strandell A, Lindhard U, Waldenström J, et al: Hydrosalpinx and IVF outcome: a prospective, randomized multicentre trial in Scandinavia on salpingectomy prior to IVF. Hum Reprod 1999;14:2762–2769. **(Ib, A)**
8. Strandell A, Lindhard A, Waldenström U, Thorburn J: Hydrosalpinx and IVF outcome: cumulative results after salpingectomy in a randomized controlled trial. Hum Reprod 2001;16:2403–2410. **(Ib, A)**
9. Scott RT, Opsahl MS, Leonardi MR, et al: Life table analysis of pregnancy rates in a general infertility population relative to ovarian reserve and patient age. Hum Reprod 1995;10:1706–1701. **(IIa, B)**
10. Hendriks DJ, Broekmans FJ, Bancsi LF, et al: Repeated clomiphene citrate challenge testing in the prediction of outcome in IVF: a comparison with basal markers for ovarian reserve. Hum Reprod 2005;20:163–169. **(IIa, B)**
11. Jain T, Soules MR, Collins JA: Comparison of basal follicle-stimulating hormone versus the clomiphene citrate challenge test for ovarian reserve screening. Fertil Steril 2004;82:180–185. **(IIa, B)**
12. Virro MR, Larson-Cook KL, Evenson DP: Sperm chromatin structure assay (SCSA) parameters are related to fertilization, blastocyst develop-

ment, and ongoing pregnancy in in vitro fertilization and intracytoplasmic sperm injection cycles. Fertil Steril 2004;81:1289–1295. **(IIa, B)**

13. Sleptoe PC, Edwards RG: Birth after the reimplantation of a human embryo. Lancet 1978;12:366. **(III, B)**

14. MacDougall MJ, Tan SL, Hall V, et al: Comparison of natural with clomiphene citrate stimulated cycles in in vitro fertilization: a prospective randomized trial. Fertil Steril 1994;61:1052–1057. **(Ib, A)**

15. Barbieri RL, Hornstein MD: Assisted reproduction–in vitro fertilization success is improved by ovarian stimulation with exogenous gonadotropins and pituitary suppression with gonadotropin-releasing hormone analogues. Endocr Rev 1999;20:249–252. **(III, B)**

16. Palagiano A, Nesti E, Pace L: FSH: urinary and recombinant. Eur J Obstet Gynecol Reprod Biol 2004;8:419–430. **(III, B)**

17. Daya S, Gumby J: Recombinant versus urinary follicle stimulating hormone for ovarian stimulation in assisted reproduction. Hum Reprod 1999;14:2207–2215. **(Ia, A)**

18. Albuquerque LE, Saconato H, Maciel MC, et al: Depot versus daily administration of GnRH agonist protocols for pituitary desensitization in assisted reproduction cycles: a Cochrane Review. Hum Reprod 2003;18:2008–2017. **(Ia, A)**

19. Hughes EG, Fedorkow DM, Daya S, et al: The routine use of gonadotropin-releasing hormone agonists prior to in vitro fertilization and gamete intrafallopian transfer: a meta-analysis of randomized controlled trials. Fertil Steril 1992;58:888–896. **(Ia, A)**

20. Coccia ME, Comparetto C, Bracco GL, Scarselli G: GnRH antagonists. Eur J Obstet Gynecol Reprod Biol 2004;115(Suppl):S44–S56. **(III, B)**

21. Pope CS, Cook EK, Arny M, et al: Influence of embryo transfer depth on in vitro fertilization and embryo transfer outcomes. Fertil Steril 2004;81:51–58. **(IIa, B)**

22. Sallam HN, Sadek SS: Ultrasound-guided embryo transfer: a meta-analysis of randomized controlled trials. Fertil Steril 2003; 80:1042–1046. **(Ia, A)**

23. Buckett WM: A meta-analysis of ultrasound-guided versus clinical touch embryo transfer. Fertil Steril 2003;80:1037–1041. **(IIb, B)**

24. Coroleu B, Barri PN, Carreras O, et al: The usefulness of ultrasound guidance in frozen-thawed embryo transfer: a prospective randomized clinical trial. Hum Reprod 2002;17:2885–2890. **(Ib, A)**

25. Pritts EA, Atwood AK: Luteal phase support in infertility treatment: a meta-analysis of the randomized trials. Hum Reprod 2002; 17:2287–2299. **(Ia, A)**

26. Bergh PA, Navot D: Ovarian stimulation syndrome: a review of pathophysiology. J Assist Reprod Genet 1992;9:429–438. **(III, B)**

27. Blankstein J, Shalev J, Saadon T, et al: Ovarian hyperstimulation syndrome: prediction by number and size of preovulatory ovarian follicles. Fertil Steril 1987;47:597–602. **(IIa, B)**

28. McArdle C, Siebel M, Hann LE, et al: The diagnosis of ovarian hyperstimulation (OHS): the impact of ultrasound. Fertil Steril 1983; 39:464–467. **(IIb, B)**

29. Pride SM, James CSJ, Yuen BH: The ovarian hyperstimulation syndrome. Semin Reprod Endocrinol 1990;8:247–260. **(III, B)**

30. Tollan A, Holst N, Forsdahl F, et al: Transcapillary fluid dynamics during ovarian stimulation for in vitro fertilization. Am J Obstet Gynecol 1990;162:554–558. **(IIb, B)**

31. Goldsman MP, Pedram A, Domingues CE, et al: Increased capillary permeability induced by human follicular fluid: a hypothesis for an ovarian origin of the hyperstimulation syndrome. Fertil Steril 1995; 63:268–272. **(IIb, B)**

32. Levin ER, Rosen GF, Cassidenti DL, et al: Role of vascular endothelial cell growth factor in ovarian hyperstimulation syndrome. J Clin Invest 1998;102:1978–1985. **(IIb, B)**

33. Pellicer A, Albert C, Mercader A, et al: The pathogenesis of ovarian hyperstimulation syndrome: in vivo studies investigating the role of interleukin-1, interleukin-6, and vascular endothelial growth factor. Fertil Steril 1999;71:482–489. **(IIa, B)**

34. Whelan JG III, Vlahos NF: The ovarian hyperstimulation syndrome. Fertil Steril 2000;73: 883–896. **(III, B)**

35. Golan A, Ron-el R, Herman A, et al: Ovarian hyperstimulation syndrome: an update review. Obstet Gynecol Surv 1989;44:430–440. **(III, B)**

36. Borenstein R, Elhalah U, Lunenfeld B, Schwartz ZS: Severe ovarian hyperstimulation syndrome: a reevaluated therapeutic approach. Fertil Steril 1989;51:791–795. **(III, B)**

37. Rizk B, Aboulghar M: Modern management of ovarian hyperstimulation syndrome. Hum Reprod 1991;6:1082–1087. **(III, B)**

38. Al-Shawaf T, Zosmer A, Hussain S, et al: Prevention of severe ovarian hyperstimulation syndrome in IVF with or without ICSI and embryo transfer: a modified "coasting" strategy based on ultrasound for identification of high-risk patients. Hum Reprod 2001;16:24–30. **(III, B)**

39. Ulug U, Gahceci M, Erden HF, et al: The significance of coasting duration during ovarian stimulation for conception in assisted fertilization cycles. Hum Reprod 2002;17:310–313. **(IIa, B)**

40. Aboulghar M, Evers JH, Al-Inany H: Intravenous albumin for preventing severe ovarian hyperstimulation syndrome: a Cochrane review. Hum Reprod 2002;17:3027–3032. **(Ia, A)**

41. De Mouzon J, Lancaster P: World Collaborative Report on in vitro fertilization, preliminary data for 1995. J Assist Reprod Genet 1997; 14(Suppl):251–265. **(III, B)**

42. Petterson B, Nelson K, Watson L, Stanley F: Twins, triplets, and cerebral palsy in births in Western Australia in the 1980s. BMJ 1993; 307:1239–1243. **(IIa, B)**

43. Yokohama Y, Shimizu T, Hayakawa K: Prevalence of cerebral palsy in twins, triplets and quadruplets. Int J Epidemiol 1995;24:943–948. **(IIa, B)**

44. Van Royen E, Mangelschots K, De Neubourg D, et al: Characterization of top quality embryo, a step towards single-embryo transfer. Hum Reprod 1999;14:2345–2349. **(IIa, B)**

45. Vilska S, Tiitinen A, Hyden-Granskog C, Hovatta O: Elective transfer of one embryo results in an acceptable pregnancy rate and eliminates the risks of multiple birth. Hum Reprod 1999;14:2392–2395. **(IIa, B)**

46. Evans MI, Dommergues M, Wapner RJ, et al: International collaborative experience of 1978 patients having multifetal pregnancy reduction: a plateauing of risks and outcomes. J Soc Gynecol Invest 1996;3:23–26. **(III, B)**

47. Blake D, Proctor M, Johnson N, Olive D: Cleavage stage versus blastocyst stage embryo transfer in assisted conception. Cochrane Database Syst Rev 2002;(2):CD002118. **(Ia, A)**

48. Boldt J, Cline D, McLaughlin D: Human oocyte cryopreservation as an adjunct to IVF-embryo transfer cycles. Hum Reprod 2003; 18:1250–1255. **(IIa, B)**

49. Cohen J, Inge KL, Suzmann M: Video-cinematography of fresh and cryopreserved embryos: a retrospective analysis of embryonic morphology and implantation. Fertil Steril 1989;51:820–827. **(III, B)**

50. Hellebaut S, De Sutter P, Dozortsev D, et al: Does assisted hatching improve implantation rates after in vitro fertilization or intracytoplasmic sperm injection in all patients? J Assist Reprod Genet 1996;13:19–22. **(III, B)**

51. Nakayama T, Fujiwara H, Yamada S, et al: Clinical application of a new assisted hatching method using a piezomicromanipulator for morphologically low-quality embryos in poor-prognosis infertile patients. Fertil Steril 1999;71:1014–1018. **(III, B)**

52. Obruca A, Strohmer H, Sakkas D: Use of lasers in assisted fertilization and hatching. Human Reprod 1949;9:1723–1726. **(III, B)**

# Chapter 54

# Male Infertility

## Mohit Khera, MD, MBA, MPH, and Larry I. Lipshultz, MD

### KEY POINTS

- From 40% to 50% of infertile couples are infertile because of a significantly impaired male factor.
- Approximately 20% of couples are infertile *solely* because of a male factor.
- Etiologies for male infertility can be simply classified as pretesticular, testicular, and post-testicular causes.
- The advancement of assisted reproductive technologies not only has revolutionized the field of male infertility, but now also offers reproductive options to men who could not have conceived several years ago.

Infertility is defined as the inability to conceive after 1 year of unprotected, adequately timed intercourse. Approximately 15% of all couples are infertile. In up to 50% of these infertile couples, the infertility has a male factor component; 20% of couples will not be able to conceive solely because of a male factor.

Traditionally, the initial evaluation of the male was performed only when the couple had been unable to conceive after 1 year of unprotected intercourse. However, because many couples are now postponing parenthood, and because the risk of a female's infertility increases as she passes age 35, most male infertility evaluations are performed on initial presentation (six months of unprotected intercourse). A detailed history and physical examination and a semen analysis are essential initial steps in diagnosing the infertile male. With the advancement of assisted reproductive technologies (ARTs), a variety of treatment options are now available for the infertile couple.

## ETIOLOGY

Causes of male infertility can be simply classified into three categories: pretesticular, testicular, and post-testicular. Pretesticular causes of infertility are generally associated with endocrinopathies. These endocrinopathies, which include multi-organ syndromes, androgen receptor and conversion disorders, neoplasms, and exogenous hormones, have numerous causes. Testicular causes of infertility include genetic disorders, varicoceles, gonadotoxins, cryptorchidism, androgen synthesis disorders, impaired sperm motility, and certain acquired disorders. Finally, post-testicular causes of infertility involve obstruction of sperm passage, ejaculatory dysfunction, and erectile dysfunction. It is important to remember that the etiology of infertility is unknown in 25% of infertile males.

## Pretesticular Causes of Infertility

### Endocrinopathies

Causes of endocrinopathies include congenital disorders, neoplasms, systemic diseases, use of exogenous steroids, and certain androgen disorders (Table 54-1). Note that except for androgen disorders, which are associated with hypergonadotropic hypogonadism, most endocrinopathies are associated with hypogonadotropic hypogonadism. To understand how endocrine disorders can lead to infertility, one must first have a basic understanding of how the hypothalamic-pituitary-gonadal (HPG) axis functions and how it affects the testis.

### Hypothalamic-Pituitary-Gonadal Axis

The hypothalamus receives input from the central nervous system in the form of neurotransmitters (dopamine, serotonin, acetylcholine, and norepinephrine) and neuropeptides (endogenous opioids). It also receives feedback from the testes and adrenal glands in the form of steroids (i.e., estradiol and testosterone) and protein hormones (i.e., inhibin). In turn, the hypothalamus secretes gonadotropin-releasing hormone (GnRH) in a pulsatile fashion from the preoptic and arcuate nucleus. GnRH is released into the portal hypophyseal venous system that leads into the anterior pituitary (Fig. 54-1).

The anterior pituitary secretes luteinizing hormone (LH) and follicle-stimulating hormone (FSH) in response to GnRH. LH binds to receptors on Leydig cells in the testis to cause the release of testosterone. Testosterone enters the circulation and can be converted to either dihydrotestosterone (DHT), by the enzyme $5\alpha$-reductase, or to estradiol. Testosterone, DHT, and estradiol act independently to modulate LH secretion. It is believed that testosterone acts at the hypothalamic level while estrogen acts at the pituitary level, and both cause negative feedback inhibition. The initiation and maintenance of spermatogenesis by the seminiferous tubules is dependent on testosterone as well as on the binding of FSH to receptors on Sertoli cells. Sertoli cells release inhibin and activin, which provide negative and positive feedback, respectively, to the hypothalamus and to the anterior pituitary.

Prolactin has several effects on the HPG axis. Hyperprolactinemia has been shown to inhibit GnRH secretion as well as inhibit the effects of testosterone. Patients with elevated prolactin and low testosterone levels do not show improvement in libido and sexual function when given testosterone supplementation. In addition, these patients have low LH levels, indicating that the hypothalamus does not respond to the low testosterone levels. Finally, hyperprolactinemia has been shown to alter the production of DHT. It is therefore important to

# Reproductive Endocrinology and Infertility

| Table 54-1 Pretesticular Causes of Infertility: Endocrinopathies | |
|---|---|
| **Congenital** | **Acquired** |
| **Multiorgan syndromes** | **Neoplasms** |
| Kallmann syndrome | Pituitary adenomas |
| Prader-Willi syndrome | Leukemia and lymphoma |
| Fertile eunuch syndrome | Germinomas |
| Laurence-Moon-Biedl syndrome | Prolactinomas |
| Pituitary hypoplasia or aplasia | Gliomas |
| | Craniopharyngiomas |
| **Gene mutations** | |
| | **Systemic diseases** |
| DAX 1 gene mutation | |
| PC1 gene mutation | Renal failure |
| | Liver failure |
| **Androgen receptor disorder** | Anorexia/starvation |
| | Hypoparathyroidism |
| Testicular feminization | |
| Lub syndrome | **Infiltrative and infectious disease of** |
| Rosewater's syndrome | **the hypothalamus and pituitary** |
| Reifenstein's syndrome | |
| | Sarcoidosis |
| **Androgen conversion disorders** | Tuberculosis |
| | Syphilis |
| 5α-reductase deficiency | Hemochromatosis |
| | Abscess |
| | **Trauma, postsurgery, postirradiation** |
| | **Exogenous hormones and drugs** |
| | See Table 54-2 |

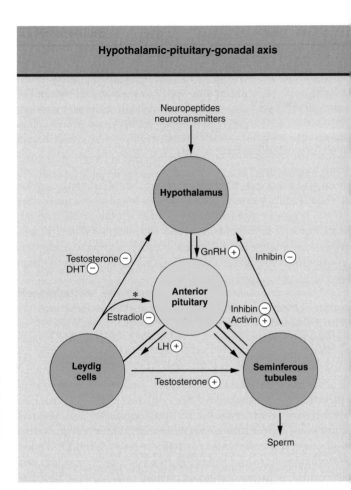

**Figure 54-1 Hypothalamic-pituitary-gonadal axis.** Testosterone is aromatized (*) to estradiol in the brain and peripheral circulation. Note that testosterone may also have a small inhibitory effect on the anterior pituitary to decrease luteinizing hormone secretion.

check prolactin levels in all infertile males when an endocrine problem is suspected.

### Congenital Disorders

Kallmann syndrome occurs in approximately 1 in 10,000 to 1 in 60,000 live births and is the most common X-linked disorder associated with male infertility. Most occurrences, however, are of the "sporadic" type. Kallmann syndrome consists of congenital, isolated idiopathic hypogonadotropic hypogonadism and anosmia. Other clinical features may also include congenital deafness, cleft palate, cerebellar dysfunction, renal abnormalities, cryptorchidism, and diabetes mellitus. The *KAL1* gene, located on chromosome Xp22.3, is responsible for the X-linked form of this syndrome. This gene encodes the protein anosmin, which plays a critical role in the migration of GnRH neurons and olfactory nerves to the hypothalamus. Because these patients lack FSH and LH stimulation to the testis, testosterone production and spermatogenesis are absent. Through hormone replacement therapy with FSH and human chorionic gonadotropin (hCG), many of these patients can become fertile.

Prader-Willi syndrome is associated with idiopathic hypogonadotropic hypogonadism, mild to moderate mental retardation, obesity, and infantile hypotonia. The syndrome is caused by a mutation or deletion on the short arm of chromosome 15 when it is inherited from the patient's father, or less commonly, when two chromosomal copies of this locus are inherited from the patient's mother. Treatment involves hormone replacement therapy with FSH and hCG.

Gene mutations associated with hypogonadotropic hypogonadism include mutations in the *DAX1* and *PC1* genes. The

*DAX1* gene is found on the X chromosome and encodes for a nuclear hormone receptor that has a critical role in the development of the hypothalamus, adrenals, pituitary, and gonads. This gene also appears to function in maintaining the epithelial integrity of the testis and spermatogenesis.[1] Mutations with the *DAX1* gene are associated with congenital adrenal hyperplasia and idiopathic hypogonadotropic hypogonadism. The *PC1* gene, a convertase-1 gene, influences GnRH secretion by the hypothalamus. Mutations in this gene are associated with idiopathic hypogonadotropic hypogonadism, obesity, and diabetes mellitus.

### Neoplasms

Neoplasms such as pituitary adenomas and prolactinomas have been associated with hypogonadotropic hypogonadism and infertility. Pituitary adenomas can cause a decrease in gonadotropin release via direct compression of the portal system or by decreased LH/FSH secretion. These patients may present with peripheral visual field defects, headaches, and decreased libido. A pituitary adenoma must be considered in any patient experiencing these symptoms and a decreased testosterone level along with a low serum LH level. A magnetic resonance imaging

(MRI) scan of the head should be obtained for these patients. Large lesions are generally treated via transsphenoidal surgical resection.

Prolactin microadenomas cause an elevation of prolactin and a subsequent inhibition of LH and FSH secretion. Hyperprolactinemia can also result in altered DHT production, leading to impaired spermatogenesis. Management may consist of surgical excision of the adenoma or medications. Most patients are treated medically with cabergoline (Dostinex) or bromocriptine (Parlodel).

### Systemic Disease

Hypogonadotropic hypogonadism has been associated with systemic diseases such as renal and liver failure and primary hypothyroidism. Renal failure and associated uremia can lead to impotence, altered spermatogenesis, and decreased libido. These changes may be related to estrogen excess, elevated prolactin levels, or elevated parathyroid hormone and usually will be corrected by successful renal transplantation. Liver failure results in decreased testosterone levels, increased testosterone binding to plasma proteins, and increased plasma estrogen levels. Finally, primary hypothyroidism is associated with an elevation in thyrotropin levels. Because thyrotropin stimulates prolactin secretion, patients may suffer from impaired gonadotropin release and altered DHT production. Thyroxine replacement usually returns thyrotropin to normal levels.

### Exogenous Steroids and Drugs

Anabolic and androgenic steroid abuse are common causes of male infertility in athletes and body builders. Exogenous androgenic steroids suppress pituitary LH release, which results in decreased intratesticular testosterone production. Because normal spermatogenesis requires intratesticular testosterone, these patients usually are azoospermic. Although the effects may be reversible, this reversibility depends on the duration and dosage of exogenous steroid use. A mistake commonly made is to prescribe testosterone supplementation to a patient who has a low serum testosterone level when the couple is trying to conceive. Other drugs that are associated with hypogonadotropic hypogonadism include selective serotonin reuptake inhibitors, which cause an increase in prolactin levels. Table 54-2 lists medications and drugs that can cause male infertility.

### Androgen Disorders

Androgen disorders can be classified as disorders of androgen synthesis, androgen receptors, or androgen conversion. Androgen receptor and conversion disorders are considered pretesticular causes of male infertility, and androgen synthesis disorders are classified as testicular causes of male infertility.

Androgen receptor disorders, also known as androgen insensitivity syndromes, are a group of X-linked disorders that include Rosewater's syndrome, Reifenstein's syndrome, testicular feminization (male pseudohermaphroditism), and Lub syndrome. These syndromes are inherited as X-linked recessive traits because the androgen receptor gene is located on the X chromosome at Xq11–12. Complete androgen insensitivity leads to a female phenotype with intra-abdominal testes; incomplete androgen insensitivity leads to ambiguous genitalia, hypospadias, and micropenis.

| Table 54-2 Gonadotoxic Agents | |
|---|---|
| **Medications and Drugs** | **Other** |
| **Inhibitors of testosterone synthesis** | **Direct effect on spermatogenesis** |
| Ketoconazole | Radiation |
| Ethanol | >600 rads: permanent germ cell |
| Cryptoterone | damage |
| Spironolactone | >3000 rads: permanent interstitial |
| Sulfasalazine | cell damage |
| Exogenous steroids (indirectly) | Environmental toxins |
| SSRIs (indirectly) | DDT |
| | Fungicides |
| **Stimulators of estradiol synthesis or activity** | DBCP |
| | Solvents |
| Estrogen compounds | |
| Digoxin | **Unknown mechanism** |
| Spironolactone | |
| | Thermal exposures |
| **Direct toxin effect on testicular cells** | Hot tubs |
| Chemotherapeutic agents | |
| MOPP chemotherapy | |
| ABVD chemotherapy | |
| Cyclophosphamide | |
| Ethanol | |
| **Competition with androgen receptors** | |
| Cimetidine | |
| Flutamide | |
| Nilutamide | |
| Cryptoterone | |
| Biclutamide | |
| Spironolactone | |
| **Unknown mechanism** | |
| Cocaine | |
| Tobacco | |
| Marijuana | |
| Colchicine | |
| Allopurinol | |
| **Decreases sperm fertilization capacity** | |
| Calcium channel blockers | |

Disorders in androgen conversion disorders include 5α-reductase deficiencies. The enzyme 5α-reductase is involved in the conversion of testosterone to DHT. DHT is responsible for the development of the external male genitalia and the prostate. Newborns present as male pseudohermaphrodites with severe perineoscrotal hypospadias and a blind vaginal pouch that opens into a urogenital sinus. These patients are generally infertile because they are unable to effectively deliver sperm and their sperm counts are low. However, there has been a report of paternity by intrauterine insemination with sperm from a man with 5α-reductase deficiency.[2]

## Testicular Causes

Testicular causes of infertility are generally associated with hypergonadotropic hypogonadism. They include varicoceles, cryptorchidism, genetic abnormalities, gonadotoxins, multiorgan syndromes, androgen synthesis disorders, impaired sperm motility,

# Reproductive Endocrinology and Infertility

| Table 54-3 Testicular Causes of Infertility | |
| --- | --- |
| **Congenital** | **Acquired** |
| **Chromosomal abnormalities** | **Varicoceles** |
| Klinefelter's syndrome | |
| 46,XX male | **Orchitis** |
| 47,XYY male | Viral (mumps, HIV) |
| Mixed gonadal dysgenesis | Granulomatous (tuberculosis, leprosy) |
| **Gene mutations** | **Testicular neoplasms** |
| Y chromosome microdeletions | |
| SRY gene mutation | **Infiltrative disease** |
| | Hemochromatosis |
| **Cryptorchidism** | Amyloidosis |
| **Multiorgan syndromes** | **Gonadotoxic agents** |
| Noonan's syndrome | See Table 54-2. |
| Myotonic dystrophy | |
| Anorchia | |
| Down syndrome | |
| Niemann-Pick disease | |
| **Androgen synthesis disorders** | |
| StAR protein mutations | |
| 20,22 desmolase deficiency | |
| 3β hydroxysteroid dehydrogenase deficiency | |
| 17α-hydroxylase deficiency | |
| 17,20 desmolase deficiency | |
| 17β-hydroxysteroid dehydrogenase deficiency | |
| **Impaired sperm motility** | |
| Kartagener's syndrome | |

and certain acquired diseases that temporarily or permanently suppress spermatogenesis (Table 54-3).

## Varicoceles

Varicoceles are dilated internal spermatic veins (gonadal veins) that terminate as the pampiniform plexus and drain the testis. The dilation of these veins is thought to be secondary to incompetent venous valves. Varicoceles have an incidence of approximately 15% in the general population, increasing to up to 50% of men with primary infertility and up to 69% of men with secondary infertility.[3] These dilated veins are more commonly found on the left side or bilaterally than on the right side alone, possibly because of the greater length of the left internal spermatic vein and because of the left spermatic vein's perpendicular insertion into the left renal vein.

Many theories have been suggested to explain why varicoceles lead to impaired spermatogenesis and male infertility. One theory is that poor venous drainage leads to disruption of the countercurrent exchange of heat from the spermatic cord and thus elevates scrotal temperatures. The elevated scrotal temperatures lead to impaired spermatogenesis. Another theory is that poor venous drainage leads to impaired drainage of gonadotoxins from the testis.

Varicoceles have been shown to cause a progressive deterioration in semen parameters.[3] Subfertile males with varicoceles

have been found to have semen with decreased motility, decreased density, and abnormal morphology[4] as well as abnormal testosterone and FSH levels.[5]

## Cryptorchidism

The incidence of cryptorchidism in the full-term infant is approximately 3%. However, by age 1, 75% of these testicles will spontaneously descend and the overall incidence of cryptorchidism becomes approximately 0.8%. Testes that have not descended by the time an infant is age 6 months are not likely to descend. Patients with a history of cryptorchidism not only have decreased sperm concentrations, but they also demonstrate lower basal levels of LH and testosterone and have a worse response to GnRH stimulation.[6] These patients are also at a 40 times greater risk of developing testicular cancer.

The amount of time the cryptorchid testis is left in place can influence the degree of spermatogenesis. If the cryptorchid testis is surgically corrected postpubertally, 69% of testes will have no spermatogenesis, with either testicular agenesis, atrophy, or a Sertoli-cell-only histologic pattern.[7] Other studies have shown that if left untreated, 44% of men with unilateral cryptorchidism will be either oligospermic or azoospermic, as opposed to 100% of men with bilateral cryptorchidism.[8] In contrast, men who had an orchiopexy before puberty were found to have normal sperm densities (>20 million/mL) 62% and 30% of the time for unilateral and bilateral cryptorchidism, respectively.[9] Kumar and colleagues showed that in patients with surgically corrected cryptorchid testes, fertility rates ranged from 84% in those with unilateral cryptorchidism to 60% in those with bilateral cryptorchidism.[10]

## Genetics

### Karyotype Abnormalities

Karyotype abnormalities have been found in 12% of azoospermic and severely oligospermic males.[11] Klinefelter's syndrome (47,XXY or 46,XY/XXY) is the most common sex chromosomal abnormality, occurring in approximately 1 in 650 live male births; it accounts for up to 11% of all cases of azoospermia.[11,12] This syndrome is due to paternal or maternal sex chromosomal nondisjunction during meiosis. Roughly 8% of patients will have a mosaic 46,XY/XXY karyotype, and approximately 92% will have the 47,XXY karyotype.[11] These patients present with some or all of the following: small firm testis, infertility, obesity, diabetes mellitus, decreased intelligence, decreased Leydig cell function, increased height, and an increased risk of leukemia, extragonadal germ cell tumors, and breast cancer. These patients are hypogonadotropic with low-normal serum testosterone levels. They have variable amounts of sperm production and are generally unable to conceive naturally.

Several other sex chromosomal defects occur less commonly. All of these can occur in phenotypically normal males. Men with the XYY chromosome pattern, occurring in approximately 1 in 850 live births, are phenotypically normal except for increased height.[12] Although some of these men may be fertile, most men are shown to have Sertoli-cell-only or maturation arrest histology on testicular biopsy. Males with 46,XX karyotype (XX male syndrome) also have a normal phenotype but are infertile. This syndrome occurs in approximately 1 in 9000 live births.[12] It is believed that these patients suffer from a translocation of the

*SRY* gene on the Y chromosome to the homologous region on the X chromosome. These patients exhibit Sertoli-cell-only histology on testis biopsy and are azoospermic. They can be born with ambiguous genitalia or hypospadias. Finally, patients with mixed gonadal dysgenesis can present as phenotypic males, females, or with ambiguous genitalia. They commonly have a 45,X/46,XY mosaic karyotype, although 33% may present with a normal karyotype. This mosaic pattern is thought to be due to loss of the Y chromosome early in development. Most patients have a testis and a streak gonad, which is at risk for later developing gonadoblastoma. Normal Leydig and Sertoli cells are usually present within the testis, but the seminiferous tubules lack germ cells.

### Gene Mutations or Deletions

The Y chromosome is the smallest chromosome in the human genome. The short arm (Yp) is associated with the *SRY* gene, or the testis-determining factor. An absent or deficient *SRY* gene results in a 46,XY female. The long arm of the Y chromosome (Yq11) contains the azoospermia factor *(AZF)* region. Three distinct regions *(AZFa, AZFb, AZFc)* are responsible for encoding proteins involved in spermatogenesis. Microdeletions in any or all of these three regions will be found in infertile males. Pryor and colleagues showed that 7% of infertile males and 2% of normal males had an *AZF* microdeletion and that the size and position of the deletion did not correlate with the severity of spermatogenic failure.[13]

### Gonadotoxins

Some gonadotoxins have been discussed earlier in this chapter. It is important to remember that recreational drugs, such as alcohol, cocaine, marijuana, and tobacco, have all been implicated as gonadotoxic agents. Thermal exposures, such as hot tubs, as well as radiation, chemotherapy, and environmental toxins have also all been shown to impair spermatogenesis. Table 54-2 provides a comprehensive listing of gonadotoxic agents.

### Multiorgan Syndromes

Noonan's syndrome is one example of a multiorgan syndrome that causes hypergonadotropic hypogonadism. These patients have features similar to those found with Turner's syndrome, such as webbed neck, low-set ears, ptosis, hypertelorism, cubitus valgus, short stature, congenital heart disease, and hypogonadism. Most patients with Noonan's syndrome are infertile due to primary testicular failure. Table 54-3 lists other multiorgan syndromes causing hypergonadotropic hypogonadism.

### Androgen Synthesis Disorders

Androgen synthesis is a complex process that involves the transport of cholesterol into the mitochondria. This first rate-limiting step is under the regulation of the steroidogenic acute regulatory protein (StAR). Mutations of the StAR protein result in congenital lipoid adrenal hyperplasia. Patients with this disorder have external female genitalia, irrespective of karyotype, and suffer from a severe salt-wasting form of adrenal hyperplasia. The disease is lethal if glucocorticosteroids are not administered.

The synthesis of testosterone from cholesterol requires five enzymes. A deficiency in any of the first three enzymes (20,22-desmolase, 3β-hydroxysteroid dehydrogenase, 17α-hydroxylase)

results in congenital adrenal hyperplasia. Patients presenting with this deficiency have incomplete virilization due to defective androgen synthesis. A deficiency in the last two enzymes (17, 20-desmolase and 17β-hydroxysteroid dehydrogenase) leads to pseudohermaphroditism in males with ambiguous genitalia or completely feminized genitalia with cryptorchid testes.

### Motility

Poor sperm motility, or asthenospermia, is most often seen with defects in sperm morphology, or teratospermia. However, 20% of patients will have isolated asthenospermia. Factors that can contribute to poor sperm motility are infections, varicoceles, antisperm antibodies, and certain genetic abnormalities. The classic syndrome associated with immotile sperm is Kartagener's syndrome, which consists of the triad of situs inversus, bronchiectasis, and chronic sinusitis. Kartagener's syndrome is a form of immotile cilia syndrome, which is associated with structural defects in the axoneme, the basic structure of the spermatozoon tail. Immotile cilia syndrome occurs in approximately 1 in 20,000 live births, and there have been reports of successful fertilization with in vitro fertilization (IVF) and intracytoplasmic sperm injection (ICSI) in patients with Kartagener's syndrome.[14]

### Acquired Disorders

Certain acquired disorders can cause testicular damage and lead to hypergonadotropic hypogonadism. These acquired disorders include trauma to the testicles, testicular neoplasms, history of orchitis, and exposure to gonadotoxic agents (see Table 54-2). These disorders are generally associated with decreased spermatogenesis.

## Post-Testicular Causes

### Obstruction

Approximately 40% of azoospermic men have an obstructed ductal system.[15] Obstruction of sperm delivery can occur anywhere from the efferent ducts to the ejaculatory ducts. Causes of epididymal obstruction include chronic or recurrent epididymitis, orchiopexy, hydrocelectomy, and other scrotal surgeries. Epididymal obstruction also is seen in men with Young's syndrome, which is characterized by bronchiectasis and inspissated epididymal secretions, causing gradual epididymal obstruction. The most frequent causes of vasal obstruction include any type of pelvic or inguinal surgery, such as herniorrhaphy and vasectomy (Fig. 54-2). Vasectomy is the leading cause of vasal obstruction in this country. Ejaculatory duct obstruction can be caused by a cyst (often a müllerian remnant), a wolffian duct malformation, prior prostatic inflammation and scarring (i.e., due to infection or trauma), prostate cancer, and stones or calcifications (Table 54-4).

Semen analysis and transrectal ultrasound (TRUS) are helpful in making the diagnosis. Because the seminal vesicles are responsible for making fructose and alkalinizing the seminal fluid, complete obstruction of the ejaculatory ducts will result in a low-volume, acidic, fructose-negative ejaculate. TRUS will support the diagnosis by showing dilated ejaculatory ducts and seminal vesicles. The seminal vesicles can be aspirated at this time to confirm the diagnosis.

In some cases, sperm passage is inhibited because of congenital bilateral absence of the vas deferens (CBAVD). CBAVD

# Reproductive Endocrinology and Infertility

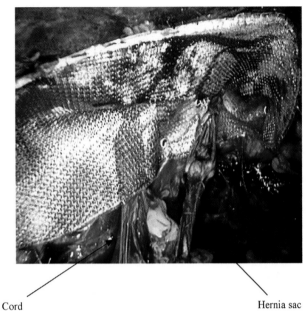

Cord        Hernia sac

**Figure 54-2    Hernia mesh causing vasal obstruction.**

is found in 2% of infertile males and in more than 90% of patients with cystic fibrosis. It is thought that CBAVD alone may in fact represent a milder form of cystic fibrosis. Cystic fibrosis is caused by a genetic mutation of the cystic fibrosis transmembrane conductance regulator *(CFTR)* gene; therefore, men with CBAVD and their wives should be screened for *CFTR* mutations and be referred to genetic counseling.

## Ejaculatory Dysfunction

Ejaculatory dysfunction can be due to retrograde ejaculation or anejaculation. In order for a male to ejaculate, semen must be deposited in the prostatic urethra (emission). Coordinated

| Table 54-4 Post-testicular Causes of Infertility | |
|---|---|
| **Congenital** | **Acquired** |
| **Obstruction** | **Obstruction** |
| Young's syndrome | Vasectomy |
| Congenital bilateral absence of the vas deferens (CBAVD) | Inflammation/scarring |
| |     Pelvic/inguinal/scrotal surgery |
| |     Trauma |
| | Ejaculatory duct obstruction |
| |     Cystic mass |
| |     Calcifications |
| | **Ejaculatory dysfunction** |
| | Retrograde ejaculation |
| |     Medications |
| |     Transurethral or bladder neck surgery |
| |     Neurologic disease |
| | Anejaculation |
| |     Psychological |
| |     Retroperitoneal surgery |
| |     Neurologic disease |
| | **Erectile dysfunction** |

closure of the bladder neck and contraction of the pelvic floor and periurethral muscles are also necessary. Emission is controlled by the sympathetic nerves T10–L2 that course through the paravertebral sympathetic ganglion. The pudendal nerve (S2–S4) is responsible for contractions of the pelvic floor and periurethral muscles.

Retrograde ejaculation may be caused by pharmacologic, anatomic, or neurologic conditions. Medications that cause retrograde ejaculation include alpha-adrenergic antagonists used to treat benign prostatic hyperplasia and antihypertensive medications, such as prazosin and terazosin. Anatomic causes of retrograde ejaculation involve disruption of the bladder neck or internal sphincter; these are often iatrogenic following transurethral or bladder neck surgeries. Riehmann and colleagues showed that 68% of patients undergoing a transurethral resection of the prostate developed retrograde ejaculation.[16] Neurologic conditions that can lead to retrograde ejaculation include diabetes mellitus, spinal cord injury, and multiple sclerosis.

Anejaculation is typically seen with spinal cord injury or following retroperitoneal surgery; it can also have a psychological etiology. Ninety-five percent of spinal cord–injured patients have ejaculatory failure due to their nerve injury. Depending on the level of their spinal cord lesion, they can ejaculate through stimulation of their sympathetic nerves with electroejaculation or vibratory stimulation. Most retroperitoneal surgeries, such as a retroperitoneal lymph node dissection for testicular cancer, involve the risk of injuring the sympathetic nerves T10–L2. Injury to these nerves results in failure of emission. Finally, a psychological cause for anejaculation must be considered for any patient who suddenly is unable to ejaculate and for whom no other causes of ejaculatory dysfunction can be identified.

## Erectile Dysfunction

Erectile dysfunction is defined as the persistent inability to achieve and maintain an erection sufficient for intercourse. Although erectile dysfunction can occur at any age, most men by age 45 have experienced erectile dysfunction at least some of the time. According to the Massachusetts Male Aging Study, complete impotence increases from 5% among men age 40 to 15% among men age 70 and older.[17]

The penis is composed of two dorsal cavernosal bodies and a ventral corpus spongiosum, which encompasses the urethra. Through central and peripheral stimulation, the parasympathetic nerves are activated, and the cavernosal muscles relax to allow blood to fill the cavernosal sinusoids. The expanding sinusoids compress the subtunical venous plexuses and prevent the outflow of blood. This corporal tumescence increases the intracavernosal pressure and allows for a rigid erection.

Erectile dysfunction has numerous causes, including neurogenic, endocrine, vascular, iatrogenic, and trauma-related causes. Vasculogenic impotence can be caused by arterial insufficiency, seen in patients with atherosclerosis and diabetes, or by venous leaks, when the subtunical venous plexus is inadequately compressed to prevent the outflow of blood. Neurogenic disorders include spinal cord injury, Parkinson's disease, strokes, and peripheral neuropathy, as seen in chronic alcoholics and diabetics. Most endocrine disorders, as previously noted, can lead to decreased testosterone production and therefore decreased libido. Pelvic fractures and perineal trauma have also been associated with erectile dysfunction because of arterial damage. Iatrogenic causes of impotence include surgical procedures such as radical prostatectomies or cystectomies, lumbar laminectomies, and abdominoperineal resections. Other iatrogenic causes of erectile dysfunction include pelvic irradiation and the use of certain medications, such as sympatholytics, anticholinergics, antiandrogens, and centrally acting agents such as tricyclic antidepressants and alcohol.

## DIAGNOSIS

Evaluation of the infertile male starts with a detailed history and physical examination. Because of the vast number of etiologies of male infertility, we advocate a systematic approach using a standard evaluation form (Fig. 54-3).

### History

Many diagnoses of male infertility can be made on the basis of a detailed history alone. It is important to inquire how long the couple has been trying to conceive, whether there is a history of pregnancy with the current or previous partners, and about frequency and timing of intercourse. When possible, a female history should be taken directly from the patient's partner. Often neither partner understands the menstrual cycle nor how to calculate the optimal time for intercourse. Patients should be instructed to have intercourse every 48 hours around the time of ovulation. This pattern is suggested because sperm have been shown to be viable for approximately 2 days in the cervical mucus and crypts. The use of lubricants should be discussed because products such as Lubifax, Surgilube, Keri Lotion, and K-Y Jelly have all been shown to decrease sperm motility in vitro; if needed, vegetable oil can be recommended.[18]

A complete childhood and developmental history is important in evaluating the subfertile male. Patients should be asked about the history of cryptorchidism, testicular torsion, testicular trauma, and the onset of puberty. Several studies have confirmed abnormal sperm production after testicular torsion, showing overall that 37% of patients had low sperm density, 56% had poor sperm motility, and 53% had poor sperm morphology.[19] Delayed puberty can often be a sign of an underlying endocrinopathy. A history of postpubertal mumps is also important because this can lead to orchitis in roughly 25% of males and cause severe testicular atrophy in up to 55% of these patients.[20]

Surgical procedures such as orchiopexy, retroperitoneal surgery, transurethral prostate surgery, herniorrhaphy, and Y-V plasty of the bladder neck have all been associated with male infertility. Most of these procedures will lead to ductal obstruction, anejaculation, or retrograde ejaculation.

The patient should be asked about any recent infections, particularly febrile viral illnesses, because these can impair spermatogenesis for up to 3 months. It takes approximately 74 days for type B spermatogonia to develop into mature spermatozoa and be seen in the ejaculate.[21] The clinician should elicit a family history and inquire about cystic fibrosis, testosterone deficiencies, and any first-degree infertile relatives. Finally, a thorough review of systems, questioning such symptoms as headaches, impaired visual field defects, anosmia, respiratory infections, and galactorrhea, can help diagnose other endocrinopathies.

### Physical Examination

Almost any systemic illness can impair spermatogenesis; therefore, every infertile patient should have a thorough physical examination, with focus on the male genitalia. The normospermic male has a testicular length greater than 4 cm and a volume of at least 20 mL[3]. Because 85% of the testis is involved in spermatogenesis, a decrease in testicular size indicates impaired spermatogenesis.[22] The epididymis should be palpated for any induration or irregularities. The spermatic cord should be carefully examined to identify the presence of a varicocele and the presence or absence of the vas deferens. Varicoceles are graded according to size on a scale from 1 to 3 (Table 54-5). Grade 1 varicoceles are often difficult to detect; a scrotal ultrasound can help with a suspected diagnosis. The penile meatus should be examined to identify any ulcerative lesions indicating infection or the presence of a hypospadias, which could lead to impairment of sperm delivery to the cervix. Finally, signs of gynecomastia and inadequate virilization, such as decreased body hair, should lead the clinician to consider an endocrine abnormality.

### Laboratory Evaluation

#### Semen Analysis

The initial laboratory assessment includes semen analysis. Ideally, a minimum of two semen samples should be obtained after 2 to 3 days of sexual abstinence. Longer periods of abstinence are associated with decreased sperm motility, and shorter periods of abstinence result in low volume and density. The specimen can be obtained by masturbation or by intercourse with special condoms that do not contain any spermicidal agents. Although samples can be collected at home, ideally they should be collected in the office, because the specimens need to be analyzed within 30 minutes to 1 hour after collection. It is always important to ask the patient if the entire specimen was collected, because partial sample loss can erroneously lead to reports of low semen volume and other impaired parameters.

Most laboratories use the set of standards established by the World Health Organization (WHO) to describe the minimal limits of semen parameters adequate for establishing a pregnancy[23] (Table 54-6). The five main semen parameters evaluated are ejaculate volume, sperm density, percent motility, forward progression (qualitative movement), and morphology. Statistically, fertility rates decrease as sperm counts fall below 20 million/mL. Many laboratories now use morphologic criteria described by Kruger as opposed to the WHO standards. Kruger's strict criteria involve evaluating each sperm's size and shape, the size of the acrosome, and the absence of cytoplasmic droplets. Kruger and colleagues noted that men with less than 4% normal morphologic spermatozoa had IVF success rates of 7.6%, whereas patients with normal sperm morphology between 4% and 14% had IVF success rates of 63.9%.[24]

Semen fructose level should also be measured in azoospermic men. Fructose is produced by the seminal vesicles, and the absence of fructose in the ejaculate indicates ejaculatory duct obstruction, seminal vesicle dysfunction, or hypoplasia.

#### Semen Function Tests

##### Sperm Viability Testing

A test commonly used to check for sperm viability is the hypo-osmotic swelling test. Spermatozoa are placed in a hypo-osmotic

**BAYLOR COLLEGE OF MEDICINE**
**SCOTT DEPARTMENT OF UROLOGY**
*Male Infertility Initial Consultation*

DATE ____ / ____ / ____
M      D      Y

NAME _____     Referring M.D. _____
Last          First

## HISTORY

_____ y.o. M     Trying _____ yrs     Married _____ yrs
Previous pregnancies

**Previous Evaluation and Treatment:**
Physician
SA
Hormones
Other
IUI/IVF

Intercourse frequency     _____ x/wk
Lubricants
Previous contraception

## FEMALE EVALUATION

_____ y.o. F     Doctor _____
_____

**Previous Evaluation and Treatment:**
G_____     P_____     A_____
Menses (regular/irregular)
HSG
Laparoscopy
Medications

Intercourse frequency     _____ x/wk
Lubricants
Previous contraception

## Allergies

Medications

Past Medical History

Past Surgical History

Social History
TOB
ETOH
Occupation

## REVIEW OF SYSTEMS

| + | − | SYSTEMS |
|---|---|---|
|   |   | Chemicals |
|   |   | Toxins |
|   |   | Radiation |
|   |   | Fevers > 102°F |
|   |   | Trauma |
|   |   | Torsion |
|   |   | Varicocele |
|   |   | Mumps |
|   |   | Epididymitis |
|   |   | STD |
|   |   | Family hx of infertility |
|   |   | Prostatitis |
|   |   | Other |

## REVIEW OF SYSTEMS (General)

| + | − | SYSTEMS |
|---|---|---|
|   |   | Constitutional systems |
|   |   | HEENT |
|   |   | Cardiovascular |
|   |   | Respiratory |
|   |   | Gastrointestinal |
|   |   | Genitourinary |
|   |   | Musculoskeletal |
|   |   | Integumentary/skin |
|   |   | Neurological |
|   |   | Psychiatric |
|   |   | Endocrine |
|   |   | Hematology/lymphatic |
|   |   | Allergy/immunology |

## EXAMINATION

|  | R | L |
|---|---|---|
| **Testes**  Size |  |  |
| Consistency |  |  |
| **Vas/epididymis** |  |  |
| **Varicocele** |  |  |
| **Phallus** |  |  |
| **Rectal** |  |  |

## GENERAL EXAMINATION

| + | − | SYSTEMS |
|---|---|---|
|   |   | Abdomen |
|   |   | Genitalia/pelvic |
|   |   | Rectal/prostate |
|   |   | Neurologic |
|   |   | HEENT |
|   |   | Neck |
|   |   | Chest/lungs |
|   |   | Heart |
|   |   | Breast |
|   |   | Back |
|   |   | Extremities |
|   |   | Lymphatic |

## IMPRESSION

## URINALYSIS

## PLAN

**Hormones:**
_____ FSH
_____ LH
_____ Testosterone
_____ Prolactin
_____ Estradiol
_____ IGF-1
_____ PSA

## SEMEN ANALYSIS

_____ IMB
_____ WBC
_____ SM
_____ Other SPA
_____ Semen C&S
_____ Cryopreservation
_____ Wash (Percoll/Chymotrypsin)
_____ Pellet

LIL/eb (08/31/2000)

**Figure 54-3   Infertile male evaluation form.**

| Table 54-5 | |
|---|---|
| **Grading of Varicoceles** | |
| Grade | Findings |
| I (small) | Palpable only with Valsalva maneuver |
| II (moderate) | Palpable without the Valsalva maneuver |
| III (large) | Visible through the scrotal skin |

medium where viable sperm will absorb the fluid and swell, causing a curling of their tails. Nonviable sperm will not manifest these signs. The hypo-osmotic swelling test does not have any toxic effects on the sperm and is used to select viable sperm for ICSI. Another test of sperm viability is the use of stains such as eosin Y and trypan blue to determine whether the plasma membrane is intact.

#### Sperm Penetration Assay

The sperm penetration assay (SPA) measures the fertilization potential of the sperm. This in vitro test, performed with hamster oocytes that have had their zona pellucida enzymatically removed, enables interspecies generation of the sperm into the oocyte. This assay evaluates the sperm's ability to undergo capacitation, the acrosome reaction, and fusion with the oocyte. Many feel the SPA is an invaluable test for screening patients before they undergo IVF due to the high cost of this high-technology assisted reproduction procedure. Studies have shown a correlation between positive SPA results and improved IVF outcomes.[25]

#### Postcoital Testing

The postcoital test, also known as the cervical mucous penetration assay, is designed to evaluate impaired male factors such as hyperviscosity, abnormal penile anatomy, decreased semen volume despite good sperm density, and unexplained infertility. The postcoital test is performed by examining the cervical mucus several hours after intercourse, ideally around the periovulatory phase of the female. The cervical mucus is smeared on a slide and examined microscopically for the presence of ferning within the mucus and for the quantitative presence of sperm and forward sperm motility. The role of the postcoital test continues to be a point of debate.

| Table 54-6 | |
|---|---|
| **WHO Criteria: Minimal Limits for Adequate Fertilization** | |
| Volume | ≥2.0 mL |
| pH | 7.2–7.8 |
| Density | ≥20 million/mL |
| Total sperm count | ≥40 million |
| Motility | ≥50% with normal morphology |
| Morphology | ≥30% normal forms |

#### Acrosome Reaction Test

For fertilization to occur, the sperm must undergo the acrosome reaction. The acrosome is a membrane-bound organelle covering most of the head of the sperm. On interaction with the zona pellucida of the ova, the sperm releases proteolytic enzymes from the acrosome to penetrate and enter the ova. This acrosome reaction may be insufficient, or absent, in some infertile males. Pampiglione and colleagues showed that an acrosome response of less than 31.3% predicted fertilization failure in 100% of cases.[26] In the laboratory, the acrosome reaction can be induced with a calcium ionophore. The acrosome generally is examined with electron microscopy but can also be evaluated with monoclonal antibodies to the acrosome or by utilizing triple-stain techniques.

### Additional Semen Tests

#### Leukocyte Testing

Most evidence suggests that leukocytes impair sperm function and motility. Pyospermia has been associated with abnormal results on SPA and the inability to fertilize with IVF. However, it is difficult to differentiate between leukocytes and immature germ cells on a standard semen analysis. To evaluate for pyospermia, the patient's ejaculate is mixed with peroxidase test working solution and placed into a hemocytometer, where it is examined under high magnification. Peroxidase-positive cells will stain brown; this helps differentiate between leukocytes and germ cells. Pyospermia may be indicative of an infection and should be treated with a semen culture and appropriate antibiotics. More commonly pyospermia is due to an inflammatory process causing the release of oxidants (reactive oxygen species, ROS) from the defective sperm. Use of an anti-inflammatory medication is usually curative.

#### Sperm Antibody Testing

Antisperm antibodies have been associated with lower pregnancy rates and are present in nearly 13% of males presenting to an infertility clinic.[27] Clumping of sperm, decreased sperm motility, and a poor postcoital test result may all indicate the presence of antisperm antibodies. A postcoital test will often show immotile sperm with a characteristic shaking motion. Risk factors for antisperm antibodies include vasal obstruction, genital infections, cryptorchidism, and genital trauma. The immunobead test is the most accurate assay in identifying antisperm antibodies. This assay utilizes polyarylamide beads linked to rabbit antihuman antibodies. Immunoglobulin A (IgA) or IgG antibodies can bind freely to the sperm, and a result showing that greater than 20% to 50% of sperm demonstrate immunobead binding is believed to be clinically significant.

### Hormone Assays

Indications for a hormone evaluation in a subfertile male include signs of decreased sexual function (i.e., decreased libido), low sperm density (<10 million sperm/mL), and suspected endocrinopathies (i.e., hypothyroidism). Serum FSH and testosterone levels can identify up to 99% of all endocrinopathies in men with soft testes and less than 1 million sperm/mL. Standard hormone assays undertaken in completely evaluating the infertile male also should include LH and prolactin levels. Many causes of endocrinopathies can initially be identified by these

# Reproductive Endocrinology and Infertility

| Table 54-7<br>Hormone Findings in Male Infertility | | | | |
|---|---|---|---|---|
| | **FSH** | **LH** | **Testosterone** | **Prolactin** |
| Normal spermatogenesis | Normal | Normal | Normal | Normal |
| Hyperprolactinemia | Normal/↓ | Normal/↓ | ↓ | ↑ |
| Hypogonadotropic hypogonadism | ↓ | ↓ | ↓ | Normal |
| Hypergonadotropic hypogonadism (primary testicular failure) | ↑ | ↑ | Normal/↓ | Normal |
| Impaired spermatogenesis | ↑/Normal | Normal | Normal | Normal |
| Exogenous androgens | Normal/↑ | ↓ | ↑ | Normal |

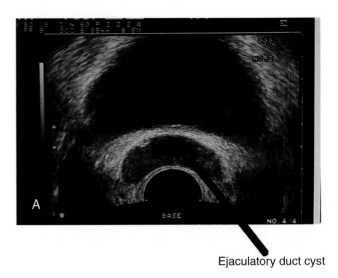

Ejaculatory duct cyst

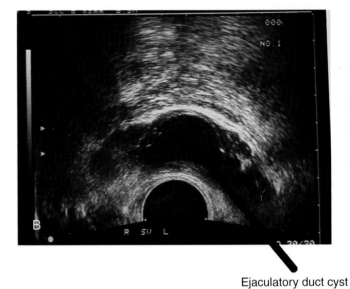

Ejaculatory duct cyst

**Figure 54-4    Ejaculatory duct cyst extending from distal (A) to proximal (B) prostatic urethra.** (Courtesy of Linda Scherefred, Sonographer, Scott Department of Urology, Baylor College of Medicine, Houston.)

four hormone assays: LH, FSH, prolactin, and testosterone (Table 54-7). Some advocate also checking estradiol levels, because elevated testosterone-to-estradiol ratios (T/E ratios) have been shown to result in decreased spermatogenesis in some infertile males.

## Radiologic Evaluation
### Ultrasound
The transrectal ultrasound (TRUS) and the scrotal ultrasound are invaluable tools in helping to diagnose the infertile male. TRUS is particularly useful when evaluating a patient with a low-volume, acidic, fructose-negative ejaculate or when there is a high suspicion for ejaculatory duct obstruction (Fig. 54-4). Seminal vesicles larger than 15 mm in thickness are suggestive of ejaculatory duct obstruction; the seminal vesicles can be aspirated at this time to confirm the diagnosis, which can be done by finding a large number of sperm (Fig. 54-5). TRUS can also be helpful in identifying a unilateral absence of the seminal vesicles, which is frequently associated with absence of the ipsilateral vas deferens and kidney (Fig. 54-6). The scrotal ultrasound is used to evaluate patients with suspected varicoceles as well as to evaluate testicular and epididymal masses. A scrotal Doppler ultrasound showing reversal of blood flow within a spermatic vein greater than 3 mm in diameter is a diagnostic indicator of a varicocele (Fig. 54-7). Finally, patients without vas deferens should have a renal ultrasound because approximately 20% of them will have renal malformations.[28]

### Vasography
Vasography is a useful tool in diagnosing patients with obstruction. It is indicated in azoospermic patients with the presence of sperm documented on testis biopsy. Vasography should be performed at the time of reconstructive surgery because of the risk of vasal injury. Vasography involves injecting contrast into the proximal vas deferens toward the ejaculatory ducts. Contrast should not be injected in the direction of the epididymis because of the risk of epididymal injury associated with this procedure. Radiographic imaging is then used to delineate the point of vasal obstruction (Fig. 54-8).

## Genetic Evaluation
Routine testing for genetic abnormalities is not generally performed. However, patients with severe oligospermia (<10 million sperm/mL) and nonobstructed azoospermia should have a karyotype and determination of Y chromosome microdeletion performed, because 12% of azoospermic and severely oligospermic males are found to have a genetic abnormality.[11] Most laboratories use polymerase chain reaction assays or gel electrophoresis to identify Y chromosome microdeletions. Patients with bilateral and unilateral absence of the vas deferens should be tested for mutations in the *CFTR* gene and for mutations in the 5T allele as well. Up to 86% of patients with CBAVD have an identifiable *CFTR* mutation. Finally, mutations in the *KAL* gene have also been frequently found in patients suspected of having Kallmann syndrome.

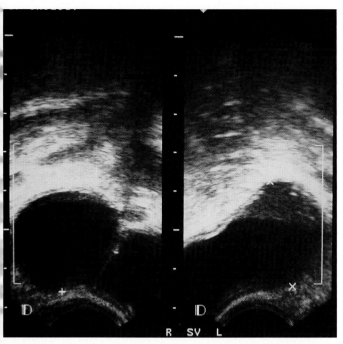

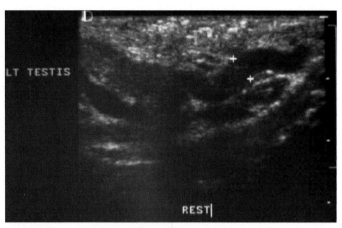

Figure 54-7 A 32-year-old male with a left-sided varicocele measuring 3.4 mm, noted between + signs. (Courtesy of Linda Scherefred, Sonographer, Scott Department of Urology, Baylor College of Medicine, Houston.)

Figure 54-5 A patient with an ejaculatory duct cyst and bilaterally dilated seminal vesicles, each measuring approximately 22 mm in diameter. (Courtesy of Linda Scherefred, Sonographer, Scott Department of Urology, Baylor College of Medicine, Houston.)

## Testicular Biopsy

A testicular biopsy is indicated in azoospermic patients to differentiate between those with obstructed and nonobstructed azoospermia. Multiple diagnostic biopsies (testicular mapping) should be performed on both testes if present. Patients with suspected nonobstructed azoospermia (small testis and FSH levels 2 times normal) who desire to proceed with ART should not have a testicular biopsy for diagnostic purposes only. These patients should undergo a therapeutic procedure (testicular

mapping or micro-testicular sperm extraction [TESE]) for sperm retrieval with subsequent IVF or ICSI.

Testicular biopsies can be performed through a percutaneous needle biopsy, fine-needle aspiration for cytology, or through an open surgical approach (Fig. 54-9). With the open surgical approach, the biopsy specimen can be sent for a frozen section or an intraoperative "touch prep" can be made. The touch preparation involves gently moving the specimen across a microscope slide with fine tissue forceps. An intraoperative evaluation can rapidly assess whether sperm are present or if another area of the testis should be biopsied.

There are six main histologic patterns seen on testicular biopsy: normal, hypospermatogenesis, Sertoli-cell-only, maturation arrest, sclerosis, and a mixed type (Fig. 54-10). Up to 40% of patient with Sertoli-cell-only histology have occasional rare foci of spermatogenesis. Other mixed histological findings

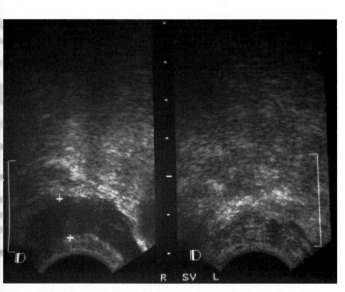

Figure 54-6 Absent left seminal vesicle in a patient also found to have an absent left kidney on abdominal ultrasound.

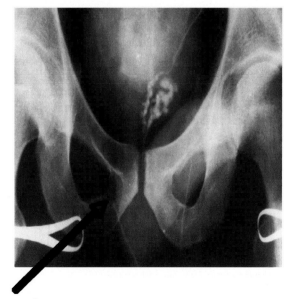

Vasal obstruction

Figure 54-8 Vasogram showing right-sided vasal obstruction.

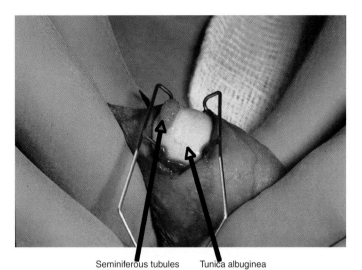

Figure 54-9    Testicular sperm extraction using the "window technique."

Seminiferous tubules    Tunica albuginea

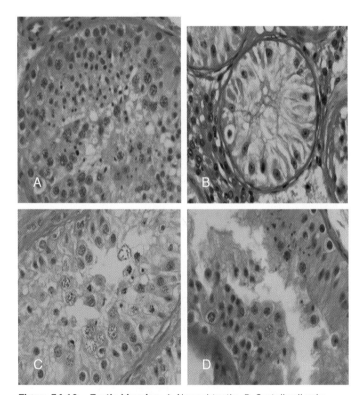

**Figure 54-10    Testis biopsies.** *A*, Normal testis. *B*, Sertoli-cell-only. *C*, Maturation arrest. *D*, Hypospermatogonia. (Courtesy of Dr. Thomas Wheeler, Department of Pathology, Baylor College of Medicine, Houston.)

can include complex pathologic patterns, with some tubules representing Sertoli-cell-only and others with maturation arrest.

# TREATMENT

## Pretesticular Causes of Infertility
### Endocrinopathies
Most endocrinopathies are treated with hormone replacement, treatment of the underlying disease, or cessation of certain

drugs or gonadotoxins. In the case of pituitary adenomas and prolactinomas, surgery may be required. Recent studies have shown that some men will present with a decreased T/E ratio. Aromatase inhibitors prevent the peripheral conversion of testosterone to estradiol and androstenedione to estrone. Treatment with aromatase inhibitors has been shown to result in significant increases in sperm concentration and motility in some of these oligospermic males.[29] Mainly for this reason, estradiol levels are now included in most infertility hormone assays.

## Testicular Causes of Infertility
### Varicoceles
Indications for varicocele repair include abnormal semen parameters in the subfertile male, persistent testicular pain, and testicular atrophy. Semen parameters most likely to improve after varicocele repair are sperm motility and sperm density. Some studies have shown improvements in sperm morphology and penetration assays as well as return of sperm to the ejaculate of previously azoospermic men.[30] Varicoceles can be repaired surgically or nonsurgically. Nonsurgical repairs consist of radiographic embolization of the spermatic veins using coils, balloons, or sclerotherapy. These percutaneous procedures have a higher recurrence rate than traditional open surgical procedures and are advocated in cases of recurrent varicoceles. Surgical repairs by most urologic reproductive surgeons involve microsurgical techniques that preserve the internal spermatic arteries and lymphatics.

Correction of varicoceles has been shown to improve not only semen motility, density, and morphology, but also serum FSH and testosterone levels.[5] A study by Marks and colleagues showed approximately 41% improvement in sperm motility and morphology and 21% improvement in sperm forward progression.[31] These investigators also found that men who had a varicocele repair had a 45% pregnancy rate in 1 year as opposed to a 26% rate in those treated empirically with clomiphene citrate for idiopathic infertility. In a randomized prospective trial of varicocelectomies, 10% of men randomized to no therapy were able to achieve spontaneous pregnancies in 1 year compared to 60% of men who underwent a varicocele repair.[32]

### Genetic Disorders
The treatment of genetic causes of infertility varies depending on the type of disorder. Most commonly, patients with genetic disorders have primary testicular failure resulting in azoospermia or severe oligospermia. In some of these patients a combination of TESE with ICSI is successful. However, the patient and his partner must be properly counseled about the risks of passing on the genetic disorder before proceeding with ART. In certain instances, such as with patients with CBAVD and cystic fibrosis, the patient's partner should also undergo genetic testing.

## Post-Testicular Causes of Infertility
### Vasal Obstruction
#### Microsurgical Reconstruction
A variety of microsurgical techniques exist to bypass obstructions of the vas deferens or the epididymis. These operations are among the most technically challenging procedures that urologists perform and should be done only by a well-trained and experienced microsurgeon. Vasovasostomy involves reanastomosis

Epididymovasostomy is an extremely challenging operation that involves performing an end-to-side anastomosis between the vas deferens and an epididymal tubule (Fig. 54-12). Because sperm maturation and motility occur in the epididymis, some believe that the anastomosis should be performed as low/distal as possible on the epididymis. Spontaneous pregnancy rates after an epididymovasostomy range from 23% to 43% for unilateral and bilateral repair, respectively.[34]

A study from Baylor has shown that the location of a vasectomy can influence the type of microsurgical reconstruction performed later during vasectomy reversal. Patients with vasectomies performed close to the testicle were twice as likely to have an epididymovasostomy as those who had a more distal occlusion site. These findings suggest that vasectomies should be performed as far away from the testicle as possible to improve the success of potential later reversal.

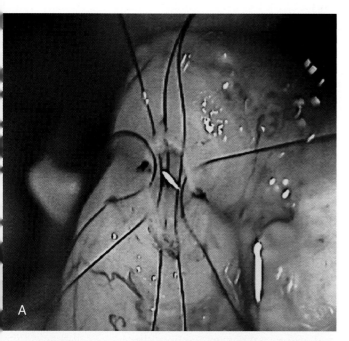

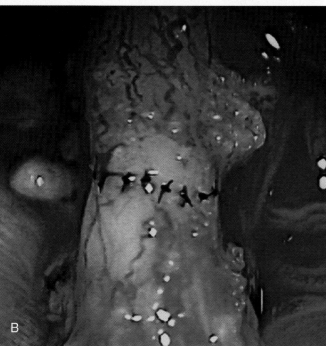

**Figure 54-11** **Vasovasostomy performed using the standard two-layer closure.** *A,* Inner layer. *B,* Outer layer.

of the vas deferens under high magnification using 9-0 and 10-0 sutures (Fig. 54-11). Most vasovasostomies are performed on patients desiring a vasectomy reversal because of a change in marital status. The success rate of a vasovasostomy depends on the experience of the surgeon and duration of obstruction. One study showed that men with vasal obstruction lasting less than 3 years had a 76% spontaneous pregnancy rate following vasectomy reversal as compared with 30% in men in whom the obstruction lasted longer than 15 years.[33]

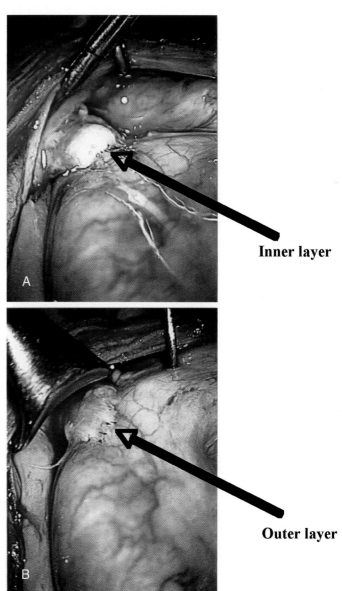

**Inner layer**

**Outer layer**

**Figure 54-12** *A and B,* **Epididymovasostomy repair in a man desiring vasectomy reversal.** This patient's contralateral side was able to be repaired through a vasovasostomy.

# Reproductive Endocrinology and Infertility

### Transurethral Resection of the Ejaculatory Duct

Patients with ejaculatory duct obstruction are treated with transurethral resection of the ejaculatory ducts (TURED). This procedure can be made easier with simultaneous TRUS or injection of colored dye into the seminal vesicles or vas deferens. In a series of 24 patients undergoing TURED, 50% had an increase in sperm density and 29% of patients were able to achieve spontaneous pregnancies.[35] Other options in treating ejaculatory duct obstruction are laser drilling and balloon dilation of the ejaculatory ducts, but these procedures are performed much less frequently.

### Epididymal Sperm Aspiration

Microsurgical epididymal sperm aspiration, or MESA, is indicated for sperm retrieval when vasal obstruction cannot be repaired following a previously failed microsurgical reconstruction and in cases of CBAVD. The procedure involves opening the epididymal tubules and aspirating spermatozoa (Fig. 54-13). Percutaneous epididymal sperm aspiration, or PESA, is a fast, inexpensive way to also obtain sperm from the epididymis. However, MESA is the preferred method for obtaining larger numbers of motile sperm for cryopreservation or ICSI. Patients must be willing to undergo IVF or ICSI after MESA or PESA.

### Testicular Sperm Extraction and Aspiration

Testicular sperm extraction is used for therapeutic sperm retrieval. TESE involves open excisional biopsies of the testis and is often used in conjunction with ICSI. The specimen is examined under a microscope; this procedure can be done either in the operating room or the office to make a rapid assessment of the presence of sperm. If no sperm are present, another area of the testis can be biopsied at that time. Su and colleagues demonstrated that nearly 60% of men with nonobstructed azoospermia will have some sperm found in their testicular biopsy.[36] They also showed that when TESE was combined with ICSI they were able to achieve a 55% clinical pregnancy rate.

Another alternative to TESE is testicular sperm aspiration, or TESA. TESA involves percutaneous aspiration of sperm by inserting a needle directly into the testicular parenchyma. Although TESA is faster and less expensive than TESE, it offers

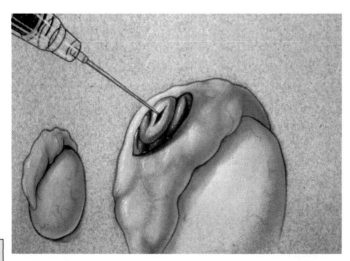

**Figure 54-13    Microscopic epididymal sperm aspiration (MESA).**

significantly less sperm than TESE. TESA has also been associated with a higher rate of hematoma formation due to the blind passage of the aspiration needle.

### *Ejaculatory Disorders*

Patients with retrograde ejaculation can be treated with medications or retrieval of their sperm from their postejaculate urine. Sympathomimetics, such as imipramine and pseudoephedrine, are known to close the bladder neck and enhance emission. If these medications fail, sperm can be retrieved from an alkalinized postejaculate urine and used for intrauterine insemination (IUI) or IVF cycles. Postejaculate urine examination should also be performed on males with an ejaculatory volume of less than 1 mL.

Patients with anejaculation can benefit from electroejaculation or vibratory stimulation. Electroejaculation involves inserting a rectal probe and stimulating the sympathetic nerves with an electrical current. Vibratory stimulation involves placing a vibrator on the frenulum of the glans penis. For vibratory stimulation to induce ejaculation, the ejaculatory reflex arc in the thoracolumbar spinal cord must be intact. Therefore, spinal cord–injured patients with lesions above T10 will benefit from vibratory stimulation while those with lesions below T10 will need electroejaculation.[37]

## Idiopathic Infertility

Empiric treatment of idiopathic infertility initially centers around pharmacologic therapy. Clomiphene citrate (Clomid), an estrogen antagonist, is one of the most widely used drugs in treating idiopathic oligospermia. The estrogen antagonist interferes with the negative feedback of estrogen, which causes an increase in gonadotropin secretion. Although some studies have shown improvements in semen parameters after clomiphene citrate treatment, most randomized controlled trials have shown no improved benefit in taking this drug. Exogenous GnRH has also been tried with disappointing results. The medication has to be administered every 2 hours to simulate pulsatile release. High costs and poor efficacy have led many clinicians to abandon this therapy. Finally, mesterlone, a synthetic androgen widely used in Europe, has been used to treat idiopathic male infertility. However, double-blinded controlled trials have failed to show any significant benefit of the drug over placebo.

## Treatment Algorithms

Many treatment algorithms have been designed to help the clinician in evaluating and treating the subfertile male. However, the most common algorithms used are the ones to evaluate and treat low volume (<1.5 mL) and normal volume (>1.5 mL) azoospermia. The initial evaluation of the azoospermic male involves repeating the semen analysis with centrifugation of the specimen. The pellet is then examined under a microscope and if sperm are present, an oligospermia workup is initiated. If sperm are absent and the vas deferens are palpable, the patient is further evaluated for either low-volume or normal-volume azoospermia. If the vas deferens are not palpable and the patient has testes of normal size and normal FSH levels, epididymal aspiration with ART can be performed. However, these patients will need to be tested for *CFTR* gene and 5T allele mutations before proceeding with ART.

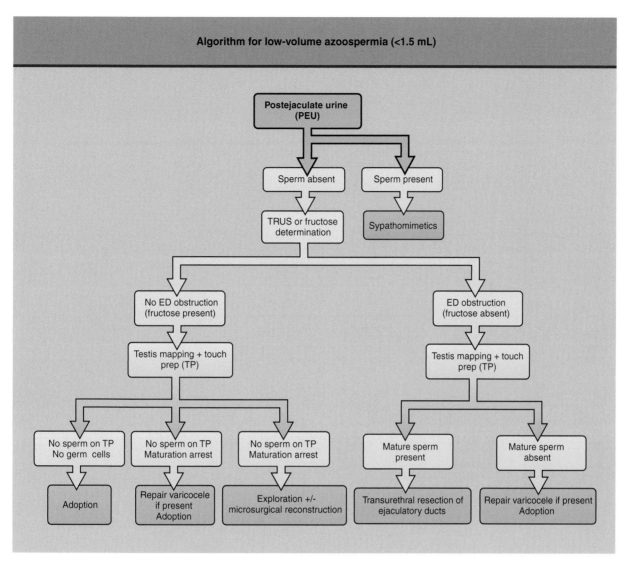

**Figure 54-14** Algorithm for low-volume azoospermia (<1.5 mL).

The low-volume azoospermic evaluation involves first checking the patient's postejaculate urine (Fig. 54-14). If spermatozoa are absent, the presence of seminal fructose is assessed or a TRUS is performed to determine the presence of ejaculatory duct obstruction. If no obstruction is found, testicular mapping is performed and further treatment is based on these biopsy results.

When patients have normal-volume azoospermia or abnormal hormone levels, further evaluation by the hormone assay findings is dictated (Fig. 54-15). If the patient is found to have an elevated prolactin level, an MRI or computed tomographic scan of the hypothalamus and pituitary is performed and a tumor evaluation is initiated. If prolactin levels as well as LH and FSH levels are low, an endocrine cause for hypogonadotropic hypogonadism (see Fig. 54-1) is investigated and the patient generally is treated with hormone therapy. When FSH and LH levels are normal or elevated and testosterone levels are normal or decreased, patients will undergo a testicular biopsy and further definitive treatment will be based on these results. Similarly, a normal-volume azoospermic male with normal FSH, LH, and

testosterone levels will also be initially evaluated with a biopsy and touch preparation. On the basis of these results, further treatment options can be decided (see Fig. 54-15).

### Assisted Reproductive Technologies
With the advancement of ART, many more reproductive options are now available for the subfertile male. Procedures such as IVF and ICSI have revolutionized the field of male infertility and now offer hope to men who could not have conceived just over 10 years ago. A full description of ART is covered in Chapter 52.

## SUMMARY

Treatment and understanding of male infertility is a rapidly evolving field, with new technologies and procedures constantly being developed. Yet, 25% of males still present with idiopathic infertility. The etiology for male infertility is vast, and the clinician must learn to take a detailed history and perform a thorough physical examination. In addition, the clinician should be familiar with the appropriate radiologic and laboratory tests

# Reproductive Endocrinology and Infertility

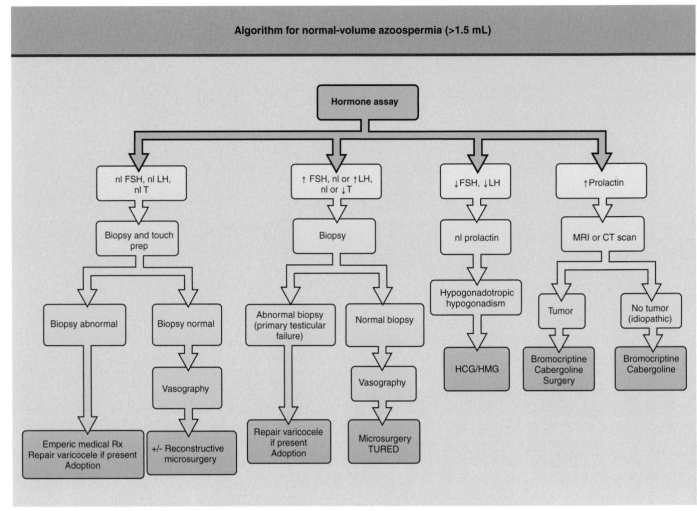

**Figure 54-15    Algorithm for normal-volume azoospermia (>1.5 mL).**

needed to make an accurate diagnosis. Surgical treatment of male infertility, especially when it involves microsurgery, should only be performed by highly skilled, experienced surgeons to offer the best outcome to these patients. In half of all infertile couples, male infertility will be a component. Only after the male partner has been completely evaluated can these couples be offered the most cost-effective and productive treatment options.

## REFERENCES

1. Yu RN, Ito M, Saunders TL, et al: Role of AHCH in gonadal development and gametogenesis. Nat Genet 1998;20:353–357. **(IIa, B)**
2. Katz MD, Kligman I, Cai LQ, et al: Paternity by intrauterine insemination with sperm from a man with 5α-reductase-2 deficiency. N Engl J Med 1997;336:994–997. **(III, B)**
3. Witt MA, Lipshultz LI: Varicocele: a progressive or static lesion? Urology 1993;42:541–543. **(IIa, B)**
4. Greenberg SH, Lipshultz LI, Wein AJ: Experience with 425 subfertile male patients. J Urol 1978;119:507–510. **(IIb, B)**
5. Cayan S, Kadioglu A, Orhan I, et al: The effect of microsurgical varicocelectomy on serum follicle stimulating hormone, testosterone and free testosterone levels in infertile men with varicocele. BJU Int 1999;84:1046–1049. **(IIb, B)**
6. Job JC, Toublanc JE, Chaussain JL, et al: The pituitary-gonadal axis in cryptorchid infants and children. Eur J Pediatr 1987;146(Suppl 2): S2–S5. **(IIa, B)**
7. Rogers E, Teahan S, Gallagher H, et al: The role of orchiectomy in the management of postpubertal cryptorchidism. J Urol 1998;159:851–854. **(IIb, B)**
8. Chilvers C, Dudley NE, Gough MH, et al: Undescended testis: the effect of treatment on subsequent risk of subfertility and malignancy. J Pediatr Surg 1986;21:691–696. **(III, B)**
9. Lipshultz LI: Cryptorchidism in the subfertile male. Fertil Steril 1976;27:609–620. **(IIb, B)**
10. Kumar D, Bremner DN, Brown PW: Fertility after orchiopexy for cryptorchidism: a new approach to assessment. Br J Urol 1989; 64:516–520. **(IIb, B)**
11. De Braekeleer M, Dao TN: Cytogenetic studies in male infertility: a review. Hum Reprod 1991;6:245–250. **(III, B)**
12. Nielsen J, Wohlert M: Chromosome abnormalities found among 34,910 newborn children: results from a 13-year incidence study in Arhus, Denmark. Hum Genet 1991;87:81–83. **(IIa, B)**
13. Pryor JL, Kent-First M, Muallem A, et al: Microdeletions in the Y chromosome of infertile men. N Engl J Med 1997;336:534–539. **(IIa, B)**
14. Cayan S, Conaghan J, Schriock ED, et al: Birth after intracytoplasmic sperm injection with use of testicular sperm from men with Kartagener/immotile cilia syndrome. Fertil Steril 2001;76:612–614. **(III, B)**
15. Jarow JP, Espeland MA, Lipshultz LI: Evaluation of the azoospermic patient. J Urol 1989;142:62–65. **(IIb, B)**

16. Riehmann M, Knes JM, Heisey D, et al: Transurethral resection versus incision of the prostate: a randomized, prospective study. Urology 1995;45:768–775. **(Ib, A)**

17. Feldman HA, Goldstein I, Hatzichristou DG, et al: Impotence and its medical and psychosocial correlates: results of the Massachusetts Male Aging Study. J Urol 1994;151:54–61. **(III, B)**

18. Goldenberg RL, White R: The effect of vaginal lubricants on sperm motility in vitro. Fertil Steril 1975;26:872–873. **(IIb, B)**

19. Anderson JB, Williamson RC: Fertility after torsion of the spermatic cord. Br J Urol 1990;65:225–230. **(III, B)**

20. Werner C: Mumps orchitis and testicular atrophy. Ann Intern Med 1950;32:1066. **(IIb, B)**

21. Heller CH, Clermont Y: Kinetics of the germinal epithelium in man. Recent Prog Horm Res 1964;20:545–575. **(IIb, B)**

22. Lipshultz LI, Corriere JN II: Progressive testicular atrophy in the varicocele patient. J Urol 1977;117:175–176. **(IIa, B)**

23. World Health Organization: WHO Laboratory Manual for the Examination of Human Semen and Sperm–Cervical Mucus Interaction, 4th ed. Cambridge, UK: Cambridge University Press, 1999. **(IV, C)**

24. Kruger TF, Acosta AA, Simmons KF, et al: Predictive value of abnormal sperm morphology in in vitro fertilization. Fertil Steril 1988;49:112–117. **(IIa, B)**

25. Smith RG, Johnson A, Lamb D, et al: Functional tests of spermatozoa. Sperm penetration assay. Urol Clin North Am 1987;14:451–458. **(IIa, B)**

26. Pampiglione JS, Tan SL, Campbell S: The use of the stimulated acrosome reaction test as a test of fertilizing ability in human spermatozoa. Fertil Steril 1993;59:1280–1284. **(IIa, B)**

27. Sinisi AA, Di Finizio B, Pasquali D, et al: Prevalence of antisperm antibodies by SpermMARtest in subjects undergoing a routine sperm analysis for infertility. Int J Androl 1993;16:311–314. **(IIb, B)**

28. Augarten A, Yahav Y, Kerem BS, et al: Congenital bilateral absence of vas deferens in the absence of cystic fibrosis. Lancet 1994;344:1473–1474. **(IIb, B)**

29. Pavlovich CP, King P, Goldstein M, et al: Evidence of a treatable endocrinopathy in infertile men. J Urol 2001;165:837–841. **(IIa, B)**

30. Kim ED, Leibman BB, Grinblat DM, et al: Varicocele repair improves semen parameters in azoospermic men with spermatogenic failure. J Urol 1999;162:737–740. **(IIb, B)**

31. Marks JL, McMahon R, Lipshultz LI: Predictive parameters of successful varicocele repair. J Urol 1986;136:609–612. **(IIa, B)**

32. Madgar I, Weissenberg R, Lunenfeld B, et al: Controlled trial of high spermatic vein ligation for varicocele in infertile men. Fertil Steril 1995;63:120–124. **(Ib, A)**

33. Belker AM, Thomas AJ II, Fuchs EF, et al: Results of 1,469 microsurgical vasectomy reversals by the Vasovasostomy Study Group. J Urol 1991;145:505–511. **(IIb, B)**

34. Kim ED, Winkel E, Orejuela F, et al: Pathological epididymal obstruction unrelated to vasectomy: results with microsurgical reconstruction. J Urol 1998;160:2078–2080. **(IIb, B)**

35. Meacham RB, Hellerstein DK, Lipshultz LI: Evaluation and treatment of ejaculatory duct obstruction in the infertile male. Fertil Steril 1993;59:393–397. **(IIb, B)**

36. Su LM, Palermo GD, Goldstein M, et al: Testicular sperm extraction with intracytoplasmic sperm injection for nonobstructive azoospermia: testicular histology can predict success of sperm retrieval. J Urol 1999;161:112–118. **(IIb, B)**

37. Sonksen J, Ohl DA: Penile vibratory stimulation and electroejaculation in the treatment of ejaculatory dysfunction. Int J Androl 2002;25:324–332. **(III, B)**

## KEY POINTS

- A complete evaluation for recurrent pregnancy loss will reveal a possible cause in 70% of cases.
- A complete evaluation (genetic, endocrinologic, anatomic, immunologic, microbiologic, and thrombophilic) should be initiated when the decision to evaluate a couple is made.
- Couples with primary recurrent pregnancy loss have identifiable causes just as frequently as couples with secondary recurrent pregnancy loss; therefore, both types of couples should be evaluated.
- Women with two losses have identifiable problems just as frequently as women with three or more losses; thus, an evaluation for causes can be initiated after two losses.
- If no cause is identified after a complete evaluation, 65% of couples will have a successful subsequent pregnancy.

## EPIDEMOLOGY, RISK FACTORS, AND PATHOGENESIS

Recurrent pregnancy loss is a devastating problem to couples seeking parenthood and a difficult challenge to their physician. Whereas spontaneous abortion occurs in approximately 15% of clinically diagnosed pregnancies, recurrent pregnancy loss occurs in about 1% to 2% of this same population.[1] Great strides have been made in characterizing the incidence and diversity of this heterogeneous disorder, and a definite cause of pregnancy loss can be established in approximately two thirds of couples after a thorough evaluation.[2] A complete evaluation will include investigations into genetic, endocrinologic, anatomic, immunologic, microbiologic, thrombophilic, and iatrogenic causes. In cases of idiopathic recurrent miscarriage, intense supportive care is indicated and successful outcomes will occur in more than two thirds of all couples.[3]

### Definition of Recurrent Pregnancy Loss

The traditional definition of recurrent pregnancy loss included those couples with three or more consecutive spontaneous miscarriages. However, several studies have indicated that the causes of miscarriage that can be identified after two consecutive pregnancy losses are similar to the causes that can be identified after three consecutive pregnancy losses. Thus, it has been recommended that couples with two or more consecutive spontaneous miscarriages warrant an evaluation to identify any factor that may be associated with their poor reproductive history.[4,5] Miscarriages are considered to be any loss before 20 gestational weeks and can be further divided into embryonic, defined as a pregnancy that fails before 10 weeks' gestation, and fetal, defined as a pregnancy that fails at or after 10 weeks' gestation. Those couples with primary recurrent miscarriage have never had an ongoing pregnancy beyond 20 weeks' gestation, and those with secondary recurrent miscarriage have previously had a pregnancy that progressed beyond 20 weeks' gestation followed by three or more consecutive spontaneous miscarriages.

### Recurrence Risk

The risk of recurrence depends on several factors, including maternal age, the number of previous miscarriages, and the history of previous term deliveries. Studies that evaluated the frequency of pregnancy loss, based on highly sensitive tests for quantitative human chorionic gonadotropin, indicated that the risk of miscarriage, both clinical and preclinical, in women age 20 to 30 is approximately 25%. The risk of miscarriage in women age 40 or older is at least double that figure.[6,7] Similarly, a greater number of prior miscarriages are associated with a higher risk of subsequent miscarriage in most studies. A patient with two prior losses has a recurrence risk of at least 25%; after four losses, that figure is at least doubled. Most studies have indicated a more favorable prognosis in women with secondary recurrent pregnancy loss.

### Etiology of Miscarriage

Numeric chromosomal abnormalities as a cause of miscarriage have been studied extensively. Based on seven studies, in which 7182 miscarriages were successfully cytogenetically analyzed, it is estimated that nearly 50% of miscarriages in the general population are due to numeric chromosomal abnormalities.[8] Approximately 56% of such abnormalities are trisomies, 20% are polyploidies, 18% are monosomy X, and 6% are other genetic defects. Approximately one third of all trisomies are trisomy 16. All pregnancies with trisomy 16 end in first-trimester miscarriage. Only pregnancies with trisomy 21, 18, and 13 have been reported to survive to birth, although the probability of this is 22%, 5%, and 38%, respectively. Sex chromosome trisomies, including XXY, XXX, and XYY, have a higher likelihood of survival, estimated at 55%, 70%, and 100%, respectively.

The gestational age of demise does have some bearing on the frequency and specificity of chromosomal abnormalities. Approximately 70% of preclinical miscarriages (<6 weeks' gestation) have a numeric chromosomal abnormality.[9] Approximately 46% of clinically recognized miscarriages have a numeric chromosomal abnormality, whereas only 5% of stillbirths are abnormal.[8,10] Advancing maternal age highly impacts the likelihood of preclinical and clinical miscarriage because of an increased likelihood of errors in maternal meiosis, resulting in trisomic pregnancies.

A numeric chromosomal abnormality in a previous miscarriage does not increase the risk in a subsequent pregnancy. Therefore, such abnormalities are random occurrences, although advancing maternal age is a confounder.

Cytogenetic analysis is an important test to perform in a couple with a history of miscarriage. Conventional chromosome banding does have its limitations, including a failure rate of 10% to 40% because of tissue culture failure and/or maternal contamination. Comparative genomic hybridization supplemented with flow cytometry appears to be a promising alternative for cytogenetic analysis. This technique is more accurate, is less labor intensive, has a lower failure rate because tissue culturing is not required, and has less risk of maternal contamination.

## DIAGNOSIS AND TREATMENT OF RECURRENT PREGNANCY LOSS

In addition to random miscarriage, noncytogenetic factors may be associated with a history of recurrent pregnancy loss. These factors may increase the recurrence risk of miscarriage; therefore, evaluation of couples with recurrent pregnancy loss is warranted. Management based on sound scientific evidence is paramount, with randomized, controlled trials being the gold standard for determining effectiveness of treatment.

### Structural Genetic Factors

A structural genetic factor is found in either partner in 3% to 5% of couples with recurrent pregnancy loss. The most common structural factor is a balanced reciprocal translocation. In recurrent pregnancy loss, this abnormality is found more frequently in the female partner, at a ratio from 2:1 to 3:1 (female:male). Other structural genetic factors occur less frequently, such as a robertsonian translocation, an inversion, or a supernumerary chromosome. Genetic counseling is key because the impact of such structural genetic factors depends on the chromosomes involved. Prenatal diagnosis by amniocentesis or chorionic villus sampling can identify whether an ongoing pregnancy is affected. Donor gametes or preimplantation genetic diagnosis may be considered, but cytogenetic documentation of miscarriages should be confirmed before proceeding with such advanced reproductive technology.

### Endocrinologic Factors
#### Luteal Phase Deficiency
Progesterone produced from the corpus luteum is necessary for successful implantation and maintenance of early pregnancy until progesterone production by the placenta takes over. Luteal phase deficiency has been described as a cause of recurrent pregnancy loss. Classically, the definition of a luteal phase deficiency was based on two mid- to late luteal phase endometrial biopsies, which revealed two or more days of histologic delay. More recently, a midluteal progesterone level of less than 10 ng/mL has been suggested to be diagnostic. Women with out-of-phase endometrial biopsies are unable to maintain endo-

metrial progesterone receptors and have abnormal expression of the $\alpha_V\beta_3$ integrin, a biomarker of uterine receptivity.[11] The $\alpha_V\beta_3$ integrin normally appears in the endometrium glands on cycle days 20 to 21, during the "window of implantation." The majority of these patients, when treated with supplemental progesterone or low-dose clomiphene citrate, will have restoration of normal histologic endometrium and normal $\alpha_V\beta_3$ expression. Late implantation of the embryo has also been associated with an increased miscarriage rate.[12]

### Untreated Hypothyroidism
Untreated hypothyroidism may increase the risk of miscarriage. A recent study of more than 700 patients with recurrent pregnancy loss identified hypothyroidism in 7.6%.[13] Hypothyroidism is easily diagnosed with a sensitive thyrotropin stimulation test; patients should be treated to become euthyroid before attempting a pregnancy.

### Insulin Resistance
Patients with poorly controlled diabetes are known to have an increased risk of spontaneous miscarriage. This risk can be reduced to normal if the patient is treated appropriately and becomes euglycemic preconceptually.[6] It is known that women with polycystic ovary syndrome (PCOS) have an increased risk of miscarriage. The high prevalence of insulin resistance in women with PCOS may account for the increased risk of miscarriage in this group.[14] Testing for fasting insulin and glucose is simple, and treatment with insulin-sensitizing agents can reduce the risk of recurrent miscarriage.[15]

### Elevated Day 3 Follicle-Stimulating Hormone Levels
Elevated day 3 follicle-stimulating hormone (FSH) levels (>12 mIU/mL) have been associated with decreased pregnancy rates in women undergoing in vitro fertilization. Although the frequency of elevated day 3 FSH levels in women with recurrent miscarriage is similar to the frequency in the infertile population, the prognosis for a successful pregnancy outcome in women with recurrent miscarriage and an elevated day 3 FSH is decreased.[16] Some clinicians recommend that testing should be performed in women over age 35 with recurrent pregnancy loss, and that these women may produce embryos with a high rate of aneuploidy.[17] One study identified a higher rate of aneuploidy in women with recurrent miscarriage compared to women undergoing similar analysis for sex-linked disorders (70.7% vs. 45.1%) using preimplantation genetic diagnosis at the time of in vitro fertilization. Women with recurrent miscarriage and elevated day 3 FSH levels should have appropriate counseling.

### Anatomic Factors
#### Congenital Uterine Anomalies
Congenital uterine anomalies associated with müllerian fusion defects have been associated with an increased risk of pregnancy loss.[18] The most common abnormality associated with pregnancy loss is the septate uterus. Uncontrolled studies suggest that resection of the uterine septum results in higher delivery rates than in women without treatment. Other congenital abnormalities, such as bicornuate and unicornuate uterus, are more frequently associated with later trimester losses or preterm delivery, rather than recurrent miscarriage.

## Acquired Uterine Abnormalities

Intrauterine adhesions or synechiae (Asherman's syndrome) have been associated with recurrent miscarriage. Intrauterine synechiae are most commonly secondary to uterine curettage at the time of abortion or a postpartum curettage. The adhesions are thought to interfere with normal placentation. They can be excised hysteroscopically. Intrauterine cavity abnormalities, such as leiomyomas and polyps, can contribute to pregnancy loss by interfering with implantation. Until recently, it was felt that only submucous leiomyomas should be surgically removed before subsequent attempts at pregnancy. However, several studies investigating the implantation rate in women undergoing in vitro fertilization have clearly demonstrated decreased implantation with intramural myomas in the range of 30 mm.[19] When smaller myomas are identified, it is unclear if myomectomy is beneficial in patients undergoing in vitro fertilization.[20]

## Immunologic Factors
### Autoimmune Factors
#### Antiphospholipid Antibodies

Autoantibodies to phospholipids, thyroid antigens, nuclear antigens, and other substances have been investigated as possible causes for pregnancy loss.[13] Antiphospholipid antibodies include both the lupus anticoagulant and anticardiolipin antibodies. The occurrence of recurrent pregnancy loss, fetal death, and/or thrombosis in conjunction with antiphospholipid antibodies is termed the *antiphospholipid antibody syndrome*[21] (Table 55-1). Controversy still exists concerning testing for other phospholipids, but an increasing number of studies suggest that antibodies to phosphatidyl serine are also associated with pregnancy loss.[22] In the past, treatment with low-dose steroids was advocated; however, subsequent studies indicate that this treatment significantly increases maternal and fetal complications without enhancing live birth rate.[23,24] Independent, prospective investigations have indicated the efficacy of subcutaneous heparin and low-dose (81 mg/day) aspirin for the treatment of antiphospholipid antibody syndrome.[25–27]

#### Antithyroid Antibodies

Antithyroid antibodies (antithyroid peroxidase, antithyroglobulin) have been reported in increased frequency in women with recurrent pregnancy loss. However, if the patient is euthyroid, the presence of antithyroid antibodies does not affect pregnancy outcome.[28] Women who have positive antithyroid antibodies and are euthyroid are at an increased risk for hypothyroidism during and after pregnancy. These women should have their thyrotropin levels tested during each trimester and postpartum for thyroiditis.[29]

#### Antinuclear Antibodies

Approximately 10% to 15% of all women will have detectable antinuclear antibodies regardless of their history of pregnancy loss. Their chance of successful pregnancy outcome is not dependent on the presence or absence of antinuclear antibodies. Treatments such as steroids have been shown to increase the maternal and fetal complications without benefiting live births[24]; thus, routine testing and treatment for antinuclear antibodies is not indicated.

### Alloimmune Factors
#### Human Leukocyte Antigens, Embryotoxic Factors, and Immunophenotypes

Alloimmune factors have been suggested to be associated with recurrent pregnancy loss. Previously, sharing of human leukocyte antigen (HLA) between partners was thought to be associated with recurrent pregnancy loss, based on a decreased maternal immune response to paternal HLA antigens and, thus, decreased production of blocking antibodies. Recent large studies, however, reveal no association between HLA (and HLA-DQα), homozygosity, and recurrent pregnancy loss.[30] Other investigators have implicated certain embryotoxic factors, such as tumor necrosis factor-α and interferon-δ, identified in the supernatants of peripheral blood lymphocytes from women with pregnancy loss; however, this has not been confirmed by independent studies. Immunophenotypes of endometrial cells from women with recurrent pregnancy loss demonstrate altered natural killer cell (CD56+) populations. Some have suggested that increased natural killer cells are associated with pregnancy loss; others have indicated that decreased natural killer cells are associated with pregnancy loss. None of these factors have been clearly associated with pregnancy loss; thus, there are no recommended tests or treatments at this time.[31]

Despite the lack of diagnostic tests to identify an alloimmune factor association with a history of recurrent pregnancy loss, there is abundant evidence that there are immunologic interactions between the mother and her allogeneic pregnancy.[32–34] On the basis of this evidence, active and passive immunotherapies have been offered to many couples with otherwise unexplained recurrent pregnancy loss.

#### Active and Passive Immunotherapy

Active immunotherapy, in the form of either paternal or third-party mononuclear cell immunization, has been extensively evaluated since the initial controlled trial published in 1985.[35] Subsequent trials, all with small numbers of patients enrolled, had inconsistent results.[36,37] In 1999, a multicenter, randomized, double-blind, placebo-controlled trial supported by the National

**Table 55-1**
**Clinical and Laboratory Characteristics of Antiphospholipid Antibody Syndrome**

| Clinical | Laboratory |
|---|---|
| **Pregnancy morbidity** | |
| ≥1 unexplained death at ≥10 weeks | IgG aCL (≥20 GPL) |
| Delivery at ≤34 weeks with severe PIH | IgM aCL (≥20 MPL) |
| 3 or more losses before 10 weeks | Positive lupus anticoagulant test |
| **Thrombosis** | |
| Venous | |
| Arterial, including stroke | |

GPL, IgG phospholipid units; MPL, IgM phospholipid units; PIH, pregnancy-induced hypertension.
Patients should have at least one clinical and one laboratory feature at some time in the course of their disease. Laboratory tests should be positive on at least two occasions more than 6 weeks apart.
Modified from Wilson WA, Ghavari AK, Piette JC: International classification criteria for antiphospholipid syndrome: synopsis of a post-conference workshop held at the Ninth International (Tours) APL Symposium. Lupus 2001;10:457–460.

Institutes of Health showed that paternal mononuclear cell immunization did not improve pregnancy outcome in couples with unexplained recurrent pregnancy loss.[30]

The first randomized, controlled trial assessing the efficacy of passive immunotherapy using intravenous immunoglobulin for treatment of unexplained recurrent miscarriage was published in 1994.[38] Three subsequent trials showed encouraging results for couples with unexplained secondary recurrent pregnancy loss.[39-41] A multicenter, randomized, controlled trial is currently in progress.

### Microbiologic Factors

Certain infectious agents have been identified more frequently in cultures from women who have had sporadic miscarriages.[42] These include *Ureaplasma urealyticum, Mycoplasma hominis, Chlamydia,* and other less common pathogens. Although no studies have associated any infectious agent with recurrent pregnancy loss, it is unlikely that many clinicians would leave a patient untreated to determine this association. Because of the clear association with sporadic pregnancy losses and the ease of diagnosis, women with recurrent pregnancy loss should be cultured for these organisms and both partners should be treated if positive.

### Thrombophilic Factors

Attention has been focused on certain inherited disorders that may predispose to arterial and/or venous thrombosis and their possible association with pregnancy complications.[43,44] These include the group of mutations leading to a hypercoagulable state, such as factor V Leiden (G1691A), factor II–prothrombin mutation (G20210A), and hyperhomocysteinemia (thermolabile MTHFR C677T). Other possible abnormalities leading to hypercoagulable states that may be associated with recurrent miscarriage include the antithrombin III deficiency, protein C deficiency, protein S deficiency, and elevated factor VIII (Table 55-2).

Although such inherited thrombophilias are established causes of thrombosis, they have only recently been associated with adverse pregnancy outcomes, including fetal demise. Subanalysis of individual inherited thrombophilias has confirmed an association with recurrent pregnancy loss and factor V Leiden.[45] Other associations have been suggested between many inherited thrombophilias and adverse pregnancy outcomes, including but not limited to recurrent pregnancy loss, fetal demise, fetal growth restriction, gestational hypertension, and abruption. Subanalysis of individual inherited thrombophilias and an individual adverse pregnancy outcome suggests but has not confirmed such associations.

It seems clear that some of these inherited thrombophilias are found more commonly in women with recurrent early pregnancy losses.[43,46] Although outcome studies of patients with recurrent pregnancy loss and a positive test for an inherited thrombophilia are limited and conflicting, a case-control study suggests that the presence of factor V Leiden is significantly associated with a lower live birth rate.[45] Hyperhomocysteinemia has been reported in early pregnancy losses and is treated with 1 to 2 mg/day of folic acid supplementation.[47]

Currently prophylactic or therapeutic heparin has been advocated by some researchers when an inherited thrombophilia is found in association with unexplained recurrent pregnancy loss,[44] although there have been no prospective controlled studies. Ideally, randomized, controlled trials will be performed to determine whether thromboprophylaxis improves the live birth rate in such patients.

### Lifestyle Issues

Tobacco use of more than 15 cigarettes a day has been associated with a 1.5-fold to 2-fold increased risk of pregnancy loss; alcohol consumption of greater than five drinks per week is associated with a similar increased risk.[48] When both personal habits are present in the same individual, the risk of pregnancy loss may increase fourfold. Couples should be counseled appropriately and be strongly encouraged to discontinue such use before attempting another pregnancy.

## CLINICAL COURSE AND PROGRESSION

### Course of Evaluation

When the clinician makes the decision to initiate an evaluation for recurrent pregnancy loss, it is recommended that complete diagnostic testing be performed. This obviously includes a detailed history, including documentation of prior pregnancies, any pathologic tests that were performed on prior miscarriages, any evidence of chronic or acute infections or diseases, any

---

**Table 55-2**
**Common Thrombophilias Possibly Associated with Recurrent Pregnancy Loss**

| Thrombophilia | Inheritance | Prevalence* | Risk of DVT |
|---|---|---|---|
| Factor V Leiden G1691A mutation (activated protein C resistance) | Autosomal dominant | 2%–15% | 3–8x |
| Factor II G20210A mutation (prothrombin mutation) | Autosomal dominant | 2%–3% | 3x |
| MTHFR C677T mutation (hyperhomocysteinemia) | Autosomal recessive | 11% | 2.5–4x |
| Antithrombin deficiency | Autosomal dominant | 0.02% | 25–50x |
| Protein C deficiency | Autosomal dominant | 0.2%–0.3% | 10–15x |
| Protein S deficiency | Autosomal dominant | 0.1%–0.2% | 2x |
| Elevated factor VIII | X-linked | 5%–15% | 5x |

DVT, deep vein thrombosis.

*Prevalence is in the general population; however, significant ethnic differences are known. Risk of DVT in the nonpregnant individual with the listed thrombophilia compared with a nonpregnant individual without the thrombophilia.

**Table 55-3**
**Standard Evaluation and Management of Recurrent Pregnancy Loss**

| Etiology | Diagnostic Evaluation | Abnormal Result | Therapy |
|---|---|---|---|
| Structural genetic | Cytogenetic analysis of both partners | 3%–5% | Genetic counseling, donor gametes |
| Anatomic | Hysterosalpingogram, hysteroscopy, or sonohysterography (saline-infused sonogram) | 15%–20% | Hysteroscopic septum resection, myomectomy, lysis of adhesions |
| Endocrinologic | Midluteal progesterone<br>Thyrotropin<br>Prolactin<br>Fasting insulin:glucose<br>Day 3 FSH, estradiol | 8%–12% | Progesterone<br>Levothyroxine<br>Bromocriptine, cabergoline<br>Metformin<br>Counseling |
| Immunologic | Lupus anticoagulant<br>Anticardiolipin antibodies<br>?Embryotoxicity assay<br>?Immunophenotyping | 15%–20% | Aspirin<br>Heparin + aspirin<br>?Intravenous immunoglobulin |
| Microbiologic | Cervical cultures | 5%–10% | Antibiotics |
| Thrombophilic | ?Antithrombin III<br>?Protein C, Protein S<br>Factor V Leiden mutation<br>?Factor II (prothrombin) mutation<br>Hyperhomocysteinemia | 8%–12% | <br><br>Heparin<br><br>Folic acid |
| Psychological | Interview<br>Questionnaire | Varies | Support groups<br>Counseling |
| Iatrogenic | Tobacco, alcohol use<br>Exposure to toxins, chemicals | 5% | Eliminate consumption<br>Eliminate exposure |

recent physical or emotional trauma, a history of cramping or bleeding with a previous miscarriage, any family history of pregnancy loss, and any previous gynecologic surgery or complicating factor. A summary of the diagnosis and management of recurrent pregnancy loss includes an investigation of genetic, endocrinologic, anatomic, immunologic, microbiologic, iatrogenic, and thrombophilic causes (Table 55-3).

### Outcome of Evaluation
In approximately 70% of all cases of recurrent pregnancy loss, a complete evaluation will reveal a possible etiology.[2] If no cause can be found, the majority of couples will eventually have a successful pregnancy outcome with supportive therapy alone.[3] Couples who have experienced recurrent pregnancy loss want to know what caused the miscarriage. Unexplained reproductive failure can lead to anger, guilt, and depression. Anger may be directed toward their physician for not being able to solve their reproductive problems. Feelings of grief and guilt following an early loss are often as intense as those following a stillbirth, and parents experience a grief reaction similar to that associated with the death of an adult. The couple should be assured that exercise, intercourse, and dietary indiscretions do not cause miscarriage. Any questions or concerns that the couple may have about personal habits should be discussed.

Women who suffer recurrent pregnancy loss have already begun to prepare for their baby, both emotionally and physically, as compared to couples with infertility who have never conceived. When a miscarriage occurs, a couple may have great difficulty informing friends or family about the loss. Feelings of

hopelessness may continue long after the loss. Patients may continue to grieve and have episodes of depression on the expected due date or the date of the pregnancy loss. Participation in support groups or referral for grief counseling may be beneficial in many cases.[49]

## REFERENCES

1. Kutteh WH: Recurrent pregnancy loss. In Rebar RW (ed): Precis: An Update in Obstetrics and Gynecology: Reproductive Endocrinology, 2nd ed. Washington, DC: American College of Obstetrics and Gynecology, 2002, pp 151–161. **(IV, C)**
2. Stephenson M: Frequency of factors associated with habitual abortion in 197 couples. Fertil Steril 1996;66:24–29. **(III, B)**
3. Brigham SA, Conlon C, Farguharson RG: A longitudinal study of pregnancy outcome following idiopathic recurrent miscarriage. Hum Reprod 1999;14:2868–2871. **(III, C)**
4. Branch DW, Silver RM: Antiphospholipid syndrome. ACOG Educational Bull 1998;244:302–211. **(IV, C)**
5. Carson SA, Branch DW: Management of recurrent early pregnancy loss. ACOG Practice Bull 2001;24:1–12. **(IV, C)**
6. Mills JL, Simpson JL, Driscoll SG, et al: Incidence of spontaneous abortion among normal women and insulin-dependent diabetic women whose pregnancies were identified within 21 days of conception. N Engl J Med 1998;319:1617–1623. **(IIa, B)**
7. Clifford K, Rai R, Regan L: Future pregnancy outcome in unexplained recurrent first trimester miscarriage. Hum Reprod 1997;12:387–389. **(IIa, B)**
8. Jacobs PA, Hassold TJ: Chromosome abnormalities: origin and etiology in abortions and livebirths. In Vogel R, Sperling K (eds): Human Genetics. Berlin: Verlag, 1987, pp 233–244. **(III, B)**

9. Ohno M, Maeda T, Matsunobu A: A cytogenetic study of spontaneous abortions with direct analysis of chorionic villi. Obstet Gynecol 1991; 77:394–398. **(III, B)**

10. Simpson JL: Incidence and timing of pregnancy losses: relevance to evaluating safety of early prenatal diagnosis. Am J Med Genet 1990; 35:165–173. **(III, B)**

11. Castelbaum AJ, Lessy BA: Infertility and implantation defects. Infertil Reprod Med Clin No Amer 2001;12:427–446. **(IIa, B)**

12. Wilcox AJ, Baird DD, Weinberg CR: Time of implantation of the conception and loss of a pregnancy. N Engl J Med 1999;340:1796–1799. **(IIb, B)**

13. Ghazeeri GS, Clark DA, Kutteh WH: Immunologic factors in implantation. Infertil Reprod Med Clin No Amer 2001;12:315–337. **(IV, C)**

14. Craig LB, Ke RW, Kutteh WH: Increased prevalence of insulin resistance in women with a history of recurrent pregnancy loss. Fertil Steril 2002;78:487–490. **(IIa, B)**

15. Sills ES, Perloe M, Palermo GD: Correction of hyperinsulinemia in oligo-ovulatory women with clomiphene-resistant polycystic ovary syndrome: a review of therapeutic rationale and reproductive outcomes. Eur J Obstet Gynecol Reprod Biol 2000;91:135–141. **(IIb, B)**

16. Hoffman GE, Khoury J, Thie J: Recurrent pregnancy loss and diminished ovarian reserve. Fertil Steril 2000;74:1192–1195. **(III, B)**

17. Rubio C, Simon C, Vidal F, et al: Chromosomal abnormalities and embryo development in recurrent miscarriage couples. Hum Reprod 2003;18:182–188. **(IIa, B)**

18. Lin PC: Reproductive outcomes in women with uterine anamalies. J Women's Health 2004;13:33–39. **(IIb, B)**

19. Stovall DW, Parrish SB, Van Voorhis BJ, et al: Uterine leiomyomas reduce the efficacy of assisted reproduction cycles: results of a matched follow-up study. Hum Reprod 1998;13:192–197. **(IIa, B)**

20. Surrey ES, Lietz AK, Schoolcraft WB: Impact of intramural leiomyomata in patients with a normal endometrial cavity on in vitro fertilization–embryo transfer cycle outcome. Fertil Steril 2001; 75:405–410. **(III, B)**

21. Wilson WA, Ghavari AK, Piette JC: International classification criteria for antiphospholipid syndrome: synopsis of a post-conference workshop held at the Ninth International (Tours) APL Symposium. Lupus 2001;10:457–460. **(IV, C)**

22. Franklin RD, Kutteh WH: Antiphospholipid antibodies and recurrent pregnancy loss: treating a unique APA-positive population. Hum Reprod 2002;17:2981–2985. **(IIa, B)**

23. Cowchock FS, Reece EA, Balaban D: Repeated fetal losses associated with antiphospholipid antibodies: a collaborative randomized trial comparing prednisone with low-dose aspirin treatment. Am J Obstet Gynecol 1992;166:1318–1323. **(Ib, A)**

24. Laskin CA, Bombardier C, Hanna ME, et al: Prednisone and aspirin in women with autoantibodies and unexplained recurrent fetal loss. N Engl J Med 1997;337:148–153. **(Ib, A)**

25. Kutteh WH: Antiphospholipid antibody-associated recurrent pregnancy loss: treatment with heparin and low dose aspirin is superior to low dose aspirin alone. Am J Obstet Gynecol 1996;174:1584–1589. **(IIa, A)**

26. Rai R, Cohen H, Dave M, et al: Randomized controlled trial of aspirin and aspirin plus heparin in pregnant women with recurrent miscarriage associated with phospholipid antibodies. Br Med J 1997;314:253–257. **(Ib, A)**

27. Empson M, Lassere M, Craig JC, et al: Recurrent pregnancy loss with antiphospholipid antibody: a systematic review of therapeutic trials. Obstet Gynecol 2002;99:135–144. **(I, A)**

28. Rushworth FH, Bakos M, Rai R, et al: Prospective pregnancy outcome in untreated recurrent miscarriers with thyroid antibodies. Hum Reprod 2000;15:1637–1639. **(III, B)**

29. Esplin MS, Branch DW, Silver R, et al: Thyroid antibodies are not associated with recurrent pregnancy loss. Am J Obstet Gynecol 1998; 179:1583–1586. **(III, B)**

30. Ober C, Karrison T, Odem RR, et al: Mononuclear-cell immunisation in prevention of recurrent miscarriages: a randomised trial. Lancet 1999; 354:365–369. **(Ib, A)**

31. Laird SM, Tuckerman EM, Cork BA, et al: A review of immune cells and molecules in women with recurrent miscarriage. Human Reprod Update 2003;9:163–174. **(IV, C)**

32. Wegmann TG, Lin H, Guilbert L, Mosmann TR: Bidirectional cytokine interactions in the maternal-fetal relationship: is successful pregnancy a Th2 phenomenon? Immunol Today 1993;14:353–356. **(IV, C)**

33. Clark DA, Vince G, Flanders KC, et al: CD56+ lymphoid cells in human first trimester pregnancy decidua as a source of novel TGF-$\beta_2$-related immunosuppressive factors. Hum Reprod 1994;9:2270–2277. **(IIb, B)**

34. Szekeres-Bartho J, Autran B, Debre P, et al: Immuno-regulatory effects of a suppressor factor from healthy pregnant women's lymphocytes after progesterone induction. Cell Immunol 1989;122:281–294. **(III, B)**

35. Mowbray JF, Liddel H, Underwood JL, et al: Controlled trial of treatment of recurrent spontaneous abortion by immunization with paternal cells. Lancet 1985;i:941–943. **(IIa, B)**

36. Ho HN, Gill TJ, Hsieh HJ, et al: Immunotherapy for recurrent spontaneous abortions in a Chinese population. Am J Reprod Immunol 1991;25:10–15. **(Ib, A)**

37. Cauchi MN, Lim D, Young DE, et al: Treatment of recurrent aborters by immunization with parental cells—controlled trial. Am J Reprod Immunol 1991;25:16–17. **(IIa, B)**

38. German RSA/IVIG Group: Intravenous immunoglobulin in the prevention of recurrent miscarriage. Br J Obstet Gynaecol 1994; 101:1072–1077. **(Ib, A)**

39. Coulam CB, Krysa L, Stern J, Bustillo M: Intravenous immunoglobulin for treatment of recurrent pregnancy loss. Am J Reprod Immunol 1995;34:333–337. **(IIa, B)**

40. Christiansen OB, Mathiesen O, Husth M, et al: Placebo-controlled trial of treatment of unexplained secondary recurrent spontaneous abortions with i.v. immunoglobulin. Hum Reprod 1995;10:2690–2695. **(IIa, B)**

41. Stephenson MD, Dreher K, Houlihan E, Wu V: Prevention of unexplained recurrent spontaneous abortion using intravenous immuno-globulin: A prospective, randomized, double-blinded, placebo-controlled trial. Am J Reprod Immunol 1998;39:82–88. **(Ib, A)**

42. Penta M, Lukic A, Conte MP, et al: Infectious agents in tissues from spontaneous abortions in the first trimester of pregnancy. New Microbiol 2003;26:329–337. **(III, B)**

43. Kovalevsky G, Garcia CR, Berlin JA, et al: Evaluation of the association between hereditary thrombophilias and recurrent pregnancy loss: a meta-analysis. Arch Intern Med 2004;164:558–563. **(Ia, A)**

44. Regan L, Rai R: Thrombophilia and pregnancy loss. J Reprod Immunol 2002;55:163–180. **(IV, C)**

45. Rai R, Bakos M, Elgaddal S, et al: Factor V Leiden and recurrent miscarriage—a prospective outcome of untreated pregnancy. Hum Reprod 2002;17:442–445. **(IIb, B)**

46. Rey E, Kahn SR, David M, Shriver I: Thrombophilic disorders and fetal loss: a meta-analysis. Lancet 2003;361:901–908. **(Ia, A)**

47. Quéré I, Mercier E, Bellet H, et al: Vitamin supplementation and pregnancy outcome in women with recurrent early pregnancy loss and hyperhomocysteinemia. Fertil Steril 2001;75:823–825. **(IIb, B)**

48. Ness RB, Grisso JA, Hirschinger N, et al: Cocaine and tobacco use and the risk of spontaneous abortion. N Engl J Med 1999;340:333–339. **(IIa, B)**

49. SHARE, Pregnancy and Infant Loss Support, Inc., St. Joseph Health Center, 300 First Capitol Drive, St. Charles, MO 63301, 1-800-821-6819. www.nationalshareoffice.com **(IV, C)**

# Chapter 56 Hyperprolactinemia

Jeremy A. King, MD, and Howard A. Zacur, MD, PhD

---

## KEY POINTS

- Diagnosis of pathologic hyperprolactinemia should be made only after all known causes of physiological or iatrogenic hyperprolactinemia are excluded.
- Management of hyperprolactinemia depends on the presence and size of a prolactinoma and the patient's desire for fertility.
- Dopamine agonists are highly effective for treating microprolactinomas, macroprolactinomas, and idiopathic hyperprolactinemia.
- Although all dopamine agonists are effective, cabergoline is often more effective and better tolerated than bromocriptine.
- Because more data are available for bromocriptine use during pregnancy, bromocriptine should be the drug of choice when pregnancy is desired.
- In general, surgical resection of prolactinomas should be a last resort.

---

The existence of a human prolactin molecule was proven in 1971.[1] Prior to this discovery it was assumed that biological activities that depended on prolactin in other animals were mediated by growth hormone in the human. Once its existence in the human was established, assays were developed and normal plasma concentrations defined. As a consequence, abnormal concentrations were soon identified and the diagnosis of hyperprolactinemia was made for many patients with previously unexplained amenorrhea or impotence.

Prolactin is a polypeptide hormone secreted primarily by lactotrophs in the anterior pituitary gland. In humans, it has lactogenic, steroidogenic, and immunoregulatory functions. Hyperprolactinemia, simply defined as circulating plasma prolactin concentrations exceeding the upper limit of normal, may be caused by a variety of physiological, iatrogenic, or pathologic conditions. An understanding of the physiology and regulation of prolactin is required to distinguish pathologic conditions from physiological responses.

## EPIDEMIOLOGY

The prevalence of hyperprolactinemia ranges from 0.4% in an unselected adult population to 17% of patients with polycystic ovary syndrome (PCOS).[2] An incidence of 5% has been reported among women of reproductive age[3] and 14% among women with secondary amenorrhea.[4] Pituitary microadenomas have been found in 1.5% to 26.7% of autopsies in subjects not known to have had pituitary lesions while alive.[5] Macroadenomas, on the other hand, are very rarely encountered in postmortem studies.

## PHYSIOLOGY

Human prolactin is a 199–amino acid protein with a molecular weight (MW) of 23,000 daltons. Larger prolactin-like molecules can also be found in the circulation. Big prolactin (MW 48,000 to 56,000 daltons) and big, big prolactin (100,000 daltons) are immunologically active but have less biologic activity than the small prolactin monomer. These larger prolactin molecules may represent dimers or tetramers of the native hormone, or may consist of prolactin molecules bound by immunoglobulin G.[6]

The known biologic actions of prolactin in humans are lactogenesis, steroidogenesis, and immunoregulation. The prolactin receptor, encoded by a single gene located on chromosome 5, is expressed in a variety of organ systems. During pregnancy, breast tissue is primed by estrogen and progesterone. The elevated estrogen level during gestation results in proliferation of lactotrophs and increased prolactin production. Prolactin initiates the synthesis of casein, whey, lactoglobulin, and lactalbumin within the breast. However, lactation is not initiated until the high estrogen concentration of pregnancy is reduced postpartum. Breast milk production continues in response to exposure to prolactin secreted as a result of nipple stimulation during breastfeeding.

In the ovary human prolactin has been shown to influence the secretion of progesterone from luteinized human granulosa cells in culture. Conditions of prolactin excess or deficiency in the culture medium are associated with marked decreases in progesterone production. Prolactin receptors and prolactin itself are expressed by luteinized granulosa cells.[7] Prolactin receptors have also been demonstrated within the human adrenal gland. Adrenal stimulation by prolactin affects the secretion of cortisol, aldosterone, and dehydroepiandosterone from adrenal cell cultures.

Prolactin also appears to play a role in the maintenance of immunocompetence.[8] Receptors for the hormone have been identified on human T and B lymphocytes. The ability of prolactin to stimulate proliferation of lymphoma cells from Nb2 rats provides the basis for current biologic assays. Cyclosporine, an immunosuppressive agent, has been shown to displace prolactin from its receptors. A role for prolactin in the etiology of human autoimmune diseases is currently being investigated.

Regulation of prolactin production and secretion is multifactorial. The primary regulatory mechanism is chronic inhibition by dopamine. Dopamine secreted by neurons in the hypothalamus and the infundibulum of the uterine tube reaches the

# Reproductive Endocrinology and Infertility

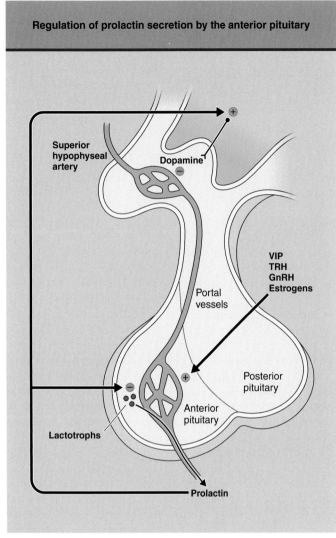

**Regulation of prolactin secretion by the anterior pituitary**

Labels in figure: Superior hypophyseal artery; Dopamine; VIP TRH GnRH Estrogens; Portal vessels; Posterior pituitary; Anterior pituitary; Lactotrophs; Prolactin

**Figure 56-1    Regulation of prolactin secretion by the anterior pituitary.**

anterior pituitary via the portal circulation. Stimulation of $D_2$ receptors on lactotroph cell membranes results in the lowering of intracellular adenylate cyclase activity. Lower levels of intracellular cyclic adenosine monophosphate result in diminished prolactin release. Prolactin may also inhibit its own release by providing negative feedback at the level of the lactotroph or by stimulating the release of hypothalamic dopamine. Several substances are known to stimulate prolactin secretion. These include epidermal growth factor, vasoactive intestinal peptide, thyrotropin-releasing hormone (TRH), gonadotropin-releasing hormone (GnRH), and estrogens (Fig. 56-1).

There are currently five recognizable dopamine receptors, each of which belongs to the superfamily of G-protein receptors. They are classified into the $D_1$ group (comprised of the $D_1$ and $D_5$ receptors) and the $D_2$ group (consisting of the $D_2$, $D_3$, and $D_4$ receptors). The $D_2$ receptor is the dopamine receptor displayed by lactotrophs. Not all lactotrophs express equally functioning dopamine receptors. The difference in responsiveness to dopamine is evidence of a phenomenon termed *lactotroph*

*heterogeneity*. This heterogeneity is of clinical importance because a subset of hyperprolactinemic patients is resistant to dopamine agonist therapy.

## CLINICAL FEATURES

Premenopausal women with hyperprolactinemia may present with menstrual disturbances, infertility, and/or galactorrhea. Table 56-1 lists the most common complaints. Galactorrhea refers to nipple discharge, either spontaneous or expressed, that contains milk. The diagnosis can be made simply by viewing fat globules in a droplet of discharge under light microscopy. When galactorrhea alone is identified, prolactin levels will be normal in up to 85% of cases. However, when both galactorrhea and amenorrhea are experienced, the chance of being hyperprolactinemic is 90%.[9]

Hyperprolactinemia accounts for 10% to 38% of secondary amenorrhea. The cause of gonadal dysfunction is suppression of GnRH release by excess stimulation of prolactin receptors in the hypothalamus. The hypogonadism associated with hyperprolactinemia can result in hot flushes, vaginal dryness, and decreased bone density due to subnormal levels of circulating estradiol.

Diminished bone mineral density associated with hyperprolactinemia has been described in multiple studies. One study of premenopausal women with prolactinomas found a relative risk for osteoporosis of 4.5 compared to healthy controls.[10] Up to 80% of women will have osteoporosis or osteopenia of the lumbar spine, femoral neck, or both at the time of diagnosis.[11] Bone mineral density is significantly decreased in hyperprolactinemic women with amenorrhea but not in those with normal menstruation.[12,13] Bone loss is greater in women with amenorrhea associated with hyperprolactinemia than in those with amenorrhea and normal prolactin levels.[14,15] Bone mineral loss may be reversed after successful treatment of hyperprolactinemia, but bone density does not return to baseline levels.[11,12,15] Hyperprolactinemia in adolescents with menstrual disturbances warrants prompt attention because virtually all of these young women will demonstrate osteopenia or osteoporosis at the time of diagnosis.[11]

## CAUSES OF HYPERPROLACTINEMIA

Hyperprolactinemia is defined simply as the elevation of circulating prolactin hormone above the normal level (usually 20 ng/mL in women). Diagnosis of "pathologic" hyperprolactinemia requires exclusion of other physiologic or iatrogenic causes of excess

| Table 56-1 |
| Most Common Symptoms of Hyperprolactinemia |
| --- |
| Oligomenorrhea |
| Amenorrhea |
| Galactorrhea |
| Infertility |
| Headache |
| Visual Impairment |
| Hypopituitarism |

**Table 56-2**
**Causes of Hyperprolactinemia**

| Physiologic | Pharmacologic | Pathologic |
|---|---|---|
| Stress | Neuroleptics | Prolactinoma |
| Sleep | SSRIs | Nonfunctioning pituitary |
| Lunch or dinner | H$_2$-receptor blockers | tumors |
| Chest wall stimulation | Methyldopa | Empty sella syndrome |
| Pregnancy | Verapamil | Infiltrative disorders or |
| | Reserpine | CNS masses |
| | Metoclopramide | Hypothyroidism |
| | Protease inhibitors | Renal failure |
| | | Idiopathic |

prolactin secretion. Table 56-2 lists many of the causes of hyperprolactinemia.

## Physiologic Variation

The level of circulating prolactin is subject to a variety of physiologic influences, which must be considered. Acute physical or emotional stress will cause transient hyperprolactinemia. Sleep causes prolactin levels to rise. Food ingestion at lunch or dinner (but not breakfast) will also cause a transient elevation of prolactin values.

Stimulation or irritation of the chest wall by suckling, breast implants, herpes zoster, or local trauma can cause prolactin to increase. Conflicting data are available regarding the impact of a clinical breast examination on prolactin secretion. Pregnancy can cause an elevation of prolactin levels to as high as 600 ng/mL. This elevation is believed to result from increased serum estrogen stimulation of the hypothalamus and pituitary.

## Pharmacologic Hyperprolactinemia

Medications that prevent the release of, or block the action of, dopamine are common causes of hyperprolactinemia. All conventional antipsychotics block D$_2$ receptors and can elevate prolactin levels up to tenfold.[16] Overall, 65% of reproductive-age women taking antipsychotics experience hyperprolactinemia (mean value of 69 ng/mL).[17] Newer "prolactin-sparing" antipsychotics such as clozapine, quetiapine, and olanzapine may cause no change or even a small decrease in prolactin levels.[18,19] Selective serotonin reuptake inhibitors, tricyclic antidepressants, H$_2$ receptor blockers, methyldopa, verapamil, reserpine, metoclopramide, and protease inhibitors can all cause elevations of prolactin.

## Pathologic Hyperprolactinemia

Pathologic hyperprolactinemia can be caused by lactotroph adenomas, decreased inhibition of prolactin secretion, or underlying medical conditions. Any process involving the hypothalamus and/or pituitary that interrupts the normal secretion of dopamine in the portal circulation can cause hyperprolactinemia. Examples include nonfunctioning pituitary tumors, craniopharyngiomas, sarcoidosis, trauma, or seizures. Other endocrine conditions such as acromegaly or primary hypothyroidism are associated with hyperprolactinemia. TRH can stimulate prolactin release. Renal failure is frequently associated with hyperprolactinemia, but any degree of chronic renal insufficiency may also cause elevated prolactin levels due to impaired clearance of the hormone or of a prolactin-stimulating factor.[20,21]

Prolactin-secreting pituitary lesions are not true adenomas and are thus most appropriately termed *prolactinomas.* Such lesions are found in at least 40% of hyperprolactinemic patients. Over 90% are confined to the sella and rarely increase in size over time.[22,23] They are almost always benign.

## EVALUATION

Diagnosis of pathologic hyperprolactinemia is made only after other causes have been ruled out. More than one blood sample should be used to verify the diagnosis. Collection is ideally performed in the fully awake, fasting state and in the follicular phase of the menstrual cycle (if ovulatory). Occasionally levels of prolactin that are normal or only moderately elevated are reported when high levels are suspected clinically. This can be caused by the *hook effect,* a falsely low reading due to oversaturation of some immunoradiometric or chemiluminometric assays.[24] If such an effect is suspected, a sample should be reevaluated with serial dilutions.

In other cases prolactin concentrations that are several times normal may be found in patients without any symptoms of hyperprolactinemia. This may occur when the majority of excess circulating hormone is in the form of big, big prolactin. This condition is termed *macroprolactinemia.* Approximately 25% of hyperprolactinemic serum samples are accounted for by the presence of macroprolactin (big, big prolactin).[6,25] Although some macroprolactinemic patients present with amenorrhea, galactorrhea, or infertility, macroprolactin is less biologically active than the prolactin monomer and the majority of patients are asymptomatic. Many asymptomatic women with hyperprolactinemia due to macroprolactin have undergone costly and unnecessary evaluations and treatments.

Most commercial assays do not differentiate between macroprolactin and the prolactin monomer. Polyethylene glycol (PEG) precipitation can be used to identify macroprolactin when this condition is suspected.[6,26] Figure 56-2 demonstrates the difference in serum prolactin concentrations after PEG treatment of samples with and without macroprolactin. For the asymptomatic patient with macroprolactinemia, neither pituitary imaging nor treatment is required. A complete evaluation, however, is indicated if symptoms are present.

When an elevation of serum prolactin levels has been confirmed and careful history has excluded other known causes, laboratory evaluation consists of measurement of serum thyrotropin, human chorionic gonadotropin, blood urea nitrogen, and creatinine. When such testing fails to identify a cause for confirmed hyperprolactinemia, a central lesion should be sought (Fig. 56-3).

Imaging of the pituitary is indicated at any degree of unexplained hyperprolactinemia (as opposed to waiting until the serum level exceeds a given cutoff value). Some 40% of hyperprolactinemic patients will have a detectable pituitary abnormality even when prolactin levels are only mildly elevated.[27] As demonstrated in Figure 56-4, prolactin levels tend to correlate with prolactinoma size,[28] although exceptions do occur. Nonfunctioning adenomas or other lesions may be large despite

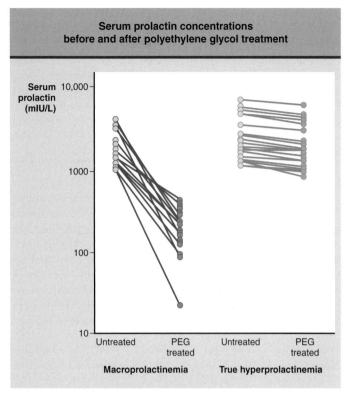

**Figure 56-2** **Serum prolactin concentrations before and after treatment with polyethylene glycol (PEG) in patient with either macroprolactinemia or true hyperprolactinemia.** (From Suliman AM, Smith TP, Gibney J, McKenna TJ: Frequent misdiagnosis and mismanagement of hyperprolactinemic patients before the introduction of macroprolactin screening: application of a new strict laboratory definition of macroprolactinemia. Clin Chem 2003;49:1504–1509.)

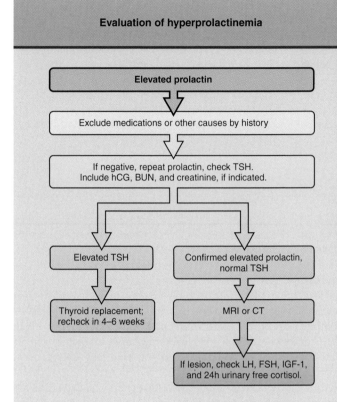

**Figure 56-3** **Evaluation of hyperprolactinemia.**

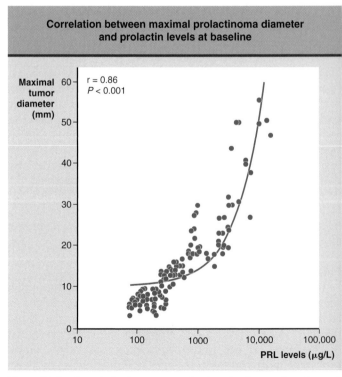

**Figure 56-4** **Correlation between maximal prolactinoma diameter and prolactin levels at baseline.** (From Colao A, Sarno AD, Cappabianca P, et al: Gender differences in the prevalence, clinical features and response to cabergoline in hyperprolactinemia. Eur J Endocrinol 2003;148:325–331.)

relatively low levels of excess prolactin secretion. If a suspected explanation for hyperprolactinemia exists, such as the administration of neuroleptics, but prolactin levels are very elevated (>200 ng/mL), imaging should be performed because such levels may be associated with a prolactinoma. Magnetic resonance imaging (MRI) is the most sensitive diagnostic modality, although contrast-enhanced computed tomography scanning may also be employed.[29] If a lesion within the pituitary gland measures less than 10 mm in diameter, it is termed a *microadenoma.* Lesions 1 cm or larger are *macroadenomas.* If the tumor extends beyond the sella turcica or is adjacent to the optic chiasm, ophthalmologic referral should be made for visual field testing.

Almost half of all pituitary lesions secrete prolactin. However, pituitary lesions are capable of secreting any pituitary hormone. At times nonprolactin-secreting lesions may cause hyperprolactinemia secondarily by blocking the inhibitory influence of the hypothalamus on pituitary lactotrophs. Therefore, when lesions are identified, screening tests should be performed to rule out the secretion of other hormones. A 24-hour urine free cortisol level and a serum insulin-like growth factor 1 (IGF-1) will exclude a corticotropin-secreting lesion and a somatotropin-secreting lesion, respectively. Follicle-stimulating hormone, luteinizing hormone, and thyrotropin levels should also be evaluated to exclude gonadotropic or thyrotropic adenomas. If the pituitary lesion is shown to secrete prolactin only, further management will depend on the size of the lesion, the patient's desire to conceive, and concern about hypoestrogenism.

Women with galactorrhea who have a normal serum prolactin level do not require pituitary gland imaging. However, these women should be screened for somatotropin disturbances because elevated somatotropin levels may stimulate milk secretion. Hyperhidrosis, glucose intolerance, arthritis, neuropathy, hypertension, heart disease, and acral and soft tissue overgrowth may be signs and symptoms of acromegaly in addition to galactorrhea.

# MANAGEMENT

Management options include observation, medication, and surgery. The goals of management depend on the degree of clinical symptoms, the presence and size of a pituitary adenoma, the patient's fertility desires, and concern about bone density.

## Observation

Observation is a valid option in the patient with nontumoral hyperprolactinemia or a microprolactinoma not causing neurologic signs or symptoms. It has been reported that 90% to 95% of microadenomas remain stable or shrink over time.[23,30] In approximately 34% of cases an elevated prolactin concentration will spontaneously normalize within 5 years.[22,31,32] It is unlikely that a prolactinoma will grow significantly without an associated increase in serum prolactin levels. Most patients can be safely monitored with serial prolactin levels, with repeat imaging reserved for cases of significant serum elevations or development of neurologic symptoms.

When observation is selected it is important to advise the patient that osteopenia or osteoporosis may result from prolonged hypoestrogenism and hyperprolactinemia. Estrogen therapy or an estrogen-containing contraceptive should be considered.

## Medical Therapy

The goals of treatment are suppression of excess prolactin secretion, elimination of clinical symptoms, reduction in tumor size, and preservation of normal pituitary function. Medical therapy is directed at stimulating dopamine receptors, which inhibit prolactin production and secretion and lactotroph mitosis. Options include the ergot-derived bromocriptine, cabergoline, and pergolide and the apomorphine-derived quinagolide. Table 56-3 outlines current preparations. Bromocriptine and cabergoline are the only medications currently approved by the Food and Drug Administration (FDA) for the treatment of primary hyperprolactinemia. Bromocriptine carries the additional indication of ovulation induction.

### Bromocriptine

Bromocriptine mesylate (Parlodel) was the first dopamine agonist used with widespread success. If taken as directed, bromocriptine allows resumption of regular ovulation and cyclic menses in over 90% of women with gonadal dysfunction.[33,34] Prolactin levels will become normal in 70% to 90% of treated women, depending on lesion size.[33-35] After the start of therapy 70% of macroprolactinomas begin to shrink within 6 weeks and up to 100% within 6 months.[35] Approximately half of macroprolactinomas shrink at least 50% in size. Tumor shrinkage may continue for several years.[34] If present, visual changes often resolve within days of initiating treatment.[35]

Bromocriptine reaches peak serum levels within 3 hours of oral administration. It has a half-life of 3.3 hours and is capable of lowering prolactin concentrations for 9 hours. Oral dosing is

## Table 56-3
### Medications Used to Treat Hyperprolactinemia

| Medication | Recommended Dosage | Common Side Effects |
|---|---|---|
| Bromocriptine (Parlodel) | 2.5–10 mg/day, divided PO, 2.5 mg/day PV | Nausea, dizziness, headache, syncope, nasal congestion, orthostatic hypotension, (fewer GI effects when given vaginally) |
| Bromocriptine (Parlodel SRO)* | 2.5–15 mg/day | Similar to bromocriptine |
| Bromocriptine (Parlodel LA)* | 50–100 mg q month IM | Similar to bromocriptine; milder or more transient |
| Cabergoline (Dostinex) | 0.25–1 mg q week or twice weekly | Similar to bromocriptine Hypotension more common |
| Quinagolide (Norprolac)* | 0.025–0.15 mg/day | Similar to bromocriptine, but less common, milder, and more transient |
| Pergolide (Permax) | 0.025–0.5 mg/day | Similar to bromocriptine Fever, nasal congestion, hypotension more common |
| Hydergine | 6–12 mg/day, divided | Similar to bromocriptine |
| Pramipexole (Mirapex) | 0.125–0.3 mg/day | Nausea, postural hypotension |
| Ropinirole (Requip) | 0.08–2.5 mg/day, divided | Nausea, postural hypotension |
| Lisuride (Dopergin) | 0.1–1.2 mg/day, divided | Similar to bromocriptine Nausea, dizziiness, drowsiness more common |
| Terguride | 0.25–1.5 mg/day, divided | Similar to bromocriptine Transient CNS effects more common |

*Not available in the United States.
Adapted from Bankowski BJ, Zacur HA: Dopamine agonist therapy for hyperprolactinemia. Clin Obstet Gynecol 2003;46:349–362.

# Reproductive Endocrinology and Infertility

thus required two to three times a day. A long-acting injectable form and a slow-release oral form of bromocriptine are available outside the United States. The slow-release oral form is administered daily, and the injectable is given every 28 days. The side effect profiles of all forms of bromocriptine are similar.

Bromocriptine stimulates $D_2$ receptors but binds to $D_1$ receptors as well, which results in adrenergic side effects such as nausea, vomiting, postural hypotension, dizziness, syncope, headache, constipation, and nasal congestion. Approximately half of all patients experience at least one adverse effect, and up to 12% of patients will not tolerate the drug.[36] A low starting dose with gradual dosage increases may help prevent many adverse effects. Treatment is usually initiated with one half of a 2.5 mg bromocriptine tablet taken with food at night. The dose is then increased by one half to one tablet every few days as needed. Dosages greater than 2.5 mg three times a day are rarely required. Response to bromocriptine is assessed by checking the level of circulating prolactin several days after initiating therapy and after each dose adjustment. Vaginal administration of 2.5 to 5 mg daily is also effective and may be used to reduce side effects.[37,38]

When used for ovulation induction, an alternative to daily dosing is intermittent bromocriptine administration. Taking bromocriptine only during the follicular phase results in ovulation and pregnancy rates similar to continuous administration while resulting in decreased cost and improved compliance.[39]

## Cabergoline

Cabergoline (Dostinex) was approved by the FDA for the treatment of hyperprolactinemia in 1996. It is effective in normalizing prolactin levels and restoring ovulation in over 85% and 90% of women, respectively. It has a high affinity and selectivity for $D_2$ receptors, allowing for once- or twice-weekly dosing and decreased side effects compared to bromocriptine. Dopaminergic

side effects are similar to those observed with bromocriptine, but overall tolerability with cabergoline is superior.[40]

Cabergoline suppresses prolactin levels in a dose-dependent fashion. In a placebo-controlled, multicenter study 74% of hyperprolactinemic patients had normal prolactin levels within 4 weeks of therapy with 0.5 mg twice weekly. A dosage of 1 mg twice weekly resulted in normalization in 95% of subjects. All dosages ranging from 0.125 mg to 1 mg twice weekly were successful at restoring menses in 82% of amenorrheic women.[41] Cabergoline and bromocriptine were compared in a large, multicenter, double-blind trial for the treatment of hyperprolactinemic, amenorrheic women.[36] A dosage of 0.5 to 1 mg of cabergoline twice a week was more effective than 2.5 to 5 mg of bromocriptine twice a day at restoring ovulatory cycles (72% vs. 52%). Stable normoprolactinemia was achieved in 83% and 58% in the cabergoline and bromocriptine groups, respectively. Figure 56-5 shows the mean prolactin concentrations in both groups. Cabergoline was also better tolerated, with only 3% discontinuing therapy versus 12% of the bromocriptine group (Fig. 56-6). Another trial, by Di Sarno and colleagues, showed that serum prolactin concentration was normalized and tumor size reduced in 82% of macroprolactinomas and 90% of microprolactinomas (compared to 46% and 57%, respectively, in a cohort of subjects treated with bromocriptine).[42]

Cabergoline is often effective treatment for patients who are intolerant or resistant to bromocriptine. Verhelst showed a normalization of prolactin concentration in 86% and 70% of patients with bromocriptine intolerance or resistance, respectively.[43] Colao and colleagues found that cabergoline is effective in treating many patients with macroprolactinomas who received previous treatment with other dopamine agonists but that it is most effective in agonist-naive patients.[44] They prospectively evaluated 110 patients with macroprolactinomas treated with cabergoline; 26 patients had not had any prior therapy, and the

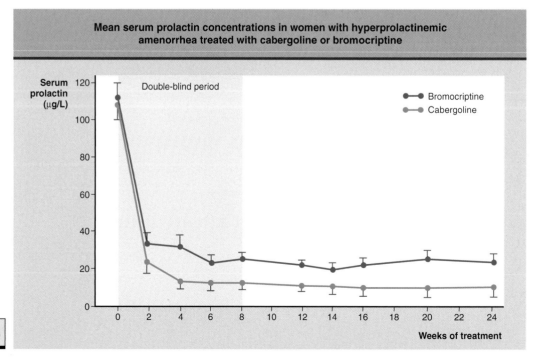

**Mean serum prolactin concentrations in women with hyperprolactinemic amenorrhea treated with cabergoline or bromocriptine**

**Figure 56-5   Mean (+/− SE) serum prolactin concentrations in women with hyperprolactinemic amenorrhea treated with cabergoline or bromocriptine.** (From Webster J, Piscitelli G, Polli A, et al: A comparison of cabergoline and bromocriptine in the treatment of hyperprolactinemic amenorrhea. Cabergoline Comparative Study Group: N Engl J Med 1994;331:904–909.)

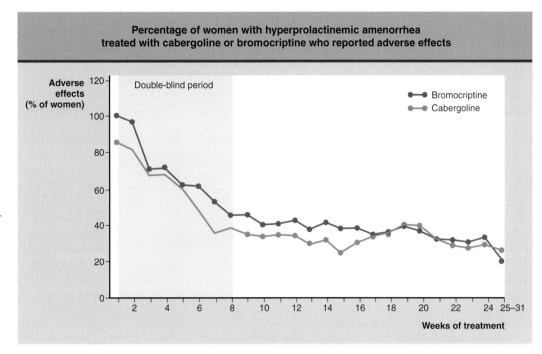

**Figure 56-6    Percentage of women with hyperprolactinemic amenorrhea treated with cabergoline or bromocriptine who reported adverse effects.** (From Webster J, Piscitelli G, Polli A, et al: A comparison of cabergoline and bromocriptine in the treatment of hyperprolactinemic amenorrhea. Cabergoline Comparative Study Group: N Engl J Med 1994;331:904–909.)

rest had been treated previously with bromocriptine or other dopamine agonists. Nineteen were intolerant, 37 resistant, and 28 responsive (but had discontinued therapy for various reasons). Normal prolactin levels were achieved in virtually all patients (109/110), but higher doses and a longer treatment time were required to achieve normalization in the resistant group. In addition, 30% of the resistant patients went on to experience recurrent mild hyperprolactinemia. Figure 56-7 shows that

shrinkage was greatest among the agonist-naive group, with an average reduction of 92%. Average shrinkage was 66%, 58%, and 59% in the intolerant, resistant, and responsive groups, respectively.

Cabergoline is a long-acting agonist capable of inhibiting pituitary prolactin secretion for more than 7 days after a single dose.[45] Oral dosing is started at 0.25 mg twice a week or 0.5 mg weekly. This dosage is often sufficient to normalize prolactin

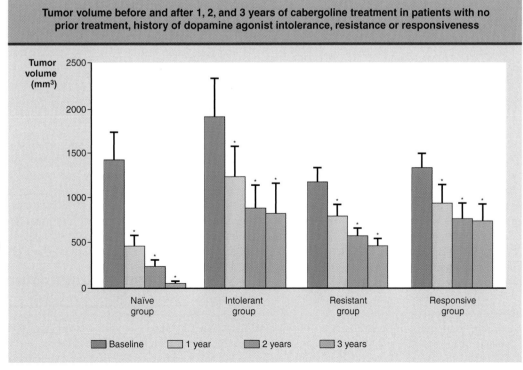

**Figure 56-7    Tumor volume before and after 1, 2, and 3 years of cabergoline treatment in patients with no prior treatment, history of dopamine agonist intolerance, resistance, or responsiveness.** (From Colao A, DiSarno A, Landi ML, et al: Macroprolactinoma shrinkage during cabergoline treatment is greater in naïve patients than in patients pretreated with other dopamine agonists: a prospective study in 110 patients: J Clin Endocrinol Metab 2000;85:2247–2252.)

# Reproductive Endocrinology and Infertility

levels.[43] If nausea or vomiting are significant, vaginal administration of 0.5 mg twice weekly is safe and effective.[46]

Data on safety of cabergoline in pregnancy is limited. Reports are available for more than 300 conceptions occurring concomitant with cabergoline administration without evidence of teratogenic risk.[47] Small series suggest that the rate of pregnancy loss is equal to that of the general population.[40,48] However, because data are limited, it is currently recommended that cabergoline be discontinued at least 1 month before attempting conception.

### Pergolide

Pergolide (Permax) is a synthetic ergot derivative currently approved by the FDA for the treatment of parkinsonism but has been used successfully to treat hyperprolactinemia. It is the least expensive dopamine agonist available. Pergolide requires only once-daily dosing. Administration is generally begun at 25 μg orally in the evening. The dose can be increased every 3 to 4 days by 25 μg increments as needed up to 500 μg.

Randomized, controlled trials have shown pergolide to be as effective as bromocriptine at lowering prolactin levels, reducing galactorrhea, and restoring normal menstruation.[49,50] Two recent series of patients with macroprolactinomas showed an average reduction of 88% to 97% in serum prolactin levels.[51,52] The combined results of these series showed shrinkage of 50% or more in 36 of 44 cases, and 75% or more in 19 of 44. Visual field defects were completely restored in 15 of 18 subjects. The incidence of adverse dopaminergic effects is similar to bromocriptine, although patients taking pergolide experience more flulike symptoms, fever, and vasodilation.

### Other Agents

Quinagolide (Norprolac, CV 205-502) is a $D_2$ agonist derived from apomorphine. It is currently available only in Europe. With a half-life of 22 hours, it is given once daily. Oral dosing is begun at 25 μg. Quinagolide returns prolactin to normal levels in 82% of hyperprolactinemic subjects.[53] Patients who are unable to tolerate bromocriptine are better able to tolerate quinagolide.[54,55] When compared in clinical trials quinagolide is similar to cabergoline in its ability to reduce prolactin concentration.[56,57] However, cabergoline is better tolerated and induces greater tumor suppression than quinagolide.[57]

Hydergine, another ergot derivative, is approved by the FDA for treatment of dementia. It has been used to lower prolactin levels and induce ovulation in hyperprolactinemic women with oral doses of 2 mg three times a day.[58] It has not been compared directly to other dopamine agonists.

Pramipexole (Mirapex) and ropinirole (Requip) are nonergot dopamine agonists that are approved by the FDA for the treatment of Parkinson's disease. Both have been shown in small studies to lower prolactin levels.[59,60] Dopaminergic side effects are common and are similar to those for other dopamine agonists. Other similar agents have been found to treat hyperprolactinemia in a limited number of studies and are included in Table 56-3.

### Surgery

Prior to the availability of dopamine agonists, surgical resection of prolactinomas was the mainstay of therapy. It is most often accomplished as a transsphenoidal partial hypophysectomy.

Neurosurgeons have recommended surgical resection in the presence of pituitary apoplexy, macroadenoma, intolerance or resistance to medication, patient preference, or risk of enlargement during pregnancy.[61,62] Because long-term cure rates are highest and complication rates lowest after resection of microadenomas, others have suggested that primary surgery be considered as an alternative to medical therapy for patients with small lesions.[63–65]

Complication rates of transsphenoidal pituitary surgery can be high. These include pituitary insufficiency (19%), diabetes insipidus (18%), cerebrospinal fluid fistulas (4%), carotid artery injury, loss of vision, and meningitis (1% to 2%).[66] Morbidity for prolactinoma resection is often lower than for other pituitary lesions, especially when lesions are small. In recent years an endonasal approach using a rigid endoscope has been used successfully while incurring less morbidity.[67,68] A randomized trial comparing endonasal endoscopy with sublabial transsphenoidal microsurgery reported similar cure rates (normoprolactinemia in 66% and 75% of patients, respectively) with a mean follow-up of 3.5 years. The complication rate was only 4.5% among the endoscopic group, versus 27% in the open group.[69]

Surgical therapy frequently fails to cure hyperprolactinemia. A recent review of 120 microadenomas and macroadenomas treated surgically reported an initial cure rate (postoperative prolactin of <20 ng/mL) of 64%. However, there was a 16.9% recurrence of hyperprolactinemia within 50 months. High preoperative prolactin levels were most predictive of recurrence.[65] These results are similar to other studies. A summary of 34 published series, including a total of 2600 surgical resections showed that 73.7% of microadenomas and 32.4% of macroadenomas had normal prolactin levels within 1 to 12 weeks of surgery. Recurrence rates were 21% for microadenomas and 19.8% for macroadenomas.[30]

The incidence of malignancy in prolactinomas is rare.[70] Current data do not support surgery for the purpose of excluding malignancy. It therefore appears that, in general, surgery should be considered only as a last resort for treatment of prolactinomas. Clear indications include pituitary apoplexy and lesions that grow despite dopamine agonist therapy. Patients with prolactinomas who are undergoing concurrent treatment with neuroleptics or those who are intolerant of or unwilling to undergo chronic medical therapy may also be offered surgery.

### Irradiation

Irradiation of the pituitary has been used in various forms to treat prolactinomas, but cure rates are inconsistent. Irradiation achieves reduction and control of prolactin secretion in 44% to 70% of patients.[71] Side effects include hypopituitarism, increased risk of cerebrovascular accident, and vision loss. Furthermore, if subsequent surgery becomes necessary it is often complicated by radiation-induced fibrosis. Currently gamma knife radiotherapy is employed on a limited basis to treat residual lesions.[72]

## INDIVIDUALIZING MANAGEMENT RECOMMENDATIONS

There are no official guidelines for treatment of hyperprolactinemia. Proper management is guided by the findings on pituitary imaging and the patient's desire for fertility.

## No Prolactinoma—Pregnancy Not Desired

Two therapeutic choices are available for the patient without a detectable pituitary abnormality who does not desire pregnancy. These are observation and dopamine agonist therapy. If observation is selected the patient should be informed of the potential for negative impact on bone density. Oral contraceptives (OCs) can usually be safely taken. However, estrogen is known to stimulate pituitary prolactin secretion. Estrogen in combination OCs has been implicated in the formation or expansion of pituitary adenomas in some individuals. Some early reports suggested a relationship between OC use and development of prolactinomas. However, more recent attempts to link OCs to elevated prolactin levels and adenoma growth have not supported a correlation.[73] A prospective study of 16 patients (8 with idiopathic hyperprolactinemia and 8 with microprolactinomas) failed to show any increase in prolactin levels or growth of adenomas after 2 years of combination OC use.[74] Corenblum and Donovan reported on 38 women with hyperprolactinemia and amenorrhea with and without prolactinomas who were taking either combination OCs for up to 2.8 years or conjugated estrogens and medroxyprogesterone acetate for up to 4 years. Prolactin levels and adenoma size remained unchanged or decreased in all groups.[75]

Prolactin levels should be checked yearly after normalization has been achieved. If normal prolactin levels are not attained or dopamine agonist therapy is not tolerated, changing to another agonist may be effective.

## Prolactinoma Present—Pregnancy Not Desired

Other hormone-producing adenomas should be excluded when a pituitary lesion is visualized. In most cases microadenomas do not enlarge over time. Patients should be offered medical therapy or observation. Either dopamine agonist is appropriate, but cabergoline is often better tolerated and may be more effective. Periodic monitoring by MRI is recommended, with more frequent assessment if a macroprolactinoma is present. Combination OCs can generally be taken safely in the presence of microprolactinomas and may protect against bone loss. Women with prolactinomas should be counseled about the risks of OCs and other estrogen-containing products. In addition to pituitary imaging, patients not receiving medical therapy should undergo periodic bone density monitoring. Because macroadenomas have a higher incidence of expansion, medical therapy is indicated. Dopamine agonists are effective at normalizing prolactin levels and reducing macroprolactinoma volume. Prolactin levels drop dramatically within days to weeks of therapy, but tumor shrinkage may take weeks to years.[44] A repeat MRI 6 months after initiating therapy is appropriate.

If a macroprolactinoma threatens to compromise the optic nerve and does not respond to medical therapy, surgical resection should be considered. External radiation may be a necessary adjunct to surgery if substantial tumor bulk remains.

## No Prolactinoma—Pregnancy Desired

When pregnancy is desired by the hyperprolactinemic patient, bromocriptine is the first line of therapy. Normalization of prolactin levels and resumption of menses typically occur within 8 weeks of therapy. The drug is discontinued when pregnancy is diagnosed. Discontinuation does not increase the chance of pregnancy loss. Children conceived during bromocriptine administration are not at increased risk for congenital malformation.[76] Due to the normal elevation and variation of prolactin levels in pregnancy there is no clinical utility in measuring serum values.

Some hyperprolactinemic, anovulatory patients fail to respond to dopamine agonists or cannot tolerate the side effects. In such cases clomiphene citrate or gonadotropins may be used for ovulation induction. Although cabergoline is also effective at restoring normal gonadotropic activity, there are only limited data about the impact of the medication on early pregnancy.[48,77]

## Prolactinoma Present—Pregnancy Desired

Identification of pituitary hormone secretion other than prolactin from pituitary lesions is essential. After this has been accomplished, the patient is managed in a manner similar to that described for the hyperprolactinemic patient who does not have a lesion. Dopamine agonists or ovulation induction agents may be used. Patients should be counseled about the risks of pregnancy. Gland and adenoma enlargement may occur under the influence of elevated estrogen levels. The chance of developing neurologic symptoms such as headache or visual changes is only 1% to 5% for women with microadenomas but as high as 36% when a macroadenoma is present. When suprasellar extension of a macroadenoma is present, there is a 15% to 35% chance of tumor enlargement during pregnancy.[35]

When pregnancy is achieved, dopamine agonists are discontinued by tapering the daily dose to avoid adenoma infarction. A baseline neuro-opthalmologic examination is recommended. When a macroprolactinoma is present, visual field testing is performed each trimester to detect gland or lesion enlargement. Measurement of prolactin levels during pregnancy is not useful for predicting prolactinoma growth. Any suggestion of optic nerve compression should prompt MRI evaluation. Dopamine agonist therapy may be restarted if optic nerve compromise is confirmed.

Breastfeeding is not contraindicated. Dopamine agonists can be administered during lactation if neurological symptoms occur. Occasionally spontaneous infarction of an adenoma occurs postpartum. This can result in lowered prolactin levels and resumption of normal menses. If breastfeeding does not occur following delivery, prolactin levels rapidly fall to normal at the end of the first postpartum week. If breastfeeding occurs, prolactin concentrations may remain elevated for a prolonged time, depending on the frequency, duration, and intensity of the suckling stimulus.

# CONTROVERSIES

## Duration of Medical Therapy

Lifelong dopamine agonist therapy may not be necessary for all hyperprolactinemic patients. Early investigations of the effect of agonist withdrawal found that hyperprolactinemia recurred in 70% to 90% of patients. A shortcoming of these studies was a lack of criteria for determining when to attempt withdrawal. Another factor contributing to the poor withdrawal results was the limited duration of therapy in some studies. Regrowth of prolactinomas was particularly likely if therapy was limited to 1 year or less. However, more recent evidence suggests that

# Reproductive Endocrinology and Infertility

withdrawal of medications in properly selected patients can be successful. This may be due to morphologic changes of the lesion, such as fibrosis, cellular atrophy, and necrosis, that occur after long-term dopamine agonist therapy.[78,79]

In the largest study of bromocriptine withdrawal to date Passos and colleagues studied 62 patients with microprolactinomas and 69 with macroprolactinomas who had achieved normoprolactinemia prior to withdrawal. Normal prolactin levels persisted in 20.6% for a median of 44 months of follow-up (range, 3 to 240 months). There was no tumor regrowth observed. The authors attempted to identify variables that could predict successful withdrawal; however, none of the variables studied, including gender, age, tumor size, pretreatment prolactin levels, treatment duration, or initial dose, was predictive of stable normoprolactinemia.[80]

Patients treated with cabergoline may be especially amenable to withdrawal. In a prospective study of 39 patients taking cabergoline for just 1 year, 17% remained euprolactinemic for 12 months of follow-up.[57] In the same study, none of the 39 subjects withdrawn from quinagolide maintained normoprolactinemia.

Colao and colleagues prospectively observed more than 300 patients taking cabergoline as primary therapy for at least 2 years (median, 3 years). Criteria used to consider withdrawal were a normal prolactin concentration, MRI showing no tumor or at least 50% reduction of an existing tumor, and availability for follow-up. In this group, 200 patients discontinued therapy and were followed for 2 to 5 years. Elevated prolactin levels recurred in only 24% of nontumoral patients, 31% of those with microprolactinomas, and 38% of those with macroprolactinomas. None of the 175 patients with lesions before starting therapy experienced tumor regrowth. The risk of recurrent hyperprolactinemia increased 19% for each millimeter increment in diameter of the residual tumor.[81]

It therefore appears safe to consider medication withdrawal in patients with or without prolactinomas who have achieved normal prolactin levels. Ideally patients should be asymptomatic for 2 years and have demonstrated a reduction in tumor size, if present. Patients should be monitored for recurrence of hyperprolactinemia or corresponding symptoms. An appropriate schedule for checking serum prolactin is 3, 6, and 12 months after cessation. An MRI should be repeated every 6 months for the first year, then annually thereafter (or sooner if clinically indicated).

## REFERENCES

1. Hwang P, Hardy J, Friesen H, Wilansky D: Biosynthesis of human growth hormone and prolactin by normal pituitary glands and pituitary adenomas. J Clin Endocrinol Metab 1971;33:1–7. **(IIa, B)**
2. Biller BM, Luciano A, Crosignani PG, et al: Guidelines for the diagnosis and treatment of hyperprolactinemia. J Reprod Med 1999;44(12 Suppl):1075–1084. **(IIb, B)**
3. Luciano AA, Sherman BM, Chapler FK, et al: Hyperprolactinemia and contraception: a prospective study. Obstet Gynecol 1985;65:506–510. **(IIb, B)**
4. Reindollar RH, Novak M, Tho SP, McDonough PG: Adult-onset amenorrhea: a study of 262 patients. Am J Obstet Gynecol 1986; 155:531–543. **(IIb, B)**
5. Molitch ME, Russell EJ: The pituitary "incidentaloma." Ann Intern Med 1990;112:925–931. **(IIb, B)**
6. Leslie H, Courtney CH, Bell PM, et al: Laboratory and clinical experience in 55 patients with macroprolactinemia identified by a simple polyethylene glycol precipitation method. J Clin Endocrinol Metab 2001;86:2743–2746. **(IIb, B)**
7. Vlahos NP, Bugg EM, Shamblott MJ, et al: Prolactin receptor gene expression and immunolocalization of the prolactin receptor in human luteinized granulosa cells. Mol Hum Reprod 2001;7:1033–1038. **(IIa, B)**
8. Gala RR: Prolactin and growth hormone in the regulation of the immune system. Proc Soc Exp Biol Med 1991;198:513–527. **(IIa, B)**
9. Kleinberg DL, Noel GL, Frantz AG: Galactorrhea: a study of 235 cases, including 48 with pituitary tumors. N Engl J Med 1977;296:589–600 **(IIb, B)**
10. Vartej P, Poiana C, Vartej I: Effects of hyperprolactinemia on osteoporotic fracture risk in premenopausal women. Gynecol Endocrinol 2001;15:43–47. **(IIa, B)**
11. Colao A, Di Somma C, Loche S, et al: Prolactinomas in adolescents persistent bone loss after 2 years of prolactin normalization. Clin Endocrinol (Oxf) 2000;52:319–327. **(IIa, B)**
12. Biller BM, Baum HB, Rosenthal DI, et al: Progressive trabecular osteopenia in women with hyperprolactinemic amenorrhea. J Clin Endocrinol Metab 1992;75:692–697. **(IIa, B)**
13. Klibanski A, Biller BM, Rosenthal DI, et al: Effects of prolactin and estrogen deficiency in amenorrheic bone loss. J Clin Endocrinol Metab 1988;67:124–130. **(IIb, B)**
14. Schlechte JA, Sherman B, Martin R: Bone density in amenorrheic women with and without hyperprolactinemia. J Clin Endocrinol Metab 1983;56:1120–1123. **(IIa, B)**
15. Schlechte J, el-Khoury G, Kathol M, Walkner L: Forearm and vertebral bone mineral in treated and untreated hyperprolactinemic amenorrhea J Clin Endocrinol Metab 1987;64:1021–1026. **(IIa, B)**
16. Wieck A, Haddad PM: Antipsychotic-induced hyperprolactinaemia in women: pathophysiology, severity and consequences. Selective literature review. Br J Psychiatry 2003;182:199–204. **(IIa, B)**
17. Kinon BJ, Gilmore JA, Liu H, Halbreich UM: Hyperprolactinemia in response to antipsychotic drugs: characterization across comparative clinical trials. Psychoneuroendocrinol 2003;28(Suppl 2):69–82. **(Ib, A)**
18. Volavka J, Czobor P, Cooper TB, et al: Prolactin levels in schizophrenia and schizoaffective disorder patients treated with clozapine, olanzapine, risperidone, or haloperidol. J Clin Psychiatry 2004;65:57–61. **(Ib, A)**
19. Arvanitis LA, Miller BG: Multiple fixed doses of Seroquel (quetiapine) in patients with acute exacerbation of schizophrenia: a comparison with haloperidol and placebo. The Seroquel Trial 13 Study Group. Biol Psychiatry 1997;42:233–246. **(Ib, A)**
20. Hou SH, Grossman S, Molitch ME: Hyperprolactinemia in patients with renal insufficiency and chronic renal failure requiring hemodialysis or chronic ambulatory peritoneal dialysis. Am J Kidney Dis 1985, 6:245–249. **(IIb, B)**
21. Sievertsen GD, Lim VS, Nakawatase C, Frohman LA: Metabolic clearance and secretion rates of human prolactin in normal subjects and in patients with chronic renal failure. J Clin Endocrinol Metab 1980, 50:846–852. **(IIa, B)**
22. Schlechte J, Dolan K, Sherman B, et al: The natural history of untreated hyperprolactinemia: a prospective analysis. J Clin Endocrinol Metab 1989;68:412–418. **(IIb, B)**
23. Sisam DA, Sheehan JP, Sheeler LR: The natural history of untreated microprolactinomas. Fertil Steril 1987;48:67–71. **(IIb, B)**
24. St-Jean E, Blain F, Comtois R: High prolactin levels may be missed by immunoradiometric assay in patients with macroprolactinomas. Clin Endocrinol (Oxf) 1996;44:305–309. **(IIa, B)**
25. Smith TP, Suliman AM, Fahie-Wilson MN, McKenna TJ: Gross variability in the detection of prolactin in sera containing big big prolactin (macroprolactin) by commercial immunoassays. J Clin Endocrinol Metab 2002;87:5410–5415. **(IIb, B)**
26. Suliman AM, Smith TP, Gibney J, McKenna TJ: Frequent misdiagnosis and mismanagement of hyperprolactinemic patients before the introduction of macroprolactin screening: application of a new strict laboratory definition of macroprolactinemia. Clin Chem 2003;49:1504–1509. **(IIa, B)**

27. Brenner SH, Lessing JB, Quagliarello J, Weiss G: Hyperprolactinemia and associated pituitary prolactinomas. Obstet Gynecol 1985; 65:661–664. **(IIb, B)**

28. Colao A, Sarno AD, Cappabianca P, et al: Gender differences in the prevalence, clinical features and response to cabergoline in hyperprolactinemia. Eur J Endocrinol 2003;148:325–331. **(IIb, B)**

29. Naidich MJ, Russell EJ: Current approaches to imaging of the sellar region and pituitary. Endocrinol Metab Clin North Am 1999;28:45–79. **(IIb, B)**

30. Molitch M: Prolactinoma. In Melmed S (ed): The Pituitary, 2nd ed. Malden, Mass.: Blackwell Publishing, 2002, pp 455–495. **(IIb, B)**

31. Sluijmer AV, Lappohn RE: Clinical history and outcome of 59 patients with idiopathic hyperprolactinemia. Fertil Steril 1992;58:72–77. **(IIb, B)**

32. Jeffcoate WJ, Pound N, Sturrock ND, Lambourne J: Long-term follow-up of patients with hyperprolactinaemia. Clin Endocrinol (Oxf) 1996; 45:299–303. **(IIb, B)**

33. Vance ML, Evans WS, Thorner MO: Drugs five years later. Bromocriptine. Ann Intern Med 1984;100:78–91. **(Ib, A)**

34. Bevan JS, Webster J, Burke CW, Scanlon MF: Dopamine agonists and pituitary tumor shrinkage. Endocr Rev 1992;13:220–240. **(Ia, A)**

35. Molitch ME, Elton RL, Blackwell RE, et al: Bromocriptine as primary therapy for prolactin-secreting macroadenomas: results of a prospective multicenter study. J Clin Endocrinol Metab 1985;60:698–705. **(IIb, B)**

36. Webster J, Piscitelli G, Polli A, et al: A comparison of cabergoline and bromocriptine in the treatment of hyperprolactinemic amenorrhea. Cabergoline Comparative Study Group. N Engl J Med 1994; 331:904–909. **(Ib, A)**

37. Kletzky OA, Vermesh M: Effectiveness of vaginal bromocriptine in treating women with hyperprolactinemia. Fertil Steril 1989; 51:269–272. **(IIb, B)**

38. Jasonni VM, Raffelli R, de March A, et al: Vaginal bromocriptine in hyperprolactinemic patients and puerperal women. Acta Obstet Gynecol Scand 1991;70:493–495. **(IIb, B)**

39. Parra A, Crespo G, Coria I, Espinosa de los Monteros A: Clinical and hormonal response to short-term intermittent versus continuous oral bromocriptine in hyperprolactinemic women. Int J Fertil Menopausal Stud 1995;40:96–101. **(Ib, A)**

40. Ciccarelli E, Giusti M, Miola C, et al: Effectiveness and tolerability of long term treatment with cabergoline, a new long-lasting ergoline derivative, in hyperprolactinemic patients. J Clin Endocrinol Metab 1989;69:725–728. **(IIa, B)**

41. Webster J, Piscitelli G, Polli A, et al: Dose-dependent suppression of serum prolactin by cabergoline in hyperprolactinaemia: a placebo controlled, double blind, multicentre study. European Multicentre Cabergoline Dose-finding Study Group. Clin Endocrinol (Oxf) 1992; 37:534–541. **(Ib, A)**

42. Di Sarno A, Landi ML, Cappabianca P, et al: Resistance to cabergoline as compared with bromocriptine in hyperprolactinemia: prevalence, clinical definition, and therapeutic strategy. J Clin Endocrinol Metab 2001;86:5256–5261. **(IIa, B)**

43. Verhelst JA: Toward the establishment of a clinical prediction rule for response of prolactinomas to cabergoline. J Clin Endocrinol Metab 1999;84:4747. **(III, B)**

44. Colao A, Di Sarno A, Landi ML, et al: Macroprolactinoma shrinkage during cabergoline treatment is greater in naive patients than in patients pretreated with other dopamine agonists: a prospective study in 110 patients. J Clin Endocrinol Metab 2000;85:2247–2252. **(IIb, B)**

45. Ferrari C, Barbieri C, Caldara R, et al: Long-lasting prolactin-lowering effect of cabergoline, a new dopamine agonist, in hyperprolactinemic patients. J Clin Endocrinol Metab 1986;63:941–945. **(IIa, B)**

46. Motta T, de Vincentiis S, Marchini M, et al: Vaginal cabergoline in the treatment of hyperprolactinemic patients intolerant to oral dopaminergics. Fertil Steril 1996;65:440–442. **(III, B)**

47. Webster J: Clinical management of prolactinomas. Baillieres Best Pract Res Clin Endocrinol Metab 1999;13:395–408. **(IIb, B)**

48. Ricci E, Parazzini F, Motta T, et al: Pregnancy outcome after cabergoline treatment in early weeks of gestation. Reprod Toxicol 2002;16:791–793. **(III, B)**

49. Lamberts SW, Quik RF: A comparison of the efficacy and safety of pergolide and bromocriptine in the treatment of hyperprolactinemia. J Clin Endocrinol Metab 1991;72:635–641. **(Ib, A)**

50. Kletzky OA, Borenstein R, Mileikowsky GN: Pergolide and bromocriptine for the treatment of patients with hyperprolactinemia. Am J Obstet Gynecol 1986;154:431–435. **(Ib, A)**

51. Freda PU, Andreadis CI, Khandji AG, et al: Long-term treatment of prolactin-secreting macroadenomas with pergolide. J Clin Endocrinol Metab 2000;85:8–13. **(III, B)**

52. Orrego JJ, Chandler WF, Barkan AL: Pergolide as primary therapy for macroprolactinomas. Pituitary 2000;3:251–256. **(IIb, B)**

53. Webster J: A comparative review of the tolerability profiles of dopamine agonists in the treatment of hyperprolactinaemia and inhibition of lactation. Drug Saf 1996;14:228–238. **(Ib, A)**

54. Glaser B, Nesher Y, Barziliai S: Long-term treatment of bromocriptine-intolerant prolactinoma patients with CV 205-502. J Reprod Med 1994;39:449–454. **(III, B)**

55. Vilar L, Burke CW: Quinagolide efficacy and tolerability in hyperprolactinaemic patients who are resistant to or intolerant of bromocriptine. Clin Endocrinol (Oxf) 1994;41:821–826. **(IIb, B)**

56. Giusti M, Porcella E, Carraro A, et al: A cross-over study with the two novel dopaminergic drugs cabergoline and quinagolide in hyperprolactinemic patients. J Endocrinol Invest 1994;17:51–57. **(Ib, A)**

57. Di Sarno A, Landi ML, Marzullo P, et al: The effect of quinagolide and cabergoline, two selective dopamine receptor type 2 agonists, in the treatment of prolactinomas. Clin Endocrinol (Oxf) 2000;53:53–60. **(IIa, B)**

58. Tamura T, Satoh T, Minakami H, Tamada T: Effect of hydergine in hyperprolactinemia. J Clin Endocrinol Metab 1989;69:470–474. **(IIa, B)**

59. Acton G, Broom C: A dose rising study of the safety and effects on serum prolactin of SK&F 101468, a novel dopamine $D_2$-receptor agonist. Br J Clin Pharmacol 1989;28:435–441. **(IIa, B)**

60. Schilling JC, Adamus WS, Palluk R: Neuroendocrine and side effect profile of pramipexole, a new dopamine receptor agonist, in humans. Clin Pharmacol Ther 1992;51:541–548. **(Ib, A)**

61. Wilson CB: Surgical management of pituitary tumors. J Clin Endocrinol Metab 1997;82:2381–2385. **(IV, C)**

62. Laws ER II, Thapar K: Pituitary surgery. Endocrinol Metab Clin North Am 1999;28:119–131. **(IV, C)**

63. Turner HE, Adams CB, Wass JA: Trans-sphenoidal surgery for microprolactinoma: an acceptable alternative to dopamine agonists? Eur J Endocrinol 1999;140:43–47. **(IIb, B)**

64. Tyrrell JB, Lamborn KR, Hannegan LT, et al: Transsphenoidal microsurgical therapy of prolactinomas: initial outcomes and long-term results. Neurosurg 1999;44:254–263. **(IIa, B)**

65. Losa M, Mortini P, Barzaghi R, et al: Surgical treatment of prolactin-secreting pituitary adenomas: early results and long-term outcome. J Clin Endocrinol Metab 2002;87:3180–3186. **(IIb, B)**

66. Ciric I, Ragin A, Baumgartner C, Pierce D: Complications of transsphenoidal surgery: results of a national survey, review of the literature, and personal experience. Neurosurg 1997;40:225–237. **(IV, C)**

67. Jho HD, Carrau RL: Endoscopic endonasal transsphenoidal surgery: experience with 50 patients. J Neurosurg 1997;87:44–51. **(IIb, B)**

68. Koren I, Hadar T, Rappaport ZH, Yaniv E: Endoscopic transnasal transsphenoidal microsurgery versus the sublabial approach for the treatment of pituitary tumors: endonasal complications. Laryngoscope 1999;109:1838–1840. **(IIb, B)**

69. Cho DY, Liau WR: Comparison of endonasal endoscopic surgery and sublabial microsurgery for prolactinomas. Surg Neurol 2002; 58:371–376. **(Ib, A)**

70. Ragel BT, Couldwell WT: Pituitary carcinoma: a review of the literature. Neurosurg Focus 2004;16:E7. **(IIb, B)**

71. Becker G, Kocher M, Kortmann RD, et al: Radiation therapy in the multimodal treatment approach of pituitary adenoma. Strahlenther Onkol 2002;178:173–186. **(IIb, B)**

72. Landolt AM, Lomax N: Gamma knife radiosurgery for prolactinomas. J Neurosurg 2000;93(Suppl 3):14–18. **(IIb, B)**

73. Fahy UM, Foster PA, Torode HW, et al: The effect of combined estrogen/progestogen treatment in women with hyperprolactinemic amenorrhea. Gynecol Endocrinol 1992;6:183–188. **(IIb, B)**

74. Testa G, Vegetti W, Motta T, et al: Two-year treatment with oral contraceptives in hyperprolactinemic patients. Contraception 1998; 58:69–73. **(IIb, B)**

75. Corenblum B, Donovan L: The safety of physiological estrogen plus progestin replacement therapy and with oral contraceptive therapy in women with pathological hyperprolactinemia. Fertil Steril 1993; 59:671–673. **(IIb, B)**

76. Molitch ME: Pregnancy and the hyperprolactinemic woman. N Engl J Med 1985;312:364–370. **(IIb, B)**

77. Robert E, Musatti L, Piscitelli G, Ferrari CI: Pregnancy outcome after treatment with the ergot derivative, cabergoline. Reprod Toxicol 1996; 10:333–337. **(III, B)**

78. Landolt AM, Osterwalder V: Perivascular fibrosis in prolactinomas: is it increased by bromocriptine? J Clin Endocrinol Metab 1984; 58:1179–1183. **(IIa, B)**

79. Gen M, Uozumi T, Ohta M, et al: Necrotic changes in prolactinomas after long term administration of bromocriptine. J Clin Endocrinol Metab 1984;59:463–470. **(III, B)**

80. Passos VQ, Souza JJ, Musolino NR, Bronstein MD: Long-term follow-up of prolactinomas: normoprolactinemia after bromocriptine withdrawal. J Clin Endocrinol Metab 2002;87:3578–3582. **(IIb, B)**

81. Colao A, Di Sarno A, Cappabianca P, et al: Withdrawal of long-term cabergoline therapy for tumoral and nontumoral hyperprolactinemia. N Engl J Med 2003;349:2023–2033. **(IIb, B)**

# Secondary Amenorrhea

## Elizabeth E. Puscheck, MD

## KEY POINTS

- Pregnancy is the most common cause of secondary amenorrhea in reproductive age women.
- After pregnancy, the next five most common causes are polycystic ovary syndrome (PCOS), hypothalamic amenorrhea, thyroid dysfunction, hyperprolactinemia, and ovarian failure.
- Chronic anovulation is a risk factor for endometrial hyperplasia and carcinoma without treatment.
- PCOS patients are at additional increased risk for type 2 diabetes, hypertension, and myocardial infarction.
- Mild elevation in prolactin may occur with hypothyroidism, and the thyroid-stimulating hormone (TSH) level should be measured to rule out thyroid disease. Treating the thyroid disease is likely to normalize the prolactin level.
- Prolactin normally increases with pregnancy.
- Hyperprolactinemia can lead to hypoestrogenism and osteopenia/osteoporosis.
- Forty percent of pituitary adenomas are prolactinomas, and 90% of prolactinomas are microadenomas.
- Hypoestrogenism from hypogonadotropic hypogonadism or hypergonadotropic hypogonadism left untreated increases the likelihood of low peak bone mass/osteopenia/osteoporosis.
- Differentiating hypoestrogenism from hypogonadotropic (hypothalamic) amenorrhea or hypergonadotropic hypoestrogenism is best achieved by the measurement of follicle-stimulating hormone (FSH). In the former case, FSH is normal or low, and in the latter case, FSH is high (>40 mIU/mL).
- Premature ovarian failure deserves rapid and full evaluation and treatment; psychological counseling is also important.
- Up to 25% of hypergonadotropic hypogonadal women with a karyotype containing an intact (or a portion of the) Y chromosome may have a propensity for a gonadal tumor, and the gonad should be removed.
- The most common cause of intrauterine adhesions is uterine curettage performed during or shortly after a pregnancy.

Additionally, the hypothalamic-pituitary-ovarian (HPO) axis must be intact to allow for normal pubertal milestones to be met and result in the initial menses prior to the onset of secondary amenorrhea, effectively ruling out primary causes of hypogonadotropic hypogonadism. The pathologic conditions resulting in secondary amenorrhea cover a broad list of etiologies: anatomic, endocrine, genetic, systemic disease, exogenous factors, and iatrogenic causes (see Table 57-3). Some etiologies for amenorrhea such as pregnancy, lactation, and menopause are normal, while others are pathologic and can have a significant impact on overall health. It is best to use a systematic approach to identify the etiology of secondary amenorrhea. One such approach is the World Health Organization (WHO) classification system of amenorrhea[3] (Table 57-2).

Alternatively, a review of the menstruation process and the hypothalamic-pituitary-ovarian-uterine axis is helpful in determining a logical physiologic approach to the etiology of secondary amenorrhea; it is easy to remember and assists in directing an evaluation.

A brief review of the normal menstruation process is important to identify when abnormal cycles or amenorrhea deserve evaluation. The normal menstrual cycle is orchestrated by a complex array of signals involving the hypothalamic-pituitary-ovarian-uterine axis. These signals consist of endocrine, paracrine, and autocrine mechanisms. The brief review will address only some of the endocrine signals. The hypothalamus contains an area within the medial basal portion called the arcuate nucleus, and this area consists of specialized neurosecretory cells that produce gonadotropin-releasing hormone (GnRH) in a pulsatile fashion. These GnRH signals are released at 60- to 90-minute intervals into a portal connection with the anterior pituitary.[4] The pituitary gonadotroph cells synthesize gonadotropins in response to the GnRH signals.[5] Gonadotropins consist of follicle-stimulating hormone (FSH) and luteinizing hormone (LH). The amplitude and frequency of the GnRH signals regulates the type and amount of gonadotropins synthesized. These gonadotropins are released into the bloodstream and are detected by FSH receptors and LH receptors in the ovarian follicles. The ovarian follicles initially respond to FSH by producing estrogen, which is released into the bloodstream where the uterus has receptors and responds by proliferating the endometrial lining. The estrogen also feeds back to the hypothalamus and the pituitary. When a sufficient amount of estrogen is made for an appropriate amount of time, the pituitary responds with a spike in LH secretion, called the LH surge. Approximately 24 hours after the peak LH surge, ovulation occurs. The ovarian follicle releases the oocyte and the follicle converts into a corpus luteum and produces progesterone. The uterus responds to the progesterone secretion by decidualizing the endometrium in preparation for

Secondary amenorrhea is a common problem of reproductive age women. It is defined as the cessation of menses, after at least one or more menstrual cycles, for a minimum of three cycles or 6 months[1,2] (Table 57-1). By the presence of at least one menses the reproductive organs must be initially intact, effectively ruling out congenital urogenital anomalies (e.g., imperforate hymen, transverse vaginal septum, cervical agenesis, uterine agenesis).

Reproductive Endocrinology Infertility

**Table 57-1**
**Diagnostic Criteria for Secondary Amenorrhea**

- Normal pubertal milestones
- Initial onset of menses
- Cessation of menses for 3 cycles (if regular cycles) or 6 months (if irregular cycles are present)

an embryo to implant. If no embryo is formed, the corpus luteum stops producing progesterone about 14 days later (±2 days). The waning progesterone levels result in sloughing of the endometrium to the basal layer of the uterus. The sloughing endometrium exits the uterus via its three openings (two fallopian tube ostia and cervical canal) with the assistance of uterine contractions. Since the cervical canal is generally larger and more distensible, most endometrial tissue and blood exit via the vagina in the form of a menstrual period. A majority of women are believed to normally have some retrograde blood flow into the abdominal cavity at the time of menstruation that is later absorbed.[6] Although this physiologic explanation is grossly oversimplified, it helps in addressing issues and approaches in secondary amenorrhea.

The first portion of the menstrual cycle, the follicular phase, begins at the onset of menstruation and continues until ovulation. The duration of the follicular phase varies among women and between cycles in the same woman, and may range from 8 to 21 days. As a woman ages, this phase of the menstrual cycle may shorten. This fact may lead to a shortening of the entire menstrual cycle (e.g., from 29 to 22 days, or a similar shortening when there is a shorter follicular phase and an unchanged luteal phase). The next portion of the menstrual cycle, which describes the time period after ovulation until the onset of the next menses, is called the luteal phase. The luteal phase is fairly consistent from cycle to cycle within women and between women; the duration is usually 12 to 14 days. Consequently, adding the duration of the two phases yields the length of the entire normal menstrual cycle; normal menstrual cycle lengths may vary from 21 to 35 days. When cycle durations are shorter than 21 days or longer than 35 days, it is likely that the patient is not ovulating. Longer cycles may also occur naturally when a pregnancy occurs and the corpus luteum persists in response to the hCG signal.

Secondary amenorrhea is defined as no menstruation for three cycles or 6 months.[1,2] Three cycles may be as short as 63 days to as long as 105 days or longer according to the information stated above. In women with irregular or erratic cycles, 6 months is the arbitrary cutoff when an evaluation should be initiated.

## EPIDEMIOLOGY

Secondary amenorrhea, not including pregnancy or other normal physiologic causes, affects an estimated 3% to 4% of women from the general population.[7–10] During the first few years after menarche (the first period), it is not uncommon for girls to have anovulatory cycles that later become regular cycles. Close monitoring is warranted but intervention at this point is not required. Once beyond these first few years, oligomenorrhea and secondary amenorrhea should be evaluated. Prior texts have recommended that an evaluation begin at age 16 when other secondary sexual characteristics are present. However, recent published reports of pubertal data on U.S. girls suggest that this evaluation should begin earlier, at about 14 years of age in developed countries, since 90% of U.S. girls menstruate by age 13.75; in less well developed countries the age may be lowered only to 15 or left at 16.[11–15] For the time being, the standard of care for the United States is dictated by the American Society for Reproductive Medicine (ASRM) Practice Committee, which recommends that this evaluation occur at 15 years of age with secondary sexual characteristics and 13 years of age without breast development, or within 5 years after breast development if that occurs before age 10.[2]

Etiologies for secondary amenorrhea are listed in Table 57-3.[9,10,16] Pregnancy should always be ruled out first. Even patients who have a history of amenorrhea may ovulate unexpectedly and conceive. Either a urine or a serum β-human chorionic gonadotropin (hCG) concentration is an adequate test. Most over-the-counter urine kits measure an hCG level over 50 mIU/mL as positive and some go as low as 25 mIU/mL. Serum β-hCG can be measured down to less than 5 mIU/mL. By the time of a missed period, the hCG level should be about 100 mIU/mL and will double every 2 days in 66% of cases.[17] Adolescents, in general, may not be forthcoming regarding sexual activity and should be offered pregnancy testing.[13] Amenorrhea due to pregnancy (normal or not) is not the focus of this chapter. Besides pregnancy, cases of secondary amenorrhea will likely be due to one of five etiologies: polycystic ovary syndrome (PCOS), thyroid dysfunction, hyperprolactinemia, hypothalamic amenorrhea, and ovarian failure. The remaining etiologies are much less common.

## CLINICAL FEATURES

Any patient with secondary amenorrhea or even oligomenorrhea deserves a diagnostic evaluation. Initially, a thorough history and physical examination should be performed. In secondary amenorrhea, developmental milestones for growth and secondary sexual characteristics (breast and pubic hair development)

**Table 57-2**
**World Health Organization (WHO) Classification of Secondary Amenorrhea**

| WHO Class | Estradiol | Follicle-stimulating Hormone (FSH) | Prolactin | Other | Diagnosis |
|---|---|---|---|---|---|
| WHO 1 | Low | Normal or low | Normal | No hypothalamic or pituitary mass | Functional hypothalamic amenorrhea |
| WHO 2 | Normal | Normal | Normal | – | Eugonadal |
| WHO 3 | Low | High | Normal | – | Ovarian failure |

**Table 57-3**
**Etiologies of Secondary Amenorrhea**

| Anatomic Site | Etiologies of Amenorrhea |
|---|---|
| Hypothalamus (hypogonadotropic hypogonadism) | Stress (physical or emotional) <br> Eating disorder <br> Excessive exercise <br> Obesity <br> Excessive weight loss <br> Chronic systemic disease <br> Idiopathic hypogonadotropic hypogonadism (IHH) <br> CNS tumor |
| Pituitary | Thyroid disease (hyper- or hypo-) <br> Pituitary adenoma <br> Hyperprolactinemia (drug-induced, physiologic, idiopathic, etc) <br> Craniopharyngioma <br> Other pituitary tumors <br> Hypopituitarism <br> Empty sella <br> Pituitary infarct |
| Ovary | Polycystic ovary syndrome <br> Premature ovarian failure <br> Ovarian neoplasm |
| Uterus | Pregnancy <br> Endometrial atrophy (drug-induced) <br> Endometrial damage (infection) <br> Asherman's syndrome (intrauterine adhesions) |
| Cervix | Cervical stenosis or obstruction |
| Adrenal | Cushing's syndrome <br> Adrenal adenoma <br> Late-onset congenital adrenal hyperplasia |
| Systemic | Chronic systemic disease |
| Exogeneous | Contraceptives, depot leuprolide |

should be reviewed and most likely will be normal, unlike the case in some patients with primary amenorrhea. Occasionally, a patient may have what initially sounds like secondary amenorrhea, but upon review of developmental milestones, may reveal that puberty did not occur normally but was induced by hormonal therapy and amenorrhea occurred when she stopped the cyclic hormonal therapy. This type of case should be classified as primary and not secondary amenorrhea (see Chapter 31).

A detailed history should review the patient's general health looking for chronic diseases such as diabetes, renal failure, seizures, inflammatory bowel disease, hypertension, depression, or any form of malabsorption or nutritional deficiency.[2,18] Any chronic illness that is not diagnosed or is not well controlled may affect the menstrual cycle.[19] In some circumstances the medical therapy for a chronic illness may be the cause of the menstrual irregularity (e.g., antidepressant, dopamine antagonist, phenothiazines, reserpine derivative).[20] Use of illicit drugs, such as opiates or amphetamines, may affect the menstrual cycle. Trauma to the head, breast, or pelvis may affect the HPO axis and subsequently the menstrual cycle. Similarly, tumors of the central nervous system (CNS) may cause an HPO axis disturbance and result in amenorrhea. Additionally, significant weight changes (gain or loss) often impacts the menstrual cycle. Significant weight gain and obesity have been associated with anovulation and amenorrhea.[21,22] Significant weight loss, either

voluntary or iatrogenic (e.g., gastric bypass surgery), has also been associated with secondary amenorrhea. It is important to consider anorexia nervosa in the differential diagnosis. Anorexia nervosa criteria include onset before 25 years of age, loss of at least 25% of original body weight, distorted attitude toward eating (weight overrides hunger, admonitions, reassurance, and threats), denial of illness, enjoyment in losing weight, desired body image of extreme thinness, unusual handling of food, no known medical cause to account for the weight loss, no other psychiatric diagnosis, and at lease two of the following: amenorrhea, lanugo, persistent bradycardia ($\leq$ 60 beats per minute), periods of overactivity, episodes of bulimia, and vomiting.[23] A few questions regarding diet, exercise (frequency and intensity), and stress are warranted.[24–26]

A clinical history of change in hair quality (coarser or finer; increased loss) may point to an endocrine disturbance. Increased hair growth may be associated with hypothyroidism, hirsutism, PCOS, Cushing's syndrome, and late-onset congenital adrenal hyperplasia. Rapid increases in terminal hair growth or the onset of virilization should raise suspicion of an androgen-secreting tumor, most likely of ovarian or adrenal origin.[27] The clinical history and physical examination are often sufficient to suspect the diagnosis. The measurement of serum androgens can help clinch the diagnosis and identify the likely source of the tumor. Occasionally, a patient comes in with secondary amenorrhea and a new diagnosis of Cushing's syndrome is made; most have additional symptoms such as hypertension, central obesity, and purplish striae.[28]

A detailed review of the patient's gynecologic history is important. Irregular periods since the onset of menarche are more common in PCOS syndrome and late-onset congenital adrenal hyperplasia, whereas a later onset after menarche may indicate new-onset thyroid disease, a PCOS variant, or other cause. Secondary amenorrhea associated with a history of hot flashes suggests the presence of ovarian failure, which occurs in 1% to 5% of women under 40 years of age.[29,30] Abnormal Papanicolaou (Pap) smears, sexually transmitted diseases, pelvic infections, and gynecologic procedures (either cervical or uterine) may be of consequence. Infrequently, secondary amenorrhea results after surgical procedures, such as cryosurgery, cone biopsy, dilation and curettage (D&C; particularly D&C associated with pregnancy, as in missed abortion, elective termination, or postpartum hemorrhage), or hysteroscopic procedures (e.g., myoma resection, intrauterine adhesiolysis). These procedures may result in cervical stenosis, which blocks the outflow of menstruation and is often associated with significant dysmenorrhea, or may result in lack of endometrial development due to intrauterine adhesions, causing hypomenorrhea or amenorrhea without other symptoms.[31] Secondary amenorrhea is uncommon after uterine artery embolization; however, there have been two such case reports.[32,33] In these cases, the amenorrhea occurs immediately after the surgical procedure and the time course is evident. Rarely, after an obstetric delivery associated with significant bleeding, the patient may note no lactation and later amenorrhea resulting from an insult to the pituitary, causing Sheehan's syndrome (hypopituitarism). Intentional (iatrogenic) secondary amenorrhea may follow endometrial ablation.

Occasionally, secondary amenorrhea occurs after stopping the birth control pill (postpill amenorrhea) or after stopping depot

# Reproductive Endocrinology Infertility

medroxyprogesterone acetate. Patients with postcontraceptive amenorrhea deserve an evaluation if amenorrhea persists beyond 6 months after the last birth control pill or 12 months after the last medroxyprogesterone injection. The incidence of postpill amenorrhea is 0.7% to 0.8%[7] and is a diagnosis of exclusion. The past menstrual history prior to contraceptive therapy alerts the physician as to whether amenorrhea is a new, progressive, or recurring problem (such as may occur in PCOS).

Additionally, progestational agents, hormonal contraceptives, and GnRH agonists may be used to induce a medical secondary amenorrhea to treat significant endometriosis symptoms or other causes of dysmenorrhea. One case report exists of two individuals with secondary amenorrhea as a result of occupational exposure to microparticles of estrogens/progestins while working in an oral contraceptive manufacturing plant.[34]

Close attention during the physical examination can help elucidate some of these etiologies and narrow the differential diagnosis. The vital signs may reveal the bounding and rapid pulse of hyperthyroidism, the slow pulse associated with hypothyroidism, or the hypertension of Cushing's syndrome. The body habitus and body mass index (>25 = overweight, >30 = obesity, and <21 = underweight) may yield extremes of weight. Skin color and consistency can also be indicators of appropriate nutrition or other endocrine etiologies (such findings as soft, moist skin with a rapid, bounding pulse may suggest hyperthyroidism, whereas dry skin with mild hirsutism may suggest hypothyroidism or hypoestrogenism). Skin lesions such as acanthosis nigricans may indicate insulin resistance, or striae may indicate the presence of Cushing's syndrome. Hair type and distribution may indicate hirsutism (associated with PCOS syndrome) or lanugo (suggestive of a nutritional disorder). The breast examination may reveal a bilateral, cloudy white nipple discharge, which appears as multiple fat cells on microscopy and is consistent with galactorrhea. Frequently, galactorrhea is associated with hyperprolactinemia. The abdominal and pelvic examinations serve to rule out a mass or infection. Ovarian masses or a hematometra may be present. In the latter case, the patient usually has a tender mass on pelvic examination and possibly on abdominal examination. If a hematometra results from cervical stenosis, then probing the cervical canal with a uterine sound during the physical examination may both diagnose and cure the problem; more commonly cervical dilation is needed or an ultrasound-guided D&C in severe cases. Decreased pubic hair and decreased vaginal rugae with pinkish-red shiny mucosa suggests hypoestrogenism. The patient may also note decreasing breast size, hot flashes, and vaginal dryness when asked. A swab of the vaginal side wall rolled on a microscope slide and stained with a nuclear stain can reveal a maturation index consistent with a higher percentage of parabasal cells than intermediate or superficial cells, which also indicates hypoestrogenism.

## DIAGNOSIS

During the initial visit for secondary amenorrhea, it is important to reassure the patient that the etiology will likely be determined by a thorough history, physical examination, ultrasound examination, and a few blood tests.[35] The history and physical and ultrasound examinations may guide the diagnostic testing so that

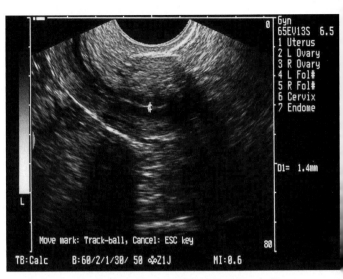

**Figure 57-1  Transvaginal ultrasonogram of the uterus.** The endometrial stripe (≠) is very thin, consistent with hypoestrogenism.

fewer tests are needed. If an ultrasound machine is available in the office, a quick assessment at the time of the physical examination may indicate whether estrogen is being produced, by the thickness of the endometrium and the size of the uterus. Transvaginal ultrasound can be quite helpful during this initial assessment.[36] Ovaries with rare follicles and a uterus with a thin endometrial stripe (Fig. 57-1) on ultrasound suggest ovarian failure. Ovaries with several small follicles and a thin endometrial stripe also indicate a hypoestrogenic state. Ovaries with many (>10) small follicles each (Fig. 57-2) and an endometrium with a trilaminar pattern (Fig. 57-3) suggest chronic anovulation and possibly PCOS.[37] Overly thickened endometrium (>14 mm) may be associated with early pregnancy or may suggest endometrial hyperplasia or worse; nonpregnant individuals in this

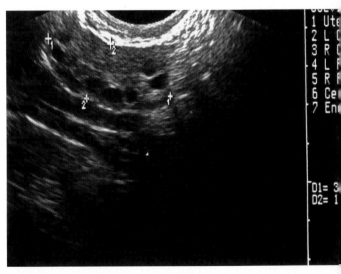

**Figure 57-2  Transvaginal ultrasonogram of an ovary.** This ovary has multiple small follicles that can be normal in the early part of the menstrual cycle or consistent with polycystic ovary syndrome (PCOS). In addition, the small follicles are displaced to the periphery, which is consistent with the "pearl necklace" sign commonly seen in PCOS.

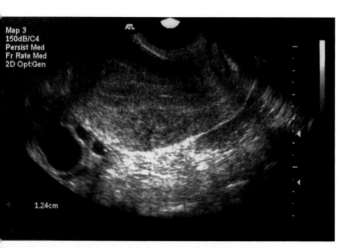

**Figure 57-3    Transvaginal ultrasonogram of the uterus.** The endometrial stripe is thickened and has a trilaminar appearance. This finding is normal in the proliferative phase, and this image also shows an enlarged ovarian follicle, consistent with the proliferative phase. Chronic anovulation can also present with a trilaminar, thickened endometrial stripe because of the unopposed estrogen effect.

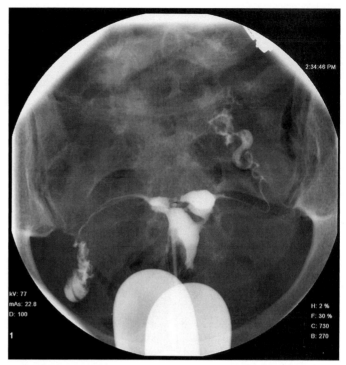

**Figure 57-5    Hysterosalpingogram of the uterus.** An intrauterine adhesion or synechia is noted by the displaced contrast material.

situation deserve an endometrial biopsy. Secondary amenorrhea with unopposed endogenous estrogen may have an increased risk for progression to complex hyperplasia with atypia or endometrial cancer. Lastly, irregular areas of thin endometrium within thicker endometrium may suggest intrauterine adhesions or Asherman's syndrome.[38] Transvaginal ultrasound is only about 52% accurate in making the diagnosis of intrauterine adhesions alone.[39] Saline infusion sonohysterography is a technique by which saline is injected into the uterine cavity through a catheter with a balloon or acorn plug to block backflow through the cervix (Fig. 57-4). This technique allows for improvement in the diagnosis of intrauterine synechiae to about 90% to 100%.[39] A hysterosalpingogram (HSG) may also reveal the diagnosis of

synechiae (Fig. 57-5). Pelvic ultrasound yields more information than HSG especially regarding the appearance of the ovaries and the endometrial stripe, which can help guide the amenorrhea assessment. In addition, a hematometra is easily detected by pelvic ultrasound as well as by computed tomography (CT) (Fig. 57-6) or magnetic resonance imaging (MRI).

At a minimum the evaluation tests (Table 57-4) should include a pregnancy test, TSH level, and prolactin level in a

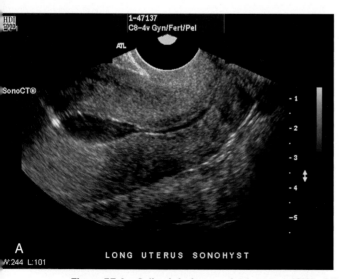

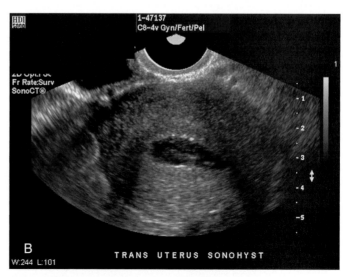

**Figure 57-4    Saline infusion sonohysterogram (SIS) of the uterus.** A, The transvaginal ultrasonogram of the uterus in the longitudinal position is shown. The hypoechoic area within the uterine cavity is saline, which was injected during the SIS procedure. B, The transvaginal ultrasonogram of the transverse uterus near the fundus is shown with saline within the uterine cavity.

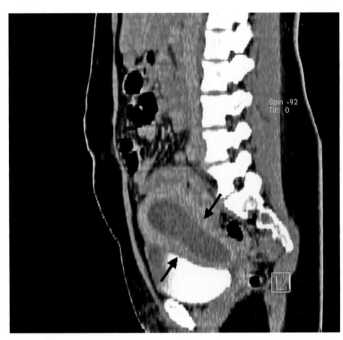

**Figure 57-6    CT scan of the uterus.** This sagital CT scan with contrast is notable for a uterus that is distended with blood, also known as hematometra, due to cervical stenosis. The arrows demonstrate the position of the uterocervical junction. Both the uterus and the cervical canal were distended after a prior loop electrical excision procedure. The bladder contains contrast material and is anterior to the uterus.

reproductive-aged woman. If there are concerns about hypoestrogenism, then FSH and estradiol measurements are warranted. An elevated FSH with a low estradiol suggests ovarian failure. This test should be repeated a month later to confirm this diagnosis. Most of these women will have hot flashes if they have been exposed to endogenous estrogen previously (as is presumed in secondary amenorrhea). A normal or low FSH with a low estradiol suggests hypothalamic amenorrhea; this group of patients rarely complain of other symptoms besides secondary amenorrhea.

The third-generation TSH test is a highly sensitive test that can detect hyper- or hypothyroidism. In the case of hypothyroidism there may be a concurrent elevation in prolactin levels in 0% to 40% of cases, and 85% of hypothyroid patients with hyperprolactinemia normalize the prolactin levels with thyroid therapy.[40] A case of pituitary gland hyperplasia in primary hypothyroidism regressed with aggressive thyroid hormone therapy.[41] Control of thyroid disease can result in resolution of anovulation and resumption of normal menstrual cycling.

Hyperprolactinemia deserves further evaluation. Multiple causes need to be considered. A mild elevation in prolactin maybe due to hypothyroidism, pregnancy, or a poorly timed test. Certain medications (e.g., antidepressants) may elevate the prolactin level and make the laboratory interpretation difficult. First, the prolactin level should be retested in the ideal setting: fasting, morning, follicular phase, and prior to any exercise, sex, or breast manipulation.[42] If the prolactin level is still elevated, even mildly, then MRI of the head is recommended to determine the presence or absence of a pituitary tumor. Fifty to sixty

percent of women with hyperprolactinemia, regardless of level, have a pituitary tumor. MRI can also determine whether there is extension of a pituitary tumor into the bony structures above the sella turcica to rule out potential compression of the optic nerve or, conversely, another CNS lesion may be compressing the pituitary stalk and indirectly cause hyperprolactinemia.

Pituitary tumors are designated as microadenomas when their size is less than 10 mm and as macroadenomas when their size is greater than 10 mm (Fig. 57-7). Approximately 90% of prolactinomas are small.[43] It is rare for a microadenoma to progress to a macroadenoma even without treatment.[44] On the other hand, all macroadenomas must have been microadenomas at one point in time, though macroadenomas are much rarer.[45] Macroadenomas increase in size about 20% to 33% of the time.[46]

The most common pituitary tumor is the prolactin-secreting pituitary adenoma or prolactinoma, and it makes up about 40% of all pituitary tumors.[43] Nonsecreting pituitary tumors make up another 30% to 40%, followed by ACTH-secreting tumors and GH-secreting tumors at 2% to 10% each, and lastly by TSH-secreting tumors at 1%.[45,47] Nonsecreting pituitary tumor patients may secrete excess α- or β-subunit FSH as measured by radioimmunoassays.[48] Occasionally, a nonpituitary tumor or mass compressing the pituitary stalk or distorting the pituitary anatomy may result in hyperprolactinemia without a prolactinoma being present. In autopsy reports, 3% to 27% of asymptomatic patients were found to have occult pituitary tumors and about 10% of normal live human volunteers had pituitary tumors of 3 to 6 mm size on MRI of the pituitary[49]—these asymptomatic tumors are referred to as incidentalomas. Another study showed that 88% of asymptomatic individuals with "incidentalomas"

| Table 57-4 | |
|---|---|
| **Diagnostic Evaluation for Secondary Amenorrhea** | |
| **Routinely Performed Tests** | **Excluded Disorder** |
| Urine or serum hCG | Pregnancy |
| TSH | Hypo- or hyperthyroidism |
| PRL | Hyperprolactinemia |
| FSH and estradiol | Hyper- or hypogonadotropic hypogonadism |
| Ultrasound | Ovarian and uterine abnormalities (neoplasms, polycystic-appearing ovaries, leiomyomas, endometrial hyperplasia, pregnancy, intrauterine adhesions, hematometrium) |
| **Tests Performed Based on Presentation or History** | **Excluded Disorder** |
| 17-hydroxyprogesterone | Nonclassical congenital adrenal hyperplasia |
| Dexamethasone suppression test or 24-hour urine free cortisol | Cushing's syndrome |
| MRI of head or abdomen/pelvis | Neoplasms (cerebral, pituitary, ovarian or adrenal) |
| Progesterone withdrawal test | Hypoestrogenism (less reliable and unnecessary if FSH and estradiol are measured) |

FSH, follicle-stimulating hormone; hCG, human chorionic gonadotropin; MRI, magnetic resonance imaging; PRL, prolactin; TSH, thyroid-stimulating hormone.

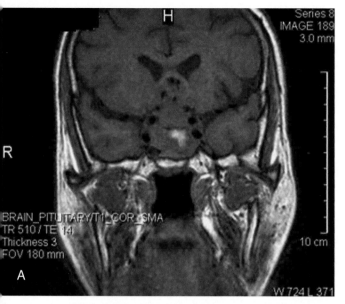 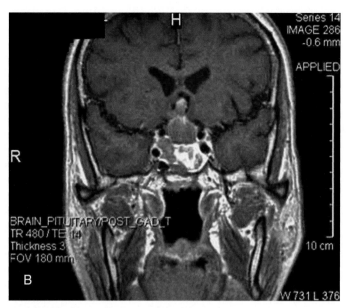

**Figure 57-7    MRI of the head.** *A,* MRI focuses on the pituitary gland without gadolinium. *B,* MRI after gadolinium. Note the enhancement of the pituitary macroadenoma after the gadolinium. (Courtesy of Dr. Alvaro Magalaes.)

ranging in size between 5 and 25 mm could be followed without surgery and that these tumors are benign.[50] Other etiologies in this differential diagnosis include craniopharyngiomas, meningiomas, arachnoid cysts, granulomatous diseases, gliomas, metastatic tumors, chordomas, germ cell tumors, and other cell rest tumors and benign lesions.[27,45,47] Most hormone over-secreting tumors have few clinical symptoms and typically are subtle and slowly progressive clinically.[45] In addition to the above screening, clinical screening for hormone oversecretion is indicated and should include insulin-like growth factor 1 (most sensitive for acromegaly) or growth hormone (GH) level after an oral glucose load (normal GH level <2 ng/L) and a test for Cushing's disease (24-hour urinary free cortisol or an overnight dexamethasone suppression test).

## Polycystic Ovary Syndrome, Nonclassical Adrenal Hyperplasia, and Hyperandrogenism

The diagnosis of PCOS is a clinical diagnosis after exclusion of other etiologies with similar symptoms of anovulation, hyper-androgenism, and possibly obesity (e.g., hypothyroidism, late-onset or nonclassical congenital adrenal hyperplasia, and hyperprolactinemia). Nonclassical congenital adrenal hyperplasia can be screened for via a basal 17-hydroxyprogesterone level; elevation over 200 ng/dL requires further testing with an ACTH stimulation test.[51] The clinical diagnosis of PCOS is based on a triad of symptoms and signs: oligomenorrhea/amenorrhea, hyperandrogenism (by clinical examination or laboratory values), and polycystic-appearing ovaries on ultrasound, according to the last consensus statement.[52] Hyperandrogenism may consist of hirsutism and acne or may have no external symptoms, just elevated androgens in reproductive-aged women (elevated or high normal total testosterone or free testosterone or other androgen).[53] Asians are more likely to have elevated androgen levels than hirsutism or acne when the diagnosis is PCOS syndrome. Other groups may be similar. Polycystic-appearing ovaries on ultrasound (see Fig. 57-2) consists of multiple small

follicles (>10 follicles per ovary that are less than 10 mm in size). These small preantral follicles may be aligned along the cortical border of the ovary, called the "pearl necklace" sign. The diagnosis of PCOS does not rely on the LH:FSH ratio, although this ratio may be elevated at or over 2:1. Some PCOS patients have normal LH:FSH ratios. A subset of patients with PCOS syndrome has insulin resistance, and this should be evaluated. Skin findings of acanthosis nigricans suggest the presence of insulin resistance.[53] There are several ways to diagnose insulin resistance: an elevated fasting insulin level, an increased ratio of insulin to glucose, or increased levels of insulin during a glucose challenge test. These patients are at increased risk for type 2 diabetes and should be screened with a fasting glucose level regularly. Two fasting glucose levels on separate occasions that are greater than 126 mg/dL indicate the presence of type 2 diabetes, according to the American Diabetes Society.

Highly elevated androgens (total testosterone >200 ng/dL or dehydroepiandrosterone sulfate [DHEA-S] >700 µg/dL) with rapidly worsening hirsutism or virilization may be indicators of a tumor in the ovary or adrenal gland. Elevated total testosterone with normal DHEA-S suggests that the tumor likely originates in the ovary and not the adrenal gland. Occasionally, PCOS presents with a high testosterone and a pelvic ultrasound is indicated to evaluate the ovaries for the presence of a neoplasm. If both the total testosterone and the DHEA-S levels are elevated, the tumor is more likely to be in the adrenal gland. MRI of the abdomen/pelvis and possibly the head is warranted to confirm the diagnosis. MRI is preferred over CT because it can visualize soft tissue structures better (pituitary, ovaries, etc.) without artifacts from bony structures.

If symptoms of Cushing's syndrome are present, a 24-hour urine free cortisol test or a dexamethasone suppression test is indicated to make the diagnosis. A dexamethasone suppression test is performed by giving 1 mg dexamethasone at about 10 or 11 PM and then measuring the fasting morning cortisol level the next morning at 8 AM, which should be suppressed (<5 mg/dL).

Reproductive Endocrinology Infertility

An elevated cortisol deserves further evaluation for Cushing's syndrome or other sources of cortisol production with either a long dexamethasone suppression test or MRI.

## TREATMENT BY DIAGNOSIS AND OUTCOME

The treatment for secondary amenorrhea depends on the etiology.

### Hypothalamic Amenorrhea

In hypothalamic amenorrhea, the patient is not making much estrogen or progesterone because there is no stimulus from the hypothalamus and thus the rest of the HPO axis is not activated. It is important to identify and treat the cause whenever possible. Ninety-four percent of these patients have reversible causes, and only 6% have irreversible conditions.[16] Causes may be stress, eating disorders, excessive exercise, or organic disease, such as CNS tumors.[25,26,54] MRI should be performed to rule out a CNS lesion prior to any medical therapy. CNS lesions causing hypothalamic amenorrhea may need surgical intervention and deserve referral to a neurosurgeon for assessment. Once a CNS tumor is ruled out, it is important to treat any identified causes (e.g., reduce stress, deal with eating disorders, meet nutritional needs, and reduce excessive exercise). Treating the cause leads to ovulatory cycles within 12 months, but as many as 30% remain amenorrheic.[5] Despite therapy, patients with eating disorders often replace their eating problem with excessive exercise, which continues the hypothalamic amenorrhea. Amenorrhea due to excessive exercise may be, in part, due to inadequate nutritional replacement. Increased exercise increases the nutritional requirements. Yet, protein, fat, and total caloric intake are often lower than needed in relation to the increased energy demands of exercise in amenorrheic athletes.[24] Body composition and psychological stress may also be playing a role. The initial therapy for excessive exercise is to reduce the amount of exercise and to modify dietary intake appropriately; this is usually sufficient for resumption of menstrual cycles. In addition, patients with anorexia nervosa benefit from participation of a team of experts in their therapy. This team may consist of a medical physician or gynecologist, nutritionist, and psychiatrist.

Hypothalamic amenorrhea has the greatest detrimental impact on bone when it occurs during adolescence. These individuals are at increased risk of not achieving their normal peak bone mass. With a lower peak bone mass, they will be at increased risk of osteopenia and osteoporosis later in adult life.[55,56] The amount of bone loss is directly proportional to the duration of hypoestrogenism.[55] The minimum level of estradiol to maintain bone mineral density is estimated to be 60 pg/mL.[24]

Concurrent hormonal supplementation and calcium and vitamin supplements are warranted in patients with hypothalamic amenorrhea to protect against rapid bone loss. Hormonal supplementation may be given in a variety of ways: cyclically to mimic a menstrual cycle or continuously to maintain the amenorrhea, yet treat the bone loss issue. Cyclically, a conjugated estrogen (0.625 mg/day) or ethinyl estradiol (1–2 mg/day) is given daily and a progestin (5–10 mg) or progesterone (100–200 mg) is given for 12 to 14 days per month. It is usually easiest to pick an easy-to-remember day like the first of each month to start the progestin or progesterone therapy. Continuously, hormones may be given with the same dose of estrogenic compound but a lower dose of progestin (e.g., 2.5 mg) per day. Alternatively, higher dose hormones, such as birth control pills or the contraceptive vaginal ring or patch may be administered to achieve the same purpose.[57] In the reproductive-age group, some women prefer one of the hormonal contraceptive methods, whether or not they are sexually active, since their peers may be using contraceptive therapy and the patients may perceive it as more acceptable. In situations such as amenorrhea due to anorexia nervosa or excessive exercise the patient may prefer a continuous regimen of hormonal contraceptives without using the placebo pills and without breaks in treatment in the hope of maintaining the amenorrhea (iatrogenically) but lessening the adverse sequelae of hypoestrogenism. Prolonged therapy with a progestin-dominant drug as in hormonal contraceptive therapy leads to endometrial atrophy and amenorrhea. Over time some of these individuals may have breakthrough bleeding, which responds to a short course of supplemental estrogen. Beside the possible minor side effect if breakthrough bleeding, there is no known medical contraindication to continuous use of oral contraceptives, vaginal rings, or patches, even for years at a time. This regimen has been a common practice for women with pelvic pain and endometriosis.[58] A number of athletes and dancers (e.g., ballerinas) appreciate the medically induced amenorrhea. It is a wonderful approach in the right patient.

### Fertility with Hypothalamic Amenorrhea

Women with persistent hypogonadotropic hypogonadism (i.e., hypothalamic amenorrhea) who wish to conceive usually receive pretreatment with estradiol and progesterone cyclically for at least 1 month (1–2 mg ethinyl estradiol or 0.625–2.5 mg conjugated estrogen daily overlapping the last 10–14 days with 5–10 mg medroxyprogesterone or 100–200 mg progesterone). This hormonal pretreatment up-regulates the gonadotropin receptors, and then these patients are given gonadotropin therapy. It is possible to override most causes of hypothalamic amenorrhea with gonadotropin therapy, but it is better to address the underlying cause of the hypothalamic amenorrhea first. For these patients, pharmacologic doses of gonadotropins (a combination of FSH and LH) are used as injectable therapy to directly stimulate the ovaries. Since the ovaries and uterus are physiologically normal, the ovaries respond with follicular growth and the uterine lining proliferates in response to the ovarian follicular estradiol production. These patients will rarely respond to the milder oral fertility drug clomiphene citrate. Clomiphene citrate requires an intact and functioning HPO axis, since it works like an antiestrogen and indirectly stimulates the hypothalamus to stimulate the pituitary to secrete FSH and LH, which then stimulate the ovaries. Once these patients ovulate, they have similar pregnancy rates as their age-matched cohorts,[59] and they will need luteal progesterone support to maintain the pregnancy. They are still at increased risk for multiple gestation and ovarian hyperstimulation with gonadotropin therapy.

Alternatively, these patients could be treated with GnRH therapy with 90% success for ovulation.[5] GnRH therapy is administered with an intravenous or subcutaneous pulsatile pump, which allows only one or two follicles to mature and ovulate. Again, the luteal phase after ovulation needs to be supplemented, either with the GnRH pump or with progesterone supplementation. These GnRH pump–treated patients have a lower risk of multiple gestation. This treatment can be effective in the compliant and dedicated patient with a closely monitoring physician. However, it is cumbersome in the daily life of the patient and is prone to difficulties (e.g., clotting of the catheter, catheter falling out, infection, moving the site every few days). Due to its low level of use in the United States, the pharmaceutical company that made the GnRH pump voluntarily took it off the market, and therefore it is difficult to find. Research is currently under way to consider alternative routes of administration. Perhaps there may be a GnRH patch in the near future that will be easier to use and this therapy will become more popular. Psychological support in the form of counseling may also benefit these patients.

## Hypergonadotropic Hypoestrogenism

Hypergonadotropic hypoestrogenism specifically describes patients with amenorrhea due to elevated gonadotropins (FSH >30 or 40 mIU/mL, depending on the laboratory, and performed on at least two occasions separated by 1 month or more) and low estrogen (<50 pg/mL). In patients with amenorrhea due to hypergonadotropic hypoestrogenism and under 40 years of age, the diagnosis is premature ovarian failure (POF). The incidence is approximately 1%.[30] This disorder can occur in patients with primary or secondary amenorrhea. It is more common for patients with secondary amenorrhea to have the associated hot flashes than for those with primary amenorrhea (85.6% vs 22.2%).[60]

Chromosomal abnormalities occurred in 13.3% of women with secondary amenorrhea due to premature ovarian failure.[16] Trisomy, mosaicism, balanced translocations, and monosomy have all been reported.[60] Individuals with an abnormal karyotype and the presence of a Y chromosome or a portion of the Y chromosome may be at increased risk of a gonadal tumor formation (most often a gonadoblastoma), and the gonads should be excised.[61,62] To date, there are no reported cases of secondary amenorrhea in patients with POF and a karyotype containing a Y chromosome. In the case of Turner's mosaic (45,X; 46,XY), the gonads may be difficult to completely identify either by laparoscopy or laparotomy, since these gonads are streaks (unless a tumor is present). These streaks may extend anywhere along the ovarian suspensory ligament to the upper infundibular pelvic ligament, at or above the pelvic brim. If the karyotype does not include a portion of the Y chromosome, then the gonads do not need to be extirpated. Occasionally, a true Turner's syndrome patient has secondary amenorrhea[63]; the majority have primary amenorrhea, delayed puberty, and other stigmata (e.g., short stature, webbed neck, increased carrying angle, low hairline).

Immune disturbances are fairly common in this POF group (17.4%) and consist of a majority of thyroid disorders and rarely vitiligo, hypoparathyroidism, Addison's disease, insulin-dependent diabetes mellitus, and polymyositis. Other common causes of POF are iatrogenic: chemotherapy, radiation therapy (even if irradiation is not to the pelvis but focused above the diaphragm), or ovarian surgery. Approximately 3.5% of patients developed POF after infection with chickenpox, shigellosis, malaria, or an undefined viral syndrome.[60] POF may also occur with a systemic disease (e.g., galactosemia). About 28% of POF patients have a familial history of POF.[29] There have been isolated reports of resumption of menses, some with reported pregnancies, in patients with POF; however, there are no tests to predict who will have resumption of menses. Resumption of menses is estimated to occur in 10% of cases and less than 1% of these patients have conceived. Withdrawal bleeding in response to progestin occurred in about 50% of these patients, again indicating that progestin withdrawal is not an accurate test. Laparoscopic ovarian biopsies are also unreliable; Rebar and Connolly[60] reported on three patients with no ovarian follicles on biopsy specimens who later resumed menses and ovulated. There is no medical reason to perform a biopsy on these ovaries, and laparoscopy should not be part of this workup. These patients are also at risk for accelerated bone loss and osteopenia.

The initial evaluation should include a full workup for any of the potentially serious disorders associated with hypergonadotropic hypoestrogenic amenorrhea, including complete blood count with differential, sedimentation rate, total serum protein, albumin/globulin ratio, rheumatoid factor, antinuclear antibody, fasting blood sugar, morning fasting cortisol, serum calcium and phosphorus, free thyroxine, TSH, antithyroglobulin antibodies, antimicrosomal antibodies, thyroid-stimulating immunoglobulins, and karyotype. There is no reason to look for ovarian antibodies, except on a research protocol. A baseline dual-energy X-ray absorption (DEXA) test of the hip and lumbar spine can be considered, particularly if the patient has been hypoestrogenic for a long period of time.

The treatment for patients with POF is to alleviate the hypoestrogenic symptoms (hot flashes, vaginal dryness, etc.) and to decrease bone loss. Therapy can be given as hormone replacement therapy or contraceptive hormones, similar to the treatment for hypothalamic amenorrhea described above. Some patients require a higher dose of estrogen to relieve their menopausal symptoms (particularly hot flashes). The dose may range from 0.625 to 2.5 mg/day of conjugated estrogens or from 1 to 2 mg/day of ethinyl estradiol. Typically, it takes approximately a month to reach a steady state. Progestins, as noted above, should be given to anyone who still has an intact uterus to avoid the increased risk of endometrial hyperplasia or carcinoma. The progestins may be given cyclically, continuously, or every 3 months. Contraceptive hormones are also effective in reducing menopausal symptoms and protecting against bone loss.[57] Either therapy is acceptable. POF is often an emotional situation for patients. Counseling should be recommended. A small percentage of these patients develop "polyglandular syndrome type II." In this syndrome, other endocrine glands may become hypofunctioning over time. Consequently, these individuals should be tested every 1 to 2 years for endocrinopathies and immune disorders. Any identified abnormalities should be further assessed and treated.

Since it is unpredictable who will and who will not ovulate in POF, hormone replacement therapy given in a cyclic fashion will mimic a natural cycle and will not suppress any natural ovulations, should they occur. Some patients like to have this opportunity. Obviously, if ovulation occurs, there will likely be bleeding at an unexpected time, or less likely, persistent amenorrhea during an expected withdrawal bleed owing to conception.[64] One retrospective study noted that patients with

# Reproductive Endocrinology Infertility

secondary ovarian failure had an 11.1% chance of ovulating on estradiol replacement and a 4.8% chance of conception.[65] There is really no treatment that predictably reverses this ovarian failure process or induces ovulation effectively and reliably. A few prospective randomized studies investigated the down-regulation of FSH and LH levels by use of a GnRH agonist for endogenous gonadotropin suppression followed by treatment with gonadotropins to stimulate ovulation without significant success.[66,67] These findings offer little hope for conception with a patient's oocytes. However, these patients are excellent candidates to be egg donor recipients, once the endometrium is adequately prepared. Pregnancy rates in these patients with donor oocytes are high (currently ranging from 40% to 70% per cycle, depending on the center). However, the decision to use donor oocytes may be a difficult hurdle to overcome. A special note regarding Turner's syndrome patients: donor egg programs have been successful at getting Turner's syndrome patients pregnant but there is an increased risk of aortic dissection and a half-dozen Turner's syndrome patients have died as a result.[68] There is controversy over whether Turner's syndrome patients should proceed with donor oocyte programs. Certainly, an echocardiogram and aortic assessment are indicated prior to conception and possibly periodically during the pregnancy.

When hypergonadotropic hypogonadism occurs at 40 years of age or older, it is referred to as early menopause. Again, hormone therapy is indicated to treat symptoms and to protect against accelerated bone loss. These individuals are less likely to have as high a risk for immunologic or endocrine disorders than younger patients; routine general health screening is indicated. Again, these patients are good candidates for donor oocyte programs but have a low likelihood of conception with their own oocytes.

## Pituitary Causes: Hyperprolactinemia

Hyperprolactinemia that results in secondary amenorrhea also is associated with hypoestrogenism. It is important to correct the hyperprolactinemia and thus reverse the hypoestrogenism and stop the accelerated bone loss. Prolactin-secreting micro- and macroadenomas both are initially treated medically with a dopamine agonist, such as bromocriptine or cabergoline. This medication is slowly titrated upward until it brings the prolactin level into the normal range. Slow titration of oral doses or vaginal placement of oral tablets may help reduce side effects. The side effects of bromocriptine are often more prevalent than of cabergoline. The types of side effect are similar for the two medications and include nausea, headache, and dizziness; other side effects have less than 10% incidence. Within a few months after the prolactin level is under control, menstrual cycling often recurs. If a couple is interested in conceiving, they can then try. In the event that conception occurs, medical therapy is discontinued in the case of microadenomas, since microadenomas are rarely aggressive. In the case of macroadenomas, the medication is continued throughout pregnancy. Bromocriptine and cabergoline are Pregnancy Category B drugs. The surgical approach for macroadenomas is reserved for those tumors which are resistant to medical therapy and for those patients who cannot tolerate the side effects of the medication. Medical therapy can reduce the size of macroadenomas by 10%, but close followup with radiologic evaluation every 6 to 12 months

is required. Observation is another alternative for macroadenomas without visual field defects, since only about 33% increase in size; again close observation with frequent MRI is indicated. If tumor growth occurs or if there are visual field defects, surgery is indicated. Surgical treatment may not totally remove the tumor, and medical therapy may be needed postsurgically.

If the patient is not interested in conceiving and has a microadenoma, it is likely that she will decrease her dose of dopamine agonist (bromocriptine or cabergoline) after a year or two of therapy. When she is tapered off the therapy, she may continue menstrual cycling and the prolactin level may remain normal.

Alternatively, a patient with a prolactin-secreting microadenoma may choose not to use dopamine agonist therapy to control her hyperprolactinemia, but to use only hormone therapy (estradiol and progestin) to treat the hypoestrogenism resulting from the hyperprolactinemia. Hormonal therapy alone is perfectly acceptable when a patient has a microadenoma because it rarely progresses in size. Bone mineral density loss is a significant medical concern in these patients, so they should be treated with either hormonal replacement or reversal of the hyperprolactinemia to avoid significant bone loss. Bone mineral density monitoring is indicated.

## Thyroid Disease: Either Primary Hypothyroidism or Hyperthyroidism

The initial screening test for thyroid disease is a serum TSH measurement. Most laboratories measure a highly sensitive or third-generation TSH level, which can detect both hypothyroidism (elevated TSH) and hyperthyroidism (low TSH). If serum TSH is abnormal, it should be repeated and a free thyroxine (tetraiodothyronine or $T_4$) level added. Hypothyroidism is much more common than hyperthyroidism. Primary hypothyroidism or hypothyroidism originating in the thyroid gland is diagnosed by an elevated TSH and a low free thyroxine ($T_4$) level. It is treated with daily oral levothyroxine therapy that is started at 0.05 mg/day and increased slowly over 6- to 8-week intervals to bring the serum levels into the normal range; typically the replacement dose is 0.1 to 0.2 mg/day (or 100 to 200 μg/day). This medication is usually well tolerated. Jitteriness, sweats, and palpitations may occur if the dose is started too high or moved up too quickly. These patients should be followed every 6 to 8 weeks until the thyroid function tests normalize and are stable, and then every 6 to 12 months with laboratory evaluations.

Subclinical hypothyroidism is diagnosed by an elevated TSH and a normal free $T_4$ concentration. In patients who desire to conceive soon, it is reasonable to treat subclinical hypothyroidism with low doses of levothyroxine (usually <100 μg/day is needed to control TSH level). If fertility is not a present concern, no treatment is necessary; the patient is followed up with repeat laboratory assessment in 6 to 12 months and treated when clinically significant hypothyroidism occurs.

Other thyroid disorders may figure in the etiology of secondary amenorrhea (see Chapter 63). Again briefly, if both TSH and free $T_4$ levels are low, secondary hypothyroidism or hypothyroidism due to a pituitary origin may be present and further evaluation with MRI and other pituitary function testing are indicated.

Hyperthyroidism deserves further evaluation with laboratory tests for antithyroid antibodies, possibly thyroid ultrasound, and radioiodine uptake screening. Thyroid nodules may require fine needle aspiration or biopsy. Medical therapy for hyperthyroidism consists of methimazole or propylthiouracil (PTU). Radioactive iodine therapy is often the procedure of choice for hyperthyroidism but may leave the patient hypothyroid and then thyroid replacement therapy is indicated. There is also a role for surgical therapy in some cases of hyperthyroidism and thyroid carcinoma. Occasionally, hyperthyroidism results from overtreatment of hypothyroidism. Whatever the cause of hyperthyroidism, it will have a significant negative impact on bone metabolism, resulting in increased bone loss, if it is not corrected.

## Polycystic Ovary Syndrome

PCOS is a common disorder that is diagnosed clinically by the triad of oligomenorrhea/amenorrhea, hyperandrogenism, and polycystic-appearing ovaries. Treatment is directed at either inducing ovulation or giving a progestational agent. Prolonged time periods without progestin treatment expose the patient to unopposed estrogen, which can eventually cause endometrial carcinoma. In patients with a history of chronic anovulation without treatment, an endometrial biopsy is warranted, prior to initiating therapy, to rule out endometrial carcinoma or precancer (e.g., complex hyperplasia with atypia). Once this is ruled out, a patient may be treated monthly (or at least every 3 months) with progestin or progesterone. The progestin regimen may consist of medroxyprogesterone at 5 to 10 mg/day for 7 to 14 days. This therapy will induce a withdrawal bleed within 2 weeks of the completion of therapy, when endogenous estrogen production has been present to develop an endometrial lining. Alternative therapies to medroxyprogesterone include progesterone vaginal cream or progesterone 100 to 200 mg/day for 10 to 14 days, vaginal micronized progesterone gel 4% to 8% every other day for 6 doses, or a 100-mg injection of progesterone in oil. Some practitioners use this progesterone withdrawal therapy to confirm the presence of estrogen production in lieu of measuring estradiol and FSH levels, but this test is less reliable. Alternatively, patients may choose oral contraceptives or contraceptive rings or patches for treatment. The latter two treatments are also progestin-dominant therapies that cause the endometrium to atrophy and additionally offer contraceptive benefits. For couples trying to conceive, a mild oral fertility therapy may be used. The traditional therapy is clomiphene citrate at 50 to 150 mg/day for 5 days (cycle days 3–7 or 5–9) to induce ovulation. It is effective for ovulation induction in about 60% to 80% of these patients.[69] Patients typically ovulate about 7 days after the last pill. However, there is enough variability in women that instruction in the use of an ovulation predictor kit (OPK) is helpful, and OPKs should be used on cycle days 10 to 20. A positive OPK measures the presence of urinary LH metabolites and indicates when an LH surge is present. Ovulation typically occurs 10 to 48 hours after an LH surge is detected by an OPK. The oocyte has about 12 to 24 hours after ovulation to be fertilized, and sperm survive about 2 days, on average, in the human body after ejaculation. Timing intercourse for the day before and/or the day of ovulation offers the best pregnancy rates.[70] Counseling the patient to have intercourse the day of the surge and daily (or at least every other day) for 3 days should be sufficient exposure to allow optimal opportunities for conception.

In PCOS patients with insulin resistance, an insulin sensitizer may be used. Several reports note the resumption of menstrual cycles and ovulation while this therapy is being used.[71] In the United States, metformin is the current drug of choice. This medication is started at 500 mg/day, or every other day if the gastrointestinal side effects are bothersome. The dose is increased every few weeks to a treatment range of 1500 to 2000 mg/day in divided doses (500 mg three times a day, 875 or 1000 mg twice a day). A typical mistake is to undertreat this disorder. Once the patient is in the treatment range, cycles tend to resume within a few months if they are going to resume at all. Carmina and Lobo gave metformin in a randomized placebo-controlled trial to nonandrogenic, anovulatory women at a dose of 1500 mg daily for 3 months, and the study resulted in ovulatory cycles in 58% of patients randomized to the treatment arm.[72] Clomiphene citrate can be given in addition to metformin, and ovulation results in 90% of cases, even in patients previously resistant to clomiphene citrate alone.[73,74] The main side effects are gastrointestinal disturbances (gas, diarrhea, etc.). Liver function tests (LFTs) should be monitored prior to therapy and periodically after therapy. Liver dysfunction as a result of this medication is rare; however, if LFTs increase to two times the normal limit, the medication should be discontinued.

An alternative, off-label-use, oral fertility therapy is aromatase inhibitors. Aromatase inhibitors, such as letrozole and anastrozole, have been studied in a limited number of patients in non-randomized prospective trials that report improved ovulation rates. In patients who had inadequate response to clomiphene citrate, letrozole 2.5 mg for 5 days (cycle days 3 to 7) resulted in 75% ovulation and 25% pregnancy rates.[75] Anastrozole 1 mg/day on cycle days 3 to 7 may also be used for ovulation induction, and if not successful, the dose is doubled.[76] A randomized, double-blind comparison study using letrozole and anastrozole showed improved ovulation rates (84.4% vs 60%, respectively) and improved pregnancy rates (18.8% per cycle vs 9.7% per cycle, respectively).[76] The side effects of these medications are better tolerated than those of clomiphene citrate. Only one or two follicles mature and ovulate (average, 1.5), resulting in similar pregnancy rates to clomiphene citrate but lower multiple gestation rates.

Lastly, if the PCOS patient is resistant to oral therapy, gonadotropin therapy is the next step. Over 90% of PCOS patients respond to gonadotropin therapy with ovulation. Typically, the starting dose for PCOS patients is lower than that given to patients with other diagnoses because of the increased risk of overstimulation and potential cancellation. These patients need to be closely monitored and counseled. After ovulation, these patients are also at increased risk for multiple gestation and ovarian hyperstimulation syndrome. Ovarian hyperstimulation syndrome (OHSS) is a phenomenon that occurs after ovulation induction. The syndrome is described in mild to severe levels. The main characteristics are weight gain, abdominal distention, enlarged multicystic ovaries, abdominal discomfort, hemoconcentration, hyponatremia, and hyperkalemia. As the syndrome worsens, the patient may have shortness of breath, ascites, pleural effusions, elevated liver function tests, worsening electrolytes, and dehydration. This syndrome resolves within 2 to 4 weeks with treatment consisting of aggressive hydration, bed rest with deep venous thrombosis (DVT) prophylaxis, protein supplementation, and possible paracentesis or culdocentesis. Rarely thoracentesis is necessary. Pregnancy may exacerbate OHSS and prolong its duration.

Owing to the risks of multiple gestation and particularly high-order multiple gestation, the PCOS patient may opt for in vitro fertilization (IVF). In this process the ovaries are stimulated with gonadotropin therapy, the LH surge is suppressed with either a GnRH agonist or a GnRH antagonist, and hCG is usually used to mature the follicles. The oocytes are removed just prior to ovulation by ultrasound-guided transvaginal needle aspiration. After insemination with sperm and incubation, one to three cleaved embryos (or four to five embryos in older patients) are transferred into the endometrial cavity depending on the patient's age, clinical situation, and national recommendations. Controlling the number of embryos being transferred decreases the risk of high-order multiple gestation.

Another alternative treatment for PCOS is surgical therapy with ovarian drilling. This technique consists of making small (2–3 mm) holes in the ovarian cortex with laser or electrocautery. Ovarian drilling technique is based on the historical wedge resection, which resulted in spontaneous ovulation for a limited time period. Approximately one third of patients from Stein's original report[77] continued to have regular periods for more than 6 years.[78] A randomized controlled trial comparing the effectiveness of laparoscopic electrocautery drilling of the ovaries to ovulation induction protocols[79] showed a cumulative pregnancy rate with electrocautery alone at 34%, whereas the cumulative pregnancy rates with clomiphene citrate and gonadotropins were 49% and 67%, respectively. The latter two ovulation induction treatments did not vary whether they were given alone or after electrocautery drilling. Multiple gestations are reduced if gonadotropin therapy is avoided, but the risks of surgery must be considered.

After delivery of a baby, most PCOS patients resume their anovulatory pattern and require long-term progestational therapy. Additionally, PCOS patients are at increased risk for hypertension and type 2 diabetes mellitus (non-IDDM) and should be screened regularly.[78,80]

### Late-onset or Nonclassical Congenital Adrenal Hyperplasia

Patients with late-onset or nonclassical congenital adrenal hyperplasia (CAH) typically have premature adrenarche or with a polycystic ovary–like syndrome. The clinical findings consist of oligomenorrhea or amenorrhea, hirsutism, and no virilization (classical CAH presents as ambiguous genitalia). On laboratory evaluation the 17-hydroxyprogesterone level is definitely elevated or is just over 200 ng/dL. In the latter case, an ACTH stimulation test should be performed. A baseline 17-hydroxyprogesterone level is drawn, 100 µg of ACTH (cosyntropin) is given, and a repeat 17-hydroxyprogesterone is drawn 1 hour after the ACTH is given. The baseline and stimulated results are compared with the reference normograms.[81] Typically, the 1-hour 17-hydroxyprogesterone level is in the thousands and the diagnosis of nonclassical CAH is made. Heterozygotes may not have as high a level of 17-hydroxyprogesterone. This disorder is caused by partial or complete enzyme deficiency, and 21-hydroxylase

deficiency is the most common cause. Treatment is merely to replace the deficiency in the end product—cortisol—usually using the oral form: prednisone, dexamethasone, or other equivalent. Occasionally, the patient may need a mineralocorticoid such as fluorocortisone; this is more common in the early-onset or classic form of CAH. All these patients need genetic counseling and should be offered genetic testing prior to conceiving to determine their risk for transmitting this disorder to future offspring and to discuss their need for future prenatal testing and therapy.

### Cushing's Syndrome

Cushing's syndrome may have many features that overlap with PCOS: anovulation, hirsutism, and obesity. In addition, Cushing's patients may have a "buffalo hump," striae, and hypertension. The standard diagnostic tests include the 24-hour urine free cortisol and the dexamethasone suppression test. An elevated 24-hour urine free cortisol level is abnormal, and further evaluation for a source of excess cortisol production is indicated. In the dexamethasone suppression test, 1 mg of dexamethasone is given at 10 or 11 PM and the fasting cortisol level is drawn the next morning at 8 AM. The normal response is suppression of the morning fasting cortisol level (<5 ng/dL). If the cortisol is elevated, the diagnosis is made. Further evaluation prior to therapy is indicated and may consist of a prolonged dexamethasone suppression test and MRI to localize the source of steroid production.

### Ovarian and Adrenal Neoplasms

Ovarian or adrenal neoplasms that are producing androgens are often suspected by the clinical history of rapid progression of hirsutism and virilization. Elevated total testosterone (>200 ng/dL) and DHEA-S (>700 ng/dL) levels may indicate the presence of an ovarian or an adrenal secreting tumor. Since similar amounts of testosterone are produced in the ovary and the adrenal gland, this test alone cannot specify an ovarian tumor. Both test results are needed. Since 99% of DHEA-S is produced in the adrenal, if both laboratory tests are elevated, an adrenal tumor is likely. If only the testosterone level is elevated, then the ovary is the likely culprit for an androgen-producing tumor. Ovarian neoplasms are typically best detected by ultrasound and adrenal tumors by MRI. However, very small ovarian tumors may not be detected by ultrasound, and MRI may be helpful. MRI of the abdomen and pelvis may be needed to determine whether an ovarian or adrenal neoplasm is present. If neither technique is helpful, selective catheterization may help locate the source. These neoplasms are typically treated surgically.

## OUTFLOW CAUSES OF SECONDARY AMENORRHEA AND TREATMENT

### Uterus

Pregnancy is the most common cause of amenorrhea and is normal. It is treated expectantly.

Endometrial atrophy due to progestational agents can be easily corrected by estradiol supplementation, in the form of oral, patch, gel, or vaginal ring preparations. The estradiol enables a small amount of endometrium to proliferate and stop the bleeding due to atrophy. Alternatively, the progestational agent may be stopped for a period of time to allow natural estradiol to be produced.

Endometritis (particularly pelvic tuberculosis) may cause abnormal bleeding and may result in adhesions with hypomenorrhea or amenorrhea over time. Acute endometritis needs to be treated with antibiotics—usually broad spectrum.

Asherman's syndrome results from intrauterine adhesions or synechiae due to a prior intrauterine procedure (e.g., D&C, hysteroscopic myomectomy) or infection (e.g., endometritis). It may be diagnosed on transvaginal ultrasound, saline infusion sonohysterogram, or hysterosalpingogram, as noted above. The standard approach to remove intrauterine adhesions, if the patient is interested in conceiving, is hysteroscopic adhesiolysis under direct vision and posttreatment with an intrauterine balloon for a few days, with estrogen therapy to proliferate the endometrium over previously scarred areas, followed by progesterone or a progestin for a withdrawal bleed. If the patient is not interested in conceiving, no therapy is necessary. She may remain hypomenorrheic or amenorrheic once a diagnosis is established. Since these patients are euestrogenic, there is no risk for accelerated bone loss.

## Cervix

Cervical stenosis is an uncommon cause of secondary amenorrhea. It typically results from a prior cervical procedure, such as cryosurgery or a cervical cone biopsy. It is a rare result of a loop excision electrocautery procedure (LEEP). Patients typically have amenorrhea and pelvic/abdominal pain. Ultrasonography, CT, or MRI reveals a hematometra (see Fig. 57-6). Cervical dilatation is all that is needed for menstruation to resume. This treatment may be performed in some cases with a uterine sound alone, while in others, full cervical dilation is needed. In difficult situations, the cervix does not have an identifiable cervical os or the canal is irregular. Intraoperative ultrasound guidance can be helpful. Rarely, the cervical stenosis is so severe that it cannot be corrected despite the above measures. In cases with evidence of infection or cases of prolonged hematometra, pretreatment with antibiotics before surgical correction of the cervical stenosis is indicated.

Once the cervical stenosis is corrected, these patients may still need assistance in conceiving because the cervical canal glands are likely to be scarred and not produce sufficient mucus for the sperm to swim through to the uterus. These patients tend to respond well to timed intrauterine inseminations with or without superovulation therapy.

Some patients with cervical stenosis also have a very short cervix, particularly after an aggressive cone biopsy, which may have been necessary because of an abnormal Pap smear but is problematic for maintaining a pregnancy. In such cases, the obstetrician would like to be aware of the problem early so that cerclage therapy may be considered.

## BONE HEALTH

In most situations where hypoestrogenism exists for prolonged time periods, there is significant risk for bone loss. Whether the hypoestrogenism is due to hypogonadotropism (hypothalamic amenorrhea) or to hypergonadotropism (premature ovarian failure), the impact on bone is similar. If the hypoestrogenism occurs during adolescence, the peak bone mass may not be attained. The duration of hypoestrogenism directly correlates with the amount of bone loss. Consequently, there should be a low threshold for starting hormone (replacement) therapy. Estrogen therapy has a direct impact on bone metabolism and on absorption of calcium through the gastrointestinal system.

In addition to appropriate replacement of estrogen, sufficient dietary intake of calcium and vitamin D is important. Calcium supplementation should be on the order of 1200 to 1500 mg/day in divided doses. For bone health, vitamin D intake should be higher than currently supplied in multivitamins; vitamin D supplements should total 400 to 800 IU/day or greater.

## SUMMARY

In general, patients with secondary amenorrhea should be evaluated by a thorough history, physical examination, and ultrasound examination to narrow the differential diagnosis and to direct the laboratory and radiologic evaluations to help identify the etiology. The hypothalamic-pituitary-ovarian-uterine axis approach as outlined above is a logical approach to assessing and treating secondary amenorrhea. The WHO classification system is another usable approach. Once a diagnosis is identified, it is important to treat the cause (e.g., hypothyroidism, pituitary adenoma, infection, stress, outflow tract scarring, or obstruction).

If the patient has persistent anovulation, treatment with a progestational agent is indicated to reduce the risk for endometrial hyperplasia. If there has been a prolonged time period of unopposed estrogen exposure, an endometrial biopsy is warranted before therapy. If the patient desires conception, begin treatment with ovulation induction. The progesterone that is produced during pregnancy as well as the pregnancy itself will prevent endometrial hyperplasia. If the patient is not interested in pregnancy at this time, treatment with hormonal contraceptives or cyclic progestins is the therapy of choice.

In patients with hypoestrogenic amenorrhea (i.e., hypothalamic amenorrhea or hypergonadotropic hypogonadism), estrogen production needs to be induced by treatment of the cause or to be replaced by estrogen supplementation. The estrogen therapy along with calcium and vitamin D supplementation are needed to prevent bone loss. Patients will also need progesterone therapy to avoid the "unopposed estrogen" situation that predisposes to endometrial hyperplasia or carcinoma. Hormonal replacement therapy or oral contraceptive therapy is recommended. When patients with hypothalamic amenorrhea wish to conceive and have not resumed menstrual cycling, they will need either gonadotropin therapy or pulsatile GnRH therapy for ovulation and then luteal support to allow for conception. In patients with hypergonadotropic hypogonadism (premature ovarian failure), the only method to reliably achieve pregnancy is with an oocyte donation program.

In patients with hypoestrogenic amenorrhea due to ovarian failure, estrogen supplementation is important to relieve hot flashes and vaginal dryness and maintain bone mineral density among other benefits. Again, hormone replacement therapy or hormonal contraception is appropriate. It is only this group of patients with POF who are unlikely to be fertile in the future despite any therapy. Luckily, less than 1% of women under age 40 have premature ovarian failure. Unfortunately, less than 10% of these women will ovulate again in their lifetime.[60]

# REFERENCES

1. Gallinelli A, Matteo ML, Volpe A, et al: Autonomic and neuro-endocrine responses to stress in patients with functional hypothalamic secondary amenorrhea. Fertil Steril 2000;73:812–816. **(IIa, B)**

2. Practice Committee of the American Society for Reproductive Medicine: Current evaluation of amenorrhea. Fertil Steril 2004;82: 266–272. **(IV, C)**

3. Insler V: Gonadotropin therapy: new trends and insights. Int J Fertil 1988;33:85–97. **(IV, C)**

4. Adashi EY, Hennebold JD: Single-gene mutations resulting in reproductive dysfunction in women. N Engl J Med 1999;340:709–718. **(III, B)**

5. Marshall JC, Eagleson CA, McCartney CR: Hypothalamic dysfunction. Mol Cell Endocrinol 2001;183:29–32. **(IV, C)**

6. Blumenkrantz MJ, Gallagher GN, Bashore RA, Tenckhoff H: Retrograde menstruation in women undergoing chronic peritoneal dialysis. Obstet Gynecol 1981;57:667–670. **(III, B)**

7. Pettersson F, Fries H, Nillius SJ: Epidemiology of secondary amenorrhea. 1. Incidence and prevalence rates. Am J Obstet Gynecol 1973;117: 80–86. **(III, B)**

8. Bachmann GA, Kemmann E: Prevalence of oligomenorrhea and amenorrhea in a college population. Am J Obstet Gynecol 1982;144: 98–102. **(IIb, B)**

9. Mavroudis K: Clinical syndromes of secondary amenorrhea. Ann N Y Acad Sci 1997;816:241–249. **(IV, C)**

10. Hernandez I, Cervera-Aguilar R, Vergara MD, et al: [Prevalence and etiology of secondary amenorrhea in a selected Mexican population]. Ginecol Obstet Mex 1999;67:374–376. **(III, B)**

11. Anderson SE, Dallal GE, Must A: Relative weight and race influence average age at menarche: results from two nationally representative surveys of US girls studied 25 years apart. Pediatrics 2003;111(Pt 1): 844–850. **(III, B)**

12. Chumlea WC, Schubert CM, Roche AF, et al: Age at menarche and racial comparisons in US girls. Pediatrics 2003;111:110–113. **(III, B)**

13. Slap GB: Menstrual disorders in adolescence. Best Pract Res Clin Obstet Gynaecol 2003;17:75–92. **(IV, C)**

14. Herman-Giddens ME, Slora EJ, Wasserman RC, et al: Secondary sexual characteristics and menses in young girls seen in office practice: a study from the Pediatric Research in Office Settings network. Pediatrics 1997;99:505–512. **(III, B)**

15. Parent AS, Teilmann G, Juul A, et al: The timing of normal puberty and the age limits of sexual precocity: variations around the world, secular trends, and changes after migration. Endocr Rev 2003;24:668–693. **(IV, C)**

16. Reindollar RH, Novak M, Tho SP, et al: Adult-onset amenorrhea: a study of 262 patients. Am J Obstet Gynecol 1986;155:531–543. **(III, B)**

17. Kadar N, Caldwell BV, Romero R: A method of screening for ectopic pregnancy and its indications. Obstet Gynecol 1981;58:162–166. **(III, B)**

18. Bisaga K, Petkova E, Cheng J, et al: Menstrual functioning and psychopathology in a county-wide population of high school girls. J Am Acad Child Adolesc Psychiatry 2002;41:1197–1204. **(III, B)**

19. la Marca A, Morgante G, De Leo V: Evaluation of hypothalamic-pituitary-adrenal axis in amenorrhoeic women with insulin-dependent diabetes. Hum Reprod 1999;14:298–302. **(IIb, B)**

20. Kinon BJ, Gilmore JA, Liu H, et al: Prevalence of hyperprolactinemia in schizophrenic patients treated with conventional antipsychotic medications or risperidone. Psychoneuroendocrinology 2003;28:55–68. **(IIb, B)**

21. Kiddy DS, Hamilton-Fairley D, Bush A, et al: Improvement in endocrine and ovarian function during dietary treatment of obese women with polycystic ovary syndrome. Clin Endocrinol (Oxf) 1992; 36:105–111. **(IIb, B)**

22. Clark AM, Thornley B, Tomlinson L, et al: Weight loss in obese infertile women results in improvement in reproductive outcome for all forms of fertility treatment. Hum Reprod 1998;13:1502–1505. **(IIb, B)**

23. Sherman B, Halmi K, Zamudio R: J Clin Endocrinol Metab 1975;41: 135–142. **(III, B)**

24. Chen EC, Brzyski RG: Exercise and reproductive dysfunction. Fertil Steril 1999;71:1–6. **(IV, C)**

25. Golden NH: Eating disorders in adolescence and their sequelae. Best Pract Res Clin Obstet Gynaecol 2003;17:57–73. **(IV, C)**

26. Ferin M: Clinical review 105: stress and the reproductive cycle. J Clin Endocrinol Metab 1999;84:1768–1774. **(IV, C)**

27. Kallenberg GA, Pesce CM, Norman B, et al: Ectopic hyperprolactinemia resulting from an ovarian teratoma. JAMA 1990;263: 2472–2474. **(III, B)**

28. Tomlinson JW, Draper N, Mackie J, et al: Absence of Cushingoid phenotype in a patient with Cushing's disease due to defective cortisone to cortisol conversion. J Clin Endocrinol Metab 2002;87:57–62. **(III, B)**

29. Vegetti W, Marozzi A, Manfredini E, et al: Premature ovarian failure. Mol Cell Endocrinol 2000;161:53–57. **(III, B)**

30. Coulam C, Adamson S, Annegers JF: Incidence of premature ovarian failure. Obstet Gynecol 1986;67:604–606. **(III, B)**

31. Schenker JG, Margalioth EJ: Intrauterine adhesions: an updated appraisal. Fertil Steril 1982;37:593–610. **(IV, C)**

32. Amato P, Roberts AC: Transient ovarian failure: a complication of uterine artery embolization. Fertil Steril 2001;75:438–439. **(IV, C)**

33. Davies C, Gibson M, Holt EM, et al: Amenorrhoea secondary to endometrial ablation and Asherman's syndrome following uterine artery embolization. Clin Radiol 2001;57:317–318. **(IV, C)**

34. Karosi M, Swamy M: Secondary occupational amenorrhea. Int J Gynecol Obstet 2004;87:48–49. **(III, B)**

35. Alzubaidi NH, Chapin HL, Vanderhoof VH, et al: Meeting the needs of young women with secondary amenorrhea and spontaneous premature ovarian failure. Obstet Gynecol 2002;99(Pt 1):720–725. **(III, B)**

36. Khalid A: Irregular or absent periods—what can an ultrasound scan tell you? Best Pract Res Clin Obstet Gynaecol 2004;18:3–11. **(IV, C)**

37. Lakhani K, Seifalian AM, Atiomo WU, et al: Polycystic ovaries. Br J Radiol 2002;75:9–16. **(III, B)**

38. Coccia ME, Becattini C, Bracco GL, et al: Pressure lavage under ultrasound guidance: a new approach for outpatient treatment of intrauterine adhesions. Fertil Steril 2001;75:601–606. **(III, B)**

39. Salle B, Gaucherand P, de Saint Hilaire P, et al: Transvaginal sonohysterographic evaluation of intrauterine adhesions. J Clin Ultrasound 1999;27:131–134. **(III, B)**

40. Raber W, Gessl A, Nowotny P, et al: Hyperprolactinaemia in hypothyroidism: clinical significance and impact of TSH normalization. Clin Endocrinol (Oxf) 2003;58:185–191. **(III, B)**

41. Sarlis NJ, Brucker-Davis F, Doppman JL, et al: MRI-demonstrable regression of a pituitary mass in a case of primary hypothyroidism after a week of acute thyroid hormone therapy. J Clin Endocrinol Metab 1997;82:808–811. **(III, B)**

42. Yazigi RA, Quintero CH, Salameh WA: Prolactin disorders. Fertil Steril 1997;67:215–225. **(IV, C)**

43. Schlechte JA: Clinical practice: prolactinoma. N Engl J Med 2003;349: 2035–2041. **(IV, C)**

44. Schlechte J, Dolan K, Sherman B, et al: The natural history of untreated hyperprolactinemia: a prospective analysis. J Clin Endocrinol Metab 1989;68:412–418. **(III, B)**

45. Molitch ME: Clinical review 65: evaluation and treatment of the patient with a pituitary incidentaloma. J Clin Endocrinol Metab 1995; 80:3. **(IV, C)**

46. Donovan LE, Corenblum B: The natural history of the pituitary incidentaloma. Arch Intern Med 1995;155:181–183. **(III, B)**

47. Katznelson L, Alexander JM, Klibanski A: Clinical review 45: clinically nonfunctioning pituitary adenomas. J Clin Endocrinol Metab 1993;76: 1089–1094. **(IV, C)**

48. Katznelson L, Alexander JM, Bikkal HA, et al: Imbalanced follicle-stimulating hormone beta-subunit hormone biosynthesis in human pituitary adenomas. J Clin Endocrinol Metab 1992;74:1343–1351. **(IIb, B)**

49. Hall WA, Luciano MG, Doppman JL, et al: Pituitary magnetic resonance imaging in normal human volunteers: occult adenomas in the general population. Ann Intern Med 1994;120:817–828. **(IIb, B)**

50. Reincke M, Allolio B, Saeger W, et al: The "incidentaloma" of the pituitary gland. Is neurosurgery required? JAMA 1990;263:2772–2776. **(III, B)**

51. Azziz R, Hincapie LA, Knochenhauer ES, et al: Screening for 21-hydroxylase-deficient nonclassic adrenal hyperplasia among hyperandrogenic women: a prospective study. Fertil Steril 1999;72: 915–925. **(IIa, B)**

52. Revised 2003 consensus on diagnostic criteria and long-term health risks related to polycystic ovary syndrome. Fertil Steril 2004;81:19–25. **(IV, C)**

53. Barbieri RL, Ryan KJ: Hyperandrogenism, insulin resistance, and acanthosis nigricans syndrome: a common endocrinopathy with distinct pathophysiologic features. Am J Obstet Gynecol 1983;147: 90–101. **(IV, C)**

54. Warren MP, Goodman LR: Exercise-induced endocrine pathologies. J Endocrinol Invest 2003;26:873. **(IV, C)**

55. Miller KK, Klibanski A: Clinical review 106: amenorrheic bone loss. J Clin Endocrinol Metab 1999;84:1775–1783. **(IV, C)**

56. Munoz MT, Argente J: Anorexia nervosa in female adolescents: endocrine and bone mineral density disturbances. Eur J Endocrinol 2002;147:275–286. **(IV, C)**

57. Grinspoon SK, Friedman AJ, Miller KK, et al: Effects of a triphasic combination oral contraceptive containing norgestimate/ethinyl estradiol on biochemical markers of bone metabolism in young women with osteopenia secondary to hypothalamic amenorrhea. J Clin Endocrinol Metab 2003;88:3651–3656. **(Ib, A)**

58. Adashi E: Long-term gonadotrophin-releasing hormone agonist therapy: the evolving issue of steroidal 'add-back' paradigms. Hum Reprod 1994; 9:1380–1397. **(IV, C)**

59. Balen AH, Braat DD, West C, et al: Cumulative conception and live birth rates after the treatment of anovulatory infertility: safety and efficacy of ovulation induction in 200 patients. Hum Reprod 1994;9: 1563–1570. **(IIb, B)**

60. Rebar RW, Connolly HV: Clinical features of young women with hypergonadotropic amenorrhea. Fertil Steril 1990;53:804. **(III, B)**

61. Manuel M, Katayama PK, Jones HW Jr: The age of occurrence of gonadal tumors in intersex patients with a Y chromosome. Am J Obstet Gynecol 1976;124:293–300. **(III, B)**

62. Troche V, Hernandez E; Neoplasia arising in dysgenetic gonads. Obstet Gynecol Surv 1986;41:74–99. **(IV, C)**

63. Pasquino AM, Passeri F, Pucarelli I, et al: Spontaneous pubertal development in Turner's syndrome. Italian Study Group for Turner's Syndrome. J Clin Endocrinol Metab 1997;82:1810–1813. **(III, B)**

64. Laml T, Huber J, Albrecht A, et al: Unexpected pregnancy during hormone-replacement therapy in a women with elevated follicle-stimulating hormone levels and amenorrhea. Gynecol Endocrinol 1999;13: 89–92. **(IV, C)**

65. Kreiner D, Droesch K, Navot D, et al: Spontaneous and pharmacologically induced remissions in patients with premature ovarian failure. Obstet Gynecol 1988;72:926. **(III, B)**

66. Rosen G, Stone S, Yee B: Ovulation induction in women with premature ovarian failure: a prospective, crossover study. Fertil Steril 1992; 57:448–449. **(Ib, A)**

67. van Kasteren YM, Hoek A, Schoemaker J: Ovulation induction in premature ovarian failure: a placebo-controlled randomized trial combining pituitary suppression with gonadotropin stimulation. Fertil Steril 1995;64:273–278. **(Ib, A)**

68. Karnis M, Zimon A, Lalwani S, et al: Risk of death in pregnancy achieved through oocyte donation in patients with Turner syndrome: a national survey. Fertil Steril 2003;80:498–501. **(III, B)**

69. Bayram N, van Wely M, Kaaijk EM, et al: Using an electrocautery strategy or recombinant follicle stimulating hormone to induce ovulation in polycystic ovary syndrome: randomized controlled trial. BMJ 2004;328:192–196. **(Ib, A)**

70. Wilcox A, Weinberg C, Baird D: Timing of sexual intercourse in relation to ovulation: effects on the probability of conception, survival of the pregnancy, and sex of the baby. N Engl J Med 1995;333:1517–1521. **(III, B)**

71. Knowler WC, Barrett-Connor E, Fowler SE, et al: Reduction in the incidence of type 2 diabetes with lifestyle intervention or metformin. N Engl J Med 2002;346:393–403. **(Ib, A)**

72. Carmina E, Lobo R: Does metformin induce ovulation in normoandrogenic anovulatory women? Am J Obstet Gynecol 2004;191: 1580–1584. **(Ib, A)**

73. Nestler JE, Jakubowicz DJ, Evans WS, et al: Effects of metformin on spontaneous and clomiphene-induced ovulation in the polycystic ovary syndrome. N Engl J Med 1998;338:1876–1880. **(Ib, A)**

74. Vandermolen DT, Ratts VS, Evans WS, et al: Metformin increases the ovulatory rate and pregnancy rate from clomiphene citrate in patients with polycystic ovary syndrome who are resistant to clomiphene citrate alone. Fertil Steril 2001;75:310–315. **(II, B)**

75. Mitwally MF, Casper RF: Use of an aromatase inhibitor for induction of ovulation in patients with an inadequate response to clomiphene citrate. Fertil Steril 2001;75:305–309. **(III, B)**

76. Al-Omari W, Sulaiman W, Al-Hadithi N: Comparison of two aromatase inhibitors in women with clomiphene-resistant polycystic ovary syndrome. Int J Gynaecol Obstet 2004;85:289–2891. **(III, B)**

77. Stein IS: Duration of fertility following ovarian wedge resection—Stein-Leventhal syndrome. West J Surg Obstet Gynecol 1964;72: 237–242. **(III, B)**

78. Dahlgren E, Johansson S, Lindstedt G, et al: Women with polycystic ovary syndrome wedge resected in 1956 to 1965: a long-term follow-up focusing on natural history and circulating hormones. Fertil Steril 1992;57:505. **(IIb, B)**

79. Bayram N, van Wely M, van der Veen F: Pulsatile gonadotrophin releasing hormone for ovulation induction in subfertility associated with polycystic ovary syndrome: randomized controlled trial. BMJ 2004;382: 192–196. **(Ib, A)**

80. Solomon CG, Hu FB, Dunaif A, et al: Long or highly irregular menstrual cycles as a marker for risk of type 2 diabetes mellitus. JAMA 2001;286:2421–2426. **(III, B)**

81. New M, Lorenzen F, Lerner A, et al: Genotyping steroid 21-hydroxylase deficiency: hormonal reference data. J Clin Endocrinol Metab 1983;57:320–326. **(III, B)**

## Ronald T. Burkman, MD, Kristin L. Dardano, MD, and Patricia E. Bailey-Sarnelli, MD

### KEY POINTS

- Approximately 50% of pregnancies in the United States are unintended or unplanned.
- Contraceptive methods with the highest typical use failure (pregnancy) rates require either daily use or use at the time of intercourse.
- Most hormonal methods, including the levonorgestrel-releasing intrauterine contraceptive system, have noncontraceptive health benefits.
- Barrier methods, particularly condoms, protect against some sexually transmitted infections.
- Successful use of a contraceptive method requires counseling on proper use, risks, and side effects.

The introduction of oral contraceptives (OCs) in 1960 defines the major starting point for today's contraceptive methods. Although some methods clearly preceded the "Pill," such as barrier methods and early forms of the intrauterine contraceptive devices (IUDs), the publicity around the availability of OCs increased awareness about contraception both for potential users and the health care profession. Yet, despite the introduction of OCs and the development of many new or improved methods of contraception, unintended or unplanned pregnancies continue to be a major problem in the United States. According to the 1995 National Survey of Family Growth, there were a total of 6.3 million pregnancies in the United States, with 49.2% unintended.[1,2] Among the unintended pregnancies, nearly one half result in a pregnancy termination and more than 10% in spontaneous abortion. Approximately 40% of unintended pregnancies occur among women who do not desire pregnancy yet do not use a method of contraception. About 60% of unintended pregnancies occur among women using some form of birth control, with about 1 million of these pregnancies occurring in OC users. Thus, despite more than 40 years' experience with modern contraceptives, substantial challenges still remain relative to identifying women or couples who can be successful with a given method as well as assisting them in proper use of the method.

When evaluating contraceptive methods, efficacy is narrowly defined as the frequency of pregnancy prevention while a method is being used correctly and consistently. Effectiveness of a contraceptive method usually reflects typical use rates of unintended pregnancy, which would include method or perfect use failures as well as user failure (e.g., not using the method correctly or consistently).[3] Most method or typical use rates are calculated using either the Pearl Index or a life-table analysis. The Pearl Index is calculated by dividing the number of unintended pregnancies by the total months or menstrual cycles of exposure; the result is multiplied by 1200 if months are used and 1300 if menstrual cycles are used. The result is expressed in number of pregnancies per 100 women–years of exposure. The majority of the efficacy rates expressed in this chapter are calculated by the Pearl Index and express rates occurring during the first year of use. The major problem with this index is that it does not account for duration of exposure; the Pearl Index is reasonably reflective of contraceptive failure if duration of use is short (i.e., 6 to 12 months) and most users use the method for about the same period of time. In a life-table analysis, a separate failure rate is calculated for each month of use such that varying durations of use are not problematic. However, the life-table calculations are often more tedious than those for the Pearl Index, leading to less use of this approach except among researchers. Factors that affect efficacy results in clinical trials include not only methodological issues such as choice of method to calculate efficacy, but also subject characteristics such as frequency of intercourse and motivation.

## CONTRACEPTIVE METHODS

### Barrier Methods and Spermicides

Barrier methods are designed to either block the introduction of spermatozoa into the vagina or their ascent from the vagina into the uterine cavity.[4] Among the contraceptive methods available, they also have the benefit of providing some protection against some sexually transmitted infections (STIs). Because barrier methods require motivation at the time of intercourse and given erratic contraceptive compliance (correct use of a method) in the United States, one can understand why barrier methods have higher typical use pregnancy rates than other contraceptive methods.

#### Condoms

The most common material used for male condom manufacture is latex, although there are also condoms available made from polyurethane material and lamb cecums.

Most condoms are lubricated with silicone or a water-soluble lubricant; some also use a spermicide as a lubricant. In addition to male condoms, there are female condoms, which consist of a rim that holds the condom against the vulva, a sheath of polyurethane material, and a ring that helps anchor the vaginal portion.

The primary mechanism of action of the condom is to capture seminal fluid and sperm within the device at the time of ejaculation. Condoms lubricated with a spermicide can also inactivate or destroy sperm. Use of petroleum jelly (Vaseline) as a lubricant should be avoided because it may destroy the latex. Successful use of male condoms requires that they not be stored at high temperature; that they be handled gently to avoid damage; that they be rolled down the length of the penis before use, leaving a reservoir at the tip of the penis; that users withdraw the penis immediately after intercourse when the penis is still erect while holding the condom; and that the condom be carefully inspected to ensure there is no leakage. Similarly, female condoms should be inspected for leakage after intercourse. If leakage is discovered or the condom breaks during intercourse, spermicide should be inserted into the vagina immediately and emergency contraception started as soon as possible.

In well-motivated couples, pregnancy rates as low as 3 to 5 pregnancies per 100 women–years can be achieved. However, typical use rates are substantially higher, at 10 to 30 pregnancies per 100 women–years.[5]

The primary risk with condom use is hypersensitivity of the skin or vagina to the material or lubricants. Individuals with known latex allergy should use polyurethane condoms.

The major noncontraceptive benefit of condoms is protection against STIs, such as gonorrhea, syphilis, herpes, and human immunodeficiency virus (HIV). In addition, condoms reduce the risk of acute salpingitis or pelvic inflammatory disease (PID).

### Female Diaphragm

The diaphragm is circular with a rim that can be compressed along its length (coiled spring version) or compressed at specific sites (arcing spring); diaphragms are also made with a a flat spring design, which is similar to the coiled spring diaphragm except the rim is thinner. After fitting by a health care professional, when inserted into the vagina the diaphragm should fit under the symphysis pubis and cover the uterine cervix. Before insertion, spermicide is placed on the side that opposes the cervix and along the rim. Thus, the diaphragm both acts as a barrier to ascent of sperm and provides spermicidal activity. Potential users should be instructed that the device can be inserted up to 6 hours before intercourse and should be left in place for at least 6 hours after intercourse. If intercourse occurs more than once, the device should not be removed but rather more spermicide should be inserted into the vagina. Because successful use requires the device to be held in place by the women's bony pelvis, cervix, and pelvic musculature, conditions such as pelvic relaxation with uterine prolapse and cystocele and/or rectocele, sharply anteverted or retroverted uterus, shortened vagina, poor muscle tone, or prior vaginal injury are potential contraindications to the use of a diaphragm. Fitting is essentially done by trial and error. One inserts the index and middle fingers of the examining hand into the vagina, then estimates the distance from the inferior margin of the symphysis pubis to the posterior cul-de-sac behind the uterine cervix. This distance is used to size a diaphragm. After showing the user how to compress the diaphragm's rim and insert the device into the vagina, one lets the user practice until she is comfortable with both inserting and removing the device.

The perfect use failure rates are about 6 pregnancies per 100 women–years; typical use rates climb to about 15 to 20 pregnancies per 100 women–years.[5]

A potential noncontraceptive benefit is reduced risk of some STIs. The most commonly reported risk is cystitis; voiding after intercourse may reduce its frequency of occurrence. In addition, a few cases of toxic shock syndrome have been reported among users of diaphragms. Sensitivity to the diaphragm's material or spermicide may also occur.

### Cervical Cap

The Prentif cervical cap, the only cap currently distributed in the United States, is made of latex rubber and is shaped like a thimble. It comes in four sizes, with internal diameters ranging from 2.2 to 3.1 cm. Held in place against the cervix by suction, its mode of action is as a barrier to the ascent of sperm. A health care professional must fit the cap and teach the user how to attach it to the cervix. In general, it requires somewhat more skill to successfully place compared to a diaphragm, such that it has been estimated that only about 50% to 80% of potential users feel they can use it successfully or be properly fitted. It should be left in place for at least 6 hours after the last act of intercourse. However, unlike the diaphragm, it does not require a spermicide and can be left in place for 24 to 48 hours.

It has been estimated that perfect use failure rates range from about 9 pregnancies per 100 women–years in nulliparous users to 26 pregnancies per 100 women–years in multiparas. Typical use rates are about 16 per 100 women–years and 32 per 100 women–years for nulliparas and multiparas, respectively.[5]

As with other barrier methods, users of a cervical cap may have a reduced risk of some STIs. Cervical erosion leading to spotting may occur if the device is left in place too long or if it is ill fitting. Although toxic shock syndrome is theoretically possible, no cases have been reported in association with use of cervical caps. Some women may note a vaginal discharge with prolonged use; some may also experience an allergic reaction to the latex.

### Spermicides

The only spermicide available in the United States is nonoxynol-9, which is a long-chain surfactant with the chemical name nonylphenoxypolyethoxy ethanol. Its mode of action is to penetrate the cell membranes of spermatozoa to produce sperm death or loss of motility. Similar activity may occur with vaginal epithelial cells, leading to irritation. If used alone, spermicide is inserted high into the vagina no sooner than 30 minutes before intercourse. One should not use other lubricants in conjunction with a spermicide. Douching should be avoided for at least 8 hours after intercourse.

The perfect use failure rate is about 15 pregnancies per 100 women–years; typical use rate is about 30 pregnancies per 100 women–years.[5,6]

An advantage of spermicides is that they may reduce the risk of some STIs, although they do not prevent the transmission of HIV infections.[7] In fact, due to the action of nonoxynol-9 on epithelial cells, women with HIV infection or at risk for such infection should not use spermicides containing nonoxynol-9. In addition, condoms lubricated with this spermicide should not be used by such at-risk women. The only other risks relative to spermicide use are possible hypersensitivity and an increased risk of urinary tract infections.

## Intrauterine Contraceptive Device

Although only about 1% of U.S. women using contraception use IUDs, among all users of contraception, IUD users are perhaps the happiest with their method.[8] Further, the efficacy rate is better than many methods, including OCs, barrier methods, and even tubal ligation. In countries such as Sweden and Germany, 15% to 20% of married women use the IUD as their contraceptive method. The reasons women in the United States use this method less frequently relates to misperceptions about mechanism of action (e.g., acts as an abortifacient), infection risk, ectopic pregnancy risk, and the whole litigious atmosphere associated with the Dalkon Shield. However, with the introduction of new IUDs such as the Copper T 380 A and the levonorgestrel-releasing system, it is anticipated that the frequency of use of this method in the United States may increase.

### Copper Device

The Copper T 380 A is a T-shaped device about 36 mm in length and 32 mm in diameter. It is wound with fine copper wire, 300 mm$^2$ on its vertical arm and 40 mm$^2$ on each side arm. Attached to the base of the vertical arm are two monofilament strings. This IUD has a useful life span of at least 10 years. Although IUDs have been used for many decades, little scientific evidence documents an exact mechanism of action. A few small studies suggest that this IUD may be spermicidal and that all IUDs interfere with either normal development of ova or the fertilization of ova. Also, this IUD has activity on the endometrium that leads to leukocyte infiltration, a circumstance that leads to phagocytosis of sperm and may impede sperm migration or capacitance. It has been suggested that by making the endometrium a "hostile" environment, the IUD interferes with implantation and thus may act as an abortifacient. However, studies have failed to document rises in human chorionic gonadotropin levels in the second half of menstrual cycles when implantation would occur among IUD users. In the past, IUDs were associated with an increased risk for PID around the time of insertion. However, by restricting use to mutually monogamous couples and couples currently at low risk of STIs, the absolute risk of PID in association with IUD use is almost negligible. Women at risk for HIV infection or who are already infected are still candidates for use of this device. Because this IUD has a duration of action of at least 10 years, it is intended for couples who want long-term contraception. Other ideal candidates are women in whom combination hormonal contraception is contraindicated, such as women with prior thrombosis, smokers older than age 35, and lactating women. As is true of any contraceptive method, symptoms such as abnormal bleeding or discharge should be evaluated before initiating the method. One should document the informed consent process using the materials provided by the manufacturer. Included in the discussion are the risks and benefits of the method as well as how to feel for the strings once insertion has occurred. To ensure successful placement and reduce risk of expulsion, the uterine cavity should not be distorted and be between 6 and 9 cm in depth. Currently, IUDs available in the United States are inserted under aseptic conditions using a modification of the withdrawal technique, which reduces the risk of uterine perforation. Training is required from a skilled practitioner to learn the proper technique and avoid complications. After insertion, users should be instructed to contact their provider if they miss a menstrual period, experience an abnormal discharge or bleeding, experience pelvic pain or fever, have an exposure to STIs, or cannot feel the string.

The perfect use failure rate with the Copper T380 A is 0.6 pregnancies per 100 women–years; typical use failure rate is approximately 0.8 per 100 women–years.[5] The obvious reason for the two rates being similar is that the IUD does not require motivation either at intercourse or on a frequent basis to use it effectively. However, unlike other methods, such as barriers and most forms of hormonal contraception, users have less individual control relative to stopping use. Over a 10-year period, failure rates range between 2 and 3 pregnancies per 100 women–years, roughly equivalent to the rates achieved by tubal sterilization.

The major risks that have been reported in association with use of this IUD include ectopic pregnancy, spontaneous abortion, uterine perforation, expulsion, and PID. Although 5% to 8% of pregnancies that occur with use of this IUD are ectopic, overall, because of the high effectiveness of this device, the absolute risk of ectopic pregnancy in users is substantially less than that experienced by nonusers of contraception. In addition, if a user becomes pregnant with a device in place, the risk of a spontaneous abortion is about 50%. Removing the device when the strings can be readily identified will reduce this risk by about one half. If an intrauterine pregnancy is confirmed but strings are not seen and the IUD is identified in the uterus (usually by ultrasound), users should be apprised that there is an increased risk of premature rupture of the membranes and preterm delivery. Uterine perforation, which occurs at the time of insertion, has been reported at a rate of 1 to 2 events per 1000 insertions. This risk is minimized by a careful preinsertion pelvic examination to determine the position of the uterus and by use of a tenaculum to straighten the uterine axis during insertion. Expulsion of the device is more common in the first few weeks of use, with rates of about 5%. Improper placement of the device may contribute to expulsion. Over a 5-year time span of use, cumulative expulsion rates are approximately 11%. PID appears to be associated primarily with the insertion of the device, not with its duration of use. Currently, with appropriately selected users, the rate of infection is about 1 case per 1000 insertions. Minor side effects include abnormal bleeding and cramping. Women using this particular device tend to have regular menstrual periods, but the amount of flow is increased by about one third. Use of nonsteroidal anti-inflammatory agents often will reduce the overall amount of flow. In addition, some women experience increased dysmenorrhea, particularly in the first few months of use. Overall, complaints related to bleeding and pain result in about 12% of women discontinuing use in the first year.

A not-infrequent issue with IUD use is the management of missing strings. First, the patient should be encouraged to use a backup contraceptive method until the patient is evaluated. If the IUD strings cannot be seen even with gentle probing of the endocervical canal, one should perform a pregnancy test, if indicated, and consider ordering a transvaginal ultrasound to determine if the IUD is intrauterine, intraperitoneal, or has been expelled (most likely). If the patient is pregnant, an ectopic pregnancy must be excluded. If the IUD is determined to be in an intraperitoneal location, removal is usually indicated due to likely peritoneal irritation by the device.

### Levonorgestrel-releasing System

Although technically considered a hormonal contraceptive, the levonoregestrel-releasing IUD or system (LNg-20 IUS) is discussed here. The LNg-20 IUS, a more recently developed IUD, also uses a T-shaped frame but has a reservoir on the vertical arm that releases 20 µg of the progestin levonorgestrel daily. A single string attached to the vertical arm differentiates it from the T 380 A, which has two strings. Blood levels of levonorgestrel among users are about 25% of that seen among users of oral contraceptives containing this progestin and about one half the levels seen among users of Norplant, the implanted contraceptive that releases levonorgestrel. In contrast to the Copper T 380 A device, the LNg-20 has a life span of 5 years in clinical trials. The LNG-20 IUS's primary mechanisms of action are to thicken cervical mucus to impede ascent of sperm and to alter uterotubal fluid to interfere with sperm migration. Some available data indicate that this IUS causes anovulation in about 10% to 15% of cycles. It also changes the characteristics of the endometrium to reduce the likelihood of implantation. Candidates for use of this IUS fit the same profile as those who would consider use of the Copper T 380 A. The insertion technique also uses a modified withdrawal approach. However, because the technique used differs from that used with the Copper T 380 A, training is required to ensure appropriate placement. Overall, the counseling is similar except for additional information about bleeding.

The LNg-20 IUS has been shown to be highly effective in clinical trials, with both perfect use and typical use pregnancy rates being 0.1 pregnancies per 100 women–years after 1 year of use.[5] Further, the cumulative pregnancy rate over 5 years is 0.7 pregnancies per 100 women–years. Approximately 50% of the pregnancies that occur are ectopic, but, as with the Copper T 380 A device, the absolute risk of ectopic pregnancy is still substantially lower than that experienced by nonusers of contraception.[9]

Because this device releases a potent progestin at the endometrial level, the bleeding pattern is substantially different from that seen with the Copper T 380 A. During the initial 3 to 4 months of use, some women will experience irregular bleeding, which at times may be heavy. However, after a few months of use, most women experience a significant decrease in menstrual flow—by as much as 70%. In some studies, 20% to 25% of users become amenorrheic in the second year of use. In addition, dysmenorrhea tends to improve with use of this device. Because of the effectiveness of the LNg-20 IUS in reducing menstrual blood flow, it has been used as a treatment for menorrhagia. Results in clinical trials to date indicate that it is an effective treatment modality which even approaches the results achieved with endometrial ablation.[10] Thus, this is the first IUS to have significant noncontraceptive benefits. Major risks with this IUS are similar to those noted for the Copper T 380 A. The one

exception is PID. Because one of the effects of the LNg-20 IUS is to thicken cervical mucus, this leads to interference with ascent of bacteria. In addition, the reduced blood flow associated with this device results in an environment that is less likely to enhance bacterial growth. The minor side effects of bleeding and cramping are less frequent with this device, except for irregular bleeding patterns during the first few months of use. Some women have reported headache, acne, or mastalgia, which could be related to the systemic effects of the progestin. Management of possible pregnancy and missing strings is similar to the approach used with the Copper T 380 A.

## Hormonal Contraceptives

The introduction of the oral contraceptive about 1960 initiated the modern era of hormonal contraception. Hormonal contraception is broadly defined as the use of steroidal hormones (estrogens, progestins, androgens) to alter normal physiological function to inhibit fertility. At this time, all clinically available forms are directed toward altering female physiology. Although experimental studies suggest that use of high-dose androgens may inhibit spermatogenesis, there are no products on the market for clinical use. Of particular note, the 21st century brought the introduction of two new delivery systems for hormonal contraception, the transdermal patch and the vaginal ring.

Adolescents present significant challenges relative to motivating them to use effective contraception correctly and to practice safe sex. Use of interactive counseling regarding the risks of pregnancy, including medical, social, and economic consequences and the importance of condom use to prevent STIs and HIV infection can be effective. Because many young adolescents fear pelvic examinations, deferring such examinations in asymptomatic or low-risk women until a subsequent visit will allow contraception to be initiated promptly for those at risk for pregnancy. Finally, in an effort to improve compliance, some practitioners start hormonal methods such as OCs on the same day as the initial office visit, as opposed to menstrual cycle day 1 or a Sunday start. This approach, termed *Quick Start*, allows women to initiate contraception immediately and facilitates getting refills because it is much more likely that the last pill in a pack will be taken on a weekday, when the office is open. When using this approach, women need to be advised that they may experience irregular bleeding for the first few weeks and that they need to use backup contraception until the second package of oral contraceptives is started.

### Combination Oral Contraceptives

Combination OCs provide both an estrogen and progestin in each pill during the active phase of the oral contraceptive cycle. Most packages contain 21 pills containing hormones and 7 pills that are placebos. Virtually all preparations contain ethinyl estradiol as the estrogen, in doses ranging from 20 µg to 50 µg per pill. However, in general use, most preparations contain 35 µg or less. The most commonly used progestins in the United States are the estranes: norethindrone and norethindrone acetate; the gonanes: levonorgestrel, desogestrel, and norgestimate; and a spironolactone analog, drospirenone. In general, with the dosages utilized in combination OCs, the estranes are less potent relative to their effects on the endometrium than the other progestins. Further, it should also be noted that the overall dosages of estrogen and progestins in combination OCs have been reduced by a factor of two to five over the past 40 years, resulting in an improved safety profile. Depending on the preparation, dosages may remain constant throughout a pill cycle or be used in a phasic pattern. More recently, an extended-use formulation that has users take active pills for 84 days followed by a week of placebos, has been introduced in the United States.[11] The intent of this formulation is to reduce the frequency of menstrual periods. All users of OCs are instructed to start OC use on either the first day of their menstrual cycle or on the Sunday following the first day of their menstrual period. The latter approach helps some women keep track of their pill use better. If using the Sunday start approach, use of backup contraception for the first week is recommended if the start date is more than 5 days from the start of the menstrual period. Although most women are candidates for combination OCs, there are some contraindications. These include current or past history of thromboembolism, myocardial infarction, stroke, breast cancer and other estrogen-dependent tumors, lupus, gall-bladder disease, poorly controlled hypertension, diabetes with vascular complications, severe migraine headaches, lactation, and women over age 35 who smoke or who have cardiovascular risk factors.

Combination OCs suppress ovulation by diminishing the frequency of gonadotropin-releasing hormone pulses and eliminating the luteinizing hormone surge at midcycle. They also change the consistency of cervical mucus, resulting in less sperm penetration; make the endometrial lining less receptive to implantation; and alter tubal transport of both sperm and oocytes. The perfect use pregnancy rate is about 0.3 pregnancies per 100 women–years, although there is substantial variation due to use of differing methodology in clinical trials.[5] The typical use failure rate ranges from 3 to 8 pregnancies per 100 women–years. Incorrect pill taking unfortunately leads to contraceptive failure. In a study of 103 students who kept a pill-taking diary and who also were provided with an electronic pill pack to record when pills were removed from the pack, the electronic pack recorded missed pills at rates two to three times higher than those study subjects recorded in their diaries.[12] Other factors that also affect typical use effectiveness include perceived convenience, cost, and motivation.

A number of health benefits are associated with combination OC use. Table 58-1 outlines noncontraceptive health benefits associated with combination OCs. Benefits that are reasonably well established include reduction in risk of ovarian and endometrial cancer, ectopic pregnancy, PID, menstrual disorders, benign breast disease, and acne. Emerging benefits include protection against bone mineral density loss, development of colorectal cancer, and progression of rheumatoid arthritis.

Multiple observational studies have demonstrated that combination OCs have a protective effect against development of ovarian cancer, with between a 40% and 80% overall decrease in risk among users compared to nonusers.[13] The protection begins approximately 1 year after initiating use and conveys about a 10% to 12% decrease in risk for each year of use. In addition, protection persists for 15 to 20 years after the patient has discontinued use of OCs. This protective effect primarily involves epithelial tumors of the ovary. The mechanisms by which OCs may produce their protective effects include suppression

| Table 58-1 |
| --- |
| **Health Benefits of Oral Contraceptives** |

**Reasonably established decline in risk for**

Ovarian cancer
Endometrial cancer
Ectopic pregnancy
Pelvic inflammatory disease
Menstrual disorders
   Abnormal bleeding
   Dysmenorrhea
Benign breast disease
Ovarian cysts
Acne

**Potential effect on**

Bone mineral density loss
Colorectal cancer
Rheumatoid arthritis

of ovulation, thus resulting in a reduced frequency of "injury" to the ovarian capsule, and the suppression of gonadotropins. A recent theory based on a primate model suggests that induction of ovarian apoptosis, which in turn eliminates surface epithelium inclusion cysts, may play a role in reducing ovarian cancer risk among OC users.[14]

A number of studies have demonstrated that use of combination OCs conveys protection against endometrial cancer.[15] Overall, these studies suggest up to a 50% reduction in risk that begins about 1 year after initiation of use. Protection appears to increase with duration of use; indeed, some data indicate that the protection persists up to 20 years after OC use is discontinued. Protection has been demonstrated for adenocarcinoma, adenosquamous tumors, and adenoacanthomas. However, the strength of the protective effect has varied in studies for women with potential risk factors, such as obesity and nulliparity. The purported protective mechanism is a reduction in the mitotic activity of endometrial cells by the action of the progestin component of OCs.

Based on results of various epidemiologic studies, combination OCs convey an approximately 90% reduction in risk of ectopic pregnancy. The likely mechanism is through suppression of ovulation, an effect that obviously prevents all types of pregnancy.

The use of OCs has been associated with a reduction of risk of acute salpingitis or PID by 50% to 80% compared to use of no contraception or use of barrier methods in a number of studies. A more recent multicenter study, in contrast, failed to show a protective effect of combination OC use.[16] Interestingly, there is no protective effect against the acquisition of lower genital tract STIs, including *Chlamydia trachomatis* and *Neisseria gonorrhoeae* infections of the uterine cervix. Purported mechanisms by which OCs exert protection include progestin-induced changes to cervical mucus, making it thick and viscous such that ascent of bacteria is substantially inhibited. Additional theories include reduced menstrual flow such that there is less retrograde menstrual flow to the fallopian tubes, resulting in a less favorable environment for promoting growth of bacterial organisms, and possible changes in uterine contractility such that ascent of organisms is less likely.

# Reproductive Endocrinology and Infertility

It is well accepted that combination OCs reduce menstrual blood loss. In addition, recent data indicates that combination OCs can be used effectively in the treatment of abnormal bleeding. For example, a randomized clinical trial demonstrated that both the investigators' and subjects' perceptions of the amount of reduction in blood loss were similar.[17] More importantly, the combination OC reduced blood loss substantially more than the comparative placebo. The mechanism of action is probably a stabilization effect of the estrogen and progestin combination on the endometrium. Dysmenorrhea has also been shown to be reduced through use of combination OCs. These preparations remain one of the mainstays in the treatment of primary dysmenorrhea. Combination OCs may reduce pain by reducing the prostaglandin content of menstrual fluid, leading to less local vasoconstriction and ischemia, and by reducing uterine contractility.

Results of several studies reveal a significant decrease in the incidence of benign fibrocystic conditions of the breast with oral contraceptive use, with a 30% to 50% decrease overall. The occurrence of fibroadenomas, specifically, decreases among women younger than age 45. These effects are mainly seen in current and recent long-term users of combination OCs. The likely mechanism is through suppression of ovulation, and, therefore, inhibition of the breast cell proliferation that normally occurs in the first half of an ovulatory menstrual cycle.

Randomized, placebo-controlled clinical trials have demonstrated that some combination OCs will reduce acne lesions. Although it is likely that many formulations will lead to acne reduction, the data to date are not well controlled. The mechanisms by which combination OCs achieve these effects include elevation of sex hormone–binding globulin, which binds and decreases available testosterone; suppression of the enzyme that converts testosterone to dihydrotestosterone; and suppression of gonadotropins, resulting in decreased levels of ovarian androgens. In addition, combination OCs appear to improve BMD in many studies, although other studies have shown no effect. No studies have demonstrated a negative effect on BMD. It appears that combination OCs are most effective at preventing bone loss during times of low estrogen and have a further protective effect with increased duration of use. Women who have used OCs for 5 to 10 years or longer are afforded the greatest protection. One study has shown a 25% reduction in hip fracture risk.[18] Estrogens act on bone by increasing calcium absorption, decreasing calcium loss, and directly inhibiting bone reabsorption through inhibition of osteoclasts.

Several observational studies have suggested that combination OCs may protect against colorectal cancer. Potential mechanisms of action leading to the protective effect include reduction of bile acid production and concentration and effects on colonic mucosa or flora. A large meta-analysis has also suggested that combination OCs may prevent progression of rheumatoid arthritis to the more severe varieties.[19] However, this protective effect was noted in hospital-based studies but not population-based studies, which suggests the possibility of confounding or bias.

The major risks associated with combination OCs, although uncommon, relate to cardiovascular events (venous thromboembolism, myocardial infarction [MI], stroke) and possibly breast cancer.[20] Tables 58-2 and 58-3 provide estimates of the

risk of cardiovascular morbidity and mortality for combination OC users in women age 24 or younger. As shown, use of most current combination OCs roughly triples a user's risk of venous thromboembolism, although some studies of formulations containing desogestrel suggest that the risk could climb as high as sevenfold. However, it is important to recognize that even with the worst-case scenarios, the attributable risk annually is about 18 additional events per 100,000 users compared with nonusers of combination OCs. Venous thromboembolism risk is enhanced by risk factors such as recent leg trauma, pelvic surgery, stasis (but not varicose veins), and the presence of the mutation known as factor V Leiden. Although the presence of this latter clotting abnormality markedly elevates a user's risk of venous thromboembolism, the absolute risk is still low such that routine screening for the disorder among all potential oral contraceptive users would not be cost effective.[21] Obesity is also inconsistently cited as a risk factor; smoking, hypertension, and diabetes are not risk factors that increase the risk of venous thromboembolism among OC users. MI is a rare condition in reproductive-age women. This disorder occurs among

**Table 58-2**
**Incidence* of Cardiovascular Disease Among Low-Dose Oral Contraceptive† Users by Progestin Type, Ages 20–24 Years**

| | | Oral Contraceptive Type | |
| | | Levonorgestrel/ | Gestodene/ |
| Condition | None | Norethindrone | Desogestrel |
|---|---|---|---|
| Venous thromboembolism | 3.0 | 9.6 | 7.7–21.1 |
| Stroke | | | |
| Ischemic | 1.0 | 2.5 | 2.5 |
| Hemorrhagic | 2.0 | 2.0 | 2.0 |
| Myocardial infarction | 0.2 | 0.5 | 0.2 |

*Incidence per 100,000 annually.
†Less than 50 μg of estrogen, with most at 35 μg or less.
Adapted from International Federation of Fertility Societies: Consensus conference on combination oral contraceptives and cardiovascular disease. Fertil Steril 1999;71(Suppl 3): S1–S6.

**Table 58-3**
**Mortality* from Cardiovascular Disease Among Low-Dose Oral Contraceptive† Users by Progestin Type, Ages 15–24 Years**

| | | Oral Contraceptive Type | |
| | | Levonorgestrel/ | Gestodene/ |
| Condition | None | Norethindrone | Desogestrel |
|---|---|---|---|
| Venous thromboembolism | 0.1 | 0.3 | 0.2–0.7 |
| Stroke | 1.0 | 1.5 | 1.5 |
| Myocardial infarction | 0.1 | 0.3 | 0.1 |

*Incidence per 100,000 annually.
†Less than 50 μg of estrogen with most at 35 μg or less.
Adapted from International Federation of Fertility Societies: Consensus conference on combination oral contraceptives and cardiovascular disease. Fertil Steril 1999;71(Suppl 3): S1–S6.

combination OC users only in the presence of risk factors such as hypertension, diabetes, severe dyslipidemia and, in particular, cigarette smoking. In fact, it has been estimated that 80% of the cases of MI among combination OC users are directly attributable to cigarette smoking. Age above 35 years and smoking also act synergistically to increase risk; prescription of combination OCs is not recommended to women over age 35 who smoke. However, even with a 20- to 30-fold relative risk of MI among smoking combination OC users, this risk only equates to a maximum of 500 to 600 events per million women–years. However, unlike venous thromboembolism, in which the case-fatality rate in the reproductive age group is less than 1%, the case-fatality rate for MI is about 50%. Stroke is also a rare condition among women in the reproductive age group, with hemorrhagic stroke being somewhat more common than ischemic stroke. Among nonsmoking women, the rates range from 6 to 46 events per million women–years; combination OC use increases that risk only if risk factors are present. The major risk factors include age, cigarette smoking, migraine headaches (for ischemic but not hemorrhagic stroke), and especially hypertension. Overall, the relative risk of stroke varies between twofold and tenfold, depending on the number of risk factors present.

For several decades, concern has been expressed regarding the possible association between OC use and breast cancer. Unfortunately, many epidemiologic studies reported conflicting results. The discrepancies probably related to how well potential biases and confounding were addressed in the individual studies. In 1996, a collaborative project representing a reanalysis of most of the better epidemiologic studies in the literature was published.[22] In total, 54 studies were included in the analysis, representing 53,297 women with breast cancer and 100,239 control subjects. For current users of OCs, the relative risk of breast cancer compared with those who had never used OCs was 1.24. This small increase in risk persisted for about 10 years after OC use was discontinued, with the risk essentially disappearing after that time. In addition, there was no overall effect of OC use by dosage, specific formulation, duration of use, age at first use, age at time of cancer diagnosis, or by family history of breast cancer. The comparison of ever-users of OCs with never-users revealed that the relative risk for tumors that had spread as opposed to localized disease was 0.88. Thus, although OC users face a modest increase in risk of breast cancer, the disease tends to be localized. In addition, the pattern of disappearance of risk after 10 years coupled with the tendency toward localized disease suggests that the overall effect may represent detection bias or perhaps a promotional effect. More recently, a large population-based case-control study from the United States analyzed risk of breast cancer among women aged 35 to 64.[23] Neither current nor past use of any type of OC increased the risk of breast cancer compared to population-based controls. Further, the results did not vary according to potential risk factors, such as estrogen dose, duration of use, family history of breast cancer, or age at initiation of use. Thus this study also indicates that breast cancer risk associated with OC use is negligible for most women.

Minor side effects reported in association with combination OC use include abnormal bleeding, nausea, breast tenderness, headache, and weight gain. Effective management of these problems markedly improves the overall compliance with this method. Whether women start combination OCs for prevention of pregnancy or regulation of their menstrual cycles, a significant proportion have abnormal bleeding after initiation. Abnormal bleeding patterns on OCs are associated with improper pill taking, although fully compliant users also can experience changes in bleeding patterns. Patients need to be counseled to expect some change in their bleeding and be reassured that it does not indicate a gynecologic cancer. Lower doses of estrogen have been associated with an increase in breakthrough bleeding. Therefore, in patients with a particular concern about abnormal bleeding, a 30- to 35-mg ethinyl estradiol content may be indicated. Although extended-use OCs were introduced in an effort to reduce the frequency of menstrual periods, initial data suggests that abnormal bleeding or spotting is common as one approaches the end of the extended-use time period, although the effect is somewhat ameliorated with time. Persistent abnormal uterine bleeding on OCs should be investigated. The initial evaluation should include assessment for cervicitis or cervical neoplasia. The evaluation may also include an endometrial biopsy and sonohysterography.

Up to half of women report a feeling of nausea on initiation of combination OCs; many fewer experience vomiting. The incidence of these side effects has decreased with the decrease in the estrogen content of the pill under 50 mcg, but it is still frequently experienced. Anecdotal reports suggest a 50-mcg daily dose of vitamin $B_6$ may be effective for amelioration of symptoms. Other strategies include taking the pill with meals or at bedtime, decreasing the dose to 20 mcg, or switching to a progestin-only contraceptive. Reassuring the patient of the likely transient nature of the nausea is an important part of contraceptive counseling. There is no evidence that combined OCs directly cause weight gain. Users should be counseled that eating and exercise patterns are major contributors to weight gain.

Estrogens are known to stimulate breast tissue and lead to increased growth and tenderness. This side effect seems to decrease in frequency with continued use as endogenous levels of estrogen and progesterone are suppressed. Lower levels of ethinyl estradiol, as in the 20-mcg combination pills, could theoretically decrease this side effect. If patients are experiencing increased breast tenderness immediately before the pill-free interval, they may actually benefit from a higher-dose estrogen combination pill that more effectively inhibits ovulatory cycles. Patients should be reassured that the tenderness is not evidence of growth of a breast cancer, and that with time the overall incidence of benign breast disease will decrease.

Headache is a common complaint among reproductive-age women. Unfortunately, there are few controlled data on the incidence of headache in OC users or on the potential interaction with dose, formulation, or duration of use. One study indicated that the frequency of headache overall has not changed with the introduction of the new lower-dose formulations, suggesting that the occurrence of many headaches is independent of OC use. From an overall management standpoint, careful history taking should allow one to differentiate between tension-like headache and migraine headache. If one suspects migraine headache, combination OCs should be used with care. Although there are no conclusive data on differences in stroke risk for migraine with or without aura, OC use in the former circumstance should

# Reproductive Endocrinology and Infertility

be considered only if other contraceptive methods cannot be used and only after detailed counseling. If migraine occurs without aura and if other risk factors are not present, most women can be given a trial of oral contraceptives. Follow-up should be initiated within the first 2 to 3 months to assess frequency and severity of headaches. If there is a slight increase in frequency during the trial, a change in formulation might be considered. If headache occurs more frequently in the hormone-free interval, the physician might consider the use of daily continuous OCs without a hormone-free interval. However, if the headaches become significantly more severe or frequent, OCs should be discontinued and other contraceptive approaches used.

### Transdermal Patch

The transdermal contraceptive patch is 20 cm$^2$, roughly the size of a small Post-It pad. The patch consists of a matrix in three layers: an outer polyester protective layer, which is light tan in color; a middle layer containing an adhesive and the contraceptive steroids; and an inner clear polyester liner that is removed before applying the patch to the skin. The transdermal contraceptive patch is designed to deliver 150 μg of norelgestromin and 20 μg of ethinyl estradiol daily for a 7-day period. Norelgestromin, also known as 17-deacetylnorgestimate, is the active metabolite of norgestimate, a progestin contained in certain OCs. Ethinyl estradiol is the estrogen component of most OCs. After 7 days are completed, the patch is removed and a new one is applied to another skin site. Three consecutive 7-day patches are applied in a typical cycle followed by a 7-day patch-free period to allow withdrawal bleeding. Data also indicates that the efficacy of the transdermal contraceptive patch would be maintained even if a scheduled change was missed for as long as 2 full days.[24] Application sites that have been determined in clinical trials to be therapeutically equivalent include the buttocks, lower abdomen, upper outer arm, and upper torso except for the breasts. Because this is a combination steroid preparation, the same contraindications noted for combination OC use apply.

The efficacy of the transdermal contraceptive patch, as determined in three clinical trials, demonstrated a method use and typical use rate of 0.70 and 0.88 pregnancies per 100 women–years, respectively.[24,25] These rates are comparable to pregnancy rates achieved with current oral contraceptives. Further, the similarity of the two rates suggests that the ability to use the method correctly is high. This finding was confirmed in compliance studies, which showed that about 90% of women across all age groups used the method correctly.[26] However, a failure rate approaching the typical use failure rate seen with combination OC users was noted for women using the patch who weigh over 198 pounds.

Since this method was introduced, no reports have documented rates of serious adverse events. Until such data are available, one should assume that the events and risks will be similar to those noted for combination OCs. Similarly, there are no data available on noncontraceptive benefits, although one might assume that some of the benefits seen with combination OC users would accrue to patch users as well. The frequency of side effects such as headache and nausea is similar to that seen among combination OC users. Contraceptive patch users in clinical trials have application site reactions, more breast symptoms (only during the first two cycles), and more dys-

menorrhea than combination OC users. The pattern of breakthrough bleeding (bleeding requiring more than one pad or tampon daily) and spotting with the transdermal contraceptive patch is similar to that demonstrated in combination OC trials. Based on data from a placebo-controlled, randomized clinical trial over 9 months, there is no evidence that use of the patch influences body weight.

Women without contraindications to combination OC use constitute the initial set of potential users of the transdermal patch. However, women with a history of significant skin allergy or exfoliative dermatologic disorders may not be ideal candidates. Obese women also need to be counseled about the potential for reduced efficacy. Reminder systems to ensure appropriate weekly changing of the patch, using a different site for the next application, and avoiding use of lotions or occlusive dressings needs to be stressed during counseling. An obvious important attribute of any transdermal delivery system is its ability to remain adherent during the course of the dosing schedule. In the various trials, 1.8% of transdermal patches required replacement for complete detachment and 2.9% became partially detached. Detachment rates were similar for women living in warm, humid climates and for women who engaged in vigorous exercise, swimming, and sauna use. When patches do become detached, users should attempt to re-attach them if possible, without using ancillary adhesives or tape. If detachment is noted to last 24 hours or less, the cycle continues as usual, with the patch being changed on the previously determined change day. If detachment has lasted for longer than 24 hours, a new patch should be applied and backup contraception should be used for 1 week. The day the new patch is applied would then become the patch change day. When a new patch cycle is delayed beyond the scheduled start day, the user should apply a patch as soon as they remember and use backup contraception for at least 1 week. Further, the day the user applies the patch becomes the new patch change day. If a user forgets to change the first or second patch on time, various strategies can be employed to help get back on schedule and avoid an unplanned pregnancy. If a user changes the patch within 9 days of application, the patch change day remains the same and there is no need for backup contraception. Failure to replace a patch after this extra 2-day time period increases the risk for contraceptive failure. Therefore, users will need to use backup contraception or in some instances, emergency contraception if this occurs. In addition, the day she remembers to apply the patch becomes the new change day. Forgetting to remove the third patch on time carries less risk. The user should remove it when she remembers; the change day is not altered. Finally, if the user wishes to switch to a new patch change day, this should be done during the last week of a cycle, when patches are not usually used. The FDA has recently required a change in labeling, with a black box warning regarding adverse effects.

### Vaginal Ring

The contraceptive vaginal ring is flexible, about 5 cm in diameter and 4 mm in thickness. It releases ethinyl estradiol at a rate of 15 μg daily and etonogestrel, the active metabolite of desogestrel, at 120 μg daily.[27] The ring is worn for 3 weeks out of 4, although there is enough contraceptive steroid content in the ring's reservoir for about 14 more days. The ring maintains its efficacy even if removed for up to 3 hours, although it is designed to be left in place even during intercourse. If removed for longer time periods, use of a backup method for 7 days is recommended while the user continues ring use. Users are instructed to insert it high into the vagina; fitting by a health professional is not required. In a large clinical trial, the overall pregnancy rate over 1 year of use was 0.65 pregnancies per 100 women–years.[28]

As with the transdermal contraceptive patch, there is no published data to indicate rates of major side effects or potential noncontraceptive benefits. However, because the vaginal ring contains steroids that are utilized in combination OCs, rates of serious side effects may be similar and some of the noncontraceptive benefits may accrue to users of this method. Minor side effects are similar to those seen with users of combination OCs. Of particular note, however, is the low frequency of breakthrough bleeding and spotting occurring in 2.6% and 6.4% of cycles, respectively, in a noncomparative trial conducted over 13 cycles.[28] The pattern is relatively constant for all cycles as opposed to the usual declining incidence seen in most OC trials. As with the transdermal patch, about 90% of users use the vaginal ring according to the instructions. Approximately 10% to 15% of users report vaginal-related symptoms such as slight discomfort, a sensation of a foreign body, leukorrhea, vaginitis, or coital problems.

When starting use, the vaginal ring can be inserted during the first 5 days of a menstrual period. However, backup contraception should be used for the first 7 days of ring use. Regardless of when use of the vaginal ring is initiated, as noted previously, if it is removed for more than 3 hours, backup contraception should be used. Also the vaginal ring has enough hormone content for up to 35 days of use. Therefore, failure to remove the ring on time is not a major issue with this method.

## Progestin-only Hormonal Contraception

Progestin-only contraceptives are ideal for women for whom estrogen is contraindicated. Particularly ideal candidates include women with seizure disorders (metabolism of OC components are affected by many seizure medications), sickle cell anemia, mental retardation (if using an injectable or implant), migraine headache, hypertension, or systemic lupus erythematosus; older women who smoke; and those who are breastfeeding.

### Depot Medroxyprogesterone Acetate

Depot medroxyprogesterone acetate (DMPA) has been utilized as a contraceptive in the United States for at least 40 years, although Food and Drug Administration approval did not take place until 1992. DMPA is an aqueous suspension of 17-acetoxy-6-methyl progesterone.[29] The usual dose is 150 mg administered intramuscularly into the gluteus maximus or deltoid every 3 months. DMPA's mechanisms of action include suppression of ovulation by suppressing the surge of gonadotropins, thickening cervical mucus to impede ascent of sperm, and thinning of the endometrium such that implantation of a blastocyst is less likely. Although labeled by the manufacturer as effective for up to 13 weeks, the contraceptive activity actually persists for about 4 months after an injection, such that some practitioners will allow a "grace period" of 1 to 2 weeks after the previous administration for the next injection. Others schedule the follow-up injections at about 11 weeks from the last injection

to allow greater latitude to reschedule missed visits yet reduce the chance of unintended pregnancy. During 1 year of use, the perfect use failure rate is 0.3 pregnancies per 100 women–years, and the typical use failure rate is 3 pregnancies per 100 women–years.

There are health benefits associated with use of DMPA. The risk of ectopic pregnancy is significantly lower among users compared to women not using contraception. In studies conducted by the World Health Organization, the risk of endometrial cancer was reduced by as much as 80%. As with use of OCs, the risk reduction for endometrial cancer is long term and is greater for women who use DMPA for prolonged periods. Although no protective effect has been demonstrated relative to ovarian or breast cancer, neither is there evidence of an increase in risk with use of this agent. Studies have shown as much as a 70% reduction in the frequency of sickle cell crises; the mechanism for this effect is not known. Finally, some women with endometriosis have improvement of symptoms with use of DMPA.

There is no evidence that DMPA or other progestin-only contraceptives increase the risk for arterial or venous disease. The most significant potential risk associated with DMPA use is a reduction in bone mineral density. Although several observational studies have demonstrated such changes, most lack rigorous study designs that would allow one to adjust for other risk factors or clearly determine duration effects. Overall, in studies that are prospective and at least 1 year in duration, a maximum reduction of 1.5% to 2.3% in bone mineral density has been shown. A cross-sectional study showed reductions in the range of 2.2% to 2.5%, depending on site. However, this study also noted that the decreases were greater among younger users. No studies to date have shown any increase in fracture risk. Finally, retrospective studies have shown improvement in bone mineral density when DMPA is discontinued. Until further data become available, adequate calcium intake should be encouraged for DMPA users, particularly young patients and longer term users. The most frequently cited side effects are menstrual pattern alterations, mood disturbances, weight change, and delay in restoration of fertility after discontinuation. For the first 6 months of use, irregular spotting and prolonged menstrual flow is not uncommon. However, with continued use, many women become amenorrheic. By 3 months of use, 20% of DMPA users are amenorrheic; at 1 year up to 70% experience no menses. Mood change and depression have been reported in association with DMPA use. However, most studies are uncontrolled. Studies that have attempted to use some type of comparison group have yielded conflicting results. Thus, it is unclear whether DMPA use is associated with either depression or mood change. Although earlier studies suggested DMPA users may gain on average 5 pounds after 1 year of use, a recent randomized clinical trial demonstrated that DMPA is not associated with significant weight gain or changes in variables that might lead to weight gain.[30] Finally, when DMPA users stop injections in an effort to achieve pregnancy, the return to baseline fertility may take on average 10 months.

Patient instructions relate to ensuring that users return for their re-injections. Specially designed calendars can be used to aid in scheduling re-injections on time. After injection, DMPA users should not rub the injection site because that may distribute the drug more rapidly than intended and can lead to

# Reproductive Endocrinology and Infertility

decreased efficacy near the end of the 3-month cycle. Because menstrual patterns are altered with DMPA, proactive counseling to alleviate future concerns is important.

### Implants

Currently, there are no implantable contraceptives available in the United States. However, research is under way in the United States with a single-rod implant that is 4 cm long and 2 mm in diameter.[31] This system releases etonogestrel, the major metabolite of desogestrel, at a rate of 67 µg daily. It maintains its efficacy for up to 3 years. The system is usually inserted in the upper arm using a trocar; removal, although requiring an incision, is easier than with other implants because of the single-rod system. The likely mechanism of action is similar to DMPA. Overall efficacy is extremely high, with no reported pregnancies in more than 70,000 cycles of use. No major complications have been reported to date. Side effects include menstrual abnormalities and weight gain. For example, up to 19% of women will develop amenorrhea over 1 year; irregular bleeding, although not infrequent, was not cited as a significant issue for most users. In a 3-year study, mean body mass index increased by 3.5%, but about 20% of users experienced increases in body mass index of more than 10% compared to baseline.

### Minipill

Available progestin-only oral contraceptives (the "minipill") contain either 0.35 mg of norethindrone or 0.075 mg of norgestrel in packs of 28 pills without placebos. The mechanism of action is the same as for other progestin-only contraceptives. However, because dosing is daily, these actions may dissipate if the pills are not taken on schedule. Candidates for use of the minipill are the same as those for other progestin-only contraceptives. However, in the United States, the group who most widely use this method are lactating women. Perfect use failure rates are about 0.3 pregnancies per 100 women–years; typical use rates rise to 8 pregnancies per 100 women–years.

As with other progestin-only contraceptives, no major cardiovascular complications with use of this method have been reported. Irregular spotting and occasional amenorrhea are the side effects most frequently reported. Reduction of endometrial cancer is the only major noncontraceptive benefit that may accrue to users of this method.

For lactating women, in general the medication is started at the 6-week postpartum visit if the breastfeeding pattern is well established because lactational amenorrhea alone is effective as a "contraceptive" during the first few weeks postpartum. At the time that the decision to wean is made or when additional foods are added to the infant's diet, the patient can then switch to combination OCs if she is a candidate.

### Emergency Contraception

Emergency contraception is an approach to prevent pregnancy after unprotected intercourse or with known failure of a contraceptive method, such as a leaking condom.[32] The major methods used for emergency contraception include combination OCs containing the progestin levonorgestrel, levonorgestrel tablets, or the Copper T 380 A IUD. The hormonal methods prevent pregnancy by delaying or inhibiting ovulation or by disrupting the function of the corpus luteum. The IUD may inhibit implantation or possibly interfere with sperm function. The usual combination hormonal formulation consists of 100 µg of ethinyl estradiol and 500 to 600 µg levonorgestrel in several tablets administered twice, 12 hours apart. Currently it is recommended that the first dose be administered within 72 hours of intercourse. The levonorgestrel-alone formulation requires the administration of 750 µg of the progestin twice, also 12 hours apart. Initial dosing within 72 hours is currently recommended by many authorities, although there is data to suggest this approach may be effective as long as 5 days after intercourse. Further, data suggests that a single dose of 1500 µg of levonorgestrel may be as effective as the two-dose regimen. The Copper T 380 A is inserted within 7 days from the time of unprotected intercourse.

Emergency contraception, if used appropriately, can reduce the risk of unintended pregnancy by as much as 75%. One midcycle episode of unprotected intercourse carries a pregnancy risk of about 8%. Use of the combination hormonal method, the levonorgestrel-only method, and the Copper T 380 A IUD reduce this rate to 2%, 1%, and 0.5%, respectively. Data suggests that the earlier one initiates emergency contraception, particularly the combination hormonal approach, the more effective it will be.

Nausea is seen in about 50% and vomiting in 20% of users of combination hormonal emergency contraception. Administration of an antiemetic such as meclizine an hour before may reduce this effect. Levonorgestrel-only emergency contraception is associated with rates of nausea and vomiting that are 50% and 70% lower, respectively, than those experienced with combination emergency contraception. Women selecting the Copper T 380 A IUD will have side effects and risks as noted in the discussion of this method but will have the added advantage of initiating a highly effective long-term method at the same time.

## SUMMARY

With approximately one half of pregnancies in the United States being unintended or unplanned, there is a need for safe and effective contraceptive methods. Currently, many methods are available, each with their advantages and disadvantages. Further, emergency contraception is a highly effective backup method when methods fail or when it is known they have not been used correctly. Table 58-4 outlines some of the differences among methods. Regardless of the method selected, successful use requires that health care providers counsel on proper use of the method as well as expected risks, side effects, and possible noncontraceptive health benefits.

**Table 58-4**
**Characteristics of Contraceptive Methods**

| | Barriers and Spermicides | IUD | | Combination Oral Contraceptives | Contraceptive Patch | Vaginal Ring | Progestin-only | | | Emergency Contraception |
|---|---|---|---|---|---|---|---|---|---|---|
| | | *Copper* | *Levonorgestrel* | | | | *DMPA* | *Implant* | *Minipill* | |
| Typical use failure rates (per 100 woman–years) | 10–32 | 0.8 | 0.1 | 3–8 | 0.9 | 0.7 | 3 | <1 | 8 | 0.5–2 |
| Dosing frequency | At time of intercourse | 10 years | 5 years | Daily | Weekly | Monthly | Every 3 months | 3 years | Daily | After intercourse |
| Immediately reversible | Yes | Yes | Yes | Yes | Yes | Yes | No | Yes | Yes | Yes |
| Noncontraceptive health benefits | Yes | No | Yes | Yes | Probable | Probable | Yes | Probable | No | No |
| Office visits | Varies | Insertion and removal | Insertion and removal | Prescription | Prescription | Prescription | Every 3 months | Insertion and removal | Prescription | Prescription (usually) |
| User control* | Yes | No | No | Yes | Yes | Yes | No | No | Yes | Yes |
| Discreet† | Yes | Yes | Yes | Yes | Sometimes | Yes | Yes | Sometimes | Yes | Yes |

*Ability of user to immediately discontinue method.
†Whether method can be seen by someone other than the user.

# REFERENCES

1. Henshaw SK: Unintended pregnancy in the United States. Fam Plann Perspect 1998;30:24–29. **(III, B)**

2. Piccinino LJ, Mosher WD: Trends in contraceptive use in the United States: 1982–1995. Fam Plann Perspect 1998;30:4–10. **(III, B)**

3. Dardano KL, Burkman RT: Contraceptive compliance. Obstet Gynecol Clin North Am 2000;27:933–941. **(IIa, B)**

4. Gilliam ML, Derman RJ: Barrier methods of contraception. Obstet Gynecol Clin North Am 2000;27:841–858. **(IIa, B)**

5. Trussell J, Vaughan B: Contraceptive failure, method-related discontinuation and resumption of use: results from the 1995 National Survey of Family Growth. Fam Plann Perspect 1999;31:64–72. **(III, B)**

6. Raymond EG, Chen PL, Luoto J: Contraceptive effectiveness and safety of five nonoxynol-9 spermicides: a randomized trial. Obstet Gynecol 2004;103:430–439. **(Ib, A)**

7. Roddy RE, Zekeng L, Ryan KA, et al: A controlled trial of nonoxynol-9 film to reduce male-to-female transmission of sexually transmitted diseases. N Engl J Med 1998;339:504–510. **(Ib, A)**

8. Dardano KL, Burkman RT: The intrauterine contraceptive device: an often-forgotten and maligned method of contraception. Am J Obstet Gynecol 1999;181:1–5. **(IIa, B)**

9. Backman T, Rauramo I, Huhtala S, Koskenvuo M: Pregnancy during the use of levonorgestrel intrauterine system. Am J Obstet Gynecol 2004; 190:50–54. **(III, B)**

10. Marjoribanks J, Lethaby A, Farquhar C: Surgery versus medical therapy for heavy menstrual bleeding. Cochrane Database Syst Rev 2003: CD003855. **(Ib, A)**

11. Anderson FD, Hait H: A multicenter, randomized study of an extended cycle oral contraceptive. Contraception 2003;68:89–96. **(Ib, A)**

12. Potter L, Oakley D, de Leon-Wong E, Canamar R: Measuring compliance among oral contraceptive users. Fam Plann Perspect 1996; 28:154–158. **(III, B)**

13. Hankinson SE, Colditz GA, Hunter DJ, et al: A quantitative assessment of oral contraceptive use and risk of ovarian cancer. Obstet Gynecol 1992;80:708–714. **(IIb, B)**

14. Rodriguez GC, Walmer DK, Cline M, et al: Effect of progestin on the ovarian epithelium of macaques: cancer prevention through apoptosis? J Soc Gynecol Investig 1998;5:271–276. **(IIb, B)**

15. Schlesselman JJ: Risk of endometrial cancer in relation to use of combined oral contraceptives. A practitioner's guide to meta-analysis. Hum Reprod 1997;12:1851–1863. **(IIa, B)**

16. Ness RB, Soper DE, Holley RL, et al: Hormonal and barrier contraception and risk of upper genital tract disease in the PID Evaluation And Clinical Health (PEACH) study. Am J Obstet Gynecol 2001; 185:121–127. **(III, B)**

17. Davis A, Lippman J, Godwin A, et al: Triphasic norgestimate/ethinyl estradiol oral contraceptive for the treatment of dysfunctional uterine bleeding. Obstet Gynecol 2000;96:913–920. **(Ib, A)**

18. Michaelsson K, Baron JA, Farahmand BY, et al: Oral contraceptive use and risk of hip fracture: a case-control study. Lancet 1999; 353:1481–1484. **(IIa, B)**

19. Spector TD, Hochberg MC: The protective effect of the oral contraceptive pill on rheumatoid arthritis: an overview of the analytic epidemiological studies using meta-analysis. J Clin Epidemiol 1990; 43:1221–1230. **(IIa, B)**

20. Burkman RT: Cardiovascular issues with oral contraceptives: evidenced-based medicine. Int J Fertil Womens Med 2000;45:166–174. **(IIa, B)**

21. Winkler UH: Blood coagulation and oral contraceptives. A critical review. Contraception 1998;57:203–9 **(IV, C)**

22. Collaborative Group on Hormonal Factors in Breast Cancer: Breast cancer and hormonal contraceptives: collaborative reanalysis of individual data on 53,297 women with breast cancer and 100,239 women without breast cancer from 54 epidemiological studies. Lancet 1996;347:1713–1727 **(IIa, B)**

23. Marchbanks PA, McDonald JA, Wilson HG, et al: Oral contraceptives and the risk of breast cancer. N Engl J Med 2002;346:2025–2032. **(IIa, B)**

24. Audet MC, Moreau M, Koltun WD, et al: Evaluation of contraceptive efficacy and cycle control of a transdermal contraceptive patch vs. an oral contraceptive: a randomized controlled trial. JAMA 2001; 285:2347–2354. **(Ib, A)**

25. Sibai BM, Odlind V, Meador ML, et al: A comparative and pooled analysis of the safety and tolerability of the contraceptive patch (Ortho Evra/Evra). Fertil Steril 2002;77:S19–S26. **(Ia, A)**

26. Archer DF, Bigrigg A, Smallwood GH, et al: Assessment of compliance with a weekly contraceptive patch (Ortho Evra/Evra) among North American women. Fertil Steril 2002;77:S27–S31. **(Ia, A)**

27. Timmer CJ, Mulders TM: Pharmacokinetics of etonogestrel and ethinyl estradiol released from a combined contraceptive vaginal ring. Clin Pharmacokinet 2000;39:233–242. **(III, B)**

28. Roumen FJ, Apter D, Mulders TM, Dieben TO: Efficacy, tolerability and acceptability of a novel contraceptive vaginal ring releasing etonogestrel and ethinyl oestradiol. Hum Reprod 2001;16:469–475. **(III, B)**

29. Kaunitz AM: Current concepts regarding use of DMPA. J Reprod Med 2002;47:785–789. **(IIa, B)**

30. Pelkman C: Hormones and weight change. J Reprod Med 2002; 47:791–794. **(IIb, B)**

31. Meckstroth KR, Darney PD: Implant contraception. Semin Reprod Med 2001;19:339–354. **(IIb, B)**

32. Westhoff C: Clinical practice. Emergency contraception. N Engl J Med 2003;349:1830–1835. **(IIa, B)**

## KEY POINTS

- The *menstrual cycle* is the term used to refer to the process by which the primate ovary produces and releases an ovum. In primates, ovarian cyclicity is signaled by uterine bleeding. The "typical" menstrual interval is roughly 29 days. Regular uterine bleeding is often taken as evidence of reproductive competence, although this is clearly not always the case. Nonetheless, the cyclic nature of the menstrual interval due to the pattern of ovarian function is indeed a prerequisite for female fertility.
- Coordination of the ovarian–uterine cycle requires appropriate interplay between the hypothalamic gonadotropin-releasing hormone "pulse generator," pituitary gonadotropin release, and ovarian steroids and peptides.
- Hypothalamic, pituitary, and ovarian action differ during the three phases of the cycle, which are termed *follicular*, *ovulation*, and *luteal* when referring to ovarian events and *proliferative* and *secretory* when referring to endometrial events.
- The follicular phase is the first half of the cycle, during which the dominant follicle is selected from a pool of recruited follicles, estradiol levels rise, and the endometrium proliferates.
- Ovulation involves the release of the oocyte from the dominant follicle and the genesis of the corpus luteum in the ovarian follicle.
- The luteal phase is the second half of the cycle, during which the corpus luteum produces high levels of estradiol and progesterone to support a potential pregnancy and the endometrium is transformed to a secretory state to facilitate implantation.
- In the absence of pregnancy, menstruation occurs as the luteal phase terminates with decreasing estradiol and progesterone due to corpus luteum deterioration and the next wave of follicular recruitment and selection begins.
- Understanding of the physiology of the menstrual cycle is best achieved by examining the dynamics of each component of the hypothalamic-pituitary-ovarian axis at each phase of the cycle (Fig. 59-1).

## OOCYTE

Each oocyte is encircled by granulosa cells, which in turn are surrounded by theca cells and stroma in the ovarian cortex; this spherical ovarian structure is termed the *follicle*. In the embryo, germ cells migrate from yolk sac endoderm to the gonadal ridge by 7 weeks of gestation. Peak ovarian oocyte quantity of 6 to 7 million occurs by 16 to 20 weeks of gestation. Approximately 400 of these oocytes will be released; the remainder undergo atresia via programmed cell death (i.e., apoptosis). After their genesis in fetal development, the oocytes remain as dormant primordial follicles, each composed of an ovum arrested in the diplotene stage of meiotic prophase surrounded by a single epithelial layer of flattened granulosa cells (Fig. 59-2).

Gonadotropin-independent growth from primordial follicle (0.05 mm) to preantral follicle (0.2 mm) occurs by yet to be fully defined mechanisms in both ovulatory and anovulatory states from infancy to perimenopause (Fig. 59-3). During each cycle from puberty to menopause, a cohort of oocytes compete to be the dominant ovulatory follicle. The cohort's journey begins 3 months before ovulation with gonadotropin-independent follicular development. Cohort selection and continued follicular development requires gonadotropin exposure. Antral follicles (2 mm) are either selected, and thus become part of the preovulatory cohort, or become atretic (Fig. 59-4). From the preovulatory cohort of antral follicles emerges the dominant graafian follicle (Fig. 59-5) that will be released at ovulation.

Menopause occurs when the primordial follicle count is depleted to approximately 1000. The average age for menopause is 51.7 or 52 years (Fig. 59-6).

## HYPOTHALAMUS

The neurons that secrete gonadotropin-releasing hormone (GnRH) are located in the arcuate nucleus of the mediobasal hypothalamus at the base of the third ventricle. These cells that comprise the GnRH pulse generator migrate from the olfactory placode during early gestation; the pulse generator is active by 20 weeks of fetal life.

### CLINICAL CORRELATION

GnRH deficiency leading to primary hypothalamic amenorrhea associated with anosmia, or Kallmann syndrome, results from insufficient GnRH neuron migration to the hypothalamus from the olfactory placode. The more common X-linked recessive form affects men, whereas an autosomal dominant form affects men and women. Mutations in genes affecting pituitary gonadotropins can also cause idiopathic hypogonadotropic hypogonadism; these patients are normosmic.[1]

Afferent input to the hypothalamic GnRH neurons includes neural signals located in the brain stem, limbic lobe, and frontal

# Reproductive Endocrinology and Infertility

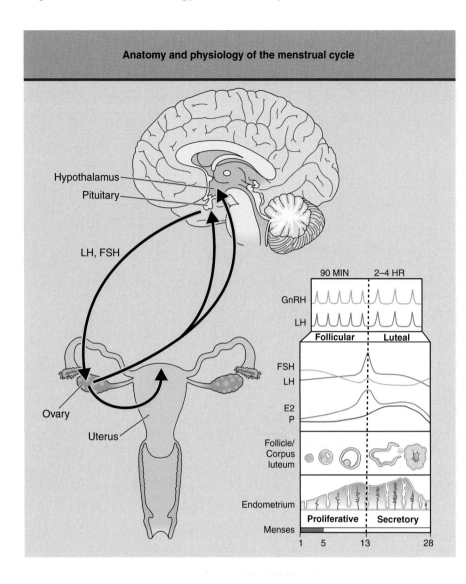

**Anatomy and physiology of the menstrual cycle**

**Figure 59-1    Anatomy and physiology of the menstrual cycle.** (From Berga SL: Menstrual cycle. In Knobil E, Neill JD [eds]: Encyclopedia of Reproduction, Vol. 3. San Diego, Academic Press, 1998: pp 189–194.)

cortex. Putative central neuromodulators include corticotropin releasing hormone, endogenous opioids, γ-amino butyric acid (GABA), dopamine, norepinephrine, neuropeptide Y, and serotonin. GnRH neurons receive peripheral signals from the circulation via the fenestrated blood-brain barrier.

## Pulsatile Nature of GnRH Release

Gonadotropin-releasing hormone is produced by neurons located in the ventral and anterior hypothalamus. GnRH is released in a pulsatile fashion into the hypophyseal portal circulation to stimulate the anterior pituitary to release the gonadotropins, follicle-stimulating hormone (FSH), and luteinizing hormone (LH). The pulsatile nature of GnRH release and its effect on pituitary gonadotropin release is of central importance to the regulation of the ovarian cycle (Fig. 59-7).[2] Because GnRH has a short half-life and is therefore not measurable in the peripheral circulation, GnRH pulse frequency is inferred by measuring LH pulses in the circulation. LH, and therefore GnRH pulse frequency, changes with menstrual cycle phase. In the follicular phase, LH is released at a frequency of one pulse every 60 to 90 minutes, with an increase in frequency preceding ovulation. LH pulse amplitude decreases in the midfollicular phase. In the

luteal phase, GnRH pulse frequency decreases from one pulse every 60 to 90 minutes to one pulse every 2 to 4 hours. This may be due in part to the induction of endogenous opioidergic modulation of GnRH.[3] The result is slowing of LH pulse frequency but amplification of LH pulse amplitude.

In the first months after birth, pulsatile GnRH secretion permits FSH secretion. Then, hypothalamic GnRH drive becomes suppressed until puberty. GnRH secretion resumes again at puberty, resulting in increases in pituitary gonadotropins, first at night and then around the clock. Neuropeptide Y and GABA are two factors that may act to restrain GnRH secretion from infancy to puberty. Increasing leptin levels associated with increasing body fat may permit the resumption of pulsatile GnRH release.[4]

Disruptions in GnRH pulse frequency lead to anovulation and subsequent infertility. Endogenous or exogenous opiate administration causes a slowing in GnRH pulsation that can be reversed with the opioid antagonist naloxone. The slowing of the GnRH pulse frequency with increase in pulse amplitude in the luteal phase is in part mediated by endogenous opiates, because it is reversible with naloxone. GnRH agonists given intramuscularly occupy the pituitary GnRH receptor in a sustained

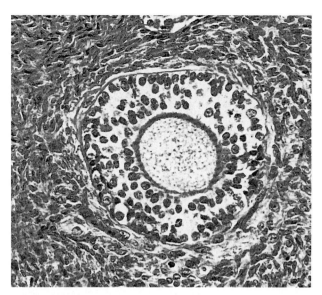

**Figure 59-3    Preantral follicle.** Oocyte surrounded by several layers of granulosa cells. (From Clement PB: Anatomy and histology of the ovary. In Kurman RJ [ed]: Blaustein's Pathology of the Female Genital Tract, 5th ed. New York: Springer-Verlag, 2002, pp 649–673.)

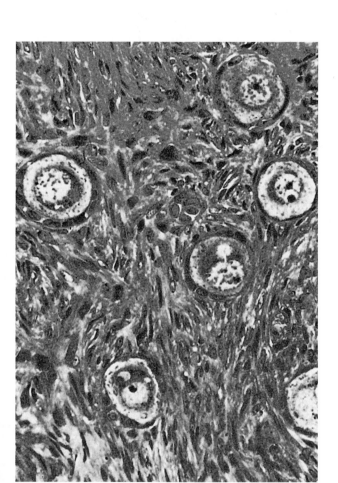

**Figure 59-2    Primordial follicles.** Primary oocytes surrounded by single layer of flattened granulosa cells. (From Clement PB: Anatomy and histology of the ovary. In Kurman RJ [ed]: Blaustein's Pathology of the Female Genital Tract, 5th ed. New York: Springer-Verlag, 2002, pp 649–673.)

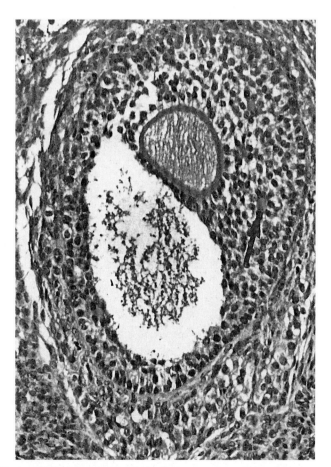

**Figure 59-4    Antral follicle. Fluid-filled cavity lined by granulosa cells.** (From Clement PB: Anatomy and histology of the ovary. In Kurman RJ [ed]: Blaustein's Pathology of the Female Genital Tract, 5th ed. New York: Springer-Verlag, 2002, pp 649–673.)

# Reproductive Endocrinology and Infertility

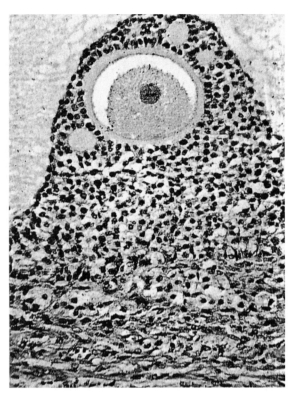

**Figure 59-5   Graafian follicle.** Proliferating granulosa cells form the cumulus oophorus, which contain the oocyte and project into the antrum. (From Clement PB: Anatomy and histology of the ovary. In Kurman RJ [ed]: Blaustein's Pathology of the Female Genital Tract, 5th ed. New York: Springer-Verlag, 2002, pp. 649–673.)

nonpulsatile fashion. These agonists have high binding affinity to the receptor and a longer half-life. Prolonged occupation of the GnRH receptors causes their evolution. Thus GnRH agonist use "desensitizes" the pituitary gonadotropes to endogenous GnRH drive. When given in a depot formulation or continuous fashion, GnRH agonists initially cause GnRH and gonadotropin secretion to rise, an effect which is often termed a *flare.* Thereafter, pituitary GnRH receptors involute and profound suppression of gonadotropin release ensues.

## CLINICAL CORRELATION

- In clinical practice, GnRH agonists are used to suppress ovarian and menstrual cyclicity and decrease estradiol production to treat estrogen-dependent pathology such as fibroids or endometriosis.
- GnRH pulse frequency is increased causing LH to exceed FSH in polycystic ovary syndrome (PCOS), a syndrome characterized by chronic anovulation and androgen excess. However, PCOS involves a constellation of metabolic adjustments, and treatment may involve targeting insulin resistance.
- GnRH pulse frequency is suppressed in functional hypothalamic amenorrhea, a syndrome characterized by decreased pituitary gonadotropins, anovulation, and estrogen deficiency. However, functional hypothalamic amenorrhea is more than an isolated disorder of GnRH drive because other neuroendocrine perturbations accompany the reproductive compromise.

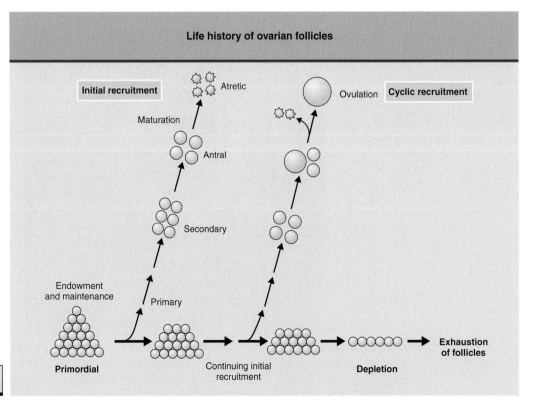

**Figure 59-6   Life history of ovarian follicles.** Gonadotropin-independent initial recruitment from primordial to antral follicle. Gonadotropin-dependent cyclic recruitment rescues some of the antral follicles from atresia to proceed toward ovulation. Eventual depletion of follicles leads to menopause. (From McGee EA, Hsueh AJ: Initial and cyclic recruitment of ovarian follicles. Endocr Rev 2000;21:200–214. Copyright 2000, The Endocrine Society.)

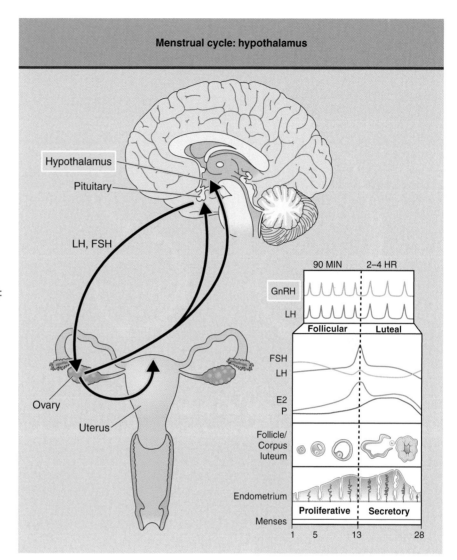

**Figure 59-7    GnRH pulses from the hypothalamus stimulate luteinizing hormone (LH) and follicle-stimulating hormone (FSH) secretion.** (From Berga SL: Menstrual cycle. In Knobil E, Neill JD [eds]: Encyclopedia of Reproduction, Vol. 3. San Diego: Academic Press, 1998, pp 189–194.)

In animals that breed seasonally, melatonin from the pineal gland synchronizes the GnRH pulsatility to the ambient light-dark cycle, so that parturition occurs at a time when the environment is supportive (a link to metabolism). Humans are only weakly seasonal, although they are highly circadian, and melatonin may serve to gate the timing of the LH surge. There is no evidence that melatonin per se can disrupt human reproduction. Nocturnal secretion of melatonin is increased in women with hypothalamic amenorrhea; however, secretion has not been found to vary with menstrual cycle phase in normal control subjects.[5,6] In contrast to normal control subjects, subjects with premenstrual dysphoric disorder exhibit decreased nocturnal melatonin concentrations during the luteal phase that change with therapeutic light therapy.[7] From this, it has been postulated that melatonin rhythms signal altered states of neuroendocrine "imprinting."

## Pituitary

The anterior pituitary gonadotropins, LH and FSH, are composed of distinct beta subunits combined with a common alpha subunit also shared by human chorionic gonadotropin (hCG)

and thyrotropin. The anterior pituitary releases FSH and LH in a pulsatile manner in response to GnRH pulses from the hypothalamus (Fig. 59-8). FSH pulses are not detectable in the circulation because FSH has a long 4-hour half-life. LH pulses are detectable because LH has a shorter 20-minute half-life. GnRH has an ephemeral (2-minute) half-life, which provides a lower signal-to-noise ratio when the GnRH pulse frequency is slower; therefore, LH pulse frequency is utilized as a reliable indicator of GnRH release.

The rise of FSH during the early follicular phase of the menstrual cycle stimulates ovarian granulosa cell growth and induces aromatase. LH stimulates the theca cells to produce androgens. Androgens are aromatized in the granulosa cells to make estradiol. Initially estradiol exerts negative feedback on the pituitary FSH release. When rising exponentially and at peak levels, estradiol exerts positive feedback at the level of the pituitary and probably hypothalamus to create the ovulatory LH surge (Fig. 59-9). That estradiol exerts its feedback on gonadotropin secretion at the level of the pituitary is supported by studies of ovariectomized rhesus monkeys with hypothalamic lesions who, despite absence of functioning hypothalamus or

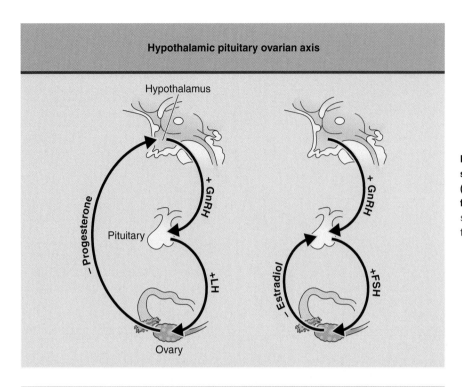

**Figure 59-8    The pituitary responds to GnRH stimulation by releasing follicle-stimulating hormone (FSH) and luteinizing hormone (LH) to stimulate follicular development in the ovary.** The ovary secretes estradiol and progesterone that provides feedback to the pituitary and hypothalamus.

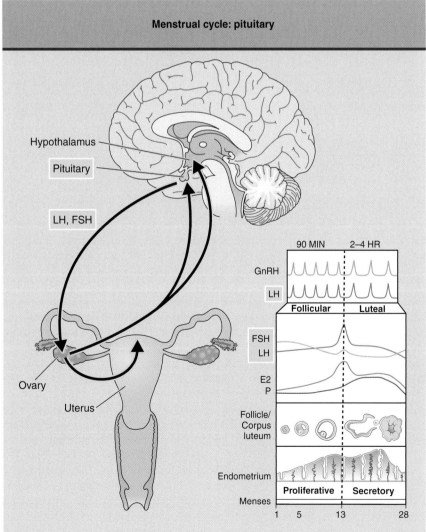

**Figure 59-9    The pituitary releases follicle-stimulating hormone (FSH) and luteinizing hormone (LH) to stimulate follicle development.** The LH surge triggers ovulation of the dominant follicle. LH supports progesterone release from the corpus luteum. (From Berga SL: Menstrual cycle. In Knobil E, Neill JD [eds]: Encyclopedia of Reproduction, Vol. 3. San Diego: Academic Press, 1998, pp 189–194.)

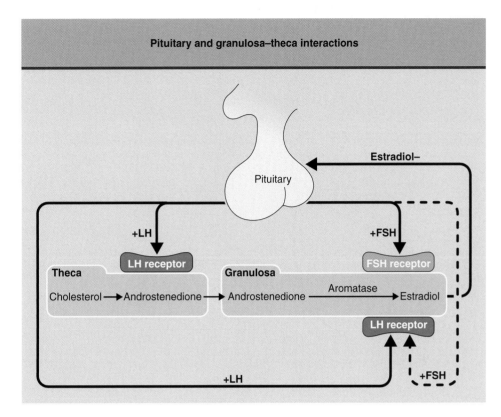

**Pituitary and granulosa–theca interactions**

**Figure 59-10  Pituitary luteinizing hormone (LH) stimulates the theca to produce androgens.** FSH stimulates the granulosa to aromatize androgens to estradiol and induces LH receptors on the granulosa. Estradiol provides feedback to the pituitary.

ovary, exhibited an LH surge when given exogenous GnRH followed by estradiol administration.[8] However, there may be a concomitant GnRH surge that reinforces the pituitary response.

# OVARY

The central importance of the dynamic interactions between the hypothalamus and pituitary is their effect on the ovary and ovulation. The changes in ovarian hormonal milieu intrinsic with each phase of the menstrual cycle are best illustrated by examining interactions between individual granulosa and theca cells.

The follicle is an oocyte surrounded by estradiol-producing granulosa cells, which, in turn, are surrounded by androgen-secreting theca cells. In the follicular phase, FSH stimulates the granulosa cells to become cuboidal and multiply. The surrounding thecal layers differentiate from stromal cells. The theca cell responds to LH by secreting androstenedione; only the granulosa cells have sufficient aromatase to actively convert androstenedione to estradiol (Fig. 59-10). Androstenedione is the predominant androgen secreted by the ovary. The granulosa cell lacks the enzyme to produce sufficient quantities of androgen, but has abundant aromatase to convert the androgens produced by the theca into estradiol. Estradiol and FSH increase production of follicular fluid, which accumulates into a cavity, thereby delineating the antral follicle stage.

Granulosa cells of small follicles (<10 mm in diameter) favor conversion of androstenedione to dihydrotestosterone. Higher levels of FSH than LH early in the cycle are therefore needed to increase aromatization and create an estradiol-rich environment. Granulosa cells of larger follicles (>10 mm in diameter)

preferentially convert androstenedione to estradiol. The preovulatory theca and granulosa compartments in the larger follicles therefore collaborate to produce the requisite rapid rise of estradiol seen in the late follicular phase (Fig. 59-11).[9]

Ovulation occurs 36 hours after initiation of the LH surge. The corpus luteum develops in the ruptured ovarian follicle. The length of the luteal phase is dictated by the longevity of the corpus luteum. Progesterone release from the corpus luteum is LH dependent. Progesterone slows GnRH drive, which secondarily leads to reduced LH and FSH release by the pituitary. This gonadotropin suppression, along with the suppression of pituitary FSH by high estradiol levels, prevents further follicular development during the luteal phase.

## Dominant Follicle

Selection of the dominant preovulatory or graafian follicle occurs in the mid- to late follicular phase. The dominant follicle must continue to mature while inhibiting the growth of other follicles. FSH induces aromatase within the granulosa cells, resulting in rising estradiol levels and subsequently declining circulating FSH concentrations. The follicle that is best able to produce estradiol from the available androgens and become FSH independent will become the dominant follicle. Follicles that are less able to convert androgens succumb to atresia as FSH levels decline. Thus, the rise in estradiol by the most mature follicle suppresses FSH and starves the other follicles.[10,11] Healthy oocytes are more likely to be found in follicles with the highest number of granulosa cells and estradiol levels and lowest androgen-to-estrogen ratio. Atretic oocytes are more likely to be found in follicles with low granulosa cell number, low estradiol level, and high ratio of androgen to estrogen.[12]

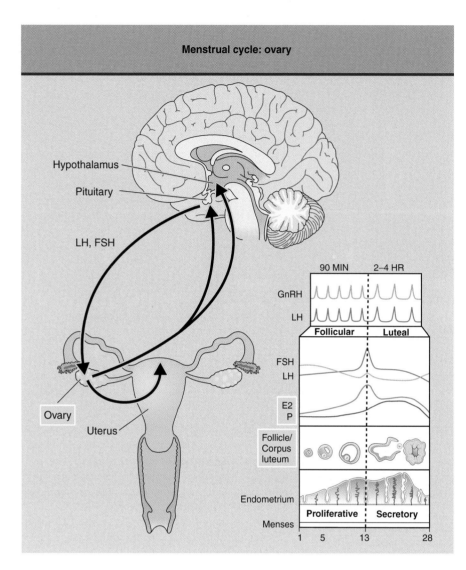

**Menstrual cycle: ovary**

Hypothalamus

Pituitary

LH, FSH

Ovary

Uterus

90 MIN    2–4 HR

GnRH

LH

**Follicular** | **Luteal**

FSH
LH

E2
P

Follicle/
Corpus
luteum

Endometrium

Menses

**Proliferative** | **Secretory**

1    5    13    28

**Figure 59-11**   **Ovarian follicular development stimulated by the pituitary gonadotropins results in rising estradiol levels, peaking at ovulation.** The corpus luteum supported by pituitary LH produces progesterone in the luteal phase. (From Berga SL: Menstrual cycle. In Knobil E, Neill JD [eds]: Encyclopedia of Reproduction, Vol. 3. San Diego: Academic Press, 1998, pp 189–194.)

Follicle-stimulating hormone also induces LH receptors on the granulosa cells that activate the same intracellular cyclic adenosine monophosphate pathway as FSH receptors. Women undergoing ovulation induction with FSH stimulation were randomized to subsequently receive FSH, LH, or saline once the lead follicle diameter reached 14 mm. Estradiol levels continued to rise in both the LH- and FSH-treated groups.[13] Thus, FSH-stimulated granulosa cells in the maturing dominant follicle acquire the ability to respond to LH and survive declining FSH concentrations.[10]

The LH receptors acquired by the granulosa cells will also facilitate response to the LH surge. Sustained administration of late follicular estradiol followed by GnRH elicits gonadotropin release in a dose-dependent fashion.[14] At midcycle, the rise in estradiol from the mature dominant follicle is exponential, with peak levels around 300 to 400 pg/mL. This pattern and amount of estradiol elicits a pituitary LH surge. The LH receptors on the granulosa cells then permit the corpus luteum to secrete progesterone during the luteal phase and during early pregnancy.

Rising estradiol levels intrinsic to the follicular phase are important not only for follicular development and ovulation,

but also for preparation for successful fertilization. Estradiol promotes endometrial proliferation and progesterone receptor induction as well as changes of the cervical mucus to a watery consistency to facilitate motile sperm penetration.

### Inhibin, Activin, and Follistatin

Inhibin, activin, and follistatin are peptides synthesized by the granulosa cells; their roles in cycle regulation are beginning to be delineated.[15] Inhibin has two forms, inhibin A and B, that share a common alpha subunit but different beta subunits. Inhibin B predominates in the early follicular phase, falling in the late follicular and luteal phase; inhibin B rises rapidly during the luteal–follicular transition and is found in higher concentration in follicular fluid. Inhibin A rises in the late follicular phase, peaking at the midluteal phase (Fig. 59-12).[16] Inhibin B levels have been suggested to reflect the growth of the follicular cohort, and inhibin A levels to reflect secretion from the dominant follicle.[15] Inhibin acts on the pituitary to inhibit FSH secretion by many mechanisms, including blockade of FSH synthesis and release and decrease in pituitary sensitivity to GnRH.[17] In the follicular phase, FSH induces granulosa cel

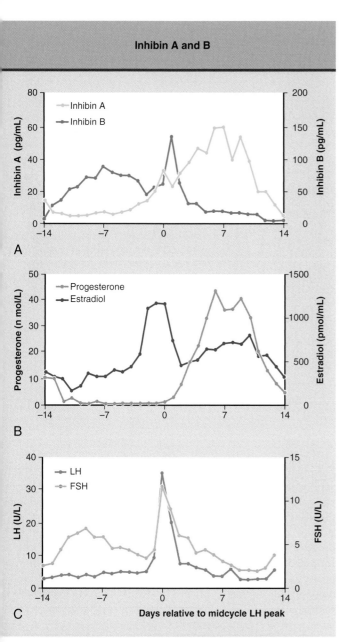

**Figure 59-12** Plasma concentrations of inhibin A and B *(A)*, estradiol and progesterone *(B)*, and luteinizing hormone (LH) and follicle-stimulating hormone (FSH) *(C)* during the menstrual cycle. (Groome NP, Illingworth PJ, O'Brien M, et al: Measurement of dimeric inhibin B throughout the human menstrual cycle. J Clin Endocrinol Metab 1996;81:1401–1405.)

Activin combines the two beta subunits of inhibin to create three forms—activin A, AB, and B. Despite similar structure, activin exerts opposing action to inhibin, augmenting FSH action at the level of the ovary and stimulating FSH secretion from the pituitary.

Follistatin suppresses FSH by inhibiting pituitary synthesis and secretion. It decreases activin activity by binding and thereby sequestering it.

In the early follicular phase, FSH induces granulosa cell secretion of inhibin and activin. Activin up-regulates granulosa cell proliferation, increases FSH receptors and aromatization, but inhibits thecal cell production of androgens. Inhibin up-regulates thecal cell androgen production (Fig. 59-13).[19] As the follicular phase progresses, activin enhances LH receptor expression on the granulosa cells, thereby enhancing inhibin production despite declining FSH concentrations.

### Insulin-like Growth Factors

Insulin-like growth factors (IGFs) have received much attention as potential intraovarian gonadotropin modulators that augment FSH action on the granulosa cell.[20] The primary insulin-like growth factor in the ovary is IGF-2, which is synthesized in the theca of small antral follicles and in the granulosa of large dominant follicles.[21] FSH stimulates IGF-2 expression; IGF-2 stimulates steroidogenesis and estradiol secretion. IGF-binding proteins inhibit IGF-2 action. Granulosa cell-derived IGF-binding proteins are modified by FSH in a dose- and time-dependent manner.[22] Androgen-dominant follicles have high inhibitory IGF-binding protein levels with subsequently lower bioavailable IGF and less estradiol production associated with follicular atresia. In estradiol-dominant follicles, IGF-binding proteins are depleted, enhancing IGF availability and estradiol production.[23]

## OVULATION

Ovulation occurs 36 hours after the onset of the LH surge that induces oocyte maturation. Two to three days before ovulation, the dominant follicle expands and estradiol levels rise rapidly. Granulosa cells produce more fluid, thecal vascularity increases, and the follicle reaches 20 mm in diameter before enzymatic digestion of the basal lamina facilitates follicular rupture and oocyte release. The granulosa cells closest to the oocyte, referred to as the *cumulus layer*, remain adherent to the oocyte after the release and are the first layer the inseminating sperm must pass through to initiate binding of the egg. The first meiotic division of the oocyte with extrusion of the first polar body is completed before ovulation. Completion of meiosis requires fertilization, at which time the second polar body is extruded with reduction to the haploid DNA complement.

Sustained exponential estradiol elevation is required to initiate the midcycle gonadotropin surge. The LH surge following increases of estradiol alone is of shorter duration than in natural cycles. The addition of progesterone is required to restore the normal dimension of the surge.[24] Therefore, progesterone in low doses after estradiol priming facilitates the LH surge. Progesterone administered before estradiol or in high doses inhibits the LH surge and subsequent ovulation by suppressing GnRH drive.

secretion of inhibin. Inhibin feedback to the pituitary decreases FSH secretion. The suppression of the pituitary by inhibin facilitates selection of the dominant follicle, which remains capable of continued steroidogenesis despite declining FSH levels. Inhibin B concentrations are lower in women with diminished ovarian reserve, evident by elevated FSH concentrations. Lower inhibin B concentrations are thought to result from less robust granulosa cells associated with the aging follicle.[18]

Reproductive Endocrinology and Infertility

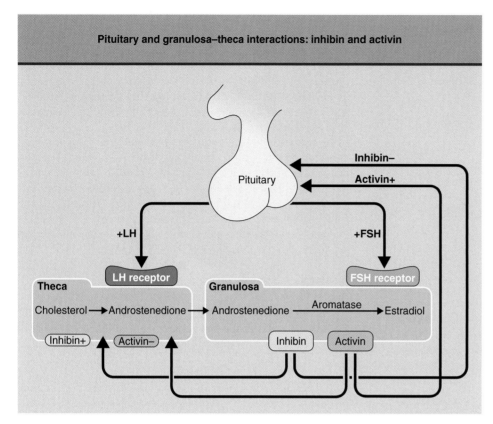

**Pituitary and granulosa–theca interactions: inhibin and activin**

**Figure 59-13    Inhibin, produced by the granulosa cell, acts locally to up-regulate thecal androgen synthesis and inhibits follicle-stimulating hormone (FSH) secretion.** Activin, produced by the granulosa cell, inhibits the production of androgens by the theca and stimulates FSH secretion.

## CLINICAL CORRELATION

- The ability of progesterone (progestin) to inhibit the LH surge and subsequent ovulation, when administered in high doses before peak estrogen, is one mechanism by which emergency contraception preparations decrease risk of unwanted conception when administered prior to the LH surge.[25]
- Follicle rupture and oocyte release by ovarian smooth muscle depends on prostaglandin production to induce enzymatic digestion of the follicular wall. Therefore, nonsteroidal anti-inflammatory drugs should be avoided at midcycle by women attempting conception.

## LUTEAL PHASE

After ovulation, the follicular remnant closes around the antrum. The granulosa, theca, and stromal cells become large and fill with cholesterol, new blood vessels occupy the area, and steroidogenesis begins. The resulting structure is the *corpus luteum*, from the Latin "yellow body," which produces estradiol, progesterone, and inhibin A in response to LH. Estradiol, progesterone, and inhibin in turn suppress FSH release to prevent follicular development during the luteal phase. The life of the corpus luteum includes 10 days of maximal function followed by 3 to 4 days of regression if pregnancy does not occur. Menses occurs with the drop in progesterone, estradiol, and inhibin that follow the demise of the corpus luteum. In the days preceding menses,

FSH begins to rise after release from estradiol and inhibin suppression, and follicular recruitment resumes. In fertile cycles, the corpus luteum is rescued by hCG made by the developing pregnancy; hCG sustains luteal progesterone production until 8 to 12 weeks of gestation, when the placenta takes over. Progesterone domination of the luteal phase prepares the uterus for pregnancy. Progesterone causes secretory endometrium, suppresses uterine contractions, increases cervical mucous viscosity, induces development of breast tissue, and increases body temperature.

## CLINICAL CORRELATION

The increase in body temperature secondary to progesterone release after ovulation is the basis for the basal body temperature charting method of tracking ovulation.

## ENDOMETRIUM

The endometrium proliferates during the estrogen-dominated follicular phase. The endometrial lining develops from 1 mm in thickness early in the follicular phase to 8 to 12 mm at the time of implantation (Fig. 59-14). When progesterone rises in the luteal phase, the endometrium differentiates to become secretory (Fig. 59-15). Progesterone from the corpus luteum prevents the endometrial lining from shedding. Decreases in estradiol, progesterone, and inhibin from the dissolution of the corpus luteum trigger menstruation (Figs. 59-16 and 59-17).

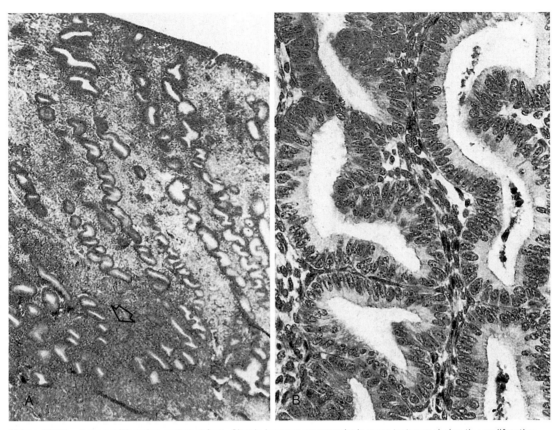

**Figure 59-14    Late proliferative endometrium.** Glands become progressively more tortuous during the proliferative phase *(arrow)*. (From Mutter GL, Ferenczy A: Anatomy and histology of the uterine corpus. In Kurman RJ [ed]: Blaustein's Pathology of the Female Genital Tract, 5th ed. New York: Springer-Verlag, 2002, pp 383–419.)

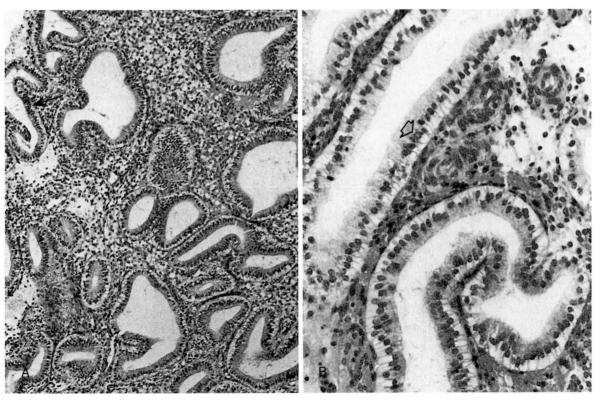

**Figure 59-15    Postovulatory, secretory endometrium.** Subnuclear vacuolization push the nuclei to the center of the cell, producing nuclear palisading *(arrows)*. (From Mutter GL, Ferenczy A: Anatomy and histology of the uterine corpus. In Kurman RJ [ed]: Blaustein's Pathology of the Female Genital Tract, 5th ed. New York: Springer-Verlag, 2002, pp 383–419.)

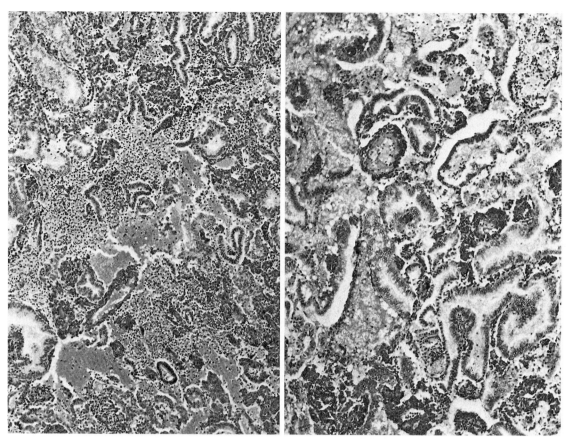

**Figure 59-16 Menstrual endometrium.** Collapsed stroma and ruptured glands are seen as the mucosa degenerates and is expelled. (From Mutter GL, Ferenczy A: Anatomy and histology of the uterine corpus. In Kurman RJ [ed]: Blaustein's Pathology of the Female Genital Tract, 5th ed. New York: Springer-Verlag, 2002, pp 383–419.)

## MENSTRUAL CYCLE VARIATIONS

Within the overall structure of the menstrual cycle there are variations. A withdrawal bleed does not always confirm a preceding ovulation (Fig. 59-18). If the dominant follicle was not of sufficient quality to become FSH independent, ovulation will not occur, but bleeding may result from fluctuations in estradiol levels as the follicle succumbs to atresia. During the anovulatory cycle depicted in Figure 59-18B, a low-amplitude estradiol rise and fall triggers uterine bleeding, but the gonadotropin surge and luteal rise in progesterone characteristic of an ovulatory cycle, as seen in Figure 59-18C, are absent.

The luteal phase is described as being 14 days in duration; however, poor progesterone production due either to an inadequate LH surge or poor corpus luteum development can result in shorter luteal phases (<10 days) or normal-duration luteal phases with inadequate progesterone production. Either pattern is referred to as a *luteal phase deficiency* or *luteal insufficiency*. During the luteal phase deficiency cycle depicted in Figure 59-18A, the follicular phase is lengthened and the luteal phase progesterone is of lower amplitude and duration than seen in the ovulatory cycle (see Fig. 59-18C).

An inadequate luteal phase can be seen in perimenopausal women due to dysfunction of the follicular apparatus consistent with incipient ovarian failure. Perimenopausal women exhibit a shortened follicular phase in ovulatory cycles, with periods of anovulation as well as higher estrogen excretion throughout the ovulatory cycles and lower luteal progesterone excretion.[26]

An inadequate luteal phase can also be seen in chronic exercisers; the mechanism is primarily a decrease in GnRH drive. A rigorous study of regularly menstruating women found a higher frequency of luteal phase deficiency and anovulation in recreational women runners compared to sedentary women. Luteal–follicular transition FSH elevation was lower in exercising women with luteal phase defect, potentially leading to the lower early follicular estradiol and luteal phase progesterone excretion. Energy availability was lower in anovulatory cycles.[27] Recreational runners with evidence of luteal phase defect also exhibit evidence of a hypometabolic state, including decreased serum total $T_3$, leptin, and insulin.[28] Decreases in LH pulse frequency and increases in LH pulse amplitude are seen during periods of decreased energy availability; this effect is more pronounced in women with shorter luteal phases.[29]

Energy availability has also been linked to likelihood of conception, pregnancy duration, and resumption of menstrual cyclicity postpartum. Studies of Lese horticulturalist women reveal lower salivary progesterone and estradiol levels during weight loss in the preharvest season that results in a seasonal conception pattern. Similar low salivary progesterone is seen in Polish farm women during times of increased agricultural

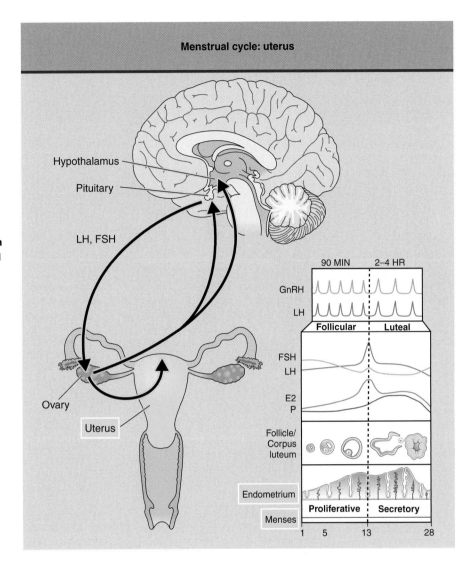

**Figure 59-17** **Endometrium exhibits proliferation during the estrogen-dominant follicular phase and secretory changes during the progesterone-dominated luteal phase.** (From Berga SL: Menstrual cycle. In Knobil E, Neill JD [eds]: Encyclopedia of Reproduction, Vol. 3. San Diego: Academic Press, 1998, pp 189–194.)

workload.[30] These less robust menstrual cycles decrease conception rates during times of inadequate energy supply. The independent role of psychogenic variables is difficult to gauge; however, high levels of cortisol, regardless of cause, induce metabolic demands. Thus, psychogenic stress, with or without weight loss, has the potential to disrupt GnRH drive and produce anovulation.[31]

## SUMMARY

Understanding the roles and interactions of the hypothalamus, pituitary, ovary, and uterus in the menstrual cycle facilitates diagnosis-driven treatment of menstrual cycle alterations. Before appreciation of the different causes of menstrual irregularity, patients with menstrual dysfunction were either treated with

oral contraceptives for cycle regulation or clomiphene for fertility enhancement. This approach did not address the underlying cause of the dysfunction or the associated morbidities. Knowledge of the connection between polycystic ovary syndrome (PCOS), hyperinsulinemia, and the metabolic syndrome, discussed in Chapter 62, allows the clinician to more completely treat the disease and assist the patient in initiating lifestyle modifications to prevent cardiac morbidity and improve longevity as well as fertility. Awareness of the hypoestrogenic state resulting from hypothalamic amenorrhea, which is discussed in Chapter 57, allows one to focus therapy on osteoporosis prevention while helping patients initiate lifestyle modifications that treat the underlying energy imbalance.[32] Through knowledge of the menstrual cycle, health care providers can delineate the appropriate diagnosis and tailor treatment to prevent the related negative sequelae and best facilitate fertility.

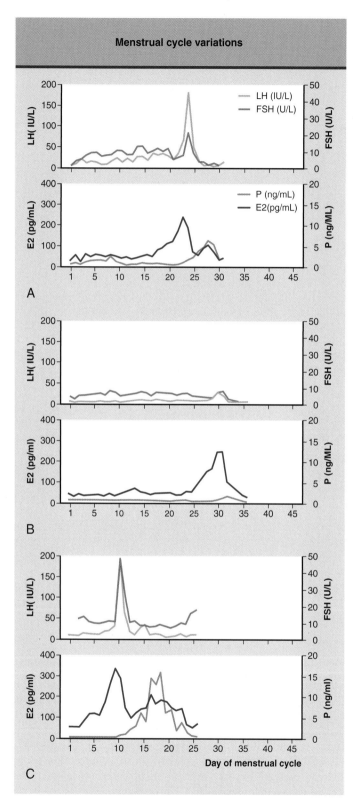

**Figure 59-18** **Three women who reported regular cyclic menses.**
*A,* Luteal phase insufficiency. The LH surge is present, but the luteal progesterone is lower and the luteal length is shorter. *B,* Anovulatory cycle. The LH surge is absent, but a rise and fall in estradiol level produces bleeding consistent with an anovulatory cycle. *C,* Normal ovulatory menstrual cycle. (From Berga SL, Daniels TL: Use of the laboratory in disorders of reproductive neuroendocrinology. J Clin Immunoassay 1991;14:23–28.)

## REFERENCES

1. Layman LC: Genetic causes of human infertility. Endocrinol Metab Clin North Am 2003; 32:549–572. **(IV, C)**
2. Knobil E: The neuroendocrine control of the menstrual cycle. Recent Prog Horm Res 1980;36:53–88. **(IV, C)**
3. Genazzani AR, Petraglia F, Gamba O, et al: Neuroendocrinology of the menstrual cycle. Ann N Y Acad Sci 1997;816:143–150. **(IV, C)**
4. Plant TM, Barker-Gibb ML: Neurobiological mechanisms of puberty in higher primates. Hum Reprod Update 2004;10:67–77. **(IV, C)**
5. Berga SL, Mortola JF, Yen SS: Amplification of nocturnal melatonin secretion in women with functional hypothalamic amenorrhea. J Clin Endocrinol Metab 1988;66:242–244. **(IIa, B)**
6. Berga SL, Yen SSC: Circadian pattern of plasma melatonin concentrations during four phases of the human menstrual cycle. Neuroendocrinol 1990;51:606–612. **(III, B)**
7. Parry BL, Berga SL, Mostofi N, et al: Plasma melatonin circadian rhythms during the menstrual cycle and after light therapy in premenstrual dysphoric disorder and normal control subjects. J Biol Rhythms 1997;12:47–64. **(Ib, A)**
8. Nakai Y, Plant TM, Hess DL, et al: On the sites of the negative and positive feedback actions of estradiol in the control of gonadotropin secretion in the rhesus monkey. Endocrinol 1978;102:1008–1014. **(IV, C)**
9. McNatty KP, Makris A, Reinhold VN, et al: Metabolism of androstenedione by human ovarian tissues in vitro with particular reference to reductase and aromatase activity. Steroids 1979;34:429–443. **(IV, C)**
10. Zeleznik AJ: Follicle selection in primates: "many are called, but few are chosen." Biol Reprod 2001;65:655–659. **(IV, C)**
11. Zeleznik AJ: Modifications in gonadotropin signaling: a key to understanding cyclic ovarian function. J Soc Gynecol Invest 2001;8:S24–S25. **(IV, C)**
12. McNatty KP, Smith DM, Makris A, et al: The microenvironment of the human antral follicle: interrelationships among the steroid levels in antral fluid, the population of granulosa cells, and the status of the oocyte in vivo and in vitro. J Clin Endocrinol Metab 1979;49:851–860. **(IV, C)**
13. Sullivan MW, Stewart-Akers A, Krasnow JS, et al: Ovarian responses in women to recombinant follicle-stimulating hormone and luteinizing hormone (LH): a role for LH in the final stages of follicular maturation. J Clin Endocrinol Metab 1999;84:228–232. **(Ib, A)**
14. Young JR, Jaffe RB: Strength–duration characteristics of estrogen effects on gonadotropin response to gonadotropin-releasing hormone in women. II. Effects of varying concentrations of estradiol. J Clin Endocrinol Metab 1976;42:432–442. **(IIa, B)**
15. Welt CK: The physiology and pathophysiology of inhibin, activin, and follistatin in female reproduction. Curr Opin Obstet Gynecol 2002; 14:317–323. **(IV, C)**
16. Groome NP, Illingworth PJ, O'Brien M, et al: Measurement of dimeric inhibin B throughout the human menstrual cycle. J Clin Endocrinol Metab 1996;81:1401–1405. **(IV, C)**
17. Luisi S, Florio P, Reis FM, et al: Inhibins in female and male reproductive physiology: role in gametogenesis, conceptions, implantation, and early pregnancy. Hum Repro Update 2005;11:123–135. **(IV, C)**
18. Hofmann GE, Danforth DR, Seifer DB: Inhibin-B: the physiologic basis of the clomiphene citrate challenge test for ovarian reserve screening. Fertil Steril 1998;69:474–477. **(IIa, B)**
19. Muttukrishna S, Tannetta D, Groome N, Sargent I: Activin and follistatin in female reproduction. Mol Cell Endocrinol 2004;225:45–46. **(IV, C)**
20. Adashi EY: Insulin-like growth factors as determinants of follicular fate. J Soc Gynecol Invest 1995;2:721–726. **(IV, C)**
21. El-Roeiy A, Chen X, Roberts VJ, et al: Expression of insulin-like growth factor-I (IGF-I) and IGF-II and the IGF-I, IGF-II, and insulin receptor genes and localization of the gene products in the human ovary. J Clin Endocrinol Metab 1993;77:1411–1418. **(IV, C)**

22. Adashi EY, Resnick CE, Hurwitz A, et al: Ovarian granulosa cell-derived insulin-like growth factor binding proteins: modulatory role of follicle-stimulating hormone. Endocrinol 1991;128:754–760. **(IV, C)**

23. Giudice LC: Insulin-like growth factor family in graafian follicle development and function. J Soc Gynecol Invest 2001;8:S26–S29. **(IV, C)**

24. Liu JH, Yen SSC: Induction of midcycle gonadotropin surge by ovarian steroids in women: a critical evaluation. J Clin Endocrinol Metab 1983;57:797–802. **(IV, C)**

25. Croxatt HB, Devoto L, Durand M, et al: Mechanism of action of hormonal preparations used for emergency contraception: a review of the literature. Contraception 2003;63:111–121. **(IV, C)**

26. Santoro N, Rosenberg Brown J, Adel T, et al: Characterization of reproductive hormonal dynamics in the perimenopause. J Clin Endocrinol Metab 1996;81:1495–1501. **(IV, C)**

27. DeSouza MJ, Miller BE, Loucks AB, et al: High frequency of luteal phase deficiency and anovulation in recreational women runners: blunted elevation in follicle-stimulating hormone observed during luteal–follicular transition. J Clin Endocrinol Metab 1998;83:4220–4232. **(IV, C)**

28. DeSouza MJ, Van Heest J, Demers LM, et al: Luteal phase deficiency in recreational runners: evidence for a hypometabolic state. J Clin Endocrinol Metab 2003;88:337–346. **(IV, C)**

29. Loucks AB, Thuma JR: Luteinizing hormone pulsatility is disrupted at threshold of energy availability in regularly menstruating women. J Clin Endocrinol Metab 2003;88:297–311. **(I, A)**

30. Ellison P: Energetics and reproductive effort. Am J Hum Biol 2003;15:342–351. **(IV, C)**

31. Berga SL, Daniels TL, Giles DE: Women with functional hypothalamic amenorrhea but not other forms of anovulation display amplified cortisol concentrations. Fertil Steril 1997;67:1024–1030. **(IV, C)**

32. Berga SL, Marcus MD, Loucks TL, et al: Recovery of ovarian activity in women with functional hypothalamic amenorrhea who were treated with cognitive behavior therapy. Fertil Steril 2003;80:976–981. **(Ib, A)**

# Chapter 60

# Menopause

## Robert L Reid, MD, FRCSC

## KEY POINTS

- Menopause is a natural process, tolerated well by many women, which may be attended by obvious adverse symptomatology (vasomotor symptoms or urogenital atrophy) or insidious disease processes (accelerated osteoporosis and cardiovascular disease) that, when revealed by adverse events, have the potential to significantly reduce quality of life.
- Counseling is essential to allow women to arrive at correct decisions about the lifestyle changes and medical options that will promote well-being and delay onset of disease.
- Hormone replacement therapy remains a safe and effective treatment for vasomotor symptoms and urogenital atrophy and will maintain bone while being used systemically.
- Available evidence suggests little if any increased risk for breast cancer with hormone replacement therapy (either estrogen alone or combined estrogen-progestin) for less than 5 years' duration. A small increase in the risk of breast cancer is seen with longer use of hormone therapy; this risk is comparable to the risk of breast cancer associated with several other lifestyle variables, such as delayed parenting, lack of breastfeeding, postmenopausal obesity, excessive alcohol ingestion, and lack of exercise.
- Hormone replacement therapy has not been shown to delay the onset or slow the progression of cardiovascular disease, stroke, or dementia when started several to many years after the menopause (the effect of early initiation of hormone therapy at the time of menopause on these conditions remains controversial).
- Women with spontaneous or induced premature menopause are at risk for premature cardiovascular disease and osteoporosis. Whether hormone replacement therapy in such women will avoid the increased cardiovascular disease risk is unknown, but it will delay the development of osteoporosis.

The "baby boomers" have finally reached the age of menopause. Estimates suggested that in the late 20th century one female baby boomer was entering menopause every 10 seconds, resulting in a postmenopausal population in excess of 50 million when the world celebrated the turn of the century (Fig. 60-1).

Now, more than ever, the health concerns of the aging population in developed countries focus on health promotion, disease prevention, and maintenance of a high quality of life. Health care providers to menopausal women will be called on to counsel the worried well, to determine who is truly at risk for disease and to suggest appropriate preventive strategies for these women, to offer effective interventions for those with established disease(s), and to provide care that is both compassionate and comprehensive to an increasingly dependent population in the final years of their lives.

## EPIDEMIOLOGY, RISK FACTORS, AND PATHOGENESIS

### Physiologic Changes of Menopause

During the reproductive years the main source of circulating estrogen is the developing ovarian follicle, in which the ovarian androgens, androstenedione and testosterone from the theca cell layer, are aromatized by granulosa cells within the follicle into estrone and estradiol, respectively. Inhibin B, also a product of the granulosa cells, feeds back to suppress follicle-stimulating hormone (FSH) released from the pituitary.

With advancing age the number of primordial follicles within the ovary is progressively depleted, resulting in reduced negative feedback by inhibin B, elevated FSH, and increased estradiol production from the remaining follicles. Eventually antral follicle count is sufficiently reduced such that even the elevated FSH cannot maintain regular follicular development with release of estrogen into the circulation. Typically this process is intermittent in the perimenopausal transition, resulting in periods of amenorrhea and typical menopausal vasomotor symptoms interspersed with episodes of menstrual cyclicity during which symptoms abate. In the postmenopausal years the elevated luteinizing hormone drives the interstitial cells of the ovary to produce androgens. These androgenic steroids may have a positive effect on energy and libido in the postmenopausal woman. In the periphery, particularly in fat cells, ovarian and adrenal androstenedione can be converted to the weak estrogen, estrone, which may, in turn, ameliorate estrogen deficiency symptoms to some extent in obese women.

### Cultural Differences with the Experience of Menopause

In cultures where high value is placed on youth, many women see menopause as one further sign of aging—a sign that is attended by distressing symptoms that foreshadow age-related deterioration in health and quality of life. In cultures where elders are revered, menopause is often seen as a sign of maturity and experience—the elderly woman or "crone" being a source of wisdom and guidance in the community. Although there has been speculation that these cultural differences may exert a strong influence on the perception or expression of menopausal symptoms, cross-cultural studies confirm the presence of similar menopausal symptoms in women from different ethnic and cultural backgrounds.

859

# Reproductive Endocrinology and Infertility

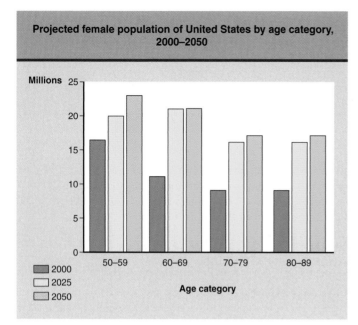

**Figure 60-1    Projected female population of the United States by age category, 2000–2050.** (Adapted from U.S. Census Bureau data from *http://www.encsus.gov/cgi.*)

## CLINICAL FEATURES

### Overview

The onset of menopause heralds a time of diminished estrogen exposure, which may have both acute and chronic effects on health and quality of life. However, it is important to remember that estrogen deficiency cannot be blamed for all the ills occurring in the menopausal woman. Menopause typically occurs at a time in life when women are dealing with teenage children and/or ailing parents. In addition, work-related transitions, marital discord, and/or ill health of a life partner are all common reasons for mood disruption at the time of menopause.

Estrogen deficiency symptoms may be categorized as acute (vasomotor flushes, night sweats, palpitations, headache, irritability, or mood swings) or chronic (urogenital atrophy with vaginal dryness, dyspareunia, vaginal itching or burning, urinary frequency, urgency, or nocturia). Other chronic degenerative diseases of advancing age may have clear links to estrogen deficiency (i.e., osteoporosis) or may be suggested by epidemiologic evidence (i.e., cardiovascular disease, cognitive impairment, impaired vision due to macular degeneration).

### Diagnosis

Amenorrhea by itself will not establish a diagnosis of menopause nor will the presence of vasomotor flushes. Although vasomotor flushes have long been considered the hallmark of the menopausal transition, flushes that appear identical from a physiological perspective have been documented in the luteal and menstrual phases of the cycle in most women reporting premenstrual syndrome.[1] FSH measurements fluctuate during the perimenopausal transition so that a single high FSH, though suggestive, is not diagnostic of menopause. Researchers are studying whether the fall of antimüllerian hormone, which

reflects the pool of primary, secondary, and antral follicles, may afford a more predictive measure of incipient menopause than measures of FSH, inhibin B, or ultrasound-determined antral follicle count, each of which correlates only with the number of antral follicles.

At present menopause is a retrospective diagnosis that can be made with reasonable certainty in the presence of elevated FSH or vasomotor symptoms in a woman after 12 months of amenorrhea. Typically menopause occurs around the mean age of 51.5 years, with a wide range from age 40 to 58. A mother's age at menopause shows a modest correlation to her daughter's age at menopause, suggesting genetic determinants, although cigarette smoking and prior hysterectomy can advance the normal age when ovarian estrogen production stops by 2 to 5 years.

### Early Estrogen Deficiency Symptoms
#### Menopausal Hot Flashes

The majority of women report hot flashes developing with increasing severity in the menopausal transition (a period of intermittent ovarian activity lasting on average 5 years before menopause) and becoming incessant in the years following the last menstrual period. These hot flashes have been linked to estrogen withdrawal that results initially from intermittent ovarian activity and ultimately from the complete loss of ovarian follicular estrogen production.

Typically these hot flashes (or flushes) are associated with an increased pulse rate, a rise in skin temperature, peripheral vasodilatation and sweating, and a gradual fall in core temperature. For some this means nothing more than an occasional transient sensation of warmth; however, others experience hourly waves of heat, drenching sweats, and increased heart rate. Cold chills by themselves or following a "heat wave" are reported by some women. In addition, sleep may be disrupted by night sweats several times a night, resulting in fatigue and irritability. Frequent hot flashes may be disabling, with attendant social, psychological, and economic consequences. Anecdotal reports suggest that alcohol, caffeine, and spicy foods may trigger hot flashes; women often report that hot flashes are less severe if the ambient temperature is kept cool.

Observational studies suggest that as many as 75% of women will experience hot flashes after menopause. Left untreated, most women will have spontaneous cessation of hot flashes within 5 years, although some women continue to experience distressing symptoms for 30 years or more (Fig. 60-2). Hot flashes are the primary reason approximately 50% of menopausal women seek medical treatment.

#### Sleep Disturbance

Sleep disturbance is frequently reported in the menopausal years; although many women perceive that sleep is disrupted by the occurrence of night sweats, sleep laboratory data do not confirm a tight correlation between vasomotor symptoms and recorded sleep disruption.[2] In any event it is clear that frequent nighttime awakenings may contribute to daytime fatigue, irritability, and mood change in some postmenopausal women.

#### Changes in Mood, Cognition, and Memory

Abrupt loss of estrogen has been associated with development of depression in some circumstances, and the clinical response

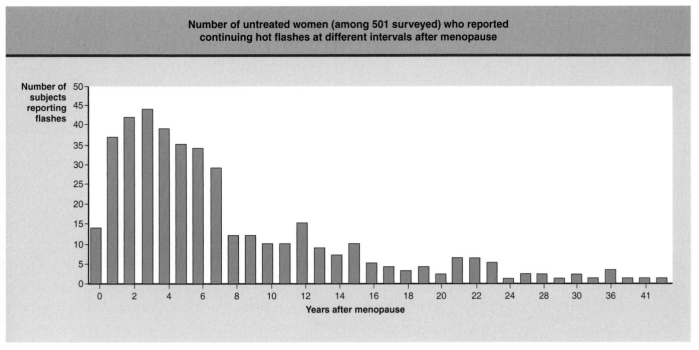

**Number of untreated women (among 501 surveyed) who reported continuing hot flashes at different intervals after menopause**

**Figure 60-2** Number of untreated women (among 501 surveyed) who reported continuing hot flashes at different intervals after menopause. (Reproduced with permission from Kronenberg F: Hot flashes: epidemiology and physiology. Ann NY Acad Sci 1990;592:52–86.)

to estrogen in perimenopausal depression supports a causative relationship.[3] Several lines of investigation suggest that estrogen also has important beneficial effects on attention, oral reading, and short-term memory.[4] Some, but not all, studies have suggested a role for estrogen loss in accelerating the age-related decline in memory.

### Delayed Estrogen Deficiency Changes

#### Urogenital Atrophy

Loss of estrogen in the menopausal years results in gradual thinning of the vaginal epithelium and a decrease in vaginal secretions. Manifestations of this may include vaginal irritation, itching, or burning and frictional dyspareunia. A variety of senescent bladder symptoms, including urinary frequency, urgency, and recurrent urinary infections, have been linked to hypoestrogenism (Fig. 60-3).

Pelvic organ prolapse is common in elderly postmenopausal women; however; the role of estrogen deprivation remains under study. Although hormone therapy (HT) use does not appear to correlate with the incidence of prolapse, certain estrogen receptor modulators have been associated with either increased or decreased rates of genital prolapse.

#### Skin Aging

Several investigations have documented increased collagen content and skin thickness in estrogen users compared to nonusers, suggesting a role for estrogen in the maintenance of skin integrity and health.

#### Eye Diseases

Observational studies in humans seem to indicate that estrogen loss at menopause is one factor contributing to lens opacities

(cataracts) associated with aging. Macular degeneration, the major cause of bilateral central retinal blindness in the elderly, also appears to occur with greater frequency in women who have not used estrogen replacement during the menopausal years. Maturational changes are induced in corneal cells by estrogen;

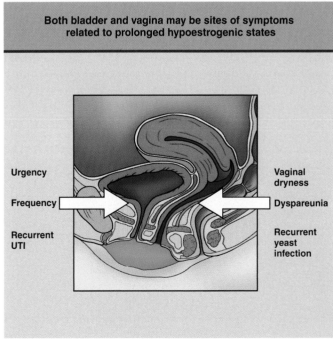

**Both bladder and vagina may be sites of symptoms related to prolonged hypoestrogenic states**

Urgency

Frequency

Recurrent UTI

Vaginal dryness

Dyspareunia

Recurrent yeast infection

**Figure 60-3** Both bladder and vagina may be sites of symptoms related to prolonged hypoestrogenic states.

this may account for the observed increase in complaints of "dry eye" syndrome in women on hormone therapy.

### Osteoporosis

Osteoporosis is characterized by low bone mass, increased skeletal fragility, and susceptibility to fractures. Osteoporotic spinal compression fractures (affecting 20% of white women over age 60), fractures of the forearm (10 times more common in menopausal women than in their male counterparts), and hip fractures (increasing in frequency from 0.3 per 1000 at age 45 to 20 per 1000 at age 85) are major causes of pain, disability, and/or death in the postmenopausal woman. The cost to manage osteoporotic fractures and to provide care for women who have sustained them was estimated at $14 billion in the United States in 1995; this cost is expected to soar exponentially as the older population grows in the next few decades.

Bone mass, measured as bone mineral density (BMD), has been known for some time to be inversely related to the risk for fracture. More recently bone quality (specifically the microarchitecture of bone) is being recognized as an equally important determinant of risk for fragility fractures. Of course most fragility fractures result from falls, so that BMD must be considered in the context of a person's age and propensity to fall when trying to determine overall risk for osteoporotic fracture.

Peak bone mass in women is reached around age 30, and it is from this level that losses of bone reduce overall BMD. Accordingly, peak bone mass is an important determinant of subsequent fracture risk. A variety of factors are known to contribute to the risk of fragility fractures in postmenopausal women (Table 60-1).

An age-related decline in bone mass occurs until, in women, estrogen deprivation induces an accelerated rate of decline (Fig. 60-4). Estrogen deficiency increases bone turnover; biochemical markers of bone resorption increase by 90% in the years just after menopause while markers of bone formation increase by only 45%.[5] Premature loss of ovarian function (due to premature ovarian failure, oophorectomy, or medical ovarian suppression with gonadotropin-releasing hormone agonists) produces the same accelerated rate of bone loss. This accelerated loss of bone lasts from 4 to 8 years and is then followed by a return to the more gradual age-related decline once again (see Fig. 60-4). The rapid loss of bone in the early menopausal period means that postmenopausal women move more rapidly toward

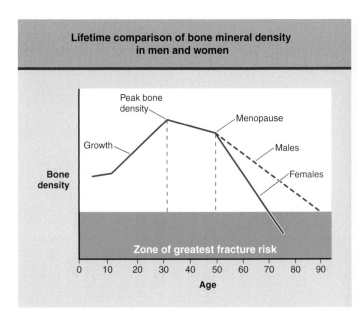

**Figure 60-4** Lifetime comparison of bone mineral density in men and women.

the fracture threshold (the level of BMD at which fracture risk increases). Although much attention has been focused on hip fractures as a cause of morbidity and mortality, recent evidence shows that the much more prevalent vertebral fractures can have a major negative influence on quality of life, morbidity, and mortality (Fig. 60-5).[6]

### Cardiovascular Disease

Due, in part, to successful breast cancer prevention campaigns, many women still believe that breast cancer is the leading cause of death in women. The number of deaths from breast cancer relative to deaths from other (mostly cardiovascular causes) is dramatically displayed in Figure 60-6. Heart disease is the leading cause of death in women, accounting for some 500,000 deaths annually in North America.

| Table 60-1 Risk Factors for Osteoporosis-Related Fractures | |
|---|---|
| **Nonmodifiable** | **Modifiable** |
| Female sex | Low bone mineral density |
| Advanced age | Low body weight |
| White race | Cigarette smoking |
| History of fracture as adult | Low calcium intake |
| Family history of osteoporosis | Vitamin D deficiency |
| Premature loss of ovarian function | Sedentary lifestyle |
| | Use of certain medications (e.g., glucocorticoids, heparin) |
| | Current estrogen deficiency |
| | Increased risk for falls |

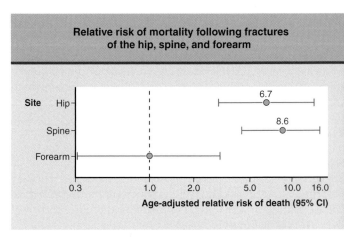

**Figure 60-5** **Relative risk of mortality following fractures of the hip, spine, and forearm.** (Reproduced with permission from Cauley JA, Thompson DE, Ensrud KC, et al: Risk of mortality following clinical fractures. Osteoporosis Int 2000;11:556–561.)

| Age | Cases of Breast Cancer /1000 | Breast Cancer deaths /1000 | All causes death /1000 |
|---|---|---|---|
| 40 | 15 | 2 | 21 |
| 50 | 28 | 5 | 55 |
| 60 | 37 | 7 | 126 |
| 70 | 43 | 9 | 309 |
| 80 | 35 | 11 | 670 |

Chance of development and death from breast cancer, compared to other causes of death, for women per decade

**Figure 60-6    Chances of development of breast cancer and death from breast cancer, compared to other causes of death, for women per decade.** (Reproduced by permission from Fletcher SW, Elmore JG: Mammographic screening for breast cancer. New Engl J Med 2003;348:1672–1680.)

More women than men die from this disease, and the gap continues to widen, with approximately $30 million spent annually in the United States for treatment of heart disease in women. The incidence of cardiovascular diseases increases with advancing age, and while there is little doubt that these complications are an inevitable consequence of aging there is biologic and epidemiologic evidence to suggest that these conditions are accelerated by loss of estrogen.

Menopause is marked by an increase in total cholesterol, low-density lipoprotein cholesterol, and lipoprotein(a), all known risk factors for cardiovascular disease, and by a concomitant reduction in high-density lipoprotein cholesterol, a known cardioprotective factor. Estrogen-dependent genomic and nongenomic mechanisms that favorably modulate endothelial function and vascular tone become less active, potentially contributing to increased vascular resistance and hypertension, the incidence of which rises sharply in the early postmenopausal years. Postmenopausal women tend to gain weight, with a shift in distribution from gynecoid (peripheral) to android (central), which also is an established marker for cardiovascular disease. Android fat distribution may exert this effect by leading to increased insulin resistance, which is known to increase progressively after menopause. Hemostatic factors are also altered after menopause, with increased levels of procoagulant factor VII, fibrinogen, and plasminogen activator inhibitor-1.

Numerous observational studies have reported higher rates of cardiovascular disease in women with premature hypoestrogenism compared to those whose ovaries function normally until the usual age of menopause.[7]

# COUNSELING AND INTERVENTIONS FOR MENOPAUSAL WOMEN

## Therapy for Vasomotor Symptoms
Women who experience distressing hot flashes should initially be advised to avoid situations (hot environments) and triggers (hot drinks, spicy foods) that provoke these symptoms whenever possible. Although exercise has been suggested as a means to reduce the frequency and severity of hot flashes, randomized clinical trial data indicates that the effectiveness of this approach is limited.[8] In contrast there is unambiguous clinical trial data demonstrating that systemic estrogen or estrogen-progestin therapy can dramatically reduce both the frequency and severity of flashes—an effect that can be seen at a range of doses by 4 weeks.[9] Progestin alone given in adequate dosage can also alleviate hot flashes.

Several nonhormonal agents have been reported to reduce hot flashes; these include Bellergal (a combination of phenobarbital, ergotamine, and belladonna), clonidine, vitamin E, and soy supplementation, but prospective, randomized clinical trials have demonstrated that these agents are only moderately more effective than placebo and may be associated with significant toxicity. Selective serotonin reuptake inhibitors have been shown to afford modest benefit for hot flashes in women trying to avoid estrogen (such as breast cancer survivors). Gabapentin has been used with some success for women with hot flashes who wish to avoid hormone exposure. This medication is very sedating, and its long-term safety in this situation has not been established.

In recent years aggressive marketing of "natural" or "nonhormonal" remedies for menopausal symptoms has led to widespread use of these compounds. Most of the initial reports on effectiveness of these agents were limited to uncontrolled trials in patients with mild symptoms. As more rigorous comparative trials have been performed, it is clear that few of these agents have significant benefits for vasomotor symptoms[10,11] and that many may have significant adverse interactions with other medications, particularly around the time of surgery.[12]

Phytoestrogens are nonsteroidal compounds derived from plants that are structurally similar to estradiol. They exhibit both estrogenic and antiestrogenic activity. The main classes of phytoestrogens are isoflavones, lignans, and coumestans. Isoflavones, which include genistein and daidzein, are found in soybeans, soy products, lentils, chickpeas, and red clover. Genistein and daidzein are believed to be responsible for the estrogen-like effects of soy. Lignans, which include enterodiol and enterolactone, are found in many fruits, vegetables, and cereals. Coumestans can be isolated in high concentrations from bean sprouts and fodder crops, such as alfalfa.

Mirroring the conclusion of the North American Menopause Society consensus panel,[11] a later meta-analysis of 22 randomized, controlled trials concluded that neither whole soy products nor isoflavone extracts were better than placebo at improving hot flush frequency or severity.[13]

## Sleep Disturbance
Research has suggested that the same hypothalamic trigger that incites the hot flush also triggers awakening. Not surprisingly, estrogen treatment has been shown to improve sleep and reduce daytime fatigue and irritability in symptomatic postmenopausal women. Estrogen therapy shortens the time between lights out and sleep onset (sleep latency), improves the quality of sleep by increasing the amount of rapid eye movement sleep and in some women may even improve sleep-disordered breathing such as sleep apnea.

# Reproductive Endocrinology and Infertility

## Vaginal Atrophic Symptoms and Urinary Symptoms

Estrogen therapy, whether systemic or local (intravaginal), has been shown to promptly relieve vaginal atrophy and associated symptoms of itching, burning, and frictional dyspareunia.[14] It is important to differentiate vulvar disease (lichen sclerosis) from vaginal atrophic symptoms because the former generally responds well to topical application of high-potency corticosteroids but not to topical estrogen. Estrogen replacement has been shown to improve tissue elasticity, to maintain urethral mucosal integrity, and to increase alpha-adrenergic sensitivity—all effects that, in theory, might reduce urinary incontinence. A meta-analysis found that estrogen alone afforded some benefit for urge incontinence.[15] Nevertheless, controlled trials in women with stress incontinence and urge incontinence have not shown improvement after HT.[16] Estrogen replacement is frequently recommended before surgery for genuine stress incontinence to improve blood flow, tissue quality, and healing.

## Sexual Function

Estrogen is required for normal blood flow to the vulva and vagina, to thicken and moisten the vaginal epithelium, and to make pelvic tissues resilient for comfortable intercourse. Estrogen may influence nerve transmission and sensory perception as well as promoting the activity of nitric oxide synthase—an enzyme responsible for mediating labial and clitoral engorgement.[17] Estrogen seems to have little direct impact on sexual arousal or sexual frequency—rather this function is subserved by testosterone from the ovaries and adrenal glands. Bioavailable testosterone, derived from free- and albumin-bound testosterone in circulation, seems to play an important role in maintaining a sense of energy and vitality and is the biologic component most responsible for female sexual interest and motivation.

Observational studies have demonstrated decreases in sexual responsiveness, libido, and sexual frequency along with increased vaginal dyspareunia and partner sexual problems in women around the time of menopause. Health and interpersonal factors appear to be as important as the hormonal changes of menopause on many of these problems. Many perimenopausal women are using selective serotonin reuptake inhibitors for depression, and many of these drugs are known to delay or inhibit orgasm. When diminished libido is the primary concern and factors such as depression, ill health of the woman or her partner, pelvic pain, and use of medications known to inhibit sexual function have been ruled out, consideration should be given to hormonal explanations. Total and free testosterone levels decline with age in premenopausal women such that women in their forties have half of the free testosterone of women in their twenties. Levels of testosterone (total and free) remain relatively stable into menopause but may show a further decline as adrenal function diminishes with advancing age. When hormonal therapies are being considered for the menopausal woman with diminished libido, adequate estrogenization of the vagina should be ensured before using supplemental androgens.[18] Topical moisturizers alone may be sufficient to relieve vaginal dryness in some women; however, local intravaginal hormone replacement (or systemic therapy if this is indicated for other reasons) is also highly effective for relief of vaginal dryness, itching, and dyspareunia. Transdermal estrogen replacement may be preferable when systemic hormone therapy is indicated because this results in less liver production of sex-hormone–binding globulin and less reduction of bioavailable testosterone. Placebo-controlled trials have confirmed that in surgically menopausal women in whom ovarian androgen production has been lost and in premenopausal women with ovaries intact but complaints of diminished libido, androgen replacement was associated with greater sexual frequency, pleasure/orgasm, and feelings of well-being than was use of a placebo.

### Osteoporosis

Ideally strategies to reduce the numbers of osteoporotic fractures in postmenopausal women should be started early in life and maintained. These include such lifestyle initiatives as participation in a regular program of exercise, avoidance of prolonged hypothalamic amenorrhea (due to eating disorders, excessive exercise, or medications that suppress estrogen production), ingestion of adequate amounts of calcium and vitamin D, and avoidance of cigarette smoking and excessive ingestion of alcohol. When women reach menopause they should be encouraged to continue a regular program of exercise because this has been shown to reduce bone loss somewhat while improving muscle strength and balance, which are equally critical to the prevention of fractures. Women should consider supplements of calcium and vitamin D if they are not getting the daily equivalent of 1000 mg calcium and 400 to 800 IU vitamin D up to age 65 with 1500 mg calcium and 800 IU vitamin D per day thereafter. Most studies have shown that calcium and vitamin D alone have little impact on the accelerated bone loss in the early postmenopausal years, although they may retard the more gradual age-related bone loss that occurs in the later postmenopausal years.[19] Smoking cessation should be encouraged and assistance provided with counseling and substitution therapy as necessary.

If history reveals that the postmenopausal woman may be at risk for osteoporosis because she was exposed to adverse lifestyle variables or if she has other risk factors (see Table 60-1), she should be considered for BMD assessment to predict fracture risk and to chart an appropriate course of therapy to halt bone loss and prevent future fractures. Assessment of bone microarchitecture at this time requires bone biopsy, which is not practical in a clinical setting. Biochemical markers of bone turnover, while valuable in clinical research, are not presently recommended for routine assessment of women at risk for osteoporosis.

Although a variety of techniques for determination of bone mass have been employed (dual x-ray absorptiometry, quantitative computed tomography [central or peripheral], quantitative ultrasonometry, and radiographic absorptiometry) dual x-ray absorptiometry, measured at the hip, remains the single strongest predictor of fractures at all other sites. The World Health Organization (WHO) has established diagnostic criteria to assist with the interpretation of BMD readings taken at the hip. The BMD measurements are given as a T-score (which refers to the number of standard deviations from the young adult mean BMD; Table 60-2). When osteoporosis is identified, certain laboratory tests such as complete blood count, serum creatinine (to exclude renal disease), calcium (to exclude hyperparathyroidism), phosphate, alkaline phosphatase, thyroid function, and protein electrophoresis in women over age 60 may help to exclude secondary causes.

| Table 60-2 World Health Organization Diagnostic Categories for Osteoporosis in Postmenopausal Women | |
| --- | --- |
| Category | Criteria |
| Normal | T-score above −1 |
| Osteopenia | T-score between −1 and −2.5 |
| Osteoporosis | T-score at or below −2.5 |

**Table 60-3**
**Strategies to "Fall Proof" Living Areas for the Elderly**

Ensure adequate lighting
Suggest sensible footwear with soles that ensure traction
Obtain orthopedic supports if foot problems contribute to instability
Avoid throw rugs and loose electrical cords
Install railings along walkways and steps
Add white tape to highlight edges of any steps
Wear appropriate outer footwear, especially in wet or icy conditions
Provide care worker assistance and appropriate supports (cane or walker) as
   necessary

The risk for fragility fractures depends not only on BMD and bone microarchitecture, but also on the age of the woman and her propensity to fall.[20] Women with alcoholism, those who use certain medications (such as sedatives); those who are frail, of advanced age; or with slow gait, foot problems, or inappropriate footwear; those with impaired cognition and balance or bad eyesight; and those with neurologic disease or past stroke are at increased risk for falls and may benefit from "fall proofing" of their homes (Table 60-3).

### Hormone Therapy

The efficacy of estrogen replacement therapy in preventing menopausal bone loss and osteoporotic fractures has been well documented in both retrospective and prospective studies (Figs. 60-7 and 60-8). Bone loss in women who continue HT is rare; women who use HT for control of vasomotor symptoms early in menopause can usually expect protection from the accelerated bone loss that typically occurs at this time. BMD declines at a modest pace after discontinuation of HT[21]; on average, 3 years after cessation of HT mean vertebral BMD remains significantly higher than at baseline. Most studies suggest, however, that for HT to be effective in reducing osteoporotic fractures it needs to be taken for at least 10 years after menopause. Estrogen therapy is effective in reducing bone loss even if given in lower than standard doses or if started many years after menopause, although, ideally, therapy should commence when hypoestrogenism first appears. Women who do not use HT at menopause or who stop HT after symptoms subside need to be particularly vigilant about monitoring BMD at intervals of 1 to 2 years to detect evidence of osteopenia and to take appropriate steps with alternative therapies (such as selective estrogen receptor modulators [SERMs], bisphosphonates, or calcitonin) to retard this process before the risk of osteoporotic fractures rises further.

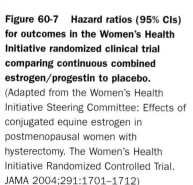

**Figure 60-7** Hazard ratios (95% CIs) for outcomes in the Women's Health Initiative randomized clinical trial comparing continuous combined estrogen/progestin to placebo. (Adapted from the Women's Health Initiative Steering Committee: Effects of conjugated equine estrogen in postmenopausal women with hysterectomy. The Women's Health Initiative Randomized Controlled Trial. JAMA 2004;291:1701–1712)

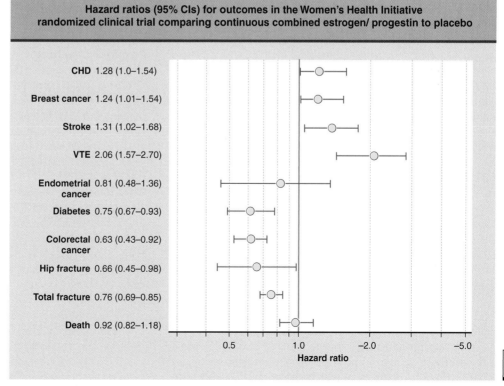

Hazard ratios (95% CIs) for outcomes in the Women's Health Initiative randomized clinical trial comparing continuous combined estrogen/ progestin to placebo

CHD 1.28 (1.0–1.54)
Breast cancer 1.24 (1.01–1.54)
Stroke 1.31 (1.02–1.68)
VTE 2.06 (1.57–2.70)
Endometrial cancer 0.81 (0.48–1.36)
Diabetes 0.75 (0.67–0.93)
Colorectal cancer 0.63 (0.43–0.92)
Hip fracture 0.66 (0.45–0.98)
Total fracture 0.76 (0.69–0.85)
Death 0.92 (0.82–1.18)

0.5   1.0   −2.0   −5.0
Hazard ratio

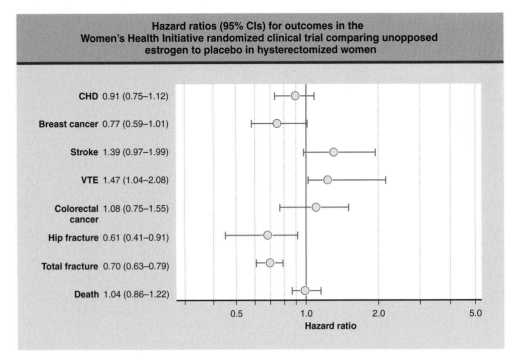

**Hazard ratios (95% CIs) for outcomes in the Women's Health Initiative randomized clinical trial comparing unopposed estrogen to placebo in hysterectomized women**

| | |
|---|---|
| CHD | 0.91 (0.75–1.12) |
| Breast cancer | 0.77 (0.59–1.01) |
| Stroke | 1.39 (0.97–1.99) |
| VTE | 1.47 (1.04–2.08) |
| Colorectal cancer | 1.08 (0.75–1.55) |
| Hip fracture | 0.61 (0.41–0.91) |
| Total fracture | 0.70 (0.63–0.79) |
| Death | 1.04 (0.86–1.22) |

Hazard ratio

**Figure 60-8    Hazard ratios (95% CIs) for outcomes in the Women's Health Initiative randomized clinical trial comparing unopposed estrogen to placebo in women with hysterectomies.** (Adapted from the Women's Health Initiative Steering Committee: Effects of conjugated equine estrogen in postmenopausal women with hysterectomy. The Women's Health Initiative Randomized Controlled Trial. JAMA 2004;291:1701–1712.)

### Selective Estrogen Receptor Modulators

Selective estrogen receptor modulators exert selective agonist and antagonist effects on various estrogen target tissues. In postmenopausal women with osteoporosis raloxifene decreases bone resorption marked by a decrease in markers of bone turnover (by 30% to 40%) after 1 year and an increased BMD by 2% to 3% after 3 years. The 50% decrease in vertebral fractures in women using raloxifene is comparable to the benefit seen with other agents such as bisphosphonates, which increase BMD by as much as 9%, suggesting that at least part of the benefit of raloxifene is through its modulation of bone microarchitecture.[22] Studies to date have demonstrated that unlike unopposed estrogen therapy raloxifene does not cause uterine bleeding and is not associated with any increase in endometrial cancer. In those studies raloxifene users had a 76% decrease in estrogen receptor–positive breast cancers. Like hormone therapy raloxifene has been associated with a slight increase in venous thromboembolism. Although raloxifene has favorable effects on markers of cardiovascular disease in experimental studies and has been shown to reduce cardiovascular risk in women at highest risk, its role as an agent for primary cardioprotection remains under investigation.

### Bisphosphonates

Bisphosphonates bind to mineralized bone surfaces and inhibit osteoclast activity that would normally remove bone during the bone remodeling process—hence their designation as *antiresorptive agents*.

Etidronate, a non-nitrogen-containing bisphosphonate given cyclically, has been shown to reduce both vertebral and hip fractures. The major drawback with this agent is its tendency for poor absorption and gastrointestinal irritation. Alendronate and risedronate are nitrogen-containing bisphosphonates that are 1000 and 3000 times more potent, respectively, than etidronate.

When given continuously in low daily doses or in a slightly larger once-weekly dose, they have proven highly effective for prevention of bone loss in postmenopausal women and less irritating to the gastrointestinal tract.

### Calcitonin

Calcitonin, available as a nasal spray, is an effective therapy to prevent further vertebral compression fractures in those with osteoporosis while suppressing the back pain often associated with this complication. Its side effect profile is favorable, with some women reporting rhinitis, flushing, or nasal dryness.

### Parathyroid Hormone

Teriparatide is another addition to the therapeutic armamentarium for management of severe osteoporosis. This synthetic parathyroid hormone is indicated for treatment of severe osteoporosis that has failed to respond to conventional therapies. Initial studies have shown striking increases in BMD of as much as 10% by 18 months of treatment and a concomitant 40% reduction in subsequent fracture risk.

## Cardiovascular Disease

The mainstay for cardiovascular disease prevention remains a lifelong pattern of healthy living, incorporating a balanced diet, moderate exercise, weight control, and avoidance of smoking, limited use of alcohol, and attention to treatment of known risk factors such as hypertension if these arise. Randomized, controlled trial data confirm that an intervention involving diet and exercise can slow the progression of thickening of the intima-media layer of the carotid during the menopausal transition—an established early marker for coronary artery disease.[23] Known cardioprotective medications, including aspirin, statins, and beta-adrenergic antagonists, should be used where appropriate (indications for their use are beyond the scope of this chapter).

A variety of epidemiologic studies, observational studies, and clinical trials have provided support for the premise that estrogen has a cardioprotective role in women.[24–27] Exogenous estrogen has been found to have a favorable impact on lipids and lipoproteins, direct anti-atherosclerotic effects, antiplatelet-aggregating properties, and positive changes on endothelium-dependent vasodilation while exerting certain prothrombotic and pro-inflammatory effects (increases in C-reactive protein after oral administration) that may be greatest in the first years after estrogen is started.[28] Women on HT have a smaller increase in systemic blood pressure over time than do women not using hormones.[29] Observational trials have suggested that "ever-use" of estrogen was associated with a 30% to 40% reduction in the risk of cardiovascular events and cardiovascular mortality compared to nonuse of hormone therapy.[30]

Randomized clinical trials, however, have not confirmed the cardiovascular benefits reported in observational trials. The first large scale secondary prevention clinical trial was the Heart and Estrogen/Progestin Replacement Study (HERS) trial.[31] This randomized, placebo-controlled trial, which involved 2763 elderly women with documented coronary artery disease over a 4.1-year follow-up, showed no benefit from daily conjugated equine estrogen and medroxyprogesterone acetate started immediately following a myocardial infarction (MI) or coronary angioplasty, for the first time challenging the promising results of hormones for secondary prevention reported in earlier observational trials. Neither oral nor transdermal hormone replacement was found to delay progression of angiographically proven coronary artery lesions in randomized clinical trials comparing hormone therapy to placebo in older postmenopausal women with established cardiovascular disease.[32–34] Combined, these observations make a strong case for not starting women with known cardiovascular disease on hormone therapy as a means to delay progression of the disease.

The data on the role of hormone therapy for primary prevention of cardiovascular disease are more limited and have been the focus of ongoing debate. Clarkson's data in the nonhuman primate supports the notion that hormone therapy started early after loss of ovarian estrogen production may have significant benefits in terms of prevention of coronary artery disease.[35] Other data lend support to this notion. In the Estrogen in the Prevention of Atherosclerosis Trial, a randomized, double-blind, placebo-controlled trial involving 222 healthy postmenopausal women, hormone therapy started early in menopause was shown to delay the progression of subclinical cardiovascular disease (as determined by ultrasound measurement of carotid intima-media thickness).[36]

The Women's Health Initiative (WHI), described by its authors as a primary prevention trial, is the largest randomized, controlled trial to evaluate the risks and benefits of hormone therapy in postmenopausal women. This trial reported no cardiovascular disease benefit in "generally healthy" women randomized either to continuous combined conjugated equine estrogen and medroxyprogesterone acetate (combination HT) versus placebo[37] (or conjugated equine estrogen versus placebo in a separate trial for women with prior hysterectomy).[38] Although the initial WHI publication on the combination HT arm generated much public consternation by suggesting that hormone therapy actually increased rates of coronary artery events, when the "adjudicated" findings were subsequently published there was no statistically significant overall increase in cardiovascular events or mortality in hormone users (see Fig. 60-7). There was, however, a significant elevation in cardiovascular events in combination HT users compared to women on placebo in the first year of therapy (nonfatal MIs, attributable risk 21/10,000 women-years—no significant differences after year one.[37] There was a very small increase in the risk of nonfatal ischemic stroke in women receiving combination HT (attributable risk, 7/10,000 women-years)[39] (see Fig. 60-7). In the conjugated equine estrogen arm of the WHI there was no increase or decrease in coronary artery events in estrogen users compared to women on placebo (see Fig. 60-8). There was a slight increase in the risk of nonfatal ischemic stroke in older postmenopausal women (only in those older than age 60) on estrogen alone (attributable risk, 9/10,000 women-years; see Fig. 60-8).

Those who accept that the results of the WHI effectively contradict numerous observational and clinical studies suggesting cardioprotective effects of HT point out that observational studies are potentially fraught with bias. In the case of hormone therapy it is known that women who seek hormones are better educated and from higher socioeconomic status; thus they have greater access to other health care resources where they may receive treatment for other cardiovascular risk factors such as diabetes, hypertension, or high cholesterol. In fact for many of the years covered by the observational studies these conditions, which increased the risk of cardiovascular disease, were considered relative contraindications to the use of hormone therapy. Those who adhered to hormones for their putative merits in disease prevention were more likely to adhere to other wellness advice—they tended to be leaner, to exercise more often, and to consume more alcohol, which, by itself, afforded a degree of cardioprotection. Women who became sick with comorbid conditions were more likely to stop hormones so that there would appear to be more deaths in nonusers or past users than in current users of hormone therapy. These and other biases of observational studies, they claim, could explain the discrepant findings of the WHI, which failed to confirm a cardioprotective benefit of hormone therapy in menopausal women.

However, many within the scientific community, while acknowledging the potential for bias in observational studies, do not agree that randomized clinical trial data is available that refutes the preponderance of experimental and clinical trial data suggesting cardioprotective benefits for hormone therapy when started early in postmenopausal women. They have challenged the premise that the WHI was a primary prevention trial because of the older ages of participants and the duration of elapsed time since loss of ovarian estrogen production (an average of 13 years).[40] Time since menopause has been shown to correlate with extent of subclinical atherosclerosis.[41] Clearly with close to 70% of women over age 60 at enrollment there must have been a large proportion of women with pre-existing subclinical cardiovascular disease in the trial—making it more of a secondary prevention trial. The first-year increase in cardiovascular events with no overall difference in cardiovascular mortality in this context is similar to the effect of hormone therapy started in older women in the other secondary prevention trial—the HERS trial. The prothrombotic or plaque-destabilizing effects of hormone therapy in women with established coronary artery disease probably account for the initial small absolute increase in coronary artery events reported in the conjugated equine estrogen arm of the WHI.

A truer picture of the risk for early cardiovascular events in newly menopausal women emerged when investigators pooled data from two large randomized trials that had been conducted for reasons other than examining cardiovascular endpoints. In these pivotal trials, in which all cardiovascular events were carefully documented, no cases of MI were reported in younger postmenopausal women on hormone therapy during the first year of hormone use.[42] This data examines only the first year of therapy and does not follow subjects long enough to determine if there were long-term cardioprotective benefits or risks associated with hormone therapy. Another meta-analysis, however, examined the impact of HT on mortality in populations of younger and older postmenopausal women and concluded that HT reduced total mortality in trials in which women had a mean age younger than 60 but had no impact on mortality if the mean age exceeded this.[43]

The research challenge now is to confirm with an appropriate clinical trial whether early initiation of HT does indeed have cardioprotective effects for menopausal women. To conduct such a study would require very large numbers of newly menopausal women followed for a significant period of time—a type of study that is challenging for a number of reasons. Newly menopausal women are more likely to be symptomatic and many may not agree to be randomly assigned to hormone or placebo; long-term adherence is likely to be a problem because a recent survey of U.S. households revealed that only 3% of women on combination HT (10% for estrogen alone in women who have had a hysterectomy) stayed on their hormones for more than 5 years.[44] The challenges and costs of such an initiative would be staggering. At the present time clinicians are left to decide in the absence of good clinical trial data whether epidemiological and experimental data supporting the use of hormones for primary cardioprotection in newly menopausal women justifies the potential risks of long-term hormone replacement. Women with premature loss of ovarian function probably represent a special situation because exogenous hormone therapy generally results in exposure to a lower total dose of hormone than would have resulted from normal ovarian function until the time of menopause.

### Venous Thromboembolism

Population-based studies have shown that venous thromboembolism increases with advancing age (Table 60-4). Numerous observational studies and two randomized, controlled trials involving older postmenopausal women (HERS and WHI) have indicated that use of oral hormone therapy, either combined estrogen/progestin or estrogen alone, results in a twofold to fourfold increased relative risk of developing a venous thromboembolism.[45] In the older HERS population, this translated into an attributable risk of 2.3/1000 women-years. In WHI, women age 50 to 59 had half the risk for venous thromboembolism of women age 60 to 69 and about one quarter the risk for women age 70 and older. Obesity, a prevalent finding in the WHI population, was associated with a threefold increased risk for venous thromboembolism. Normal-weight women age 50 to 59 had

| Table 60-4 Age-related Changes in Risk for Venous Thromboembolism | |
|---|---|
| Age (years) | Venous Thromboembolic Events per 1000 Person–Years |
| <20 | .01 |
| 20–40 | 0.1 |
| 41–75 | 1.0 |
| >75 | 10 |

From Gomes MPV, Deitcher SR: Risk of venous thromboembolic disease associated with hormonal contraceptives and hormone replacement therapy. Arch Intern Med 2004; 164:1965–1976.

an attributable risk for venous thromboembolism of 0.8/1000 women-years.[46] Most studies have shown the risk of venous thromboembolism to be greatest in the first year of HT—perhaps because initiation of therapy unmasks some women with an heritable thrombophilia. Limited data suggest that transdermal hormone therapy may be associated with lower rates of venous thromboembolism.[47]

### Cognitive Function and Dementia

Whether estrogen will reduce age-related cognitive decline remains controversial. Neurobiologists have demonstrated in animal models that estrogen can stimulate growth of neurons, increase synaptic connections, enhance neurotransmitters involved in memory, and stimulate cytokines responsible for repair of damaged neurons. Observational studies indicate that the incidence of Alzheimer's disease may be reduced by HT, with the greatest effect in those women who started it earliest and used it the longest. HT, however, affords no benefit to women who already have Alzheimer's disease.[48] As part of the WHI, selected women over age 65 were recruited to participate in studies on memory and cognition (the WHI Memory Study: WHIMS, and the WHI Study of Cognition and Aging: WHISCA). The results of the conjugated equine estrogen/medroxyprogesterone acetate (combination HT) and conjugated equine estrogen alone arms of the WHI have been similar. In women over age 65 rates of "probable dementia" were increased slightly in women receiving hormone therapy compared to those on placebo (attributable risks: conjugated equine estrogen, 12/10,000 women-years, combination HT, 23/10,000 women-years).[49] It is quite possible that elderly women with pre-existing atherosclerotic vascular disease became more vulnerable to minivascular accidents when started on hormones after age 65. The WHIMS authors remark that although the differences in performance between women on hormone therapy and those on placebo were statistically significant, the magnitude of the differences were "too small to have relevance in clinical practice." Nevertheless, this randomized clinical trial data shows clearly that hormone therapy should not be started in older postmenopausal women with the intent of reducing the incidence or severity of cognitive decline. Unresolved is the question of whether starting hormone therapy at the time of menopause might have long-term protective effects on neurovascular function, resulting in less cognitive impairment and dementia as the population ages.[50]

## Diabetes Mellitus

Consistent with the HERS trial, in which HT users had a 6.2% incidence of diabetes compared to 9.5% in placebo users, a secondary analysis of the WHI data also found a lower incidence of diabetes in HT users compared to placebo users (3.5% vs. 4.2%).[51] Given the economic and health impact of this disease in our aging population, these differences may be important.

# HORMONE THERAPY AND CANCER

## Breast Cancer

Until the recent publication of the WHI study, the best data on hormone therapy and breast cancer came from the reanalysis of data from the Collaborative Group on Hormonal Factors in Breast Cancer (CGHFBC) published in 1997.[52] This research, which examined all prior publications on hormone therapy (most of which would have involved conjugated equine estrogen alone) and breast cancer reported that use of conjugated equine estrogen for 5 years or less did not influence breast cancer risk. Very small increases in breast cancer risk appeared in women using hormone therapy for longer durations—an absolute increase of 0.2 cancers per 100 women after 5 years, 0.6 cancers per 100 women after 10 years, and 1.2 cancers per 100 women after 15 or more years of use between ages 50 and 70. The worst-case scenario that they reported was basically a 1% absolute increase with long-term use of conjugated equine estrogen—a risk that is similar to the breast cancer risk of being overweight, drinking excessive amounts of alcohol, failing to exercise regularly, having first birth after age 35, or failing to breastfeed.[53]

Shortly thereafter a qualitative review of all the published information on HT and breast cancer risk was published.[54] This is a different way to evaluate the data—which looks at the direction of change in situations where a cause-and-effect relationship is suspected. For example, all research on the value of seatbelts for preventing injury in car accidents points to a beneficial effect, just as all studies on the effects of cigarette smoking on lung cancer point to an increased risk. The data on HT and breast cancer are mixed, with as many studies reporting a decreased risk as reporting an increased risk. The conclusion of that analysis was as follows:

> The evidence did not support the hypotheses that estrogen use increases the risk of breast cancer and that combined hormone replacement therapy increases the risk more than estrogen only. Additional observational studies are unlikely to alter this conclusion. Although a small increase in breast cancer risk with long duration of use (15 years or more) cannot be ruled out, the likelihood of this is small, given the large number of studies conducted to date.[54]

Subsequently a large observational study (The Million Women Study) reported that both estrogen alone and combined estrogen/progestin increased the risk of new breast cancers in 830,000 women being followed with mammographic screening in the United Kingdom.[55] This study has been widely criticized for potential inclusion/exclusion biases that could have significantly altered the findings as well as for systematic under-estimation of the years of hormone use in establishing "duration of use" categories. The rapid development of tumors within a mean of 1.2 years of enrollment in that report seems biologically implausible based on known tumor biology and indicates a strong likelihood that many of the breast cancers detected during follow-up were in fact pre-existing.

More important to this question has been the WHI, a large randomized trial that evaluated breast cancer incidence in two separate arms—one in which the active drug was combined estrogen and progestin (combined HT) and one in which women who had undergone a hysterectomy received either estrogen alone or placebo. In the combination HT arm the 75% of women who had not used hormone therapy before enrollment showed no increase in the rate of breast cancer during the 5 years of the study—consistent with the results shown in the 1997 CGHFBC reanalysis. Also consistent with prior publications, the 25% of women who had previously received hormones had a slight increase in breast cancer after the 5 years of additional hormone therapy in the study (attributable risk for combination HT, 8/10,000 user per year). In the estrogen alone arm there was a lower rate of breast cancer diagnosis in the estrogen-treated women than in the placebo-treated women that just failed to achieve statistical significance (see Fig. 60-7). Together these findings should reassure women and their health care providers about the relative safety of hormone therapy for distressing vasomotor symptoms in the early menopausal years.

### Hormone Therapy in Women with Benign Breast Disease

Women with benign breast disease have a 1.8-fold to 3.6-fold increased risk of breast cancer, depending on whether past biopsies showed cellular atypia. The use of HT, even long term, by women with previous biopsy-proven benign breast disease had no further impact on breast cancer risk.[56] Similarly, it seems that HT does not interact with other known risk factors for breast cancer (e.g., benign breast disease, alcohol, parity, body mass index) to augment the overall risk of breast cancer.[57]

### Hormone Therapy with a Positive Family History for Breast Cancer

A common question faced by practitioners is whether a positive family history of breast cancer precludes use of HT. Family history by itself can provide useful information about a woman's personal risk for breast cancer. Women with a single first-degree family member (mother, sister, daughter) affected by breast cancer over age 50 have little increase in risk over the general population (approximately 12%). Those with two affected first-degree relatives over age 50 have an approximate doubling of their lifetime risk (to approximately 24%), and those with affected first-degree relatives under age 50 have a risk from 24% to 48%, depending on whether the number of affected first-degree relatives was 1 or 2, respectively. In a study designed to address the question about the safety of hormone therapy in women with a positive family history, the use of hormones was not associated with an increase in the overall risk for breast cancer yet was associated with a reduced overall mortality.[58]

### Hormone Therapy in Symptomatic Breast Cancer Survivors

Some 30,000 premenopausal women with a diagnosis of breast cancer are rendered acutely symptomatic subsequent to chemotherapy-induced ovarian failure each year in North America. There are more than 2.5 million breast cancer survivors in North America, many of whom have been unable to achieve a satisfactory quality of life because alternative approaches to vasomotor symptoms remain largely unsatisfactory.

A limited number of observational studies have reported on outcomes in women who choose to use HT after breast cancer compared to those who do not. When compared to "low-risk" controls, women on HT in these studies have not had a worse outcome.[59] Many people have now forgotten that high-dose estrogen once was a treatment for metastatic breast cancer. When tamoxifen was shown in a randomized clinical trial from the Mayo Clinic[60] to have equal benefit with fewer side effects, it became the mainstay of therapy in this circumstance. A recent report with a 20-year follow-up of the original trial participants revealed two surprising findings.[61] First, the diethylstilbestrol (DES)-treated participants survived longer than tamoxifen-treated women (35% of DES vs. 16% of tamoxifen-treated group were alive at 5 years; $P = 0.03$). Secondly, 30% of women who failed to respond to tamoxifen went on to show a clinical improvement when switched to DES treatment. A possible mechanism for this effect has been recently uncovered with the discovery that in vitro estrogen treatment of previously estrogen-deprived breast cancer cells promotes rapid cell death.[62]

Data from the first randomized clinical trials to examine this issue have recently appeared. The HABITS trial from Scandinavia found that women who used hormones after a diagnosis of breast cancer had a higher recurrence risk than did women assigned to placebo. Among 434 randomized to the study there were 26 recurrences in women assigned to hormone therapy and 6 recurrences in women receiving placebo.[63] Surprisingly a concurrent study conducted in Sweden failed to find any adverse effect of hormone therapy, leaving this issue unresolved. Both studies were stopped prematurely on the basis of the HABITS trial findings and the concern that ongoing recruitment would no longer be possible because of the adverse publicity about the preliminary findings.

Women who wish to consider HT for quality of life issues after a diagnosis of breast cancer should understand that a definitive answer to the question of whether HT will influence prognosis is lacking. Observational studies, which are fraught with potential biases, have been reassuring; however, a single, randomized, controlled trial suggested that HT had an adverse effect on recurrence rates. Alternative nonhormonal therapies exist for many menopausal symptoms (such as SSRIs for hot flashes and topical estrogen for urogenital atrophy). If these options are unsuitable and quality of life is seriously impaired, individual women with low risk of tumor recurrence may still wish to explore the option of HT.

## Uterine Cancer

The absolute risk of endometrial cancer in an untreated postmenopausal woman is approximately 1/1000 per year such that her lifetime risk after menopause is in the order of 2% to 3%. To put this risk into perspective, it is worth noting that merely being overweight by 25 to 50 pounds can produce a comparable increase in risk for endometrial cancer. Persson and colleagues, following a cohort of 23,244 patients for 6 years, reported a threefold increase in the relative risk for developing endometrial cancer in women using estrogen alone. In the PEPI trial, unopposed estrogen was associated with a significantly increased risk of adenomatous or atypical hyperplasia (35% vs. 1% com-

pared to women receiving progestational supplementation) and of subsequent hysterectomy (6% vs. 1% compared to the same group). Cure rates for estrogen-associated endometrial cancer are excellent, exceeding 95% in properly treated cases. Although annual office endometrial biopsy remains the gold standard, vaginal ultrasound monitoring of endometrial thickness may provide needed reassurance if the combined endometrial thickness is less than 5 mm.

To avoid the increased risks of endometrial hyperplasia and cancer associated with unopposed estrogen, most physicians prescribe combination HT to women who have a uterus. Progestins have multiple effects that impede endometrial growth. First, progestins decrease estrogen receptor number, decrease DNA synthesis, and modify growth factors, all of which impede estrogen-mediated transcription of oncogenes.[64] Second, progestins induce the enzyme estradiol 17β-dehydrogenase, resulting in enhanced local endometrial conversion of the more potent estradiol to the weaker estrogen, estrone. Finally, exposure to progestin will result in secretory transformation of the endometrium that may or may not be associated with endometrial sloughing, depending on whether the progestin is administered cyclically or continuously. Although the move toward using lower doses of estrogen for protection against postmenopausal bone loss may have merit[65] and may be less likely to induce endometrial hyperplasia, vigilance is required in any woman with unscheduled bleeding. Newer approaches are examining the possibility that progestin-releasing intrauterine systems or intravaginal progestin creams could achieve endometrial inhibitory concentrations of progestin without the same systemic progestin exposure that occurs with oral progestin therapy.

## Colorectal Cancer

Several past observational studies reported reduced rates of colorectal cancer in women on combined HT. In the WHI, combined HT (but not estrogen alone) was associated with a small reduction in the rate of colorectal cancer.

## CLINICAL MANAGEMENT OF POSTMENOPAUSAL WOMEN

Postmenopausal women need individual assessment and counseling. The factors that motivate consultation for different women and that determine an individual's propensity to seek treatment may be very different. Some women are motivated to obtain relief from their own symptoms, whereas others are driven more by fear that they will suffer the fate of a mother or relative who struggled with cancer, heart disease, or dementia. Positive lifestyle choices should be encouraged long before the menopause; however, when the onset of menopause creates an opportunity to discuss maintenance of health and disease prevention, strategies such as smoking cessation, moderation of alcohol intake, weight control, and regular exercise should be reinforced.

Clinicians should be aware of the fact that most women will have tried alternative therapies before seeking medical assistance and should make enquiries about the approaches that have been tried. While keeping an open mind to such approaches, it is also wise to be armed with available information and evidence that examines the effectiveness of such approaches to facilitate a balanced and informed interaction. Several excellent articles are available that have examined the claims and effectiveness of alternative therapies for menopausal vasomotor symptoms.[11]

The first issue in counseling is to determine and document any reasons to consider HT. Issues such as distressing hot flashes, night sweats, sleep disturbance, daytime fatigue and irritability, vaginal dryness, or dyspareunia might all be reasonable grounds to consider starting some form of hormone therapy. This should be followed by a brief but thorough discussion, again well documented, about potential benefits and potential risks of hormone therapy (Table 60-5).

It is important to remember that the risks reported in the media since the recent publications from the WHI have been average risks for a population of old and young women combined. As pointed out in the editorial that accompanied the WHI publication on the conjugated equine estrogen alone arm, "Women in their 50s have half the (baseline) risk of women in their 60s and one quarter the risk of women in their 70s." Accordingly it is likely that younger, newly menopausal women will have risk profiles that are even lower than the small overall risks reported for hormone users in the WHI reports. For example, the risk of stroke in the conjugated equine estrogen alone arm of the WHI was reported to be increased by 39% overall (44/10,000 in estrogen users vs. 32/10,000 in placebo users), yet in women under age 60 the rate for women suffering stroke was identical for both estrogen users and women on placebo (16/10,000).

To assist health care providers in explaining risks attributable to medical interventions the WHO convened a panel of experts

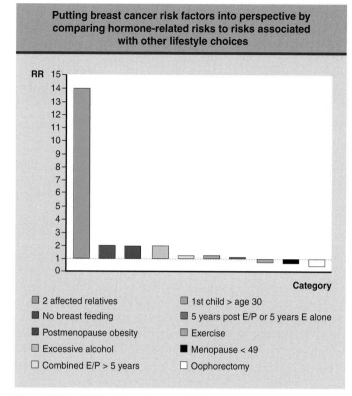

**Figure 60-9   Putting breast cancer risk factors into perspective by comparing hormone-related risks to risks associated with other lifestyle choices.** E, estrogen; P, progestin.

to develop standardized nomenclature to describe the risk for adverse events. The Council for International Organizations of Medical Sciences (CIOMS) task force released its report in 1998—providing a strict form of risk categorization to assist health care professionals and the public when interpreting risk.[66] According to the CIOMS classification, risks occurring in less than 1/1000 people, like all the risks reported by the WHI, are considered "rare."

Another effective way to put risks into context is to compare them with risks related to other lifestyle choices or other commonly prescribed medications. The risks of breast cancer associated with failure to exercise, postmenopausal obesity, excessive alcohol ingestion, delayed parenting, and failure to breastfeed probably all outweigh the risks associated with short-term hormone replacement[54] (Fig. 60-9).

Aspirin is widely prescribed and extensively utilized for prophylaxis against MI. Not generally recognized is the fact that this use of aspirin is associated with an absolute increase in the risk of hemorrhagic stroke of 12 per 10,000 individuals (more than the risk of heart attack or stroke reported in the WHI). The benefits of this intervention are assumed to outweigh this potential risk for most individuals (with an absolute risk reduction in MIs of 137 per 10,000 users, and in ischemic strokes of 39 per 10,000 users).[67]

If, on balance, the health care provider and the menopausal woman agree that the potential benefits outweigh potential risks, the second issue in counseling is to decide whether she needs

| Table 60-5 Summary of Risks and Benefits of Hormone Therapy | |
|---|---|
| **Benefits** | **Risks** |
| Effective control of hot flashes, night sweats, and associated sleep disturbance | **Systemic hormone therapy** |
| Improved energy and sense of well-being | Increased venous thromboembolic disease with oral estrogen (0.8/1000 with combination HT; Cushman 2004) but not transdermal estrogen (Scarabin 2003) |
| Preservation of bone and reduction in fragility fractures (56/10,000) | Increased risk of biliary tract surgery (absolute increase 1/185 treated women; Simon 2001) |
| Maintenance of vaginal and urinary health | |
| Improved sexual functioning | **Combination hormone therapy** |
| Diminished skin aging | Stroke—WHI, 8/10,000 per year overall (4/10,000 per year under age 60) |
| Less central weight gain | Breast cancer—WHI, 8/10,000 per year after 5 years |
| Reduced colorectal cancer (6/10,000 with combination hormone therapy) | Probable dementia—over age 65 WHIMS, 23/10,000 |
| | **Estrogen replacement** |
| | Stroke—WHI, 8/10,000 overall (no increase under age 60) |
| | Breast cancer—no significant change after 7 years |
| | Probable dementia—no significant change |

combined HT or estrogen alone. The only reason to use combination HT is if the uterus is intact. Women who have had an endometrial ablation usually continue to require progestin therapy because the possibility remains that there is some sequestered endometrium that could become cancerous under the influence of unopposed estrogen. In the absence of a uterus, progestin therapy is not indicated. In those with hysterectomy and bilateral salpingo-oophorectomy estrogen alone may be supplemented with an androgen-containing product in selected circumstances where estrogen alone has been inadequate to restore satisfactory sexual drive and enjoyment and other relationship and health issues have been excluded as contributory factors. Normally this decision would not be made until a 3-month trial of estrogen replacement had been completed.

Once a woman has decided that she wishes to try hormone therapy her input should be sought in determining the most appropriate regimen for her. The third issue to discuss, then, is whether she is prepared for or prefers to have regular periods or whether she wishes amenorrhea (and understands there may be some unpredictable bleeding until this is achieved). Some women early in menopause prefer to stick with a familiar monthly bleeding pattern, whereas others are just happy that menstruation is "over." This will determine if continuous estrogen and sequential progestin (for the first 12 to 14 days each month) or continuous combined therapy is optimal.

A fourth issue is which route of delivery (Table 60-6) appeals to her (oral, vaginal, transdermal [patch or gel], or intramuscular). Evidence suggests that a woman's participation in the choice of delivery route is critical to adherence to the prescribed regimen.

Follow-up is essential after 2 months to provide reassurance and to determine if symptom control and bleeding are acceptable. Sometimes persistent symptoms with an oral route may dictate the need for a switch to a transdermal route or persistent vaginal dryness may indicate the need for additional local vaginal estrogen therapy.

**Table 60-6**
**Options for Hormone Therapy**

**Oral**

Estrogen alone
Progestin alone
Estrogen/progestin combination (continuous or sequential)

**Transdermal**

Patch
    Estrogen alone
    Estrogen/progestin combination
    Testosterone
Gel or emulsion

**Vaginal**

Systemic
    Tablet (estrogen alone)
    Gel (progesterone alone)
Local
    Cream, tablet, ring (estrogen alone)

## REFERENCES

1. Hahn PM, Wong J, Reid RL: Menopausal-like hot flashes reported in women of reproductive age. Fertil Steril 1998;70:913–918. **(III, B)**
2. Freedman RR, Roehrs TA: Lack of sleep disturbance from menopausal hot flashes. Fertil Steril 2004;82:138–144. **(Ib, A)**
3. Soares CN, Almeida OP, Joffe H, et al: Efficacy of estradiol for the treatment of depressive disorders in perimenopausal women: a double-blind, randomized, placebo-controlled trial. Arch Gen Psychiatry 2001; 58:529–534. **(Ib, A)**
4. Shaywitz SE, Naftolin F, Zelterman D, et al: Better oral reading and short term memory in midlife, postmenopausal women taking estrogen. Menopause 2003;10:420–426. **(Ib, A)**
5. Garnero P, Somay-Rendu E, Chapuy MC, et al: Increased bone turnover in late postmenopausal women is a major determinant of osteoporosis. J Bone Miner Res 1996;11:337–349. **(II, B)**
6. Cauley JA, Thompson DE, Ensrud KC, et al: Risk of mortality following clinical fractures. Osteoporosis Int 2000;11:556–561. **(III, B)**
7. Joakimsen O, Bonnaa K, Stensland-Bugge E, et al: Population based study of age at menopause and ultrasound assessed carotid atherosclerosis. J Clin Epidemiol 2000;53:525–530. **(IIa, B)**
8. Lindh–Astrand L, Nedstrand E, Wyon Y, et al: Vasomotor symptoms and quality of life in previously sedentary postmenopausal women randomized to physical activity or estrogen therapy. Maturitas 2004; 48:97–105. **(Ib, A)**
9. MacLennan A, Lester S, Moore V: Oral estrogen replacement therapy versus placebo for hot flushes: a systematic review. Climacteric 2001; 4:58–74. **(Ia, A)**
10. Huntley AL, Ernst E: A systematic review of herbal medicinal products for the treatment of menopausal symptoms. Menopause 2003; 10:465–476. **(Ia, A)**
11. North American Menopause Society: Treatment of menopause-associated vasomotor symptoms: position statement. Menopause 2004;11:11–33. **(Ia, A)**
12. Ang-Lee MK, Moss J, Yuan CS: Herbal medicines and perioperative care. JAMA 2001;286:208–216. **(III, B)**
13. Krebs EE, Ensrud EB, MacDonald R, et al: Phytoestrogens for treatment of menopausal symptoms: a systematic review. Obstet Gynecol 2004;104:824–836. **(Ia, A)**
14. Cardozo L, Bachmann G, McClish D, et al: Meta-analysis of estrogen therapy in the management of urogenital atrophy in postmenopausal women: second report of the Hormones and Urogenital Committee. Obstet Gynecol 1998;92:722–727. **(Ia, A)**
15. Moehrer B, Hextall A, Jackson S: Oestrogens for urinary incontinence in women. Cochrane Database of Systematic Reviews 2003, Vol. 2. CD 001405. **(Ia, A)**
16. Nygaard IE, Heit M: Stress urinary incontinence. Obstet Gynecol 2004;104:607–620. **(IV, C)**
17. Bachmann GA, Leiblum SR: The impact of hormones on menopausal sexuality: a literature review. Menopause 2004;11:120–130. **(IV, C)**
18. Goldstat R, Briganti E, Tran J, et al: Transdermal testosterone therapy improves well-being, mood, and sexual function in premenopausal women. Menopause 2003;10:390–398. **(Ib, A)**
19. Miller PD, Siris ES, Barrett-Connor E, et al: Prediction of fracture risk in postmenopausal white women with peripheral bone densitometry: evidence from the National Osteoporosis Risk Assessment. J Bone Miner Res 2002;17:2222–2230. **(III, B)**
20. Hui SL, Slemenda CW, Johnston CC II: Age and bone mass as predictors of fracture in a prospective study. J Clin Invest 1988; 81:1804–1809. **(II, B)**
21. Greendale GA, Espeland M, Slone S, et al, for the PEPI Safety Follow-up Study Investigators: bone mass response to discontinuation of long-term hormone replacement therapy. Arch Intern Med 2002; 162:665–672. **(II, B)**
22. Riggs BL, Hartmann LC: Drug therapy: selective estrogen-receptor modulators—mechanisms of action and application to clinical practice. N Engl J Med 2003;348:618–629. **(IV, C)**

23. Wildman RP, Schott L, Brockwell S, et al: A dietary and exercise intervention slows menopause-associated progression of subclinical atherosclerosis as measured by intima-media thickness of the carotid arteries. J Am Coll Cardiol 2004;44:579–585. **(Ib, A)**

24. Collins P: Vascular effects of hormones. Maturitas 2001;38:45–50. **(IV, C)**

25. The PEPI Investigators: The Postmenopausal Estrogen/Progestin Interventions (PEPI) trial. Effects of estrogen estrogen or estrogen/progestin regimens on heart disease risk factors in postmenopausal women. JAMA 1995;273:199–208. **(Ib, A)**

26. Grodstein F, Stampfer MJ, Colditz GA, et al: Postmenopausal hormone therapy and mortality. N Engl J Med 1997;336:1769–1775. **(IIb, B)**

27. Mendelsohn ME, Karas R: The protective effects of estrogen on the cardiovascular system. N Engl J Med 1999;340:1801–1811. **(IV, C)**

28. Miller J, Chan BKS, Nelson HD: Postmenopausal estrogen replacement and risk for venous thromboembolism: a systematic review and meta-analysis for the U.S. Preventive Services Task Force. Ann Intern Med 2002;136:680–690. **(Ia, A)**

29. Scuteri A, Bos AJG, Brant LJ, et al: Hormone replacement therapy and longitudinal changes in blood pressure in postmenopausal women. Ann Intern Med 2001;135:229–238. **(IIa, B)**

30. Grodstein F, Manson JE, Colditz GA, et al: A prospective observational study of postmenopausal hormone therapy and primary prevention of cardiovascular disease. Ann Intern Med 2001;133:933–941. **(IIb, B)**

31. Hulley S, Grady D, Bush T, et al: Randomized trial of estrogen plus progestin for secondary prevention of coronary heart disease in postmenopausal women. Heart and Estrogen/progestin Replacement Study (HERS) Research Group. JAMA 1998;280:605–613. **(Ib, A)**

32. Hodis HN, Mack WJ, Azen SP, et al: Hormone therapy and the progression of coronary artery atherosclerosis in postmenopausal women. N Engl J Med 2003;349:535–545. **(Ib, A)**

33. Nair GV, Herrington DM: The ERA trial: findings and implications for the future. Climacteric 2000;3:227–232. **(Ib, A)**

34. Clarke SC, Kelleher J, Lloyd-Jones H, et al: A study of hormone replacement therapy in postmenopausal women with ischemic heart disease: the Papworth HRT Atherosclerosis Study. Br J Obstet Gynaecol 2002;109:1056–1062. **(Ib, A)**

35. Clarkson TB: The new conundrum: do estrogens have any cardiovascular benefits? Int J Fertil Womens Med 2002;47:61–68. **(IV, C)**

36. Hodis HN, Mack WJ, Lobo RA, et al, for the Estrogen in the Prevention of Atherosclerosis Trial Research Group: Estrogen in the prevention of atherosclerosis. A randomized, double-blind, placebo-controlled trial. Ann Intern Med 2001;135:939–953. **(Ib, A)**

37. Manson JE, Hsia J, Johnson KC, et al: Estrogen plus progestin and the risk of coronary heart disease. N Engl J Med 2003;349:523–534. **(Ib, A)**

38. Anderson GL, Limacher M, Assaf AR, et al: Effects of conjugated equine estrogen in postmenopausal women with hysterectomy: the Women's Health Initiative randomized controlled trial. JAMA 2004; 291:1701–1712. **(Ib, A)**

39. Wassertheil-Smoller S, Hendrix SL, Limacher M, et al: Effect of estrogen and progestin on stroke in postmenopausal women. The Women's Health Initiative: a randomized trial. JAMA 2003; 289:2673–2684. **(Ib, A)**

40. Naftolin F, Taylor HS, Karas R, et al: The Women's Health Initiative could not have detected cardioprotective effects of starting hormone therapy during the menopausal transition. Fertil Steril 2004; 81:1498–1501. **(IV, C)**

41. Mack WJ, Slater CC, Xiang M, et al: Elevated subclinical atherosclerosis associated with oophorectomy is related to time since menopause rather than type of menopause. Fertil Steril 2004; 82:391–397. **(IIa, B)**

42. Lobo RA: Evaluation of cardiovascular event rates with hormone therapy in healthy, early menopausal women: results from two large clinical trials. Arch Intern Med 2004;164:482–484. **(Ia, A)**

43. Salpeter SR, Walsh JME, Greyber E, et al: Mortality associated with hormone replacement therapy in younger and older women: a meta-analysis. J Gen Intern Med 2004;19:791–804. **(Ia, A)**

44. Brett KM, Reuben CA: Prevalence of estrogen or estrogen-progestin hormone therapy use. Obstet Gynecol 2003;102:1240–1249. **(IIb, B)**

45. Gomes MPV, Deitcher SR: Risk of venous thromboembolic disease associated with hormonal contraceptives and hormone replacement therapy. Arch Intern Med 2004;164:1965–1976. **(III, B)**

46. Cushman M, Kuller LH, Prentice R, et al: Estrogen plus progestin and risk of venous thrombosis. JAMA 2004;292:1573–1580. **(Ib, A)**

47. Scarabin PY, Oger E, Plu-Bureau G, for the Estrogen and THromboEmbolism Risk (ESTHER) Study Group: Differential association of oral and transdermal oestrogen-replacement therapy with venous thromboembolism risk. Lancet 2003;362:428–432. **(IIa, B)**

48. Mulnard RA, Cotman CW, Kawas C, et al, for the Alzheimer's Disease Co-operative Study: Estrogen replacement therapy for the treatment of mild to moderate Alzheimer's disease. JAMA 2000;283:1007–1015. **(Ib, A)**

49. Shumaker SA, Legault C, Kuller L, et al, for the Women's Health Initiative Memory Study Investigators: Conjugated equine estrogens and incidence of probable dementia and mild cognitive impairment in postmenopausal women. Women's Health Initiative Memory Study. JAMA 2004;291:2947–2958. **(Ib, A)**

50. Birge S: The WHI and the brain: what have we learned? Sex Reprod Menopause 2004;2:71–75. **(IV, C)**

51. Margolis KL, Bonds DE, Rodabough RJ, et al, for the Women's Health Initiative Investigators: Effect of oestrogen plus progestin on the incidence of diabetes in postmenopausal women: results from the Women's Health Initiative Hormone Trial. Diabetologia 2004;47:1175–1187. **(Ib, A)**

52. Collaborative Group on Hormonal Factors in Breast Cancer: Breast cancer and hormone replacement therapy: collaborative reanalysis of data from 51 epidemiological studies of 52,705 women with breast cancer and 108,411 women without breast cancer. Lancet 1997; 350:1047–1059. **(IIa, B)**

53. Reid RL: Double jeopardy: hormone therapy on trial again. JOGC 2004;26:541–543. **(IV, C)**

54. Bush TL, Whiteman M, Flaws JA: Hormone replacement therapy and breast cancer: a qualitative review. Obstet Gynecol 2001;98:498–508. **(IIb, B)**

55. Million Women Study Collaborators: Breast cancer and hormone-replacement therapy in the Million Women Study. Lancet 2003; 362:419–427. **(Ib, B)**

56. Byrne C, Connolly JL, Colditz GA, et al: Biopsy proven benign breast disease, postmenopausal use of exogenous female hormones and breast carcinoma risk. Cancer 2000;89:2046–2052. **(IIa, B)**

57. Ursin G, Tseng CC, Paganini-Hill A, et al: Does menopausal hormone replacement interact with known factors to increase risk of breast cancer? J Clin Oncol 2002;20:699–706. **(IIa, B)**

58. Sellars TA, Mink PJ, Gerhan JR, et al: The role of hormone replacement therapy in the risk for breast cancer and total mortality in women with a family history of breast cancer. Ann Intern Med 1997; 127:973–890. **(IIa, A)**

59. Col NF, Hirota LK, Orr RK, et al: Hormone replacement therapy after breast cancer: a systematic review and quantitative assessment of risk. J Clin Oncol 2001;19:2357–2363. **(III, B)**

60. Ingle JN, Ahmann DL, Green SJ, et al: Randomized clinical trial of diethylstilbestrol versus tamoxifen in postmenopausal women with advanced breast cancer. N Engl J Med 1981;304:16–21. **(Ib, B)**

61. Peethambaram PP, Ingle JN, Suman VJ, et al: Randomized trial of diethylstilbestrol vs tamoxifen in postmenopausal women with metastatic breast cancer. An updated analysis. Breast Cancer Res Treat 1999;54:117–122. **(Ib, A)**

62. Song RX, Mor G, Naftolin F, et al: Effect of longterm estrogen deprivation on apoptotic responses of breast cancer cells to 17beta-estradiol. J Natl Cancer Inst 2001;93:1714–1723. **(Ib, B)**

63. Holmberg L, Anderson H, for the HABITS steering and data monitoring committees: HABITS (Hormonal replacement therapy After Breast cancer—is IT Safe?), a randomised comparison: trial stopped. Lancet 2004;363:453–455. **(Ib, A)**

**873**

64. Persson I, Adami HO, Bergkvist L, et al: Risk of endometrial cancer after treatment with oestrogens alone or in conjunction with progestogens: results of a prospective study. Br Med J 1989;289:147–151. **(III, B)**

65. Ettinger B, Ensrud KE, Wallace R, et al: Effects of ultralow-dose transdermal estradiol on bone mineral density: a randomized clinical trial. Obstet Gynecol 2004;104:443–451. **(Ib, A)**

66. Council for International Organizations of Medical Sciences (CIOMS): Guidelines for Preparing Core Clinical-Safety Information on Drugs, 2nd ed. Geneva: CIOMS, 1998. **(III, B)**

67. He J, Whelton PK, Vu B, et al: Aspirin and risk of hemorrhagic stroke: a meta-analysis of randomized controlled trials. JAMA 1998; 280:1930–1935. **(Ia, A)**

## CLASSIC CASE PRESENTATION

A 42-year-old female bank executive comes in for a well-woman examination. She complains of increasing menstrual irregularity over the past 6 months. In addition, she states that she has experienced several episodes of hot flashes at night and is not sleeping well. As a result, she has noticed increasing irritability that has affected her job performance. She is quite disturbed by these occurrences and seeks advice regarding therapy.

## INTRODUCTION

The preceding case scenario is a classic presentation of perimenopausal symptoms. Physicians and the lay public have long recognized menopause as a defined state of female transition from reproductive to postreproductive years. However, only in the relatively recent past has the importance of symptom recognition, evaluation of pathophysiology, and treatment of perimenopause been recognized and addressed as a biologic process distinct from the menopause.

With the aging of the "baby boom" population, the number of women aged 50 to 59 years will increase by 50% by 2006. As life expectancy increases, a female may expect to spend approximately one third of her life as a postmenopausal person. There were an estimated 42.9 million women over the age of 50 in the United States in 2000. By 2020, the number of women over age 55 is estimated to increase to 45.9 million (Table 61-1).[1] A woman who reaches age 54 today may expect to survive to age 84.3 years. About two thirds of the U.S. population may survive to age 85 or longer. No data exist on how many women will reach menopause in a given year. Based on assumptions about spontaneous, premature, surgical, and induced menopause, it is estimated that approximately 4200 women become menopausal per day in the United States.

The transition defined by perimenopause and menopause may be viewed as a problematic period of menstrual, emotional, and physiologic changes. Beginning with perimenopausal changes in hormones, females may begin the common degenerative process of aging, which includes the possibility of cardiovascular disease, diabetes, and osteoporosis, among other diseases. However, medically, perimenopause may present an opportunity for improvement of health screening, recognition of otherwise silent disease, and motivation for a healthier life style for the rest of the patient's life.

This chapter describes the pathophysiology, clinical signs and symptoms, and therapy of perimenopause (Table 61-2).[2]

## DEFINITIONS AND TERMINOLOGY

In 2001, the Stages of Reproductive Aging Workshop (STRAW), sponsored by the North American Menopause Society (NAMS), and others addressed nomenclature and staging of menopause. A continuum was devised; however, it was recognized that some women may "seesaw" between or skip some stages[1] (Fig. 61-1). Menopause is the anchor point defined as 12 months of amenorrhea following the final menstrual period (FMP).[1] Menopause occurs at an average age of 51.4 years with a Gaussian distribution of 40 to 58 years.

Perimenopause (peri = around) is defined as beginning with stage 2 (see Fig. 61-1) and ending 12 months after the FMP. STRAW suggests using climacteric as synonymous with perimenopause. STRAW recommends use of perimenopause and climacteric only with patients or in the lay press; however, owing to widespread usage in the medical community and NAMS, the term is used in its stated context in this chapter. Postmenopause is the span of time dating from the FMP whether spontaneous or induced. It is early (stage +1) within 5 years of FMP and late (stage +2) when more than 5 years after FMP.

# Reproductive Endocrinology and Infertility

**Table 61-1**
**Increase in the Number of Postmenopausal Women in the United States**

| Age | July 1, 1999 | July 1, 2000 | Percentage Change | Postmenopausal |
|---|---|---|---|---|
| Age 50+ | 41,000,000 | 42,189,280 | +2.9 | 39,944,824 |
| Age groups | | | | |
| Age 40–44 | 11,188,000 | 11,312,761 | +1.1 | 1,134,000 |
| Age 45–49 | 9,832,000 | 10,202,898 | +3.8 | 2,017,600 |
| Age 50–54 | 8,439,000 | 8,977,824 | +6.4 | 6,733,368 |

Data from U.S. Census Bureau, 2000 Census; and Stages of Reproductive Aging Workshop (STRAW): Menopause 2001;8:402–407.

**Table 61-2**
**Most Common Signs and Symptoms of Perimenopause**

| | |
|---|---|
| Cycle irregularities | Physical discomfort |
| Hot flashes | Reduced libido |
| Menorrhagia | Sexual dysfunction |
| Menstrual changes | Spotting |
| Night sweats | Vasomotor disturbances |

From Association of Professors of Gynecology and Obstetrics: Managing the Perimenopause. APGO Educational Series on Women's Health Issues. Washington, DC, APGO, 2001, pp 1–20.

## PATHOPHYSIOLOGY

### Ovarian Follicles

The pathophysiology of perimenopause is directly related to the aging ovary. The human ovary contains approximately 7 million oocytes at the fifth week of gestation. After this time, the number is reduced by atresia to approximately 1 to 2 million at birth and 400,000 by menarche. By menopause, only a few hundred oocytes remain (Figs. 61-2 and 61-3). During reproductive life, only 300 to 400 follicles will grow to ovulatory status. Follicular atresia occurs on a monthly basis, as a cohort of up to 50 follicles may be recruited, resulting in one dominant follicle proceeding to ovulation while the others are absorbed. However, 80% of follicular atresia may be due to a gonadotropin-independent process.

### Endocrine Changes

Although the exact nature of the endocrine changes occurring in perimenopause are not totally understood, variation and finally persistent elevation of, first, follicle-stimulating hormone (FSH) and then luteinizing hormone (LH) and loss of ovarian secretion of inhibin characterize this period. The age of menopause appears to have changed little since early Grecian times. The perimenopausal transition may begin as early as the fourth decade (late 30s) and may vary between 2 and 8 years in length. The Massachusetts Women's Health Study (MWHS)[4] and a longitudinal study by Treloar[5] are two of the classic studies most often quoted when defining the age of onset and duration of

**Stages/nomenclature of normal reproductive aging in women**

| Stages: | −5 | −4 | −3 | −2 | −1 | 0 (FMP) | +1 | +2 |
|---|---|---|---|---|---|---|---|---|
| Terminology: | Reproductive | | | Menopausal transition | | | Postmenopause | |
| | Early | Peak | Late | Early | Late* | | Early* | Late* |
| | | | | Perimenopause | | | | |
| Duration of stage: | Variable | | | Variable | | ⓐ 1 yr | ⓑ 4 yrs | Until demise |
| Menstrual cycles: | Variable to regular | Regular | | Variable cycle length (>7 days different from normal) | 2 skipped cycles and an interval of amenorrhea (60 days) | Amen. x 12 mos | None | |
| Endocrine: | Normal FSH | | ↑ FSH | ↑ FSH | | | ↑ FSH | |

*Stages most likely to be characterized by vasomotor symptoms.

**Figure 61-1   Stages/nomenclature of normal reproductive aging in women.** (From Stages of Reproductive Aging Workshop (STRAW). Menopause 2001;8:402–407.)

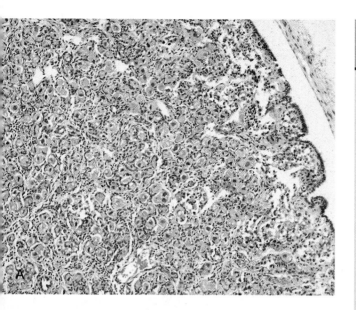

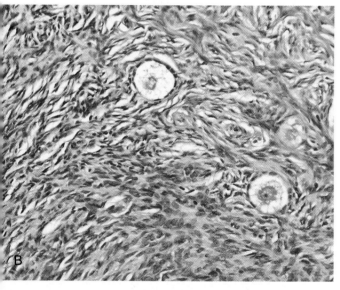

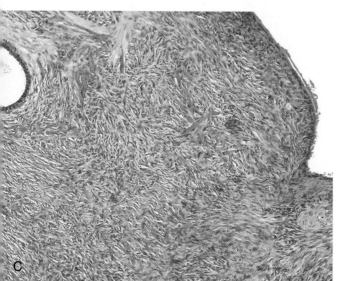

**Figure 61-2   Stages of ovarian senescence.** *A,* Newborn. *B,* Age 25. *C,* Age 50.

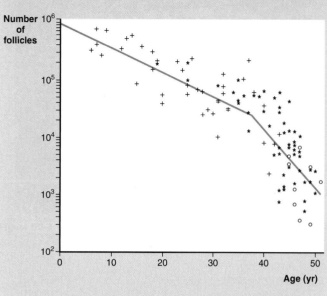

### Age-related decrease in primordial follicles from birth to menopause

Bi-exponential model of declining follicle numbers in pairs of human ovaries from neonatal age to 51 years old. Data were obtained from the studies of Block (1952, 1953) ($\times$, *n* = 6; +, *n* = 43), Richardson et al. (1987) (○, *n* = 9) and Gougeon (unpublished) (⋆ *n* = 52)

**Figure 61-3   The age-related decrease in the total number of primordial follicles (PFs) within both human ovaries from birth to the menopause.** As a result of recruitment (initiation of PF growth), the number of PFs decreases progressively from about 1 million at birth to 25,000 at 37 years. At 37 years, the rate of recruitment increases sharply, and the number of PFs declines to 1000 at menopause (about 51 years of age). (From Faddy MJ, Gosden RG, Gougeon A, et al: Accelerated disappearance of ovarian follicles in mid-life: implications for forecasting menopause. Hum Reprod 1992;7:1342–1346.)

the menopause. The MWHS followed 2570 women aged 45 to 55 years over a 5-year period. The median age at onset for perimenopause was 47.5 years and median age of FMP was 51.3 years (Fig. 61-4).[4] Only 10% of women cease menses without any menstrual irregularity. In the study by Treloar, the average age of menopause was 50.7 years and the range was 44 to 56 years. Treloar prospectively studied the record of 2700 women constituting 25,825 woman years. He demonstrated an age-related shortening of menstrual cycle length of median 28 days at age 20, to 26 days at age 40. The shortened cycle length is due to a progressive shortening of the follicular phase without a significant change in the luteal phase. The overall decreased cycle length continues to approximately age 43, when both average cycle length and interval begin to increase.

### Inhibin

The secretion of FSH is mainly influenced by inhibin. Inhibin is a family of glycoprotein hormones produced by the granulosa cells of the ovary. The two inhibin species found in humans, A and B, are composed of a common $\alpha$-subunit and one of two

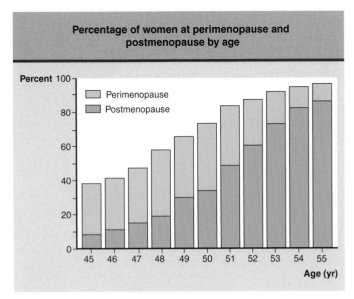

**Figure 61-4** **Percentage of women at perimenopause (yellow) and postmenopause (green) by age.** Median age of onset for the perimenopause was 47.5 years; median age for the menopause was 51.3 years. (From McKinlay SM, Brembilla DJ, Posner JG: The normal menopause transition. Maturitas 1992;14:107.)

β-subunits, βa and βb. The physiologic role of inhibin is due to the β-subunits, which show functional, structural, and molecular differences. Males make only inhibin B while females produce both inhibins A and B. While estradiol appears to be mainly produced by the dominant follicle, inhibin is produced by follicles in both ovaries. These hormones act both in vitro and in vivo to suppress FSH secretion. Plasma levels of the α-subunit are high; however, it is biologically inactive in FSH suppression. In the menstrual cycle, inhibin B is produced by antral follicles, but little is produced by the dominant follicle or corpus luteum. Inhibin A is produced by both the developing and the dominant follicle and corpus luteum. Inhibin A concentrations remain stable throughout much of the follicular phase of the cycle and increase in the first half of the luteal phase followed by a decline as menses approaches (Fig. 61-5).[6] Functionally, inhibin exerts negative feedback on regulation of pituitary FSH secretion. FSH administration stimulates inhibin production, and inhibin levels are inversely correlated with FSH concentrations. Inhibin B is important in FSH regulation in the follicular phase of the cycle, whereas inhibin A is dominant in the luteal phase. Inhibin B levels correlate with serum FSH during the early stages of the menstrual cycle, which suggest inhibin B is under FSH regulation. In the later follicular phase, inhibin B levels increase while FSH falls, which supports feedback of inhibin on FSH secretion. FSH is elevated in the cycles of perimenopausal women and is associated with a decrease in inhibin B but not in inhibin A. This decreased serum inhibin B is attributed to decreased follicle count and competency. Inhibin is undetectable after both normal and premature menopause.

### FSH, LH, Estrogen, and Progesterone Levels

Perimenopause is marked by changes in the secretion of gonadotropins. Urinary FSH, LH, estrogen, and progesterone levels

were studied in a group of 6 cycling women, 47 years or older, for 6 months (Fig. 61-6).[7] Perimenopausal women had shorter cycles due to an attenuated follicular phase. Estrone excretion was greater in perimenopausal than in mid-reproductive-aged women, both overall and in the follicular and luteal phases of the cycle. Basal pregnanediol concentrations did not differ between perimenopausal and control groups; however, overall they were lower in the perimenopausal group.

FSH and LH levels, especially FSH, were elevated in the early follicular phase of the cycle. Mean follicular-phase FSH was elevated in perimenopausal women (median, 14 IU/g creatinine) compared with mid-reproductive-aged women (median, 4 IU/g creatinine). LH was also elevated though less markedly. In contrast, age-appropriate postmenopausal women demonstrated

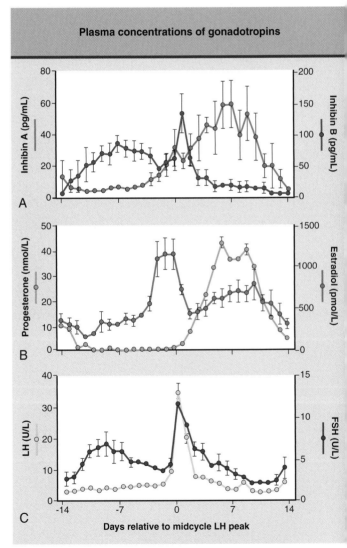

**Figure 61-5** **Plasma concentrations of inhibin A and B (A); progesterone and estradiol (B); and luteinizing hormone (LH) and follicle-stimulating hormone (FSH) (C) during the menstrual cycle.** Data displayed with respect to the day of the midcycle LH peak. (From Groome NP, Illingworth PJ, O'Brien M, et al: Measurement of dimeric inhibin B throughout the human menstrual cycle: J Clin Endocrinol Metab 1996;81:1401–1405.)

## Urinary gonadotropin and sex steroid excretion patterns

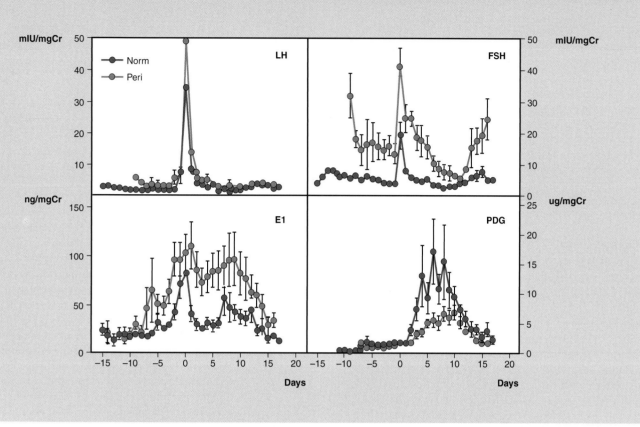

**Figure 61-6** **Mean ± SEM daily urinary gonadotropin and sex steroid excretion patterns in 11 perimenopausal women aged 43 to 52 years** *(red circle)* **compared with those in 11 mid-reproductive-aged women** *(blue circle).* Data are standardized to day 0, the putative day of ovulation, as described in the test. $E_1$, estrone conjugates. (From Santoro N, Brown JR, Adel T, et al: Characterization of reproductive hormonal dynamics in the perimenopause. J Clin Endocrinol Metab 1996;81:1495–1501.)

little variation in gonadotropins and estrogen. FSH and LH were clinically elevated and estrone conjugate excretion was low (hypergonadotropic-hypoestrogenism; see Fig. 61-6).[7]

The elevation of estrone conjugates suggests that although follicular numbers are decreasing, the ability of the ovary to produce estrogen continues. This finding is consistent with the observed increase in uterine myoma size, endometrial hyperplasia, and dysfunctional bleeding noted in these women, which are commonly attributed to anovulation.

However, hyperestrogenism was noted even in ovulatory cycles. The decline in luteal-phase progestin may aggravate the already relatively unopposed estrogen state noted in these women. Therefore, from an endocrine point of view, management of the perimenopausal woman should be viewed as treatment of a hyperestrogenic, hypoprogestogenic state. These data also appear to negate concerns about potential bone loss and decreased estrogen.

Perimenopausal women in the study also demonstrated occasional periods of hypogonadotropic hypoestrogenism interspersed with periods of cyclic ovulatory and anovulatory activity. As expected, the periods of hypoestrogenism became more frequent with proximity to menopause. This implies that progression from reproductive life to postmenopause represents not a continuous but a discontinuous process of intermittent ovulation and anovulation.

### Physiologic Menstrual Irregularity

Our understanding of menstrual irregularity is largely due to the classic studies of Treloar.[5] Volunteers were initially recruited in the 1930s and asked to record menstrual cycles until menopause. Initial reports were in 2702 women representing 25,825 woman-years of menstrual experience with the later addition of longer term data. The mean age of menopause was 49.8 years and duration of menstruation was 35.9 years. Cycle variability began 6 years prior to menopause in 10% to 15% of women, with an increase in variability in another 30% 2 to 3 years prior to menopause. The data demonstrated a wide variability in menstrual cycle length associated with defective luteal function increasing from 8% of cycles at 31 to 35 years to 36% at 40 to 50 years. Also, the study demonstrated an increase in anovulation from 8% at 31 to 35 years to 16% of cycles at 45 to 50 years.

# Reproductive Endocrinology and Infertility

A recent Scandinavian study[8] examining 1616 women aged 45 to 54 confirmed that irregular cycles increased from 58.3% at age 45 to 46 years to 100% at 53 to 54 years. Irregularity was accompanied by both increased variation in length and subjective assessment of heaviness of bleeding episodes in individuals and between women. Spotting and prolonged bleeding were common. Heaviness of bleeding episodes was higher in women with regular cycles.

The relationship of menstrual variability to menopause was addressed in a recent study in a group of 326 menstruating women with irregular perimenopausal periods.[9] Of six definitions of menstrual variability, "60+ days of amenorrhea" showed the best balance of sensitivity (94%) and specificity (91%) for ascertained menopause within 2 years. Specificity was 90% or better with all the definitions of "more than 90 days since LMP," "60+ days amenorrhea" and "cycles too variable to represent a usual length" for ascertained menopause within 2 years and within 4 years, respectively.

## Abnormal Uterine Bleeding

While physiologic alteration in menstrual pattern is the hallmark of perimenopause, abnormal uterine bleeding accounts for more than two thirds of office visits to the gynecologist. Examples of abnormal bleeding include heavier than usual bleeding, prolonged bleeding, menses more often than every 3 weeks, bleeding or spotting between menses, and postcoital bleeding. A differential diagnosis for abnormal bleeding is listed in Table 61-3.[10]

Ruling out bleeding related to unexpected pregnancy is the first order of business, followed by evaluation of possible endometrial neoplasia resulting from unopposed estrogen (Table 61-4).[11] Risk factors associated with endometrial neoplasia are listed in Table 61-5.[10]

---

**Table 61-4**

**Mechanism of Increased Endometrial Estrogen Exposure**

Anovulatory menses (lack of luteal-phase progesterone)
Increased precursor androgen (functional or nonfunctional endocrine tumors, liver disease)
Increased aromatization (obesity, hyperthyroidism, liver disease)
Increased direct secretion of estrogens (ovarian tumors)
Decreased levels of sex hormone–binding globulin leading to increased levels of free estrogen
Iatrogenic (nonjudicious use of prescribed unopposed estrogen)

From Menopause and the perimenopausal transition. In Speroff L, Glass RH, Kase NG (eds): Clinical Gynecologic Endocrinology and Infertility, 6th ed. Philadelphia, Lippincott Williams & Wilkins, 1999, pp 643–724.

---

### Evaluation of Abnormal Uterine Bleeding

In a patient with abnormal uterine bleeding, a detailed history is mandatory. Data regarding the last episode of bleeding, length, character, duration, and amount of flow are important. Ascertain not only when the last episode of bleeding occurred but also the pattern of bleeding over the previous 6 months to 1 year to establish whether the bleeding is abnormal or a variation in the normal perimenopausal pattern.

The history should include possible interruption of normal daily activities, contraception type and possible relation to bleeding (e.g., intrauterine device, depot medroxyprogesterone acetate), current medications and concomitant disease states. Laboratory testing including pregnancy assessment (serum hCG), prolactin, thyroid-stimulating hormone, complete blood count, and coagulation studies should be obtained depending on the patient's history.

Farquhar[12] reviewed a laboratory data base of 1033 endometrial samples over a 30-month period from 1995 through

---

**Table 61-3**

**Possible Causes of Abnormal Uterine Bleeding in Perimenopausal Women**

Anovulation (dysfunctional uterine bleeding)

Benign reproductive tract conditions
  Pregnancy
  Leiomyomata uteri
  Endometrial or endocervical polyps
  Adenomyosis
  Endometritis
  Pelvic inflammatory disease: vaginal or cervical infection

Endometrial neoplasia
  Endometrial hyperplasia without atypia
  Endometrial hyperplasia with atypia
  Endometrial adenocarcinoma

Systemic diseases
  Coagulation disorders (thrombocytopenia, von Willebrand's disease, leukemia)
  Hypothyroidism
  Liver disease

Iatrogenic causes
  Hormone therapy
  Contraceptive devices or injections

From Kaunitz AM: Gynecologic problems of the perimenopause: evaluation and treatment. Obstet Gynecol Clin North Am 2002;29:455–473.

---

**Table 61-5**

**Risk Factors for Endometrial Neoplasia\* in Premenopausal Women Aged 17 to 50 Years with Abnormal Uterine Bleeding**

| Risk Factor | Odds Ratio[†] (95% CI) | P Value |
|---|---|---|
| Age ≥45 yr | 3.1 (1.5–6.1) | 0.0016 |
| Weight ≥90 kg | 5.5 (2.9–10.6) | <0.0001 |
| History of infertility | 3.6 (1.3–9.9) | 0.0127 |
| Family history of colon cancer | 5 (1.3–19.1) | 0.0182 |
| Nulliparity | 2.8 (1.1–7.2) | 0.0267 |
| Family history of endometrial cancer | NS | NS |

CI, confidence interval; NS, not significant.
\*Endometrial hyperplasia or carcinoma.
[†]Multivariate analyses.
Adapted from Farquhar CM, Lethaby MA, Sowter M, et al: An evaluation of risk factors for endometrial hyperplasia in premenopausal women with abnormal menstrual bleeding. Am J Obstet Gynecol 1999;181:525–529; and Kaunitz AM: Gynecologic problems of the perimenopause: evaluation and treatment. Obstet Gynecol Clin North Am 2002;29:455–473.

1997 to determine clinical risk factors for endometrial hyperplasia in perimenopausal women. Forty-six cases of endometrial hyperplasia and 6 cases of endometrial cancer were diagnosed. The following factors were independently associated with risk of endometrial hyperplasia or presence of carcinoma: age ≥ 45 (odds ratio [OR] 3.1, 95% confidence interval [CI] 1.5–6.1), weight ≥ 90 kg (OR 5.5, CI 2.9–10.6), history of infertility (OR 3.6, 95% CI 1.3–99), family history of colonic carcinoma (OR 5.0, 95% CI 1.3–19.1) and nulliparity (OR 2.8, 95% CI 1.1–7.2). The authors noted no increased association of endometrial hyperplasia on the basis of menstrual cycle irregularity or duration of menstrual bleeding. Overall the rate of hyperplasia or carcinoma in women who underwent endometrial biopsy for abnormal uterine bleeding was 5%. Ash[13] reported a rate of 6.7% in a similar study. In light of the greater than 60% rate of overweight and obesity currently epidemic in the United States, the finding that body mass index (BMI) and weight gain are independent risk factors for endometrial cancer is significant. A body weight equal to or greater than 90 kg is the most important risk factor in the current study,[13] probably based on peripheral conversion of estrogen precursors.

Outpatient office sampling of the endometrial cavity is fundamental to the evaluation of abnormal uterine bleeding. Traditional dilation and curettage (D&C) under anesthesia and biopsy by rigid Novak curette has been replaced by flexible cannula biopsy (e.g., Pipelle cannula and Milex cannula). The device may usually be placed without requirement of cervical dilation and causes brief and minimal discomfort. If it is difficult to insert the 3 mm cannula secondary to cervical stenosis in a nulliparous or elderly patient, 1% lidocaine may be utilized to infiltrate the cervix in a circumferential fashion. Small Pratt or Hagar dilators starting with 1 mm may then be utilized to explore the cervical canal and axis of the endometrial cavity. Once the axis of the upper cervical canal is noted, the cervix may be safely dilated to 4 mm to accommodate the flexible biopsy cannula. In general, more than 90% of patients may be safely sampled in the office without significant discomfort. If small graduated dilators are not available, a standard Papanicolaou (Pap) smear brush may be utilized to give an assessment of cervical axis and patency. An attempt should be made to sample the endometrial cavity in a 360-degree rotation, and adequate sampling is usually obtained.

Transvaginal ultrasound has replaced abdominal ultrasound as the standard technique of initial pelvic anatomy and endometrial evaluation. Goldstein et al[14] reviewed 433 women who had abnormal uterine bleeding in perimenopause. Sixty-five percent were able to be adequately evaluated by transvaginal study. The remainder underwent saline-infused sonohysterography secondary to endometrium greater than 5 mm or inadequate assessment. The author recommended hysteroscopic biopsy if an abnormality was demonstrable.

Saline infusion sonohysteroscopy and hysteroscopy are currently playing a larger role in the evaluation of perimenopausal women with abnormal bleeding. Hysteroscopic biopsy has been considered the gold standard of comparison; however, it requires an anesthetic or at least conscious sedation to provide adequate comfort for the patient. Bernard and colleagues[15] prospectively reviewed 233 perimenopausal and postmenopausal patients, finding a sensitivity of 85.7% and specificity of 95.4% in the

diagnosis of polyps and submucous myomas. A review of sonohysterography findings in 100 asymptomatic women 30 years of age or older matched to 80 similar women with abnormal bleeding by Clevenger-Hoeft et al[16] revealed a higher incidence of polyps, intracavitary myomas, and intramural myomas.

Bronz et al,[17] deVries et al,[18] and Farquhar et al[19] have compared transvaginal sonography, saline-infused sonography (SIS), and hysteroscopy in the evaluation of perimenopausal women with abnormal bleeding. Bronz and deVries found specificity was significantly improved by saline infusion (95% vs 21%). Farquhar performed a review of 19 studies, finding that while all studies were accurate in detection of intrauterine pathology, SIS and hysteroscopy performed better than transvaginal sonography in detecting submucous fibroids. Transvaginal sonography was noted to be a sensitive test for the diagnosis of endometrial hyperplasia in perimenopausal women when the endometrial thickness was equal to or greater than 12 mm.

DeVries et al[18] studied 62 patients who underwent transvaginal ultrasonography (TVS), SIS, and finally hysteroscopy for abnormal uterine bleeding. Most of these women were perimenopausal (mean age, 44 years; range, 36 to 54). SIS demonstrated higher accuracy in the diagnosis of intracavitary abnormalities than did TVS.

The study also reviewed accuracy of TVS in diagnosis of endometrial hyperplasia in premenopausal women. Previously, cutoff levels of 8 mm, 10 mm, and 12 mm had been proposed. However, in the study, endometrial measurement alone provided poor diagnostic results. TVS definition of an abnormality (i.e., endometrial thickness of >5 mm) yielded sensitivity of 85% and specificity of 21%, but would have resulted in many unnecessary D&Cs or hysteroscopic procedures. If SIS had been used as the triage method in the study, diagnostic hysteroscopy would have been avoided in 72% of cases. SIS was also able to distinguish characteristics of the myometrium and therefore would have been more suitable for defining the degree of extension of myomas. In fact, Widrich and coworkers[20] found diagnostic accuracy of SIS to be similar to that of hysteroscopy (Table 61-6).[18–20] The authors concluded that SIS was the diagnostic tool of choice in evaluation of perimenopausal women with abnormal uterine bleeding (sensitivity of 88% to 100%, specificity of 76% to 98%) for diagnosing intracavitary abnormalities.

Kaunitz[10] has recommended an algorithm for the evaluation of perimenopausal abnormal uterine bleeding. A thorough history and physical examination are performed. Pregnancy and other intrauterine causes of bleeding are ruled out, and an in-office endometrial biopsy is then performed. If the histology study is benign, medical management is instituted. If medical management does not result in a satisfactory bleeding profile, the next step is transvaginal sonography. If measurements are greater than 5 mm, saline-infused sonohysterography is the next step.

Hysteroscopy may be utilized as an alternative to SIS and permits direct visualization of polyps and submucous myomas and may be performed in an appropriate office setting[21]; however, it requires local anesthesia and or conscious sedation to avoid significant patient discomfort. Goldstein et al[14] and Kaunitz[10] recommend reserving hysteroscopy for the patient with an unclear diagnosis, recurrent bleeding after treatment of other findings, and with lesions requiring biopsy or excision that are

# Reproductive Endocrinology and Infertility

**Table 61-6**
**Findings in Studies Using Saline Infusion Sonography to Diagnose Endometrial Abnormalities**

| First Author | Year | No. of Patients (Status) | Reference Test | Transvaginal Sonography | | Saline Infusion Sonography | |
|---|---|---|---|---|---|---|---|
| | | | | Sensitivity (%) | Specificity (%) | Sensitivity (%) | Specificity (%) |
| Goldstein[14] | 1997 | 21 (Premenopausal) | Suction curettage, surgical procedure | — | — | 100 | 90 |
| Gauscherand | 1995 | 36 (Pre- and postmenopausal) | Hysteroscopy, surgical treatment | 85 | 97 | 94 | 98 |
| Widrich[20] | 1996 | 113 (Pre- and postmenopausal) | Hysteroscopy | — | — | 96 | 88 |
| Bronz[17] | 1997 | 139 (Pre- and postmenopausal) | Hysteroscopy | 92* | 22* | 92 | 86 |
| Bernard[15] | 1997 | 109 (Pre- and postmenopausal) | Hysteroscopy, hysterectomy | — | — | 99 | 76 |
| Williams | 1998 | 39 (Pre- and postmenopausal) | Hysteroscopy, hysterectomy | 67 | 93 | 100 | 86 |
| O'Connell | 1998 | 104 (Postmenopausal) | Hysteroscopy, D&C | 79 | 57 | 88 | 96 |
| de Vries[18] | 2000 | 62 (Premenopausal) | Hysteroscopy | 60 | 93 | 89 | 95 |
| | | | | 85† | 21† | — | — |

*Endometrial thickness cutoff level, 8 mm.
†Endometrial thickness cutoff level, 5 mm.
From deVries LD, Dijkhuizen FP, Mol BWJ, et al: Comparison of transvaginal sonography, saline infusion sonography, and hysteroscopy in premenopausal women with abnormal uterine bleeding. J Clin Ultrasound 2000;28:217–223.

noted on SIS. Figure 61-7 demonstrates one of several logical schema for management of abnormal bleeding in the perimenopausal female.

## MEDICAL MANAGEMENT OF ABNORMAL UTERINE BLEEDING

If the evaluation outlined previously reveals no evidence of pathology requiring surgical excision or correction, a variety of options exist for therapy of hormonally induced bleeding.

Proliferative endometrium or hyperplasia without atypia may be treated with cyclic or acyclic progestational agents or oral contraceptives (OCs). Medroxyprogesterone acetate 10 mg daily for at least 10 days per month, or micronized progesterone 200 mg daily at bedtime, should result in menstrual cycle regulation and reversal of hyperplasia. If abnormal bleeding does not resolve, then hysteroscopy and D&C should be considered to rule out malignancy.

### Oral Contraceptives

In the nonsmoking, nonhypertensive patient without a history of deep vein thrombosis or other contraindication, combination estrogen/progesterone contraceptives are ideal for control of menstrual irregularity. Some currently available options are listed in Table 61-7.[14] Kaunitz[22] has recently reviewed use of OCs in menopause. The American College of Obstetricians and Gynecologists Practice Bulletin recommends OC formulations as the treatment of choice for anovulatory uterine bleeding.[23]

A variety of preparations including triphasic[24] and low-dose monophasic OCs are effective in correction of anovulatory bleeding. However, to date no OC has received FDA approval for this purpose. Many clinicians prefer formulations containing 20 µg of ethinyl estradiol (EE) for perimenopausal women. However, cycle control may not be as good with lower estrogen

doses. Newer, 25 µg EE triphasic low-dose OC formulations provide good cycle control.[25] Other options including transdermal contraceptive patches and vaginal rings have been used with good success.

Hormone therapy regimens used for postmenopausal therapy have been utilized in some women. However, these regimens do not suppress ovulation and may make bleeding worse.[22] Kaunitz[26] has reviewed use of oral or transdermal estradiol and depot medroxyprogesterone acetate in these women as opposed to standard postmenopausal hormone therapy. The combination suppresses ovulation, produces amenorrhea, and treats vasomotor symptoms commonly encountered in this group. Another option is use of fixed-dose hormone therapy combinations containing estradiol 1 mg plus norethindrone acetate 0.5 mg or ethinyl estradiol 5 µg plus norethindrone acetate 1 mg. The preceding

**Table 61-7**
**Contraceptive Formulations**

**Cyclical formulations**

Low estrogen dose (≤35 µg) combination oral contraceptives
Weekly transdermal contraceptive patch: 150 µg norelgestromin/20 µg ethinyl estradiol daily (Ortho Evra)
Three-week contraceptive vaginal ring: ~120 µg etonogestrel/15 µg ethinyl estradiol per day (NuvaRing)
Three-month depot medroxyprogesterone acetate injection: 150 mg per injection (Depo-Provera) plus oral or transdermal estradiol
Levonorgestrel intrauterine device (Mirena) plus oral estrogen

**High progestin dose combination menopausal formulations**

Norethindrone acetate 0.5 mg/estradiol 1 mg (Activella)
Norethindrone acetate 1 mg/ethinyl estradiol 5 µg (femhrt)

From Kaunitz AM: Gynecologic problems of the perimenopause: evaluation and treatment. Obstet Gynecol Clin North Am 2002;29:455–473.

**Evaluation and treatment of uterine bleeding**

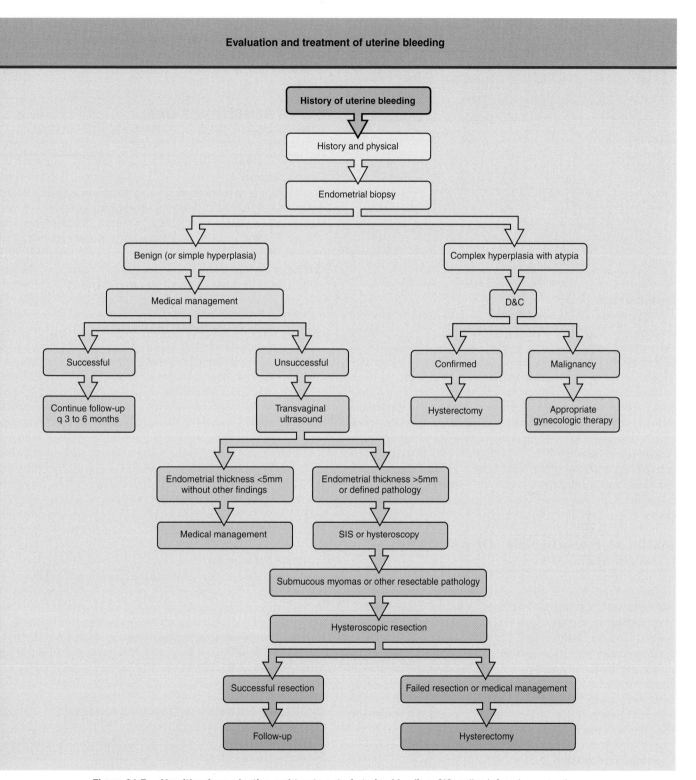

**Figure 61-7    Algorithm for evaluation and treatment of uterine bleeding.** SIS, saline-infused sonography.

regimen may then be continued for menopausal therapy if indicated.

## Progestin Therapy

Cyclic oral progestin therapy has been long utilized for treatment of dysfunctional uterine bleeding. Table 61-8 lists doses that may be used for 12 to 14 days per month and yield good results. Cyclic progestins are especially useful in the obese patient who exhibits excess estrogen from peripheral aromatization. Endometrial protection should be documented by biopsy. Use of danazol, while successful in reducing menstrual flow, is limited by significant side effects of hirsutism, weight gain, and acne.

**Table 61-8**
**Oral Cyclic Progestin-only Regimens for Treatment of Abnormal Uterine Bleeding in Perimenopausal Women**

| Progestin | Tablet Strength | Daily Dose* |
|---|---|---|
| Medroxyprogesterone acetate | 2.5, 5, 10 mg | 5–10 mg |
| Norethindrone acetate | 5 mg | 2.5–5 mg[†] |
| Norethindrone | 0.35 mg | 0.7–1 mg[†] |
| Danazol | 50, 100, 200 mg | 200 mg |

*Administered for 12–14 days each month.
[†]0.5–1 tablet/day.
[†]2–3 tablet/day.
From Kaunitz AM: Gynecologic problems of the perimenopause: evaluation and treatment. Obstet Gynecol Clin North Am 2002;29:455–473.

## Intrauterine Systems

A levonorgestrel-containing intrauterine system (IUS) has been available in the United States for a number of years. Several older studies and a Cochrane review[27] have established that the IUS is as effective in menstrual control as norethindrone and allows some women considering surgical therapy to continue medical therapy of dysfunctional uterine bleeding. Hurskainen et al[28] established that the IUS resulted in patient satisfaction and allowed hysterectomy to be avoided in a study group. Hubacher and Grimes[29] reviewed the literature of non-contraceptive benefits of IUSs and concluded that the levonorgestrel intrauterine system may treat a variety of gynecologic disorders, including menorrhagia and anemia. Use of non-hormonal IUSs was associated with a decrease in endometrial cancer.

## SURGICAL MANAGEMENT OF ABNORMAL UTERINE BLEEDING

Hysterectomy is the second most common surgical procedure performed in reproductive age women in the United States, most commonly for leiomyomata. Utilization of laparoscope-assisted vaginal hysterectomy (LAVH), laparoscopic subtotal hysterectomy, and laparoscopic total hysterectomy have supplemented the standard options of vaginal or transabdominal hysterectomy. When hysterectomy is indicated for medically unresponsive bleeding, the surgeon should utilize the procedure best indicated by his or her experience, the disease process, and the patient's clinical circumstances.

## Endometrial Ablation

Various laser-focused endometrial ablation techniques have gradually been replaced by thermal balloon ablation and other types of thermal ablation including bipolar, microwave, and cryoablation. These techniques have a shorter learning curve and reasonable rates of decreased uterine bleeding and amenorrhea. Several issues should be kept in mind when choosing these techniques. First, malignancy should be ruled out by endometrial sampling prior to use. Second, the techniques do not adequately treat intrauterine pathology such as polyps. Therefore, it is wise to evaluate the endometrial cavity with hysteroscopy or SIS and

remove the lesion prior to therapy. Third, pretreatment with danazol or a gonadotropin-releasing hormone (GnRH) analog should be considered although Lissak and colleagues[30] noted no difference in response between immediate and delayed therapy.

## OTHER BENEFITS OF ORAL CONTRACEPTIVES FOR PERIMENOPAUSAL WOMEN

### Contraception

The most obvious benefit of OCs to perimenopausal women is birth control. Although fertility significantly decreases in perimenopause, ovulation frequently continues. Data suggest that 80% of women aged 40 to 49 may potentially conceive. Data from the National Survey of Family Growth showed that 51% of pregnancies occurring in women 40 years of age or older were unintended and 65% of those resulted in abortion.[31] Women over age 35 can use OCs or transdermal contraceptives provided they do not smoke or have other cardiovascular risk factors (Table 61-9).[32] Most authors recommend use of lower dose OCs in perimenopausal women; however, the major difference in risk of venous thromboembolic events appears to occur between 50 g EE pills and those containing 30 to 35 µg. Until 1995, the conventional wisdom held that risk of thrombosis in OCs was related to the estrogen component and the progestin component was not thought to affect clinical thrombosis. In 1995, three papers reported an increase in thrombosis associated with two new progestins (desogestrel and gestodene). Follow-up studies reported both increased and unchanged rates of thromboembolism. Two recent reviews of third-generation progestins concluded that the risk of venous thromboembolism was higher than second-generation products.[33,34] For a complete discussion of general oral contraceptive risks and benefits, see Chapter 58.

### Fracture Prevention

Bone mass peaks in females at approximately age 22. After age 40, bone loss may approach 1% per year and increase to 3% to 5% per year in postmenopausal women. Women who take OCs have been shown to preserve bone mass, and a study by Michaelssson of women in their 40s who took OCs showed a decreased risk of hip fracture of 30% compared with those who had never used OCs (Table 61-10).[35]

**Table 61-9**
**Risk Factors for Cardiovascular Disease**

Androgen excess states
Cigarette smoking
Diabetes mellitus
Dyslipidemias
Family history of early onset of cardiovascular disease
Hypertension
Obesity
Pregnancy-induced hypertension

From Archer D: Use of contraceptives for older women. In Lobo RA (ed): Treatment of the Postmenopausal Woman: Basic and Clinical Aspects, 2nd ed. Philadelphia, Lippincott Williams & Wilkins, 1999, pp 83–92.

**Table 61-10**
**Decreased Risk of Hip Fracture with Oral Contraceptive Use**

| Age at Oral Contraceptive Use | Odds Ratio (95% CI) | |
| --- | --- | --- |
| | Multivariate (Any Oral Contraceptive) | ≥50 µg Ethinyl Estradiol Oral Contraceptive |
| Never used | 1.0 (referent) | 1.0 (referent) |
| <30 yr | 1.3 (0.88–2.1) | 1.1 (0.6–2.0) |
| 30–39 yr | 0.8 (0.6–1.2) | 0.8 (0.5–1.1) |
| ≥40 yr | 0.7 (0.5–0.9) | 0.6 (0.4–0.9) |

CI, confidence interval.

Adapted from Michäelsson K, Baron JA, Farahmand BY, et al: Oral-contraceptive use and risk of hip fracture: a case-control study. Lancet 1999;353:1481–1484. © 1999 by The Lancet Ltd; and Kaunitz AM: Injectable contraception: new and existing options. Obstet Gynecol Clin North Am 2000;27:741–780.

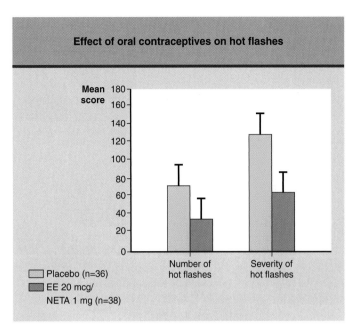

**Effect of oral contraceptives on hot flashes**

Placebo (n=36)
EE 20 mcg/ NETA 1 mg (n=38)

**Figure 61-8    Oral contraceptives decrease the number and severity of hot flashes in perimenopausal women in a randomized, double-blind, placebo-controlled, six-cycle trial.** EE, ethinyl estradiol; NETA, norethindrone acetate. (Adapted with permission from Casper RF, Dodin S, Reid RL, and Study Investigators: The effect of 20 µg ethinyl estradiol/l mg norethindrone acetate [Minestrin], a low-dose oral contraceptive, on vaginal bleeding patterns, hot flashes, and quality of life in symptomatic perimenopausal women. Menopause 1997;4:139–147.)

## Lipid Profile

Table 61-11[36] shows the results of a recent study of triphasic OCs on the lipid profile of a group of perimenopausal women. Whether these results have significant clinical implications for the average perimenopausal female is unknown. It appears, however, that OCs do not have a unfavorable effect in the clinically low-risk individual.

## Vasomotor Symptoms

Approximately 85% of perimenopausal women experience vasomotor instability with marked variation in frequency, duration, and intensity.[37] Studies reviewing treatment of hot flashes and other perimenopausal symptomatology are difficult to perform secondary to a 30% placebo effect. However, placebo-controlled, double-blind, randomized studies of OCs have shown approximately 50% fewer hot flashes in the treatment group (Fig. 61-8).[38] Not only was the frequency of hot flashes decreased but the severity also was decreased by 50% compared with placebo. However, because of the significant placebo effect, the differences were not statistically significant.

### Endometrial and Ovarian Cancer

OCs have been shown to decrease the incidence of both endometrial and ovarian cancer presumably owing to progestin action on the endometrium and prevention of ovulation. Endometrial and ovarian cancer is reduced by 40% in a variety of studies. In addition, the effect appears to continue for 15 years following one or more years' use. Perhaps more importantly, the effect appears applicable to women with a family history of breast and ovarian cancer.[39]

### Miscellaneous Benefits

The incidence of pregnancy is obviously reduced in perimenopausal women taking OCs; likewise, the incidence of ectopic pregnancy is decreased. In addition, OCs have been shown to reduce the incidence of ovarian cysts.

### Pelvic Inflammatory Disease

Older studies indicated that women on OCs may be at increased risk for cervical *Chlamydia* infection. However, other studies indicate that the incidence of pelvic inflammatory disease (PID) and the clinical and laparoscopic severity of PID are reduced

**Table 61-11**
**Impact of Low-dose Oral Contraceptives on Lipid Profiles in Premenopausal Women***

| Lipid | Median Change (%) | |
| --- | --- | --- |
| | Triphasic norgestimate/35 µg ethinyl estradiol | Norethindrone estradiol acetate/20 µg ethinyl estradiol |
| High-density lipoprotein cholesterol | 4.5%† | –4% |
| HDL₂ | 25%† | 13.3% |
| Apo A-1 | 17.9%† | 9.8% |

HDL₂, high-density lipoprotein variant 2.

*Randomized, open-label, six-cycle trial in women aged 18–50 years; lipid changes baseline to final visit.

† P <0.001.

† P <0.004.

Adapted from Sulak P, Lippman J, Siu C, et al: Clinical comparison of triphasic norgestimate/35 µg ethinyl estradiol and monophasic norethindrone acetate/20 µg ethinyl estradiol: cycle control, lipid effects, and user satisfaction. Contraception 1999;59:161–166. © 1999, Elsevier Science; and Kaunitz AM: Oral contraceptive use in perimenopause. Am J Obstet Gynecol 2001;185:S32–S37.

# Reproductive Endocrinology and Infertility

by 40% to 60% in patients taking OCs. The mechanism may be the effect of progestins on cervical mucus or modification of the immune response. Perimenopausal women taking OCs have shorter and lighter menses. In addition, endometrial atrophy affected by conceptive pills and decreased uterine contractility may decrease movement of bacteria into the upper genital tract. While in vitro studies indicate that progestins may inhibit the growth of gonorrhea, animal studies indicate that estrogen and progestin may facilitate the ascent of *Chlamydia trachomatis* into the upper tract. Ness et al[40] appear to have confirmed this hypothesis in an animal model. A summary of oral contraceptive benefits is shown in Table 61-12.[5]

## Vasomotor Symptoms and Sleep Disturbances

Vasomotor symptoms, including hot flashes (hot flushes) and night sweats, are reported by women of all ages. While common in the postmenopausal period, hot flash occurrences become more frequent during perimenopause, peak about the time of the last menstrual period, and decline after menopause, as reported in the MWHS.[4] Women who had long perimenopausal transitions reported more prominent hot flashes than women who had short transitions to menopause.

The "hot flash" describes a sudden onset of erythema affecting the upper body, chest, and head, accompanied by a feeling of intense body heat and sweating. Hot flashes may be frequent or rare and vary from several seconds to one hour in duration. They are most disturbing when occurring at night and cause marked lack of sleep and subsequent problems in daily functioning secondary to fatigue. A cool environment may mitigate the effects of hot flashes.

Hot flashes are not confined to postmenopausal women. In the MWHS, the incidence was 10% in premenopausal women; 37% to 50% in perimenopausal women, 50% at about the time of the last menstrual flow; and 20% to 62% in postmenopausal women. By 4 years after menopause, the incidence had decreased to 20%.

The physiology of hot flashes is incompletely understood. They are most commonly related to decreased or fluctuating estrogen levels encountered in the peri- and postmenopausal time period. However, not all hot flashes are due to estrogen deficiency. Other conditions such as diabetes and thyroid disease that first manifest in the perimenopausal age group also may mimic hot flashes. A differential diagnosis of hot flashes is listed in Table 61-13.[10]

| Table 61-13 |
|---|
| **Medical Conditions That Mimic Hot Flashes** |

**Systemic diseases**

Thyroid disease
Pheochromocytoma
Carcinoid syndrome
Systemic mast cell disease
Leukemia
Pancreatic tumors
Renal cell carcinoma

**Neurologic causes**

Stress and anxiety
Brain tumors
Orthostatic hypotension
Migraines
Parkinson's disease
Spinal cord injury

**Emotional flushing**

**Alcohol**

**Drug use**

Vasodilators, calcium channel blockers, bromocriptine, tamoxifen, raloxifene, gonadotropin-releasing hormone agonists

**Food additives**

Nitrites, sulfites, red pepper, capsaicin

**Eating**

From Kaunitz AM: Gynecologic problems of the perimenopause: evaluation and treatment. Obstet Gynecol Clin North Am 2002;29:455–473.

Estrogen and progestins in combination (for women with a uterus) or estrogen alone has long shown reasonable efficacy in relief of hot flashes in postmenopausal women. However, use of standard hormone therapy for perimenopausal women is controversial. Shulman and Harari[41] studied 22 consecutive menstruating perimenopausal women with vasomotor symptoms in an open-label observational study over 12 months. All patients received estradiol 0.025 mg/day administered through a transdermal weekly patch for 12 months. The authors administered unopposed estrogen feeling that in women who continue to menstruate, unopposed estrogen is unlikely to prove a risk to the endometrium. Forty-five percent of patients reported complete relief and an additional 27% moderate relief of symptoms in this study. Other authors recommend periodic administration of progestin if exogenous estrogen is used in perimenopausal women, menstruating or not (see Chapter 60).

## Sexual Dysfunction and Vulvovaginal Changes

Sexual dysfunction, most often vulvovaginal dryness secondary to decreased estrogen or decreased libido, is common in perimenopause. In addition, irregular menses, hot flashes, and sleep disturbances have an adverse effect on sexuality at this time. Weight gain and emotional issues about body image, marital relations, and social relations also are common. Nachtigall[37] and others have written extensively regarding physiologic changes in perimenopause that may adversely affect sexual function.

| Table 61-12 |
|---|
| **Benefits of Oral Contraceptive Use in Perimenopausal Women** |

Effective contraception (if needed)
High bone density/fewer fractures
Prevention of ovarian and endometrial cancers
Reduction in vasomotor symptoms
Treatment of acne
Treatment of irregular menses/dysfunctional uterine bleeding, menorrhagia, and/or dysmenorrhea

From Kaunitz AM: Oral contraceptive use in perimenopause. Am J Obstet Gynecol 2001;185:S32–S37.

Vulvovaginal dryness, irritation, and dyspareunia are common. Even though estradiol levels may be elevated, vaginal dryness (75%) and decreased vaginal lubrication are frequently reported. Kaunitz[42] summarized recommendations in this regard and a recent meta-analysis[43] has shown that vaginal low-dose estrogen is as effective as systemic estrogen in relief of symptoms. Compared with systemic estrogen, local therapy may even be more effective[44] for relief of vaginal symptoms. Vaginal creams are often not well accepted secondary to soiling of bed linens and clothing. However, estradiol vaginal tablets and rings are efficacious.[45,46] Many women begin experiencing increasing urinary incontinence in this age range, whether overflow, urge, or mixed incontinence. Until recently, both oral and vaginal estrogen have been recommended for improvement of these symptoms. Both older and current studies, e.g., the heart and estrogen progestin replacement study HERS,[47] found no improvement in urinary incontinence associated with systemic hormone therapy.

## OSTEOPOROSIS IN PERIMENOPAUSAL WOMEN

More than 60 years ago it was recognized that postmenopausal women developed vertebral fractures leading to pain, disfigurement, and dysfunction. It is now estimated that the annual cost of osteoporosis in the United States exceeds $14 billion and affects 28 million persons. The morbidity and mortality associated with a hip fracture are significant, and only 15% of those affected women return to their previous lifestyle. Females exhibit maximal bone mass in their early 20s, with maintenance and remodeling until approximately the time of menopause. Perimenopause and associated symptoms give gynecologists the opportunity to be effective in screening and treatment of this significant disease.

Risk factors for osteoporosis are listed in Table 61-14[48] (see Chapter 1). Women at risk for osteoporosis should be screened when they exhibit signs of estrogen deficiency or if they are at high risk by other criteria. If osteopenia or osteoporosis are detected, therapy should be initiated in the same fashion as for the postmenopausal female.

## DEPRESSION IN PERIMENOPAUSAL WOMEN

The perimenopausal period is often associated with depression. Granted, it is a time of physiologic and hormonal change, but also it is a time of peak performance in careers with accompanying job stress and of balancing career aspirations with family and possibly caregiving to aging parents. Any of the foregoing may cause enough turmoil to elicit depression in a susceptible individual. However, contrary to popular assumptions, while depression is more common in women at all ages than in men, the perimenopausal and menopausal time period is not itself a major risk factor for depression. In fact, most studies indicate that a history of previous depression is the strongest predictor of future depression. In the MWHS,[4] a diagnosis of depression at study entry was the strongest predictor of depression at the close of the study 25 months later. The MWHS noted that the highest incidence of depression occurred in those who remained perimenopausal throughout the period of observation (Fig. 61-9).[4] Increased depression appeared to be related to the continued presence of menopausal symptoms rather than the menopausal status per se (Fig. 61-10).[4] Therefore, the physician should be aware of the possibility of depression in perimenopausal females, especially those who have had symptoms for a longer period of time and those with a previous history of depression (Table 61-15).

Depressive-type symptoms coinciding with the onset of perimenopausal symptoms in the patient without a history of previous depression should raise suspicion of hormone-related episodes. In these persons, a trial of hormone therapy may be considered.

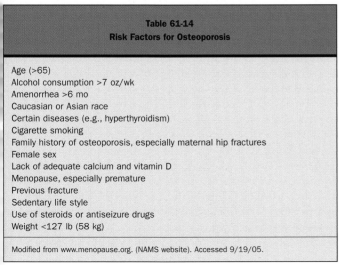

| Table 61-14 |
| --- |
| Risk Factors for Osteoporosis |

Age (>65)
Alcohol consumption >7 oz/wk
Amenorrhea >6 mo
Caucasian or Asian race
Certain diseases (e.g., hyperthyroidism)
Cigarette smoking
Family history of osteoporosis, especially maternal hip fractures
Female sex
Lack of adequate calcium and vitamin D
Menopause, especially premature
Previous fracture
Sedentary life style
Use of steroids or antiseizure drugs
Weight <127 lb (58 kg)

Modified from www.menopause.org. (NAMS website). Accessed 9/19/05.

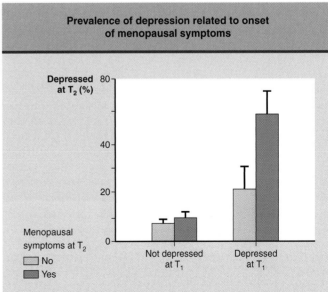

**Figure 61-9** **An increased prevalence of depression was related to the onset of menopausal symptoms.** Study subjects were evaluated for depression at the beginning of the study ($T_1$) and again 27 months later ($T_2$). (From Avis NE, Brambilla D, McKinlay SM, Vass K: A longitudinal analysis of the association between menopause and depression: results from the Massachusetts Women's Health Study. Ann Epidemiol 1994;4:217.)

# Reproductive Endocrinology and Infertility

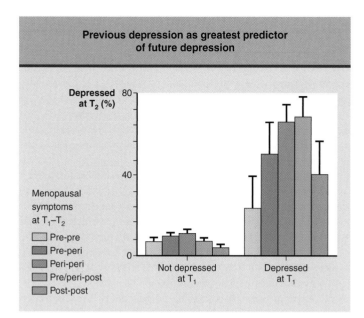

**Figure 61-10    Previous depression is the greatest predictor of future depression.** Women at different stages in the menopausal transition were evaluated for depression at the beginning of the study ($T_1$) and again 27 months later ($T_2$). This illustration reports the rate of depression among women at premenopausal, perimenopausal, and postmenopausal stages. For women across all stages, those who were depressed at the beginning of the study ($T_1$) had higher rates of depression 27 months later ($T_2$). For women who were not depressed at $T_1$, rates of depression increased slightly among women who moved from the premenopausal stage into the perimenopausal stage and were highest for women who remained at the perimenopausal stage for at least 27 months. In the same group, depression began to decrease as women became postmenopausal and was lowest among those who were postmenopausal for at least 27 months. (From Avis NE, Brambilla D, McKinlay SM, Vass K: A longitudinal analysis of the association between menopause and depression: results from the Massachusetts Women's Health Study. Ann Epidemiol 1994;4:217.)

It is unclear whether there is a relationship between hormones and changes in neurotransmitters that may be related to depression. However, estrogens have been shown to potentiate the efficacy of fluoxetine therapy for depression.

In addition to exogenous job and family-related stress, women may encounter self-image stress during perimenopause.

### Table 61-15
### Risk Factors for Depression

Concurrent illness
Concurrent substance abuse
Fatigue, malaise, irritability, or sadness
Lack of social support
Personal or family history of depression, bipolar disorder, or suicide attempts
Prior depression
Recent stressful life event

From Association of Professors of Gynecology and Obstetrics: Managing the Perimenopause. APGO Educational Series on Women's Health Issues. Washington, DC, APGO, 2001, pp 1–20.

### Table 61-16
### American Psychiatric Association Criteria* for Diagnosis of Major Depression

Depressed mood most of the day, nearly every day
Diminished interest in most activities most of the day, nearly every day
Significant weight loss or gain
Insomnia or hypersomnia
Psychomotor agitation or retardation
Fatigue
Feelings of worthlessness or guilt
Indecisiveness
Recurrent thoughts of death or suicide

*At least 5% of the preceding criteria, including either of the first two most of the time for at least 2 weeks.
From Association of Professors of Gynecology and Obstetrics: Managing the Perimenopause. APGO Educational Series on Women's Health Issues. Washington, DC, APGO, 2001, pp 1–20.

Realization of the end of reproductive years and the "empty nest syndrome" may be particularly troublesome to some individuals. It is therefore incumbent upon the physician to inquire about the preceding issues in a caring and sensitive fashion to ascertain whether a significant potential for depression exists and if it requires therapy. The American Psychiatric Association has established criteria for diagnosis of major depression (Table 61-16).

## FERTILITY IN PERIMENOPAUSAL WOMEN

Secondary to changes in career orientation, marriage, and the aging "baby boom" generation, the proportion of older primiparous women (>35 years) is expected to exceed 25% in Western countries in 2005. Although uncommon, spontaneous pregnancies occur even into the fifth and sixth decade of life. How old is old then in relation to fertility? In the United States, it is estimated that rates of infertility are 10% at 20 to 29 years of age, 25% at 30 to 39 years of age, and 50% over 40 years of age. The estimated rate of a spontaneous pregnancy is 2% at age 42 and almost zero after 45 years. The implantation rate also drops from 20% at age 30 to less than 4% at age 40, as do birth rates. Age 41 is generally considered the time when fertility stops, and menopause occurs approximately 10 years after loss of conception potential. The percentage of women who do not succeed in conceiving after 1 years' time increase from 5% at less than 25 years of age to 30% at more than 35 years of age.

Fertility has been studied in several stable, fertile populations, most notably the Hutterites (Fig. 61-11 and Table 61-17).[49,50] In this population, the height of fertility was between 18 and 30, but fertility was present in 86% of women at age 36, 66% at age 40, and 13% at age 45.

As previously indicated, ovarian reserve decreases with advancing age from 4 to 7 million oocytes at 20 weeks of gestation to 400,000 at birth. The pool of follicles declines exponentially, and from age 35 forward, accelerated loss occurs so that by age 38 a woman may have only 25,000 follicles; at age 40, 1500; at age 45, 5000; and in the early 50s, only a few hundred. Furthermore, polymorphisms of genes and a decrease

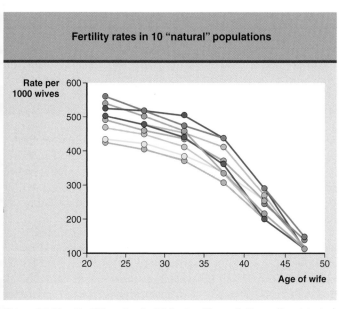

**Figure 61-11    Fertility rates in 10 "natural" populations.** (Reprinted with permission from Menken J, Trussell J, Larsen U: Age and infertility. Science 1986;233:1389–1394. ©1986 American Association for the Advancement of Science.)

in the quality of oocytes may occur, as indicated by the increased number of oocyte aneuploides noted in women greater than 37 years of age undergoing in vitro fertilization (IVF). Therefore, in the perimenopausal woman, oocyte aneuploides reduce the chance of successful fertilization, implantation, and development. Interestingly, juvenile and adult mouse ovaries possess mitotically active germ cells that, based on rates of oocyte degeneration (atresia) and clearance, are needed to continuously replenish the follicle pool. These data tentatively established the existence of proliferative germ cells that sustain oocytes and follicle production in the postnatal mammalian ovary. These data are contrary to the basic doctrine of mammalian development that has been accepted for many years.[51]

By most epidemiologic data, the probability of pregnancy in perimenopause is low and the spontaneous abortion rate in clinically recognized pregnancies increases from 10% before age 30 to 34% at age 40, and to 50% to 75% at after age 45 years.

| Table 61-17 Estimated Percentage of Sterile Couples of Specified Ages in the Hutterite Population | |
| --- | --- |
| Age of Wife (yr) | Percentage Sterile |
| <25 | 3.5 |
| 30 | 7 |
| 35 | 11 |
| 40 | 33 |
| 45 | 87 |
| 50 | 100 |

From the American Society for Reproductive Medicine; and Klein J, Sauer MV: Assessing fertility in women of advanced reproductive age. Am J Obstet Gynecol 2001;185:758–770.

In addition, some fetuses are noted to have chromosomal anomalies.

After age 40 the likelihood of a successful response to assisted reproductive technology decreases and most women are considered to have a poor prognosis for successful fertility. In couples undergoing IVF/embryo transfer therapy, implantation, clinical pregnancy, and live birth rates drop with advancing age. The quoted implantation rate is less than 6% after age 40, and the live birth rate is less than 3.5% after age 45 and 8% between ages 40 and 45 (Fig. 61-12).[52]

Oocyte donation was used initially in women with inherited defects but now has been applied to those wishing to extend child-bearing potential into later years. These pregnancies have a significantly higher success rate than conventional IVF (Fig. 61-13). For example, in the United States in 1999 (the last year for which such data are available), 5844 donor oocyte cycles resulted in a live birth rate of 41.1%, whereas in women undergoing IVF, the rate was 9.7%. In the United States more than 70% of all assisted reproductive technology cycles at age 46 involve donor eggs. If oocytes are donated by young women to older women, implantation and pregnancy rates are normal in the recipients regardless of age. Therefore, the limiting factor appears to be largely the condition of oocytes and not necessarily the uterus of the woman. However, pregnancies after donation incur a higher risk of obstetric complications including vaginal bleeding (12% to 50%), pregnancy-induced hypertension (16% to 40%), premature rupture of membranes (6%), and premature labor (13% to 56%).[53] The interested reader is referred to the Klein and Sauer[50] review of this material.

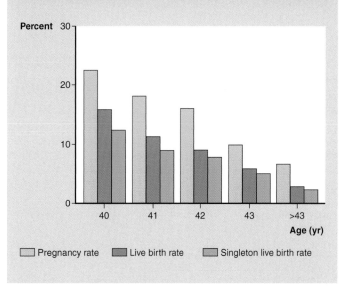

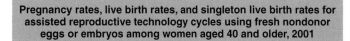

**Figure 61-12    Pregnancy rates, live birth rates, and singleton live birth rates for assisted reproductive technology (ART) cycles using fresh nondonor eggs or embryos among women aged 40 years and older, 2001.** (From Ventura SJ, Abma JC, Mosher WD: Revised pregnancy rates, 1990–97, and new rates for 1998–99: United States. Natl Vital Stat Rep 2003;52:1–16.)

# Reproductive Endocrinology and Infertility

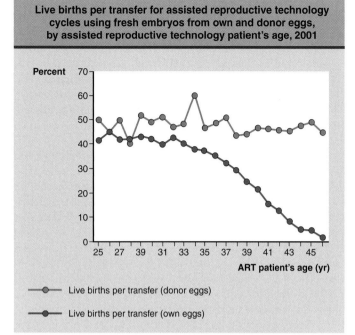

Live births per transfer for assisted reproductive technology cycles using fresh embryos from own and donor eggs, by assisted reproductive technology patient's age, 2001

Percent

ART patient's age (yr)

— Live births per transfer (donor eggs)
— Live births per transfer (own eggs)

**Figure 61-13** Live births per transfer for assisted reproductive technology (ART) cycles using fresh embryos from own and donor eggs, by ART patient's age, 2001. (From Ventura SJ, Abma JC, Mosher WD: Revised pregnancy rates, 1990–97, and new rates for 1998–99: United States. Natl Vital Stat Rep 2003;52:1–16.)

| Table 61-18 Health Screening Recommendations for Perimenopausal Women | |
| --- | --- |
| **Evaluation** | **Frequency** |
| **Medical history** Family and personal history | Annually |
| **Physical examination** Including blood pressure and breast, pelvic and rectovaginal, and skin examinations | Annually |
| **Laboratory and other screening tests** | |
| Cholesterol | Every 5 years |
| Urinalysis | Review yearly |
| Pap smear | At physician's discretion after three annual consecutive normal tests in low-risk patient |
| **Mammogram** | Every 1 to 2 years before age 50; annually after age 50 |
| **Colon cancer screening** | |
| Fecal occult blood test | Annually |
| Sigmoidoscopy | Every 3 to 5 years after age 50 |
| **Bone density evaluation** | Review yearly |
| **Flu vaccine** | Review yearly |

From ACOG Technical Bulletin. Health maintenance for perimenopausal women. No. 210, Aug 1995. Int J Gynaecol Obstet 1995;51:171–181.

## HEALTH MAINTENANCE AND SCREENING

Evaluation and treatment of the patient's problems are obviously the most important task in caring for the perimenopausal woman. However, equally important is screening for pathophysiologic conditions that may not be apparent to the patient and encouraging health maintenance. The current epidemic of overweight and obesity associated with "metabolic syndrome," diabetes, and heart disease promise to have a major impact on health care in the next 20 to 50 years in the United States. Therefore, it is incumbent upon the gynecologist to perform proper health screening and make recommendations for prevention or correction of conditions that may compromise the patient in the future.

At the time of the annual well-woman examination, the patient should be asked about smoking, alcohol intake, diet and exercise habits, and stress. A review of personal and family history of chronic and inheritable diseases should be obtained. Standard health screening and laboratory testing appropriate for that age group should be performed (Table 61-18).[54] In addition, the physician should screen for signs of depression.

## LIFESTYLE INTERVENTION: CARDIOVASCULAR DISEASE

Patients need to understand the physiologic consequences of aging and loss of estrogen in the menopausal transition. Despite the new data regarding lack of cardiovascular protection by hormone therapies in older women, younger females (i.e., those who are still menstruating) continue to have low relative rates of apparent cardiovascular disease. Therefore, screening for risk factors of elevated serum lipids, lack of exercise, and improper nutrition is important. Proper nutrition serves to maintain desirable body weight and reduces predisposition to insulin resistance, impaired insulin secretion, hyperglycemia, and reduced pulmonary function. General recommendations should include taking adequate calcium and minerals, increasing fiber intake, limiting alcohol and caffeine, and avoiding high-fat foods. Absorption of dietary calcium is more efficient than from supplements; however, if dietary screening indicates low calcium intake, supplements of 1000 mg/day for women under 51 years and 1200 mg/day for those over 51 years are recommended by the National Osteoporosis Foundation. Calcium, whether from diet or supplements, is best absorbed when taken in amounts of 500 mg or less. Calcium carbonate is best absorbed when taken with food, while calcium citrate may be taken at any time.

Older women, especially those in northern climates where activities take place indoors for much of the year, should be encouraged to add supplements containing vitamin D to their diet. Skin has a decreased ability to synthesize the active form of vitamin D as aging occurs, and lack of exposure to sunlight, especially during the winter, compounds the problem. There is no clear evidence that addition of vitamin D is beneficial in younger, perimenopausal women; however, screening for the recommended daily allowance of 400 IU is encouraged. While vitamin D doses of 400 to 800 IU/day are desirable, women should not consume over 800 IU/day.

## HORMONE THERAPY

Beginning in 1998 with the publication of the HERS and estrogen replacement atherosclerosis (ERA) studies and culminating with data from the Women's Health Initiative (WHI), researchers and patient attitudes regarding the use of hormone replacement therapy have dramatically changed. Hormone therapy (HT), as it is now called, recognizes that according to current convention, a hormone is not being replaced, as is done with the thyroid. Hormones in the form of OCs and conventional hormone therapy have a place in management of the perimenopausal female.[55]

The goals of hormone therapy for perimenopausal and post-menopausal women differ and as do the agents utilized. One major goal in perimenopausal women is to control menstrual irregularity and menorrhagia or metrorrhagia due to hormonal causes. However, many of these same women are also affected by common menopausal symptoms such as irritability, hot flashes, and night sweats. In addition, at least some concern must be given to the inevitable onset of cardiovascular disease, increased vulvovaginal symptoms, and osteoporosis common after hormone production ceases.

If the patient does not have any of the standard contra-indications (smoking, history of deep venous thrombosis, etc), it is generally accepted that she may use OCs containing equal to or less than 35 µg EE for menstrual irregularity and dysfunctional bleeding. The obvious advantage of these agents is gonadotropin suppression and contraception.

The use of standard HT is more controversial. Since the standard dose of HT is approximately 25% of the amount of estrogen in a 20 µg contraceptive, some authors argue that hormone levels may continue to fluctuate and result in further bleeding. In addition, an Association of Professors in Gynecology and Obstetrics (APGO)[2] publication states that use of progester-one alone may fail to control menstrual irregularity, since it may not fully suppress FSH and estradiol fluctuation. In addition, the data from the WHI have resulted in a dramatic decrease in HT utilization of all types. Women are now reluctant to begin HT secondary to concern about breast cancer, stroke, and heart disease. Even the long-touted potential of HT to decrease Alzheimer's disease and dementia has been seriously questioned by the WHI.

OCs may be reasonably utilized for those who meet criteria until menopause is established. At that time, the decision must be made whether to change to standard HT or to stop therapy. APGO[2] advocates continuation of OCs until approximately age 50 to 52. OCs may be arbitrarily stopped at that time and the patient followed or transferred to HT. Use of gonadotropin measurements (FSH) to determine the proper timing is contro-versial. In the past some have advocated day 3 or 7 of the pill-free week to obtain an FSH level. A consistent level of FSH equal to or greater than 20 mIU/mL indicates that menopause has occurred, especially if LH is consistently elevated also. Nevertheless, other authors have utilized HT in perimenopause for therapy of vasomotor symptoms with good results.[41]

There appears to be agreement among most organizations regarding indications of HT. Recommendations from a recent North American Menopause Society (NAMS)[48] statement on use of HT in peri- and postmenopausal women is summarized in Table 61-19. The currently understood risks and benefits of

**Table 61-19**
**North American Menopause Society Recommendations for Estrogen and Progesterone in Peri- and Postmenopausal Women**

Treatment of moderate to severe menopausal symptoms
Treatment of vulvovaginal atrophy
Progestins for endometrial protection in women with a uterus
No hormone therapy for primary or secondary prevention of coronary heart disease
Progestins may be associated with increased risk of breast cancer
Hormone therapy is effective for prevention of osteoporosis, but other agents should be considered
Hormone therapy is not recommended for prevention of dementia after age 65
Data from WHI and HERS should be extrapolated with caution to women younger than age 50 who initiate hormone therapy
Use of hormone therapy should be limited to shortest duration consistent with treatment goals of the individual woman
Lower than standard dose of hormone therapy should be considered

From Estrogen and progestogen use in peri- and postmenopausal women: September 2003 position statement of the North American Menopause Society. Menopause 2003;10:497–506.

HT in the postmenopausal woman are discussed in detail in Chapter 60.

### Acknowledgment

Many thanks to my wife, Teresa Snyder, for her assistance in preparation and editing of this chapter.

## REFERENCES

1. Stages of reproductive aging workshop (STRAW): executive summary. Menopause 2001;8:402–407. **(IV, C)**
2. Association of Professors of Gynecology and Obstetrics: Managing the Perimenopause. APGO Educational Series on Women's Health Issues. Washington, DC, APGO, 2001, pp 1–20. **(IV, C)**
3. Faddy MJ, Gosden RG, Gougeon A, et al: Accelerated disappearance of ovarian follicles in mid-life: implications for forecasting menopause. Hum Reprod 1992;7:1342–1346. **(IIa, B)**
4. McKinlay SM, Brambilla DJ, Posner JG: The normal menopause transition. Maturitas 1992;14:103–115. **(IIa, B)**
5. Treloar AE: Menstrual cyclicity and the pre-menopause. Maturitas 1981;3:249–264. **(III, B)**
6. Groome NP, Illingworth PJ, O'Brien M, et al: Measurement of dimeric inhibin B throughout the human menstrual cycle: J Clin Endocrinol Metab 1996;81:1401–1405. **(IIa, B)**
7. Santoro N, Brown JR, Adel T, et al: Characterization of reproductive hormonal dynamics in the perimenopause. J Clin Endocrinol Metab 1996;81:1495–1501. **(IIa, B)**
8. Astrup K, Olivarius NF, Møller S, et al: Menstrual bleeding patterns in pre- and perimenopausal women: a population-based prospective diary study. Acta Obstet Gynecol Scand 2004;83:197–202. **(IIa, B)**
9. Taylor SM, Kinney AM, Kline JK: Menopausal transition: predicting time to menopause for women 44 years or older from simple questions on menstrual variability. Menopause 2004;11:40–48. **(IIa, B)**
10. Kaunitz AM: Gynecologic problems of the perimenopause: evaluation and treatment. Obstet Gynecol Clin North Am 2002;29:455–473. **(III, B)**
11. Menopause and the perimenopausal transition. In Speroff L, Glass RH, Kase NG (eds): Clinical Gynecologic Endocrinology and Infertility, 6th ed. Philadelphia, Lippincott Williams & Wilkins, 1999, pp 643–724. **(IV, C)**
12. Farquhar CM, Lethaby A, Sowter M, et al: An evaluation of risk factors for endometrial hyperplasia in premenopausal women with abnormal menstrual bleeding. Am J Obstet Gynecol 1999;81:525–529. **(III, B)**

13. Ash SJ, Farrell SA, Flowerden G: Endometrial biopsy in DUB. J Reprod Med 1996;41:892–896. **(IIa, B)**

14. Goldstein SR, Zeltser I, Horan CK, et al: Ultrasonography-based triage for perimenopausal patients with abnormal uterine bleeding. Am J Obstet Gynecol 1997;177:102–108. **(IIa, B)**

15. Bernard JP, Rizk E, Camatte S, et al: Saline contrast sonohysterography in the preoperative assessment of benign intrauterine disorders. Ultrasound Obstet Gynecol 2001;17:145–149. **(IIa, B)**

16. Clevenger-Hoeft M, Syrop CH, Stovall DW, et al: Sonohysterography in premenopausal women with and without abnormal bleeding. Obstet Gynecol 1999;94:516–520. **(IIa, B)**

17. Bronz L, Suter T, Rusca T: The value of transvaginal sonography with and without saline instillation in the diagnosis of uterine pathology in pre- and postmenopausal women with abnormal bleeding or suspect sonographic findings. Ultrasound Obstet Gynecol 1997;9:53–58. **(IIa, B)**

18. deVries LD, Dijkhuizen FP, Mol BWJ, et al: Comparison of transvaginal sonography, saline infusion sonography, and hysteroscopy in premenopausal women with abnormal uterine bleeding. J Clin Ultrasound 2000;28:217–223. **(IIa, B)**

19. Farquhar C, Ekeroma A, Furness S, et al: A systematic review of transvaginal ultrasonography, sonohysterography and hysteroscopy for the investigation of abnormal uterine bleeding in premenopausal women. Acta Obstet Gynecol Scand 2003;82:493–504. **(IIa, B)**

20. Widrich T, Bradley LD, Mitchinson AR, et al. Comparison of saline infusion sonography with office hysteroscopy for the evaluation of the endometrium. Am J Obstet Gynecol 1996;174:1327–1334. **(IIa, B)**

21. Valle RF: Office hysteroscopy. Clin Obstet Gynecol 1999;42:276–289. **(III, C)**

22. Kaunitz AM: Oral contraceptive use in perimenopause. Am J Obstet Gynecol 2001;185:S32–S37. **(III, C)**

23. American College of Obstetricians and Gynecologists: Management of Anovulatory Bleeding. ACOG Practice Bulletin No. 14. Washington, DC, ACOG, 2000; pp 434–441. **(III, C)**

24. Davis A, Godwin A, Lippman J, et al: Triphasic norgestimate-ethinyl estradiol for treating dysfunctional uterine bleeding. Obstet Gynecol 2000;96:913–920. **(III, B)**

25. Kaunitz AM: Efficacy, cycle control, and safety of two triphasic oral contraceptives: Cyclessa (desogestrel-ethinyl estradiol) and Ortho-Novum 7/7/7 (norethindrone/ethinyl estradiol): a randomized trial. Contraception 2000;61:295–302. **(III, B)**

26. Kaunitz AM: Injectable contraception: new and existing options. Obstet Gynecol Clin North Am 2000;27:741–780. **(IV, C)**

27. Lethaby AE, Cooke I, Rees M: Progesterone/progestogen releasing intrauterine systems versus either placebo or any other medication for heavy menstrual bleeding (Cochrane Review). Available at www.cochrane.org/cochrane/revabstr/mainindex.htm. Accessed 5/30/05. **(IV, C)**

28. Hurskainen R, Teperi J, Rissanen P, et al: Quality of life and cost-effectiveness of levonorgestrel-releasing intrauterine system versus hysterectomy for treatment of menorrhagia: a randomized trial. Lancet 2001;357:273–277. **(IV, C)**

29. Hubacher D, Grimes DA: Noncontraceptive health benefits of intrauterine devices: a systematic review. Obstet Gynecol Surv 2002;57:120–128. **(IV, C)**

30. Lissak A, Fruchter O, Mashiach S, et al: Immediate versus delayed treatment of perimenopausal bleeding due to benign causes by balloon thermal ablation. J Am Assoc Gynecol Laparosc 1999;6:145–150. **(III, B)**

31. Henshaw SK: Unintended pregnancy in the United States. Fam Plann Perspect 1998;30:24–29,46. **(IV, C)**

32. Archer D: Use of contraceptives for older women. In Lobo RA (ed): Treatment of the Postmenopausal Woman: Basic and Clinical Aspects, 2nd ed. Philadelphia, Lippincott Williams & Wilkins, 1999, pp 83–92. **(IV, C)**

33. Kemmeren JM, Algra A, Grobbee DE: Third generation oral contraceptives and risk of venous thrombosis: meta-analysis. BMJ 2001; 323:131–134. **(IV, C)**

34. Jick H, Kaye JA, Vasilakis-Scaramozza C, et al: Risk of venous thromboembolism among users of third generation oral contraceptives compared with users of oral contraceptives with levonorgestrel before and after 1995: cohort and case-control analysis. BMJ 2000;321:1190–1195. **(IIa, B)**

35. Michaelsson K, Baron JA, Farahmand BY, et al: Oral-contraceptive use and risk of hip fracture: a case-control study. Lancet 1999; 353:1481–1484. **(IIa, B)**

36. Sulak P, Lippman J, Siu C, et al: Clinical comparison of triphasic norgestimate/35 µg ethinyl estradiol and monophasic norethindrone acetate/20 µg ethinyl estradiol: cycle control, lipid effects, and user satisfaction. Contraception 1999;59:161–166. **(IIa, B)**

37. Nachtigall LE: The symptoms of perimenopause. Clin Obstet Gynecol 1998;41:921–927. **(IV, C)**

38. Casper RF, Dodin S, Reid RI, and Study Investigators: The effect of 20 µg ethinyl estradiol/1 mg norethindrone acetate (Minestrin), a low-dose oral contraceptive, on vaginal bleeding patterns, hot flashes, and quality of life in symptomatic perimenopausal women. Menopause 1997;4:139–147. **(IIa, B)**

39. Narod SA, Risch H, Moslehi R, et al: Oral contraceptives and the risk of hereditary ovarian cancer. Hereditary Ovarian Cancer Clinical Study Group. N Engl J Med 1998;339:424–428. **(Ib, B)**

40. Ness RB, Keder LM, Soper DE, et al: Oral contraception and the recognition of endometritis. Am J Obstet Gynecol 1997;176:580–585. **(III, B)**

41. Shulman LP, Harari D: Low-dose transdermal estradiol for symptomatic perimenopause. Menopause 2004;11:34–39. **(IV, C)**

42. Kaunitz AM: Sexual pain and genital atrophy: breaking down barriers to recognition and treatment. Menopause Management 2001;10:22–32. **(IV, C)**

43. Cardozo L, Bachmann G, McClish D, et al: Meta-analysis of estrogen therapy in the management of urogenital atrophy in postmenopausal women: second report of the Hormones and Urogenital Therapy Committee. Obstet Gynecol 1998;92:722–727. **(IV, C)**

44. Freedman M: Sexuality in post-menopausal women. Menopausal Med 2000;8:1–5. **(IV, C)**

45. Rioux JE, Devlin MC, Gelfand MM, et al: 17-Beta-estradiol vaginal tablet versus conjugated equine estrogen vaginal cream to relieve menopausal atrophic vaginitis. Menopause 2000;7:156–161. **(IIa, B)**

46. Notelovitz M: Urogenital atrophy and low-dose vaginal estrogen therapy (editorial). Menopause 2000;7:140–142. **(IV, C)**

47. Grady D, Brown JS, Vittinghoff E, et al, for the HERS Research Group: Postmenopausal hormones and incontinence: the Heart and Estrogen/Progestin Replacement Study. Obstet Gynecol 2001; 97:116–120. **(Ib, A)**

48. Estrogen and progestogen use in peri- and postmenopausal women: September 2003 position statement of the North American Menopause Society. Menopause 2003;10:497–506. **(IV, C)**

49. Menken J, Trussell J, Larsen U: Age and infertility. Science 1986; 233:1389–1394. **(IIb, B)**

50. Klein J, Sauer MV: Assessing fertility in women of advanced reproductive age. Am J Obstet Gynecol 2001;185:758–770. **(IV, C)**

51. Johnson J, Canning J, Kaneko T, et al: Germline stem cells and follicular renewal in the postnatal mammalian ovary. Nature 2004;428:145–150. **(IIb, B)**

52. Ventura SJ, Abma JC, Mosher WD: Revised pregnancy rates, 1990–97, and new rates for 1998–99: United States. Natl Vital Stat Rep 2003; 52:1–16. **(IIb, B)**

53. Tarlatzis BC, Zepiridis L: Perimenopausal conception. Ann N Y Acad Sci 2003;997:93–104. **(IV, C)**

54. American College of Obstetricians and Gynecologists: Health maintenance for perimenopausal women. ACOG Technical Bulletin No. 210, Aug 1995, pp 169–177. Int J Gynaecol Obstet 1995;51:171–181. **(IV, C)**

55. Herringon DS, Reboussin D, Brosninan K, et al: Effects of estrogen replacement in progression of coronary artery disease. N Engl J Med 2000;343:522–529. **(IV, C)**

# Chapter 62

# Polycystic Ovary Syndrome

## Ertug Kovanci, MD, and John E. Buster, MD

---

## KEY POINTS

- Polycystic ovary syndrome (PCOS) is the most common endocrine disorder in reproductive-aged women.
- PCOS is a lifelong disease beginning in fetal life and extending into the postmenopausal period.
- Hyperinsulinemia is the pivotal factor in the pathogenesis.
- PCOS is an inherited disorder that follows an autosomal dominant inheritance pattern although the gene or genes involved are unknown.
- Hyperandrogenemia with or without hyperandrogenism along with oligomenorrhea are the hallmark features of PCOS.
- Anovulation resulting in infertility is a common presentation.
- Obesity worsens metabolic abnormalities such as hyperinsulinemia and hyperandrogenemia.
- Diabetes, lipid disorders, heart disease, and endometrial cancer are metabolic sequelae of PCOS.
- Insulin-sensitizing agents have dramatically changed the management of PCOS. Metformin, an insulin-sensitizing agent, is now the first choice for the treatment of anovulation in PCOS. Weight loss and exercise are the best long-term therapy to decrease the metabolic sequelae of PCOS.

---

PCOS is a lifelong, multisystem genetic disorder. Although manifestations of PCOS may be present at birth, they are traditionally first noticed in puberty as menstrual irregularities and weight gain. PCOS evolves throughout life into a series of disorders characterized by insulin resistance, premature adrenarche, infertility, hyperandrogenemia, dyslipidemia, and can be related to heart disease, diabetes mellitus, endometrial hyperplasia, and cancer. However, PCOS is best known and most extensively studied as a cause of anovulatory infertility in reproductive-aged women. Patients with PCOS represent a heterogeneous population with different subtypes of the disease. These women have various symptoms depending on their age and the manifestations of the disease. Therefore, numerous diagnostic criteria are used in the literature to detect women with PCOS. Although various short-term symptomatic therapies are available, the best long-term management strategies have not been established. Taken together, all these factors make PCOS a challenging disorder to diagnose, treat, and study.

## EPIDEMIOLOGY, RISK FACTORS, AND PATHOGENESIS

PCOS is most extensively studied as an endocrine disorder of reproductive-aged women. Most studies reporting the prevalence of PCOS are not reliable because of the various diagnostic criteria used for patient selection in each study. However, three well-designed studies have found similar results in different reproductive-aged patient populations.[1-3] The first examined unselected white and African American women who were being evaluated for employment at a large institution and found that 4.7% of whites and 3.4% of blacks had PCOS as defined by 1990 National Institutes of Health (NIH) consensus criteria.[1] Two other studies using similar methods reported a prevalence of 6.8% and 6.5%, respectively, in unselected populations from the Greek island of Lesbos and from Spain.[2,3] In the United States, it is estimated that PCOS afflicts approximately 3 million reproductive-aged women.[4] PCOS is therefore the most common endocrine disorder in the reproductive-aged woman.

Although the principal molecular defect that causes PCOS is still unknown, insulin resistance seems pivotal. Dysfunctional gonadotropin metabolism and excessive androgen production are now believed to be downstream consequences of insulin resistance.

### Insulin Resistance

An association between insulin resistance and hirsutism has been known for decades. The first report describing diabetes in bearded women appeared in 1921 by Achard and Thiers.[5] Burghen et al described the association of hyperinsulinemia with PCOS in 1980.[6] These investigators demonstrated that obese PCOS patients had elevated glucose and insulin levels on a 3-hour glucose tolerance test (GTT) compared with the obese non-PCOS controls. Almost a decade later another study reported that not only obese but also nonobese or lean PCOS patients had greater insulin resistance than weight-matched controls.[7] Now it is generally accepted that 50% to 80% of women with PCOS have at least some insulin resistance. A correlation between serum insulin and androgen levels has been reconfirmed in many studies.

There is compelling evidence that hyperinsulinemia precedes the hyperandrogenism. Suppression of androgens does not restore normal insulin sensitivity.[8,9] Conversely, androgen administration does not produce insulin resistance of the same magnitude as seen in PCOS.[10] Several mechanisms are implicated in insulin-augmented androgen production in the ovary and adrenal gland. Insulin induces pituitary luteinizing hormone (LH) secretion and LH-stimulated androgen synthesis in the ovarian theca cells.[11] Insulin also affects ovarian androgen production directly.[12] Suppression of insulin levels reduces circulating androgens.[13] Adrenal steroidogenesis is also augmented by insulin through increased sensitivity to adrenocorticotropic hormone (ACTH).[14] These findings support the pivotal role of insulin resistance in PCOS (Fig. 62-1).

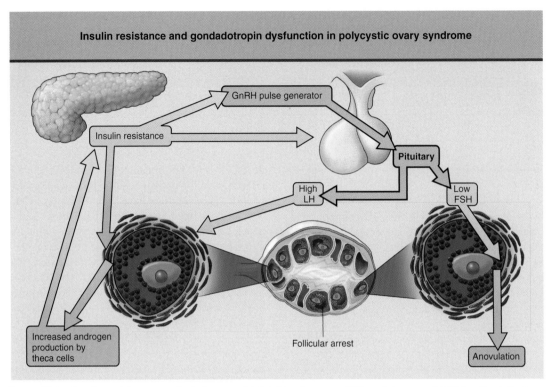

**Figure 62-1** **Insulin resistance results in increased luteinizing hormone (LH) and decreased follicle-stimulating hormone (FSH) secretion.** Gonadotropin dysfunction leads to follicular arrest and increased androgen production.

The underlying mechanism of insulin resistance is unknown. Insulin receptor number or binding affinity has been shown to be normal in PCOS. No mutations have been identified in the insulin receptor gene. One explanation for the insulin resistance in PCOS is decreased insulin receptor (INSR) tyrosine autophosphorylation along with increased serine phosphorylation.[15] INSR has been shown to be inactivated when serine residues are phosphorylated rather than tyrosine residues (Fig. 62-2). This finding suggests a postbinding defect in insulin receptor signaling. Suppressed insulin receptor substrate-1-associated kinase activity has also been reported in some PCOS patients with decreased skeletal muscle glucose uptake compared with matched controls.[16] All these findings are consistent with an obesity-independent insulin receptor–signaling defect. However, obesity increasingly fuels insulin resistance and in turn hyperandrogenemia. Weight loss alone can improve insulin sensitivity and may result in resumption of regular cycles. However, not all PCOS patients have insulin resistance. Furthermore, many women with type 2 diabetes do not have PCOS. Therefore, hyperinsulinemia alone also is an insufficient explanation for the development of PCOS.

## Dysfunctional Gonadotropin Metabolism

Both lean and obese women with PCOS have overall increased LH secretion. Elevated 24-hour levels of LH, increased LH pulse frequency, and greater pulse amplitude are normally characteristic of these women.[17] However, single-sample basal concentrations of LH are highly variable. The elevated LH of PCOS is probably not causative but rather a result of another underlying pathology. Thus, in one transgenic mouse system, pituitary LH secretion was extremely sensitive to exogenous

gonadotropin-releasing hormone (GnRH) stimulation when the *INSR* gene was knocked out in the central nervous system.[18] The same animals were also obese and had elevated triglyceride and insulin levels. These findings strongly suggest that elevated LH levels in PCOS may be secondary to insulin resistance.

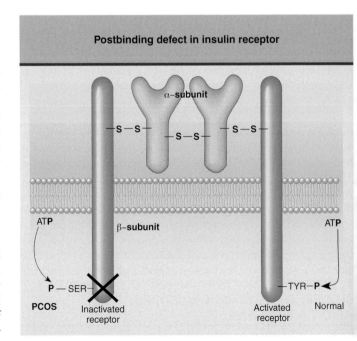

**Figure 62-2** **Increased insulin receptor serine phosphorylation results in a postbinding defect leading to insulin resistance.**

## Obesity and polycystic ovary syndrome

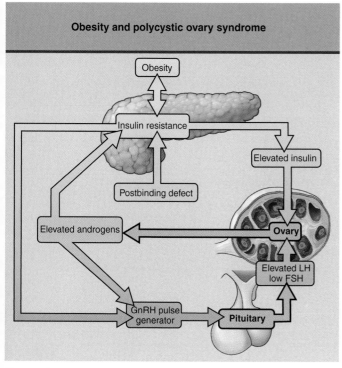

**Figure 62-3** Insulin resistance aggravated by obesity impairs the hypothalamic-pituitary-ovarian axis, resulting in anovulation.

Both lean and obese women with PCOS have overtly decreased follicle-stimulating hormone (FSH) secretion. One could thus argue that insufficient levels of FSH might cause an arrest in follicle maturation and result in decreased aromatase activity in granulosa cells. Thus, low $E_2$ and elevated androgen production might be expected. However, follicles in polycystic ovaries are responsive to exogenous FSH, and clomiphene induces FSH secretion sufficiently to enable mature follicle development.[4] Therefore, the suppressed FSH is most likely a secondary phenomenon in PCOS (Fig. 62-3).

### Excessive Androgen Production

Increased androgen production and its manifestations are hallmark features of PCOS.

In normal women, adrenal glands and ovaries both contribute to circulating androgens. Dehydroepiandrosterone (DHEA) and androstenedione are the major androgen products of the ovary. Adrenals and ovaries equally contribute to androstenedione production, whereas one half of circulating DHEA is secreted by adrenals and about 20% comes from the ovary. The remaining 30% is produced in peripheral tissues from dehydroepiandrosterone sulfate (DHEAS) intracellularly.[19] DHEAS is almost exclusively produced by the adrenal gland and is converted in peripheral tissues to biologically active androgens. Thus, one half of testosterone arises from peripheral conversion of androstenedione and the other half is secreted equally by the ovary and the adrenal (Fig. 62-4). Testosterone is converted by the intracellular 5α-reductase in androgen responsive tissues to form intracellular dihydrotestosterone (DHT), the most potent androgen. Androstenedione and DHEAS are weak androgens with no receptors and are frequently considered "prehormones."

Androstenedione and testosterone are biosynthesized in the theca cells and converted to estrone and estradiol in the granulosa cells by aromatase (Fig. 62-5).

The majority (69% to 79%) of testosterone molecules in serum are bound to sex hormone–binding globulin (SHBG) which is a β-globulin. Approximately 20% to 30% of testosterone is albumin-bound, and 1% is found free in serum. This small unbound, or free, portion constitutes the biologically active hormone. Free testosterone levels are determined by the amount of androgen production and the circulating levels of SHBG. Hyperthyroidism, pregnancy, and estrogens increase SHBG levels, whereas corticoids, androgens, progestins, growth hormone, insulin, and insulin-like growth factor-1 (IGF-1) decrease SHBG. Thus, insulin increases the bioavailability of testosterone. Androgen production including testosterone, DHEA, and DHEAS declines significantly with age. Free testosterone levels also decrease in older women as the percentage of free testosterone does not change with age. Six cytochrome P-450 (CYP) enzymes are involved in steroidogenesis including members of the CYP11, CYP17, CYP19, and CYP21 enzyme families. CYP11A, or cholesterol side-chain cleavage enzyme, participates in the conversion of cholesterol to pregnenolone. CYP17A (P450c17) possesses 17-hydroxylase and 17,20-lyase activities, which catalyze 17α-hydroxylation of pregnenolone and progesterone and oxidation of their side chains (Fig. 62-6). CYP21A or 21-hydroxylase participates in the biosynthesis of glucocorticoids and mineralocorticoids from progesterone and 17-hydroxyprogesterone. Another important steroidogenic enzyme is 3β-hydroxysteroid dehydrogenase, which belongs to the short-chain dehydrogenase/reductase enzyme family. This enzyme catalyzes the conversion of pregnenolone and DHEA to progesterone and androstenedione, respectively.

In women with PCOS, production rates of androgens are approximately four-fold increased over normal controls.[20] Thus, clinical hyperandrogenism is a major component of PCOS. Approximately 80% of PCOS diagnosed by NIH consensus criteria demonstrates elevated androgen levels. Hyperandrogenemia is directly accountable for the traditional signs and symptoms of PCOS: hirsutism, acne, and anovulation. Major sources of androgen excess in PCOS are the ovary, primarily theca cells, and the zona reticularis of the adrenal cortex. It is well documented in vitro that isolated theca cells from women with PCOS produce significantly higher levels of DHEA, androstenedione, and 17-hydroxyprogesterone at baseline and in response to LH or forskolin compared with control theca cells.[21] Theca cells from PCOS patients also exhibit increased activity of steroidogenic enzymes such as CYP11A, CYP17, and 3β-hydroxysteroid dehydrogenase after forskolin stimulation.[21] Therefore, increased steroidogenic enzyme activity is in part responsible for ovarian hyperandrogenism. Persistence of increased enzyme activity in long-term cultured theca cells suggests an intrinsic defect in theca cells that may contribute to the pathogenesis of PCOS.

Adrenal androgen production is also increased in many women with PCOS. One proposed mechanism is an increase in cortisol clearance that leads to compensatory stimulation of ACTH. This, in turn, induces excessive androgen production by the reticularis zone of the adrenal gland. Cortisol is inactivated in an irreversible fashion by 5α-reductase and 5β-reductase.

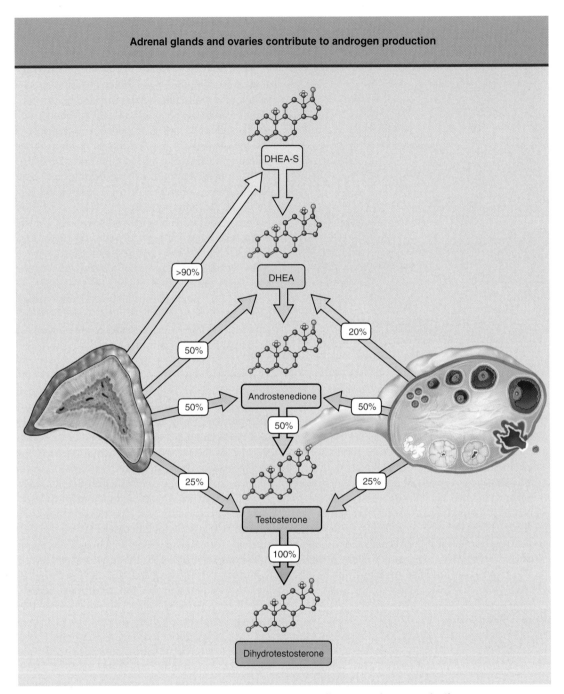

**Adrenal glands and ovaries contribute to androgen production**

DHEA-S

DHEA

>90%

50%

20%

Androstenedione

50%

50%

50%

25%

25%

Testosterone

100%

Dihydrotestosterone

**Figure 62-4    The adrenal gland and ovary contribute to androgen production.**

Women with PCOS have higher levels of urinary 5α-cortisol metabolites compared with controls.[22] It is known that androgens augment the enzymatic activity of 5α-reductase, thereby inducing the inactivation of cortisol. Additionally, the activity of 11β-hydroxysteroid dehydrogenase-1, the enzyme that converts inactive cortisone into active cortisol, has been shown to be reduced in women with PCOS.[23] This may also contribute to the increased ACTH stimulation and augmented androgen production by the zona reticularis.

Insulin resistance has been reported following exogenous testosterone administration and in other hyperandrogenemic disorders such as nonclassical congenital adrenal hyperplasia (CAH).[24] However, insulin resistance probably is not caused by hyperandrogenemia in PCOS, since suppressing androgens does not completely restore normal insulin sensitivity.[8,9] Furthermore, insulin resistance produced by androgen administration does not have the same magnitude as that seen in PCOS.[10]

### Anovulation in Polycystic Ovary Syndrome

Dysfunctional gonadotropin metabolism, characterized by increased LH and suppressed FSH, leads to follicular arrest and anovulation. Hyperandrogenemia and steady mid-follicular levels of estradiol also contribute to anovulation through potentiation of dysfunctional gonadotropin secretion. Hyperinsulinemia also

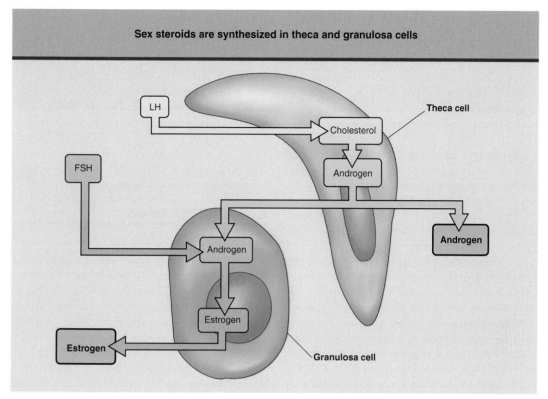

**Figure 62-5** **Androgens produced by theca cells under the control of luteinizing hormone (LH) are aromatized to estrogens in granulosa cells and by peripheral conversion.** Follicle-stimulating hormone (FSH) stimulates follicular maturation and granulosa cell growth.

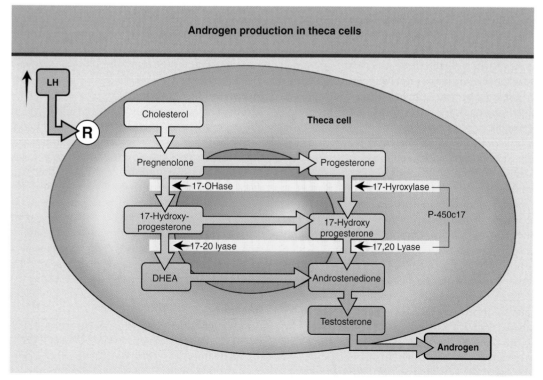

**Figure 62-6** **Androgens are produced in theca cells from cholesterol following steroidogenic pathways.**

# Reproductive Endocrinology and Infertility

triggers increased LH pulse amplitude and pulse frequency in response to GnRH stimulation. It also sensitizes granulosa cells to LH. Granulosa cells from women with PCOS are more responsive to LH than granulosa cells from size-matched follicles obtained from normal women.[25] This hyperresponsiveness to LH has been suggested as a possible major mechanism for anovulation. Hyperandrogenemia may further aggravate the effects of hyperinsulinemia and elevated LH secretion.

## Polycystic Ovary Syndrome as an Inherited Disorder

PCOS is an inherited disorder. Pedigree studies have consistently suggested an autosomal dominant inheritance pattern with elevated androgen levels in about 50% of sisters of women with PCOS. Only a few studies suggested X-linked or polygenic inheritance. One well-designed, controlled study showed that approximately 22% of sisters of women with PCOS also had PCOS as defined by hyperandrogenemia and oligomenorrhea, and another 24% of these sisters had hyperandrogenemia alone.[26] The segregation ratio for overall hyperandrogenemia was 0.46, which is consistent with an autosomal dominant inheritance. The risk of hyperandrogenemia in sisters of PCOS women was approximately three-fold increased compared with controls in this study. However, androgen levels are also highly heritable independent of PCOS.[27] Moreover, a large twin study of PCOS failed to support a strong genetic component.[28] The male phenotype expected from these genetic studies has been also elusive. A recent study showed that male-pattern balding score did not differ between controls and male relatives of PCOS patients.[29] However, a higher incidence of insulin resistance and impaired glucose tolerance has been found among male and female relatives of women with PCOS.[30] Thus, pancreatic β-cell dysfunction may be a heritable phenotype.

Familial aggregations of PCOS led investigators long ago to search for candidate genes. Logically, the genes involved in steroid hormone biosynthesis, carbohydrate metabolism, and gonadotropin action and regulation were investigated. Therefore, early studies focused on CYP11A, CYP17, and CYP21, which are important enzymes in steroidogenesis. Although initial studies suggested an association between these genes and PCOS, later studies did not confirm the initial findings. Follistatin, a glycoprotein, suppresses pituitary FSH production. This glycoprotein's locus, thought to be associated with PCOS in an early study,[31] was not linked to PCOS as shown by later studies.[32] Neither overexpression nor granulosa cell–specific inactivation of follistatin in mice resulted in features similar to those of PCOS.[33,34] A variable number tandem repeat (VNTR) locus, upstream of the insulin gene, regulates insulin expression. Thus, Waterworth et al suggested an association between alleles of this locus and PCOS.[35] Further studies, however, failed to confirm this linkage.[31] Insulin receptor gene mutations cause insulin resistance similarly to PCOS. However, several studies did not find changes in the sequence of the insulin receptor gene in PCOS patients. Tucci et al reported a significant association between PCOS and an insulin receptor gene marker D19S884.[36] This marker is about 1 Mbp telomeric to the *INSR* gene. The authors concluded that the susceptibility gene may be the *INSR* itself or a closely related gene. Unfortunately, a later study failed to confirm an association between marker D19S884 and PCOS in women from Spain and Italy.[37] Microarray technology can detect differential expressions of up to 45,000 genes. With this new technique, Wood et al compared gene expression profiles of normal and PCOS theca cells using oligonucleotide microarray chips.[38] These investigators identified approximately 400 genes that were either up- or down-regulated in PCOS theca cells. Genes that are involved in retinoic acid synthesis, such as retinol dehydrogenase and aldehyde dehydrogenase, and genes that encode transcription factors, such as GATA6, were selected by the authors as candidate genes that might have an impact on theca cell steroidogenesis. These genes need to be investigated by further studies. This study will help researchers focus on a number of new genes that may be involved in PCOS.

## CLINICAL FEATURES

PCOS is a lifelong disease which traditionally manifests in puberty with premature adrenarche, obesity, and menstrual irregularity. Sequelae later in life include infertility, diabetes mellitus, cardiovascular disease, and gynecologic cancers (Fig. 62-7).

In reproductive-aged women, the main features of PCOS are oligomenorrhea, hirsutism, acne, obesity, and infertility. None of these features is pervasive and universal except oligomenorrhea, which is a diagnostic criterion by 1990 NIH consensus. Reproductive-aged women with PCOS usually come in for one of the following three reasons: (1) symptoms of androgen excess, (2) menstrual irregularity, and/or (3) infertility.

### Androgen Excess

Hirsutism is subjective, and not every woman with elevated androgen levels is hirsute. Hair growth depends on the number of hair follicles and 5α-reductase activity. For instance, hirsutism is milder in Asian women. It is considered normal in some Mediterranean women. The number of hair follicles, thickness, and pigmentation of individual hairs in the hormone-dependent areas such as upper lip, chin, chest, back, upper abdomen, thighs, and arms are increased in hirsutism. Acne and seborrhea are the other common signs of androgen excess in PCOS. Male pattern baldness and clitoromegaly are infrequently encountered.

### Menstrual Irregularity

Erratic ovulation with breakthrough bleeding results in oligomenorrhea in many women with PCOS. The onset of oligomenorrhea is usually peripubertal and continues through the first two decades of reproductive life. However, menstrual regularity improves after age 30, and the majority of women with PCOS have regular cycles by age 40.[39] Regular menstrual cycles commonly return between ages 35 and 43. This phenomenon may be related to the decline of the follicle cohort and decreased ovarian androgen production with age. These women do not necessarily have gynecologic or reproductive problems after age 35, and diabetes and heart disease are diagnosed later in life (Fig. 62-8).

### Infertility

Anovulation is the underlying mechanism for infertility in women with PCOS in reproductive years. Thus, PCOS accounts for 75% of anovulatory infertility.[40] Although the precise mechanism of anovulation in PCOS has not been determined, inadequate FSH stimulation and tonic levels of LH are believed to impair follicle

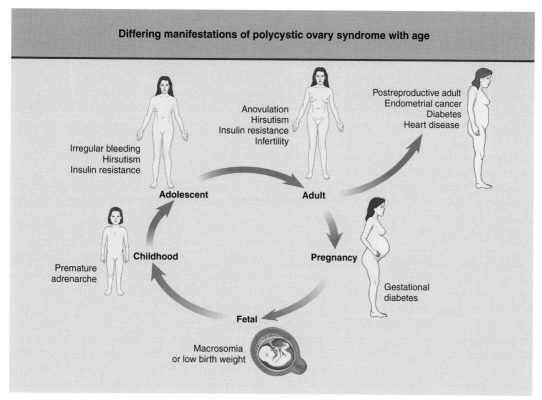

**Differing manifestations of polycystic ovary syndrome with age**

Anovulation
Hirsutism
Insulin resistance
Infertility

Postreproductive adult
Endometrial cancer
Diabetes
Heart disease

Irregular bleeding
Hirsutism
Insulin resistance

**Adolescent**

**Adult**

**Childhood**

**Pregnancy**

Premature
adrenarche

Gestational
diabetes

**Fetal**

Macrosomia
or low birth weight

**Figure 62-7** Polycystic ovary syndrome (PCOS) is a lifelong disease with differing manifestations evolving over the different stages of a woman's life.

maturation and ovulation. Although women with PCOS may ovulate incidentally and become pregnant spontaneously, they frequently require ovulation induction. Ovulation induction, however, is challenging in these women because many do not respond predictably to ovulation induction agents. Unfortunately, when they do respond, ovarian hyperstimulation and multiple gestation often occur.

## Other Clinical Features

Other clinical features of PCOS include obesity, acanthosis nigricans, and morphologic appearance of polycystic ovaries on

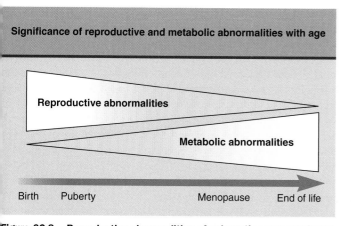

**Significance of reproductive and metabolic abnormalities with age**

Reproductive abnormalities

Metabolic abnormalities

Birth    Puberty          Menopause    End of life

**Figure 62-8** Reproductive abnormalities of polycystic ovary syndrome decrease with advancing age, whereas metabolic abnormalities such as diabetes and heart disease become more significant.

ultrasound. Although many women with PCOS are obese, they may be lean with wide variability among patient populations. Approximately 30% to 60% of women with PCOS have a body mass index (BMI) greater than 30. These obese women frequently have central or android body fat distribution. The prevalence of abdominal body fat distribution is also higher in lean PCOS patients, which contributes to their increased risk for metabolic abnormalities. Obesity fuels androgen production and hyperinsulinemia and decreases SHBG production, resulting in elevated free testosterone.

Acanthosis nigricans is an abnormal thickening of the epidermis associated with hyperpigmentation and hyperkeratosis. It is usually encountered in severe insulin resistance and type 2 diabetes along with HAIR-AN syndrome. Hyperandrogenism (HA), insulin resistance (IR) and acanthosis nigricans (AN) is considered a subtype of PCOS and commonly caused by mutations in the *INSR* gene.[41]

One of the most controversial features of PCOS is the ultrasound morphology of polycystic ovaries. The typical polycystic ovary is defined ultrasonographically by more than 12 subcapsular follicles measuring 2 to 9 mm and hyperechogenic stroma representing stromal hyperplasia. About 20% of women with normal menstrual cycles and no hirsutism have this morphology on ultrasound, whereas only 70% of women with hirsutism and oligomenorrhea have such ultrasound findings. Therefore ultrasound findings alone are not diagnostic, although it is commonly used as a diagnostic criterion in Europe. PCOS most likely represents a heterogeneous disorder with different subtypes. Therefore, patients have differing degrees of metabolic and gonadotropic abnormalities.

# Reproductive Endocrinology and Infertility

## Polycystic Ovary Syndrome in Adolescence

There is increasing evidence that PCOS manifests before birth and continues throughout life. Some studies report a significant relationship between low birth weight and development of PCOS later in life,[42] whereas others show an association between high birth weight and PCOS.[42] These findings suggest a U-shaped relationship between birth weight and PCOS caused by different subtypes of the disease. Peripubertal girls with pubarche before age 8, obesity, and irregular cycles are at risk for PCOS and so should be followed closely. Clinical features of PCOS in adolescent girls are similar to those of adult women. These adolescent girls have obesity, irregular cycles secondary to anovulation, and hirsutism and acne as a result of hyperandrogenemia. Another clinical feature that has recently been linked to adolescent PCOS is premature pubarche or adrenarche, which is defined as pubic hair development before the age of 8 years. Girls with premature pubarche have been shown to develop insulin resistance and hyperandrogenemia during puberty.[43] Therefore, premature pubarche has been proposed as an early marker of PCOS. Insulin resistance and obesity seem to precede hyperandrogenemia, which is usually seen after menarche. Acanthosis nigricans is also a common finding in pubertal girls with obesity and insulin resistance. Pubertal physiologic anovulation has been challenged. Some investigators suggest that oligomenorrhea in adolescence may be an early sign of PCOS rather than a physiologic maturation process. Treatment of these girls with insulin-sensitizing agents is controversial at this time, although initial studies showed improved metabolic parameters in treated girls.

## Diabetes Mellitus

Insulin resistance combined with the worsening effect of accompanying obesity makes PCOS a major risk factor for type 2 diabetes in adolescents and premenopausal women. Several studies reported increased prevalence of type 2 diabetes in women with PCOS. About 15% of PCOS patients develop diabetes, based on current evidence.[44] The Nurses' Health Study II investigated the relative risk of diabetes among women with a cycle length greater than 40 days, between ages 18 and 22 years, who were followed prospectively for over 8 years.[45] The total number of women who participated in this study was 101,703 of whom 7.6% had a cycle length greater than 40 days or too irregular to estimate. The relative risk (RR) of diabetes was 2.08 (95% confidence interval [CI] 1.62–2.66) among oligomenorrheic women, and this risk was further increased by high BMI (RR 3.86, 95% CI 2.33–6.38). In this study, hirsutism and/or severe acne during teenage years and family history of diabetes were also important predictors for the development of type 2 diabetes. Similarly, the incidence of PCOS among women with type 2 diabetes has been shown to be higher than in the general population, although these studies are small and used ultrasound appearance as a diagnostic marker.

## Cardiovascular Disease

The association between lipid abnormalities and PCOS has been known since the mid-1980s. Several studies have shown that women with PCOS have higher levels of low-density lipoprotein (LDL) and triglycerides, and lower levels of high-density lipoprotein (HDL) compared with weight-matched controls.

LDL and HDL are good predictors of coronary heart disease. Small LDL particles are strongly associated with coronary heart disease, and PCOS patients have significantly smaller LDL particle size than regularly cycling women.[46] LDL particle size is associated with SHBG levels, which are inversely correlated with insulin levels. In the light of these findings, women with PCOS seem to be more likely to have coronary artery abnormalities. Several studies support this conclusion. For instance, women with PCOS are more likely to have coronary artery calcification than age- and weight-matched controls.[47] Women with extensive coronary artery disease on coronary angiography are also more likely to have PCOS on ultrasound.[48] These women are at greater risk for developing hypertension than are age-matched controls.[49] Syndrome X, or metabolic syndrome, which is associated with atherosclerosis and CHD, is characterized by hypertension, hypertriglyceridemia, low HDL, insulin resistance, and obesity. Approximately 45% of women with PCOS demonstrate features of the metabolic syndrome at a relatively young age.[50] Surprisingly, it is not clear whether cardiovascular events are more common in women with PCOS. One study found no increase in the death rate due to the circulatory disease among women with PCOS.[51] This study, however, lacked controls and the diagnosis was made based on ovarian wedge resection. A prospective cohort study with large numbers is necessary to answer whether cardiovascular events are associated with PCOS.

## Gynecologic Cancers

Several studies suggest an association between PCOS and gynecologic cancers. The first report suggesting an association between endometrial cancer and PCOS was published in 1949, 14 years after the classical description by Stein and Leventhal in 1935. However, no controlled studies have appeared since the first report. Most studies that examined the relationship between PCOS and a variety of cancers lack control groups and suffer from poor study design and inconsistent diagnostic criteria.

Although the risk of endometrial cancer is increased with exposure to unopposed estrogens, the association between PCOS and endometrial cancer is not clear. Six studies show an increased risk of endometrial cancer. However, all these studies were retrospective and most lacked control groups. Probably the most frequently cited study by Coulam et al found an RR of 3.1 (95% CI 1.1–7.3) for the development of endometrial carcinoma in women with a diagnosis of chronic anovulation.[52] Escobedo et al reported an increased risk of endometrial cancer in women with ovarian factor infertility,[53] whereas Dahlgren et al showed a significant relationship between endometrial cancer and such variables as hirsutism, parity, BMI, diabetes mellitus, and smoking.[54] Gallup and Stock found that about 31% of endometrial cancer patients who are younger than 40 years of age had polycystic ovaries and tended to be more overweight than older patients.[55] Two recent studies evaluated women with infertility. One was a retrospective cohort study by Wild et al, which found the odds ratio for endometrial cancer in women with PCOS to be 5.3.[56] The other study was also retrospective and looked at endometrial biopsy findings in infertile women.[57] Four of 2573 endometrial biopsy specimens from women with PCOS showed endometrial cancer. However, all these studies used stigmata of PCOS rather than an actual diagnosis. Therefore, their results cannot be extrapolated to all women with PCOS. Nonetheless, they suggest that the incidence of clinical features of PCOS is higher in younger women with endometrial cancer although these patients are only a small number of all women with endometrial cancer. Moreover, PCOS may not be an independent risk factor, and specific endocrine or metabolic abnormalities occurring as a result of PCOS, such as obesity, may play a more important role in the development of endometrial cancer. Although a few studies failed to find an association between PCOS and endometrial cancer, intuitively it seems likely that these women are at risk for endometrial cancer because of the stimulatory effects of unopposed estrogen secretion in PCOS. Moreover, there is strong evidence that risk of premalignant atypical endometrial hyperplasia is increased in PCOS. Thus, women with PCOS should be counseled for a probable increased risk of endometrial cancer.

Risk for breast cancer may also be increased in PCOS. However, evidence linking the two is circumstantial. PCOS carries potential risk factors for postmenopausal breast cancer including obesity, infertility, and elevated androgen levels. However, the evidence is not strong. Two studies from the same group of investigators found an increased risk for breast cancer in women with elevated androgen and estrogen levels.[58,59] However, four large population-based studies failed to show this association.[60-62] This is in line with findings from the Women's Health Initiative (WHI), because breast cancer risk did not increase in the estrogen-only arm of this study.[63] It seems that progesterone is necessary for estrogens to increase breast cancer risk, and progesterone levels are significantly low in women with PCOS. Currently, there is not enough evidence to suggest an association between breast cancer and PCOS. A subset of women with PCOS may be at risk for breast cancer, since elevated hormone levels and obesity may act in a complex manner in breast cancer. Further studies are needed to resolve this issue.

The risk for ovarian cancer does not appear increased. Intuitively, women with PCOS would be protected against ovarian cancer owing to the elimination of uninterrupted ovulation, which is one of the risk factors for ovarian cancer. However, a retrospective case-control study suggests that PCOS patients may be at increased risk for epithelial ovarian cancer.[64] In this study, history of PCOS was determined by self-report. Endocrine testing, ultrasound scanning, or medical record review were not performed to confirm the diagnosis. The adjusted odds ratio for ovarian cancer was 2.4 (95% CI 1.0–5.9). Animal data also suggest that increased LH may be associated with ovarian tumorigenesis.[65] Overexpression of LH in transgenic mice leads to infertility, polycystic ovaries, and granulosa cell tumors. However, LH levels in these animals were 12 to 14 times greater than in controls, which is much higher than LH levels encountered in women with PCOS. Further studies are necessary, but evidence linking the two is lacking.

## DIAGNOSIS

The most commonly used diagnostic criteria are based on the 1990 NIH/National Institute of Child Health and Human Development (NICHD) consensus: (1) chronic anovulation, (2) clinical and/or biochemical signs of hyperandrogenism, and (3) exclusion of other etiologies such as congenital nonclassical

**Table 62-1**
**Diagnostic Criteria for Polycystic Ovary Syndrome***

1. Oligo- or anovulation
2. Clinical and/or biochemical signs of hyperandrogenism
3. Polycystic ovaries
4. Exclusion of other etiologies such as congenital adrenal hyperplasia, androgen-secreting tumors, and Cushing's syndrome

ASRM, American Society for Reproductive Medicine; ESHRE, European Society of Human Reproduction and Embryology.
*The presence of two of the first three criteria is sufficient for diagnosis.
Rotterdam ESHRE/ASRM–Sponsored PCOS Consensus Workshop Group: Revised 2003 consensus on diagnostic criteria and long-term health risks related to polycystic ovary syndrome. Fertil Steril 2004;81:19–25. Copyright 2004. Reprinted with permission from the American Society for Reproductive Medicine.

adrenal hyperplasia, Cushing's syndrome, androgen-secreting tumors, and hyperprolactinemia. The presence of polycystic ovaries on ultrasound is not one of the NIH consensus criteria. These criteria were revised by the Rotterdam European Society of Human Reproduction and Embryology (ESHRE)/American Society for Reproductive Medicine (ASRM)-sponsored PCOS consensus workshop group in 2004.[66] New criteria include (1) oligo-ovulation or anovulation, (2) clinical and/or biochemical signs of hyperandrogenism, (3) polycystic ovaries, and (4) exclusion of other etiologies. The presence of two of the first three criteria is sufficient for diagnosis when other etiologies are ruled out (Table 62-1). This workshop combined European and North American diagnostic approaches; however, it may not diminish the use of different diagnostic criteria in the literature, which may be partly responsible for divergent findings in various studies. Another point that should be emphasized is that neither obesity nor insulin resistance is necessary for diagnosis by either consensus.

### History

History is essential in establishing the diagnosis. A long-standing history of oligomenorrhea (cycles >35 days) indicates chronic anovulation. Hair growth and skin changes such as acne are consistent with hyperandrogenism. Onset, severity, and rapidity of these symptoms are crucial for the exclusion of other etiologies. Thus, rapidly progressing, severe androgen excess should suggest an androgen-secreting tumor. Severe hyperandrogenism in postmenopausal women or women with a recent history of regular cycles is also suggestive of a tumor. If the onset of androgen excess coincides with puberty, PCOS and nonclassical CAH are likely diagnoses. A history of galactorrhea is consistent with hyperprolactinemia in women with oligomenorrhea. Regular cycles and normal testosterone levels in a woman with hair growth are indicative of idiopathic hirsutism.

### Physical Examination

Physical examination is paramount. Classical findings of PCOS are hirsutism and central obesity. The Ferriman-Gallwey score may be useful to quantify hirsutism objectively, but it is most beneficial to determine response to treatment. (The Ferriman-Gallwey scoring system consists of five grades based on densities and areas involved for each of nine hormonal sites including upper lip, chin, chest, upper back, lower back, upper abdomen, lower abdomen, arm, and thigh.) Seborrhea, acne, and alopecia

# Reproductive Endocrinology and Infertility

may also be seen. Virilization defined as clitoromegaly, deepening of the voice, and temporal balding is rarely encountered in PCOS. Virilization suggests an androgen-secreting tumor, although a severe variant of PCOS, hyperthecosis, may cause clitoromegaly. A palpable ovarian mass in a woman with virilization implies an androgen-secreting tumor. Signs of insulin resistance such as acanthosis nigricans are consistent with PCOS. Hyperprolactinemia is strongly suspected when galactorrhea is detected during the physical examination. Centripetal obesity, moon face, hirsutism, purple striae, and plethora indicate Cushing's syndrome.

## Laboratory Testing

The goal of laboratory testing is exclusion of other etiologies. It is not essential to rule in the diagnosis of PCOS. High levels of total testosterone, above 200 ng/dL, are usually encountered in the presence of an androgen-secreting tumor. A mildly elevated total testosterone level in the serum is consistent with PCOS. Basal LH levels are highly variable and may be elevated in PCOS. Thus, LH/FSH ratio may be reversed to 2:1. However, this finding is only supportive and not required for the diagnosis. The FSH level may be helpful to rule out hypergonadotropic or hypogonadotropic hypogonadism. Serum prolactin (PRL) and thyroid-stimulating hormone (TSH) levels should be obtained on all patients with oligomenorrhea to rule out hyperprolactinemia and thyroid disorders. Androgen levels including total testosterone, DHEA and DHEAS may be elevated in women with hyperprolactinemia. Conversely, mildly increased PRL levels may be found in PCOS. Hypothyroidism reduces the levels of SHBG and thus may cause hyperandrogenism. A morning serum 17-hydroxyprogesterone level is helpful to rule out nonclassical CAH especially in woman of Ashkenazi Jewish, Hispanic, and central European descent. If the 17-hydroxyprogesterone level is elevated, an ACTH stimulation test should be performed to diagnose nonclassical CAH. However, the clinical importance of a nonclassical CAH diagnosis is debatable. Women with this disorder respond well to antiandrogen therapy and ovulatory agents that are standard therapies for PCOS. However, this is an autosomal recessive disorder, and patients should be counseled appropriately. These women also have a theoretic risk for adrenal insufficiency in case of surgery and trauma, although this has never been reported.[67] A serum cortisol level immediately following a 1-mg dexamethasone suppression test is a helpful screening method if Cushing's syndrome is suspected. When an adrenal tumor is suspected, DHEAS levels may be highly elevated, which is an indication for adrenal imaging. Although the presence of insulin resistance is not required for diagnosis, insulin resistance and glucose intolerance should be assessed in obese women with PCOS. Although indices calculated using fasting glucose and insulin such as the homeostasis model assessment (HOMA), quantitative insulin sensitivity check index (QUICKI), and the fasting glucose to insulin ratio (G/I) may be helpful in determining insulin resistance, no clinical tests are validated for accurate detection of insulin resistance. The 2-hour glucose level after a 75-g oral glucose load is preferred to determine glucose intolerance over the fasting plasma glucose level. A 2-hour glucose level between 140 and 199 mg/dL indicates impaired glucose tolerance, and a level above 199 mg/dL is diagnostic for type 2 diabetes mellitus. A fasting lipid profile also

**Table 62-2**
**Diagnostic Evaluation for Polycystic Ovary Syndrome**

| Tests Performed Routinely | Excluded Disorder |
| --- | --- |
| TSH | Hypo- or hyperthyroidism |
| PRL | Hyperprolactinemia |
| FSH | Premature ovarian failure |
| LH | Increased in PCOS—too variable to be useful |

| Tests Performed Based on Presentation and History | Excluded Disorder |
| --- | --- |
| 17-Hydroxyprogesterone | Nonclassical congenital adrenal hyperplasia |
| Total testosterone | Androgen-secreting tumors |
| DHEAS | Adrenal adenoma |
| Dexamethasone suppression test | Cushing's syndrome |

DHEAS, dehydroepiandrosterone sulfate; FSH, follicle-stimulating hormone; LH, luteinizing hormone; PRL, prolactin; TSH, thyroid-stimulating hormone.

may be obtained. Assessment of glucose intolerance and lipid levels is crucial for patient counseling and long-term management in obese women with PCOS.

Routine measurement of TSH, PRL, and FSH levels is recommended in women with oligomenorrhea and hyperandrogenism. Other laboratory tests including 17-hydroxyprogesterone, total testosterone, DHEAS, and the dexamethasone suppression test should be performed to exclude nonclassical CAH, androgen-secreting tumors, and Cushing's syndrome if the clinical presentation is suggestive or the prevalence in the patient's ethnic background is high (Table 62-2).

## Imaging Studies

Imaging of ovaries and adrenals should be performed when a tumor is suspected. Transvaginal ultrasound is the preferred method to rule out an adnexal mass. Typically, polycystic ovaries appear enlarged with 12 or more subcapsular follicles measuring less than 10 mm around dense hyperechoic stroma. However, some women with PCOS do not have these findings, whereas normal women may have polycystic ovaries on ultrasound. Therefore, ultrasound findings are not diagnostic. Abdominal CT or MRI should be performed if an adrenal tumor is suspected.

# TREATMENT

## Treatment of Infertility

Traditionally, clomiphene citrate (CC) has been the first-line agent followed by gonadotropin stimulation when CC is unsuccessful. Overall understanding about the role of insulin resistance has dramatically changed this tradition, and insulin sensitizers, for example, metformin are now used as first-line agents by many clinicians. However, it is always prudent to recommend weight loss and exercise to reduce insulin resistance and resume ovulation (Table 62-3).

### Weight Loss and Exercise

Obesity and PCOS have synergistic negative impact on insulin resistance and hyperandrogenemia. Studies on weight loss have

**Table 62-3**
**Treatment of Polycystic Ovary Syndrome**

| Therapy | Benefit |
| --- | --- |
| Weight loss: diet and exercise | Prevention of long-term sequelae such as diabetes, resumption of ovarian function |
| Insulin-sensitizing agents | Resumption of ovulation, prevention of long-term sequelae, possible improvement of hirsutism |
| Clomiphene citrate | Ovulation induction |
| Gonadotropins | Ovulation induction |
| Oral contraceptive pills | Suppression of hyperandrogenism, prevention of endometrial hyperplasia and cancer |
| Progestin | Prevention of endometrial hyperplasia and cancer |
| Spironolactone, flutamide, finasteride, cyproterone acetate, GnRH analogs | Suppression of hyperandrogenism |

GnRH, gonadotropin-releasing hormone.

consistently showed an improvement in insulin resistance, hyperandrogenemia, menstrual irregularity, and anovulation. As little as 5% loss of the starting weight causes a significant decrease in insulin resistance, as defined by reduction in insulin levels after fasting and in response to 75 g oral glucose.[68] This decline in insulin is accompanied by an increase in SHBG levels and a decrease in free testosterone, which may lead to improvement of hirsutism. Weight loss also restores reproductive function as indicated by regular cycles, increased pregnancy rates, and greater efficacy of ovulation induction agents. Improved pregnancy outcome after weight loss is perhaps the most important benefit.[69] Spontaneous ovulation may resume in up to 90% of obese women after 10% decline in BMI.[70]

Weight loss is an effective therapy with no side effects. Therefore, all patients should be strongly encouraged to lose weight. However, in today's clinical environment this is difficult to achieve even though patients are strongly driven to conceive. This is in part because effective medical treatment options are available, and weight loss is more arduous and may take longer.

### Insulin-Sensitizing Agents

The strong association between hyperinsulinemia and PCOS has led to use of insulin-sensitizing agents such as metformin, thiazolidinediones, and D-chiro-inositol as ovulation induction agents. Of these medications, metformin is the most extensively studied.

### Metformin

The first reported use of metformin for the management of PCOS, by Velazquez et al, appeared in 1994.[71] Metformin is a biguanide that is a well-established oral antidiabetic agent. Interestingly, biguanide compounds are also used as chemical sanitizers in swimming pools and as topical antiseptics such as contact lens cleansing solutions. Metformin decreases hepatic glucose production and increases peripheral glucose uptake by muscle and adipose tissue. The molecular mechanism of metformin action is still unknown, although the drug was developed in the 1950s. Metformin does not stimulate insulin secretion, but it does decrease fasting plasma insulin levels and improves insulin-mediated glucose metabolism, that is, insulin sensitivity. Therefore, it does not cause hypoglycemia. The most frequently used dose is 500 mg orally three times a day. Some investigators also used an oral 850 mg, twice-a-day regimen. The optimal dose range for ovulation induction has not been studied formally. Seven randomized, controlled studies investigated the efficacy of metformin on ovulation induction. Moghetti et al showed improved menstrual regularity and ovulation along with reduced hyperinsulinemia and hyperandrogenemia.[72] In this study, 50% of patients started having regular cycles. Vandermolen et al showed that addition of metformin to CC increased ovulation and pregnancy rates in CC-resistant patients compared with placebo (75% vs. 27% and 55% vs. 7%, respectively).[73] Nestler et al found that 34% of women who were placed on CC ovulated spontaneously, as opposed to 4% of women in the placebo group.[74] When metformin was combined with CC in women unresponsive to CC, the ovulation rate increased to 90% compared with 2% in the CC-plus-placebo group. The area under the insulin curve after an oral GTT also decreased significantly in the metformin group compared with placebo. Ng et al failed to find a significant improvement in ovulation rate with metformin treatment in a small randomized study.[75] There were only 10 patients in each metformin and placebo group, which limits the reliability of their findings. Kocak et al found that metformin therapy decreased hyperandrogenism and insulin resistance and improved ovulation rates in 56 CC-resistant patients who were randomized to receive metformin or placebo.[76] Fleming et al conducted the largest randomized, controlled trial to date.[77] They reported that metformin treatment improved ovulation frequency (23% in the metformin group vs. 13% in the placebo group, $P < 0.05$) and HDL levels in their 94 randomized patients. Treatment efficacy was inversely correlated with BMI. Sturrock et al also investigated the efficacy of metformin treatment on ovulation rates in their randomized, placebo-controlled, double-blind, cross-over study in 19 patients.[78] These patients did not benefit from metformin therapy. In summary, the majority of the randomized, controlled trials reported higher ovulation rates and improved insulin resistance with metformin therapy. Small randomized, controlled trials that failed to confirm the beneficial effects of metformin probably suffered from a subset of patients who were not insulin resistant. A large, multicenter, randomized, controlled study comparing metformin with CC or CC plus metformin is currently under way. The authors routinely use metformin as the first-line agent in ovulatory dysfunction with PCOS and have achieved a 42% pregnancy rate in our case series.[79] This was the first study to report pregnancy as an endpoint.

Beneficial effects of metformin use during pregnancy such as decreased first trimester spontaneous abortion rate and decreased gestational diabetes prevalence have been suggested by retrospective or no-control trials. Randomized, controlled studies are needed to determine the effects of metformin on pregnancy outcome.

Side effects of metformin include diarrhea, nausea, vomiting, abdominal bloating, flatulence, and anorexia. Approximately

30% more women experienced these symptoms compared with women who received placebo. Some investigators suggest starting with 500 mg daily and increasing the dose by 500 mg increments every week up to maximum of 2.5 g daily to reduce side effects. Hepatotoxicity is uncommon. Cessation of the therapy is warranted if liver function tests are found to be elevated. The most serious but rare side effect of metformin is lactic acidosis, which is fatal in 50% of the patients in whom it develops. The risk factors for lactic acidosis are not the usual circumstances of PCOS: impaired renal function, chronic liver and lung disease, and older age. Intravascular administration of radiocontrast media can also induce reduction in renal function and result in accumulation of metformin and lactic acidosis in patients with elevated serum creatinine, since metformin is excreted unchanged through the kidneys.

### Thiazolidinediones

Thiazolidinediones improve insulin resistance and decrease insulin levels presumably through binding to the peroxisome proliferator activator receptor gamma (PPARγ). Troglitazone, pioglitazone, and rosiglitazone are the three commercially available thiazolidinediones. Troglitazone is the most extensively studied therapeutic agent of the three. However, it was withdrawn from the market in March 2000 owing to reports of idiosyncratic hepatic injury. There are limited data on the effects of pioglitazone and rosiglitazone in inducing ovulation. These agents are also associated with embryotoxicity in animal studies.

### Clomiphene Citrate

CC is an orally active nonsteroidal agent that contains a mixture of two isomers: zuclomiphene and enclomiphene. Its structure is similar to estrogens and it has mixed estrogen agonist and antagonist effects. In animal models, CC acts as an estrogen antagonist in the presence of estrogen and is a weak estrogen agonist in the absence of estrogen. The main mechanism of its action is thought to be its antagonistic effects on the hypothalamic-pituitary axis and stimulation of GnRH secretion. CC also has antiestrogenic effects on the uterus, cervix, and vagina.

The initial dose of CC is 50 mg daily for 5 days between cycle days 3 and 7 or 5 and 9. The ovulatory LH surge usually occurs 7 days after the last pill. Approximately 75% of pregnancies occur in the first three treatment cycles, and 50% of patients conceive at the 50 mg dose.[80] If ovulation does not occur at the starting dose, dosage is increased by 50-mg increments up to 200 to 250 mg daily. It has been reported that 15% of patients who require higher doses of 150 and 200 mg become pregnant. However, doses above 100 mg have antiestrogenic effects and may not be efficient at producing pregnancy. If patients do not conceive within the first 6 months after the initiation of CC, prolongation of treatment does not improve the outcome. It is not possible to predict which patients will respond to CC. High BMI and elevated levels of androgens and PRL are associated with CC resistance. Dexamethasone may help women with high levels of androgens. The usual dose of dexamethasone is 0.5 mg at bedtime every day in addition to CC at the starting dose of 50 mg. Patients with elevated PRL levels may benefit from bromocriptine, a dopamine agonist that directly inhibits PRL secretion by the pituitary. The initial dose is 2.5 mg at bedtime. Some anovulatory women with normal PRL levels who did

not become pregnant with CC treatment may benefit from bromocriptine although this is controversial. Weight loss and insulin-sensitizing agents are the choice of treatment for hyperinsulinemic women with high BMI.

Side effects of CC are hot flashes, nausea and vomiting, headache, breast discomfort, abdominal bloating, hair changes, and visual symptoms. These side effects are not dose-dependent. Hot flashes are the most common side effect and are seen in about 10% of patients. They are thought to be due to the antiestrogenic effect of CC on the hypothalamic-pituitary axis. Visual symptoms including visual spots or flashes and blurry vision are considered a reason to discontinue CC. Liver function tests should be checked in women with symptoms or a history of liver disease.

### Gonadotropins

When the previously mentioned treatment options fail, the next step is to administer gonadotropins. However, anovulatory women with PCOS are prone to ovarian hyperstimulation syndrome (OHSS) and multiple pregnancies as a result of gonadotropin treatment. Many investigators have looked at the optimal ovulation induction protocols with gonadotropins including the type of the gonadotropins, dosing, and length of the treatment. Low-dose, step-up gonadotropin therapy with small starting doses for 14 days and a small incremental dose change thereafter has the highest pregnancy rates and lowest OHSS and multiple pregnancy rates.[81] Routine addition of GnRH agonists or antagonists is not recommended. However, addition of insulin-sensitizing agents may moderate hyperstimulation and is recommended by some investigators.

### Aromatase Inhibitors

Aromatase inhibitors have recently been suggested as an ovulation induction agent. They suppress the conversion of androgens to estrogens and thus decrease the negative feedback of estrogens on the hypothalamic-pituitary axis, similarly to CC. However, the current data are derived from only small preliminary studies.[82,83]

### D-Chiro-inositol

An initial randomized, controlled pharmaceutical-supported study reported that D-chiro-inositol was effective in improving insulin resistance and ovulatory function in 22 women with PCOS. However, phase II clinical trials failed to show this benefit.[84]

### Corticosteroids

Women with high serum androgen levels are likely resistant to CC. Women with elevated serum DHEAS levels may benefit from the addition of dexamethasone. In one randomized, controlled study in anovulatory, CC-resistant women with normal DHEAS levels, the addition of 2 mg dexamethasone to CC increased the ovulation rate compared with CC plus placebo (80% vs. 20%, respectively).[85] Although it is believed that a decline in adrenal androgen production improves responsiveness to CC, corticosteroids may also have direct effects on follicle development, cytokines such as IGF-1, and the hypothalamic-pituitary-ovarian axis. Dexamethasone treatment, 0.5 to 2 mg at bedtime, in addition to CC may be considered in CC-resistant women. However, prolonged use of dexamethasone in excess of

0.5 mg/day may induce iatrogenic Cushing's syndrome and is no longer recommended. The addition of metformin is now preferred by most clinicians.

### Combination Therapy with Insulin-sensitizing Agents

Metformin in combination with other ovulation induction agents may improve pregnancy rates. When CC was used in conjunction with metformin in women who are unresponsive to either drug alone, pregnancy rates improved and ovulation was achieved at lower doses of CC.[86] Metformin also appears to suppress hyperresponsiveness of the ovary to FSH. However, randomized studies with sufficient power are needed in order to make definitive conclusions.

### Surgery

Ovarian wedge resection for ovulation induction was first developed by Stein and Leventhal. It was abandoned years later because of the risk of postoperative peritubal and paraovarian adhesion formation although many patients resumed ovulation after wedge resection. With the advent of laparoscopy, a less invasive technique, laparoscopic ovarian drilling, has emerged. This technique employs puncturing of the ovary using electrocautery or laser. The ovary is usually punctured at 5 to 10 different places, which are approximately 10 mm deep and 1 mm in diameter. The purpose of ovarian drilling is similar to that of wedge resection: removal or destruction of hormone-producing tissue. Thus, it results in decreased testosterone and inhibin levels, leading to a rise in FSH and resumption of normal folliculogenesis. A randomized, controlled study comparing ovarian drilling to FSH for ovulation induction showed that ovarian drilling alone yielded lower pregnancy rates compared with recombinant FSH alone (37% vs. 75%, respectively).[87] Addition of FSH injections to ovarian drilling improved pregnancy rates to be similar to those of FSH alone. One advantage of ovarian drilling was the reduced rate of multiple pregnancy (rate ratio 0.11, CI 0.01–0.88). This procedure may be considered for patients who are adverse to risk of multiple pregnancy or are unresponsive to other conservative therapies.

## Treatment of Symptoms Unrelated to Infertility

The main goal of treatment for women who do not desire fertility is the prevention of long-term sequelae.

### Type 2 Diabetes Mellitus

Three large randomized, controlled studies report that significant reductions in the incidence of diabetes can be obtained through intensive lifestyle changes.[88–90] Diet and exercise in high-risk groups such as people with a first-degree diabetic relative, history of gestational diabetes, or impaired glucose tolerance are beneficial. One randomized, controlled study compared metformin therapy to lifestyle intervention and placebo.[91] Although both metformin and intensive lifestyle intervention reduced type 2 diabetes incidence, metformin was not as effective as lifestyle changes only (31% vs. 58%, respectively). As noted previously, weight loss as low as 5% alone may improve metabolic parameters and measurably decrease diabetes risk. A low-calorie, low-fat diet combined with moderate exercise has been successful. However, extensive one-on-one counseling is needed to reinforce the behavioral changes. Weight loss also facilitates

spontaneous ovulation and the effectiveness of ovulation induction agents.

### Cardiovascular Disease

Because women with PCOS exhibit known risk factors for cardiac disease such as obesity, diabetes, and dyslipidemia, therapies directed toward prevention of these comorbidities may reduce the heart disease risk. Diet and exercise are the mainstay of preventative therapy. Currently, there are insufficient data to recommend insulin-sensitizing agents as a means of cardiovascular protection. However, indirect evidence including decreased cardiovascular events in diabetic patients on metformin and improvement of metabolic parameters such as triglyceride and LDL levels warrants further investigation.

### Endometrial Hyperplasia/Cancer

Although efficacy is unknown, intuitively accepted practice is to induce withdrawal bleeding with a progestin at least four times a year. A well-established prevention method for endometrial cancer is oral contraceptive pills (OCPs). At least a 1-year use of OCPs decreases the risk of endometrial cancer between ages 40 and 55 years by 50%. However, there are concerns about altered carbohydrate metabolism in women on OCPs. Progestins increase plasma insulin and decrease glucose tolerance. However, to date, studies have failed to find a significant relationship between diabetes and currently used combined OCP formulations.[92] Another concern is the increased risk of cardiovascular disease among OCP users. A large study conducted by the World Health Organization (WHO) reported that OCPs increase myocardial infarction risk only in women with known cardiovascular risk factors such as smoking and hypertension.[93] A Dutch study found an increased risk of myocardial infarction in women on second-generation OCPs but not in women on third-generation OCPs.[94] Several other studies in the literature showed increased risk of myocardial infarction only in women who smoke and use OCPs. Randomized, controlled studies are needed to investigate the effects of OCPs on the development of diabetes and heart disease in women with PCOS.

Intuitively, insulin-sensitizing medications may protect the endometrium in women who resume regular cycles on these drugs.

### Hirsutism and Acne

Treatment directed to the suppression of androgen production and its peripheral action may prevent new hair growth and enhance cosmetic removal of existing hairs. Several medications can be used to achieve this goal.

#### Oral Contraceptive Pills

The most commonly used medication for hirsutism is OCPs. They suppress LH and FSH secretion, which decreases ovarian androgen production. Estrogens in OCPs also increase SHBG levels, which in turn decreases free testosterone levels. Progestins such as norethindrone may inhibit 5α-reductase activity in the skin. Intuitively, progestins with low androgenic activity including gestodene, desogestrel, and norethindrone acetate are preferred. Therapy should be continued for at least 6 months before an improvement can be expected. The hair growth cycle is approximately 6 months long.

# Reproductive Endocrinology and Infertility

### Spironolactone

Spironolactone is an aldosterone antagonist diuretic. It is also a competitive androgen receptor antagonist and directly inhibits 5α-reductase activity. Spironolactone is generally accepted as a potent agent for the treatment of hirsutism although there are only a few randomized, controlled trials that investigated the effectiveness of this medication in hirsutism. A review of all randomized, controlled studies in the literature reported that spironolactone treatment achieved significant subjective and objective improvement in hair growth compared with placebo.[95] It was also superior to finasteride and low-dose cyproterone acetate in one randomized, controlled study.[96] The effective dose is usually 200 mg daily. Side effects include metrorrhagia, urticaria, polyuria, nocturia, and dyspepsia. Hyperkalemia is a potential complication of the treatment that can occur in the elderly, persons with diabetes, and women taking a potassium-saving diuretic.

### Flutamide

Flutamide is a nonsteroidal androgen receptor antagonist that is used as adjuvant treatment for prostate cancer. Hair growth is directly inhibited at a starting dose of 250 mg daily. However, in randomized comparison studies, flutamide was not superior to spironolactone or finasteride.[97] Moreover, hepatotoxicity is a rare but potentially serious complication.

### Finasteride

Finasteride is a 5α-reductase inhibitor; it blocks conversion of testosterone to dihydrotestosterone. Finasteride is approved for the treatment of benign prostate hyperplasia and hair loss in men. The usual dose is 5 mg daily. It has not been shown to be more effective than flutamide or cyproterone acetate.[98] However, the lack of side effects makes finasteride a favorable option for the treatment of hirsutism.

### Cyproterone Acetate

This is a potent progestin that inhibits pituitary LH secretion and thus ovarian androgen production. Cyproterone acetate also blocks the androgen receptors and reduces the activity of skin 5α-reductase. The most commonly used form is called Diane-35 in Europe and Canada, and Dianette in Great Britain. It contains 2 mg cyproterone acetate and 35 μg ethinyl estradiol and is taken by mouth daily. Another method is the reversed sequential regimen with high-dose cyproterone acetate. In this regimen, 50 or 100 mg cyproterone acetate is given for the first 10 days of the cycle with 30 or 50 μg ethinyl estradiol given for 21 days. However, a dose-ranging study did not find a significant difference in treatment effectiveness among different dose regimens of cyproterone acetate (i.e., 2, 20, and 100 mg) after 6 months of therapy, although higher doses showed an improvement 3 months after the initiation of therapy.[99] When cyproterone acetate is compared with other antiandrogenic medications such as flutamide, spironolactone, and finasteride, no significant difference has been demonstrated.[100] Cyproterone acetate appears to be safe as side effects include headache, mood changes, and decreased libido.

### GnRH Analogs

Long-acting GnRH agonists such as leuprolide and nafarelin have been used for the treatment of hirsutism since the mid-1980s. They suppress pituitary LH secretion and thus decrease ovarian androgen production. Higher doses of GnRH agonists are required to inhibit androgen secretion compared with estradiol secretion. In a randomized study, OCPs alone were as effective as GnRH agonist alone or GnRH agonist plus OCPs, although women in the latter groups had a faster clinical response.[101] Women taking a GnRH agonist alone had significant bone loss, which was not seen in the other two groups. On the contrary, another randomized study showed that the combination of a GnRH agonist and OCPs resulted in greater improvement of hirsutism compared with GnRH alone or OCPs alone.[102] GnRH agonist therapy is as effective as high-dose cyproterone acetate and its effect lasts longer.[103] However, GnRH agonists are relatively expensive and should be used in conjunction with OCPs to prevent bone loss. Therefore, their use is recommended in women with severe insulin resistance and hyperthecosis that is unresponsive to other medical therapies.

### Insulin-Sensitizing Agents

The efficacy of metformin in hirsutism is not well characterized despite the fact that it reduces serum androgens significantly. There are conflicting studies in the literature some of which cannot be used to evaluate hirsutism because of the short follow-up periods. Some studies showed a significant improvement especially in adolescent girls, whereas others did not find a significant reduction. Large randomized studies with a long follow-up period are needed to establish the efficacy of metformin in hirsutism.

### Other Drugs

Ketoconazole inhibits androgen synthesis through the suppression of the cytochrome P-450 system. The high incidence of side effects such as elevated liver enzymes prevents ketoconazole's widespread use, although it is efficacious in the treatment of hirsutism. Cimetidine is a weak androgen receptor blocker and clinically is not effective. Dexamethasone is used only in women with adrenal enzyme deficiency.

## SUMMARY

PCOS is a lifelong inherited disease that evolves with age. Diagnosis may be challenging, since PCOS is a heterogeneous disorder with various manifestations including reproductive and metabolic abnormalities. Although insulin-sensitizing agents have revolutionized treatment, molecular studies will unveil the pathophysiology of PCOS and allow clinicians to develop new treatment strategies.

## REFERENCES

1. Knochenhauer ES, Key TJ, Kahsar-Miller M, et al: Prevalence of the polycystic ovary syndrome in unselected black and white women of the southeastern United States: a prospective study. J Clin Endocrinol Metab 1998;83:3078–3082. **(III, B)**
2. Diamanti-Kandarakis E, Kouli CR, Bergiele AT, et al: A survey of the polycystic ovary syndrome in the Greek island of Lesbos: hormonal and metabolic profile. J Clin Endocrinol Metab 1999;84:4006–4011. **(III, B)**

3. Asuncion M, Calvo RM, San Millan JL, et al: A prospective study of the prevalence of the polycystic ovary syndrome in unselected Caucasian women from Spain. J Clin Endocrinol Metab 2000;85:2434–2438. (III, B)

4. Guzick DS: Polycystic ovary syndrome. Obstet Gynecol 2004; 103:181–193. (IV, C)

5. Achard EC, Thiers J: Le virilisme pilaire et son association à l'insuffisance glycotique (diabète des femmes à barbe). Bulletin de l'Académie Nationale de Médecine, Paris 1921;86:51–56. (III, B)

6. Burghen GA, Givens JR, Kitabchi AE: Correlation of hyperandrogenism with hyperinsulinism in polycystic ovarian disease. J Clin Endocrinol Metab 1980;50:113–116. (III, B)

7. Dunaif A, Segal KR, Futterweit W, et al: Profound peripheral insulin resistance, independent of obesity, in polycystic ovary syndrome. Diabetes 1989;38:1165–1174. (IIa, B)

8. Geffner ME, Kaplan SA, Bersch N, et al: Persistence of insulin resistance in polycystic ovarian disease after inhibition of ovarian steroid secretion. Fertil Steril 1986;45:327–333. (IIb, B)

9. Dunaif A, Green G, Futterweit W, et al: Suppression of hyperandrogenism does not improve peripheral or hepatic insulin resistance in the polycystic ovary syndrome. J Clin Endocrinol Metab 1990; 70:699–704. (IIb, B)

10. Polderman KH, Gooren LJ, Asscheman H, et al: Induction of insulin resistance by androgens and estrogens. J Clin Endocrinol Metab 1994; 79:265–271. (IIb, B)

11. Nestler JE, Jakubowicz DJ, de Vargas AF, et al: Insulin stimulates testosterone biosynthesis by human thecal cells from women with polycystic ovary syndrome by activating its own receptor and using inositolglycan mediators as the signal transduction system. J Clin Endocrinol Metab 1998;83:2001–2005. (IIa, B)

12. Dunaif A, Graf M: Insulin administration alters gonadal steroid metabolism independent of changes in gonadotropin secretion in insulin-resistant women with the polycystic ovary syndrome. J Clin Invest 1989;83:23–29. (IIa, B)

13. Nestler JE, Barlascini CO, Matt DW, et al: Suppression of serum insulin by diazoxide reduces serum testosterone levels in obese women with polycystic ovary syndrome. J Clin Endocrinol Metab 1989; 68:1027–1032. (IIb, B)

14. Moghetti P, Castello R, Negri C, et al: Insulin infusion amplifies 17 alpha-hydroxycorticosteroid intermediates response to adrenocorticotropin in hyperandrogenic women: apparent relative impairment of 17,20-lyase activity. J Clin Endocrinol Metab 1996;81:881–886. (IIa, B)

15. Dunaif A, Xia J, Book CB, et al: Excessive insulin receptor serine phosphorylation in cultured fibroblasts and in skeletal muscle: a potential mechanism for insulin resistance in the polycystic ovary syndrome. J Clin Invest 1995;96:801–810. (IIa, B)

16. Dunaif A, Wu X, Lee A, et al: Defects in insulin receptor signaling in vivo in the polycystic ovary syndrome (PCOS). Am J Physiol Endocrinol Metab 2001;281:E392–E399. (IIa, B)

17. Morales AJ, Laughlin GA, Butzow T, et al: Insulin, somatotropic, and luteinizing hormone axes in lean and obese women with polycystic ovary syndrome: common and distinct features. J Clin Endocrinol Metab 1996;81:2854–2864. (IIa, B)

18. Bruning JC, Gautam D, Burks DJ, et al: Role of brain insulin receptor in control of body weight and reproduction. Science 2000; 289:2122–2125. (IIa, B)

19. Burger HG: Androgen production in women. Fertil Steril 2002; 77(Suppl 4):S3–S5. (III, B)

20. Aiman J, Edman CD, Worley RJ, et al: Androgen and estrogen formation in women with ovarian hyperthecosis. Obstet Gynecol 1978;51:1–9. (III, B)

21. Nelson VL, Legro RS, Strauss JF III, et al: Augmented androgen production is a stable steroidogenic phenotype of propagated theca cells from polycystic ovaries. Mol Endocrinol 1999;13:946–957. (IIa, B)

22. Stewart PM, Shackleton CH, Beastall GH, et al: 5 Alpha-reductase activity in polycystic ovary syndrome. Lancet 1990;335:431–433. (III, B)

23. Rodin A, Thakkar H, Taylor N, et al: Hyperandrogenism in polycystic ovary syndrome: evidence of dysregulation of 11 beta-hydroxysteroid dehydrogenase. N Engl J Med 1994;330:460–465. (IIa, B)

24. Speiser PW, Serrat J, New MI, et al: Insulin insensitivity in adrenal hyperplasia due to nonclassical steroid 21-hydroxylase deficiency. J Clin Endocrinol Metab 1992;75:1421–1424. (IIa, B)

25. Willis DS, Watson H, Mason HD, et al: Premature response to luteinizing hormone of granulosa cells from anovulatory women with polycystic ovary syndrome: relevance to mechanism of anovulation. J Clin Endocrinol Metab 1998;83:3984–3991. (IIa, B)

26. Legro RS, Driscoll D, Strauss JF III, et al: Evidence for a genetic basis for hyperandrogenemia in polycystic ovary syndrome. Proc Natl Acad Sci U S A 1998;95:14956–14960. (IIa, B)

27. Hong Y, Gagnon J, Rice T, et al: Familial resemblance for free androgens and androgen glucuronides in sedentary black and white individuals: the HERITAGE Family Study. Health, Risk Factors, Exercise Training and Genetics. J Endocrinol 2001;170:485–492. (IIa, B)

28. Jahanfar S, Eden JA, Warren P, et al: A twin study of polycystic ovary syndrome. Fertil Steril 1995;63:478–486. (III, B)

29. Legro RS, Kunselman AR, Demers L, et al: Elevated dehydroepiandrosterone sulfate levels as the reproductive phenotype in the brothers of women with polycystic ovary syndrome. J Clin Endocrinol Metab 2002;87:2134–2138. (IIa, B)

30. Colilla S, Cox NJ, Ehrmann DA: Heritability of insulin secretion and insulin action in women with polycystic ovary syndrome and their first degree relatives. J Clin Endocrinol Metab 2001;86:2027–2031. (IIb, B)

31. Urbanek M, Legro RS, Driscoll DA, et al: Thirty-seven candidate genes for polycystic ovary syndrome: strongest evidence for linkage is with follistatin. Proc Natl Acad Sci U S A 1999;96:8573–8578. (IIa, B)

32. Urbanek M, Wu X, Vickery KR, et al: Allelic variants of the follistatin gene in polycystic ovary syndrome. J Clin Endocrinol Metab 2000; 85:4455–4461. (IIa, B)

33. Guo Q, Kumar TR, Woodruff T, et al: Overexpression of mouse follistatin causes reproductive defects in transgenic mice. Mol Endocrinol 1998;12:96–106. (IIa, B)

34. Jorgez CJ, Klysik M, Jamin SP, et al: Granulosa cell–specific inactivation of follistatin causes female fertility defects. Mol Endocrinol 2004; 18:953–967. (IIa, B)

35. Waterworth DM, Bennett ST, Gharani N, et al: Linkage and association of insulin gene VNTR regulatory polymorphism with polycystic ovary syndrome. Lancet 1997;349:986–990. (IIa, B)

36. Tucci S, Futterweit W, Concepcion ES, et al: Evidence for association of polycystic ovary syndrome in Caucasian women with a marker at the insulin receptor gene locus. J Clin Endocrinol Metab 2001; 86:446–449. (IIa, B)

37. Villuendas G, Escobar-Morreale HF, Tosi F, et al: Association between the D19S884 marker at the insulin receptor gene locus and polycystic ovary syndrome. Fertil Steril 2003;79:219–220. (IIa, B)

38. Wood JR, Nelson VL, Ho C, et al: The molecular phenotype of polycystic ovary syndrome (PCOS) theca cells and new candidate PCOS genes defined by microarray analysis. J Biol Chem 2003; 278:26380–26390. (IIa, B)

39. Elting MW, Korsen TJ, Rekers-Mombarg LT, et al: Women with polycystic ovary syndrome gain regular menstrual cycles when aging. Hum Reprod 2000;15:24–28. (III, B)

40. Balen AH, Braat DD, West C, et al: Cumulative conception and live birth rates after the treatment of anovulatory infertility: safety and efficacy of ovulation induction in 200 patients. Hum Reprod 1994; 9:1563–1570. (IIb, B)

41. Barbieri RL, Ryan KJ: Hyperandrogenism, insulin resistance, and acanthosis nigricans syndrome: a common endocrinopathy with distinct pathophysiologic features. Am J Obstet Gynecol 1983;147:90–101. (IV, C)

42. Ibanez L, Potau N, François I, et al: Precocious pubarche, hyperinsulinism, and ovarian hyperandrogenism in girls: relation to reduced fetal growth. J Clin Endocrinol Metab 1998;83:3558–3562. (IIa, B)

43. Ibanez L, Potau N, Virdis R, et al: Postpubertal outcome in girls diagnosed of premature pubarche during childhood: increased frequency of functional ovarian hyperandrogenism. J Clin Endocrinol Metab 1993;76:1599–1603. **(IIa, B)**

44. Dahlgren E, Johansson S, Lindstedt G, et al: Women with polycystic ovary syndrome wedge resected in 1956 to 1965: a long-term follow-up focusing on natural history and circulating hormones. Fertil Steril 1992;57:505–513. **(IIb, B)**

45. Solomon CG, Hu FB, Dunaif A, et al: Long or highly irregular menstrual cycles as a marker for risk of type 2 diabetes mellitus. JAMA 2001;286:2421–2426. **(III, B)**

46. Dejager S, Pichard C, Giral P, et al: Smaller LDL particle size in women with polycystic ovary syndrome compared to controls. Clin Endocrinol (Oxf) 2001;54:455–462. **(IIa, B)**

47. Christian RC, Dumesic DA, Behrenbeck T, et al: Prevalence and predictors of coronary artery calcification in women with polycystic ovary syndrome. J Clin Endocrinol Metab 2003;88:2562–2568. **(IIa, B)**

48. Birdsall MA, Farquhar CM, White HD: Association between polycystic ovaries and extent of coronary artery disease in women having cardiac catheterization. Ann Intern Med 1997;126:32–35. **(III, B)**

49. Elting MW, Korsen TJ, Bezemer PD, et al: Prevalence of diabetes mellitus, hypertension and cardiac complaints in a follow-up study of a Dutch PCOS population. Hum Reprod 2001;16:556–560. **(III, B)**

50. Glueck CJ, Papanna R, Wang P, et al: Incidence and treatment of metabolic syndrome in newly referred women with confirmed polycystic ovarian syndrome. Metabolism 2003;52:908–915. **(IIa, B)**

51. Pierpoint T, McKeigue PM, Isaacs AJ, et al: Mortality of women with polycystic ovary syndrome at long-term follow-up. J Clin Epidemiol 1998;51:581–586. **(III, B)**

52. Coulam CB, Annegers JF, Kranz JS: Chronic anovulation syndrome and associated neoplasia. Obstet Gynecol 1983;61:403–407. **(III, B)**

53. Escobedo LG, Lee NC, Peterson HB, et al: Infertility-associated endometrial cancer risk may be limited to specific subgroups of infertile women. Obstet Gynecol 1991;77:124–128. **(IIb, B)**

54. Dahlgren E, Johansson S, Oden A, et al: A model for prediction of endometrial cancer. Acta Obstet Gynecol Scand 1989;68:507–510. **(IIb, B)**

55. Gallup DG, Stock RJ: Adenocarcinoma of the endometrium in women 40 years of age or younger. Obstet Gynecol 1984;64:417–420. **(III, B)**

56. Wild S, Pierpoint T, Jacobs H, et al: Long-term consequences of polycystic ovary syndrome: results of a 31 year follow-up study. Hum Fertil (Camb) 2000;3:101–105. **(III, B)**

57. Kurabayashi T, Kase H, Suzuki M, et al: Endometrial abnormalities in infertile women. J Reprod Med 2003;48:455–459. **(III, B)**

58. Secreto G, Toniolo P, Berrino F, et al: Serum and urinary androgens and risk of breast cancer in postmenopausal women. Cancer Res 1991;51:2572–2576. **(III, B)**

59. Berrino F, Muti P, Micheli A, et al: Serum sex hormone levels after menopause and subsequent breast cancer. J Natl Cancer Inst 1996;88:291–296. **(IIa, B)**

60. Gammon MD, Thompson WD: Polycystic ovaries and the risk of breast cancer. Am J Epidemiol 1991;134:818–824. **(III, B)**

61. Anderson KE, Sellers TA, Chen PL, et al: Association of Stein-Leventhal syndrome with the incidence of postmenopausal breast carcinoma in a large prospective study of women in Iowa. Cancer 1997;79:494–499. **(III, B)**

62. Pierpoint T, McKeigue PM, Isaacs AJ, et al: Mortality of women with polycystic ovary syndrome at long-term follow-up. J Clin Epidemiol 1998;51:581–586. **(III, B)**

63. Anderson GL, Limacher M, Assaf AR, et al: Effects of conjugated equine estrogen in postmenopausal women with hysterectomy: the Women's Health Initiative randomized controlled trial. JAMA 2004;291:1701–1712. **(Ib, A)**

64. Schildkraut JM, Schwingl PJ, Bastos E, et al: Epithelial ovarian cancer risk among women with polycystic ovary syndrome. Obstet Gynecol 1996;88:554–559. **(III, B)**

65. Risma KA, Clay CM, Nett TM, et al: Targeted overexpression of luteinizing hormone in transgenic mice leads to infertility, polycystic ovaries, and ovarian tumors. Proc Natl Acad Sci U S A 1995; 92:1322–1326. **(IIa, B)**

66. Revised 2003 consensus on diagnostic criteria and long-term health risks related to polycystic ovary syndrome. Fertil Steril 2004;81:19–25. **(IV, C)**

67. Azziz R, Hincapie LA, Knochenhauer ES, et al: Screening for 21-hydroxylase-deficient nonclassic adrenal hyperplasia among hyperandrogenic women: a prospective study. Fertil Steril 1999;72:915–925. **(IV, C)**

68. Kiddy DS, Hamilton-Fairley D, Bush A, et al: Improvement in endocrine and ovarian function during dietary treatment of obese women with polycystic ovary syndrome. Clin Endocrinol (Oxf) 1992; 36:105–111. **(IIb, B)**

69. Clark AM, Thornley B, Tomlinson L, et al: Weight loss in obese infertile women results in improvement in reproductive outcome for all forms of fertility treatment. Hum Reprod 1998;13:1502–1505. **(IIb, B)**

70. Clark AM, Thornley B, Tomlinson L, et al: Weight loss in obese infertile women results in improvement in reproductive outcome for all forms of fertility treatment. Hum Reprod 1998;13:1502–1505. **(IIb, B)**

71. Velazquez EM, Mendoza S, Hamer T, et al: Metformin therapy in polycystic ovary syndrome reduces hyperinsulinemia, insulin resistance, hyperandrogenemia, and systolic blood pressure, while facilitating normal menses and pregnancy. Metabolism 1994;43:647–654. **(IIb, B)**

72. Moghetti P, Castello R, Negri C, et al: Metformin effects on clinical features, endocrine and metabolic profiles, and insulin sensitivity in polycystic ovary syndrome: a randomized, double-blind, placebo-controlled 6-month trial, followed by open, long-term clinical evaluation. J Clin Endocrinol Metab 2000;85:139–146. **(Ib, A)**

73. Vandermolen DT, Ratts VS, Evans WS, et al: Metformin increases the ovulatory rate and pregnancy rate from clomiphene citrate in patients with polycystic ovary syndrome who are resistant to clomiphene citrate alone. Fertil Steril 2001;75:310–315. **(Ib, A)**

74. Nestler JE, Jakubowicz DJ, Evans WS, et al: Effects of metformin on spontaneous and clomiphene-induced ovulation in the polycystic ovary syndrome. N Engl J Med 1998;338:1876–1880. **(Ib, A)**

75. Ng EH, Wat NM, Ho PC: Effects of metformin on ovulation rate, hormonal and metabolic profiles in women with clomiphene-resistant polycystic ovaries: a randomized, double-blinded placebo-controlled trial. Hum Reprod 2001;16:1625–1631. **(Ib, A)**

76. Kocak M, Caliskan E, Simsir C, et al: Metformin therapy improves ovulatory rates, cervical scores, and pregnancy rates in clomiphene citrate-resistant women with polycystic ovary syndrome. Fertil Steril 2002;77:101–106. **(Ib, A)**

77. Fleming R, Hopkinson ZE, Wallace AM, et al: Ovarian function and metabolic factors in women with oligomenorrhea treated with metformin in a randomized double blind placebo-controlled trial. J Clin Endocrinol Metab 2002;87:569–574. **(Ib, A)**

78. Sturrock ND, Lannon B, Fay TN: Metformin does not enhance ovulation induction in clomiphene resistant polycystic ovary syndrome in clinical practice. Br J Clin Pharmacol 2002;53:469–473. **(Ib, A)**

79. Heard MJ, Pierce A, Carson SA, et al: Pregnancies following use of metformin for ovulation induction in patients with polycystic ovary syndrome. Fertil Steril 2002;77:669–673. **(III, B)**

80. Gysler M, March CM, Mishell DR Jr, et al: A decade's experience with an individualized clomiphene treatment regimen including its effect on the postcoital test. Fertil Steril 1982;37:161–167. **(III, B)**

81. Christin-Maitre S, Hugues JN: A comparative randomized multicentric study comparing the step-up versus step-down protocol in polycystic ovary syndrome. Hum Reprod 2003;18:1626–1631. **(Ib, A)**

82. Fafemi HM, Kolibianakis E, Tournaye H, et al: Clomiphene citrate versus letrozole for ovarian stimulation. A pilot study. Reprod Biomed Online 2003;7:543–546. **(IIa, B)**

83. Mitwally MF, Casper RF: Use of an aromatase inhibitor for induction of ovulation in patients with an inadequate response to clomiphene citrate. Fertil Steril 2001;75:305–309. **(IIb, B)**

84. Insmed discontinues internal development of INS-1 for diabetes and polycystic ovary syndrome (PCOS). News release, business wire, Sept 10, 2002.

85. Parsanezhad ME, Alborzi S, Motazedian S, et al: Use of dexamethasone and clomiphene citrate in the treatment of clomiphene citrate-resistant patients with polycystic ovary syndrome and normal dehydroepiandrosterone sulfate levels: a prospective, double-blind, placebo-controlled trial. Fertil Steril 2002;78:1001–1004. **(Ib, A)**

86. Nestler JE, Jakubowicz DJ, Evans WS, et al: Effects of metformin on spontaneous and clomiphene-induced ovulation in the polycystic ovary syndrome. N Engl J Med 1998;338:1876–1880. **(Ib, A)**

87. Bayram N, Van Wely M, Kaaijk EM, et al: Using an electrocautery strategy or recombinant follicle stimulating hormone to induce ovulation in polycystic ovary syndrome: randomised controlled trial. BMJ 2004;328:192–196. **(Ib, A)**

88. Knowler WC, Barrett-Connor E, Fowler SE, et al: Reduction in the incidence of type 2 diabetes with lifestyle intervention or metformin. N Engl J Med 2002;346:393–403. **(Ib, A)**

89. Tuomilehto J, Lindstrom J, Eriksson JG, et al: Prevention of type 2 diabetes mellitus by changes in lifestyle among subjects with impaired glucose tolerance. N Engl J Med 2001;344:1343–1350. **(Ib, A)**

90. Pan XR, Li GW, Hu YH, et al: Effects of diet and exercise in preventing NIDDM in people with impaired glucose tolerance. The Da Qing IGT and Diabetes Study. Diabetes Care 1997;20:537–544. **(Ib, A)**

91. Knowler WC, Barrett-Connor E, Fowler SE, et al: Reduction in the incidence of type 2 diabetes with lifestyle intervention or metformin. N Engl J Med 2002;346:393–403. **(Ib, A)**

92. Chasan-Taber L, Willett WC, Stampfer MJ, et al: A prospective study of oral contraceptives and NIDDM among U.S. women. Diabetes Care 1997;20:330–335. **(IIa, B)**

93. Acute myocardial infarction and combined oral contraceptives: results of an international multicentre case-control study. WHO Collaborative Study of Cardiovascular Disease and Steroid Hormone Contraception. Lancet 1997;349:1202–1209. **(III, B)**

94. Tanis BC, van den Bosch MA, Kemmeren JM, et al: Oral contraceptives and the risk of myocardial infarction. N Engl J Med 2001; 345:1787–1793. **(IIb, B)**

95. Farquhar C, Lee O, Toomath R, et al: Spironolactone versus placebo or in combination with steroids for hirsutism and/or acne. Cochrane Database Syst Rev 2003;CD000194. **(Ia, A)**

96. Lumachi F, Rondinone R: Use of cyproterone acetate, finasteride, and spironolactone to treat idiopathic hirsutism. Fertil Steril 2003; 79:942–946. **(Ib, A)**

97. Moghetti P, Tosi F, Tosti A, et al: Comparison of spironolactone, flutamide, and finasteride efficacy in the treatment of hirsutism: a randomized, double blind, placebo-controlled trial. J Clin Endocrinol Metab 2000;85:89–94. **(Ib, A)**

98. Fruzzetti F, Bersi C, Parrini D, et al: Treatment of hirsutism: comparisons between different antiandrogens with central and peripheral effects. Fertil Steril 1999;71:445–451. **(Ib, A)**

99. Barth JH, Cherry CA, Wojnarowska F, et al: Cyproterone acetate for severe hirsutism: results of a double-blind dose-ranging study. Clin Endocrinol (Oxf) 1991;35:5–10. **(Ib, A)**

100. Van der Spuy ZM, le Roux PA: Cyproterone acetate for hirsutism. Cochrane Database Syst Rev 2003;CD001125. **(Ia, A)**

101. Carr BR, Breslau NA, Givens C, et al: Oral contraceptive pills, gonadotropin-releasing hormone agonists, or use in combination for treatment of hirsutism: a clinical research center study. J Clin Endocrinol Metab 1995;80:1169–1178. **(Ib, A)**

102. Heiner JS, Greendale GA, Kawakami AK, et al: Comparison of a gonadotropin-releasing hormone agonist and a low dose oral contraceptive given alone or together in the treatment of hirsutism. J Clin Endocrinol Metab 1995;80:3412–3418. **(Ib, A)**

103. Carmina E, Lobo RA: Gonadotrophin-releasing hormone agonist therapy for hirsutism is as effective as high dose cyproterone acetate but results in a longer remission. Hum Reprod 1997;12:663–666. **(IIa, B)**

# Chapter 63

# Thyroid Function and Disorders

Kristiina Parviainen, MD, Hyagriv N. Simhan, MD, MSCR, and Thomas P. Foley, Jr., MD

## KEY POINTS

- Normal thyroid function is essential for optimal reproductive function and pregnancy outcome.
- Failure to diagnose or to appropriately treat hypothyroidism in pregnancy can have significant impact on the neurologic development of the child.
- Most women with pregestational hypothyroidism will require a dosage increase in order to maintain euthyroid status.
- Radioactive iodine ($^{131}$I) is contraindicated in pregnancy owing to potential for ablation of the fetal thyroid gland.
- Neonatal screening for congenital hypothyroidism is mandatory in the United States.

Thyroid disorders are among the most common endocrine disorders affecting women. Thyroid dysfunction may be associated with menstrual irregularity, infertility, and adverse pregnancy outcomes. It is therefore essential that the clinician be well versed in the diagnosis and treatment of thyroid disorders. Diagnosis in pregnancy is particularly important owing to associated pregnancy complications and potentially significant adverse fetal and neonatal sequelae.

Hypothyroidism, defined as inadequate thyroid hormone production, has an incidence of 2.5% in pregnancy.[1] Risk factors for hypothyroidism include history of thyroid surgery, history of head/neck irradiation, family history of thyroid disorders, drug uses (lithium carbonates, amiodarone, aminoglutethimide, interferon, thalidomide, iodides, and stavudine), and pituitary and hypothalamic disorders. Other high-risk populations are the elderly, postpartum women, and individuals with autoimmune disorders including type 1 diabetes mellitus, adrenal insufficiency, and premature ovarian failure. Increased incidence is also reported among individuals with Down syndrome and Turner's syndrome.[2] Although rare in the United States, iodine deficiency is the foremost cause of hypothyroidism worldwide.[3] Goiters are commonly seen in pregnancy in iodine-deficient regions but rarely in the United States.

Hyperthyroidism, defined as excess production of, release of, or exposure to thyroid hormone, and thyrotoxicosis, caused by hyperfunctioning of the thyroid gland, are much less common in pregnancy with a reported incidence of 0.2%.[1] Ninety-five percent of all hyperthyroidism in pregnancy is due to Graves' disease, which is an autoimmune disease characterized by the presence of thyroid-stimulating immunoglobulins (TSIs). Thyroid-stimulating hormone–binding inhibitory immuno-globulins (TBIs) also may be present in treated cases and may cause hypothyroidism in mother and fetus.[4] Thyroid crisis or storm resulting from the sudden release of thyroxine from the thyroid gland is a medical emergency, with a 2% incidence in pregnancy among thyrotoxic women.

Postpartum thyroiditis is a diagnosis of particular interest to the obstetrician, with a reported incidence of 5% to 9%.[1] This condition usually presents as transient thyrotoxicosis followed by hypothyroidism that by definition occurs within 1 year of childbirth.

Hashimoto's thyroiditis, or chronic lymphocytic thyroiditis, is an autoimmune disease caused by antibody-dependent cell-mediated cytotoxicity. Affected women usually are euthyroid, though approximately 20% are hypothyroid, and may have diffuse thyromegaly, or goiter. It is the most common cause of acquired hypothyroidism in women.

The incidence of thyroid cancer among pregnant women is 1 per 1000 thyroid nodules detected.[5] Clinicians must therefore be cognizant of this rare but serious condition when evaluating women for possible thyroid pathology.

Congenital hypothyroidism (CH) is the most common treatable cause of mental retardation, with an incidence of 1 in 4000 newborns in iodine-sufficient regions of the world. Most of these cases result from permanent thyroid disease that requires lifelong therapy with thyroid hormone. Approximately 15% of CH may be attributed to genetic causes including inherited disorders that cause defects in thyroid hormone synthesis, metabolism, and rarely thyroid embryogenesis.

## PHYSIOLOGY

The thyroid gland consists of a spherical orientation of follicular cells that surround colloid composed of thyroglobulin, the glycoprotein substrate for synthesis of iodothyronines. Thyroid function is regulated by the hypothalamic-pituitary axis through thyrotropin-releasing hormone (TRH) production by the paraventricular nucleus of the hypothalamus that stimulates the production of thyroid-stimulating hormone (TSH) by the pituitary thyrotrophs.

TSH is a glycoprotein that shares the $\alpha$ subunit with follicle-stimulating hormone (FSH), luteinizing hormone (LH), and human chorionic gonadotropin (hCG). TSH regulates thyroid gland production of thyroxine ($T_4$) and triiodothyronine ($T_3$). Iodide trapping is mediated by the sodium iodide symporter (NIS) and is the rate-limiting step in thyroid hormone synthesis. The unbound or free $T_4$ ($FT_4$) circulates in the serum and is converted peripherally to $T_3$ by monodeiodination. $T_3$ has

# Reproductive Endocrinology and Infertility

| Table 63-1 Thyroid Function, Values in Pregnancy, Hyper- and Hypothyroidism Compared to Healthy Nonpregnant Women | | | | | |
|---|---|---|---|---|---|
| Condition | TSH | Free $T_4$ | Total $T_4$ | Total $T_3$* | $rT_3U$ |
| Pregnancy | Normal | Normal | Elevated | Elevated | Decreased |
| Hyperthyroidism | Decreased | Elevated | Elevated | Elevated | Elevated |
| Hypothyroidism | Elevated | Decreased | Decreased | Normal/decreased | Decreased |

$rT_3U$, resin $T_3$ uptake.
*Total and free $T_3$ values may not be elevated when there is coexisting nonthyroidal illness syndrome or low $T_3$ syndrome.

greater biologic activity than $T_4$ owing to the increased affinity for nuclear receptors. On binding of $T_3$ to specific receptors attached to DNA, $T_3$ stimulates transcription and translation of proteins, which results in an elevated metabolic rate at the cellular level.

Circulating thyroid hormone, dopamine, and somatostatin cause a negative feedback by inhibition on pituitary TSH secretion.

Thyroid function changes in early pregnancy as a consequence of (1) increased iodine uptake by the thyroid gland, (2) increased estrogen-mediated production (twofold increase) and decreased clearance of thyroid binding globulin by the liver, and (3) hCG stimulation of the TSH receptor. These effects cause a mild increase in $FT_4$ that in turn may cause transient gestational thyrotoxicosis.[6] $FT_4$ concentrations, however, remain essentially stable during pregnancy provided there is normal thyroid function and adequate iodine substrate. Expected changes in thyroid function values in normal pregnancy as compared with the nonpregnant state are depicted in Table 63-1. Maternal blood levels of iodine are decreased in pregnancy owing to an increase in the glomerular filtration rate, provided that it is not accompanied by an increase in iodine intake. The recommended daily iodine intake in pregnancy is 200 μg.[3]

The thyroid gland develops during the first trimester, whereas maturation of the hypothalamic-pituitary-thyroid feedback system and peripheral action of the thyroid hormones continues throughout fetal life into early postnatal life. The thyroid originates from an outpouching of the anterior pharyngeal floor at the base of the tongue (foramen caecum) and migrates to an anterior midline position by 7 weeks' gestation. Iodine trapping is detected by 10 to 12 weeks and thyroxine production by week 14. Normal adult levels of $T_4$ are achieved by 36 weeks' gestation,[7] continue to increase until delivery, and remain greater than adult levels during infancy. Serum $T_3$ levels are low during fetal life compared with adult levels, but surge shortly after birth to concentrations above adult levels in response to the abrupt surge of TSH immediately after birth.[8]

## PATHOLOGY

Graves' disease is the most common cause of thyroid gland hyperfunction, with stimulation of the gland mediated by TSIs. The mechanisms for the immune-mediated autoantibody production are unknown.

Thyroid crisis is a severe and life-threatening form of thyrotoxicosis resulting from release of thyroxine stores. Precipitating events include surgery, trauma, infection, and labor.

Hyperemesis gravidarum is a pregnancy-associated, hCG-mediated condition in which uncontrolled nausea and vomiting leads to weight loss and electrolyte imbalance. These symptoms and the typically depressed TSH level seen with hyperemesis gravidarum can make the distinction from hyperthyroidism difficult.

Molar pregnancy/trophoblastic disease with the associated markedly elevated hCG levels can also cause an hCG-mediated hyperthyroid syndrome. This diagnosis should always be considered when symptoms of thyrotoxicosis appear for the first time in the presence of a positive pregnancy test. Molar pregnancy may also be accompanied by elevated blood pressure and thus mimic preeclampsia.

Most cases of hypothyroidism in the United States are caused by primary dysfunction of the thyroid gland. In Hashimoto's thyroiditis, a diffuse lymphocytic infiltrate and lymphoid follicles fill the thyroid parenchyma. Circulating autoantibodies are also detected in serum.[2] Significant sequelae of unrecognized or inadequately treated severe maternal hypothyroidism include low birth weight, congenital anomalies, stillbirth, and neurologic impairment, including impaired cognitive development, in the progeny of women with mild to moderate hypothyroidism during pregnancy.[9,10]

Postpartum thyroiditis is caused by autoimmune lymphocytic infiltration and inflammation of the thyroid gland. The inflammatory process causes injury to the thyroid follicles, release of preformed $T_4$ and $T_3$ contained therein, and mild thyrotoxicosis. A hypothyroid phase ensues during healing and recovery of normal thyroid gland architecture and function.

Fetal hyperthyroidism is caused by transplacental passage of thyroid-stimulating immunoglobulins, which stimulate the fetal thyroid gland to secrete excessive amounts of thyroxine. The incidence of neonatal Graves' disease is approximately one clinically affected infant born to 70 women with Graves' disease. The risk for clinical expression of Graves' disease in the newborn is thought to be related to the maternal titer of TSIs and the binding affinity of TSI for the TSH receptor. However, since exact clinical correlation is yet to be determined, the application of TSI titers to clinical practice remains controversial.[11]

Fetal hypothyroidism can also be seen in women with Graves' disease and/or Hashimoto's thyroiditis through the action of the TBIs that block the fetal TSH receptor.

There are several causes of primary CH. The most common category is thyroid dysgenesis, which includes agenesis or dysgenesis of the fetal thyroid gland, familial disorders of thyroid hormone synthesis, and iodine deficiency. Transient iatrogenic hypothyroidism may also be the consequence of overtreatment with antithyroid drugs. Maternal hypothyroidism secondary to iodine deficiency and compounded by other trace metal deficiencies is the most significant risk factor for congenital hypothyroidism and cretinism worldwide. Less common causes are genetic and developmental defects that affect the embryogenesis of the fetal hypothalamus, pituitary, and thyroid that include inactivating mutations of the genes for the synthesis of hormones, receptors, and transcription factors.[12]

## CLINICAL FEATURES

Since routine laboratory screening is currently not recommended in asymptomatic adults, timely diagnosis requires vigilance on the part of the clinician. The signs and symptoms of hyperthyroidism and those specific for Graves' disease are listed in Tables 63-2 and 63-3, respectively. Proptosis and external ocular muscle palsy are distinguishing features of Graves' disease—a direct result of infiltrating ophthalmopathy—but are present in only 30% of cases. Of note, some of the features of hyperthyroidism including tachycardia, heat intolerance, fatigue, anxiety, emotional lability, nausea, and weight loss are not infrequently seen in early pregnancy, potentially resulting in a delay in diagnosis.

The differential diagnosis for goiter in pregnancy includes Graves' disease, Hashimoto's thyroiditis, iodine deficiency, excessive iodine intake, lymphocytic thyroiditis, thyroid cancer, lymphoma, and iatrogenic hypertrophy secondary to treatment with lithium or thioamides.

**Table 63-2**
**Clinical Signs and Symptoms of Hyperthyroidism**

- Excessive sweating
- Frequent stools
- Goiter
- Heat intolerance
- Hypertension
- Insomnia
- New-onset atrial fibrillation
- Oligomenorrhea or hypomenorrhea
- Palpitations
- Tachycardia
- Tremors
- Weight loss

**Table 63-3**
**Clinical Signs and Symptoms Specific to Graves' Disease**

- Dermopathy
- Lid lag
- Lid retraction
- Pretibial myxedema
- Proptosis
- Thyroid acropathy

**Table 63-4**
**Clinical Signs and Symptoms of Hypothyroidism**

- Carpal tunnel syndrome
- Cold intolerance
- Constipation
- Edema
- Fatigue
- Hair loss
- Hypercholesterolemia
- Insomnia
- Intellectual slowness
- Menorrhagia
- Muscle cramps
- Prolonged relaxation of deep tendon reflexes
- Voice changes
- Weight gain

Thyroid storm is a known complication of hyperthyroidism in pregnancy. The classic signs of thyroid crisis are hyperthermia, tachycardia, hypertension, altered mental status, and diarrhea, but the diagnosis should be considered when any of these signs are present in a patient with known hyperthyroidism.

The clinical features of hypothyroidism are depicted in Table 63-4. The symptoms can be subtle and are often dismissed by the patient and clinician as normal changes of pregnancy.

Most infants with congenital hypothyroidism are asymptomatic at birth. Fetal hypothyroidism is rare among cases of congenital hypothyroidism, since the clinical features are often partially masked in utero by the transplacental passage of maternal thyroxine. Congenital hypothyroidism is associated with an increased incidence of congenital anomalies, including cardiac anomalies. Clinical findings of CH in the newborn include lethargy, slow movement, hoarse cry, constipation, large fontanels, hypotonia, and prolonged jaundice.[13] Cretinism, the most dramatic form of congenital hypothyroidism, is characterized by mental retardation, small stature, and neurologic disorders.

Fetal hyperthyroidism is characterized by tachycardia, intrauterine growth restriction, and craniosynostosis.[14] Neonatal findings include diffuse goiter, vomiting, diarrhea, poor weight gain, hepatosplenomegaly, thrombocytopenia, hypertension, cardiac arrhythmia, and exophthalmos.

## DIAGNOSIS

Clinical suspicion is the key to diagnosis of thyroid disorders, as it leads to appropriate laboratory tests to confirm or refute the diagnosis. Symptoms of hypothyroidism, hyperthyroidism, or anterior cervical discomfort, for example, warrant further evaluation. TSH is typically the initial test recommended, with current TSH assays demonstrating improved sensitivities at or below 0.01 mU/L. Results from analysis of the National Health and Nutrition Examination Survey (NHANES III) data demonstrate that the normal upper range for TSH in adults in the United States is 2.5 to 3.5 mU/L.[15] In patients with clinical suspicion, monoclonal TSH assay has 98% sensitivity and 92% specificity.[16] It is important to remember, however, that a low TSH value based on older TSH normal range data is found in up to 15% of normal pregnancies in the first trimester. Furthermore, recent data in pregnant women suggest that the upper limit for TSH and other thyroid function varies with gestational age.[6,17]

A careful examination of the thyroid gland may also suggest the need for additional evaluation. For example, a firm, lumpy, irregularly shaped, enlarged thyroid gland is most often associated with autoimmune/Hashimoto's thyroiditis. A soft, spongy goiter is more commonly seen in patients with Graves' disease, inherited disorders of thyroid hormone synthesis, or iodine deficiency but may also be seen in autoimmune thyroiditis in adolescents and young adults. Serum thyroid antibodies, especially the thyroid peroxidase antibodies (TPOAbs), are the diagnostic test for autoimmune thyroid disease (Hashimoto's thyroiditis), since they are present in 95% of cases. By contrast only 60% of these patients will have positive thyroglobulin antibodies (TGAbs).[15]

Among women with known hypothyroidism prior to pregnancy who receive L-thyroxine therapy, 35% to 62% with autoimmune hypothyroidism will require a dosage increase; and 70% to 100% of athyreotic women with congenital athyreosis, following [131]I ablation therapy or thyroidectomy, require a dosage increase. In fact, some thyroidologists recommend that women with established hypothyroidism receiving L-thyroxine therapy increase their $T_4$ dose by 30% as soon as they suspect that they are pregnant.[18]

Since the thyroid immunoglobulins are IgG subclass 1 and can therefore readily cross the placenta from mother to fetus, the TSIs can cause fetal and neonatal thyrotoxicosis,[19] whereas the TBIs may affect fetal and neonatal hypothyroidism.[20,21] Most cost-effective TSH receptor antibody (TRAb) assays, however, do not distinguish between a TSH-receptor stimulating immunoglobulin, or antibody (TSI), as seen in active Graves' disease with hyperthyroidism[19] and a TSH-receptor blocking antibody (TBI), as seen in Hashimoto's thyroiditis with hypothyroidism.[21] Therefore, although the potential consequences of the transmission of these antibodies across the placenta to the fetus are significant,[20] the utility of immunoglobulin titers in the clinical surveillance of pregnancy is uncertain. The American College of Obstetricians and Gynecologists (ACOG) 2002 Practice Bulletin on thyroid disease in pregnancy states that testing for TRAb (refers to an assay that measures TSI, TBI, and TBII) titers remains controversial.[11]

Although mild thyroid enlargement is commonly seen in pregnancy, a thyroid nodule should be evaluated in the same manner as in the nonpregnant state. An ultrasound-guided, fine-needle aspiration biopsy of the nodule, serum TSH, and $FT_4$ are the preferred initial tests to determine whether the nodule is benign or malignant.[22]

Newborn screening programs for hypothyroidism include testing for TSH alone (primary TSH screening), $T_4$ as the primary test and TSH as a confirmatory test on the lowest percentile of $T_4$ values (usually the lowest 10%), or TSH and $T_4$ initially. The screening tests are performed on blood from a heel prick that is applied to a filter paper specimen that is collected from 24 hours to 3 days after delivery. The goal of newborn screening is to detect and treat neonates with primary hypothyroidism (high TSH, low $T_4$) as early as possible to prevent impaired intellectual development and neurobehavioral disabilities. Every infant with an abnormal TSH screen should have

a serum TSH to confirm the diagnosis, and a serum $FT_4$ to assess the degree of hypothyroidism to determine the appropriate dose of L-thyroxine. Therapy should be initiated pending confirmation, and may be discontinued if the test returns normal. Most physicians also obtain an imaging study, most commonly a thyroid ultrasound, to diagnose possible causes such as an absent thyroid gland (athyreosis), small thyroid (hypoplasia), thyroid tissue in another location that is usually in the cervical region (ectopia), or a normal or enlarged thyroid as seen with inherited disorders of thyroid hormone synthesis.

Some programs that include $T_4$ as a screening test also include further tests to detect central (hypothalamic/pituitary) hypothyroidism with the findings of a low $T_4$ and a TSH that is not elevated as expected in primary hypothyroidism. These additional tests, however, require recalling approximately 3% of the population for an uncommon group of diseases that occurs in approximately 1 in 20,000 infants in Europe and 1 in 50,000 infants in North America.

## TREATMENT

Hyperthyroidism during pregnancy is typically treated with thioamide drugs (propylthiouracil [PTU] and methimazole [MTZ] in the United States and also carbimazole [CBZ]) in other parts of the world. CBZ is functionally the same as MTZ, since the former is enzymatically converted to MTZ in vivo. Their primary mechanisms of action are competitive inhibition of thyroglobulin iodination and iodothyronine biosynthesis. PTU also inhibits conversion of $T_4$ to $T_3$.[23]

PTU has been traditionally preferred to MTZ in the United States in pregnant women owing to reportedly more limited passage across the placenta, inhibition of conversion of $T_4$ to $T_3$, and the reported link between aplasia cutis and methimazole. There is evidence, however, to suggest that both drugs are safe and effective in pregnancy.[24] The goal of therapy in pregnancy is to achieve control with minimal drug dosage, and the target maternal $FT_4$ should be in the high-normal range. PTU therapy is prescribed in divided doses, with a reasonable initial regimen being 100 to 150 mg three times daily. Often the dose can be deceased in the third trimester. Possible side effects of PTU therapy (1% to 5% incidence) include rash, itching, fever, hepatitis, bronchospasm, and the most serious complication of agranulocytosis and hepatitis.[25] Both PTU and MTZ are compatible with breastfeeding.[26]

The thioamides are not effective in the treatment of the thyrotoxic phase of postpartum thyroiditis, since this is not caused by an overproduction of thyroid hormone but rather by excessive release from the disrupted thyroid gland. β-Blockers such as metoprolol and atenolol can, however, be utilized in the treatment of symptomatic tachycardia, tremors, and anxiety.

Thyroidectomy is a possible therapeutic option for severe thyrotoxicosis during pregnancy. However, despite considerable advances in anesthesia, thyroidectomy during pregnancy is associated with a higher perioperative complication rate owing to increased vascularity of the thyroid gland. Short-term potassium iodide therapy can be utilized in combination with PTU and β-blockers in the treatment of severe thyrotoxicosis and during the preoperative preparation of the patient to decrease vascularity.[27]

Radioactive iodine treatment, which is the most commonly used therapy for Graves' disease because of its efficacy and cost effectiveness, is *contraindicated* and not a therapeutic option in pregnancy owing to the potential for fetal thyroid ablation. Women who have been treated with radioiodine for hyperthyroidism should avoid pregnancy for 1 year after treatment.[28]

Thyroid crisis is a very rare complication of Graves' disease. It requires prompt treatment with β-blockers (the most important therapeutic modality), sodium iodide infusion, PTU, and hypothermia. β-Blockers are utilized to reverse the hyperadrenergic state and to control the heart rate and thereby to improve cardiac output and also inhibit the peripheral conversion of $T_4$ to $T_3$. PTU may be administered acutely by mouth or nasogastric tube. Sodium iodide is administered intravenously to inhibit thyroid release.[29] Acetaminophen is the drug of choice for treatment of pyrexia because salicylates can displace $T_3$ and $T_4$ from TBG.[30] A hypothermic blanket and maintenance of fluid and electrolyte balance and normovolemia are most important. A schematic for treatment of thyroid crisis in pregnancy is depicted in Figure 63-1.[29]

Hypothyroidism in pregnancy should be treated as soon as the diagnosis is made in order to minimize fetal and neonatal sequelae. Thyroxine should be initiated at a dose of 2.0 μg/kg of pregnancy weight once daily.[31] TSH should be repeated in 2 to 4 weeks and the dose adjusted until the TSH is in the target range. Patients should be informed that iron included in prenatal vitamins and calcium tablets (e.g., Tums) can interfere with thyroxine absorption in the gastrointestinal tract, and thyroid supplement intake should be timed accordingly.

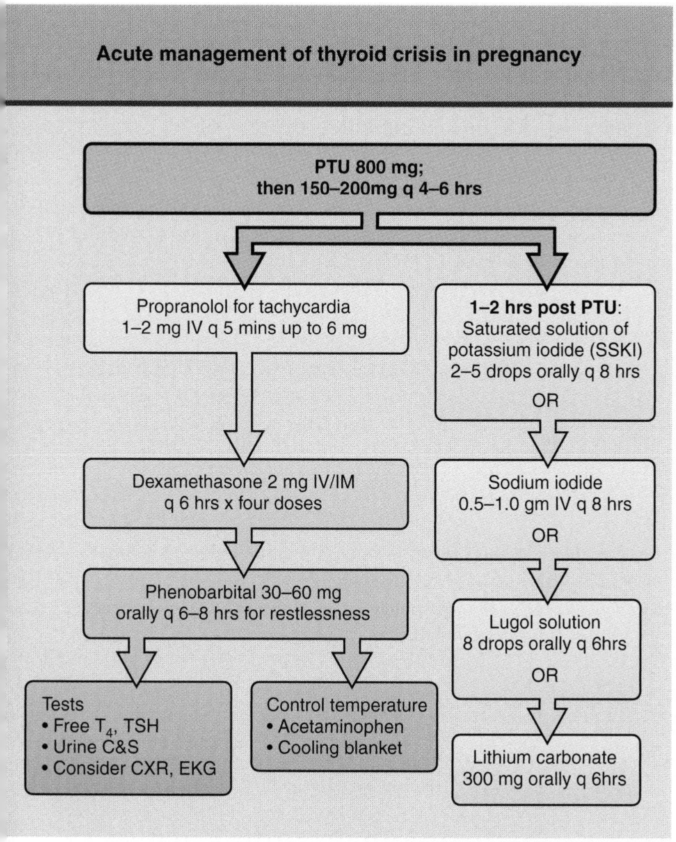

In cases of pregestationally diagnosed hypothyroidism, women should continue to take thyroxine. An increase in thyroxine dose is usually necessary with advancing pregnancy. TSH testing should be repeated 2 to 4 weeks after a dose change and every 8 to 12 weeks thereafter in women who are euthyroid at initial assessment.

Postpartum thyroiditis requires treatment only if symptomatic. The transient hyperthyroid phase is treated with β-blockers and the hypothyroid phase with thyroxine replacement.

Women who have thyroid carcinoma are treated surgically, optimally in the second trimester. Delay until the postpartum period is also an acceptable option in cases of well-differentiated papillary and selected cases of follicular thyroid carcinoma without evidence of extrathyroidal extension or distant metastasis.[5]

## CLINICAL COURSE AND PROGRESSION

Diagnosis and appropriate treatment of pregestational hypothyroidism are essential for optimal pregnancy outcome for mother and child. Programs that ensure adequate maternal iodine intake are crucial in the effort to reduce the incidence of fetal hypothyroidism and cretinism worldwide.[3] In iodine-sufficient populations, undiagnosed or inadequately treated maternal hypothyroidism during pregnancy has been associated with adverse pregnancy outcomes and suboptimal neuropsychological development in the euthyroid children.[8]

Hyperthyroidism in pregnancy is associated with increased risk of preterm labor, spontaneous abortion, low birth weight, preeclampsia, and heart failure. PTU dosing should be adjusted frequently to minimize fetal effects by utilizing the lowest dose that maintains $T_4/FT_4$ in the high-normal and TSH in the low-normal range. The dose can often be reduced or therapy discontinued in the third trimester.

Utilizing the minimal dose is important because of the reported association between PTU dose and clinical neonatal hypothyroidism, with 50% incidence of neonatal hypothyroidism in infants of mothers treated with PTU dose greater than 300 mg/day.[24]

The incidence of neonatal Graves' disease is 1% to 5% in newborns of mothers with hyperthyroidism secondary to maternal Graves' disease.[32] The low incidence is thought to be secondary to the combination of stimulatory and inhibitory immunoglobulins that cross the placenta.[33] Findings of neonatal hyperthyroidism include high baseline heart rate, goiter, advanced bone age, and craniosynostosis. With regard to follow-up of the neonate, it is important to remember that thioamides are cleared more rapidly than the stimulatory TSH-receptor antibodies. Furthermore, infants of euthyroid women treated with surgery or radioactive iodine in the past may still be at significant risk for neonatal Graves' disease, since immunoglobulin production may still be present.

As previously mentioned, clinical signs and symptoms of CH can be masked, in part, during the early newborn period by the presence of maternal thyroxine. However, transplacentally acquired maternal thyroxine does not completely normalize

**Figure 63-1** Acute management of thyroid crisis in pregnancy. (From Winkler CL, Davis LD: Endocrine emergencies. In Dildy GA, Belfort MA, Saade GR, et al [eds]: Critical Care Obstetrics, 4th ed. Malden, Mass, Blackwell Science, 2004, pp 423–428.)

**Acute management of thyroid crisis in pregnancy**

PTU 800 mg; then 150–200mg q 4–6 hrs

Propranolol for tachycardia 1–2 mg IV q 5 mins up to 6 mg

1–2 hrs post PTU: Saturated solution of potassium iodide (SSKI) 2–5 drops orally q 8 hrs
OR

Dexamethasone 2 mg IV/IM q 6 hrs x four doses

Sodium iodide 0.5–1.0 gm IV q 8 hrs
OR

Phenobarbital 30–60 mg orally q 6–8 hrs for restlessness

Lugol solution 8 drops orally q 6hrs
OR

Tests
• Free $T_4$, TSH
• Urine C&S
• Consider CXR, EKG

Control temperature
• Acetaminophen
• Cooling blanket

Lithium carbonate 300 mg orally q 6hrs

neonatal thyroid function in infants with CH, with the possible exception of very low birth weight (VLBW) infants. If CH is unrecognized and untreated, cretinism can ensue. For this reason, neonatal screening is mandated in the 50 states and the District of Columbia.

## PITFALLS AND CONTROVERSIES

The diagnosis of hyperthyroidism may be difficult to make in early pregnancy as a result of the clinical overlap of signs and symptoms with those of normal early pregnancy and because TSH can be suppressed by hCG-mediated stimulation of the TSH receptor. If the TSH result is depressed in the first trimester, it should be repeated in the second trimester.

Normal values for TSH in pregnancy are rarely provided by commercial laboratories for reference.

The application of antibody titer levels to clinical practice in pregnancy surveillance remains controversial.

Universal screening of women before or during pregnancy, although an attractive idea, is currently not recommended.

## REFERENCES

1. Lazarus JH: Epidemiology and prevention of thyroid disease in pregnancy. Thyroid 2002;12:861–865. (IV, C)
2. Roberts CG, Ladenson PW: Hypothyroidism. Lancet 2004;363:793–803. (IV, C)
3. Delange F, de Benoist B, Pretell E, Dunn JT: Iodine deficiency in the world: where do we stand at the turn of the century? Thyroid 2001; 11:437–447. (IV, C)
4. Jameson JL, Weetman AP: Disorders of the thyroid gland. In Braunwald E, Fauci AS, Kasper DL, et al (eds): Harrison's Principles of Internal Medicine, 15th ed. New York, McGraw-Hill, 2001, pp 2060–2084. (IV, C)
5. Moosa M, Mazzaferri EL: Outcome of differentiated thyroid cancer diagnosed in pregnant women. J Clin Endocrinol Metab 1997; 82:2862–2868. (III, B)
6. Vernmiglio F, Lo Presti VP, Castagna MG, et al: Increased risk of maternal thyroid failure with pregnancy progression in an iodine deficient area with major iodine deficiency disorders. Thyroid 1999; 9:19–24. (III, B)
7. Thorpe-Beeston JG, Nicolaides KH, Felton CV, et al: Maturation of the secretion of thyroid hormone and thyroid-stimulating hormone in the fetus. N Engl J Med 1991;324:532–536. (IIa, B)
8. Fisher DA: Disorders of the thyroid in the newborn and infant. In Sperling MA (ed): Pediatric Endocrinology, 2nd ed. Saunders/Elsevier Science, Philadelphia, 2002, pp 161–185. (IV, C)
9. Haddow JE, Palomaki GE, Allan WC, et al: Maternal thyroid deficiency during pregnancy and subsequent neuropsychological development of the child. N Engl J Med 1999;341:549–555. (IIb, B)
10. Pop VJ, Brouwers EP, Vulsma T, et al: Maternal hypothyroxemia during early pregnancy and subsequent child development: a 3-year follow-up study. Clin Endocrinol 2003;59:282–288. (IIa, B)
11. American College of Obstetricians and Gynecologists: Thyroid disease in pregnancy. ACOG Practice Bulletin. Clinical Management Guidelines for Obstetrician-Gynecologists. No. 37, August 2002. Obstet Gynecol 2002;100:387. (IV, C)
12. De Felice M, Di Lauro R: Thyroid disorders and its development: genetics and molecular mechanisms. Endocr Rev 2004;25:722–746. (IV, C)
13. LaFranchi S: Congenital hypothyroidism: etiologies, diagnosis and management. Thyroid 1999;9:735–740. (IV, C)
14. Becks GP, Burrow GN: Thyroid diseases and pregnancy. Med Clin North Am 1991;75:121–150. (IV, C)
15. Hollowell JG, Staehling NW, Flanders WD, et al: Serum TSH, $T_4$ and thyroid antibodies in the United States population (1988 to 1994): National Health and Nutrition Examination Survey (NHANES III). J Clin Endocrinol Metab 2002;87:489–499 (IIa, B)
16. U.S. Preventive Services Task Force: Screening for thyroid disease: recommendation statement. Ann Intern Med 2004;140:125–127. (IV, C)
17. Mandel SJ, Spencer CA, Hollowell JG: Are detection and treatment of thyroid insufficiency in pregnancy feasible? Thyroid 2005;15:44–53. (III, B)
18. Alexander EK, Marqusee E, Lawrence J, et al: Timing and magnitude of increases in levothyroxine requirements during pregnancy in women with hypothyroidism. N Engl J Med 2004;351:241–249. (III, B)
19. Foley TP Jr, White C, New A: Juvenile Graves' disease: the usefulness and limitations of thyrotropin receptor antibody determinations. J Pediatr 1987;110:378–386. (IV, C)
20. Foley TP Jr: Maternally transferred thyroid disease in the infant: recognition and treatment. In Bercu BB, Schulman DI (eds): Advances in Perinatal Thyroidology. New York, Plenum Press, 1991, pp 209–226. (IV, C)
21. Brown RS, Belissario RL, Botero D, et al: Incidence of transient congenital hypothyroidism due to maternal thyrotropin receptor-blocking antibodies in over one million babies. J Clin Endocrinol Metab 1996;81:1147–1151. (III, B)
22. Tan GH, Gharib H, Goellner JR, et al: Management of thyroid nodules in pregnancy. Arch Intern Med 1996;156:2317–2320. (IV, C)
23. Mandel SJ, Cooper DS: The use of antithyroid drugs in pregnancy and lactation. J Clin Endocrinol Metab 2001;86:2354–2359. (IV, C)
24. Wing DA, Millar LK, Koonings PP, et al: A comparison of propylthiouracil versus methimazole in the treatment of hyperthyroidism in pregnancy. Am J Obstet Gynecol 1994;170:90–95. (IIa, B)
25. Cooper DS: The side effects of antithyroid drugs. Endocrinologist 1999;9:457–467. (III, B)
26. Briggs GG, Freeman RK, Yaffe SJ: Drugs in Pregnancy and Lactation: A Reference Guide to Fetal and Neonatal Risk. Baltimore, Md, Williams & Wilkins, 1998. (III, B)
27. Burrow GN, Fisher DA, Larsen PR: Maternal and fetal thyroid function. N Engl J Med 1994;331:1072–1078. (IV, C)
28. Ayala C, Navarro E, Rodriguez JR, et al: Conception after iodine-131 therapy for differentiated thyroid cancer. Thyroid 1998;811:1009–1011 (IV, C)
29. Winkler CL, Davis LD: Endocrine emergencies. In Dildy GA, Belfort MA, Saade GR, et al (eds): Critical Care Obstetrics, 4th ed. Malden, Mass, Blackwell Science, 2004, pp 423–428. (IV, C)
30. Larsen PR: Salicylate-induced increases in free triiodothyronine in human serum: evidence of inhibition of triiodothyronine binding to thyroxine-binding globulin and thyroxine-binding prealbumin. J Clin Invest 1972;51:1125–1134. (IIb, B)
31. Montoro MN: Management of hypothyroidism during pregnancy. Clin Obstet Gynecol 1997;40:65–80. (IV, C)
32. Weetman AP: Medical Progress: Graves' disease. N Engl J Med 2000; 343:1236–1248. (IV, C)
33. Laurberg P, Nygaard B, Glinoer D, et al: Guidelines for TSH-receptor antibody measurements in pregnancy: results of an evidence-based symposium organized by the ETA. Eur J Endocrinol Metab 1998; 139:584–590. (IV, C)

# Chapter 64

# Disorders of the Adrenal Gland

## Carla P. Roberts, MD, PhD

### KEY POINTS

- The adrenal gland is responsible for the production of cortisol, aldosterone, and the adrenal androgens.
- Exogenous corticosteroids may result in adrenal suppression within a relatively short time frame, so cortisol deficiency states should always be suspected and evaluated.
- Acute adrenal insufficiency is an emergency.
- Chronic adrenal insufficiency can become an emergency in the setting of superimposed stress or illness without adequate corticosteroid replacement.
- Late-onset congenital adrenal hyperplasia may masquerade as polycystic ovary syndrome. This enzymatic deficiency should be ruled out.

## INTRODUCTION

The anatomy of the adrenal glands was described 450 years ago by Bartholomeo Eustacius; however, a functional role for the adrenal glands was not defined until the pioneering work of Thomas Addison in 1855. Table 64-1 demonstrates the remarkable pathway of the history of the adrenal gland that allows us to manipulate and manage the steroidogenic disorders discussed in this chapter. A review of mineralocorticoids, pheochromocytomas, and other disorders of endocrine hypertension is not included in this discussion.

The control of adrenocortical function by a pituitary factor was demonstrated in the 1920s, and this led to the isolation of sheep adrenocorticotropic hormone (ACTH) in 1943. Such a concept was supported through clinical studies, notably in 1932 by Harvey Cushing, who associated his original clinical observations of 1912 (a "polyglandular syndrome" caused by pituitary basophilism) with adrenal hyperactivity. The neural control of pituitary ACTH secretion by corticotropin-releasing hormone (CRH) was defined by Harris and other workers in the 1940s, but CRH was not characterized and synthesized until 1981 in the laboratory of Wylie Vale.

Located on top of the kidneys, the adrenal glands are triangular shaped and measure approximately a half-inch in height and 3 inches in length. The inner adrenal medulla secretes epinephrine and norepinephrine, which affect blood pressure, heart rate, and sweating. The outer cortex secretes hormones as well as mineralocorticoids (Fig. 64-1). Three main types of hormones are produced by the adrenal cortex: glucocorticoids (cortisol, corticosterone), mineralocorticoids (aldosterone, deoxycorticosterone [DOC]), and sex steroids (mainly andro-

gens). All steroid hormones are derived from the cyclopentanoperhydrophenanthrene structure, that is, three cyclohexane rings and a single cyclopentane ring. Figure 64-2 depicts the steroidogenic pathway found in the adrenal gland. Steroidogenesis in the adrenal gland involves a coordinated action of several enzymes, including a series of cytochrome P-450 enzymes. Most of these enzymes have been cloned and characterized, and mutations in the genes encoding these enzymes result in human disease, so some understanding of the underlying pathways and steroid precursors is required (Table 64-2). Recent studies have confirmed the importance of a 30-kd protein, steroidogenic acute regulatory protein (StAR), in mediating this effect. StAR is induced by an increase in intracellular cyclic adenosine monophosphate after the binding of ACTH to its receptor, providing the first important rate-limiting step in adrenal steroidogenesis.

ACTH is the principal hormone stimulating adrenal glucocorticoid biosynthesis and secretion. ACTH has 39 amino acids but is synthesized within the anterior pituitary as part of a much larger 241–amino acid precursor, pro-opiomelanocortin (POMC). POMC is cleaved in tissue-specific fashion to yield smaller peptide hormones. In the anterior pituitary this results in the secretion of β-lipoprotein and pro-ACTH, the latter being further cleaved to an N-terminal peptide, joining peptide, and ACTH itself (Fig. 64-3). The functions of the N-terminal peptide and β-lipoprotein are unknown, although they have weak steroidogenic activity of their own and may augment the effect of ACTH, particularly on stimulating adrenal growth. The first 24 amino acids of ACTH are common to all species, and synthetic ACTH 1 to 24 (cosyntropin) is available commercially for clinical testing of the hypothalamic-pituitary-adrenal (HPA) axis and assessment of adrenal glucocorticoid reserve. Melanocyte-stimulating hormones (MSH-α, -β, and -γ) are also cleaved products from POMC.

CRH is the principal stimulus for ACTH secretion. The peak response of ACTH to CRH does not differ throughout the day, but it is affected by endogenous function of the HPA axis in that responsiveness is reduced in subjects treated with corticosteroids but increased in subjects with Cushing's disease. ACTH is secreted in pulsatile fashion with a circadian rhythm so that levels are highest on waking and decline throughout the day, reaching lowest values in the evening. ACTH pulse frequency is higher in normal adult men than in women (on average 18 pulses vs. 10 pulses per 24 hours), and the circadian ACTH rhythm appears to be mediated principally by an increased ACTH pulse amplitude between 5 and 9 AM but also by a reduction in ACTH pulse frequency between 6 and 12 PM. Food ingestion is a further stimulus to ACTH secretion. Circadian rhythm is dependent on both day-night and sleep-wake patterns and is disrupted by alternating day-night shift working patterns and by

# Reproductive Endocrinology and Infertility

**Table 64-1**
**Milestones in Clinical Adrenal Medicine**

| | |
|---|---|
| 1563 | Eustachius describes the adrenals (published by Lancisi in 1714) |
| 1849 | Thomas Addison, while searching for the cause of pernicious anemia, "stumbles" on a bronzed appearance associated with the adrenal glands—"melasma suprarenale" |
| 1855 | Thomas Addison describes the clinical features and autopsy findings of 11 cases of diseases of the suprarenal capsules, at least 6 of which were tuberculous in origin |
| 1856 | In adrenalectomy experiments, Brown-Séquard demonstrates that the adrenal glands are essential for life |
| 1896 | William Osler gives an oral glycerine extract derived from pig adrenals and demonstrates clinical benefit in patients with Addison's disease |
| 1905 | Bulloch and Sequeria describe patients with congenital adrenal hyperplasia |
| 1929 | Liquid extracts of cortical tissue are used to keep adrenalectomized cats alive indefinitely (Swingle and Pfiffner); subsequently, this extract was used successfully to treat a patient with Addison's disease (Rowntree and Greene) |
| 1932 | Harvey Cushing associates the "polyglandular syndrome" of pituitary basophilism first described by himself in 1912 with hyperactivity of the pituitary-adrenal glands |
| 1936 | Concept of stress and its effect upon pituitary-adrenal function described by Seyle |
| 1937–1952 | Isolation and structural characterization of adrenocortical hormones (Kendall, Reichstein) |
| 1943 | Li and colleagues isolate pure adrenocorticotropic hormone from sheep pituitary |
| 1950 | Hench, Kendall, and Reichstein share Nobel Prize in Medicine for describing the anti-inflammatory effects of cortisone in patients with rheumatoid arthritis |
| 1953 | Isolation and analysis of the structure of aldosterone (Simpson and Tait) |
| 1956 | Conn describes primary aldosteronism |
| 1981 | Characterization and synthesis of corticotropin-releasing hormone (Vale) |
| 1980–present | The "molecular era": cloning and functional characterization of steroid receptors, steroidogenic enzymes, and adrenal transcription factors; definition of the molecular basis for human adrenal diseases |

From Larsen PR, Kronenberg HM, Melmed S, et al: (eds): Williams Textbook of Endocrinology, 10th ed. Philadelphia, WB Saunders, 2002, p 492.

**Anatomy of the adrenal glands**

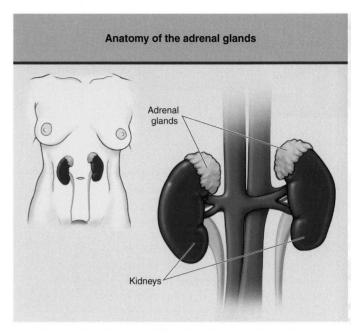

**Figure 64-1    Anatomy of the adrenal glands.** (From A.D.A.M.)

The effects of ACTH on the adrenal include both immediate and chronic effects; the end result is the stimulation of adrenal steroidogenesis and growth. Acutely, steroidogenesis is stimulated through a StAR-mediated increase in cholesterol delivery to the CYP11A1 enzyme in the inner mitochondrial membrane. Chronically (within 24 to 26 hours of exposure), ACTH acts to increase the synthesis of all steroidogenic CYP enzymes (CYP11A1, CYP17, CYP21A2, CYP11B1) in addition to adrenodoxin, effects that are mediated at the transcriptional level. ACTH also increases synthesis of the low-density lipoprotein (LDL) and high-density lipoprotein (HDL) receptors and possibly also 3-hydroxy-3-methylglutaryl coenzyme A reductase, the rate-limiting step in cholesterol biosynthesis. ACTH increases adrenal weight by inducing both hyperplasia and hypertrophy. Adrenal atrophy is a feature of ACTH deficiency.[2]

**Table 64-2**
**Gene Location for Adrenal Steroidogenic Enzymes**

| Enzyme Name | Gene | Chromosome |
|---|---|---|
| Cholesterol side-chain cleavage (SCC) (desmolase) | CYP11A1 | 15q23–q24 |
| 3β-Hydroxysteroid dehydrogenase (3β-HSD) (type II isozyme) | HSD3B2 | 1p13.1 |
| 17α-Hydroxylase/17,20 lyase | CYP17 | 10q24.3 |
| 21-Hydroxylase | CYP21A2 | 6p21.3 |
| 11β-Hydroxylase | CYP11B1 | 8q24.3 |
| Aldosterone synthetase | CYP11B2 | 8q24.3 |

From Larsen PR, Kronenberg HM, Melmed S, et al: (eds): Williams Textbook of Endocrinology, 10th ed. Philadelphia, WB Saunders, 2002, p 495.

long-distance travel across time zones. It may take up to 2 weeks for circadian rhythm to reset to an altered day-night cycle.

An important aspect of CRH and ACTH secretion is the negative feedback control exerted by glucocorticoids themselves. Glucocorticoids inhibit POMC gene transcription in the anterior pituitary and CRH messenger RNA (mRNA) synthesis and secretion in the hypothalamus. This negative feedback effect is dependent on the dose, potency, half-life, and duration of administration of the glucocorticoid and has important physiologic and diagnostic consequences. Suppression of the HPA axis by pharmacologic corticosteroids may persist for many months after cessation of therapy, and adrenocortical insufficiency should be anticipated.[1]

## Adrenal steroid pathway

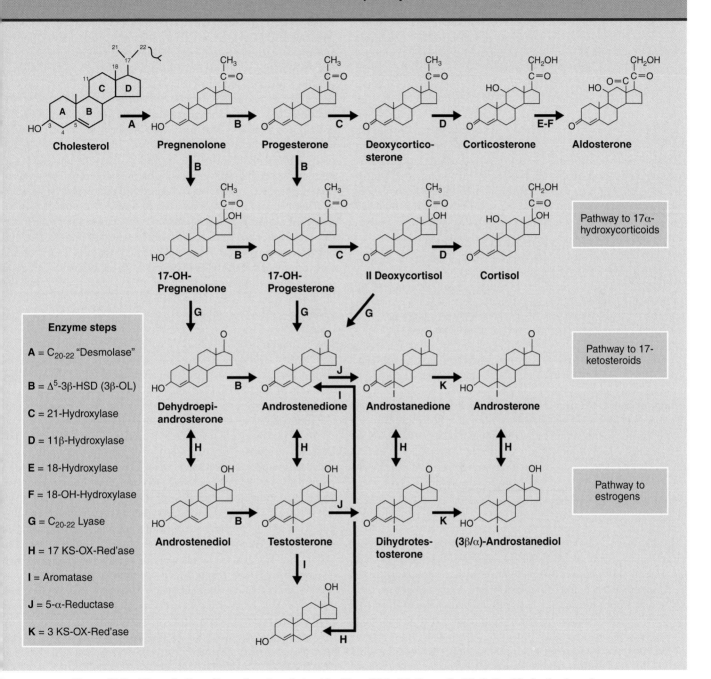

**Figure 64-2 Biosynthetic pathway for adrenal steroids.** (From White PC, Pescovitz OH, Cutler GB: Synthesis and metabolism of corticosteroids. In Becker KL, Bilezikian JP, Hung W, et al [eds]: Principles and Practice of Endocrinology and Metabolism, 2nd ed. Philadelphia, JB Lippincott, 1995, p 650.)

## Mineralocorticoid Secretion: Renin-Angiotensin-Aldosterone Axis

Aldosterone is secreted from the zona glomerulosa under the control of angiotensin II, potassium, and to a lesser extent ACTH. Other factors, notably somatostatin, heparin, atrial natriuretic factor, and dopamine, can directly inhibit aldosterone synthesis. The secretion of aldosterone and its intermediary 18-hydroxylated metabolites is restricted to the zona glomerulosa because of the zona-specific expression of CYP11B2 (aldosterone synthase). Corticosterone and DOC, although synthesized in both the zona fasciculata and the zona glomerulosa, can act as mineralocorticoids; this becomes significant in some clinical diseases, notably, some forms of congenital adrenal hyperplasia (CAH) and adrenal tumors. Similarly, it is now established that cortisol can act as a mineralocorticoid in the setting of impaired metabolism to cortisone carried out by the enzyme 11β-hydroxysteroid

# Reproductive Endocrinology and Infertility

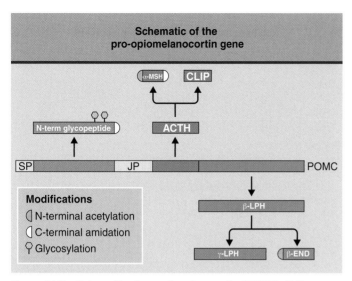

**Figure 64-3  Schematic of pro-opiomelanocortin (POMC).** CLIP, corticotropin-like intermediate lobe peptide; β-END, β-endorphin; JP, joining peptide; β-LPH, β-lipotropin; γ-LPH, γ-lipotropin; α-MSH, α–melanocyte-stimulating hormone; SP, signal peptide. (From White PC, Pescovitz OH, Cutler GB: Synthesis and metabolism of corticosteroids. In Becker KL, Bilezikian JP, Hung W, et al [eds]: Principles and Practice of Endocrinology and Metabolism, 2nd ed. Philadelphia, JB Lippincott, 1995, p 1489.)

dehydrogenase (HSD); this is important in patients with hypertension, ectopic ACTH syndrome, and renal disease.

The rate-limiting step in the renin-angiotensin system is the secretion of renin, which is also controlled through a negative feedback loop. Renin is secreted from juxtaglomerular epithelial cells within the macula densa of the renal tubule in response to underlying renal arteriolar pressure, oncotic pressure, and sympathetic drive. Thus, low perfusion pressure or low tubular fluid sodium content, as seen in hemorrhage, renal artery stenosis, dehydration, or salt loss, increases renin secretion. Conversely, secretion is suppressed by a high-salt diet and by factors that increase blood pressure. Autoregulation is therefore maintained because the increase in renin secretion stimulates angiotensin II and aldosterone production; the concomitant increase in blood pressure and renal sodium retention results in feedback inhibition of renin secretion.

Hypokalemia increases and hyperkalemia decreases renin secretion; in addition, potassium exerts a direct effect on the adrenal cortex to increase aldosterone secretion. The sensitivity of the renin-angiotensin system to changes in circulating potassium is high, with changes in potassium concentrations of only 0.1 to 0.5 mmol/L producing marked changes in aldosterone concentrations. Potassium concentrations also determine the sensitivity of the aldosterone response to a given infusion of angiotensin II, with high potassium intake increasing responsiveness.

The effect of ACTH on aldosterone secretion is modest and differs in the acute and chronic situations. An acute bolus of ACTH increases aldosterone secretion, principally by stimulating the early pathways of adrenal steroidogenesis, but circulating levels increase by no more than 10% to 20% above baseline values. ACTH has no effect on *CYP11B2* gene transcription or

enzyme activity. Chronic continual ACTH stimulation has either no effect or an inhibitory effect on aldosterone production, possibly because of receptor down-regulation or suppression of angiotensin II–stimulated secretion because of a mineralocorticoid effect of cortisol, DOC, or corticosterone. Dopamine and atrial natriuretic peptide inhibit aldosterone secretion, as does heparin.

The separate control of glucocorticoid biosynthesis through the HPA axis and mineralocorticoid synthesis through the renin-angiotensin system has important clinical consequences. Patients with primary adrenal failure invariably have both cortisol and aldosterone deficiency, whereas patients with ACTH deficiency related to pituitary disease have glucocorticoid deficiency but normal aldosterone concentrations because the renin-angiotensin system is intact.

## Adrenal Androgen Secretion

Adrenal androgens represent an important component (>50%) of circulating androgens in premenopausal females. In males this contribution is much smaller because of the testicular production of androgens, but adrenal androgen excess even in males may be of clinical significance, notably in patients with CAH. The adult adrenal secretes dehydroepiandrosterone (DHEA) at approximately 4 mg/day, dehydroepiandrosterone sulfate (DHEAS) at 7 to 15 mg/day, androstenedione at 1.5 mg/day, and testosterone at 0.05 mg/day. DHEA is a weak sex steroid but can be converted to androgens and estrogens through the activities of 3β-HSD, a superfamily of 17β-HSD isozymes, and aromatase, expressed in peripheral target tissues, and this is of clinical importance in many diseases.

ACTH stimulates androgen secretion; DHEA (but not DHEAS because of its increased plasma half-life) and androstenedione demonstrate a similar circadian rhythm to cortisol. However, there are many discrepancies between adrenal androgen and glucocorticoid secretion, which has led to the suggestion of an additional androgen-stimulating hormone. Many putative androgen-stimulating hormones have been proposed including POMC derivatives such as joining peptide, prolactin, and insulin-like growth factor-1 (IGF-1), but conclusive proof is lacking. Adrenal androgen steroidogenesis is dependent on the relative activities of 3β-HSD and 17α-hydroxylase and in particular on the 17,20-lyase activity of 17α-hydroxylase. Factors that determine whether 17-hydroxylated substrates, 17-hydroxypregnenolone and 17-hydroxyprogesterone (17-OHP), undergo 21-hydroxylation to form glucocorticoid or side-chain cleavage by 17α-hydroxylase to form DHEA and androstenedione are unresolved and seem likely to be important in defining the activity of any putative androgen-stimulating hormone.[3]

## THERAPEUTIC CORTICOSTEROIDS

Since the anti-inflammatory effect of cortisone was first demonstrated in the 1950s, a series of synthetic corticosteroids have been developed for therapeutic purposes. These are used to treat a diverse variety of human diseases and rely principally on their anti-inflammatory and immunologic actions. The main corticosteroids used in clinical practice, together with their relative glucocorticoid and mineralocorticoid potencies, are shown in Table 64-3.

**Table 64-3**
**Potency Equivalents for Synthetic Steroids**

| Steroid | Anti-inflammatory Action | Hypothalamic-Pituitary-Adrenal Suppression | Salt Retention |
|---|---|---|---|
| Cortisol | 1 | 1 | 1 |
| Prednisolone | 3 | 4 | 0.75 |
| Methylprednisolone | 6.2 | 4 | 0.5 |
| Fludrocortisone | 12 | 12 | 125 |
| $\Delta^1$ Fludrocortisone | 14 | — | 225 |
| Triamcinolone | 5 | 4 | 0 |
| Dexamethasone | 26 | 17 | 0 |

Modified from Axelrod L: Adrenal corticosteroids. In Miller RR, Greenblatt DJ (eds): Handbook of Drug Therapy. New York, Elsevier North-Holland, 1979, p 809; and Axelrod L: Glucocorticoids. In Kelly WN, Harris ED Jr, Ruddy S, Sledge CB (eds): Textbook of Rheumatology, 4th ed. Philadelphia, WB Saunders, 1993, p. 779.

## Chronic Corticosteroid Therapy, Hypothalamic-Pituitary-Adrenal Axis Suppression, and Steroid Withdrawal

The negative feedback control of the HPA axis by endogenous cortisol was discussed earlier. Synthetic corticosteroids similarly suppress the function of the HPA axis through a process that is dependent on both dose and duration of treatment. As a result, sudden cessation of corticosteroid therapy may result in adrenal failure. This may also occur after treatment with high doses of the synthetic progestagen medroxyprogesterone acetate, which possesses glucocorticoid agonist activity. In patients taking any steroid dose for less than 3 weeks, clinically significant suppression of the HPA axis is rarely a problem and patients can withdraw from steroids suddenly with no ill effect. The possible exception is the patient who receives frequent short courses of corticosteroid therapy, for example, patients with recurrent episodes of severe asthma. Conversely, suppression of the HPA axis is invariable in patients taking the equivalent of 15 mg or more of prednisolone per day chronically. In patients taking lower doses of corticosteroid chronically (prednisolone 5 to 15 mg/day or equivalent), suppression of the HPA axis is variable. Defects

in response of the HPA axis to insulin-induced hypoglycemia or exogenous ACTH have been reported in patients taking prednisolone doses as low as 5 mg/day, but clinically significant suppression at these doses is debatable. Alternate-day therapy is associated with less suppression of the HPA axis.

All patients treated chronically with corticosteroids should be treated in a similar fashion to patients with chronic ACTH deficiency; they should carry steroid cards and be offered Steroid Alert bracelets or necklaces. In the event of an intercurrent stress (infection, surgery), supplemental steroid coverage should be given, equivalent to hydrocortisone at 100 to 150 mg/day. If the patient is unable to take drugs orally, parenteral therapy is required.

Recovery from suppression may take 6 to 9 months. CRH secretion returns to normal, and within a few weeks ACTH levels begin to increase and indeed rise above normal values until adrenal steroidogenesis recovers. In the interim, and without replacement therapy, patients may experience symptoms of glucocorticoid deficiency including anorexia, nausea, weight loss, arthralgia, lethargy, skin desquamation, and postural dizziness. To avoid symptoms of glucocorticoid deficiency, steroids should be withdrawn cautiously over a period of months if the clinical course of the underlying disease permits a reduction. The dose should be reduced from a pharmacologic to a physiologic level (equivalent to prednisolone at 7.5 mg/day) over a few weeks. Thereafter doses should be reduced by 1 mg/day prednisolone every 2 to 4 weeks depending on the patient's clinical symptoms. An alternative approach is to change to hydrocortisone at 20 mg/day and reduce the daily dose by 2.5 mg/day every week to 10 mg/day. Nighttime doses should be avoided, since they result in greater suppression of early morning ACTH secretion.[4]

After 2 to 3 months of these reduced doses of corticosteroids, endogenous function of the HPA axis can be assessed through a corticotropin (ACTH, cosyntropin) stimulation test or an insulin-induced hypoglycemia test. A normal response to either of these tests indicates adequacy of function of the HPA axis, and corticosteroid therapy can be safely withdrawn. In patients taking physiologic doses of prednisolone (less than 5 to 7.5 mg/day) or equivalent, a corticotropin stimulation test 12 to 24 hours after having omitted steroid therapy will provide an immediate answer about whether sudden or gradual withdrawal of steroid therapy is indicated (Table 64-4).

**Table 64-4**
**Method to Determine Whether Synthetic Steroid Administration Requires Tapering Before Stopping to Prevent Adrenal Insufficiency**

| Dose (mg Prednisolone/day) | ≤3 weeks | >3 weeks | | |
|---|---|---|---|---|
| ≥7.5 mg | Stop steroid | Reduce rapidly e.g., 2.5 mg every 3–4 days then | | |
| 5–7.5 mg | Stop steroid | Reduce by 1 mg every 2–4 wk | or | Convert 5 mg prednisolone to hydrocortisone 20 mg and decrease by 2.5 mg/wk to 10 mg for 2–3 mo |
| <5 mg | Stop steroid | Reduce by 1 mg every 2–4 wk | | Cortrosyn stimulation test or insulin tolerance test Alternatively administer If pass, withdraw steroid If fail, continue steroid tapering |

From Larsen PR, Kronenberg HM, Melmed S, et al: (eds): Williams Textbook of Endocrinology, 10th ed. Philadelphia, WB Saunders, 2002, p 508.

# DISORDERS OF GLUCOCORTICOID EXCESS

The first case of glucocorticoid excess was described in 1912 by Cushing. The patient was a 23-year-old woman with obesity, hirsutism, and amenorrhea. Glucocorticoid excess is most prevalent in adults between the ages of 20 and 50; it occurs when too much cortisol is produced in the adrenal glands. It can also be caused by excessive or prolonged use of exogenous steroids.

Prolonged natural production of cortisol can be linked to various sources, the most common of which is a tumor of the pituitary gland. The tumor stimulates overproduction of ACTH, which in turn stimulates growth and activity of the adrenal glands. This pituitary hypersecretion of ACTH accounts for 75% to 85% of all Cushing's cases. The other 15% to 25% are due to adrenocortical tumors. The term *Cushing's syndrome* is used to describe all causes, while Cushing's disease is reserved for cases of pituitary-dependent Cushing's syndrome.

Cushing's sufferers can be identified by their characteristic "moon" facies (round and full) and "buffalo" humps (fat collected between the shoulders). The disorder is marked by many other symptoms, the most common of which are obesity (90%), hypertension (80%), diabetes (80%), weakness (80%), excessive body hair (70%), and menstrual abnormalities/sexual dysfunction (70%).[2]

Cushing's syndrome comprises the symptoms and signs associated with prolonged exposure to inappropriately elevated levels of free plasma glucocorticoids (Table 64-5).

## Cushing's Syndrome

The classical features of Cushing's syndrome of centripetal obesity, moon face, hirsutism, and plethora are well known following Cushing's initial descriptions in 1912. Weight gain and obesity are the most common sign, and at least in adults this is invariably centripetal in nature. Interestingly, generalized obesity is more common in the general population than in patients with Cushing's syndrome except in childhood when glucocorticoid excess may result in generalized obesity. In addition to centripetal obesity, patients develop fat depots over the thoracocervical

---

**Table 64-5**
**Common Signs and Symptoms of Cushing's Syndrome**

- Weight gain, particularly around your midsection and upper back
- Severe fatigue
- Muscle weakness
- Rounding of face (moon face)
- Facial flushing
- Fatty pad or hump between shoulders (buffalo hump)
- Thinning of arms and legs
- Pink or purple stretch marks on the skin of abdomen, thighs, breasts, and arms
- Thin and fragile skin that bruises easily
- Slow healing of cuts, insect bites, and infections
- Depression, anxiety, and irritability
- Thicker or more visible body hair (hirsutism)
- Acne
- Irregular or stopped menstrual periods in females
- Erectile dysfunction in males
- High blood pressure

---

spine ("buffalo hump"), in the supraclavicular region, and over the cheeks and temporal regions, giving rise to the rounded moon-like facies. The epidural space is another site of abnormal fat deposition, and this may lead to neurologic deficits.

Gonadal dysfunction is common, with menstrual irregularity in females and loss of libido in both sexes. Hirsutism is frequently found in female patients, as is acne. The most common form of hirsutism is vellus hypertrichosis on the face and should be distinguished from darker terminal differentiated hirsutism, which may occur but usually signifies concomitant androgen excess. Hypogonadism occurs because of a direct inhibitory effect of cortisol on gonadotropin-releasing hormone pulsatility and LH or FSH secretion and is reversible on correction of the hypercortisolism.[3]

Psychiatric abnormalities occur in approximately 50% of patients with Cushing's syndrome regardless of cause. Agitated depression and lethargy are among the most common problems, but paranoia and overt psychosis are also well recognized. Memory and cognitive function may also be affected, and increased irritability may be an early feature. Insomnia is common, and both rapid eye movement and delta wave sleep patterns are reduced. Lowering of plasma cortisol by medical or surgical therapy usually results in a rapid improvement in the psychiatric state.[5]

In childhood the most common presentation is with poor linear growth and weight gain. Many patients with long-standing Cushing's syndrome have lost height because of osteoporotic vertebral collapse. This can be assessed by measuring the patient's height and comparing it with the patient's span; in normal subjects these measurements should be equal. Pathologic fractures, either spontaneous or after minor trauma, are not uncommon. Rib fractures, in contrast to those of the vertebrae, are often painless. The radiographic appearances are typical, with exuberant callus formation at the site of the healing fracture. In addition, aseptic necrosis of the femoral and humeral heads, a recognized feature of high-dose exogenous corticosteroid therapy, can occur in endogenous Cushing's syndrome.

Hypercortisolism results in skin thinning, separation, and exposure of the subcutaneous vascular tissue. On examination, wrinkling of the skin on the dorsum of the hand may be seen resulting in a "cigarette paper" appearance (Liddle's sign). Minimal trauma may result in bruising, which frequently resembles "senile purpura." The plethoric appearance of the patient with Cushing's syndrome is secondary to the thinning of the skin combined with loss of facial subcutaneous fat and is not due to true polycythemia. Acne and papular lesions may occur over the face, chest, and back.

The typical, almost pathognomonic red-purple livid striae greater than 1 cm in diameter are most frequently found on the abdomen but may also be present on the upper thighs, breasts, and arms. They are common in younger patients and less so in those older than 50 years. They must be differentiated from the paler, less pigmented striae that occur postpartum (striae gravidarum) or in association with rapid weight loss. Increased skin pigmentation is rare in Cushing's disease but common in the ectopic ACTH syndrome and arises because of overstimulation of melanocyte receptors by ACTH.

Myopathy and bruising are two of the most discriminatory features of the syndrome. The myopathy of Cushing's syndrome involves the proximal muscles of the lower limb and the shoulder girdle. Complaints of weakness such as inability to climb stairs or get up from a deep chair are relatively uncommon, but testing for proximal myopathy by asking the patient to rise from a crouching position often reveals the problem.

Hypertension is another prominent feature, occurring in up to 75% of cases; even though epidemiologic data show a strong association between blood pressure and obesity, hypertension is more common in patients with Cushing's syndrome than in those with simple obesity. This, together with the established metabolic consequences of the disease (diabetes, hyperlipidemia) is thought to explain the increased cardiovascular mortality in untreated cases. In addition, thromboembolic events may be more common in Cushing's patients.

Infections are more common in patients with Cushing's syndrome. In many instances these are asymptomatic and occur because the normal inflammatory response is suppressed. Reactivation of tuberculosis has been reported and has even been the presenting feature in some cases. Fungal infections of the skin (notably tinea versicolor) and nails may occur, as may opportunistic fungal infections. Bowel perforation is more common in patients with extreme hypercortisolism, and the hypercortisolism may mask the usual symptoms and signs of the condition. Wound infections are more common and contribute to poor wound healing.

Glucose intolerance occurs, and overt diabetes mellitus is present in up to one third of patients in some series. Hepatic lipoprotein synthesis is stimulated, and increases in circulating cholesterol and triglycerides may be found. Hypokalemic alkalosis is found in 10% to 15% of patients with Cushing's disease but in more than 95% of patients with ectopic ACTH syndrome. Several factors may contribute to this mineralocorticoid excess state, including corticosterone and DOC excess, but the principal culprit is thought to be cortisol itself. Depending on the prevailing cortisol production rate, cortisol swamps the normal metabolizing enzyme, 11β-HSD type 2 in the kidney, to act as a mineralocorticoid. Hypokalemic alkalosis is more common in ectopic ACTH syndrome because cortisol production rates are higher than in patients with Cushing's disease. This can be diagnosed by documenting an increase in the ratio of urinary cortisol to cortisone metabolites.

Ocular effects include raised intraocular pressure and exophthalmos (increased retro-orbital fat deposition). Cataracts, a well-recognized complication of corticosteroid therapy, seem to be uncommon except as a complication of diabetes.

## Cushing's Disease

When iatrogenic causes are excluded, the most common cause of Cushing's syndrome is Cushing's disease, accounting for approximately 70% of cases (Table 64-6). The adrenal glands in these patients show bilateral adrenocortical hyperplasia with widening of the zona fasciculata and zona reticularis. The hypothalamic theory states that ACTH-secreting adenomas arise because of dysfunctional regulation of corticotrophs through chronic stimulation by CRH, but other studies provide data to support a primary pituitary defect as the cause of the condition. The hypothalamus may have an initiating role, but the overwhelming evidence is that, at presentation, the condition is pituitary dependent. The majority of tumors are small micro-

| Table 64-6 |
| Classification of Causes of Cushing's Syndrome |

**ACTH-dependent**

Cushing's disease (pituitary-dependent)
Ectopic ACTH syndrome
Ectopic CRH syndrome
Macronodular adrenal hyperplasia
Iatrogenic (treatment with ACTH 1–24)

**ACTH-independent**

Adrenal adenoma and carcinoma
Primary pigmented nodular adrenal hyperplasia and Carney's syndrome
McCune-Albright syndrome
Aberrant receptor expression (gastric inhibitory polypeptide, interleukin-1β)
Iatrogenic (e.g., pharmacologic doses of prednisolone, dexamethasone)

**Pseudo-Cushing's syndromes**

Alcoholism
Depression
Obesity

ACTH, adrenocorticotrophic hormone; CRH, corticotropin-releasing hormone.
From Larsen PR, Kronenberg HM, Melmed S, et al: (eds): Williams Textbook of Endocrinology, 10th ed. Philadelphia, WB Saunders, 2002, p 509.

adenomas, but larger macroadenomas occur in up to 10% of cases and usually signify a more invasive tumor.[6] Selective surgical removal of a microadenoma results in cure with a low recurrence rate. However, it is possible, particularly in cases with no identifiable pituitary adenoma, that Cushing's disease may be heterogeneous with different subtypes. A key biochemical hallmark of the disease is a relative resistance of ACTH secretion to normal glucocorticoid feedback inhibition.[7,8]

### Ectopic Adrenocorticotropic Hormone Syndrome

In 15% of cases, Cushing's syndrome may be associated with nonpituitary tumors secreting ACTH—the ectopic ACTH syndrome. Clinically, this condition comprises two entities: cases occurring in the setting of highly malignant tumors, such as small cell carcinoma of the bronchus, and more indolent cases occurring in patients with underlying neuroendocrine tumors, such as bronchial carcinoids (Table 64-7). Circulating ACTH concentrations and cortisol secretion rates can be extremely high. As a result, the duration of symptoms from onset to presentation is short (<3 months); patients commonly have characteristic pigmentation, and the metabolic manifestations of glucocorticoid excess are often rapid and progressive. Weight loss, myopathy, and glucose intolerance are prominent signs and symptoms. The association of these features with hypokalemic alkalosis and peripheral edema should alert the clinician to the diagnosis.[9]

### Cortisol-secreting Adrenal Adenoma and Carcinoma

With the exclusion of iatrogenic Cushing's syndrome, adrenal adenomas are responsible for about 10% to 15% of cases and carcinomas for less than 5%. By contrast, in children 65% of cases of Cushing's syndrome have an adrenal etiology (15% adenoma, 50% carcinoma). Onset of clinical features is gradual in patients with adenomas but often rapid in adrenal carcinoma. In addition

Reproductive Endocrinology and Infertility

**Table 64-7**
**Tumors Associated with Ectopic Adrenocorticotropic Hormone Syndrome**

| Tumor Type | Approximate Incidence (%) |
| --- | --- |
| Small cell lung carcinoma | 50 |
| Non–small cell lung carcinoma | 5 |
| Pancreatic tumors (including carcinoids) | 10 |
| Thymic tumors (including carcinoids) | 5 |
| Lung carcinoids | 10 |
| Other carcinoids | 2 |
| Medullary carcinoma of thyroid | 5 |
| Pheochromocytoma and related tumors | 3 |
| Rare carcinomas of prostate, breast, ovary, gallbladder, colon | 10 |

From Larsen PR, Kronenberg HM, Melmed S, et al: (eds): Williams Textbook of Endocrinology, 10th ed. Philadelphia, WB Saunders, 2002, p 513.

to the features of hypercortisolism, patients may complain of loin or abdominal pain and a tumor may be palpable. The tumor may secrete other steroids, such as androgens or mineralocorticoids. Thus, in females, there may be features of virilization, with hirsutism, clitorimegaly, breast atrophy, deepening of the voice, temporal recession, and severe acne. With "pure" cortisol-secreting adenomas, hirsutism is uncommon.

### McCune-Albright Syndrome

In McCune-Albright syndrome, fibrous dysplasia and cutaneous pigmentation may be associated with pituitary, thyroid, adrenal, and gonadal hyperfunction. The most common manifestation is of sexual precocity and GH excess, but Cushing's syndrome has been reported. The underlying abnormality is a somatic mutation in the α subunit of the stimulatory G protein that is linked to adenyl cyclase. The mutation results in the G protein being constitutively activated, mimicking constant ACTH stimulation at the level of the adrenal. ACTH levels are suppressed, and adrenal adenomas may occur.[10]

### Iatrogenic Cushing's Syndrome

Development of the features of Cushing's syndrome depends on the dose, duration, and potency of the corticosteroid used in clinical practice. ACTH is rarely prescribed but chronically also results in cushingoid features. Some features such as increased intraocular pressure, cataracts, benign intracranial hypertension, aseptic necrosis of the femoral head, osteoporosis, and pancreatitis are more common in iatrogenic than in endogenous Cushing's syndrome, whereas other features, notably hypertension, hirsutism, and oligomenorrhea or amenorrhea, are rarer.

### Pseudo-Cushing's Syndromes

A pseudo-Cushing's state can be defined as some or all of the clinical features of Cushing's syndrome together with some evidence of hypercortisolism. Resolution of the underlying cause results in disappearance of the cushingoid state. Several causes have been described.

#### Alcohol

In the original description of this syndrome, urinary and plasma cortisol levels were elevated and not suppressed by dexamethasone. Plasma ACTH has been found to be normal or suppressed. The condition is rare but should be suspected in a patient with an ongoing history of heavy alcohol intake and biochemical or clinical evidence of chronic liver disease. Chronic liver disease of any cause is associated with impaired cortisol metabolism, but in alcoholics this is associated with an increase in cortisol secretion rate rather than concomitant suppression in the presence of impaired metabolism. In some studies, alcohol has directly stimulated cortisol secretion; alternatively, vasopressin levels are elevated in patients with decompensated liver disease and may stimulate the HPA axis. With abstinence from alcohol the biochemical abnormalities rapidly revert to normal.[5]

#### Depression

It is well recognized that patients with depression may exhibit the hormonal abnormalities of patients with Cushing's syndrome. These abnormalities are reversible on correction of the psychiatric condition. Conversely, patients with Cushing's syndrome are frequently depressed, and a careful clinical and endocrinologic assessment is required.[5]

#### Obesity

Patients with obesity have mildly increased cortisol secretion rates, and the data suggest that this is due to activation of the HPA axis. However, circulating cortisol concentrations are invariably normal and urinary free cortisol concentrations are either normal or only slightly elevated. The stimulus for the increased secretion rate appears to be increased peripheral metabolism and hence clearance of cortisol.[2]

### Diagnosis of Cushing's Syndrome

Diagnosis of Cushing's syndrome is based on medical history, physical examination, and laboratory tests to determine cortisol overproduction. Patients are usually asked to collect a 24-hour urine sample to be screened for high levels of the hormone. In normal subjects, plasma cortisol levels are at their highest first thing in the morning and reach a nadir at about midnight (<50 nmol/L, or 2 µg/dL, in a nonstressed subject). This circadian rhythm is lost in patients with Cushing's syndrome so that in the majority of patients the 9 AM plasma cortisol is normal but nocturnal levels are raised. Random morning plasma cortisol levels are therefore of little value in making the diagnosis, and a midnight cortisol level greater than 200 nmol/L (7 µg/dL) indicates Cushing's syndrome. However, various factors such as stress of venipuncture, intercurrent illness, and admission to the hospital may result in false-positive results. Ideally, patients should be hospitalized for 24 to 48 hours before cortisol is measured at midnight, but some centers have reported discriminant results from measurements of midnight values on an outpatient basis. Salivary cortisol concentrations may offer a sensible alternative in patients who are unable to go to the hospital.

For many years the diagnosis of Cushing's syndrome was based on the measurement of urinary metabolites of cortisol (24-hour urinary 17-hydroxycorticosteroid or 17-oxogenic steroid excretion, depending on the method used). However, the sensitivity and specificity of these methods are poor, and most centers have replaced these assays with the more sensitive measurement of urinary free cortisol excretion. Urinary free cortisol is an integrated measure of plasma free cortisol; as cortisol secretion increases, the binding capacity of corticosteroid-binding globulin (CBG) is exceeded, resulting in a disproportionate rise in urinary free cortisol. Normal values are less than 220 to 330 nmol (80 to 120 μg) per 24 hours depending on the assay used.

Patients should make two or three complete consecutive collections to account for error in collecting samples and episodic cortisol secretion, notably from adrenal adenomas. Simultaneous creatinine excretion (which differs by no more than 10% on a day-to-day basis) may be used to ensure adequacy of collection. Urinary free cortisol is a useful screening test, but it is accepted that urinary free cortisol may be normal in up to 8% to 15% of patients with Cushing's syndrome. Conversely, moderately elevated results should always be endorsed by further testing before a diagnosis of Cushing's syndrome is made.[2,11,12]

### Low-Dose and Overnight Dexamethasone Suppression Tests
In normal subjects, the administration of a supraphysiologic dose of glucocorticoid results in suppression of ACTH and cortisol secretion. In Cushing's syndrome of any cause there is failure of this suppression when low doses of the synthetic glucocorticoid dexamethasone are given. The overnight test is a useful outpatient screening test. Various doses of dexamethasone have been used, but 1 mg of dexamethasone is usually given at midnight. A normal response is a plasma cortisol of less than 140 nmol/L (5 μg/dL) between 8 and 9 AM the following morning. The outpatient overnight test has high sensitivity (95%) but low specificity, and further investigation is often required.

In the 48-hour low-dose dexamethasone test, plasma cortisol is measured at 9 AM on day 0 and 48 hours later following dexamethasone given at a dose of 0.5 mg every 6 hours for 48 hours. Using a postdexamethasone plasma cortisol concentration of less than 50 nmol/L (2 μg/dL), this test is reported as having a 97% to 100% true-positive rate and a false-positive rate less than 1%. Sensitivity is higher if plasma rather than urinary cortisol is measured.

Certain drugs (phenytoin, rifampin) may increase the metabolic clearance rate of dexamethasone and lead to false-positive results. Simultaneous measurement of plasma dexamethasone may be useful in this case and also detects patients who failed to take the drug.[2,11,12]

## Determining the Cause of Cushing's Syndrome
### 9 AM Plasma ACTH
Ideally, ACTH should be measured by a modern, two-site immunoradiometric assay that differentiates ACTH-dependent from ACTH-independent causes. In Cushing's disease, 50% of patients have a 9 AM ACTH within the normal reference range (2 to 12 pmol/L [9 to 54 pg/mL]); in the remainder it is modestly elevated. ACTH levels in the ectopic ACTH syndrome are high (usually > 20 pmol/L [90 pg/mL]) but nevertheless overlap values seen in Cushing's disease in 30% of cases and cannot therefore be used to differentiate these two conditions. The most discriminatory time of day to measure ACTH is actually between 11 PM and 1 AM, when ACTH-cortisol secretion is at the nadir; it has been advocated that ACTH be measured with cortisol in the circadian rhythm studies. A midnight ACTH

result greater than 5 pmol/L (23 pg/mL) in a patient with biochemical hypercortisolism confirms that the underlying disease is ACTH-dependent. The measurement of ACTH precursors (pro-ACTH, POMC) is not routinely available but may be more useful in detecting an ectopic source of ACTH; more data are required on patients with occult tumors causing the syndrome. In patients with adrenal tumors, plasma ACTH is invariably undetectable (<1 pmol/L [4.5 pg/mL]). This can also occur with degradation of ACTH; as a result, nonhemolyzed blood samples should be taken on ice and immediately separated.[2]

### Plasma Potassium
Hypokalemic alkalosis is present in more than 95% of patients with the ectopic ACTH syndrome but is present in fewer than 10% of patients with Cushing's disease. Patients with the ectopic syndrome usually have higher cortisol secretion rates that saturate the renal protective 11β-HSD type 2 enzyme, resulting in cortisol-induced, mineralocorticoid hypertension. In addition, these patients have higher levels of the ACTH-dependent mineralocorticoid DOC.[2,11]

### High-Dose Dexamethasone Suppression Test
The rationale for the high-dose dexamethasone suppression test is that in Cushing's disease there is a resetting of the negative feedback control of ACTH to a higher level than normal. Thus, cortisol levels are not suppressed with low-dose but are suppressed with high-dose dexamethasone. The original test introduced by Liddle was based on giving dexamethasone at 2 mg every 6 hours for 48 hours and demonstrating a greater than 50% fall in urinary 17-hydroxycorticosteroids after dexamethasone. In the modern test, plasma or urinary free cortisol, or both, are measured at 0 and +48 hours and a greater than 50% suppression of plasma cortisol in comparison with the baseline sample defines a positive response. In all cases, response is graded and dependent upon the original cortisol secretion rate; greater suppression is often observed in patients with lower basal cortisol values.

In Cushing's disease about 90% of patients have a positive 48-hour test in comparison with 10% with the ectopic ACTH syndrome. The test has 100% specificity for diagnosing pituitary disease if more than 90% suppression in urinary free cortisol is used. Up to 50% of patients with ectopic ACTH syndrome related to indolent bronchial carcinoid tumors exhibit some suppression after high-dose dexamethasone. Conversely, some patients with Cushing's disease, usually those with large invasive ACTH-secreting pituitary macroadenomas, may show no suppression after high-dose dexamethasone.[2]

### Metyrapone Test
Metyrapone blocks the conversion of 11-deoxycortisol to cortisol and DOC to corticosterone by inhibiting 11β-hydroxylase. This effect lowers plasma cortisol and, through negative feedback control, increases plasma ACTH. This, in turn, stimulates an increase in the secretion of adrenal steroids proximal to the block. When metyrapone is given in doses of 750 mg every 4 hours for 24 hours, patients with Cushing's disease exhibit an exaggerated rise in plasma ACTH with 11-deoxycortisol levels at 24 hours exceeding 1000 nmol/L (35 μg/dL). In most patients with the ectopic ACTH syndrome there is little or no response, but

occasional patients (possibly those producing both ACTH and CRH) have an 11-deoxycortisol response that may be similar to that observed in Cushing's disease.

The metyrapone test was originally used to distinguish patients with Cushing's disease from those with a primary adrenal cause. However, these can be more reliably distinguished by measuring plasma ACTH with subsequent computed tomography (CT) scanning of the adrenals.[2]

### Corticotropin-releasing Hormone Test

CRH is a 41–amino acid peptide identified by Vale in 1981 from ovine hypothalami. The ovine sequence differs by seven amino acid residues from that of the human but, despite this, is slightly more effective in stimulating the release of ACTH in humans. The test involves the intravenous injection of either ovine or human CRH in a dose of 1 μg/kg body weight or a single dose of 100 μg. The test can be performed in the morning or afternoon, and after basal sampling, blood samples for ACTH and cortisol are taken every 15 minutes for 1 to 2 hours following the administration of CRH.

In normal subjects, CRH produces a rise in ACTH and cortisol (approximately 15% to 20%), but this response is exaggerated in Cushing's disease, where typically an ACTH rise greater than 50% and a cortisol rise greater than 20% over baseline values are seen. No response is seen in the ectopic ACTH syndrome, but false-positive results have been reported. In distinguishing pituitary-dependent Cushing's from the ectopic ACTH syndrome, the response of ACTH and cortisol to CRH has a specificity and sensitivity of approximately 90%. However, with an ACTH test, an increase of 100% or a cortisol rise of 50% over baseline values, a positive response effectively eliminates a diagnosis of ectopic ACTH syndrome, and this is the real benefit of this test. Up to 10% of patients with Cushing's disease do not respond to CRH.[12]

### Inferior Petrosal Sinus Sampling and Selective Venous Catheterization

The most robust test to distinguish Cushing's disease from the ectopic ACTH syndrome is inferior petrosal sinus sampling (IPSS). As blood from each half of the pituitary drains into the ipsilateral inferior petrosal sinus, catheterization and venous sampling of both sinuses simultaneously can distinguish a pituitary from an ectopic source. In virtually all patients with the ectopic ACTH syndrome, the ratio of ACTH concentrations between the inferior petrosal sinus and simultaneously drawn peripheral venous level is less than 1.4:1. In contrast, in Cushing's disease this ratio is elevated at greater than 2.0. However, because of the problem of intermittent ACTH secretion, it is useful to make measurements before and at intervals (e.g., at 2, 5, and 15 minutes) after intravenous injection of 100 μg of synthetic ovine CRH. With this approach, an ACTH petrosal sinus/peripheral ratio greater than 3.0 after CRH has a sensitivity of 97% and specificity of 100% for the diagnosis of Cushing's disease.

IPSS may also be of value in lateralizing a pituitary tumor in a patient in whom imaging techniques have failed to demonstrate a microadenoma. Coadministration of desmopressin with CRH may help in localizing the tumor. However, it should be remembered that many tumors are central and may drain into both sinuses; current evidence suggests that it would unwise to base the surgical procedure on the results of IPSS studies alone. IPSS is a useful technique for establishing the differential diagnosis of ACTH-dependent Cushing's syndrome. However, it is technically demanding, has been associated with complications (referred aural pain, thrombosis), and is expensive. Rarely, selective catheterization of vascular beds may be required to identify the source of ectopic ACTH secretion, for example, from a small pulmonary carcinoid or thymic tumor.[2]

### Imaging Studies

High-resolution, thin-section, contrast-enhanced imaging using either CT or magnetic resonance imaging (MRI) has revolutionized the investigation of Cushing's syndrome. However, the results of any imaging technique must always be interpreted alongside the biochemical results if mistakes are to be avoided. In imaging the adrenals, asymmetric nodular hyperplasia may lead to a false diagnosis of adrenal adenoma. Because of the presence of pituitary incidentalomas, pituitary CT or MRI scanning may produce false-positive results, particularly for lesions less than 5 mm in diameter.

Pituitary MRI is the investigation of choice when the biochemical tests suggest Cushing's disease, with a sensitivity of 70% and specificity of 87%. About 90% of ACTH-secreting pituitary tumors are microadenomas (i.e., less than 10 mm in diameter). The classical features of a pituitary microadenoma are a hypodense lesion after contrast, associated with deviation of the pituitary stalk and a convex upper surface of the pituitary. With such small tumors it is not surprising that the sensitivity of CT scanning is relatively low (20% to 60%) with a similar specificity.[13]

By contrast, for adrenal imaging, CT rather than MRI is the investigation of choice, offering better spatial resolution, but MRI scanning may provide diagnostic information in patients with suspected adrenal carcinoma. Once again, it is stressed that adrenal incidentalomas are present in up to 5% of normal subjects (see section on Cortisol-secreting Adrenal Adenoma and Carcinoma), and thus adrenal imaging should not be performed unless biochemical investigation suggests a primary adrenal cause (undetectable ACTH concentrations).[14] Adrenal carcinomas are large and often associated with metastatic spread at presentation.

In patients with occult ectopic ACTH syndrome, high-definition CT or MRI scanning of thorax, abdomen, and pelvis with images every 0.5 cm may be required to detect small ACTH-secreting carcinoid tumors.[13]

### Scintigraphy Studies

Scintigraphy is of value in certain patients with primary adrenal pathology. The most commonly used agent is [131]I-labeled 6β-iodomethyl-19-norcholesterol. This is a marker of adrenocortical cholesterol uptake. In patients with adrenal adenomas, the isotope is taken up by the adenoma but not by the contralateral suppressed adrenal. Adrenal scintigraphy is useful for suspected adrenocortical macronodular hyperplasia, for which CT scanning may be misleading by suggesting unilateral pathology, whereas with isotope scanning the bilateral adrenal involvement is identified.

Many neuroendocrine tumors giving rise to the ectopic ACTH syndrome express somatostatin receptors and can be imaged by administering radiolabeled analogs of somatostatin (most commonly [111]In-labeled octreotide). This technique can detect tumors only a few millimeters in diameter and should be considered for patients with ACTH-dependent Cushing's syndrome in whom pituitary disease has been excluded.[2]

## Treatment of Cushing's Syndrome

### Adrenal Causes

Adrenal adenomas should be removed by unilateral adrenalectomy, which has a 100% cure rate. With the increasing experience of laparoscopic adrenalectomy, this has become the surgical treatment of choice for unilateral tumors, reducing surgical morbidity and postoperative hospital stay compared with traditional open approaches. After surgery, it may take many months or even years for the contralateral suppressed adrenal to recover. Thus, it is necessary to give slightly suboptimal replacement therapy with dexamethasone at 0.5 mg in the morning, with intermittent measurement of morning plasma cortisol. When the morning plasma cortisol is above 180 nmol/L (6 µg/dL), dexamethasone can be stopped. A subsequent insulin tolerance test may then demonstrate whether the response to stress is normal. In the interim, all patients should carry a Steroid Alert card and increase their dose of replacement therapy in the event of an intercurrent illness.

Adrenal carcinomas have a poor prognosis, and most patients are dead within 2 years of diagnosis. It is usual practice to try to remove the primary tumor even though metastases may be present so as to enhance the response to the adrenolytic agent o,p'-dichlorodiphenyldichloroethane (o,p'-DDD, mitotane). Radiotherapy to the tumor bed and to some metastases, such as those in the spine, may be of limited value.

### Pituitary-Dependent Cushing's Syndrome

The treatment of Cushing's disease has been significantly enhanced through transsphenoidal surgery conducted by an experienced surgeon. Before the selective removal of a pituitary microadenoma, the treatment of choice was bilateral adrenalectomy. This had an appreciable mortality even in the best centers (up to 4%) and significant morbidity. The major risk was the subsequent development of Nelson's syndrome (postadrenalectomy hyperpigmentation with a locally aggressive pituitary tumor), which was attributed to loss of any negative feedback after adrenalectomy. In an attempt to avoid this, pituitary irradiation was often carried out at the time of bilateral adrenalectomy. In addition, these patients required lifelong replacement therapy with hydrocortisone and fludrocortisone. Today, bilateral adrenalectomy is rarely indicated for patients with Cushing's disease but may be performed when pituitary surgery has failed or when the condition has recurred.

The surgical outcome for transsphenoidal hypophysectomy is center-dependent and related to surgical expertise. In optimal centers, cure rates are 80% to 90% for microadenomas and 50% for macroadenomas. Rates for hypopituitarism and permanent diabetes insipidus postoperatively depend on how aggressive the surgeon has been in removing pituitary tissue. The ideal outcome is a cured patient with intact pituitary function, but this may not be possible in a patient with Cushing's disease in whom a pituitary adenoma was not identified preoperatively or during the operation itself.

At the time of surgery, patients should be treated with corticosteroids as for any other potential or confirmed deficit of the HPA axis. Postoperatively, hydrocortisone can be withdrawn to maintenance replacement doses, usually within 3 to 7 days.[7,8]

### Ectopic Adrenocorticotropic Hormone Syndrome

Treatment of the ectopic ACTH syndrome depends on the cause. If the tumor can be found and has not spread, then its removal can lead to cure (e.g., bronchial carcinoid or thymoma). However, the prognosis for small cell lung cancer associated with the ectopic ACTH syndrome is poor. The cortisol excess and associated hypokalemic alkalosis and diabetes mellitus can be corrected by medical therapy. The treatment of the small cell tumor itself also, at least initially, produces improvement. Sometimes, if the ectopic source of ACTH cannot be found, it may be necessary to perform bilateral adrenalectomy and then observe the patient carefully before the primary tumor becomes apparent.[9]

### Medical Treatment

Several drugs have been used in the treatment of Cushing's syndrome. Metyrapone inhibits 11β-hydroxylase and has been most commonly given, often to lower cortisol concentrations prior to definitive therapy or while awaiting benefit from pituitary radiation. The daily dose has to be determined by measuring either plasma or urinary free cortisol. The aim should be to achieve a mean plasma cortisol of about 300 nmol/L (11 µg/dL) during the day or a normal urinary free cortisol. The drug is usually given in doses ranging from 250 mg twice daily to 1.5 g every 6 hours.

Aminoglutethimide is a more toxic drug that, in high doses, blocks earlier enzymes in the steroidogenic pathway and thus affects the secretion of steroids other than cortisol. In doses of 1.5 to 3 g daily (start with 250 mg every 8 hours) it commonly produces nausea, marked lethargy, and a high incidence of skin rash. It is commonly prescribed as combination therapy with metyrapone.[15,16]

Ketoconazole is an imidazole that has been widely used as an antifungal agent but causes abnormal liver function tests in about 15% of patients. Ketoconazole blocks a variety of steroidogenic cytochrome P-450–dependent enzymes and thus lowers plasma cortisol levels. For effective control of Cushing's syndrome, 400 to 800 mg daily has been required.[17]

Mitotane is an adrenolytic drug that is taken up by both normal and malignant adrenal tissue, causing adrenal atrophy and necrosis. Because of its toxicity, it has been used mainly in the management of adrenal carcinoma. Doses of up to 10 to 20 g/day are required to control glucocorticoid excess, although evidence that it causes tumor shrinkage or improves long-term survival is lacking. The drug also produces mineralocorticoid deficiency, and concomitant glucocorticoid and mineralocorticoid replacement therapy may be required. Side effects are common and include fatigue, skin rashes, and gastrointestinal disturbance.[9]

## Prognosis of Cushing's Syndrome

Studies carried out before the introduction of effective therapy indicated that 50% of patients with untreated Cushing's syndrome died within 5 years, principally from vascular disease.

## Reproductive Endocrinology and Infertility

Even with modern management, an increased prevalence of cardiovascular risk factors persists for many years after an apparent cure. Paradoxically, upon correction of the hypercortisolism, patients may feel worse. Skin desquamation, steroid withdrawal arthropathy, profound lethargy, and mood changes may occur and take several weeks or months to resolve.

Features of Cushing's syndrome disappear over a period of 2 to 12 months. Hypertension and diabetes mellitus improve but, as with other secondary causes, may not resolve completely. The osteopenia of Cushing's syndrome improves rapidly in the first 2 years after treatment but resolves more slowly thereafter. Vertebral fractures and aseptic necrosis are irreversible, and permanent deformity results. Visceral obesity and myopathy are both reversible features. Reproductive and sexual functions return to normal within 6 months provided anterior pituitary function was not compromised.[9]

## DISORDERS OF GLUCOCORTICOID DEFICIENCY

Primary hypoadrenalism is glucocorticoid deficiency occurring in the setting of adrenal disease; secondary hypoadrenalism arises from deficiency of ACTH. A major distinction between these two is that mineralocorticoid deficiency invariably accompanies primary hypoadrenalism but does not occur in secondary hypoadrenalism because only ACTH is deficient with the latter, the renin-angiotensin-aldosterone axis is intact. A further important cause of adrenal insufficiency where there may be dissociation of glucocorticoid and mineralocorticoid secretion is CAH.

### Primary Hypoadrenalism: Addison's Disease

This condition was first described by Thomas Addison in 1855. It is a rare condition with an estimated incidence in the developed world of 0.8 cases per 100,000 and prevalence of 4 to 11 cases per 100,000 population. It is associated with significant morbidity and mortality, but when the diagnosis is made it can be easily treated. The causes of Addison's disease are listed in Table 64-8.

#### Autoimmune Adrenalitis

Autoimmune adrenalitis accounts for over 70% of all cases of Addison's disease. In this condition, the adrenal glands are atrophic, with loss of most of the cortical cells, but the medulla is usually intact. In 75% of cases, adrenal autoantibodies can be detected. Fifty percent of patients with this form of Addison's disease have an associated autoimmune disease (Table 64-9), thyroid disease being the most common. Conversely, only 1% to 2% of patients with more common autoimmune diseases such as insulin-dependent diabetes mellitus and thyrotoxicosis have anti-adrenal autoantibodies and adrenal disease. This figure is higher in patients with autoimmune hypoparathyroidism (16%).

These autoimmune polyendocrine syndromes (APSs) are classified as two distinct variants. APS type I is inherited as an autosomal recessive condition and comprises Addison's disease, chronic mucocutaneous candidiasis, and hypoparathyroidism. Other autoimmune conditions such as pernicious anemia, thyroid disease, chronic active hepatitis, and gonadal failure may occur but are rare. APS II is more common and comprises Addison's disease, autoimmune thyroid disease, diabetes mellitus, and

---

| Table 64-8 |
|---|
| **Etiology of Adrenocortical Insufficiency** |

**Primary (Addison's disease)**

Autoimmune
  Sporadic
  Autoimmune polyendocrine syndrome type I: Addison's disease, chronic mucocutaneous candidiasis, hypoparathyroidism, dental enamel hypoplasia, alopecia, primary gonadal failure
  Autoimmune polyendocrine syndrome type II (Schmidt's syndrome): Addison's disease, primary hypothyroidism, primary hypogonadism, insulin-dependent diabetes, pernicious anaemia, vitiligo
Infection
  Tuberculosis
  Fungal infection
  Cytomegalovirus
  HIV
Metastatic tumor
Infiltrations
  Amyloid
  Hemochromatosis
Intra-adrenal hemorrhage (Waterhouse-Friderichsen syndrome) after meningococcal septicemia
Adrenoleukodystrophies
Congenital adrenal hypoplasia
  *DAX-1* mutations
  *SF-1* mutations
ACTH resistance syndromes
  Mutations in *MC2-R*
  Triple A syndrome
Bilateral adrenalectomy

**Secondary**

Exogenous glucocorticoid therapy
Hypopituitarism
Selective removal of ACTH-secreting pituitary adenoma
Pituitary tumors and pituitary surgery, craniopharyngiomas
Pituitary apoplexy
Granulomatous disease: tuberculosis, sarcoid, eosinophilic granuloma
Secondary tumor deposits (breast, bronchus)
Postpartum pituitary infarction (Sheehan's syndrome)
Pituitary irradiation (effect usually delayed for several years)
Isolated ACTH deficiency
Idiopathic
Lymphocytic hypophysitis
POMC processing defect
POMC gene mutations

ACTH, adrenocorticotropic hormone; HIV, human immunodeficiency virus; POMC, pro-opiomelanocortin.
From Larsen PR, Kronenberg HM, Melmed S, et al: (eds): Williams Textbook of Endocrinology, 10th ed. Philadelphia, WB Saunders, 2002, p 526.

---

hypogonadism. This condition has an inherited basis with linkage to the human leukocyte antigen (HLA) major histocompatibility complex, notably HLA-DR3 and HLA-DR4. Autoantibodies to 21-hydroxylase are usually present and are predictive of the development of adrenal destruction. Other features may accompany APS I and APS II. Patients with APSs are more likely to be female (70%); however, patients with isolated autoimmune adrenalitis are usually male.[18]

Worldwide, infectious diseases are the most common cause of primary adrenal insufficiency and comprise tuberculosis, fungal infections (histoplasmosis, cryptococcosis), and cytomegalovirus infection. Adrenal failure may also occur in the acquired immunodeficiency syndrome (AIDS). Tuberculous Addison's disease results from hematogenous spread of the infection from

**Table 64-9**
**Other Endocrine and Autoimmune Diseases Associated**
**with Autoimmune Adrenalitis**

| Disease | Incidence (%) |
|---|---|
| Thyroid disease | |
| Hypothyroidism | 8 |
| Nontoxic goiter | 7 |
| Thyrotoxicosis | 7 |
| Gonadal failure | |
| Ovarian | 20 |
| Testicular | 2 |
| Insulin-dependent diabetes mellitus | 11 |
| Hypoparathyroidism | 10 |
| Pernicious anemia | 5 |

From Larsen PR, Kronenberg HM, Melmed S, et al: (eds): Williams Textbook of Endocrinology, 10th ed. Philadelphia, WB Saunders, 2002, p 526.

elsewhere in the body, and extra-adrenal disease is usually evident.

The adrenals are frequently involved in patients with AIDS; adrenalitis may occur after infection with cytomegalovirus or atypical mycobacterium, and Kaposi's sarcoma may result in a requirement for adrenal replacement. The onset is often insidious, but if tested, over 10% of patients with AIDS demonstrate a subnormal cortisol response following an ACTH stimulation test. Adrenal insufficiency may be precipitated through administration of anti-infectives such as ketoconazole (inhibits cortisol synthesis) or rifampin (increases cortisol metabolism).[18,19]

### Other Causes of Addison's Disease

With the exception of tuberculosis and autoimmune adrenal failure, other causes of Addison's disease are rare. Adrenal metastases (the most common primary being lung and breast) are often found at postmortem examination, but adrenal insufficiency resulting from these is uncommon, perhaps because over 90% of the adrenal cortex needs to be compromised before symptoms and signs become apparent. Necrosis of the adrenals related to intra-adrenal hemorrhage should be considered in any severely sick patient, particularly those with underlying infection, trauma, or coagulopathy. Intra-adrenal bleeding may be found with any cause of severe septicemia, particularly in children, in whom a common cause is infection with *Pseudomonas aeruginosa*. When Addison's disease is caused by meningococcus, the association with adrenal insufficiency is known as the Waterhouse-Friderichsen syndrome. Adrenal deficiency may also occur with amyloidosis and hemochromatosis.

Adrenal hypoplasia congenita is an X-linked disorder comprising congenital adrenal insufficiency and hypogonadotropic hypogonadism. The condition is caused by mutations in the dose-sensitive sex reversal, adrenal hypoplasia congenita, X-chromosome factor (*DAX-1*) gene, a member of the nuclear receptor family of unknown function that is expressed in the adrenal cortex, gonads, and hypothalamus. Mutations in another transcription factor, steroidogenic factor-1, also results in adrenal insufficiency related to lack of development of a functional

adrenal cortex. The transcriptional regulation of many P-450 steroidogenic enzymes is dependent on steroidogenic factor-1.

### Secondary Hypoadrenalism
### (Adrenocorticotropic Hormone Deficiency)

Secondary hypoadrenalism is a common clinical problem and is most often due to sudden cessation of exogenous glucocorticoid therapy. Such therapy suppresses the HPA axis with consequent adrenal atrophy, and this may last for months after glucocorticoid treatment ceases. Adrenal atrophy and subsequent deficiency should be anticipated in any patient who has taken more than the equivalent of 30 mg of hydrocortisone per day orally (7.5 mg/day prednisolone or 0.75 mg/day dexamethasone) for more than 3 weeks. In addition to the magnitude of the dose of glucocorticoid, the timing of administration of the dose may affect the degree of adrenal suppression. Thus, prednisolone in a dose of 5 mg given last thing at night and 2.5 mg in the morning produces more marked suppression of the HPA axis than does 2.5 mg at night and 5 mg in the morning because the larger evening dose blocks the early morning surge of ACTH. Secondary hypoadrenalism may also occur after failure to give adequate glucocorticoid replacement therapy for intercurrent stress in a patient who has received long-term glucocorticoid therapy.

Other causes of secondary adrenal insufficiency reflect inadequate ACTH production by the anterior pituitary gland. In these patients, other pituitary hormones are deficient in addition to ACTH and there is partial or complete hypopituitarism. Secondary hypoadrenalism also is observed in patients with Cushing's disease after successful and selective removal of the ACTH-secreting pituitary adenoma. The function of adjacent "normal" pituitary corticotrophs is suppressed and may remain so for many months after surgery.

### Clinical Features of Adrenal Insufficiency

Patients with primary adrenal failure usually have both glucocorticoid and mineralocorticoid deficiency (Table 64-10). In contrast, those with secondary adrenal insufficiency have an intact renin-angiotensin-aldosterone system. This accounts for differences in salt and water balance in the two groups of patients, which in turn results in different clinical presentations. The most obvious feature that differentiates primary from secondary hypoadrenalism is skin pigmentation, which is nearly always present in primary adrenal insufficiency (unless of short duration) and absent in secondary insufficiency. The pigmentation is seen in sun-exposed areas rather than old scars, in the axillae, nipples, palmar creases, pressure points, and mucous membranes (buccal, vaginal, vulval, anal). The cause of the pigmentation has long been debated, but it is thought to reflect increased stimulation of the melanocortin-2 receptor by ACTH itself. In autoimmune Addison's disease there may be associated vitiligo.

The clinical features are related to the rate of onset and severity of adrenal deficiency. In many cases, the disease has an insidious onset and a diagnosis is made only when the patient comes in with an acute crisis during an intercurrent illness. Acute adrenal insufficiency or an adrenal or addisonian crisis is a medical emergency manifesting as hypotension and acute circulatory failure (Table 64-11). Anorexia may be an early feature,

# Reproductive Endocrinology and Infertility

| Table 64-10 Clinical Features of Primary Adrenal Insufficiency | |
|---|---|
| Symptom, Sign, or Laboratory Finding | Frequency (%) |
| **Symptom** | |
| Weakness, tiredness, fatigue | 100 |
| Anorexia | 100 |
| Gastrointestinal symptoms | 92 |
|   Nausea | 86 |
|   Vomiting | 75 |
|   Constipation | 33 |
|   Abdominal pain | 31 |
|   Diarrhea | 16 |
| Salt craving | 16 |
| Postural dizziness | 12 |
| Muscle or joint pains | 6–13 |
| **Sign** | |
| Weight loss | 100 |
| Hyperpigmentation | 94 |
| Hypotension (<110 mm Hg systolic) | 88–94 |
| Vitiligo | 10–20 |
| Auricular calcification | 5 |
| **Laboratory finding** | |
| Electrolyte disturbances | 92 |
|   Hyponatremia | 88 |
|   Hyperkalemia | 64 |
|   Hypercalcemia | 6 |
| Azotemia | 55 |
| Anemia | 40 |
| Eosinophilia | 17 |

Modified from Baxter JD, Tyrrell JB. In Felig P, Baxter JD, Frohman LA (eds): Endocrinology and Metabolism, 3rd ed. New York, McGraw-Hill, 1995.

| Table 64-11 Clinical Features of Adrenal Crisis |
|---|
| • Dehydration, hypotension, or shock out of proportion to severity of current illness |
| • Nausea and vomiting with a history of weight loss and anorexia |
| • Abdominal pain, so-called acute abdomen |
| • Unexplained hypoglycemia |
| • Unexplained fever |
| • Hyponatremia, hyperkalemia, azotemia, hypercalcemia, or eosinophilia |
| • Hyperpigmentation or vitiligo |
| • Other autoimmune endocrine deficiencies, such as hypothyroidism or gonadal failure |

Modified from Baxter JD, Tyrrell JB. In Felig P, Baxter JD, Frohman LA (eds): Endocrinology and Metabolism, 3rd ed. New York, McGraw-Hill, 1995.

nervosa. These features regress on treatment with replacement corticosteroids.

In secondary adrenal insufficiency associated with hypopituitarism, the presentation may be related to deficiency of hormones other than ACTH, notably, LH or FSH (infertility, oligomenorrhea or amenorrhea, poor libido) and TSH (weight gain, cold intolerance). Fasting hypoglycemia occurs because of loss of the gluconeogenic effects of cortisol. It is rare in adults unless there is concomitant alcohol abuse or additional GH deficiency. However, hypoglycemia is a common presenting feature of ACTH or adrenal insufficiency in childhood. In addition, patients with ACTH deficiency present with malaise, weight loss, and other features of chronic adrenal insufficiency.

## Diagnosis of Primary Adrenal Insufficiency

In established primary adrenal insufficiency, hyponatremia is present in about 90% of cases and hyperkalemia in 65%. The blood urea concentration is usually elevated. Hyperkalemia occurs because of aldosterone deficiency and is therefore usually absent in patients with secondary adrenal failure. Hyponatremia may be depletional in an addisonian crisis, but in addition vasopressin levels are elevated, resulting in increased free water retention. Thus, in secondary adrenal insufficiency there may be a dilutional hyponatremia with normal or low blood urea. Reversible abnormalities in liver transaminases frequently occur. Hypercalcemia occurs in 6% of all cases and may be particularly marked in patients with coexisting thyrotoxicosis. However, free thyroxine concentrations are usually low or normal but TSH values are frequently moderately elevated. This is a direct effect of glucocorticoid deficiency and reverses with replacement therapy. Persistent elevation of TSH in association with positive thyroid autoantibodies suggests concomitant autoimmune thyroid disease.

In primary hypoadrenalism, mineralocorticoid deficiency usually occurs with elevated plasma renin activity and either low or low normal plasma aldosterone. The investigation of zona glomerulosa activity is frequently neglected in Addison's disease as compared with assessment of zona fasciculata function. In secondary adrenal insufficiency, the renin-angiotensin-aldosterone system is intact.

Clinical suspicion of the diagnosis should be confirmed with definitive diagnostic tests. Basal plasma cortisol and urinary free

which progresses to nausea, vomiting, diarrhea, and sometimes abdominal pain. Fever may be present, and hypoglycemia may occur. Patients presenting acutely with adrenal hemorrhage have hypotension; abdominal, flank, or lower chest pain; anorexia; and vomiting. The condition is difficult to diagnose, but evidence of occult hemorrhage (rapidly falling hemoglobin), progressive hyperkalemia, and shock should alert the clinician to the diagnosis.

Alternatively, the patient may have vague features of chronic adrenal insufficiency—weakness, tiredness, weight loss, nausea, intermittent vomiting, abdominal pain, diarrhea or constipation, general malaise, muscle cramps, arthralgia, and symptoms suggestive of postural hypotension. Salt craving may be a feature, and there may be a low-grade fever. Supine blood pressure is usually normal, but almost invariably there is a fall in blood pressure on standing. Although adrenal androgen secretion is lost, this is clinically more apparent in women, who may complain of loss of axillary and pubic hair. Psychiatric symptoms may occur in long-standing cases and include memory impairment, depression, and psychosis. Patients may be inappropriately diagnosed as suffering from chronic fatigue syndrome or anorexia cortisol levels are often in the low normal range and cannot be used to exclude the diagnosis. However, a basal cortisol value greater than 400 nmol/L (15 μg/dL) invariably indicates an intact HPA axis. All patients suspected of having adrenal insufficiency should have an ACTH stimulation test, although in patients with an addisonian crisis treatment should be instigated immediately and stimulation tests conducted at a later stage.[20]

The ACTH stimulation test involves intramuscular or intravenous administration of 250 μg of cosyntropin (Cortrosyn), which is made up of the first 24 amino acids of normally secreted ACTH 1 to 39. Plasma cortisol levels are measured at 0 and 30 minutes after ACTH, and a normal response is defined by a peak plasma cortisol level greater than 525 nmol/L (19 μg/dL). Response is unaffected by the time of day of the test, and the test can be performed in patients who have commenced corticosteroid replacement therapy provided this is of short duration and does not include hydrocortisone (which would cross-react in the cortisol assay).

A prolonged ACTH stimulation test, involving the administration of depot or intravenous infusions of cosyntropin for 24 to 48 hours, differentiates primary from secondary hypoadrenalism. In normal subjects the plasma cortisol at 4 hours is greater than 1000 nmol/L (36 μg/dL), and beyond this time there is no further increase. Patients with secondary hypoadrenalism show a delayed response with usually a much higher value at 24 and 48 hours than at 4 hours, but in primary hypoadrenalism there is no response at either time. However, the test is now rarely required if plasma ACTH has been appropriately measured at baseline. In primary adrenal insufficiency, the ACTH level is disproportionately elevated in comparison with plasma cortisol.

Radioimmunoassays to detect autoantibodies such as those against the 21-hydroxylase antigen are available and should be analyzed in patients with primary adrenal failure. In autoimmune Addison's disease, it is also important to look for evidence of other organ-specific autoimmune disease. A CT scan may reveal enlarged or calcified adrenals, suggesting an infective, hemorrhagic, or malignant diagnosis. A chest radiograph, tuberculin testing, and early morning urine samples cultured for *Mycobacterium tuberculosis* should be obtained if tuberculosis is suspected. A CT-guided adrenal biopsy specimen may reveal an underlying diagnosis in patients with suspected malignant deposits in the adrenal. Adrenoleukodystrophy can be diagnosed by measuring circulating levels of very long chain fatty acids. Finally, appropriate investigations, including pituitary MRI scans and an assessment of anterior (pituitary) function, are required for patients suspected of having secondary hypoadrenalism who are not receiving corticosteroid therapy.[21,22]

## Treatment of Acute Adrenal Insufficiency

Acute adrenal insufficiency is a life-threatening emergency, and treatment should not be delayed for definitive proof of diagnosis (Table 64-12). However, in addition to measurement of plasma electrolytes and blood glucose, appropriate samples for ACTH and cortisol should be taken before corticosteroid therapy is given. If the patient is not critically ill, an acute ACTH stimulation test can be performed.

Intravenous hydrocortisone should be given in a dose of 100 mg every 6 hours. If this is not possible, the intramuscular route should be used. In the shocked patient, 1 L of normal

**Table 64-12**
**Treatment of Adrenal Crisis**

**Emergency measures**

1. Establish intravenous access with a large-gauge needle
2. Draw blood for stat serum electrolytes and glucose and routine measurement of plasma cortisol and ACTH
   *Do not wait for laboratory results*
3. Infuse 2 to 3 L of 154 mmol/L NaCl (0.9% saline) solution or 50 g/L (5%) dextrose in 154 mmol/L NaCl (0.9% saline) solution as quickly as possible
   Monitor for signs of fluid overload by measuring central or peripheral venous pressure and listening for pulmonary rales
   Reduce infusion rate if indicated
4. Inject intravenous hydrocortisone (100 mg immediately and every 6 hr)
5. Use supportive measures as needed

**Subacute measures after stabilization of the patient**

1. Continue intravenous 154 mmol/L NaCl (0.9% saline) solution at a slower rate for next 24 to 48 hr
2. Search for and treat possible infectious precipitating causes of the adrenal crisis
3. Perform a short ACTH stimulation test to confirm the diagnosis of adrenal insufficiency, if patient does not have known adrenal insufficiency
4. Determine the type of adrenal insufficiency and its cause if not already known
5. Taper glucocorticoids to maintenance dosage over 1 to 3 days, if precipitating or complicataing illness permits
6. Begin mineralocorticoid replacement with fludrocortisone (0.1 mg by mouth daily) when saline infusion is stopped

ACTH, adrenocorticotropic hormone.
Modified from Baxter JD, Tyrrell JB. In Felig P, Baxter JD, Frohman LA (eds): Endocrinology and Metabolism, 3rd ed. New York, McGraw-Hill, 1995.

saline should be given intravenously over the first hour. Because of possible hypoglycemia, it is usual to give 5% dextrose saline. Subsequent saline and dextrose therapy depends on biochemical monitoring and the patient's condition. Clinical improvement, especially in the blood pressure, should be seen within 4 to 6 hours if the diagnosis is correct. It is important to recognize and treat any associated condition, such as an infection, which may have precipitated the acute adrenal crisis.

After the first 24 hours the dose of hydrocortisone can be reduced, usually to 50 mg intramuscularly every 6 hours, and then, if the patient can take it by mouth, to oral hydrocortisone, 40 mg in the morning and 20 mg at 6 PM. This can then be rapidly reduced to a more standard replacement dose of 20 mg on wakening and 10 mg at 6 PM.

### Chronic Replacement Therapy

The aim is to give replacement doses of hydrocortisone to mimic the normal cortisol secretion rate (Table 64-13). Most patients can be maintained with less than 84 μmol/day (30 mg/day; 15 to 25 mg/day in divided doses). Doses are usually given on wakening, with a smaller dose in the late afternoon, but some patients may feel better with dosing three times daily. In primary adrenal failure, cortisol day curves with simultaneous ACTH measurements may provide some insight into the adequacy of replacement therapy, but unfortunately there are no good objective tests in secondary adrenal failure. Decisions about doses of replacement therapy are largely based on crude but nevertheless important endpoints such as weight, well-being, and blood

# Reproductive Endocrinology and Infertility

pressure. Bone mineral density may be reduced with conventional hydrocortisone doses of 30 mg/day, highlighting the need to strive for the lowest effective dose.[23]

In primary adrenal failure, mineralocorticoid replacement is usually also required in the form of fludrocortisone (or $9\alpha$-fluorinated hydrocortisone) at 0.05 to 0.2 mg/day. The mineralocorticoid activity of this treatment is about 125 times that of hydrocortisone. After the acute phase has passed, the adequacy of mineralocorticoid replacement should be assessed by measuring electrolytes and supine and erect blood pressure and plasma renin activity; too little fludrocortisone may cause postural hypotension with elevated plasma renin activity, and too much may cause the opposite.[24]

Patients receiving glucocorticoid replacement therapy should be advised to double the daily dose in the event of intercurrent febrile illness, accident, or mental stress such as an important examination. If the patient is vomiting and cannot take medi-

cation by mouth, parenteral hydrocortisone must be given. For minor surgery, 50 to 100 mg of hydrocortisone hemisuccinate is given with the premedication. For major operations, this is then followed by the same regimen as for acute adrenal insufficiency. Pregnancy proceeds normally in patients taking replacement therapy, but daily doses of hydrocortisone are usually increased modestly (5 to 10 mg/day) in the last trimester. During labor, patients should be well hydrated with a saline drip and receive hydrocortisone at 50 mg intramuscularly every 6 hours until delivery. Thereafter, doses can be rapidly tapered off to usual maintenance regimens.

Every patient receiving glucocorticoid therapy should be advised to register for a Medic Alert bracelet or necklace and must carry a Steroid Alert card.

For patients with both primary and secondary adrenal failure, beneficial effects of adrenal androgen replacement therapy with DHEA at 25 to 50 mg/day have been reported. To date, the reported benefit is principally confined to female patients and includes improvement in sexual function and well-being.[25]

## Congenital Adrenal Hyperplasia

These inherited syndromes are caused by deficient adrenal corticosteroid biosynthesis. In each case, there is reduced negative feedback inhibition of cortisol and, depending on the steroidogenic pathway involved, alteration in adrenal mineralocorticoid and androgen secretion (Table 64-14).

### 21-Hydroxylase Deficiency

Ninety percent of cases of CAH are due to 21-hydroxylase deficiency. The incidence varies from 1 in 5000 to 1 in 15,000 live births. The condition arises because of defective conversion of $17\alpha$-hydroxyprogesterone to 11-deoxycortisol. Reduced cortisol biosynthesis results in reduced negative feedback drive and increased ACTH secretion; as a consequence, adrenal androgens are produced in excess (see Fig. 64-2). Seventy-five percent of cases include mineralocorticoid deficiency because of the failure to convert progesterone to DOC in the zona glomerulosa. Clinically, several distinct variants of 21-hydroxylase deficiency have been recognized (Table 64-15).

### Simple Virilizing Form

The enhanced ACTH drive to adrenal androgen secretion in utero leads to virilization of an affected female fetus. Depending on the severity, clitoral enlargement, labial fusion, and development of a urogenital sinus may occur, leading to sexual ambiguity at birth and even inappropriate sex assignment. Rarely, the diagnosis is missed in the neonatal period, especially in boys, who may be phenotypically normal at birth. Such patients may present in early childhood with sexual precocity and pubic hair development. Initially, linear growth is accelerated because of premature androgen excess that, left untreated, stimulates epiphyseal closure and compromises final adult height.

### Salt-Wasting Form

Seventy-five percent of cases in both sexes also have concomitant aldosterone deficiency. In addition to the preceding clinical features, neonates may have a salt-wasting crisis and hypotension in the first week of life. Indeed, this may alert the clinician to the diagnosis in a male, but unfortunately the diag-

**Table 64-14**
**Features of Gene-specific Defects of Congenital Adrenal Hyperplasia**

| Feature | 21-Hydroxylase Deficiency | 11β-Hydroxylase Deficiency | 17α-Hydroxylase Deficiency | 3β-Hydroxysteroid Deficiency | Lipoid Hyperplasia | Aldosterone Synthetase Deficiency |
|---|---|---|---|---|---|---|
| Defective gene | CYP21 | CYP11B1 | CYP17 | HSD3B2 | StAR | CYP11B2 |
| Chromosomal localization | 6p21.3 | 8q24.3 | 10q24.3 | 1p13.1 | 8p11.2 | 8q24.3 |
| Ambiguous genitalia | +(Female) | +(Female) | +(Male) Absent puberty (female) | +(Male) Mild in female | +(Male) Absent puberty (female) | No |
| Acute adrenal insufficiency | + | Rare | No | + | ++ | Salt wasting only |
| Incidence | 1:15,000 | 1:100,000 | Rare | Rare | Rare | Rare |
| Hormones | | | | | | |
| Glucocorticoids | Reduced | Reduced | Reduced | Corticosterone normal | Reduced | Normal |
| Mineralocorticoids | Reduced | Increased | Reduced | Increased | Reduced | Reduced |
| Androgens | Increased | Increased | Reduced | Reduced (male) Increased (female) | Reduced | Normal |
| Elevated metabolite | 17-Hydroxyprogesterone | DOC, 11-deoxycortisol | B, DOC | DHEA, 17Δ$^5$-pregnenolone | None | B, 18-OHB |
| Blood pressure, sodium balance | Decreased | Increased | Decreased | Increased | Decreased | Decreased |
| Potassium | Increased | Decreased | Increased | Decreased | Increased | Increased |

B, corticosterone; DHEA, dehydroepiandrosterone; DOC, deoxycorticosterone; 18-OHB, 18-hydroxycorticosterone.
Modified from White CW, Pescovitz OH, Cutler GB: Synthesis and metabolism of corticosteroids. In Becker KL, Bilezikian JP, Hung W, et al (eds): Principles and Practice of Endocrinology and Metabolism, 2nd ed. Philadelphia, JB Lippincott, 1995, p 687.

nosis is still delayed in many cases and the condition carries a significant neonatal mortality rate.

### Late-Onset 21-Hydroxylase Deficiency

These patients present with premature pubarche or with a phenotype that may masquerade as polycystic ovary syndrome (PCOS). Indeed, late-onset CAH is a recognized secondary cause of PCOS and appears to be more common than the classical variety. In some series from tertiary referral centers, late-onset 21-hydroxylase deficiency may account for up to 12% of all patients with PCOS, but more realistic prevalence rates are probably 1% to 3%. Females have hirsutism and primary or

**Table 64-15**
**Different Forms of 21-Hydroxylase Deficiency**

| Phenotype | Classical Salt Wasting | Simple Virilizing | Nonclassical |
|---|---|---|---|
| Age at diagnosis | Newborn to 6 mo | Newborn to 2 yr (female) 2–4 yr (male) | Child to adult |
| Genitalia | Males normal, females ambiguous | Males normal, females ambiguous | Males normal, females virilized |
| Incidence | 1:20,000 | 1:60,000 | 1:1000 |
| Hormones | | | |
| Aldosterone | Reduced | Normal | Normal |
| Renin | Increased | Normal or increased | Normal |
| Cortisol | Reduced | Reduced | Normal |
| 17-Hydroxyprogesterone | >5000 nmol/L | 2500–5000 nmol/L | 500–2500 nmol/L (ACTH stimulation) |
| Testosterone | Increased | Increased | Variable, increased |
| Growth | –2 to 3 SD | –1 to 2 SD | Probably normal |
| 21-Hydroxylase activity (% of wild type) | 0% | 1% | 20% to 50% |
| Typical CYP21A2 mutations | Deletions, conversions, nt656g G110Δ8nt, R356W 1236N, V237E, M239K, Q318X | 1172N nt656g | V281L P30L |

ACTH, adrenocorticotropic hormone; SD, standard deviation.
From Larsen PR, Kronenberg HM, Melmed S, et al: (eds): Williams Textbook of Endocrinology, 10th ed. Philadelphia, WB Saunders, 2002, p 534.

secondary amenorrhea or anovulatory infertility. Androgenic alopecia and acne may be other presenting features.

### Heterozygote Deficiency

Salt-wasting, simple virilizing, and late-onset 21-hydroxylase deficiencies are all caused by homozygous or compound heterozygous mutations in the human CYP21A2 gene, whereas in the carrier heterozygote state, only one allele is mutated. The clinical significance of the heterozygote state is uncertain; it does not appear to affect reproductive capability but may cause signs of hyperandrogenism in women.

A diagnosis of 21-hydroxylase deficiency should be considered in any infant with genital ambiguity, salt wasting, or hypotension. Hyponatremia and hyperkalemia with raised plasma renin activity are found in salt wasters. In later life, adrenal androgen excess (DHEAS, androstenedione) is found in patients with sexual precocity or a PCOS-like phenotype. 17-OHP is invariably elevated, and clinically useful nomograms have been developed comparing circulating concentrations of 17-OHP before and 60 minutes after exogenous ACTH. This separates patients with classical and nonclassical 21-hydroxylase deficiency from heterozygote carriers and normal subjects, but there is some overlap between values seen in heterozygotes and normal people. 17-OHP is measured basally and then 60 minutes after 250 µg of cosyntropin. Stimulated values are invariably grossly elevated in patients with classical and nonclassical varieties (in excess of 35 nmol/L [11 µg/dL]). Heterozygote patients usually have stimulated values between 10 and 30 nmol/L (3 to 9 µg/dL). Stimulation tests are not always required to make a diagnosis; for example, a basal 17α-OHP concentration less than 5 nmol/L in the follicular phase of the menstrual cycle effectively excludes late-onset 21-hydroxylase deficiency. Androgen excess in 21-hydroxylase deficiency is readily suppressed after glucocorticoid administration.

Prenatal diagnosis of 21-hydroxylase deficiency has been advocated because treatment of an affected female may prevent masculinization in utero. 17-OHP can be assayed in amniotic fluid, but the most robust approach is the rapid genotyping of fetal cells obtained by chorionic villus sampling in early gestation. Unlike hydrocortisone, which is inactivated by placental 11β-HSD, maternally administered dexamethasone can cross the placenta to suppress the fetal HPA axis. One approach is to advocate dexamethasone therapy as soon as pregnancy is confirmed in high-risk cases and to continue this until the diagnosis is excluded in the fetus. If the fetus is affected, only those of female sex require dexamethasone therapy during gestation. Therapy must be initiated before 8 to 10 weeks of gestation to be effective. However, because only one in eight patients treated in this way have an affected female fetus, the use of steroid therapy in this setting has been questioned. Dexamethasone can lead to maternal cushingoid effects in pregnancy and may in turn have long-term, deleterious effects on the fetus.

In patients with known 21-hydroxylase deficiency requesting fertility (be they male or female), determination of 17-OHP levels by means of a cosyntropin test in the partner before conception occurs uncovers late-onset or heterozygote cases and provides the endocrinologist or geneticist with some assignment of risk before pregnancy.

## Treatment of Congenital Adrenal Hyperplasia

The treatment strategies have subtle variations depending on the age of the patient. In childhood the overall goal is to replace glucocorticoids and mineralocorticoids, thereby preventing further salt-wasting crises, and also to suppress adrenal androgen secretion so that normal growth and skeletal maturation can proceed. Accurate replacement is essential, since glucocorticoids in excess suppress growth, and inadequate replacement results initially in accelerated linear growth but ultimately in short stature because of premature epiphyseal closure. Response is best monitored through growth velocity and bone age, with biochemical markers (17-OHP, DHEAS, testosterone) being useful adjuncts. Corrective surgery is frequently required (clitoral reduction, vaginoplasty) during childhood. In late childhood and adolescence, appropriate replacement therapy is equally important. Overtreatment may result in obesity and delayed menarche or puberty with sexual infantilism, whereas under-replacement results in sexual precocity. Compliance with regular medication is often an issue through adolescence. Problems in adulthood are related to fertility concerns, hirsutism, and menstrual irregularity in women, obesity and impact of short stature, sexual dysfunction, and psychological problems; counseling is often required in addition to endocrine support.

Usual starting doses of hydrocortisone in childhood are 10 to 25 mg/m$^2$ per day in divided doses. Reverse-phase therapy may be appropriate, giving the largest dose of hydrocortisone at night to suppress early morning ACTH secretion. Long-acting steroids such as dexamethasone are more effective in this regard, but care should be taken to avoid oversuppression and reduction in linear growth. Fludrocortisone is required for patients with salt wasting (although this may improve spontaneously with age); doses of 0.1 to 0.2 mg/day should be given and blood pressure, electrolytes, and supine-erect plasma renin activity monitored to assess response.

In women with hyperandrogenism and untreated late-onset CAH, there is no evidence that final height is affected. In this setting, glucocorticoid suppression in isolation rarely controls hirsutism and additional antiandrogen therapy is often required (cyproterone acetate, spironolactone, flutamide together with an oral estrogen contraceptive pill). However, ovulation induction rates with gonadotropin therapy are improved after suppression of nocturnal ACTH levels with 0.25 to 0.5 mg of dexamethasone.

### 11β-Hydroxylase Deficiency

11β-Hydroxylase deficiency accounts for 7% of all cases of CAH with an incidence of 1 per 100,000 live births. The condition arises because of mutations in the CYP11B1 gene that result in loss of enzyme activity and a block in the conversion of 11-deoxycortisol to cortisol. There is loss of negative cortisol feedback and enhanced ACTH-mediated adrenal androgen excess. Clinical features are therefore similar to those reported in the simple virilizing form of CAH (virilized female fetus, sexual ambiguity), and again milder cases can present later in childhood or even young adulthood. The principal difference compared with 21-hydroxylase deficiency is hypertension, and this is thought to be secondary to the mineralocorticoid effect of DOC excess.[26,27]

## 17α-Hydroxylase Deficiency

Fewer than 150 cases of 17α-hydroxylase deficiency have been reported. Mutations within the CYP17 gene result in the failure to synthesize cortisol (17α-hydroxylase activity), adrenal androgens (17,20-lyase activity), and gonadal steroids. Thus, in contrast to 21-hydroxylase and 11-hydroxylase deficiencies, 17α-hydroxylase deficiency results in adrenal and gonadal insufficiency. Loss of negative feedback results in increased secretion of steroids proximal to the block, and mineralo-corticoid synthesis is enhanced.

The diagnosis is usually made at the time of puberty when patients come in with hypertension, hypokalemia, and hypogonadism, the latter occurring because of lack of CYP17 expression within the gonad and impaired gonadal steroidogenesis. As a result, LH and FSH levels are elevated. Female patients (46,XX) have primary amenorrhea with absent sexual characteristics, and males (46,XY) have complete pseudohermaphroditism with female external genitalia but absent uterus and fallopian tubes. The intra-abdominal testes should be removed, and such patients are usually reared as female. Glucocorticoid replacement reverses the DOC-induced suppression of the renin-angiotensin system and lowers blood pressure. Additional sex steroid replacement is required from puberty onward.[26,27]

## 3β-Hydroxysteroid Dehydrogenase Deficiency

In this rare form of CAH, the secretion of all classes of adrenal and ovarian steroids is impaired because of mutations within the HSD3B2 gene encoding 3β-HSDII. The disorder usually presents in early infancy with adrenal insufficiency. Loss of mineralocorticoid secretion results in salt wasting, although this is absent in 30% to 40% of cases. As with 21-hydroxylase deficiency, absence of salt wasting may delay the presentation until childhood or puberty. The spectrum of genital development is variable in both sexes. In males, because the 3β-HSDII enzyme is also expressed within the gonad, male pseudo-hermaphroditism may occur, with female external genitalia. In milder cases, hypospadias may be found or even normal male genitalia. In females, genital development can be normal but there is usually evidence of mild virilization, presumably because of enhanced adrenal secretion of DHEA, which is converted peripherally to testosterone. A late-onset form has been described in patients with premature pubarche and a PCOS-like phenotype (hirsutism, oligomenorrhea, amenorrhea).

Because activity of the 3β-HSDI enzyme present in skin and other peripheral tissues is intact, circulating Δ4 steroid levels (progesterone, 17α-hydroxyprogesterone, androstenedione) may be normal (or even increased). However, a diagnosis is established by demonstrating an increased ratio of Δ5 steroids (pregnenolone, 17α-hydroxypregnenolone, DHEA) to Δ4 steroids in plasma or urine. ACTH stimulation may be required to detect a late-onset presentation. Treatment is with replacement glucocorticoids, fludrocortisone (if indicated), and sex steroids from puberty onward.

## Steroidogenic Acute Regulatory Protein Deficiency

Mutations in the gene encoding StAR result in a failure of transport of cholesterol from the outer to the inner mitochondrial membrane in steroidogenic tissues; as a result, there is deficiency of all adrenal and gonadal steroid hormones. Presentation is of acute adrenal insufficiency in the neonatal period, and males exhibit pseudohermaphroditism because of absent gonadal steroids. The condition is fatal in infancy in two thirds of cases. The adrenal glands are often massively enlarged and lipid laden; prior to the characterization of StAR, the condition was termed *congenital lipoid hyperplasia* and the candidate gene was thought to be cholesterol side-chain cleavage (CYP11A1). In fact, to date, no mutations have been reported in the CYP11A1 gene; such mutations are thought to be lethal in utero.[28]

## REFERENCES

1. Bornstein SR, Chrousos GP: Adrenocorticotropin ACTH- and non-ACTH-mediated regulation of the adrenal cortex: neural and immune inputs. J Clin Endocrinol Metab 1999;84:1729–1736. **(Ib, A)**
2. Newell-Price J, Trainer P, Besser M, Grossman A: The diagnosis and differential diagnosis of Cushing's syndrome and pseudo-Cushing's states. Endocr Rev 1998;19:647–672. **(Ib, A)**
3. Chrousos GP, Torpy DJ, Gold PW: Interactions between the hypothalamic-pituitary-adrenal axis and the female reproductive system: clinical implications. Ann Intern Med 1998;129:229–240. **(Ib, A)**
4. Jeffcoate WJ, Silverstone JT, Edwards CRW, et al: Psychiatric manifestations of Cushing's syndrome: response to lowering of plasma cortisol. Q J Med 1979;48:465–472. **(III, B)**
5. Biller BM: Pathogenesis of pituitary Cushing's syndrome: pituitary versus hypothalamic. Endocrinol Metab Clin North Am 1994; 23:547–554. **(Ib, B)**
6. Guilhaume B, Bertagna X, Thomsen M, et al: Transsphenoidal pituitary surgery for the treatment of Cushing's disease: results in 64 patients and long term follow-up studies. J Clin Endocrinol Metab 1988; 66:1056–1064. **(IIa, B)**
7. Bochicchio D, Losa M, Buchfelder M, et al: Factors influencing the immediate and late outcome of Cushing's disease treated by trans-sphenoidal surgery: a retrospective study by the European Cushing's Disease Survey Group. J Clin Endocrinol Metab 1995;80:3114–3120. **(III, B)**
8. Howlett TA, Drury PL, Perry L, et al: Diagnosis and management of ACTH-dependent Cushing's syndrome: comparison of the features in ectopic and pituitary ACTH production. Clin Endocrinol (Oxf) 1986; 24:699–713. **(Ib, A)**
9. Weinstein LS, Shenker A, Gejman PV, et al: Activating mutations of the stimulatory G protein in McCune-Albright syndrome. N Engl J Med 1991;325:1688–1695. **(III, B)**
10. Mengden T, Hubmann P, Muller J, et al: Urinary free cortisol versus 17-hydroxycorticosteroids: a comparative study of their diagnostic value in Cushing's syndrome. Clin Invest 1992;70:545–548. **(III, B)**
11. Yanovski JA, Cutler GB Jr, Chrousos GP, Nieman LK: Corticotropin-releasing hormone stimulation following low-dose dexamethasone administration: a new test to distinguish Cushing's syndrome from pseudo-Cushing's states. JAMA 1993;269:2232–2238. **(III, B)**
12. Escourolle H, Abecassis JP, Bertagna X, et al: Comparison of computerized tomography and magnetic resonance imaging for the examination of the pituitary gland in patients with Cushing's disease. Clin Endocrinol (Oxf) 1993;39:307–313. **(III, B)**
13. Axelrod L: Glucocorticoid therapy. Medicine (Baltimore) 1976; 55:39–65 **(Ib, A)**
14. Laudat MH, Cerdas S, Fournier C, et al: Salivary cortisol measurement: a practical approach to assess pituitary-adrenal function. J Clin Endocrinol Metab 1988;66:343–348. **(III, B)**
15. McCance DR, Hadden DR, Kennedy L, et al: Clinical experience with ketoconazole as a therapy for patients with Cushing's syndrome. Clin Endocrinol (Oxf) 1987;27:593–599. **(III, B)**

16. Carey RM.: The changing clinical spectrum of adrenal insufficiency. Ann Intern Med 1997;127:1103–1105. **(Ib, A)**

17. Betterle C, Greggio NA, Volpato M: Autoimmune polyglandular syndrome type 1. Clinical Review 93. J Clin Endocrinol Metab 1998; 83:1049–1055. **(Ib, A)**

18. Clark PM, Neylon I, Raggatt PR, et al: Defining the normal cortisol response to the short Synacthen test: implications for the investigation of hypothalamic-pituitary disorders. Clin Endocrinol (Oxf) 1998; 49:287–292. **(III, B)**

19. Stewart PM, Corrie J, Seckl JR, et al: A rational approach for assessing the hypothalamo-pituitary-adrenal axis. Lancet 1988;1:1208–1210. **(Ib, A)**

20. Abdu TA, Elhadd TA, Neary R, Clayton RN: Comparison of the low dose short Synacthen test (1 μg), the conventional dose short Synacthen test (250 μg) and the insulin tolerance test for assessment of the hypothalamo-pituitary-adrenal axis in patients with pituitary disease. J Clin Endocrinol Metab 1999;84:838–843. **(III, B)**

21. Howlett TA: An assessment of optimal hydrocortisone replacement therapy. Clin Endocrinol (Oxf) 1997;46:263–268. **(Ib, A)**

22. Smith SJ, Markandu ND, Banks RA, et al: Evidence that patients with Addison's disease are undertreated with fludrocortisone. Lancet 1984; 1:11–14. **(Ib, A)**

23. Arlt W, Callies F, van Vlijmen JC, et al: Dehydroepiandrosterone replacement in women with adrenal insufficiency. N Engl J Med 1999; 341:1013–1020. **(Ib, A)**

24. Klingensmith GJ, Garcia SC, Jones HW, et al: Glucocorticoid treatment of girls with congenital adrenal hyperplasia: effects on height, sexual maturation, and fertility. J Pediatr 1977;90:996–1004. **(Ib, A)**

25. Azziz R, Dewailly D, Owerbach D: Nonclassic adrenal hyperplasia: current concepts. Clinical Review 56. J Clin Endocrinol Metab 1996; 78:810–815. **(Ib, A)**

26. Miller WL: Gene conversions, deletions, and polymorphisms in congenital adrenal hyperplasia. Am J Hum Genet 1988;42:4–7. **(III, B)**

27. Kloos RT, Gross MD, Francis IR, et al: Incidentally discovered adrenal masses. Endocr Rev 1995;16:460–484. **(IIb, A)**

28. Baxter JD, Tyrrell JB: In Felig P, Baxter JD, Frohman LA (eds): Endocrinology and Metabolism, 3rd ed. New York, McGraw-Hill, 1995. **(Ib, A)**

# Section 9　Coding and Office Management

## Chapter 65

# Coding Tips for the Busy Physician

### Philip N. Eskew, Jr., MD

## KEY POINTS

- Be involved in the coding process.
- Learn to use history templates.
- For "complaint" visits, examine only what is clinically relevant.
- Learn the difference between a consultation and counseling.
- Compare your use of the five established patient visits codes with those used by your partners, then audit each other's charts.
- Document only what you do, code for only what you documented.

Medicine has changed! Most physicians want to just take care of patients and enjoy the challenge of diagnosing, treating, and modifying behaviors toward an improvement in their patients' overall health. However, physicians must also learn and participate in the *business* of medicine—coding, documentation, reimbursement, contracting, compliance, and risk management. Physicians are busy and most do not want to learn about coding and documentation, but these basic skills will create a better medical record, improve billings and collections, and decrease their level of anxiety regarding fraud and abuse.

The process of reimbursement for physician services involves utilizing coding and documentation principles. Insurance plans and managed care plans reimburse based on the submission, by the physician, of proper CPT (Current Procedural Terminology) and ICD-9 (International Classification of Diseases, ninth edition) codes.

CPT codes are used to record services provided by the physician. Those services include surgical procedures, hospital care, critical care, and office visits. CPT codes are five-digit numbers that indicate to the insurance company what services were provided to the patient (Example 1). ICD-9 codes are three-, four-, or five-digit numbers used to define the diagnosis for the services provided (Example 2).

## EXAMPLE I

99223 Initial hospital care, per day, for the evaluation and management of a patient, which requires these three key components:
　a comprehensive history
　a comprehensive examination
　medical decision making of high complexity

Counseling and/or coordination of care with other providers or agencies are provided consistent with the nature of the problem(s) and the patient's and/or family's needs. Usually the problem(s) requiring admission are of high severity. Physicians typically spend 70 minutes at the bedside and on the patient's hospital floor or unit.

This information is in the CPT book under the listing of the code. Information is also provided under the category heading of Initial Hospital Care.

> When the patient is admitted to the hospital as an inpatient in the course of an encounter in another site of service (e.g., hospital emergency department, observation status in a hospital, physician's office, nursing facility), all evaluation and management services provided by that physician in conjunction with that admission are considered part of the initial hospital care when performed on the same date as the admission. The inpatient care level of service reported by the admitting physician should include the services related to the admission he or she provided in the other sites of service as well as in the inpatient setting.
>
> Evaluation and management services on the same date provided in sites that are related to the admission "observation status" should not be reported separately. For a patient admitted and discharged from observation or inpatient status on the same date, the services should be reported with codes 99234–99236 as appropriate.

## EXAMPLE 2

Diabetes with renal manifestations
　Use additional code to identify manifestation, as:
　　Diabetic:
　　　Nephropathy NOS (583.81)
　　　Nephrosis (581.81)
　　　Intercapillary glomerulosclerosis (581.81)
　　　Kimmelstiel-Wilson syndrome (581.81)

There is a reminder in the book that a fifth digit is required. Use of a fifth digit makes the code more specific and frequently will provide additional information indicating the severity of the condition.

The following fifth-digit subclassification is for use with category 250:
[Category 250 is diabetes mellitus and excludes gestational diabetes (648.8), hyperglycemia NOS (790.6), neonatal diabetes mellitus (775.1), and nonclinical diabetes (790.2)]
　0 type II (non-insulin-dependent type) (NICCM type) (adult-onset type) or unspecified type, not stated as uncontrolled

## Coding and Office Management

Fifth-digit 0 is for use with type II, adult-onset diabetic patients, even if the patient requires insulin

1  type I (insulin-dependent type) (IDDM) (juvenile type), not stated as uncontrolled

2  type II (non-insulin-dependent type) (NIDDM type) (adult-onset type) or unspecified type, uncontrolled

Fifth-digit 2 is for use with type II, adult-onset diabetic patients, even if the patient requires insulin

3  type I (insulin-dependent type) (IDDM) (juvenile type), uncontrolled

The physician's responsibility does not end with the selection of the proper CPT and ICD-9 codes. All insurance companies require that the documentation on the patient's chart accurately reflect the physician work involved in the patient encounter. Each encounter requires the physician to document the history obtained from the patient, the amount of the physical examination performed, and the medical decision making involved in the encounter.

This process may sound simple, but most physicians have developed short cuts, abbreviated forms, and handwritten notes that do not meet documentation guidelines. In other situations, some physicians will make up a diagnosis that will allow the patient's encounter to be reimbursed by the insurer. This can be dangerous, since the patient's medical history may reflect an inaccurate diagnosis that could affect their ability to obtain health insurance in the future. Far too many physicians have been charged with fraud for falsifying insurance claims with procedures that were not performed or for providing inaccurate documentation to justify the insurance claim.

The history obtained from the patient should begin at the initial visit and require the patient to complete a comprehensive intake history form. Many such forms are available that are comprehensive in nature and meet the requirements for a comprehensive history. It is important for the physician to review the history with the patient and sign the history form in addition to asking for the patient's signature. Several insurance and managed care companies inform the patient that to call the company if they feel the physician has over-charged for the visit, and the company will request the medical records for documentation of the visit. This same comprehensive intake history form can be reviewed by the patient, signed, and dated, and countersigned and dated by the physician the next year.

The patient does not have to fill out a new form each year. However, some physicians ask patients to fill out an interval history form if they return within the year for a visit other than an annual examination. At this visit the interval history form can simply ask the patient what changes in their health, family, or medication status have taken place since the last visit. It is appropriate to put on this form a sentence such as "I apologize for having you fill out this form, but most insurance companies require it." This will make up for the inconvenience and frustration that some patients feel when asked to fill out one more form.

In addition to these forms, the physician must record, either on a form or by dictation or in handwriting, the chief complaint, history of present illness, and any pertinent changes in the patient's history since the last visit, to document the reason for the encounter (Example 3).

## EXAMPLE 3

Chief Complaint:        "I have a pain in my belly."
History of Present Illness:        The patient complains of an <u>intense</u>, constant, <u>sharp</u> pain in the upper right quadrant that is only <u>relieved by lying down</u>. This <u>began three days ago</u>.

Example 3 provides the Chief Complaint and six components of the History of Present Illness. A detailed or comprehensive history requires only four components. The eight components are location, severity, duration, timing, quality and context, modifying factors, signs and symptoms.

This form provides a good medical record that can easily be understood by the physician's partner or the insurance company or serve as an excellent source for the physician when the patient returns. Physicians are required to go back to basics—to use the history-taking methods learned in medical school and residency training—in meeting the requirements of today's insurers. Templates are acceptable and can serve as a reminder for the physician but also create a comprehensive history.

Most physicians have their own format for dictation of a complete physical examination. The physician can utilize a check-off form for the physical examination as long as each individual item is individually checked. A physician who prefers dictation to document the physical examination must mention each body area actually examined. Whichever method the physician utilizes, the medical record must contain documentation of the clinically relevant body areas examined relative to the patient's diagnosis.

The key to reimbursement is for the physician to only perform an examination of "clinically relevant" body areas. Performing a comprehensive physical examination will not allow the physician to be reimbursed more when the patient's symptoms require only an abbreviated examination. However, physicians place themselves at risk if they submit a claim for a patient encounter that does not document the physical examination required for that CPT code.

The most difficult area of the patient encounter to document is the medical decision-making component. This requires physicians to document their thought processes regarding how they are managing the patient's diagnosis, which tests they are ordering and why, prescriptions written, procedures planned, and diagnoses considered and ruled out (Example 4). With each patient encounter, the physician should devote a portion of their dictation or written narrative to the documentation of what conditions the patient complains of and what tests or procedures the physician is considering to help with the diagnosis and treatment of the complaint.

## EXAMPLE 4

| | |
|---|---|
| Impression: | Pneumonia |
| Labs: | CBC |
| Tests ordered: | Chest x-ray |
| Prescriptions: | Antibiotic, expectorant |
| Plan: | Follow-up in 7 days, force fluids, report worsening of symptoms |

When a patient is hospitalized, the physician must record the services performed in the hospital—either surgical or medical care—and submit that information to his or her office billing clerk. Each patient has a hospital face sheet with insurance information on which the physician should record the date(s) of service along with the appropriate CPT and ICD-9 codes for each day of hospitalization.

Consultation services should be carefully documented following the requirements prescribed by CPT. A request for a consultation means that another physician wants your advice or opinion. In some cases, this service can be provided on your own patient (Example 5). During a consultation encounter you may order tests, write prescriptions, or provide therapy. The main requirements are for documentation in the chart of the physician who requested the consultation and documentation of a letter sent to that requesting physician.

## EXAMPLE 5

I was asked to see Mrs. Smith in consultation regarding the status of her hypertension prior to undergoing an abdominal hysterectomy for uterine leiomyomata and persistent menorrhagia.

The relative value units for a consultation are much higher than for a new patient visit, so whenever your opinion or advice is requested, use a consultation code.

Many patients come to your office for their "annual physical." An age-appropriate comprehensive physical examination should be performed. A review of the patient's intake history form with the patient will meet the requirements for a comprehensive history. It is appropriate to review the patient's status with regard to several ongoing clinical conditions, refill or adjust medications, and order appropriate screening tests. It is a general rule that if greater than 50% of that visit is related to performing an "annual examination," then bill it as an "annual examination." If the patient comes into the office with a new complaint that requires significant physician work, then the visit should be billed at the appropriate established patient level code. If you discover or suspect a new condition, you may order tests to confirm or rule out the condition as long as greater than 50% of your time is spent performing an "annual examination."

Each physician should take the time to become involved in the coding and billing portion of his or her practice. This means that the physician should meet regularly (weekly or biweekly) with the insurance or billing person in the office. Discussions as to why claims were questioned, denied, or returned for more information by the insurer will help educate the physician in the documentation phase of the patient encounter. Several medical journals and subscription newsletters regularly publish helpful hints regarding coding, billing, and documentation information. Physicians should read these and share them with office personnel. Attendance at coding postgraduate courses by physicians and office staff are valuable in helping everyone understand the importance of coding and documentation.

How accurately the physician codes each patient encounter can affect the amount of money earned in the practice. Some practices divide the financial profits based on a productivity principle. Each physician's productivity is based on the relative value units assigned to each procedure and each office encounter. The relative value unit total for the individual physician's work determines his or her productivity for that time period (Example 6). If a physician incorrectly records a lower level office visit than is actually documented, the relative value unit total will be affected when profits are split.

## EXAMPLE 6

| Medicare Reimbursement Unit for 2005 is $37.8974 | | | |
|---|---|---|---|
| **New Patient Encounters** | | **Established Patient Encounters** | |
| 99201 | 0.97 | 99211 | 0.57 |
| 99202 | 1.72 | 99212 | 1.02 |
| 99203 | 2.56 | 99213 | 1.39 |
| 99204 | 3.62 | 99214 | 2.18 |
| 99205 | 4.58 | 99215 | 3.17 |
| **Outpatient Consultation** | | **Inpatient Consultation** | |
| 99241 | 1.33 | 99251 | 0.95 |
| 99242 | 2.43 | 99252 | 1.91 |
| 99243 | 3.24 | 99253 | 2.61 |
| 99244 | 4.56 | 99254 | 3.75 |
| 99245 | 5.90 | 99255 | 5.17 |
| **New Patient Annual Examination** | | **Established Patient Annual Examination** | |
| 99385 | 3.14 | 99395 | 2.57 |
| 99386 | 3.69 | 99396 | 2.85 |
| 99387 | 4.00 | 99397 | 3.13 |

Each year CPT and ICD-9 publish a book with updates that add, delete, or edit some codes. The physician and office staff need to obtain the new book each year and review the changes. Several publications summarize these changes in articles or newsletters, and physicians can share this information at their regular office staff or business meetings. The Coding Institute publishes a Coding Alert for each specialty offering helpful hints and explanations for the physician and the office staff. The AMA publishes The CPT Assistant, which has helpful articles answering coding questions.

The practice of medicine now requires the physician to not only learn about new procedures and techniques but also how to document the appropriate amount of history, physical examination, and medical decision making for each patient encounter. The challenge for busy physicians is to assess how well they are doing, educate themselves and their office staff about coding principles, and take steps to improve coding, documentation, and compliance. Perform a self-audit of the office visit codes during the past 2 months for each physician. Compare the bar graphs, and then multiply the total number of each level by the relative value units. This can be an eye-opening experience and the beginning of improved coding, documentation, compliance, and comfort.

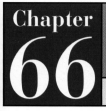

# Chapter 66

# Federal Regulations

Joseph Sanfilippo, MD, MBA, and Ira R. Horowitz, MD, MHCM

## HIPAA COMPLIANCE

The Health Insurance Portability and Accountability Act (HIPAA) is federal legislation that was passed in 1996. It provides guidelines for patient privacy in a medical practice focused on three main areas:

- Insurance portability
- Administrative focus
- Privacy and security

HIPAA is designed to establish the minimum necessary standard to make a reasonable effort to limit use, disclosure, and requests for patient information.

The insurance portability segment of HIPAA focuses on the patient's ability to maintain health insurance coverage when one makes a decision to change health plans. It is designed to prevent denial of coverage based on a "preexisting" condition.

The administrative segment is predicated on development of standards for the process of information exchange, especially electronically. This aspect of HIPAA also requires health care professionals to implement policies designed to protect patient privacy and confidentiality.

The privacy and security segment addresses the medical record and the effort to keep patient information private and secure from inappropriate access.

The Health Insurance Portability and Accountability Act applies to all health care professionals. It is our responsibility to comply with HIPAA privacy rules and regulations.

### Minimum Necessary Information

The *minimum necessary* rule is designed to provide patient information on a need-to-know basis and applies to all uses, disclosures, and requests for information by individuals and/or industrial organizations that utilize such information to perform health care–related operations. This would include the following:

- Payment for services
- Administrative purposes
- Request for information from other covered entities for their payment or administrative-related activities
- Research purposes

HIPAA includes all aspects of patient information access: written, verbal, and electronic.

Protected health information includes the following:

- Patient name and address
- Social Security number
- Date of birth
- Medical record number

- Medical history
- Diagnosis
- Plan of management
- Medications

### HIPAA Highlights

- Sign-in sheets should only have patient name and not reason for the visit.
- Patients must sign a document that they want to be reminded about a visit as, for example, "annual examination."
- Be discreet about discussing patient information in public areas.
- Never leave patient charts unattended.
- Close the curtain in semiprivate rooms, and ask visitors to step out.
- Position the computer screen such that patient information cannot be viewed easily.
- Do not keep screen up when the computer is unattended.
- Obtain patient authorization before releasing any information not related to billing or collections.
- When finished with confidential information, place in paper shredder.
- Have appropriate security measures in place when e-mailing personal health information.
- When faxing, do not leave patient information unattended.
- Confirm that the fax was received.

### Implementing HIPAA Regulations

To implement HIPAA regulations:

- Identify an individual in the office responsible for implementation of rules and regulations.
- Limit access to patient information.
- Identify individuals who need access to patient information. This can be stated as an all-encompassing policy regarding medical employees (i.e., all involved in the patient's treatment).
- Establish policies and procedures that limit access to patient's medical information. This can be accomplished by establishing a protocol.
- The Minimum Necessary Standard does not apply to disclosures or requests for treatment purposes. This means you may disclose the entire medical record to another provider or request an entire medical record for treatment purposes without documenting on the patient's chart the specific justification.
- Front desk sign-in sheets as well as calling out of patient's name in the waiting room are permitted. Discretion is required if discussing patient information in an open area.

- Patients should be escorted to the examination room and not left to find it on their own.
- Leaving the patient's record outside the door of the examination room is permissible. If the patient's name can be identified, it must be placed facing the wall to protect privacy.
- Make use of a Business Associate Agreement (Fig. 66-1).

**Protocol for Implementation of HIPAA**

Identify the individuals who may receive or record information on the patient's chart, which may include the following:

- Nursing staff
- Medical assistants
- Clerical personnel employed by the office

# BUSINESS ASSOCIATE AGREEMENT

Date: _____

Name of Company: _____

Representative Name: (Print) _____

Reason for Records: _____

We are furnishing you and your Company with Patient Confidential Information. Use of Private Patient Information must meet the guidelines of The Health Insurance Portability and Accountability Act (HIPAA).

I (We) understand the information provided is subject to federal privacy regulations (HIPAA 1996 and codified at 45 C.F.R. parts 160 and 164–the Privacy Rule). The purpose of this agreement is to enter into compliance with the Privacy Rule. The information released to you/your company may be used for collection or audit of records, insurance, research, or legal purposes. IT IS YOUR RESPONSIBILITY TO KEEP THESE RECORDS PRIVATE. THE INTENDED PURPOSE IS EXCLUSIVELY AS NOTED ABOVE.

I (We) agree to appropriate safeguards to prevent use or disclosure of the Protected Health Information. All subcontractors and agents that receive the information must agree to the same restrictions.

I am in agreement with the stipulations.

Sincerely,

_____

Representative/Company: _____

**Figure 66-1   Business Associate Agreement.**

Specify the type of information that may be accessed, which may include the following:

- History and physical examination information
- Progress notes
- Orders
- Medication sheets
- Phone calls
- E-mails related to the patient
- Medical transcription

List who may receive information and state the purpose, such as a claims processor and/or billing and collection personnel.

Educate office personnel with regard to HIPAA rules and regulations.

Do not leave the photocopier unattended when making a copy of information covered under the protected health information.

Confirm information regarding fax number before sending. Include a cover sheet stating that this is confidential information. Verify that the fax was received.

Develop a plan to monitor implementation and compliance in the practice.

Office redesign is not necessary, but privacy protection must include segregating or locking file cabinets or using a password to gain access to patient information in the case of electronically recorded medical records.

The individual in charge must decide on a case-by-case basis regarding provision of protected information to an individual or corporation. Then only the Minimum Necessary Information may be supplied.

### Retention of Records

All medical records must be retained for a minimum of 6 years to comply with HIPAA regulations.

### Release of Protected Information

To release protected health information when it is not being used for health care–related reasons, (e.g., treatment, payment), proceed as follows.

The following information must be recorded:

- Patient's name
- Reason for requesting information
- Name, agency to receive the information
- Name of practice providing the information
- Patient's consent to release the information, including his or her signature
- Provision of minimal but appropriate amount of information

### Research

If patient information is planned to be used in research, the patient must supply specific consent. This would also hold true for retrospective studies.

### Minors

Minors may provide their own authorization for contraception, pregnancy-related care, venereal disease evaluation and treatment, or other reportable medical conditions.

### Posting of Notice of Privacy

The Notice of Privacy Practices (Fig. 66-2) is to be displayed in an area that patients have ready access to. The waiting room is the ideal location for listing of such information.

### Patient Aspect

Patients are to receive the Notice of Privacy Practices document for their signature. If the practice chooses to communicate via e-mail, a separate consent form should be obtained (Figs. 66-3 and 66-4).

Patients may review their medical records, but a request should be obtained in writing. Ideally it should state the reason the request is being made. Patients may be denied access if the record provides information related to psychotherapy or court proceedings, or if the health care provider makes a judgment call regarding information "not in the patient's best interest" (i.e., knowledge of the information could result in life-threatening circumstances).

Sale of a patient list, as, for example, to a pharmaceutical company is not permitted by HIPAA regulations.

### Discussions with Other Health Care Professionals

Such discussion is permitted, but discretion is advised.

In semiprivate locations appropriate judgment is recommended (e.g., close the curtain, ask family members to step out of the room, be discreet in discussions outside of the patient's room).

## Violations of HIPAA

Violations of HIPAA can result in both civil and criminal penalties. Civil penalties of $100 per violation, with a cap up to $25,000 in 1 year, can be imposed. In addition criminal penalties ranging from $50,000 to $250,000 as well as imprisonment for up to 10 years can be imposed. Enforcement of HIPAA regulations is under the jurisdiction of the U.S. Department of Health and Human Services, Office for Civil Rights.

### Reporting of Complaints

The Secretary of the U.S. Department of Health and Human Services may be contacted directly.

You are referred to the U.S. Department of Health and Human Services for further information.

HIPAA Federal regulations information can be accessed at: http://aspe.hhs.gov/admnsimp/final/PvcTxt01.htm

The Office for Civil Rights document regarding HIPAA can be accessed at: http://www.hhs.gov/ocr/hipaa/privacy.html

## CLINICAL LABORATORY IMPROVEMENT AMENDMENTS OF 1988

In 1988, Congress passed the Clinical Laboratory Improvement Amendments (CLIA) Act. The initial motivation was to standardize all laboratory testing. One impetus for this amendment was to ensure quality assurance on tests performed for diagnosis, prevention, and treatment. This need was demonstrated in the latter part of 1980, when medical organizations and the media highlighted concerns about "Pap smear mills" with questionably reproducible results. Under CLIA, all laboratories

# HIPAA PRIVACY AWARENESS

## The Health Insurance Portability and Accountability Act (HIPAA) is Federal Legislation concerning the following areas:

## Insurance
## Administrative Activities
## Privacy and Security

- **There is limited access to your medical records in your office.**
- **The appropriate Minimal Information is provided for billing purposes.**
- **Your Protected Health Information includes your Name-Address-Social Security Number-Medical Record Number-Date of Birth and Medical Record.**
- **Any concerns you have about Violation of HIPAA Privacy can be directed to the United States Department of Health and Human Services, Office for Civil Rights.**

**Figure 66-2    Notice of Privacy Practices.**

performing analysis on human specimens must be certified by the Secretary of the U.S. Department of Health and Human Services (HHS).

Presently more than 40 tests have been approved for a Certificate of Waiver through CLIA (http://www.fda.gov/cdrh/clia). CLIA Laboratory Certification as well as Certificates of Waiver are certified by the U.S. Secretary of HHS, the Centers for Disease Control and Prevention (CDC), and the Food and Drug Administration (FDA). CMS (the Centers for Medicare and Medicaid Services) administers CLIA certification for the HHS Secretary. To qualify for a Certificate of Waiver, it is imperative that the FDA and CDC deem a laboratory test simple enough that the risk of erroneous results is minimal An example would be the use of urine pregnancy tests in the office setting. The complete list of CLIA waived procedures as well as manufacturers is located at http://www.cms.hhs.gov/clia/waivetbl.pdf.

# PATIENT HIPAA AWARENESS DOCUMENT

The Health Insurance Portability and Accountability Act (HIPAA) is Federal legislation designed to protect the privacy of your health care information. Every effort is made to protect your privacy and the information regarding your medical care.
This means access to your medical records is restricted to those directly involved in your medical care. The minimum appropriate information is provided to individuals involved with billing. We are careful to be discrete and confidential so that others do not hear when talking to you about your medical care. Our workforce is educated with regard to HIPAA and the implementation of it. Privacy and Security are an integral part of how we deal with your medical record.

I consent to obtain notification of visits via mail or other means.

If you request additional information regarding guidelines for release of Protected Health Information, it can be obtained from my health care professional.

NAME: _____

DATE: _____

SIGNATURE: _____

Figure 66-3   Patient HIPAA Awareness Document.

Currently waived analytes used in laboratory test systems waived laboratories are shown in Figure 66-5 and at http://www.accessdata.fda.gov/scripts/cdrh/cfdocs/cfClia/analyteswaived.cfm. The complete list of CLIA-waived procedures as well as manufacturers is located at http://www.cms.hhs.gov/clia/waivetbl.pdf. To obtain a CLIA Certificate of Waiver one must complete the form CMS 116, which can be obtained at http://www.cms.hhs.gov/forms/cms116.pdf.

In addition to CLIA Certificate of Waivers, it is imperative that obstetricians and gynecologists also apply for the Provider-Performed Microscopy Procedure (PPMP) Laboratory Certification. The PPMP certificate permits a laboratory to have physicians, midlevel practitioners, or dentists perform moderately complex tests utilizing a microscope. The certificate permits the laboratory to also perform waived tests (Fig. 66-6).

### Quality Problems in Laboratories

Since the inception of the Certificate of Waiver in 1992, as the number of waived tests has grown, the number of Certificate of Waiver laboratories has grown, from 20% to 55% of the total 174,504 laboratories enrolled. In addition, PPMP laboratories make up 22% of all laboratories; this results in a total of 77% of laboratories not having any oversight. These led to a desire to examine the safey of laboratories.

In 2000–2001 several pilot studies were performed to evaluate CLIA Certificate of Waiver and PPMP laboratories. The

# E-MAIL CONSENT FORM

NAME: _____

ADDRESS: _____

_____

TELEPHONE NUMBER: _____

E-MAIL ADDRESS: _____

DATE OF BIRTH: _____

I consent to use of e-mail for communication regarding my health care.

I am aware of the Patient Privacy Protected Health Information (HIPAA–Health Insurance Portability and Accountability Act).

I agree to provide my **full name and date of birth with each e-mail** communication for proper identification.

I will clearly **state the reason for the e-mail:**

- Medical question
- Medication question
- Billing question
- Request for appointment

I understand the Internet may not always be secure and thus an unauthorized party may inadvertently obtain information regarding my medical care.

I understand there is no guarantee of privacy but that every effort will be made to protect the privacy of my health care information.

I understand that if it is permitted and I receive information regarding my health care at my place of employment, it may not be as secure compared to my home e-mail.

I agree to use of information regarding my medical record for purposes of reimbursement from insurance-related third parties.

I agree not to use e-mail as the method of communication for an emergency circumstance.

I agree to contact the practice directly if my e-mail is not responded to in a timely manner.

I consent to having a copy of my e-mails incorporated into my medical record.

Any changes in my e-mail address will be conveyed in a timely manner.

I may revoke my consent to communication via e-mail by providing a written statement requesting such.

I agree that no liability on the part of this practice will ensue for anyone inadvertently receiving my e-mail information.

I fully understand the information provided in this consent form and have had all questions answered.

SIGNATURE: _____

DATE: _____

WITNESS: _____

**Figure 66-4    E-Mail Consent Form.**

ALANINE AMINOTRANSFERASE (ALT) (SGPT)
ALBUMIN, URINARY
ALCOHOL, SALIVA
AMINES
AMPHETAMINES
ASPARTATE AMINOTRANSFERASE (AST) (SGOT)
B-TYPE NATRIURETIC PEPTIDE (BNP)
BARBITURATES
BENZODIAZEPINES
BLADDER TUMOR ASSOCIATED ANTIGEN
CANNABINOIDS (THC)
CATALASE, URINE
CHOLESTEROL
COCAINE METABOLITES
COLLAGEN TYPE I CROSSLINK, N-TELOPEPTIDES (NTX)
CREATININE
ERYTHROCYTE SEDIMENTATION RATE, NONAUTOMATED
ESTRONE-3 GLUCURONIDE
ETHANOL (ALCOHOL)
FECAL OCCULT BLOOD
FERN TEST, SALIVA
FOLLICLE STIMULATING HORMONE (FSH)
FRUCTOSAMINE
GASTRIC OCCULT BLOOD
GASTRIC pH
GLUCOSE
GLUCOSE MONITORING DEVICES (FDA CLEARED/HOME USE)
GLUCOSE MONITORING DEVICES (PRESCRIPTION USE ONLY)
GLUCOSE, FLUID (APPROVED BY FDA FOR PRESCRIPTION HOME USE)
GLYCATED HEMOGLOBIN, TOTAL
GLYCOSYLATED HEMOGLOBIN (Hgb A1c)
HCG, URINE
HDL CHOLESTEROL
HELICOBACTER PYLORI
HELICOBACTER PYLORI ANTIBODIES
HEMATOCRIT
HEMOGLOBIN
HEMOGLOBIN BY COPPER SULFATE, NONAUTOMATED
HEMOGLOBIN, SINGLE ANALYTE INSTRUMENTS W/SELF-CONTAINED...
HIV-1 AND HIV-2 ANTIBODIES
HIV-1 ANTIBODY
INFECTIOUS MONONUCLEOSIS ANTIBODIES (MONO)
INFLUENZA A
INFLUENZA A/B
INFLUENZA B
KETONE, BLOOD

**Figure 66-5   Currently waived analytes used in laboratory test systems.** (http://www.accessdata.fda.gov/scripts/ cdrh/cfdocs/cfClia/analyteswaived.cfm)

*Continued*

KETONE, URINE
LACTIC ACID (LACTATE)
LDL CHOLESTEROL
LITHIUM
LUTEINIZING HORMONE (LH)
LYME DISEASE ANTIBODIES (BORRELIA BURGDORFERI ABS)
METHADONE
METHAMPHETAMINE/AMPHETAMINE
METHAMPHETAMINES
METHYLENEDIOXYMETHAMPHETAMINE (MDMA)
MICROALBUMIN
MORPHINE
NICOTINE AND/OR METABOLITES
OPIATES
OVULATION TEST (LH) BY VISUAL COLOR COMPARISON
OXYCODONE
pH
PHENCYCLIDINE (PCP)
PLATELET AGGREGATION
PROTHROMBIN TIME (PT)
RESPIRATORY SYNCYTIAL VIRUS
SEMEN
SPUN MICROHEMATOCRIT
STREPTOCOCCUS, GROUP A
THYROID STIMULATING HORMONE (TSH)
TRICHOMONAS
TRICYCLIC ANTIDEPRESSANTS
TRIGLYCERIDE
URINE DIPSTICK OR TABLET ANALYTES, NONAUTOMATED
URINE HCG BY VISUAL COLOR COMPARISON TESTS
URINE QUALITATIVE DIPSTICK ASCORBIC ACID
URINE QUALITATIVE DIPSTICK BILIRUBIN
URINE QUALITATIVE DIPSTICK BLOOD
URINE QUALITATIVE DIPSTICK CHEMISTRIES
URINE QUALITATIVE DIPSTICK CREATININE
URINE QUALITATIVE DIPSTICK GLUCOSE
URINE QUALITATIVE DIPSTICK KETONE
URINE QUALITATIVE DIPSTICK LEUKOCYTES
URINE QUALITATIVE DIPSTICK NITRITE
URINE QUALITATIVE DIPSTICK pH
URINE QUALITATIVE DIPSTICK PROTEIN
URINE QUALITATIVE DIPSTICK SPECIFIC GRAVITY
URINE QUALITATIVE DIPSTICK UROBILINOGEN
VAGINAL pH

**Figure 66-5,cont'd**

---

**List of PPMP Procedures**

**Q0111**—Wet mounts, including preparations of vaginal, cervical, or skin specimens

**Q0112**—All potassium hydroxide (KOH) preparations

**Q0113**—Pinworm examinations

**Q0114**—Fern test

**Q0115**—Postcoital direct, qualitative examinations of vaginal or cervical mucus

**81015**—Urinalysis; microscopic only

**81000**—Urinalysis, by dipstick or tablet reagent for bilirubin, glucose, hemoglobin, ketones, leukocytes, nitrite, pH, protein, specific gravity, urobilinogen, any number of these constituents; nonautomated, with microcopy

**81001**—Urinalysis, by dipstick or tablet reagent for bilirubin, glucose, hemoglobin, ketones, leukocytes, nitrite, pH, protein, specific gravity, urobilinogen, any number of these constituents; automated, with microscopy (NOTE: May only be used when the laboratory is using an automated dipstick urinalysis instrument approved as waived.)

**81020**—Urinalysis; two or three glass test

**89055**—Fecal leukocyte examination (effective 1 January 2004)

**G0027**—Semen analysis; presence and/or motility of sperm, excluding Huhner

**89190**—Nasal smears for eosinophils

---

**Figure 66-6    List of PPMP procedures.** (http://www.cms.hhs.gov/clia/ppmplst.asp)

---

following were the results of this pilot study, which examined laboratories in 10 states (Certificate of Waiver laboratories and PPMP laboratories were considered separately):

Quality problems in waived laboratories included the following:

- 32% failed to have current manufacturer's instructions on hand
- 32% didn't perform quality control as required by manufacturer or the CDC
- 16% failed to follow current manufacturer's instructions
- 7% did not perform calibration as required by manufacturer
- 23% had certificate issues (i.e., change of name, director, or address)
- 20% cut occult blood cards and urine dipsticks
- 19% had personnel who were neither trained nor evaluated
- 49% did not follow manufacturer's storage and handling instructions
- 56% were using expired reagents/kits

Quality problems in PPMP laboratories included the following:

- 38% had no quality control (did not evaluate test accuracy 2 times a year)
- 36% had no microscope/centrifuge maintenance
- 28% had no director-approved standard-operating procedure manual
- 25% did not document personnel competency (QA)
- 23% had certificate issues

**Recommendations**

It was felt that in 2002 CMS should have the ability to perform independent inspections of these laboratories (http://www.cms.hhs.gov/clia/ppmpfr2001.pdf). On completion of the pilot studies, the following recommendations were made:

- To provide educational programs for all waived laboratories
- For all Certificate of Waiver and PPMP laboratory staff to take educational programs

## SELF-ASSESSMENT CHECKLIST FOR THE PHYSICIAN'S OFFICE EXEMPT LAB

Laboratory Name _____ Address _____
Physician/Director _____ Lab Contact _____ Phone _____
Tests _____
_____

CLIA certificate type: Waiver, PPMP, Compliance, or Accreditation _____ and # 29D _____

Current State of Nevada Physician's License _____

**1. NAC 652.155 (1)** THIS PROVISION **ONLY** APPLIES TO A PHYSICIAN PERFORMING **ALL** OF THE TESTS – WITHOUT ASSISTANCE – ON HIS OWN PATIENTS.
Does a Nevada State licensed physician perform and read 100 % of the test (s)?
If "No", proceed below. If "Yes", the rest of the regulations do not apply.

**2. NAC 652.155 (2)(a)** APPLIES TO ASSISTANTS PERFORMING WAIVED TESTING FOR A PHYSICIAN'S PRACTICE.
Are office personnel (other than the physician) performing CLIA Waived tests *only–* for the physician or associates of the physician's private practice? If "Yes", proceed to NAC 652.155 (2)(b).
**Note:** **The answer is "No" if an APN or a PA is performing microscopic procedure for KOH and Wet Prep, or if one or more office personnel (other than the physician) is performing non-CLIA waived test, such as tests defined by CLIA as moderate or high complexity tests. The facility needs to apply for a Registered Lab and will not qualify as an Exempt Lab.**

**3. NAC 652.155 (2)(b)(1)** THE LAB DIRECTOR OR DESIGNEE VERIFIES THAT THE PERSON IS COMPETENT TO PERFORM TESTING
Documented training for each test performed in the office (*training and competency assessment of all testing personnel for all tests performed must be documented and signed by the lab director or designee*).

**4. NAC 652.155 (2)(b)(2)** ENSURES THAT TESTS ARE PERFORMED ACCORDING TO MANUFACTURER'S INSTRUCTIONS
Step by step procedures are followed. Written procedures available at *bench (test manufacturer's package inserts are acceptable).*
Proper storage of reagents/kits: temperatures monitored, maintained and documented
room _____ refrigerator _____ (*daily temperature monitoring logs maintained*)
Expiration dates not exceeded or modified upon opening, when applicable (*No expired reagents/supplies in-use with in-use date noted on the vial or log, or expired modified on the vial or log*)

**5. NAC 652.155 (2)(b)(3)** CONTROLS USED FOR VALIDATION AND VERIFICATION
Positive and negative controls for each day of use (*2 levels of external or internal controls, performed and documented each day of testing, or used per manufacturer's directions*)

**6. SAFETY NAC 652.155 (3)(a)** SAFETY CONTROLS
Written policy prohibits eating, drinking, smoking and storage of food in lab area (*Universal Precautions policies and procedures developed and enforced*)
Proper disposal of bio-hazardous waste
Sharps container appropriate
Eye wash available (*portable or fixed eyewash station*)
Adequate ventilation, temperatures controlled
Proper disinfection of lab areas

**7. NAC 652.155 (3)(b)** CERTIFIED OR LICENSED BY STATE AS OFFICE LABORATORY ASSISTANT
*All non-physician testing personnel (M.A., LPN, RN, APN, PA, CNA) performing testing,* **must apply** for *personnel certification as an office laboratory assistant.*

**REVIEW BY DIRECTOR**
Training _____ Safety Policy _____ Written Procedures/Product Package Inserts _____ Control logs ____

This is intended to be used as a tool and is not intended to replace any regulation in
NAC 652 – Medical Laboratories

**Figure 66-7** **Self-assessment checklist for the physician's office exempt laboratory.**

- To survey a percentage of Certificate of Waiver and PPMP laboratories annually
- To develop self-assessment tools for PPMP laboratories
- To provide appropriate information of CLIA requirements to new Certificate of Waiver and PPMP laboratories

Although testing is not mandatory, it is imperative that the directors of the Certificate of Wavier and PPMP laboratories ensure that all of the clinicians performing these tests have been appropriately tested and evaluated for competency. As a result of the preceding pilot data, CMS will inspect approximately 2% of Certificate of Wavier laboratories. The purpose will be to provide education to Certificate of Wavier laboratories and improve quality of care. Several states have recommended self-assessments for Certificate of Wavier and PPMP laboratories. Figure 66-7 is a copy of the self-assessment checklist for physician offices in the State of Nevada.

# Index

Note: Page numbers followed by f indicate figures; those followed by t indicate tables.